I0885522

BARNHILL'S

Dermatopathology Challenge

Self-Assessment & Review

NOTICE

BARNHILL'S

Dermatopathology Challenge

Self-Assessment & Review

Garrett T. Desman, MD

Assistant Professor of Pathology and Dermatology
Icahn School of Medicine at Mount Sinai
New York, New York
Attending Physician, Dermatopathology Services
Mount Sinai Hospital
New York, New York

Raymond L. Barnhill, MD, MSc

Professor
Department of Pathology
Institut Curie
Paris, France

Mc Graw Hill Education

New York Chicago San Francisco Athens London Madrid Mexico City Milan
New Delhi Singapore Sydney Toronto

Barnhill's Dermatopathology Challenge: Self-Assessment & Review

1 2 3 4 5 6 7 8 9 0 DSS/DSS 20 19 18 17 16

ISBN 978-0-07-148922-5
MHID 0-07-148922-3

This book was set in Minion Pro 10/12 pt by MPS Limited.
The editors were Karen G. Edmonson, and Peter J. Boyle.
The production supervisor was Catherine H. Saggese.
Project management was provided by Ruchika Abrol, MPS Limited.
The designer was Eve Siegel.

Library of Congress Cataloging-in-Publication Data

Names: Desman, Garrett T., author. | Barnhill, Raymond L., author.
Title: Barnhill's dermatopathology challenge : self-assessment & review / Garrett T. Desman, Raymond L. Barnhill.
Other titles: Dermatopathology challenge
Description: New York : McGraw-Hill Education, [2016] | Includes bibliographical references and index.
Identifiers: LCCN 2015041103 | ISBN 9780071489225 (pbk.) | ISBN 0071489223 (pbk.)
Subjects: | MESH: Skin Diseases—diagnosis—Examination Questions. | Diagnosis, Differential—Examination Questions. | Skin—pathology—Examination Questions.
Classification: LCC RM328 | NLM WR 18.2 | DDC 616.5/075076—dc 3 LC record available at http://lccn.loc.gov/2015041103

To my longtime colleague and best friend Dr. Lurmag Orta
—GTD

To Claire
—RLB

Contents

Foreword 1

Over the course of my academic career, I have been directly and indirectly involved in the training of hundreds of young physicians in the field of dermatology. The importance of dermatopathology to the practicing dermatologist cannot be overstated. We now have an increased understanding of which mechanisms contribute to the various clinical and histopathological findings associated with specific conditions. Practicing dermatopathologists and dermatologists must be cognizant of not only their respective differential diagnoses, but also the possible pathological mechanisms at hand and how this information may impact the diagnosis and treatment plan. In this modern era, there is a need to teach dermatopathology on a scale that encompasses the intricacies of pathogenesis in addition to clinicopathologic correlation.

Barnhill's Dermatopathology Challenge: Self-Assessment & Review, a companion to Dr. Barnhill's *Dermatopathology,* 3rd ed., is a unique and effective teaching tool that takes advantage of numerous clinical and histopathological images, combining many resources concerning dermatology and dermatopathology into one easy to use volume. Drs. Desman and Barnhill have drawn on years of experience to create a comprehensive and engaging guide to cutaneous clinicopathologic correlation with an emphasis of current concepts of pathogenesis. Each vignette is used to emphasize the prototypes of various conditions and the differential permutations of related entities, thus providing a well-rounded mechanistic approach to clinicopathologic correlation. Highlights include summary tables, quick fact guides, an index of key terms, and options for differential diagnosis surrounding each case studied.

This book will be useful to doctors at various levels of experience in that it can function both as a programmed instruction and a reference guide. Whether you are reviewing for an upcoming dermatopathology fellowship, studying for dermatology or pathology board certification, or simply referring back to an uncommon entity in clinical practice, this edition will be helpful in building perspective in pathology and treatment of cutaneous diseases.

Mark Lebwohl, MD
Professor and System Chair, Department of Dermatology
Icahn School of Medicine at Mount Sinai
President, American Academy of Dermatology

Foreword 2

This new text, *Barnhill's Dermatopathology Challenge: Self-Assessment & Review,* by Garrett T. Desman and Raymond L. Barnhill is original in its conception.

It is, to date, the first book of its kind in dermatopathology, which has been written in the form of "lessons" with a clinical and microscopic approach to a precise topic and self-assessment exercises, followed by a summary and broad synthesis by experts in the field. The work is comprehensive as more than 700 entities and 400 illustrated questions have been included.

This type of case-oriented presentation has been written especially for trainees (residents and fellows) in dermatology, pathology, and dermatopathology who are preparing for their "speciality" board examinations. This work also directly addresses the educational exigencies of medical school educational programs in the United States and Europe. It can also serve as a valuable source of knowledge for medical students and as well as more senior medical doctors, particularly, dermatologists, pathologists, and even dermatopathologists who need to continually update their clinical training and ongoing medical education.

The authors are both experts in dermatopathology. Garrett Desman, still early in his career, has envisioned the need for this type of book, and he is already a gifted author, teacher, and dermatopathologist. Raymond Barnhill is an internationally recognized dermatopathologist and professor who has taught medical students, residents, fellows, and practicing physicians for almost 30 years in the United States and France. His broad experience has led him to initiate this necessary evolution from his previous dermatopathology textbooks.

In our time of deep social integration with the internet, the publication of such a book is also an act of faith. As a senior pathology professor trained in dermatology, I am convinced that in university training there is still a place for such complete, concise, and "student-friendly" books.

Professor Anne Janin, MD, PhD
Pathology Department, Hôpital Saint Louis, Paris
Director of Inserm Research Unit University Paris 7

Preface

Our goal in writing this textbook is to provide a unique teaching tool that tests the reader's fund of knowledge in cutaneous clinicopathologic correlation through a series of hypothetical clinical vignettes. This type of resource is currently not available for dermatopathology. Use of this book provides self-assessment and a comprehensive review of the pertinent clinical and histopathological conditions encountered in community and academic dermatopathology practice. We view this work as an engaging middle-ground text and atlas that includes a large number of standard clinical and pathology images drawn from many sources into a single volume. These images are typical of those shown on board certification examinations in dermatology, pathology, and dermatopathology, as well as conditions commonly encountered by dermatologists and dermatopathologists in clinical practice.

In conjunction with many supplementary images, the text uses hundreds of photomicrographs from *Dermatopathology*, 3rd ed., Raymond L. Barnhill, Editor-in-Chief, widely acknowledged as the best resource for a conceptual approach and differential diagnosis in this field. Additionally, this work is used as an organizational framework for the content included within each chapter. We would like this textbook to be used as a testing/teaching tool *and* a reference guide for routine clinical practice, and thus we have included a searchable index that references various keywords and phrases (shown in bold) within the body of the text. Each question is accompanied by a detailed explanation discussing essential clinical and histopathological differential diagnoses for quick access and ease of use. The text contains more than 400 illustrated questions encompassing over 700 diagnostic entities, many of which include a summary table for rapid review or small "quick fact" tables highlighting important diagnostic findings. The images included in the questions and answers throughout this textbook are hypothetical and do not necessarily come from the same patient. In addition to the clinical scenarios applied to these case studies, each may not reflect the real-life clinical presentation or clinical course experienced by the patient shown in the images. However, they are typical or "classic" presentations of each corresponding condition.

The target audience for this book includes dermatopathology fellows, dermatology and pathology residents, medical students, and more generally dermatologists, pathologists, and dermatopathologists.

We would like to acknowledge the associate editors of the third edition of *Dermatopathology*, Drs. Crowson, Magro, and Piepkorn, whose contributions have had significant influence directly and indirectly on the content of *Barnhill's Dermatopathology Challenge*. In addition, we acknowledge and thank all the contributors of *Dermatopathology* in its previous editions and any influences they have had on this new work. We would also like to thank Dr. Andrea Suarez, Department of Dermatology, Weill Cornell Medical College, for contributing various tables containing mnemonics and acronyms. Lastly, we would like to acknowledge the editors and contributors of *Fitzpatrick's Dermatology in General Medicine*, 8th ed., for the numerous clinical photographs included in this new book. We are enormously grateful to these individuals and thank them most sincerely.

Garrett T. Desman, MD
Raymond L. Barnhill, MD, MSc

CHAPTER 1

Inflammatory Diseases of the Epidermis

QUESTION 1-1.

Which of the following statements regarding this lesion is INCORRECT?

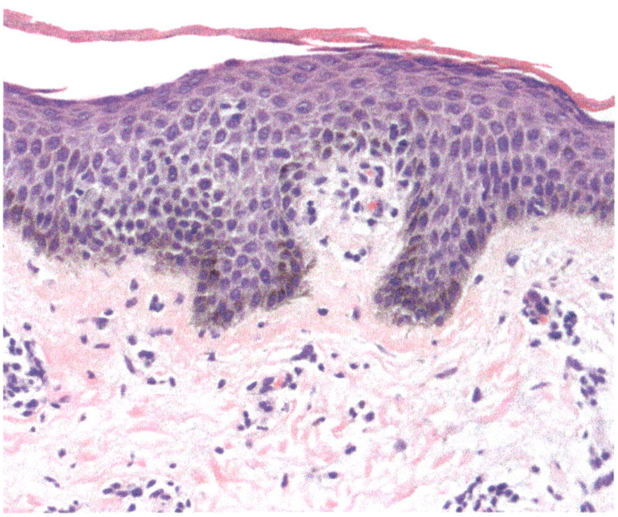

A) It is characterized by intercellular edema that results in impaired cohesion between epidermal keratinocytes. This finding represents a nonspecific inflammatory reaction pattern with little correlation to etiology.
B) The clinical and histological appearances vary depending on the etiology, duration, location, and superimposed secondary changes (ie, excoriation).
C) The eruption always represents a type IV hypersensitivity reaction to an exogenous antigen.
D) It is divided into acute, subacute, and chronic stages.
E) A PAS stain should be considered to exclude dermatophyte infection.

QUESTION 1-2.

Which sequence of events CORRECTLY describes the acute phase of allergic contact dermatitis?

1) Extracellular edema
2) Stretching and rupture of desmosomes and keratinocyte membranes
3) Langerhans cells present foreign antigen to presensitized T lymphocytes that become activated and, along with keratinocytes, secrete various cytokines.
4) Reticular degeneration
5) Lymphocytes marginate from the superficial vascular plexus with subsequent papillary dermal edema. Occasional eosinophils may be present.
6) Increased exocytosis of lymphocytes
7) Slight exocytosis of lymphocytes
8) Expansion in volume of the epidermis
9) Intracellular edema

A) 5, 3, 1, 2, 4, 7, 6, 9, 8
B) 3, 5, 7, 9, 1, 2, 6, 4, 8
C) 5, 1, 2, 3, 6, 4, 8, 7, 9
D) 3, 5, 7, 1, 9, 2, 6, 4, 8

QUESTION 1-3.

Which of the following is NOT a feature of chronic spongiotic dermatitis?

A) There are intraepidermal Langerhans cell–rich microvesicles and transepidermally eliminated spongiotic vesicles producing serum-imbued parakeratotic scale crusts.
B) Spongiosis gradually decreases in chronic lesions.
C) Irregular psoriasiform epidermal hyperplasia

D) Papillary dermal hyperplasia
E) Hypergranulosis and thick hyperkeratosis (orthokeratosis and parakeratosis)

QUESTION 1-4.

Which of the following statements regarding irritant contact dermatitis is INCORRECT?

A) It is caused by the direct noxious effect of substances such as acid, alkali, or organic solvents.
B) It will occur in all persons exposed to an offending agent in sufficient concentration.
C) Phototoxicity is the result of direct tissue and cellular injury following UVR-induced activation of a phototoxic agent.
D) Generalized irritant contact dermatitis is always attributed to hypersensitivity against systemically administered substances in individuals who have been presensitized to the substance.

QUESTION 1-5.

A 27-year-old male presents with a well-circumscribed, erythematous, scaly lesion involving the full circumference of a finger. He reports that the finger lesion appeared approximately 15 days ago when he started wearing his grandfather's ring. Five days ago he developed a widespread, erythematous and pruritic eruption on the chest and upper back. Biopsies of the finger and back are performed and the findings are illustrated below, respectively (C & D). Which of the following statements regarding this condition is INCORRECT?

A) The eruptions on the finger, chest, and upper back are most likely attributed to a type IV delayed hypersensitivity reaction directed against a substance present within his grandfather's ring.
B) Substances that are known to cause this type of reaction include nickel, urushiol, and topical medications.
C) The eruption on the chest and back is most likely unrelated to the eruption on the finger.
D) The patient should be referred for patch testing.

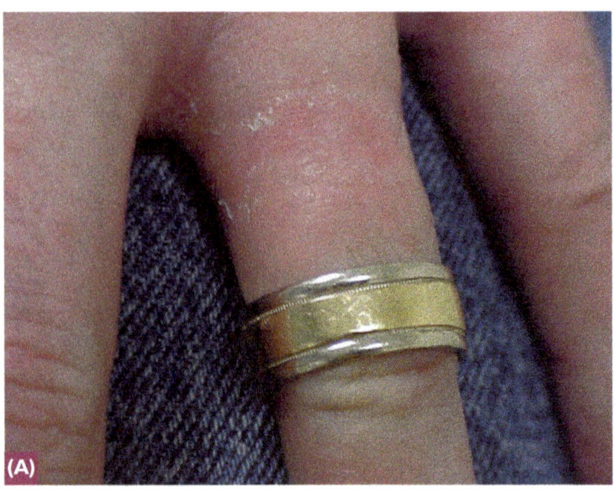
(A)

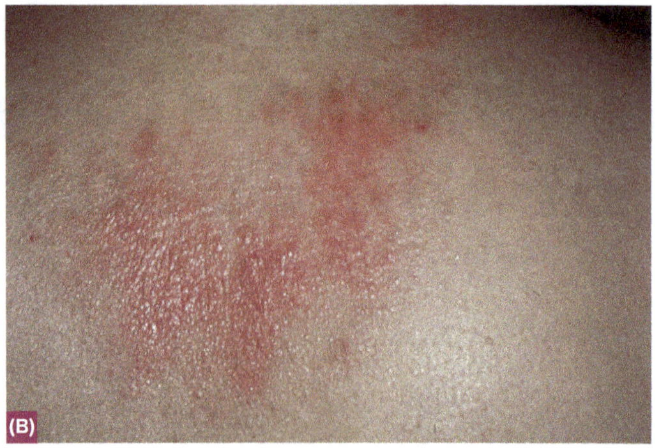
(B)

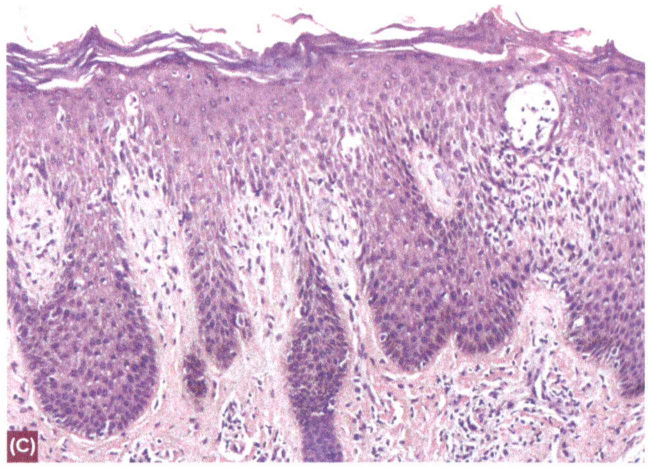
(C)

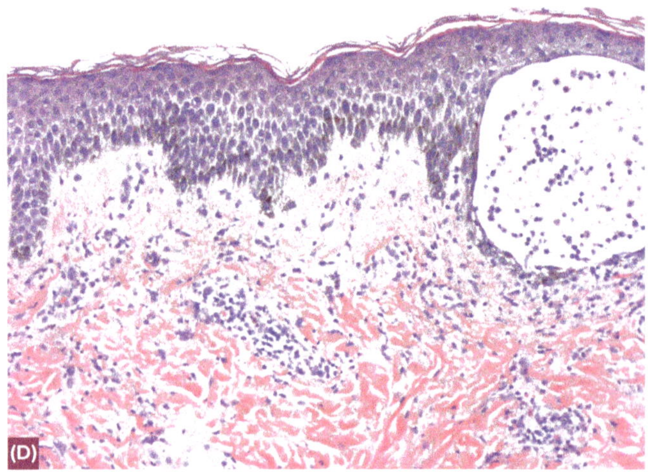
(D)

(A) Reproduced with permission from Milgrom EC et al: *Practical Allergy*. Philadelphia, PA: Elsevier; 2004. **(B)** Reproduced, with permission, from Goldsmith LA, Katz SI, Gilchrest BA, Paller AS, Leffell DJ, Wolff K, eds. *Fitzpatrick's Dermatology in General Medicine*. 8th ed. New York, NY: McGraw-Hill Education; 2012.

QUESTION 1-6.

A 60-year-old Park Ranger presents with pruritic erythematous papulovesicles around her eyes, antecubital fossae, axilla, eyelids, sides of the neck, and genitalia. During the physical examination a few papulovesicles arranged in a linear distribution are noted on the lateral aspects of the fingers. She had recently spent the day hiking through the forest, and has a prior history of a similar eruption on the fingers during the last camping season. One of the finger lesions is biopsied. Which of the following statements regarding these lesions is INCORRECT?

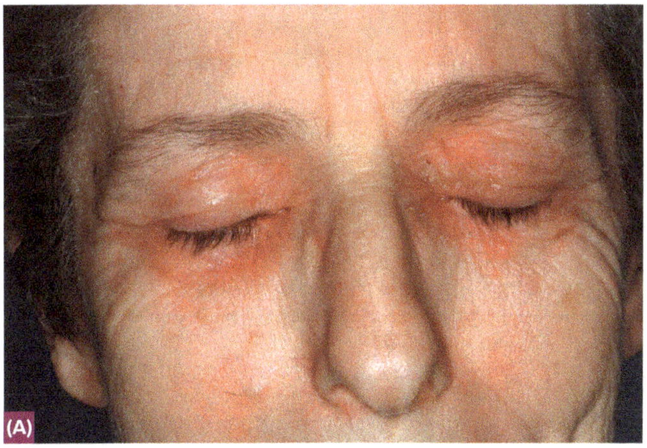
(A)

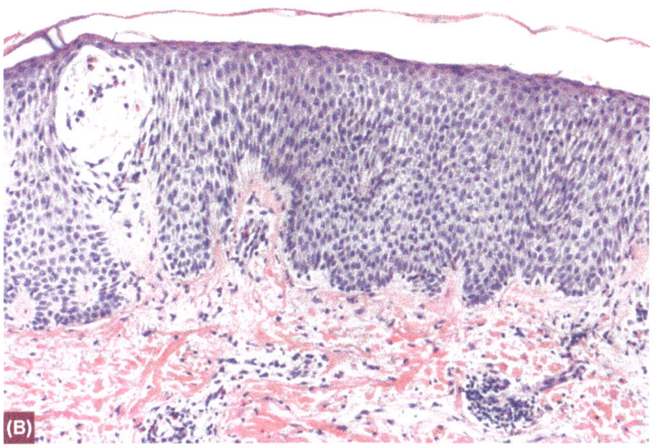
(B)

A) This dermatitis is most likely related to poison ivy exposure.
B) All persons exposed to this offending agent in sufficient concentration will develop an inflammatory response.
C) The presence of eosinophils within spongiotic vesicles and dermis suggests an allergic-based etiology.
D) A generalized systemic form of this dermatitis may be seen in individuals who ingest oral antibiotics, antihistamines, and various food products.
E) The lesions around the eyes and genitalia are most likely attributed to direct inoculation of an offending substance from the fingers.

QUESTION 1-7.

A 27-year-old female presents with red exudative patches on the central chest. She states the lesions stings. Prior to developing this rash, she had been applying an over-the-counter shampoo to her chest for 10 hours at a time, in an effort to self-treat a fungal infection. A biopsy is performed and the findings are illustrated below. Which of the following statements regarding this eruption is INCORRECT?

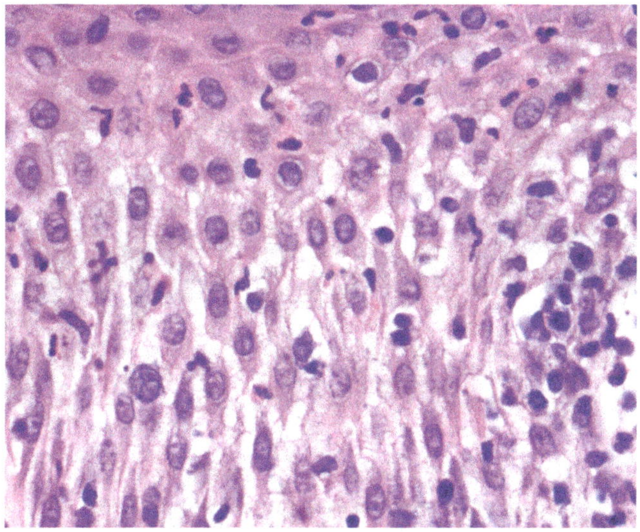

A) Once the eruption has resolved, she can continue using the shampoo, but should not leave it on the skin for more than a few minutes.
B) The findings are most consistent with an allergic-based etiology.
C) Although the upper-most layers of the epidermis are not visualized in the image, the granular and corneal layers will most likely reveal necrotic and hydropic superficial keratinocytes admixed with serum and neutrophils.
D) All persons who expose their skin to prolonged contact with this shampoo will develop an inflammatory response.
E) A PAS stain should be ordered to rule out a dermatophyte infection.

QUESTION 1-8.

A 60-year-old patient, who just returned from a summer at the family beach home presents with ill-defined, erythematous papulovesicles and thickened, scaly, plaques on the hands, face, and V-area of the neck. There is relative sparing of the submental area, upper eyelids, and postauricular area. His medications include hydrochlorothiazide for hypertension. You perform a biopsy of one of the lesions, but forget to provide the clinical history. The diagnosis comes back as,

SUBACUTE SPONGIOTIC DERMATITIS. Which of the following statements regarding this condition is INCORRECT?

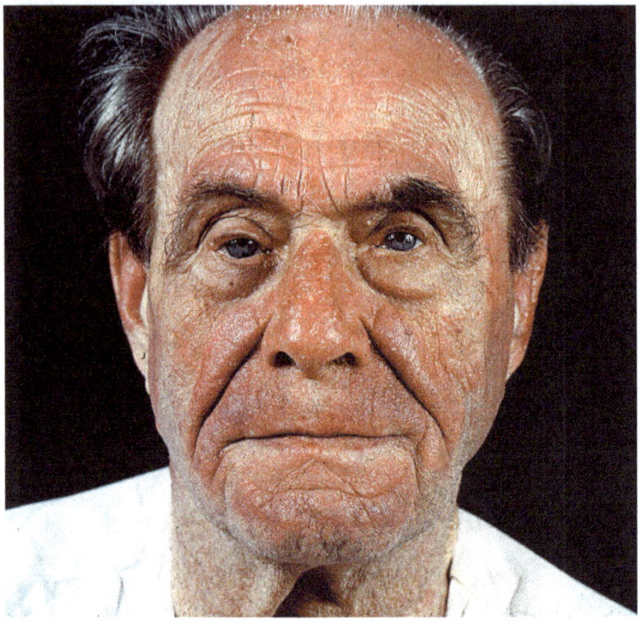

A) Similar localized lesions have been reported in some individuals who are exposed to the sun and wear cosmetics that contain sandalwood oil, bergamot oil, and musk ambrette.
B) This condition frequently spreads to sun-protected areas.
C) These eruptions may develop within seconds or as long as 3 months after UV exposure.
D) If exposure to light is ceased, the lesions always rapidly resolve and do not evolve into chronic lesions.
E) The presence of superficial and deep perivascular and interstitial inflammatory infiltrate suggests an allergy-based etiology to a systemic circulating antigen.

QUESTION 1-9.

A 24-year-old male medical student presents to the clinic with symmetric, erythematous, greasy, yellow, flaking scales covering the scalp, nasolabial folds, and eyebrows for the past 2 months. A biopsy is performed and the findings are illustrated below. Which of the following statements regarding this entity is INCORRECT?

A) These lesions tend to arise in areas with high concentrations of sebaceous glands.
B) The patient should be questioned for risk factors for HIV infection, stress, and mood changes.
C) In patients with Parkinson disease, these lesions frequently contain confluent parakeratosis, intraepidermal apoptotic keratinocytes, and dermal plasma cell infiltrates.
D) The pathogenesis for this condition is unknown; however, *Malassezia* spp (*Pityrosporum*) have been implicated since patients frequently respond to oral and topical ketoconazole.

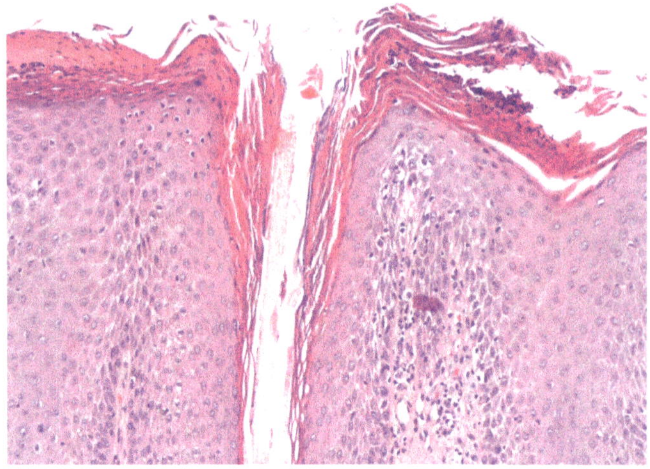

QUESTION 1-10.

An elderly woman with a long-standing history of stasis dermatitis reports gradual worsening of edema, pruritus, and multiple punctate, superficial, excoriated ulcers overlying the medial malleoli (Image A). Nine days after the ulcers appeared, she developed an acute, extremely pruritic, erythematous,

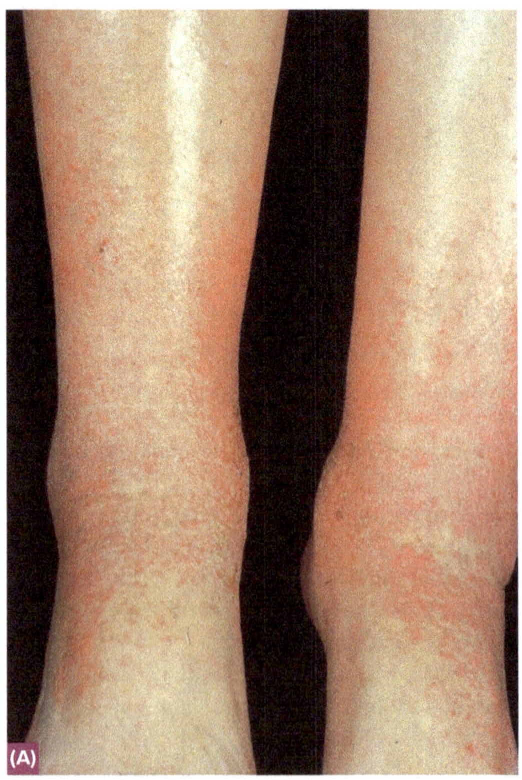

(A)

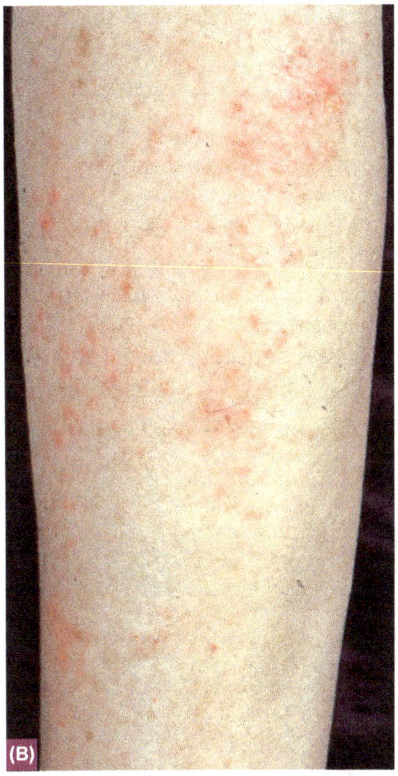

(B)

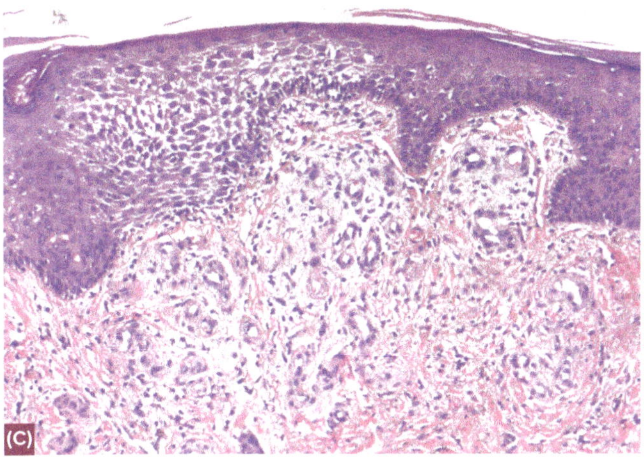

(C)

(A), (B) Reproduced, with permission, from Goldsmith LA, Katz SI, Gilchrest BA, Paller AS, Leffell DJ, Wolff K, eds. *Fitzpatrick's Dermatology in General Medicine*. 8th ed. New York, NY: McGraw-Hill Education; 2012.

papulovesicular eruption over the forearms, which progressively involved the hands, upper arms, and upper torso (Image B). Physical examination reveals that the acute papulovesicular dermatitis also involves the lower extremities and can be noted overlying the chronic stasis dermatitis. Biopsies are performed of both lower and upper extremities. The findings of the lower extremity biopsy are illustrated in image C. Which of the following statements regarding this condition is INCORRECT?

A) The upper extremity biopsy will most likely reveal subacute spongiotic dermatitis with marked subepidermal edema and few eosinophils.
B) A similar phenomenon of distant and delayed secondary eruptions may occur in patients with scabies, radiation dermatitis, and tinea pedis.
C) The upper extremity lesions most likely arise due to activated T lymphocytes and/or cytokines generated from the lower extremity eruption.
D) The upper extremity biopsy will also reveal dense dermal fibrosis, thick-walled vessels in clusters, hemosiderin-laden macrophages, and overlying epidermal attenuation.

QUESTION 1-11.

A 1-year-old infant with a history of allergic rhinitis and asthma presents with crusted, pruritic, erythematous plaques and small vesicles on the face, diaper area, and extensor surfaces of the extremities. There is circumoral sparing. The patient's mother reports that these lesions follow a waxing and waning course. Additionally, she reports to have a similar condition that has afflicted her throughout her entire life. Which of the following statements regarding this condition is INCORRECT?

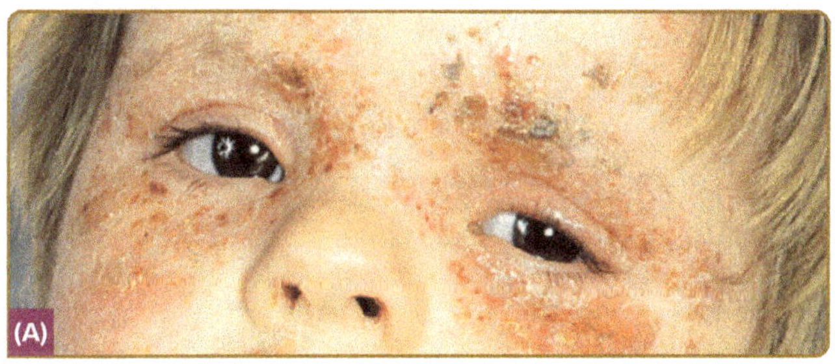

(A)

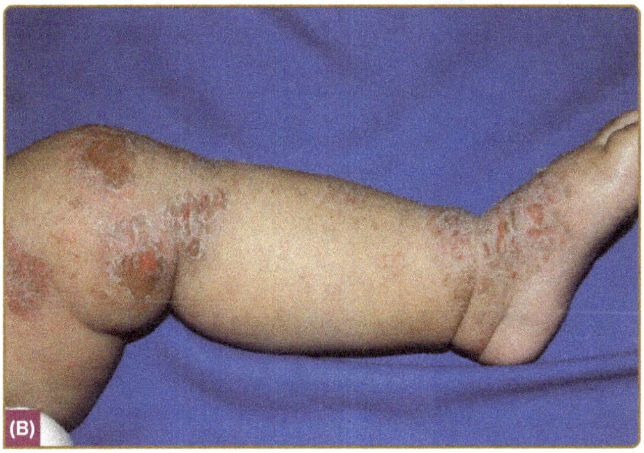

(B)

Reproduced, with permission, from Goldsmith LA, Katz SI, Gilchrest BA, Paller AS, Leffell DJ, Wolff K, eds. *Fitzpatrick's Dermatology in General Medicine*. 8th ed. New York, NY: McGraw-Hill Education; 2012.

A) A biopsy of the child's eruption will reveal acute spongiotic dermatitis characterized by a superficial perivascular lymphocytic infiltrate, possibly rare scattered eosinophils, spongiosis, and normal thickness epidermis.
B) These patients frequently have variable degrees of immunosuppression against viral infections such as molluscum contagiosum and herpes simplex and may develop extensive generalized infections.
C) The vast majority of these patients will have elevated circulating IgA antibodies.
D) The normal appearing skin of these patients contains higher concentrations of dermal eosinophils than the general population.
E) KOH of the scale crust will reveal hyphae, as this condition is caused by dermatophytes.

QUESTION 1-12.

A 23-year-old female patient presents with multiple, coin-sized, well-demarcated, erythematous plaques and vesicles on the dorsum of the forearms, hands, shins, and ankles. A few of the vesicles have burst, leaving behind scale crust. She has a history of asthma and allergic rhinitis. There are exacerbations during the cold winter months. She recently completed a course of topical antifungal medication with no improvement. Which of the following statements regarding this entity is INCORRECT?

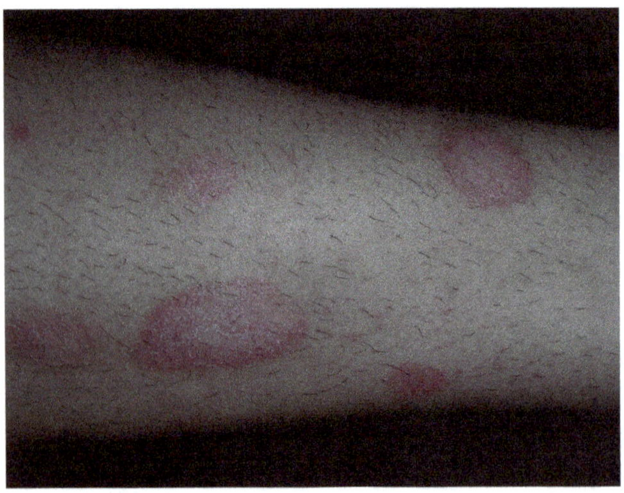

Reproduced, with permission, from Usatine RP, Smith MA, Mayeaux EJ Jr, Chumley HS, eds. *Color Atlas of Family Medicine*. 2nd ed. New York, NY: McGraw-Hill Education; 2012.

A) The precise etiology is unknown.
B) The histomorphologic features of this condition mimic those of allergic contact dermatitis at the various stages of evolution.
C) Male patients tend to present in middle to late age.
D) Patients frequently have a history of severe allergic contact dermatitis to nickel.

QUESTION 1-13.

A 3-year-old patient presents with two vaguely erythematous, round macules on the face with indistinct borders. One of the lesions around the mouth measures 2 cm and appears to be resolving with a fine scale and lighter discoloration than the adjacent skin. The lesions are asymptomatic. A biopsy is performed. The pathologist renders a diagnosis of SUBACUTE SPONGIOTIC DERMATITIS. Which of the following microscopic findings is LEAST likely to be present in this patient's biopsy?

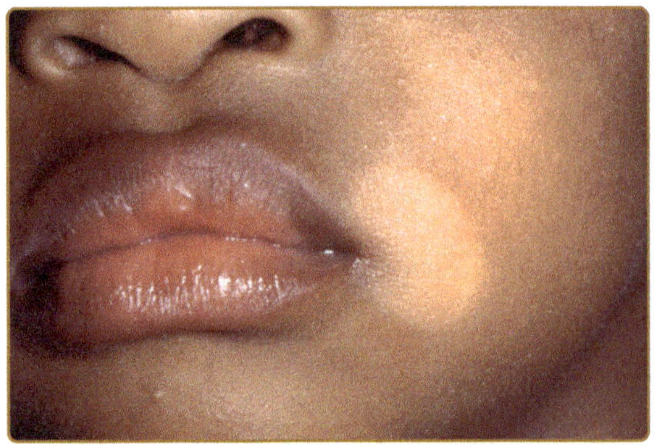

Reproduced, with permission, from Goldsmith LA, Katz SI, Gilchrest BA, Paller AS, Leffell DJ, Wolff K, eds. *Fitzpatrick's Dermatology in General Medicine*. 8th ed. New York, NY: McGraw-Hill Education; 2012.

A) Melan-A stain will reveal a complete absence of melanocytes along the dermal-epidermal junction.
B) Rare scattered melanophages will be present in the papillary dermis.
C) The amount of melanin pigment within the basal layer keratinocytes is less than that of adjacent normal skin.
D) Electron microscopy of the biopsy will reveal degenerative changes within melanocytes and a reduced number of melanosomes in the keratinocytes.
E) There is predominantly infundibular spongiosis with follicular plugging and atrophic sebaceous glands.

QUESTION 1-14.

A 24-year-old patient presents with recurrent crops of deep-seated vesicles on the sides of the fingers. Full body examination reveals erythematous patches with scaling, fissures, and maceration in the toe web spaces. A KOH test of the finger lesions is negative for fungi; however, numerous hyphae are identified from the toes. One of the lesions on the fingers is biopsied. Which of the following regarding this condition is INCORRECT?

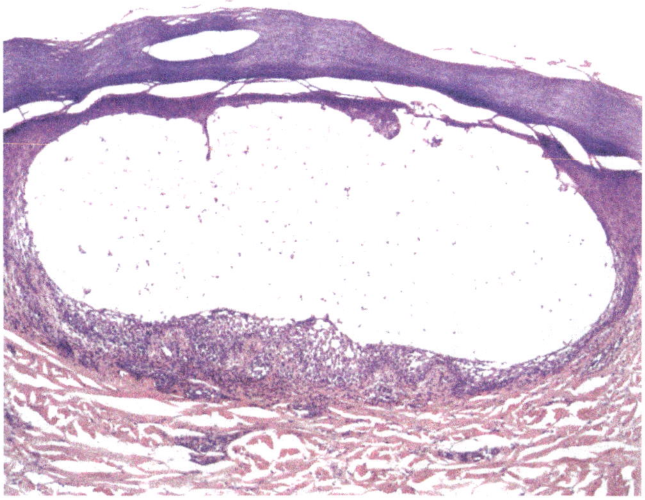

- **A)** These lesions have been associated with several putative casual factors such as allergens and stasis.
- **B)** The exact mechanism of this eruption is unknown; however, it frequently associated with hyperhidrosis and anxiety.
- **C)** Histopathologically, the acrosyringia are not typically involved by the spongiotic process.
- **D)** The positive KOH test from the toes for fungal forms is an incidental finding and not significant in formulating this diagnosis.

QUESTION 1-15.

A 63-year-old woman with a history of multiple deep vein thromboses presents with chronic bilateral edema and bronze discoloration of the lower extremities on the medial aspects of the leg above the malleolus. Fissuring and scaling of the epidermis is noted. Which of the following statements regarding this condition is INCORRECT?

- **A)** The epidermis may exhibit a spectrum of changes from a spongiotic and variable hyperplastic epidermis with parakeratosis and scale crust to changes of lichen simplex chronicus.
- **B)** There is papillary and upper reticular dermal edema with perivascular inflammatory infiltrates of variable density, extravasated red blood cells, and siderophages.
- **C)** There is thickening of the walls of small veins and venules with a tortuous and glomeruloid appearance. There are clusters of thick-walled venules in the subepidermal regions.
- **D)** Eosinophilic infiltrates within the dermis are never seen.

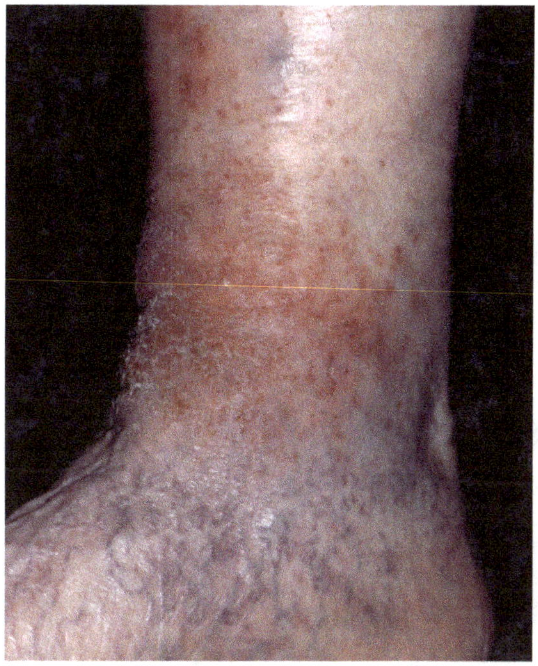

Reproduced, with permission, from Wolff K, Johnson RA, Saavedra AP. *Fitzpatrick's Color Atlas and Synopsis of Clinical Dermatology*. 7th ed. New York, NY: McGraw-Hill Education; 2013.

QUESTION 1-16.

A 13-year-old patient presents with a generalized eruption on the trunk and proximal extremities following the Langer lines of cleavage. The eruption is characterized by discrete, 1 cm, oval, salmon-pink scaly plaques with pinpoint vesiculation. Some of the lesions exhibit a peripheral collarette of scale with central clearing. This generalized eruption was preceded 10 days by an initial 5 cm, oval, salmon-pink plaque on the flank (arrow). A biopsy is performed on one of the smaller plaques. Which of the following is the MOST likely microscopic description?

- **A)** There is acanthosis with irregular and elongated rete ridges, neutrophil exocytosis, and mounds of parakeratosis centered on follicular ostia with follicular plugging.
- **B)** There is acanthosis with irregular, elongated, and pointed rete ridges. The epidermis is spongiotic with lymphocyte and neutrophil exocytosis and overlying thick parakeratotic scale crust containing neutrophils. A band-like lymphoplasmacytic infiltrate is present along the dermal epidermal junction with scattered dyskeratotic basilar keratinocytes. The dermal inflammatory infiltrate extends into the deep dermis with extension along adnexal structures and nerve bundles. Endothelial cells are swollen and protrude into the vascular lumens.
- **C)** There are focal areas of acanthosis with spongiosis and lymphocyte exocytosis directed toward the suprapapillary plates. Mounds of parakeratosis are present

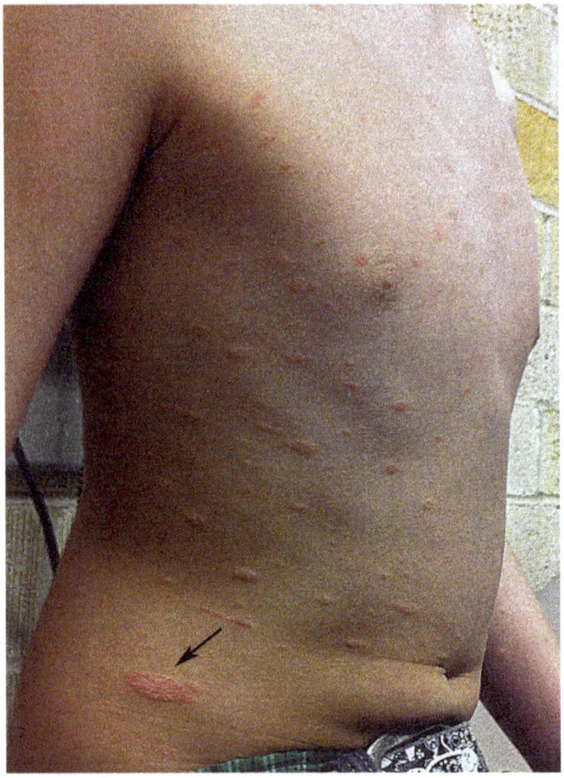

Reproduced, with permission, from Usatine RP, Smith MA, Mayeaux EJ Jr, Chumley HS, eds. *Color Atlas of Family Medicine*. 2nd ed. New York, NY: McGraw-Hill Education; 2012.

overlying the foci of spongiosis. Rare lymphocytes are present in close apposition to the dermal epidermal junction. No lymphocyte atypia is present. A few rare dyskeratotic basilar keratinocytes are noted. Superficial perivascular lymphocytic infiltrates are present. Extravasated red blood cells are present within the epidermis and dermis.

D) There is acanthosis with irregular and elongated rete ridges. The epidermis is spongiotic with marked lymphocyte exocytosis into the upper spinous layers. Intraepidermal clusters of lymphocytes and Langerhans cells are noted. A broad parakeratotic scale containing degenerating inflammatory cells surmounts the epidermis. A superficial and deep dermal lymphocytic infiltrate is present with basal layer vacuolization and numerous dyskeratotic basilar keratinocytes. Intraepidermal and dermal extravasated red blood cells are present.

E) There is acanthosis with irregular elongated rete ridges, minimal spongiosis, and hypergranulosis with alternating areas of orthokeratosis and parakeratosis. Thick papillary dermal fibrosis is present with collagen bundles oriented perpendicular to the epidermal surface. Superficial perivascular lymphocytic infiltrates and scattered eosinophils are present.

QUESTION 1-17.

A 7-year-old female patient presents with abrupt onset of monomorphic, skin-colored to pink, edematous papules that are distributed symmetrically on the face, buttocks, and extensor elbows and knees. The child had been kept home from school for the past 5 days due to having "flu-like" symptoms. A biopsy of one of the buttock lesions is performed. Which of the following microscopic findings below is NOT associated with this condition?

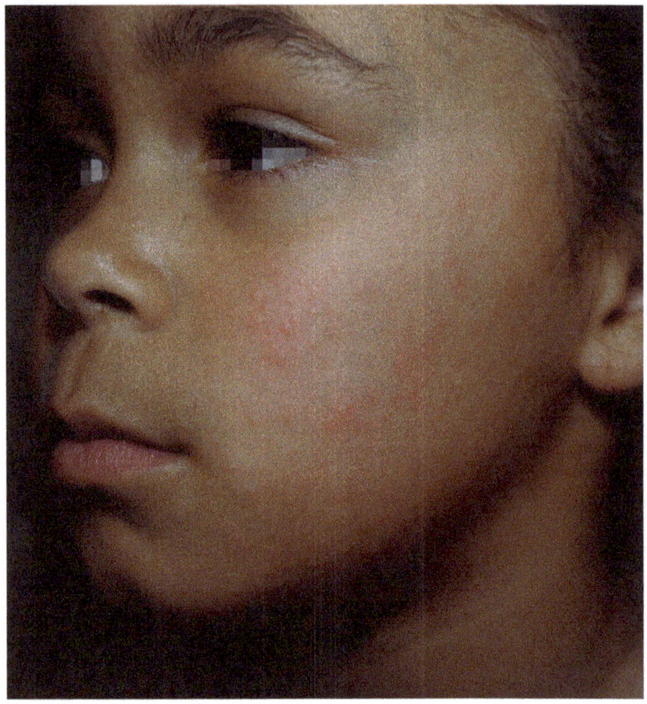

Reproduced, with permission, from Wolff K, Johnson RA, Saavedra AP. *Fitzpatrick's Color Atlas and Synopsis of Clinical Dermatology*. 7th ed. New York, NY: McGraw-Hill Education; 2013.

A) Red blood cell extravasation
B) Nonspecific immunoreactant profile on direct immunofluorescence
C) Lymphocyte-predominant small vessel vasculitis containing fibrin thrombi and fibrinoid necrosis of vessel walls
D) Slight epidermal acanthosis and spongiosis with focal lymphocyte exocytosis
E) Sparse vacuolar interface dermatitis with rare dyskeratotic basilar keratinocytes

QUESTION 1-18.

A newborn female infant presents with small vesicles in a background of erythema. The lesions are most prominent on the extremities and arranged in a whorled pattern following Blaschko lines (image A). The mother reports a history of several miscarriages in the past. A quick examination of the mother reveals hypopigmented atrophic lesions following Blaschko lines on the legs (image B). A biopsy is performed on one of the infant's lesions and the findings are illustrated below (image C). Which of the following diagnoses is CORRECT?

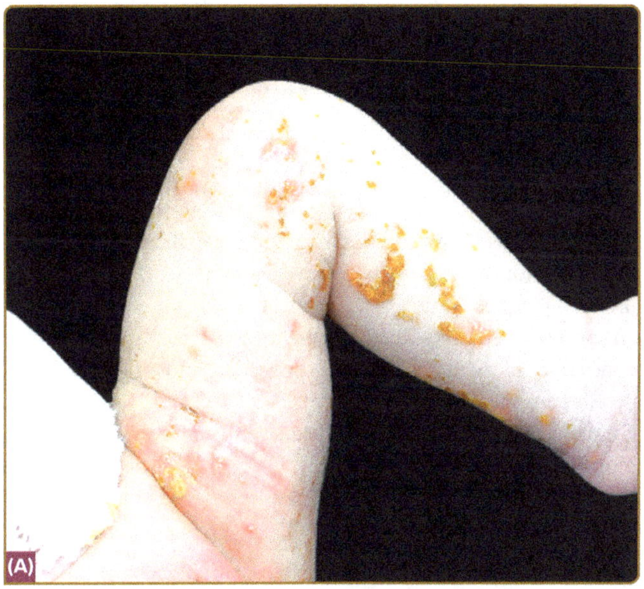
(A)

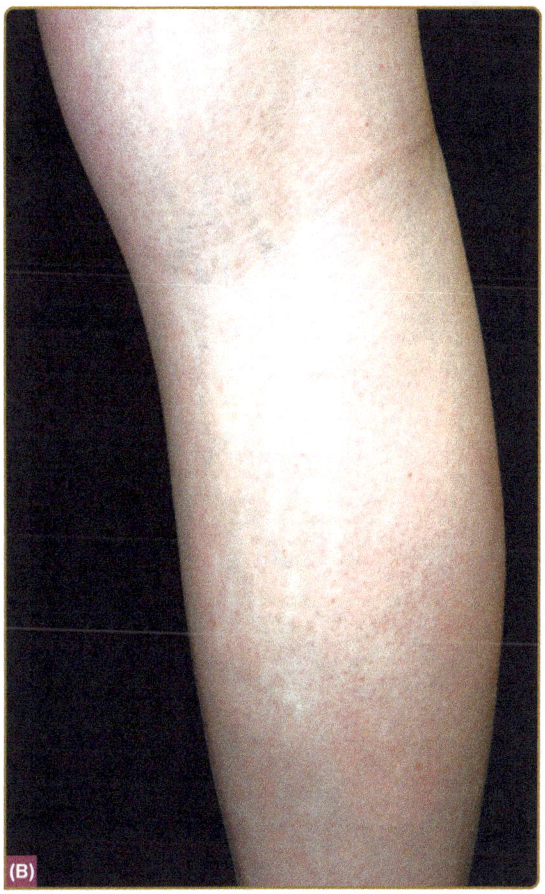
(B)

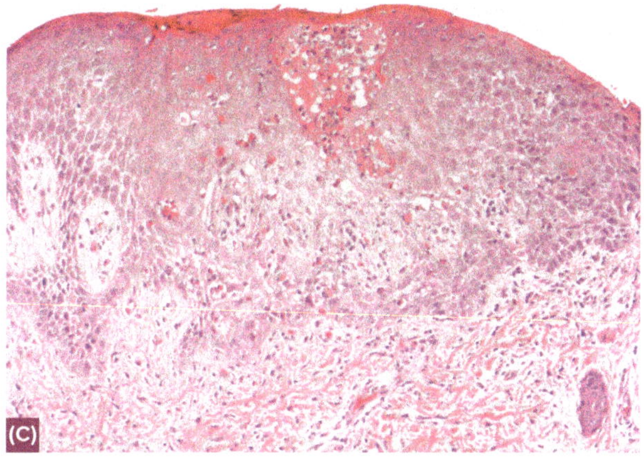
(C)

(A), (B) Reproduced, with permission, from Goldsmith LA, Katz SI, Gilchrest BA, Paller AS, Leffell DJ, Wolff K, eds. *Fitzpatrick's Dermatology in General Medicine*. 8th ed. New York, NY: McGraw-Hill Education; 2012.

A) Incontinentia pigmenti
B) Eosinophilic pustular folliculitis
C) Erythema toxicum neonatorum
D) Transient neonatal pustular melanosis
E) Infantile acropustulosis

QUESTION 1-19.

Which of the following dermatitides is LEAST likely to exhibit exocytosis of eosinophils?

A) Allergic contact dermatitis
B) Photoallergic contact dermatitis
C) Atopic dermatitis
D) Arthropod bite reactions
E) Urticarial stage of bullous pemphigoid
F) Pruritic and urticarial papules and plaques of pregnancy
G) Urticarial stage of pemphigus vulgaris
H) Virus-associated pityriasis rosea

QUESTION 1-20.

Which of the following dermatitides with spongiosis is LEAST likely to exhibit exocytosis of neutrophils?

A) Psoriasis
B) Reactive arthritis
C) Seborrheic dermatitis
D) Phototoxic dermatitis
E) IgA pemphigus
F) Toxic shock syndrome
G) Acute generalized exanthematous pustulosis (AGEP)
H) Infantile acropustulosis
I) Transient neonatal pustular melanosis
J) Incontinentia pigmenti

QUESTION 1-21.

Which of the following features of interface dermatitis is INCORRECT?

A) Band of T lymphocytes at the dermal epidermal junction extending upward into the basal layer of the epidermis

B) Cell death of individual keratinocytes, referred to as "dyskeratotic cells or dyskeratinocytes" when confined to the epidermis

C) Spillage of keratinocyte intracellular contents into the intercellular space producing edema and exacerbating damage to neighboring cells

D) Vacuolar degeneration characterized by tiny vacuoles on both sides of the basement membrane

E) Melanin containing macrophages in the superficial dermis

QUESTION 1-22.

There are multiple ways to categorize interface dermatitis. Two important and distinct pathophysiologic processes regarding interface dermatitis are lichenoid interface dermatitis versus vacuolar interface dermatitis (acute cytotoxic damage). All of the following statements distinguish lichenoid interface dermatitis from vacuolar interface dermatitis, EXCEPT…

A) In lichenoid interface dermatitis, the band of lymphocytes at the dermal epidermal junction is dense and persistent, inducing vacuolar degeneration and keratinocyte apoptosis.

B) In lichenoid interface dermatitis, the dense infiltrate erodes the rete ridges and may create cleft-like spaces (Max-Joseph space) in the basal layer; however, the intercellular spaces of the upper epidermal layers become narrowed.

C) In lichenoid interface dermatitis, the apoptotic keratinocytes are not eliminated transepidermally and instead drop down into the papillary dermis as colloid bodies.

D) In lichenoid interface dermatitis, the dense infiltrate erodes the rete ridges and may create cleft-like spaces (Max-Joseph space) in the basal layer and may even extend into the lower spinous layer, resulting in widened intercellular spaces of the upper epidermis.

E) In lichenoid interface dermatitis, associated epidermal changes include squamatization of the basal cells, accumulation of eosinophilic "glassy" cytoplasm of the spinous layer cells, wedge-shaped hypergranulosis, and compact orthohyperkeratosis of the stratum corneum.

QUESTION 1-23.

Which of the following statements regarding premature terminally differentiated keratinocytes in lichenoid interface dermatitis is INCORRECT?

A) Upper spinous layer keratinocytes express filaggrin and involucrin.

B) Spinous layer keratinocytes express keratins 1 and 10.

C) Lower spinous layer keratinocytes express keratins 6 and 16.

D) Disruption of the $\alpha5\beta1$ fibronectin receptor in basal cells induces premature terminal differentiation.

E) The epidermal basal keratinocytes become eosinophilic, the granular layer becomes thickened, and the stratum corneum contains compact orthokeratosis.

QUESTION 1-24.

A female patient who recently received a hepatitis B vaccination presents with multiple pruritic erythematous to violaceous papules and plaques on the extensor surfaces. A few lesions are present on the vulva. No scale is present; however, surface changes consisting of white lines or grooves are noted. Lacy white patches are seen on the buccal mucosa. Dystrophic nail changes characterized by ridging and distal splitting are also noted. A biopsy of a wrist lesion is performed. Which of the following is the MOST likely microscopic description of the biopsy?

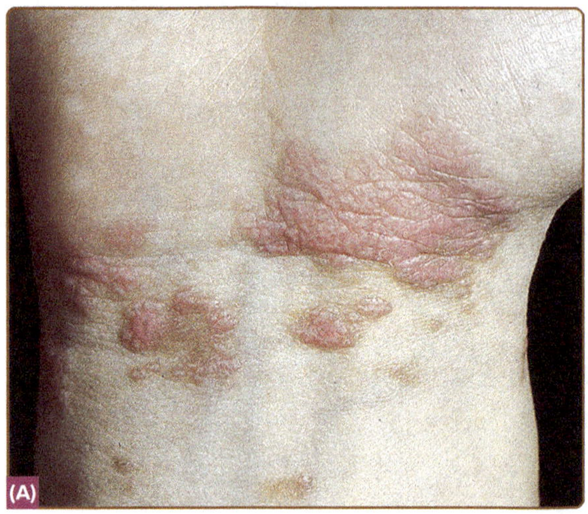

(A)

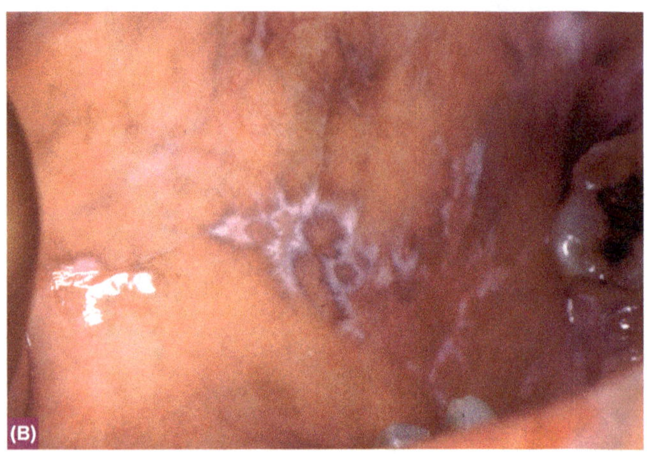

(B)

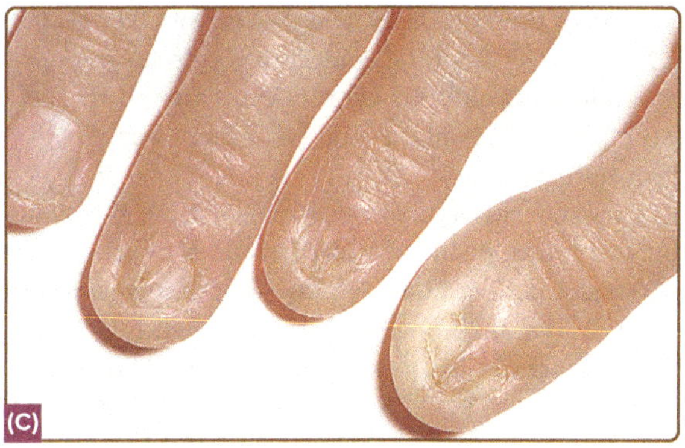

(A), (C) Reproduced, with permission, from Goldsmith LA, Katz SI, Gilchrest BA, Paller AS, Leffell DJ, Wolff K, eds. *Fitzpatrick's Dermatology in General Medicine*. 8th ed. New York, NY: McGraw-Hill Education; 2012. **(B)** Reproduced, with permission, from Wolff K, Johnson RA, Saavedra AP. *Fitzpatrick's Color Atlas and Synopsis of Clinical Dermatology*. 7th ed. New York, NY: McGraw-Hill Education; 2013.

A) A dense band-like lymphocytic infiltrate is present in the superficial dermis obscuring the dermal epidermal junction with exocytosis into the basal cell layer accompanied by keratinocyte apoptosis. Squamatization of the basal cell layer with saw-tooth rete ridges, wedge-shaped hypergranulosis, and orthohyperkeratosis is present.

B) A dense band-like lymphocytic infiltrate obscures the dermal epidermal junction with exocytosis into the basal cell layer accompanied by keratinocyte apoptosis. The epidermis exhibits partial thickness keratinocyte atypia, a diminished granular cell layer, and thick parakeratosis.

C) A band-like lymphocytic infiltrate of moderately density is present along the dermal epidermal junction with vacuolar alteration of the basal layer and outer root sheath epithelium. The epidermis is atrophic with hypergranulosis and orthohyperkeratosis. Follicular ostia are dilated and contain compact keratin plugs. The dermal lymphocytic infiltrate is superficial and deep and clusters around vessels, hair follicles, and eccrine ducts. There is thickening of the basement membrane and increased dermal mucin.

D) A dense band-like lymphocytic infiltrate obscures the dermal epidermal junction with exocytosis into the basal cell layer accompanied by keratinocyte apoptosis. The epidermis is surfaced by orthokeratosis and parakeratosis and contains markedly elongated and thin rete ridges. The dermal infiltrate also contains plasma cells and extends into the deep dermis with accentuation around blood vessels, adnexal structures, and nerve bundles.

E) A dense band-like lymphocytic infiltrate obscures the dermal epidermal junction with exocytosis into the basal cell layer accompanied by keratinocyte apoptosis. The infiltrate also contains eosinophils and plasma cells and extends into the mid- to deep dermis with accentuation around blood vessels. There is squamatization of the basal cell layer with saw-tooth rete ridges, a normal granular cell layer, and delicate laminated hyperkeratosis with focal parakeratosis.

QUESTION 1-25.

A patient's biopsy reveals the findings illustrated below. Alcian blue stain is negative for dermal mucin. Which of the following statements regarding the lesion illustrated below is INCORRECT?

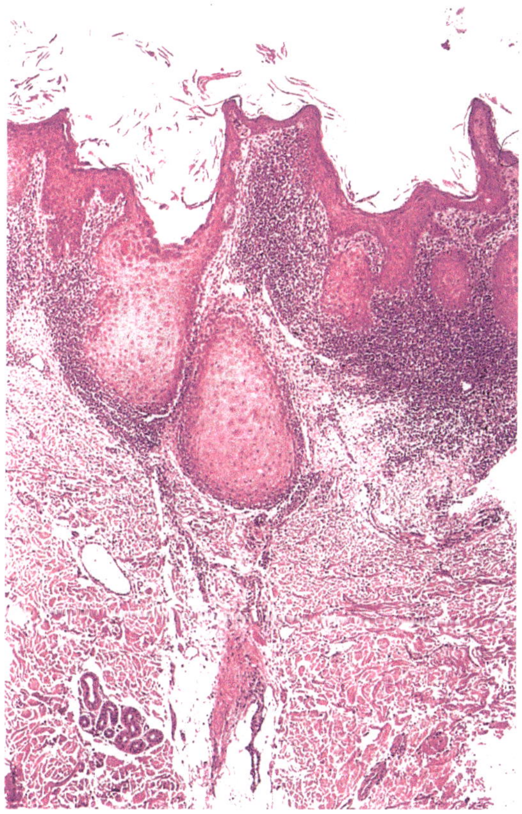

A) Direct immunofluorescence studies reveal shaggy fibrin deposition along the basement membrane zone and large globules of immunoglobulin and complement deposition in the papillary dermis.

B) This is a rare and extremely pruritic condition that usually occurs on the lower legs.

C) This condition preferentially involves sun-exposed skin and is associated with hyperpigmentation and antinuclear antibodies.

D) This condition may occasionally exhibit parakeratosis, spongiosis, necrotic keratinocytes above the basal cell layer, and eosinophils and plasma cells in the dermal infiltrate.

E) The dermal lymphocytic infiltrate is composed of predominantly CD3+ and CD4+ T cells that secrete various cytokines affecting epidermal keratin expression, whereas intraepidermal lymphocytes express CD3 and CD8 and induce keratinocyte apoptosis.

QUESTION 1-26.

A 19-year-old patient, recently diagnosed with herpes labialis, presents with multiple blanching discrete target-shaped erythematous and pruritic papulovesicles with central gray discoloration on the palms and soles and dorsal hands. The peripheral aspect of one of the lesions is biopsied. Which of the following is the MOST likely microscopic description of the biopsy?

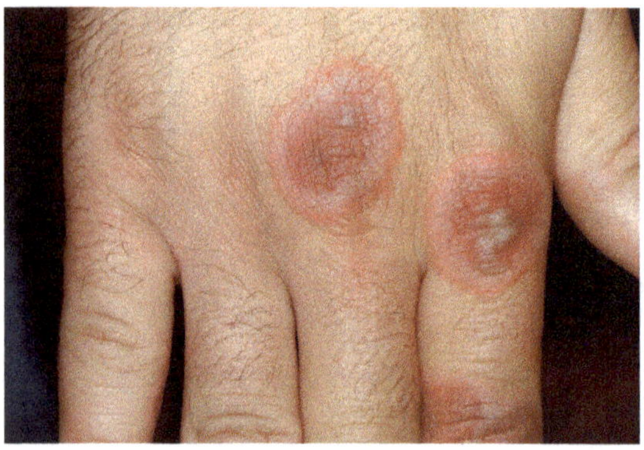

A) There is a superficial and deep dermal perivascular and interstitial inflammatory infiltrate of lymphocytes, eosinophils, neutrophils, and melanophages. There are lymphocytes along the dermal-epidermal junction with vacuolar alteration of the basal layer, dyskeratotic keratinocytes at all levels of the epidermis, acanthosis, mild hypergranulosis, and hyperkeratosis.

B) There is a superficial dermal perivascular and interstitial lymphocytic infiltrate with vacuolar alteration of the basal layer, epidermal atrophy, hyperorthokeratosis, eosinophilic homogenization of the basement membrane, and increased dermal mucin.

C) There is a dense superficial and deep dermal perivascular lymphocytic infiltrate of lymphocytes with vacuolar alteration of the basal layer, rare dyskeratotic keratinocytes within the lower epidermis, mild spongiosis, intraepidermal Langerhans cell clusters, exocytosis of lymphocytes into the upper levels of the epidermis, and thick parakeratosis containing degenerating inflammatory cells. Additionally, there are dermal and intraepidermal extravasated red blood cells.

D) There is a sparse superficial dermal perivascular and interstitial infiltrate with lymphocytes along the dermal epidermal junction, papillary dermal edema, vacuolar alteration of the basal layer, and dyskeratotic keratinocytes at all levels of the epidermis. Lymphocytes surrounding dyskeratotic keratinocytes are noted. The stratum corneum contains normal "basket-weave" orthokeratosis.

E) There are superficial and deep lymphocytic and plasma cellular infiltrates with vacuolar alteration of the dermal epidermal junction. The rete ridges of the epidermis are elongated. The inflammatory infiltrate extends along adnexal structures and nerve bundles into the deep dermis.

QUESTION 1-27.

A 37-year-old professional photographer with a history of treated hypertension presents with pruritic, violaceous, and polygonal papules on the extensor surfaces of the hands and fingers with a thin scale. Additionally, tiny confluent papules with similar morphology are present diffusely on the chest and back. You photograph the diffuse lesions and prescribe topical steroids. The patient is lost for clinical follow-up, and 1 year later returns to clinic stating that he has changed professions and that routine exercise and modified diet have controlled his hypertension. He no longer takes any medications and reports to never filling your topical steroid prescription. On clinical examination you notice that his lesions have completely resolved. Which of the following microscopic findings would LEAST likely be present on a biopsy taken from the previous diffuse eruption illustrated below?

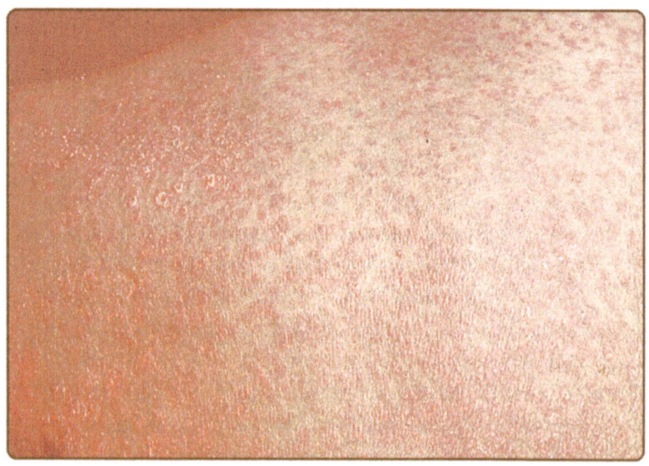

Reproduced, with permission, from Goldsmith LA, Katz SI, Gilchrest BA, Paller AS, Leffell DJ, Wolff K, eds. *Fitzpatrick's Dermatology in General Medicine*. 8th ed. New York, NY: McGraw-Hill Education; 2012.

A) Rare dyskeratinocytes may be seen within all levels of the epidermis.

B) Mixed superficial and deep perivascular infiltrates with eosinophils are present.

C) A corneal scale composed of compact orthokeratosis and focal parakeratosis is present.
D) A sparse superficial dermal-epidermal infiltrate with vacuolar degeneration, spared rete ridges, and increased dermal mucin are present.
E) Mild spongiosis may be present.

D) Rare inciting triggers include contact with dormex and exotic woods containing quinonoids, such as rosewood, ebony, and pao ferro.
E) This condition represents a form of progressive deregulated epithelial injury and frequently results in patient death when greater than 30% of the skin surface is involved.

QUESTION 1-28.

Which of the following statements regarding the lesion illustrated below is INCORRECT?

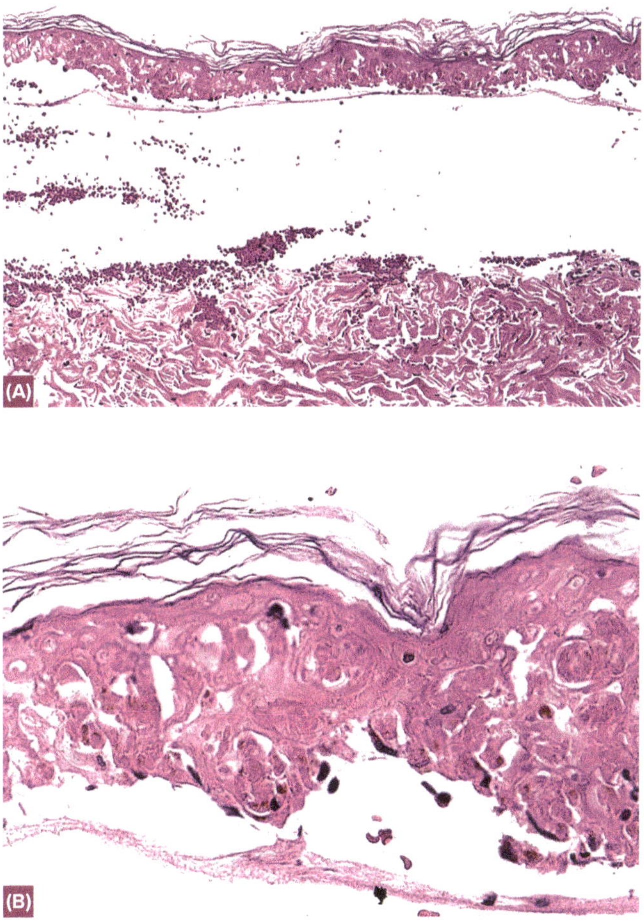

A) Patients may present with diffuse erythema, necrosis, and sloughing of the cutaneous and mucosal surfaces triggered by an exogenous antigen such as medications, including sulfonamides, anticonvulsants, allopurinol, and NSAIDs.
B) The lesion is frequently associated with exotoxins A and B released by *Staphylococcus aureus*.
C) The lymphocytes within the epidermis are of the CD8-positive cytotoxic phenotype with MHC class I restricted cytotoxicity toward keratinocytes.

QUESTION 1-29.

A 17-year-old patient was reportedly given acetaminophen for fever and developed an ovoid erythematous patch on the penis that gradually became hyperpigmented over a 4-week period. The patient now presents months later with a recurrent lesion in the same location. The mother admits to recently giving the patient acetaminophen again for a headache. The lesion is biopsied and illustrated below. Numerous scattered eosinophils, neutrophils, and melanophages are noted within the superficial and deep dermis. Which of the following regarding this lesion is INCORRECT?

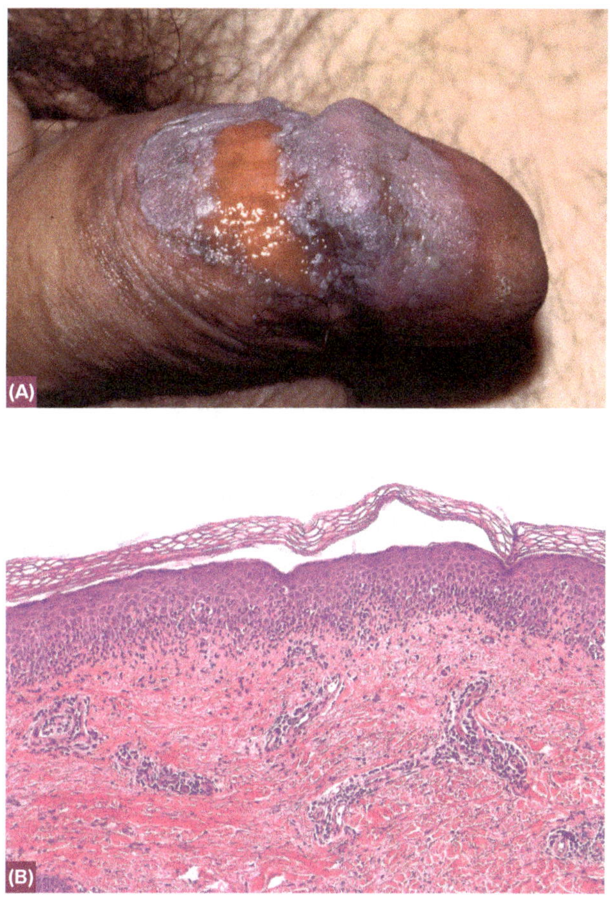

A) These lesions are associated with the administered medication and may remain inflamed for up to 10 days after exposure.

B) These lesions are associated with infection by a herpes virus and may reappear transiently throughout life.
C) The T lymphocytes present at the periphery of the lesion are mostly CD4+, while the T lymphocytes in the center of the lesion are mostly CD8+.
D) Individuals with darker pigmentation may develop postinflammatory hypopigmented macules once the lesions have resolved.
E) This eruption most commonly affects the lips, genitalia, and occasionally the oral mucosa.

QUESTION 1-30.

An otherwise healthy 21-year-old patient presents with multiple crops of painless papules on the neck and chin. Some of them are hemorrhagic and ulcerated. She reports that the lesions rapidly developed 3 weeks ago, and some have spontaneously resolved. During the examination, it is noted that some of these lesions have healed to form shallow scars. Which of the following diagnoses is CORRECT?

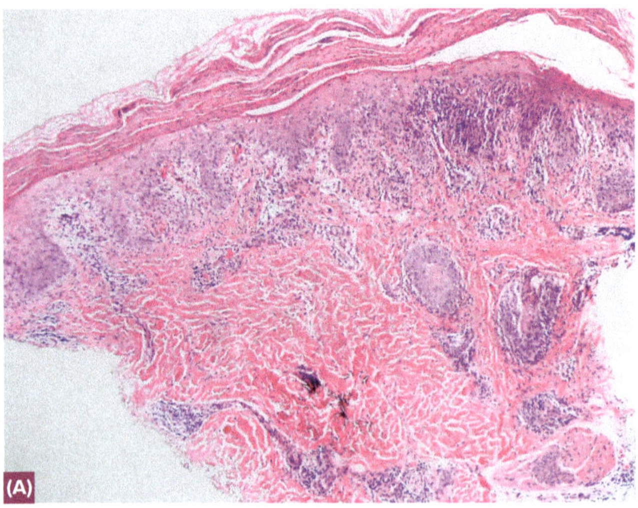
(A)

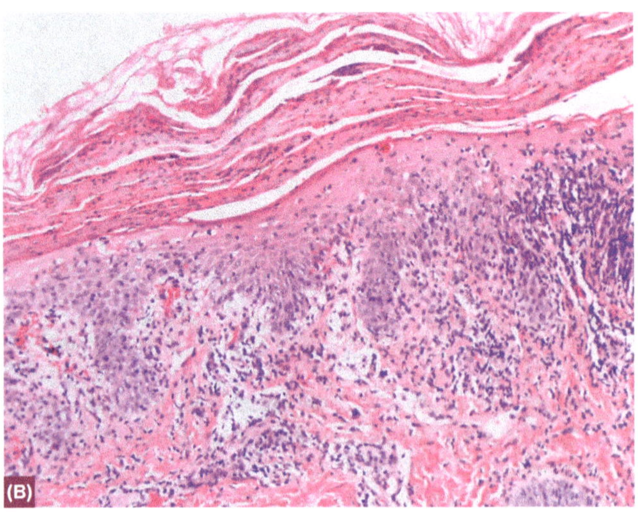
(B)

A) Pityriasis rosea
B) Pityriasis lichenoides et varioliformis acuta
C) Lichen planus
D) Herpes zoster (shingles)
E) Lichenoid drug eruption

QUESTION 1-31.

All of the following are microscopic features that distinguish pityriasis lichenoides et varioliformis acuta (PLEVA) from pityriasis lichenoides chronica (PLC) EXCEPT...

A) Evolved lesions of PLEVA exhibit endothelial swelling, extravasation of red blood cells, and frequent ulceration with small amounts of fibrin within the underlying vessel walls. Severe vascular damage with fibrinoid necrosis of vessel walls is rare.
B) Evolved lesions of PLEVA exhibit dense wedge-shaped superficial and deep dermal lymphocytic infiltrates that are band like at the dermoepidermal junction.
C) In PLEVA, extensive vacuolar degeneration and dyskeratotic keratinocytes rimmed by lymphocytes are seen in all levels of the epidermis and may form confluent clusters.
D) Both intact and ulcerated lesions of PLEVA may exhibit broad tapered mounds of parakeratosis with degenerating inflammatory cells.
E) The lymphocytes of PLEVA may occasionally exhibit mild nuclear contour irregularity, reduced expression of pan T-cell markers (ie, CD7), and clonality via T-cell-receptor rearrangement analysis.

QUESTION 1-32.

The biopsy imaged below reveals a sparse superficial dermal infiltrate composed of lymphocytes interfacing with the dermal epidermal junction. Other inflammatory cell types are absent. Which of the following statements regarding this inflammatory reaction pattern is LEAST likely?

A) When lesions are typically confined to the palms and soles, a proposed mechanism of action involves lymphocytes directed toward keratinocytes presenting non-self-antigens and the activation of the apoptotic pathway via gamma interferon.
B) The lymphocytic infiltrate at the dermal epidermal junction is composed of various mixtures of CD8+ cytotoxic T cells, CD4+ helper T cells, and natural killer cells.
C) When lesions are typically confined to the palms and soles, there is a strong association with herpes simplex viral infection, various medications, and other infectious agents, such as *Mycoplasma pneumoniae.*
D) This is most likely a solitary lesion on the genitalia that is associated with various medications, most commonly

naproxen, and recurs in the exact same location with each repeated exposure.

E) These findings may be seen in diffuse cutaneous eruptions of patients within the first 100 days following bone marrow transplantation.

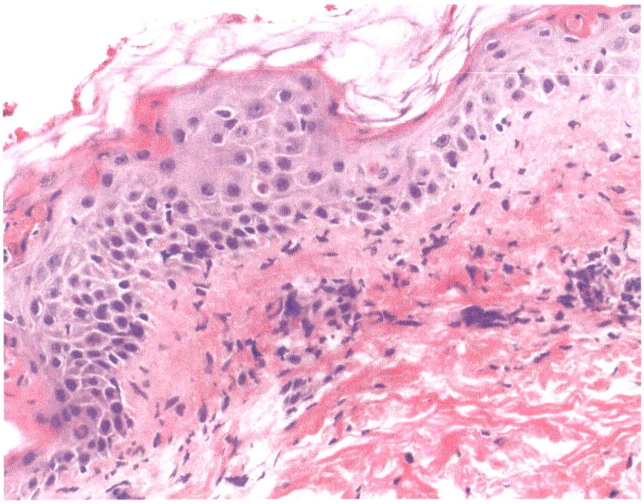

QUESTION 1-33.

A patient presents with multiple confluent erythematous macules on the chest and back with minute follicular papules. He reports undergoing emergency surgery 14 days ago for a stab injury. The patient has an extremely rare blood type and received several units of nonirradiated blood. Which of the following regarding this patient's skin condition is INCORRECT?

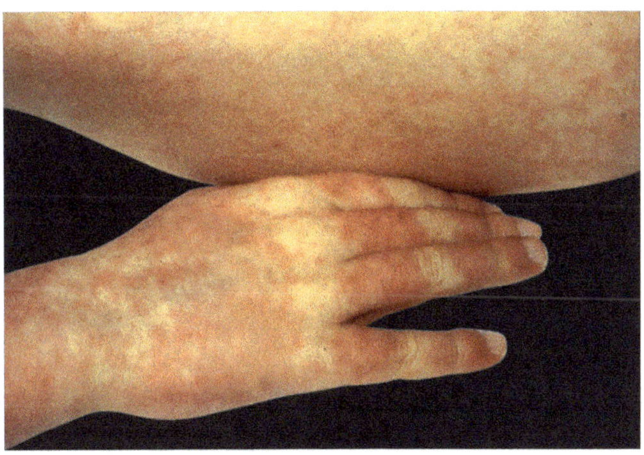

Reproduced, with permission, from Goldsmith LA, Katz SI, Gilchrest BA, Paller AS, Leffell DJ, Wolff K, eds. *Fitzpatrick's Dermatology in General Medicine*. 8th ed. New York, NY: McGraw-Hill Education; 2012.

A) The acute form of this condition may be microscopically indistinguishable from erythema multiforme.

B) These lesions are characterized by a sparse dermal-epidermal lymphocytic infiltrate with occasional partial premature terminal differentiation of the epidermis.

C) These lesions frequently contain prominent vacuolar degeneration of the sweat ducts and hair follicles with overlying parakeratosis and parakeratotic follicular plugs.

D) Dyskeratotic keratinocytes with closely apposed lymphocytes (aka "satellite cell necrosis") is a specific feature of this condition.

E) Severe forms of this condition may result in subepidermal blister formation and sloughing of skin.

QUESTION 1-34.

A patient with acute myelogenous leukemia who was treated with chemotherapy and allogenic bone marrow transplantation presents 110 days later with purple, flat-topped papules with secondary pigmentary alteration. Alopecia, mucositis, and nail changes are also present. A biopsy is performed. Which of the following microscopic descriptions is LEAST likely to be correct?

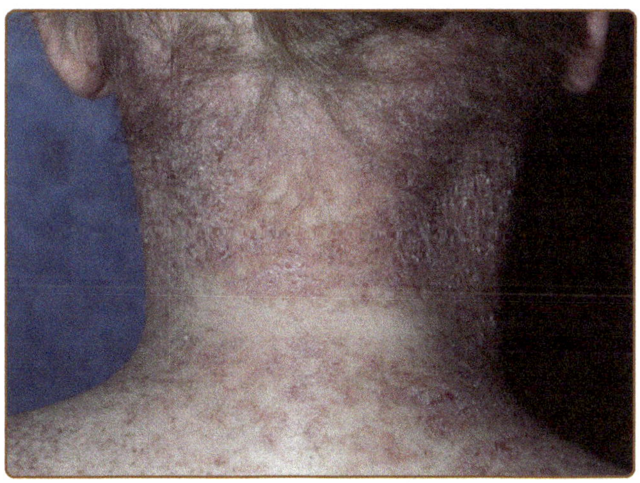

Reproduced, with permission, from Goldsmith LA, Katz SI, Gilchrest BA, Paller AS, Leffell DJ, Wolff K, eds. *Fitzpatrick's Dermatology in General Medicine*. 8th ed. New York, NY: McGraw-Hill Education; 2012.

A) Numerous dyskeratotic keratinocytes surrounded by lymphocytes are scattered throughout a necrotic epidermis that has separated from the underlying dermis.

B) A sparse band-like dermal-epidermal lymphocytic infiltrate is present with premature terminal differentiation of the epidermis and absent transepidermally eliminated dyskeratotic keratinocytes.

C) There is vacuolar degeneration of the basal layer with colloid bodies and wedge-shaped foci of hypergranulosis overlying acrosyringia occasionally exhibiting squamous metaplasia.
D) Perivascular, interstitial, and interface infiltrates containing lymphocytes and variable numbers of eosinophils and plasma cells are present.
E) Dense dermal sclerosis is focally present.

QUESTION 1-35.

A female patient presents with diffuse erythematous macules and patches with photoaccentuation involving the cheeks. Serological studies reveal positive antinuclear antibodies against double-stranded DNA and hypocomplementemia. A biopsy is performed and the findings are illustrated below. Alcian blue stain reveals increased dermal mucin. Direct immunofluorescence reveals intense granular deposits of IgG, C3, and C5b-9 along the dermal epidermal junction. Which of the following is the CORRECT diagnosis?

A) Viral exanthem
B) Reticular erythematous mucinosis
C) Scleromyxedema
D) Dermatomyositis
E) Acute systemic lupus erythematosus
F) Lichen planus

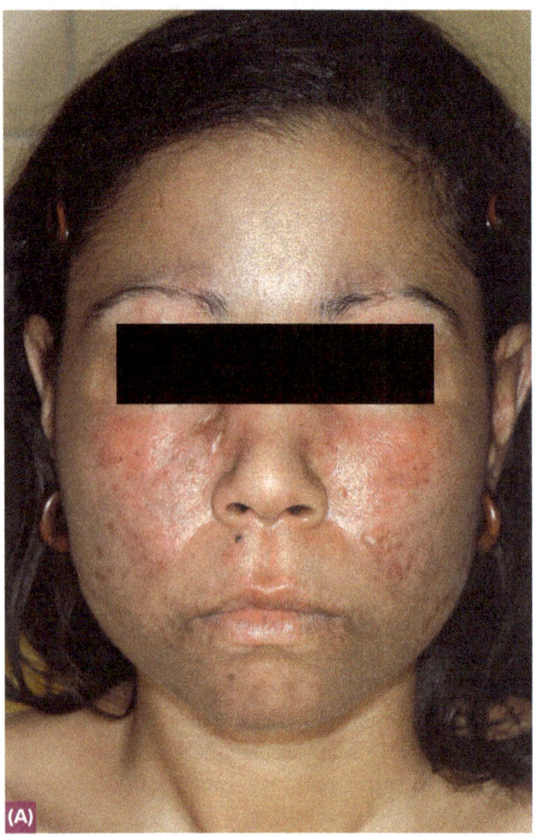
(A)

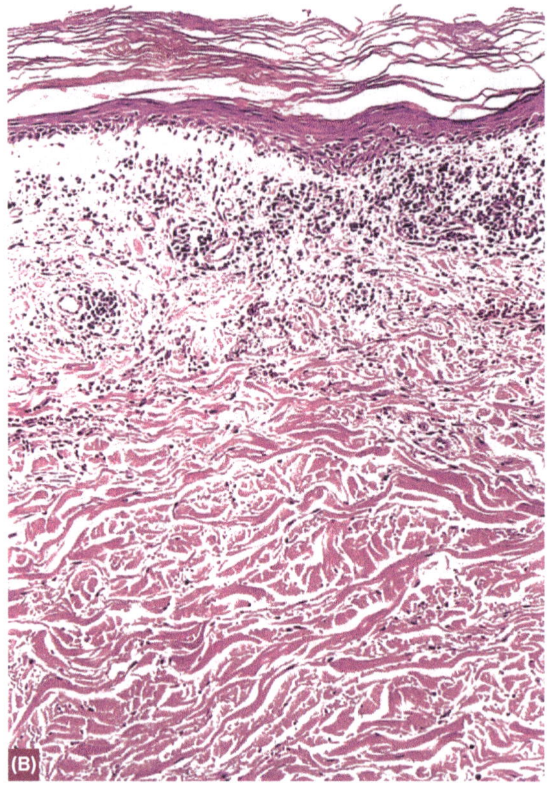
(B)

QUESTION 1-36.

A previously healthy patient presents with the sudden onset of widely scattered, erythematous-to-violaceous, scaling, well-demarcated annular plaques on the shoulders, extensor surface of the arms, dorsal surface of the hands, upper back, and V-neck area of the upper chest. He reports that the eruption presented a few days ago while on a beach vacation in the Bahamas. The emergency room doctor there told him that he had psoriasis. Your review of systems reveals mild fatigue,

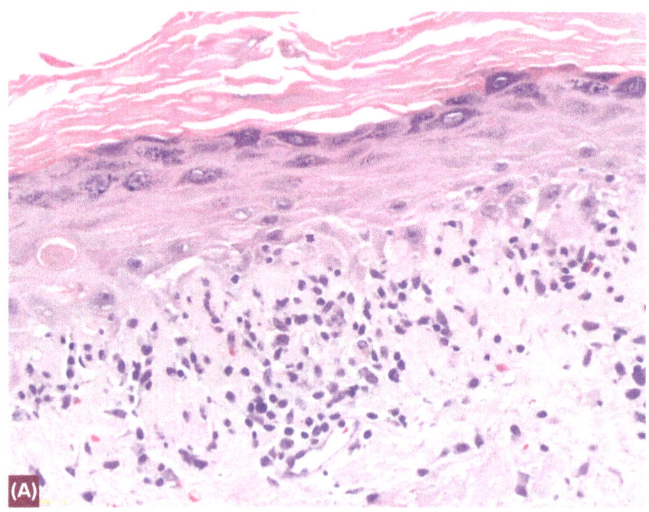
(A)

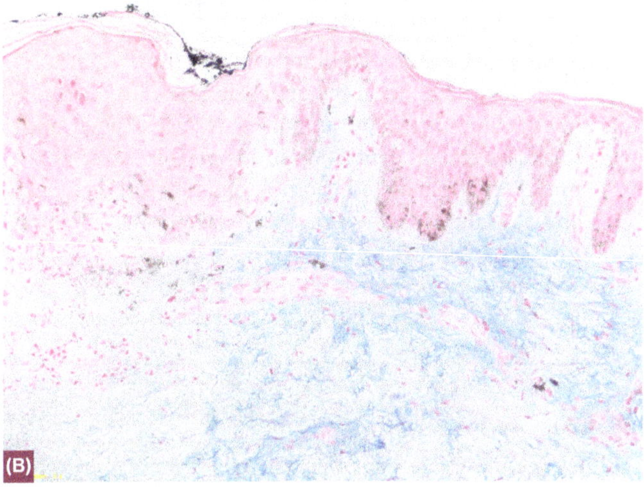

malaise, some arthralgia, and a fever of unknown origin. He is currently taking no prescribed medications. Serological studies reveal antibodies to Ro (SS-A) and La (SS-B) and high levels of circulating immune complexes. Direct immunofluorescence of lesional skin reveals intense granular IgM, IgG, C3, and C5b-9 deposition along the dermal epidermal junction as well as granular labeling of keratinocytes. A biopsy is performed and the findings of the H&E and Alcian blue stained sections are illustrated below. Which of the following diagnoses is CORRECT?

A) Dermatomyositis
B) Psoriasis
C) Subacute lupus erythematosus
D) Secondary syphilis
E) Polymorphous light eruption
F) Pityriasis lichenoides et varioliformis acuta (PLEVA)

QUESTION 1-37.

A female patient presents with a sharply circumscribed erythematous plaque of alopecia with an atrophic firm hypopigmented center on the forehead. Immunohistochemical stains reveal the epidermis, follicular epithelium, and scattered inflammatory cells to be positive for human myxovirus resistance protein 1 (MXA). The lesion is biopsied and the findings are illustrated below. Which of the following statements regarding this lesion is INCORRECT?

A) These lesions are a result of both autoantibodies and cell-mediated cytotoxicity.
B) Patients with this eruption have circulating antinuclear antibodies (ANA) in the majority of cases.
C) An Alcian blue stain may be helpful in diagnosing this condition.
D) A PAS stain may be helpful in diagnosing this condition.
E) Direct immunofluorescence usually reveals immunoglobulin and complement deposition along the dermal epidermal junction and C5b-9 frequently found within venular walls.

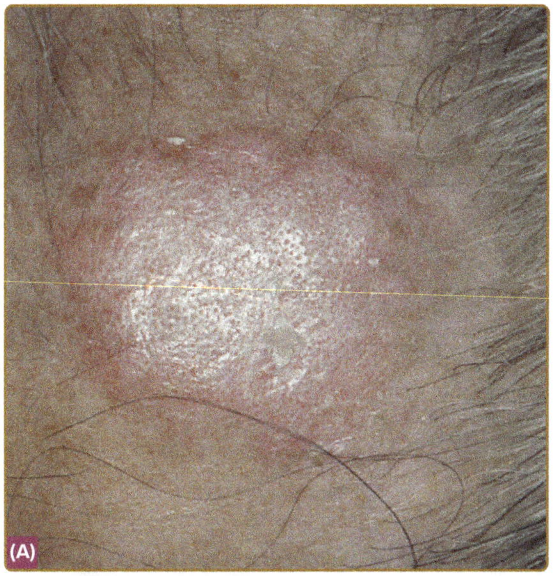

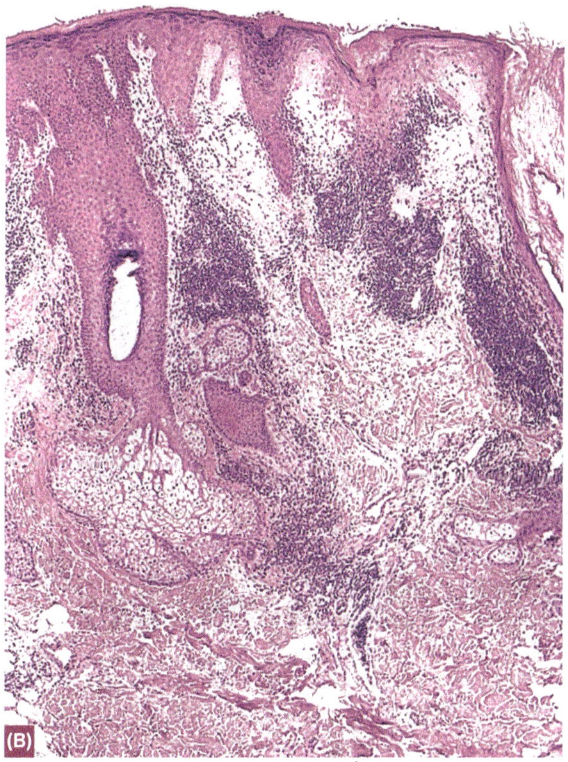

(A) Reproduced, with permission, from Goldsmith LA, Katz SI, Gilchrest BA, Paller AS, Leffell DJ, Wolff K, eds. *Fitzpatrick's Dermatology in General Medicine*. 8th ed. New York, NY: McGraw-Hill Education; 2012.

QUESTION 1-38.

A 60-year-old female patient presents with erythema on the face with periorbital accentuation assuming a violaceous hue. Additionally, atrophic papules with scale on the knuckles and periungual erythema and dystrophic cuticles are present. The patient reports the recent onset of symmetrical weakness of proximal limb muscles and anterior neck flexors plus dyspnea and dysphagia. Serological studies reveal a positive antinuclear antibody titer and elevated levels of creatine kinase. Skin and skeletal muscle biopsies are performed. Which of the following statements regarding this condition is INCORRECT?

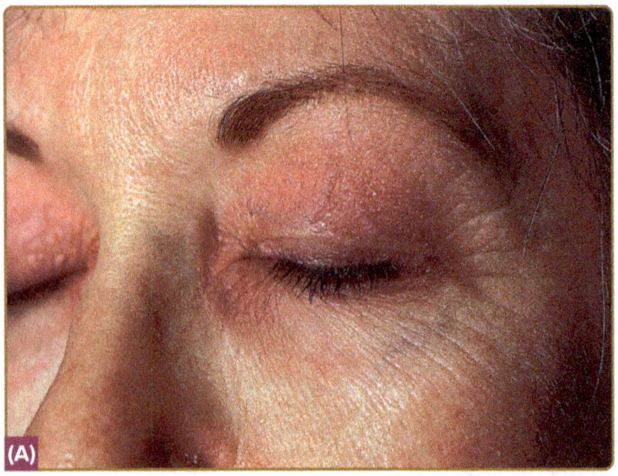

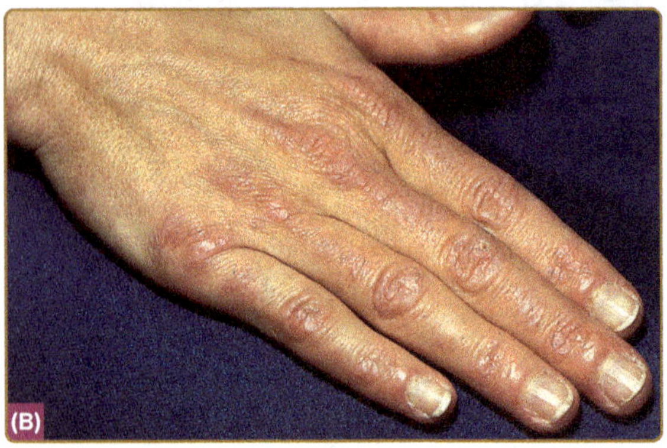

(A), (B) Reproduced, with permission, from Goldsmith LA, Katz SI, Gilchrest BA, Paller AS, Leffell DJ, Wolff K, eds. *Fitzpatrick's Dermatology in General Medicine*. 8th ed. New York, NY: McGraw-Hill Education; 2012.

A) In adult patients, a careful search for visceral malignancy and pulmonary function tests for restrictive lung disease are necessary if their signs are not apparent at the time of diagnosis.
B) Leukocytoclastic vasculitis, digital ulcerations, periungual infarcts, mouth ulcers, and severe calcinosis cutis often accompany the juvenile form of this disease.
C) A highly sensitive finding for this condition is the presence of granular deposits of immunoglobulin (IgG, IgA, and/or IgM) and complement along the dermal-epidermal junction via direct immunofluorescence of lesional skin.
D) Skin biopsies often reveal mild degrees of lymphocytic inflammation in the upper dermis with overlying epidermal atrophy, vacuolar interface change, and increased mucin deposition in the dermis. Skeletal muscle changes include both degenerative and regenerative features in addition to a focal chronic inflammatory cell infiltrates.
E) Autoantibodies, such as anti-Jo-1 and anti-Mi-2, have a low sensitivity but high specificity for this condition.

QUESTION 1-39.

A 17-year-old female patient presents with facial erythema, heliotrope, acral telangiectases, cutaneous fibrosis, dysphagia, dyspnea, polyarthritis, and proximal muscle weakness. Serological studies reveal high-titer antinuclear antibodies with antibodies to ribonucleoprotein (RNP). Direct immunofluorescence reveals reactivity of epidermal keratinocytes for IgG and C5b9 along with prominent vascular deposits of C5b9. A biopsy is performed and the findings are illustrated below. Which of the following diagnoses is CORRECT?

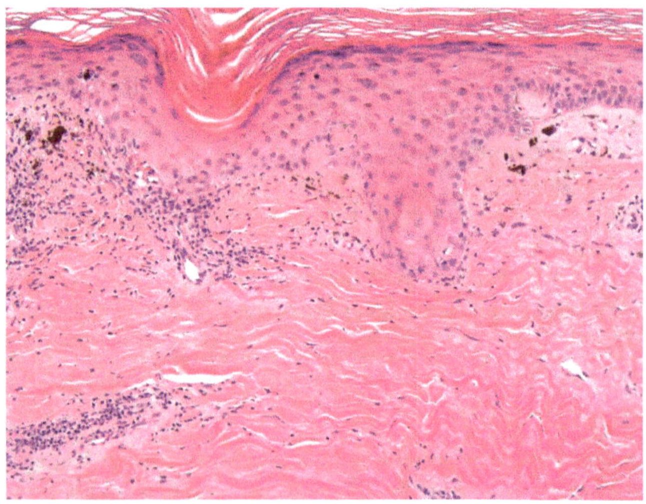

A) Scleroderma
B) Subacute lupus erythematosus
C) Juvenile variant of dermatomyositis
D) Mixed connective tissue disease
E) Rheumatoid arthritis

QUESTION 1-40.

Below is the illustration of a biopsy taken from a chronic vulvar lesion of an otherwise healthy 27-year-old patient. Which of the following statements regarding this condition is INCORRECT?

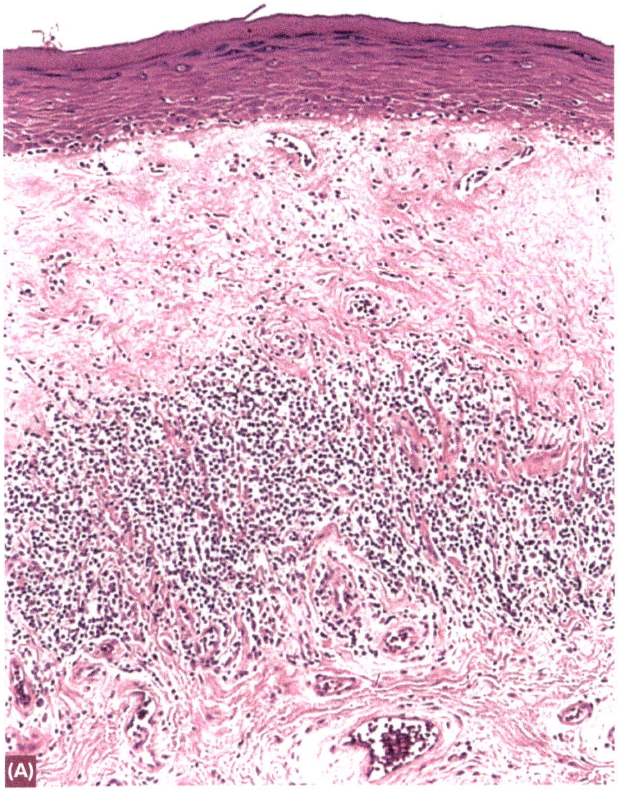

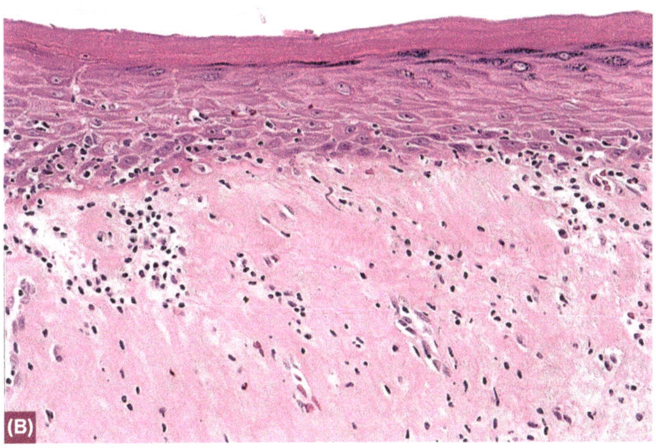

A) Clinically, lesions present as an erythematous patch or plaque, often with an edematous center. This central zone may display pallor and thus impart a white color.
B) There is a reported association between squamous cell carcinoma and chronic forms of this condition on the vulva, with the incidence estimated at 3% to 4%.
C) Microscopically, early lesions reveal a papillary and upper reticular dermis with marked edema, imparting a light, airy, and indistinct quality to the collagen bundles. Occasional subepidermal bullae may occasionally be present.
D) High power microscopic examination of the dermis will reveal bizarre pleomorphic fibroblasts and thickened waxy blood vessel walls.
E) Elastic stains will reveal a paucity of elastic fibers in the bright eosinophilic superficial dermis and a compressed band of elastic fibers at the base with admixed lymphoplasmacytic infiltrates.

QUESTION 1-41.

The histopathological findings illustrated below correspond with clinical patches of atrophic skin with shiny fine "cigarette paper–like" wrinkles and variable melanin content, imparting a mottled hyper- and hypopigmented appearance. Ectatic papillary dermal vessels are responsible for a faint erythema and/or distinct telangiectasias. Which of the following conditions is LEAST likely to present with these combined clinical and histopathological findings?

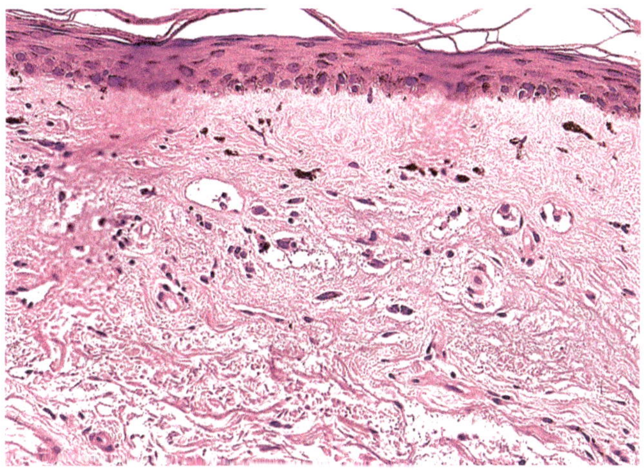

A) Chronic radiation dermatitis
B) Poikiloderma of Civatte
C) Rothmund-Thomson syndrome
D) Bloom syndrome
E) Dyskeratosis congenita
F) Anetoderma
G) Dermatomyositis
H) Mycosis fungoides

QUESTION 1-42.

A 14-year-old male presents with multiple discrete 1- to 2-mm, skin-colored to minimally erythematous papules in clustered groups on the penis and acral skin. A biopsy is performed and the findings are illustrated below. Which of the following is the MOST likely diagnosis?

A) Lichen striatus
B) Lichen planus

C) Secondary syphilis
D) Pityriasis lichenoides et varioliformis acuta
E) Lichen nitidus

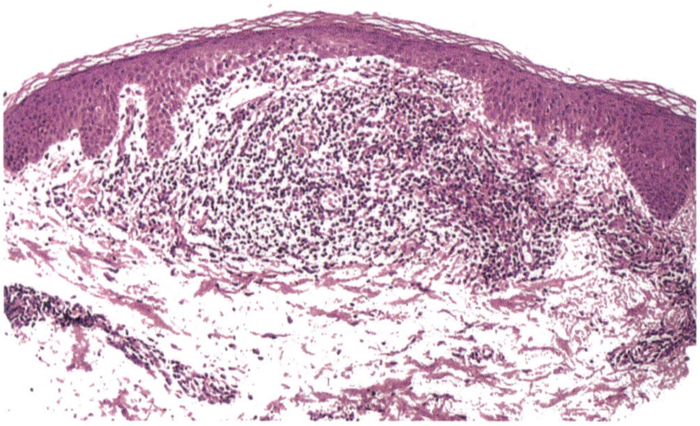

QUESTION 1-43.

A 12-year-old patient presented with a linear array of closely set skin-colored to erythematous papules with little or no scale. The eruption originally presented as progressively lengthening collections of erythematous papules beginning on the proximal portion of the right lower extremity and eventually extended over several months to the acral surface. No systemic abnormalities are identified. You perform a biopsy but do not prescribe any treatment. As mysteriously as the eruption began, it spontaneously resolved after a few months, leaving behind only areas of variable dyspigmentation. Which of the following diagnoses is CORRECT?

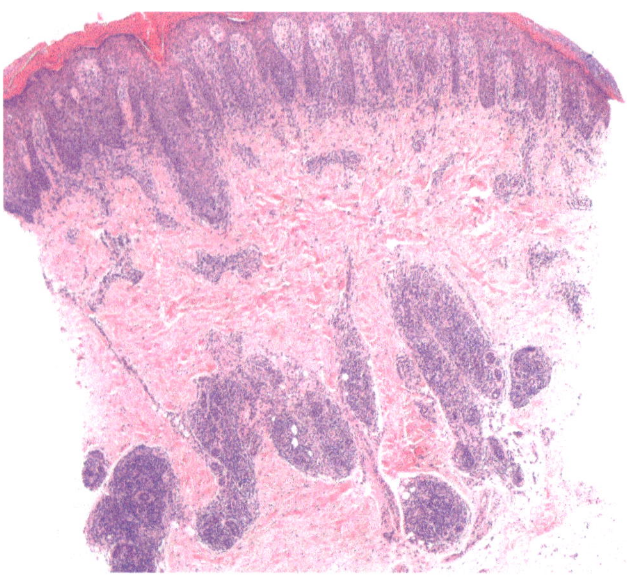

A) Lichen planus
B) Inflammatory linear verrucous epidermal nevus (ILVEN)
C) Lichen striatus
D) Lichen nitidus
E) Allergic contact dermatitis

QUESTION 1-44.

Which of the following features of psoriasiform dermatitis is INCORRECT?

A) There is epidermal hyperplasia characterized by elongation of the rete ridges, thinning of the suprapapillary plates, and hyperkeratosis usually of the parakeratotic type.
B) There is increased keratinocyte proliferation due to more rapid turnover of stem cells or an increased pool of proliferating cells, resulting in mitotic figures frequently present above the basal layer.
C) The distribution and composition of inflammatory cells and quality of the scale allow the various forms of psoriasiform dermatitis to be distinguished from each other.
D) Mild to moderate spongiosis is usually superimposed within these lesions.
E) Vacuolar interface dermatitis with scattered basilar dyskeratotic keratinocytes is a constant feature.

QUESTION 1-45.

A patient presents with multiple sharply demarcated erythematous plaques covered with a thick silvery scale on the extensor surfaces. Pinpoint areas of bleeding are noted when the scale of a plaque is scratched. The fingernails exhibit pitting of the nail plate as well as yellow/brown discoloration under the nail plate, distal onycholysis, and subungual hyperkeratosis. A biopsy is performed on one of the scales on the knee. Which of the following is the MOST likely microscopic description of the biopsy?

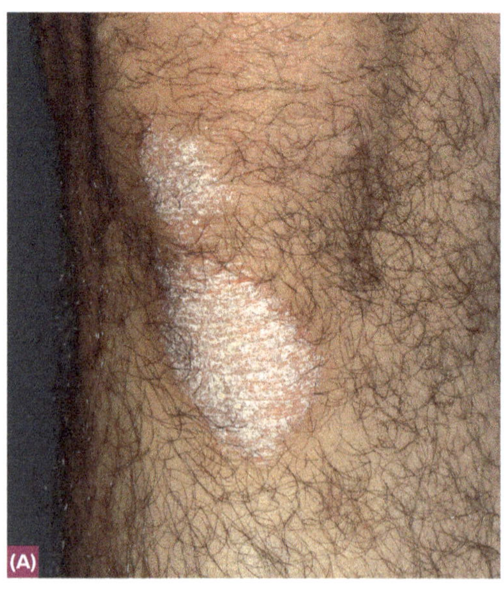

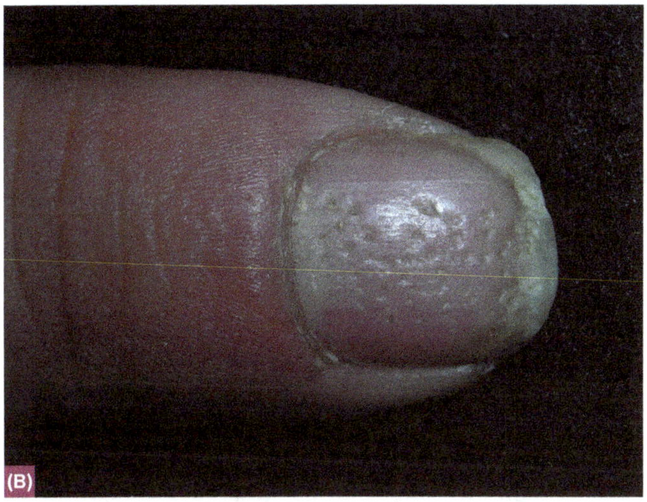

(B) Reproduced, with permission, from Usatine RP, Smith MA, Mayeaux EJ Jr, Chumley HS, eds. *Color Atlas of Family Medicine*. 2nd ed. New York, NY: McGraw-Hill Education; 2012.

A) There is irregular elongation of the rete ridges with epidermal acanthosis, spongiosis, and hypogranulosis. Foci of parakeratosis are present overlying follicular ostia. The superficial dermal inflammatory infiltrate is composed of lymphocytes and eosinophils.

B) There is elongation and fusion of the rete ridges with marked spongiosis including vesiculation composed of lymphocytes and Langerhans cells. There is acanthosis, variable hypogranulosis. There is parakeratosis containing serum and degenerating lymphocytes and Langerhans cells. The dermal inflammatory infiltrate is composed of lymphocytes and eosinophils.

C) There is prominent irregular elongation and thickening of the rete ridges with pointed tips, marked acanthosis, and hypergranulosis. There is hyperkeratosis of both orthokeratotic and parakeratotic types. The papillary dermis shows thickened collagen fibers oriented perpendicular to the epidermal surface. There is a sparse lymphocytic infiltrate within the dermis.

D) There is irregular elongation of the rete ridges with sharp pointed tips, acanthosis, and variable hypogranulosis. There is hyperkeratosis of both orthokeratotic and parakeratotic types. The hyperkeratotic scale contains serum and neutrophils. Rare scattered dyskeratotic keratinocytes are present along the dermal epidermal junction. There is a superficial and deep perivascular and perineural infiltrate composed of lymphocytes and plasma cells. The endothelial cells are swollen and protrude into the vascular lumens.

E) There is regular elongation of the rete ridges with epidermal acanthosis and thinning of the suprapapillary plates. The dermal papillae underlying these thin suprapapillary plates contain dilated and congested vessels. There is hypogranulosis and broad confluent parakeratosis without serum. Clusters of neutrophils are present within the epidermis and within the stratum corneum. Mild spongiosis is present; however, Langerhans cell–rich microvesicles are not present. Several mitoses are identified above the basal layer. The dermal inflammatory infiltrate is composed of lymphocytes.

QUESTION 1-46.

The lesion illustrated below contains inflammatory infiltrates composed of lymphocytes and neutrophils. Which of the following clinical presentations is LEAST likely to be associated with these histopathological findings?

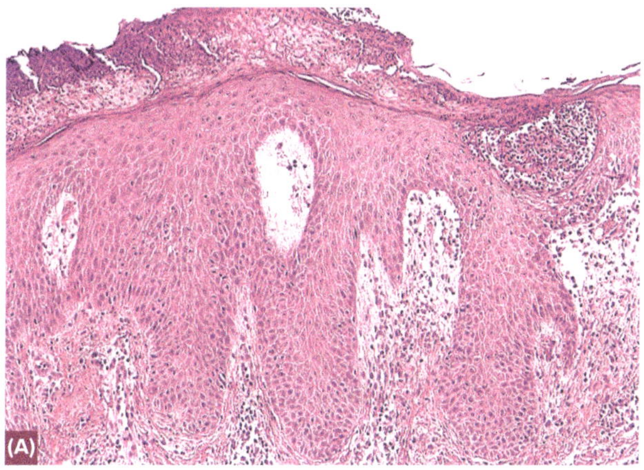

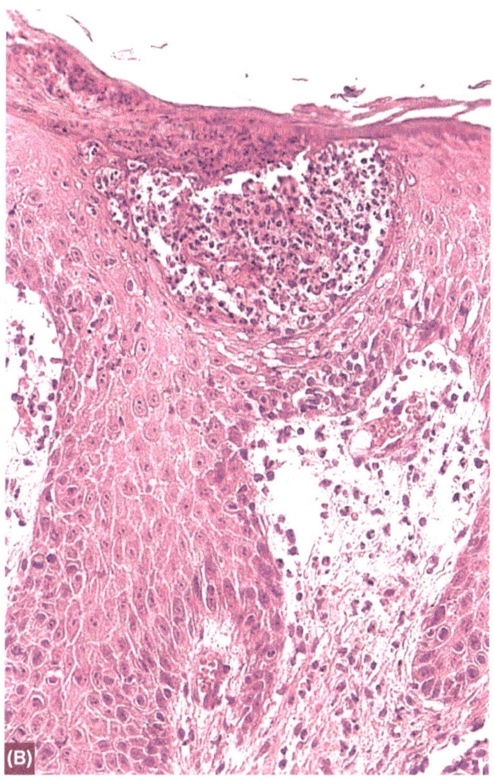

A) This condition may present with the sudden eruption of 2- to 3-mm, sterile pustules tending toward confluence with a distribution over the trunk and extremities and sparing of the face. There is an accompanying fever, leukocytosis, hypocalcemia, hypoalbuminemia, and arthralgias lasting several days. The eruption is frequently precipitated by systemic corticosteroids.
B) This condition may present with pustules localized to the palms and soles.
C) This condition may present as an acute eruption during pregnancy characterized by erythematous patches whose margins are studded with pustules originating in the flexural areas but may spread centrifugally and become generalized. The face, palms, and soles are commonly spared. Onset of the eruption is accompanied by constitutional symptoms of fever, chills, malaise, diarrhea, nausea, and arthralgias. Rarely, tetany, delirium, and convulsions may occur if hypocalcemia is severe.
D) This condition may present with relapsing periungual and subungual pustules with onycholysis, which may lead to permanent loss of nails and scarring.
E) This condition may present as an acute febrile eruption characterized by numerous, tiny, sterile, nonfollicular pustules arising within large areas of erythema, preferentially involving the face and trunk. The eruption typically occurs 5 days after the ingestion of antibiotics. Facial edema, peripheral eosinophilia, and hepatitis are common concomitant findings.

QUESTION 1-47.

The biopsy illustrated below contains infiltrates of lymphocytes and neutrophils. PAS stain is negative for hyphae (not illustrated). Which of the following patients is LEAST likely to have these histopathological findings?

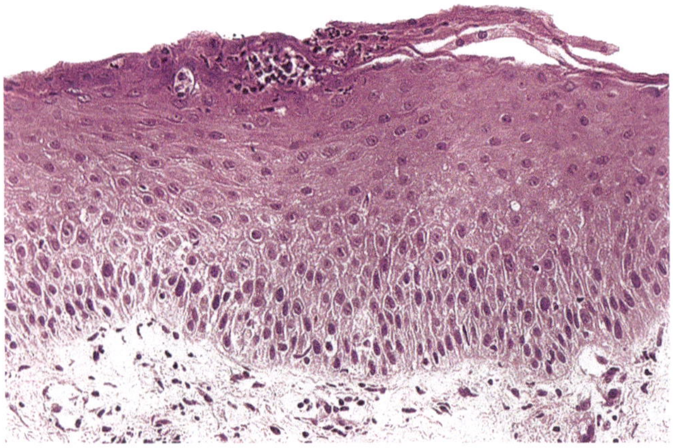

A) A young child presents with the abrupt onset of small, discrete, erythematous, scaling papules that tend to coalesce on the trunk and proximal extremities following a pharyngeal streptococcal infection.
B) An adult patient presents with well-demarcated plaques without overlying scale that appear beefy-red and located in the intertriginous regions where it is warm and moist. There is a history of sharply demarcated erythematous plaques covered with a thick silvery scale on the extensor surfaces.
C) A patient presents with the rapid onset of generalized vivid red erythema and fine branny scales, without loss of scalp and body hair. There is onycholysis of the nails. The patient feels hot and cold, shivers, and has fever.
D) A young patient from the local high school wrestling team presents with annular and serpiginous plaques with scale across an active erythematous border. The border contains vesicles and is advancing centrifugally. The center of the plaque contains areas of clearing without scale. He reports that one of his teammates has a similar condition.

QUESTION 1-48.

Which of the following statements regarding the pathogenesis of psoriasis is INCORRECT?

A) There is evidence that psoriasis represents a low-grade neoplastic process based on a low concordance for disease in monozygotic twins.
B) There is evidence for genomic imprinting in the inheritance of psoriasis.
C) The pathogenesis involves a complex interaction between inflammatory cells and keratinocytes. Th1-cell activation and cytokines (IL-2, IFN-γ, IL-17, and IL-12/23) are involved in epidermal proliferation, and cytokines produced by activated keratinocytes (IL-1α, IL-1β, and TNF-α) are thought to induce keratinocyte proliferation and lymphocyte migration.
D) One hypothesis is that genetic susceptibility coupled with an inflammatory process that may be triggered by activation of T cells by bacterial superantigens leads to the development of psoriasis.
E) A total of nine chromosomal loci (PSORS1-PSORS9) have now been linked to psoriasis susceptibility, with PSORS1 being the most important genetic determinant for heritability.

QUESTION 1-49.

A 22-year-old sailor presents with conjunctivitis and red-to-brown papules, vesicles, and pustules with central erosion, crusting, and peripheral scaling on the dorsolateral and plantar feet. Full body examination also reveals moist, well-demarcated erosions with a slightly raised micropustular circinate border on the glans penis, erosive oral lesions, and subungual pustules associated with onycholysis. Review of systems reveals painful urination and arthritis for over the past 4 weeks. He admits to recent high-risk sexual behavior. Which of the following statements regarding this condition is CORRECT?

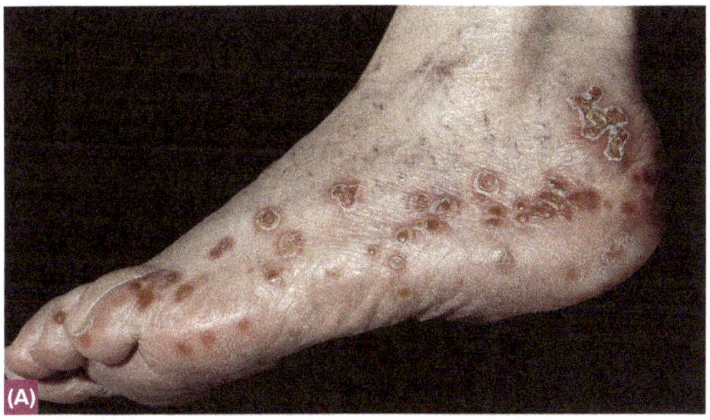

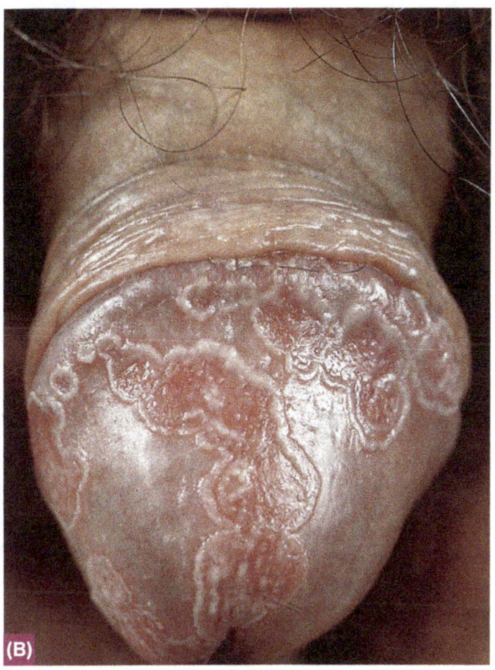

(A), (B) Reproduced, with permission, from Wolff K, Johnson RA, Saavedra AP. *Fitzpatrick's Color Atlas and Synopsis of Clinical Dermatology*. 7th ed. New York, NY: McGraw-Hill Education; 2013.

A) Patients who are HLA-B27 positive have a milder course, with significantly less sacroiliitis, uveitis, and carditis.
B) A triad of urethritis, arthritis, and conjunctivitis must be present to meet the criteria for this condition.
C) The histopathological features of the foot and penile lesions are essentially identical to those of pustular psoriasis.
D) Urethral swab culture will most likely grow *Neisseria gonorrhoeae*.
E) This patient's mucocutaneous lesions represent a rare presentation of this condition.

QUESTION 1-50.

An adult patient presents with a generalized reddish orange scaling dermatitis with sharply demarcated islands of unaffected skin. The nails are noted to exhibit a distal yellow-brown discoloration, nail plate thickening, splinter hemorrhages, and subungual hyperkeratosis. The patient reports that the eruption began 2 months ago as follicular-based hyperkeratotic papules that eventually spread in a cephalocaudal direction to cover the entire body. Hair and teeth are normal. There is no prior history of dermatitis, asthma, or allergic rhinitis. The only medication the patient has taken in the last 6 months is metformin. Lymphadenopathy is not appreciated clinically. Peripheral blood analysis reveals leukocytosis with a 2:1 CD4 to CD8 ratio. The buffy coat reveals 1% of the lymphocytes to have cerebriform nuclei. T-cell-receptor rearrangement analysis is pending. Serial blood cultures are negative for infection. A biopsy is performed and the findings are illustrated below. The dermal inflammatory infiltrate contains scattered lymphocytes and rare eosinophils. Which of the following is the CORRECT diagnosis?

A) Erythrodermic psoriasis
B) Atopic dermatitis
C) Drug-induced erythroderma
D) Pityriasis rubra pilaris
E) Sézary syndrome

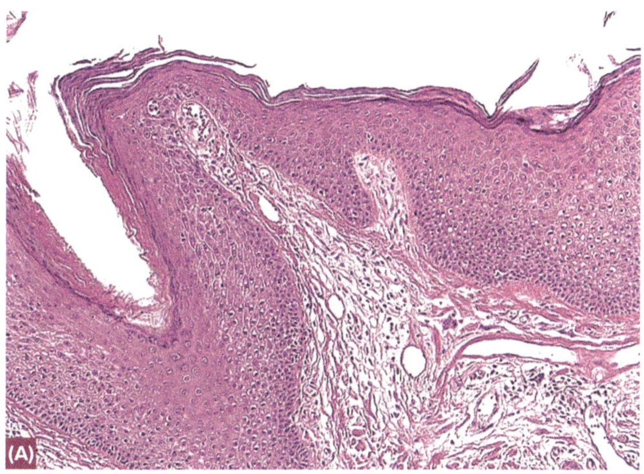

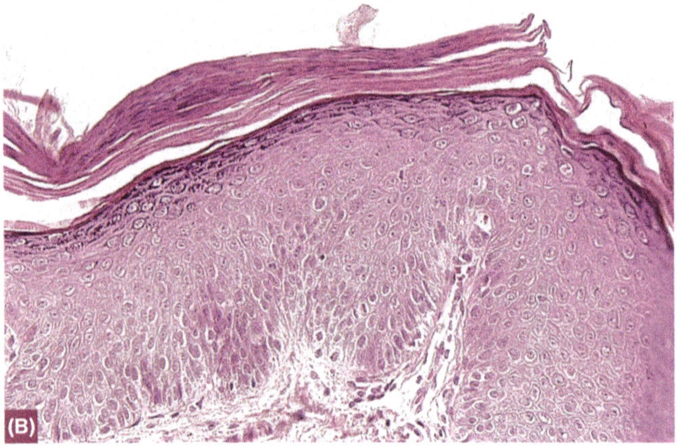

QUESTION 1-51.

A patient presents with a well-demarcated, scaly, focally excoriated, pruritic plaque on the upper extremity. A biopsy is performed and the findings are illustrated below. Which of the following diagnoses is CORRECT?

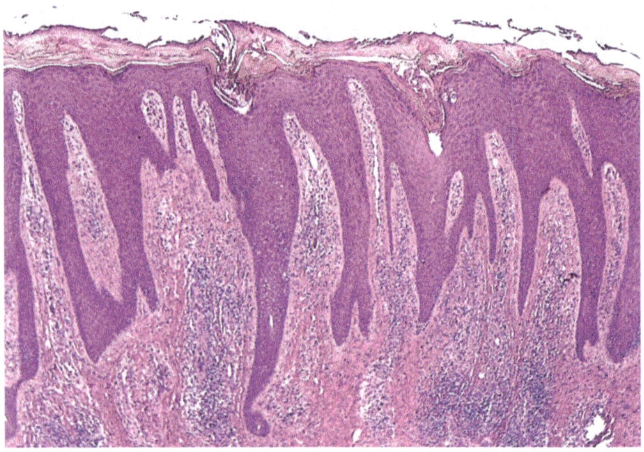

A) Secondary syphilis
B) Lichen simplex chronicus
C) Psoriasis vulgaris
D) Seborrheic dermatitis
E) Scabies

QUESTION 1-52.

A 60-year-old male patient presents with numerous round to oval discrete patches and very thin plaques, mainly on the flank. The lesions are asymptomatic, measure less than 5 cm in diameter, and are covered with fine scale. The eruption first appeared over a year ago and has remained stable. A biopsy is performed and the findings are illustrated below. Which of the following regarding this condition is INCORRECT?

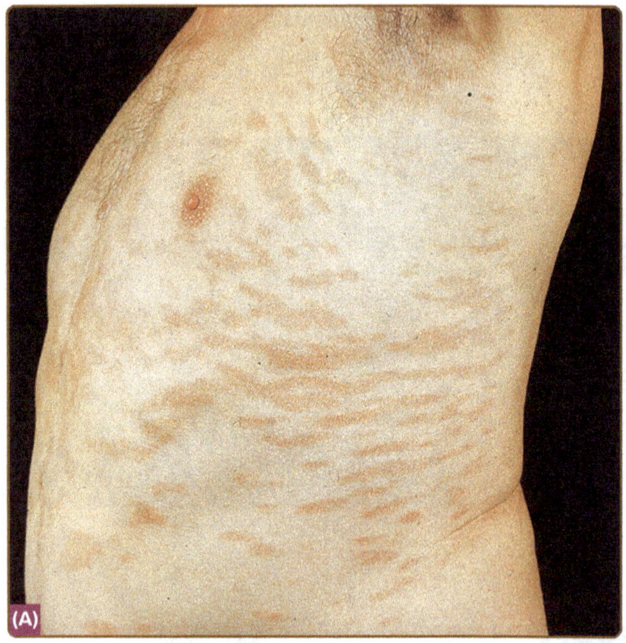

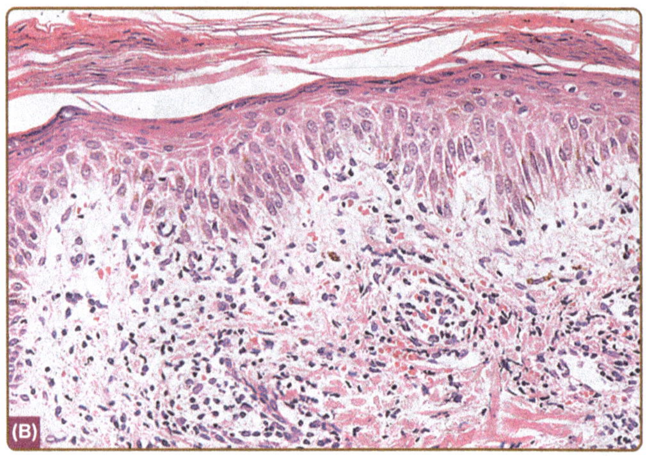

Reproduced, with permission, from Goldsmith LA, Katz SI, Gilchrest BA, Paller AS, Leffell DJ, Wolff K, eds. *Fitzpatrick's Dermatology in General Medicine*. 8th ed. New York, NY: McGraw-Hill Education; 2012.

A) Immunohistochemical staining of these lesions will reveal expression of CD3, CD5, and CD7 within the lymphocytic infiltrate. There is a dominance of CD4 over CD8 expression.
B) T-cell-receptor rearrangement studies will reveal polyclonality.
C) A PAS stain should be ordered to rule out dermatophyte infection.

D) These lesions have a high probability to evolve into mycosis fungoides.
E) High-power magnification will reveal lymphocytes with minimal to absent nuclear contour irregularity.

QUESTION 1-53.

An otherwise healthy adult patient presents with intense pruritus and numerous excoriations in the interdigital webs, sides of fingers, volar aspects of the wrists and lateral palms, elbows, axillae, scrotum, and genitalia. The head and neck are spared. Closer inspection of the fingers reveals areas with thin, thread-like, linear scale that end in a tiny fluid filled vesicle. After rubbing a black felt-tip marker across an affected area and wiping away the ink with an alcohol pad, the structures appear darker than the surrounding skin. A biopsy is performed and the findings are illustrated below. The dermis contains scattered lymphocytes and eosinophils. Which of the following is the CORRECT diagnosis?

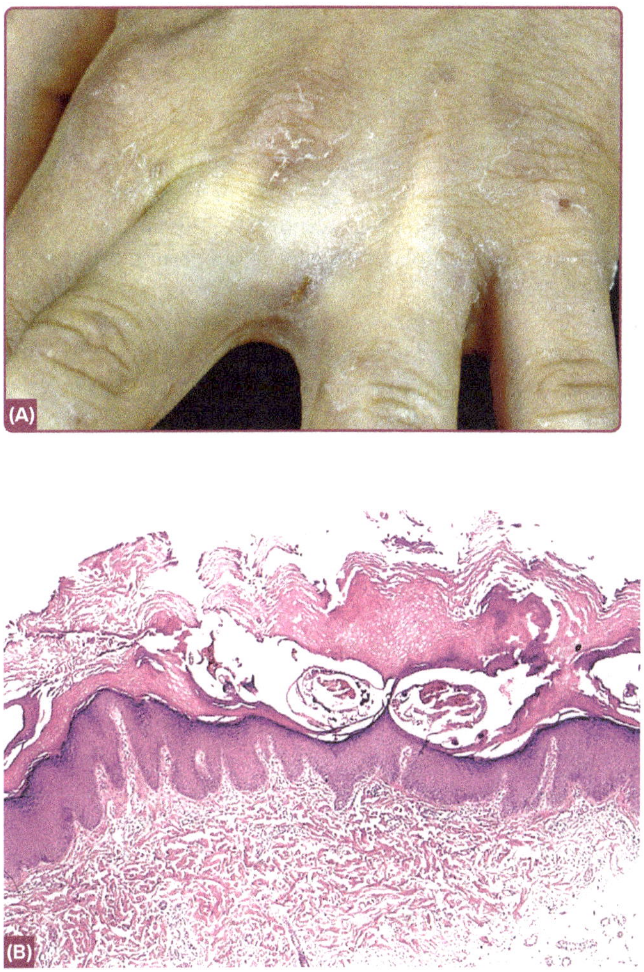

Reproduced, with permission, from Goldsmith LA, Katz SI, Gilchrest BA, Paller AS, Leffell DJ, Wolff K, eds. *Fitzpatrick's Dermatology in General Medicine*. 8th ed. New York, NY: McGraw-Hill Education; 2012.

A) Dyshidrotic eczema
B) Allergic contact dermatitis
C) Dermatitis herpetiformis
D) Lichen planus
E) Scabies

QUESTION 1-54.

An adult patient presents with grouped verrucous papules in a linear arrangement on the lower extremity. Lesions follow the lines of Blaschko and are pruritic with waxing and waning intensity. The lesions have been present since early infancy. One of the lesions is biopsied and the findings are illustrated below. Which of the following diagnoses is CORRECT?

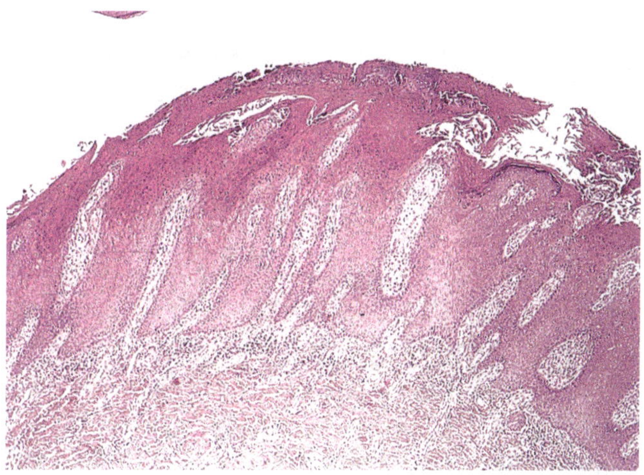

A) Clear cell acanthoma
B) Inflammatory linear verrucous epidermal nevus
C) Linear Darier disease
D) Linear psoriasis
E) Porokeratosis

QUESTION 1-55.

A patient presents with an initial eruption characterized by symmetrical, painful, erythematous, pruritic patches in a photodistribution. The skin becomes progressively more edematous, and several days later evolved into vesicles and bullae, which rupture leaving behind crusted erosions and brown scales. Over time, the skin thickens into sharply demarcated, keratotic, hyperpigmented plaques. The dorsum of the hands is extensively involved and extends proximally, more on the radial than ulnar side. Painful fissures develop in the palms and soles, resembling goose skin. A butterfly distribution of lesions is apparent on the face that extends from the nose to the cheeks, chins, and lips. Confluent areas are noted in the upper central portion of the chest and neck. Mucous membrane involvement consisting of cheilitis, angular stomatitis, a red tongue, and ulceration of the buccal mucosa is present. There is a history of diarrhea and mental status changes. A biopsy of one of the sharply demarcated, keratotic, and hyperpigmented plaques is performed and the findings are illustrated below. Which of the following diagnoses is CORRECT?

A) Pellagra
B) Acrodermatitis enteropathica
C) Necrolytic migratory erythema
D) Necrolytic acral erythema
E) Friction blister

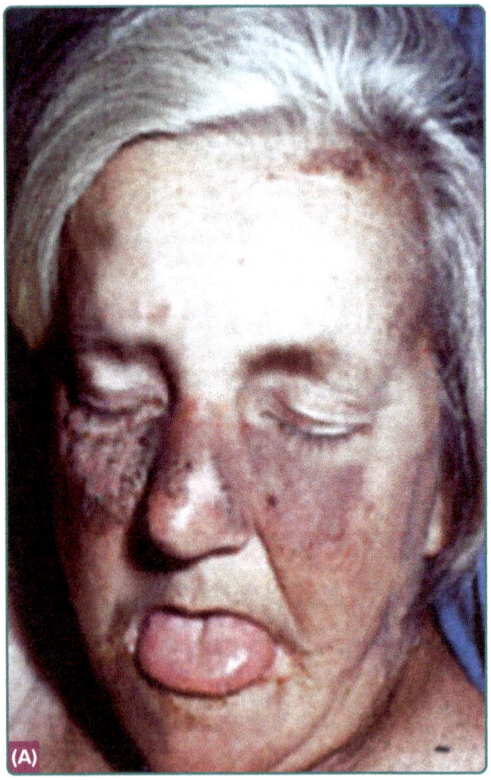

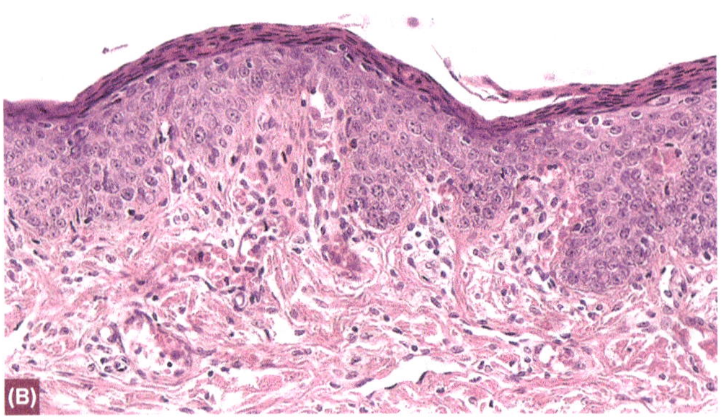

(A) Courtesy of Dr. Ian McColl

ANSWERS

ANSWER 1-1: C.

Spongiotic dermatitis is a nonspecific inflammatory reaction pattern (histopathologic diagnosis) that corresponds to the clinical **eczematous dermatoses.** The eczematous dermatoses differ in their pathophysiology. They can result from immune dysregulation (**atopic dermatitis**), delayed type IV hypersensitivity (**allergic contact dermatitis**), or direct epidermal injury/innate immune reaction (**irritant contact dermatitis**).

Common Eczematous Dermatoses

EXOGENOUS	ENDOGENOUS
Allergic contact dermatitis	Atopic dermatitis
Irritant contact dermatitis	Dyshidrotic eczema
Photoallergic dermatitis	Nummular dermatitis
Phototoxic dermatitis	Stasis dermatitis
Dermatophyte	Spongiotic pigmenting purpura
Id reaction	

The unifying microscopic feature is a sponge-like appearance of the epidermis due to intraepidermal edema with widened spaces between keratinocytes. This is the result of **exocytosis** of T lymphocytes into the epidermis with release of proinflammatory cytokines and induction of keratinocyte apoptosis through "killer molecules." Keratinocyte adhesion molecules (ie, E-cadherin) are subsequently destroyed and there is accumulation of extracellular fluid in the widened intracellular spaces.

Quick Fact

Spongiotic dermatitis with neutrophils could be TINEA. So order a PAS stain!!!!

There is significant variability in the clinical and histopathologic appearance of spongiotic dermatitis depending on the duration, etiology, location, and presence of superimposed secondary changes such as excoriation. Most examples evolve through a course of acute, subacute, and chronic stages; however, not all lesions do this. Histopathologically, lesions of **acute spongiotic dermatitis** exhibit pronounced superficial dermal and intraepidermal edema with lymphocyte exocytosis and intraepidermal vesicles that contain clusters of Langerhans cells admixed with lymphocytes. The corresponding clinical presentation is of edematous, inflamed, oozing papules and plaques, often with visible vesicles. As the lesions evolve into **subacute spongiotic dermatitis**, there are varying degrees of acanthosis (hyperplasia) with foci of **serum-imbued parakeratosis** resulting from the transepidermal elimination of the spongiotic vesicles. This correlates clinically with the presence of scale crust. As this occurs, there is also decreased superficial dermal and intraepidermal edema. Lesions of **chronic spongiotic dermatitis** exhibit acanthosis, hypergranulosis, and compact hyperkeratosis (para- and orthokeratosis) with minimal superficial dermal and intraepidermal edema. Papillary dermal fibrosis is usually present. The corresponding clinical presentation is of firm papules and plaques with accentuation of skin lines and often with **postinflammatory pigmentary alteration**. The dermal inflammatory infiltrates of acute, subacute, and chronic lesions vary depending on the underlying etiology. **Exogenous allergic** forms tend to contain robust eosinophilic infiltrates, whereas **exogenous irritant** and **infectious** forms tend to contain neutrophils. **Endogenous** forms tend to contain fewer eosinophils and possibly rare neutrophils. Cutaneous fungal infections (**dermatophytosis**) can manifest as spongiotic dermatitis; therefore a PAS stain should be considered in these cases, especially those with neutrophilic infiltrates.

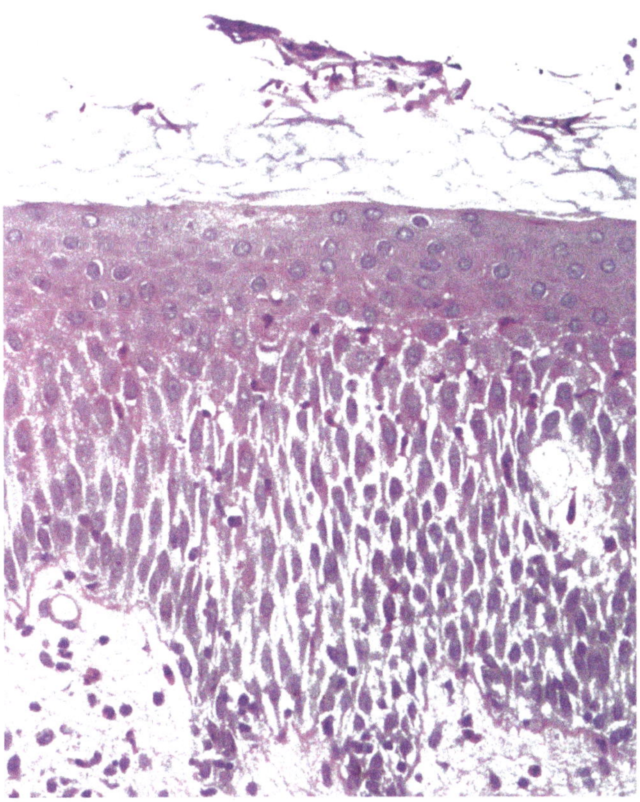

Dermatophytosis (PAS stain). Spongiosis with neutrophil exocytosis and fungal hyphae within the stratum corneum.

ANSWER 1-2: B.

Allergic contact dermatitis is the prototype for the spongiotic reaction pattern. Eczematous eruptions are dynamic and lesions can be biopsied at any stage. Normally, there are a small number of T lymphocytes in the epidermis that function in ongoing immunologic surveillance. Offending antigens are presented to a presensitized T lymphocyte by a Langerhans cell. The antigen can be introduced to the Langerhans cell by topical inoculation (ie, allergic contact) or via systemic administration (ie, ingested medication). Activated T cells and keratinocytes then secrete various cytokines that induce migration of lymphocytes and macrophages from the superficial vascular plexus into the dermis. This migration results in vascular dilatation and papillary dermal edema, manifesting clinically as erythema. Exocytosis of a small number of lymphocytes into the epidermis occurs and exaggerates the reaction. First, intracellular edema of spinous-layer keratinocytes occurs followed by intercellular edema. Desmosomes between keratinocytes initially limit intercellular edema. As the process evolves, lymphocytes migrate into the epidermis, and increasing intracellular edema leads to rupture of keratinocytes and keratinocyte desmosomes (referred to as **cytolysis**). This leads to widening of the extracellular space and **spongiotic vesiculation** containing plasma, antigen presenting Langerhans cells, lymphocytes, and keratinocytic debris (**Langerhans cell–rich microvesicles**). Confluence of these vesicles with multiloculation is referred to as **reticular degeneration**. During this acute phase, the stratum corneum maintains a normal basket-weave appearance. Overall, there is an increase in volume of the epidermis (mostly edema), which correlates with papules and papulovesicles seen clinically with these acute lesions.

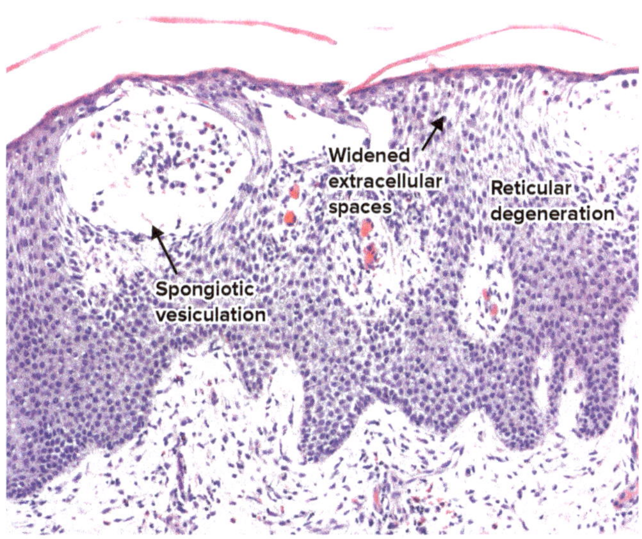

Acute spongiotic dermatitis. Marked epidermal intercellular edema with spongiotic microvesicles and superficial perivascular lymphocytic infiltrate. The stratum corneum shows normal basket weave pattern.

Acute Eczema: "Red, Weepy, Wet"

Erythema
- Lymphocytes and macrophages to the dermis
- Vascular dilatation
- Papillary dermal edema

Vesicles
- Reticular degeneration

Papulovesicles
- Increased edema in the epidermis

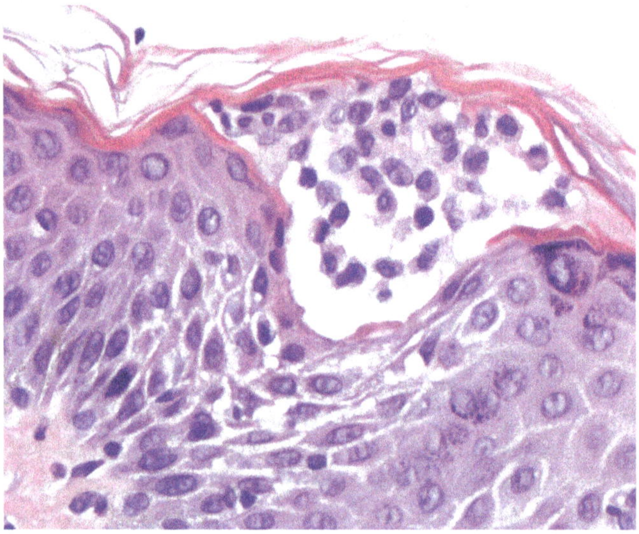

Langerhans cell microvesicles with adjacent epidermal spongiosis.)

ANSWER 1-3: A.

In the face of persistent inflammation, lesions progress from a subacute to a chronic stage of spongiotic dermatitis. Initially, spinous-layer keratinocytes are preferentially damaged by spongiosis, inducing a compensatory adaptive response of hyperplasia (**acanthosis**). Parakeratosis is a result and signifies a rapid increase in cellular proliferation/cellular turnover. The weeping spongiotic vesicles of acute spongiosis are gradually eliminated transepidermally resulting in the serum-imbued scale crusts of **subacute spongiosis** (choice A). Additionally, a phenomenon equivalent to hypertrophy occurs where keratinocytes increase their intracellular keratin content, resulting in hypergranulosis and compact orthokeratosis. Erythema is still present in chronic lesions since the perivascular lymphocytic infiltrates are present. Spongiosis gradually decreases in chronic lesions, and may even be absent. The hyperplastic epidermis forms elongated rete ridges that are markedly irregular in terms of length and width, unlike the regular elongated rete ridges seen in **psoriasis** (ie, rack of test tubes). The papillary dermis becomes hyperplastic with increased collagen deposition along the contours of the rete ridges. Often the collagen bundles appear to run perpendicular to the epidermal surface. **Lichen simplex chronicus** is synonymous with chronic spongiotic dermatitis, but with less inflammation clinically and microscopically.

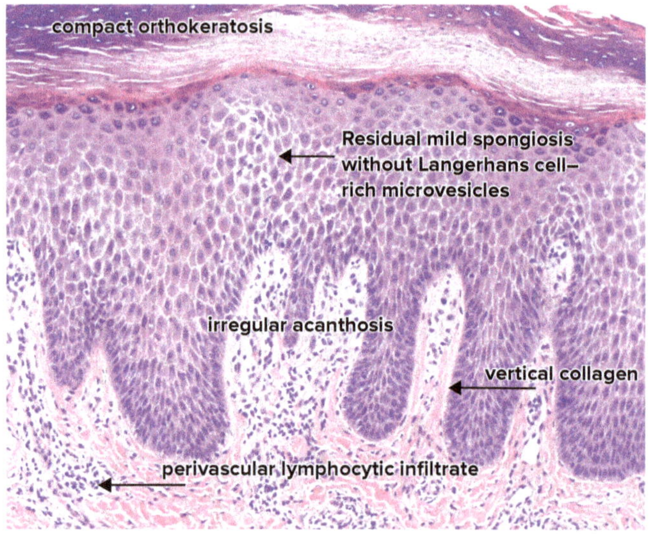

Chronic spongiotic dermatitis. Marked compact hyperkeratosis and parakeratosis, epidermal acanthosis, minimal spongiosis, and superficial perivascular lymphocytic infiltrate.

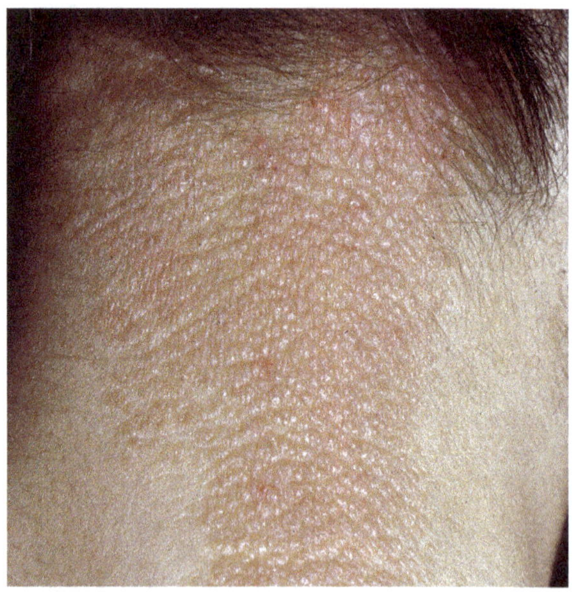

Lichen simplex chronicus. Confluent, papular, follicular eczema, creating a plaque of lichen simplex chronicus of the posterior neck and occipital scalp. Condition had been present for many years as a result of chronic rubbing of the area. (Reproduced, with permission, from Wolff K, Johnson RA, Saavedra AP. *Fitzpatrick's Color Atlas and Synopsis of Clinical Dermatology*. 7th ed. New York, NY: McGraw-Hill Education; 2013.)

Histopathologic Features in Spongiotic Dermatitis

	ACUTE	SUBACUTE	CHRONIC
Stratum corneum	Often normal; sometimes parakeratosis, scale crust	Parakeratosis and scale crust	Hyperkeratotic orthokeratosis
Epidermal acanthosis	None to minimal	Mild to moderate	Moderate to marked
Spongiosis	Mild to marked	Mild to moderate	Minimal to absent
Intraepidermal microvesicles	Yes ± macrovesicles	Yes	No
Dermal perivascular inflammation	Lymphocytes and eosinophils	Lymphocytes and eosinophils	Lymphocytes and histiocytes
Papillary dermal edema	Minimal to marked	Minimal	No
Papillary dermal thickening	No	No	Yes

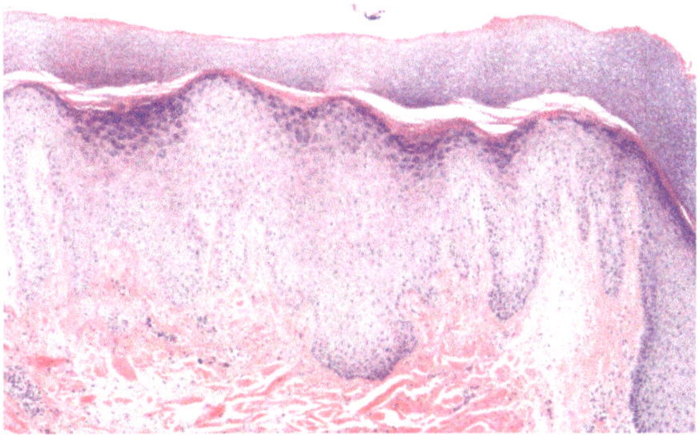

Lichen simplex chronicus. Marked compact hyperkeratosis, hypergranulosis, irregular epidermal acanthosis, and fibrosis of the superficial dermis with sparse inflammation.

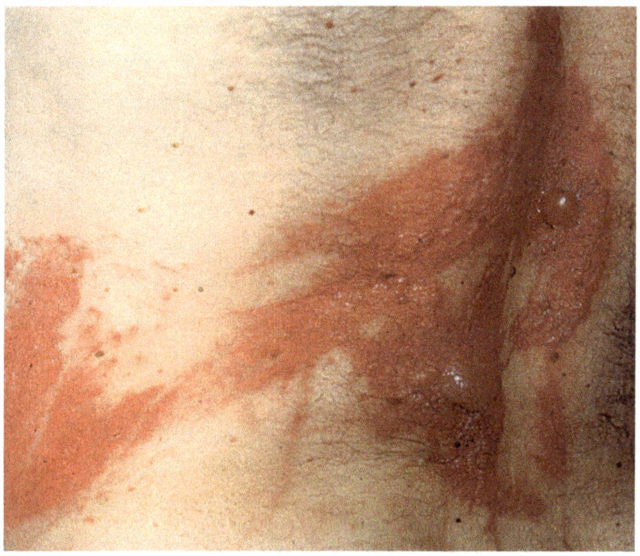

Irritant contact dermatitis. The streaky pattern indicates an "outside job." The eruption is characterized by massive erythema with vesiculation and blister formation and is confined to the sites exposed to the toxic agent. (Reproduced, with permission, from Wolff K, Johnson RA, Saavedra AP. *Fitzpatrick's Color Atlas and Synopsis of Clinical Dermatology*. 7th ed. New York, NY: McGraw-Hill Education; 2013.)

ANSWER 1-4: D.

There are two types of contact dermatitis: irritant and allergic. In **irritant contact dermatitis**, anyone exposed to offending substances in high enough concentrations for long enough duration will result in direct keratinocyte damage and the subsequent spongiotic inflammatory reaction pattern. Common offending substances include detergents, solvents, sunscreens, acids, alkalis, adhesives, metalworking fluids, and friction. Clinically, the lesions of irritant contact dermatitis are often well demarcated with a glazed surface. There may be redness, itching, swelling, blistering, and scaling.

Quick Fact

- ✓ Spongiosis with eosinophils favors allergic contact dermatitis.
- ✓ Neutrophils and ballooning keratinocytes irritant dermatitis.

The extent of keratinocyte necrosis varies and neutrophils are frequently seen within the epidermis along with the classic spongiotic reaction pattern. There is prominent papillary dermal edema with lymphohistiocytic aggregates surrounding the superficial vascular plexus.

Choice D describes **systemic allergic contact dermatitis**, which requires prior sensitization of T lymphocytes to illicit an immune response. Although localized contact dermatitis is more common, generalized forms may also occur. Allergic contact dermatitis can occur with ingested antigen and dissemination through the blood (systemic allergic contact dermatitis) or through widespread external inoculation.

Additionally, diffuse eruptions can have an irritant-based etiology (generalized irritant contact dermatitis). **Phototoxic dermatitis** is related to irritant dermatitis when the offending substance absorbs UV light and lowers the threshold of UV light exposure needed for keratinocyte damage. The reaction pattern for phototoxic dermatitis is similar to irritant contact dermatitis, but contains numerous dyskeratotic **"sunburn" cells** throughout the epidermis.

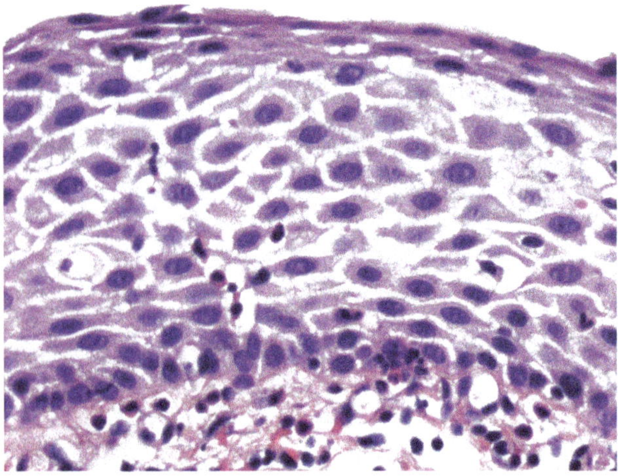

Irritant contact vulvitis. Spongiosis with neutrophil exocytosis.

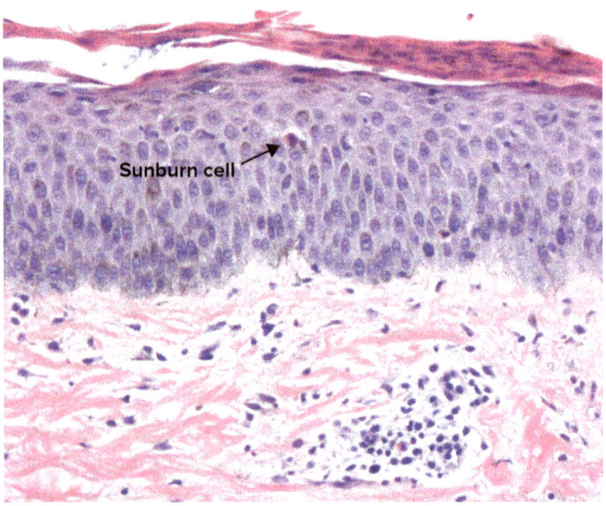

Photoirritant, or phototoxic, dermatitis. There are features of irritant contact dermatitis with dyskeratotic "sunburn" keratinocytes throughout the epidermis.

The damage may be so severe that full-thickness coagulative necrosis of the epidermis may be seen. The diffuse exaggerated erythema or "sunburn" seen in individuals taking doxycycline, tetracyclines, or sulfonamides is an example of a **systemic phototoxic dermatitis** caused by a circulating ingested substance.

ANSWER 1-5: C.

This is a classic example of **allergic contact dermatitis** with secondary **autoeczematization** (aka **id reaction**). The well-circumscribed, erythematous, vesicular, and scaly eruption on the finger with a band-like circumferential distribution correlates with the area where metal jewelry would come into contact with the skin. Nickel is a notorious metal for causing allergic contact dermatitis. The biopsy of the finger reveals epidermal acanthosis, spongiosis with Langerhans cell–rich microvesicles containing eosinophils, and superficial perivascular lymphocytic and eosinophilic infiltrates. These findings are consistent with **subacute spongiotic dermatitis**. The biopsy of the upper back reveals mild acanthosis, marked intraepidermal edema with large Langerhans

Common Allergens in Allergic Contact Dermatitis

- Metals (nickel, cobalt, gold sodium thiosulfate, potassium dichromate)
- Preservatives (thimerosal, quaternium-15, formaldehyde, diazolidinyl urea)
- Antibiotics (neomycin, bacitracin)
- Fragrance (balsam of Peru)
- Components of rubber products (mercaptobenzothiazole, carba mix)
- Hair dye (p-Phenylenediamine)

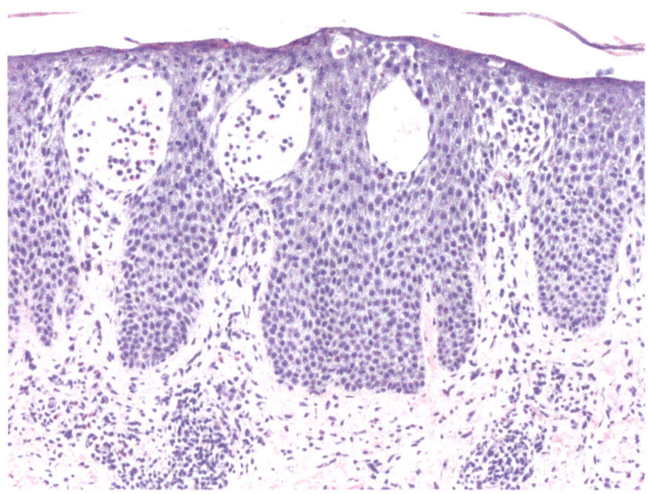

Allergic contact dermatitis. Epidermal acanthosis, spongiosis with microvesicles containing eosinophils, and superficial perivascular and interstitial lymphocytic and eosinophilic infiltrates.

cell-rich microvesicles, and superficial perivascular lymphocytic and eosinophilic infiltrates, consistent with **acute spongiotic dermatitis**. The diffuse eruption on the chest and upper back represents **autoeczematization** (aka **id reaction**), which probably occurs because inflammatory processes at the primary site travel distally and thus facilitate the development of a second eczematous reaction. With **id reactions**, both eruptions will have similar histopathologic findings. All patients with severe allergic contact dermatitis should undergo **patch testing** to elucidate the offending antigen.

Allergic Contact Dermatitis

Clinical Features
- Delayed hypersensitivity reaction (type IV)
- All ages affected except below age 5 years and the elderly
- Rash occurs at the site of exposure in previously sensitized host
- Morphology of rash is eczematous—acute, subacute, or chronic

Histopathologic Features
- Acute
  - Spongiosis often with formation of clinically evident intraepidermal vesicles, superficial perivascular lymphocytic infiltrate usually rich in eosinophils, migration of inflammatory cells into the epidermis
- Subacute
  - Epidermal hyperplasia with spongiosis, superficial perivascular lymphocytic and eosinophilic infiltrate with variable exocytosis
- Chronic
  - Psoriasiform hyperplasia with a superficial perivascular lymphocytic and eosinophilic infiltrate; spongiosis is minimal to absent

Differential Diagnosis
- Many forms of eczematous dermatitis
- Irritant and photoallergic reactions
- Scabetic infestation
- Drug reactions
- Bullous pemphigoid
- Parasitic infestations

ANSWER 1-6: B.

This patient is experiencing a cell-mediated allergic reaction to **poison ivy**. This is an example of **allergic contact dermatitis** and not **irritant contact dermatitis**. These lesions may appear identical to irritant dermatitis by clinical inspection; therefore clinical history may be the biggest clue. Regions of thickened skin, such as the palms and soles, are frequently resistant to this inflammatory reaction pattern, unlike the thin skin around the eyelids. This individual most likely developed these lesions by direct inoculation of the **allergen** from the fingers to the skin around the eyes. In general, the lesions of contact dermatitis are distributed on exposed parts or in bizarre asymmetric patterns, and consist of erythematous macules, papules, and vesicles. The affected area is often hot and swollen, with an exudation and crusting, simulating (and at times complicated by) infection. The pattern of the eruption may be diagnostic (ie, typical linear streaked vesicles on the extremities in poison oak or ivy dermatitis). Allergic contact dermatitis is the prototype of spongiotic dermatitis. In allergic contact dermatitis, eosinophils are frequently present, whereas neutrophils are more common in irritant contact dermatitis. Remember, in allergic contact dermatitis individuals must be presensitized to the allergen, and while high concentrations may increase the likelihood of developing an immune response, the substance does not directly damage the skin.

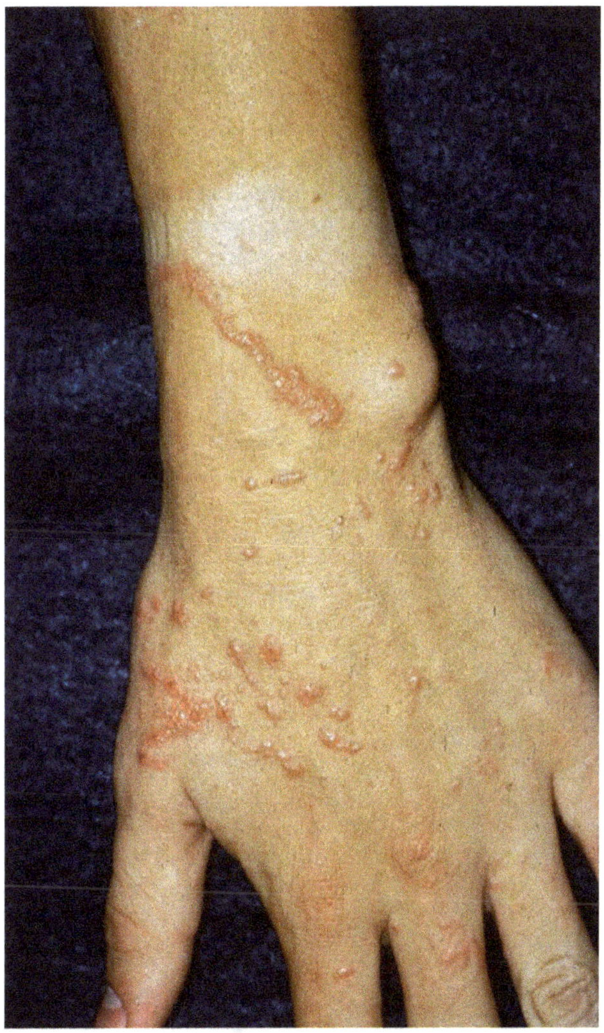

Poison ivy allergic contact dermatitis. There are numerous erythematous vesicles with linear pattern due to poison ivy. (Used, with permission, from Berger TG, Dept. Dermatology, UCSF.)

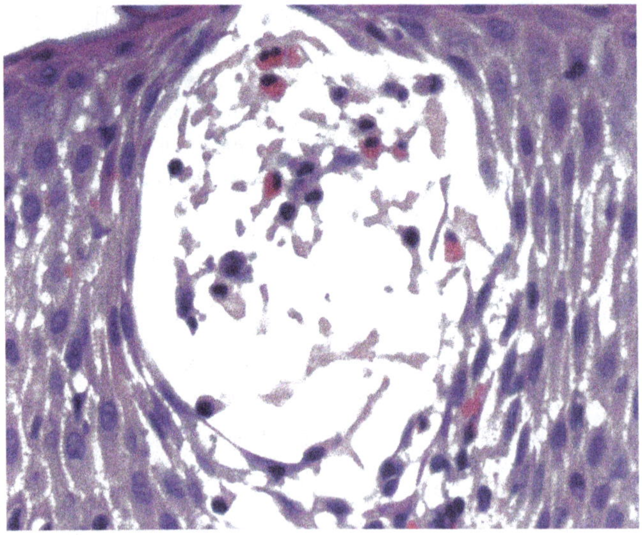

Eosinophilic spongiosis. Intraepidermal microvesicle with eosinophils and mononuclear cells.

A diffuse dermatitis may occur following systemic exposure to a chemical to which the patient has had a prior contact allergy. This so-called **systemic allergic contact dermatitis** reaction is due to a delayed T-cell-mediated immune response. When the offending allergen is a medication, the eruption is referred to as an **eczematous drug eruption**. Historically, one of the most common examples of systemic contact dermatitis was the patient with a history of allergic contact dermatitis to ethylenediamine who then developed a diffuse dermatitis secondary to intravenous aminophylline, which contains ethylenediamine. Other causes of systemic contact dermatitis include antibiotics, plants/plant products, propylene glycol, sorbic acid, and metals.

Topical Allergens That May Result in Systemic Contact Dermatitis After Systemic Exposure

TOPICAL ALLERGEN	SYSTEMIC EXPOSURE
Ethylenediamine hydrochloride	Aminophylline, hydroxyzine/cetirizine
Poison ivy	Cashews, mangoes
Fragrance (balsam of Peru)	Foods (tomatoes, citrus), sodas, mouthwashes, spices
Sorbic acid	Preservative in food
Nickel and other metal salts	Nickel/metal salts in food, nickel from catheter hub
Quinolones	Oral antibiotics
Ampicillin	Surgical solutions
Neomycin	Streptomycin, kanamycin
Thiuram	Disulfiram (Antabuse)

Eczematous Drug Reactions

Clinical Features
- Erythematous, papular, or vesicular eruption in patients exposed to an agent to which they were previously sensitized
- Sites often correspond to those previously affected

Histopathologic Features
- Spongiosis and intraepidermal vesiculation
- Moderately dense dermal lymphocytic and eosinophilic infiltrate with variable exocytosis

Differential Diagnosis
- Other delayed-type hypersensitivity reactions of diverse cause

ANSWER 1-7: B.

The biopsy reveals spongiosis with intraepidermal neutrophils. This is a classic example of **irritant contact dermatitis** and is the result of a direct toxic effect due to prolonged application of a chemical substance (in this case shampoo) to the skin. Lesions of irritant contact dermatitis tend to burn or sting, rather than itch; however, they are often indistinguishable clinically from allergic contact dermatitis. Irritants include everyday things such as water, detergents, solvents, acids, alkalis, adhesives, metalworking fluids, and friction. Often several of these act together to injure the skin. The histopathologic findings of irritant contact dermatitis can also be similar to those of allergic contact dermatitis. In fact, many cases of allergic contact dermatitis will have superimposed changes of irritation due to constant rubbing and scratching. Both lesions may progress from an acute to chronic spongiotic dermatitis. Unlike allergic contact dermatitis, this condition requires exposure in a specific concentration and duration. Histopathologic features that favor **irritant contact dermatitis** over **allergic contact dermatitis** include necrosis and hydropic swelling (balloon cell change) of superficial keratinocytes accompanied by dermal and intraepidermal neutrophils. Solitary lymphocytes and neutrophils permeate the epidermis without large vesicle formation. Neutrophils have polylobated nuclei and pink cytoplasm. The presence of eosinophils, marked spongiosis, and Langerhans cell–rich microvesicles favors allergic contact dermatitis. A PAS stain should be ordered to rule out a dermatophyte infection, as the histopathology for both conditions may be identical on H&E sections.

Mechanisms of Toxicity of Irritants

IRRITANT	TOXICITY
Detergents	Barrier disruption, protein denaturation, membrane toxicity
Acids	Protein denaturation
Alkalis	Barrier lipid denaturation, cellular swelling
Oils	Disrupt lipid barrier organization
Organic solvents	Solubilize membrane lipids
Oxidants	Cytotoxic
Reducing agents	Keratolysis
Water	Epidermal cell swelling

ANSWER 1-8: D.

This is an example of **photoallergic dermatitis**, which is a hypersensitivity reaction to an allergen activated or produced by the effect of light on a drug (or its metabolite). Photoallergic dermatitis may be localized or generalized depending on the route of allergen administration (topical versus systemic, respectively). The lesions are mediated by UV-induced immediate type I and/or delayed type IV hypersensitivity. Just like allergic contact dermatitis, individuals must be presensitized to the allergen. The histopathologic reaction pattern is identical to **allergic contact dermatitis**; however, there is a tendency to form both superficial and deep perivascular lymphocytic and eosinophilic infiltrates when the antigen is circulating through the blood stream. In this patient, note the sparing under the nose and under the lower lip; areas which are relatively shaded from sun exposure. Common topical offenders include sunscreens, bergamot "perfume" oil, and antibacterial agents such as chlorhexidine. This patient is experiencing **systemic photoallergic dermatitis**, most likely due to hydrochlorothiazide. Unlike **photoirritant/phototoxic contact dermatitis,** photoallergic lesions tend to resolve without hyperpigmentation and may occasionally persist and/or progress to chronic forms even after the cessation of UV light exposure. Microscopically, photoirritant/phototoxic dermatitis presents with changes identical to irritant contact dermatitis with additional findings of atypical intraepidermal necrotic/apoptotic keratinocytes ("sunburn cells"), postinflammatory pigmentation, clusters of melanin pigment within the stratum corneum, and overall less spongiosis.

Quick Fact

- ✓ Eosinophilic spongiosis and necrotic keratinocytes: **topical photoallergic**
- ✓ Eosinophilic spongiosis and necrotic keratinocytes, plus superficial and deep inflammatory infiltrates: **systemic photoallergic**
- ✓ Sunburn keratinocytes and pallor of superficial keratinocytes, neutrophils, and melanin pigment in the stratum corneum and melanophages: **phototoxic**

Common Phototoxic and Photoallergic Agents

PHOTOTOXIC	PHOTOALLERGIC
• **Antiarrhythmics** – Amiodarone – Quinidine • **Triazole antifungals** – Voriconazole • **Diuretics** – Furosemide – Thiazides • **NSAIDs** – Nabumetone – Naproxen – Piroxicam • **Phenothiazines** – Chlorpromazine – Prochlorperazine • **Psoralens** – 5-methoxypsoralen – 8-methoxypsoralen – 4,5',8-trimethylpsoralen • **Quinolones** – Ciprofloxacin – Lomefloxacin – Nalidixic acid • **St John wort (hypericin)** • **Sulfonamides** • **Sulfonylureas** • **Tar (topical)** • **Tetracyclines** – Doxycycline – Demeclocycline	***TOPICAL AGENTS*** • **Sunscreens (oxybenzone)** • **Fragrances** – 6-methylcoumarin – Musk ambrette – Sandalwood • **Antimicrobial agents** – Bithionol – Chlorhexidine – Fenticlor – Hexachlorophene • **NSAIDs** – Diclofenac – Ketoprofen • **Phenothiazines** – Chlorpromazine – Promethazine ***SYSTEMIC AGENTS*** • **Antiarrhythmics** – Quinidine • **Antimalarials** – Quinine • **Antifungals** – Griseofulvin • **Antimicrobials** – Quinolones (eg, enoxacin, lomefloxacin) • **NSAIDs** – Ketoprofen – Piroxicam

Photosensitivity Drug Reactions

Clinical Features

Erythematous macular, papular, or vesicular eruptions in a photodistribution, sparing submental and retroauricular areas

Photosensitivity Drug Reactions (*continued*)

Phototoxic: occur 5-20 hours after exposure to drug and light
Photoallergic: occur within 24 hours of repeat antigenic challenge with drug and sunlight and may occur on non–sun-exposed skin
Combined phototoxic/photoallergic eruptions common

Histopathologic Features
- Phototoxic
  - Keratinocyte injury (apoptosis or reticular degeneration) at all levels with architectural disarray and dysmaturation
  - Neutrophilic epidermotropism at sites of injury
  - Perivascular lymphocytic infiltrate in dermis
  - Superficial vasculature ectatic with endothelial swelling
- Photoadaptive: hypergranulosis, hyperkeratosis, and melanocytic hyperplasia
- Photoallergic
  - Spongiosis and vesiculation with adherent scale crust
  - Mixed lymphohistiocytic and eosinophilic dermal infiltrate
- Papillary dermal edema

Differential Diagnosis
- Phototoxic
  - Viral exanthemata
  - Erythema multiforme
  - Graft versus host disease
- Photoallergic: delayed-type hypersensitivity reactions of diverse cause

ANSWER 1-9: C.

This patient has **seborrheic dermatitis**, a common disorder that presents with erythematous, flaky, yellow-brown, greasy scales of the scalp, ears, nasolabial folds, eyebrows, central chest, and intertriginous areas. These "seborrheic areas" have a high concentration of sebaceous glands; however, patients with seborrheic dermatitis may have normal sebum production and those with excessive sebum production are often free of seborrheic dermatitis. Thus, the amount of sebum produced alone does not appear to be the decisive risk factor. The pathogenesis of this condition is unknown; however, a *Malassezia* species (*Pityrosporum*) has been implicated. Exacerbations may be associated with stress, HIV disease, Parkinson disease, and mood disorders. Histopathologically, the lesions show overlapping features of a spongiotic and psoriasiform dermatitis including hyperkeratosis, parakeratosis, psoriasiform epidermal hyperplasia, spongiosis, and neutrophils. Langerhans cell–rich microvesicles may be present as well as dermal eosinophilic infiltrates. The most specific feature for **seborrheic dermatitis** is the presence of focal parakeratosis surrounding follicular ostia resulting in follicular plugging. In the setting of HIV-associated immune dysregulation, seborrheic dermatitis can show confluent parakeratosis with necrotic and dyskeratotic squamous cells combined with dermal plasma cell infiltrates. Unlike seborrheic dermatitis in immunocompetent patients, the lesional skin of HIV-infected patients characteristically expresses heat shock proteins (HSP65 and HSP72). The significance of this is unknown.

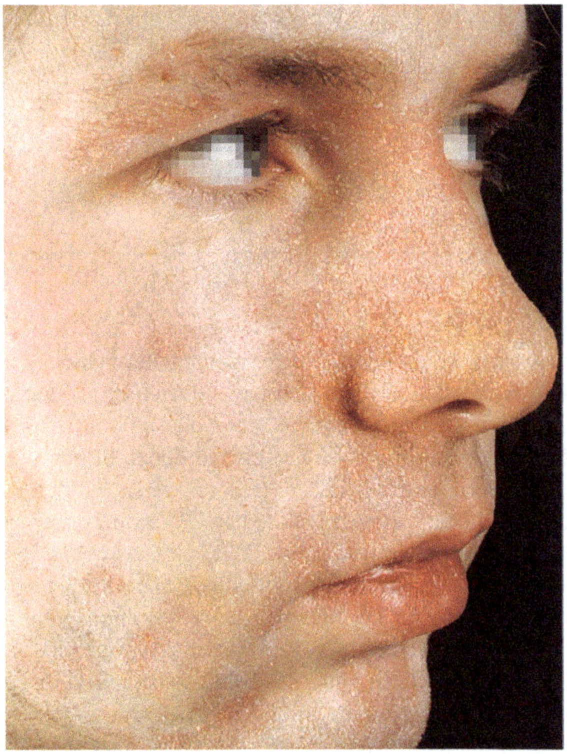

Seborrheic dermatitis. Yellow, greasy scales involving the nasolabial folds, cheeks, eyebrows, and nose. (Reproduced, with permission, from Goldsmith LA, Katz SI, Gilchrest BA, Paller AS, Leffell DJ, Wolff K, eds. *Fitzpatrick's Dermatology in General Medicine*. 8th ed. New York, NY: McGraw-Hill Education; 2012.)

Seborrheic Dermatitis

Clinical Features
- Common disorder affecting the scalp, face, upper chest, and back
- Greasy, scaly, red-brown patches
- Often pruritic
- Dandruff is one type of seborrheic dermatitis

Histopathologic Features
- Psoriasiform hyperplasia
- Hyperkeratosis and parakeratosis, especially parafollicular

Seborrheic Dermatitis (*continued*)

Spongiosis
Neutrophilic exocytosis
Superficial perivascular lymphocytic infiltrates, often with eosinophils

Differential Diagnosis

Psoriasis
Eczematous dermatitis
Impetigo
Dermatophytosis
Secondary syphilis
Gyrate erythemas
Pityriasis rosea
Irritant contact dermatitis
Drug reaction

ANSWER 1-10: B.

This patient's clinical and histopathologic findings are consistent with lower extremity **stasis dermatitis** with secondary upper extremity **id reaction. Id reactions** are diffuse and symmetric, papular, eczematous eruptions that occur at distant sites from a known long-standing localized eczematous eruption of known etiology. Common primary localized eruptions that frequently give rise to id reactions include **dermatophyte infection, scabies infestation, acute allergic contact dermatitis, stasis dermatitis,** and **ionizing radiation**. The id reaction usually has a nonspecific distribution that occurs days, weeks, months, or even years after the initial localized dermatitis. Both lesions will demonstrate similar histopathology. One histopathologic finding in the "id" lesions that is frequently unique from the primary histopathology is the presence of prominent papillary dermal edema. In stasis dermatitis, an endogenous for eczema, biopsy specimens display an acute, subacute, or chronic spongiotic pattern, as well as signs of chronic venous hypertension: clusters of dilated capillaries surrounded by cuffs of fibrin, hemosiderin deposits, and hyperplastic (and at times thrombotic) venules. In later stages, there is fibrosis of the dermal connective tissue and sclerosis of adipose tissue. These dermal changes are separate from spongiosis and will not be present in the subacute secondary id eruption.

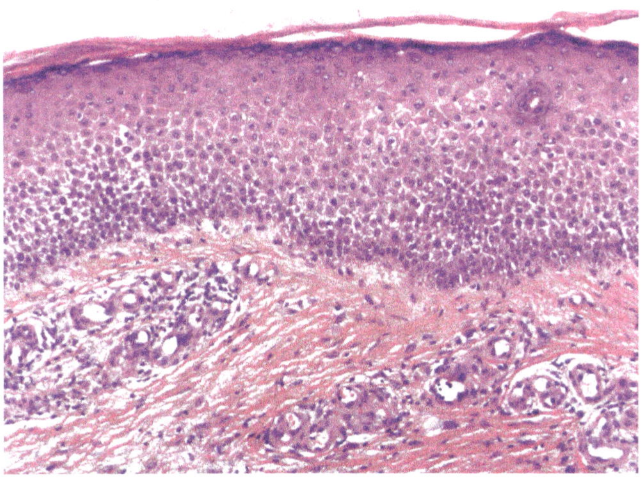

Stasis dermatitis. Epidermal acanthosis, spongiosis, and lobular proliferation of blood vessels with fibrosis in the dermis.

ANSWER 1-11: C.

These patients (mother and child) both have **atopic dermatitis**, which is an **endogenous eczematous dermatitis** of unknown etiology affecting approximately 1%-2% of the population. About half of patients also report **allergic rhinitis** and **asthma** and 75% of cases have a family history of atopy. Lesions tend to develop first in infancy with characteristic facial involvement. The diaper region and extensor surfaces of

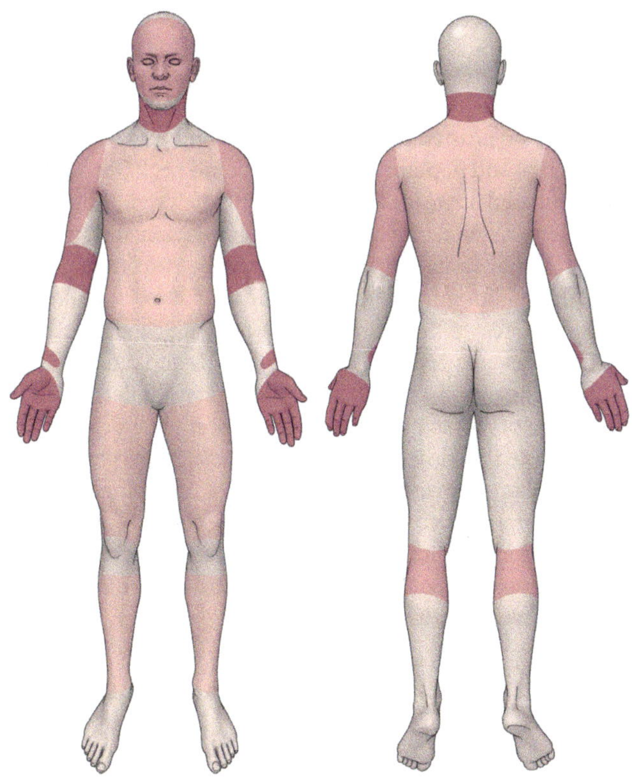

Predilection sites of atopic dermatitis. (Reproduced with permission from Wolff K, Johnson RA, Saavedra AP. *Fitzpatrick's Color Atlas and Synopsis of Clinical Dermatology*. 7th ed. New York, NY: McGraw-Hill Education; 2013.)

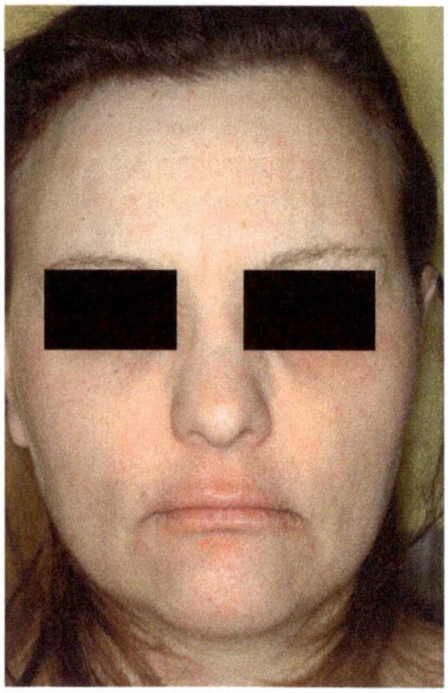

Atopic dermatitis. The patient demonstrates ill-defined, diffuse xerosis (dryness and fine scaling); erythema; and slight edema of the face. There is an accentuation of skin cleavage lines.

the extremities are also frequently affected. The lesions manifest as pruritic plaques of erythema with small vesicles that frequently rupture and crust. Circumoral sparing is typical in infants. In late childhood, lesions are lichenified (chronic) with weeping and crusted papules that most commonly involve the antecubital and popliteal fossae, wrists, and neck (flexural surfaces). In adults, the lesions are similar with weeping and crust being less frequent. Some authors refer to atopic dermatitis as the "itch that rashes" due to the extensive pruritic nature of these lesions that frequently precedes any clinical cutaneous findings. Greater than 90% of patients with atopic dermatitis have elevated levels of serum IgE. Morphologically these lesions range from acute to chronic eczematous dermatitis. In one study of atopic patients, clinically normal appearing skin was biopsied to reveal minimal epidermal hyperplasia, mild intercellular edema, and sparse dermal inflammatory infiltrates containing eosinophils, reflecting subclinical disease. Atopy is generally regarded as an inherent form of immune dysregulation, since there is a higher incidence of cutaneous viral infections in these patients.

Atopic Dermatitis

Clinical Features

- Common disorder of all ages
- Associated with allergic rhinitis and/or asthma
- Family history of atopy common
- Marked pruritus associated with a variety of lesions
  - Erythematous, scaling areas
  - Edematous, oozing, weepy areas
  - Lichenified areas
  - Dry fissured scaly areas
- Skin of patients generally lackluster, pruritic, and irritable
- Abnormalities of vascular and immune responses

Histopathologic Features

- Acute pattern
  - Spongiosis, sometimes spongiotic vesiculation, a usually superficial perivascular lymphocytic and eosinophilic infiltrate, epidermis of normal thickness
- Subacute pattern
  - Thickened epidermis (usually psoriasiform type), spongiosis, a usually superficial perivascular lymphocytic and eosinophilic infiltrate, variable fibrosis of papillary dermis
- Chronic pattern
  - Psoriasiform hyperplasia, spongiosis minimal to absent, vascular ectasia, a usually superficial perivascular lymphocytic infiltrate with eosinophils, variable fibrosis of the papillary dermis

Differential Diagnosis

- All other types of eczematous dermatitis
- Clinicopathologic correlation largely determines the diagnosis
- Pathologic diagnosis is usually expressed as acute, subacute, or chronic eczematous dermatitis

ANSWER 1-12: E.

The patient has **nummular dermatitis**, which is an **idiopathic eczematous dermatitis** in which coin-shaped, well-demarcated, and erythematous plaques and vesicles develop on dry scaly skin. **Dermatophytosis** is on the differential diagnosis and a KOH should be performed; however, **tinea** is not the causative agent of **nummular eczema**. It is regarded as a particular clinical presentation rather than a specific disease. It occurs most frequently in young women (15-30 years old) and in both middle-aged and elderly men and women. Nummular lesions of dermatitis are frequently associated with contact sensitization as well as with xerosis and venous hypertension. Clinical and laboratory signs of atopy are absent in "true" nummular dermatitis. Cold temperatures and certain medications (ie, gold) are associated with exacerbations. The microscopic features are similar to other spongiotic dermatitides at comparable chronological stages of evolution.

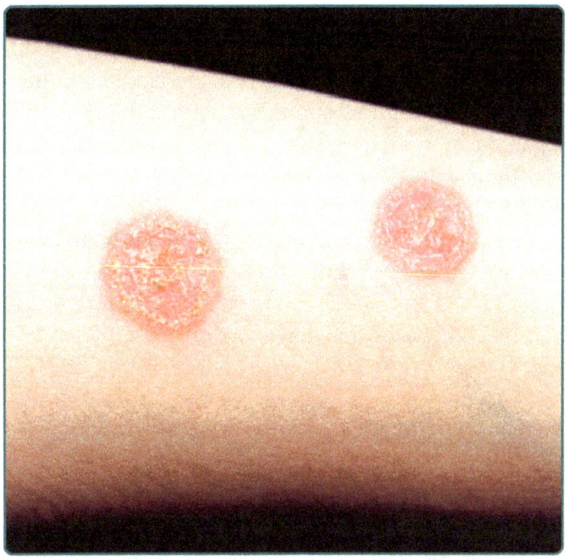

Nummular eczema. (Reproduced, with permission, from Goldsmith LA, Katz SI, Gilchrest BA, Paller AS, Leffell DJ, Wolff K, eds. *Fitzpatrick's Dermatology in General Medicine*. 8th ed. New York, NY: McGraw-Hill Education; 2012. Illustration by Glen Hintz, MS. Dermatology Lexicon Project.)

Nummular (Discoid) Dermatitis

Clinical Features
Coin-shaped, pruritic, erythematous patches on the hands, forearms, and legs
Patches may have tiny vesicles or erosions, which can evolve to form annular plaques or dry scaly areas
Tends to affect men and women 55 years and older as well as women 15-30 years old

Histopathologic Features
Varies according to the lesion biopsied: acute, subacute, and chronic eczematous patterns

Differential Diagnosis
All types of eczematous dermatitis
Dermatophytosis
Figurate erythemas
Seborrheic dermatitis

ANSWER 1-13: A.

This patient has **pityriasis alba**, an idiopathic, localized, hypopigmented eczematous dermatitis of childhood. Regarded as a minor feature of atopic dermatitis, typically there are only one to two lesions. The lesions are most common on the face and may be slightly pruritic. They present as faintly erythematous, round macules with indistinct borders. As parts of the lesion resolve, the erythema fades, leaving behind a hypopigmented region surfaced by a fine, "furfuraceous" scale. Histopathologically, there is mild spongiotic dermatitis with mild to moderate orthokeratosis and parakeratosis. The spongiosis can be folliculocentric with follicular plugging and atrophy of the sebaceous glands. There is mild papillary dermal edema and a sparse superficial

Pityriasis Alba

Clinical Differential Diagnosis

- Progressive macular hypomelanosis
- Pigmenting pityriasis alba
- Postinflammatory hypopigmentation
- Vitiligo
- Tinea versicolor
- Hypomelanosis of Ito
- Nevus anemicus
- Nevus depigmentosus
- Mycosis fungoides
- Pharmacologic nevi (benzoyl peroxide, topical/intralesional steroids)

Skin Diseases With Follicular Spongiosis

Atopic dermatitis
Infundibulofolliculitis
Fox-Fordyce disease (apocrine miliaria)
Pityriasis alba
Infectious folliculitis
Eosinophilic folliculitis
Follicular mucinosis

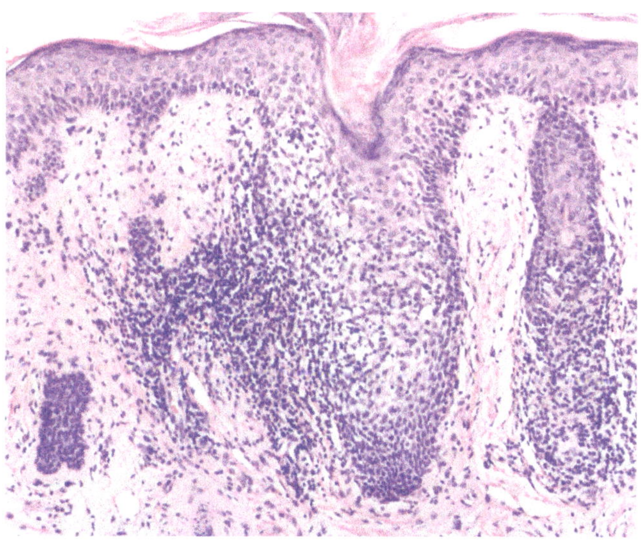

Follicular spongiosis. The outer root sheath epithelium reveals lymphocyte exocytosis and intercellular edema.

perivascular lymphomonocytic infiltrate. Rare scattered melanophages may be present in the papillary dermis. Compared to nonlesional skin, the basal keratinocytes contain a reduced amount of melanin pigment, due to a decrease in the number of functionally active melanocytes within the basal layer with a decreased amount of melanin transferred to the basal layer keratinocytes. There is no dysfunction in melanosome transfer. Melan-A stain will reveal only a slight reduction in total melanocyte concentration along the dermal epidermal junction.

ANSWER 1-14: D.

Pompholyx (aka **dyshidrotic eczema**) is characterized by a recurrent and intensely pruritic, vesicular eruption on the fingers, palms, and soles.

Allergic Contact Dermatitis, Rather Than Pomphylox, If:

✓ Epidermal spongiosis adjacent to a microvesicle
✓ Intraepidermal eosinophils

Exogenous factors, such as contact dermatitis or, as in this case, dermatophyte infection, may trigger episodes. These antigens may act as haptens with a specific affinity for palmoplantar proteins of the stratum lucidum of the epidermis. Flares of pompholyx are associated with emotional anxiety and hyperhidrosis; however, the acrosyringium is typically not involved. Distinguishing between an **id reaction** involving the palms or soles and **dyshidrotic eczema** can sometimes be difficult and some clinicians view them as overlapping entities. Histopathologically, minimal spongiosis within the epidermis is accompanied by macrovesicles. Vesicles can develop into pustules, with prominent neutrophil exocytosis, and raises the differential diagnosis of **pustular psoriasis** or **pustular dermatophytosis**. A PAS stain should be performed in all cases. Eosinophils are characteristically few or absent. A thickened stratum corneum is consistent with the acral location. Clinical correlation is essential for this diagnosis.

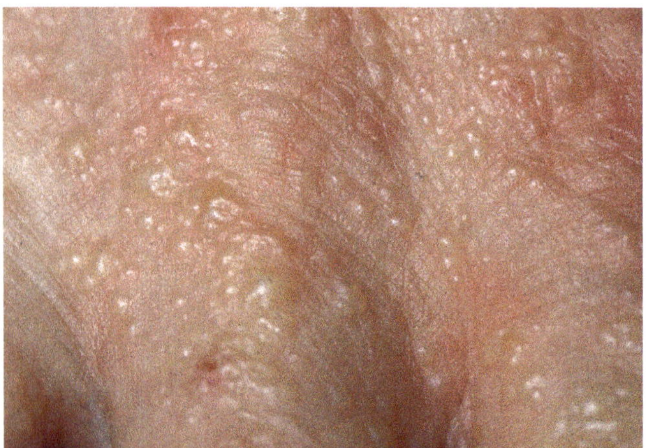

Dyshidrotic eczematous dermatitis. Confluent tapioca-like vesicles and crusted (excoriated) erosions on the dorsum of fingers and finger webs. (Reproduced, with permission, from Wolff K, Johnson RA, Saavedra AP. *Fitzpatrick's Color Atlas and Synopsis of Clinical Dermatology*. 7th ed. New York, NY: McGraw-Hill Education; 2013.)

Dyshidrotic Dermatitis

Clinical Features
Itchy tense vesicles on the digits, palms, and soles
Histopathologic Features
Intraepidermal spongiotic vesicles usually on epidermis of normal or increased thickness
Variable amount of superficial perivascular lymphocytic infiltrate
Differential Diagnosis
Atopic dermatitis
Allergic contact dermatitis
Dermatophytosis
Miliaria
Other types of acute vesicular eczematous eruptions

ANSWER 1-15: D.

Stasis dermatitis is a manifestation of chronic venous insufficiency with edema of the lower extremities and bronze (hemosiderin) staining of the medial aspects of the legs above the malleolus. There is a strong correlation with patients who have had a history of deep vein thrombosis. The lesions may be fissured, scaly, and intensely pruritic. Histopathologically, the most distinctive features are independent of spongiosis with dermal changes consisting of small veins and venules with thickened walls, often with a tortuous and glomerular architecture. Frequently there are clusters of thick-walled vessels in the subepidermal region. Red blood cell extravasation and siderophages are typically present in an edematous papillary and reticular dermis. Variable perivascular inflammatory infiltrates may be seen. Pruritus and dryness frequently prompts the patient to apply various over-the-counter creams or ointments, home remedies, and topical medication. Therefore, patients with chronic venous insufficiency more often than not exhibit multiple contact allergies, and a concomitant **allergic contact dermatitis** with abundant eosinophils. The epidermis exhibits a spectrum of changes ranging from subacute spongiotic dermatitis to lichen simplex chronicus.

Stasis Dermatitis

Clinical Features
- Legs, especially the inner aspects
- Red, edematous, scaling lesions
- Variable oozing
- Evidence of stasis, such as brown pigmentation, ulcers, varicose veins, and atrophic scars

Histopathologic Features
- Acute, subacute, or chronic eczematous pattern with lobular proliferation of capillaries, hemorrhage, hemosiderin deposition, and fibrosis

Differential Diagnosis
- Granulation tissue next to a leg ulcer
- Kaposi sarcoma

ANSWER 1-16: C.

Pityriasis rosea (PR) is a mild, acute, self-limited papulosquamous eruption that favors otherwise healthy adolescents and young adults. A viral etiology is proposed, but this remains unproven. There is an increased incidence in the fall and spring. Approximately 80% of cases begin with a solitary, oval, 2-10 cm, salmon-pink plaque on the trunk or proximal extremity, referred to as the "herald patch." The course is followed 7-14 days later by a generalized eruption of small 1 cm plaques on the trunk and proximal extremities along Langer lines of cleavage, resulting in the characteristic "fir-tree" distribution. The condition gradually resolves within 6 to 8 weeks. Lesions less commonly present on the face, scalp, genitalia, palms, soles, and oral cavity. Inverse PR is when lesions predominate on the extremities over the trunk.

Choices A, B, D, and E describe **seborrheic dermatitis, secondary syphilis, pityriasis lichenoides et varioliformis acuta,** and **lichen simplex chronicus**, respectively. PR exhibits areas of slight acanthosis with spongiosis and lymphocyte exocytosis directed toward the sides of rete ridges and acrosyringia (areas with high concentrations of antigen presenting

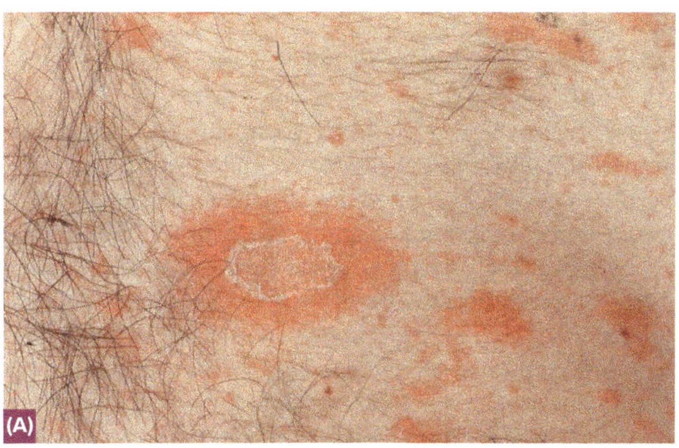

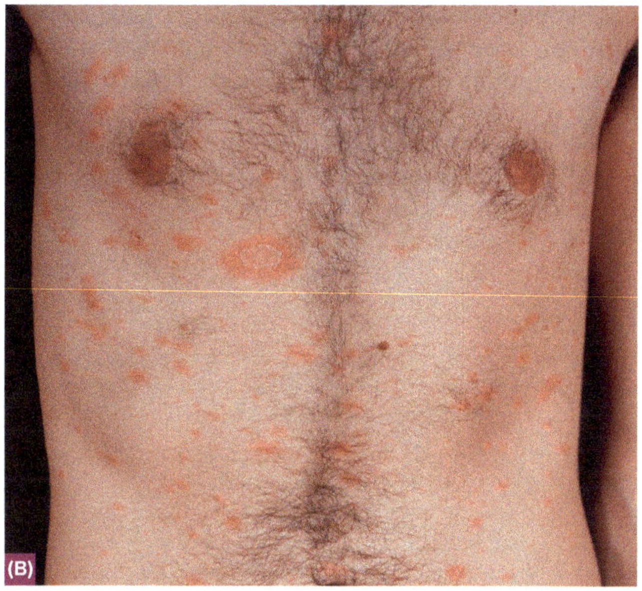

Pityriasis rosea. (A) Herald patch. An erythematous (salmon-red) plaque with a collarette scale on the trailing edge of the advancing border. Collarette means that scale is attached at periphery and loose toward the center of the lesion. **(B)** Overview of exanthem of pityriasis rosea with the herald patch shown in part A. There are papules and small plaques with oval configurations that follow the lines of cleavage. The fine scaling of the salmon-red papules cannot be seen at this magnification, while the collarette of the herald patch is obvious. (Reproduced, with permission, from Wolff K, Johnson RA, Saavedra AP. *Fitzpatrick's Color Atlas and Synopsis of Clinical Dermatology*. 7th ed. New York, NY: McGraw-Hill Education; 2013.)

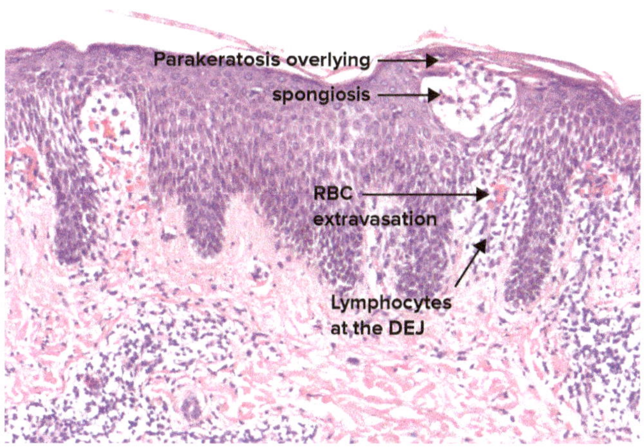

Pityriasis rosea. Slight epidermal hyperplasia, spongiosis, mounds of parakeratosis, with lymphocyte and erythrocyte exocytosis.

Langerhans cells). Discrete mounds of parakeratosis are present overlying these foci of epidermal injury. Lymphocytes may be seen along the dermal epidermal junction with only rare or absent dyskeratotic keratinocytes. Lymphocyte atypia characterized by nuclear contour irregularity (cerebriform) is never present, distinguishing PR from **large plaque parapsoriasis**. Extravasated red blood cells are present within the dermis and frequently within the epidermis. Superficial perivascular lymphocytic infiltrates are present usually without eosinophils. Lesions containing a large number of dermal eosinophils suggest a **pityriasis rosea-like drug eruption**, most commonly associated with angiotensin-converting enzyme inhibitors, gold, and barbiturates.

Pityriasis Rosea

Clinical Features
- Duration of disease: less than 10 weeks
- Herald patch
- Generalized eruption, usually on trunk
- Multiple salmon-colored macules with fine scale
- "Fir-tree" pattern
- Atypical pityriasis rosea may exhibit vesicles, pustules, urticarial lesions, purpura
- Inverse pityriasis rosea refers to a rash that is distributed on the extremities instead of the trunk
- Drug eruptions may result in a pityriasis rosea–like eruption

Histopathologic Features
- Mild subacute spongiotic dermatitis often with focal parakeratosis (which may tilt upward)
- Perivascular lymphocytic infiltrate with variable exocytosis
- Sometimes a microvesicle containing mononuclear cells in the epidermis
- Atypical forms tend to show vesicles, dyskeratosis, more parakeratosis and inflammation, hemorrhage, and eosinophils

Differential Diagnosis
- Drug reactions
- Eczematous dermatitis
- Chronic superficial dermatitis (parapsoriasis)
- Pityriasis lichenoides
- Guttate psoriasis
- Dermatophytosis

Drugs Associated With Pityriasiform Reactions (PR-Like Drug Eruptions)

- Acetylsalicylic acid
- Griseofulvin
- Metronidazole
- Captopril
- Clonidine
- Gold
- Arsenic

ANSWER 1-17: C.

Gianotti-Crosti syndrome is a self-limited cutaneous response to various infections, and is often preceded by an upper respiratory tract infection. It is characterized by multiple 1- to 5-mm symmetrical, flesh-colored to erythematous, edematous papules of the face, buttocks, and extensor surfaces of the extremities, usually sparing the trunk.

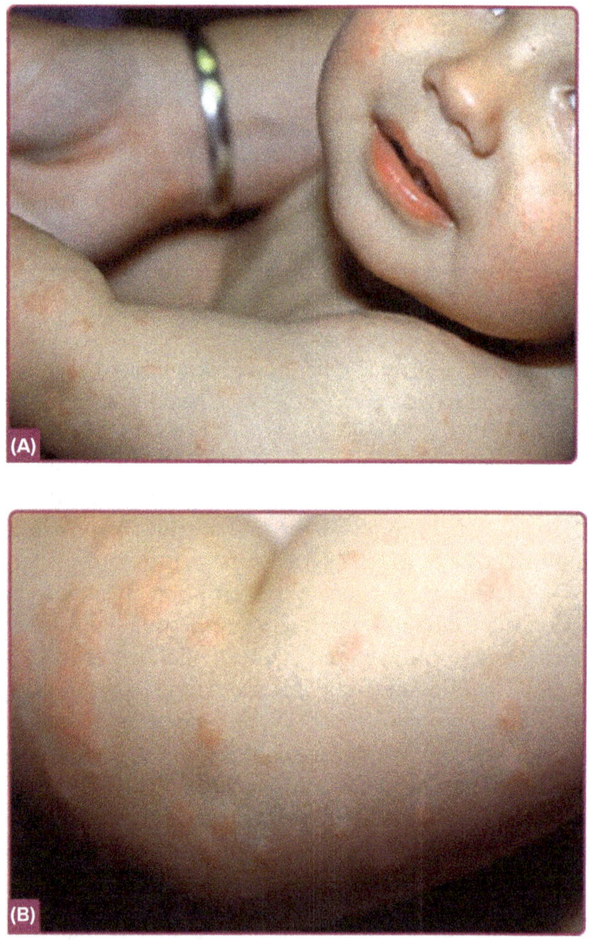

Gianotti-Crosti syndrome (A), (B). Erythematous, edematous but uniform papules in a toddler with Gianotti-Crosti syndrome that developed 1 month after hepatitis B vaccination. (Reproduced, with permission, from Goldsmith LA, Katz SI, Gilchrest BA, Paller AS, Leffell DJ, Wolff K, eds. *Fitzpatrick's Dermatology in General Medicine*. 8th ed. New York, NY: McGraw-Hill Education; 2012.)

Histopathologic features of **Gianotti-Crosti syndrome** are variable and nonspecific, but typically show a superficial perivascular lymphocytic infiltrate, as seen in most **morbilliform viral exanthems**. Slight epidermal acanthosis, mild spongiosis, and focal lymphocyte exocytosis can also be seen. Vacuolar interface activity may be present with rare dyskeratotic basilar keratinocytes. Papillary dermal edema with focal red blood cell extravasation and endothelial cell swelling can occur; however, true vasculitis with thrombosis and vessel necrosis is not a feature. Direct immunofluorescence studies are negative for immunoreactant deposition within vessels or within the epidermis.

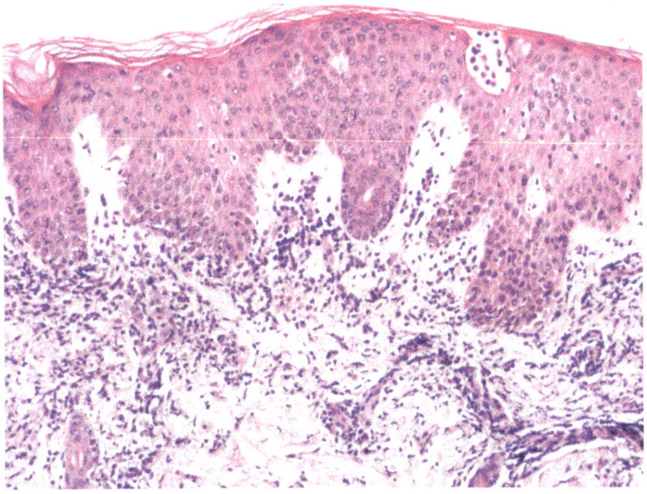

Gianotti-Crosti syndrome. Spongiotic-interface reaction pattern: Spongiosis with microvesicle formation, perivascular and interstitial lymphocytic infiltrate that focally obscures the dermoepidermal junction with lymphocyte exocytosis, and papillary dermal edema.

ANSWER 1-18: A.

This patient is presenting with stage 1 of **incontinentia pigmenti (IP)**, which is an X-linked multisystem disorder with skin lesions erupting along Blaschko lines due to functional X chromosome mosaicism. Very rarely males may inherit the condition, in which case the mutation is thought to be acquired spontaneously. It is believed that males who inherit the abnormal gene die in utero. The mother of these female patients usually reports a history of multiple miscarriages. There are typically four stages:

- Stage 1:
  At birth or within first 2 weeks of life.
  Erythema and linear vesiculation on the trunk and extremities.
  The face is characteristically spared.
  Peripheral blood leukocytosis and eosinophilia.
  Blistering stage completely resolves within 4 months.
- Stage 2:
  Uncommon and usually transitory during the second to sixth weeks of life.
  Hyperkeratotic verrucous papules and plaques most frequently found on the extremities at sites of blistering.
  Usually resolves completely by 6 months.
- Stage 3: Pathognomonic Stage
  Between the 12th and 26th weeks after birth.
  Bizarre brown to slate-gray reticulated pigmentation that appears as splashes, streaks, and whorls "Chinese lettering" on the torso and extremities.
  Hyperpigmentation of the nipples, groin, and axilla.
  The pigment follows Blaschko lines, but is independent of the blistering or verrucous lesion.
  Lesions resolve with atrophy and imperceptible pigmentation by adulthood.
- Stage 4:
  Present in adulthood.
  Only residual changes may be visible, usually on the lower extremities (atrophic, hypopigmented, hairless, reticulated patches and streaks).

The microscopic features of **stage 1 incontinentia pigmenti** consist of spongiosis with extensive eosinophilic exocytosis, eosinophilic-rich vesicles, and isolated collections of dyskeratotic keratinocytes throughout the epidermis. The vesicles are not centered at follicular ostia. The later stages generally lack spongiosis. **Stage 2 incontinentia pigmenti** exhibits acanthosis with papillomatosis, dyskeratotic keratinocytes, vacuolar degeneration along the dermal epidermal junction, and superficial dermal lymphocytic infiltrates with melanophages. Melanophages become more prominent in **stage 3 incontinentia pigmenti**.

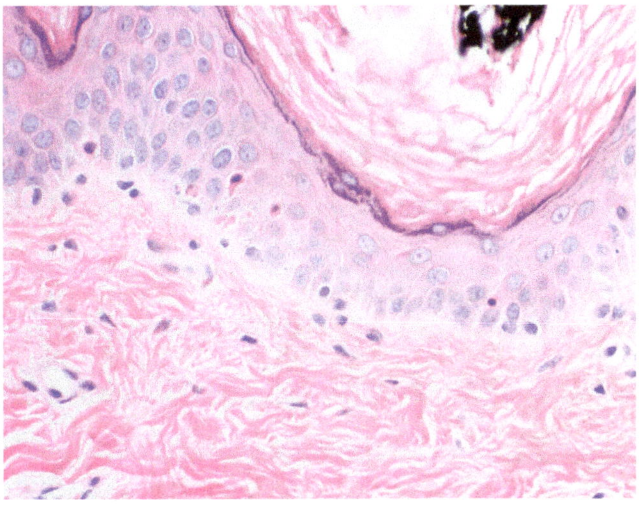

Incontinentia pigmenti, stage 2. There are random scattered dyskeratotic keratinocytes without associated lymphocyte tagging. This feature is consistent with spontaneous apoptosis.

Similar to the first stage of IP, **erythema toxicum neonatorum (ETN)** and **eosinophilic pustular folliculitis (EPF)** can show an eosinophilic pustule within the epidermis. In contrast to IP, these changes are typically folliculocentric and are not associated with epidermal spongiosis or dyskeratotic keratinocytes. In addition, cutaneous lesions of ETN resolve spontaneously. EPF in children is usually not related to HIV infection, unlike the condition in adults. Similar to ETN, it can start within the first days of life and produce follicular-based eosinophil-rich pustules. However, in contrast to ETN, the condition can persist for 3 months to 5 years. In addition, scalp and palmoplantar involvement is common in EPF. **Transient neonatal pustular melanosis** and **infantile acropustulosis** are childhood dermatoses that form pustules, which are neutrophil rich.

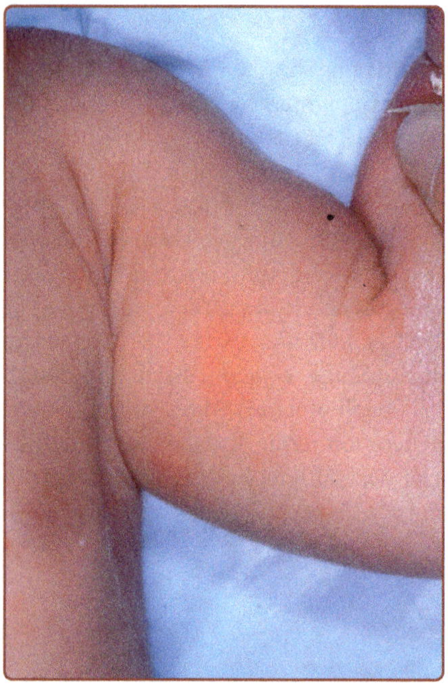

Erythema toxicum neonatorum. Erythematous macules, some with a tiny central papule or pustule, on the arm of a 1-day-old newborn. (Reproduced, with permission, from Usatine RP, Smith MA, Mayeaux EJ Jr, Chumley HS, eds. *Color Atlas of Family Medicine*. 2nd ed. New York, NY: McGraw-Hill Education; 2012.)

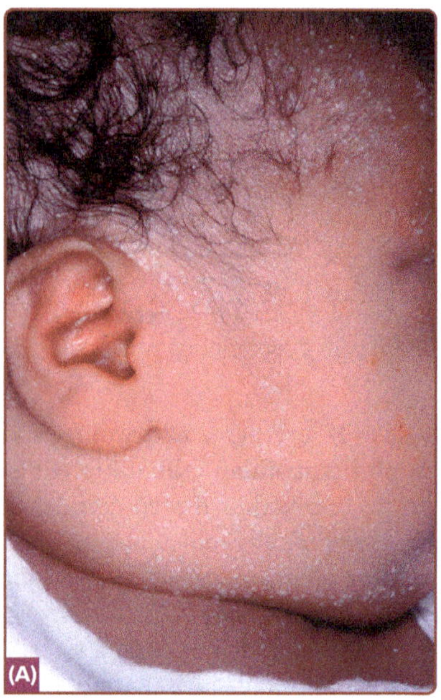

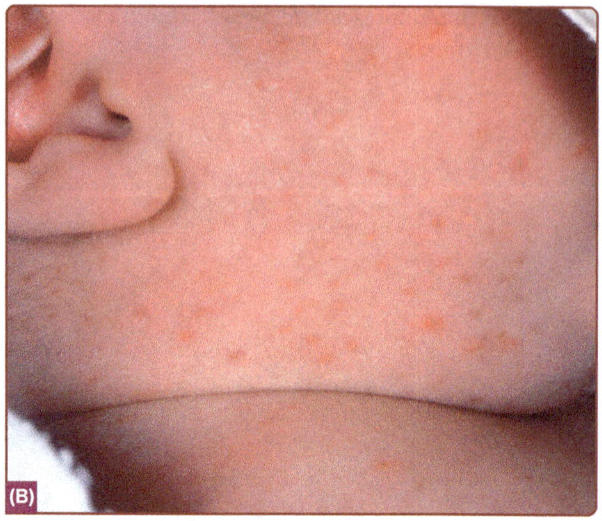

Transient neonatal pustular melanosis. (A) A newborn with congenital, thin-walled pustules that rupture easily. **(B)** Hyperpigmented macules appeared by 10 hours of age. (Reproduced, with permission, from Goldsmith LA, Katz SI, Gilchrest BA, Paller AS, Leffell DJ, Wolff K, eds. *Fitzpatrick's Dermatology in General Medicine*. 8th ed. New York, NY: McGraw-Hill Education; 2012.)

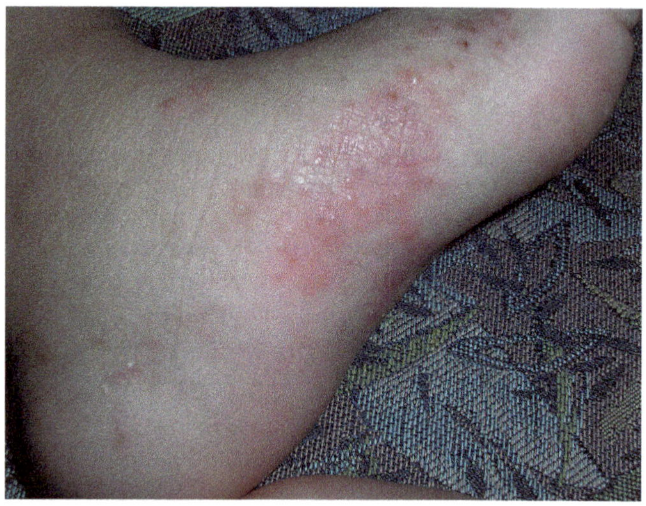

Infantile acropustulosis (acropustulosis of infancy) on the foot of a 1-year-old boy. (Reproduced, with permission, from Usatine RP, Smith MA, Mayeaux EJ Jr, Chumley HS, eds. *Color Atlas of Family Medicine*. 2nd ed. New York, NY: McGraw-Hill Education; 2012. Used with permission of Richard P. Usatine, MD.)

ANSWER 1-19: H.

Eosinophilic spongiosis is a reaction pattern in which there is exocytosis of eosinophils associated with changes of spongiosis. These changes are seen in a variety of inflammatory disorders, as listed below. Pityriasis rosea shows lymphocyte exocytosis, not eosinophil exocytosis.

Eosinophilic Spongiosis DDX

"HAPPPPIED"

Herpes gestationis
Arthropod bite
Pemphigoid (urticarial precursor)
Pemphigus (urticarial precursor)
PUPP
Photoallergic dermatitis
Incontinentia pigmenti (first stage)
Eosinophilic folliculitis
Drug reaction

ANSWER 1-20: J.

Incontinentia pigmenti has eosinophilic spongiosis. The rest show neutrophilic spongiosis.

Neutrophilic Spongiosis DDX

"TRIP SAID TIP"

Transient neonatal pustulosis
Reactive arthritis
Irritant contact dermatitis
Phototoxic dermatitis
Seborrheic dermatitis
AGEP
Impetigo
Dermatophytosis
Toxic shock syndrome
Infantile acropustulosis
Pemphigus variants (especially IgA)

ANSWER 1-21: C.

Interface dermatitis is the inflammatory reaction pattern seen when chronic inflammatory cells (predominantly T cells) marginate from the superficial vascular plexus, migrate, and coalesce along the dermal epidermal junction. The band may be dense (**lichenoid interface dermatitis**) or sparse (**vacuolar/cytotoxic interface dermatitis**). These T cells induce damage to the basal cells of the epidermis as well as structures of the underlying papillary dermis, creating tiny vacuoles on both sides of the basement membrane, referred to as vacuolar degeneration. The vacuolization imparts a ragged "saw-tooth" appearance at the base of the epidermis.

The T cells infiltrating the basal cell layer induce apoptosis of individual keratinocytes. Since these "dyskeratotic" cells are actually apoptotic bodies, the intracellular contents are not spilled into the intercellular space (unlike necrosis, commonly seen in spongiotic dermatitis). They are frequently found in direct apposition to intraepidermal lymphocytes, referred to as satellite cell necrosis (**lymphocyte satellitosis**). If these apoptotic cells drop down into the papillary dermis, they are referred to as **Civatte bodies, colloid bodies,** or **cytoid bodies**. If the process is intense and prolonged, remodeling of the basement membrane and epidermis may be seen. Dermal melanophages are almost universally present to some degree since the phagocytosed remnants of apoptotic basal keratinocytes contain the majority of the melanin pigment within the epidermis. In end-stage lesions, the only residua of an interface inflammatory process may be melanophages, referred to as **postinflammatory pigmentary alteration**. When there is sufficient vacuolar destructive interface change, subepidermal clefts may form, best exemplified by lesions of **bullous lichen planus** and grade 3 or 4 **acute graft versus host disease**.

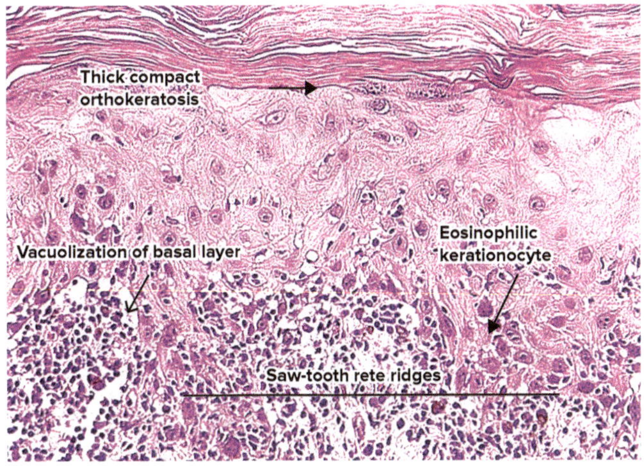

Lichenoid interface dermatitis. There is basal layer vacuolization. The epidermis is slightly acanthotic with a "saw-tooth" rete ridge pattern of the lower epidermis. Additionally there are features of premature terminal differentiation characterized by enlarged eosinophilic "glassy" basal and lower spinous keratinocytes, hypergranulosis, and thick compact orthokeratosis.

ANSWER 1-22: D.

The prototype for lichenoid interface dermatitis is **lichen planus.** This process is characterized by a dense dermal epidermal lymphocytic infiltrate that involves the basal cell layer, induces keratinocyte apoptosis, and persists for a prolonged period. This is important since the epidermis undergoes an adaptive response to the offending inflammatory assault referred to as premature terminal differentiation (analogous to cellular hypertrophy). This is characterized by squamatization of the

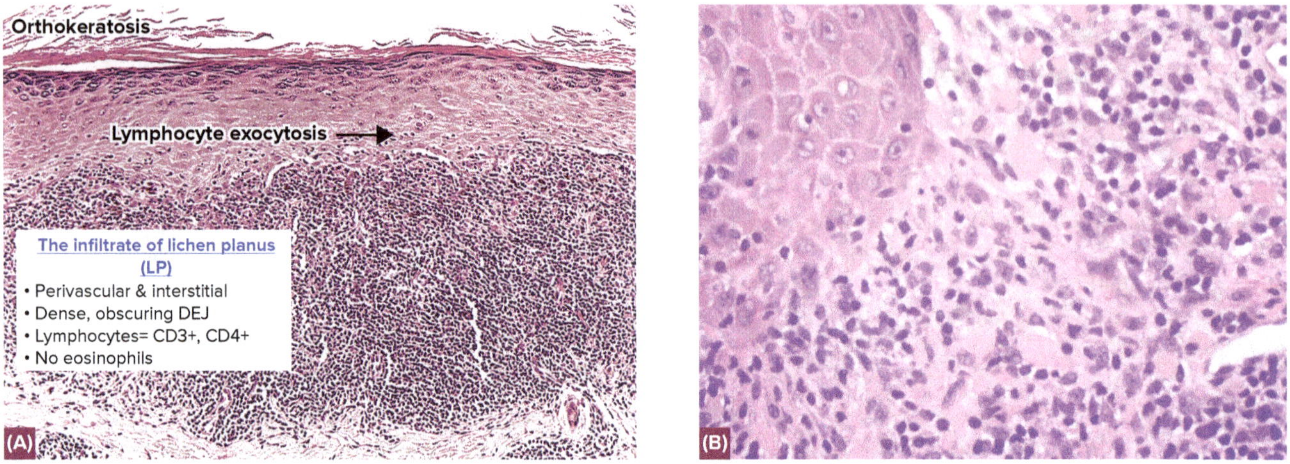

Lichen planus (lichenoid interface dermatitis). (A) This lesion shows hyperkeratosis, hypergranulosis, some acanthosis, and a band-like infiltrate that fills the papillary dermis and obscures the dermal-epidermal junction.

basal cells, accumulation of eosinophilic "glassy" cytoplasm of the lower spinous layer cells, wedge-shaped hypergranulosis, and compact orthohyperkeratosis of the stratum corneum. The rete ridges become pointed with sharply tapering tips, the so-called "saw-tooth" pattern.

Although there are cleft-like spaces (**Max-Joseph spaces**) in the basal cell layer, premature terminal differentiation results in narrowing of the intercellular spaces of the upper layers due to increased keratinocyte cytokeratin concentrations and intercellular desmosomes. As a result, apoptotic keratinocytes are not eliminated transepidermally, but instead drop down into the papillary dermis as colloid bodies. The prototype of vacuolar/cytotoxic interface dermatitis is **erythema multiforme** (EM).

Interface (IF) dermatitis

Vacuolar IF	*Lichenoid IF*
•Basal cell vacuolization •Variably dense perivascular and interstitial lymphocytic infiltrate	•Dense band-like, cell-rich infiltrate •Infiltrate overshadows vacuolization
•Examples: √EM √Fixed drug eruption √Drug eruptions √Viral exanthems √Early cutaneous LE √Dermatomyositis √Pityriasis lichenoides √Acute GVHD √Vitiligo	•Examples: √LP & variants √Lichenoid drug eruption √Lichenoid keratosis √Lichen stiratus √Lichen nitidus √Lichenoid purpura √Porokeratosis √Histologic regression of many tumors

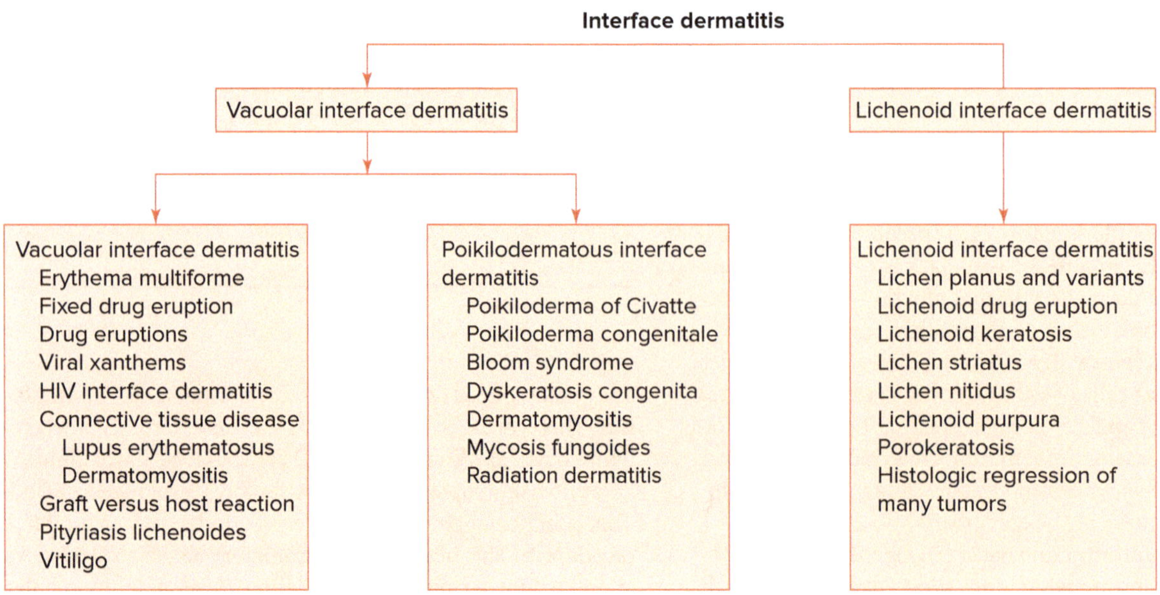

Differential diagnosis for interface dermatitis.

Unlike lichenoid interface dermatitis, this process is characterized by a sparse dermal epidermal lymphocytic infiltrate that involves the basal cell layer and induces keratinocyte apoptosis, but the lymphocytes rapidly retreat, resulting in little cellular adaptive response and minimal to no alteration in the cornification of the epidermis (preserved basket-weave stratum corneum). This is important since clusters of dyskeratotic keratinocytes may be eliminated transepidermally. Colloid bodies are usually present as well. The term **cytotoxic interface dermatitis** is sometimes used to describe **EM/Stevens-Johnson syndrome/toxic epidermal necrolysis/acute graft versus host disease,** since it represents an extreme end of the spectrum in regard to the destructive changes seen in relation to an absent epidermal adaptive response. Both processes share dermal epidermal lymphocytic infiltrates, vacuolar degeneration, dyskeratotic keratinocytes, colloid bodies, and papillary dermal edema.

ANSWER 1-23: B.

Normally the granular layer cells contain keratohyaline granules, which are composed of two proteins, profilaggrin and involucrin. **Involucrin** and **filaggrin**, which is a cleavage product of profilaggrin, are together involved in keratin aggregation within the stratum corneum. These substances are expressed in the upper spinous layer cells of lichenoid dermatitis with premature terminal differentiation. Normal spinous layer keratinocytes express keratins 1 and 10. However, premature terminally differentiated spinous layer keratinocytes express keratins 6 and 16. The process of premature terminal differentiation is initiated by the disruption of the α5β1 fibronectin receptor within the basal cells. Receptor disruption and accelerated differentiation normally occurs in the proliferative phase of wound healing. In the setting of lichenoid dermatitis, this receptor is disrupted by the inflammatory infiltrate.

Premature terminal differentiation (hypertrophy):

- Thick granular layer and compact stratum corneum (orthokeratosis)
- Increased eosinophilic cytoplasm of the spinous and basal layer keratinocytes due to increased keratin content
- Usually with dense lichenoid lymphocytic infiltrate (exception: lichenoid graft vs host disease)

Examples: LP, DLE, lichenoid drug eruptions, and lichenoid graft versus host disease (GVHD).

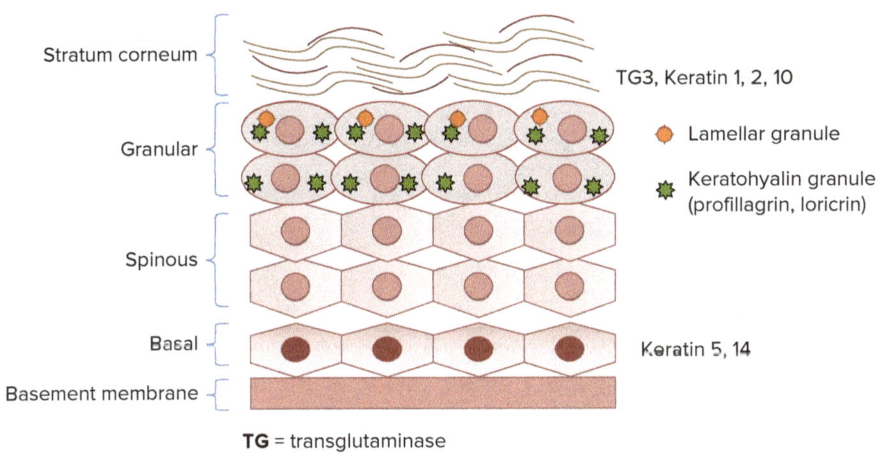

ANSWER 1-24: A.

This patient has **lichen planus**, which is the prototype of lichenoid interface dermatitis. The histological differential diagnosis includes **actinic keratosis with lichenoid inflammation, discoid lupus erythematosus, secondary syphilis,** and **lichenoid drug eruption/lichen planus-like keratosis (LPLK)** (choices B, C, D, and E, respectively). Lichen planus, an inflammatory disorder of uncertain cause, consists of variably distributed erythematous to violaceous polygonal papules and plaques, typically well defined in contour and often grouped on flexor surfaces, especially the wrists. The genitalia are frequently involved. Scale is generally absent, but surface change consisting of white lines or grooves known as **Wickham striae** are often observed. The patient frequently complains of intense pruritus. Oral and nail changes may accompany the cutaneous eruption. Nail changes include pterygium formation and longitudinal ridging and fissuring of the nail plate. Rare cases of esophageal and ocular involvement are reported. Lacy, white patches commonly involve the buccal mucosa. Associations between lichen planus and hepatitis C infection, as well as vaccination against hepatitis B, occur.

The major distinction between **LPLK** and **lichenoid drug eruption** is clinical presentation, LPLK being a solitary lesion most commonly on the chest and lichenoid drug eruption being widespread. LPLK most commonly arises in association with solar lentigines and macular seborrheic keratoses and is most commonly clinically mistaken for basal cell carcinoma. LPLK and lichenoid drug eruption are essentially histopathologically identical with a band-like lymphocytic infiltrate similar to that of lichen planus. Both entities are different from lichen planus by the presence of parakeratosis, variable hypergranulosis, and mid-dermal infiltrates containing eosinophils. Lichen planus contains a superficial band-like infiltrate, does not contain eosinophils, and may only contain plasma cells in oral lesions. Lichenoid drug eruptions tend to have a dermal inflammatory infiltrate that extends deeper into the dermis with accentuation around blood vessels; however, this feature may also be present in LPLK. It is worth mentioning that LPLK and lichenoid drug eruptions on rare occasion may present without eosinophils; therefore correlation with clinical presentation and drug history is imperative for the correct diagnosis.

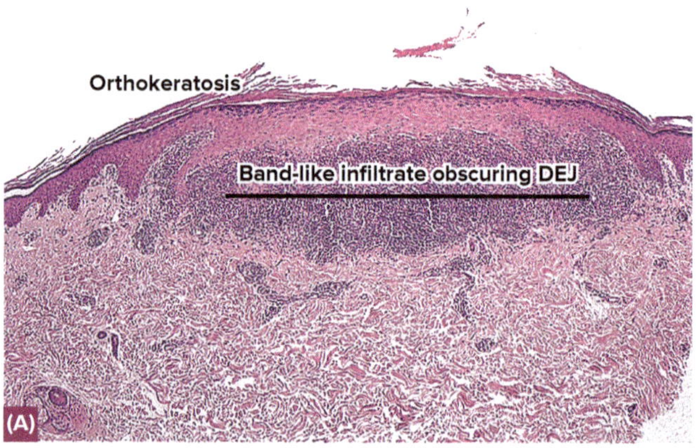

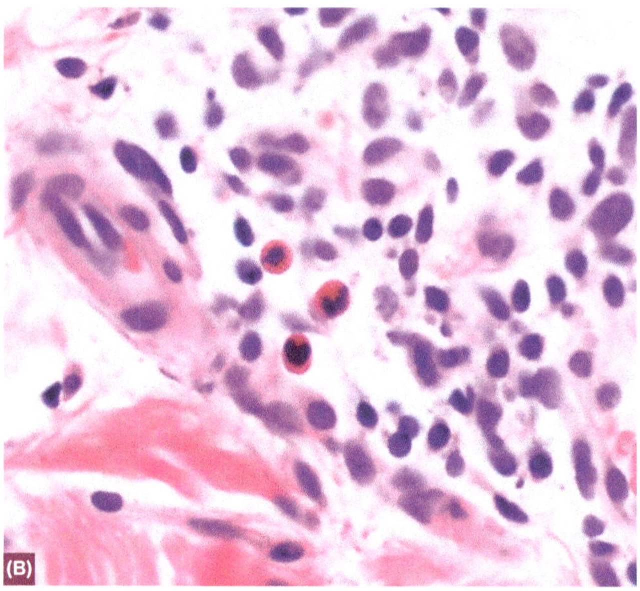

Lichen planus-like keratosis. (A) The findings are similar to that of lichen planus. There is a band-like lymphocytic infiltrate with interface activity and dyskeratotic keratinocytes limited to the lower epidermal layers. Colloid bodies are present underneath the dermal epidermal junction. Although not present in this example, LPLK frequently exhibits mild spongiosis and focal overlying parakeratosis. **(B)** Unlike lichen planus, the infiltrate contains scattered eosinophils.

Lichenoid actinic keratosis is identical to LPLK, but exhibits the partial thickness keratinocytic atypia associated with chronic solar damage. Solar elastosis is also typically present. **Secondary syphilis** presents with a wide range of clinical findings but most commonly as papulosquamous eruption of variable distribution. Involvement of the palms and soles is characteristic. The typical microscopic presentation is dense lichenoid interface dermatitis with epidermal acanthosis and markedly elongated and thinned rete ridges. The superficial and deep dermal inflammatory infiltrate contains lymphocytes and plasma cells and extends along vessels, adnexal structures, and nerve bundles. Endothelial cells are enlarged and partially or totally fill vessel lumens. The absence of plasma cells does not definitively exclude the diagnosis of syphilis. Older lesions may exhibit loose aggregates of granulomatous inflammation. Definitive diagnosis of syphilis requires a positive RPR or identification of spirochetes within vessels and the epidermis via special stains.

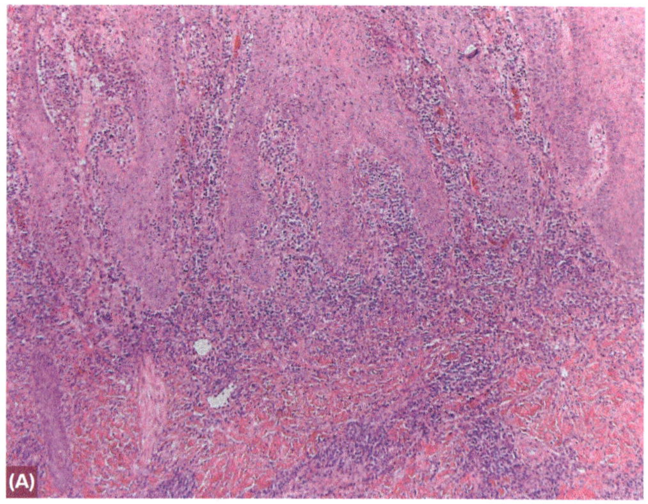

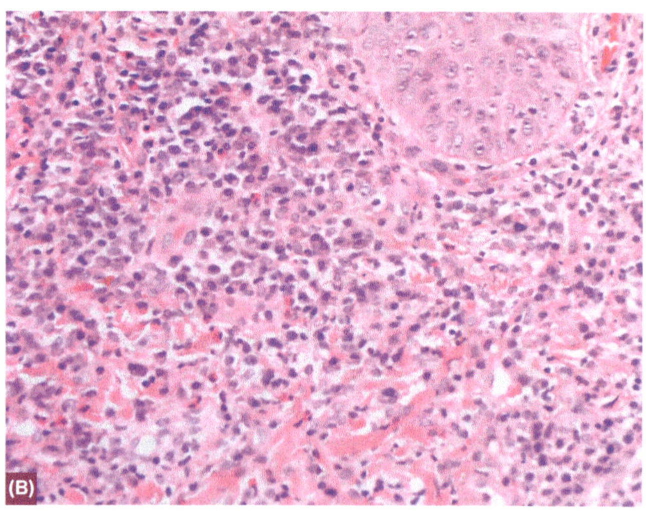

Secondary syphilis. (A) The band-like interface inflammatory infiltrate is associated with epidermal hyperplasia consisting of markedly elongated thin rete ridges. **(B)** In addition to lymphocytes, the infiltrate contains plasma cells.

LP DDX

For LP: Hypergranulosis, **No eos**, No parakeratosis

LPLK •Solitary lesion •Often with a solar lentigo or SK •Normal granular layer •+/- parakeratosis and spongiosis **•Infiltrate with eos**	**EM, TEN** Keratinocyte death>>Inflammation •Basket weave stratum corneum **•No eos**
Lichenoid drug eruption •Widespread eruption •Normal granular layer •+/- parakeratosis and spongiosis **•Deep infiltrate; eos and plasma cells**	**FDE** •Keratinocyte death >> Inflammation •Basket weave stratum corneum **•Infiltrate with eos, neuts, plasma cells** •Papillary dermal melanophages (recurrent lesion)
LE **•Lymphocytes in the eccrine coil** •Epidermal atrophy •Normal granular layer •Basement membrane thickening •Dermal mucin	**MF** •Epidermis NOT destroyed •Variable interface changes **•Cerebriform lymphocytes** •Epidermotropism

ANSWER 1-25: C.

This is a classic example of **hypertrophic lichen planus**, which is lichenoid interface dermatitis of uncertain cause presenting most commonly on the lower legs and consisting of intensely pruritic hyperkeratotic plaques. Direct immunofluorescence, just as in classic lichen planus, will reveal shaggy fibrin deposition along the basement membrane zone and immunoglobulin and complement deposition within the colloid bodies along the basal layer and within the papillary dermis. The majority of lymphocytes within the infiltrate are also CD3 and CD4 positive, consistent with a T-helper/inducer phenotype. Terminal effector mechanisms are not completely understood; however, the cytokine profile from lesional tissue may affect epidermal keratin expression, resembling that seen in wound healing, hence the features of premature terminal differentiation, and in this variant **pseudoepitheliomatous hyperplasia.**

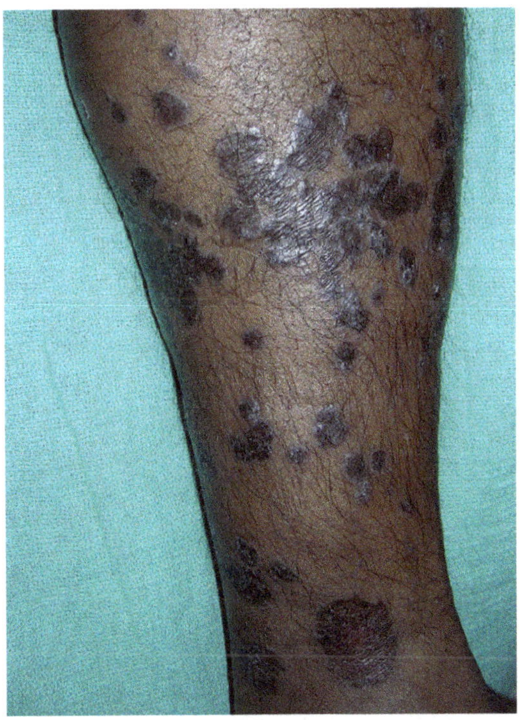

Hypertrophic lichen planus on the leg of a black man. Note the hyperpigmentation that is common when lichen planus occurs in a person with dark skin. (Reproduced, with permission, from Usatine RP, Smith MA, Mayeaux EJ Jr, Chumley HS, eds. *Color Atlas of Family Medicine*. 2nd ed. New York, NY: McGraw-Hill Education; 2012. Used with permission of Richard P. Usatine, MD.)

Several other variants of lichen planus exist including lichen planus pigmentosus, ulcerative lichen planus, lichen planus pemphigoides, bullous lichen planus, and lichen planopilaris. **Lichen planus pigmentosus** presents most commonly as pruritic pigmented dark-brown macules predominantly affecting sun-exposed skin and the flexures of dark-skinned patients. Microscopically, these lesions contain extensive pigmentary incontinence and numerous dermal melanophages. **Ulcerative lichen planus** occurs as a chronic variant affecting the fingers, hands, soles, and toes, and is frequently associated with permanent loss of the nails. Squamous cell carcinoma may complicate this ulcerative variant of lichen planus. **Lichen planus pemphigoides** is rare condition with combined features of lichen planus and bullous pemphigoid that most commonly occurs on the extremities. Microscopically, it is characterized by a lichenoid infiltrate, subepidermal blister, and linear deposition of immunoglobulin along the basement membrane zone via direct immunofluorescence. **Bullous lichen planus** is not a clinical variant but rather a histopathological finding.

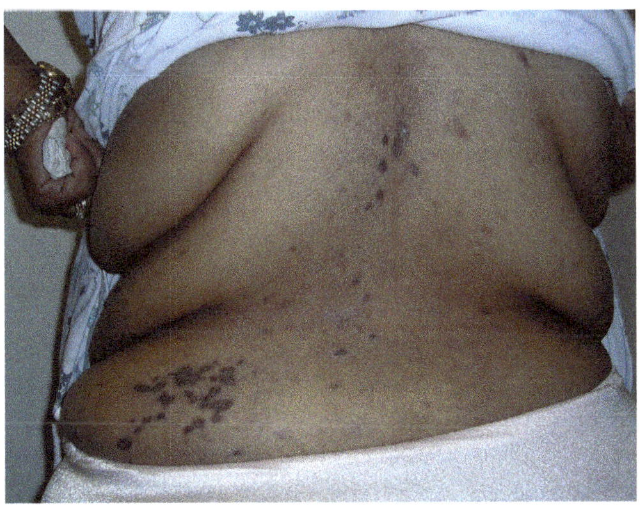

Lichen planus pigmentosus on the back proven by punch biopsy. (Reproduced, with permission, from Usatine RP, Smith MA, Mayeaux EJ Jr, Chumley HS, eds. *Color Atlas of Family Medicine*. 2nd ed. New York, NY: McGraw-Hill Education; 2012. Used with permission of Richard P. Usatine, MD.)

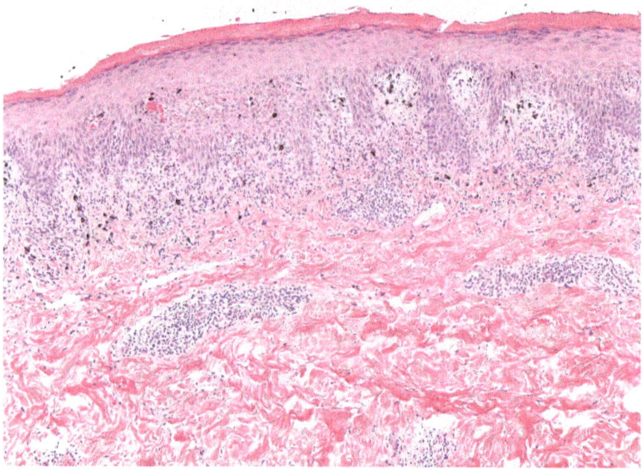

Lichen planus pigmentosus. Lichenoid interface dermatitis with extensive pigment incontinence and dermal melanophages.

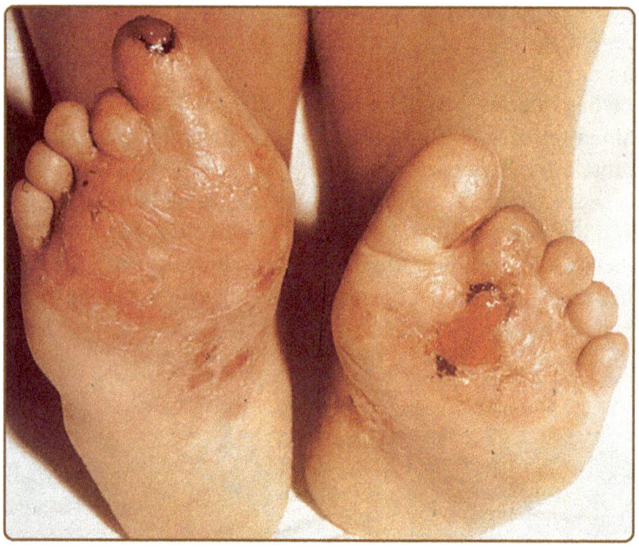

Erosive-ulcerative lichen planus showing erosions, ulcers, and granulation tissue and scarring of toes, interdigital web spaces, and soles. (Reproduced, with permission, from Goldsmith LA, Katz SI, Gilchrest BA, Paller AS, Leffell DJ, Wolff K, eds. *Fitzpatrick's Dermatology in General Medicine*. 8th ed. New York, NY: McGraw-Hill Education; 2012.)

Unlike classic lichen planus, hypertrophic LP may exhibit parakeratosis, spongiosis, apoptotic keratinocytes above the basal layer, and dermal eosinophils and plasma cells. Lichen planus is not associated with antinuclear antibodies, unlike lupus erythematosus, which may rarely histopathologically present with a band-like lymphocytic infiltrate with vacuolar alteration of the basal layer, but with deep dermal infiltrates, thickening of the basement membrane and increased dermal mucin.

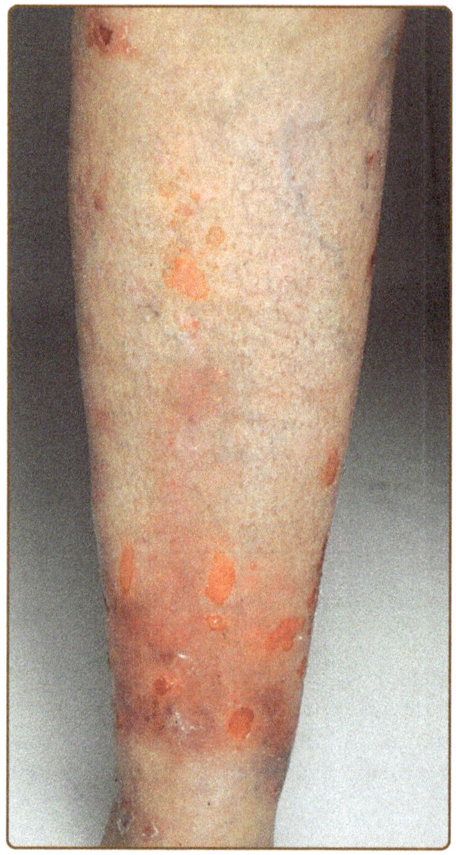

Lichen planus pemphigoides. Lichenoid maculopapular erythema, erosions, and bullae with direct immunofluorescence showing features of bullous pemphigoid. Indirect immunofluorescence was also positive for antibodies against basement membrane zone antigens. (Reproduced, with permission, from Goldsmith LA, Katz SI, Gilchrest BA, Paller AS, Leffell DJ, Wolff K, eds. *Fitzpatrick's Dermatology in General Medicine*. 8th ed. New York, NY: McGraw-Hill Education; 2012.)

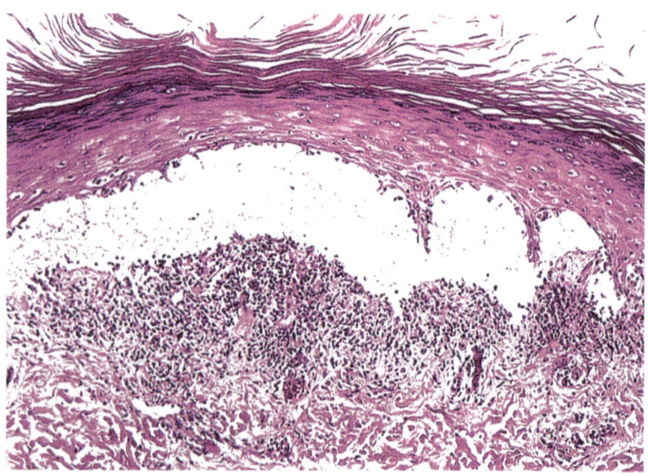

Bullous lichen planus. There is dermal-epidermal separation leading to formation of a blister cavity. Otherwise, features typical of lichen planus are present.

LP variants

1. **Actinic LP**
   - sun-exposed sites
   - epidermal atrophy
2. **Annular LP**
3. **Atrophic LP**
4. **Bullous LP**
   - confluent vacuolization → epidermis and dermis separate
5. **LP pemphigoides**
6. **Hypertrophic LP**
   - lower legs; pruritic
   - irregular acanthosis + interface
7. **Inverse LP**
8. **LP pigmentosus**
9. **Lichen planopilaris**
   - scarring alopecia
10. **Linear LP**
11. **LP-lupus erythematosus overlap**
12. **Nail LP**
13. **Oral LP**
14. **Ulcerative/erosive LP**
15. **Vulvovaginal LP (GTD)**

ANSWER 1-26: D.

This patient has **erythema multiforme** (EM), which is the prototype of **vacuolar interface dermatitis/cytotoxic interface dermatitis**. The histopathological differential diagnosis includes **Stevens-Johnson syndrome**, **toxic epidermal necrolysis**, and **acute graft versus host disease**. The histomorphology of all of these conditions is essentially identical to erythema multiforme and therefore clinical history and presentation are required for diagnostic distinction. Clinical and histopathologic subtypes of eruptions identified as erythema multiforme are likely to exist, and the description of target lesions oversimplifies the range of clinical findings. Erythema multiforme exhibits a fairly nonspecific histopathologic pattern, hence the wide clinical spectrum. The classic target lesion consists of at least three zones of color change: a peripheral rim of erythema with an inner rim of relative pallor and a central erythematous macule. This concentric pattern imparts a "bull's eye appearance." Variation from this pattern is described with erythematous patches, some with a dusky, violaceous center, but no distinct target appearance. Blisters, when present, form centrally in most cases, but a peripheral pattern may also occur. The distribution of erythema multiforme is frequently acral, with concentration on the palms and soles, but widespread lesions occur commonly. The disease is self-limited but often recurrent. Involvement of mucosal and conjunctival surfaces occurs and, if extensive, leads to classification of the disease as "major" (possibly synonymous with the term Stevens-Johnson syndrome) versus "minor" form with less severe extracutaneous disease. Universally accepted criteria distinguishing major from minor erythema multiforme and major erythema multiforme from Stevens-Johnson syndrome do not exist. The most common causes of erythema multiforme include herpes simplex virus infection, medications, and other infectious agents, especially *Mycoplasma pneumoniae*. Typical target lesions were associated more frequently with herpes simplex virus infection and "atypical" lesions with drug etiology in one study.

Drugs Associated With Erythema Multiforme and Stevens-Johnson Syndrome

Pyrazolone derivatives including phenylbutazone and oxyphenbutazone
Penicillins
Slowly excreted sulfonamides
Ampicillin
Salicylates
Salazopyrin
Barbiturates
Phenobarbital
Hydantoins
Carbamazepine
Phenothiazine derivatives
D-Penicillamine

An additional histological differential diagnosis with more differential findings includes **fixed drug eruption**, **acute/subacute lupus erythematosus**, **pityriasis lichenoides et varioliformis acuta (PLEVA)**, and **secondary syphilis** (choices A, B, C, and E, respectively). In EM, the dermal infiltrate is relatively sparse with variable vacuolar degeneration and keratinocyte apoptosis (dyskeratosis) depending on the evolutionary stage of the lesion. Unlike lichenoid dermatitis, these lesions do not exhibit premature terminal differentiation; therefore whorled clusters of dyskeratotic keratinocytes may be eliminated transepidermally and seen at all levels of the epidermis. Additionally, clusters of dyskeratotic keratinocytes may be seen plugging acrosyringia. The overlying stratum corneum is unaltered and exhibits a normal basket-weave configuration.

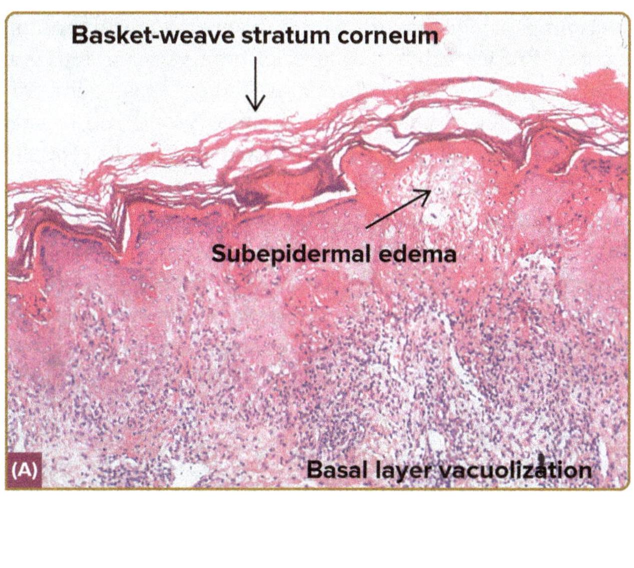

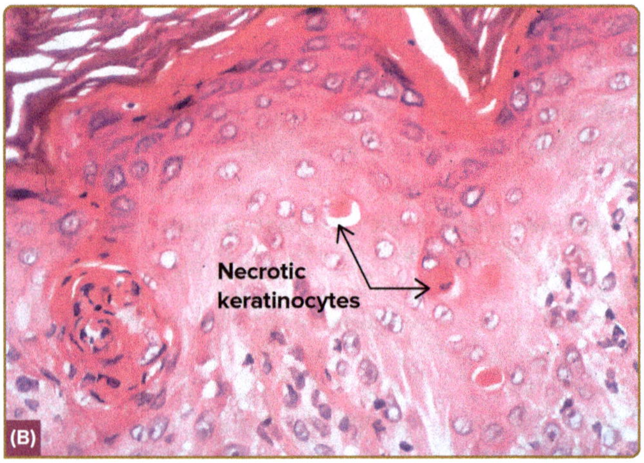

Erythema multiforme. There is cytotoxic interface dermatitis with basal layer vacuolization, subepidermal edema, and a predominantly lymphocytic infiltrate in the superficial dermis. Note the numerous dyskeratotic keratinocytes throughout all of the epidermal layers. The epidermis does not exhibit an adaptive response and the overlying stratum corneum exhibits a normal basket-weave configuration. (Reproduced, with permission, from Goldsmith LA, Katz SI, Gilchrest BA, Paller AS, Leffell DJ, Wolff K, eds. *Fitzpatrick's Dermatology in General Medicine*. 8th ed. New York, NY: McGraw-Hill Education; 2012.)

In more advanced lesions, destruction of the dermal epidermal junction may be extensive and result in vesicle or bullae formation. Regional anoxia from this clefting may result in epidermal necrosis, which corresponds clinically with the gray discoloration in the center of the lesion. **Fixed drug eruptions** and PLEVA tend to have robust superficial and deep dermal inflammatory infiltrates, unlike EM. Fixed drug eruptions contain mixed inflammatory infiltrates with eosinophils, neutrophils, and melanophages. Additionally, there is epidermal acanthosis, variable hypergranulosis, and hyperkeratosis. The infiltrates of **lupus erythematosus** range from extremely sparse to dense band like (similar to that of lichenoid dermatitis); however, the degree of keratinocyte destruction is substantially less than EM. The epidermis in lupus is atrophic with overlying orthohyperkeratosis. Increased dermal mucin and variable thickening of the basement membrane are distinguishing features. **PLEVA** exhibits features of both vacuolar interface dermatitis and spongiotic dermatitis. There is broad parakeratosis containing degenerating inflammatory cells and dermal and intraepidermal hemorrhage. **Secondary syphilis** typically exhibits robust cellular infiltrates of lymphocytes, plasma cells, and occasionally eosinophils. The infiltrate extends into the deep dermis along adnexal structures and nerve bundles. The epidermis exhibits variable changes of spongiosis and premature terminal differentiation; however, a somewhat unique finding is the presence of unusually elongated rete ridges.

ANSWER 1-27: D.

This is an example of a **lichenoid drug eruption**. Substances such as gold, thiazide diuretics, β-blockers, penicillamine, ACE inhibitors, and color film developing solutions are well known to induce this reaction pattern. When the eruption occurs in the distribution of UV light exposure, it is referred to as a **lichenoid photodermatitis**. These lesions clinically exhibit all of the classic features of lichenoid interface dermatitis (think Ps: pruritic, purple, polygonal, papules, or plaques), but the lesions tend to be more diffuse than those of

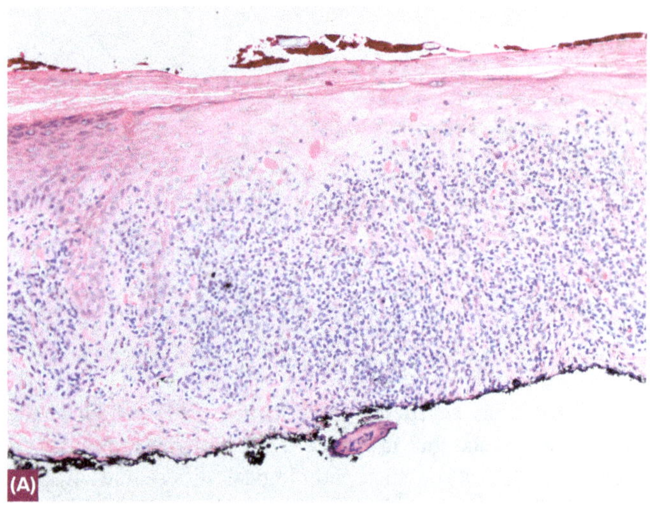

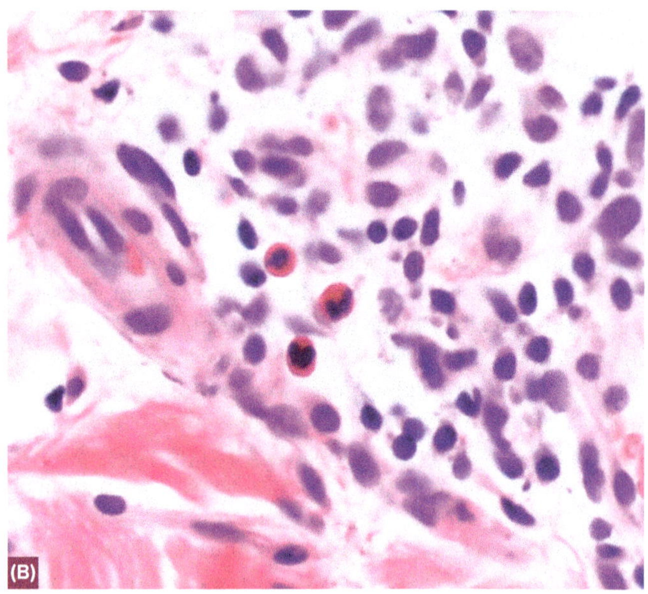

Lichenoid drug eruption. There is a band-like lymphocytic infiltrate along the dermal-epidermal junction with perivascular extension into the deep dermis. The infiltrate contains scattered eosinophils. The distinction between lichenoid drug eruption and lichen planus–like keratosis (LPLK) requires clinical correlation.

lichen planus, may be confluent, and generally do not exhibit a flexural distribution. Microscopically, there are dense dermal-epidermal infiltrates with extensive vacuolar degeneration and erosion of the rete ridges, which may result in clefting. However, unlike classic lichen planus, there are also both superficial and deep perivascular and interstitial infiltrates with lymphocytes, scattered eosinophils, and occasionally rare plasma cells. Premature terminal differentiation occurs, but it is sometimes incomplete. Therefore, unlike classic lichen planus, rare dyskeratotic cells may be eliminated transepidermally and the epidermal surface may contain both compact orthokeratosis and parakeratosis. Characteristic to the mixed histomorphology of drug eruptions, mild spongiosis may also be present. Postinflammatory pigmentary alteration (PIPA) is frequently a secondary consequence of this process. If these lesions persist, further chronic changes of epidermal atrophy, rete ridge effacement, and flattening of the dermal epidermal junction with compensatory papillary dermal fibrosis may be seen. These findings help distinguish a lichenoid drug eruption from idiopathic lichen planus; however, some cases may be identical to lichen planus. Clinical correlation is essential. Choice D describes the histopathological findings associated with collagen vascular disease (ie, lupus erythematosus or dermatomyositis).

Drugs Commonly Implicated in Lichenoid Drug Eruptions

Captopril Enalapril Labetalol Methyldopa Propanolol	ANTIHYPERTENSIVES
Chloroquine Hydroxychloroquine Quinacrine	ANTIMALARIALS
Etanercept Infliximab	TNF-α INHIBITORS
Chlorothiazide Hydrochlorothiazide	DIURETICS
Gold salts Penicillamine Quinidine	MISCELLANEOUS

ANSWER 1-28: B.

This is a classic histopathologic example of severe **cytotoxic interface dermatitis**. These findings are most commonly seen in **Stevens-Johnson syndrome (SJS)** and **toxic epidermal necrolysis (TEN),** both of which are medical emergencies and in most instances represent an idiosyncratic drug response. Common medications include sulfonamides, anticonvulsants, allopurinol, and NSAIDs. Rare inciting triggers include contactants such as dormex and exotic woods containing quinonoids, such as rosewood, ebony, and pao ferro. Histopathologically, there is sparse cytotoxic interface dermatitis with extensive epidermal dyskeratosis and blister formation with subsequent anoxic epidermal necrosis. All of these changes occur before an adaptive epidermal response can occur and a normal "basket-weave" stratum corneum is usually present. The histomorphology is essentially an exaggeration of that seen in erythema multiforme (EM). In fact, the periphery of these lesions may be indistinguishable from EM. Unlike EM, the clinical presentation of SJS/TEN is that of extensive erythema and necrosis with sloughing of the cutaneous and mucosal surfaces. Classic target lesions of EM are rarely observed.

Additionally, where EM represents a process of limited epithelial injury, SJS/TEN represents a progressive deregulated epithelial injury syndrome with a different proposed mechanism of action. It is believed that EM involves CD4+ T cells and keratinocyte apoptosis via gamma interferon, whereas SJS/TEN involves Fas ligand, tumor necrosis factor α, and CD8+ cytotoxicity toward drug hapten (peptide) bound to keratinocyte surface HLA proteins (MCH class I) rendering them antigenic. The issue remains controversial and the potential involvement of one or more pathways has not been resolved. To date, the strongest evidence suggests a key contribution of the cytotoxic molecules Fas ligand and granulysin as molecules responsible for the disseminated keratinocyte apoptosis. A diagnosis of SJS is made when two or more mucosal sites are involved and less than 10% of the skin is necrotic. A diagnosis of TEN is made when greater than 30% of the skin is necrotic. A TEN/SJS overlap syndrome is occasionally seen when 10%-30% of the skin surface is necrotic. Choice B describes **staphylococcal scalded skin syndrome (SSSS),** which histology appears as a subcorneal blister caused by exotoxins A and B (not subepidermal blister). These toxins are proteases secreted by *Staphylococcus aureus* and cleave desmoglein-1; hence the blister is confined to the stratum granulosum and stratum corneum. Full-thickness dyskeratosis and necrosis are not seen in SSSS. Like EM/SJS/TEN there are only sparse lymphocytic infiltrates in the dermis. It is worth mentioning that rare cases of severe acute graft versus host disease may also present with the histopathological findings illustrated in the biopsy in question.

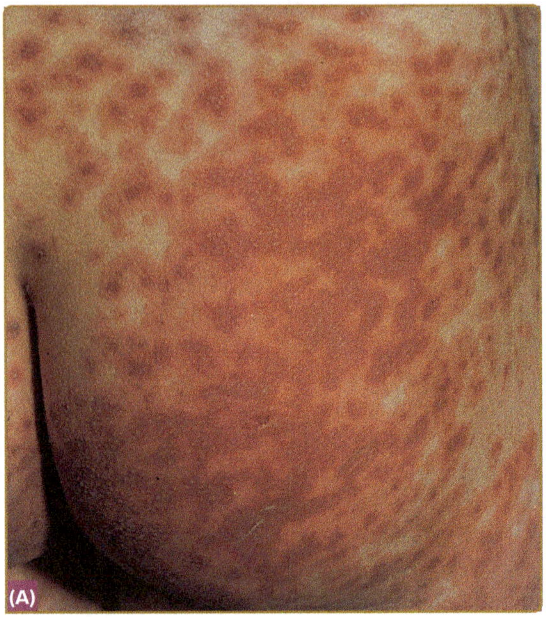

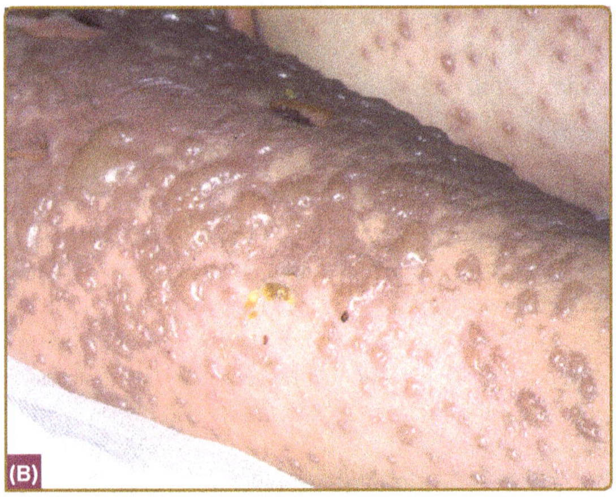

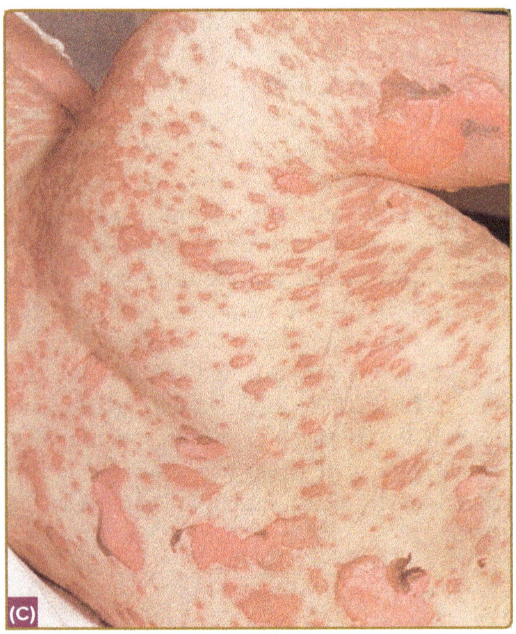

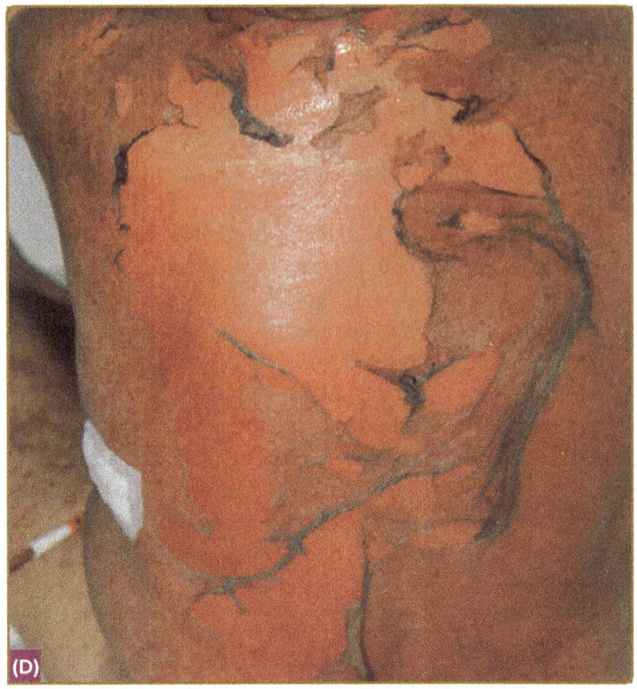

Stevens-Johnson syndrome/toxic epidermal necrolysis. (A) Early eruption. Erythematous dusky red macules (flat atypical target lesions) that progressively coalesce and show epidermal detachment. **(B)** Early presentation with vesicles and blisters, note the dusky color of blister roofs, strongly suggesting necrosis of the epidermis. **(C)** Advanced eruption. Blisters and epidermal detachment have led to large confluent erosions. **(D)** Full-blown epidermal necrolysis characterized by large erosive areas reminiscent of scalding. (Reproduced, with permission, from Goldsmith LA, Katz SI, Gilchrest BA, Paller AS, Leffell DJ, Wolff K, eds. *Fitzpatrick's Dermatology in General Medicine*. 8th ed. New York, NY: McGraw-Hill Education; 2012.)

Medications Associated With TEN "SATAN"

Sulfa antibiotics/sulfasalazine
Allopurinol
Tetracyclines/Thiacetazone
Anticonvulsants
NSAIDs/Nevirapine

Comparison of Erythema Multiforme and Toxic Epidermal Necrolysis

ERYTHEMA MULTIFORME	TOXIC EPIDERMAL NECROLYSIS
Clinical Features	
Erythematous patches with dusky centers	Diffuse erythematous patches with diffuse, full-thickness epidermal denudation
Target lesions	Mucosal and conjunctival involvement
Bullae and erosions	
Mucosal and conjunctival involvement	
Histopathologic Features	
Upper dermal interstitial infiltrate of lymphocytes	Little or no inflammation Vacuolar interface dermatitis
Basal vacuolization	Full-thickness epidermal necrosis typical
Single and clusters of necrotic keratinocytes	Scattered necrotic keratinocytes at periphery
Full-thickness epidermal necrosis possible	
Differential Diagnosis	
Toxic epidermal necrolysis	Erythema multiforme
Fixed drug eruption	Fixed drug eruption
Graft-versus-host reaction	
Viral exanthem	
Pityriasis lichenoides	

ANSWER 1-29: B.

This is an example of a **fixed drug eruption** (FDE) which is common and so named because the lesions recur at the same site with each exposure to a particular medication. In fact, patch testing with a topical medication on a different site can result in a flare in the originally affected area. The precise mechanism as to how this happens is not known. Lesions tend to occur singly and are frequently found on the lips, genitalia, oral mucosa, or limbs.

Microscopically, there are both superficial and deep perivascular and interstitial mixed infiltrates with scattered eosinophils and sometimes neutrophils. The dermal-epidermal lymphocytic infiltrates range from sparse to band like with vacuolar degeneration and clusters of dyskeratinocytes that frequently maintain their polygonal shape. Dyskeratinocytes surrounded by lymphocytes may be seen high in the spinous layer, similar to that seen in the cytotoxic interface dermatitis of **erythema multiforme, Stevens-Johnson syndrome, toxic epidermal necrolysis**, or **acute graft versus host disease**. The rete ridges tend to be elongated (psoriasiform) and spongiosis is frequently present. Severe lesions may exhibit confluent vesiculation along the dermal epidermal junction or within the epidermis (bullous FDE). Generally, these lesions rapidly evolve and devolve, resulting in little alteration to the cornification of the epidermis. Postinflammatory pigmentary alteration (PIPA) is a frequent secondary manifestation of these lesions with both epidermal pigmentation and numerous dermal melanophages. Recurrent lesions sometimes exhibit an orange discoloration due to the combination of inflammation admixed with dermal melanophages from the prior episode. Dark skinned patients may exhibit hypopigmentation once the lesions have fully resolved. The main histopathological differential diagnosis is **erythema multiforme,** which lacks eosinophils, neutrophils, and deep perivascular infiltrates. However, fixed drug eruptions may also lack these findings on occasion. Just like erythema multiforme, the T lymphocytes present at the periphery of the lesion and within the dermis are mostly CD4+, while the T lymphocytes in the center of the lesion and at the dermoepidermal junction are mostly CD8+. Clinical correlation is essential. The histopathological differential diagnosis also includes a lichenoid drug eruption, which may be impossible to distinguish from fixed drug eruptions without clinical correlation. **Lichenoid drug eruptions** also contain eosinophils, but generally contain a more robust interface infiltrate and more extensive premature terminal differentiation of the epidermis.

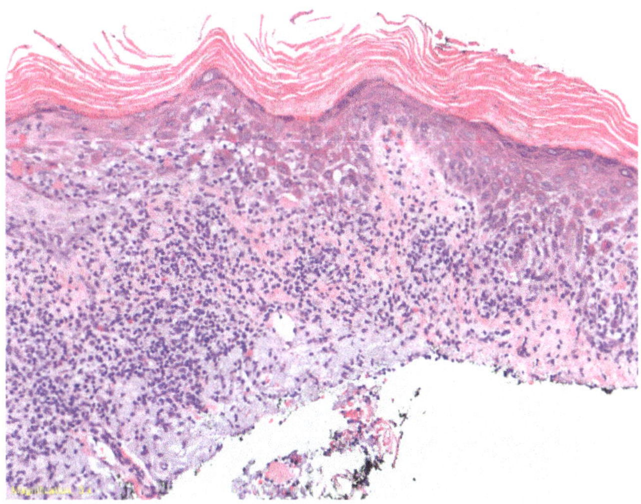

Fixed drug eruption with band-like interface infiltrate. Although the interface infiltrates are generally sparse in fixed drug eruptions, they may be band like in some cases. Dyskeratotic keratinocytes are present at all levels of the epidermis and the dermal infiltrate contains scattered eosinophils. The distinction from a lichenoid drug eruption in these cases requires clinical correlation.

Causes of FDE

"MS Barb's PeQuliar TAN"

Metronidazole
Sulfonamides
Barbiturates
Phenolphthalein
Quinine/quinidine
Tetracyclines
Acetaminophen
NSAIDs

Fixed Drug Eruption

Clinical Features
- Oval or round, sharply demarcated violaceous or dusky macule
- Arises 30 minutes to several hours after drug ingestion
- Anogenital areas, especially glans penis, and acral sites most common
- Vesiculation and blistering may ensue
- Areas of involvement tend to expand and multiply with drug rechallenge
- Postinflammatory hyperpigmentation
- Clear following drug withdrawal

Histopathologic Features
- Variably band-like lymphocytic interface infiltrate
- Basilar vacuolopathy of keratinocytes and colloid body formation, often accentuated at tips of retia
- Acanthosis more pronounced than erythema multiforme
- Patchy parakeratosis often seen
- Mixed lymphohistiocytic, eosinophilic, plasmacellular, and neutrophilic dermal infiltrate, often superficial and deep

Differential Diagnosis
- Erythema multiforme
- Viral exanthema
- Connective tissue disease
- Graft versus host disease

ANSWER 1-30: B.

This patient most likely has **pityriasis lichenoides et varioliformis acuta (PLEVA)**. These idiopathic lesions develop in otherwise healthy patients and rapidly present as crops of papules that become hemorrhagic, ulcerate, and spontaneously involute to form shallow scars. Microscopically, there is a wedge-shaped superficial and deep dermal lymphocytic infiltrate with variable interface density. Basal vacuolization and dyskeratotic keratinocytes are present. Exocytosis of lymphocytes into the upper layers of the epidermis is characteristic. Another helpful finding is the presence of cohesive collections of Langerhans cells with variable spongiosis. Unlike other forms of interface dermatitis, there is broad parakeratosis containing transepidermally eliminated leukocytes. Scattered dermal and intraepidermal red blood cell extravasation is common. A chronic form of the condition, **pityriasis lichenoides chronica (PLC)**, presents as slowly evolving red-brown papules surfaced by a scale. These lesions may persist for years and generally do not scar, but exhibit pigmentary alteration (PIPA). Both lesions (PLEVA and PLC) may be present within the same patient. In contrast to PLEVA, the microscopic features of PLC are more subtle. One observes foci of parakeratotic scale, occasional or rare necrotic keratinocytes, slight basal layer vacuolization, and a predominantly superficial perivascular infiltrate of lymphocytes. PLEVA and PLC may form part of a disease spectrum termed **pityriasis lichenoides**.

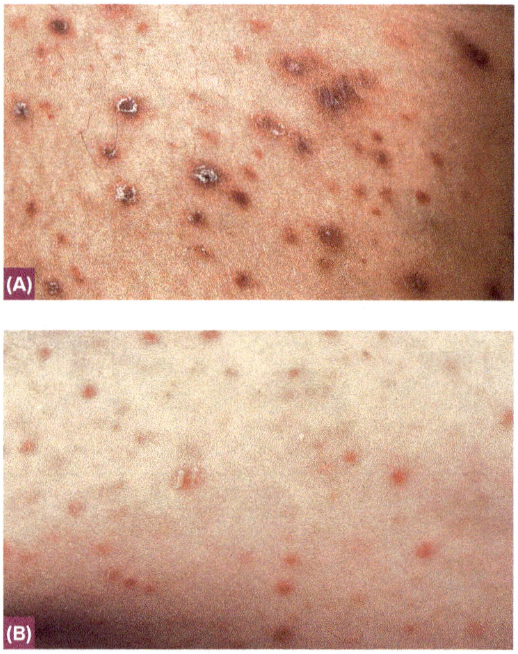

Pityriasis lichenoides. (A) PLEVA. Randomly distributed red papules of different size, some of which show hemorrhagic crusting. **(B) PLC**. Discrete papules with fine mica-like scales are present, which become more visible after slight scraping. In contrast to PLEVA there is no hemorrhagic crusting. (Reproduced, with permission, from Wolff K, Johnson RA, Saavedra AP. *Fitzpatrick's Color Atlas and Synopsis of Clinical Dermatology*. 7th ed. New York, NY: McGraw-Hill Education; 2013.)

In regard to the differential diagnosis, **pityriasis rosea (PR)** is largely a disease of older children and young adults. It is an acute, self-limiting skin eruption with a distinctive and constant course and a hypothesized viral association. Initial lesions present as erythematous, oval, macules, papules, patches, or plaques followed 1 or 2 weeks later by generalized secondary oval erythematous lesions on the trunk and upper

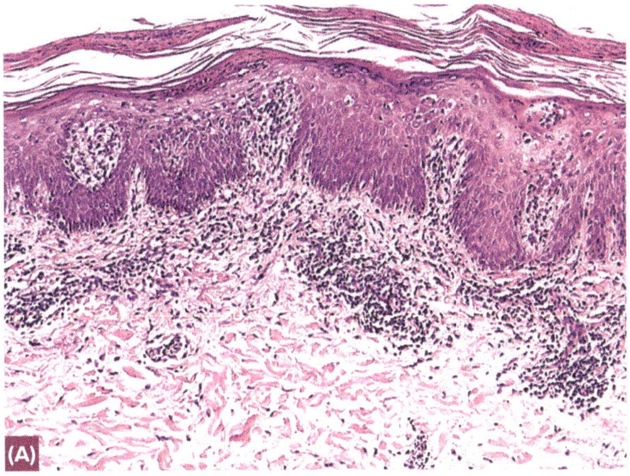

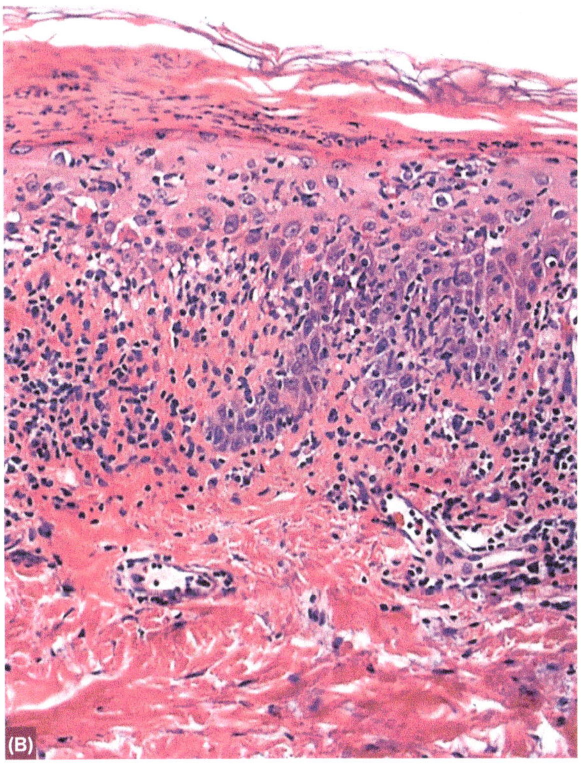

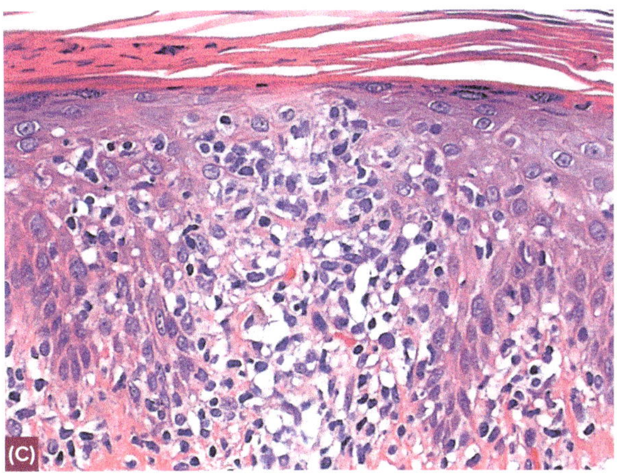

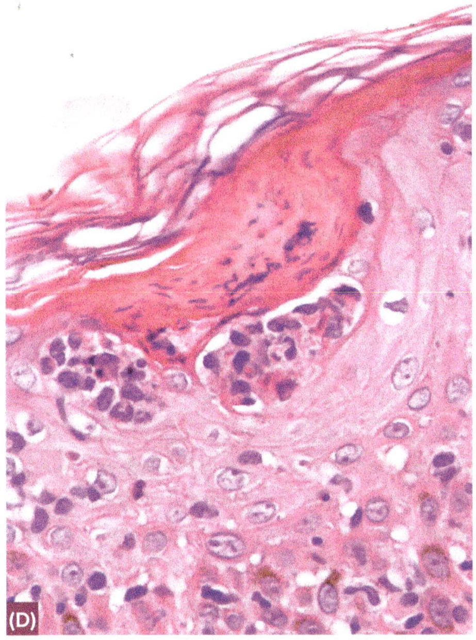

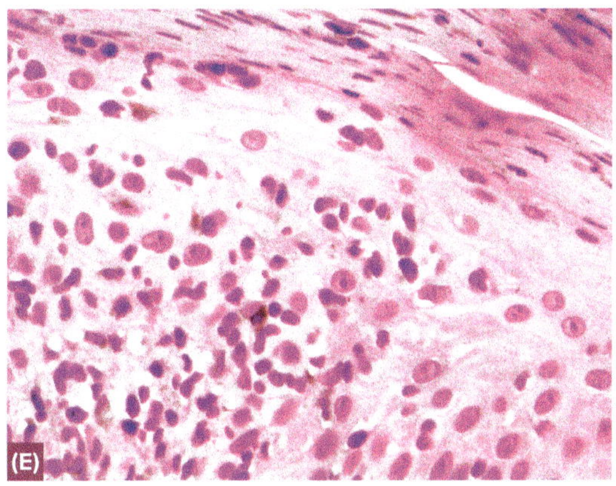

Pityriasis lichenoides et varioliformis acuta. (A) The lesion displays confluent parakeratosis, basal layer vacuolization, some exocytosis of lymphoid cells, and a perivascular lymphoid infiltrate in the dermis. **(B)** Classic changes of pityriasis lichenoides. Note the psoriasiform hyperplasia. There are classic changes of pityriasis lichenoides as defined by a psoriasiform pattern of epithelial hyperplasia and striking migration of lymphocytes to involve all layers of the epidermis with preferential localization of lymphocyte migration within the upper layers of the epidermis. Additionally, the epidermis is surmounted by a leukocyte-imbued scale crust. Extensive red cell extravasation is noted amidst a superficial interstitial and perivascular lymphocytic infiltrate. **(C)** In pityriasis lichenoides the pattern of lymphocyte migration is epidermotropic. In this particular photomicrograph there is passive migration of lymphocytes and histiocytes into the epidermis with lymphoid forms extending into the upper layers of the epidermis. Note the focal red cell extravasation and overlying parakeratotic scale. **(D)** One of the characteristic hallmarks of pityriasis lichenoides is the presence of pseudo Pautrier-like microabscesses (Langerhans cell–rich microvesicles) within the superficial layers of the epidermis. As opposed to a true Pautrier microabscess, the composition is one of small lymphocytes and histiocytes closely aggregated in contradistinction to a true Pautrier microabscess, which is composed exclusively of atypical lymphoid forms. **(E)** Lymphocyte exocytosis is present into the upper layers of the epidermis.

extremities in a "Christmas tree" distribution. The eruption heals without scaring. Microscopically, the lesions exhibit only sparse and very mild vacuolar interface activity and multiple foci of spongiosis with overlying "lens-shaped" parakeratosis (PR: spongiosis >> interface; PL: spongiosis < interface). Both PLEVA, PLC, and PR frequently contain extravasated red blood cells in the dermis and epidermis. **Lichen planus** clinically presents as multiple pruritic erythematous to violaceous papules and plaques on the extensor surfaces. Ulcerative lesions tend to follow a chronic course and are usually located on the dorsal hands, feet, and digits. Microscopically, there is a superficial heavy band-like lymphocytic infiltrate with exocytosis into only the basal and lower spinous layers resulting in papillary dermal colloid bodies and premature terminal differentiation of the epidermis. These hypertrophic epidermal changes result in hypergranulosis and compact orthokeratosis. Serum-imbued parakeratosis is characteristically absent. Lesions of **herpes zoster (shingles)** commonly occur in adults as painful eruptions characterized by vesicles confined to a dermatome distribution. Healing may occur with postinflammatory hyperpigmentation. Clinically appreciable vesiculation is unusual in PLEVA. Postherpetic lesions may fail to reveal the characteristic viral cytopathic features of herpes; however, these lesions will exhibit a mixed lymphocytic and granulomatous infiltrate that surrounds superficial and deep vessels and deep nerve bundles.

PLEVA DDX Clues

For PLEVA:

Parakeratosis, No eosinophils, # of lymphocytes roughly = keratinocytes

- •Eos → **drug eruption, arthropod bite**
- •Plasma cells, +VDRL → **syphilis**
- •TBST/Quantiferon gold+ → **papulonecrotic tuberculid**
- •Upper dermal edema → **polymorphous light eruption**
- •Follicular plugging, •Epidermal atrophy, •Basement membrane thickening, •Periadnexal inflammation, •Increased dermal mucin → **lupus erythematosus**
- •Basket weave straturm corneum, •Inflammation restricted to upper dermis, •Keratinocytes >> lymphocytes → **erythema multiforme**

ANSWER 1-31: E.

This question is very difficult as some cases of **pityriasis lichenoides chronica (PLC)** may arise within **pityriasis lichenoides et varioliformis acuta (PLEVA)** and many authors refer to both entities as pityriasis lichenoides. In general, both of these entities exhibit band-like dermal epidermal lymphocytic infiltrates of variable density but without premature terminal differentiation of the epidermis (seen in lichenoid interface dermatitis). Therefore, dyskeratinocytes may still be eliminated transepidermally and a parakeratotic scale containing leukocytes surfaces the epidermis. Often the stratum corneum contains entrapped serum, resembling the surface changes of spongiotic dermatitis.

The dense perivascular infiltrates of PLEVA are usually superficial and deep, whereas in PLC they are generally limited to the superficial dermis. Additionally, features of vasculitis with intravascular fibrin deposition are occasionally seen in PLEVA secondary to ulceration, but true vasculitis is not present and is never seen in PLC due to the absence of ulceration. Both conditions exhibit extravasation of red blood cells in the dermis and occasionally the epidermis. Foci of dyskeratotic keratinocytes rimmed by lymphocytes are more extensive in PLEVA and may coalesce to form clusters. These clusters are not seen in PLC. Spongiosis may be seen in both PLEVA and PLC, but only PLEVA may occasionally develop intraepidermal vesicles with Langerhans cell clusters. Lastly, both lesions, whether intact or ulcerated, develop confluent parakeratosis. In PLEVA, these mounds contain foci of fragmented lymphocytes and neutrophils, which are minimal to absent in PLC. T lymphocytes of PLEVA are CD3+ and CD7+ with a predominance of CD8+ cells in the infiltrate at the dermoepidermal junction. The lymphocytes of PLC may exhibit mild nuclear contour irregularity (atypia), a mild reduction in expression of

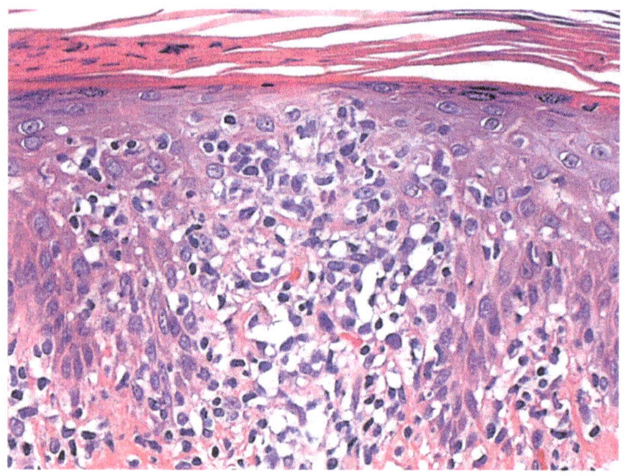

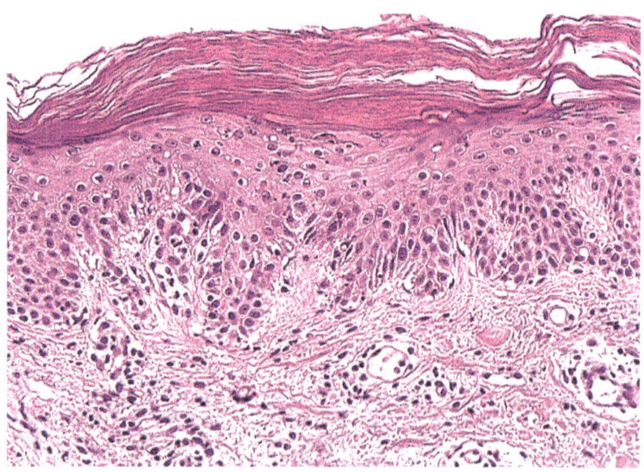

Pityriasis lichenoides chronica (PLC). This lesion exhibits prominent hyperkeratosis, occasional necrotic keratinocytes, and slight basal layer vacuolization. Note the extravasated red blood cells.

CD7, and occasional clonality via T-cell-receptor rearrangement analysis. Although PLC exhibits these atypical features, the progression to mycosis fungoides is exceptionally rare.

	PLEVA	PLC
Primary lesion	Erythematous papule → central vesiculation, pustulation, erosion, ulceration → crusts	Erythematous papule → pinpint dusky center (vesiculation or ulceration RARE)
Resolve with:	Scar	Dyspigmentation
Interface	Usually intense	Subtle
Predominant T cell	CD8	CD4
Keratinocyte necrosis	Evident	Rare
Clinical DDX	Arthropod bites, stings, infestations Leukocytoclastic vasculitis Viral exanthem Lymphomatoid papulosis Folliculitis Erythema multiforme Dermatitis herpetiformis Rickettsiosis Secondary syphilis Papulonecrotic tuberculid	Small-plaque parapsoriasis Guttate psoriasis Lichen planus Pityriasis rosea Secondary syphilis Lymphomatoid papulosis Papular dermatitis Lichenoid drug eruption Gianotti-Crosti syndrome Mycosis fungoides

ANSWER 1-32: D.

This is a classic example of cytotoxic interface dermatitis, which may be seen in **erythema multiforme (EM), Stevens-Johnson syndrome, toxic epidermal necrolysis,** and **acute graft versus host disease**. The lesions of EM present as discrete target-shaped erythematous and pruritic papulovesicles that blanch with external compression. This blanching erythema is due to vasodilatation. The eruption tends to form on acral sites with occasional mucosal involvement. There is a strong association with preexisting herpes simplex infection. In fact, herpetic antigens and DNA have been identified via immunofluorescence and PCR in lesional skin, respectively. One proposed mechanism of action is that of a type IV hypersensitivity reaction in which lymphocytes are directed against keratinocytes presenting herpetic viral antigens on MHC class I receptors and activation of the apoptotic pathway via gamma interferon. EM is also associated with various medications (sulfonamides, penicillin, barbiturates) and other infectious organisms like *Mycoplasma pneumoniae*, which theoretically could induce the same type IV hypersensitivity reaction described above. Overexpression of Fas antigen in keratinocytes may be important in drug-induced EM. The specific effector lymphocyte population is not clearly defined by immunophenotyping and the interface infiltrate is variably composed of CD8+ cytotoxic T cells, CD4+ helper T cells, and natural killer cells. No deep dermal infiltrate is present in EM. Choice D describes a **fixed drug eruption**, which exhibits a similar cytotoxic interface pattern, but contains a superficial and deep dermal mixed perivascular infiltrate composed of lymphocytes, eosinophils, neutrophils, and dermal melanophages. The epidermis of fixed drug eruptions may exhibit epidermal acanthosis with hyperkeratosis. The histomorphology of EM is identical to that seen in **acute graft versus host disease,** and a similar mechanism of action is likely with donor lymphocytes reacting against host antigens.

Causes of a Cell-Poor Interface Dermatitis

- Connective tissue disease syndromes
  - Systemic lupus erythematosus
  - Subacute cutaneous lupus erythematosus
  - Dermatomyositis
  - Mixed connective tissue disease
- Hypersensitivity reactions
  - Erythema multiforme
  - Drug reaction
  - Viral exanthem
  - Graft versus host disease

Causes of EM
"MY HOT PANS"

My*coplasma pneumoniae*

HSV1 and 2

Penicillins

Allopurinol, anticonvulsants

NSAIDs

Sulfonamides

ANSWER 1-33: D.

This is an example of **acute graft versus host disease**, which most frequently presents in patients who have received allogenic bone marrow or solid organ transplants. However, a rare but very severe and typically fatal form may develop in patients who receive nonirradiated blood transfusions. Clinically, acute GVHD presents as follicular papules and erythematous macules that may become confluent over time. As the lesions progress, scaling and vesiculation may be seen. The clinical and histopathological differential diagnosis usually includes a **drug eruption** or a **viral exanthem**.

Microscopically, early lesions may be indistinguishable from **erythema multiforme** with sparse interface infiltrates, vacuolar degeneration, and numerous dyskeratotic keratinocytes occasionally in clusters. The interface activity is especially directed toward follicular ostia and acrosyringia. However, as the lesions evolve, premature terminal differentiation of the epidermis may occur. Typically, there are prominent sweat gland and hair follicle infiltrates with overlying parakeratosis and parakeratotic follicular plugs. Some authors propose that "satellite cell necrosis" or dyskeratotic keratinocytes with closely apposed lymphocytes to be a pathognomonic feature of GVHD. However, although it is a sensitive finding, it is rather nonspecific since satellite cell necrosis may be seen in almost all forms of interface dermatitis. Occasionally the dermal infiltrate may contain rare scattered eosinophils, which may possibly reflect a component of **drug hypersensitivity** superimposed on the GVHD. **Viral exanthems** may be histopathologically identical to acute graft versus host disease. Clinical correlation with systemic findings is usually necessary for a definitive diagnosis. Patients receiving allogenic bone marrow transplants are typically pretreated with various chemotherapy agents and radiation before transfusion in efforts to rid them of the offending neoplastic cell population. This pretreatment may result in concomitant disordered epidermal maturation with significant keratinocyte atypia, mimicking squamous cell carcinoma in situ. Loss of polarity of keratinocytes resulting in disordered maturation of the epidermis from small cuboidal keratinocytes to flattened squamous epithelial cells is attributable to antineoplastic **chemotherapy effect** because these drugs disrupt the keratinocyte cell cycle. Individual keratinocyte necrosis accompanies this change; however, the cell death is metabolic and not mediated by infiltrating lymphocytes and therefore typically lacks lymphocyte satellitosis. Regardless, the diagnosis of acute GVHR is best made in unaffected portions of the epidermis, or not at all, if this change is diffusely present. Similarly, within the first 3 weeks after marrow transplant, increased numbers of necrotic keratinocytes are referable to ionizing radiation, making quantification helpful. The matter is made simpler by the requirement for significant dermal inflammation because neither **chemotherapy effect** nor **acute radiation** change is accompanied by large numbers of lymphocytes in the dermis. Other related conditions to GVHD include **lymphocyte recovery syndrome,** in which patients who have received autologous bone marrow transplants experience a rapid efflux of host lymphocytes into the skin manifesting clinically as erythematous macules. Microscopically, these lesions are typically identical to acute GVHD.

A histopathological grading scheme for acute GVHD exists by which all specimens taken for the diagnosis of acute GVHD may be classified. The minimum criteria to establish the diagnosis are codified as grade 2, namely, basal vacuolization, keratinocyte necrosis (at least four necrotic keratinocytes per linear millimeter of epidermis), and a lymphocytic infiltrate in the upper dermis with variable exocytosis. Confluence of the basal vacuoles and separation of epidermis from dermis define grades 3 and 4, respectively. Follicular epithelium is similarly involved. This cytotoxic folliculitis is the earliest manifestation in acute cutaneous GVHR, and it is advisable to study many tissue profiles from a given sample in search of this finding.

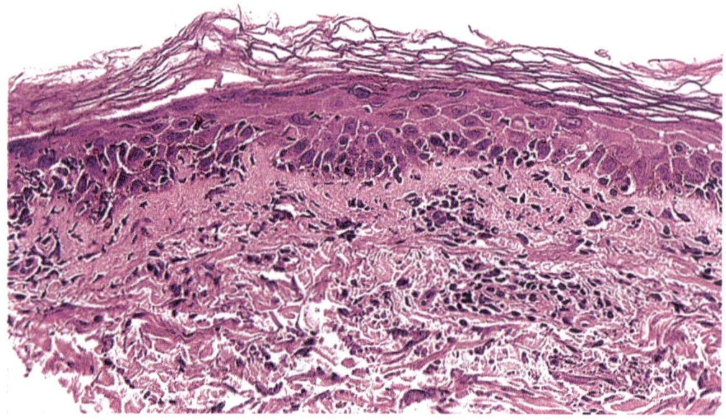

Acute graft versus host reaction, grade 2. The epidermis shows some disturbance in the maturation of keratinocytes, slight spongiosis, vacuolization of the basal layer, and a relatively scant superficial perivascular lymphocytic infiltrate.

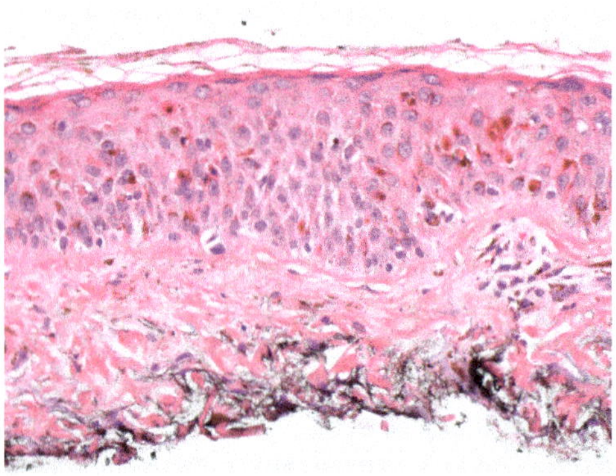

Chemotherapy/radiation effect. There are numerous dyskeratotic keratinocytes present throughout the epidermis; however, they are unaccompanied by lymphocyte satellitosis. This signifies cell death from metabolic/toxic injury compared to immunologic injury.

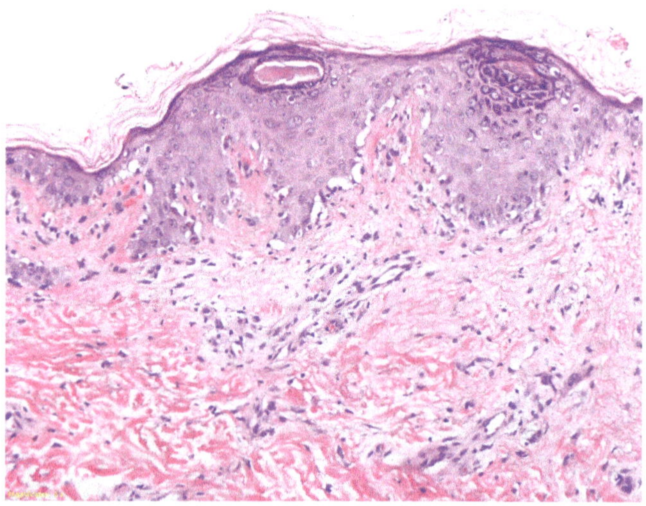

Acute graft versus host reaction, grade 3. There is confluent vacuolization along the dermal-epidermal junction and dyskeratotic keratinocytes are surrounded by lymphocytes.

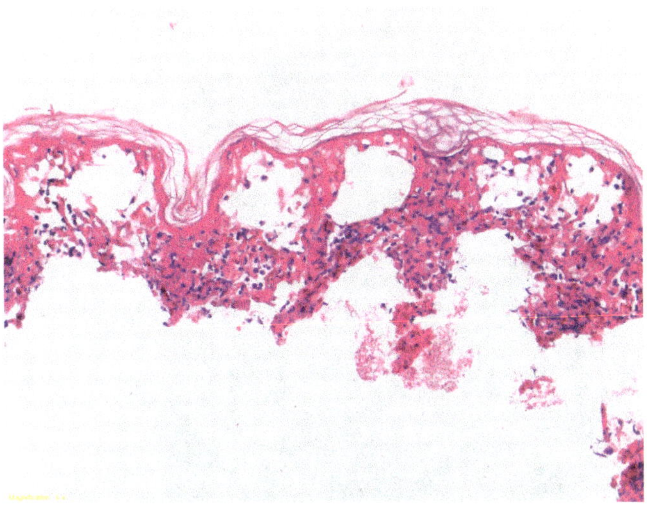

Acute graft versus host reaction, grade 4. The epidermis is completely necrotic and has separated from the dermis. There are numerous dyskeratotic keratinocytes surrounded by lymphocytes. Note the histopathological similarity with Stevens-Johnson syndrome/toxic epidermal necrolysis.

Acute Cutaneous Graft Versus Host Reaction

Grade 0	No pathologic change or diagnosis unrelated to GVHR
Grade 1	Basal vacuolization
Grade 2	Basal vacuolization, necrotic keratinocytes, dermal inflammation
Grade 3	Confluence of basal vacuoles
Grade 4	Separation of epidermis from dermis

ANSWER 1-34: A.

This is an example of **chronic lichenoid graft versus host disease (GVHD)**. In general, lesions of GVHD that present 100 days status post transplantation are considered chronic, and **chronic GVHD** is further divided into lichenoid and sclerodermoid forms. However, histopathologic changes of acute GVHD may be seen after 100 days of transplantation but the two conditions are believed to be pathophysiologically different. The development of acute GVHD predisposes to chronic GVHD, but chronic disease may arise de novo.

Early lesions of chronic GVHD are referred to as **lichenoid GVHD**, and present as purple, flat-topped papules similar to that seen in lichen planus. Alopecia, mucositis, and nail changes are usually present. Oral changes resemble those of oral lichen planus. Development of lichenoid GVHD is associated with a lower incidence of tumor relapse.

Microscopically, the lesions differ from lichen planus in that the inflammatory infiltrate is generally sparse. Therefore, the term "lichenoid" is misleading, and the infiltrate is of similar density to that seen in erythema multiforme (vacuolar interface dermatitis vs lichenoid interface dermatitis). However, the epidermal changes are similar to lichen planus with premature terminal differentiation of the epidermis, colloid bodies in the papillary dermis, absent dyskeratotic keratinocytes within the upper epidermal layers, and wedge-shaped foci of hypergranulosis overlying acrosyringia and follicular ostia. Similar to acute graft versus host disease, the inflammatory reaction preferentially targets the epidermis at follicular ostia and acrosyringia. There may be parakeratosis and compact orthokeratosis and occasional squamous metaplasia within the adnexal structures. Eosinophils and plasma cells are frequently present within the infiltrates. As in lichen planus, older lesions may exhibit effaced rete ridges, epidermal atrophy, and dense papillary dermal sclerosis.

To what extent the **chronic lichenoid GVHD** is reliably separable from **acute GVHD** is uncertain. Both conditions are interface dermatitides, with the main difference residing in the extent to which epidermal change resembles lichen planus. This distinction is important because therapy differs depending on whether the process is called acute or chronic. It is the rare biopsy specimen that fulfills all criteria for the diagnosis

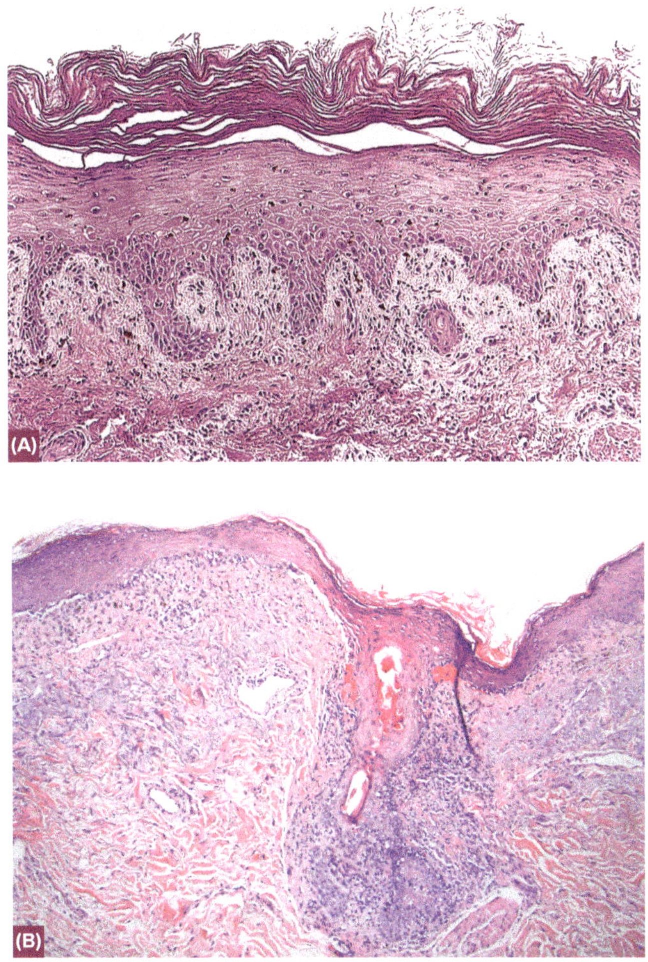

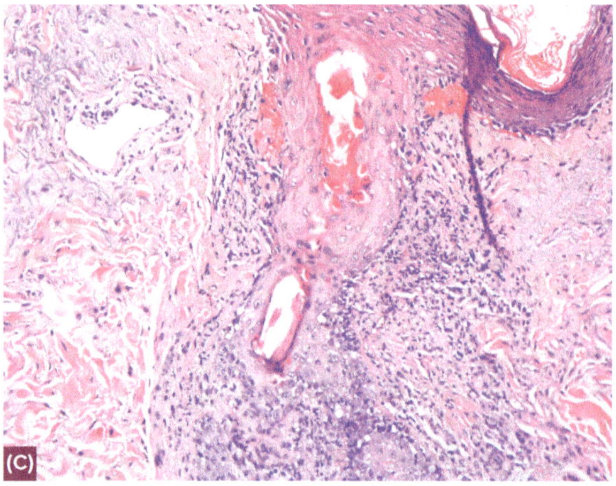

Chronic lichenoid graft versus host reaction. (A) This lesion shows hyperkeratosis, acanthosis, and a saw-tooth pattern reminiscent of lichen planus. However, a band-like infiltrate typical of lichen planus is not present. **(B)** In this case of chronic graft versus host disease there is prominent follicular involvement. **(C)** A destructive lichenoid process involves the outer root sheath epithelium with resultant thinning of the follicle.

Quick Fack

Lichenoid GVHD is actually a cell-poor lymphocytic infiltrate, but with premature terminal differentiation of the epidermis, similar to that seen in lichen planus.

of a lichenoid chronic GVHD. Therefore, when uncertain, it is advisable to make a diagnosis of "interface dermatitis consistent with graft versus host reaction" and allow the clinician to establish the final diagnosis. **Chronic sclerodermoid GVHD** typically begins 100 days or more after marrow transplantation, but again, the time of onset is variable. Progressive cutaneous sclerosis resembles systemic scleroderma. Fasciitis accompanies the skin changes and is a major cause of morbidity leading to joint contractures. Progressive cutaneous sclerosis leads to ischemia and chronic erosion and eventual ulceration of the skin—particularly the scalp and feet. Alopecia is common. Spontaneous resolution of cutaneous sclerosis with completely normal skin examination may rarely occur. In both forms of chronic GVHD, death is usually due to the accompanying smoldering immunosuppression that predisposes to frequent infectious complications, including sepsis.

Microscopically, lesions are of chronic sclerodermoid GVHD are characterized by progressive thickening of collagen bundles with loss of the normal spacing. This progression reportedly begins in the papillary dermis and extends toward the subcutis. As sclerosis progresses, there is loss of the pilosebaceous units and loss of adipose tissue around eccrine glands, so-called entrapment. Invariably, there is evidence of interface damage as well. While active inflammation is sparse, the dermal-epidermal junction will display basal vacuolization with occasional necrotic keratinocytes and upper dermal

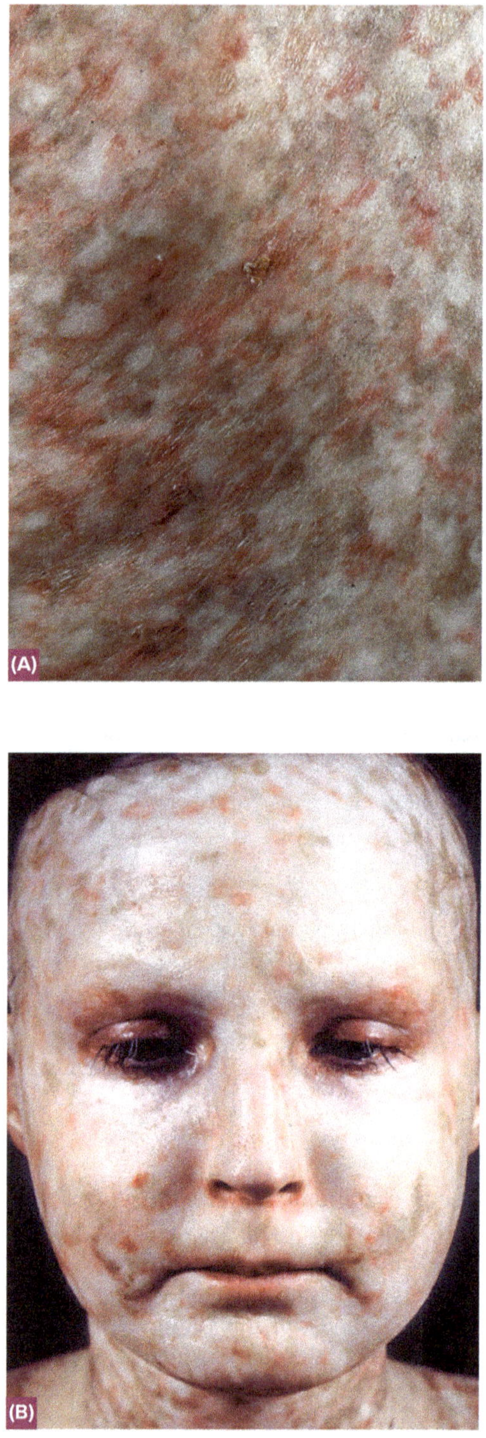

Chronic cutaneous GVHR, sclerodermoid. (A) Close-up view of the back of a patient with poikilodermatous changes (hypo- and hyperpigmentation) and telangiectasias in the sclerotic skin. **(B)** Ebony-white bound down skin and telangiectasias in the 10-year-old boy. Skin looks and feels like severe scleroderma. In this case, acute GVHR evolved directly into chronic GVHR and involved the entire skin of the head, trunk, and extremities. (Reproduced with permission from Wolff K, Johnson RA, Saavedra AP. *Fitzpatrick's Color Atlas and Synopsis of Clinical Dermatology*. 7th ed. New York, NY: McGraw-Hill Education; 2013.)

melanophages. This finding raises the interesting possibility that an epidermal cytokine mediates the pathologic collagen alteration during and after chronic damage to the interface.

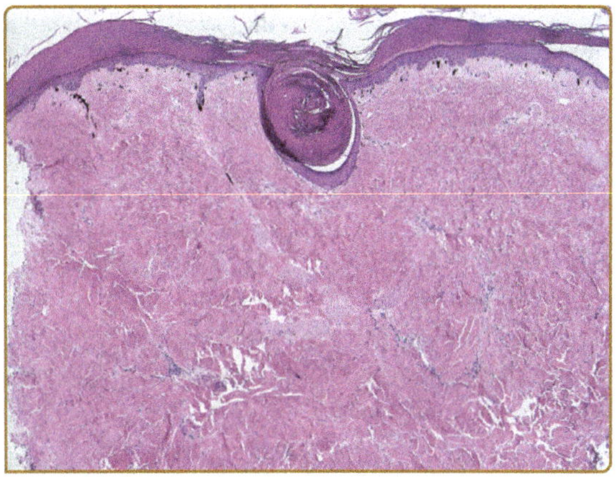

Sclerotic-type chronic GVHD. There is mild, compact hyperkeratosis or the epidermis with keratin plugging. There is hyalinization of the collagen throughout the dermis with loss of adnexal structures. (Reproduced, with permission, from Goldsmith LA, Katz SI, Gilchrest BA, Paller AS, Leffell DJ, Wolff K, eds. *Fitzpatrick's Dermatology in General Medicine*. 8th ed. New York, NY: McGraw-Hill Education; 2012.)

Acute Versus Chronic Graft Versus Host Reaction

ACUTE GVHR	CHRONIC GVHR
Clinical Features	
Variably distributed erythematous patches	Discrete erythematous to violaceous papules of variable distribution
Acral accentuation	Lacy white patches on buccal mucosa
Blisters rarely	
Histopathologic Features	
Upper dermal perivascular and interstitial infiltrate of lymphocytes, often mild	Denser band of lymphocytes in upper dermis
	Epidermal features of lichen planus
Basal vacuolization, keratinocyte necrosis	Dermal sclerosis, especially involving superficial dermis, in sclerodermoid variant
Subepidermal bullae rarely	
Differential Diagnosis	
Erythema multiforme	Lichen planus
Toxic epidermal necrolysis	Lichenoid drug eruption
Viral exanthema	Lichenoid keratosis
	Morphea/scleroderma

ANSWER 1-35: E.

Cutaneous involvement in lupus erythematosus presents with several differing clinical pictures. While photodistribution is common, any form of lupus erythematosus may display a generalized distribution of lesions. In **systemic lupus erythematosus (acute cutaneous lupus erythematosus)**, diffuse erythematous macules and patches are common combined with systemic involvement (ie, renal disease, arthritis, etc). In most cases, there is little surface change and the eruption is evanescent. Scarring and/or nonscarring alopecia may also be present. Photoaccentuation is common, leading to the malar "butterfly" distribution. Serologic tests reveal positive antinuclear antibodies in high titers. Circulating antibodies to double-stranded DNA are considered pathognomonic for systemic disease. Hypocomplementemia is common.

Direct immunofluorescence of lesional skin reveals a positive **"lupus band test,"** characterized by granular deposits of IgG, IgA, and/or IgM along with components of complement activation including C3 and C5b9 along the dermal epidermal junction. The most common and least specific form of positive lupus band test is one where there are prominent deposits of IgM within the basement membrane zone unaccompanied by other immunoglobulins. An important caveat is that IgM in isolation from other immunoglobulins can be seen in other settings including sun-exposed skin of healthy adults. Unlike the other forms of cutaneous lupus, systemic lupus erythematosus may also reveal a positive lupus band test in nonlesional sun-protected skin and significantly correlates with active renal disease.

Subtle histopathologic changes often characterize acute disease. Mild superficial dermal perivascular and interstitial infiltrates of lymphocytes are present and may exhibit little or no epidermal change, imparting a nonspecific picture. However, some degree of basal vacuolization and keratinocyte apoptosis is usually present. Atrophy of the epidermis, edema of the upper dermis, and an increase in dermal mucin are common features. Dermal mucin can be highlighted with Alcian blue and colloidal iron stains. In addition to lymphocytes, the mononuclear cells of the infiltrate show an immunophenotypic profile compatible with plasmacytoid dendritic cells exhibiting CD4, myxovirus protein (MXA), and CD123 positivity. Plasmacytoid dendritic cells secrete interferon alpha, which is a cytokine profile associated with **lupus erythematosus, dermatomyositis, lichen planus**, and **viral infections**. In aggregate, these findings allow the diagnosis of lupus erythematosus in the correct clinical setting.

The distinction between acute systemic lupus erythematosus and dermatomyositis is not possible based solely on histopathology, even with adjunct histochemical and immunohistochemical stains. Dermatomyositis frequently exhibits a negative lupus band test. Clinical correlation and serological studies are required.

Mild interface change and scant inflammation may also occur in **viral exanthems** and **phototoxic reactions**;

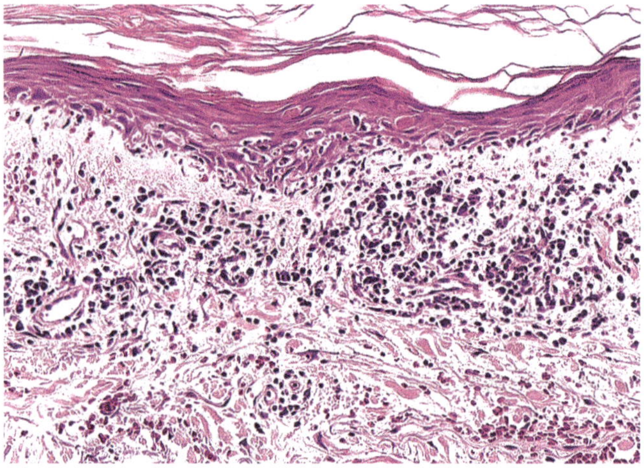

Acute lupus erythematosus. Higher magnification shows atrophy of the epidermis, basal layer vacuolization, and eosinophilic homogenization of the papillary dermis near the dermal-epidermal junction.

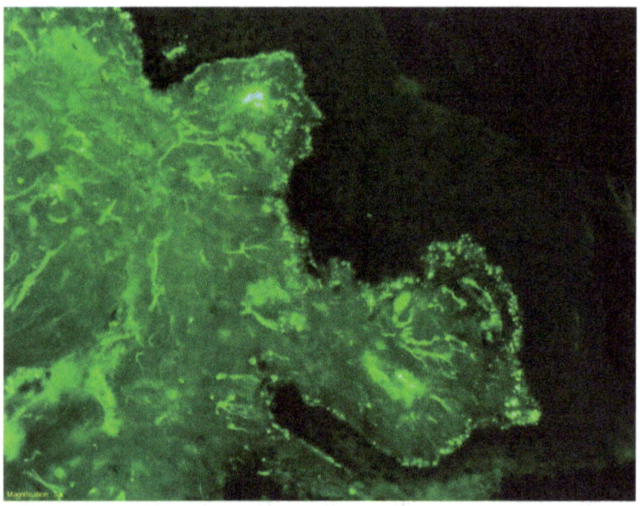

Positive lupus band test. There is granular deposition of immunoglobulin (IgG) along the dermal-epidermal junction.

however, the observation of increased dermal mucin narrows the focus to connective tissue disease. **Reticular erythematous mucinosis (REM)** is rare chronic dermatosis characterized by persistent, reticulate, urticated, macular, and sometimes papular erythema with an irregular, but well-defined border. The lesions typically occur on the central chest and upper back and are associated with photoexacerbations. A form associated with HIV infection has also been documented. The pathogenesis of REM is not well understood, but type I interferons are believed to play a role, just like in lupus erythematosus. Microscopically, REM has both mucin and mononuclear infiltrates in common with lupus erythematosus but lacks interface dermatitis and evidence of a systemic disease. Because of the similarities between REM and **tumid lupus**, the two-disease processes have often been grouped together. The remarkable overlap between the two diseases suggests that the two conditions may actually be the same disease. The mucin accumulation in **papular mucinosis** and **scleromyxedema** is accompanied by a concomitant increase in fibroblasts; this cellular proliferation is absent in lupus erythematosus. Unlike lupus, these two conditions also lack significant interface dermatitis. **Lichen planus** contains a dense band-like interface infiltrate with premature terminal differentiation of the epidermis. These features are not usual features of lupus erythematosus. Lastly, the dermis of lichen planus does not contain increased dermal mucin.

Revised Criteria of the American College of Rheumatology for the Classification of Systemic Lupus Erythematosus

1. Malar rash
2. Discoid rash
3. Photosensitivity
4. Oral ulcers
5. Arthritis
6. Serositis: (a) pleuritis or (b) pericarditis
7. Renal disorder: (a) proteinuria >0.5 g/24 h or 3+, persistently, or (b) cellular casts
8. Neurological disorder: (a) seizures or (b) psychosis (having excluded other causes, eg, drugs)
9. Hematologic disorders:
   Hemolytic anemia
   Leukopenia $<4.0 \times 10^9$/L on two or more occasions
   Lymphopenia $<1.5 \times 10^9$/L on two or more occasions
   Thrombocytopenia $<100 \times 10^9$/L
10. Immunologic disorders:
    Positive LE cell
    Raised antinative DNA antibody binding
    Anti-Sm antibody
    False-positive serologic test for syphilis, present for at least 6 months
11. Antinuclear antibody in raised titer

ANSWER 1-36: C.

This is a classic presentation of **subacute lupus erythematosus (SCLE)** where patients present with the sudden onset of widely scattered, erythematous-to-violaceous, scaling, well-demarcated plaques on the trunk, neck, and arms, mimicking the clinical appearance of **psoriasis vulgaris**. All forms of cutaneous lupus are associated with photoexacerbation.

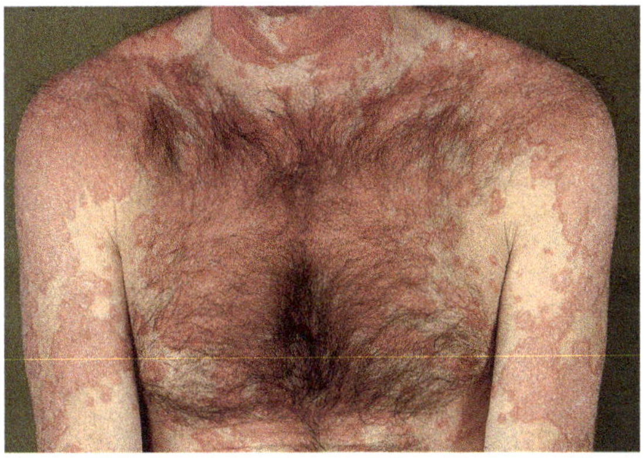

Subacute cutaneous lupus erythematosus. Widely scattered, erythematous-to-violaceous, scaling, well-demarcated plaques on the trunk, neck, and arms, mimicking the clinical appearance of psoriasis vulgaris. (Reproduced, with permission, from Wolff K, Johnson RA. *Fitzpatrick's Color Atlas & Synopsis of Clinical Dermatology*. 6th ed. New York: McGraw-Hill; 2009.)

Patients with SCLE may have some of the criteria of systemic lupus (SLE) as defined by the American Rheumatism Association, including photosensitivity, arthralgias, serositis, renal disease, and serologic abnormalities. Approximately half of patients with SCLE have SLE; however, the serious organ involvement of SLE is uncommon. Practically all have anti-Ro (SS-A) and most have anti-La (SS-B) antibodies. Exposure of keratinocytes in tissue culture to ultraviolet B (UVB) radiation results in enhanced expression of these antigens, possibly explaining the photosensitivity in this subtype.

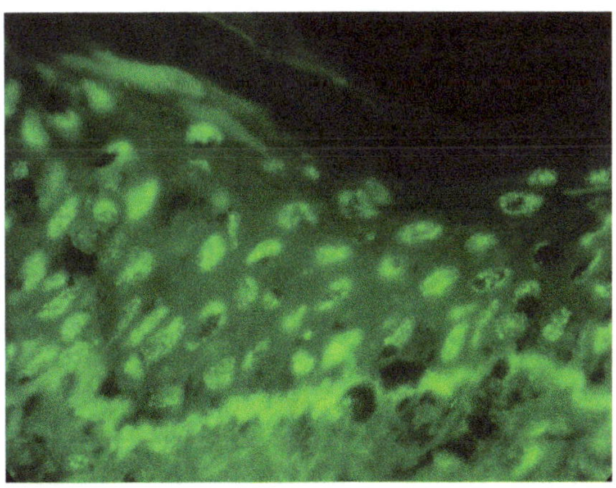

Subacute cutaneous lupus erythematosus, direct immunofluorescence. Positive staining of keratinocyte nuclei with immunoglobulins correlates strongly with antibodies to extractable nuclear antigens Ro, La, Smith, or as in this case, RNP. A similar pattern may be seen in MCTD, Sjögren syndrome, dermatomyositis, SLE, and very rare cases of DLE associated with antibodies to extractable nuclear antigens. There is also granular deposition along the dermal-epidermal junction, consistent with a positive lupus band test.

There is debate whether the clinical subtypes of cutaneous lupus erythematosus can be reliably distinguished, based on histopathologic criteria alone. The clinical skin lesions are the distinctive feature of SCLE. In contrast to the acute subtype, subacute disease displays more inflammation. A lymphocytic infiltrate is present and primarily surrounds the superficial vascular plexus, with possible extension to deeper dermal levels and the subcutis. While lymphocytes extend between collagen bundles in the upper dermis, formation of a dense band of lymphocytes is uncommon. Epidermal interface changes and increased dermal mucin are present. The lymphocytic infiltrate may extend around pilosebaceous and eccrine epithelium but generally is not as dense as in discoid disease and dilated hair follicles with keratin plugging are absent. Eosinophils are typically absent in all forms of cutaneous lupus. Thus, in comparison with acute systemic lupus erythematosus, subacute disease is characterized by a heavier lymphocytic infiltrate with a more distinct superficial perivascular and periadnexal pattern. Immunophenotypic studies will reveal CD123 positivity in scattered inflammatory cells as well as MXA staining of the epidermis, follicular epithelium, and inflammatory cells, consistent with an interferon alpha-rich microenvironment. Direct immunofluorescence of lesional skin reveals a positive lupus band test in approximately 60% of cases. Granular labeling of keratinocytes with immunoglobulin and C5b-9 is a feature that strongly correlates with anti-Ro and anti-La antibodies.

Histopathologic Criteria for Subtypes of Lupus Erythematosus

I. *Systemic lupus erythematosus*
   - Pauci-inflammatory interface dermatitis
   - Slight to absent epidermal atrophy
   - Basement membrane zone of normal thickness
   - No follicular plugging
   - Prominent papillary dermal edema and reticular dermal mucin accumulation

II. *Subacute cutaneous lupus erythematosus*
   - Prominent suprabasilar exocytosis of lymphocytes and dyskeratosis extending into upper spinous layers
   - Prominent epidermal atrophy
   - Follicular plugging or basement membrane zone thickening minimal or absent
   - Mild to moderate mononuclear cell infiltrate confined to the superficial dermis

III. *Discoid lupus erythematosus*
   - Lymphocyte-rich interface dermatitis
   - Less epidermal atrophy than SCLE; sometimes acanthosis
   - Prominent basement membrane zone thickening
   - Prominent follicular hyperkeratosis
   - Dense superficial and deep perivascular and periadnexal infiltrates with prominent follicular degeneration
   - Dermal fibrosis

Seropositivity[a] by Connective Tissue Disease Classification

	ANA	C	ss-DNA	ds-DNA	Sm	SSA/RO	SSB/La	nRNP	HISTONE	Scl70
SLE	95-100	0-10	70	70	<30[b]	40	10-20	40-50	30	0
SCLE	70	0	10-20	0	0	60-80	10	0	0	0
DLE	20-30		10-20	10-20	0	10-20	10	0	0	0
CRST	90	90	0	0	0	0	0	0	0	0
PSS	70	10	10-20	0	0	10	10	20	0	30
MCTD	95-100	0	30	0	0-5	0	0	100	0	0

Abbreviations: ANA, antinuclear antibody; C, centromere; CRST, CREST syndrome; DLE, discoid lupus erythematosus; ds-DNA, double-stranded DNA; MCTD, mixed connective tissue disease; nRNP, nuclear ribonucleoprotein; PSS, progressive systemic sclerosis/scleroderma; SCLE, subacute cutaneous lupus erythematosus; SLE, systemic lupus erythematosus; Sm, Smith; ss-DNA, single-stranded DNA.
[a]Expressed as percentage of cases.
[b]Dependent on ethnicity.

Drug Classes Associated With Drug-Induced Lupus Erythematosus

Antihypertensive
Antipsychotic
Anticonvulsant
Anti-inflammatory
Antimicrobial
Immunosuppressive
Antihormonal
Recombinant cytokines

In regard to the differential diagnosis, SCLE shares histologic features with **dermatomyositis**. Dermatomyositis is generally less heavily inflamed and lacks significant periadnexal inflammation. Clinical correlation is required for distinction. Interface dermatitis accompanied by a superficial and deep perivascular lymphocytic infiltrate also characterizes **pityriasis lichenoides et varioliformis acuta (PLEVA)** and **secondary syphilis**. Accumulation of mucin and periadnexal patterning of the infiltrate favor the diagnosis of lupus erythematosus. Furthermore, PLEVA and syphilis tend to display heavier exocytosis and more dyskeratotic keratinocytes than any variant of lupus erythematosus and are frequently surfaced by a parakeratotic scale. Secondary syphilis generally contains scattered plasma cell infiltrates. **Polymorphous light eruption** is distinguished by the presence of marked superficial dermal edema with hemorrhage, scattered eosinophils, and only minimal interface activity. Periadnexal inflammation is also not characteristic of polymorphous light eruption. **Psoriasis** is easily distinguished from the psoriasiform variant of subacute lupus erythematosus by the presence of interface dermatitis and mucin deposition in the latter entity. Occasional **photoallergic drug eruptions**, such as those induced by thiazide diuretics and antihistamines, may closely resemble and possibly induce subacute lupus erythematosus. These drug eruptions are discriminated by clinical history.

ANSWER 1-37: B.

This is a classic example of **chronic discoid lupus erythematosus**, which is one of the many cutaneous manifestations of lupus. The lesions generally present on the head and neck as sharply defined erythematous plaques with evolving central firm hypopigmented regions of atrophy. Scarring alopecia is common. In many patients, discoid lesions are the sole manifestation of the disease, whereas one in five of patients with **systemic lupus erythematosus** develops discoid lesions. The lesions of both discoid and systemic disease are mediated by combined autoantibodies and cell-mediated toxicity. In contrast to systemic lupus, patients presenting with only discoid lesions will have positive antinuclear antibody titers in a minority of cases.

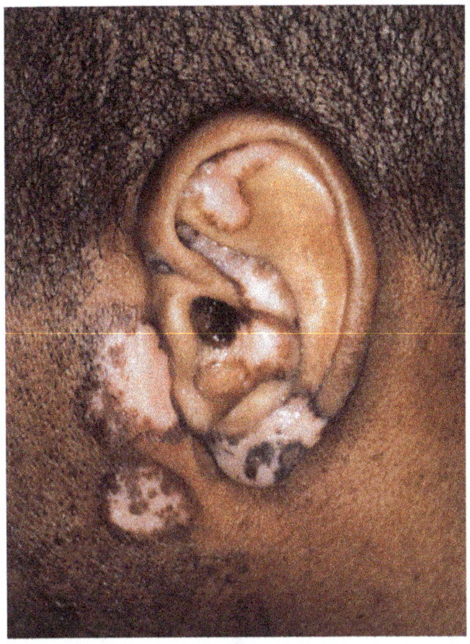

Discoid lupus erythematosus. Violaceous, hyperpigmented, atrophic plaques, often with evidence of follicular plugging, which may result in scarring, are characteristic of discoid lupus erythematosus (also called chronic cutaneous lupus erythematosus). (Reproduced with permission from Longo DL, Fauci AS, Kasper DL, Hauser SL, Jameson JL, Loscalzo J, eds. *Harrison's Principles of Internal Medicine.* 18th ed. New York, NY: McGraw-Hill Education; 2011.)

Microscopically, these evolving lesions are composed initially of superficial or combined superficial and deep perivascular lymphomonocytic infiltrates with prominent vascular ectasia, sparse interface infiltrates, and prominent vacuolar degeneration of the dermal epidermal and follicular dermal junctions. Basal dyskeratotic keratinocytes, colloid bodies, and premature terminal differentiation of the epidermis are present. The vacuolar degeneration at the perifollicular junction results in altered cornification with compact hyperkeratotic plugs.

Foci of vasculitis with fibrin thrombi are occasionally present but are not considered a characteristic feature. Lesional skin demonstrates a positive **lupus band test** by direct immunofluorescence in the majority of cases. Terminal complement components C5b-9 may also be found within the venular walls. Fully evolved lesions develop epidermal atrophy, effaced rete ridges, dermal fibrosis, and thickened basement membrane which may be highlighted with a PAS stain. The accumulation of dermal mucin in between dense collagen bundles may be highlighted with Alcian blue or colloidal iron stains. The prominent perifollicular infiltrates may result in scarring alopecia with replacement of the hair follicles with vertically scarred fibrous tracts. Occasionally, dermal infiltrates may be seen extending into the subcutaneous tissue. Immunophenotypic studies will reveal CD123 positivity in scattered inflammatory cells as well as MXA staining of the epidermis, follicular and eccrine epithelium, and inflammatory cells, consistent with an interferon alpha-rich microenvironment.

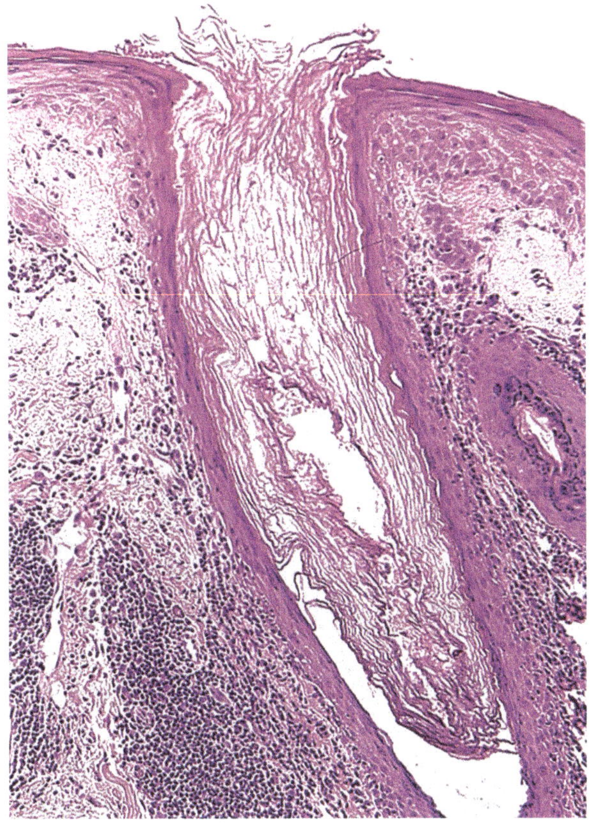

Discoid lupus erythematosus. There is prominent follicular hyperkeratosis and basement membrane thickening. Note the pale material in the dermis, consistent with dermal mucin.

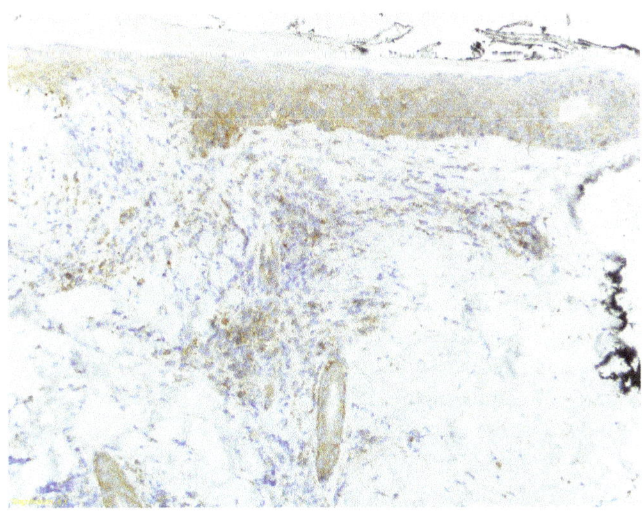

MXA immunohistochemistry in discoid lupus. There is antibody deposition within epidermal and adnexal keratinocytes as well as endothelial cells and scattered plasmacytoid dendritic cells.

Lupus Erythematosus: Comparison of Clinical and Direct Immunofluorescence Manifestations by Subtype

FEATURE	SLE	SCLE	DLE
Lesion character			
Scale	Fine, easily detached	Fine, easily detached	Thick, adherent
Follicular atrophy	Absent	Absent	Present
Photodistribution	Present	Marked	Present
Scarring	Absent	Absent	Present
Atrophy	Usually absent	Usually absent	Present—often marked
Pigmentary alteration	Slight	Slight	Often marked
Telangiectasia	Present	Present	Present
≥4ACR criteria for SLE (incidence)	100%	40%	10%
Positive Lupus Band Test			
Lesional skin	>90%	60%	90%
Nonlesional sun-protected skin	Active disease 90% Inactive disease 30%	30%	0%-10%

Abbreviations: ACR, America College of Rheumatology; DLE, discoid lupus erythematosus; SCLE, subacute cutaneous lupus erythematosus; SLE, systemic lupus erythematosus.

Lupus Erythematosus and Variants[a]

Clinical Features

Systemic lupus erythematosus
- Diffuse erythematous macules, atrophy possible
- In general, sun-exposed skin for all variants

Subacute lupus erythematosus
- Psoriasiform lesions
- Arcuate or serpiginous plaques
- Ro/La+

Discoid lupus erythematosus
- Erythematous plaques with atrophy, scarring, alopecia, and dyspigmentation

Histopathologic Features

Systemic lupus erythematosus
- Mild upper dermal perivascular and interstitial infiltrate of lymphocytes
- Mild epidermal atrophy
- Dermal mucin
- Thickened basement membrane

Subacute lupus erythematosus
- Denser lymphocytic infiltrate
- Periadnexal inflammation possible
- Dermal mucin
- Moderate regular acanthosis in psoriasiform variant

Discoid lupus erythematosus
- Hyperkeratosis, follicular plugging
- Epidermal atrophy
- Features of vacuolar interface dermatitis (above) with dense perivascular interstitial and periadnexal inflammation
- Thickened basement membrane
- Dermal mucinosis
- Loss of adnexae

Differential Diagnosis

Systemic lupus erythematosus
- Dermatomyositis
- Mixed connective tissue disease
- Viral exanthem
- Reticular erythematous mucinosis

Subacute lupus erythematosus
- Dermatomyositis
- Neonatal lupus erythematosus
- PLEVA
- Syphilis
- Lymphocytic infiltrate of Jessner
- Figurate erythemas

Discoid lupus erythematosus
- Lichen planus
- Lichen sclerosus
- Polymorphous light eruption
- Chilblains
- Deep gyrate erythema
- Pityriasis lichenoides
- Syphilis

[a]At times, dermatomyositis may resemble any variant of lupus erythematosus.

ANSWER 1-38: C.

Dermatomyositis is a syndrome consisting of variably distributed erythematous macules and plaques with photoaccentuation and inflammation of skeletal muscle. The cutaneous manifestations vary in terms of extent and location, but the typical presentation consists of erythematous infiltrated plaques usually on the face but possibly generalized. The location of the erythema on the face is often periorbital, assuming a violaceous hue, the so-called **heliotrope rash**. Atrophic papules with scale on the knuckles are characteristic and are known as **Gottron papules**. Generalized forms typically present on the upper back, shoulders, and chest and have been referred to as the **"shawl sign." Poikiloderma** as a manifestation of dermatomyositis is also common. Myositis may accompany the skin changes or may precede or follow them. Severe proximal muscle weakness may ensue, and determination of serum levels of muscle-derived enzymes and degradation products aids in diagnosis. Muscle biopsy may be necessary to establish the diagnosis. An electromyogram may also be a useful adjunct. On occasion, cutaneous findings or muscle findings may be absent, prompting the terms **polymyositis** and **dermatomyositis sine myositis**, respectively. In adult patients, there is an association with visceral malignancy. Dermatomyositis occurs in children and is unassociated with malignant neoplasms. Vasculitis and severe calcinosis cutis often accompany the juvenile form. **Drug-induced dermatomyositis**, which has a similar histopathologic appearance to classic dermatomyositis, has been reported in the literature. Medications most commonly implicated include hydroxyurea, penicillamine, and statins.

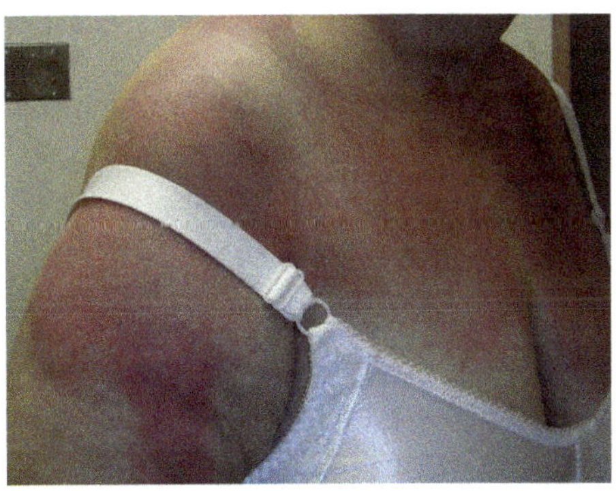

The shawl distribution of dermatomyositis. (Reproduced, with permission, from Usatine RP, Smith MA, Mayeaux EJ Jr, Chumley HS, eds. *Color Atlas of Family Medicine*. 2nd ed. New York, NY: McGraw-Hill Education; 2012. Used with permission of Richard P. Usatine, MD.)

Dermatomyositis is considered to be the result of a humoral attack against the endothelium of muscle capillaries and small arterioles. Positive antinuclear antibody titers (ANA) are common in patients with dermatomyositis, but are nonspecific. Myositis-specific autoantibodies (eg, Jo-1, Mi-2) have a low sensitivity (3.5% cases). Anti–Mi-2 antibodies are highly specific for acute-onset classic dermatomyositis and are associated with good prognosis. Anti–Jo-1 (antihistidyl transfer RNA [t-RNA] synthetase) antibodies are more common in patients with polymyositis than in patients with dermatomyositis and are associated with pulmonary involvement (interstitial lung disease).

Microscopically, the findings of dermatomyositis are nonspecific and largely indistinguishable from lupus erythematosus. Subtle findings include thickening of the basement membrane zone, best highlighted with a PAS stain. The superficial vessels are dilated and thickened, reflecting the sequelae of prior episodes of immune-based microvascular injury. Sparse vacuolar alteration along the dermal epidermal junction is usually present and dermal mucin is increased. Immunohistochemistry will reveal positivity for CD123 and MXA reflecting a microenvironment rich in type I interferons. Indirect immunofluorescence with human umbilical vein endothelial cells is commonly positive for antiendothelial antibodies. This is demonstrated by incubating the cells with the patient's serum and then tagging with fluorescent human anti-IgG antibodies. Direct immunofluorescence of lesional skin only reveals a positive lupus band test in 35% of cases; however, the vascular deposition of C5b-9 is considered a highly sensitive and specific finding.

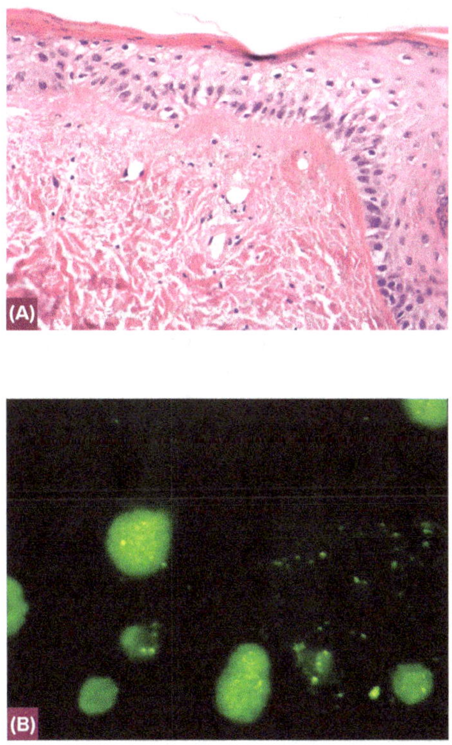

Dermatomyositis. (A) The vessels of the superficial vascular plexus exhibit ectasia and endothelial cells lining the vessels have a thickened appearance, reflecting the sequelae of prior episodes of immune-based microvascular injury. There is thickening of the basement membrane. **(B)** The presumptive basis of the vascular injury in dermatomyositis is one related to antiendothelial cell antibodies. The image is an indirect immunofluorescent assay using human umbilical vein endothelial cells as substrate. A positive reaction following incubation of the patient's serum tagged with a fluoresceinated human anti-IgG antibody.

Criteria for Myopathic Dermatomyositis

Proximal symmetric muscle weakness
Elevated serum levels of muscle-derived enzymes
Abnormal electromyogram
Abnormal muscle biopsy
Cutaneous disease compatible with dermatomyositis

ANSWER 1-39: D.

While many overlap syndromes are recognized among the connective tissue diseases, **mixed connective disease (MCTD)** is the most common, consisting of features of **systemic lupus erythematosus, scleroderma, dermatomyositis,** and **rheumatoid arthritis**. Pulmonary hypertension is a common finding which carries a poor prognosis. MCTD is characterized by a marked female predominance and typically presents in the second and third decades, but children may also be affected. Facial erythema, heliotrope, acral telangiectases, and scleroderma are the more common cutaneous manifestations. These patients possess high-titer antinuclear antibodies with antibodies to ribonucleoprotein (RNP). Microscopically, there are certain characteristic findings seen in mixed connective tissue disease. The hallmarks include an interface dermatitis which ranges in quality from areas of lichenoid inflammation to zones of cell-poor interface dermatitis in concert with variable dermal sclerosis. The direct immunofluorescence testing will demonstrate granular deposition of IgG and C5b-9 within epidermal keratinocytes along with prominent vascular deposits of C5b-9. The histopathological difference diagnosis includes chronic sclerodermoid GVHD **(chronic sclerodermoid GVHD)**, which usually can be excluded based on clinical history.

Diagnostic Criteria for Mixed Connective Tissue Disease

A diagnosis of mixed connective tissue disease (MCTD) is based on the presence of one criterion from category I, plus the criterion from category II, plus one or more criteria from category III.

I. Common symptoms:
  - Raynaud phenomenon
  - Swollen fingers or hands

II. Anti-nRNP antibody

III. Mixed findings:
  - SLE-like findings:
    - Polyarthritis
    - Lymphadenopathy
    - Facial erythema
    - Pericarditis or pleuritis
    - Leukocytopenia or thrombocytopenia
  - PSS-like findings:
    - Sclerodactyly
    - Pulmonary fibrosis, restrictive changes of the lung, or reduced diffusion capacity
    - Hypomotility or dilatation of the esophagus
  - DM-like findings:
    - Muscle weakness
    - Increased serum level of myogenic enzymes (CPK)
    - Myogenic pattern at electromyography

ANSWER 1-40: D.

Lichen sclerosus (LS) has protean clinical manifestations ranging from localized disease in the perineum to widespread erythematous plaques. The primary lesion in any site is an erythematous patch or plaque, often with an edematous center. This central zone may display pallor and thus impart a white color. Over time, dermal fibrosis ensues, resulting in the clinical impression of sclerosis resembling **scleroderma** or **morphea**. Rare lesions of LS may blister, often with hemorrhagic contents. Most commonly, LS occurs in the genital skin of women, but men and children are also affected. On the penis, LS is termed **balanitis xerotica obliterans**. There is a reported association between squamous cell carcinoma and chronic LS of the vulva. Involved vulvar skin displays a higher expression of p53 in association with increased epidermal cell proliferation. An association is reported between increased severity of disease and presence of specific IL-1 receptor alleles.

Histopathologic alterations parallel the age of the lesion. In early lesions, there is a superficial dermal perivascular and interstitial lymphocytic infiltrate immediately below the epidermis with occasional plasma cells. Overlying interface change is evident, and the epidermis may be of normal thickness. The papillary and upper reticular dermis displays edema, imparting a light, airy, and indistinct quality to the collagen bundles. As lesions evolve, this enlarging zone of alteration lies above the band of lymphocytes and usually contains ectatic vascular channels. This wispy, edematous collagen gives place over time to a more dense, homogeneous, and deeply eosinophilic collagen that continues to overlie the zone of inflammation. The epidermis is usually atrophic with hyperkeratosis and dilated and keratin-filled acrotrichial and acrosyringeal ostia. Melanophages are variably present. Elastic stain will reveal a paucity of elastic fibers in the superficial zone of dermal alteration and a compressed band of elastic fibers at the level of band-like inflammation. Fully evolved lesions may no longer contain inflammation and there is loss of pilosebaceous units and marked epidermal atrophy. Given the occasional development of squamous cell carcinoma in genital lichen sclerosus, the presence of epidermal atypia, exaggerated acanthosis, and loss of the dermal edematous-sclerotic band should be sought out, since these features are observed more commonly in the vicinity of an associated carcinoma.

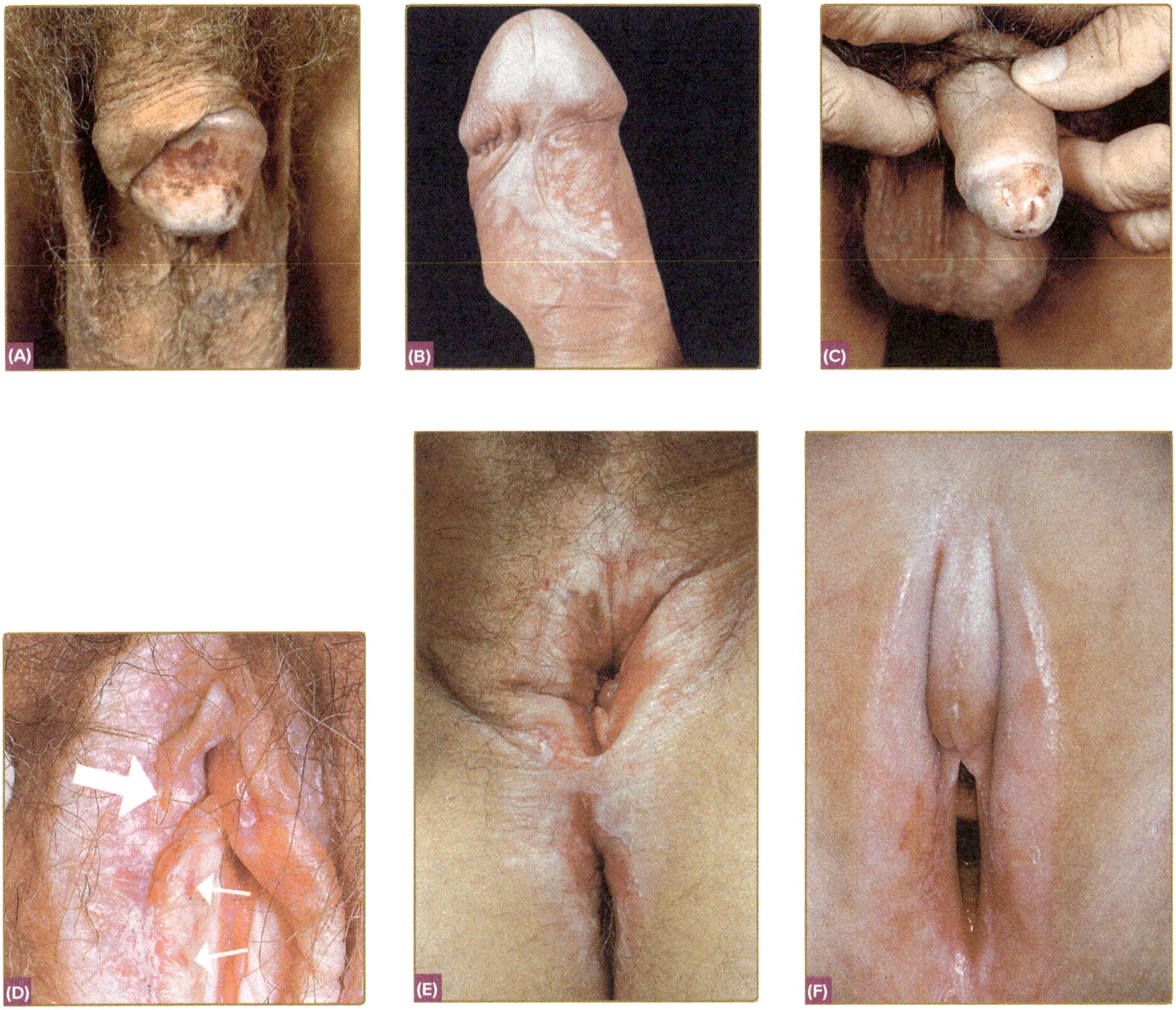

Lichen sclerosus. (A) Early sclerosis and significant hemorrhage on the glans in early lichen sclerosus. **(B)** Sclerosis of the frenulum and increased vulnerability with bleeding upon sexual intercourse. **(C)** Significant sclerosis of the glans and conglutination with the preputium in advanced lichen sclerosus. Note narrowing of the urethral orifice and hemorrhage. **(D)** In addition to the well-demarcated white vulvar plaque that is classic for lichen sclerosus, the waxy and crinkled texture, purpura (*small arrows*), and erosions (*large arrow*) are diagnostic. **(E)** Sclerotic vulva with disappearance of the smaller labia and shrinkage of the introitus. Significant erythema and erosions are seen on the vulva and the anus in a figure-8 configuration. The patient complained of severe pruritus and dyspareunia. **(F)** Erosive, sclerotic vulva in an 8-year-old girl. (Reproduced, with permission, from Goldsmith LA, Katz SI, Gilchrest BA, Paller AS, Leffell DJ, Wolff K, eds. *Fitzpatrick's Dermatology in General Medicine.* 8th ed. New York, NY: McGraw-Hill Education; 2012.)

The differential diagnosis includes **chronic radiation dermatitis**, which may closely resemble LS both clinically and histopathologically. Chronic radiation dermatitis develops months to years following radiation exposure and is associated with induration, atrophy, telangiectasia, and pigmentary changes. Late radiation necrosis can occur over bony prominences, generally beginning one or more years after exposure and often precipitated by trauma. Both conditions contain fibrotic alteration of the upper dermal collagen, vascular ectasia, and interface change. However, radiation "atypical" fibroblasts and thickened waxy blood vessel walls are absent in LS. The interstitial and band-like pattern of inflammation typical of LS is absent in radiation dermatitis.

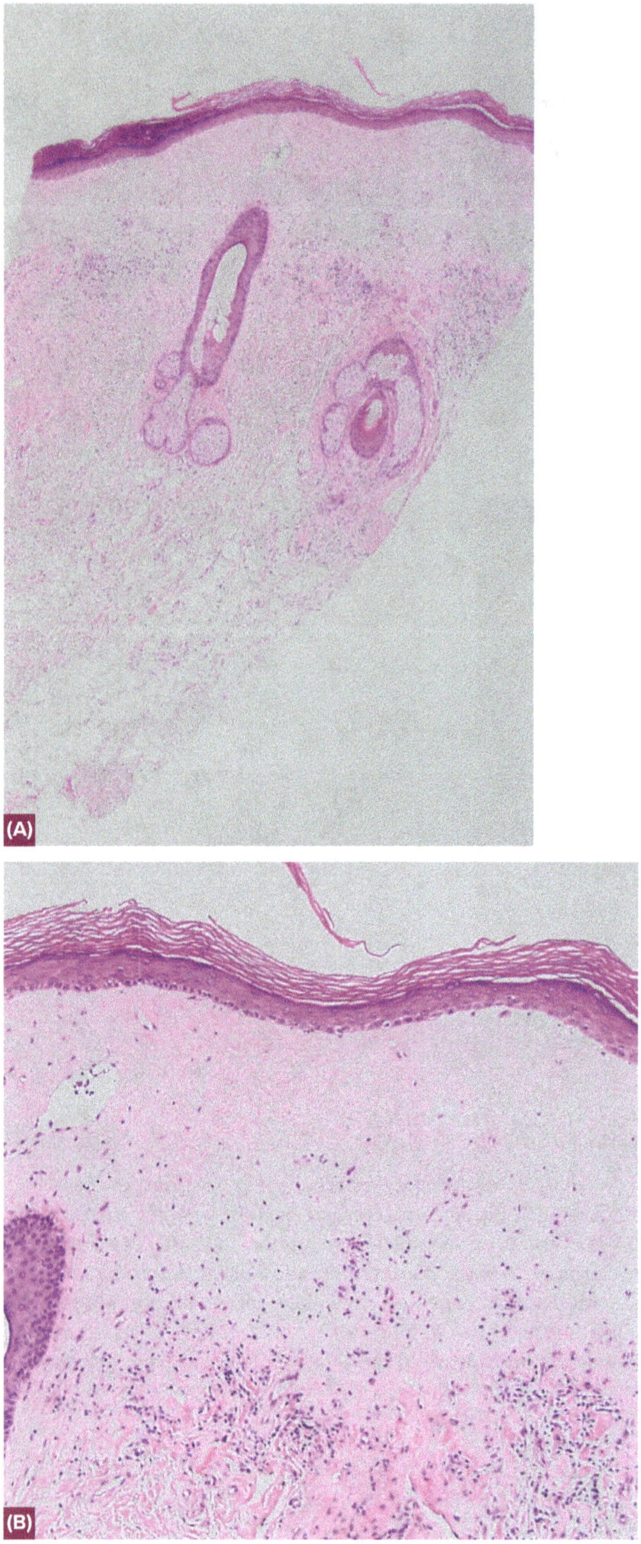

Lichen sclerosus. (A) The lesion shows typical features of lichen sclerosis, hyperkeratosis, epidermal atrophy, prominent homogenization of the papillary dermis, and a subjacent band-like lymphoid infiltrate. Note how the band-like infiltrate is centered at the base of the superficial dermal sclerosis. **(B)** Higher magnification shows the homogenous eosinophilic hyalinization of the papillary dermis with a markedly dilated vessel.

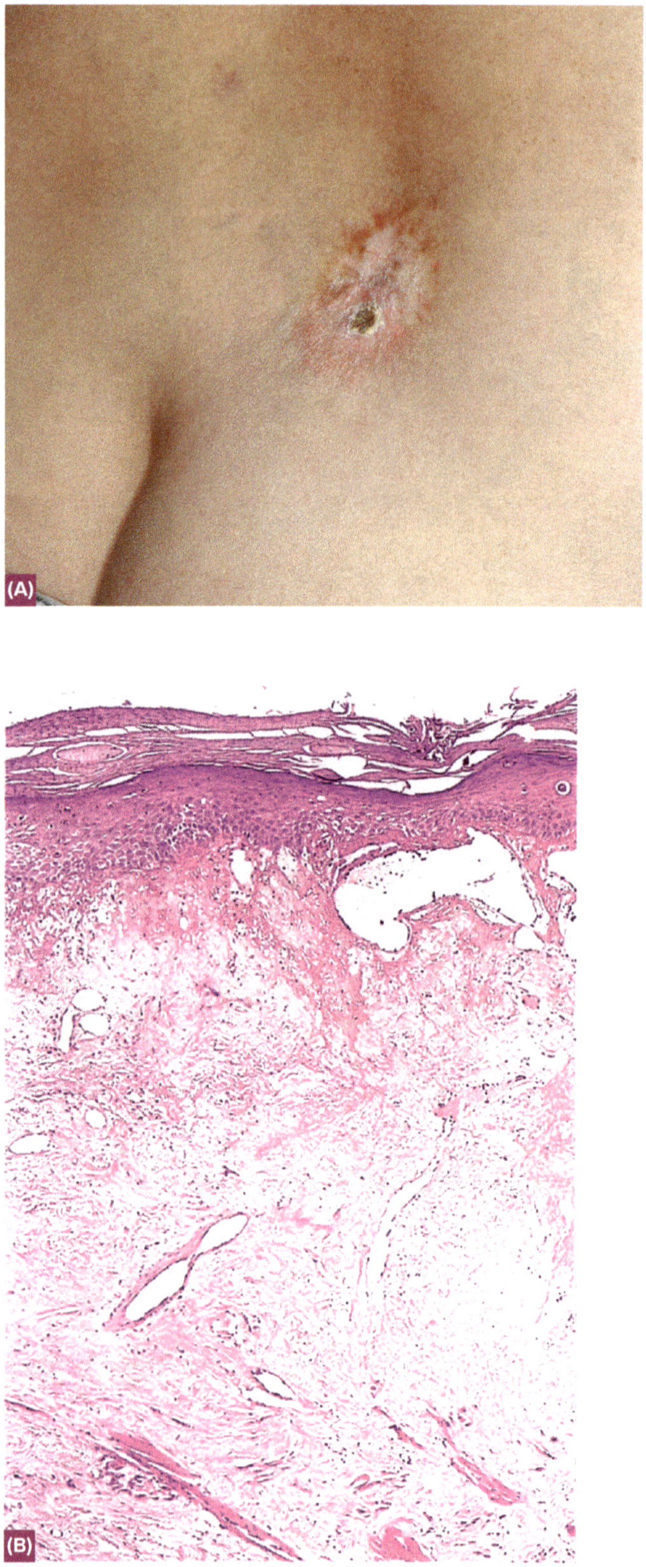

Chronic radiation dermatitis. (A) Well-defined indurated plaque demonstrating atrophy, telangiectasia, both hypo- and hyperpigmentation, and scaling. **(B)** Hyperkeratotic and parakeratotic epidermal hyperplasia with vacuolar interface change. Full-thickness dermal sclerosis with lymphatic dilation and loss of adnexa is characteristic.

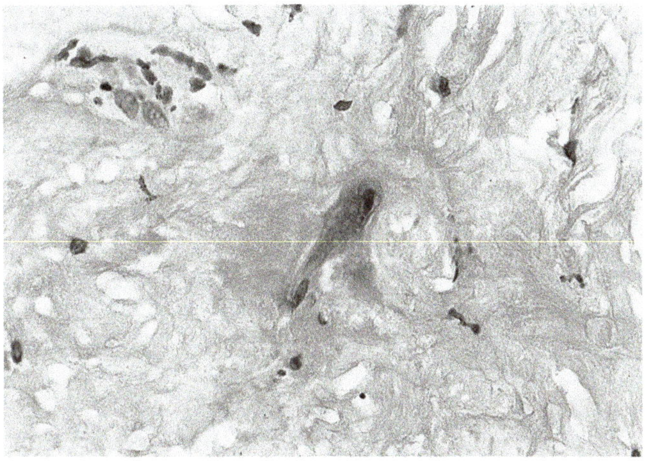

Chronic radiation dermatitis. Bizarre-appearing "stellate" fibroblast with features of radiation effect: pleomorphic hypochromatic nuclei, abundant cytoplasm, and intranuclear and intracytoplasmic vacuoles.

Radiation Dermatitis

Clinical Features
- Acute
  - Erythema
  - Hair loss
  - Vesicle formation
- Chronic
  - Atrophy
  - Telangiectasia
  - Pigmentary changes

Histopathologic Features
- Acute
  - Spongiosis
  - Epidermal necrosis
  - Dermal edema
  - Vascular ectasia and thrombosis
- Chronic
  - Epidermal hypoplasia and/or hyperplasia
  - Squamous epithelial atypia
  - Dermal sclerosis/hyalinization
  - Deeply located elastotic material in dermis
  - Loss of adnexae
  - Bizarre "radiation fibroblasts"
  - Hyalinization of vessel walls and thrombosis

Differential Diagnosis
- Scar
- Thermal burn
- Lichen sclerosus
- Morphea/scleroderma
- Chronic graft versus host reaction

ANSWER 1-41: F.

All of the listed choices exhibit **poikiloderma,** except choice F **(anetoderma)**. The term poikiloderma does not imply a specific diagnosis and is a clinical and histopathologic finding with many causes. Clinically, poikiloderma consists of patches of skin with variable melanin content, imparting a mottled or dappled hyper- and hypopigmented appearance. The epidermis is thin and may be shiny with fine "cigarette paper–like" wrinkles. Ectatic papillary dermal vessels are responsible for a faint erythema or distinct telangiectasias. The minimum criteria for the histopathologic diagnosis of poikiloderma include some element of interface change, epidermal atrophy with effacement of rete ridges, variable epidermal melanin content, dilated upper dermal vessels, and melanophages. Determining hyper- and hypopigmentation in a given skin biopsy specimen generally is not possible unless the clinician includes or identifies skin with normal pigmentation for comparison. Mild papillary dermal fibrosis often accompanies these changes. The degree of inflammation is highly variable and depends, in part, on the stage of evolution of the lesion sampled. This section will discuss entities characterized by poikiloderma. Since the histopathology alone often is not specific, clinical correlation is required for diagnosis.

Poikiloderma associated with **chronic radiation dermatitis** by convention develops later than 6 months post-radiation therapy, is insidious in onset, and usually presents many years after exposure. Ulceration is sometimes a feature and the condition may be complicated by the development of a variety of neoplasms, including **atypical fibroxanthoma (AFX),**

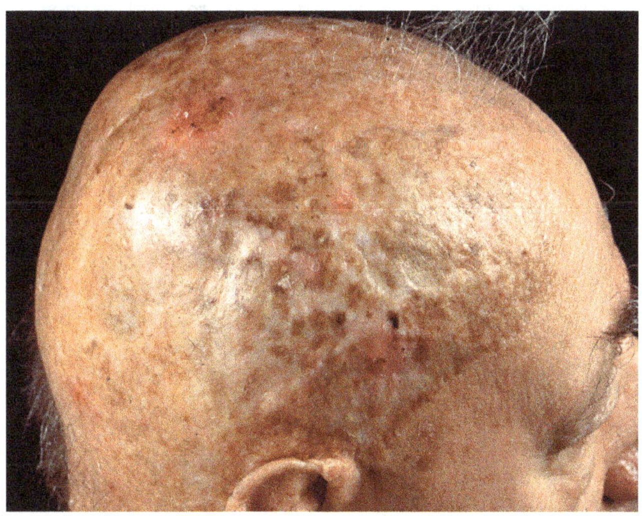

Poikiloderma associated with chronic radiation dermatitis. Poikiloderma with telangiectatic erythema, hyperpigmentation, hypopigmentation. Hairs are absent. These massive skin changes are the result of overdosed irradiation the patient received as a child for fungal infection of the scalp. He is a candidate for the development of squamous cell carcinoma in the future. (Reproduced, with permission, from Wolff K, Johnson RA, Saavedra AP. *Fitzpatrick's Color Atlas and Synopsis of Clinical Dermatology.* 7th ed. New York, NY: McGraw-Hill Education; 2013.)

angiosarcoma, basal cell carcinoma, and **squamous cell carcinoma (ie, spindle cell pseudosarcomatous variant).** Microscopically, in addition to the usual features of poikiloderma, cytological atypia of keratinocytes and dyskeratosis may be evident. A more specific feature is the presence of bizarre "radiation" fibroblasts, which may be mistaken for sarcoma if interpreted in the wrong clinical context.

Poikiloderma of Civatte occurs as patches of wrinkled skin with mottled pigmentation and telangiectasias in sun-exposed sites, frequently on the necks of women. Samples from poikiloderma of Civatte show solar elastosis and lack significant inflammation. This form of poikiloderma is poorly understood but most likely is due to chronic sun exposure.

Poikiloderma congenitale (Rothmund-Thomson syndrome) is poikiloderma of childhood onset with photosensitivity, osteosarcoma, short stature, juvenile cataracts, skeletal defects, nail dystrophy, and hypogonadism. The poikilodermatous changes typically are photodistributed and microscopically lack significant inflammation. Rothmund-Thomson syndrome is inherited in an autosomal recessive manner and is associated with mutations in the DNA helicase gene RECQL4.

Congenital telangiectatic erythema (Bloom syndrome) is characterized by facial telangiectasias beginning in infancy or early childhood with photosensitivity and progression to a poikilodermatous appearance. Skin biopsy specimens reveal interface dermatitis with some features of poikiloderma as noted earlier. Other features include short stature, genomic instability, and development of malignant neoplasms, variable immunoglobulin deficiencies, and mutations in the gene-encoding DNA helicase RECQL3. Bloom syndrome is inherited in an autosomal recessive manner and is associated with sister-chromatid exchange.

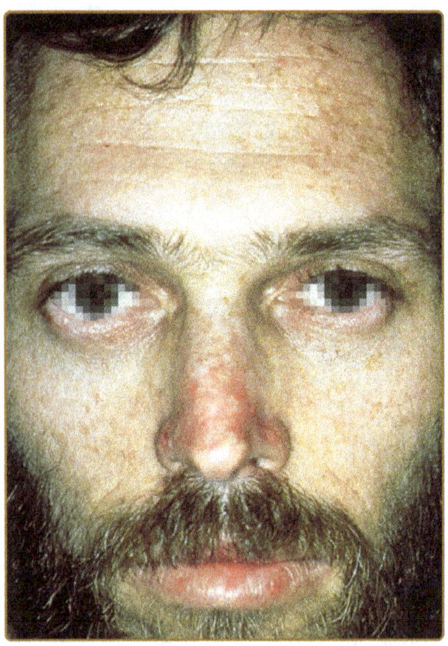

Bloom syndrome. Prominent telangiectasia in malar distribution. (Reproduced, with permission, from Goldsmith LA, Katz SI, Gilchrest BA, Paller AS, Leffell DJ, Wolff K, eds. *Fitzpatrick's Dermatology in General Medicine.* 8th ed. New York, NY: McGraw-Hill Education; 2012.)

Dyskeratosis congenita is a retiform erythema with mottled pigmentation. Recognition of this syndrome is crucial because there is a high incidence of squamous cell carcinoma arising in dysplastic oral and anal mucosal epithelium. The oral changes consist of white plaques that display variable keratinocyte atypia progressing to full-thickness dysplasia and invasive carcinoma. Skin biopsy specimens of the poikiloderma show the typical findings. Additional features of this syndrome include nail dystrophy bone marrow failure, lacrimal duct atresia, and mutation in the gene encoding dyskerin (DKC 1). Dyskeratosis congenita is inherited in an X-linked recessive manner.

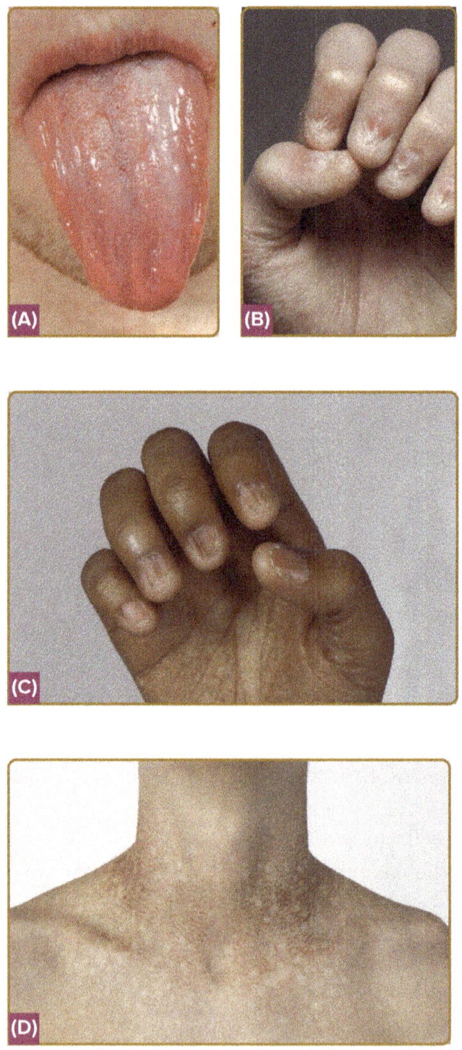

Dyskeratosis congenita. (A) Oral leukoplakia involving the tongue. **(B)** Severe atrophy of all fingernails and thickening of the palm. **(C)** Longitudinal ridging and dystrophy of several fingernails with dyspigmentation and thickening of the palm. **(D)** Poikiloderma showing reticular hypo- and hyperpigmentation of the skin of the neck and chest. (Reproduced, with permission, from Goldsmith LA, Katz SI, Gilchrest BA, Paller AS, Leffell DJ, Wolff K, eds. *Fitzpatrick's Dermatology in General Medicine.* 8th ed. New York, NY: McGraw-Hill Education; 2012.)

Poikiloderma accompanying **dermatomyositis** may represent a prominent clinical finding. The poikiloderma generally arises in long-standing plaques of erythema. The histopathology of poikiloderma in the setting of dermatomyositis is often remarkable for other changes typical of the connective tissue disorder, namely, more pronounced interface change and increased dermal mucin deposition. The biopsy illustrated in the question is from a poikilodermatous lesion of dermatomyositis.

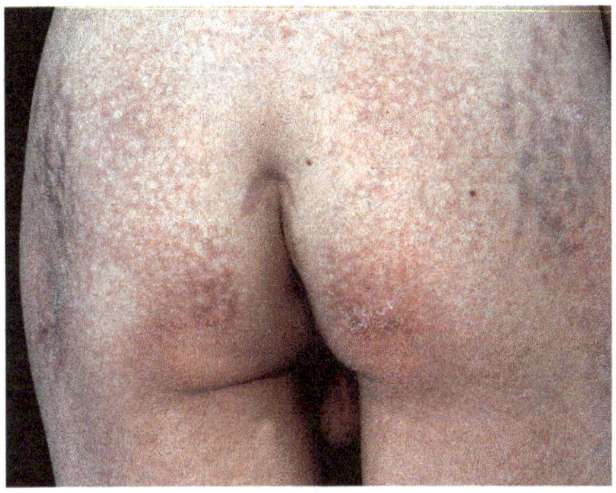

Dermatomyositis, juvenile onset, poikiloderma. There is mottled, reticular brownish pigmentation and telangiectasia plus small white scars. Note striae on trochanteric areas due to systemic glucocorticoid therapy. (Reproduced, with permission, from Wolff K, Johnson RA, Saavedra AP. *Fitzpatrick's Color Atlas and Synopsis of Clinical Dermatology.* 7th ed. New York, NY: McGraw-Hill Education; 2013.)

Poikiloderma accompanying **mycosis fungoides** as the primary clinical manifestation is rare. Many observers consider this finding to be an involutionary or regressive phase of the disease process. With any clinical description of poikiloderma, it behooves the pathologist to consider the diagnosis of cutaneous T-cell lymphoma. In addition to the constellation of findings typical of poikiloderma, the diagnosis rests mainly on identification of a band of atypical lymphocytes in the upper dermis with variable epidermotropism including the formation of Pautrier microabscesses. The epidermal changes typical of fully evolved cutaneous T-cell lymphoma are generally less pronounced in poikilodermatous forms of the disease, an argument for the resolving-lesion theory. Nonetheless, a diagnosis of cutaneous T-cell lymphoma must rest on recognition of a neoplastic T-cell population in the skin regardless of specific pattern or density of the infiltrate.

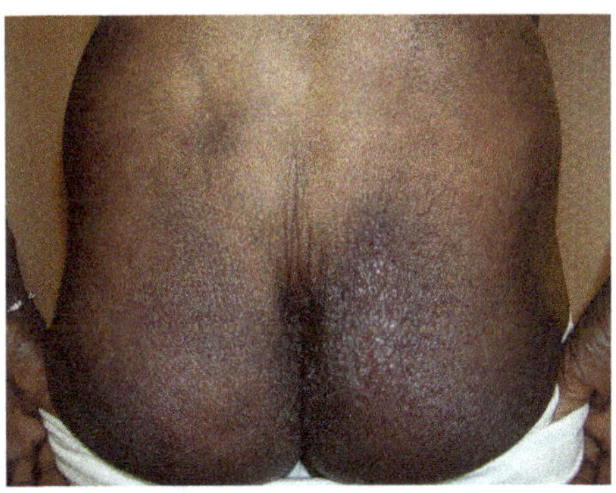

Poikiloderma of mycosis fungoides. (Reproduced, with permission, from Kaushansky K, Lichtman MA, Beutler E, Kipps TJ, Seligsohn U, Prchal JT, eds. *Williams Hematology.* 8th ed. New York, NY: McGraw-Hill Education; 2010.)

Anetoderma presents as circumscribed 1- to 2-cm areas of flaccid skin that may be elevated, macular, or depressed and reflect an absence of underlying supporting dermal substance. Circumscribed sac-like protrusions are common. Epidermal atrophy and underlying telangiectasias are not present. The examining finger sinks without resistance into a distinct pit with sharp borders as if into a hernia ring (buttonhole sign). The protrusion reappears as soon as the pressure from the finger is removed. The pathogenesis of anetoderma is unknown; however, the key findings are attributed to damage of the superficial and mid-dermal elastic fibers. Microscopically, the condition falls into the category of "invisible dermatoses" since in routinely stained sections no significant pathological findings are noticed. The findings are only revealed when elastic stains reveal a complete loss of elastic fibers within the superficial and mid-dermis. Perivascular lymphocytes are often present in all types of anetoderma and do not correlate with clinical inflammatory findings. Although **poikiloderma** also exhibits partial destruction of the elastic fiber network, it contains numerous melanophages and varying degrees of vacuolar interface activity. Lesions of anetoderma may be primary idiopathic or secondary to a preceding dermatosis in the same location such as acne and varicella. Both forms of the condition have been associated with antiphospholipid syndrome.

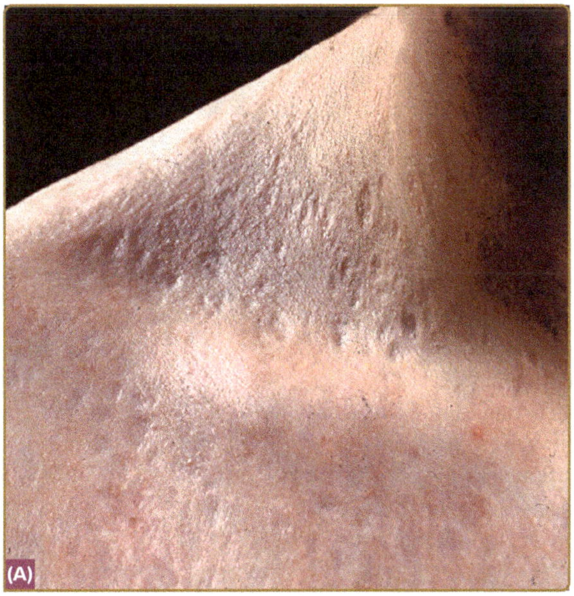

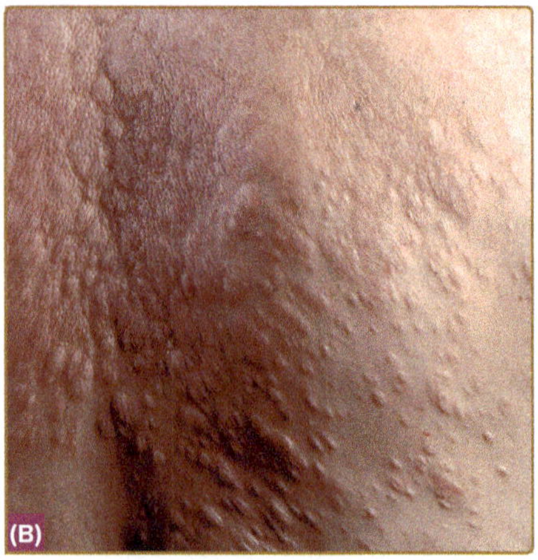

Primary anetoderma. **(A)** Multiple, sharply defined, depressed lesions that look punched out in the supraclavicular region. **(B)** Soft, sac-like protrusions on the back. When depressed, there is the buttonhole phenomenon. This is the same patient as in Part A. (Reproduced, with permission, from Goldsmith LA, Katz SI, Gilchrest BA, Paller AS, Leffell DJ, Wolff K, eds. *Fitzpatrick's Dermatology in General Medicine*. 8th ed. New York, NY: McGraw-Hill Education; 2012.)

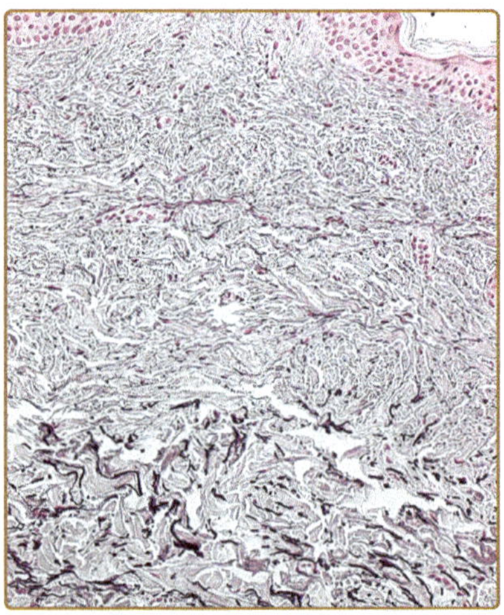

Anetoderma. Pathology shows decrease of elastic fibers in the papillary and reticular dermis (Weigert stain). (Reproduced, with permission, from Goldsmith LA, Katz SI, Gilchrest BA, Paller AS, Leffell DJ, Wolff K, eds. *Fitzpatrick's Dermatology in General Medicine*. 8th ed. New York, NY: McGraw-Hill Education; 2012. Courtesy of Victor Kokta, MD.)

Differential Diagnosis of Poikiloderma

- Large-plaque parapsoriasis
- Mycosis fungoides (poikiloderma atrophicans vasculare)
- Dermatomyositis
- Lupus erythematosus
- Chronic radiation dermatitis
- Bloom syndrome
- Rothmund-Thomson syndrome
- Dyskeratosis congenita
- Xeroderma pigmentosum

ANSWER 1-42: E.

Lichen nitidus (LN) consists of discrete 1- to 2-mm, skin-colored to minimally erythematous papules of variable distribution and extent but often grouped and located on the genital and acral skin. Lichen nitidus occurs commonly in children and is seen often on the penis. Cases of generalized lichen nitidus have been reported. The disease is self-limited. Overlap with **lichen planus** occurs, and both conditions may be recognized in a given patient. **Lichen striatus** is also common in children but presents as a linear array of closely set skin-colored to erythematous papules with little or no scale.

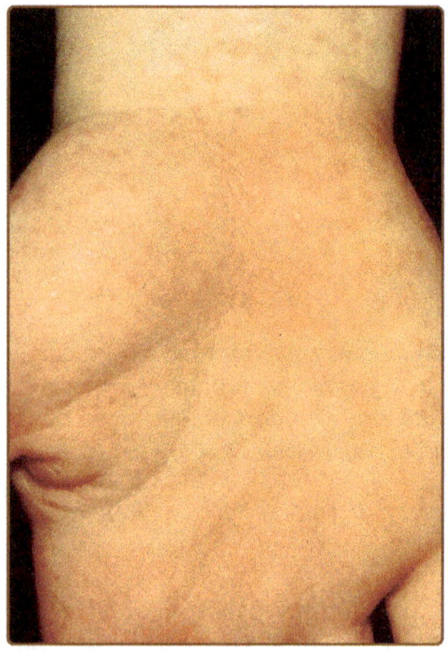

Lichen nitidus. Wrist and palmar involvement with development of hyperkeratotic lesions. (Reproduced, with permission, from Goldsmith LA, Katz SI, Gilchrest BA, Paller AS, Leffell DJ, Wolff K, eds. *Fitzpatrick's Dermatology in General Medicine*. 8th ed. New York, NY: McGraw-Hill Education; 2012.)

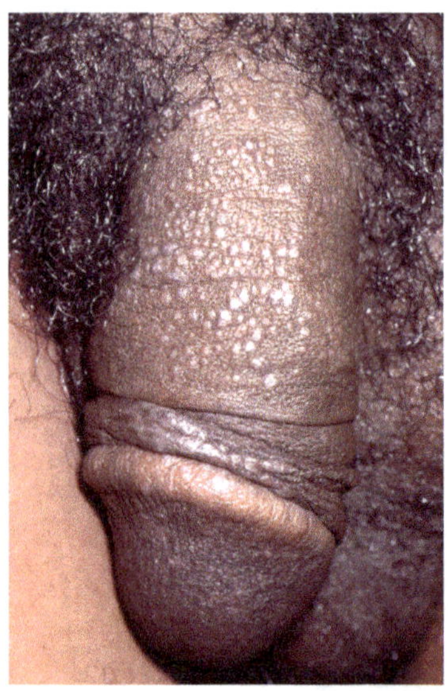

Lichen nitidus: penis Flat-topped papules on the shaft of the penis. (Reproduced, with permission, from Wolff K, Johnson RA, Saavedra AP. *Fitzpatrick's Color Atlas and Synopsis of Clinical Dermatology*. 7th ed. New York, NY: McGraw-Hill Education; 2013.)

Microscopically, **lichen nitidus (LN)** presents as discrete interstitial aggregates of lymphocytes and macrophages that expand individual dermal papillae. This expansion causes the adjacent epidermal rete ridges to bow outward and give the appearance of extension underneath the inflammatory cell aggregate as a collarette (so-called ball-and-claw effect). This discrete anatomic localization corresponds to the clinical picture of pinpoint papules and is distinct from the histopathology of **lichen planus**. The infiltrate filling two adjacent dermal papillae may fuse to form a larger lesion on occasion. Initially, the infiltrate is composed almost entirely of lymphocytes, whereas established lesions are more granulomatous with admixtures of lymphocytes and histiocytes with occasional multinucleated giant cells and melanophages. The overlying epidermis is slightly thinned and flattened with basal vacuolization and rare apoptotic keratinocytes. Parakeratotic scale often overlies these epidermal changes. Lichen nitidus represents one of the classic idiopathic eruptions associated with a lichenoid and granulomatous form of inflammation.

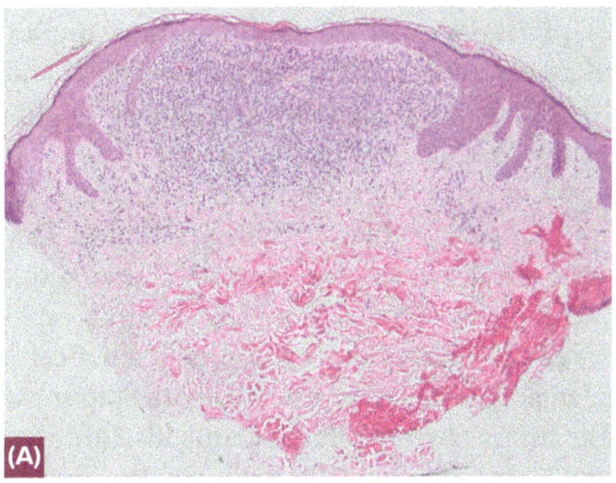

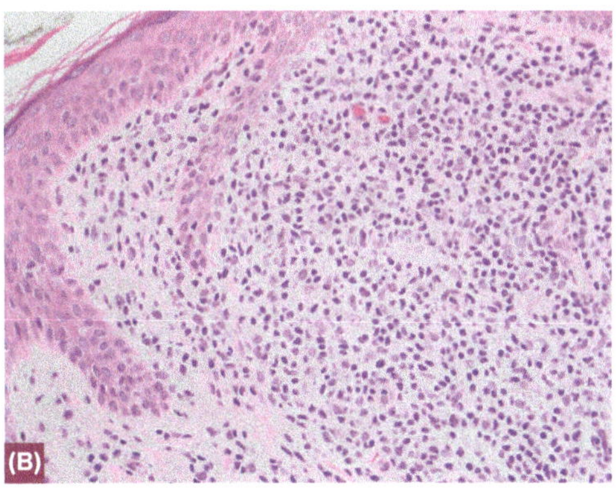

Lichen nitidus. (A) There is a circumscribed nodular lymphoid infiltrate filling the papillary dermis. The rete ridges of the epidermis surround the inflammatory infiltrate in a "ball-and-claw" configuration. **(B)** The infiltrate contains lymphocytes and macrophages.

The differential diagnosis includes **lichen striatus, lichen planus, secondary syphilis**, and **pityriasis lichenoides et varioliformis acuta (PLEVA)**. Microscopically, **lichen striatus** may reveal a band-like lymphocytic infiltrate that expands the papillary dermis in a pattern resembling both lichen planus and early lichen nitidus; however, the infiltrate is both superficial and deep and has a propensity to extend along the eccrine sweat glands. **Lichen planus** reveals superficial band-like lymphocytic infiltrates in contrast to the more nodular infiltrates of LN, which are concentrated at dermal papillae. Lichen planus lacks a granulomatous inflammatory component. **Secondary syphilis** reveals a dense band-like lymphocytic infiltrate with plasma cells that extends into the deep dermis around vessels, adnexal structures, and nerve bundles. The epidermis in secondary syphilis is acanthotic with markedly elongated and thinned rete ridges. Endothelial cells are enlarged and partially or totally obliterate vessels. Older lesions of syphilis may contain granulomatous inflammation, but the infiltrates will still be both superficial and deep, unlike LN. **Pityriasis lichenoides et varioliformis acuta (PLEVA)** reveals a wedge-shaped superficial and deep dermal lymphocytic infiltrate with variable interface density. Basal vacuolization and numerous dyskeratotic keratinocytes are present at all levels of the epidermis. Exocytosis of lymphocytes into the upper layers of the epidermis is characteristic. Another helpful finding is the presence of cohesive collections of Langerhans cells with variable spongiosis. Although LN may be surfaced by parakeratosis, the characteristic broad parakeratotic scale containing transepidermally eliminated leukocytes of PLEVA is absent. Scattered dermal and intraepidermal red blood cell extravasation is also common in PLEVA.

ANSWER 1-43: D.

This is a classic example of **lichen striatus,** which may affect individuals of any age but most commonly occurs in children. The characteristic clinical finding is a linear array of closely set skin-colored to erythematous papules with little or no scale. Almost any skin site may be affected. No associated systemic

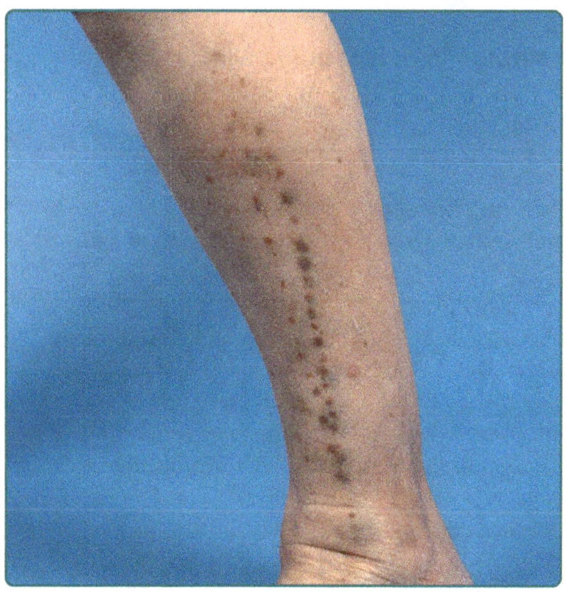

Lichen striatus. Linear configuration of slightly scaling papules in Blaschkoid distribution on the leg. (Reproduced, with permission, from Goldsmith LA, Katz SI, Gilchrest BA, Paller AS, Leffell DJ, Wolff K, eds. *Fitzpatrick's Dermatology in General Medicine.* 8th ed. New York, NY: McGraw-Hill Education; 2012.)

abnormalities occur. The eruption spontaneously involutes, leaving variable dyspigmentation.

The histopathologic features of lichen striatus are variable. Findings of a lichenoid dermatitis indistinguishable from lichen planus, lichen nitidus, or a combination may occur. Parakeratosis may be seen. Lichen striatus may also present as a spongiotic dermatitis that typically exhibits prominent dyskeratotic keratinocytes. The most classic features include lichenoid interface dermatitis with deep dermal involvement forming nodular lymphocytic infiltrates surrounding eccrine coils. Occasional cases are reported with involvement of the deep vascular plexus.

While many cutaneous diseases assume a linear patterning, lichen striatus most closely resembles **linear lichen planus** and **inflammatory linear verrucous epidermal nevus (ILVEN)**. **Linear lichen planus** displays the same histopathology as conventional lichen planus with its typical epidermal change and band of lymphocytes along the dermal epidermal junction. Lichen striatus may show fully evolved features of lichen planus but often also demonstrates parakeratosis, the "ball-and-claw" features of lichen nitidus, and deep dermal extension of the infiltrate. **Lichen nitidus** contains a lymphocytic and granulomatous infiltrate without deep dermal extension. The epidermal changes in **ILVEN** usually more closely resemble psoriasis than interface dermatitis. The significant acanthosis and hyperkeratosis that impart the verrucous appearance to ILVEN are absent in lichen striatus. **Allergic contact dermatitis** and lichen striatus may both present in a linear distribution and contain spongiosis; however, the eosinophils of allergic contact dermatitis are absent in lichen striatus. The clinical and histopathological findings of fully evolved lichen striatus are quite characteristic.

Lichen Nitidus Versus Lichen Striatus

LICHEN NITIDUS	LICHEN STRIATUS
Clinical Features	
1- to 2-mm flesh-colored papules, often genital and acral	Grouped erythematous papules in linear array
Histopathologic Features	Variable findings resembling lichen planus with deep perivascular and perieccrine inflammation at times
Discrete aggregate of lymphocytes, histiocytes, and occasional multinucleated giant cells expanding a dermal papilla	May resemble lichen nitidus
Epidermal collarette	May display spongiosis and dyskeratosis
Differential Diagnosis	
Lichen planus	ILVEN Lichen planus

ANSWER 1-44: E.

Inflammatory dermatoses can be categorized based on the pattern of inflammation and the compensatory adaptive epidermal changes. **Psoriasis vulgaris** is the prototype of the psoriasiform dermatitides and is characterized by regular elongation of the rete ridges ("rack of test tubes") with distal clubbing at the tips and frequent fusion as well as thinning of the suprapapillary plates. The epidermis shows thickening of the spinous layer (**acanthosis**) and shrinkage of the **granular** cell layer (**hypogranulosis**). There is prominent **parakeratosis** frequently containing clusters of neutrophils (**Munro microabscesses**). Mitoses may be seen in the lower to mid-spinous layers. These changes reflect an increase in cell proliferation and turnover at a rate faster than differentiation/maturation. Other inflammatory conditions can exhibit features similar to psoriasis vulgaris and include **reactive arthritis** (formerly known as Reiter Syndrome), **pityriasis rubra pilaris,** and **lichen simplex chronicus**. There are differences in the clinical appearance and pathogenesis of these entities as well as histopathological differences in the quality of scale and distribution or composition of the inflammatory infiltrate. **"Psoriasiform dermatitis"** in general represents a process of epidermal thickening that may affect all or any of the layers of the epidermis as a result from increased keratinocyte proliferation due to more rapid turnover of stem cells or increased pool of proliferating cells. Intraepidermal edema (spongiosis) is generally present to some degree in all of the forms of psoriasiform dermatitis; however, interface dermatitis with dyskeratotic keratinocytes is generally not a feature.

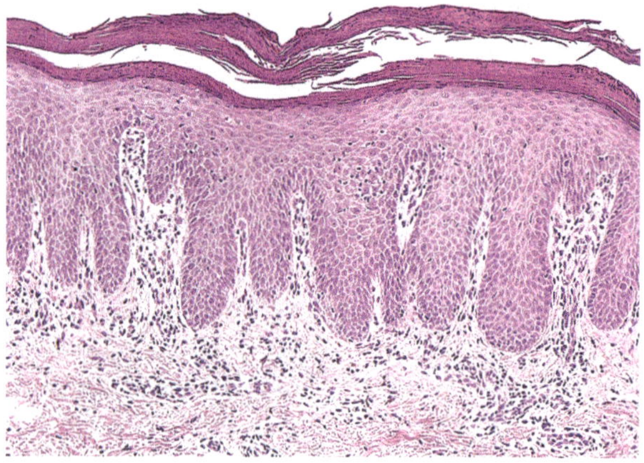

Psoriasis. The cornified layer shows horizontally confluent parakeratosis with exocytosis of neutrophils.

ANSWER 1-45: E.

This patient has **psoriasis vulgaris**, which is the prototype of psoriasiform dermatitis. Psoriasis in general is a chronic papulosquamous disease affecting 1%-2% of the US population. The disease follows a chronic relapsing course characterized by remission and exacerbation. Psoriasis is characterized by an increased epidermal turnover rate leading to thickening of the epidermis and accumulation of scale. Fingernails are involved in 50% and toenails in 35% of patients with psoriasis. Psoriasis is frequently associated with the **Koebner phenomenon (isomorphic response)** in which psoriasiform skin lesions appear at sites of injury. The histopathological differential diagnosis for psoriasis vulgaris includes **seborrheic dermatitis, subacute eczematous dermatitis, lichen simplex chronicus,** and **secondary syphilis** (choices A, B, C, and D, respectively). Psoriasis vulgaris is characterized by a regular psoriasiform pattern in which the rete ridges are thickened and elongated but are relatively uniform in size and shape (rack of test tubes) with round blunted ends. The adjacent dermal papillae contain dilated vessels in close apposition to a thinned overlying epidermal surface, referred to as the suprapapillary plates. It is these thinned suprapapillary plates and the proximity of the dilated dermal capillaries to the skin surface that produce the **Auspitz sign**, in which forcible removal of the scale produces pinpoint areas of bleeding. The hyperplastic nature of psoriasis is reflected by an increased number of mitoses, some of which may be seen one or two layers above the basal layer. Additionally, the rate of cellular turnover is faster than the rate of differentiation/maturation and reflected by the presence of hypogranulosis and parakeratosis. Collections of neutrophils with pyknotic nuclei in the parakeratotic stratum corneum, referred to as **Munro microabscesses**, are found in approximately 75% of cases. Serum is characteristically absent in the parakeratotic scale, correlating with the dry silvery scale seen clinically. Neutrophils are found less commonly in the spinous layer, where they may aggregate to form **spongiform pustules of Kogoj**. Large intraepidermal pustules are more commonly seen in the pustular forms of psoriasis. The underlying dermis is characterized by a superficial perivascular infiltrate of lymphocytes. Eosinophils are absent and plasma cells are unusual except in mucosal biopsies or in association with HIV infection/other forms of immune dysregulation. The other choices are examples of **irregular psoriasiform dermatitis** with variable size and shape and elongation of rete ridges. **Seborrheic dermatitis** may show neutrophils within parakeratotic scale but these foci contain serum and are typically situated about follicular ostia rather than the diffuse confluent-like parakeratosis of psoriasis. The dermal inflammatory infiltrate may also contain eosinophils, which is not a feature of psoriasis. The presence of marked spongiosis with Langerhans cell–rich microvesicles within rete ridges suggests a diagnosis of **subacute spongiotic dermatitis. Lichen simplex chronicus** is characterized by pointed rete ridges, hypergranulosis, and papillary dermal fibrosis, whereas psoriasis exhibits rounded rete ridges, hypogranulosis, papillary dermal edema, and dilated tortuous capillaries within the dermal papillae. The scale of lichen simplex chronicus frequently contains foci of serum. **Secondary syphilis** may show psoriasiform epidermal hyperplasia but with markedly elongated thin and pointed rete ridges, a serum-imbued scale and typically a dense

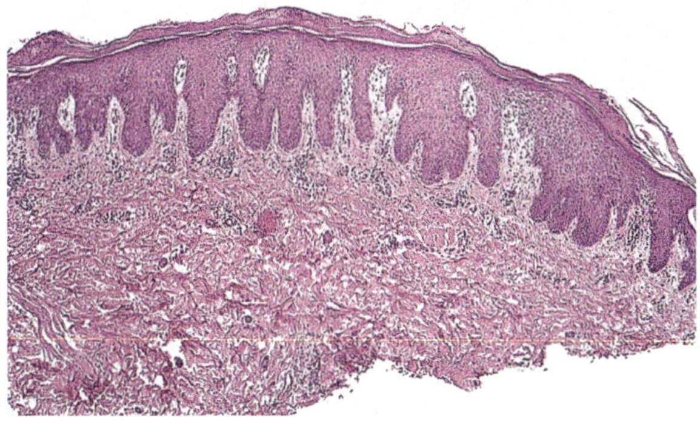

Psoriasis vulgaris. The epidermis shows regular elongation of the epidermal rete ridges, mild spongiosis, hypogranulosis, and confluent parakeratosis.

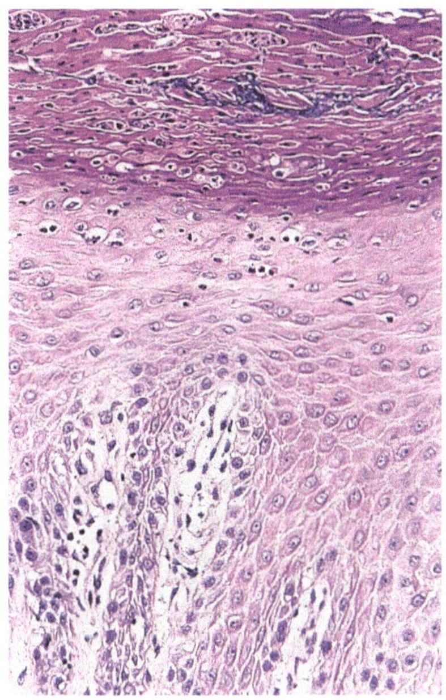

Psoriasis. The granular layer is absent, and there is prominent exocytosis of neutrophils.

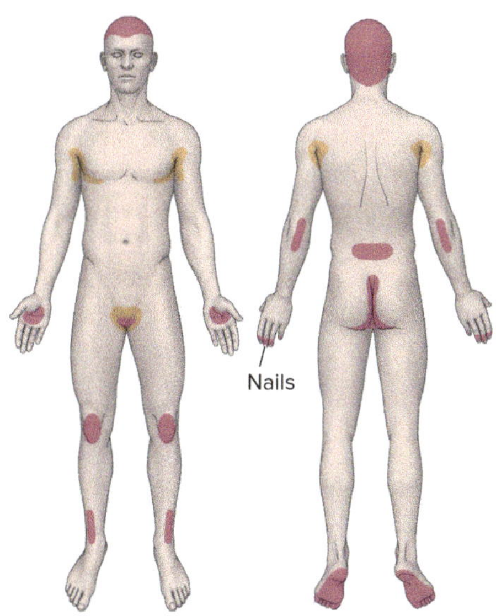

Predilection sites of psoriasis. (Reproduced, with permission, from Wolff K, Johnson RA, Saavedra AP. *Fitzpatrick's Color Atlas and Synopsis of Clinical Dermatology.* 7th ed. New York, NY: McGraw-Hill Education; 2013.)

deep dermal inflammatory infiltrate containing plasma cells around blood vessels and nerves. Interface dermatitis with scattered dyskeratotic keratinocytes along the dermal epidermal junction is a common feature of secondary syphilis. Like psoriasis, dilated blood vessels engorged with blood are present, but the endothelial cells are swollen and protrude into the vascular lumens.

Psoriasis

Clinical Features
- Sharply circumscribed plaques with silvery scale
- Auspitz sign, Koebner phenomenon
- Predilection for scalp, groin, extensor surfaces (especially elbows and knees), nails
- Inherited component

Histopathologic Features
- Hyperkeratosis with confluent parakeratosis
- Uniform elongation of rete ridges
- Papillary dermal edema with dilated tortuous capillaries
- Thinned suprapapillary plates
- Neutrophils within the stratum corneum (Munro microabscesses)
- Neutrophils within the spinous layer (spongiform pustule of Kogoj)
- Superficial perivascular lymphocytic infiltrate

Differential Diagnosis
- Chronic spongiotic (eczematous) dermatitis
- Superficial cutaneous fungal infections
- Secondary syphilis
- Reactive arthritis
- Lichen simplex chronicus

ANSWER 1-46: E.

This biopsy reveals acanthosis with prominent parakeratotic scale, a large intraepidermal neutrophilic pustule, and prominent subepidermal edema. Higher magnification reveals the intraepidermal neutrophilic pustule. This is a classic example of **pustular psoriasis**, which may occur in several settings. Occasionally, pustules may be found at the periphery of typical plaque-type lesions. Sterile pustules may be localized to the palms and soles (**palmoplantar pustular psoriasis of Barber**; choice B), to the paronychial tissues (**acrodermatitis continua of Hallopeau**; choice D), or may be generalized with associated constitutional symptoms (**pustular psoriasis of von Zumbusch**; choice A, and **impetigo herpetiformis**; choice C). The term **"palmoplantar pustulosis"** describes psoriasis in which lesions are confined to the palms and soles. Some authors separate clinical variants, such as pustular psoriasis of Barber and acrodermatitis continua of Hallopeau. We will consider these entities together because they show identical histopathologic features, although the clinical presentation and/or clinical associations may allow their discrimination. Pustular psoriasis of von Zumbusch presents as a sudden eruption of 2- to 3-mm sterile pustules tending toward confluence and a distribution over the trunk and extremities. The underlying skin shows a fiery erythema. The face is usually spared, but oral lesions are common. This process is episodic and may be accompanied by fever, leukocytosis, and arthralgias lasting several days. Nails may be shed. The average age of onset is 50 years, with males and females affected equally. Hypocalcemia may be present, possibly related to hypoalbuminemia. Pustular psoriasis of von Zumbusch has been precipitated by numerous medications, including systemic corticosteroids, iodides, salicylates, and progesterone. Impetigo herpetiformis is pustular psoriasis in association with pregnancy. Patients with impetigo herpetiformis usually have typical lesions of psoriasis elsewhere and many consider it a pregnancy presentation of pustular psoriasis of von Zumbusch. The condition is accompanied by constitutional symptoms and hypocalcemia, which may rarely result in tetany. Patients typically have no personal history or family history of psoriasis and the condition rapidly resolves postpartum. Choice E describes **acute generalized exanthematous pustulosis** (AGEP; pustular drug eruption).

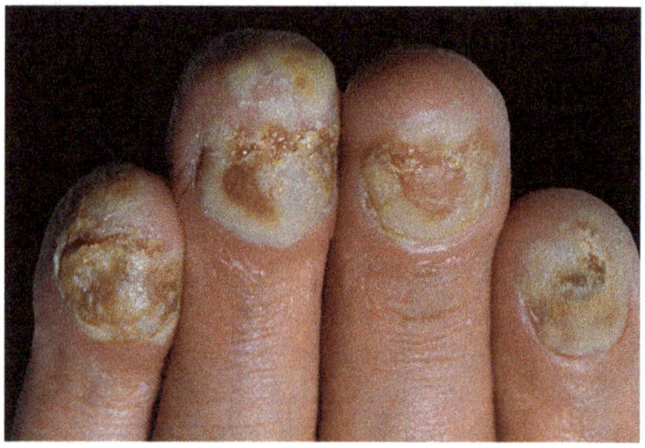

Acrodermatitis continua of Hallopeau with acral pustule formation, subungual lakes of pus, and destruction of nail plates. This may lead to permanent loss of nails and scarring. (Reproduced, with permission, from Wolff K, Johnson RA, Saavedra AP. *Fitzpatrick's Color Atlas and Synopsis of Clinical Dermatology*. 7th ed. New York, NY: McGraw-Hill Education; 2013.)

The constant histopathologic feature of pustular psoriasis is the **spongiform macropustule of Kogoj**. Neutrophils migrate from dilated, tortuous papillary dermal capillaries and collect between residual plasma membranes, accompanied by intercellular edema, producing a spongiosis within the Malpighian layer (stratum basale and stratum spinosum). Keratinocytes in the center of the spongiotic areas degenerate, leaving large unilocular pustules. With time, neutrophils arrive in the parakeratotic stratum corneum as **Munro microabscesses**. Other changes are the same as those in **psoriasis vulgaris**, namely

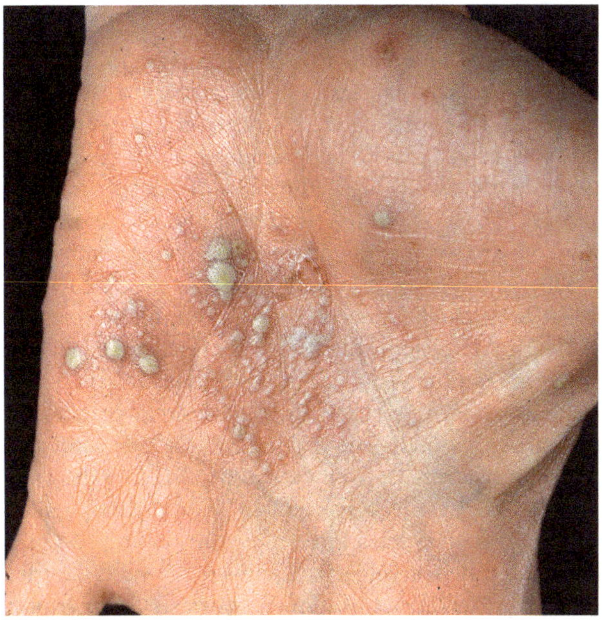

Palmar pustulosis. Creamy-yellow pustules that are partially confluent on the palm of a 28-year-old female. Pustules are sterile and pruritic, and when they get larger, become painful. At the time of this eruption there was no other evidence of psoriasis anywhere else on the body, but 2 years later the patient developed chronic stable plaque psoriasis on the trunk. (Reproduced, with permission, from Wolff K, Johnson RA, Saavedra AP. *Fitzpatrick's Color Atlas and Synopsis of Clinical Dermatology*. 7th ed. New York, NY: McGraw-Hill Education; 2013.)

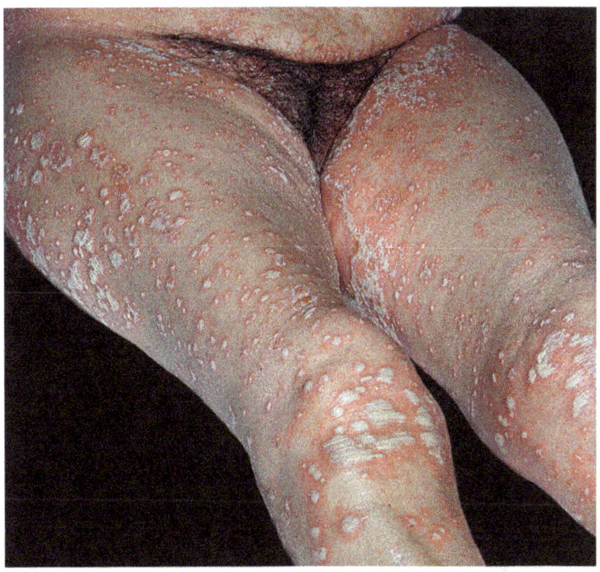

Generalized acute pustular psoriasis (von Zumbusch). This female patient was toxic and had fever and peripheral leukocytosis. The entire body was covered with showers of creamy-white coalescing pustules on a fiery-red base. Since these pustules are very superficial, they can be literally wiped off, which results in red oozing erosions. (Reproduced, with permission, from Wolff K, Johnson RA, Saavedra AP. *Fitzpatrick's Color Atlas and Synopsis of Clinical Dermatology*. 7th ed. New York, NY: McGraw-Hill Education; 2013.)

diffuse parakeratosis, hypogranulosis, regular elongation of rete ridges, papillary dermal edema, and capillary dilatation in association with a superficial perivascular infiltrate of lymphocytes and neutrophils. These findings are less well developed in eruptive lesions. On acral skin, as in palmoplantar pustular psoriasis of Barber or acrodermatitis continua of Hallopeau, pustules are large and unilocular, with the typical spongiform pattern seen primarily at the periphery of the pustule.

In regard to the differential diagnosis, a number of processes can present with spongiform or subcorneal pustules. Identification of the primary pathologic process is important

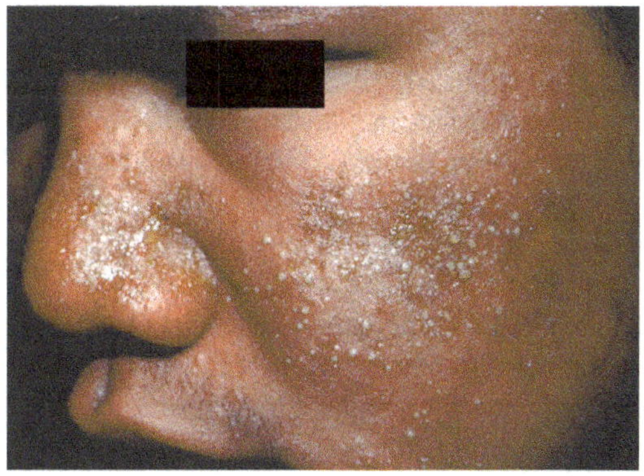

Acute generalized exanthematous pustulosis (AGEP; pustular drug eruption). The eruption is characterized by fever, a pustular eruption, and hepatitis, in a 23-year-old man after 18 days of treatment with minocycline. (Reproduced, with permission, from Goldsmith LA, Katz SI, Gilchrest BA, Paller AS, Leffell DJ, Wolff K, eds. *Fitzpatrick's Dermatology in General Medicine*. 8th ed. New York, NY: McGraw-Hill Education; 2012.)

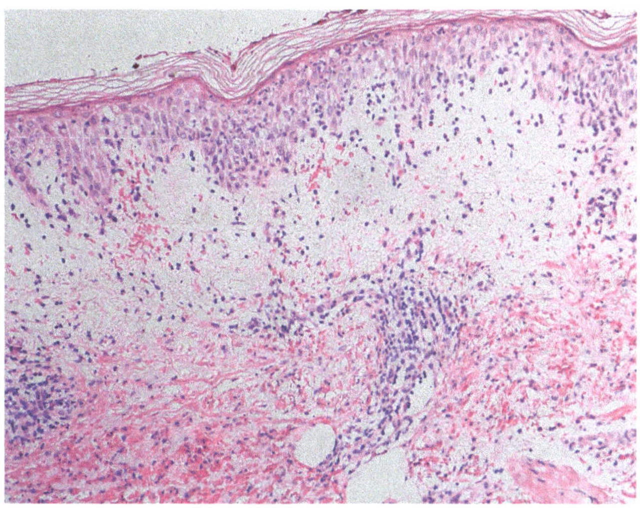

Acute generalized exanthematous pustulosis (AGEP; pustular drug eruption). There is marked papillary dermal edema and mixed perivascular inflammatory infiltrates composed of lymphocytes, neutrophils, and eosinophils. The epidermis contains neutrophilic pustules and scattered neutrophil exocytosis. The epidermis is of normal thickness and is surfaced by a normal basket-weave stratum corneum.

in differentiating these disorders. **Acute generalized exanthematous pustulosis** (AGEP; pustular drug eruption) characteristically involves the face and trunk, whereas pustular psoriasis typically spares the face. Microscopically, AGEP also contains intraepidermal pustules, neutrophil exocytosis, and papillary dermal edema. However, unlike psoriasis, the epidermis typically lacks an adaptive response and is of normal thickness and is surfaced by a basket-weave stratum corneum. An important distinguishing feature is the presence of eosinophils in pustular drug eruption, which should be absent in psoriasis. **Dyshidrotic eczema** may show intraepidermal pustules but is more spongiotic and often has eosinophils in the dermal infiltrate. The pustules of dyshidrotic eczema contain Langerhans cell–rich microvesicles and lymphocytes. Superficial fungal infections such as **candidiasis** and **dermatophytosis** may show pustules in the stratum corneum, and therefore it is imperative to order PAS stains on all cases of psoriasiform dermatitis. **Impetigo** and **subcorneal pustular dermatosis of Sneddon-Wilkinson** may all show subcorneal pustules. In these conditions, parakeratosis and epidermal hyperplasia are less developed. **Pemphigus foliaceus** and **IgA pemphigus** will have acantholytic cells within the pustule and will exhibit intercellular immunoglobulin deposition within the epidermis by direct immunofluorescence.

ANSWER 1-47: D.

The biopsy reveals the eruptive pattern of psoriasiform epidermal hyperplasia (**eruptive psoriasis**) in which marked acanthosis and elongation of rete ridges are usually not present. There is mild spongiosis, variable hypogranulosis, and focal mounds of parakeratosis containing neutrophils. In many cases, the epidermal changes are not yet apparent and the underlying dermis contains superficial perivascular lymphocytic infiltrate with rare neutrophils and extravasated erythrocytes associated with papillary dermal edema and dilated tortuous capillaries in close apposition with the epidermal surface. Only later are the suprapapillary plates thinned in association with elongation of rete ridges. In early lesions, parakeratosis is typically mounded or spotted rather than confluent. Migration of neutrophils from dermal papillae into the overlying epidermis has been referred to as squirting papillae. Neutrophils are oftentimes more numerous in eruptive psoriasis than in psoriasis vulgaris. Choices A, B, and C describe the clinical presentations of **guttate psoriasis**, **inverse psoriasis**, and **erythrodermic psoriasis,** respectively. All three of these conditions may histopathologically present with the eruptive pattern of psoriasiform dermatitis, which is relatively nonspecific without the appropriate clinical history. Choice D describes a patient with **tinea corporis gladiatorum** (ring worm), which is a dermatophytosis spread by skin-to-skin

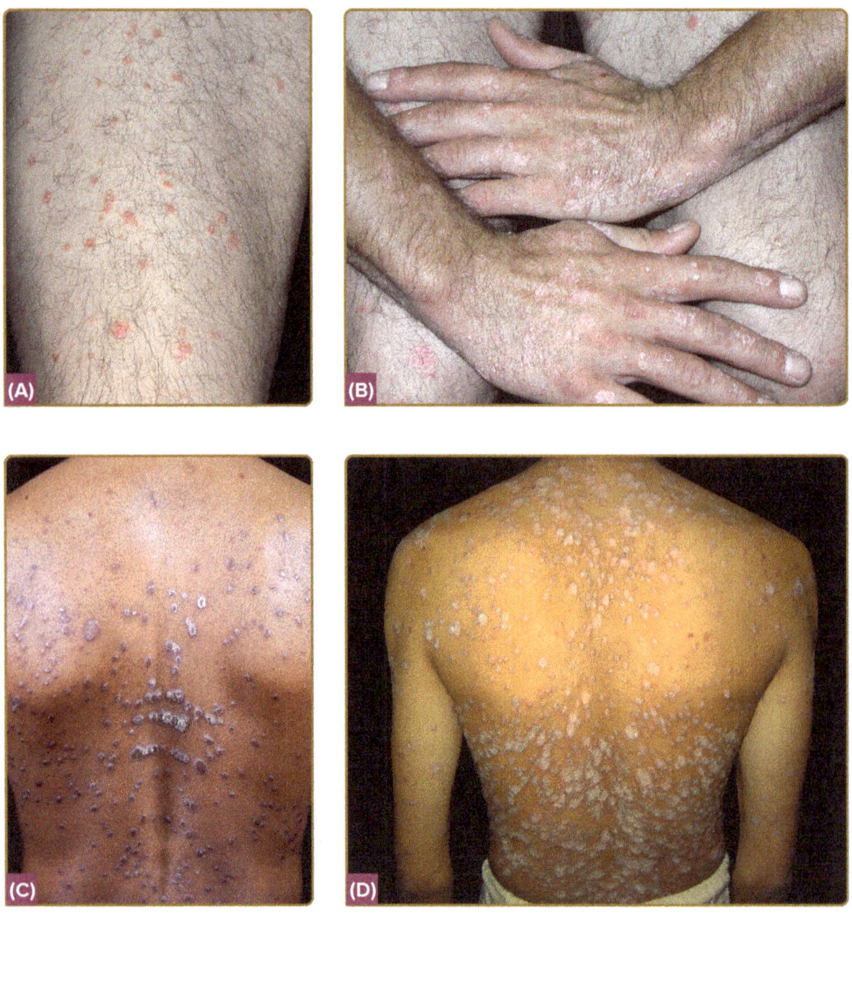

Guttate psoriasis, involving thigh (**A**), hands (**B**), and back (**C** and **D**). The patient in (**D**) went on to develop chronic plaque psoriasis. (Reproduced, with permission, from Goldsmith LA, Katz SI, Gilchrest BA, Paller AS, Leffell DJ, Wolff K, eds. *Fitzpatrick's Dermatology in General Medicine*. 8th ed. New York, NY: McGraw-Hill Education; 2012. Photos used with permission from Drs Johann Gudjonsson and Trilokraj Tejasvi, Mr Harrold Carter, and Ms Laura Vangoor.)

contact between wrestlers. This question is somewhat tricky since inverse psoriasis (choice B) may clinically resemble tinea corporis. Patients with inverse psoriasis typically have a history of psoriasis or concomitant lesions of psoriasis elsewhere. The patient in choice B has a history of plaques consistent with psoriasis vulgaris, therefore supporting a diagnosis of inverse psoriasis. A PAS stain with diastase predigestion is recommended for all cases with the histomorphology of psoriasis (eruptive, vulgaris, or pustular) in effort to adequately rule out dermatophytosis. Dermatophytosis will reveal hyphal elements within the stratum corneum. It is worth mentioning that an extremely rare form of psoriasis known as **annular psoriasis** is clinically and histopathologically identical to tinea corporis. A PAS stain must be performed to differentiate these two conditions.

Guttate psoriasis presents with an abrupt onset of small (guttate) lesions, especially on the trunk and proximal extremities, and may follow a streptococcal infection. This phenomenon is more common in children. It may be related to cross-reactive antibodies between a streptococcal and protein in human skin. **Inverse psoriasis** is characterized by involvement of the flexures. Here lesions may show less scale and exhibit a shiny erythema. **Erythrodermic psoriasis** is characterized by generalized erythema and shedding of large amounts of scale. In this setting, marked dilatation of cutaneous blood vessels adversely affects body temperature regulation.

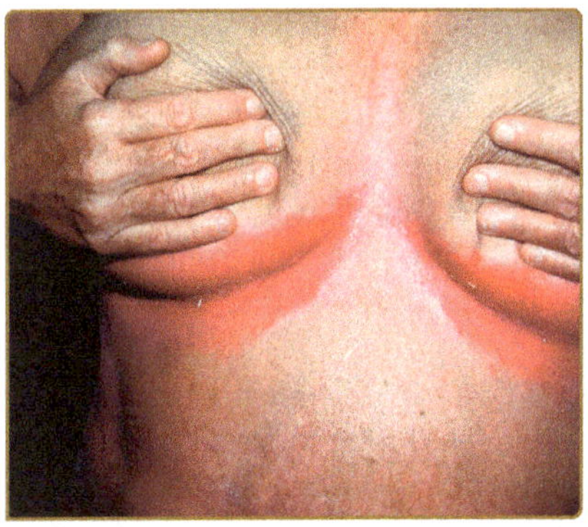

Inverse psoriasis. Note the well-demarcated, beefy-red, shiny plaques underlying the breasts. (Reproduced, with permission, from Goldsmith LA, Katz SI, Gilchrest BA, Paller AS, Leffell DJ, Wolff K, eds. *Fitzpatrick's Dermatology in General Medicine.* 8th ed. New York, NY: McGraw-Hill Education; 2012.)

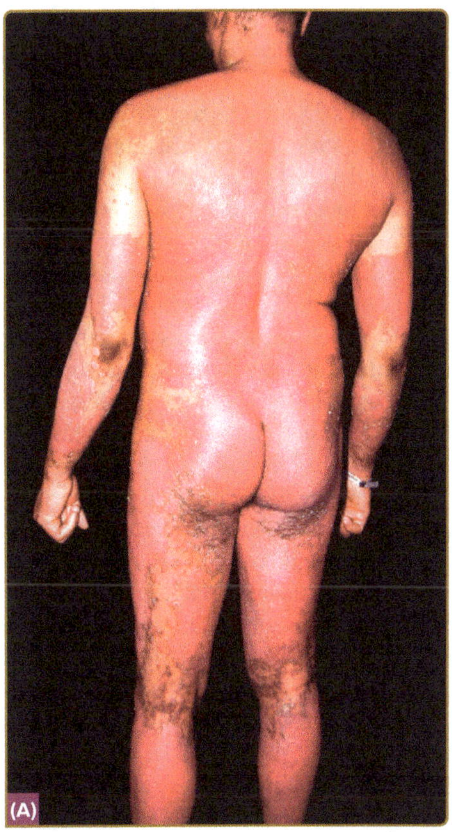

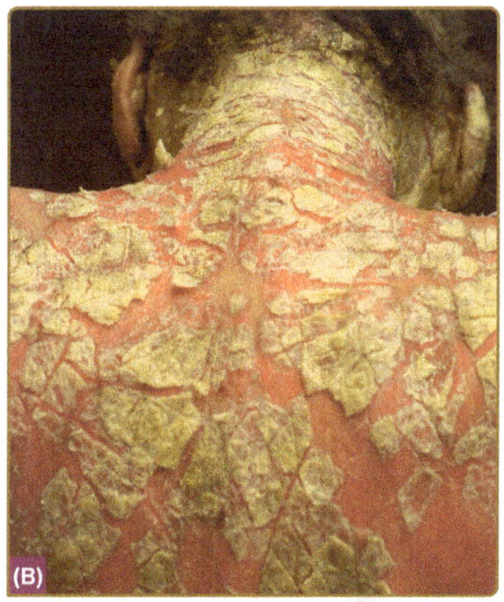

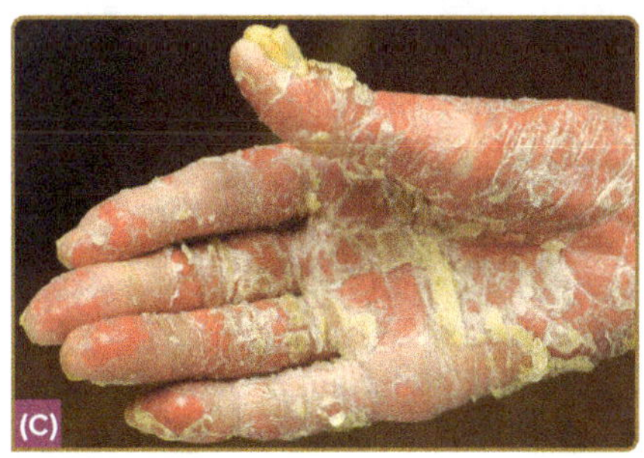

Erythrodermic psoriasis. The patient shown in panel **(A)** rapidly developed near-complete involvement and complained of fatigue and malaise. Note islands of sparing. The patient shown in panels **(B)** and **(C)** had total body involvement with marked hyperkeratosis and desquamation. These patients may occasionally have concomitant generalized lymphadenopathy; therefore, Sézary syndrome has to be excluded. Clinical history, typical psoriatic nail involvement, absence of alopecia, and biopsy verify a diagnosis of psoriasis. (Reproduced, with permission, from Goldsmith LA, Katz SI, Gilchrest BA, Paller AS, Leffell DJ, Wolff K, eds. *Fitzpatrick's Dermatology in General Medicine.* 8th ed. New York, NY: McGraw-Hill Education; 2012. Photos used with permission from Mr. Harrold Carter and Dr. Johann Gudjonsson.)

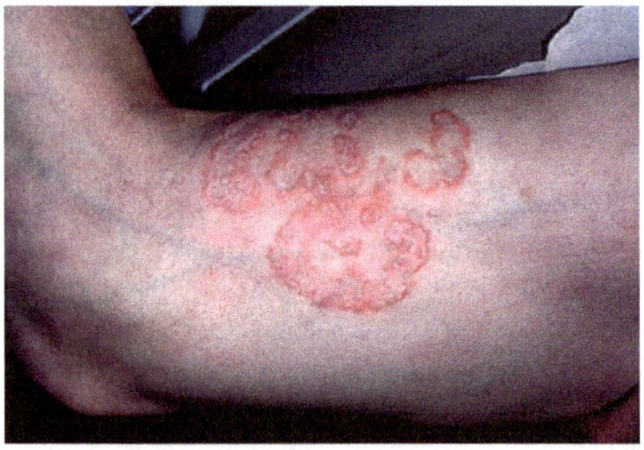

Tinea corporis. There are scaly, ring-shaped lesions with distinct borders and central clearing. A PAS stain or KOH scraping must be performed to confirm the presence of fungi. (Reproduced, with permission, from McPhee SJ, Papadakis MA, eds. *Current Medical Diagnosis & Treatment 2011.* 50th ed. New York, NY: McGraw-Hill Education; 2011. Courtesy of S. Goldstein.)

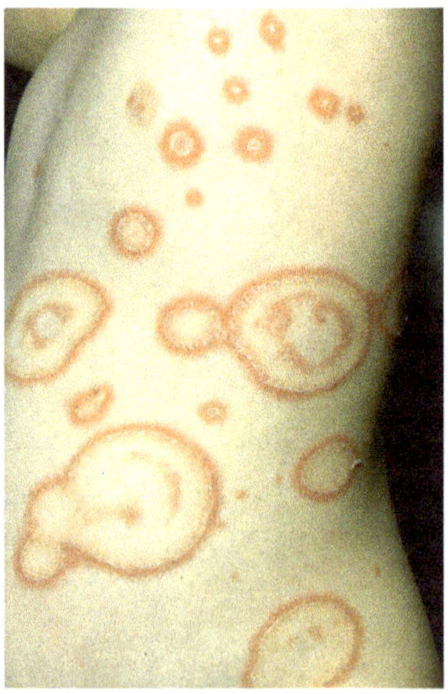

Annular psoriasis. This is an acutely eruptive process where annular lesions spread peripherally and regress in the center. The peripheral margin may be pustular and there is a collarette-like scaling. This clinical subtype of psoriasis preferentially occurs in children and can be classified as somewhere between eruptive guttate and generalized pustular psoriasis. It is clinically indistinguishable from tinea corporis or erythema annulare centrifugum.

ANSWER 1-48: A.

Psoriasis is a chronic multifactorial inflammatory skin disease that appears to be influenced by genetic and immune-mediated components. It is characterized by complex alterations in epidermal growth and differentiation and multiple biochemical, immunologic, and vascular abnormalities, and a poorly understood relationship to nervous system function. Its root cause remains unknown. Multiple theories with varying supportive data exist. The last two decades have shed enormous light on the pathogenesis of this condition; however, the initiators of the process and the precise relationship between the T-cell-driven immune reaction and keratinocyte proliferation remains unclear. Evidence for an inherited component in psoriasis includes a high concordance for disease in monozygotic twins and linkage disequilibrium with certain human lymphocyte antigen (HLA) types, especially HLA-Cw6. Linkage analysis has identified nine separate loci (PSORS1 through PSORS9) supporting a genetic susceptibility within the major histocompatability (MHC) complex. PSORS1 (HLA-Cw6) shows the strongest genetic susceptibility, being implicated in 35%-50% of cases of familial psoriasis, and is associated with psoriasis in young adults (mostly guttate psoriasis). Psoriasis vulgaris in adults over 50 years of age, pustular psoriasis, and psoriatic arthritic are not associated with PSORS1, but have a higher incidence of HLA-B27. There is also evidence for genomic imprinting in the inheritance of psoriasis, in that children of males with psoriasis are more often affected than children of females with psoriasis. The "allelic instability in mitosis" model of dominantly inherited disease, the subject of recent reviews can explain this finding and other genetic phenomena in psoriasis. The concordance rate for psoriasis in monozygotic twins ranges from 35% to 73%. This variability, and the fact that these rates do not approach 100%, supports a role for environmental factors. In fact, disease concordance decreased when patients were sampled more closely to the equator. UV light exposure is a potent inhibitor of T-cell function. Additionally, the T-cell-specific immunosuppressant cyclosporine A is highly active against psoriasis, further supporting an immunologically mediated pathogenesis. One hypothesis is that genetic susceptibility coupled with an inflammatory process that may be triggered by activation of T cells by bacterial superantigens leads to the development of psoriasis. *Streptococcal* and *staphylococcal* infections frequently precede eruptions of guttate and erythrodermic psoriasis, respectively. Below is a summary of what is currently understood regarding the immunologic pathogenesis of psoriasis.

Normal skin contains epidermal Langerhans cells (L), scattered immature dendritic cells **(D),** and skin-homing memory T cells **(T)** in the dermis.

However, nonlesional skin of patients with psoriasis exhibits slight capillary dilatation and curvature, and a slight increase in the numbers of dermal mononuclear cells and mast cells (M). A slight increase in epidermal thickness is also usually present. In chronic plaque psoriasis, the intensity of these changes may depend on distance from an established lesion.

The transition zone of a developing "eruptive" lesion is characterized by progressive increases in capillary dilatation and tortuosity, increased numbers of mast cells (M), macrophages (MP), and T cells, and mast cell degranulation (small arrows). In the epidermis, there is increasing thickness with increasingly prominent rete ridges, widening of the extracellular spaces, spotty loss of the granular layer, and parakeratosis. Langerhans cells (L) begin to exit the epidermis, and inflammatory dendritic cells (D) and $CD8^+$ T cells (8) begin to enter the epidermis.

The fully developed lesion is characterized by fully developed capillary dilatation and tortuosity with a tenfold increase in blood flow, numerous macrophages underlying the basement membrane, and increased numbers of dermal T cells (mainly $CD4^+$) making contact with maturing dermal dendritic cells (D). The epidermis of the mature lesion manifests markedly increased keratinocyte hyperplasia (approximately tenfold), further loss of the granular layer with overlying

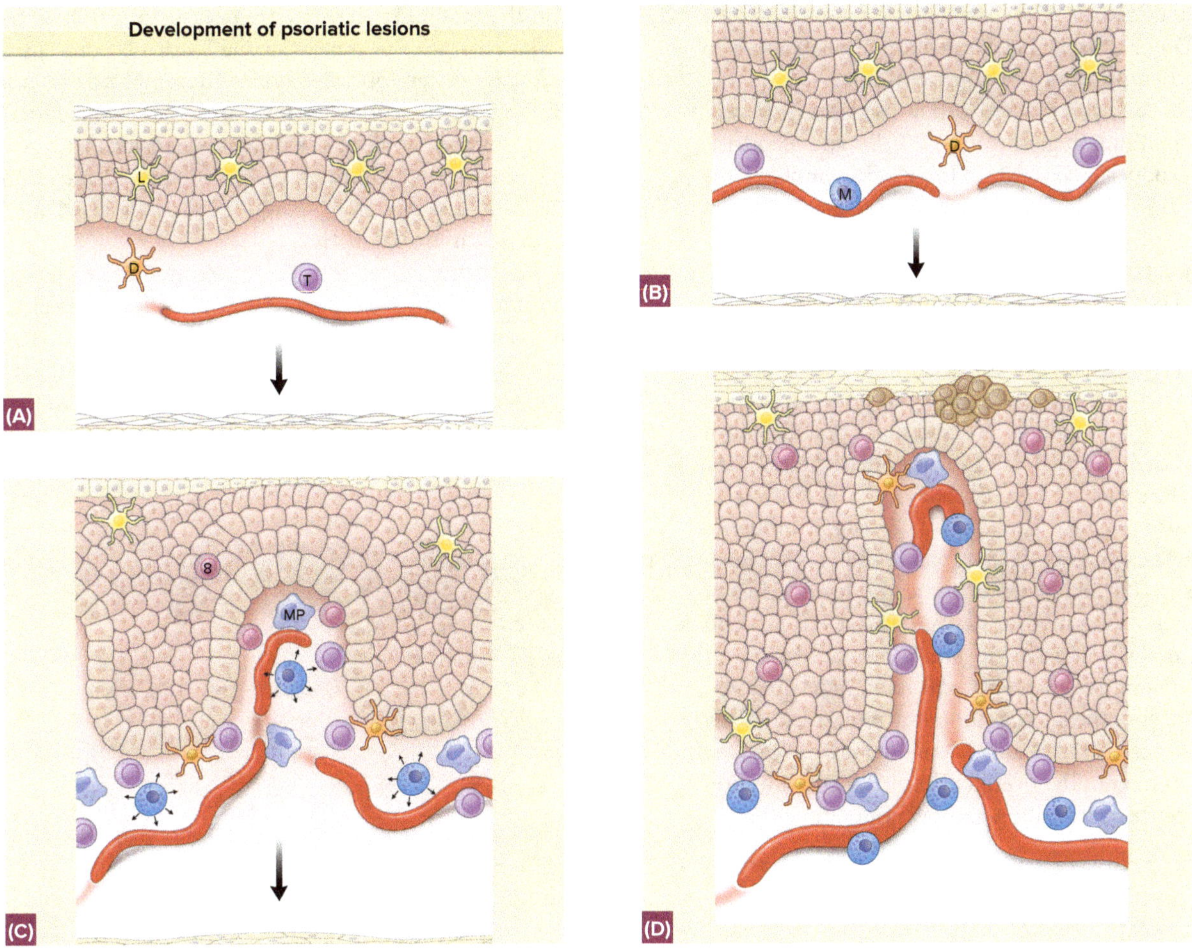

Reproduced, with permission, from Goldsmith LA, Katz SI, Gilchrest BA, Paller AS, Leffell DJ, Wolff K, eds. *Fitzpatrick's Dermatology in General Medicine*. 8th ed. New York, NY: McGraw-Hill Education; 2012.

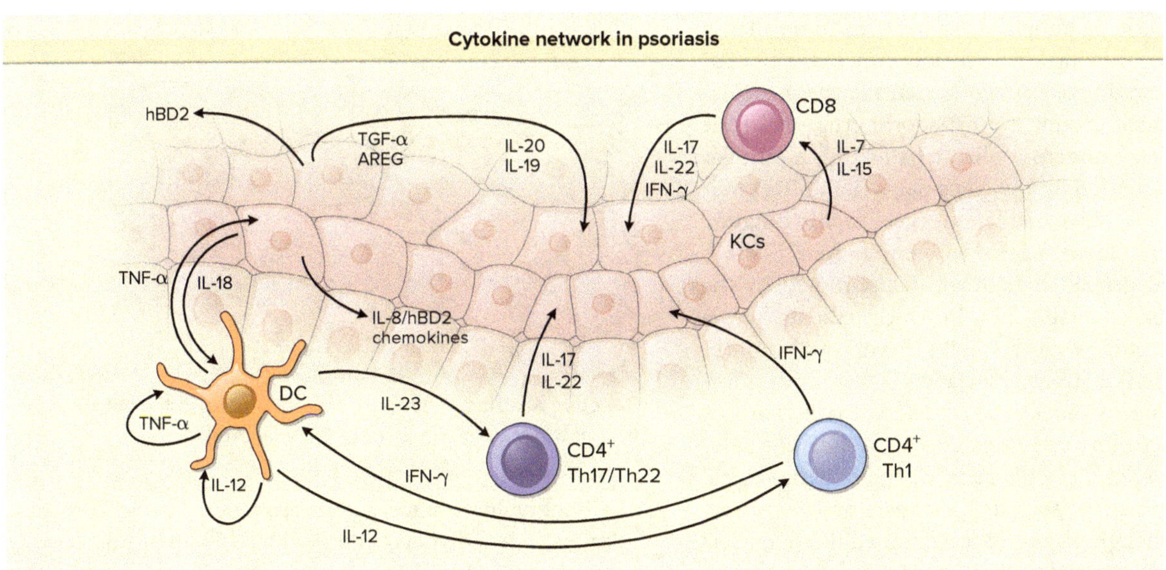

Reproduced, with permission, from Goldsmith LA, Katz SI, Gilchrest BA, Paller AS, Leffell DJ, Wolff K, eds. *Fitzpatrick's Dermatology in General Medicine*. 8th ed. New York, NY: McGraw-Hill Education; 2012.

compaction parakeratosis of the stratum corneum, increased numbers of CD8$^+$ T cells, and accumulation of neutrophils in the stratum corneum (Munro microabscesses).

In regard to the cytokine network in psoriasis, Th1 cells produce IFN-γ-stimulating activated T cells and dendritic cells (DC) to produce TNF-α. This IFN-γ also amplifies the production of IL-23 by DCs. In turn, IL-23 maintains and expands subsets of CD4$^+$ T cells, called Th17 and Th22 cells, which are characterized by production of IL-17 and IL-22, respectively. CD8$^+$ T cells are predominantly found in the epidermis, and their entry into the epidermis is necessary for lesion development. IL-17, TNF-α, IFN-γ, and IL-22 synergistically promote activation of the innate keratinocyte defense response involving secretion of antimicrobial peptides such as human-β-defensin 2 (hBD-2), IL-8 and other chemokines, and growth factors such as TGF-α, AREG, IL-19, and IL-20. Keratinocytes also produce IL-7 and IL-15, which influence the survival and turnover of CD8+ T cells, and IL-18, which via IL-12 causes DC to further increase the production of INF-γ by T cells. Keratinocyte-derived IL-1α, IL-1β, and TNF-α play a major role in angiogenesis, in recruitment of additional circulating lymphocytes, and inducing expression of a number of endothelial cell adhesion molecules. Lastly keratinocytes secrete IL-18, which is a potent chemokine for neutrophil recruitment. The overall effect is an amplification loop of keratinocyte proliferation and inflammation.

ANSWER 1-49: C.

Reactive arthritis formerly referred to as Reiter's syndrome is characterized by the triad of urethritis, arthritis, and conjunctivitis. However, only one-third of patients manifest the complete classic triad, and 40% have arthritis only. A more recent definition by the American Rheumatism Association requires "an episode of peripheral arthritis of more than 1 month's duration occurring in association with urethritis and/or cervicitis." Approximately 80% of patients have mucocutaneous lesions, which include a psoriasiform eruption of the palms and soles (**keratoderma blenorrhagicum**), a pustular or psoriasiform eruption on the glans penis (**balanitis circinata**), erosive or ulcerative oral lesions (**geographic tongue**), and subungual pustules associated with onycholysis. There is a well-established genetic component demonstrated by the strong association with HLA B27, in which patients have a more aggressive course with sacroiliitis, uveitis, and carditis. Additionally, there is a strong association with various infectious enteric pathogens (*Salmonella enteritidis, S typhimurium, S heidelberg*; *Yersinia enterocolitica, Y pseudotuberculosis*; *Campylobacter fetus*; *Shigella flexneri*) and nongonococcal genitourinary pathogens (such as *Chlamydia* or *Ureaplasma urealyticum*). Although organisms are rarely cultured, nucleic acid sequences of *Chlamydia* subspecies have been found in the synovium of affected patients. **Keratoderma blenorrhagicum** is characterized by brownish-red papules or macules mainly on the toes and soles that are occasionally topped by vesicles that enlarge. The centers of the lesions become pustular and/or hyperkeratotic and crusted resembling mollusk shells. Scaling erythematous psoriasiform plaques may arise on the scalp, elbows, and buttocks. Shallow erosions with serpiginous, micropustular borders in uncircumcised men and crusted and/or hyperkeratotic plaques in circumcised men characterize **circinate balanitis.**

The histopathological features of keratoderma blenorrhagicum and balanitis circinata are essentially identical to those of pustular psoriasis. Broad hyperkeratosis and parakeratosis with a thinned granular layer and elongated rete ridges are seen. Within the parakeratotic stratum corneum are collections of neutrophils with pyknotic nuclei (**Munro microabscesses**).

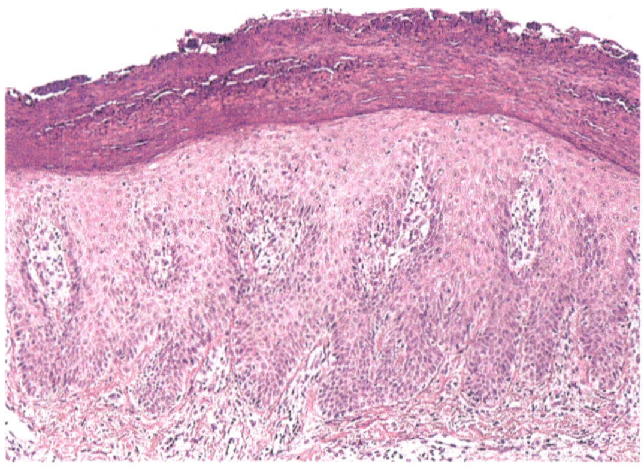

Reactive arthritis. This lesion shows a parakeratotic stratum corneum containing neutrophils that overlies psoriasiform epidermal hyperplasia.

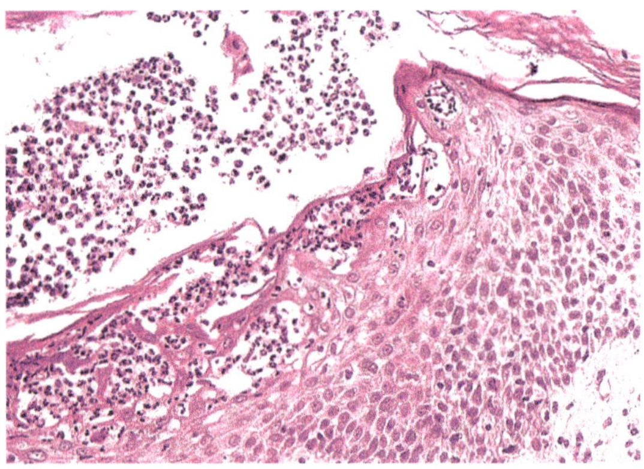

Reactive arthritis. There are spongiform pustules in the upper part of the Malpighian layer of the epidermis.

Geographic tongue shows prominent spongiform pustules with less hyperkeratosis than in cutaneous lesions. Clinical correlation may be necessary to distinguish **Reactive arthritis** from **pustular psoriasis** because the histopathologic changes may be identical.

Reactive arthritis

Clinical Features
- Triad of urethritis (negative urethral cultures), arthritis, and conjunctivitis
- Predominantly young males, HLA-B27
- Palms and soles (keratoderma blenorrhagicum)
- Penile lesions (balanitis circinata)

Histopathologic Features (identical to psoriasis)
- Hyperkeratosis with confluent parakeratosis
- Uniform elongation of rete ridges
- Papillary dermal edema with dilated tortuous capillaries
- Thinned suprapapillary plates
- Neutrophils within the stratum corneum (Munro microabscesses)
- Neutrophils within the spinous layer (spongiform pustule of Kogoj)
- Superficial perivascular lymphocytic infiltrate

Differential Diagnosis
- Psoriasis
- Chronic spongiotic (eczematous) dermatitis
- Superficial cutaneous fungal infections
- Secondary syphilis

ANSWER 1-50: D.

The biopsy reveals psoriasiform epidermal hyperplasia with broad rete ridges and a stratum corneum with an adherent scale composed of both orthokeratosis and parakeratosis. The granular layer is preserved and parakeratosis is present at the shoulder of a dilated follicular ostium containing hyperkeratosis. Neutrophils are not present in the stratum corneum. The findings are consistent with **pityriasis rubra pilaris. Exfoliative erythroderma syndrome** (**EES**) is a serious, at times life-threatening, reaction pattern of the skin characterized by generalized and uniform redness and scaling involving practically the entire skin. High blood flow to the skin may disrupt temperature regulation or lead to high-output cardiac failure. Two stages, acute and chronic, merge one into the other. In the acute and subacute phases, there is rapid onset of generalized vivid red erythema and fine branny scales; the patient feels hot and cold, shivers, and has fever. In chronic EES, the skin thickens, and scaling continues and becomes lamellar. Some 50% of patients have history of a preexisting dermatosis, which is recognizable only in the acute or subacute stages. The most frequent preexisting skin disorders are (in the order of frequency) **psoriasis, atopic dermatitis,** adverse **cutaneous drug reactions, cutaneous T-cell lymphoma (Sézary syndrome), allergic contact dermatitis,** and **pityriasis rubra pilaris (PRP)**. In most cases, these patients need to be hospitalized and worked up with appropriate laboratory and imaging studies.

Drugs Associated With Erythroderma

- Acetylsalicylic acid
- Sulfasalazine
- Fenbufen
- Oxytetracycline
- Gentamicin
- Nystatin
- Ketoconazole
- Sulfonamides
- Cotrimoxazole
- Clofazimine
- Quinidine
- Captopril
- Timolol
- Minoxidil
- Phenobarbital
- Methotrexate
- Granulocyte-macrophage colony-stimulating factor
- Etretinate

Pityriasis rubra pilaris (PRP) is a rare, idiopathic, chronic papulosquamous disease with a bimodal age of onset. There is an equal sex ratio. Some cases are familial and are transmitted as an autosomal dominant trait with expression of keratins not normally found in epidermis. As in **psoriasis**, the epidermal turnover rate is increased. PRP usually begins as asymptomatic scaling and erythema of the scalp resembling **seborrheic dermatitis**. Later, truncal lesions develop as small, orange-red, acuminate follicular papules with perifollicular erythema. These papules eventually coalesce into large plaques with fine scale and distinct borders, expanding to leave islands of uninvolved skin. The disease may progress to generalized erythroderma. Additionally, there is a yellow-red keratoderma of the palms and soles with diffuse scaling.

Follicular papules on the dorsa of fingers are said to resemble a "nutmeg grater." Nail changes include thickening of the nail plate and subungual hyperkeratosis. Oral lesions are infrequent. In the classic adult form (type I) the disease may undergo spontaneous remission within 3 years in approximately 80% of the cases, but the childhood form (type II) tends to be chronic. HIV-associated PRP may have coexisting acne conglobata or hidradenitis suppurativa.

The microscopic features of PRP include epidermal hyperplasia characterized by expansion of both the rete ridges (plate-like) and suprapapillary plates. A distinct finding is the presence of focal acantholysis and hypergranulosis surfaced by foci of parakeratosis. The stratum corneum exhibits adherent lamellar hyperkeratosis with alternating areas of parakeratosis and orthokeratosis both perpendicular and parallel to the skin surface, imparting a "checker board pattern." Parakeratotic mounds at the edges of follicular ostia, similar to that of seborrheic dermatitis, are termed "shoulder parakeratosis."

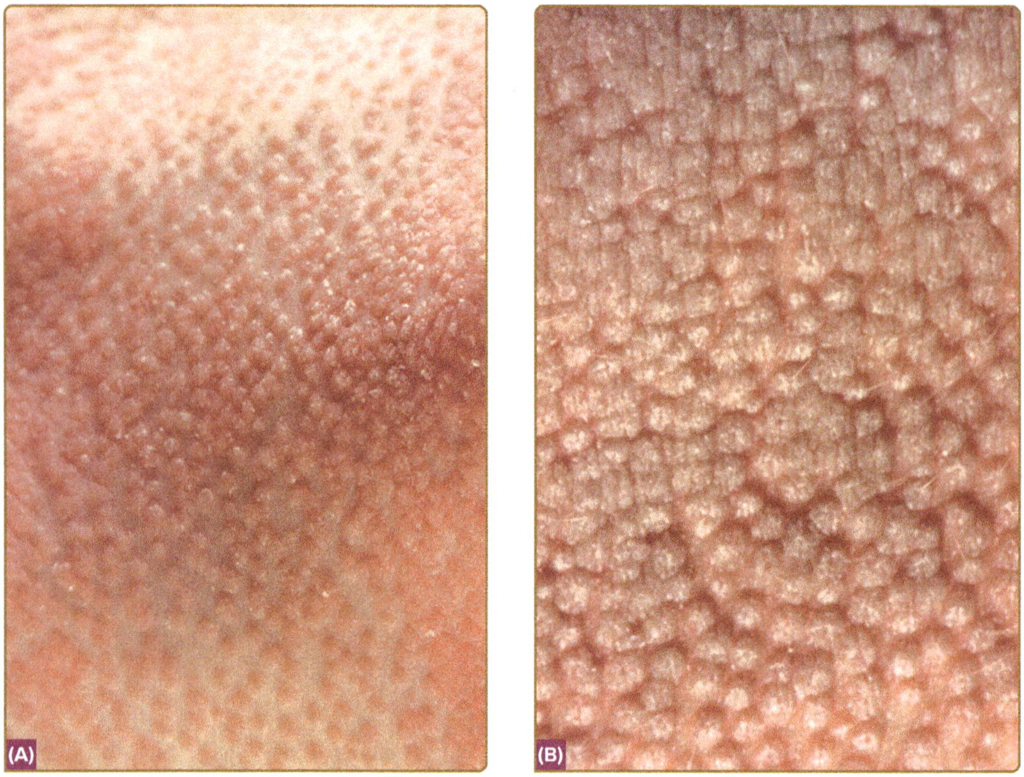

Pityriasis rubra pilaris. Numerous acuminate follicular papules close-ups of discrete **(A)** and confluent **(B)** lesions. (Reproduced, with permission, from Goldsmith LA, Katz SI, Gilchrest BA, Paller AS, Leffell DJ, Wolff K, eds. *Fitzpatrick's Dermatology in General Medicine*. 8th ed. New York, NY: McGraw-Hill Education; 2012.)

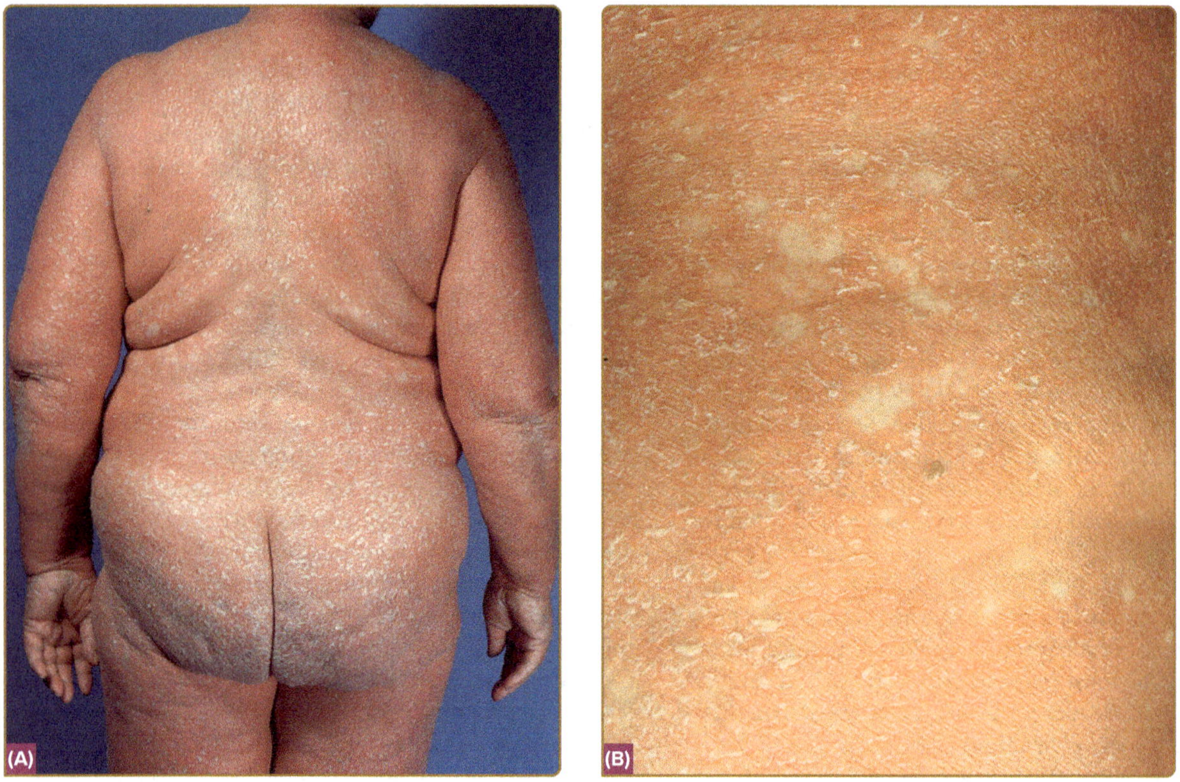

Generalized pityriasis rubra pilaris. (A) Reddish orange, scaling dermatitis, and islands of normal skin ("nappes claires"), shown in more detail in **(B)** (Reproduced, with permission, from Goldsmith LA, Katz SI, Gilchrest BA, Paller AS, Leffell DJ, Wolff K, eds. *Fitzpatrick's Dermatology in General Medicine*. 8th ed. New York, NY: McGraw-Hill Education; 2012.)

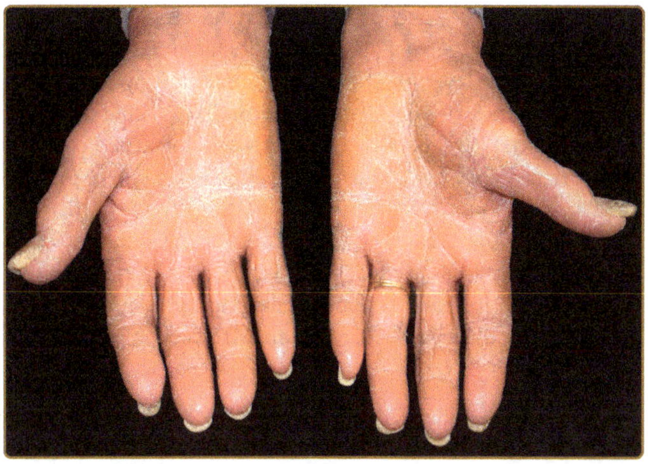

Pityriasis rubra pilaris with keratoderma. Note keratoderma with an orange hue and thickening of the thumbnails. (Reproduced, with permission, from Goldsmith LA, Katz SI, Gilchrest BA, Paller AS, Leffell DJ, Wolff K, eds. *Fitzpatrick's Dermatology in General Medicine*. 8th ed. New York, NY: McGraw-Hill Education; 2012.)

Keratotic plugs fill the follicular ostia and extend above the level of the adjacent epidermis. There is a mild superficial perivascular lymphocytic infiltrate, sometimes containing eosinophils or plasma cells. The neutrophils and Munro microabscesses of psoriasis are usually absent. Spongiosis is minimal.

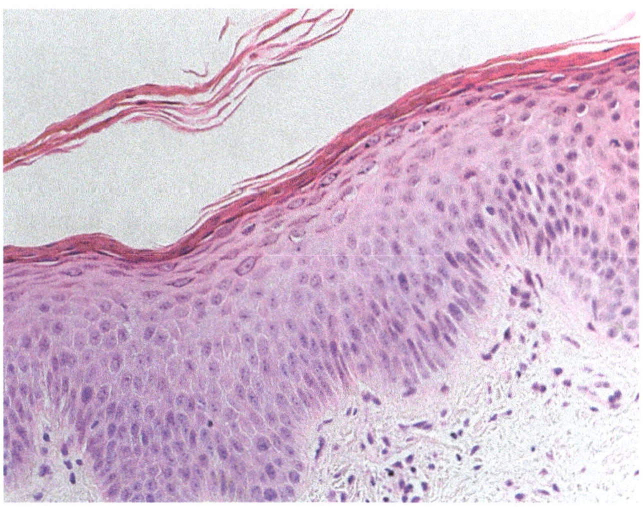

Pityriasis rubra pilaris. There is an irregular psoriasiform epidermal hyperplasia with broad rete ridges. There is hypergranulosis with an adherent overlying scale composed of alternating parakeratosis and orthokeratosis.

The clinical and histopathological differential diagnosis in **exfoliative erythroderma syndrome** can be extremely difficult. The history of the preexisting dermatosis may be the only clue. Also, pathognomonic signs and symptoms of the preexisting dermatosis may help and include dusky red color in **psoriasis** and orange-red in **pityriasis rubra pilaris**; lichenification, erosions, and excoriations in **atopic dermatitis** and eczema; diffuse, relatively nonscaling palmar hyperkeratosis with fissures in **cutaneous T-cell** lymphoma (CTCL) and **pityriasis rubra pilaris**; erythroderma with sharply demarcated patches of sparing in **pityriasis rubra pilaris**; massive hyperkeratotic scale of scalp, usually without hair loss in **psoriasis** and with hair loss in **CTCL** and **pityriasis rubra pilaris**. Many cases show no distinguishing features and may remain "idiopathic" even after biopsy. Medications associated with erythroderma include allopurinol, gold, isoniazid, phenytoin, sulfonamides, and sulfonylureas. Metformin has not been implicated in drug-associated erythroderma. Generalized lymphadenopathy with markedly enlarge lymph nodes should focus the workup on Sézary syndrome, which most commonly arises de novo without a preexisting diagnosis of mycosis fungoides. Peripheral blood analysis of **Sézary syndrome** reveals 10%-20% of lymphocytes within the buffy coat to exhibit hyperconvoluted (cerebriform) nuclei referred to as Sézary cells. The current criteria proposed by the International Society for Cutaneous Lymphoma for the diagnosis of Sézary syndrome include an absolute Sézary cell count of at least 1000 cells/mm^3; immunophenotypical abnormalities, including a CD4/CD8 ratio of 10 or higher (measured by flow cytometry) and loss of T-cell antigen (CD2, CD3, CD4, CD5, CD7) expression; or the documentation of a T-cell clonality in the blood by T-cell-receptor gene rearrangement analysis.

An objective histopathological diagnosis of PRP can be made in about 50% of cases. The most distinctive features are follicular hyperkeratosis, hypergranulosis, and shoulder parakeratosis. In **psoriasis** the parakeratosis tends to be confluent, whereas in PRP the changes are focal. Psoriasis also characteristically exhibits hypogranulosis underlying parakeratosis, whereas in PRP parakeratosis may surface a preserved granular layer. The presence of neutrophils and spongiform pustules in association with dilated, tortuous capillaries favors psoriasis and argues against the diagnosis of PRP. PRP may contain eosinophils, which are absent in psoriasis. **Chronic eczematous dermatitis** usually shows some degree of spongiosis. Follicular plugging may be seen in **keratosis pilaris**, a frequent concomitant finding in atopic patients, but keratosis pilaris does not show significant epidermal hyperplasia. Cases of **Sézary syndrome** may show atypical, cerebriform lymphocytes in the epidermis with minimal associated spongiosis. Unlike plaque stage **mycosis fungoides**, fully developed **Pautrier microabscesses** (clusters of atypical intraepidermal lymphocytes) are uncommon. **Drug eruptions** may show atypical lymphocytes along the interface and within the epidermis, leading to confusion with mycosis fungoides. In a blinded retrospective study of erythrodermic patients, histopathologic impression correlated with final diagnosis in up to 66% of cases. The authors suggest that multiple biopsies taken simultaneously may improve diagnostic accuracy.

Pityriasis Rubra Pilaris

Clinical Features
- Inherited (autosomal dominant) and sporadic forms
- Scalp involvement resembling seborrheic dermatitis
- Acuminate follicular papules
- Erythroderma with islands of sparing
- Palmoplantar keratoderma

Histopathologic Features
- Vertical and horizontal foci of orthokeratosis alternate with parakeratosis
- Parakeratotic mounds at follicular ostia (shoulder parakeratosis)
- Follicular plugging
- Rete ridges irregularly elongated and thickened
- Thickened suprapapillary plates
- Superficial perivascular lymphocytic inflammation

Differential Diagnosis
- Psoriasis
- Seborrheic dermatitis
- Keratosis pilaris

ANSWER 1-51: B.

The biopsy reveals prominent irregular psoriasiform epidermal hyperplasia with pointed rete ridges. There is overlying hyperkeratosis and hypergranulosis. Thick dermal collagen bundles are present that are oriented perpendicular to the epidermal surface. The findings are consistent with **lichen simplex chronicus (LSC),** which is produced by repetitive mechanical trauma to the skin. A number of stimuli produce pruritus and provoke scratching. When the sensation and scratching are localized, papules and plaque arise. Lesions with localized picking result in nodular lesions of **prurigo nodularis ("picker's nodule").** Psychogenic factors may be involved. Over time, the behavior may become subconscious. Identical lesions can be induced in normal skin by a minimum of 140,000 scratches. Any pruritic or eczematous dermatosis can develop secondary lichenification. We reserve the term LSC (localized neurodermatitis) for those cases in which a primary dermatosis is not apparent. Lesions of LSC are almost always pruritic and often solitary. They are chronic and most commonly involve the lower lateral legs, dorsal feet, extensor forearms, genital region, and posterior neck. Lesions of LSC are thickened, well-demarcated, scaly papules, nodules, or plaques with excoriation and lichenification. Hyperpigmentation is common and persistent. The prurigo nodularis pattern is usually multiple and symmetrically distributed on the extremities with evidence of chronicity including dyschromia and scarring.

The microscopic findings of LSC include thickening of all layers of the skin above the reticular dermis, imparting some resemblance to acral skin. Hyperkeratosis, hypergranulosis, and acanthosis are seen. When present, parakeratosis is discontinuous. The rete ridges are irregularly elongated and thickened. The epidermis may be papillomatous, and the superficial Malpighian layer may be pale as the result of glycogen accumulation. There is usually some spongiosis in the acute stage, but vesicles are rare. The papillary dermis shows thickened collagen fibers oriented perpendicular to the skin surface. There may be stellate or multinucleated fibroblasts in the superficial dermis. The superficial dermis shows vascular ectasia and a perivascular lymphocytic infiltrate with minimal exocytosis. Scattered eosinophils may be present. Prurigo nodularis has similar findings as LSC but typically reveals foci of expansive (bulbous) acanthosis.

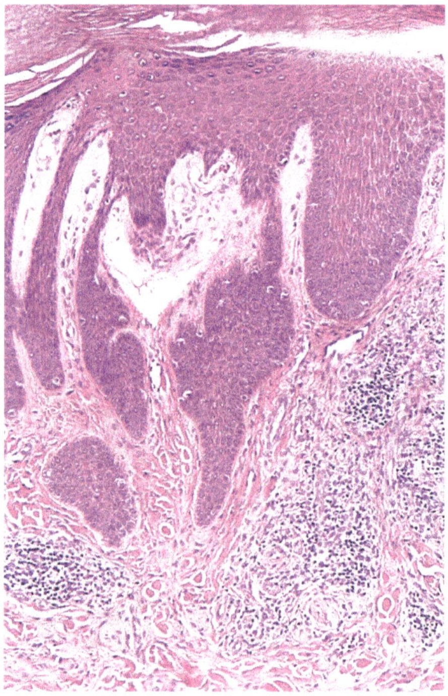

Prurigo nodularis. Note the bulbous focus of epidermal hyperplasia. There is hypergranulosis and vertical papillary dermal fibrosis identical to that of LSC.

The histopathological differential diagnosis primarily includes **psoriasis.** Changes of LSC may be seen superimposed on all forms of pruritic dermatitis. LSC may show residual intercellular edema and hypergranulosis, which are mild or absent in psoriasis. Both conditions show vascular ectasia, but vessels are more tortuous in psoriasis. Eosinophils are absent in psoriasis. Psoriasis shows more prominent parakeratosis and an edematous rather than fibrotic papillary dermis. **Seborrheic dermatitis, psoriasis,** and **chronic fungal infections** are more likely to show neutrophils within the stratum corneum. **Secondary syphilis** produces epidermal hyperplasia similar to LSC with pointed rete ridges, but syphilis exhibits lichenoid interface dermatitis and a deep dermal inflammatory infiltrate containing plasma cells. **Scabies** may produce changes identical similar to LCS also contains holes "burrows" or mites in the stratum corneum. In many cases, additional deeper levels are required to adequately investigate for scabetic infestation. A PAS stain should be ordered on all cases to exclude **dermatophytosis.** Benign keratoses and other epidermal neoplasms tend to be more sharply circumscribed.

Lichen Simplex Chronicus

Clinical Features
- Prominent pruritus
- Changes produced by repetitive scratching
- Chronic well-demarcated plaques
- Lichenification/excoriation/hyperpigmentation
- Lateral legs, posterior neck, flexures

Histopathologic Features
- Thickening of all layers of the skin above the reticular dermis
- Hyperkeratosis/hypergranulosis/acanthosis
- Papillary dermal fibroplasia
- Stellate/multinucleated fibroblasts
- Superficial perivascular lymphocytic infiltrate
- Pointed rete ridges rather than club shaped

Differential Diagnosis
- Psoriasis
- Chronic spongiotic (eczematous) dermatitis
- Superficial cutaneous fungal infections

ANSWER 1-52: D.

This patient has **small-plaque parapsoriasis (SPP),** also known as **digitate dermatosis** or **chronic superficial dermatitis**, which is a rare chronic dermatitis with a strong male predilection. **Parapsoriasis** is not a disease but a group of diseases that includes **pityriasis lichenoides, large-plaque parapsoriasis (LPP),** and **small-plaque parapsoriasis (SPP).** This group of diseases was first proposed by Brocq in an attempt to organize the inflammatory dermatoses. The diseases are essentially unrelated, except that all are idiopathic, asymptomatic (although pruritus can be a variable feature), chronic, and relatively unresponsive to therapy.

Classification of Parapsoriasis

1. Parapsoriasis en plaques
   A. Large-plaque parapsoriasis variants: poikilodermatous, retiform
   B. Small-plaque parapsoriasis variant: digitate dermatosis
2. Pityriasis lichenoides
   A. Pityriasis lichenoides chronica (Juliusberg)
   B. Pityriasis lichenoides et varioliformis acuta (Mucha-Habermann)

Reproduced, with permission, from Goldsmith LA, Katz SI, Gilchrest BA, Paller AS, Leffell DJ, Wolff K, eds. *Fitzpatrick's Dermatology in General Medicine.* 8th ed. New York, NY: McGraw-Hill Education; 2012.

SPP is clinically characterized by round to oval (finger shaped, hence *digitate dermatosis*), yellowish or fawn-colored patches and plaques with fine scale. It follows lines of cleavage of the skin and gives the appearance of a hug that left fingerprints on the trunk. The short axis of these lesions generally measures less than 5 cm; however, the long axis often measures greater than 5 cm.

Microscopically, SPP exhibits mild spongiosis with focal areas of hyperkeratosis, parakeratosis, scale crust, and lymphocyte exocytosis. In the dermis, there is a mild superficial perivascular lymphohistiocytic infiltrate and dermal edema. There is no progression of the histopathologic features toward cutaneous T-cell lymphoma (mycosis fungoides) and the lymphocytes exhibit minimal to no nuclear atypia (atypia defined as cerebriform nuclear contour irregularity). Immunohistochemical studies reveal a predominantly $CD4^+$ T-cell infiltrate with preservation of pan-T-cell markers CD3, CD5, and CD7. T-cell-receptor rearrangement (TCR) analysis reveals a polyclonal infiltrate in the vast majority of cases.

In addition to a confusing nomenclature and the difficulties in defining parapsoriasis in a reproducible fashion, considerable controversy surrounds the relationship between **large-plaque parapsoriasis (LPP)** and **mycosis fungoides (MF)**. SPP has minimal to no risk of progression to overt MF in the experience of most experts. Many authors consider LPP to be an inflammatory process that may progress to mycosis fungoides. Others consider LPP to be part of the spectrum of cutaneous T-cell lymphoma or mycosis fungoides from the outset, a low-grade malignancy that smolders in the majority of cases and follows a more aggressive course in a few. In either case, both LPP and MF may show similar abnormalities of T-cell antigen expression and monoclonality. Large-plaque parapsoriasis (LPP) is also a chronic disease, but is characterized by large (>10 cm), slightly scaly, erythematous patches and plaques with irregular outlines. The eruption is asymmetrical and affects predominantly the buttocks, flexures, and female breasts. Mucosal disease, nail changes, and acral involvement are rare. Lesions are usually asymptomatic but may be pruritic. Plaques often show epidermal atrophy manifested as fine wrinkling of the skin. The skin lesions may resemble **poikiloderma atrophicans vasculare**, which is characterized by epidermal atrophy, dyschromia, and telangiectasia. Thickening of the plaques may herald progression to overt mycosis fungoides.

Microscopically, the earliest lesions of LPP show only a superficial perivascular lymphocytic infiltrate. The epidermis initially shows mild, irregular acanthosis and mounding parakeratosis. Spongiosis is unusual. With chronicity, the infiltrate may become more dense and band like with associated papillary dermal fibrosis. Lymphocytes may be seen along the basal layer in association with vacuolar change and pigment incontinence. Unlike SPP, the lymphocytes of LPP frequently exhibit varying degrees of atypia characterized by cerebriform nuclear contour irregularity (Sézary cell). Immunohistochemical staining will reveal a predominantly CD4+ T-cell infiltrate with mild to modest reductions in CD7 expression and less frequently CD5. TCR analysis commonly reveals a monoclonal infiltrate, further blurring the lines between chronic dermatitis and mycosis fungoides.

Parapsoriasis En Plaques

Clinical Features
- Chronic disease of middle age
- Scaly erythematous patches and plaques
- Predilection for buttocks, flexures, and breasts
- Unresponsive to treatment

Histopathologic Features
- Mild irregular acanthosis
- Mounding parakeratosis
- Papillary dermal fibrosis
- Focal vacuolar change
- Superficial perivascular lymphocytic infiltrate

Differential Diagnosis
- Guttate (eruptive) psoriasis
- Mild chronic dermatitis
- Mycosis fungoides (see text)

Like all psoriasiform dermatitis, a PAS stain should be performed to rule out dermatophyte infection, which may produce similar clinical and histopathological findings.

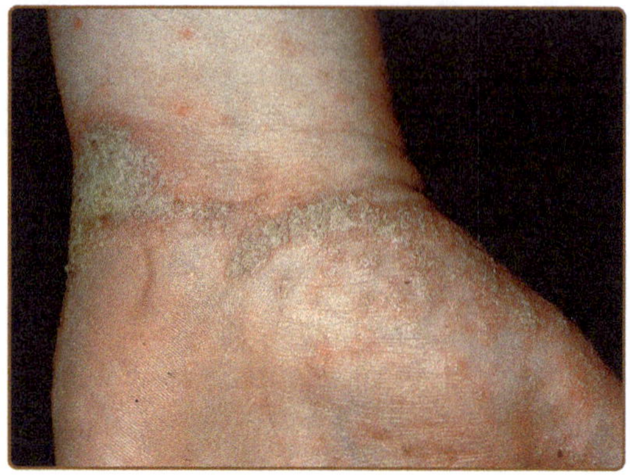

Crusted (Norwegian) scabies in a man with non-Hodgkin lymphoma. (Reproduced, with permission, from Goldsmith LA, Katz SI, Gilchrest BA, Paller AS, Leffell DJ, Wolff K, eds. *Fitzpatrick's Dermatology in General Medicine*. 8th ed. New York, NY: McGraw-Hill Education; 2012.)

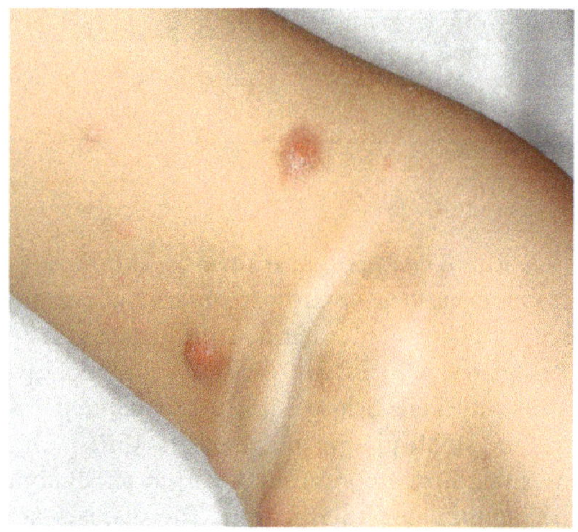

Nodular scabies. Erythematous firm nodules indistinguishable from chronic arthropod bite reactions.

ANSWER 1-53: E.

The biopsy reveals an irregular psoriasiform epidermal hyperplasia surfaced by markedly thick hyperkeratosis. The stratum corneum contains large clear spaces with concentric eosinophilic structures. The findings are consistent with scabies. **Scabies infestation** is a pruritic communicable disease caused by infestation by the human scabies mite, *Sarcoptes scabiei* var *hominis*. The itch results from sensitization to the mite or its products and subsequent cell-mediated immune response. The mite is usually transmitted by direct contact with infested individuals or, less commonly, by fomites. Mites may survive away from the human host for several days. After mating, the female mite burrows into the superficial layers of the skin and lays her eggs. The female dies after about 5 weeks; the eggs hatch, and the cycle repeats. Typically, a patient is infested with only 10 to 15 adult mites, making demonstration and diagnosis occasionally difficult. In **crusted scabies (Norwegian scabies),** however, mites are much more numerous and involvement of the face is common. Crusted scabies infestation typically occurs in the settings of mental deficiency, malnutrition, or immunosuppression. Clinically, patients present with multiple widespread, thick, gray, or yellowish scaly plaques, with numerous

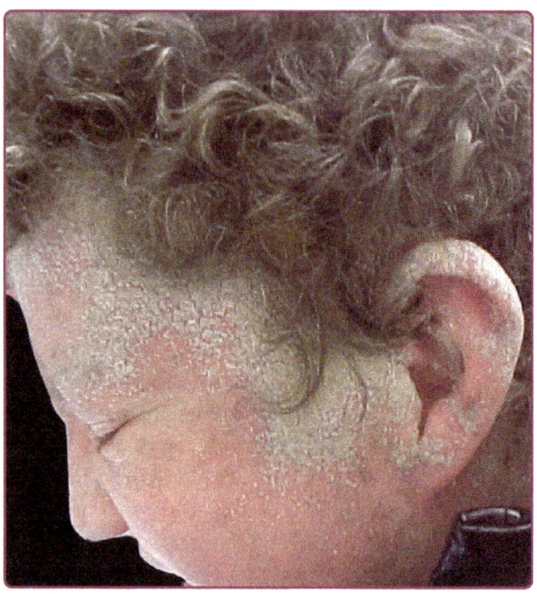

Crusted (Norwegian) scabies. Hyperkeratotic plaques populated with thousands of mites. (Reproduced, with permission, from Goldsmith LA, Katz SI, Gilchrest BA, Paller AS, Leffell DJ, Wolff K, eds. *Fitzpatrick's Dermatology in General Medicine*. 8th ed. New York, NY: McGraw-Hill Education; 2012.)

mites present within lesions. Unlike in common scabies, pruritus may be minimal. The mites are the same species as common scabies and the designation of "Norwegian" refers to the place where it was first reported. Several courses of treatment with topical permethrin, as well as keratolytics, may be necessary to cure patients. Oral ivermectin is also useful in these patients. The diagnostic clinical lesion is a linear burrow with a tiny vesicle at the blind end. Although there are typically few mites, intense pruritus and scratching may produce widespread secondary lesions. Areas of excoriation, irritant dermatitis, lichenification, or secondary infection are common. In crusted scabies, one sees hyperkeratotic or psoriasiform papules and plaques. The eruption may be diffuse, presenting as erythroderma. Because mites are numerous, these patients are highly contagious. Testing for human immunodeficiency virus (HIV) may be appropriate in patients with crusted scabies. **Nodular scabies** represents a persistent hypersensitivity response, as seen in other arthropod assaults.

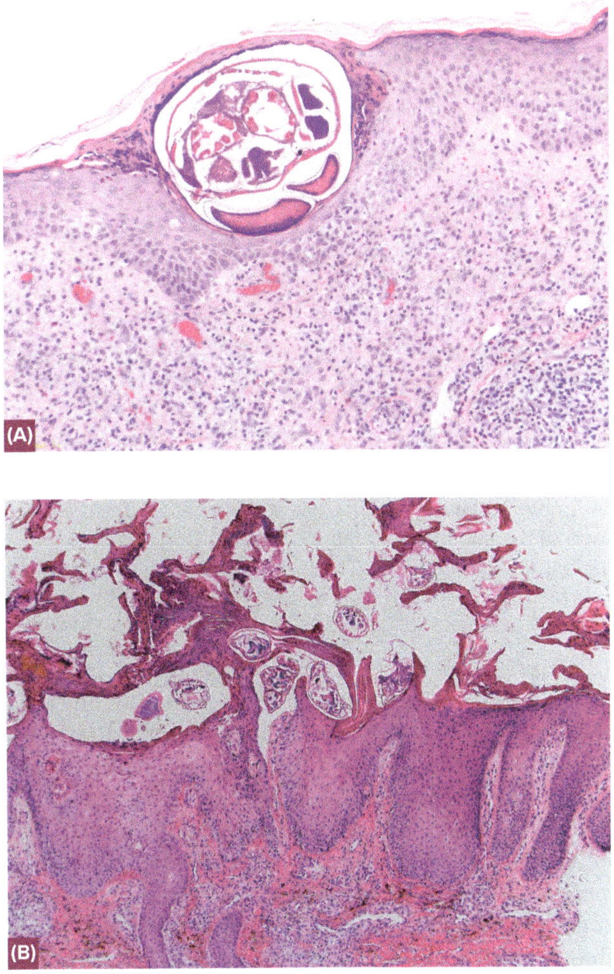

Scabies. (A) Nodular scabies with an intraepidermal mite and a robust dermal inflammatory response containing lymphocytes and eosinophils. **(B)** Crusted (Norwegian) scabies with an irregular psoriasiform epidermal hyperplasia and a thick parakeratotic crust containing burrows and mites.

Microscopically, the epidermis shows irregular acanthosis and focal spongiosis. There may be a space within or just underneath the stratum corneum corresponding to the clinical burrow. The end of the burrow extends into the superficial stratum malpighii. Step sections may reveal the female mite or its products, including eggs or fecal material (scybala). The dermis contains a superficial and deep perivascular or nodular infiltrate composed of lymphocytes and variable numbers of eosinophils (sometimes producing flame figures). The infiltrate in nodular lesions may have the picture of lymphocytoma cutis and may contain atypical lymphocytes suggesting lymphoma. In crusted (Norwegian) scabies, mites are usually numerous and easily identified within a greatly thickened stratum corneum. Mites or their products are diagnostic. A nodular dermal infiltrate with eosinophils is not seen in psoriasis.

ANSWER 1-54: B.

The biopsy reveals psoriasiform epidermal hyperplasia with alternating hyperkeratosis and parakeratosis. The combined clinical and histopathological findings are consistent with **inflammatory linear verrucous epidermal nevus (ILVEN). Epidermal nevi** are hamartomas of the epidermis or its appendages. Briefly, epidermal nevi may represent a mosaic state of disorders of cornification. For example, the acantholytic dyskeratotic variant **(acantholytic dyskeratotic epidermal nevus)** may represent a localized form of Darier disease (keratosis follicularis), and the epidermolytic variant **(epidermolytic epidermal nevus)** may represent localized epidermolytic hyperkeratosis, a disorder of keratins 1 or 10. Inflammatory linear verrucous epidermal nevus (ILVEN)

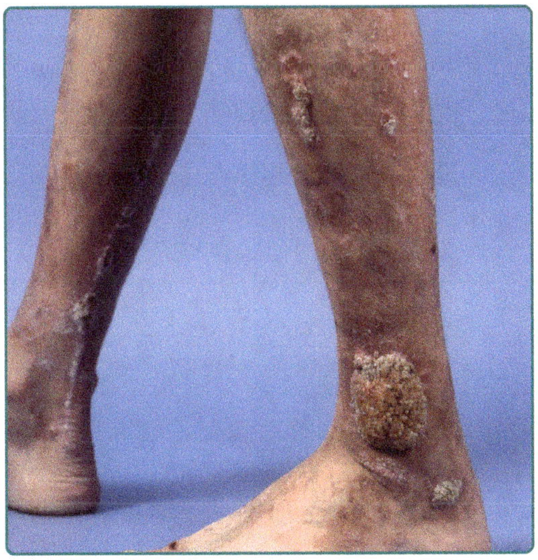

Inflammatory linear verrucous epidermal nevus showing psoriasiform erythema, scaling, and hyperkeratosis. The nodule on the left leg was a giant wart. (Reproduced, with permission, from Goldsmith LA, Katz SI, Gilchrest BA, Paller AS, Leffell DJ, Wolff K, eds. *Fitzpatrick's Dermatology in General Medicine*. 8th ed. New York, NY: McGraw-Hill Education; 2012.)

consists of grouped or coalescent lichenoid, psoriasiform, or verrucous papules in a linear arrangement, most commonly on the lower extremities. Fifty percent are present by 6 months of age and 75% by 5 years of age. Lesions follow the lines of Blaschko and are pruritic, and may wax and wane in intensity. Most cases are sporadic, but familial cases have been described. Associated skeletal malformations occur in some cases.

The classic histopathologic finding of **ILVEN** consists of broad columns of parakeratosis without an underlying granular layer, alternating in the horizontal direction with columns of compact hyperkeratosis with underlying hypergranulosis. Rete ridges are thickened and elongated with occasional slight spongiosis. Exocytosis of neutrophils as in psoriasis may occur. The superficial dermis contains a predominantly perivascular lymphocytic infiltrate.

The clinical differential diagnosis includes other linear papulosquamous lesions, such as linear psoriasis, linear Darier disease, linear porokeratosis, lichen striatus, and noninflammatory linear epidermal nevi. Clear cell acanthoma is a solitary erythematous nodule most commonly arises on the lower extremity. At the histopathological level, suprapapillary plates are thickened in **ILVEN,** whereas they are usually thinned in **psoriasis**. Parakeratosis in psoriasis is diffuse rather than arrayed in the broad columns of ILVEN. **Linear Darier disease** shows acantholysis and dyskeratosis. **Porokeratosis** is characterized by **cornoid lamellae**. Ordinary epidermal nevi show papillomatosis and are not inflammatory. **Clear cell acanthoma** is similar to psoriasis vulgaris with regular acanthosis, hypogranulosis, and confluent neutrophilic parakeratosis. The hyperplastic keratinocytes have cytologic features of outer root sheath epithelium and contain abundant glycogen-rich clear cytoplasm. A PAS stain will highlight the glycogen.

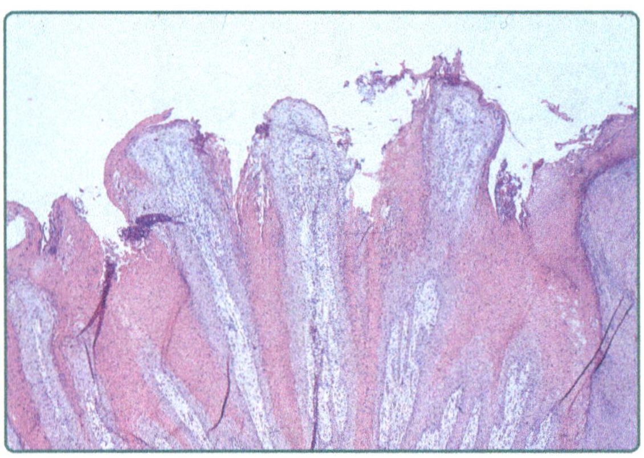

Inflammatory linear verrucous epidermal nevus (ILVEN) showing hyperkeratosis, acanthosis, papillomatosis, and elongation of rete ridges. There are alternating areas of orthokeratosis and parakeratosis. The regions with parakeratosis are associated with a complete absence of the granular layer. (Reproduced, with permission, from Goldsmith LA, Katz SI, Gilchrest BA, Paller AS, Leffell DJ, Wolff K, eds. *Fitzpatrick's Dermatology in General Medicine*. 8th ed. New York, NY: McGraw-Hill Education; 2012.)

ANSWER 1-55: A.

The biopsy reveals confluent parakeratosis, absence of the granular layer, and psoriasiform epidermal hyperplasia. The combined clinical and histopathological findings are consistent with advanced (chronic) **pellagra.** All of the listed choices have identical or extremely similar histopathological findings in both acute and chronic lesions with diagnostic distinction requiring clinical correlation and peripheral blood analysis. Acute lesions more closely resemble spongiotic dermatitis but with extensive parakeratosis overlying pallor and hydropic change (swelling) of superficial keratinocytes and eventual diffuse superficial epidermal necrosis characterized by marked reticular degeneration attributed to cytolysis. Acantholytic keratinocytes are absent. There is an adaptive irregular epidermal "psoriasiform" hyperplasia eventuating into chronic lesions. Superficial perivascular lymphocytic infiltrates are typically present.

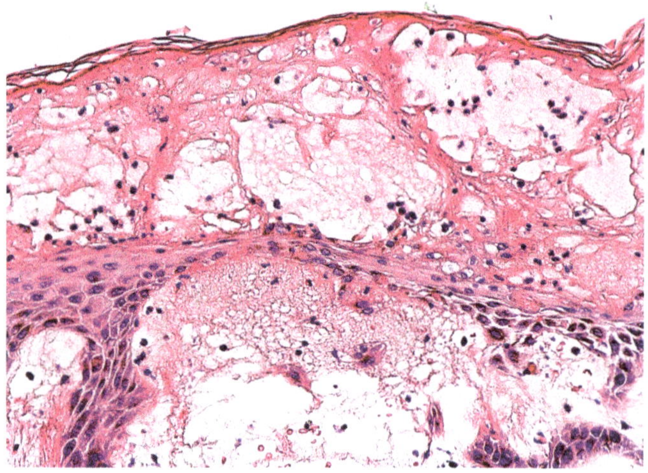

Pellagra, vesicular stage. There is striking pallor of hydropic change of the superficial keratinocytes resulting in reticular degeneration and cytolysis. The basal and lower spinous layers are normal.

Pellagra results from a systemic deficiency of **niacin** (nicotinic acid) or its precursor, the essential amino acid tryptophan. The disease is characterized by the three ***D***s—diarrhea, dementia, and dermatitis. One hypothesis holds that the clinical manifestations may be caused by increased extracellular matrix viscosity. In this model, cutaneous lesions are localized to areas of sun exposure and trauma because "mediators" cannot diffuse from the site. Increased viscosity in the gastrointestinal tract may limit absorption leading to diarrhea. Niacin deficiency may occur in the **carcinoid syndrome**, where tryptophan is converted in high quantity into serotonin (5-OH tryptophan). **Hartnup disease** is an autosomal recessive disorder characterized by an impairment of neutral amino acid transport. Tryptophan is not absorbed from the diet and is lost in the urine, leading

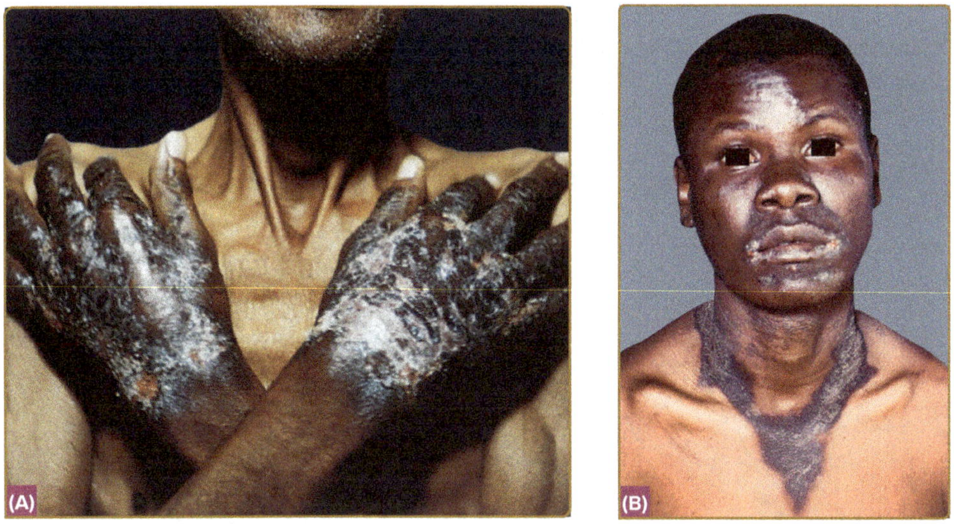

Pellagra. (A) "Glove" or "gauntlet" exudative and crusted lesions on the hands. **(B)** "Casal necklace" on the neck with facial involvement. (Reproduced, with permission, from Goldsmith LA, Katz SI, Gilchrest BA, Paller AS, Leffell DJ, Wolff K, eds. *Fitzpatrick's Dermatology in General Medicine*. 8th ed. New York, NY: McGraw-Hill Education; 2012.)

Clinical Features of Pellagra; Niacin Deficiency

- Painful pruritic dermatitis in photoexposed areas
- May be vesicular, crusted, and develops into scaly, keratotic plaques
- Dorsum of hands ("gauntlet"), neck (Casal necklace), dorsa of feet ("gaiter"); butterfly distribution in face.
- Angular stomatitis, cheilitis, glossitis
- Diarrhea, nausea, vomiting, abdominal pain, anorexia
- Insomnia, fatigue, nervousness, apathy, impaired memory, depression, psychosis, dementia

to a deficiency of niacin. Regardless of the cause of niacin deficiency, the signs and symptoms respond promptly to replacement therapy. In addition to the gastrointestinal symptoms (diarrhea) and neurologic disease, the skin eruption is characteristic. Lesions are symmetrical and involve sun-exposed skin and areas of pressure. First there is erythema and burning or itching. Early lesions may be bullous. Later hyperpigmentation, scaling, and fissuring characterize the eruption. Facial involvement may simulate the "butterfly" eruption of lupus erythematosus. The limitation to sun-exposed sites may be striking, with extremity involvement showing a glove or stocking distribution. Involvement of the neck by a sharply demarcated photoinduced rash has been termed ***Casal necklace.***

Acrodermatitis enteropathica is an autosomal recessive disease caused by a defect in dietary **zinc** absorption. The defect is not complete in that the disease may be reversed by zinc supplementation. Identical symptoms may also be produced by a diet deficient in zinc. Causes of noninherited zinc deficiency are numerous and include chronic diarrhea of any etiology, inadequate dietary content as in alcoholism or crash dieting, or renal loss as in dialysis. Also, chronic diseases with an increased catabolic rate may lead to zinc deficiency. Breast milk may have a low concentration of zinc, leading

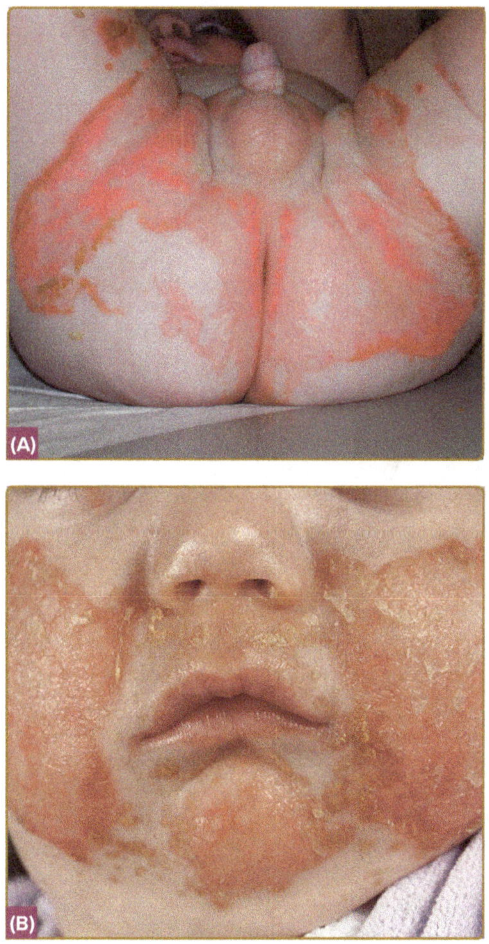

Acrodermatitis enteropathica. (A), (B) This crusted and scaly, erosive, and sharply demarcated eruption appeared shortly after weaning and resolved within 2 weeks of initiating zinc supplementation. The child was highly irritable, whining, and crying, and had diarrhea. (Reproduced, with permission, from Goldsmith LA, Katz SI, Gilchrest BA, Paller AS, Leffell DJ, Wolff K, eds. *Fitzpatrick's Dermatology in General Medicine*. 8th ed. New York, NY: McGraw-Hill Education; 2012.)

to zinc deficiency in breast-fed infants. As with the inherited form, dietary deficiency is quickly and completely reversed by supplementation with oral or parenteral zinc salts. The defective gene, *SLC39A4*, which encodes a zinc transporter named Zip4 has recently been described. The eruption typically starts as eczematous, scaly plaques on acral skin, including the scalp, paronychial folds, and perineum. Lesions may be erosive, pustular, or bullous, and secondary infection with *Candida* or bacteria is common. There may be failure to thrive. There may be alopecia or alternating light and dark banding of hair, which may be observed with polarizing light microscopy.

Clinical Features of Acrodermatitis Enteropathica; Zinc Deficiency

- Eczematous and erosive dermatitis
- Preferentially localized to periorificial and acral areas
- Alopecia
- Diarrhea
- Lethargy, irritability
- Whining and crying
- Superinfection with *Candida albicans* and *Staphylococcus aureus*

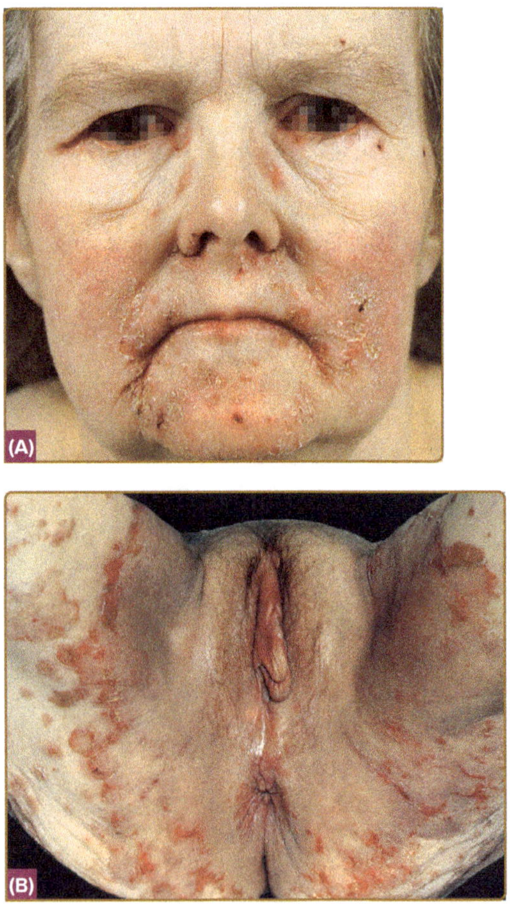

The glucagonoma syndrome, necrolytic migratory erythema. **(A)** Flaccid and papulovesicular lesions with erosions, crusting, and fissures around the orifices. **(B)** Geographic, circinate "necrolytic migratory erythema" in the groin. (A and B are not the same patient.) (Reproduced, with permission, from Goldsmith LA, Katz SI, Gilchrest BA, Paller AS, Leffell DJ, Wolff K, eds. *Fitzpatrick's Dermatology in General Medicine*. 8th ed. New York, NY: McGraw-Hill Education; 2012.)

Necrolytic migratory erythema (glucagonoma syndrome) is the result of glucagon-producing islet cell (α-cell) tumors of the pancreas. The cutaneous manifestations may be related to a hypoaminoacidemia or to the high levels of **glucagon** itself. Diagnosis is made by demonstrating increased levels of glucagon in patients with the typical syndrome. Removal of the pancreatic tumor is curative. Necrolytic migratory erythema may also occur without glucagonoma in association with hepatocellular dysfunction and hypoalbuminemia. The eruption is periorificial, acral, and flexural, often with severe glossitis. Lesions begin as erythematous papules. Later there are superficial vesicular lesions, erosions, crusting, and fissuring. Older lesions may be psoriasiform. Secondary infection with *Candida* and bacteria is common. Noncutaneous findings include stomatitis, weight loss, glucose intolerance, and diarrhea. The microscopic findings are essentially identical to pellagra and acrodermatitis enteropathica; however, this condition has also been rarely reported to show extensive suprabasilar acantholysis.

Clinical Features of Necrolytic Migratory Erythema; Elevated Glucagon

- Painful, eroded, crusted intertriginous, and facial skin eruption.
- Highly suggestive of pancreatic malignancy (glucagonoma).
- Half of tumors are metastatic at the time of diagnosis.
- Pseudoglucagonoma syndrome occurs in absence of glucagonoma.
- Skin improves with treatment of underlying nutritional aberrations.

Necrolytic acral erythema is associated with **hepatitis C infection** and clinically tends to be restricted to the dorsum of the feet, with less common involvement of the lower legs and dorsal hands. Microscopically, the findings are similar to necrolytic migratory erythema; however, vacuolar interface activity with rare scattered dyskeratotic keratinocytes along the dermal epidermal junction may be present.

Friction blisters which commonly occur on the hands and feet, however, can arise essentially anywhere. Microscopically, the findings may be similar to that of pellagra and acrodermatitis enteropathica; however, the blister cleavage plane is frequently in the stratum spinosum with a minimal inflammatory cell infiltrate. The hydropic change is frequently restricted to the blister roof.

BIBLIOGRAPHY

1. Albert MR, Mackool BT. Pityriasis rubra pilaris. *Int J Dermatol.* 1999;38:1–11.
2. Ambros-Rudolph CM, Müllegger RR, Vaughan-Jones SA, et al. The specific dermatoses of pregnancy revisited and reclassified: results of a retrospective two-center study on 505 pregnant patients. *J Am Acad Dermatol.* 2006;54:395–404.
3. Belsito DV. Autosensitization dermatitis. In: *Fitzpatrick's Dermatology in General Medicine.* 5th ed. New York, NY: McGraw-Hill; 1999:1462–1464.
4. Bennion SD, Middleton MH, David-Bajar K, et al. In three types of interface dermatitis, different patterns of expression of intercellular adhesion molecule-1 (ICAM-1) indicate different triggers of disease. *J Invest Dermatol.* 1995;105:71s-79s.
5. Bolognia JL, Orlow SJ, Glick SA. Lines of Blaschko. *J Am Acad Dermatol.* 1994;31:157–190.
6. Bonnetblanc JM. Stasis dermatitis. *Ann Dermatol Venereol.* 2002;129(1 Pt 1):98–101.
7. Brandt O, Abeck D, Gianotti R, et al. Gianotti-Crosti syndrome. *J Am Acad Dermatol.* 2006;54:136–145.
8. Broccolo F, Drago F, Careddu AM, et al. Additional evidence that pityriasis rosea is associated with reactivation of human herpesvirus-6 and -7. *J Invest Dermatol.* 2005;124:1234–1240.
9. Capon F, Munro M, Barker J, Trembath R. Searching for the major histocompatibility complex psoriasis susceptibility gene. *J Invest Dermatol.* 2002;118: 745–751.
10. Capon F, Trembath RC, Barker JN. An update on the genetics of psoriasis. *Dermatol Clin.* 2004;22:339–347.
11. Correia O, Delgado L, Barbosa IL, et al. Increased interleukin 10, tumor necrosis factor alpha, and interleukin 6 levels in blister fluid of toxic epidermal necrolysis. *J Am Acad Dermatol.* 2002;47:58–62.
12. Cosnes A, Amaudric F, Gherardi R, et al. Dermatomyositis without muscle weakness: long-term follow-up of 12 patients without systemic corticosteroids. *Arch Dermatol.* 1995;131:1381–1385.
13. Crowson AN, Brown TJ, Magro CM. Progress in the understanding of the pathology and pathogenesis of cutaneous drug eruptions: implications for management. *Am J Clin Dermatol.* 2003;4:407–428.
14. Crowson AN, Magro C. The cutaneous pathology of lupus erythematosus: a review. *J Cutan Pathol.* 2001;28(1):1–23.
15. Crowson AN, Magro CM, Mihm MC. Interface dermatitis. *Arch Pathol Lab Med.* 2008;132:652–666.
16. Crowson AN, Magro CM. The role of microvascular injury in the pathogenesis of cutaneous lesions of dermatomyositis. *Hum Pathol.* 1996;27:15–19.
17. Darmstadt GL, Donnenberg AD, Vogelsang GB, et al. Clinical, laboratory, and histopathologic indicators of the development of progressive acute graft-versus-host disease. *J Invest Dermatol.* 1992;99:397–402.
18. Drachtman RA, Alter BP. Dyskeratosis congenita. *Dermatol Clin.* 1995;13:33–39.
19. Ehrenreich M, Tarlow MM, Godlewska-Janusz E, et al. Incontinentia pigmenti (Bloch-Sulzberger syndrome): a systemic disorder. *Cutis.* 2007;79:355–362.
20. Elmore JG, Feinstein AR. Joseph Goldberger: an unsung hero of American clinical epidemiology. *Ann Intern Med.* 1994;121:372–375.
21. English JS. Current concepts of irritant contact dermatitis. *Occup Environ Med.* 2004;61:674, 722–726.
22. Farrell AM, Dean D, Millard PR, et al. Alterations in fibirillin as well as collagens I and III and elastin occur in vulva lichen sclerosus. *J Eur Acad Dermatol Venereol.* 2001;15(3):212–217.
23. Fink-Puches R, Soyer HP, Kerl H. Febrile ulceronecrotic pityriasis lichenoides et varioliformis acuta. *J Am Acad Dermatol.* 1994;30:261–263.
24. Fyhrquist-Vanni N, Alenius H, Lauerma A. Contact dermatitis. *Dermatol Clin.* 2007;25:613–623.
25. Goldman K, Don PC. Adult onset of inflammatory linear verrucous epidermal nevus in a mother and her daughter. *Dermatology.* 1994;189:170–172.
26. González LM, Allen R, Janniger CK, et al. Pityriasis rosea: an important papulosquamous disorder. *Int J Dermatol.* 2005;44:757–764.
27. Gonzalez-Lopez A, Velasco E, Pozo T, Del Villar A. HIV-associated pityriasis rubra pilaris responsive to triple antiretroviral therapy. *Br J Dermatol.* 1999;140:931–934.
28. Gottlieb GJ, Ackerman AB. The "sandwich sign" of dermatophytosis. *Am J Dermatopathol.* 1986;8:347–350.
29. Griffiths CE, Barker JN. Pathogenesis and clinical features of psoriasis. *Lancet.* 2007;370:263–271.
30. Guillet MH, Wierzbicka E, Guillet S, et al. A 3-year causative study of pompholyx in 120 patients. *Arch Dermatol.* 2007;143:1504–1508.
31. Guttman-Yassky E. Atopic dermatitis. *Curr Probl Dermatol.* 2007;35:154–172.
32. Haapalainen T, Oksala O, Kallioinen M, et al. Destruction of the epithelial anchoring system in lichen planus. *J Invest Dermatol.* 1995;105:100–103.
33. Hejazi N, Mehregen AH. Histologic study of inflammatory lesions. *Arch Dermatol.* 1975;111:37–39.

34. Hinchliffe SA, Ciftci AO, Khine MM, et al. Composition of the inflammatory infiltrate in pediatric penile lichen sclerosus et atrophicus (balanitis xerotica obliterans): a prospective, comparative immunophenotyping study. *Pediatr Pathol.* 1994;14:223–233.
35. Houck G, Saeed S, Stevens GL, et al. Eczema and the spongiotic dermatoses: a histologic and pathogenic update. *Semin Cutan Med Surg.* 2004;23:39–45.
36. Janin A, Socie G, Devergie A, et al. Fasciitis in chronic graft-versus-host disease: a clincopathologic study of 14 cases. *Ann Intern Med.* 1994;120:993–998.
37. Keat A. Reactive arthritis (review). *Adv Exp Med Biol.* 1999;455:201–206.
38. Kikuchi A, Naka W, Harada T, et al. Parapsoriasis en plaques: its potential for progression to malignant lymphoma. *J Am Acad Dermatol.* 1993;29:419–422.
39. Klemke CD, Dippel E, Dembinski A, et al. Clonal T cell receptor gamma-chain gene rearrangement by PCR-based GeneScan analysis in the skin and blood of patients with parapsoriasis and early-stage mycosis fungoides. *J Pathol.* 2002;197:348–354.
40. Kury S, Dreno B, Bezieau S, et al. Identification of *SLC39A4,* a gene involved in acrodermatitis enteropathica. *Nat Genet.* 2002;31:239–240.
41. Larcher C, Gasser A, Hattmannstorfer R, et al. Interaction of HSV-1 infected peripheral blood mononuclear cells with cultured dermal microvascular endothelial cells: a potential model for the pathogenesis of HSV-1 induced erythema multiforme. *J Invest Dermatol.* 2001;116(1):150–156.
42. Laxmisha C, Thappa DM. Generalized lichen nitidus with Down syndrome. *J Eur Acad Dermatol Venereol.* 2006;20:1156–1157.
43. LeBoit PE. Subacute radiation dermatitis: a histologic imitator of acute cutaneous graft-versus-host disease. *J Am Acad Dermatol.* 1989;20:236–241.
44. Lin RL, Janniger CK. Pityriasis alba. *Cutis.* 2005;76:21–24.
45. Lugović L, Situm M, Ozanić-Bulić S, et al. Phototoxic and photoallergic skin reactions. *Coll Antropol.* 2007;31(Suppl 1):63–67.
46. Magro CM, Crowson AN, Kovatich AJ, et al. Drug-induced reversible lymphoid dyscrasia: a clonal lymphomatoid dermatitis of memory and activated T cells. *Hum Pathol.* 2003;34:119–129.
47. Magro CM, Crowson AN, Morrison C, Li J. Pityriasis lichenoides chronica: stratification by molecular and phenotypic profile. *Hum Pathol.* 2007 Mar;38(3): 479–490. Epub 2007 Jan 19. PMID: 17239929 [PubMed—Indexed for MEDLINE].
48. Magro CM, Crowson AN. The immunoflourescent profile of dermatomyositis: a comparative study with lupus erythematosus. *J Cutan Pathol.* 1997;24(9):543–552.
49. Marinkovich MP, Botella R, Datloff J, Sangueza OP. Necrolytic migratory erythema without glucagonoma in patients with liver disease. *J Am Acad Dermatol.* 1995;32:604–609.
50. Mark BJ, Slavin RG. Allergic contact dermatitis. *Med Clin North Am.* 2006;90:169–185.
51. Marzano AV, Frezzolini A, Caproni M, et al. Immunohistochemical expression of apoptotic markers in drug-induced erythema multiforme, Stevens-Johnson syndrome and toxic epidermal necrolysis. *Int J Immunopathol Pharmacol.* 2007;20:557–566.
52. Maverakis E, Fung MA, Lynch PJ, et al. Acrodermatitis enteropathica and an overview of zinc metabolism. *J Am Acad Dermatol.* 2007;56:116–124.
53. Morgan MD, Stevens GL, Switlyk S. Benign lichenoid keratosis: a clinical and pathologic reappraisal of 1040 cases. *Am J Dermatopathol.* 2005;27:387–392.
54. Mozzanica N. Pathogenetic aspects of allergic and irritant contact dermatitis. *Clin Dermatol.* 1992;10: 115–121.
55. Muhlbauer JE, Bhan AK, Harrist TJ, et al. Immunopathology of pityriasis lichenoides acuta. *J Am Acad Dermatol.* 1984;10:783–795.
56. Mutasim DF, Meiri G. Bazex syndrome mimicking a primary autoimmune bullous disorder. *J Am Acad Dermatol.* 1999;40:822–825.
57. Nassif A, Bensussan A, Dorothee G, et al. Drug specific cytoxic T-cells in the skin lesions of a patient with toxic epidermal necrolysis. *J Invest Dermatol.* 2002;118(4):728–733.
58. Online Mendelian Inheritance in Man. http://www.ncb.inlm.nih.gov/sites/entrex?db=omn.
59. Petersel DL, Sigal LH. Reactive arthritis. *Infect Dis Clin North Am.* 2005;19:863–883.
60. Phelps RG, Miller MK, Singh F. The varieties of "eczema": clinicopathologic correlation. *Clin Dermatol.* 2003 Mar–Apr;21(2):95–100.
61. Posadas SH, Padial A, Torres MJ, et al. Delayed reactions to drugs show levels of perforin, granzyme b, and fas-l to be related to disease severity. *J Allergy Clin Immunol.* 2002;109:155–161.
62. Prieto VG, Casal M, McNutt NS. Immunohistochemistry detects differences between lichen planus-like keratosis, lichen planus, and lichenoid actinic keratosis. *J Cutan Pathol.* 1993;20:143–147.
63. Roujeau JC, Kelly JP, Naldi L, et al. Medication use and the risk of Stevens-Johnson syndrome or toxic epidermal necrolysis. *New Engl J Med.* 1995;333:1600–1607.
64. Schlesinger I, Oelrich DM, Tyring SK. Crusted (Norwegian) scabies in patients with AIDS: the range of clinical presentations. *South Med J.* 1994;87:352–356.

65. Schofield JK, De Berker D, Milligan A, et al. Keratin expression in cutaneous lichen planus. *Histopathology.* 1995;26:153–158.

66. Schwartz RA, Janusz CA, Janniger CK. Seborrheic dermatitis: an overview. *Am Fam Physician.* 2006;74:125–130.

67. Sigurgeirsson B, Lindelof B, Edhag O, et al. Risk of cancer in patients with dermatomyositis or polymositis: a population-based study. *New Engl J Med.* 1992;326:363–367.

68. Simon M, Flaig MJ, Kind P, et al. Large plaque parapsoriasis: clinical and genotypic correlations. *J Cutan Pathol.* 2000;27:57–60.

69. Sirot G. Nummular eczema. *Semin Dermatol.* 1983;2:68–74.

70. Smoller BR, Flynn TC. Immunohistochemical examination of lichen nitidus suggests that it is not a localized papular variant of lichen planus. *J Am Acad Dermatol.* 1992;27:232–236.

71. Spencer J, Silvers D, Grossman M. Pustular eruption after drug exposure: is it pustular psoriasis or a pustular drug eruption? *Br J Dermatol.* 1994;130:514–519.

72. Stein KR, Scheinfeld NS. Drug-induced photoallergic and phototoxic reactions. *Expert Opin Drug Saf.* 2007;6:431–443.

73. Stone OJ. Pellagra: increased viscosity of extracellular matrix. *Med Hypoth.* 1993;40:355–359.

74. Stur K, Karlhofer FM, Stingl G. Soluble fas ligand: a discriminating feature between drug-induced skin eruptions and viral exanthems. *J Invest Dermatol.* 2007;4:802–802.

75. Theeuwes M, Morhenn V. Allelic instability in the mitosis model and the inheritance of psoriasis (review). *Am Acad Dermatol.* 1995;32:44–52.

76. 1. Trautmann A, Disch R, Bröcker EB, et al. How does eczema arise? *J Dtsch Dermatol Ges.* 2003;1:8–11.

77. Tsankov N, Angelova I, Kazandjieva J. Drug-induced psoriasis. recognition and management. *Am J Clin Dermatol.* 2000;1:159–165.

78. Vennos EN, Collins M, James WD. Rothmund-Thomson syndrome: review of the world literature. *J Am Acad Dermatol.* 1992;27:750–762.

79. Viard I, Wehrli P, Bullani R, et al. Inhibition of toxic epidermal necrolysis by blockade of CD95 with human intravenous immunoglobulin. *Science.* 1998;282:490–493.

80. Walsh N, Prokopetz R, Tron V, et al. Histopathology in erythroderma: review of a series of cases by multiple observers. *J Cutan Pathol.* 1994;21:419–423.

81. Walsh NM, Prokopetz R, Tron VA, et al. Histopathology in erythroderma: review of a series of cases by multiple observers. *J Cutan Pathol.* 1994;21:419–423.

82. Warshaw EM, Ahmed RL, Belsito DV, et al. North American Contact Dermatitis Group. Contact dermatitis of the hands: cross-sectional analyses of North American Contact Dermatitis Group Data, 1994–2004. *J Am Acad Dermatol.* 2007;57:301–314.

83. Weinberg JM, Kristal L, Chooback L, et al. The clonal nature of pityriasis lichenoides. *Arch Dermatol.* 2002;138:1063–1067.

84. Weksberg R. Low-sister-chromatid-exchange Bloom syndrome cell lines: an important new tool for mapping the basic genetic defect in Bloom syndrome and for unraveling the biology of human tumor development. *Am J Hum Genet.* 1995;57:994–997.

85. Wood GS, Strickler JG, Abel EA. Immunohistology of pityriasis lichenoides et varioliformis acuta and pityriasis lichenoides chronia. Evidence for their interrelationship with lymphomatoid papulosis. *J Am Acad Dermatol.* 1987;16:559–570.

86. Yamamoto T, Osaki T. Characteristic cytokines generated by keratinocytes and mononuclear infiltrates in oral lichen planus. *J Invest Dermatol.* 1995;104:784–788.

87. Zelickson B, Muller S. Generalized pustular psoriasis: a review of 63 cases. *Arch Dermatol.* 1991;127: 1339–1345.

CHAPTER 2

Dermal-Based Inflammatory Diseases

QUESTION 2-1.

You are at a wedding reception and one of the guests develops the rapid onset of pruritic, diffuse, raised, edematous papules and plaques surrounded by a zone of erythema without surface alteration. There is expansion and coalescence with areas of central clearing. After a few hours, the eruption spontaneously resolves. The patient reports that a similar eruption occurred a year ago that also spontaneously resolved within several hours. The image below represents the histopathological findings associated with this condition. The epidermis is unremarkable. Which of the following regarding this patient's condition is INCORRECT?

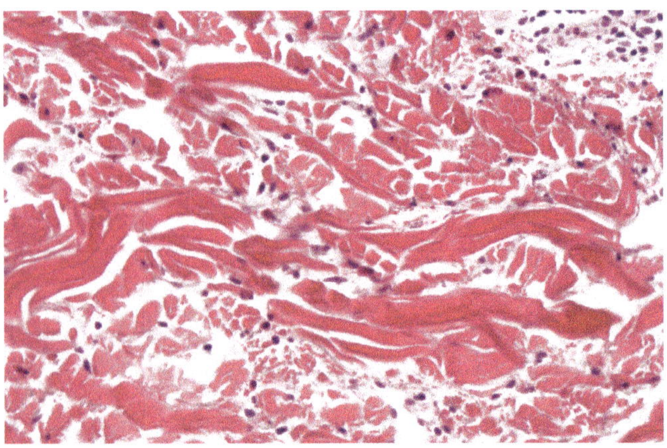

- A) Although this condition has characteristic clinical and histopathological findings, it is completely nonspecific in regards to etiology.
- B) Some chronic forms of the condition are associated with IgG autoantibodies that cross-link the alpha subunit of the high-affinity IgE receptor on mast cells and basophils.
- C) This patient most likely has the acute form of this condition since the two eruptions only lasted a few hours and occurred greater than 6 weeks apart.
- D) Common inciting triggers for the acute form of this condition include hot and cold temperatures, exposure to water and UV light, stress, exercise, and vibration and direct pressure to the skin.
- E) Severe swelling and edema of the lips, eyes, face, hands, and feet accompanied by airway obstruction is considered a medical emergency that may be treated with epinephrine.

QUESTION 2-2.

A female patient with gestational diabetes presents in her 35th week of a twin pregnancy with pruritic and erythematous papules and plaques near striae of the abdomen and proximal thighs. There is sparing of the umbilical region. A biopsy is performed. Which of the following statements regarding the histopathological findings of this condition is INCORRECT?

- A) This condition typically exhibits folliculocentric neutrophilic infiltrates and intrafollicular pustules resulting in degeneration of the outer root sheath epithelium.
- B) This condition typically exhibits superficial perivascular lymphocytic infiltrate with scattered eosinophils and papillary dermal edema.
- C) Epidermal changes of lymphocyte exocytosis and spongiosis may be seen in one-third of cases.

D) Direct immunofluorescence occasionally reveals granular deposits of IgM or IgA with complement (C3) along the dermal–epidermal junction and within vessels.

E) Leukocytoclastic debris may be present, but vascular fibrin deposition and fibrinoid necrosis of vessel walls is absent.

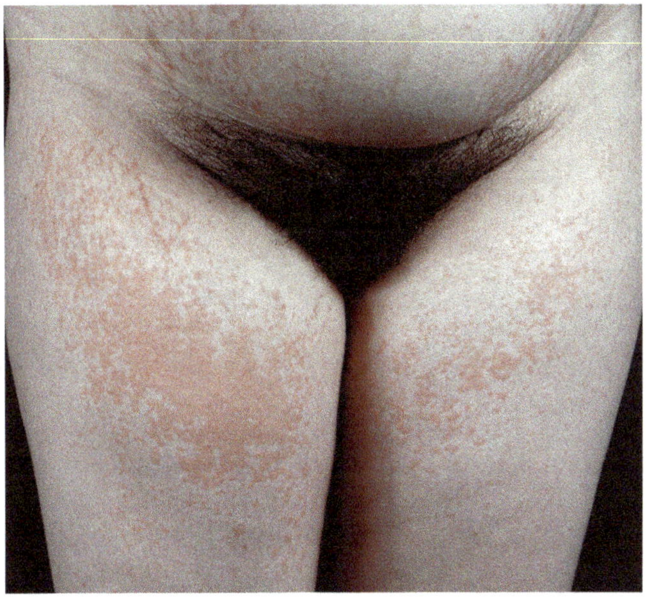

Reproduced, with permission, from Wolff K, Johnson RA, Saavedra AP. *Fitzpatrick's Color Atlas and Synopsis of Clinical Dermatology*. 6th ed. New York, NY: McGraw-Hill; 2009.

E) There is a superficial perivascular lymphocytic infiltrate with scattered eosinophils. The epidermis exhibits spongiosis with lymphocyte exocytosis and numerous large Langerhans cell–rich microvesicles.

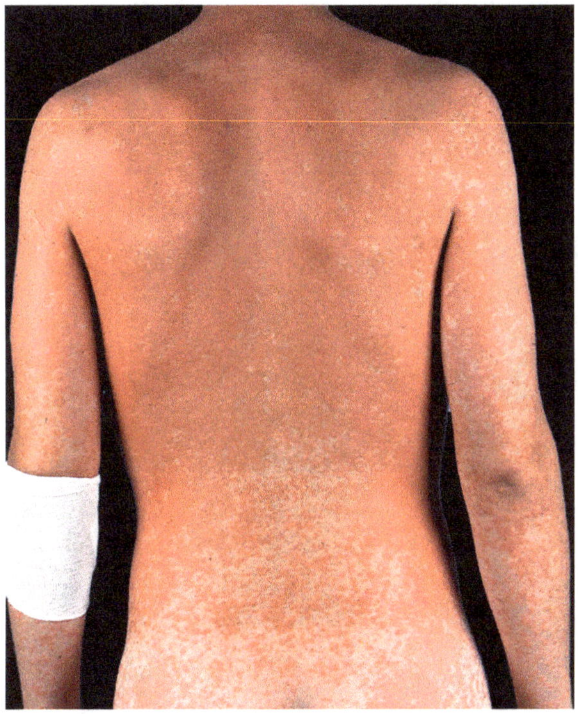

Reproduced, with permission, from Wolff K, Johnson RA, Saavedra AP. *Fitzpatrick's Color Atlas and Synopsis of Clinical Dermatology*. 6th ed. New York, NY: McGraw-Hill; 2009.

QUESTION 2-3.

A 26-year-old patient presents with a symmetric, erythematous, maculopapular eruption on the trunk and upper extremities after taking a 12-day course of amoxicillin for a sore throat. A biopsy is performed. Which of the following is the MOST likely microscopic description?

A) There is a superficial and mid dermal perivascular lymphocytic infiltrate with scattered eosinophils. The epidermis is unremarkable.

B) There is a superficial perivascular lymphohistiocytic infiltrate. The epidermis is unremarkable.

C) There is superficial dermal edema and a sparse superficial perivascular lymphocytic infiltrate with scattered interstitial neutrophils. Clusters of neutrophils are present within dilated vessels. The epidermis is unremarkable.

D) There is a sparse superficial dermal lymphocytic infiltrate with cytotoxic interface dermatitis and numerous dyskeratotic keratinocytes at all levels of the epidermis.

QUESTION 2-4.

A 27-year-old HIV positive male reports that he recently developed symmetric erythematous macules and patches on his chest, back, neck, and face. The palms and soles were not involved. The lesions have now resolved but left behind areas of hyperpigmentation. A biopsy is performed and the findings are illustrated below. Which of the following regarding this condition is INCORRECT?

A) The hyperpigmentation is a secondary reaction most likely due to a virus-associated dermal hypersensitivity reaction.

B) The pigment within the macrophages is melanin and will stain black on Fontana Masson stain.

C) The pigmented cells in the dermis will be positive for HMB45 via immunohistochemistry.

D) These lesions may also present clinically as hypopigmented macules.

E) The histopathology of the original active lesions would have most likely demonstrated superficial perivascular lymphohistiocytic infiltrates with mild vacuolar interface dermatitis or spongiosis.

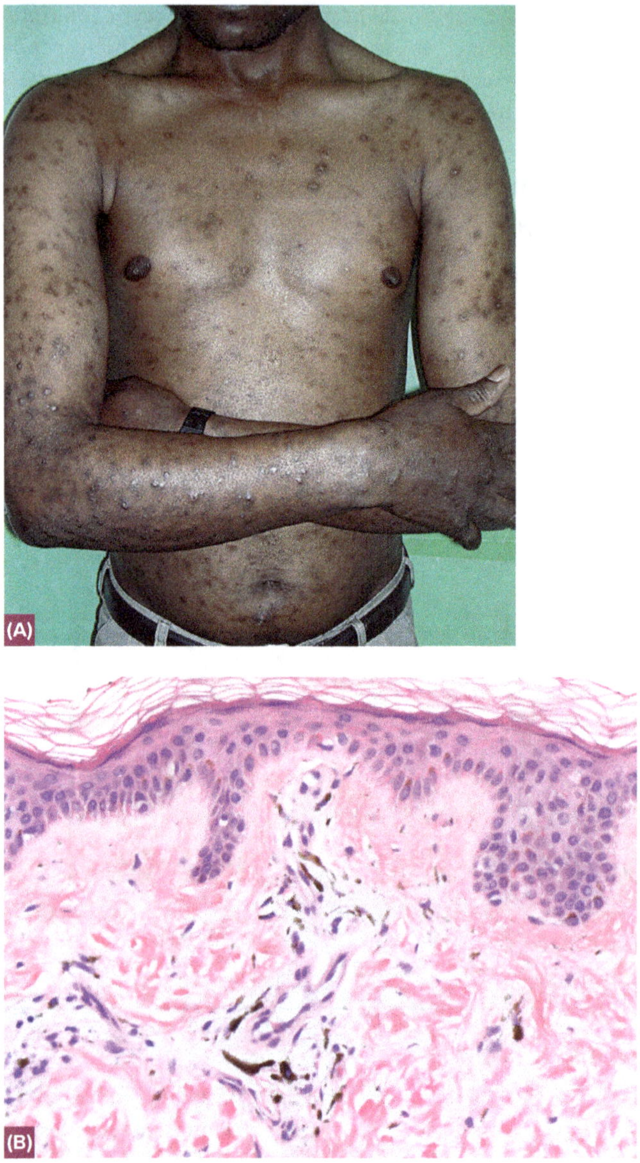

Part **(A)** reproduced, with permission, from Goldsmith LA, Katz SI, Gilchrest BA, Paller AS, Leffell DJ, Wolff K, eds. *Fitzpatrick's Dermatology in General Medicine.* 8th ed. New York, NY: McGraw-Hill Education; 2012.

QUESTION 2-5.

A 28-year-old patient presents with multiple pruritic papular lesions on the neck. Some of the lesions are excoriated. A biopsy is performed and the findings are illustrated below. Which of the following diagnoses is CORRECT?

- **A)** Eosinophilic pustular folliculitis
- **B)** Pityriasis lichenoides
- **C)** Morbilliform drug eruption
- **D)** Arthropod bite reaction
- **E)** Benign cutaneous lymphoid hyperplasia

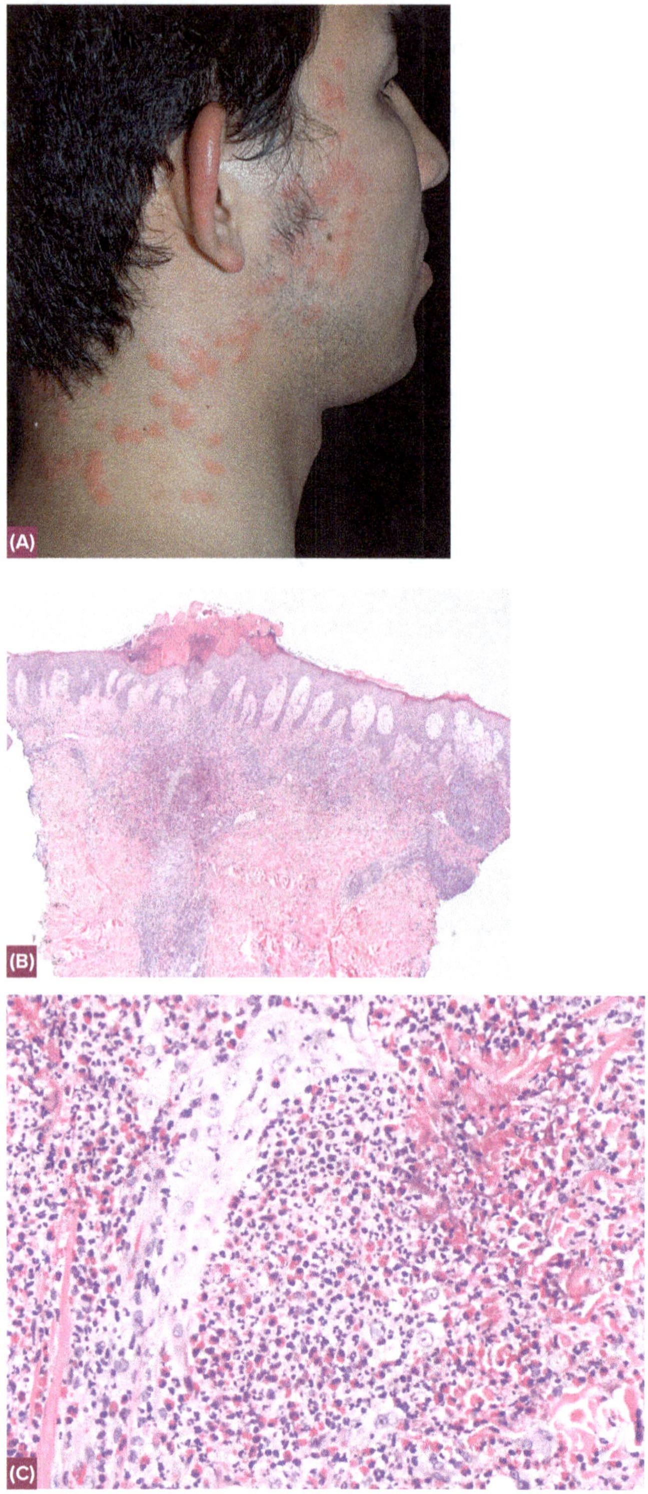

QUESTION 2-6.

A 40-year-old male patient presents with bilateral discrete clusters of pinhead-sized red flat macules and barely palpable papules confined to the distal lower extremities. Diascopy reveals pinpoint hemorrhages. The patient reports that the eruption has lasted for over 2 years. Hematologic workup is normal. A biopsy is performed. Which of the following microscopic descriptions is MOST reflective of this condition?

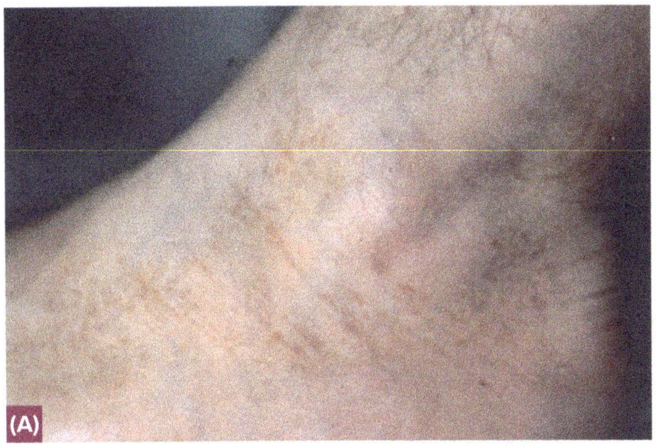

(A)

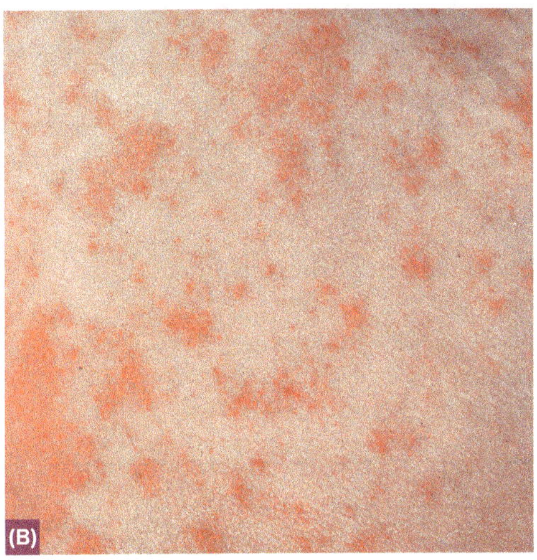

(B)

A) There are sparse superficial perivascular lymphocytic infiltrates with red blood cell extravasation and pigment containing macrophages. The pigment stains dark black on Fontana-Masson stain.
B) There are sparse superficial perivascular lymphocytic infiltrates with red blood cell extravasation and pigment containing macrophages. The pigment stains bright blue on Prussian blue stain.
C) There are superficial and deep perivascular neutrophilic infiltrates with leukocytoclasia, fibrin thrombi, fibrinoid necrosis of vessel walls, and numerous extravasated red blood cells.
D) There is a sparse superficial perivascular lymphocytic infiltrate with scattered interstitial neutrophils. No red blood cell extravasation is noted.
E) There is a superficial perivascular lymphocytic infiltrate with scattered eosinophils. The epidermis is spongiotic with lymphocyte exocytosis and Langerhans cell–rich microvesicles.

QUESTION 2-7.

A 17-year-old female cheerleader with anorexia nervosa presents with multiple, burning, erythematous to purplish papules and nodules on the toes and lateral feet. The lesions arose shortly after returning from a football game in which it was unusually cold. A biopsy is performed and the findings are illustrated below. The infiltrate is composed exclusively of lymphocytes and rare histiocytes. An alcian blue stain reveals increased deep dermal mucin with the highest concentration around the eccrine coils. Which of the following diagnoses is CORRECT?

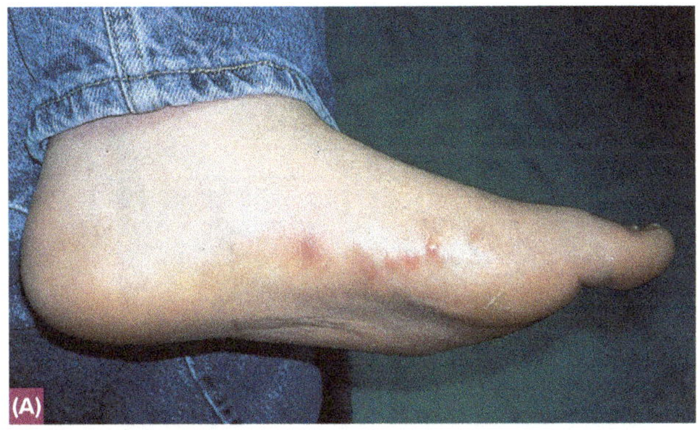

(A)

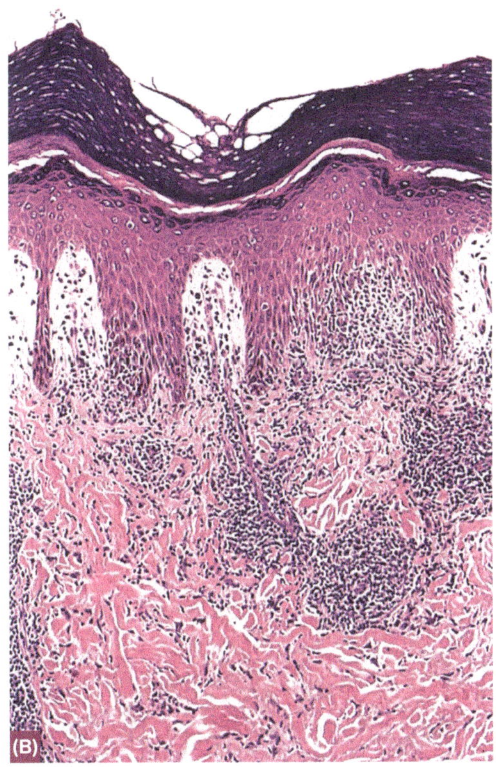

(B)

A) Leukocytoclastic vasculitis
B) Perniosis
C) Arthropod bites
D) Lichen planus
E) Polymorphous light eruption

QUESTION 2-8.

A 30-year-old female patient presents to your New York City office in late May with pruritic urticarial papules and erythematous papulovesicles on the hands, forearms, upper arms, and head and neck region. She reports that the eruption was of rapid onset and occurred shortly after spending the afternoon on her newly reopened rooftop terrace. A similar eruption occurred last spring that spontaneously resolved in a few days. Biopsies are performed and the findings are illustrated below. The inflammatory infiltrate is composed of lymphocytes, eosinophils, and neutrophils. Direct immunofluorescence reveals weak granular deposition of IgM and C3 around the superficial dermal vessels only. Serological studies are unremarkable. Which of the following diagnoses is CORRECT?

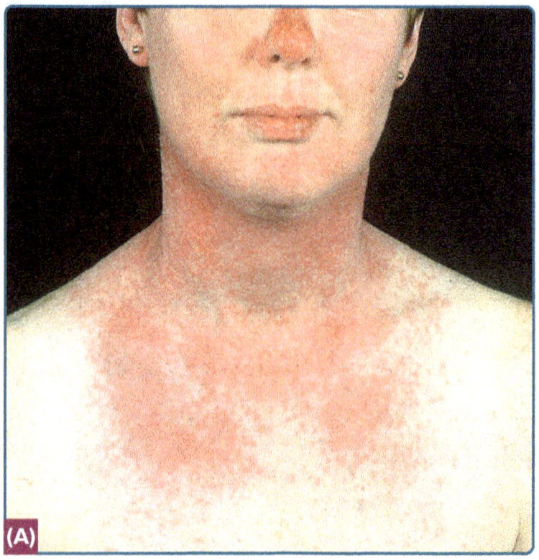

(A)

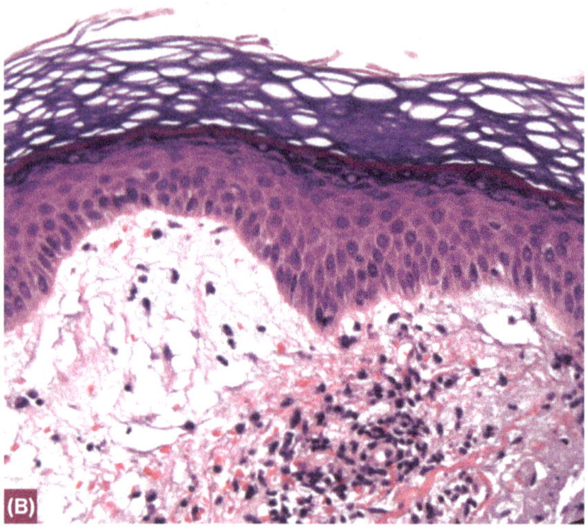

(B)

A) Bullous systemic lupus erythematosus
B) Arthropod bite reaction
C) Superficial erythema annulare centrifugum
D) Polymorphous light eruption
E) Bullous pemphigoid

QUESTION 2-9.

A 34-year-old male patient presents with persistent raised erythematous plaques on the face with a "succulent" appearance. Serological studies are unremarkable. Biopsies are performed and reveal robust superficial and deep perivascular lymphocytic infiltrates with periadnexal extension. Significant interface activity and follicular plugging are absent. Alcian blue stain reveals extensive dermal mucin deposition. Direct immunofluorescence reveals a nonspecific immunoreactant profile. Which of the following diagnoses is CORRECT?

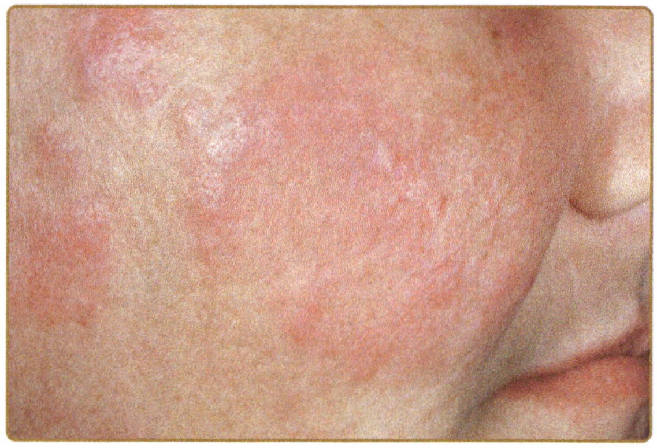

A) Erythema annulare centrifugum
B) Polymorphous light eruption
C) Morbilliform drug eruption
D) Urticaria
E) Tumid lupus erythematosus

QUESTION 2-10.

A patient who lives in New Mexico with no history of recent travel presents with a large, 5 cm, erythematous plaque with peripheral scale on a lower extremity. The lesion originally began as a pink infiltrated papule, which slowly enlarged to its current size over a period of 3 weeks. The patient reports no recent illnesses or other known conditions. A biopsy is performed and the findings are illustrated below. The infiltrate is composed of lymphocytes with rare eosinophils. Which of the following statements regarding this condition is CORRECT?

A) This eruption is associated in over 80% of cases with malignancies of parenchymal organs such as lung or kidney.
B) This eruption represents the cutaneous manifestation of a multisystem inflammatory disease associated with group A *Streptococcal* pharyngitis.
C) This eruption represents a cutaneous manifestation of stage I Lyme disease.
D) PAS stain will reveal hyphae within the stratum corneum.
E) This eruption represents a dermal hypersensitivity reaction with nonspecific etiology.

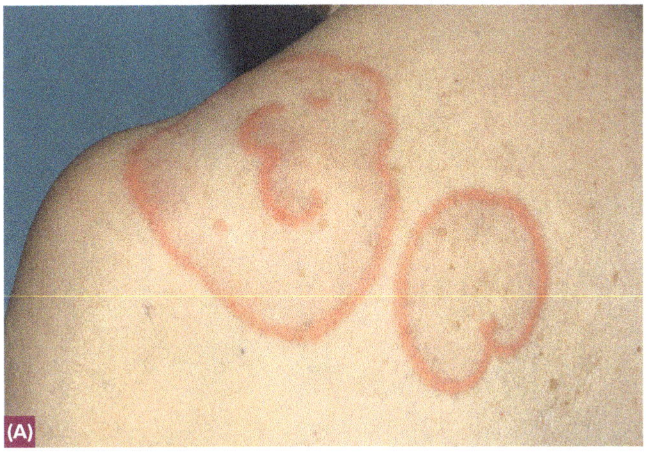

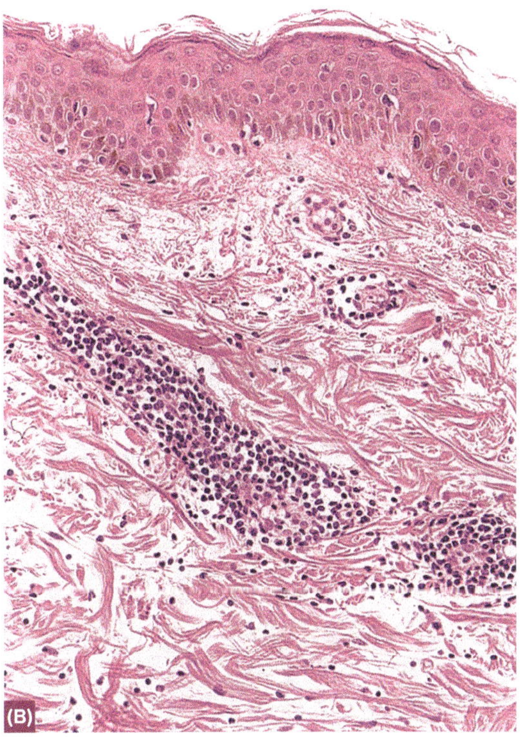

QUESTION 2-11.

Which form of gyrate erythema is associated with rheumatic fever?

A) Erythema annulare centrifugum
B) Erythema marginatum
C) Erythema migrans
D) Erythema gyratum repens

QUESTION 2-12.

Which form of gyrate erythema is associated with spirochete infection?

A) Erythema annulare centrifugum
B) Erythema marginatum
C) Erythema migrans
D) Erythema gyratum repens

QUESTION 2-13.

Which form of gyrate erythema is strongly associated with underlying malignancy?

A) Erythema annulare centrifugum
B) Erythema marginatum
C) Erythema migrans
D) Erythema gyratum repens

QUESTION 2-14.

A female patient presents with a persistently swollen upper lip, unilateral facial paralysis, and furrowed tongue. A biopsy is performed and the findings are illustrated below. Special stains for microorganisms (PAS, Gram, and Fite) are negative for microorganisms. Which of the following diagnoses is CORRECT?

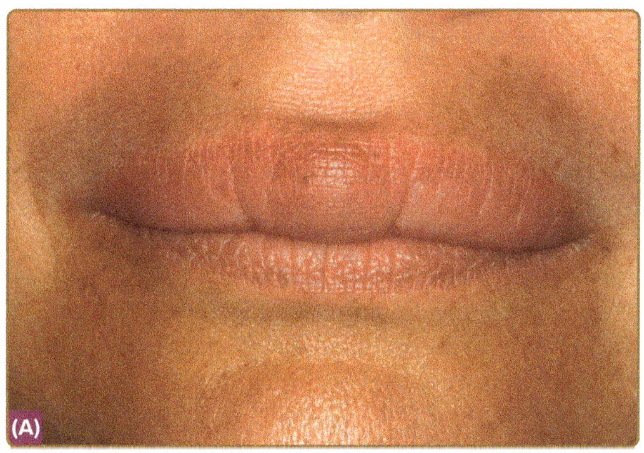

Reproduced, with permission, from Goldsmith LA, Katz SI, Gilchrest BA, Paller AS, Leffell DJ, Wolff K, eds. *Fitzpatrick's Dermatology in General Medicine*. 8th ed. New York, NY: McGraw-Hill Education; 2012.

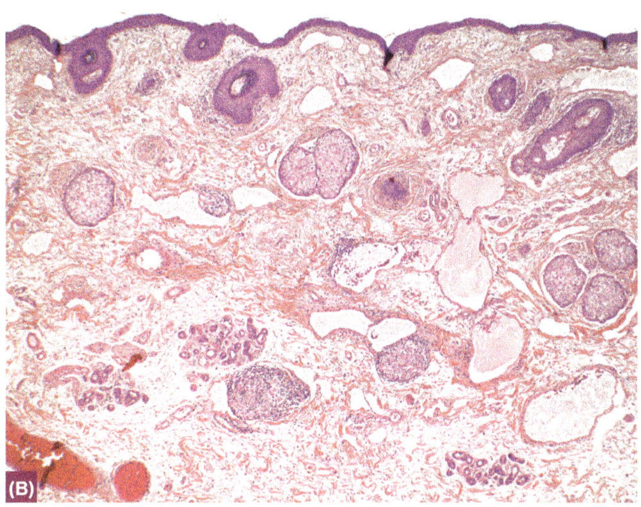

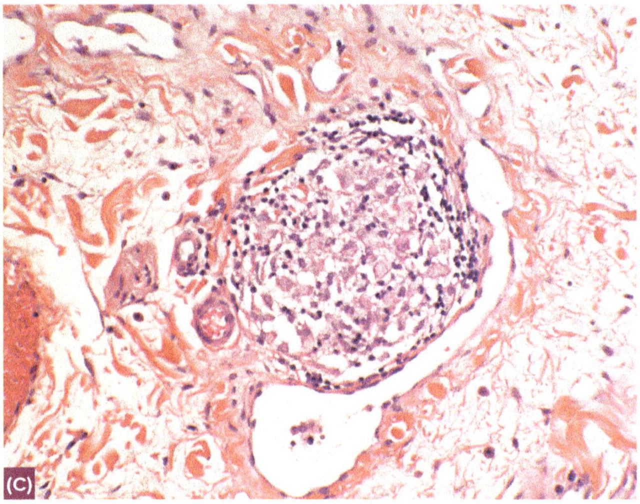

A) Granulomatous rosacea
B) Perioral dermatitis
C) Miescher-Melkersson-Rosenthal Syndrome
D) Lupus vulgaris
E) Sarcoidosis

QUESTION 2-15.

A female patient presents with deep linear "knife-cut" ulcers on the edges of the vulva with scattered aphthous ulcers on the labia majora. She has a history of chronic diarrhea, which is currently being treated with sulfasalazine. A biopsy is performed and the findings are illustrated below. The inflammatory infiltrate is composed of macrophages, lymphocytes, and plasma cells. Focal granulomatous vasculitis is noted. Special stains (PAS, Gram, and Fite) are negative for microorganisms. Which of the following diagnoses is CORRECT?

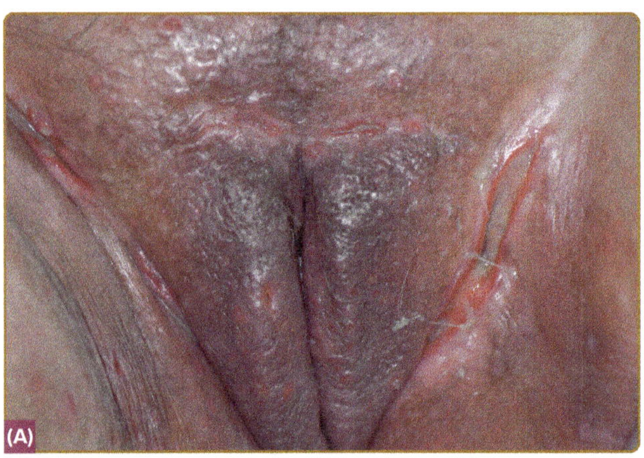

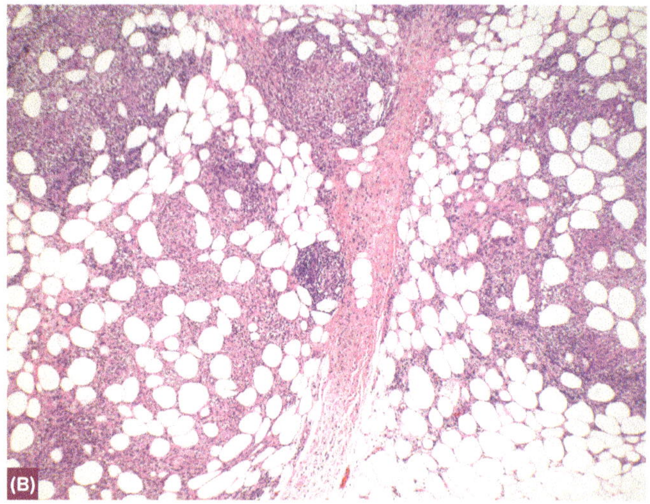

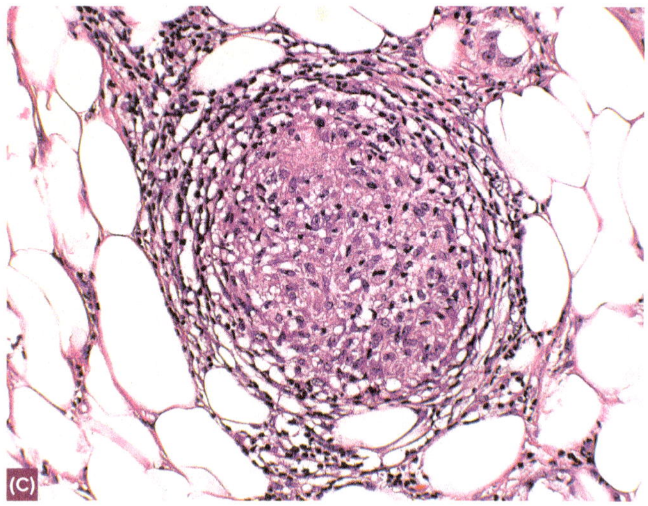

A) Hidradenitis suppurativa
B) Behçet disease
C) Cutaneous Crohn disease
D) Granulomatous slack skin disease
E) Erythema nodosum

QUESTION 2-16.

A 34-year-old African American female with pulmonary hypertension presents with a smooth-surfaced red, somewhat translucent, nodule surmounting a plaque on the upper lip. Telangiectasias are noted. A biopsy is performed and the findings are illustrated below. Special stains (PAS, Gram, and Fite) are negative for microorganisms. Which of the following statements regarding this patient's condition is INCORRECT?

A) The condition commonly presents with smooth-surfaced, violaceous nodules on the nose, cheeks, or earlobes.
B) Lesions of the scalp are commonly associated with secondary scarring alopecia.

C) Pulmonary involvement is frequently associated with elevated serum levels of angiotensin converting enzyme.
D) Occasionally, cytoplasmic positively birefringent crystals may be seen under polarized light.
E) This condition is a reaction to keratinous debris from a ruptured cyst, which may occur essentially at any site of the body.

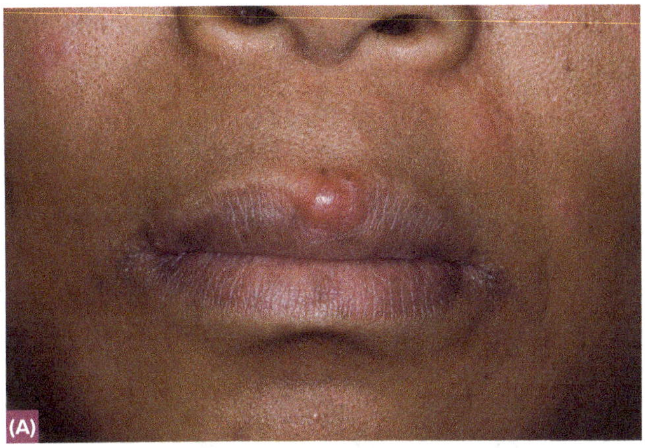

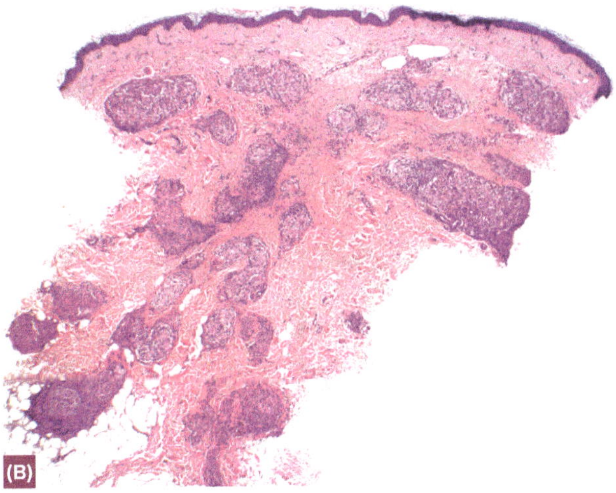

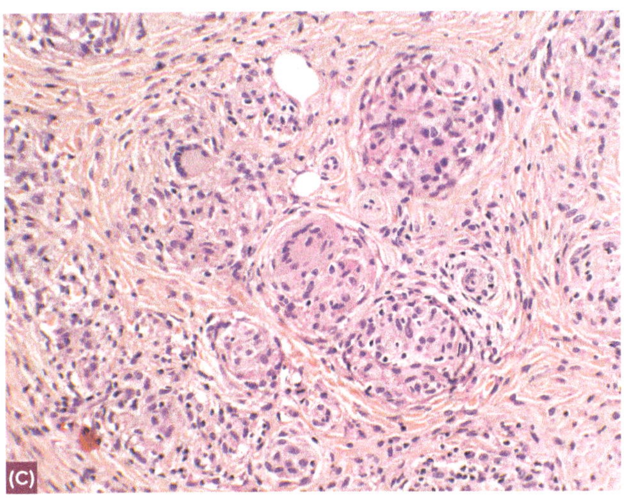

QUESTION 2-17.

A patient presents with a painful, nodular, erythematous swelling of the upper eyelid. A biopsy is performed and the findings are illustrated below. Which of the following diagnoses is CORRECT?

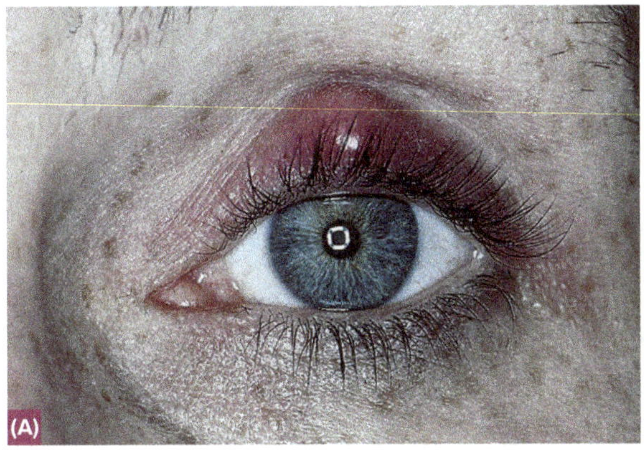

Reproduced, with permission, from Knoop KJ, Stack LB, Storrow AB, Thurman RJ. *The Atlas of Emergency Medicine*. 3rd ed. New York, NY: McGraw-Hill; 2010.

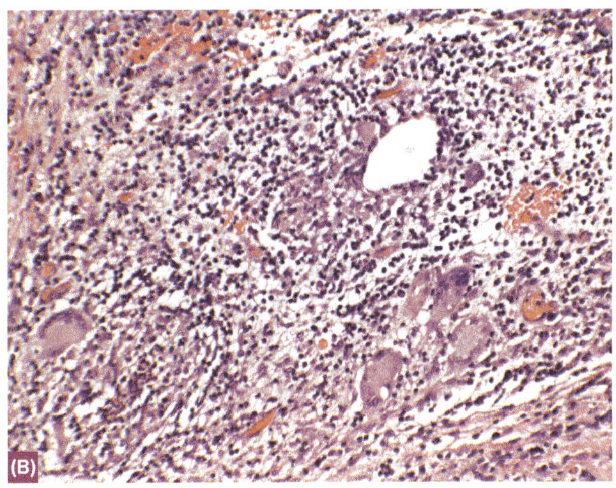

A) Chalazion
B) Sebaceous carcinoma
C) Lupus miliaris disseminatus faciei
D) Miescher-Melkersson-Rosenthal syndrome
E) Acne rosacea

QUESTION 2-18.

A patient presents with pink to erythematous coalescent papules and plaques in annular and polycyclic configurations on the dorsal surface of the ankle and foot. The lesions exhibit slightly depressed central areas. A biopsy is performed and the findings are illustrated below. Rare eosinophils are noted. An alcian blue stain reveals increased dermal mucin in the center of the lesion and in between collagen bundles. Which of the following diagnoses is CORRECT?

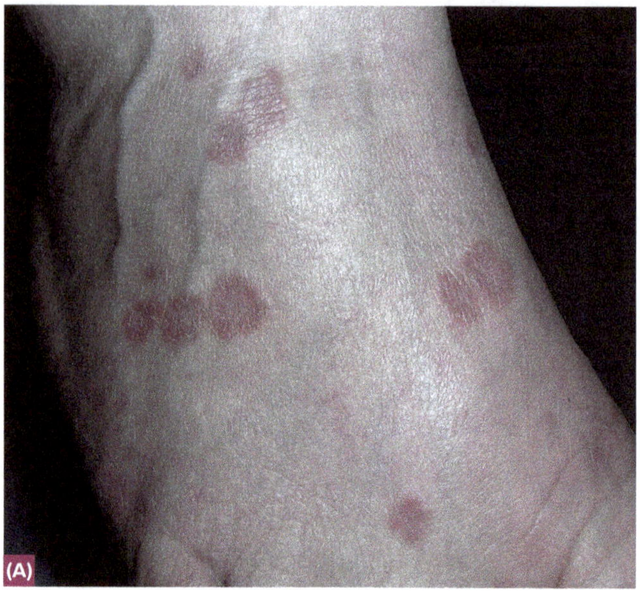

Reproduced, with permission, from Usatine RP, Smith MA, Mayeaux EJ Jr, Chumley HS, eds. *Color Atlas of Family Medicine.* 2nd ed. New York, NY: McGraw-Hill Education; 2012.

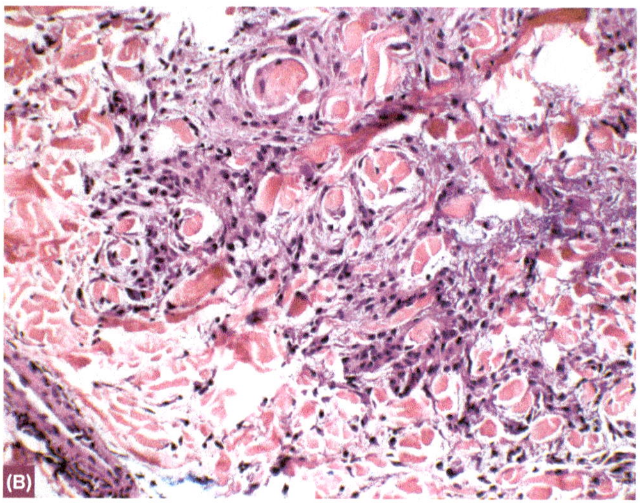

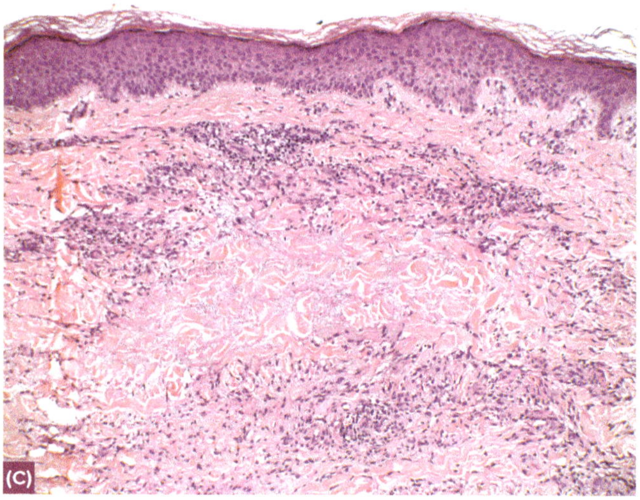

A) Interstitial granulomatous drug eruption
B) Necrobiosis lipoidica
C) Palisaded neutrophilic and granulomatous dermatitis
D) Granuloma annulare
E) Dermatofibroma

QUESTION 2-19.

A 76-year-old female patient with IgG paraproteinemia presents with indurated papules and nodules in the periorbital area and on the leg. The lesions vary in color from red–orange to violaceous and involve the dermis and subcutaneous tissue. There is central atrophy with telangiectasias. The leg lesion contains a large area of ulceration. A biopsy is performed and the findings are illustrated below. The infiltrate is composed mostly of lymphocytes, macrophages, and plasma cells. Which of the following diagnoses is CORRECT?

A) Annular elastolytic granuloma
B) Necrobiosis lipoidica
C) Xanthogranuloma
D) Necrobiotic xanthogranuloma
E) Pyoderma gangrenosum

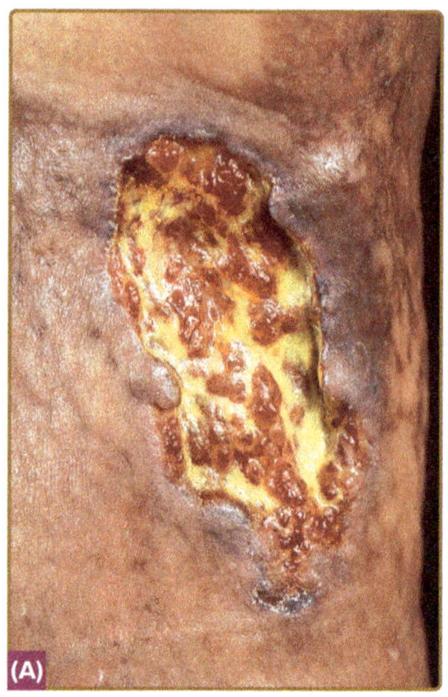

Leg. (Reproduced, with permission, from Goldsmith LA, Katz SI, Gilchrest BA, Paller AS, Leffell DJ, Wolff K, eds. *Fitzpatrick's Dermatology in General Medicine.* 8th ed. New York, NY: McGraw-Hill Education; 2012.)

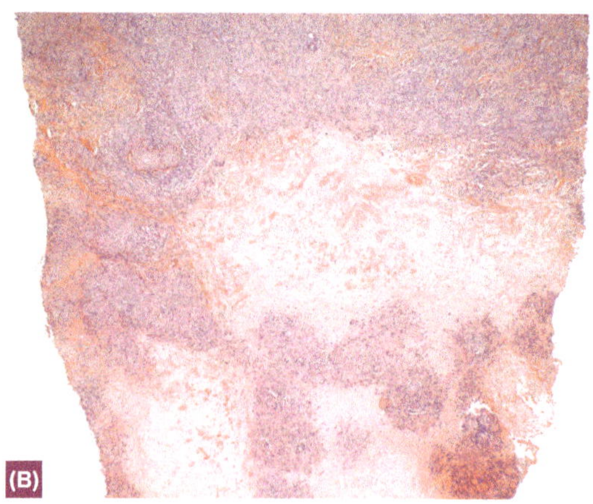

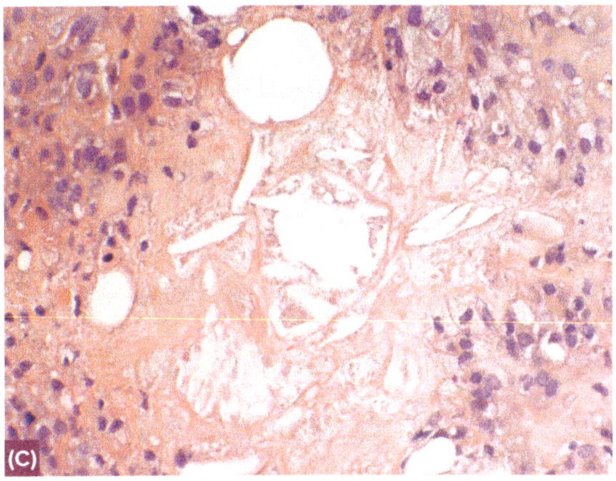
(C)

QUESTION 2-20.

A 30-year-old female presents with bilateral brown indurated plaques with prominent blood vessels on the anterior lower legs. A biopsy is performed and the findings are illustrated below. Which of the following statements regarding this condition is INCORRECT?

A) Rarely, these lesions may appear on the trunk and upper extremities and tend to have a papulonodular appearance.
B) This condition is associated with diabetes mellitus and the degree of hyperglycemia and diabetic control correlates with the onset and resolution of cutaneous lesions.
C) Alcian blue stain is typically negative for dermal mucin.
D) This condition most commonly arises in women.
E) The etiology and pathogenesis of this condition are not fully understood, but microangiopathic changes, immune complex–mediated vasculitis, and a thrombotic tendency have been implicated.

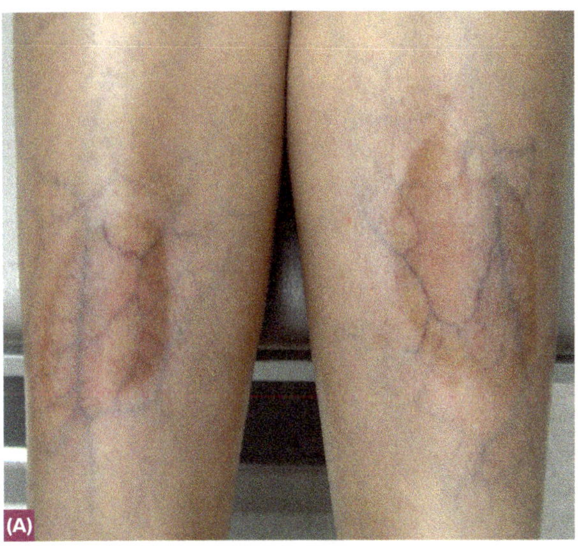
(A)

Reproduced, with permission, from Usatine RP, Smith MA, Mayeaux EJ Jr, Chumley HS, eds. *Color Atlas of Family Medicine*. 2nd ed. New York, NY: McGraw-Hill Education; 2012.

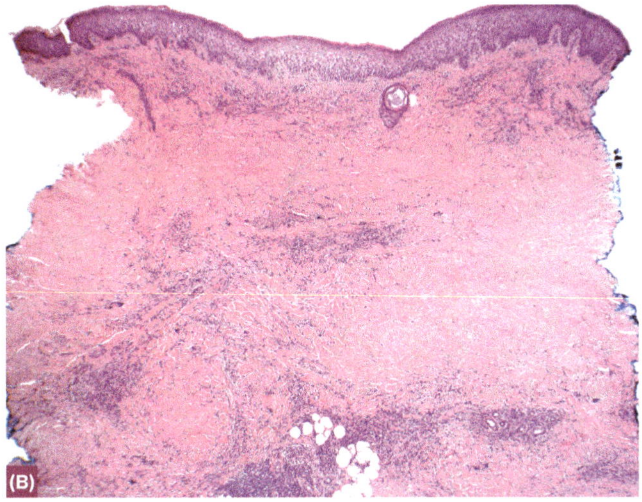
(B)

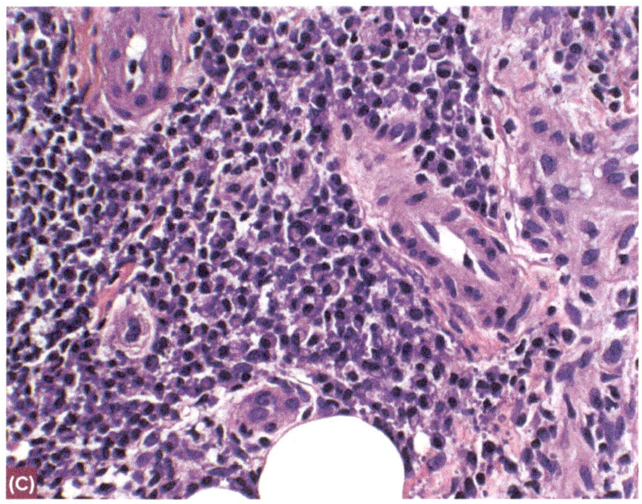
(C)

QUESTION 2-21.

A 59-year-old nurse presents to your office with a complaint of intermittent episodes of pain, stiffness, and swelling in both hands and wrists for approximately 1 year. The episodes last for several weeks and then resolve. More recently, she noticed similar symptoms in her knees and ankles. Joint pain and stiffness are making it harder for her to get out of bed in the morning and are interfering with her ability to perform her duties at work. The joint stiffness usually lasts for several hours before improving. She also reports malaise and easy fatigability for the past few months, but she denies having fever, chills, skin rashes, and weight loss. Physical examination reveals the presence of bilateral swelling, redness, and tender nodules on most proximal interphalangeal (PIP) joints, metacarpophalangeal (MCP) joints, the wrists, and the knees. A biopsy of one of the nodules is performed and the findings are illustrated below. Which of the following statements regarding this condition is INCORRECT?

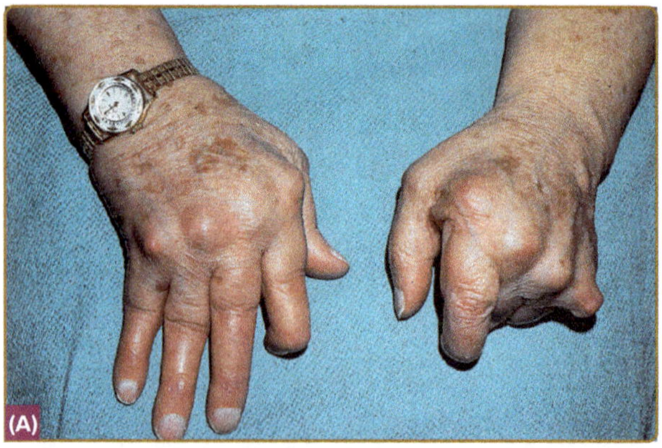

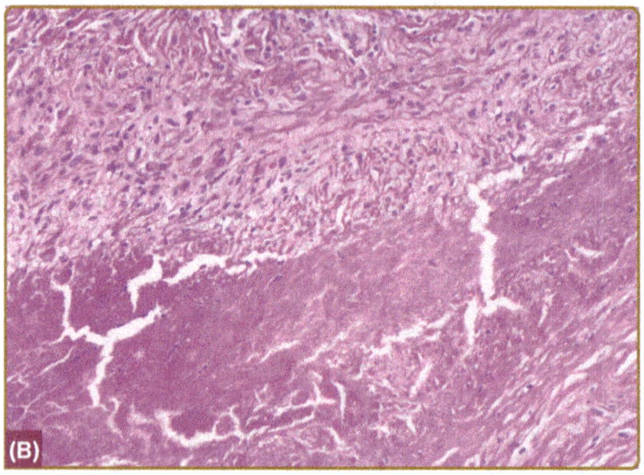

Reproduced, with permission, from Goldsmith LA, Katz SI, Gilchrest BA, Paller AS, Leffell DJ, Wolff K, eds. *Fitzpatrick's Dermatology in General Medicine*. 8th ed. New York, NY: McGraw-Hill Education; 2012.

A) The histopathologic findings reflect chronic changes associated with immune complex-mediated vasculitis.
B) Alcian blue stain will be negative for dermal mucin within the center of the lesion.
C) Similar lesions involving the myocardium may be a sequela of *Streptococcal* pharyngitis.
D) The mononuclear cells are positive for vimentin and cytokeratin.
E) Some patients with this condition may have nail fold telangiectasias, digital ulcerations, and digital pulp papules characterized histopathologically by leukocytoclastic vasculitis.

QUESTION 2-22.

A biopsy is obtained from a patient with hyperlipidemia. Which of the following clinical presentations is LEAST likely to be associated with the histopathological findings illustrated below? The overlying epidermis is unremarkable. Special stains for microorganisms are negative.

A) Asymptomatic, soft, polygonal, yellow-orange papules and plaques localized to upper and lower eyelids and around inner canthus.
B) Large yellow to skin colored subcutaneous tumors that are adherent to the Achilles tendon and extensor finger tendons.
C) Firm yellowish nodules frequently located on the elbow, hand, or over other large joints.
D) Crops of yellow or hyperpigmented papules with erythematous halos in Caucasian patients and hyperpigmented papules in African American patients.

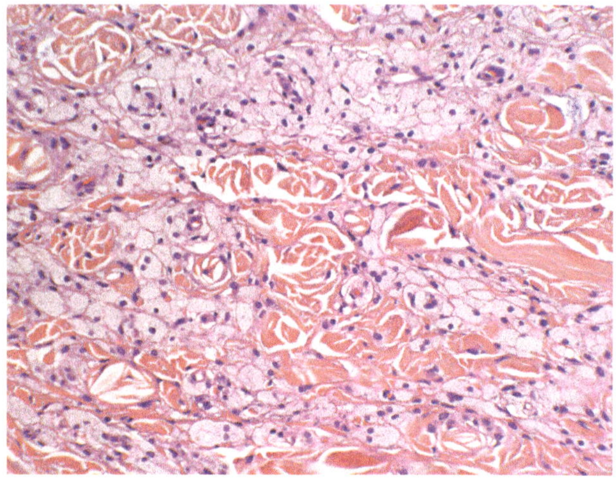

QUESTION 2-23.

Which of the following statements regarding the lesion illustrated below is INCORRECT?

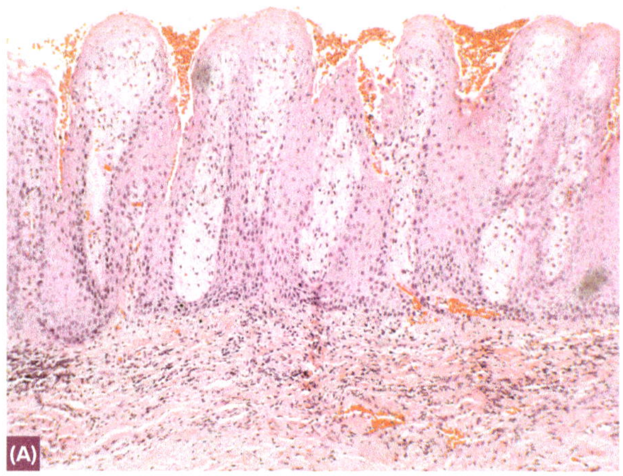

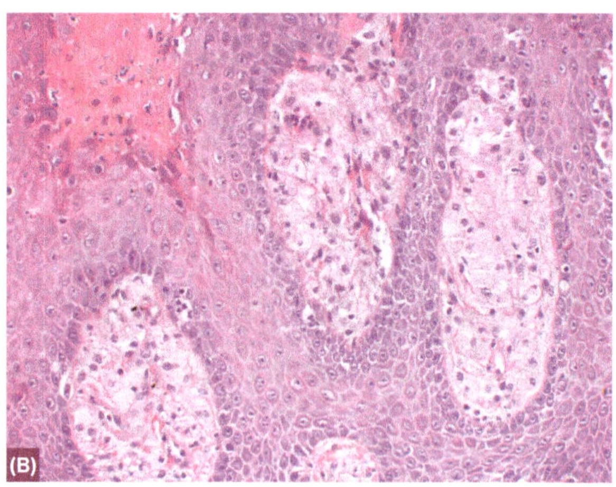

A) These lesions typically present as yellowish-red, slightly elevated plaques on the neck in patients with multiple myeloma.
B) These lesions most commonly present as yellow-red verrucous plaques on the gingiva or hard palate.
C) These lesions are not associated with diabetes or hyperlipidemia.
D) These lesions frequently present on the penis, vulva, scrotum, groin, anus, or nostril.
E) Nonmucosal lesions are a characteristic lesion in CHILD syndrome and mutations in the 3β-hydroxysteroid dehydrogenase gene.

QUESTION 2-24.

A patient presents with numerous red-brown to yellow papules that become confluent to form large plaques. Flexural areas of the neck, axillae, antecubital fossae, groin, and perianal region are preferentially affected. Oral and conjunctival lesions are present. The patient reports excessive thirst and excretion of large amounts of severely diluted urine. A biopsy is performed and the findings are illustrated below. Immunohistochemistry reveals the lesional cells to be CD68+, CD163+, S100−, and CD1a−. Which of the following diagnoses is CORRECT?

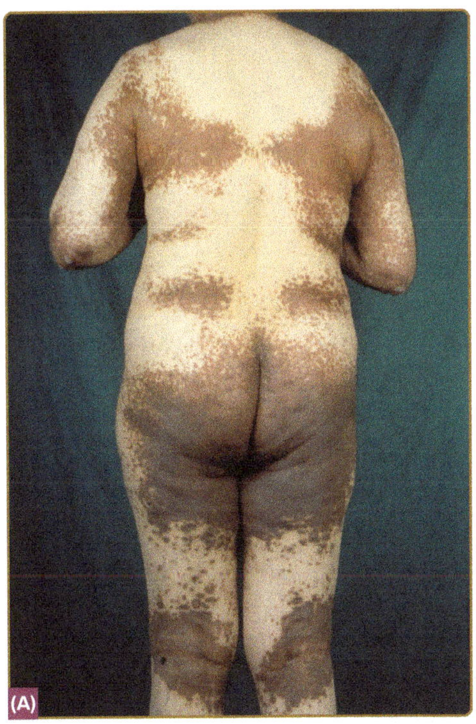
(A)

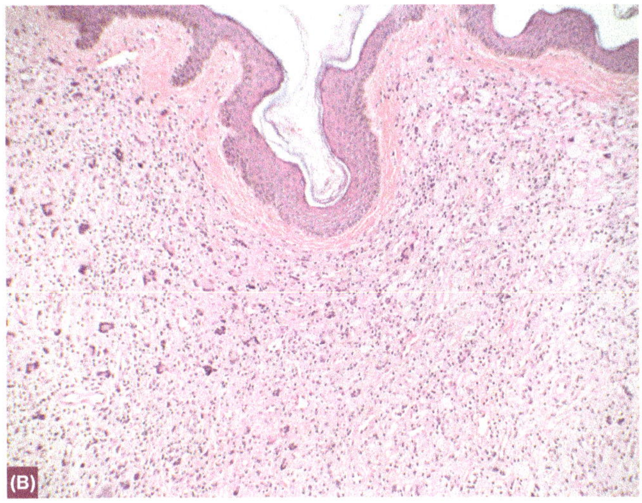
(B)

A) Xanthogranuloma
B) Benign cephalic histiocytosis
C) Generalized eruptive histiocytosis
D) Xanthoma disseminatum
E) Langerhans cell histiocytosis

QUESTION 2-25.

A female patient presents with yellow-brown cutaneous papules and nodules that are distributed over the hands and forearms. You notice a periungual arrangement of some of these nodules. Additionally, there are mucocutaneous nodules of the perioral and perinasal areas. The patient reports a history of arthritis. A biopsy of the hand is performed and the findings are illustrated below. Which of the following statements regarding this condition is INCORRECT?

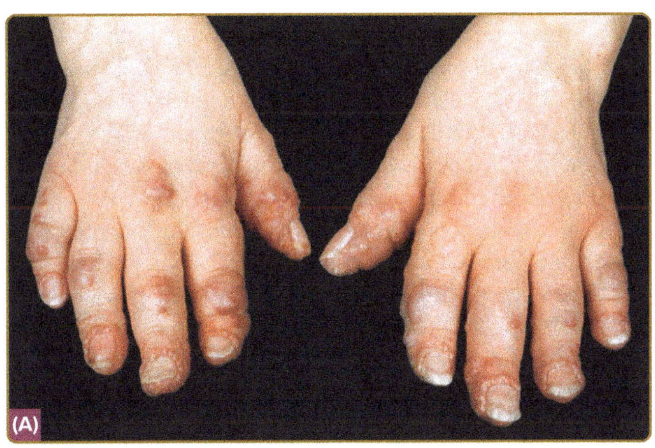
(A)

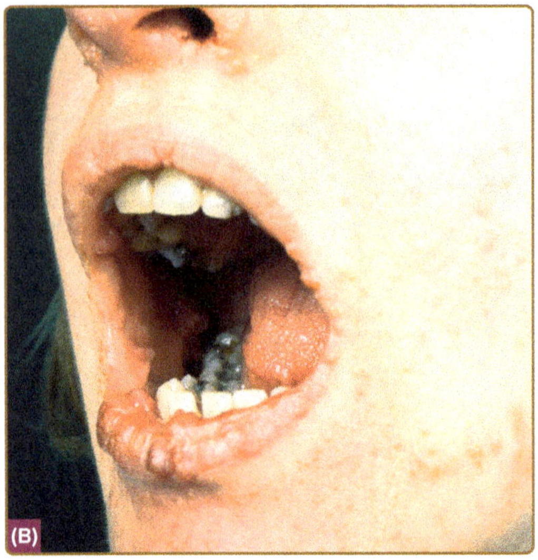

Parts **(A)** and **(B)** reproduced, with permission, from Goldsmith LA, Katz SI, Gilchrest BA, Paller AS, Leffell DJ, Wolff K, eds. *Fitzpatrick's Dermatology in General Medicine.* 8th ed. New York, NY: McGraw-Hill Education; 2012.

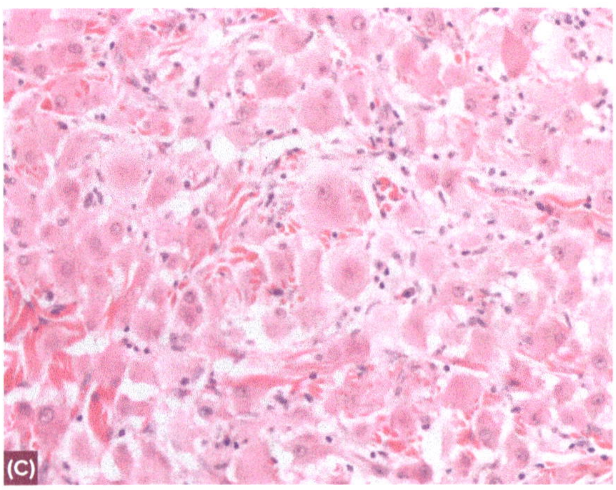

A) This condition has been associated with gastrointestinal and ovarian malignancies as well as various autoimmune diseases.
B) The large mono- and multinucleated cells with bright eosinophilic cytoplasm will be CD68+, CD163+, S100−, and CD1a− via immunohistochemistry.
C) The eosinophilic cytoplasms of the mono- and multinucleated cells are PAS-positive and diastase resistant.
D) Solitary tumors with similar histomorphology may exhibit emperipolesis of other inflammatory cells by histiocytes. These solitary tumors are not associated with arthritis.
E) This condition is much more common in males than females.

QUESTION 2-26.

A young patient presents with yellowish macules and patches, and reddish-brown papules and plaques on the neck and face. Some of the lesions are eroded and ulcerated. Massive painless bilateral cervical lymphadenopathy is appreciated. A skin biopsy is performed and the findings are illustrated below. Which of the following statements regarding this condition is INCORRECT?

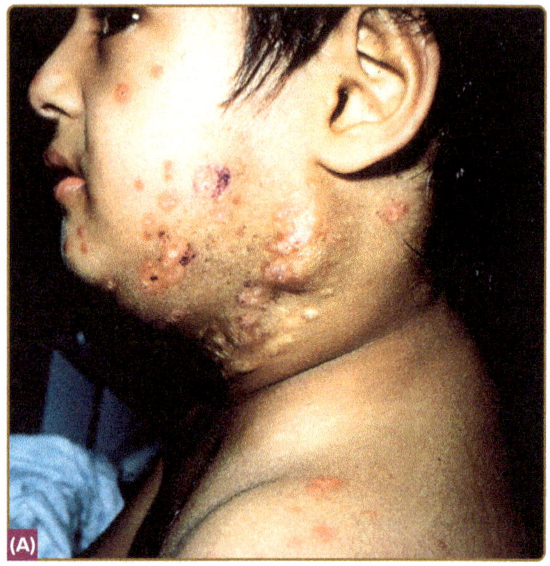

Reproduced, with permission, from Goldsmith LA, Katz SI, Gilchrest BA, Paller AS, Leffell DJ, Wolff K, eds. *Fitzpatrick's Dermatology in General Medicine*. 8th ed. New York, NY: McGraw-Hill Education; 2012.

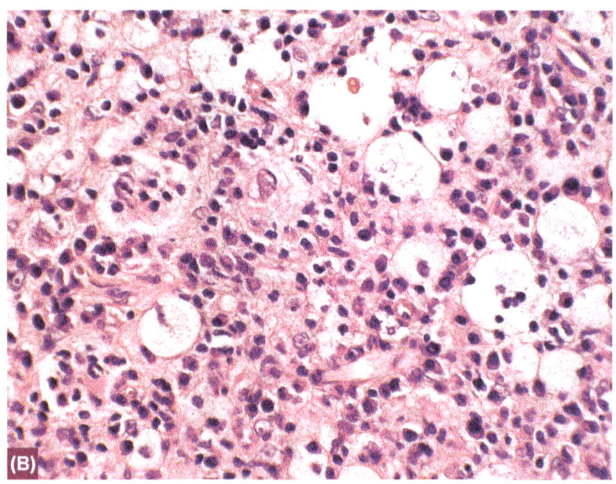

A) This is a benign generally self-limited disease confined mainly to cervical lymph nodes and only involves the skin in only 30% of cases.
B) Patients frequently present with fever, leukocytosis, hypergammaglobulinemia, and an elevated erythrocyte sedimentation rate.

C) The large multinucleated cells are CD68+, CD163+, S100+, and CD1a– via immunohistochemistry.
D) Dilated lymphatic channels with intraluminal histiocytes and thick-walled vessels surrounded by plasma cells are a distinctive finding.
E) Cytophagocytosis of red blood cells, lymphocytes, plasma cells, and neutrophils by the large histiocytes is a characteristic finding.

QUESTION 2-27.

An 81-year-old patient presents with diffuse yellow-erythematous papuloscaling and papulocrusted lesions on the trunk. Noduloulcerative lesions involving the gingival mucosa are noted. The patient reports dyspnea as well as excessive thirst and frequent urination. Physical examination reveals hepatosplenomegaly. A skin biopsy is performed and the findings are illustrated below. The mono- and multinucleated cells are CD68–, CD163–, S100+, and CD1a+ via immunohistochemistry. Which of the following diagnoses is CORRECT?

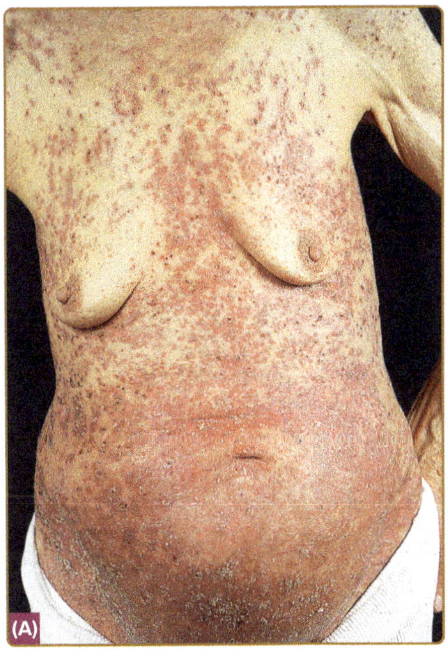
(A)

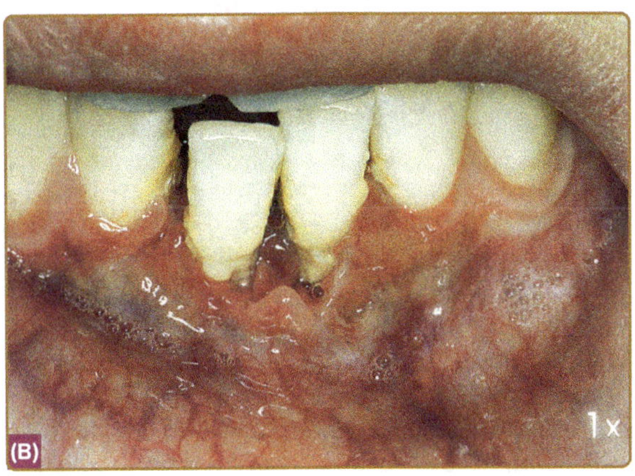
(B)

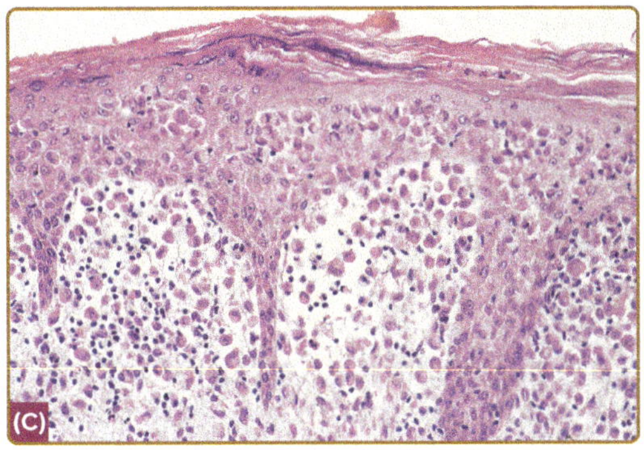
(C)

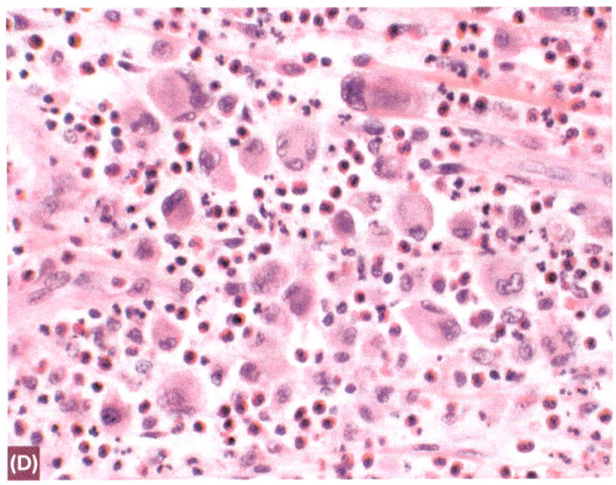
(D)

Parts **(A)**, **(B)**, and **(C)** reproduced, with permission, from Goldsmith LA, Katz SI, Gilchrest BA, Paller AS, Leffell DJ, Wolff K, eds. *Fitzpatrick's Dermatology in General Medicine*. 8th ed. New York, NY: McGraw-Hill Education; 2012.

A) Rosai–Dorfman disease
B) Xanthoma disseminatum
C) Langerhans cell histiocytosis
D) Multicentric reticulohistiocytosis
E) Anaplastic large cell lymphoma

QUESTION 2-28.

Which of the following conditions does NOT contain cutaneous infiltrates by the cell-type illustrated below?

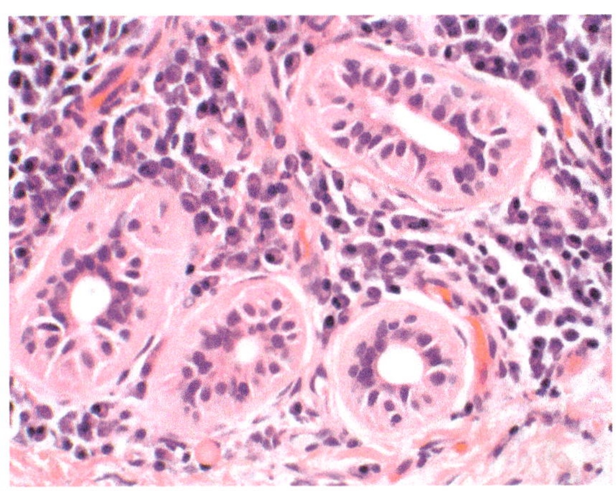

A) Urticaria pigmentosa
B) Zoon balanitis
C) Syphilis
D) Multicentric Castleman disease
E) Granuloma inguinale

QUESTION 2-29.

Which of the following clinical conditions is LEAST likely to be associated with the histopathologic findings illustrated below? The cells of the infiltrate are positive for tryptase and Giemsa staining.

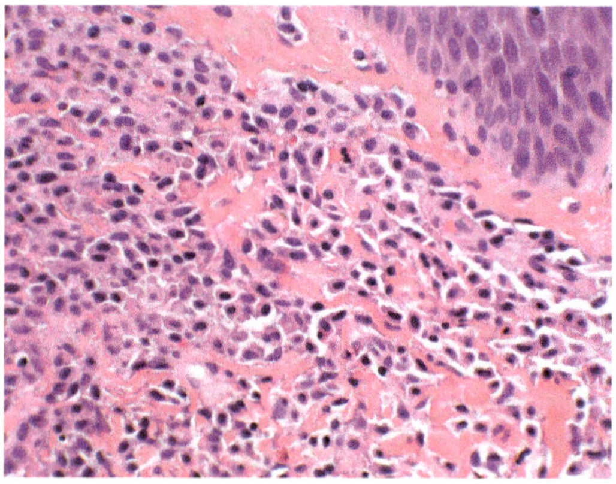

A) Urticaria pigmentosa
B) Solitary mastocytoma
C) Systemic mastocytosis
D) Telangiectasia macularis eruptiva perstans
E) Diffuse cutaneous mastocytosis

QUESTION 2-30.

A patient presents with arcuate, erythematous plaques on an extremity and abdomen. The lesions slowly resolve to form gray indurated plaques. A biopsy is performed and the findings are illustrated below. Which of the following diagnoses is CORRECT?

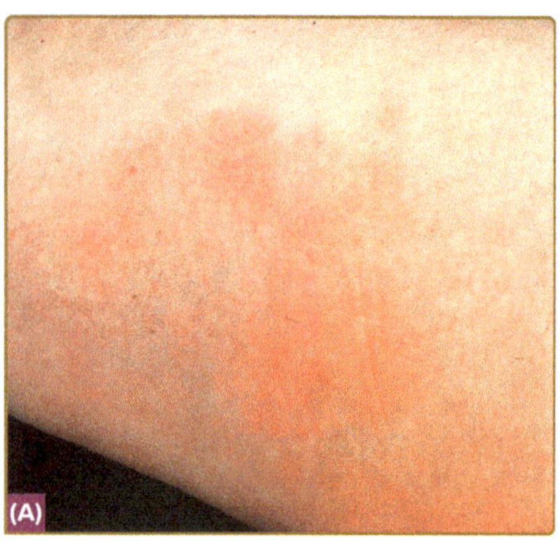

(A)

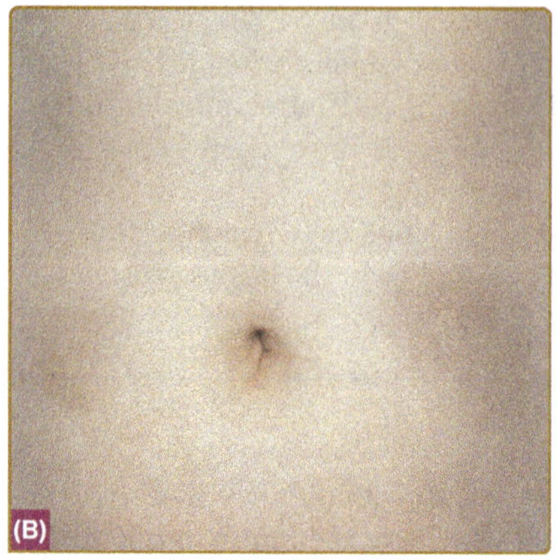

(B)

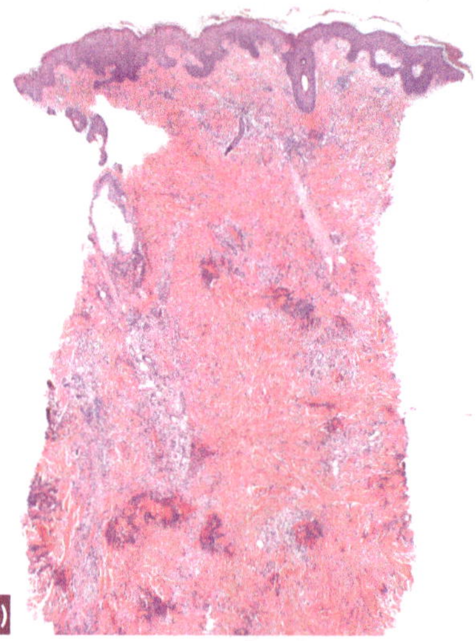

(C)

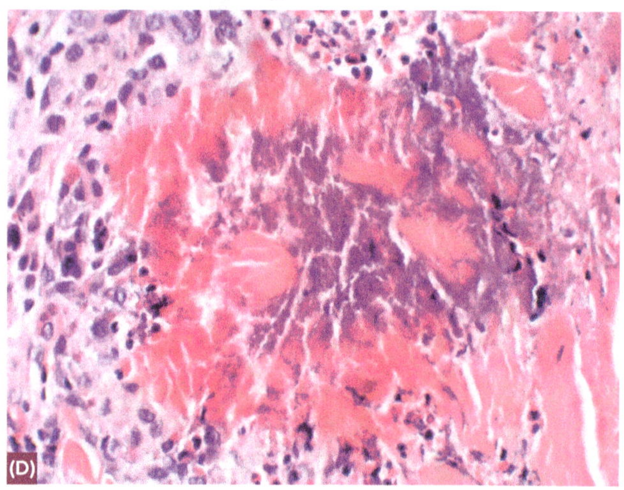

(D)

Parts **(A)** and **(B)** reproduced, with permission, from Goldsmith LA, Katz SI, Gilchrest BA, Paller AS, Leffell DJ, Wolff K, eds. *Fitzpatrick's Dermatology in General Medicine*. 8th ed. New York, NY: McGraw-Hill Education; 2012.

A) Ofuji disease
B) Tungiasis
C) Wells syndrome
D) Angiolymphoid hyperplasia with eosinophilia
E) Urticarial phase of bullous pemphigoid

ANSWERS

ANSWER 2-1: D.

The biopsy reveals a sparse perivascular lymphocytic infiltrate with scattered interstitial neutrophils and rare eosinophils. The epidermis is uninvolved (not visualized). The findings are consistent with **urticaria**. Urticarias are common, transient eruptions that affect roughly 15% of the population at some time in life. They comprise palpable erythematous papules or wheals that lack surface alteration and wax and wane without a clinical residuum. Lesions of urticaria are typically "here today and gone tomorrow," unlike urticarial rashes induced by drugs or **urticarial vasculitis**, in which the individual lesions may resemble urticaria but persist for several days. Urticarias may be acute or chronic; the latter defined as transient and fluctuating eruptions that last longer than 6 weeks. In general, **acute urticaria** typically reflects a type I (IgE-mediated) hypersensitivity response, while **chronic urticaria** has a more complex pathogenesis including physical, IgE-mediated, immune-complex-, or histamine-releasing agent-mediated types (Table 2-1A). Both immunologic and non-immunologic mechanisms may cause mast cell or basophil degranulation. The main mediators include histamine, prostaglandins, and interleukin 1 (IL-1). While patch testing may occasionally reveal the inciting antigen in acute urticaria, the majority of acute and chronic cases remain idiopathic.

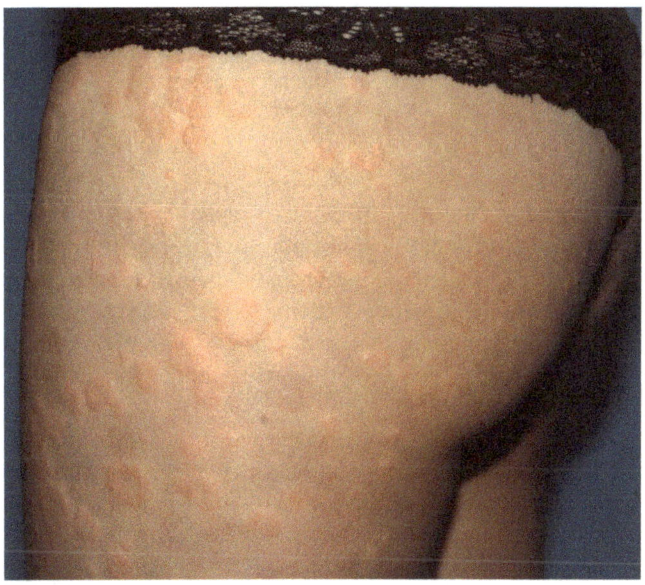

Acute urticaria. Wheals with white-to-light-pink color.

Roughly 35% of urticarias have an autoimmune basis (**autoimmune urticaria**) and are associated with other autoimmune diseases. Patients with autoantibodies tend to have more severe disease. The term "chronic urticaria" embraces **idiopathic urticaria, urticarial vasculitis**, and **physical urticaria**. Approximately one-third of all cases of chronic urticaria represent physical urticarias, defined by specific triggering stimuli and subclassified as adrenergic, aquagenic, cholinergic, cold, delayed pressure, localized heat, and solar urticarias; vibratory angioedema; **dermatographism**; and exercise-induced anaphylaxis. Some chronic autoimmune urticarias are attributed to IgG autoantibodies that cross-link the alpha subunit of the high-affinity IgE receptor (FcεRIα) on basophils and mast cells, causing their degranulation with subsequent upregulation of endothelial adhesion molecules. It is important to attempt to separate the various triggers and forms of urticaria, as both the pathogenesis and therapy may be different.

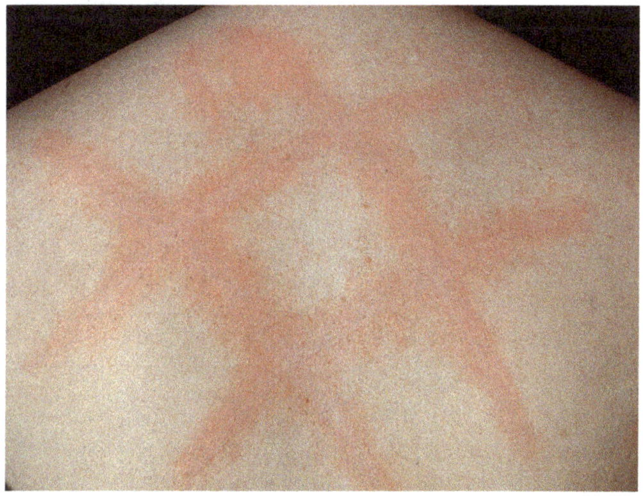

Urticaria, dermatographism. Urticaria as it appeared 5 minutes after the patient was scratched on the back. The patient had experienced generalized pruritus for several months with no spontaneously occurring urticaria. (Reproduced, with permission, from Wolff K, Johnson RA, Saavedra AP. *Fitzpatrick's Color Atlas and Synopsis of Clinical Dermatology.* 6th ed. New York, NY: McGraw-Hill; 2009.)

The **physical urticarias** typically manifest within 10 minutes of exposure to the triggering stimulus and resolve within a day. The exception is delayed pressure urticaria, which often arises several hours after an episode of sustained pressure and may last over a day.

The clinical appearance of individual lesions results from vasodilatation enhanced vascular permeability, edema, and extravasation of proteins into the dermis. There is often a surrounding erythematous flare due to an axonal reflex. Lesions may progress to form confluent plaques with an annular or arcuate morphology. **Angioedema** is a more severe yet analogous physiologic process that extends to the subcutis and subjacent soft tissues and sometimes to the upper airways with potentially fatal consequences. It may accompany acute or chronic urticaria and may relate to an absolute or relative C1 esterase-inhibitor deficiency that may be familial in some cases.

Table 2-1A. The Common Forms of Chronic Urticarias

TYPE OF URTICARIA	PRINCIPAL CLINICAL FEATURES	HISTOPATHOLOGICAL FEATURES	DIAGNOSTIC TEST
Acute and chronic idiopathic	Profuse or sparse edematous papules or wheals, often annular with itching	Absence of epidermal alteration Dermal edema Sparse perivascular infiltrate composed of lymphocytes, eosinophils, neutrophils (variable)	
Symptomatic dermatographism	Itchy, linear wheals with a surrounding bright red flare at sites of scratching or rubbing	As above	Light stroking of skin causes an immediate wheal with itching
Other physical urticarias			
Cold	Itchy pale or red swelling at sites of contact with cold surfaces or fluids	As above but neutrophils may be more prominent	10-minute application of an ice pack causes a wheal within 5 minutes of the removal of ice
Pressure	Large painful or itchy red swelling at sites of pressure lasting 24 hours or more	As above but neutrophils may be more prominent	Application of pressure produces persistent red swelling after a latent period of 1–4 hours
Solar	Itchy pale or red swelling at site of exposure to ultraviolet or visible light	As above but neutrophils may be more prominent	Irradiation by a 2.5 kW 290–690 nm source for 30–120 seconds causes wheals in 30 minutes
Cholinergic	Itchy wheals on trunk, neck, and limbs	As above but neutrophils may be more prominent	Exercise or a hot shower elicits eruption

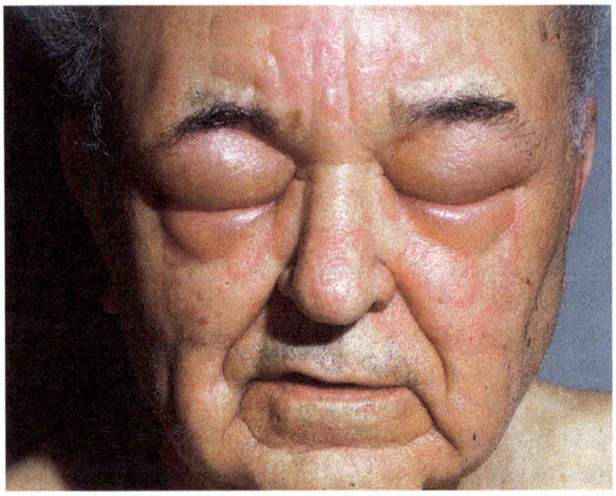

Acute urticaria and angioedema. Note that there are both superficial wheals and deep, diffuse edema. (Reproduced, with permission, from Wolff K, Johnson RA, Saavedra AP. *Fitzpatrick's Color Atlas and Synopsis of Clinical Dermatology.* 6th ed. New York, NY: McGraw-Hill; 2009.)

Roughly one in eight children with physical urticaria will develop respiratory symptoms and two-thirds will manifest angioedema. Long-term follow-up indicates that less than half will manifest complete remissions over time. **Schnitzler syndrome** is a rare form of chronic urticaria associated with IgM-*k* paraproteinemia, bone pain, hyperostosis, and pyrexia.

The histopathology reflects the age of the lesion biopsied and the type of provocative stimulus. One constant feature is edema, characterized by separation of collagen bundles. Blood vessels and lymphatics usually are dilated and show endothelial swelling. Vascular thrombosis and fibrinoid necrosis of vessel walls is absent. The upper dermis is preferentially involved, except in angioedema, which prominently involves the deep reticular dermis and subcutis. A sparse perivascular inflammatory infiltrate consisting of a variable admixture of lymphocytes, neutrophils, and occasional eosinophils characterizes the lesions. Mast cells and granulocytes are seen within the interstitium and granulocytes are present within blood vessel lumens. Degranulated mast cells resemble lymphocytes and, when present, may suggest a mononuclear cell-predominant vascular reaction (ie, lymphocytic vasculitis). The **neutrophilic urticarias** tend to have a more cellular infiltrate, often with neutrophilic packing of blood vessels. This neutrophil-rich histology may be seen in an incipient lesion of physical urticaria, which is, in its chronic state, more likely to manifest the cell-poor morphology previously described. The autoimmune and non-autoimmune urticarias have a similar histomorphology.

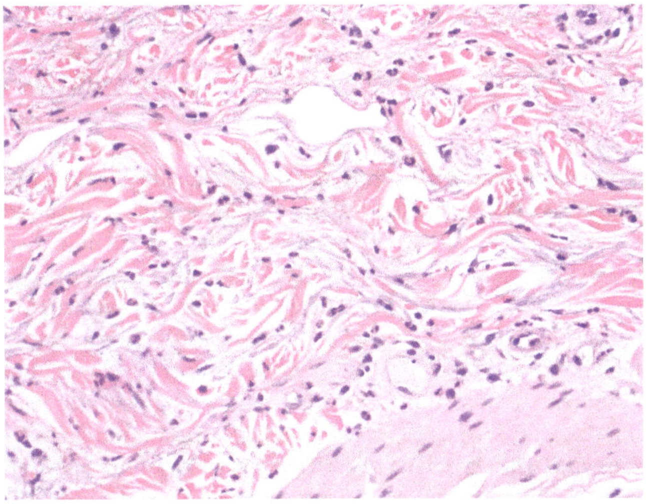

Chronic neutrophilic urticaria. There is dermal edema and a sparse lymphocytic infiltrate with robust interstitial neutrophils.

ANSWER 2-2: A.

This is a classic example of **toxic erythema of pregnancy** (aka **pruritic urticarial papules and plaques of pregnancy** or "**PUPPP**"), which is the most common dermatosis of the gravid state, occurring in 5% of pregnancies (Table 2-2A). Just as the name suggests, lesions present as pruritic urticarial papules and plaques in and near striae of the abdomen and proximal thighs. While the initial lesions are as described above, roughly half of the patients show changing morphology over time, developing polymorphous features including erythema, vesicles, and targetoid eczematous lesions. Lesions usually develop in the last few weeks of pregnancy and may spread to the extremities or become generalized. Periumbilical sparing and spontaneous resolution are characteristic findings. An association with large babies, twin and triplet pregnancies, and increased maternal weight gain raises the possibility that it relates somehow to excessive abdominal distension. It occurs in late pregnancy in 85% of cases and in the immediate postpartum period in 15% of cases.

Microscopically, the findings are nonspecific with superficial perivascular lymphocytic or mixed lymphocytic and eosinophilic infiltrates accompanied by papillary dermal edema. Interstitial neutrophils may also be present. Approximately one-third of cases reveal lymphocyte exocytosis and spongiosis. Although leukocytoclastic debris may be present, there is no evidence of vasculitis.

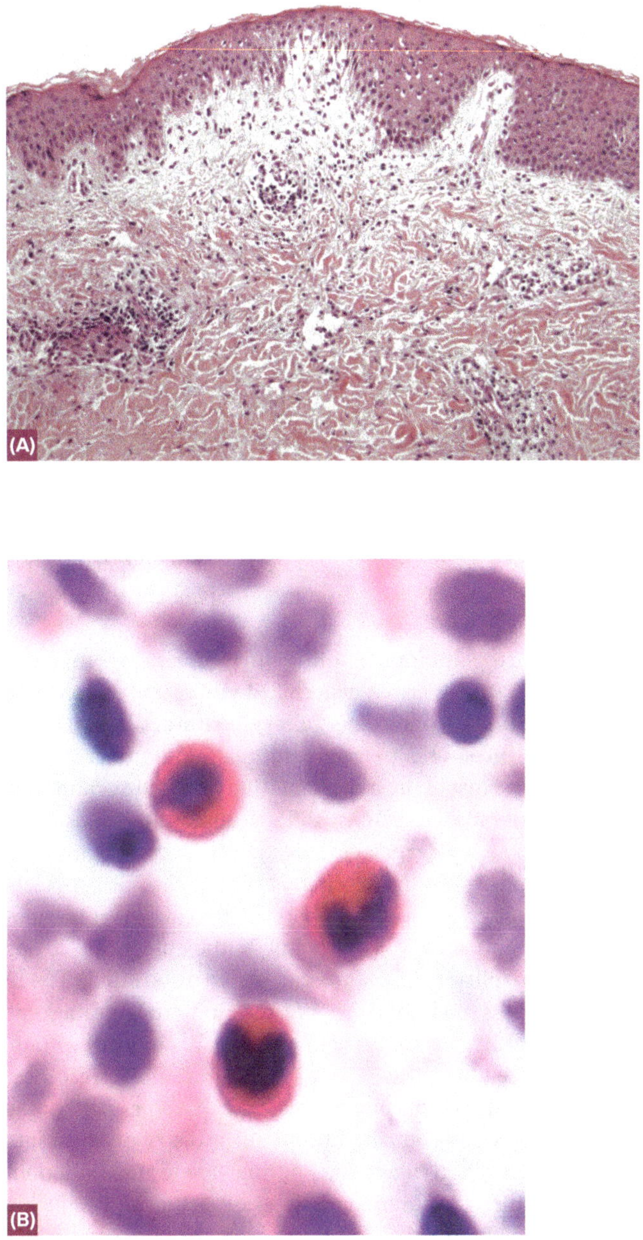

Pruritic urticarial papules and plaques of pregnancy (PUPPP). A nondescript superficial perivascular infiltrate of lymphocytes and eosinophils is present.

Although usually nonreactive by direct immunofluorescent testing, lesions of PUPPP may show granular IgM, IgA, or C3 deposition at the dermal–epidermal junction and/or

Table 2-2A. Pruritic Urticarial Papules and Plaques of Pregnancy

Clinical Features
Pruritic erythematous urticarial papules, vesicles, and plaques in and near abdominal striae
Most common dermatosis of pregnancy
Occurs classically in week 35+
Histopathologic Features
Superficial perivascular lymphocytic or Lymphocytic and eosinophilic dermal infiltrate
Exocytosis and spongiosis in one-third of cases
Differential Diagnosis
Delayed-type hypersensitivity reactions of diverse causes:
Drugs
Contactants
Insect bite reactions (including papular urticaria)
Atopic dermatitis
Herpes gestationis

within blood vessels, suggesting a delayed-type hypersensitivity reaction or possibly an immune-complex contribution to the pathogenesis.

The histopathological differential diagnosis includes **atopic dermatitis**; dermal hypersensitivity reactions to drugs (**drug eruption**), contactants (**allergic contact dermatitis**), and **insect bites**; and **pemphigoid gestationis** (aka **herpes gestationis**). Most of the **hypersensitivity reactions** cannot be reliably distinguished from PUPPP because of its nondescript histomorphology. **Herpes gestationis** can occur at any time during pregnancy and often is raised as a clinical consideration. Lesions of herpes gestationis often show subepidermal blisters accompanied by eosinophils in the epidermis, at tips of dermal papillae, and in a perivascular disposition. Tissue eosinophilia is quantitatively greater in herpes gestationis than in PUPPP. Herpes gestationis reveals circulating anti-basement membrane IgG via indirect immunofluorescence. Additionally, direct immunofluorescence of herpes gestationis reveals a linear, as compared to granular, distribution of IgG and C3 deposition along the dermal–epidermal junction. Therefore, direct immunofluorescence testing is a valuable adjunct to light microscopy in making this important distinction. Herpes gestationis is associated with increased fetal morbidity and may require systemic steroid therapy, whereas PUPPP is a self-limited eruption with no associated fetal morbidity. A less problematic diagnostic concern is that of **pruritic folliculitis of pregnancy** that manifests a follicular-based eruption characterized histopathologically by a neutrophilic folliculitis.

ANSWER 2-3: A.

This is a **morbilliform drug eruption** (aka **exanthematous drug eruption**), which is the most common adverse cutaneous reaction to medications (Table 2-3A). The eruption is characterized clinically by symmetrically arranged, brightly erythematous macules and papules, which are discrete in some areas and confluent in others (discrete on the extremities, confluent on the trunk). Clinical distinction from a **viral exanthem** may be difficult. These lesions generally present within 14 days of taking the offending medication. Drugs with a high probability of reaction include penicillin and related antibiotics, carbamazepine, allopurinol, and gold salts. There is an increased incidence of reactions in patients on allopurinol given ampicillin/amoxicillin (Table 2-3B). Up to 100% of patients with primary EBV or CMV infection (**infectious mononucleosis syndrome**) given ampicillin or amoxicillin develop a morbilliform/exanthematous drug eruption. The microscopic features are those delayed dermal hypersensitivity and are relatively nonspecific in regards to etiology. Delayed dermal hypersensitivity reactions may be divided into two basic categories based on the composition of the inflammatory infiltrate (Th1 vs Th2). **Th1 delayed dermal hypersensitivity** is characterized by variably dense superficial perivascular lymphohistiocytic infiltrates and most commonly reflects viral exanthems (choice B). Occasional mild spongiosis, vacuolar interface activity, and red blood cell extravasation may be present. **Th2 delayed dermal hypersensitivity** is characterized by variably dense superficial perivascular lymphocytic infiltrates with scattered eosinophils and most commonly reflects morbilliform drug eruptions. Mild spongiosis and vacuolar alteration of the basal layer may be present, but keratinocyte damage is minimal. When the inflammatory infiltrate extends into the deep dermis, these changes are characteristic for **arthropod bite reactions** (aka **papular urticaria**). Clinical correlation is required for definitive distinction.

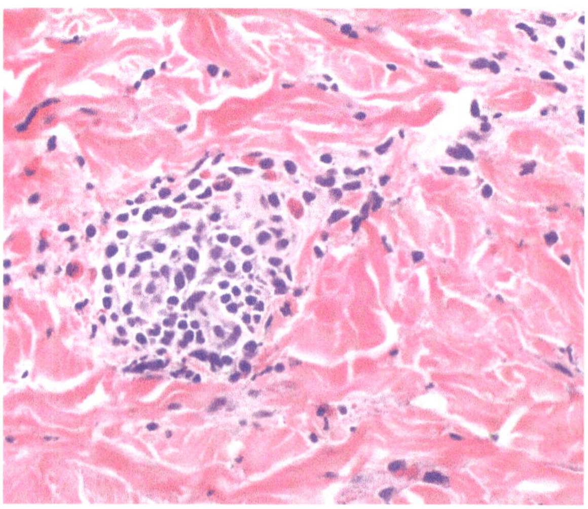

Th2 delayed dermal hypersensitivity reaction. There are superficial perivascular lymphocytic infiltrates with eosinophils. The epidermis is unremarkable (not visualized).

Table 2-3A. Morbilliform Drug Reactions

Clinical Features
Salmon-colored macular or papular eruption
Often polycyclic, gyrate, or reticular patterns
Trunk → acral areas in symmetric distribution
Dependent areas may manifest purpura
Clear following drug withdrawal
May progress to exfoliative erythroderma if drug continued
Histopathologic Features
Cell-poor lymphocytic interface dermatitis with basilar vacuolopathy
Basket-weave orthokeratosis overlying epidermis of normal thickness
Mixed lymphohistiocytic, eosinophilic, and/or plasmacellular dermal infiltrate
Papillary dermal edema
Differential Diagnosis
Viral exanthemata
Erythema multiforme

Table 2-3B. Drugs Causing Exanthematous (Morbilliform) Eruptions

Penicillin and synthetic derivatives
Phenylbutazone
Sulfonamide
Phenytoin and carbamazepine
Gold
Amphotericin B
Oral hypoglycemic agents
Thiazides
Barbiturates
Benzodiazepines
Phenothiazines
Allopurinol
Quinidine
Captopril
Nonsteroidal anti-inflammatory agents
Gentamicin
Lithium

These histopathological findings do not always correlate with the immunological response or inciting trigger, hence clinical correlation is essential in making the correct diagnosis. As an example, on rare occasion, **morbilliform drug eruption** may lack eosinophils and **viral exanthems** may contain eosinophils. In these instances, a generic diagnosis of **delayed dermal hypersensitivity** is most appropriate. Choices C, D, and E describe **urticaria, erythema multiforme**, and **acute spongiotic (eczematous) dermatitis**, respectively. **Tinea versicolor** may be histopathologically identical to morbilliform drug eruptions however characteristic "spaghetti and meatball" fungal structures are seen in the stratum corneum. A PAS stain will nicely highlight these structures. Early lesions of **erythema multiforme** may be histopathologically indistinguishable from morbilliform eruptions. Although morbilliform eruptions may have focal mild vacuolar degeneration, lesions of erythema multiforme have significant cytotoxic activity and necrosis of keratinocytes. Lastly, erythema multiforme lacks eosinophils. Morbilliform drug eruptions may also exhibit mild spongiosis however they typically do not contain the large Langerhans cell–rich microvesicles of **spongiotic dermatitis**. Cases with extensive features of spongiotic dermatitis are best classified as **eczematous drug eruptions**.

ANSWER 2-4: C.

This is an example of **post-inflammatory pigmentary alteration (PIPA)**, which is a secondary change attributed to the primary eruption. PIPA is a completely nonspecific finding associated with end-stage inflammatory processes of any kind however it is more common following interface dermatitis. Based on the clinical description of the patient's original eruption and due to the fact that there are no microscopic epidermal changes in the biopsy, the initial condition most likely represented a **viral exanthem**.

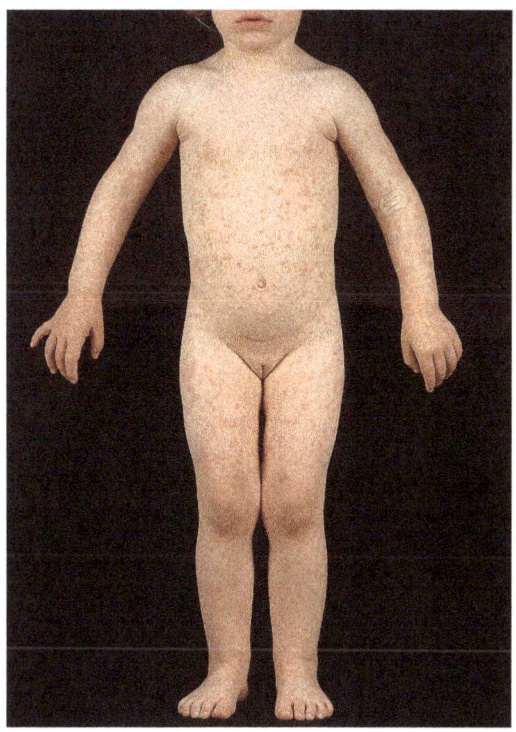

Viral exanthem. Blanching macular eruption usually spares palms and soles. (Reproduced, with permission, from Tintinalli JE, Stapczynski JS, Ma OJ, Cline DM, Cydulka RK, Meckler GD. *Tintinalli's Emergency Medicine: A Comprehensive Study Guide.* 7th ed. New York, NY: McGraw-Hill Education; 2010.)

Microscopically, PIPA is composed of superficial perivascular lymphohistiocytic infiltrates and melanin containing macrophages. **Fontana-Masson stain** highlights the pigment in black, consistent with melanin. Close histopathological inspection may reveal focal mild vacuolar degeneration or spongiosis. If there is substantial epidermal pigment incontinence and the melanophages are deep within the dermis, these lesions may appear hypopigmented. PIPA may be seen as a consequence of late spongiotic dermatitis however epidermal changes of acanthosis and a compact stratum corneum with parakeratosis would be present. PIPA may be seen as a consequence of late interface dermatitis, but epidermal changes of epidermal atrophy, effaced rete ridges, and papillary dermal fibrosis would be present. PIPA is commonly seen in **photocontact dermatitis**, especially **phototoxic dermatitis**, where random dyskeratotic keratinocytes are a constant feature. Additionally, lesions associated with photocontact dermatitis may demonstrate increased epidermal pigmentation due to increased melanogenesis and transfer of melanin pigment to keratinocytes.

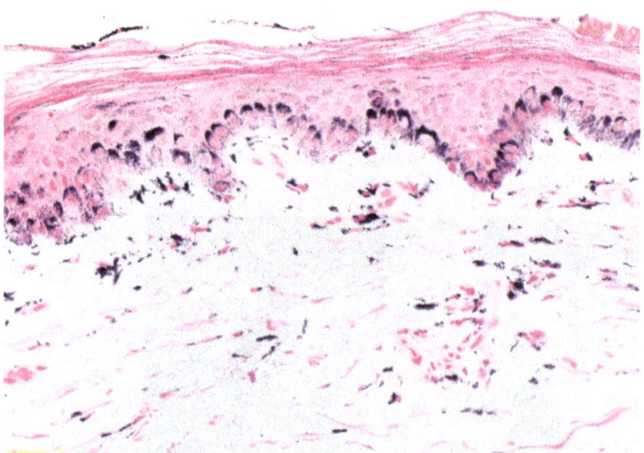

Fontana Masson stain. The black staining pigment within the basal keratinocytes and within the dermis represents melanin pigment.

Choice C describes a **blue nevus**. This form of dermal-based melanocytic nevus is characterized by a spindled cytomorphology and heavy melanin pigmentation. The distinction from melanophages may be difficult in some cases. The clinical presentation is clearly not a solitary lesion, as would characterize a nevus. Blue nevi characteristically express HMB45 via immunohistochemistry, in contrast to macrophages that are negative.

ANSWER 2-5: D.

The biopsy reveals a superficial and deep dermal inflammatory infiltrate composed of lymphocytes and numerous eosinophils. The infiltrate exhibits an almost vertical column-like distribution. There is papillary dermal edema and the overlying epidermis exhibits focal serumimbued parakeratosis. This is a classic example of an **arthropod bite** (aka **papular urticaria**). The patient in this case is the victim of a bedbug infestation. **Bedbugs** (*Cimex lectularius*) share human domains, residing in crevices of floors and walls, in beddings, and in furniture. They usually feed only once a week and less often in cold weather. Bedbugs can travel long distances in search of a human host and can survive for 6–12 months without feeding. Bite reactions occur on exposed sites such as the face, neck, arms, and hands, with two to three lesions in a row ("breakfast, lunch, dinner"). In previously unexposed individuals, bite sites typically appear as erythematous and pruritic macules. In sensitized individuals, intensely pruritic papules, papular urticaria, or vesicles/bullae may arise at the bite sites. Changes secondary to scratching include excoriations, eczematous dermatitis, and secondary infections. Close inspection may reveal a central punctum (serumimbued parakeratosis) where the arthropod mouthparts punctured the skin. The inflammatory reaction that results from a given bite depends on the nature of the offending insect and the patient's immune response.

In the acute phase, the classic microscopic findings are those of a **Th2 delayed dermal hypersensitivity reaction** characterized by a wedge-shaped superficial and deep perivascular lymphocytic infiltrate with numerous scattered eosinophils. Focal epidermal necrosis, spongiosis, and parakeratosis with plasma-rich exudate correspond with the punctum created by the arthropod mouthparts. Due to the focal nature of the punctum, some samples may lack epidermal findings altogether.

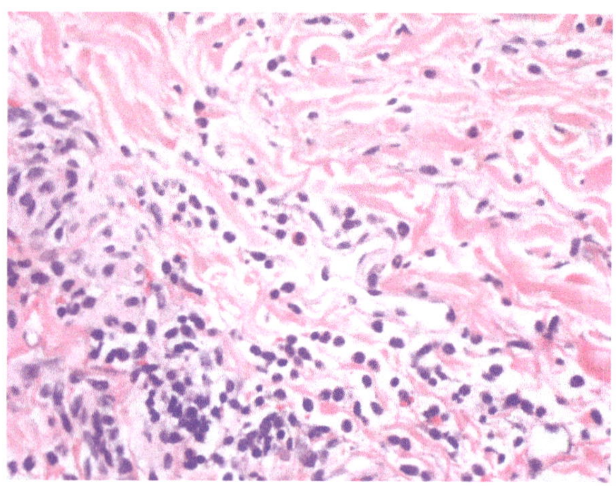

Arthropod bite reaction. Superficial and deep perivascular lymphocytic infiltrates with scattered eosinophils are present.

Neutrophils may predominate in reactions to fleas, mosquitoes, fire ants, and brown recluse spiders. Some individuals may mount exaggerated inflammatory responses with subepidermal bulla formation secondary to marked papillary edema (**bullous arthropod bite reaction**). Insect parts are rarely seen except in scabies and in tick bites where removal is incomplete. The histomorphology of **morbilliform drug eruption** may be identical to arthropod bit reaction and requires clinical correlation for distinction. Chronic lesions can appear as a **benign cutaneous lymphoid hyperplasia (B-cell pseudolymphoma)**, in which there are superficial and deep dense lymphoid infiltrates and occasional germinal center formation. Scattered eosinophils may be present in these lesions but are far outnumbered by lymphocytes. The numbers of T-cells should also outnumber B-cells and any B-cell dominant infiltrate should be worked up for a low grade B-cell lymphoma. **Pityriasis lichenoides** also clinically presents as erythematous papules, but exhibits interface dermatitis with overlying spongiotic epidermal changes and lacks eosinophils. **Eosinophilic pustular folliculitis** may reveal superficial and deep perivascular lymphocytic infiltrates with scattered eosinophils, but the infiltrate is confined to the area surrounding hair follicles, which contain large eosinophilic abscesses in the infundibular region.

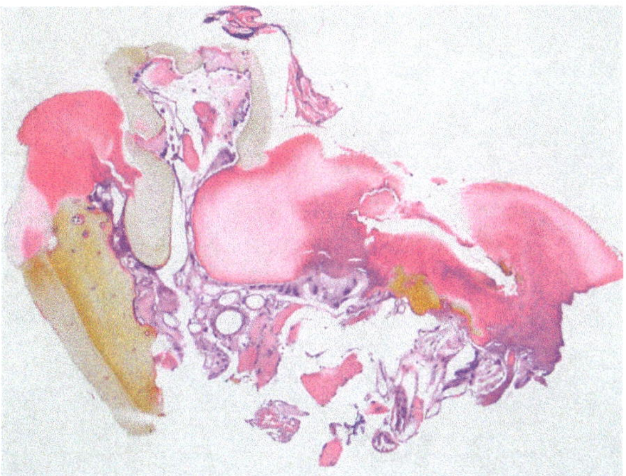

Tick. Note the bright pink mouth parts.

ANSWER 2-6: B.

This patient has **Schamberg's disease**. Pigmented purpuras are a group of idiopathic **progressively pigmented purpuric dermatoses** that may also be classified under **"lymphocytic vasculitis."** Clinically they present as macular or papular, non- or partially blanching lesions on bilateral lower extremities. Rarely they arise on the trunk and arms. The condition is chronic and may be present for years. Young to middle aged men are most commonly affected. Hematologic workup is normal. The major clinical types described are **Schamberg's disease (progressive pigmentary dermatosis), Majocchi's disease (purpura annularis telangiectodes)**, and **pigmented purpuric dermatosis of Gougerot-Blum (lichenoid purpura)**. Some believe these entities are not distinguishable and should be grouped together as **purpura pigmentosa chronica**.

It should be emphasized that the lymphocytic capillaritis characterized by sparse perivascular lymphocytic infiltrates, red blood cell extravasation, and hemosiderin-laden macrophages is nonspecific. Careful clinical correlation is required for definitive diagnosis. **Viral exanthems** may exhibit identical findings however, the pigmented macrophages usually contain melanin (choice A). In **Schamberg's** and **Majocchi's diseases**, the lesions do not exhibit epidermal changes. Only rarely may focal mild vacuolar degeneration be present. Older lesions tend to have greater concentrations of hemosiderin and hemosiderin-laden macrophages. **Prussian blue stain** may be very helpful in highlighting this feature and will stain the hemosiderin bright blue.

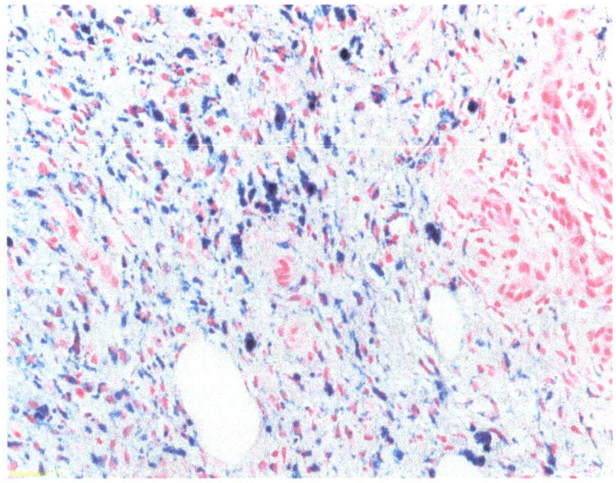

Prussian blue stain. The granular blue staining material is hemosiderin.

Despite the inflammation and extravasated red blood cells, there is no true vasculitis with fibrin thrombi or vessel necrosis. Choices C, D, and E describe **leukocytoclastic vasculitis, urticaria**, and **eczematous dermatitis**, respectively. **Leukocytoclastic vasculitis (LCV)** is clinically characterized by raised "palpable" purpura, unlike the flat macular lesions in this patient with pigmented purpuric dermatosis. Microscopically, LCV contains neutrophilic infiltrates and evidence of vascular damage in the form of fibrin thrombi and fibrinoid necrosis of the vessel walls. Simple **urticaria** is not clinically or histopathologically associated with significant hemorrhage. Additionally, urticaria contains scattered neutrophils, which are absent in pigmented purpura. Numerous fluid-filled vesicles and crusts clinically characterize **eczematous dermatitis**. A condition known as **lichen aureus** is sometimes included into the pigmented purpuric dermatosis category. These lesions are discrete or confluent lichenoid macules and papules with a golden yellow, bronze, purple, or dark brown appearance, often resembling a bruise. They are chronic lesions just like the other forms of pigmented purpuric dermatosis however are usually unilateral and are confined to only one or two locations. Microscopically, the infiltrate of lichen aureus is markedly cellular and contains a component of granulomatous inflammation, unlike the sparse lymphocytic infiltrates of classical pigmented purpura.

ANSWER 2-7: B.

The biopsy reveals a dense superficial and deep perivascular lymphocytic infiltrate associated with marked papillary dermal edema and migration of lymphocytes into retia and acrosyringia, consistent with **perniosis** (Table 2-7A). **Idiopathic perniosis (chilblains)** is a form of cold-induced injury that manifests as inflammatory red to purple macules, nodules, papules, or plaques, at times is accompanied by overlying blisters, erosions, or ulcers characteristically distributed symmetrically on acral skin. When the lesions occur on the thighs or buttocks it is referred to as **equestrian chilblains**, since historically these lesions developed in women riding horses in the cold without appropriate warm clothing. It is common in the humid climate of northwest Europe but is decreasing in frequency with modern home heating methods. A vasospastic response to cold with resulting ischemia of vessel walls is the proposed etiology, with humidity playing a role through enhanced air conductivity of temperature. Lesions clear dramatically with warming. An association with anorexia nervosa has been reported; it appears that anxiety states and the ingestion of antidepressant medications with immune dysregulating properties may play a role. Causes of **secondary perniosis** include rare childhood lesions of hyperviscosity and procoagulant states, namely, hypergammaglobulinemia, essential cryofibrinogenemia, antiphospholipid antibody syndrome, rheumatoid arthritis, Crohn disease, Behçet disease, and most commonly systemic lupus erythematosus. Lesions associated with systemic lupus are termed **chilblains lupus erythematosus** and resemble Behçet disease by virtue of the distribution of the infiltrate and the presence of vacuolar lymphocytic interface dermatitis. Patients with perniosis and cutaneous lesions of lupus (ie, subacute and discoid) are more likely to have systemic lupus or eventually develop systemic involvement.

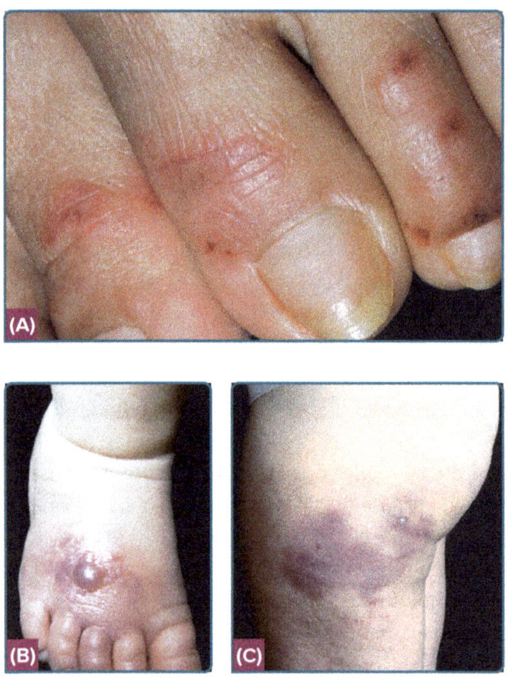

Perniosis is common at such sites as the hands and feet when they are exposed to both cooling and tight garments. **(A)** Perniosis on the toes. **(B)** Perniosis on the dorsum of the foot. Children and the elderly are most commonly affected, perhaps, because they take less care to protect themselves from cooling. **(C)** Equestrian chilblains from horse riding on a cold morning with inadequate clothing.

Microscopically, there is a dense superficial or superficial and deep perivascular lymphocytic infiltrate with exocytosis to rete ridges and acrosyringia. Dyskeratotic keratinocytes are observed occasionally. Pronounced papillary dermal edema is most characteristic. Edema of blood vessel walls accompanied by transmural lymphocytic infiltrates is also characteristic (the so-called fluffy edema of microvessels), and thrombi may be observed in dermal papillae capillaries (so-called "**lymphocytic vasculitis**"). Mucinosis around the eccrine coil and luminal fibrin thrombi localized to dermal papillae capillaries may be seen, but pandermal mucin deposition or reticular dermal vascular thrombosis is unusual. Pandermal mucinosis should prompt consideration of a systemic connective tissue disease.

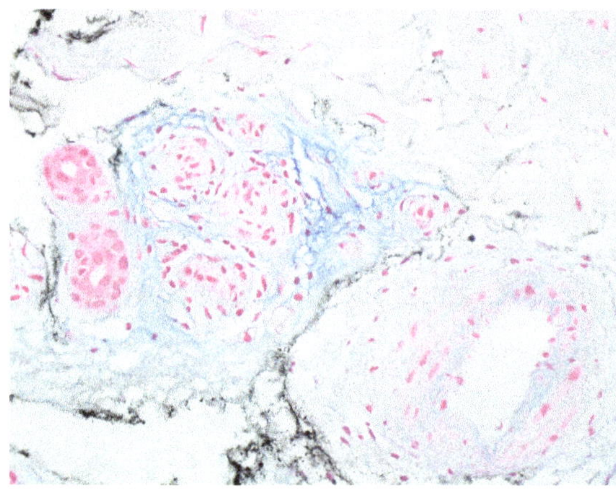

Perniosis, Alcian blue stain. There is increased dermal mucin (blue material) concentrated around the deep eccrine coil.

Table 2-7A. Perniosis (Chilblains)

Clinical Features
- Cold-induced purplish macules, papules, and nodules involving acral, thigh, or buttock skin
- Occurs in humid climates

Histopathologic Features
- Dense superficial and deep lymphocytic infiltrates with preferential migration to epidermal retia and acrosyringia
- Occasional fibrin thrombi in dermal papillae capillaries
- Transmural lymphocytic migration through blood vessel walls
- Marked papillary dermal edema
- Mucinosis around eccrine coil

Differential Diagnosis
- Connective tissue diseases, especially:
  - Chilblains lupus erythematosus
  - Mixed connective tissue disease
- Behçet disease
- Erythema multiforme
- Viral exanthems

Leukocytoclastic vasculitis is characterized by perivascular and interstitial neutrophilic infiltrates with fibrinoid necrosis of vessel walls and fibrin thrombi. **Arthropod bite reaction** may also exhibit superficial and deep perivascular lymphocytic infiltrates and occasionally marked papillary dermal edema, but they contain eosinophils and lack significant interface activity and dermal mucin. **Lichen planus** exhibits a superficial dense band-like lymphocytic infiltrate but with intense interface activity, numerous scattered dyskeratotic keratinocytes along the dermal epidermal junction, colloid bodies in the papillary dermis, and premature terminal differentiation of the epidermis. Lichen planus does not usually exhibit papillary dermal edema and dermal mucin. **Polymorphous light eruption** demonstrates many of the same findings but is usually more photo-distributed and contains mixed inflammatory cell infiltrates with neutrophils and eosinophils and lacks deep dermal mucin.

ANSWER 2-8: D.

The biopsy reveals robust papillary dermal edema and tight perivascular lymphocytic infiltrates with scattered eosinophils, neutrophils, and extravasated red blood cells. The epidermis is unremarkable. The combined clinical and histopathological findings are consistent with **polymorphous light eruption (PMLE)** (Table 2-8A). PMLE is an idiopathic photo-induced eruption likely representing the combined effects of phototoxicity and a delayed-type hypersensitivity reaction to ultraviolet (UV) light of both UVA and UVB spectra. Patients with polymorphous light eruption fail to manifest the UV-induced downregulation of epidermal CD1a+ Langerhans cells seen in normal individuals. This deviant response may be a clue to the pathogenesis as well as to diagnosis. Lesions manifest as pruritic erythematous papules, papulovesicles, or urticarial plaques that erupt 30 minutes to 3 days after UV exposure and characteristically resolve in 7-10 days. Although the clinical presentation is variable, in each patient the eruption is consistently monomorphous ("polymorphous" referring to the microscopic mixed cellular infiltrate). There is a predilection for sun-exposed areas such as the hands, forearms, upper arms, and the head and neck region. Females are preferentially affected and there is a small statistical predilection for African Americans. Roughly half of patients show decreasing photosensitivity over time. Polymorphous light eruption can be a clue to underlying seropositivity for antibodies to Ro. Patients with polymorphous light eruption may have an increased incidence of underlying autoimmune diseases, including lupus erythematosus and autoimmune thyroid disorders.

Microscopically, the most prominent finding is marked papillary and superficial reticular dermal edema accompanied in early lesions by a superficial perivascular lymphoid infiltrate and in late lesions by moderate-to-intense superficial and deep lymphocytic infiltrates, which often manifest perivascular "cuffing." Eosinophils, neutrophils, and hemorrhage are present in most cases. The epidermis may be normal or may show basal layer vacuolization, acanthosis, parakeratosis, spongiosis, vesiculation, and uncommonly, necrosis. Vascular changes consisting of mural and endothelial swelling and edema diminish in the depths of the biopsy. By direct immunofluorescence examination, perivascular IgM and C3 deposition is seen in the setting of a negative lupus band test. On occasion, patients with apparently robust clinical findings may manifest only minimal histopathologic changes.

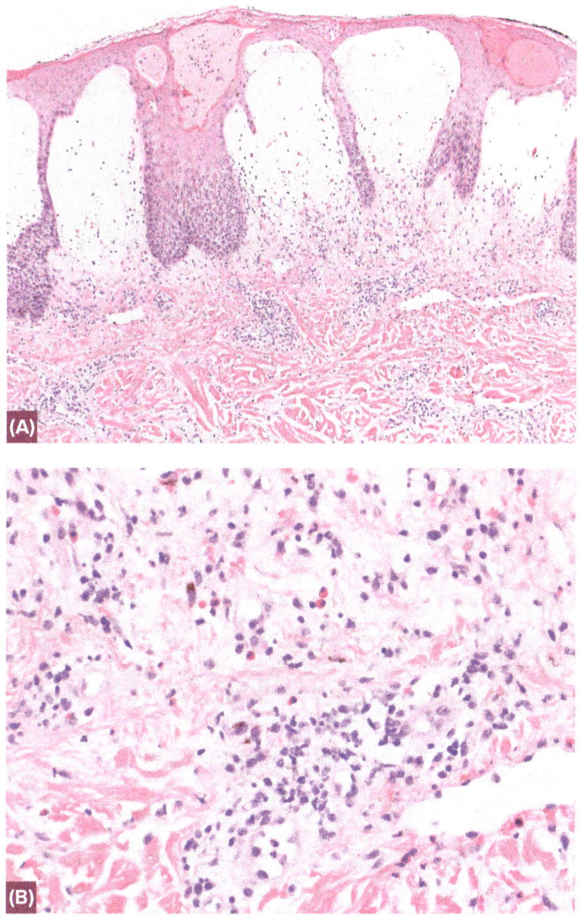

Polymorphous light eruption. (A) A superficial perivascular mixed infiltrate is associated with marked papillary dermal edema. Mild spongiosis is present and focal areas with transepidermal elimination of the edematous serum are present. **(B)** There are numerous lymphocytes, neutrophils, eosinophils, and macrophages.

The clinical and histopathological differential diagnosis includes the other **photoallergic** and **phototoxic dermatitis** (including those that are drug-related). The histopathological differential diagnosis includes **bullous systemic lupus erythematosus, immunobullous diseases, the gyrate erythemas** (particularly **superficial erythema annulare centrifugum**), and other delayed-type hypersensitivity reactions such as

rosacea, atopic dermatitis, and **insect bites**. Whereas distinction from **photoallergic eruptions** may be impossible, epidermal changes tend to be more pronounced than in polymorphous light eruption. Purely **phototoxic eruptions** show a greater degree of dyskeratotic keratinocytes. The pattern of epithelial injury in lupus erythematosus is one of vacuolopathic basal layer degeneration usually associated with atrophy. Eosinophils and neutrophils are absent. However, in **bullous systemic lupus** there is marked superficial dermal edema and a subepidermal blister where the roof is usually intact and the blister cavity contains fibrin with large numbers of neutrophils and karyorrhectic debris. Unlike classic systemic lupus, subacute lupus, and discoid lupus, the dermal infiltrate of bullous systemic lupus may contain mixed infiltrates of neutrophils and macrophages. In lupus, direct immunofluorescence will reveal a positive lupus band test with granular immunoglobulin and complement deposition along the dermal–epidermal junction. Bullous lupus will reveal linear IgG and C3 along the dermal–epidermal junction and frequently a concomitant positive IgM and IgA lupus band test. The urticarial phase of **bullous pemphigoid** may reveal identical histopathological findings however the presence of eosinophils within a spongiotic epidermis and linear deposition of immunoglobulin and complement are not present in polymorphous light eruption. The **superficial gyrate erythemas (erythema annulare centrifugum)** show mild eczematous epithelial changes, which may also be seen in polymorphous light eruption. Both are accompanied by similar patterns of dermal inflammation however gyrate erythema generally lacks the marked superficial dermal edema and neutrophilic component. **Bullous arthropod bite reaction**, in which prominent superficial edema results in subepidermal vesiculation may be identical to polymorphous light eruption. Clinical correlation is required for distinction.

Table 2-8A. Polymorphous Light Eruption

Clinical Features
- Erythematous, pruritic papules, or papulovesicles and urticarial plaques
- Eruption occurs 30 minutes to 3 days after sun exposure, and resolves in 7-10 days
- Predilection for sun-exposed sites: hands, forearms, head, and neck area

Histopathologic Features
- Perivascular infiltrates of lymphocytes, eosinophils, and neutrophils
- Exocytosis, spongiosis, vesiculation, acanthosis, and focal parakeratosis common
- Some cases show vacuolopathic interface injury pattern or no epidermal changes
- Marked papillary dermal edema classically
- Blood vessels show ectasia and endothelial swelling which preferentially affect superficial vasculature

Differential Diagnosis
- Delayed-type hypersensitivity reactions including:
  - Allergic contact reactions
  - Rosacea
  - Other photoallergic/phototoxic eruptions
  - Insect bite reactions
- Connective tissue diseases including:
  - Discoid lupus erythematosus
  - Subacute cutaneous lupus erythematosus
- Jessner lymphocytic infiltrate

ANSWER 2-9: E.

This is an example of **tumid lupus erythematosus**, which is a rare manifestation of cutaneous lupus characterized clinically by succulent, edematous, urticaria-like plaques with little surface change on the sun-exposed sites such as the face, chest, arms, and shoulders. Unlike **urticaria**, they are persistent and do not rapidly fluctuate in size and shape over a period of 24 hours. Annular and gyrate forms have been described. Unlike the other forms of lupus, there is an equal predilection for males and females. Young adults are most frequently affected. Lesions are associated with UVA and UVB exposure however an association with HIV anti-retroviral medications, estrogen, and infliximab therapy has been reported. The majority of patients lack antinuclear antibodies and rarely progress to systemic lupus.

Microscopically, the findings are similar to discoid lupus with superficial and deep perivascular and periadnexal lymphocytic infiltrates but without the epidermal changes of vacuolar interface activity, thickening of the basement membrane, or follicular plugging. There is a striking accumulation of dermal mucin. The infiltrate is composed of a mixture of CD4+ and CD8+ lymphocytes. Direct immunofluorescence usually reveals a nonspecific immunoreactant profile.

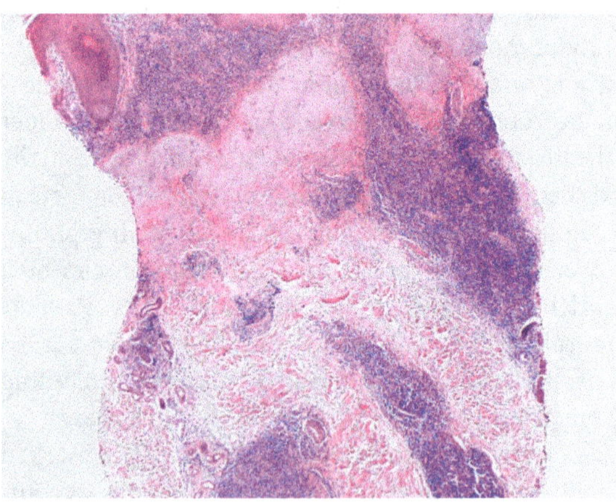

Tumid lupus erythematosus. There are robust superficial and deep perivascular and periadnexal lymphocytic infiltrates. Interface activity involving the epidermis and hair follicles is absent.

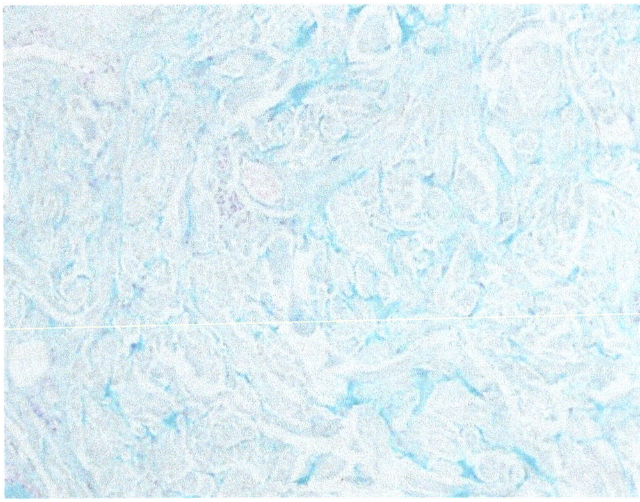

Alcian blue stain. There is increased blue material in between the collagen bundles in areas away from the inflammation. The blue material is dermal mucin.

QUICK FACT

Possible Spectrum of disease

Reticular erythematous mucinosis

(Mucin with little to no inflammation)

⇑⇓

Tumid Lupus

(Mucin with robust inflammation)

⇓⇑

Jessner's Lymphocytic Infiltrate

(Little to no mucin with robust inflammation)

The differential diagnosis includes the other forms of **cutaneous lupus**, which many feel are not reliably distinguishable based on histomorphology alone. Tumid lupus frequently lacks significant epidermal changes characteristic of lupus. **Erythema annulare centrifugum** (**EAC**) may also contain superficial and deep perivascular lymphocytic infiltrates with "cuffing" however EAC frequently contains eosinophils and lacks dermal mucin. Polymorphous light eruption is characterized by marked superficial edema and mixed inflammatory infiltrates of lymphocytes, eosinophils, neutrophils, and histiocytes. **Morbilliform drug eruption** may contain superficial and deep perivascular lymphocytic infiltrates, but also contains eosinophils and lacks dermal mucin. **Urticaria** is characterized by dermal edema and sparse superficial dermal lymphocytic infiltrates with interstitial neutrophils and eosinophils. Dermal mucin is not increased in urticaria. Distinction of tumid lupus from **Jessner's lymphocytic infiltrate** or **reticular erythematous mucinosis** based on histological examination alone may be difficult if not impossible. Jessner's lymphocytic infiltrate typically contains robust superficial and deep perivascular lymphocytic infiltrates and lacks dermal mucin and reticular erythematous mucinosis contains marked accumulations of dermal mucin and only sparse perivascular infiltrates. It has been suggested that some cases reported as lymphocytic infiltrate of Jessner or reticular erythematous mucinosis are in fact tumid lupus. In fact, these entities may represent a spectrum of single disease.

ANSWER 2-10: E.

The biopsy reveals a robust lymphocytic infiltrate that is tightly concentrated around the superficial blood vessels ("cuffing of vessels"). The epidermis is unremarkable. The combined clinical and histopathological findings are consistent with **superficial erythema annulare centrifugum (EAC)** (Table 2-10A). The **gyrate erythemas** are characterized by annular, polycyclic, often migratory erythematous macular eruptions, and include **erythema annulare centrifugum, erythema marginatum, erythema migrans**, and **erythema gyratum repens. Erythema annulare centrifugum (EAC)** consists of one or more annular fixed or migratory large (>1 cm), erythematous, scaly, indurated plaques, often with a fine peripheral scale at the advancing edge, involving the trunk and extremities. A number of triggers have been implicated however *Streptococcal* infection and Lyme's disease are not associated with EAC. Extremely rare cases have been associated with visceral and hematologic malignancies. Although lesions may be seen in the neonatal period, in which they may be a sign of maternal systemic lupus erythematosus, onset is most often in early adulthood or middle age (Table 2-10B). The initial lesion, a pink infiltrated papule, slowly enlarges to form a ring as its center fades. Some lesions reach a diameter of 8.0 cm over a 2- to 3-week period. Eccentric expansion may yield an irregular arciform pattern. Lesions may last from days to months and may be associated with purpuric or pigmented residua. The clinical differential diagnosis includes **granuloma annulare** (which more often has a beaded edge), **fungal infections, annular psoriasis, parapsoriasis, sarcoidosis, urticaria, urticarial bullous pemphigoid, connective tissue disease, atypical forms of pityriasis rosea** (particularly the **pityriasis marginatum et circinatum of Vidal variant**), and **necrolytic migratory erythema** associated with pancreatic islet cell neoplasms. The nature of the triggers associated with EAC implicates delayed-type hypersensitivity as the pathogenetic basis; internal inflammatory disease and superficial fungal infection are thought to be highly associated. However, PAS stains of lesional skin characteristically fail to reveal hyphal elements in the stratum corneum. An occasional association with the ingestion of various cheeses (ie, blue cheese) has been reported. The disorder tends to be a chronic and recurrent one despite treatment.

Table 2-10A. Erythema Annulare Centrifugum

Clinical Features
- Erythematous infiltrated papules which slowly enlarge to form annular or arciform arrays

Histopathologic Features
- Superficial EAC
  - Superficial perivascular lymphocytic or lymphocytic and eosinophilic dermal infiltrate
  - Exocytosis and spongiosis with focal parakeratosis
- Superficial and deep EAC
  - Superficial and deep perivascular lymphocytic or lymphocytic and eosinophilic dermal infiltrate with prominent "cuffing" around blood vessels

Differential Diagnosis
- Superficial EAC
  - Delayed-type hypersensitivity reactions including:
    - Allergic contact reactions
    - Atopy
    - Pityriasis rosea
    - Pityriasiform and other drug eruptions
    - Polymorphous light eruption and other photoallergic conditions
    - Insect bite reactions
  - Connective tissue diseases including:
    - Discoid lupus erythematosus
    - Subacute lupus erythematosus
    - Relapsing polychondritis
    - Sjögren syndrome
    - Mixed connective tissue disease
- Superficial and deep EAC
  - Jessner lymphocytic infiltrate
  - Connective tissue diseases including:
    - Discoid and tumid lupus erythematosus
    - Relapsing polychondritis
    - Sjögren syndrome
    - Mixed connective tissue disease
  - Delayed-type hypersensitivity reactions including:
    - Dermal contact hypersensitivity reactions (to nickel)
    - Polymorphous light eruption, deep variant
    - Insect bite reactions, and papular urticaria

Microscopically, there are two discrete forms of EAC. The **superficial variant of EAC** is characterized by superficial perivascular lymphocytic infiltrates that typically exhibit some degree of "cuffing" about blood vessels in addition to a loose scattering of lymphocytes in the papillary dermis. Frequently epidermal spongiosis, vacuolar alteration, and parakeratosis with papillary dermal edema may be present. The second form (**deep variant of EAC**) is a superficial and deep one, in which a sharply demarcated perivascular lymphoid infiltrate spares the overlying epidermis. In one series, 80% of patients had superficial EAC, and 20% had the deep form. Endothelial swelling may

Table 2-10B. Possible Trigger Factors for Erythema Annulare Centrifugum

Infective and Nondrug Hypersensitivity States
- Tinea
- Candida infection
- Ascaris infection
- Viral infection
- Ingested molds

Autoimmune Diseases
- Sjögren syndrome
- Hyperthyroidism
- Liver disease
- Immunologic disturbances

Drug-Related
- Cimetidine
- Salicylates
- Diazides
- Antimalarials

Neoplastic
- Liver disease
- Carcinoma
- Dysproteinemia
- Blood dyscrasias

be seen in both types and may be accompanied by hemorrhage, but fibrin deposition and other signs of vasculitis are absent. Eosinophils are seen in roughly 10-20% of cases (personal observation). The overall histopathological findings are nonspecific and require clinical correlation for definitive diagnosis.

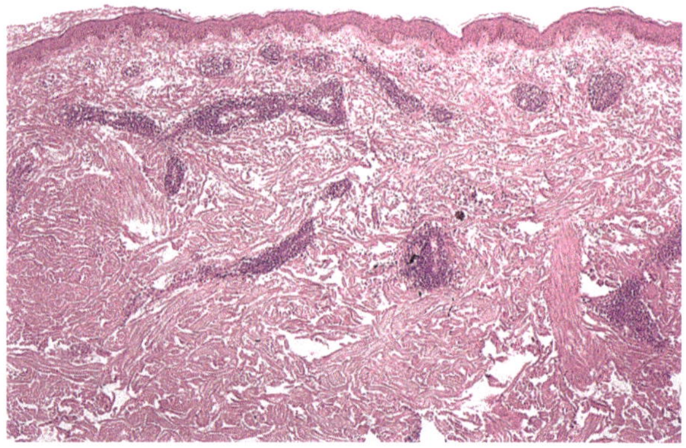

Erythema annulare centrifugum, deep variant. The dermal lymphocyte-predominant infiltrate is associated with scattered eosinophils and mural and endothelial swelling but no fibrin deposition within blood vessel walls or lumina. The epidermis is unremarkable.

The histopathological differential diagnosis of the **superficial variant of EAC** includes **allergic contact reactions, atopy, pityriasis rosea** and **pityriasiform drug eruptions, polymorphous light eruption** and **other photoallergic conditions,**

insect bite reactions, and occasional cases of **lupus erythematosus**. With respect to the **deep variant of gyrate erythema**, differential diagnostic considerations include **Jessner's lymphocytic infiltrate**, connective tissue diseases such as **discoid lupus** and **tumid lupus erythematosus, relapsing polychondritis, Sjögren syndrome**, and lesions of **mixed connective tissue disease** and **subacute cutaneous lupus erythematosus** that have been treated with topical steroids, all of which may manifest perivascular lymphocytic infiltrates without epidermal alterations. With respect to **Jessner lymphocytic infiltrate** and the aforementioned **connective tissue diseases**, eosinophils are most unusual, whereas **in tumid lupus erythematosus**, massive mucin deposition is characteristic, and the lymphocytic infiltrate usually is sparse. The **dermal contact hypersensitivity reactions**, such as those owing to nickel, may manifest perivascular lymphocytic and eosinophilic infiltrates in the absence of epidermal changes. However, these forms of contact dermatitis typically contain robust papillary dermal edema.

ANSWER 2-11: B.

Erythema marginatum is associated with rheumatic fever in less than 10% of cases and consists of erythematous macules with a raised edge and a pale center. **Rheumatic fever** is a multisystem inflammatory disease associated with group A *Streptococcal* pharyngitis. By consensus, one establishes the diagnosis clinically through the system described by T. Duckett Jones, requiring the expression of two major or one major and two minor criteria. The major criteria are carditis, migratory large joint polyarthritis, chorea, erythema marginatum, and subcutaneous nodules (**rheumatic fever nodules**), whereas the minor criteria include fever, arthralgia, an elevated erythrocyte sedimentation rate or C-reactive protein level, and an elongated P-R interval on an electrocardiogram. None of 44 patients with rheumatic fever in one study manifested erythema marginatum. Skin biopsies in erythema marginatum show superficial and deep perivascular neutrophilic, lymphocytic, and eosinophilic infiltrates with perivascular debris but absent vascular fibrin deposition.

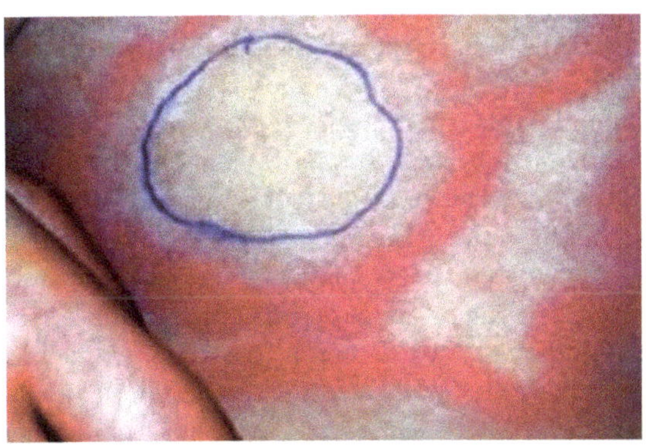

Erythema marginatum on the trunk of an 8-year-old Caucasian boy. The pen mark shows the location of the rash approximately 60 minutes previously.

The microscopic differential diagnosis includes other conditions that combine perivascular lymphocytic infiltrates with a neutrophilic and eosinophilic component in the presence of perivascular leukocytoclasia but absent or minimal fibrin deposition such as **urticaria, urticarial vasculitis, rheumatoid neutrophilic dermatosis**, and some cases of **Henoch–Schönlein purpura**.

ANSWER 2-12: C.

Erythema chronicum migrans is the distinctive cutaneous manifestation of stage I **Lyme disease**. This pathognomonic finding occurs in roughly 68% of Lyme disease cases. It is often described as a non-pruritic, maculopapular "bull's eye" eruption that typically occurs near the site of infection. The erythematous perimeter migrates outward over several days while the central area clears. Multiple lesions in different sites can develop in some individuals. Lesions can persist for 2-3 weeks if left untreated. Roughly 67% of patients will develop flu-like symptoms that can include fever, myalgias, and lymphadenopathy. Symptoms usually subside within 7-10 days.

Microscopically, the central portion of the lesion exhibits a dense superficial and deep perivascular and periadnexal mixed inflammatory infiltrate analogous to an **insect bite reaction**. The infiltrate is usually dominated by lymphocytes with smaller concentrations of neutrophils, eosinophils, histiocytes, and mast cells. Deep perineural involvement with lymphocytes and plasma cells is a frequent finding (similar to the dermal infiltrate of **secondary syphilis**). A biopsy from the periphery is nonspecific, showing a superficial and deep perivascular and interstitial infiltrate of lymphocytes, mast cells, and plasma cells. Identification of spirochetes by either silver stain (Warthin Starry) or immunohistochemistry is diagnostic.

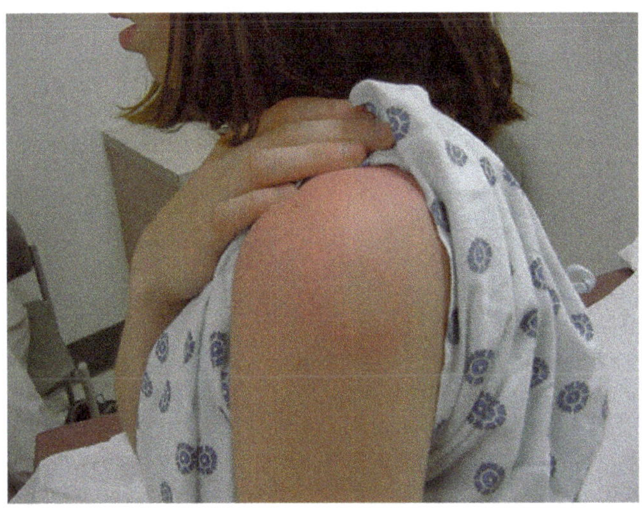

Erythema migrans. An 11-year-old girl with centrifugally advancing erythema on her shoulder. She is febrile and systemically ill.

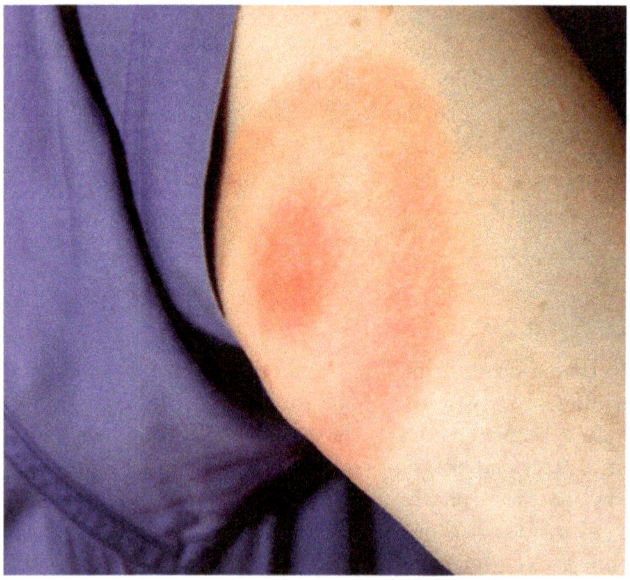

Erythema migrans due to *Borrelia burgdorferi* (Lyme disease). Note the target-shaped distribution of erythema.

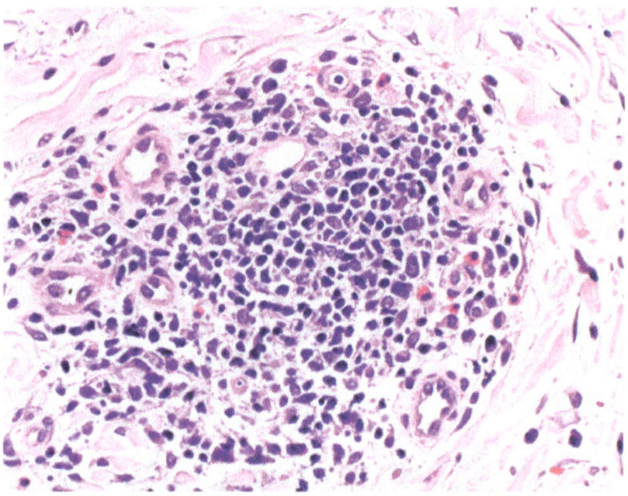

Erythema migrans. Dense superficial and deep nodular perivascular lymphoid cell infiltrates are present with many plasma cells and few eosinophils. There is a propensity for the infiltrates to track along adnexal structures and peripheral nerve bundles.

ANSWER 2-13: D.

Erythema gyratum repens manifests as broad polycyclic patches that resemble the rings on the cut surface of a tree. This eruption is associated in over 80% of cases with malignancies of parenchymal organs such as lung or kidney, tuberculosis, ichthyotic states, pityriasis rubra pilaris, hematologic dyscrasias including hypereosinophilic syndrome, and CREST syndrome. Clinical mimics include atypical cases of **autoimmune bullous dermatoses**, such as **bullous pemphigoid** or **linear IgA disease**, and **subacute cutaneous lupus erythematosus**. The pathophysiologic basis is held to reflect an autoimmune basis, although the antigen is not well characterized.

The histopathology of erythema gyratum repens comprises spongiosis with parakeratosis, focal mild perivascular lymphoid infiltrates, and variable edema or eosinophilia of the dermis. Clinical correlation is required for definitive diagnosis.

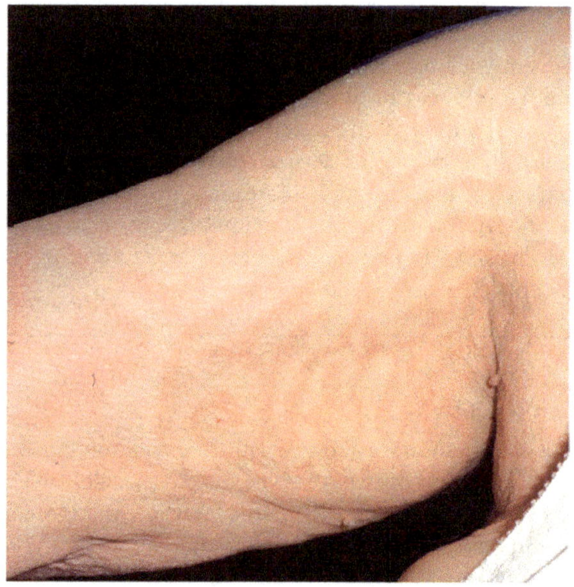

Erythema gyratum repens. Serpiginous parallel bands on axilla and arm.

ANSWER 2-14: C.

The biopsy reveals small well-formed granulomas composed of macrophages and sparse lymphocytes. The granulomas are present adjacent to lymphatic vessels with lateral compression of the vascular lumens. The combined clinical and histopathological findings are consistent with **Miescher-Melkersson-Rosenthal Syndrome**. In general, all granulomatous infiltrates require the exclusion of infectious agents and foreign material through the judicious use of special stains for microorganisms and polarization microscopy. Rarely, more sophisticated techniques will be required, such as spectrophotometric or x-ray analysis. Granulomatous infiltrates in the skin can be broadly classified as conditions in which the tissue monocytes-macrophages (histiocytes) are the predominating inflammatory cell. Because of their abundant cytoplasm, granulomatous infiltrates may have a pale appearance on scanning magnification, a clue to the granulomatous nature. In some granulomatous infiltrates, especially in early disease, the aggregations of tissue macrophages are not well-defined, so it is difficult to identify a discrete granuloma. Traditionally, granulomas have been subdivided into aggregations of tissue macrophages having no or few surrounding lymphocytes (**"naked"** or **sarcoidal**

granulomas), those rimmed by lymphocytes (**tuberculoid granulomas**), histiocytes which form around a central area of degeneration and/or necrosis (**palisading granulomas**), and granulomas containing multinucleated giant cells (**foreign-body granulomas**). These divisions have utility in defining a differential diagnosis, but there may be considerable overlap in any given patient among these particular types.

Cheilitis granulomatosa and **Miescher-Melkersson-Rosenthal Syndrome** are overlapping clinical conditions with identical histopathology (Table 2-14A). The etiology is unclear. In **Miescher-Melkersson-Rosenthal Syndrome**, patients present with a triad of lip swelling, unilateral facial paralysis, and furrowed tongue. In some cases there is more extensive facial swelling involving the eyelids. Similar swelling may affect the penis and vulva. Mono- and oligosymptomatic disease is the rule. Patients with **cheilitis granulomatosa** have lip swelling alone. Microscopically, both conditions are characterized by prominent dermal edema and noncaseating, poorly formed, "naked" granulomas adjacent to, and sometimes impinging on, dilated lymphatic channels. A perivascular lymphocytic and plasma cell infiltrate also is present.

The differential diagnosis of granulomas at oral-facial sites includes **granulomatous rosacea, perioral dermatitis, lupus miliaris disseminatus faciei**, and **sarcoidosis**. Again, in all cases of granulomatous dermatitis, special stains (PAS, Fite, Gram, etc) should be ordered to rule out an infectious etiology. **Lupus vulgaris** is a form of cutaneous tuberculosis and exhibits acid-fast mycobacteria. The pathogenesis of **acne rosacea** is unknown however a disorder of abnormal dermal vessel regulation and vasodilatory responses has been proposed. Others consider it a sebaceous gland disorder or a folliculitis. Patients present with erythematous papules, pustules, and/or telangiectasias on the central face. Long-standing cases may eventuate into **rhinophyma** or **phymas** involving other portions of the face such as the chin, forehead, or cheeks. An advanced granulomatous form (**Lewandowsky rosacea**) presents as yellow-brown nodules. Patients may give a history of blushing or flushing with consumption of hot liquids, alcohol, or spicy foods, or exposure to cold or wind.

The histopathology of **acne rosacea** depends on the stage of the disease that is biopsied. Non-pustular lesions reveal a mixed perivascular and perifollicular inflammatory infiltrate composed of lymphocytes, plasma cells, macrophages (some multinucleated), and fewer scattered neutrophils and eosinophils. In pustular lesions, the numbers of neutrophils increase, and in a variant referred to as ***pyoderma faciale*** (or ***rosacea fulminans***), perifollicular neutrophils are prominent. There is usually spongiosis of the infundibular epithelium. Pronounced granulomatous inflammation often results from rupture of involved hair follicles. In this instance, central necrosis may be present, producing caseation indistinguishable from that seen in mycobacterial infections. Although marked telangiectasia is a clinical component of acne rosacea, histopathologically this feature often is difficult to assess objectively.

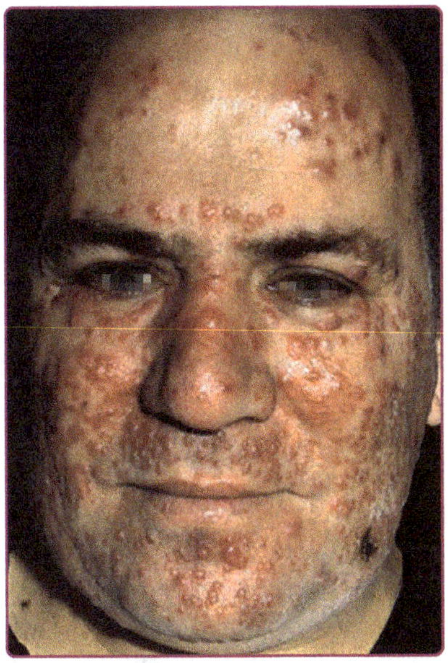

Granulomatous rosacea. There are multiple monomorphic red and yellow-brown papules that, on diascopy, show apple-jelly-like color. (Reproduced, with permission, from Goldsmith LA, Katz SI, Gilchrest BA, Paller AS, Leffell DJ, Wolff K, eds. *Fitzpatrick's Dermatology in General Medicine*. 8th ed. New York, NY: McGraw-Hill Education; 2012.)

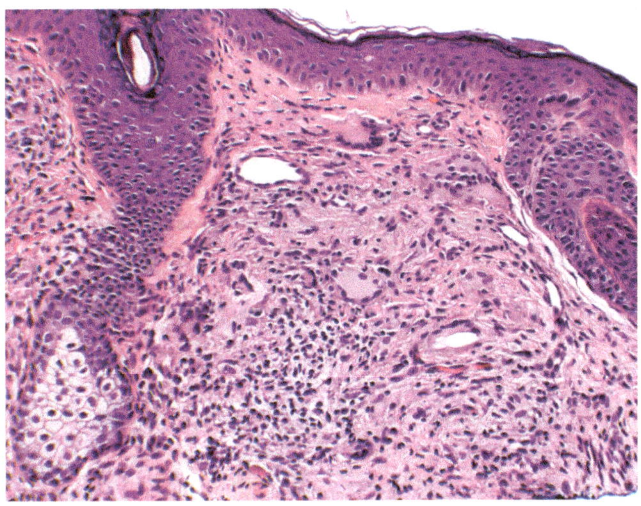

Acne rosacea, granulomatous stage. A perivascular and perifollicular granulomatous infiltrate. Note dilated, telangiectatic blood vessels.

Perioral dermatitis is seen most commonly in young women. The underlying etiology is not understood, but potent fluorinated topical steroids were implicated in the past. Some consider perioral dermatitis a distinct entity, while others consider it a form of acne rosacea. Patients present with relatively symmetric erythematous papules or pustules in a perioral distribution. Involvement of the nasolabial folds is fairly characteristic. Similar lesions may occur exclusively in a periocular distribution (**periocular dermatitis**). In general, the histopathologic features of perioral dermatitis and rosacea are identical.

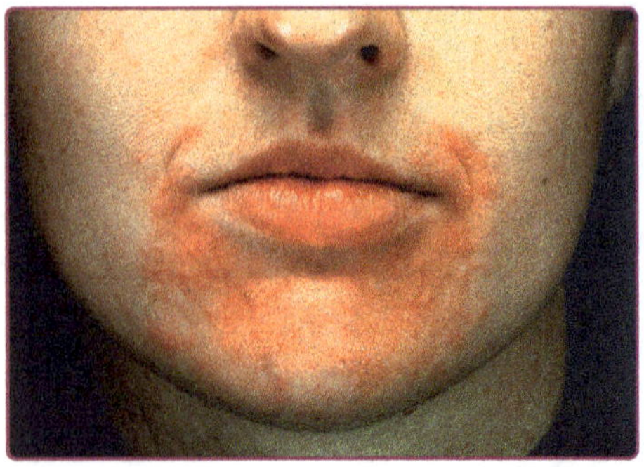

Typical perioral dermatitis. The eruption is confined to the nasolabial folds and the skin of the chin.

Lupus miliaris disseminatus faciei is probably best classified as a variant of granulomatous acne rosacea with extensive caseation necrosis. In the past, this condition was believed to be caused by mycobacterial infection however microorganisms are consistently absent. In **sarcoidosis**, the granulomas are "naked," lacking a well-developed peripheral cuff of lymphocytes. This finding is nonspecific since they may also be seen in cheilitis granulomatosa/Miescher-Melkersson-Rosenthal Syndrome. However, these "naked" granulomas of sarcoidosis are not typically situated adjacent or within lymphatics. **Cutaneous T-cell lymphomas** sometimes can demonstrate an accompanying reactive granulomatous infiltrate. On head and neck sites, the lesions of **natural killer (NK)/T-cell lymphoma** (previously known as ***lethal midline granuloma***) can feature large numbers of reactive histiocytes and NK cells that can cause misinterpretation as a reactive process.

Table 2-14A. Cheilitis Granulomatosa and Miescher-Melkersson-Rosenthal Syndrome

Clinical Features
Miescher-Melkersson-Rosenthal Syndrome
Lip swelling
Unilateral facial paralysis
Furrowed tongue
Cheilitis granulomatosa
Lip swelling, alone
Histopathologic Features
Noncaseating granulomas adjacent to and impinging on dilated lymphatics
Dermal edema
Perivascular lymphocytes and plasma cells
Differential Diagnosis
Oral-facial granulomas
Acne rosacea
Perioral dermatitis
Crohn disease
Sarcoidosis
Lupus vulgaris and other infections
Chronic granulomatous disease

ANSWER 2-15: C.

The biopsy reveals a subcutaneous inflammatory process with "naked" noncaseating granulomas (**lobular granulomatous panniculitis**). The combined clinical and histopathological findings are consistent with **cutaneous Crohn disease** (Table 2-15A). Crohn disease is a form of intrinsic inflammatory bowel disease. The pathogenesis is not understood, but it may be immunologically mediated. Unlike ulcerative colitis, all parts of the gastrointestinal tract are potentially affected, including oral and perianal areas. Clinically, oral involvement presents as cobblestoning, facial/lip swelling, or linear ulcers and may precede gastrointestinal involvement by many years. Perianal involvement presents as fistulas, sinus tracts, or ulcers. Cutaneous involvement at sites distant from the anus or mouth has been termed "**metastatic Crohn disease**," a designation that should be avoided because it implies a malignancy. These disseminated lesions present as nodules or plaques in the flexural areas and tend to ulcerate. Lesions on the lower extremities (mimicking **erythema nodosum**) and the penis are common. Vulvar disease has also been reported. Finally, in patients with colostomies, peristomal lesions may be seen. Rarely, patients may have quiescent bowel disease but active cutaneous lesions as the sole manifestation of persistent disease, even developing during sulfasalazine treatment. The cutaneous disease in these settings is very refractory to therapy.

Regardless of site, histopathology reveals noncaseating granulomatous inflammation with lymphocytes and plasma cells, often extending deeply into the subcutaneous tissue, where it may produce an extensive septal-lobular panniculitis. Palisaded granulomatous areas may be present as well as granulomatous vasculitis. On genitalia, marked edema may accompany the granulomatous changes.

In regards to the differential diagnosis, granulomas in the deep dermis or subcutis, especially with granulomatous vasculitis, should suggest Crohn disease. In oral and perioral sites, the differential diagnosis includes **cheilitis granulomatosa**, which is typified by granulomas adjacent to dilated lymphatic vessels. **Sarcoidosis** is also characterized by "naked" granulomas therefore clinical correlation is essential for diagnosis. In the perianal or vulvar areas, **hidradenitis suppurativa** enters the differential diagnosis. The granulomas of hidradenitis suppurativa are folliculocentric and usually are accompanied by suppuration. Frequently the hair follicles exhibit varying degrees of rupture and abscess formation.

Cutaneous T-cell lymphoma can exhibit granulomatous inflammation, and this is particularly true of **granulomatous mycosis fungoides** and **granulomatous slack skin disease. Granulomatous mycosis fungoides** is a histopathologic variant of mycosis fungoides that features noncaseating granulomatous inflammation in addition to usual papillary dermal and epidermal changes of mycosis fungoides. Extension into the subcutis would be highly unusual. **Granulomatous slack skin disease** is a low grade T-cell proliferation that may represent a variant of mycosis fungoides. It clinically presents as large, pendulous folds of the skin in the axillae, groin, and elsewhere. Histopathology reveals noncaseating granulomatous

Table 2-15A. Cutaneous Crohn Disease

Clinical Features
Facial or lip swelling
Oral mucosa cobblestoning/linear ulcers
Perianal ulcers, sinus tracts, fistulas
Ulcerating nodules/plaques in flexural areas, genitalia, or peri-colostomy sites
Erythema nodosum–like lesion
Histopathologic Features
Noncaseating granulomas with deep dermal and subcutaneous extension
Granulomatous panniculitis, often
Differential Diagnosis
Oral-facial granulomas
Acne rosacea
Perioral dermatitis
Cheilitis granulomatosa
Sarcoidosis
Lupus vulgaris and other infections
Chronic granulomatous disease
Hidradenitis suppurativa

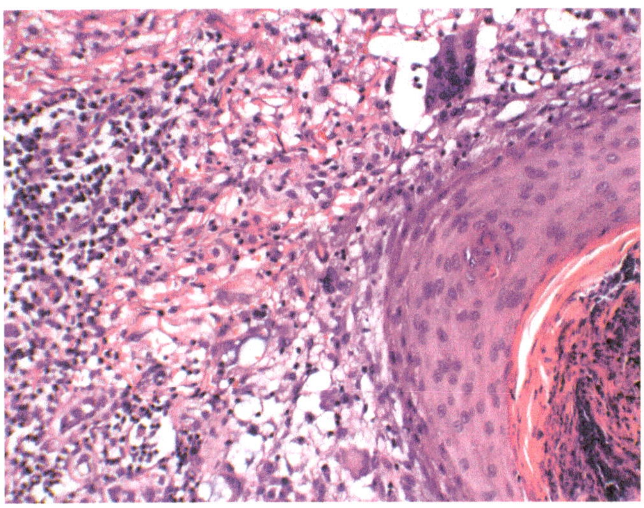

Hidradenitis suppurativa. Mixed neutrophilic and granulomatous inflammation surrounds an inflamed hair follicle, with an infundibular abscess.

inflammation with papillary dermal and epidermal changes suggesting mycosis fungoides. The multinucleated giant cells in the infiltrate are characteristic, containing large numbers of nuclei (up to 50) per cell (multinucleated giant cells). Elastic tissue stains reveal almost complete loss of connective tissue elastic fibers. Again, extension into the subcutis would be highly unusual. **Angiomatoid fibrous histiocytoma** is a soft tissue neoplasm of intermediate malignancy usually seen in childhood. Due to the combination of epithelioid and spindle-shaped cells that resemble histiocytes and accompanying lymphoid aggregates, this neoplasm superficially can resemble a reactive granulomatous infiltrate. **Behçet disease** also may present with aphthous ulcers of the oral and genital mucosa however it is histopathologically characterized by leukocytoclastic vasculitis with a robust lymphocytic infiltrate. Linear ulcerations are not characteristic.

ANSWER 2-16: E.

The biopsy reveals numerous superficial and deep "naked" granulomas without destruction of adnexal structures. The findings are consistent with **sarcoidosis** (Table 2-16A). Sarcoidosis is a systemic disease of unknown etiology that affects multiple organ systems, typically the lungs, lymph nodes, skin, and eyes. Black females are the most commonly affected patient population. Approximately 25% of patients with systemic involvement have cutaneous involvement, and rarely, the skin may be involved alone. The clinical presentation of sarcoidosis may be extremely diverse. Sarcoidosis presenting as smooth-surfaced, violaceous nodules on the nose, cheeks, or earlobes is referred to as **lupus pernio**. Other sites may show brown-purple indurated papules, nodules, or plaques with annular or serpiginous configurations. A diffuse maculopapular form also is recognized. Lesions may develop in scars or tattoos. Scalp involvement causes a secondary scarring alopecia.

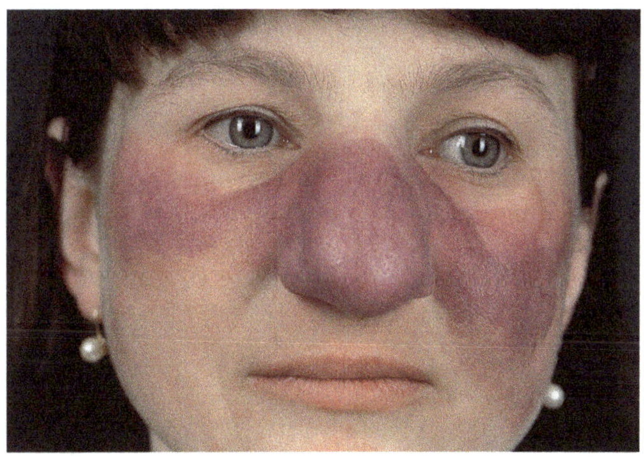

Sarcoidosis. This is the classic appearance of "lupus pernio" with violaceous, soft, doughy infiltrations on cheeks and nose, which is grossly enlarged. (Reproduced, with permission, from Wolff K, Johnson RA, Saavedra AP. *Fitzpatrick's Color Atlas and Synopsis of Clinical Dermatology*. 7th ed. New York, NY: McGraw-Hill Education; 2013.)

Microscopically, noncaseating epithelioid granulomas are typically scattered throughout the dermis without any relation to nerves, hair follicles, or blood vessels. The granulomas are usually "naked," having no or only a sparse surrounding lymphocytic infiltrate. Although not frequently described, sarcoidal granulomas may fill the papillary dermis and abut the epidermis, producing spongiosis, crusting, and irregular hyperplasia. The centers of some granulomas may

Table 2-16A. Sarcoidosis

Clinical Features
Systemic disease with lung, eye, lymph node, and skin involvement
Lupus pernio
Violaceous nodules on nose, cheeks, earlobes
Brown-purple papules, nodules, plaques
Diffuse maculopapular form, rarely
Scarring alopecia
Development of lesions in scars, tattoos
Histopathologic Features
"Naked" epithelioid granulomas, lacking well-developed lymphocyte cuff
Asteroid bodies
Schaumann bodies
Hamazaki-Wasserman bodies
Differential Diagnosis
Oral-facial granulomas
Acne rosacea
Perioral dermatitis
Cheilitis granulomatosa
Crohn disease
Chronic granulomatous disease
Foreign body granulomas
Tattoo pigments
Silicates
Zirconium
Beryllium
Infectious agents
Tuberculosis
Tuberculoid leprosy
Secondary and tertiary syphilis
Leishmaniasis
Lymphoproliferative disorders

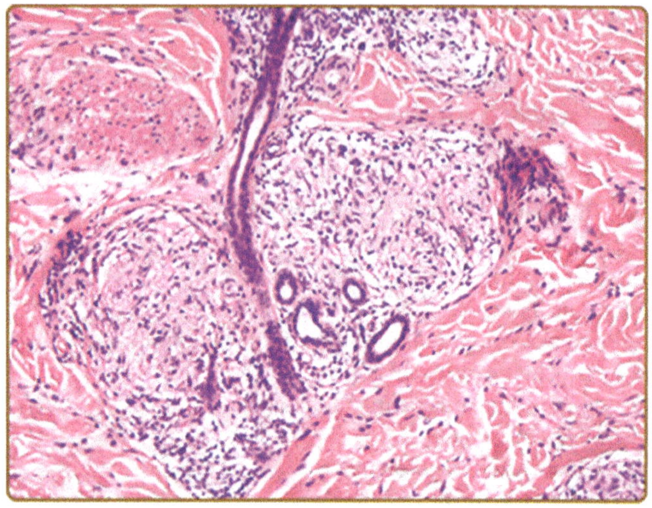

Sarcoidosis. Higher power view of "naked" epithelioid cell granulomas around a sweat duct and sweat glands. The ducts and glands are not damaged therefore the infiltrate is not a secondary response. (Reproduced, with permission, from Goldsmith LA, Katz SI, Gilchrest BA, Paller AS, Leffell DJ, Wolff K, eds. *Fitzpatrick's Dermatology in General Medicine*. 8th ed. New York, NY: McGraw-Hill Education; 2012.)

demonstrate fibrinoid degeneration and even frank caseation necrosis when the subcutaneous fat is involved. **Asteroid bodies, Schaumann bodies**, and **Hamazaki-Wasserman bodies** may be present but are nonspecific. One may see a number of cytoplasmic positively birefringent crystals on polarization, which probably are calcium oxalate and calcium carbonate degradation products of cell metabolism. Although their appearance should make one consider a diagnosis of foreign-body reaction, such crystals are a well-established phenomenon in both pulmonary and cutaneous sarcoidosis.

In regards to the differential diagnosis, lesions of **lupus pernio** on the face need to be distinguished from other forms of oral-facial granulomas, especially **acne rosacea**. Although the granulomatous stage of acne rosacea may contain "naked" granulomas, these granulomas are typically perifollicular in distribution, unlike sarcoidosis. Clinical correlation may be required for definitive diagnostic distinction. Although uncommon, an intermediate-grade soft tissue neoplasm known as ***plexiform fibrohistiocytic tumor*** can simulate a granulomatous process due to the presence of osteoclast-like multinucleated giant cells. It is usually encountered in children and young adults and is characterized by a biphasic appearance with fascicles of spindle cells merging with and surrounding small nodules composed of histiocytic cells and multinucleate osteoclast-like giant cells. When polarizable crystals are present, the differential diagnosis includes **foreign-body giant cell reactions** (Table 2-16B). Clinically, foreign-body reactions are usually solitary lesions, often with a history of prior trauma, and histopathologically, the foreign material is relatively abundant. If the clinical picture is typical, the presence of a rare crystal by polarization microscopy should not negate a diagnosis of sarcoidosis. Granulomatous inflammation frequently forms around either endogenous or exogenous material that comes in direct contact with the dermis, where it is perceived as foreign. This occurs commonly when keratin flakes or hair shaft, devoid of epithelial cloaks, are extruded into the dermis (ruptured cyst or hair follicle). A foreign-body granulomatous infiltrate, frequently with suppuration (neutrophils), forms around these structures. Injected carbon (**carbon tattoos**) is inert, and if one sees granulomatous inflammation associated with a carbon tattoo, there are additional substances present (**silica**) that are responsible for the inflammatory response. Regardless of the origin, multinucleated giant cells, usually with nuclei conglomerated centrally or at one edge of the cell, form around the structure in an attempt to phagocytize and destroy the substance. Table 2-16B lists both endogenous and exogenous foreign materials commonly encountered in skin specimens.

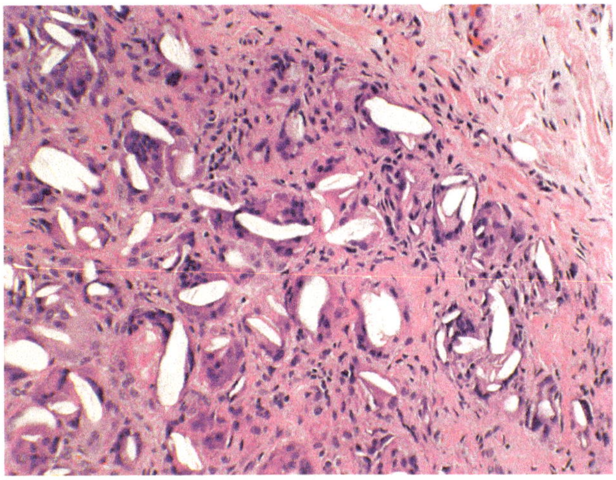

Foreign body granuloma to keratin. There are numerous multinucleated giant cells surrounding clear cleft-like spaces containing thin eosinophilic keratin flakes. This is a common finding in ruptured epidermoid cysts.

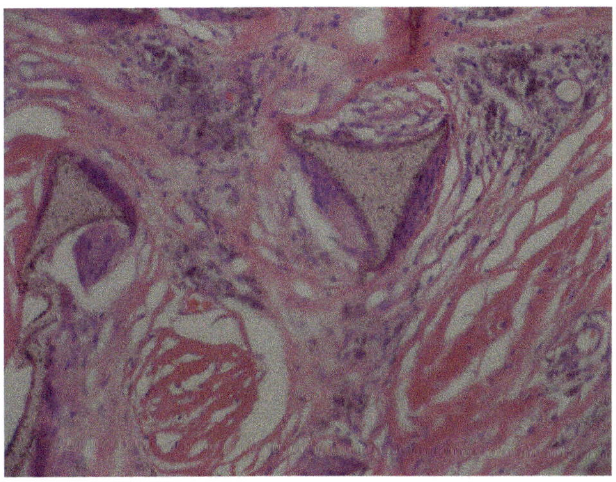

Foreign body reaction to retained surgical sponge. There is a granulomatous infiltrate with multinucleated giant cells surrounding triangular and diamond-shaped refractile material.

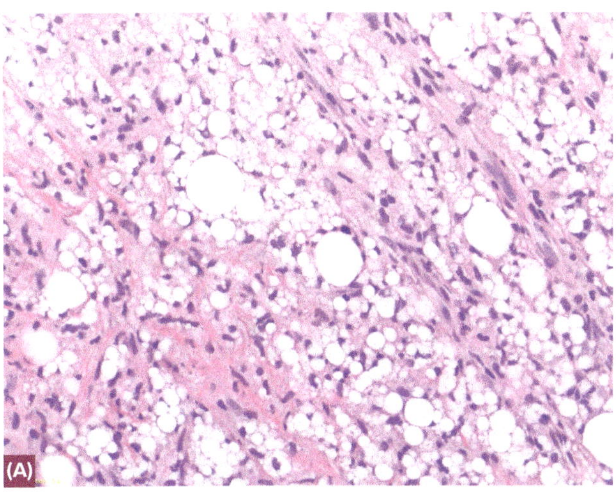

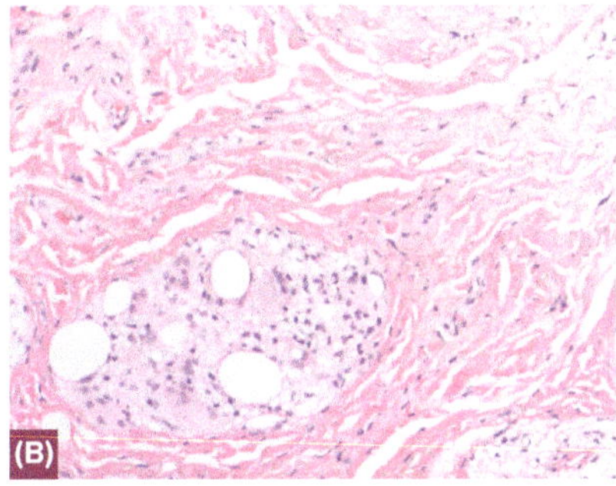

Foreign body giant cell reaction to silicone. (A) Silicone is relatively inert and may present with little inflammation. Silicone appears as clear circular spaces of varying sizes, imparting a "Swiss cheese" appearance. **(B)** There is a granulomatous infiltrate containing foreign body giant cells surrounding small round clear spaces.

ANSWER 2-17: A.

The biopsy reveals a lymphoplasmacytic and granulomatous infiltrate of the foreign-body type surrounding spherical aggregates of lipid, consistent with a **chalazion**. **Chalazia** are eyelid lesions that are the result of a foreign-body inflammatory reaction to lipid released from ruptured sebaceous glands (meibomian glands). Clinically, chalazia present as nodules of the eyelid, and they are usually painless and solitary.

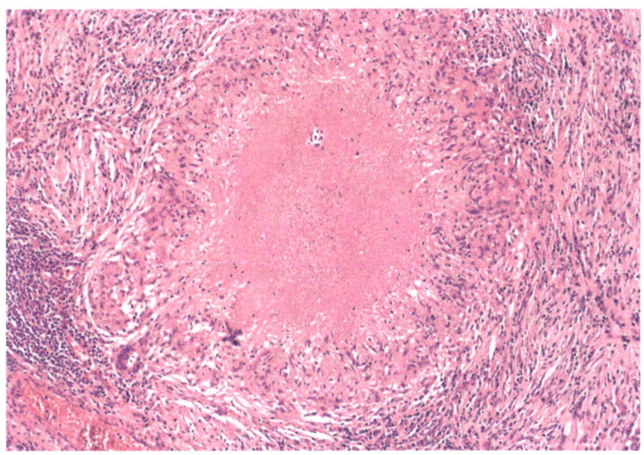

Lupus miliaris disseminatus faciei. There is a large granuloma containing central eosinophilic caseous necrosis. (Reproduced, with permission, from Brunicardi FC et al, eds. *Schwartz's Principles of Surgery*. 9th ed. New York, NY: McGraw-Hill; 2010.)

In regards to the differential diagnosis, granulomatous inflammation of the eyelid is highly suggestive of chalazion, and the presence of distinct vacuoles that represent lipid dissolved during specimen processing is distinctive. Some cases of **Miescher-Melkersson-Rosenthal Syndrome** may involve primarily the eyelid, but dilated lymphatics with perilymphatic granulomas and edema are characteristic of

Table 2-16B. Foreign-Body Granulomas

MATERIAL	H&E FEATURES	ADJUNCTIVE TECHNIQUES	CLINICAL/SOURCE
Suture material	Basophilic-yellow fibers	Polarizable	Prior surgery
Tattoo pigments	Black pigment granules		Chrome green; carbon; cobalt blue; cinnabar
Starch	10-20 μm oval, particles	Polarizable; PAS-, GMS-positive; maltese cross birefringence	Surgical glove powder; IV drug abuse
Talc (magnesium silicate)	10-20 μm particles	Polarizable, white particles; x-ray diffraction	
Oils (mineral oil, paraffin, cottenseed, sesame, camphor)	Round-ovoid clear spaces; "Swiss cheese" appearance	Sudan IV, oil red O stains reveal lipid on frozen tissue	Male genitalia (sclerosing lipogranuloma)
Silicone	Round-ovoid clear spaces; "Swiss cheese" appearance		Breast augmentation mammoplasty
Hair	Hair shaft		Interdigital web space; barbers; dog groomers
Silica (Silicon dioxide)	Sarcoidal granulomas; crystalline particles	Polarizable; spectrographic analysis	Contamination of wound from soil or glass
Zirconium	Sarcoidal granulomas	Nonpolarizable; spectrographic analysis, only	Deodorant sticks
Aluminum (adjuvant in vaccines)	Central basophilic granular material	x-ray microanalysis	Site of vaccinations
Beryllium	Sarcoidal with hyalinized central necrosis	Nonpolarizable; spectrographic analysis, only	Fluorescent light bulbs
Injectable steroid	Amphophilic granular/ amorphous material, sometimes with crystalline material	Weakly PAS-positive	Intralesional corticosteroids
Gout (sodium urate)	Amorphous amphophilic material; needle-shaped urate crystals seen in specimens fixed in alcohol	Alcohol fixation preserves crystals better than formalin; under polarized light, crystals are negatively birefringent	Big toe, helix of ear
Injectable collagen	May be sarcoidal or palisaded granulomatous	Electron microscopy	History of bovine collagen injection
Mercury	Spherical black globules with foreign body reaction, refractile brown-black granules in macrophages (up to 300 μm)		Self-injection, thermometer accidents, topical mercurial preparations

that condition. Recurrent chalazia should arouse suspicion for **sebaceous carcinoma**, but histopathologically, chalazia lack the cytologic atypia seen in sebaceous carcinoma. **Acne rosacea** may involve the lids but usually does not present as a solitary lesion. **Lupus miliaris disseminatus faciei** most likely represents a dramatic form of the granulomatous stage of acne rosacea. As with granulomatous acne rosacea, patients present with yellow-brown papules on the central face. Eyelid involvement is characteristic. Microscopically the granulomas of lupus miliaris disseminatus faciei contain caseation necrosis, which may be prominent.

ANSWER 2-18: D.

The biopsy reveals interstitial and palisading inflammation composed of histiocytes (macrophages) and lymphocytes. The palisading component forms a ring-like pattern with central bright pink and light blue material. The amorphous "smoky" blue material is mucin. The findings are consistent with **granuloma annulare**. The etiology and pathogenesis underlying granuloma annulare is unknown; however, the following mechanisms have been suggested: cell-mediated immunity, immune complex–mediated vasculitis, abnormalities of macrophage function, and primary collagen degeneration. Clinically, children and young adults are mainly affected, although the disease can occur at any age. Women are affected more often than men. Granuloma annulare presents as localized erythematous, skin-colored, and occasionally violaceous discrete and coalescent papules in annular and polycyclic configurations, mainly on the dorsal surfaces of the hands, feet, arms, and legs. The lesions often enlarge centrifugally anywhere from 1 to 5 cm and usually are not associated with pruritus or other symptoms. On occasion, large geographic patches and plaques are encountered. Generalized or widely disseminated, giant, linear, perforating, and subcutaneous forms have been described. Umbilicated clustered lesions may simulate **molluscum contagiosum**. A recently described clinical variant of granuloma annulare presents with subtle patches on the extremities and trunk.

It is important to emphasize that an incomplete, early, or interstitial granuloma annulare–type histopathologic pattern is defined as a superficial and deep perivascular lymphocytic infiltrate with histiocytes splayed between collagen bundles. The epidermis is unremarkable. This dermal reaction pattern is nonspecific and can characterize interstitial granuloma annulare or simply represent an epiphenomenon associated with other processes. For example, one can see this **interstitial granuloma annulare–type reaction** in resolving **neutrophilic dermatitides (Sweet syndrome)**, **drug reactions**, and even **insect bites** with no clinical evidence of granuloma annulare.

The fully developed lesion of granuloma annulare (**palisading GA**) displays a palisaded granulomatous dermatitis surrounding an area of degenerated collagen. Such palisading granulomas are usually focal and discrete phenomena in the dermis with intervening normal collagen. The process is typically limited to the superficial dermis however may occasionally extend along the fibrous trabeculae of the subcutaneous fat and thus constitute a septal panniculitis (**subcutaneous granuloma annulare**). Connective tissue mucin deposition within the central degenerated collagen is a near-constant finding but may require special stains (alcian blue or colloidal iron) to demonstrate. In hematoxylin and eosin (H&E)-stained sections, mucin appears as stringy and/or granular basophilic material. Uncommonly, the collagen degeneration is characterized by fully developed fibrinoid necrosis. Away from the central palisade, there is a superficial and deep perivascular inflammatory cell infiltrate of lymphocytes and macrophages. On occasion one may observe a so-called **sarcoidal variant of GA** based on the finding of aggregates of epithelioid histiocytes that mimic sarcoidosis. Lesions with overlapping feature of both GA and sarcoidosis have been described. In some instances, particularly in sun-damaged skin, the macrophages and multinucleate giant cells comprising the palisaded infiltrates are noted to contain phagocytosed elastic fibers (**elastophagocytosis**). The latter finding is nonspecific, and the demonstration of collagen degeneration with mucin deposition provides confirmatory evidence for GA. Eosinophils occur in approximately 40% of cases and may be so numerous as to suggest an **arthropod bite reaction**.

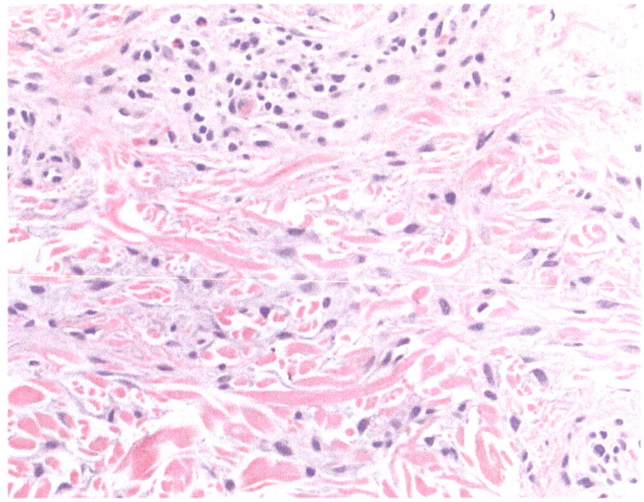

Granuloma annulare, interstitial variant. There are interstitial histiocytes scaffolding along the collagen bundles with increased dermal mucin. Note the rare scattered eosinophils.

The major differential diagnostic consideration is **necrobiosis lipoidica (NL)**. The following features help distinguish granuloma annulare from NL:

1. In GA, the dermis surrounding the primary focus of inflammation is normal. In NL, it is often altered.
2. NL features a greater degree of central collagen degeneration. Sometimes the central collagen in GA is not yet morphologically altered.

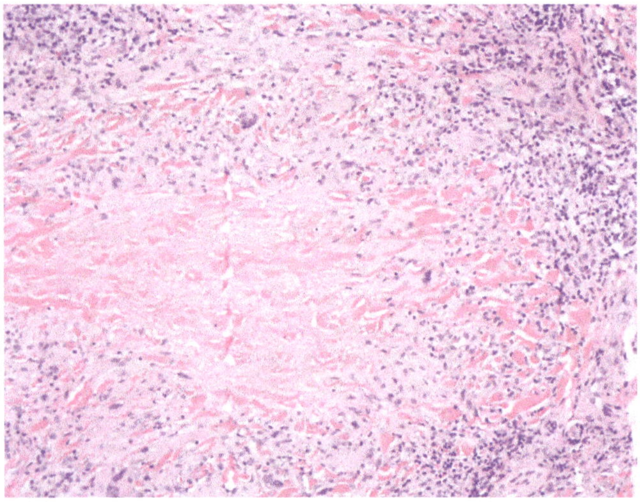

Granuloma annulare, palisaded variant. There is a "wreath" of granulomatous inflammation (including giant cells) surrounding degenerated, brightly eosinophilic, necrobiotic collagen. The pale amphophilic material is dermal mucin.

3. NL lacks central mucin deposition as a rule. Central mucin in GA usually is prominent but may require special stains for demonstration.
4. The palisades in GA are round to ovoid. In NL, they are horizontally oriented tiers (layer cake).
5. NL features prominent plasma cells, whereas GA does not and may contain eosinophils.
6. NL may demonstrate a granulomatous vasculitis not seen in GA.

QUICK FACT

Interstitial Granulomatous Drug Eruption

Interstitial GA-pattern with eosinophils + vacuolar interface dermatitis

Medications

- Ca^{2+} Channel Blockers
- ACE Inhibitors
- β-Blockers
- Statins
- Antihistamines
- Anticonvulsants
- Antidepressants

Central mucin accumulation and focal (as opposed to diffuse) dermal involvement are distinguishing features of GA. **Eruptive xanthomas** can mimic this pattern but are recognized by foamy macrophages, occasional neutrophils, extracellular lipid, no mucin, and rarely, urate-like crystals. The **interstitial granulomatous drug eruption** typically exhibits the dermal changes of interstitial granuloma annulare with eosinophils, but with sparse vacuolar interface dermatitis. Implicated drug classes include calcium channel blockers, angiotensin converting enzyme inhibitors, beta-blockers, lipid-lowering agents, antihistamines, anticonvulsants, and antidepressants.

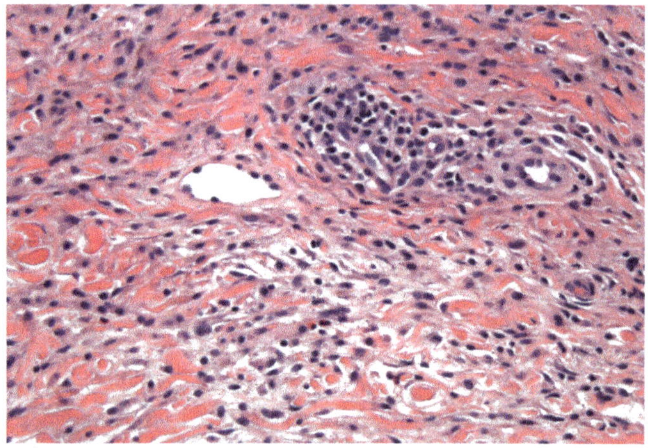

Interstitial palisading granulomatous drug reaction. The interstitium shows columns of histiocytes infiltrating between collagen bundles. Although not visualized, the epidermis most likely exhibits vacuolar interface dermatitis.

QUICK FACT

Palisaded Neutrophilic and Granulomatous Dermatitis

Interstitial GA-pattern with neutrophils, +/− leukocytoclastic vasculitis

- **Sign of systemic disease!!!!**

Palisaded neutrophilic and granulomatous dermatitis is an umbrella term suggested to encompass conditions that all share GA-like or necrobiosis lipoidica-like histology, but most likely represent an inflammatory reaction to a primary vasculopathy/vasculitis (Table 2-17A). The associated systemic diseases include **systemic lupus erythematosus, rheumatoid arthritis, Sjögren syndrome, Wegener granulomatosis** (and other **ANCA-positive vasculitides**), **inflammatory bowel disease, hepatitis, lymphoproliferative disease, myelodysplastic syndromes, cancer, thyroid disease, diabetes mellitus, drug reactions**, and **infections** (including **bacterial endocarditis, Epstein–Barr virus, HIV, *Mycoplasma pneumoniae*, parvovirus, hepatitis C**, and ***Borrelia burgdorferi***). Patients present with skin-colored to erythematous papules with overlying crust, ulceration, or umbilication. The papules are found predominantly on extremities and trunk and often are distributed symmetrically. Other clinical presentations include plaques and

Table 2-17A. Palisaded Granulomatous Dermatitis

GRANULOMA ANNULARE (GA)	NECROBIOSIS LIPOIDICA	RHEUMATOID NODULE	RHEUMATIC FEVER NODULE	PALISADED NEUTROPHILIC AND GRANULOMATOUS DERMATITIS	NECROBIOTIC XANTHOGRANULOMA	INFECTION
Clinical Features						
Annular papules	Plaques Shins	Adults with rheumatoid arthritis	Children with rheumatic fever	Many associated diseases	IgG paraproteinemia	Variable, according to specific infection
Hands, feet, arms, legs		Subcutaneous nodules	Subcutaneous nodules	Umbilicated papules	Papules, nodules, plaques	Often immuno-compromised
		Elbows, knuckles, Achilles tendon	Elbows, knuckles	Extremities	Face, periorbital	
Histopathologic Features						
Palisades	Palisades	Subcutaneous palisades	Similar to rheumatoid nodule, sometimes with neutrophils/leukocytoclasis	Early	Central cholesterol clefts	Central necrosis with numerous neutrophils
Round/oval	Horizontally oriented			GA-like, with prominent neutrophils/leukocytoclasis	Foreign-body and Touton-type giant cells	
Discrete/focal	Diffuse/full-thickness					
Central mucin	No central mucin	Central eosinophilic fibrinoid necrosis			Lymphocytes/plasma cells	
No plasma cells	Plasma cells				Lymphoid follicles, sometimes	
	Vasculitis, sometimes	No central mucin				
		Vasculitis, sometimes				
"Incomplete" form		Lipidized macrophages		Late		
Macrophages splayed between collagen fibers				Extravascular foci of degenerated stroma, mucin may be present		
Central mucin						

sometimes-linear papules, cords, and bands. Microscopically, **palisaded neutrophilic and granulomatous dermatitis** features either the interstitial or palisading granulomatous pattern, but with significant numbers of neutrophils and/or neutrophilic nuclear dust. Focal leukocytoclastic vasculitis may be present. **Granulomatous mycosis fungoides** is a histopathologic variant of mycosis fungoides that features granulomatous inflammation. The pattern of granulomatous inflammation is variable and may be diffuse or palisaded, but there are usually superimposed changes of conventional mycosis fungoides in which small, atypical lymphocytes permeate the epidermis (epidermotropism). **Dermatofibromas** also exhibit an interstitial pattern of histiocytic growth with wrapping of peripheral collagen bundles. These cells are positive for factor XIIIa. Additionally, dermatofibromas are not associated with increased dermal mucin.

ANSWER 2-19: D.

The biopsy reveals a superficial and deep palisading granulomatous dermatitis with large areas of degenerated collagen. The infiltrate is composed of lymphocytes, foamy macrophages, and plasma cells. The degenerated areas contain foci with large clear needle-shaped structures, consistent with cholesterol clefts. The findings are consistent with **necrobiotic xanthogranuloma (NXG)**. Necrobiotic xanthogranuloma occurs in association with IgG paraproteinemia (usually kappa subtype) in approximately 80% of cases. Other laboratory findings include hypocomplementemia, cryoglobulinemia, anemia, and leukopenia. Bone marrow examination may reveal plasmacytosis, and rare cases can be seen in association with **multiple myeloma** or **B-cell lymphoma**. Clinically, indurated papules, nodules, or plaques (sometimes with ulceration/atrophy) most commonly occur periobitally (85% of cases) but can involve the trunk and extremities. The oral mucosa is occasionally involved. Systemic manifestations can include hepatosplenomegaly (20% cases), arthritis/arthralgias, or neuropathy.

Microscopically, necrobiotic xanthogranuloma demonstrates broad zones of collagen degeneration and cholesterol clefts surrounded by foamy macrophages with foreign-body and Touton-type multinucleated giant cells. Numerous lymphocytes and plasma cells (sometimes with lymphoid follicle formation) are conspicuous. These changes extend throughout the dermis, sometimes into the subcutaneous fat.

In regards to the differential diagnosis, innumerable foam cells and cholesterol clefts are pathognomonic for necrobiotic xanthogranuloma. While plasma cells are seen in both **necrobiotic xanthogranuloma** and **necrobiosis lipoidica**, necrobiosis lipoidica does not involve the face and lacks numerous foam cells and cholesterol clefts. Like necrobiotic xanthogranuloma, **xanthogranuloma** (aka **juvenile xanthogranuloma**) also commonly occurs on facial skin and contains characteristic "Touton" giant cells. However, xanthogranuloma lacks the palisading growth pattern, areas of necrobiotic collagen, and cholesterol clefts. **Actinic granuloma** (aka **annular elastolytic granuloma**) is a controversial entity that also frequently presents with facial lesions. Some consider it a distinct condition. Others believe that it is simply **granuloma annulare** (**GA**) at sun-damaged sites. Like GA, its pathogenesis and inciting events are not understood. A cell-mediated immunologic reaction to altered elastotic fibers has been proposed. Adult patients present with expanding arciform papules and plaques, usually on the face, but also at other sun-exposed areas such as the chest, arms, and neck. Individual lesions tend to resolve spontaneously over time. The peripheral, "active," part of the lesion demonstrates either an interstitial collection of macrophages between individual collagen bundles (similar to the incomplete/interstitial pattern of GA) or a prominent palisaded granulomatous dermatitis arranged around elastotic material in the superficial dermis (**elastophagocytosis**). The giant cells contain blue-gray elastotic material (solar elastosis), and **asteroid bodies** may be seen. Neither prominent mucin nor degenerated collagen typically is present. The central portion of the plaque demonstrates loss of both elastotic fibers and normal elastic fibers.

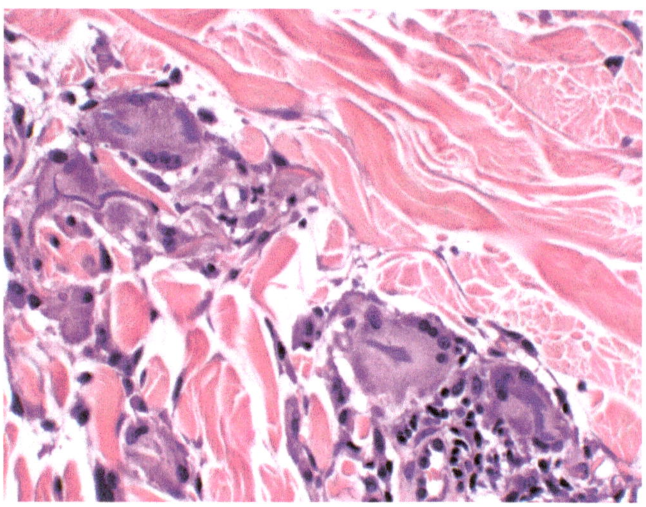

Actinic granuloma (annular elastolytic granuloma). This pattern is a granuloma annulare–type reaction on severely sun-damaged skin. There is extensive phagocytosis of elastic fibers (elastophagocytosis).

While **pyoderma gangrenosum (PG)** may present with ulcers in patients with paraproteinemia, it should really only be included in the clinical differential diagnosis. Microscopically, PG is composed of robust neutrophilic infiltrates with mild leukocytoclasia. While resolving lesions may exhibit focal areas resembling **interstitial granuloma annulare** or **palisaded neutrophilic and granulomatous dermatitis**, PG lacks the extensive areas of necrobiosis and cholesterol clefts.

ANSWER 2-20: B.

The biopsy reveals a palisaded granulomatous infiltrate alternating with degenerated collagen in a somewhat laminated array and extends in a confluent fashion from the upper reticular dermis to the subcutaneous fat. Numerous plasma cells are present around the deeper vessels. Dermal mucin is absent. This is a classic example of **necrobiosis lipoidica** (NL). Approximately two-thirds of patients with necrobiosis lipoidica have diabetes mellitus. On the other hand, in patients with diabetes mellitus, necrobiosis lipoidica occurs in less than 1%. Evidence suggests that the degree of hyperglycemia and diabetic control does not correlate with the presence of NL. The etiology and pathogenesis are not fully understood, but microangiopathic changes, immune complex–mediated vasculitis, and a thrombotic tendency have been implicated. Females are affected more often than males (3:1). Adults present with waxy, indurated, yellow-brown patches or plaques with a surrounding erythematous, raised, and expanding margin. Lesions characteristically are found on the anterior shins however 15% of patients develop lesions on the upper extremities and trunk and tend to be more papulonodular. Although pain and pruritus have been reported, most lesions are asymptomatic. Anesthesia of the plaques does occur.

Biopsies of the erythematous margin show palisaded and granulomatous dermatitis, often involving full-thickness dermis and extending into subcutaneous fat. In contrast to the circular palisades seen in **granuloma annulare**, the palisades in necrobiosis lipoidica assume a horizontal and parallel arrangement with respect to the overlying epidermis. Some have referred to this horizontal arrangement of granulomas and necrobiosis as a "layer cake." The central portion of the palisade shows marked collagen degeneration without connective tissue mucin. The dermis to the periphery of the palisaded area is usually fibrotic (in contrast to a near normal dermis seen in GA), sometimes with lipid deposition. In many instances, the interface between the dermis and subcutis is well demarcated, linear, and parallel to the skin surface. There is an accompanying superficial and deep perivascular inflammatory cell infiltrate usually demonstrating plasma cells. In some cases vessels at the junction of the dermis and subcutaneous fat show leukocytoclastic vasculitis in acute lesions and granulomatous vasculitis in chronic lesions. Involvement of the subcutis takes the form of a predominantly septal panniculitis. The atrophic centers of plaques demonstrate fibrosis.

In regards to the differential diagnosis, the main histopathological considerations include **granuloma annulare** (GA), **rheumatoid nodule**, and **necrobiotic xanthogranuloma**. Horizontally oriented arrays of palisading granulomatous dermatitis with marked collagen degeneration, diffuse as opposed to focal dermal involvement, a lack of connective tissue mucin, and the presence of plasma cells are features that distinguish necrobiosis lipoidica from **GA** and **rheumatoid**

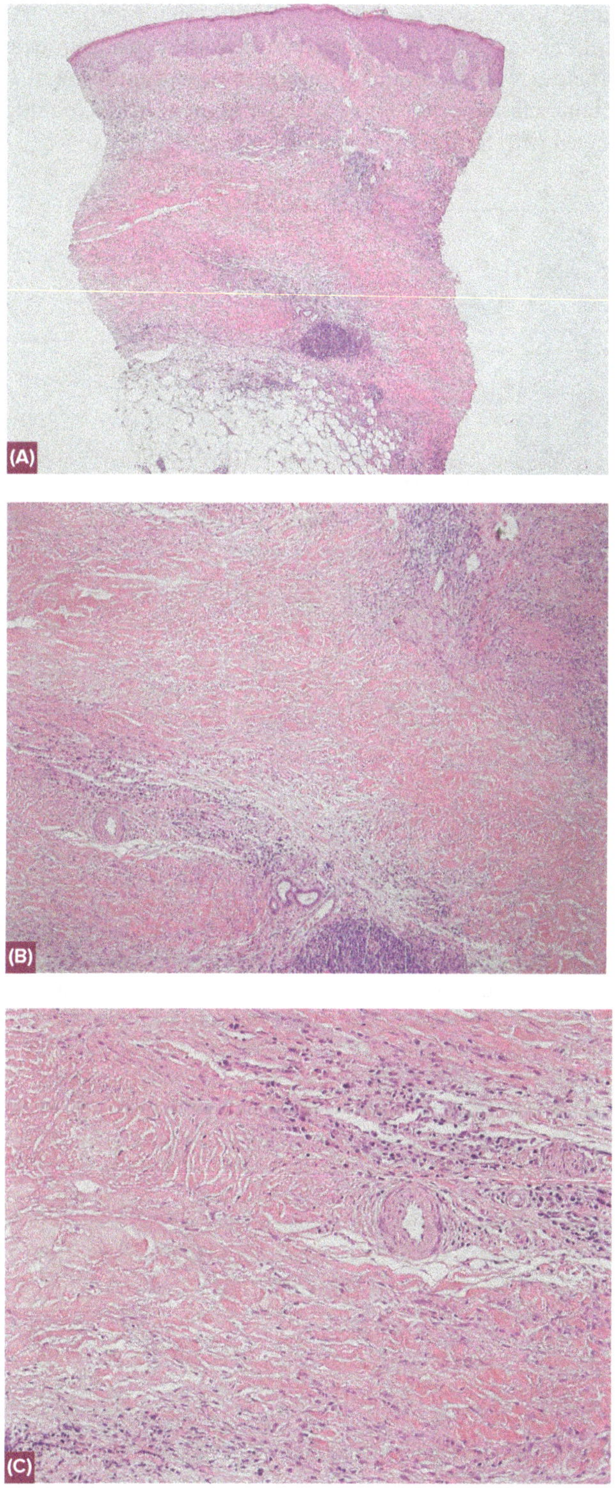

Necrobiosis lipoidica. (A) There are horizontal arrays of fibrosis and inflammation extending into the deep dermis–subcutis interface, imparting a "layer cake" configuration. **(B)** A thick horizontal band of necrobiotic collagen unaccompanied by dermal mucin is "sandwiched" between two bands of inflammatory cells. **(C)** The inflammatory infiltrate is composed of palisading granulomas admixed with plasma cells. Used with permission of Claudia Vidal, MD, PhD, St. Louis University School of Medicine.

nodule. In addition, necrobiosis lipoidica usually involves the dermis and possibly the subcutis, whereas the converse is true of rheumatoid nodule. **Necrobiotic xanthogranuloma** also contains plasma cells, but exhibits large areas of necrobiotic collagen with focal areas containing cholesterol clefts.

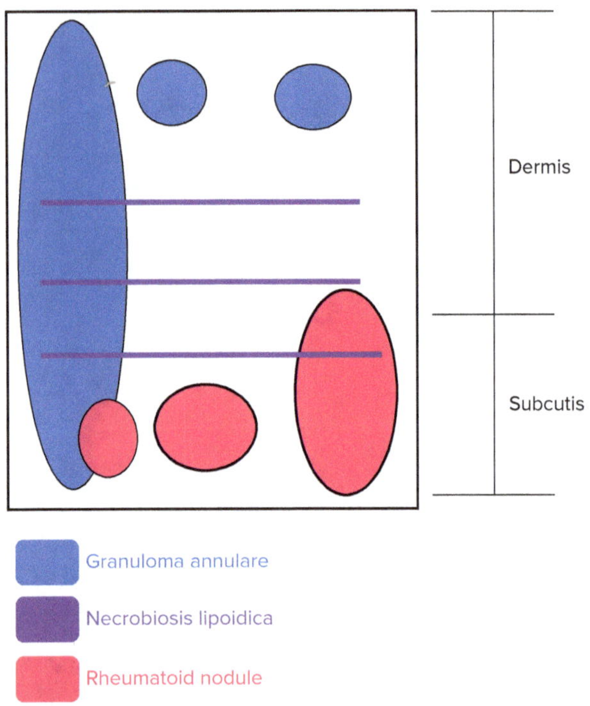

Palisaded granulomatous infiltrates. The diagram highlights the overall shape and distribution of the granulomatous infiltrates encountered in granuloma annulare, necrobiosis lipoidica, and rheumatoid nodules. Granuloma annulare is colored blue because it is the condition within the group that almost always contains dermal or subcutaneous mucin or both (blue granulomas). Although granuloma annulare most commonly involves the superficial dermis, the granulomatous inflammation may rarely extend all the way into the subcutis. Necrobiosis lipoidica demonstrates horizontal palisades of granulomatous inflammation. The nodular granulomas of rheumatoid nodule contain necrobiotic collagen without mucin (pink granulomas). Rarely both necrobiosis lipoidica and rheumatoid nodule may contain mucin.

ANSWER 2-21: D.

Rheumatoid nodules are seen in approximately 20% of adults with rheumatoid arthritis. Nodules with similar histology may be seen in visceral sites, including lung, heart, and gastrointestinal tract. The pathogenesis is most likely an immune complex–mediated vasculitis, which results in ischemic damage to subcutaneous tissues and a subsequent palisaded granulomatous inflammatory reaction. The immune complexes are typically composed of antibodies directed against other antibodies (**rheumatoid factor**). Rheumatoid nodules present in adults as subcutaneous nodules situated over joints, classically the elbows. Other common sites include the knuckles, Achilles tendon, and weight-bearing parts of the foot. Perforating variants are also known. Microscopically, within subcutaneous tissue and the lower dermis are palisaded granulomatous infiltrates surrounding a large area of homogeneous, eosinophilic fibrinoid necrosis of collagen (**necrobiosis**). The central necrobiotic area lacks pools of connective tissue mucin as a rule. Vasculitic changes with intact and degenerated neutrophils (leukocytoclastic) are usually apparent. The histopathological differential diagnosis for rheumatoid nodules includes **subcutaneous granuloma annulare, rheumatoid fever nodule**, and **epithelioid sarcoma**. The predominantly subcutaneous location and central fibrinoid necrosis (without pools of connective tissue mucin) are distinctive features of rheumatoid nodules. In general, the histology of **rheumatic fever nodule** and **rheumatoid nodule** is identical, but patients with rheumatic fever nodule have a prior or concurrent history of *Streptococcal* pharyngitis and rheumatic fever. Rheumatic fever nodules typically develop in children with a history of acute rheumatic fever. Sites of predilection include the bony prominences (humeral condyles, olecranon processes, knuckles) and occiput. Individual nodules resolve spontaneously. Similar nodules are found in the heart and are known as **Aschoff nodules**. Like rheumatoid nodules, the pathogenesis is most likely an immune complex–mediated vasculitis with subsequent ischemic damage followed by a palisaded granulomatous repair reaction. In **subcutaneous granuloma annulare**, the general architecture of the subcutaneous fat is preserved, and there are often scattered interstitial histiocytes. Granuloma annulare contains increased mucin, whereas rheumatoid arthritis almost always does not. **Epithelioid sarcoma** is a malignant soft tissue tumor that frequently demonstrates a palisaded pattern within the subcutaneous tissue. Its constituent cells may resemble macrophages, but they exhibit cytologic atypia and are positive with antibodies to cytokeratin, epithelial membrane antigen, or CD34.

QUICK FACT

- **Subcutaneous Granuloma Annulare**
  - "Blue granulomas" with mucin
- **Rheumatoid Nodule**
  - "Pink granulomas" usually without mucin
- **Rheumatic Fever Nodule**
  - Identical to rheumatoid nodule

Other cutaneous manifestations of rheumatoid arthritis include **Bywaters lesions**, which are characterized by nail fold telangiectasias, minute digital ulcerations or petechiae, and digital pulp papules. These papules are a manifestation of mild vasculitis and typically occur without systemic signs of vasculitis. The spectrum of clinical lesions reported in **rheumatoid vasculitis** is wide and varies with the size and location of the vessels involved and with the extent of the disease. Unfortunately, the presence

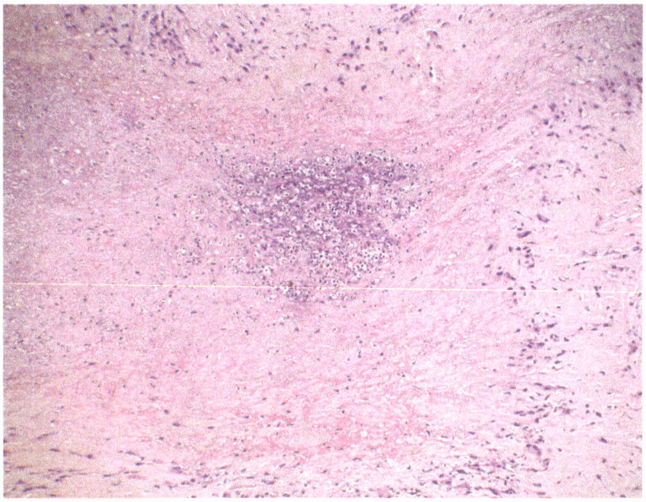

Rheumatoid nodule. Palisaded granulomatous inflammation surrounds degenerated collagen and fibrinoid material, with neutrophils and neutrophilic nuclear debris.

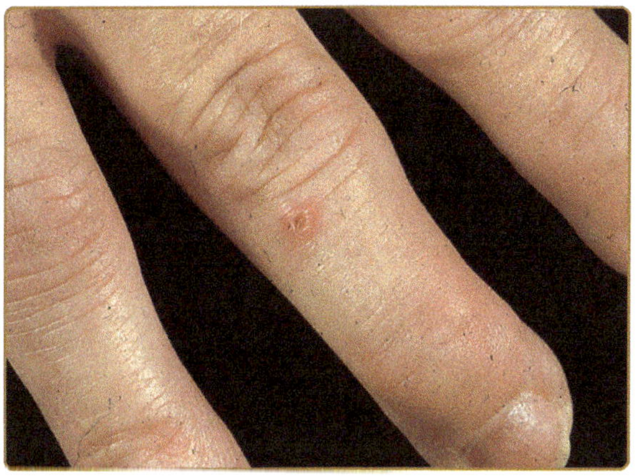

Bywaters lesions. Note the purpuric papule on the dorsal finger. (Reproduced, with permission, from Goldsmith LA, Katz SI, Gilchrest BA, Paller AS, Leffell DJ, Wolff K, eds. *Fitzpatrick's Dermatology in General Medicine.* 8th ed. New York, NY: McGraw-Hill Education; 2012.)

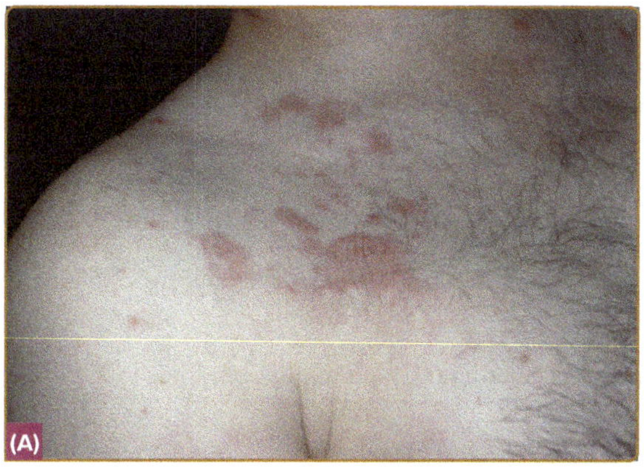

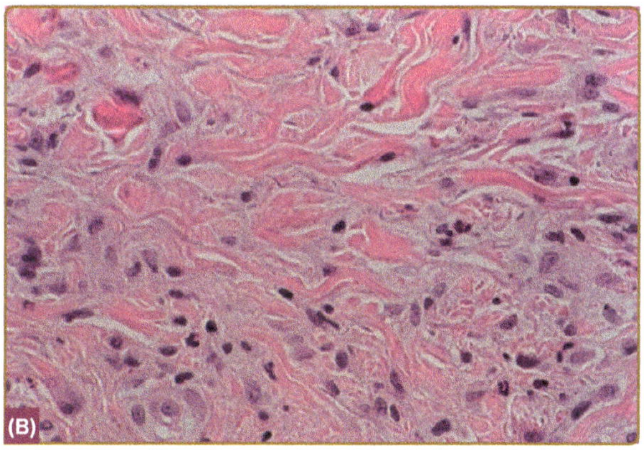

Rheumatoid neutrophilic dermatosis. (A) Lesions are erythematous urticarial papules often coalescing into plaques in a patient with rheumatoid arthritis. **(B)** Histopathologically, the changes are those of urticaria with interstitial mixed dermal infiltrates predominated by neutrophils without leukocytoclasia. This is often accompanied by papillary edema. (Reproduced, with permission, from Goldsmith LA, Katz SI, Gilchrest BA, Paller AS, Leffell DJ, Wolff K, eds. *Fitzpatrick's Dermatology in General Medicine*. 8th ed. New York, NY: McGraw-Hill Education; 2012.)

of vasculitis, especially at the onset of the disease, portends a poor outcome. Vasculitis, along with certain other extra-articular manifestations of RA (pericarditis, pleuritis, amyloidosis, and Felty syndrome) is associated with a diminished lifespan.

Rheumatoid neutrophilic dermatosis is a very rare cutaneous manifestation in patients with severe RA. These lesions are usually chronic, erythematous, and urticaria-like plaques and papules that are sharply marginated. Histopathologically, these lesions have a dense infiltrate of neutrophils without leukocytoclasia, in the setting of a mixed infiltrate and papillary dermal edema. Some authors accept **palisaded neutrophilic** and **granulomatous dermatitis** as a histopathologic finding consistent with **rheumatoid neutrophilic dermatitis**.

ANSWER 2-22: D.

The microscopic image reveals lobules and cords of foamy macrophages (pale cytoplasm) that are separated by coarse collagen bundles. **Xanthoma** (unmodified) is the generic term applied to a group of infiltrates of foamy macrophages (histiocytes) (Table 2-22A). Those associated with hyperlipidemia have characteristic sites of predilection. These xanthomas include **xanthelasma, tendinous xanthoma, tuberous xanthoma**, and **eruptive xanthoma** (answer choices A, B, C, D, respectively). The characteristic cell is the **foam cell**—a macrophage whose cytoplasm is stuffed with lipid and appears foamy in H&E-stained sections. Sites of predilection for the usual xanthoma types associated with hyperlipidemia are provided in Table 2-22A. With the exception of the eruptive type (choice D), the histopathologic appearance for all types is virtually identical. The clinical locale is most helpful in distinguishing these entities.

Table 2-22A. Xanthomas

TUBEROUS	TENDINOUS	XANTHELASMA	ERUPTIVE
Clinical Features			
Hypercholesterolemia (IIa)	Hypercholesterolemia (IIa)	Hypercholesterolemia (IIa)	Lipoprotein lipase deficiency (I)
Dyslipoproteinemia (III)	Extensor tendons of hands, feet	Dyslipoproteinemia (III)	Dyslipoproteinemia (III)
Hypertriglyceridemia (IV)	Achilles tendon	Idiopathic	Hypertriglyceridemia (IV/V)
Elbows		Eyelids	Diabetes mellitus
Knees			Buttocks and other sites
Histopathologic Features			
Foam cells arranged interstitially between collagen bundles, as small clusters, or in large nodular aggregates	Same as tuberous	Same as tuberous	Fewer foam cells More Lymphocytes Neutrophils Eosinophils
Few to no lymphocytes, eosinophils, or neutrophils			Intracellular and extracellular lipid

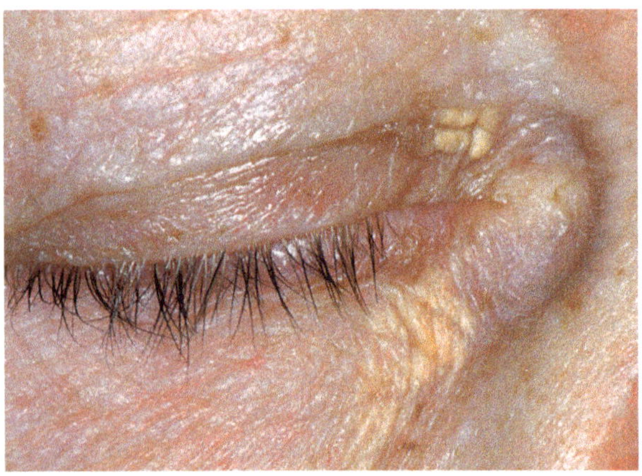

Xanthelasma. Multiple creamy-orange, slightly elevated dermal papules on the eyelids of a normolipemic individual. Hyperlipidemia is seen in approximately 50% of patients with this condition. (Reproduced, with permission, from Wolff K, Johnson RA, Saavedra AP. *Fitzpatrick's Color Atlas and Synopsis of Clinical Dermatology*. 7th ed. New York, NY: McGraw-Hill Education; 2013.)

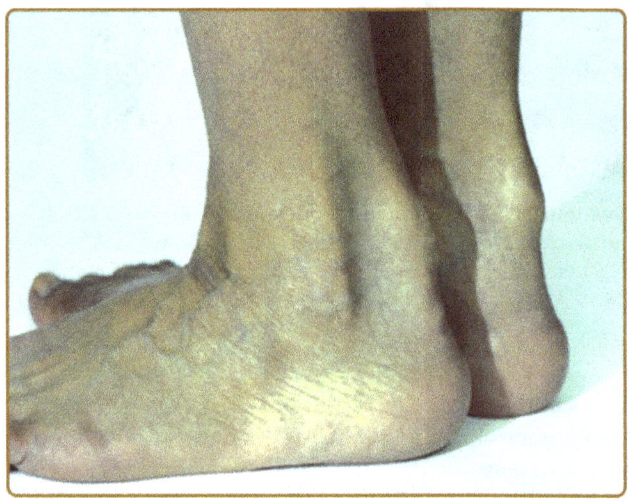

Tendinous xanthomas on the Achilles tendon of a patient with heterozygous familial hypercholesterolemia. (Reproduced, with permission, from Goldsmith LA, Katz SI, Gilchrest BA, Paller AS, Leffell DJ, Wolff K, eds. *Fitzpatrick's Dermatology in General Medicine*. 8th ed. New York, NY: McGraw-Hill Education; 2012.)

Microscopically, **tuberous xanthoma, tendinous xanthoma**, and **xanthelasma** demonstrate virtually identical histology. There is an infiltrate almost exclusively of foam cells disposed between individual collagen bundles, in small clusters, or in large nodular aggregates. Multinucleated cells are rare or absent. Lymphocytes, neutrophils, and eosinophils are completely absent or present only in small numbers. **Tuberous xanthoma** may exhibit increased collagen deposition around the xanthoma cells. **Eruptive xanthomas** are often smaller and more inflammatory clinically. They demonstrate greater

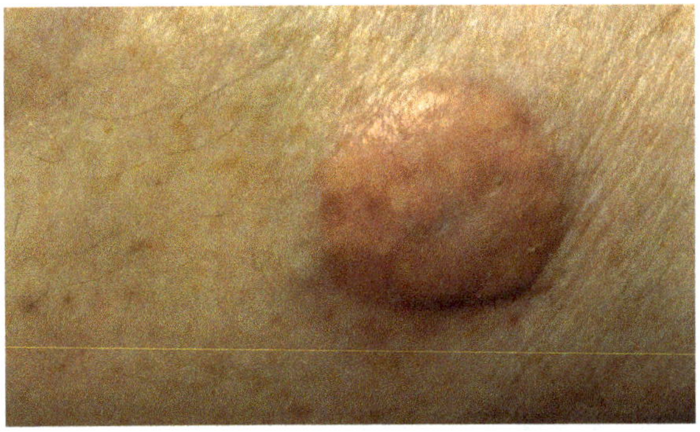

Tuberous xanthoma. Flat-topped, yellow, firm nodule. (Reproduced, with permission, from Wolff K, Johnson RA, Saavedra AP. *Fitzpatrick's Color Atlas and Synopsis of Clinical Dermatology*. 7th ed. New York, NY: McGraw-Hill Education; 2013.)

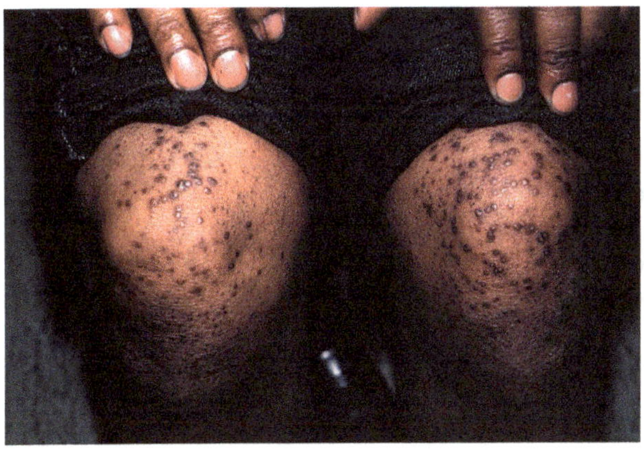

Eruptive xanthomas on the knees of a patient with hypercholesterolemia. (Reproduced, with permission, from Usatine RP, Smith MA, Mayeaux EJ Jr, Chumley HS, eds. *Color Atlas of Family Medicine*. 2nd ed. New York, NY: McGraw-Hill Education; 2012. Used with permission of Richard P. Usatine, MD. Previously published in the *Western Journal of Medicine*.)

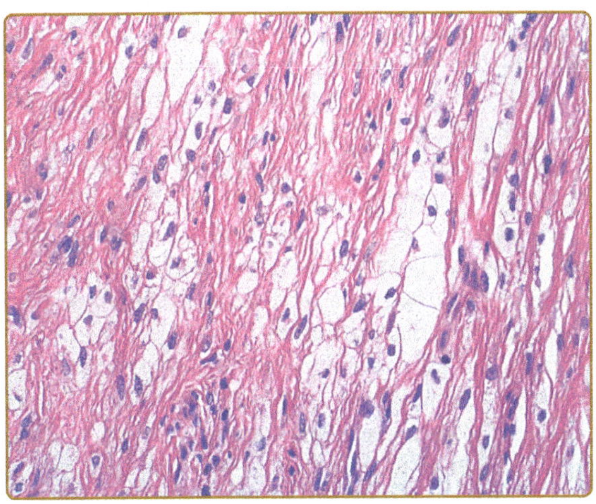

Tuberous xanthoma. There are scattered collections of foam cells embedded within a collagenous stroma. Note the absence of other inflammatory cell types. (Reproduced, with permission, from Goldsmith LA, Katz SI, Gilchrest BA, Paller AS, Leffell DJ, Wolff K, eds. *Fitzpatrick's Dermatology in General Medicine*. 8th ed. New York, NY: McGraw-Hill Education; 2012.)

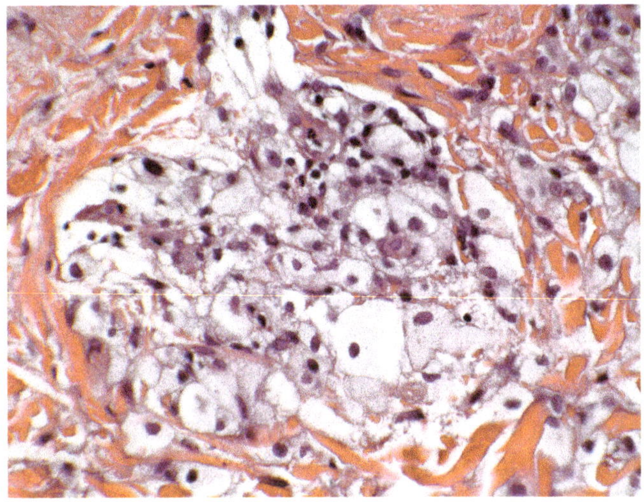

Eruptive xanthoma. A small nodular collection of foamy histiocytes within the upper dermis is accompanied by a few lymphocytes and neutrophils. Focal extracellular lipid is a common finding.

numbers of lymphocytes, neutrophils, and macrophages and fewer characteristic foam cells. One hallmark of eruptive xanthoma is the presence of both intracellular and extracellular lipid, producing a pattern similar to GA. However, the overall histopathological findings among these four different conditions are very similar and may require clinical correlation for definitive diagnosis.

The almost exclusive infiltrate of foamy histiocytes with relatively few lymphocytes, neutrophils, and eosinophils are characteristic of **hyperlipidemia-associated xanthomas** and serves to differentiate them from the other non-Langerhans cell histiocytoses. **Eruptive xanthoma** is an exception in that it exhibits an accompanying infiltrate of lymphocytes, neutrophils, and occasionally eosinophils.

ANSWER 2-23: A.

The biopsy reveals a verrucous epithelial hyperplasia with tiers of parakeratosis. There is a complete absence of the granular layer. Within an expanded submucosa (or papillary dermis), there are collections of foam cells (lipid-rich macrophages) partially enclosed by hyperplastic rete ridges. This is a classic example of **verruciform xanthoma**. Clinically, verruciform xanthoma presents as a solitary lesion encountered in the oral mucosa and occasionally at extraoral sites, such as the genitalia. The etiology is unknown, but there is no association with diabetes, hyperlipidemia, or multiple myeloma. The theorized pathogenesis involves degeneration of keratinocytes followed by a macrophage inflammatory response. Oral lesions may occur at any site, but the gingiva and hard palate are affected preferentially. They are described as soft, red, white, or yellow papules with a roughened surface. Cutaneous lesions have been described on the penis, the vulva, scrotum, groin, anus, and nostril. Although most cutaneous lesions are sporadic, these lesions are a characteristic finding in patients with congenital hemidysplasia with ichthyosiform erythroderma and limb defects **(CHILD) syndrome**. The mutation associated with CHILD syndrome is in the 3β-hydroxysteroid dehydrogenase gene.

Answer choice A describes the clinical presentation of **diffuse normolipemic plane xanthoma**, which is commonly associated with **multiple myeloma**. Other less common associations with diffuse normolipemic plane xanthoma are erythroderma, cryoglobulinemia, myelogenous leukemia, lymphomas (including mycosis fungoides), and very rarely hyperlipoproteinemia types IIA, III, and IV. Some patients have no demonstrable associated disease. Clinically, the lesions are well-demarcated yellow-orange plaques that are distributed around the eyes and on the trunk and extremities. Microscopically, in addition to perivascular lymphocytic infiltrates, there are clusters or sheets of foamy macrophages extending throughout the papillary and reticular dermis. Touton-type giant cells are variably present, resembling those of **xanthogranuloma**. Some cases may demonstrate focal collagen degeneration and cholesterol clefts, suggesting a histopathologic overlap with **necrobiotic xanthogranuloma (NXG)**. The epidermis in **plane xanthoma** is typically unremarkable and definitely lacks the verrucous hyperplasia and parakeratosis of **verruciform xanthoma**.

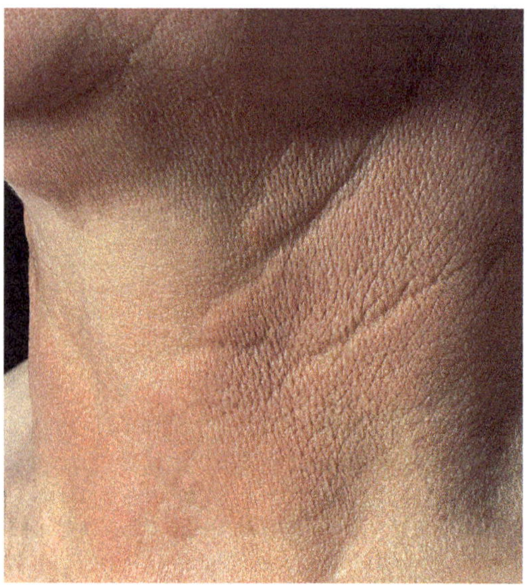

Diffuse normolipemic plane xanthoma. Yellowish-red, slightly elevated plaques on the neck, noticeable mainly because of the accentuation of the skin texture in a normolipemic patient with lymphoma. Plane xanthomas occur most commonly on the upper trunk and neck and most commonly occur in individuals with myeloma. (Reproduced, with permission, from Wolff K, Johnson RA, Saavedra AP. *Fitzpatrick's Color Atlas and Synopsis of Clinical Dermatology*. 7th ed. New York, NY: McGraw-Hill Education; 2013.)

The histopathological differential diagnosis for **verruciform xanthoma** mainly includes **inflammatory linear verrucous epidermal nevus (ILVEN)**. Both condition are characterized by a verrucous epidermal hyperplasia and striking abrupt parakeratosis with an absent granular layer. The two conditions are extremely similar except that ILVEN does not contain foamy macrophages in the papillary dermis. Verrucous forms of psoriasis (**rupioid psoriasis**) may also fall within the differential diagnosis however psoriasis also lacks these foamy macrophages.

ANSWER 2-24: D.

The biopsy reveals tissue macrophages (histiocytes) forming a diffuse infiltrate in the upper dermis accompanied by a lymphocytic infiltrate. Large numbers of Touton-type giant cells and foamy macrophages are present. The combined clinical and histopathological findings are consistent with **xanthoma disseminatum**. All of the answer choices represent normolipemic, non-Langerhans histiocytoses characterized by a CD68+, CD163+, S100−, CD1a− immunophenotype. The term "**histiocyte**" is admittedly controversial. Wood and Haber proposed that the term "histiocyte" refers to all types of bone marrow–derived macrophages and immune-related dendritic cells. Similarly, the term "**histiocytosis**" refers to any proliferative disorder exhibiting the differentiation of these cells. A similar definition is used to define the entities discussed, but in general, when the involvement remains as discrete cutaneous papules or nodules (single or multiple), the suffix *-oma* is attached (ie, **histiocytoma**, **xanthoma**). It is when lesions tend to coalesce, to progress relentlessly, and/or to involve extracutaneous sites that the suffix *-osis* is applied (ie, **histiocytosis**, **reticulohistiocytosis**). As always, there are exceptions, and some entities demonstrate overlapping clinical pictures. The histopathologic features of **xanthoma disseminatum, benign cephalic histiocytosis, generalized eruptive histiocytosis**, and **xanthogranuloma** are nearly identical. The histopathologic picture largely depends on the stage of the lesion at the time of biopsy. Early lesions demonstrate few to no Touton-type giant cells and foam cells. **Generalized eruptive histiocytosis** tends to maintain this histomorphology and not progress to the morphology seen in the later stages of **xanthogranuloma, benign cephalic histiocytosis**, or **xanthoma disseminatum**.

Mature lesions demonstrate nodular, dense, sheet-like collections of histiocytes admixed with Touton-type giant cells (giant cells with a wreath of nuclei), lymphocytes, and eosinophils. In contrast to the monotonous infiltrate of foamy macrophages seen in **hyperlipidemia-associated xanthomas** (except **eruptive xanthoma**), this group of conditions feature histiocytes with varied morphology and mixed inflammatory cellular infiltrates. In addition to foam cells (which usually constitute the majority), there are histiocytes with

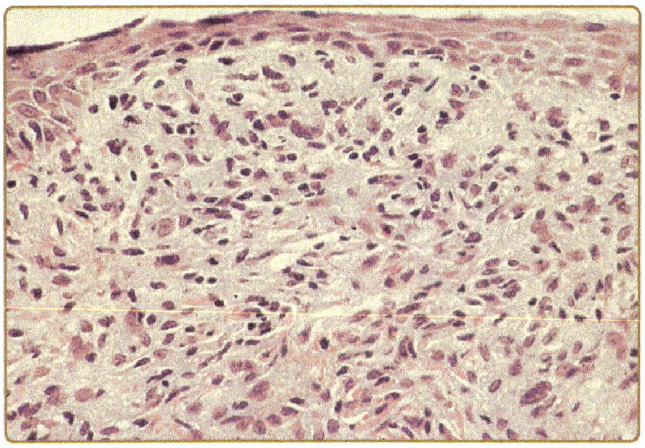

Generalized eruptive histiocytosis and early lesions of xanthoma disseminatum, benign cephalic histiocytosis, and xanthogranuloma. There is a dense monomorphous histiocytic infiltrate in the papillary and mid-dermis, intermingled with a few lymphocytes. (Reproduced, with permission, from Goldsmith LA, Katz SI, Gilchrest BA, Paller AS, Leffell DJ, Wolff K, eds. *Fitzpatrick's Dermatology in General Medicine*. 8th ed. New York, NY: McGraw-Hill Education; 2012.)

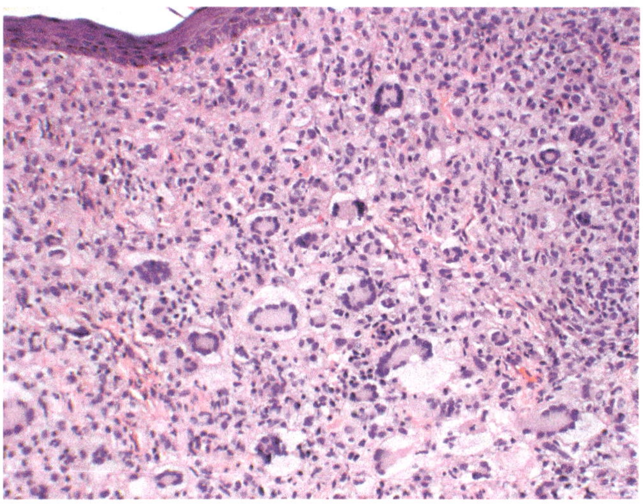

Fully evolved lesions of xanthoma disseminatum, benign cephalic histiocytosis, and xanthogranuloma. A diffuse infiltrate of macrophages, both single and multinucleate, is accompanied by a mixed inflammatory cell infiltrate of lymphocytes and scattered eosinophils. Touton-type giant cells containing a wreath of nuclei and peripheral foamy cytoplasm are present.

vacuolated cytoplasms, histiocytes with eosinophilic granular cytoplasms, and spindle-shaped histiocytes. Late lesions demonstrate areas of fibrosis. The histiocytes are positive for KP1 (CD68), CD163, and vimentin; variably positive for Factor XIIIa; and negative for S-100 and CD1a.

The patient in question has **xanthoma disseminatum**, which is a non-Langerhans cell histiocytosis that may affect all ages. It is more common in men. The etiology is unknown, but overlapping clinical and histopathological features suggest that **xanthoma disseminatum, benign cephalic histiocytosis, generalized eruptive histiocytosis**, and **xanthogranuloma** are closely related. **Xanthoma disseminatum** is also very closely related to **Erdheim-Chester disease**. There has been a recent proposal to consider Erdheim-Chester disease as a variant of xanthoma disseminatum, one in which there is bone involvement and an aggressive clinical course. Patients of any age clinically present with numerous red-brown or yellow papules that frequently become confluent to form large plaques. Flexural areas of the neck, axillae, antecubital fossae, groin, and perianal region are preferentially affected. Mucous membrane involvement is fairly common, and lesions of the buccal mucosa or larynx may cause dysphagia or breathing difficulties. The conjunctiva and cornea are additional sites of potential involvement. **Diabetes insipidus** is seen in approximately 40% of patients. Individual lesions resolve spontaneously over time. The pathognomonic bone changes of Erdheim-Chester disease are seen in the long bones (distal femur and proximal tibia and fibula) and consist of bilateral and symmetric patchy osteosclerosis involving the metaphysis and diaphysis, with epiphyseal sparing.

Juvenile xanthogranuloma is a non-Langerhans cell histiocytosis seen in infants or children usually before the age of 6 months. The etiology is not known. Although juvenile xanthogranuloma usually is limited to the skin, it may affect other organ systems. The eye is the most frequently involved extracutaneous site, but others include liver, spleen, lymph nodes, lungs, heart, testes, ovary, colon, kidneys, and bones. Adults are occasionally affected by identical lesions (**adult xanthogranuloma**). Deep subcutaneous or intramuscular forms also have been described. Clinically, cutaneous lesions present as solitary or multiple yellow-red papules or nodules on the face, neck, or upper trunk. Individual lesions regress spontaneously over time.

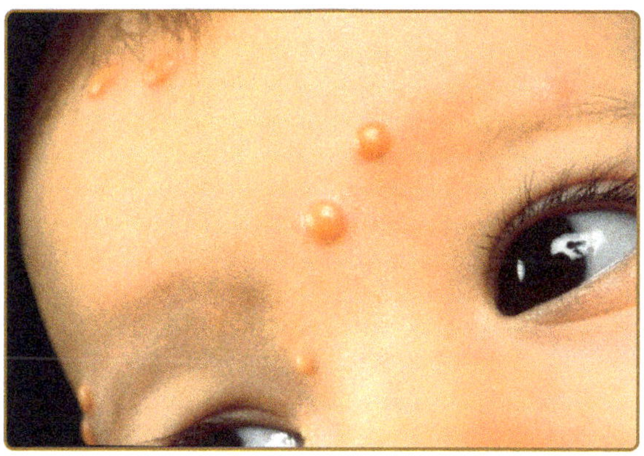

Juvenile xanthogranuloma. Papular form. (Reproduced, with permission, from Goldsmith LA, Katz SI, Gilchrest BA, Paller AS, Leffell DJ, Wolff K, eds. *Fitzpatrick's Dermatology in General Medicine*. 8th ed. New York, NY: McGraw-Hill Education; 2012.)

Benign cephalic histiocytosis is a non-Langerhans cell histiocytosis that affects infants and children younger than 3 years of age. The etiology is unknown. Clinically, infants or children younger than 3 years of age develop numerous brown-yellow papules distributed on the head, neck, and sometimes the upper trunk. Mucous membranes and viscera are spared. Individual lesions resolve spontaneously over time.

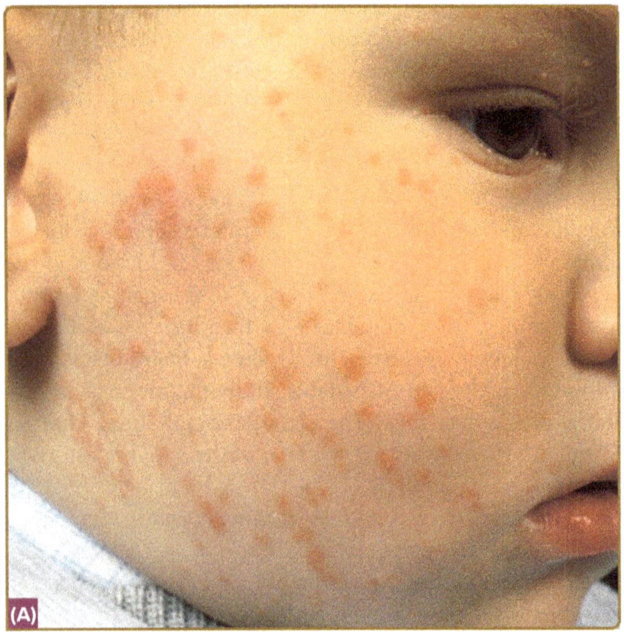

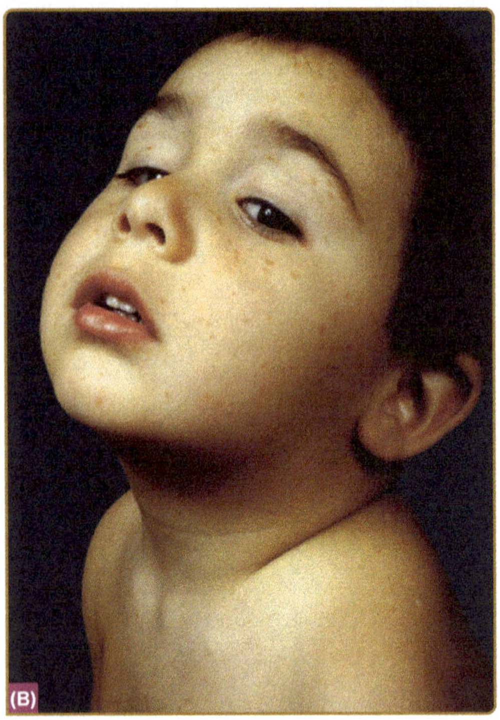

Benign cephalic histiocytosis. Note the distribution on the face **(A)** and also on the neck **(B)**. (Reproduced, with permission, from Goldsmith LA, Katz SI, Gilchrest BA, Paller AS, Leffell DJ, Wolff K, eds. *Fitzpatrick's Dermatology in General Medicine*. 8th ed. New York, NY: McGraw-Hill Education; 2012.)

Generalized eruptive histiocytosis is a non-Langerhans cell histiocytosis that affects adults. The etiology is unknown. Clinically, adult patients present with numerous, generalized, brown to dark blue papules or nodules symmetrically distributed on the trunk and extremities. Mucous membranes are involved occasionally, but there is no visceral involvement and diabetes insipidus is not a feature. Individual lesions resolve spontaneously over time. Microscopically, generalized eruptive histiocytosis tends to contain much fewer lipidized macrophages and multinucleated Touton-type giant cells compared to the other conditions in this group.

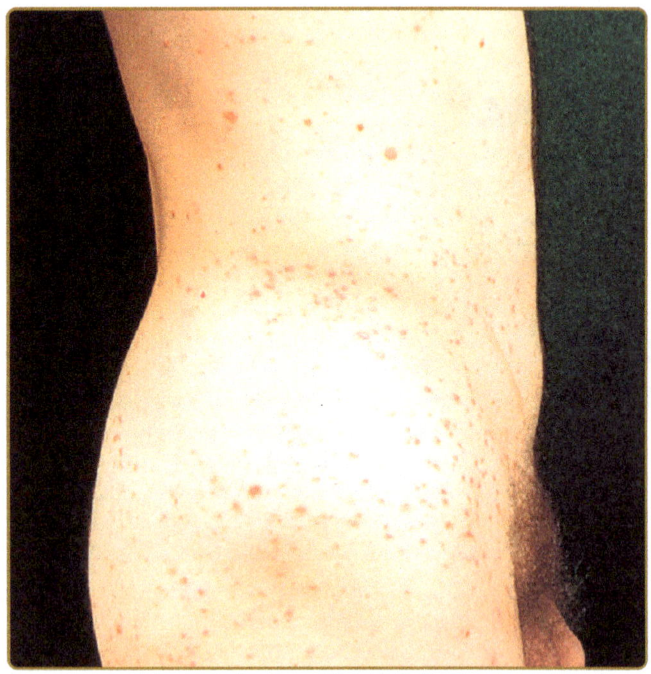

Generalized eruptive histiocytosis in an adult. (Reproduced, with permission, from Goldsmith LA, Katz SI, Gilchrest BA, Paller AS, Leffell DJ, Wolff K, eds. *Fitzpatrick's Dermatology in General Medicine*. 8th ed. New York, NY: McGraw-Hill Education; 2012.)

Langerhans cell histiocytosis may also present with widespread cutaneous and visceral involvement (including **diabetes insipidus**) however these infiltrates contain robust mixed infiltrates of eosinophils and neutrophils and lack Touton-type giant cells. Additionally, these histiocytes are CD68−, CD163−, S100+, and CD1a+.

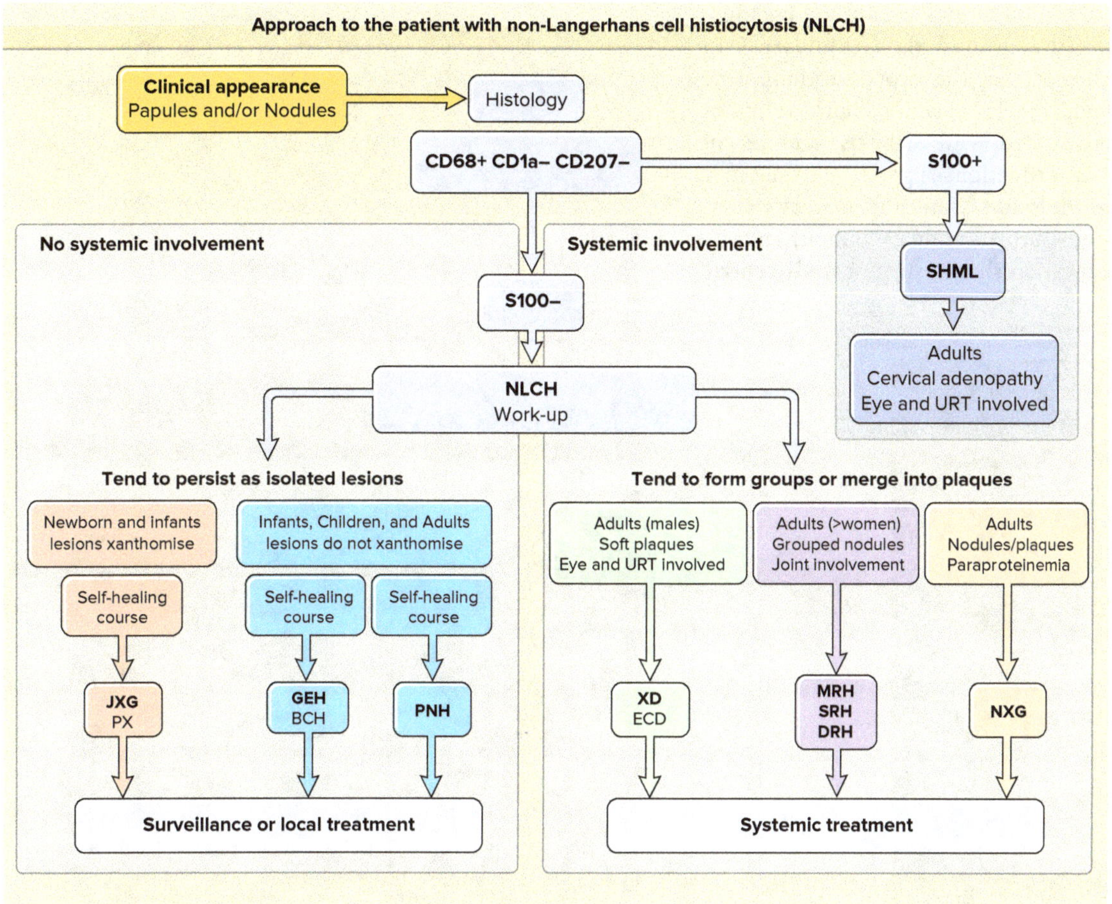

Approach to the patient with non-Langerhans cell histiocytosis (NLCH). BCH = benign cephalic histiocytosis; DRH = diffuse cutaneous reticulohistiocytosis; ECD = Erdheim–Chester disease; GEH = generalized eruptive histiocytosis; JXG = juvenile xanthogranuloma; MRH = multicentric reticulohistiocytosis; NXG = necrobiotic xanthogranuloma; PNH = progressive nodular histiocytosis; PX = papular xanthoma; SRH = solitary cutaneous reticulohistiocytosis; SHML = sinus histiocytosis with massive lymphadenopathy; URT = upper respiratory tract; XD = xanthoma disseminatum. (Reproduced, with permission, from Goldsmith LA, Katz SI, Gilchrest BA, Paller AS, Leffell DJ, Wolff K, eds. *Fitzpatrick's Dermatology in General Medicine*. 8th ed. New York, NY: McGraw-Hill Education; 2012.)

ANSWER 2-25: E.

The biopsy reveals mononuclear and multinucleated histiocytes forming a diffuse infiltrate. These multinucleated cells contain an eosinophilic ground-glass-appearing cytoplasm. Scattered lymphocytes are present. The combined clinical and histopathological findings are consistent with **multicentric reticulohistiocytosis. Multicentric reticulohistiocytosis** (aka **lipoid dermatoarthritis**) defines a distinct clinical entity in which multiple cutaneous nodules are associated with a destructive polyarthritis. The arthritis most frequently involves the interphalangeal joints of the hands, but the knees, ankles, wrists, elbows, and shoulders also may be affected. Adult females are affected more often than males, and the cutaneous nodules may precede, occur with, or postdate the onset of arthritis. In some cases multicentric reticulohistiocytosis is associated with malignancies (gastrointestinal or ovarian), thyroid disorders, tuberculosis, diabetes mellitus, dermatomyositis, celiac disease, and systemic lupus erythematosus. The etiology is unknown. Clinically, yellow-brown cutaneous papules or nodules are distributed over the hands, forearms, and face. Periungual arrays of tumor nodules is a classic presentation. The oral mucosa may be involved rarely. Microscopically, there is an interstitial and/or nodular infiltrate of histiocytes and large multinucleated giant cells with distinctive eosinophilic finely granular ("ground-glass") cytoplasm. Lymphocytes and occasional eosinophils are also present. The giant cells are relatively large (>50 μm) with randomly arranged nuclei. The cytoplasms of mono- and multinucleated cells are PAS-positive and diastase resistant.

Reticulohistiocytoma is a solitary cutaneous nodule with similar histology to that seen in **multicentric**

reticulohistiocytosis (ie, mono- and multinucleated histiocytes with characteristic ground-glass cytoplasm). In fact, prior reports indicated that the two conditions were identical histopathologically. However, solitary reticulohistiocytoma is not associated with arthritis, and recent immunohistochemical investigations suggest that they may be variants of **xanthogranulomas**. Clinically, solitary reticulohistiocytomas are yellow-brown nodules without any site predilection. An acral location should suggest **multicentric reticulohistiocytosis**.

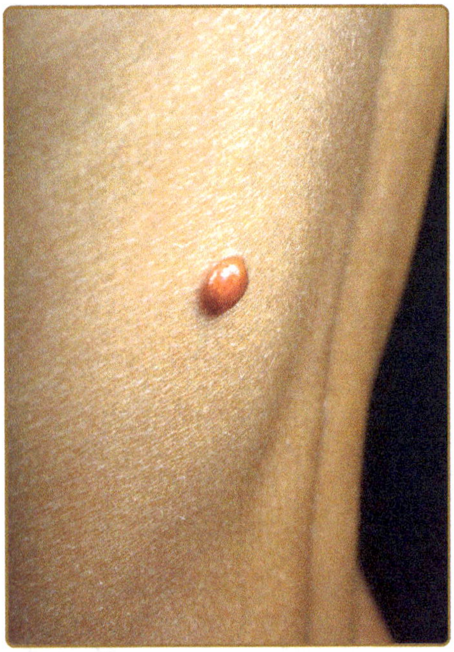

Solitary cutaneous reticulohistiocytoma. (Reproduced, with permission, from Goldsmith LA, Katz SI, Gilchrest BA, Paller AS, Leffell DJ, Wolff K, eds. *Fitzpatrick's Dermatology in General Medicine*. 8th ed. New York, NY: McGraw-Hill Education; 2012.)

Microscopically, the findings of **solitary reticulohistiocytoma** are essentially identical to those of **multicentric reticulohistiocytosis** however **emperipolesis** of other inflammatory cells by histiocytes has been observed in some cases. There are also greater numbers of Touton-type giant cells. Based on the presence of Touton-type giant cells and a minority population of vacuolated, foamy, and spindle-shaped histiocytes (ie, a heterogeneous population of histiocytes, similar to that seen in xanthogranuloma), some consider solitary reticulohistiocytoma to be a variant of xanthogranuloma.

The mono- and multinucleated cells are positive for macrophage markers CD68 and CD163 and occasionally the dermal dendritic cell marker Factor XIIIa. The cells are negative for S100 and CD1a. Although **Rosai–Dorfman disease** may exhibit **emperipolesis** of other inflammatory cells by histiocytes, the histiocytes contain clear-pale cytoplasm and are S100 positive. The cells of **Langerhans histiocytosis** express CD1a.

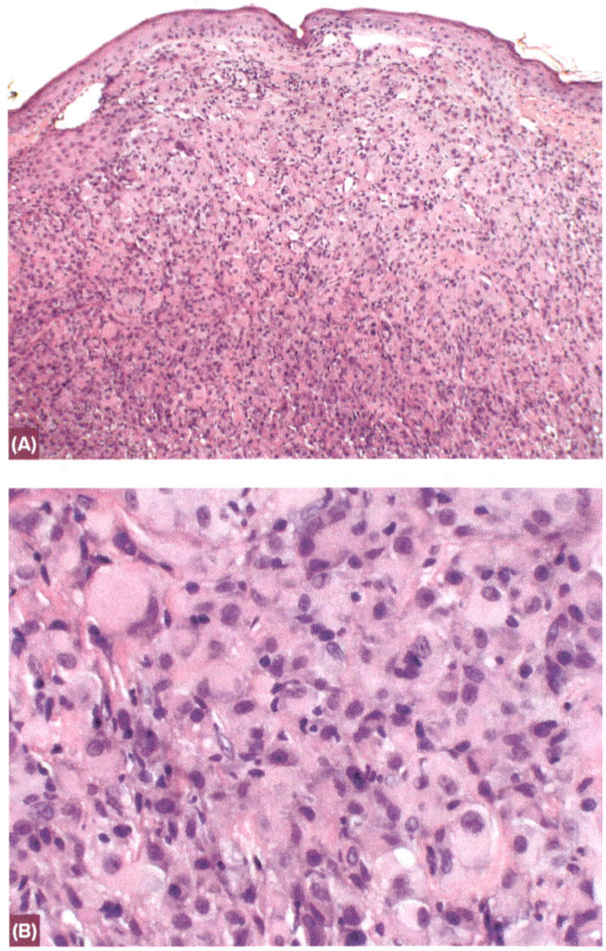

Solitary reticulohistiocytoma. (A) A discrete infiltrate of histiocytes with glassy cytoplasm and single to multiple nuclei. **(B)** They are accompanied by a mixed inflammatory cell infiltrate predominantly of lymphocytes.

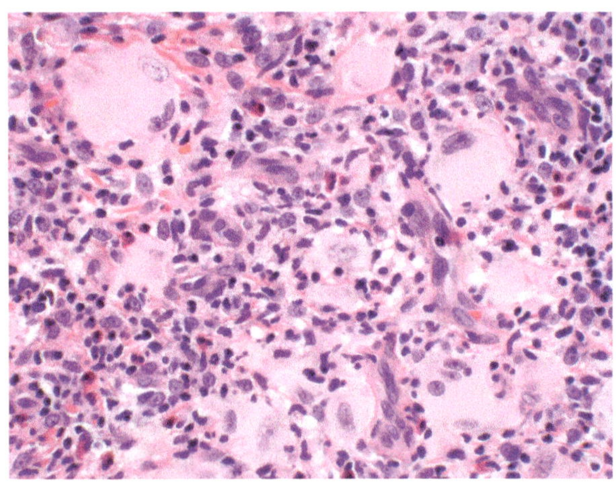

Solitary reticulohistiocytoma. Note the presence of small inflammatory cells with the cytoplasms of the large eosinophilic multinucleated histiocytes (emperipolesis).

ANSWER 2-26: E.

The biopsy reveals a mixed infiltrate of lymphocytes and plasma cells with accompanying tissue macrophages containing clear to pale cytoplasm. Many of the macrophages contain lymphocytes and plasma cells, producing the so-called beanbag appearance (**emperipolesis**). The findings are consistent with **Rosai–Dorfman disease** (aka **sinus histiocytosis with massive lymphadenopathy**). The cause of Rosai–Dorfman disease is unknown. Patients develop massive cervical lymphadenopathy accompanied by fever, leukocytosis, hypergammaglobulinemia, and an elevated erythrocyte sedimentation rate. Although painless massive bilateral cervical lymphadenopathy is the hallmark of the condition, less commonly axillary, mediastinal, inguinal, and preauricular lymph nodes may be affected. Extranodal involvement is fairly common, and the skin is the most frequent site (approximately 30% of cases), with the respiratory tract, eyes, soft tissues, bones, and genitourinary tract and nervous system less commonly affected. Cutaneous lesions may be the initial manifestation and sole presenting feature of the disease. There are also cases of skin-limited Rosai–Dorfman disease. Black patients are affected more frequently than whites, and there is a slight male predominance. The disease resolves spontaneously. In both skin-limited disease and secondary cutaneous disease, the clinical lesions are similar, with erythematous or yellow-red papules, nodules, or plaques that may be solitary or multiple.

Microscopically, **Rosai–Dorfman disease** is characterized by a dense diffuse or nodular dermal infiltrate of pale to clear histiocytes admixed with lymphocytes, plasma cells, and neutrophils. Eosinophils are seen in only small numbers. Although rare eosinophilic abscesses have been described, large numbers of eosinophils should suggest another histiocytic proliferation, especially **Langerhans cell histiocytosis**. **Emperipolesis** of lymphocytes, plasma cells, and neutrophils by histiocytes is characteristic. Emperipolesis is the passive migration of inflammatory cells through the histiocytes without phagocytic destruction. The microscopic image of this patient's biopsy reveals lymphocytes located within the histiocytes. This is contrasted with **cytophagocytosis**, where the engulfed cells are eventually incorporated into phagolysosomes and destroyed potentially resulting in peripheral cytopenias. The histiocytes have characteristic nuclei that are large, with vesicular chromatin, a delicate nuclear membrane, and prominent nucleoli. At the periphery of histiocytic nodules there are lymphoid aggregates with germinal centers and thick-walled vessels surrounded by numerous plasma cells. In the centers of histiocytic nodules, dilated lymphatics containing intraluminal histiocytes are seen. The histiocytes in Rosai–Dorfman disease are S-100+, CD1a− and lack Birbeck granules. In some cases, the subcutis, rather than the dermis, is affected primarily.

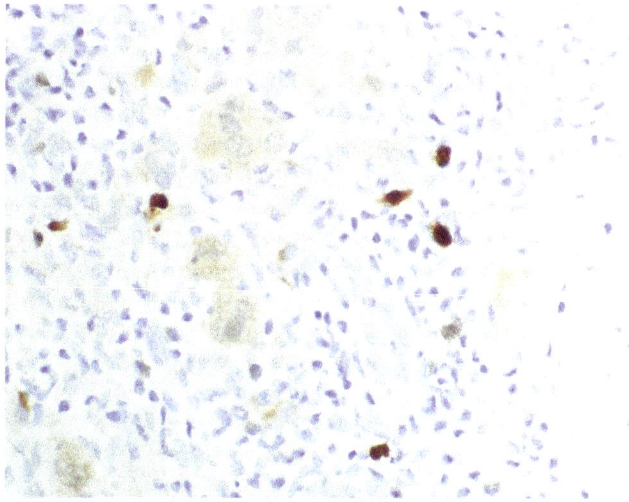

Rosai–Dorfman disease, S100 immunohistochemical stain. Note the light staining of the histiocytes for S100. The dark staining S100+ cells are most likely scattered reactive Langerhans cells.

In regards to the differential diagnosis, emperipolesis of inflammatory cells seen among an infiltrate of S-100-positive histiocytes and plasma cells is characteristic of Rosai–Dorfman disease. Additionally, dilated lymphatic channels with intraluminal histiocytes and thick-walled vessels surrounded by plasma cells are distinctive in Rosai–Dorfman disease. Some forms of **peripheral T-cell lymphoma**, particularly **subcutaneous panniculitis-like T-cell lymphomas**, are associated with benign histiocytes that engulf erythrocytes and inflammatory cells (cytophagocytosis). These patients frequently succumb to their disease due to pancytopenia attributed to cytophagocytosis. Phagocytosis of red blood cells, lymphocytes, plasma cells, neutrophils, and other inflammatory cell elements may be encountered in a variety of other conditions, including infection (most often viral but also bacterial, fungal, and parasitic), multiple myeloma, hairy cell and other leukemias, Hodgkin disease, some high-grade carcinomas, and a benign autosomal recessive familial condition.

ANSWER 2-27: C.

The term "histiocytoses" identifies a group of diseases that have in common the proliferation of cells of the mononuclear phagocyte system, including macrophages and dendritic cells. Both cells arise in the bone marrow from pluripotential stem cells, but follow different paths of differentiation. The macrophage, detectable by CD68 and CD163, is a monocyte in the peripheral blood and a macrophage in tissue. It may differentiate into a number of different giant cells, including foreign body, epithelioid, and Touton types. Dendritic cells are antigen-presenting cells that interact with T cells. The prototype dendritic cell in the skin is the **Langerhans cell (LC)**.

LCs have long cytoplasmic projections and a large almost kidney-shaped nucleus. Electron microscopy reveals the characteristic cytoplasmic organelle, the Langerhans or **Birbeck granule**, a tennis racket-shaped structure that is involved in pinocytosis and receptor-mediated endocytosis. Langerin (CD207), a receptor that permits internalization of antigen into Birbeck granules and presentation of antigen at the cell surface, is the most specific marker for LCs. LCs are also S100+ and CD1a+. Once LCs have contacted antigen, they leave the epidermis and move via the lymphatics to the T-cell rich zones of the regional lymph nodes where they are designated as **interdigitating dendritic cells** (different from **follicular dendritic cells**). There these cells present antigen to naive T-cells, activating them to proliferate if the antigen is recognized. **Indeterminate cells**, if they truly exist, are most likely immature CD1a+, S100+ Langerhans cells that lack Birbeck granules. Proliferative disorders of interdigitating and follicular-dendritic cells rarely affect the skin. **Dermal (interstitial) dendritic** cells are perivascular cells that are also capable of antigen uptake and presentation as well as secretion of various cytokines and growth factors. These cells are Factor XIIIa+ and the main lesional cell of **dermatofibromas**. Dermal macrophages are difficult to identify in the normal dermis but their numbers increase during inflammation.

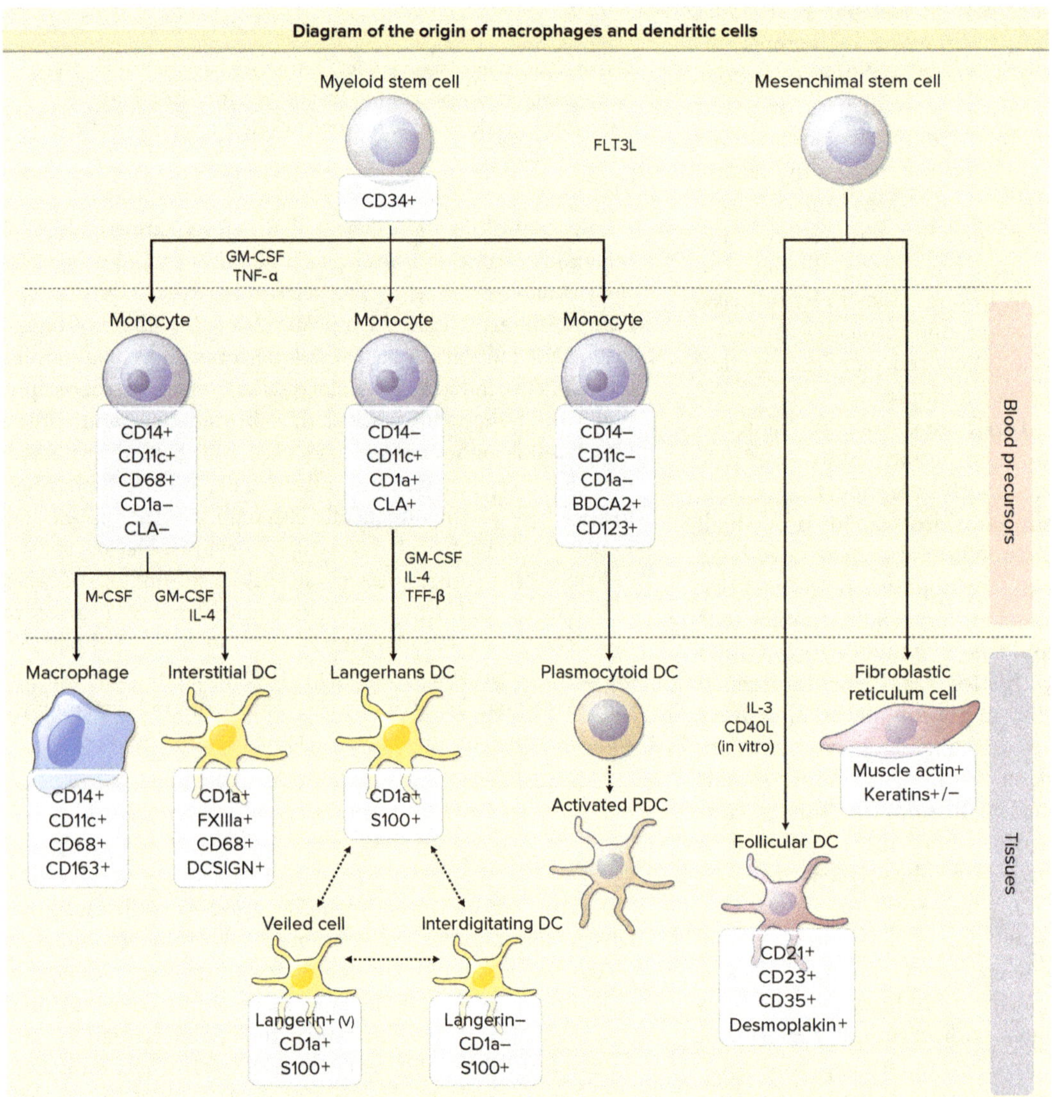

Schematic diagram of the origin of macrophages and dendritic cells. Both macrophages and dendritic cells (antigen presenting cells) are derived from a common bone marrow precursor. In contrast, follicular dendritic cells are thought to be of nonhematopoietic origin. +, most, if not all, cells positive; –, all cells negative, +/–, a minority of cells positive; v, variable intensity. (Reproduced, with permission, from Goldsmith LA, Katz SI, Gilchrest BA, Paller AS, Leffell DJ, Wolff K, eds. *Fitzpatrick's Dermatology in General Medicine*. 8th ed. New York, NY: McGraw-Hill Education; 2012. Adapted from Jaffe R et al. Histiocytic and dendritic cell neoplasms, introduction. In: SH Swerdlow et al., eds. *WHO Classification of Tumors of Haematopoietic and Lympoid Tissues*. Geneva, Lyon: WHO Press; 2008.)

Dermal macrophages, dermal dendritic cells, and Langerhans cells have a common bone marrow precursor, explaining why there are so many overlapping functions and markers.

Langerhans cell histiocytosis (LCH) is a proliferative disorder of Langerhans cells with both cutaneous and extracutaneous involvement (Table 2-27A). It is a disorder with a broad spectrum of forms: it can be local, asymptomatic with an indolent course, limited to an isolated bone lesion, or systemic and aggressive involving multiple organs and producing significant symptoms. Thus, the clinical manifestations depend on the site of the lesions and the systems involved. The nosology of Langerhans cell histiocytosis remains unsettled. Some reports, based on molecular DNA techniques, support a monoclonal proliferation and a neoplastic disorder. Others question this conclusion. The definitive answer awaits further clarification. Owing to overlapping clinical features, the classic subtypes of **Letterer–Siwe disease, Hand–Schüller–Christian disease**, and **eosinophilic granuloma** are now subsumed under the rubric of Langerhans cell histiocytosis. In 1997, experts of the Reclassification Working Group of the Histiocyte Society advocated the disuse of the eponyms. They recommended the use of the term "Langerhans cell histiocytosis" only and the stratification of patients based on the extent of disease. The classification system for histiocytosis defined by the Histiocyte Society is shown in Table 2-27A. At present, it seems realistic to describe LCH as a continuum because every patient is unique with regard to the type, number, and location of lesions.

Table 2-27A. Classification of Langerhans-Cell Histiocytosis (LCH)

Single-system Disease	
Localized (single site)	Monostotic bone involvement[a] Isolated skin involvement Solitary lymph node involvement
Multiple site	Polyostotic bone involvement[a] Multifocal bone disease (two or more different bones) Multiple lymph node involvement
Multisystem Disease	
Low-risk group	Disseminated disease with involvement of low-risk organs (skin, bone, lymph node, pituitary)
High-risk group	Disseminated disease with involvement of one or more of the high-risk organs (hematopoietic system, lungs, liver, and spleen)

[a]CNS-risk lesions: involvement of facial bones, sinuses, the maxilla, or anterior or middle cranial fossa (temporal, mastoid, sphenoidal, ethmoidal, zygomatic, orbital bones) with intracranial tumor extension. Not included are vault lesions.

Cutaneous lesions are variable and may include red-brown papules, nodules, plaques, vesicles, pustules, or ulcers. Lesions are distributed on the scalp, trunk, and intertriginous areas. Mucosal (especially gingival) involvement is characteristic. Extracutaneous involvement is frequently present in Langerhans cell histiocytosis. Commonly involved organs include bone, bone marrow, liver, spleen, hypothalamus-pituitary (producing **diabetes insipidus**), and lung. The systemic involvement separates it from **congenital self-healing Langerhans histiocytosis (Hashimoto–Pritzker disease)**. Although a misnomer, the literature has also referred to this condition as congenital self-healing reticulohistiocytosis.

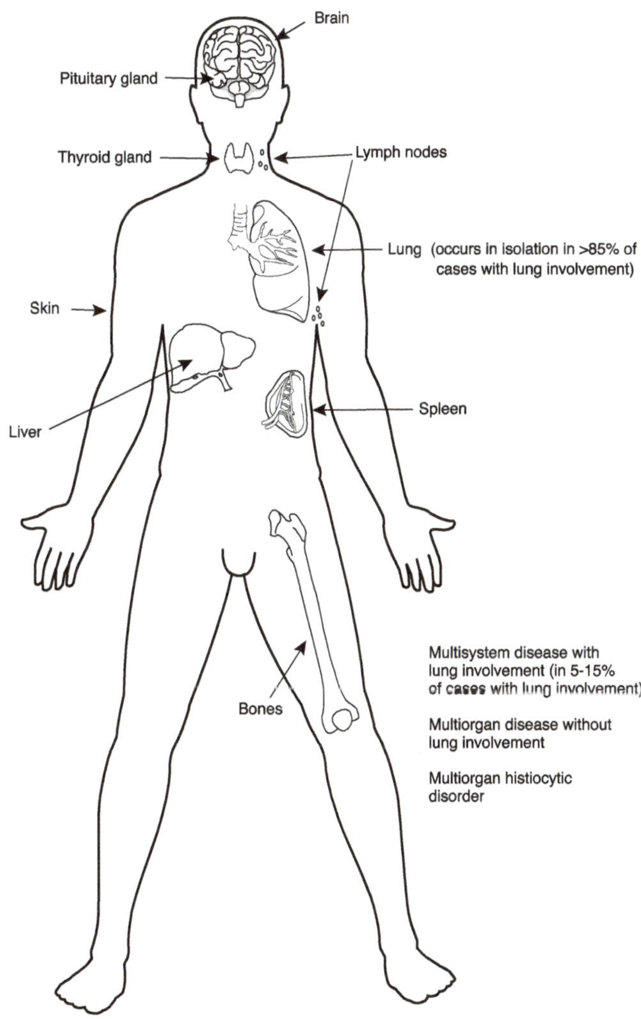

Organ involvement in Langerhans histiocytosis in adults.
(Reproduced, with permission, from Hanley ME, Welsh CH, eds. *Current Medical Diagnosis & Treatment: Pulmonary Medicine*. New York, NY: McGraw-Hill; 2003.)

Congenital self-healing Langerhans histiocytosis (Hashimoto–Pritzker disease) is a disease of infants/neonates that represents the self-limited, benign end of the spectrum of Langerhans cell proliferative disorders. The disease is confined to the skin, and there is no (or only mild) systemic involvement. The skin lesions and histopathologic features can be virtually identical to other Langerhans cell histiocytoses. Therefore, one must attempt to rule out systemic involvement through clinical evaluation of lymph nodes, liver, spleen, bone survey, complete blood count (CBC), and liver function tests. Although most cases regress spontaneously, these patients should be followed closely for the possible development of relapses or progression with skeletal involvement.

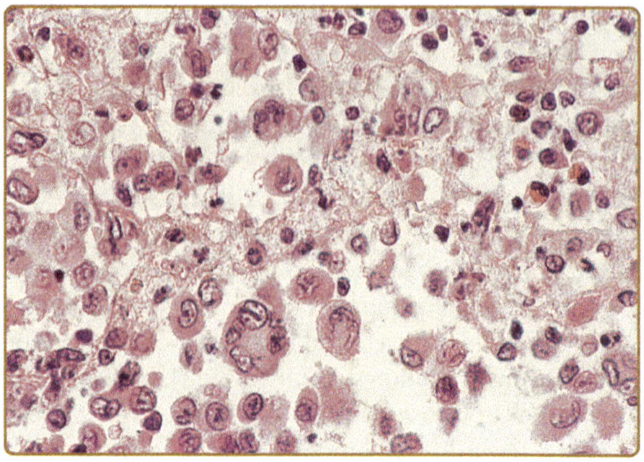

Langerhans cell histiocytosis (LCH). The granulomatous reaction consists of an aggregation of LCH cells with some multinucleated histiocytes and varying numbers of eosinophils, neutrophils, lymphocytes, and plasma cells. Note the grooved "kidney-shaped" nuclei. This type of reaction is seen in the chronic stage of the disease. (Reproduced, with permission, from Goldsmith LA, Katz SI, Gilchrest BA, Paller AS, Leffell DJ, Wolff K, eds. *Fitzpatrick's Dermatology in General Medicine*. 8th ed. New York, NY: McGraw-Hill Education; 2012.)

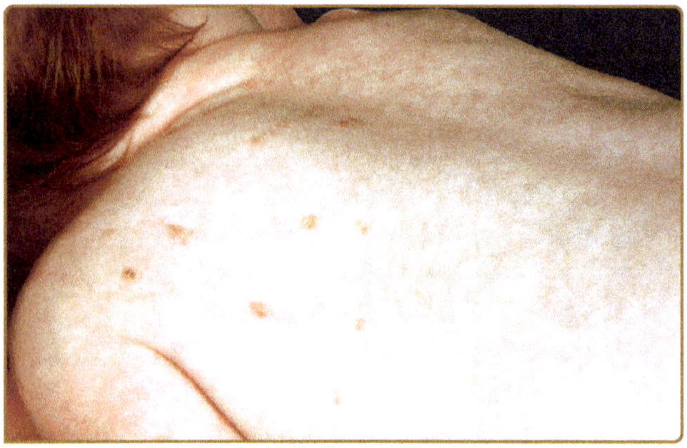

Congenital "self-healing" LCH (formerly Hashimoto–Pritzker disease). Resolving crusted reddish brown papules of congenital self-healing Langerhans cell histiocytosis with chickenpox-like lesions. (Reproduced, with permission, from Goldsmith LA, Katz SI, Gilchrest BA, Paller AS, Leffell DJ, Wolff K, eds. *Fitzpatrick's Dermatology in General Medicine*. 8th ed. New York, NY: McGraw-Hill Education; 2012.)

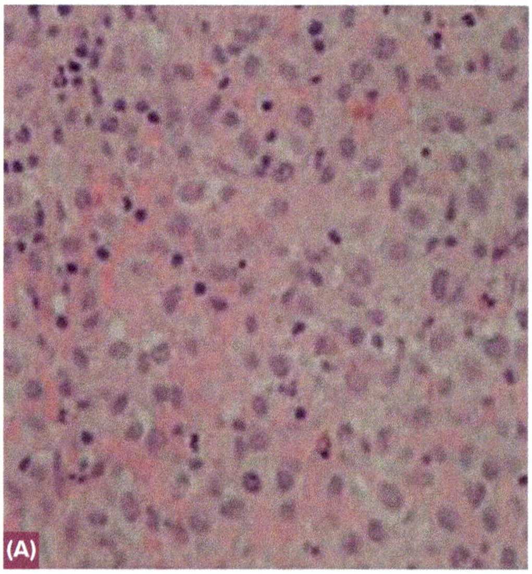

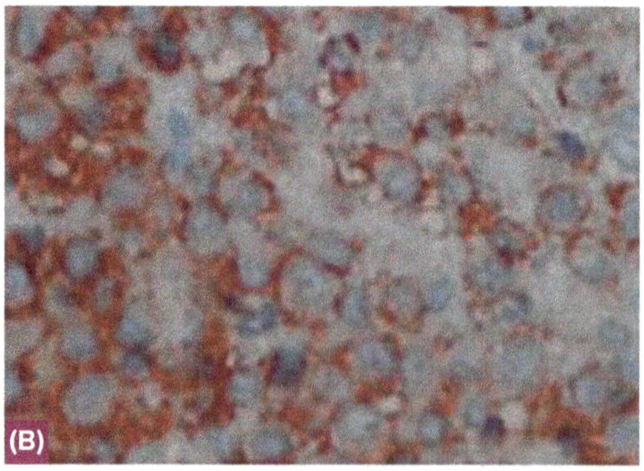

The histopathological features of **Langerhans histiocytosis** and **congenital self-healing Langerhans cell histiocytosis** are essentially identical (Table 2-27B). H&E-stained sections reveal perivascular or lichenoid infiltrates of Langerhans cells confined to the papillary and upper reticular dermis. Cytologic features are bland and characterized by cells with abundant eosinophilic or pale cytoplasms and longitudinally grooved or reniform "kidney-shaped" nuclei with small nucleoli. Epidermotropism is often seen. Eosinophils are usually prominent. Again, Langerhans cells are S-100+ and CD1a+ and contain Birbeck granules by electron microscopy. Another highly specific marker is Langerin.

In regards to the differential diagnosis, a proliferation of Langerhans cells (cytologic features described earlier) with accompanying eosinophils and epidermotropism suggest **Langerhans histiocytosis**. Identical histology may be seen in **congenital self-healing Langerhans histiocytosis**, and clinical workup to exclude extracutaneous involvement

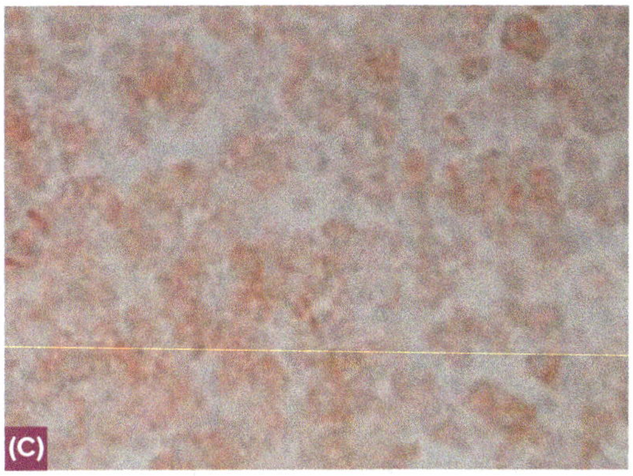

Langerhans cell histiocytosis. **(A)** H&E morphologic appearance with sheets of Langerhans cell histiocytes showing nuclear grooves. A few eosinophils are noted. **(B)** Langerhans cell histiocytes react on immunohistochemical staining for CD1a and **(C)** for the beta subunit of the protein S100. Both markers are used to identify the cells in this disorder. (Reproduced, with permission, from Lichtman MA, Shafer JA, Felgar RE, Wang N. *Lichtman's Atlas of Hematology.* New York, NY: McGraw-Hill; 2007.)

Table 2-27B. Langerhans Cell Proliferative Disorders

LANGERHANS CELL HISTIOCYTOSIS (SYSTEMIC)	CONGENITAL SELF-HEALING LANGERHANS HISTIOCYTOSIS
Clinical Features	
Cutaneous and extracutaneous disease	Cutaneous involvement only
Red-brown papules, nodules, plaques	Cutaneous lesions similar to systemic
Vesicles, pustules, ulcers Scalp, trunk, intertriginous Gingiva and other mucosal sites	Langerhans cell histiocytosis, but gingiva and other mucosal sites less commonly affected
Histopathologic Features	
Superficial perivascular or lichenoid infiltrates of Langerhans cells with grooved (reniform) nuclei	Identical to systemic Langerhans cell histiocytosis
Epidermotropism	
Eosinophils	
Langerhans cells S-100 protein, CD1a (OKT6) positive	
EM: Birbeck granules	

is required to separate the two. It must be underscored that one cannot predict the biology of Langerhans cell disease from the histopathology alone, a tenet that has been well established in clinical oncology/hematology. **Rosai–Dorfman disease** contains a mono- and multinucleated histiocytic infiltrate however the cytoplasms are typically pale/clear and the nuclei lack the characteristic grooves of the Langerhans cell. Additionally, Rosai–Dorfman exhibits emperipolesis, a finding not present in Langerhans histiocytosis. Lastly, the histiocytes in Rosai–Dorfman disease are CD68+, CD163+, S100+, and CD1a−, whereas Langerhans cells are CD68−, CD163−, S100+, and CD1a+. The histiocytes of **multicentric reticulohistiocytosis** may also contain mono- and multinucleated histiocytes with eosinophilic cytoplasm, but they lack the characteristic grooved nuclei of Langerhans cells. Reticulohistiocytes are CD68+, CD163+, Factor XIIIa+/−, S100−, and CD1a−. **Xanthoma disseminatum** may also present with widespread cutaneous disease and systemic involvement (ie, diabetes insipidus) however the infiltrates are composed of foamy macrophages and Touton-type giant cells that are CD68+, CD163+, S100−, and CD1a−. **Anaplastic large cell lymphoma** is composed of large anaplastic mononuclear T-cells admixed with small lymphocytes, macrophages, eosinophils, and neutrophils. The large anaplastic cells are CD3+, CD30+, CD68−, CD163−, S100−, and CD1a− via immunohistochemistry.

ANSWER 2-28: A.

The biopsy demonstrates a robust plasma cell infiltrate (Table 2-28A). The lower left hand corner of the image on the adjacent page reveals a bright eosinophilic **Russell body**. **Plasma cells** are characterized by eccentrically placed nuclei with peripherally placed dense chromatin ("clock face" chromatin). The cytoplasm is amphophilic with an eosinophilic **perinuclear hof** (prominent Golgi apparatus). Russell bodies are large, brightly eosinophilic, homogenous immunoglobulin-containing inclusions. All of the listed conditions are characterized by robust plasma cell infiltrates except **urticaria pigmentosa**, which is a form of **cutaneous mastocytosis**. Table 2-28A lists infectious diseases whose histopathologic pattern is typically but not exclusively composed of diffuse plasma cells.

"**Plasmacytosis mucosae**" is an encompassing term for an inflammatory accumulation of plasma cells at mucosal sites. The term "**Zoon balanitis**" is given to involvement of the prepuce or glans penis; "**plasma cell vulvitis**," to involvement of the vulva; and "**plasmacytosis circumorificialis**," to involvement of the oral mucosa, lips, gums, or tongue in both sexes. Most cases are idiopathic, but in oral mucosal lesions, immediate hypersensitivity reactions (often to chewing gum

Table 2-28A. Infectious Causes of Diffuse Lymphocytic–Plasma Cellular Infiltrates

	ORGANISM	TISSUE MORPHOLOGY	HISTOPATHOLOGIC FEATURES
Syphilis	*Treponema pallidum*	Spirochete (Warthin-Starry-positive)	Psoriasiform hyperplasia; lichenoid and granulomatous
Yaws	*T. pertenue*	Spirochete (Warthin-Starry-positive)	Spirochetes in epidermis
Pinta	*T. carateum*	Spirochete (Warthin-Starry-positive)	Spirochetes in epidermis
Chancroid	*Haemophilus ducreyi*	Gram-negative bacillus (school of fish) (Warthin-Starry- or Giemsa-positive)	Three-zone inflammation: PMNs and necrosis; granulation tissue; plasma cells
Granuloma inguinale	*Calymmatobacterium granulomatosis*	Intracellular gram-negative bacillus (Donovan bodies) (Giemsa- or Warthin-Starry-)	Organisms within macrophages
Lymphogranuloma venereum	*Chlamydia trachomatis*	1-4 μm Giemsa- or direct immunofluorescence-positive coccoid bodies	Intracellular
Rhinoscleroma	*Klebsiella rhinoscleromatis*	Intracellular gram-negative rods (Frisch bacilli) (Warthin-Starry-or PAS-positive)	Organisms within macrophages (Mikulicz cells); Russell bodies
Lyme disease	*Borrelia burgdorferi*	Spirochete (larger than *T. pallidum*)	Superficial and deep perivascular or pseudolymphoma
Necrotizing fasciitis	*Group A Strep, S. aureus*	Gram-positive cocci in chains or clusters	Blood vessel thrombosis

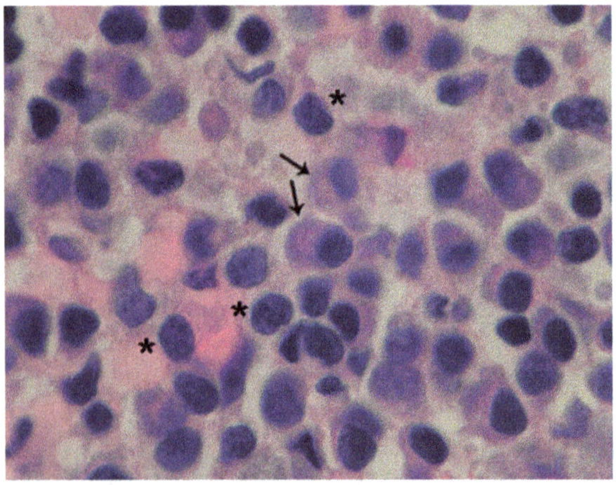

Plasma cell infiltrate in Waldenström macroglobulinemia (in lymph nodes this cellular infiltrate would be called lymphoplasmacytic lymphoma). Bone marrow biopsy shows a diffuse infiltrate of lymphocytes and Russell bodies (asterisks), and plasma cells (arrows). (Reproduced, with permission, from Lichtman MA, Shafer JA, Felgar RE, Wang N. *Lichtman's Atlas of Hematology*. New York, NY: McGraw-Hill; 2007.)

ingredients) have been implicated. The clinical presentation is similar at all three sites, consisting of well-marginated erythematous patches.

Microscopically, **plasmacytosis mucosae** are characterized by a dense, band-like, mixed mononuclear inflammatory cell infiltrate with a predominance of plasma cells. Dilated blood vessels, sometimes with red blood cell extravasation, also are seen. Varying degrees of stroma fibrosis are also typically present. The epidermis may exhibit spongiosis with exocytosis of inflammatory cells or ulceration. The heterogeneous nature of the inflammatory cell infiltrate with a predominance of plasma cells in a typical locale should suggest plasmacytosis mucosae. Immunohistochemical study for light-chain restriction may be necessary to definitively rule out plasmacytoma. Plasma cells express CD138 via immunohistochemistry.

Cutaneous plasmacytomas are monoclonal neoplastic proliferations of plasma cells. Cutaneous plasmacytomas may be primary (unassociated with multiple myeloma or extramedullary plasmacytoma) or secondary (arising in the

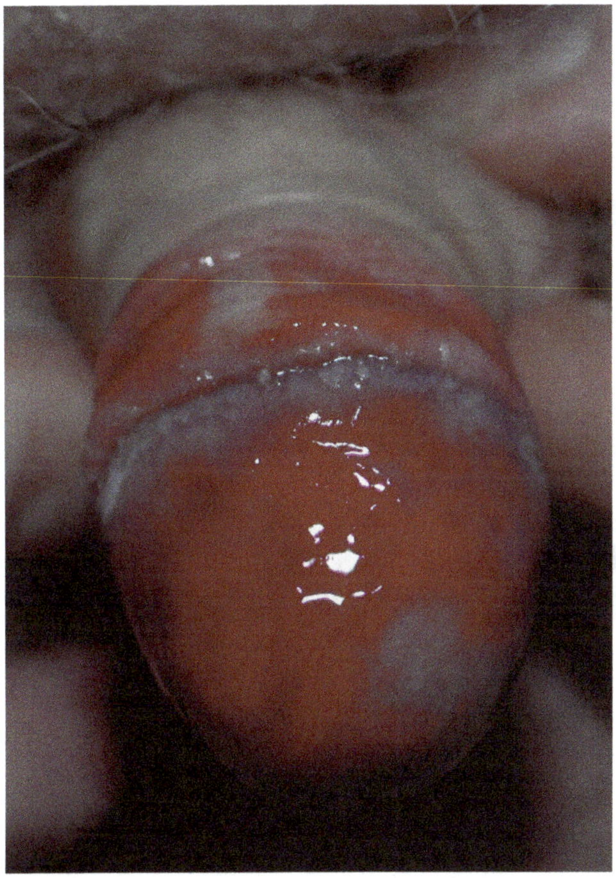

Plasma cell (Zoon) balanitis. Solitary red glistening plaque for 10 years in an uncircumcised male. (Reproduced with permission from Wolff K, Johnson RA, Saavedra AP. *Fitzpatrick's Color Atlas and Synopsis of Clinical Dermatology*. 7th ed. New York, NY: McGraw-Hill Education; 2013.)

setting of established multiple myeloma, extramedullary plasmacytoma, or plasma cell leukemia). Unlike the polyclonal infiltrates in plasmacytosis mucosae, immunohistochemical stains reveal light-chain restriction in all cases of cutaneous plasmacytoma.

In HIV-infected individuals, plasma cells may form a significant proportion of the inflammatory cell infiltrate in lesions of psoriasis, seborrheic dermatitis, and Kaposi sarcoma. Plasma cells are prominent in some cases of **nodular amyloidosis**, but nodular eosinophilic deposits of amyloid are distinctive. When the subcutis is exclusively affected by a prominent plasma cell infiltrate, the differential diagnosis includes dermatomyositis, fasciitis with eosinophilia, morphea profunda, polymyositis, Sjögren syndrome, and scleroderma. Cutaneous inflammatory pseudotumor (**plasma cell granuloma**) presents as a solitary skin tumor. Histopathologically, it is a sharply circumscribed dermal or subcutaneous nodule that exhibits varying degrees of central sclerosis accompanied by a mixed inflammatory cell infiltrate with prominent plasma cells and lymphoid follicles.

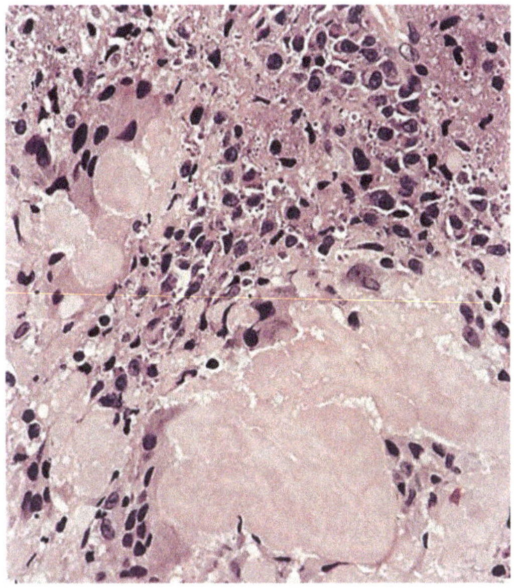

Primary nodular amyloidosis. Plasma cell myeloma with amorphous eosinophilic amyloid deposits. (Reproduced, with permission, from Lichtman MA, Shafer JA, Felgar RE, Wang N. *Lichtman's Atlas of Hematology*. New York, NY: McGraw-Hill; 2007.)

ANSWER 2-29: D.

Cutaneous mastocytosis (CM) is defined by the triad of (1) typical clinical skin lesions such as **maculopapular cutaneous mastocytosis/urticaria pigmentosa, diffuse cutaneous mastocytosis, solitary mastocytoma**, and **telangiectasia macularis eruptiva perstans (TMEP)**, (2) the histopathologic demonstration of typical focal mast cell (MC) infiltrates in the dermis, and (3) the absence of criteria for **systemic mastocytosis** (Table 2-29A).

Criteria for systemic mastocytosis include:

1. *Major:* Multifocal dense infiltrates of MCs (>15 MCs aggregating) detected in the bone marrow and/or in other extracutaneous organ(s) by tryptase-immunohistochemistry or other stains.
2. *Minor:*
   a. In MC infiltrates detected in sections of bone marrow or extracutaneous organs, more than 25% of MCs are spindle-shaped, or in bone marrow smears, atypical MCs comprise more than 25% of all MCs.
   b. Detection of a *c-kit* mutation at codon 816 in bone marrow or blood or other extracutaneous organ(s).
   c. Kit MCs in bone marrow or blood or other extracutaneous organ(s) coexpress CD2 and/or CD25.
   d. The serum total tryptase concentration is persistently greater than 20 ng/mL (in case of an associated clonal hematologic non-MC cell lineage disease, this last item is not valid).

If one major and one minor or three minor criteria are fulfilled, then the diagnosis is systemic mastocytosis.

Maculopapular cutaneous mastocytosis/urticaria pigmentosa (MPCM/UP) is the most frequent form of CM and is more common in childhood. The release of vasoactive mediators (especially histamine) leads to the clinical manifestations of urticaria, wheals, and flares with pruritus (**Darier sign**) observed in MPCM/UP. In addition to classic UP, a number of rare variants of MPCM/UP have been proposed and include plaque, nodular, and telangiectatic (TMEP) subvariants. **Diffuse cutaneous mastocytosis** may present with erythroderma. Solitary or small numbers of nodular lesions constitute **mastocytomas**. The prognosis of MPCM/UP is excellent because almost all cases begin in early childhood and regress at the end of puberty or in early adolescence. The serum tryptase level is a well-established marker of MC disease burden. In patients with CM (by definition having no systemic disease), the serum tryptase levels are within normal limits or only slightly elevated. Other laboratory studies are also unremarkable, and *c-kit* mutations are not detected in the majority of pediatric patients.

Systemic mastocytosis (SM) occurs most often in adults in whom excessive numbers of MCs may occur not only in the skin but also in the bone marrow and in the viscera, such as the gastrointestinal tract (leading to diarrhea), liver, spleen, and lymph nodes. Patients with SM often have bone marrow involvement and elevated serum tryptase levels and may develop an associated clonal hematologic non-MC lineage disease, an aggressive form of SM, and even rarely mast cell leukemia. TMEP occurs in adults and is rarely associated with systemic mastocytosis.

The cutaneous lesions of SM and MPCM/UP are reddish brown macules, papules, or nodules that may be clinically confused with melanocytic lesions. Stroking of the lesion causes MC degranulation with the development of an urticarial wheal and flare (Darier sign).

In **diffuse cutaneous mastocytosis**, the skin is uniformly erythematous (erythroderma) secondary to infiltrating mast cells with spared, white areas of normal skin. Flares of erythroderma are commonly associated with systemic symptoms such as syncope, wheezing, and diarrhea.

Solitary mastocytoma presents as a solitary, tan plaque with poorly demarcated borders on the hand of an infant. When stroked very vigorously, the lesion became red, more elevated, and a blister developed.

Telangiectasia macularis eruptiva perstans (TMEP) presents as pruritic lightly pigmented macules with surface telangiectasias distributed on the trunk and proximal extremities.

In **systemic mastocytosis, MPCM/UP, diffuse cutaneous mastocytosis, and solitary mastocytoma**, biopsy reveals either a robust perivascular or diffuses infiltrate of mast cells within the upper dermis. Mast cells in CM exhibit a mature morphology; usually they are round to oval cells with

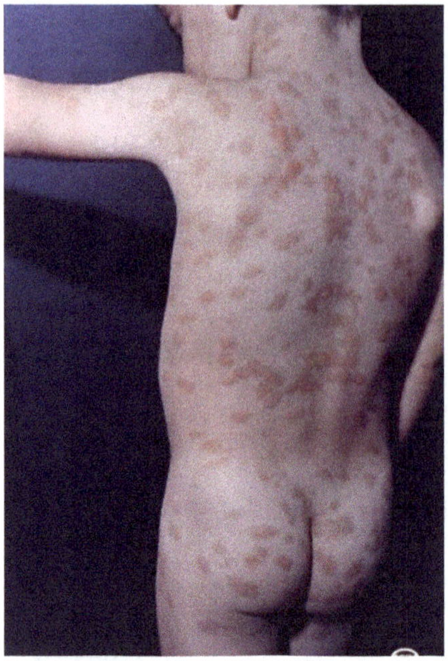

Urticaria pigmentosa (cutaneous mastocytosis). Widespread macules and plaques some with urticarial wheals. In infants and young children, this disorder is a benign dermal mastocytosis that eventually disappears by the early teens. A florid mast cell infiltrate is present in the dermis of the lesions. One can demonstrate the presumptive presence of mast cells by rubbing one of the lesions. Within a few minutes, the rubbed area becomes reddened, swollen, and itchy. This result is known as Darier sign. (Reproduced, with permission, from Lichtman MA, Shafer JA, Felgar RE, Wang N. *Lichtman's Atlas of Hematology*. New York, NY: McGraw-Hill; 2007.)

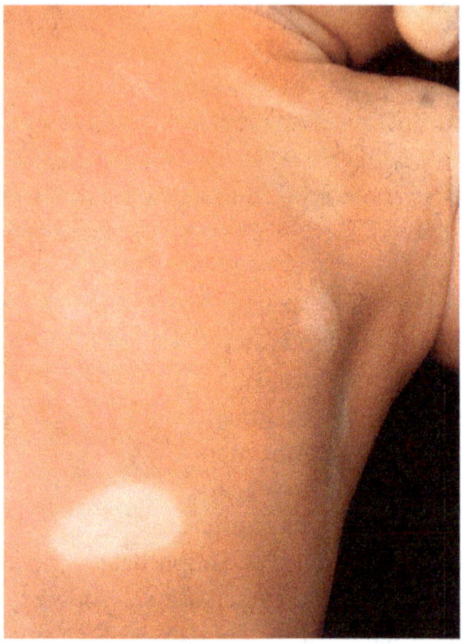

Diffuse cutaneous mastocytosis. The skin of this infant is uniformly erythematous (erythroderma) secondary to infiltrating mast cells with several spared, white areas of normal skin. (Reproduced, with permission, from Wolff K, Johnson RA, Saavedra AP. *Fitzpatrick's Color Atlas and Synopsis of Clinical Dermatology*. 7th ed. New York, NY: McGraw-Hill Education; 2013.)

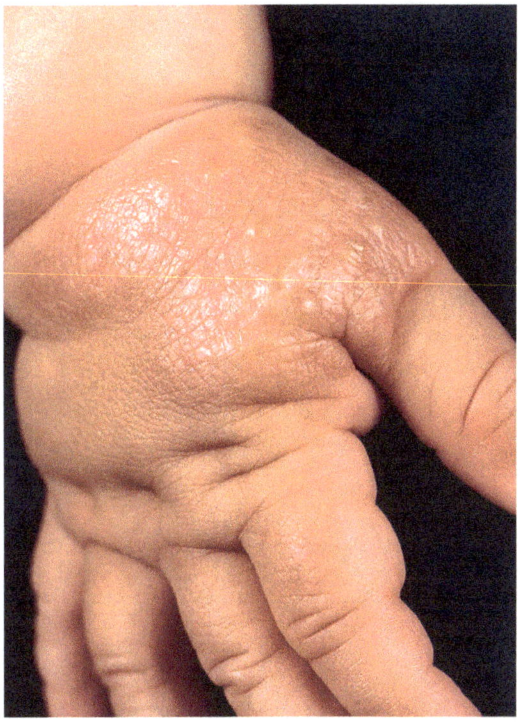

Solitary mastocytoma. There is an irregular plaque studded with erythematous papulovesicles. (Reproduced, with permission, from Wolff K, Johnson RA, Saavedra AP. *Fitzpatrick's Color Atlas and Synopsis of Clinical Dermatology.* 7th ed. New York, NY: McGraw-Hill Education; 2013.)

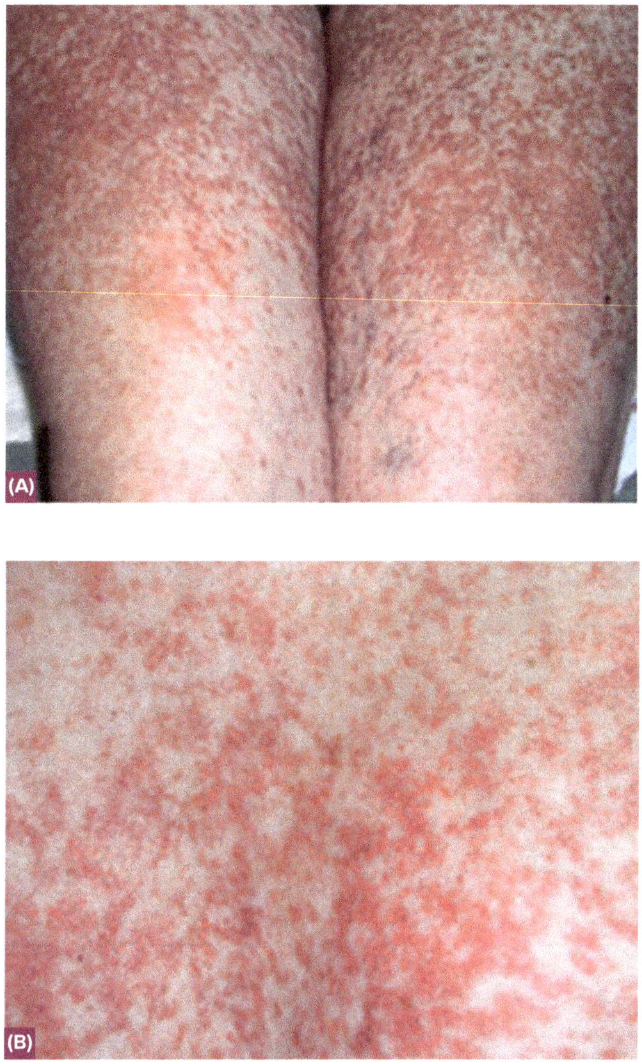

Telangiectasia macularis eruptiva perstans (TMEP). **(A)** Violaceous macules coalescing into plaques and telangiectasia. **(B)** Higher magnification of lesions revealing violaceous macules and telangiectasia. (Reproduced, with permission, from Lichtman MA, Shafer JA, Felgar RE, Wang N. *Lichtman's Atlas of Hematology.* New York, NY: McGraw-Hill; 2007.)

amphophilic-basophilic cytoplasm, centrally placed nuclei, and inconspicuous nucleoli (so-called fried-egg appearance). Mast cells stain with toluidine blue, chloracetate esterase (neutrophils are also stained), and Giemsa stains and the specific tryptase immunostain. Especially in childhood, excessive dermal edema may cause subepidermal bulla formation. Eosinophils are often present as well. Rarely, dermal fibroplasia may be observed in lesions of CM.

In **TMEP**, sparse numbers of MCs are distributed around dilated superficial dermal vessels and are elongate to spindle-shaped. Many have referred to this condition as an "**invisible dermatosis**" due to the extremely subtle histopathological findings. Without the proper clinical history, these biopsies may be mistaken for normal skin. Diffuse and nodular mast cell aggregates are not present in TMEP.

In regards to the differential diagnosis, the cells in papules and nodules are very uniform and on scanning magnification can resemble a **melanocytic nevus, histiocytes or Langerhans cells**, and **leukemic infiltrates**. The amphophilic cytoplasm and lack of nesting help to distinguish mast cell disease from melanocytic nevi. Histiocytic infiltrates may be characterized by cells with a monomorphous appearance; however, in contrast to mast cells, histiocytes usually have somewhat angulated or reniform nuclei. Plasma cells also resemble mast cells, but have eccentric nuclei, perinuclear hofs, and frequent Russell bodies. Special stains and immunohistochemistry may be needed to distinguish the latter conditions from mast cell disease.

In **TMEP**, the low-power appearance resembles normal skin. Since the histology of TMEP may be subtle, Giemsa, toluidine blue, and tryptase stains are helpful in highlighting the increased numbers of perivascular MCs. Normal skin may have up to 10 MCs per 40× field. Dermatopathologists always should keep this diagnosis in mind when dealing with "normal skin" biopsies or patients with unexplained pruritus.

Table 2-29A. Cutaneous Mastocytosis

SOLITARY MASTOCYTOMA	URTICARIA PIGMENTOSA	SYSTEMIC MASTOCYTOSIS	TMEP
Clinical Features			
Infants, neonates	Infants, neonates	Adults, usually	Adults, usually
Single red-brown macule, papule, nodule	Multiple red-brown macules, papules, nodules	Multiple red-brown macules, papules, nodules	Lightly pigmented macules with telangiectases
Vesicle, bulla, sometimes	Vesicles, bullae, often		No extracutaneous involvement usually
No extracutaneous involvement	No extracutaneous involvement	Extracutaneous involvement, as a rule	
	Rare progression to systemic mastocytosis		Rare progression to systemic mastocytosis
Histopathologic Features			
Perivascular or diffuse mast cells within upper dermis	Same as solitary mastocytoma	Same as solitary mastocytoma	Telangiectatic vessels with increased perivascular mast cells (>10 mast cells per 40× field)
Subepidermal bulla formation, sometimes			

ANSWER 2-30: C.

Wells syndrome (eosinophilic cellulitis) is an uncommon condition that is thought to be a hypersensitivity reaction (Table 2-30A). Most cases are completely idiopathic; others are associated with arthropod assaults, drug allergy, parasitic infestation, an atopic diathesis, internal malignancy, or dermatophyte infection. Wells syndrome presents as arcuate, erythematous, indurated plaques typically on the upper back, extremities, or buttocks. As the lesions evolve, they may become indurated, and complete resolution usually occurs within months.

Histopathology reveals a diffuse and, early on, massive infiltrate of eosinophils with few lymphocytes. In areas where eosinophils have degranulated, so-called **flame figures** are created. These represent dermal collagen fibers that become coated with bright red eosinophilic granules containing major basic protein surrounded by macrophages and sometimes with giant cells. Early lesions may result in subepidermal or intraepidermal vesicle/bulla formation. In later stages, macrophages with giant cells may predominate. The subcutis occasionally may be involved, one cause of eosinophilic panniculitis. In the proper clinical setting, flame figures are very suggestive of Wells syndrome, but isolated lesions of common dermatoses with numerous eosinophils may exhibit flame figures. A search to rule out associated conditions (especially internal malignancy, parasite infestation, and drug hypersensitivity) is warranted in patients with Wells syndrome.

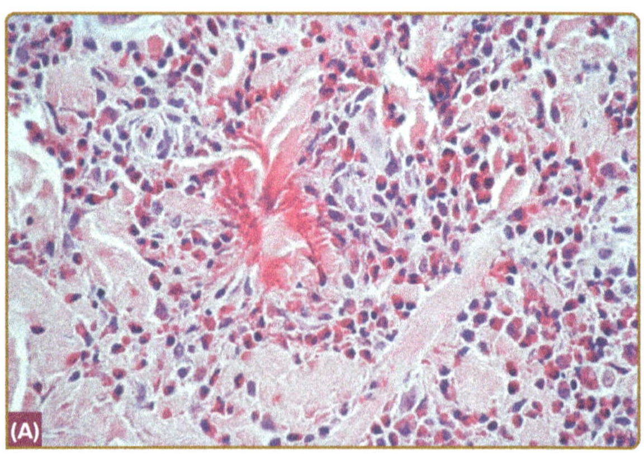
(A)

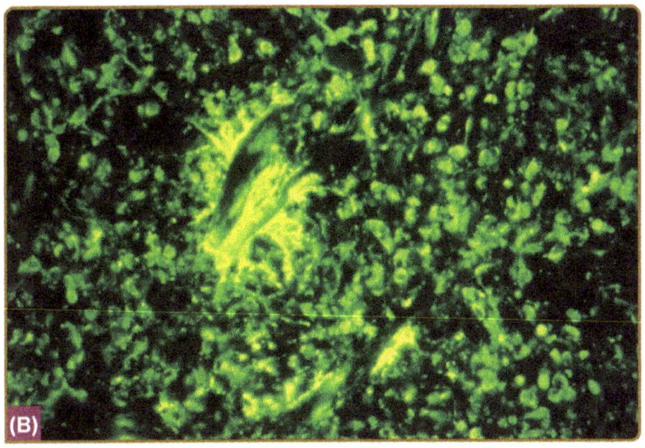

Familial Wells syndrome. **(A)** Hematoxylin- and eosin-stained section revealing numerous eosinophils and a flame figure (center). **(B)** Eosinophil granule major basic protein immunostain (of serial section to A) shows extensive granule protein deposition localized to the flame figure. (Original magnification ×400.) (Reproduced, with permission, from Goldsmith LA, Katz SI, Gilchrest BA, Paller AS, Leffell DJ, Wolff K, eds. *Fitzpatrick's Dermatology in General Medicine*. 8th ed. New York, NY: McGraw-Hill Education; 2012.)

Table 2-30A. Wells Syndrome

Clinical Features
Most cases idiopathic, but
Associations with:
Drug hypersensitivity
Parasites
Internal malignancy
Dermatophytes
Arcuate, erythematous, indurated plaques
Upper back, extremities, buttocks
Histopathologic Features
Diffuse eosinophils
Flame figures
Eosinophilic panniculitis, sometimes
Granulomas, especially in late lesions
Differential Diagnosis
Hypereosinophilic syndrome
Arthropod assault
Allergic contact dermatitis
Bullous pemphigoid
Herpes gestationis
Pruritic urticarial papules and plaques of pregnancy (PUPPP)
Urticaria

In regards to the differential diagnosis, cutaneous **arthropod assaults** owing to insects (tungiasis, myiasis, pediculosis), scabies, ticks, and spiders demonstrate dense superficial and deep perivascular and interstitial mixed-cell infiltrates with numerous eosinophils and are the most common demonstrable cause of clinical **papular urticaria**. Fortuitous sections may demonstrate embedded mouth or body parts, eggs, or excreta. Lesions of **chronic urticaria** or of **physical urticaria** demonstrate a perivascular lymphocytic infiltrate with scattered interstitial mixed-cell infiltrates composed of lymphocytes, neutrophils, and eosinophils. **Papular dermatitis (subacute prurigo)** features a relatively sparse superficial and deep perivascular lymphocytic infiltrate with scattered interstitial eosinophils and, at times, overlying epidermal spongiosis. Virtually identical appearances are seen in **papular dermatitis of HIV**.

Changes to the side of **eosinophilic folliculitis** may resemble Wells syndrome. Eosinophilic folliculitis may occur as an idiopathic condition in otherwise healthy individuals (**Ofuji disease**) or in the setting of HIV infection. Often cutting deeper into the tissue blocks of tangential samples reveals a folliculocentric infiltrate of eosinophils and lymphocytes that both surround and infiltrate the follicular epithelium, sometimes producing eosinophilic pustules. The scattered flame figures in the patient's biopsy are randomly dispersed throughout the superficial and deep dermis and are not associated with hair follicles.

Urticarial lesions of **bullous pemphigoid** may feature slight psoriasiform hyperplasia, variable spongiosis with eosinophils in the epidermis (so-called **eosinophilic spongiosis**), and eosinophils in number in a slightly edematous papillary dermis. Both **pemphigoid gestationis** and **pruritic urticarial papules and plaques of pregnancy (PUPPP)** are pregnancy-associated dermatoses that feature superficial perivascular lymphocytic infiltrates with interstitial eosinophils. Spongiosis with eosinophils is common in pemphigoid gestationis but absent in PUPPP. Additionally, the density of eosinophils is much greater in pemphigoid gestationis and bullous pemphigoid, and in PUPPP they tend to involve the reticular dermis more than the papillary dermis. While flame figures may be rarely present in these conditions, the inflammatory infiltrates are confined to the superficial dermis, whereas in Wells syndrome the inflammation involves both the superficial and deep dermis.

Angiolymphoid hyperplasia with eosinophilia (aka **epithelioid hemangioma**) is a vascular lesion that occurs most commonly on the head and neck. As its name implies, histology features a vascular proliferation with prominent endothelial cells, numerous eosinophils, and lymphoid aggregates, sometimes with germinal center formation. It is unclear as to whether this represents a reactive or neoplastic condition. Wells syndrome does not contain the characteristic vessels of angiolymphoid hyperplasia with eosinophilia.

The differential diagnosis of panniculitis with eosinophils includes erythema nodosum, vasculitis, drug reaction, atopic dermatitis, contact dermatitis, streptococcal infection, parasitic infection (*Gnathostoma* or *Toxocara canis*), atheromatous emboli, foreign-body, malignancy, or lupus erythematosus panniculitis.

BIBLIOGRAPHY

1. Aberer W, Konrad K, Wolff K. Wells' syndrome is a distinctive disease entity and not a histologic diagnosis. *J Am Acad Dermatol.* 1988;18:105.
2. Adame J, Cohen PR. Eosinophilic panniculitis: diagnostic considerations and evaluation. *J Am Acad Dermatol.* 1996;34:229.
3. Amar SM, Dreskin SC. Urticaria. *Prim Care.* 2008;35:141–157.
4. Ameen M, Chopra S, Darvay A, et al. Erythema gyratum repens and acquired ichythyosis associated with transitional carcinoma of the kidney. *Clin Exp Dermatol.* 2001;26:510–512.
5. Barnhill RL, Goldenhersh MA. Elastophagocytosis: a nonspecific reaction pattern associated with inflammatory processes in sun-protected skin. *J Cutan Pathol.* 1989;16:199.
6. Beham A, Fletcher CDM. Plexiform xanthoma: an unusual variant. *Histopathology.* 1991;19:565.
7. Boonstra HE, van Weelden H, Toonstra J, van Vloten WA. Polymorphous light eruption: a clinical, photobiologic and follow-up study of 110 patients. *J Am Acad Dermatol.* 2000;42:199–207.
8. Caputo R, Marzano AV, Passoni E, et al. Unusual variants of non-Langerhans cell histiocytoses. *J Am Acad Dermatol.* 2007;57:1031.
9. Champion RH. Annular erythemas. In: Champion RH, Burton JL, Ebling FJG, eds. *Textbook of Dermatology.* 5th ed. Oxford, England: Blackwell Scientific; 1992:1839–1842.
10. Chu P, Connolly K, LeBoit PE. The histopathologic spectrum of palisaded neutrophilic and granulomatous dermatitis in patients with collagen-vascular disease. *Arch Dermatol.* 1994;130:1278.
11. Chu P, LeBoit PE. Histologic features of cutaneous sinus histiocytosis (Rosai-Dorfman disease): study of cases both with and without systemic involvement. *J Cutan Pathol.* 1992;19:201.
12. Cooper PH. Eruptive xanthoma: a microscopic simulant of granuloma annulare. *J Cutan Pathol.* 1986;13:207.
13. Crowson AN, Magro CM. The role of microvascular injury in the pathogenesis of cutaneous lesion of dermatomyositis. *Hum Pathol.* 1996;1926:14–19.
14. Crowson AN, Magro CM. Atypical pigmentary purpura: a clinical, pathological and genotypic study of 40 cases. *Hum Pathol.* 1999;30:1104–1112.
15. David-Bajar KM. Subacute cutaneous lupus erythematosus. *J Invest Dermatol.* 1993;100:2S–8S.
16. Doria et al. Japanese diagnostic criteria for mixed connective tissue disease in Caucasian patients. *J Rheumatol* 1992;19:259–264.
17. Doutre MS, Beylot C, Beylot J, et al. Chilblain lupus erythematosus: report of 15 cases. *Dermatology.* 1992;184:26–28.
18. Elston DM, Bergfeld WF, McMahon JT. Aluminum tattoo: a phenomenon that can resemble parasitized histiocytes. *J Cutan Pathol.* 1993;20:326.
19. Ergun T, Gurbuz O, Harvell J, et al. The histopathology of pathergy: a chronological study of skin hyperreactivity in Behçet's disease. *Int J Dermatol.* 1998;37:929.
20. Eubanks LE, McBurney E, Reed R. Erythema gyratum repens. *Am J Med Sci.* 2001;321:302–305.
21. Evans MJ, Blessing K, Gray ES. Pseudorheumatoid nodule (deep granuloma annulare) of childhood: clinicopathologic features of twenty patients. *Pediatr Dermatol.* 1994;11:6.
22. Foucar E, Rosai J, Dorfman R. Sinus histiocytosis with massive lymphadenopathy (Rosai-Dorfman disease): review of the entity. *Semin Diagn Pathol.* 1993;7:19.
23. Fraser WJ, Haffejee Z, Cooper Z. Rheumatic Aschoff nodules revisited: an immunohistochemical reappraisal of the cellular component. *Histopathology.* 1995;27:457.
24. Furukawa F, Kahihara-Sawami M, Lyons MB, Norris DA. Binding of antibodies to ENA SS-A/Ro and SS-B/La is induced on the surface of human keratinocytes by UVL: implications for the pathogenesis of photosensitive cutaneous lupus. *J Invest Dermatol.* 1990;94:77–85.
25. Gianotti R, Alessi E, Caputo R. Benign cephalic histiocytosis: a distinct entity or a part of a wide spectrum of histiocytic proliferative disorders of children? A histopathological study. *Am J Dermatopathol.* 1993;15:315.
26. Gibbs NF, O'Grady TC. Progressive eruptive histiocytoma. *J Am Acad Dermatol.* 1996;35:323.
27. Goette DK. Chilblains (Perniosis). *J Am Acad Dermatol.* 1990;23:257–262.
28. Greaves MW, Tan KT. Chronic urticaria: recent advances. *Clin Rev Allergy Immunol.* 2007;33:134–143.
29. Hackzell-Bradley M, Hedbald M-A, Stephanssson EA. Metastatic Crohn's disease: report of 3 cases with special reference to histopathologic findings. *Arch Dermatol.* 1996;132:928.
30. Hanau D, Grosshans E. Monsel's solution and histological lesions. *Am J Dermatopathol.* 1981;3:418.
31. Hanno R, Callen JP. Sarcoidosis. A disorder with prominent cutaneous features and their interrelationship with systemic disease. *Med Clin North Am.* 1980;64(5):847.
32. Hill CL, Zhang Y, Sigurgeirsson B, et al. Frequency of specific cancer types in dermatomyositis and polymyositis: a population-based study. *Lancet.* 2001;357:96–100.

33. Hood AF. Superficial and deep infiltrates of the skin. In: Farmer ER, Hood AF, eds. *Pathology of the Skin.* 2nd ed. New York, NY: McGraw-Hill; 2000:327–343.

34. Jaworsky C. Connective tissue diseases. In: Elder DE, Elenitsas R, Jaworsky C, Johnson B, eds. *Lever's Histopathology of the Skin.* 8th ed. Philadelphia, PA: Lippincott-Raven; 1997:253–287.

35. Jerdan MS, Hood AF, Moore GW, Callen JP. Histopathologic comparison of the subsets of lupus erythematosus. *Arch Dermatol.* 1990;126:52–55.

36. Jorizzo JL, Abernethy JL, White WL, et al. Mucocutaneous criteria for the diagnosis of Behçet's disease: an analysis of clinicopathologic data from multiple international centers. *J Am Acad Dermatol.* 1995;32:968.

37. Jorizzo JL, Apisarnthanarax P, Subrt P, et al. Bowel-bypass syndrome without bowel bypass: bowel-associated dermatosis arthritis syndrome. *Arch Intern Med.* 1983;143:457.

38. Khakoo G, Sofianou-Katsoulis A, Perkin MR, Lack G. Clinical features and natural history of physical urticaria in children. *Pediatr Allergy Immunol.* 2008;19(4):363–366.

39. Kim KJ, Chang SE, Choi JH, et al. Clinicopathologic analysis of 66 cases of erythema annulare centrifugum. *J Dermatol.* 2002;29:61–67.

40. Kissel JT, Halterman RK, Rammohan KW, Mendell JR. The relationship of complement-mediated microvasculopathy to the histological features and clinical duration of disease in dermatomyositis. *Arch Neurol.* 1991;48:26–30.

41. Kolgen W, van Weelden H, den Hengst S, et al. CD11b+ cells and ultraviolet-B-resistant CD1a+ cells in the skin of patients with polymorphous light eruption. *J Invest Dermatol.* 1999;113:4–10.

42. Kovacs SO, Kovacs C. Dermatomyositis. *J Am Acad Dermatol.* 1998;39:899–920.

43. Kuhn A, Herrmann M, Kleber S, et al. Accumulation of apoptotic cells in the epidermis of patients with cutaneous lupus erythematosus after ultraviolet irradiation. *Arthritis Rheum.* 2006;54:939–950.

44. Lanto B, Bohm F, Maffert W, Sonnichsen N. The cytotoxic effect of anti-Ro (SS-A) antibodies and UVA light on human endothelial cells in vitro. *Dermatol Monatsschr.* 1990;176:305–311.

45. Lattanoos RL, Appleton MAC, Hughes LE, et al. Granulomatous hidradenitis suppurativa and cutaneous Crohn's disease. *Histopathology.* 1993;23:111.

46. Ledo E. Photodermatoses. *Dermatol Clin.* 1994;12: 797–803.

47. Leibold AM, Bennion S, David-Bajar K, Schleve MJ. Occurrence of positive immunofluorescence in the dermoepidermal junction of sun-exposed skin of normal adults. *J Cutan Pathol.* 1994;21:200–206.

48. Longaker MA, Frieden IJ, LeBoit PE, Sherertz EF. Congenital "self-healing" Langerhans cell histiocytosis: the need for long-term follow-up. *J Am Acad Dermatol.* 1994;31:910.

49. Lowe L, Kornfeld B, Clayman J, Golitz LE. Rheumatoid neutrophilic dermatitis. *J Cutan Pathol.* 1992;19:48.

50. Magro CM, Crowson AN. Lichenoid and granulomatous dermatitis: a novel cutaneous reaction pattern. *Int J Dermatol.* 2000;39:126–133.

51. Magro CM, Crowson AN. The cutaneous neutrophilic vascular injury syndromes: a review. *Semin Diagn Pathol.* 2001;18:47–58.

52. Marcoval J, Mana J, Moreno A, et al. Foreign bodies in granulomatous cutaneous lesions of patients with systemic sarcoidosis. *Arch Dermatol.* 2001;137:427.

53. McCalmont TH, Altemus D, Maurer T, Berger TG. Eosinophilic folliculitis: the histologic spectrum. *Am J Dermatopathol.* 1995;17:439.

54. Mehregan DA, Winkelmann RK. Necrobiotic xanthogranuloma. *Arch Dermatol.* 1992;128:94.

55. Mehregen DR, Hall MJ, Gibson LE. Urticarial vasculitis: a histopathologic and clinical review of 72 cases. *J Am Acad Dermatol.* 1992;26:441–448.

56. Michal M. Plexiform xanthomatous tumor: a report of three cases. *Am J Dermatopathol.* 1994;16:532.

57. Mutasim DF, Bridges AG. Patch granuloma annulare: clinicopathologic study of 6 patients. *J Am Acad Dermatol.* 2000;42:417.

58. Necrobiosis lipoidica vs. necrobiotic xanthogranuloma. In: Ackerman AB, White WL, Guo Y, Umbert I, eds. *Differential Diagnosis in Dermatopathology IV.* Philadelphia, PA: Lea & Febiger; 1994:38.

59. Nishimura M, Matsuda T, Muto M, Hori Y. Balanitis of Zoon. *Int J Dermatol.* 1990;29:421.

60. Oliver GF, Umbert I, Winkelmann RK. Reticulohistiocytoma cutis: review of 15 cases and an association with systemic vasculitis in two cases. *Clin Exp Dermatol.* 1990;15:1.

61. Patterson JW. Rheumatoid nodule and subcutaneous granuloma annulare: a comparative histologic study. *Am J Dermatopathol.* 1988;10:1.

62. Penneys NS, Hicks B. Unusual cutaneous lesions associated with acquired immunodeficiency syndrome. *J Am Acad Dermatol.* 1985;13:845.

63. Perez-Ordonez B, Erlandson RA, Rosai J. Follicular dendritic cell tumor: report of 13 additional cases of a distinctive entity. *Am J Surg Pathol.* 1996;20:944.

64. Peters MS, Su WPD. Panniculitis. *Dermatol Clin.* 1992;10:37.

65. Popovic K, Nyberg F, Wahren-Herlenius M, Nyberg F. A serology-based approach combined with clinical examination of 125 Ro/SSA-positive patients to define incidence and prevalence of subacute cutaneous lupus erythematosus. *Arthritis Rheum.* 2007;56:255–264.

66. Rudolph CM, Al-Fares S, Vaughan-Jones SA, et al. Polymorphic eruption of pregnancy: clinicopathology and potential trigger factors in 181 patients. *Br J Dermatol.* 2006;154:54–60.

67. Rullan E, Sigal LH. Rheumatic fever. *Curr Rheumatol Rep.* 2001;3:445–452.

68. Sabroe RA, Seed PT, Francis DM, et al. Chronic idiopathic urticaria: comparison of the clinical features of patients with and without anti-FcεRI or anti-IgE autoantibodies. *J Am Acad Dermatol.* 1999;40:443–450.

69. Sanchez RL, Raimer SS, Peltier F. Papular xanthoma: a clinical, histologic, and ultrastructural study. *Arch Dermatol.* 1985;121:626.

70. Sangueza OP, Salmon JK, White CR, Beckstead JH. Juvenile xanthogranuloma: a clinical, histopatholgic, and immunohistochemical study. *J Cutan Pathol.* 1995;22:327.

71. Saxena A. Diagnosis of rheumatic fever: current states of the Jones criteria and role of echocardiography. *Ind J Pediatr.* 2000;67:S11–S13.

72. Smith KJ, Skelton HG, Angritt P. Changes of verruciform xanthoma in an HIV positive patient with diffuse psoriasiform skin disease. *Am J Dermatopathol.* 1995;17:185.

73. Subcutaneous granuloma annulare vs. rheumatoid nodule. In: Ackerman AB, White WL, Guo Y, Umbert I, eds. *Differential Diagnosis in Dermatopathology IV.* Philadelphia, PA: Lea & Febiger; 1994:42.

74. Sweet WL, Smoller BR. Perivascular mast cells in urticaria pigmentosa. *J Cutan Pathol.* 1996;23:247.

75. Toussaint S, Kamino H. Noninfectious erythematous, papular, and squamous diseases. In: Elder D, Elenitsas R, Jaworksy C, Johnson B, eds. *Lever's Histopathology of the Skin.* 8th ed. Philadelphia, PA: Lippincott-Raven; 1997:177–178.

76. Valent P, Horny H-P, Escribano L, et al. Diagnostic criteria and classification of mastocytosis: a consensus proposal. *Leukemia Res.* 2001;25:603.

77. Vettraino IM, Merritt DF. Crohn's disease of the vulva. *Am J Dermatopathol.* 1995;17:410.

78. Walsh NMG, Hanly JG, Tremaine R, Murray S. Cutaneous sarcoidosis and foreign bodies. *Am J Dermatopathol.* 1993;15:203.

79. Walsh NMG, Murray S, D'Intino Y. Eruptive xanthoma with urate-like crystals. *J Cutan Pathol.* 1994;21:350.

80. Weigand DA. Lupus band test: anatomic regional variations in discoid lupus erythematosus. *J Am Acad Dermatol.* 1986;14:426–428.

81. Williford PM, White WL, Jorizzo JL, Greer K. The spectrum of normolipemic plane xanthoma. *Am J Dermatopathol.* 1993;15:572.

82. Willman CL, Busque L, Griffith BB, et al. Langerhans' cell histiocytosis (histiocytosis X): a clonal proliferative disease. *N Engl J Med.* 1994;331:154.

83. Wong KF, Chan JKC, Li LPK, et al. Primary cutaneous plasmacytoma: report of 2 cases and review of the literature. *Am J Dermatopathol.* 1994;16:392.

84. Wood C, Miller AC, Jacobs A, et al. Eosinophilic infiltration with flame figures: a distinctive tissue reaction seen in Well's syndrome and other diseases. *Am J Dermatopathol.* 1986;8:186.

85. Wood GS, Haber RS. Novel histiocytoses considered in the context of histiocyte subset differentiation. *Arch Dermatol.* 1993;129:210.

86. Zanolli MD, Powell BL, McCalmont T, White WL. Granuloma annulare and disseminated herpes zoster. *Int J Dermatol.* 1992;31:55.

87. Zelger B, Cerio R, Soyer HP, et al. Reticulohistiocytoma and multicentric reticulohistiocytosis: histopathologic and immunophenotypic distinct entities. *Am J Dermatopathol.* 1994;16:577.

88. Zimmer WM, Rogers RS, Reeve CM, Sheridan PJ. Orofacial manifestations of Melkersson-Rosenthal syndrome: a study of 42 patients and a review of 220 cases from the literature. *Oral Surg Oral Med Oral Pathol.* 1992;74:610.

CHAPTER 3

Vesiculobullous Diseases

QUESTION 3-1.

Many dermatologic conditions have more than one name. Please match the following diseases with their alternative designation.

1) Pemphigus foliaceus
2) Transient acantholytic dermatosis
3) Benign familial pemphigus
4) Keratosis follicularis

A) Darier disease
B) Hailey-Hailey disease
C) Grover disease
D) Fogo selvagem

QUESTION 3-2.

Which of the following statements regarding intraepidermal vesicular and pustular diseases is INCORRECT?

A) Acantholysis is defined as a disruption in cohesion between adjacent keratinocytes resulting in separated and rounded keratinocytes rimmed by a brightly eosinophilic band of keratin. Intercellular bridges are lost.
B) With spongiosis, intercellular bridges are more prominently seen due to the accumulation extracellular intraepidermal edema.
C) Cytolysis characteristically results in large numbers of acantholytic keratinocytes.
D) Pustules contain abundant inflammatory cells, usually neutrophils.
E) Traumatic or immune-mediated cytolysis may result in blister formation due to destruction of keratinocytes and their desmosomal adhesion molecules.

QUESTION 3-3.

Which of the following statements regarding the lesion illustrated below is LEAST accurate?

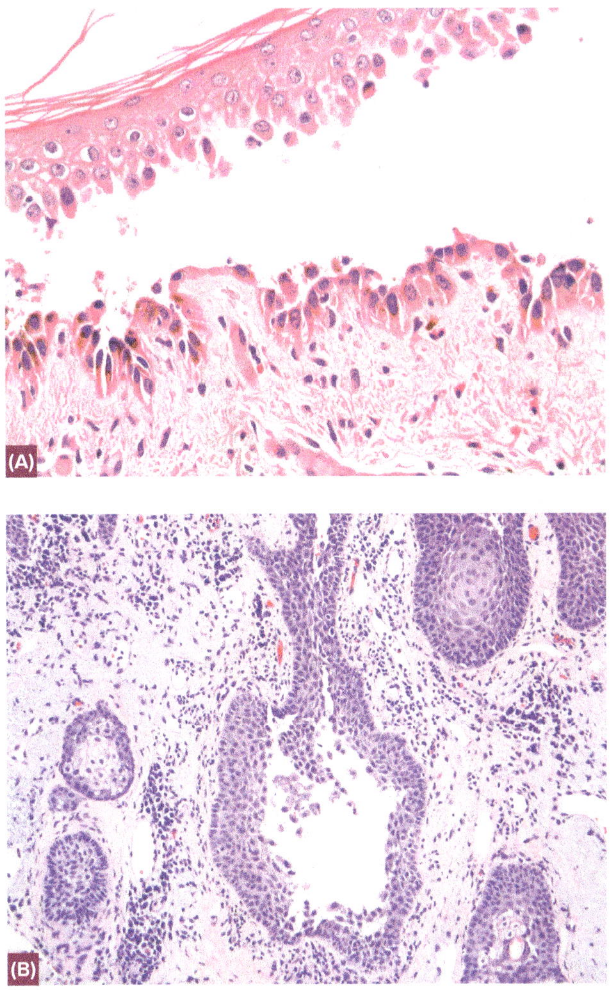

A) ELISA studies with monkey esophagus conducted on the patient's peripheral blood will be positive for antibodies directed against desmosomal cadherins. These antibody concentrations show a general correlation with disease activity.
B) Direct immunofluorescence studies will demonstrate intercellular deposition of IgG and C3d within the epidermis.
C) Oral lesions are the first manifestation in 10% to 15% of patients and almost invariably develop during the course of the disease.
D) Clinically these lesions present as persistent, small, pin-sized, skin-colored, and slightly pruritic papules arising on the upper back and chest. Mucosal involvement is absent.
E) About 30% of cases will exhibit intercellular deposition of both IgM and IgA by direct immunofluorescence studies.

QUESTION 3-4.

A 50-year-old patient presents with multiple flaccid bullae of the oral mucosa and lips as well as on the back, scalp, axilla, groin, and trunk. The patient reports that these lesions developed on normal skin without any prior erythema. The blisters extend laterally with compression. Many of the bulla on the lips and mouth are ruptured revealing underlying painful erosions. Slight rubbing of the uninvolved skin results in exfoliation of the outermost layer and the formation of a blister within minutes. A biopsy of the peripheral edge of one of the bullae is obtained. Indirect immunofluorescence using the patient's serum and monkey esophagus as a substrate is illustrated below. Which of the following is the MOST likely microscopic description for this biopsy?

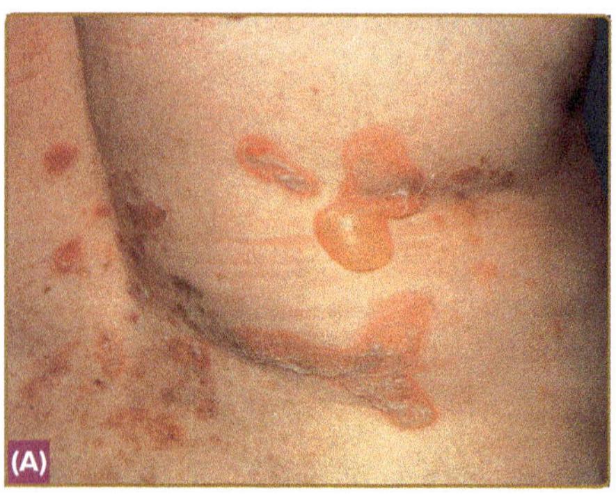
(A)

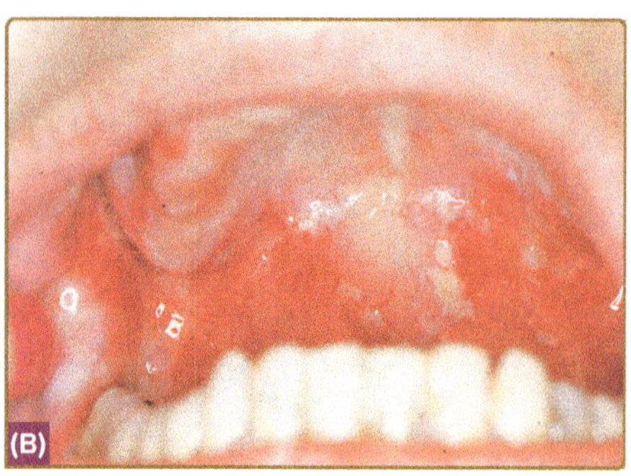
(B)

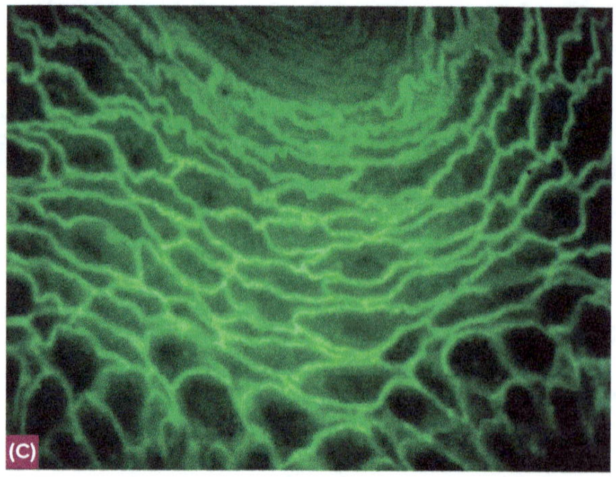
(C)

Reproduced, with permission, from Goldsmith LA, Katz SI, Gilchrest BA, Paller AS, Leffell DJ, Wolff K, eds. *Fitzpatrick's Dermatology in General Medicine*. 8th ed. New York, NY: McGraw-Hill Education; 2012.

A) There is acantholysis confined to the granular layer with loss of the stratum corneum.
B) There is an epidermal invagination filled with ortho- and parakeratotic debris. Suprabasilar acantholysis is present. Additionally, there are large keratinocytes containing perinuclear halos and clumped keratohyaline granules, as well as small seed-shaped keratinocytes with pyknotic nuclei and dense eosinophilic cytoplasm. Few inflammatory cells are present.
C) There is a subepidermal blister containing fibrin, lymphocytes, eosinophils, and Langerhans cells. At the base of the blister is a lymphocytic infiltrate with numerous eosinophils and few neutrophils.
D) There is a subepidermal blister containing fibrin, neutrophils, and rare eosinophils. At the periphery of the blister are papillary dermal neutrophilic microabscesses.
E) There is suprabasilar acantholysis involving the lower half of the epidermis. Basal cells protrude into the blister cavity, which also contains scattered lymphocytes, and eosinophils. The acantholysis extends down into hair follicles.

QUESTION 3-5.

A 32-year-old patient reports developing transient bullae in the inguinal region that evolve into erythematous papules and raised plaques studded by pustules of varying sizes. Indirect immunofluorescence using the patient's serum and monkey esophagus as a substrate reveals intercellular staining. A prolonged remission is accomplished with a low dose of corticosteroids. Which of the following statements regarding the histopathology of these lesions is INCORRECT?

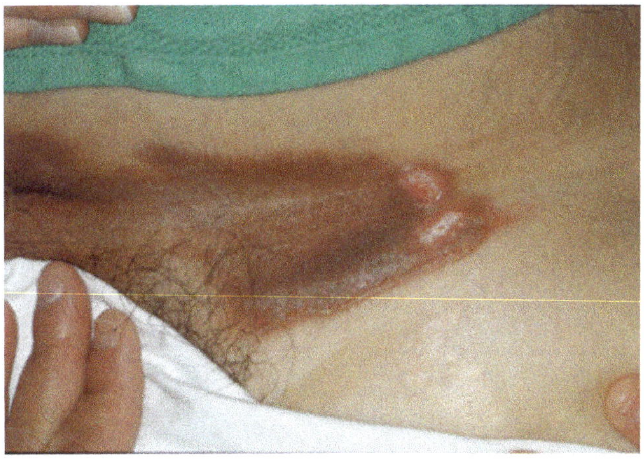

Reproduced, with permission, from Usatine RP, Smith MA, Mayeaux EJ Jr, Chumley HS, eds. *Color Atlas of Family Medicine*. 2nd ed. New York, NY: McGraw-Hill Education; 2012.

A) Initial lesions may show prominent suprabasilar acantholysis.
B) This condition is characterized by marked acanthosis with downward expansion of the rete ridges into the papillary dermis.
C) Intraepidermal abscesses and diffuse dermal infiltrates of eosinophils and lymphocytes is a constant feature.
D) Fully evolved lesions are characterized by an intraepidermal blister with a cleavage plane confined to the granular layer and large numbers of acantholytic keratinocytes.
E) Direct immunofluorescence of perilesional skin will reveal intercellular deposition of IgG and C3d.

QUESTION 3-6.

A patient with non-Hodgkin lymphoma presents with purple polygonal papules on the palms and soles and extensive painful ulcerations of the conjunctiva, lips, oral mucosa, and tongue. Biopsies are performed and the findings of the H&E-stained sections and IgG direct immunofluorescence are illustrated below. Which of the following diagnoses is CORRECT?

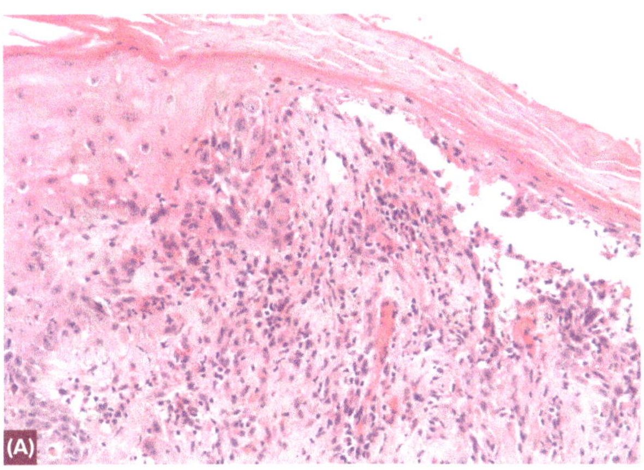

(A)

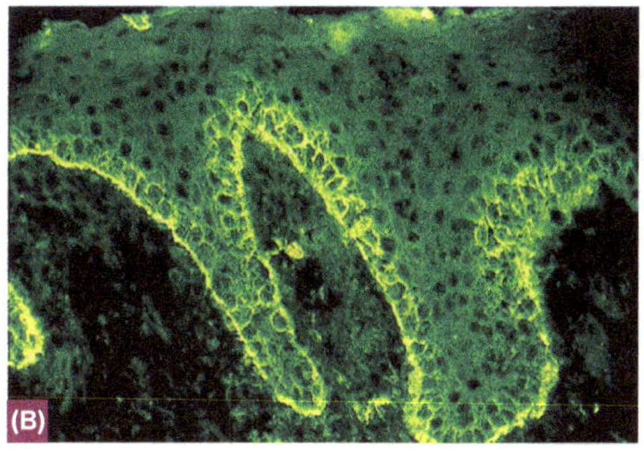

(B)

Reproduced, with permission, from Goldsmith LA, Katz SI, Gilchrest BA, Paller AS, Leffell DJ, Wolff K, eds. *Fitzpatrick's Dermatology in General Medicine*. 8th ed. New York, NY: McGraw-Hill Education; 2012.

A) Stevens-Johnson syndrome
B) Bullous lichen planus
C) Pemphigus erythematosus
D) Paraneoplastic pemphigus
E) Chronic graft versus host disease

QUESTION 3-7.

A 50-year-old patient presents with multiple erythematous oozing erosions with crust on the face, scalp, chest, and back. Closer inspection reveals that a few intact shallow bullae are present. No mucosal lesions are present. Biopsies are performed. Direct immunofluorescence of perilesional skin reveals intercellular IgG and C3d deposition within the epidermis. Which of the following regarding this condition is INCORRECT?

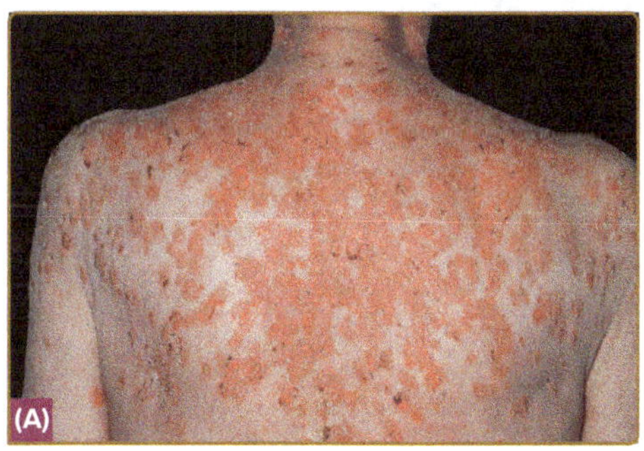

(A)

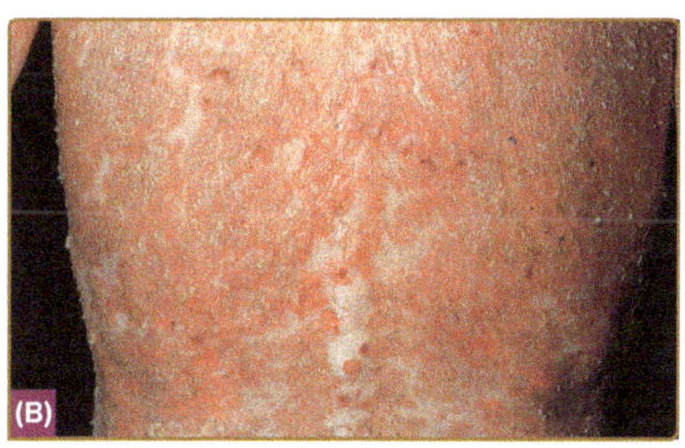

(B)

Reproduced, with permission, from Goldsmith LA, Katz SI, Gilchrest BA, Paller AS, Leffell DJ, Wolff K, eds. *Fitzpatrick's Dermatology in General Medicine*. 8th ed. New York, NY: McGraw-Hill Education; 2012.

A) This condition is characterized by acantholysis of granular layer keratinocytes.
B) Patients have autoantibodies directed against desmoglein-1 of keratinocyte desmosomes.
C) A diffuse dermal infiltrate of eosinophils and lymphocytes is present.
D) Older chronic lesions typically exhibit hypergranulosis.
E) Neutrophil-rich subcorneal pustules and clusters of gram-positive cocci within scale crusts characterize nondisrupted lesions.

QUESTION 3-8.

A 40-year-old patient presents with a pruritic vesiculopustular eruption involving the axilla, trunk, and extremities. These flaccid vesicles, pustules, and bullae are present on an erythematous base. Some of the pustules coalesce to form an annular pattern. No mucous membrane involvement is present. Biopsies are performed and the findings are illustrated below. Neutrophils are the dominant inflammatory cell type. Direct immunofluorescence of perilesional skin reveals intercellular deposition of IgA only. Which of the following diagnoses is CORRECT?

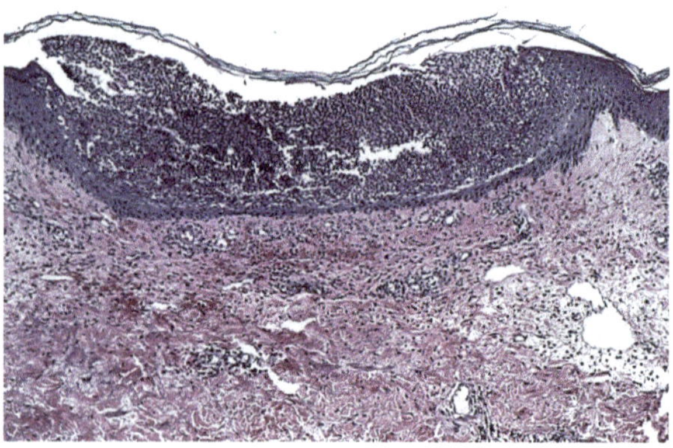

A) IgA pemphigus
B) Subcorneal pustular dermatosis (Sneddon-Wilkinson disease)
C) Pustular psoriasis
D) Impetigo
E) Acute generalized exanthematous pustulosis

QUESTION 3-9.

A patient with rheumatoid arthritis presents with a nonspecific generalized morbilliform eruption and focal blisters on scaly-crusted patches on the trunk and extremities. The patient's medication list includes penicillamine and captopril. Biopsies are performed and the findings are illustrated below. Direct immunofluorescence reveals a nonspecific immunoreactant profile without intercellular immunoglobulin or complement deposition. Culture and special stains (Gram & PAS) are negative for microorganisms. Which of the following regarding this condition is INCORRECT?

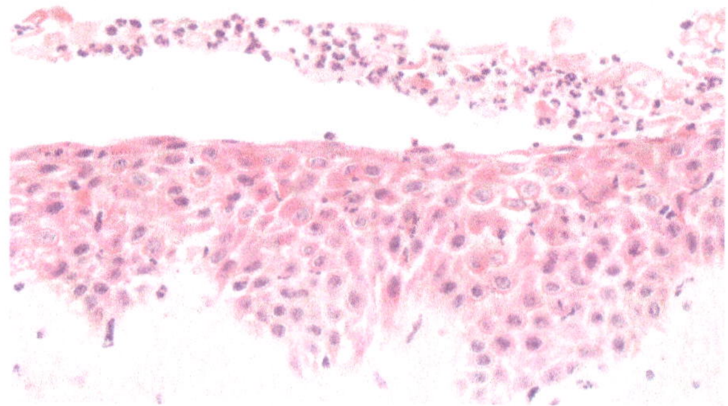

A) Circulating antibodies to desmoglein-1 and 3 and intercellular deposition of immunoreactant via direct immunofluorescence will be seen in approximately 10% of patients with this condition.
B) In early eruptions there is an acute to subacute eczematous dermatitis with occasional eosinophils.
C) The superficial acantholysis is attributed to an exotoxin.
D) One proposed mechanism for this condition is the accumulation of exogenous substances rich in sulfhydryl groups, which cleave the disulfide bonds of keratin leading to acantholysis.
E) The blister cleavage plane in some cases may involve suprabasal zones.

QUESTION 3-10.

A patient presents with erythematous plaques of the nose and malar areas. Biopsies are performed and the findings are illustrated below. Direct immunofluorescence of perilesional skin reveals intercellular deposition of IgM and C3d and granular deposition of IgM and C3 along the dermal-epidermal junction. Which of the following regarding this condition is INCORRECT?

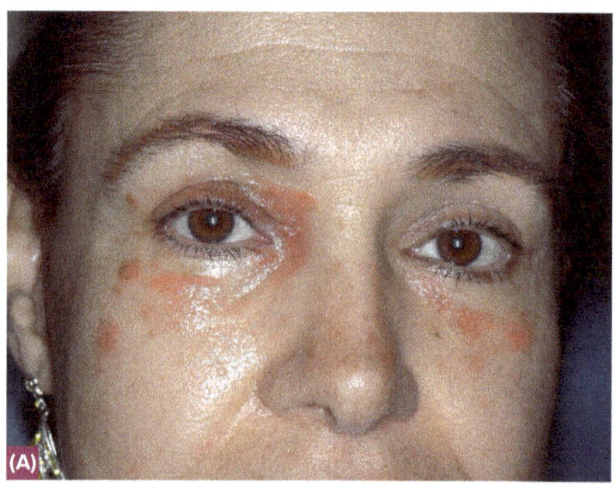

Reproduced, with permission, from Usatine RP, Smith MA, Mayeaux EJ Jr, Chumley HS, eds. *Color Atlas of Family Medicine.* 2nd ed. New York, NY: McGraw-Hill Education; 2012.

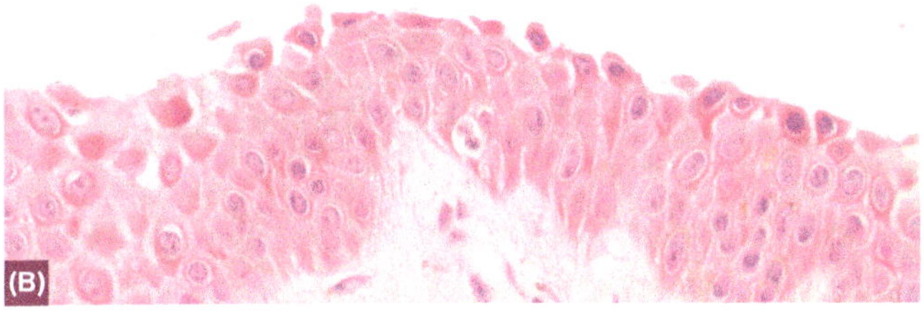

(B)

A) This condition may also exhibit eosinophilic spongiosis and abscesses.
B) This condition may also exhibit subcorneal/granular layer blisters with dyskeratotic granular cells. Vacuolar interface dermatitis may be present.
C) Approximately 30% of patients have positive antinuclear antibody titers, but rarely exhibit signs and symptoms of systemic collagen vascular disease.
D) This is a localized form of pemphigus foliaceus that may progress to a generalized distribution.
E) There is strong association with neoplasms such as non-Hodgkin lymphoma, chronic lymphocytic leukemia, Castleman disease, thymoma, sarcoma, and Waldenström macroglobulinemia.

QUESTION 3-11.

A 60-year-old female presents with right-sided facial palsy and segmental clusters of small painful vesicles with an erythematous base on the right external ear, tongue, and soft palate. The external ear eruption is band like and extends onto the lateral cheek. Some of the lesions are eroded. Tinnitus, vertigo, and deafness in the right ear are reported on review of systems. Biopsies of the tongue and external ear are performed. Which of the following regarding the microscopic description of these biopsies is INCORRECT?

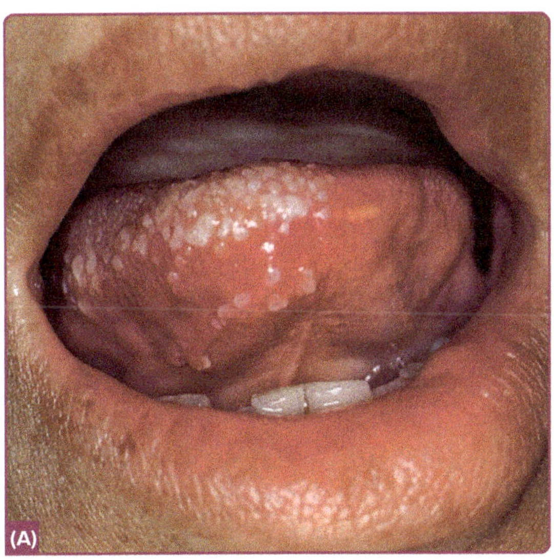

(A)

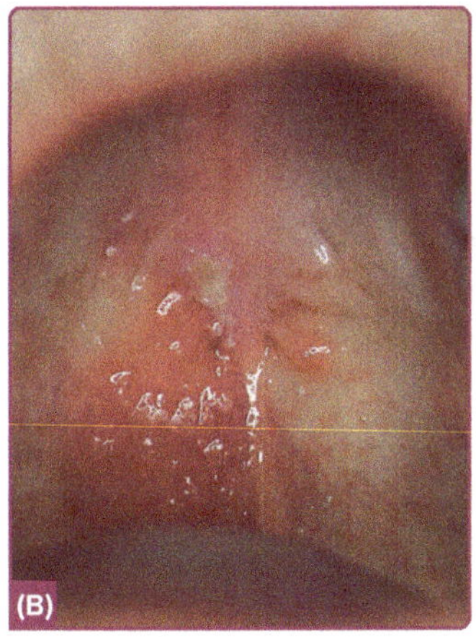

(B)

Reproduced, with permission, from Goldsmith LA, Katz SI, Gilchrest BA, Paller AS, Leffell DJ, Wolff K, eds. *Fitzpatrick's Dermatology in General Medicine.* 8th ed. New York, NY: McGraw-Hill Education; 2012.

A) Intraepidermal acantholysis with numerous dyskeratotic keratinocytes is seen.
B) The acantholytic epidermal keratinocytes exhibit enlarged pale basophilic nuclei with effaced heterochromatin and peripheral beading of the nuclear membrane.
C) Direct immunofluorescence studies reveal striking IgG and C3d deposition within the intercellular spaces of the epidermis.
D) Leukocytoclastic vasculitis and epidermal and dermal necrosis are common findings.
E) Multinucleated keratinocytes are a very common finding.

QUESTION 3-12.

A 4-year-old child presents with multiple golden crusts and pustules with an erythematous base on the hands, fingers, mouth, and intertriginous sites. The patient has a history of asthma, eczematous dermatitis, and allergic rhinitis. A biopsy is performed and the findings of the H&E and Gram stained sections are illustrated below. A PAS stain is negative for fungi. Culture results of the bullous fluid are pending. The mother reports that several other children in the child's preschool class have developed similar lesions. Which of the following regarding this entity is CORRECT?

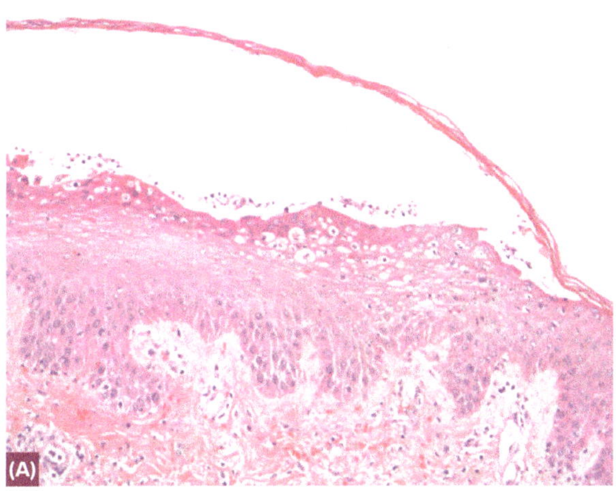

(A)

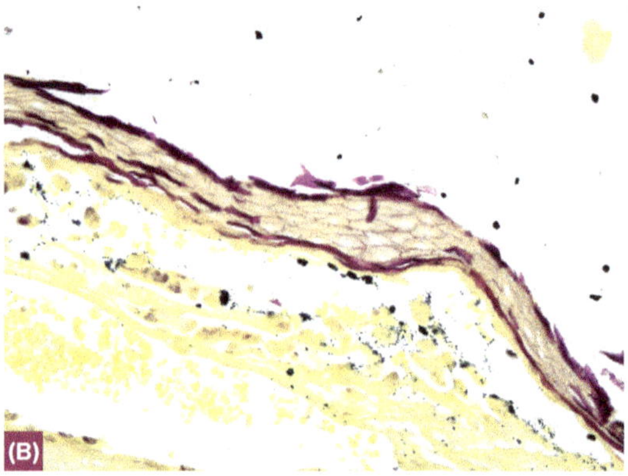

A) These lesions are caused by an exotoxin called exfoliatin.
B) This patient has classic impetigo.
C) This patient has staphylococcal scalded skin syndrome.
D) This patient has toxic epidermal necrolysis.
E) This patient has pemphigus foliaceus

QUESTION 3-13.

A 46-year-old female presents with multiple, millimeter-sized tense pustules in the groin, abdomen, and upper leg regions that coalesce in annular and circinate patterns. On physical examination you notice that the pus tends to accumulate at the lower portion of the pustules. Some of the pustules have ruptured, producing coalescent serpiginous and hyperpigmented erosions with a scaly edge. The lesions are not pruritic. The patient was recently diagnosed with multiple myeloma and has a history of both Crohn disease and rheumatoid arthritis. Biopsies are performed and the findings are illustrated below. Direct immunofluorescence reveals a nonspecific immunoreactant profile without epidermal deposition of immunoglobulin or complement. Which of the following diagnoses is CORRECT?

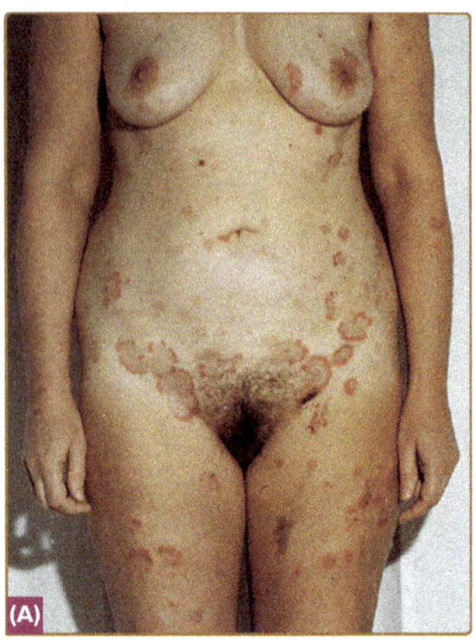

Reproduced, with permission, from Goldsmith LA, Katz SI, Gilchrest BA, Paller AS, Leffell DJ, Wolff K, eds. *Fitzpatrick's Dermatology in General Medicine*. 8th ed. New York, NY: McGraw-Hill Education; 2012.

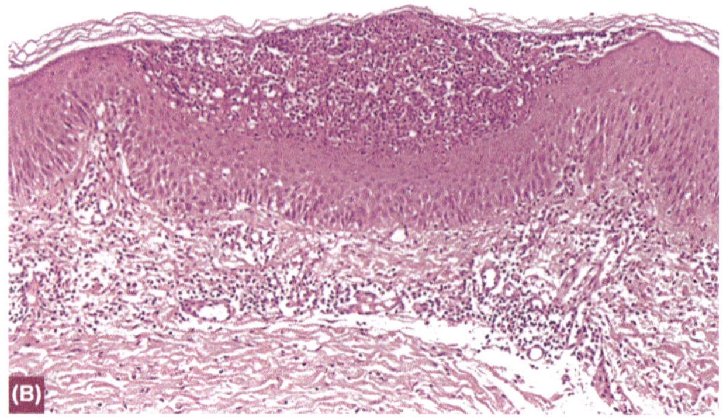

A) Sneddon-Wilkinson disease
B) IgA pemphigus
C) Pustular psoriasis
D) Dermatitis herpetiformis
E) Acute generalized exanthematous pustulosis

QUESTION 3-14.

A 42-year-old patient presents with multiple circinate, pruritic, foul-smelling, oozing, and crusted plaques on the flexural surfaces of the upper extremities, axillae, and groin. A few intact vesicles are identified on the erythematous edges of the plaques. Biopsies are performed and the findings are illustrated below. Direct immunofluorescence reveals a nonspecific immunoreactant profile. Which of the following regarding this condition is INCORRECT?

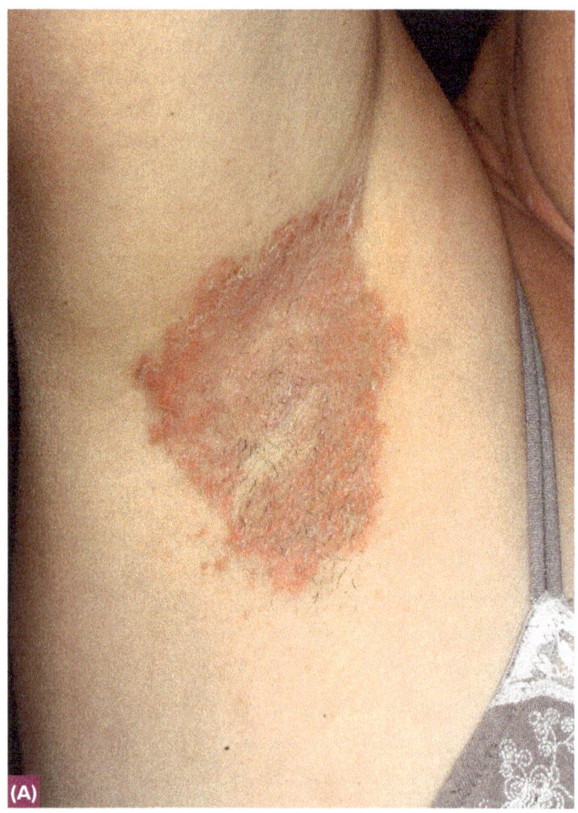

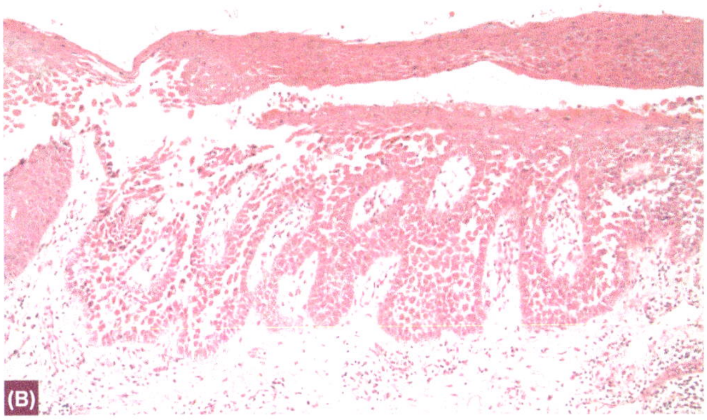

A) This condition is usually inherited in an autosomal dominant fashion.
B) The acantholysis is attributed to mutations in the *ATP2C1* gene that codes for a P-type Ca^{2+} transport ATPase.
C) Trauma has been implicated in the evolution of these lesions correlating with their typical localization to flexural surfaces.
D) The dermis may contain sparse inflammatory infiltrates composed of lymphocytes.
E) High-power examination will reveal numerous dyskeratotic keratinocytes.

QUESTION 3-15.

A patient reports developing transient, pruritic, brown papules with adherent scale that coalesce on the face and midline of the chest, upper abdomen, and back. These lesions usually arise when exposed to sunlight, heat, and humidity. Inflammatory plaques with fissures and maceration are present under the breasts. The fingernails are also dystrophic. The patient reports that the father and sibling have a similar condition. The eruption first developed in late childhood. Genetic testing reveals a mutation in the *ATP2A2* gene. A biopsy is performed. Which of the following microscopic features of this condition is INCORRECT?

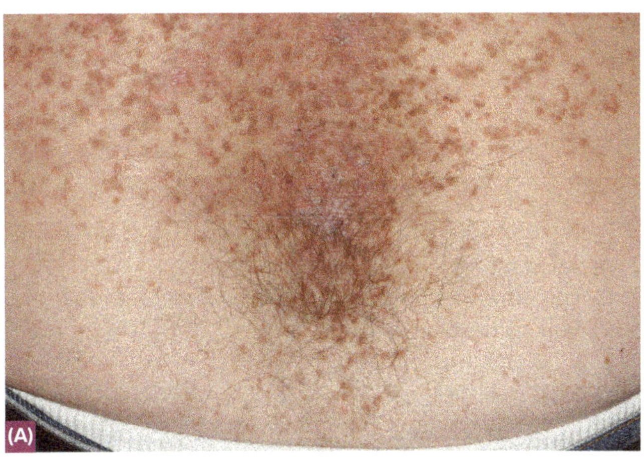

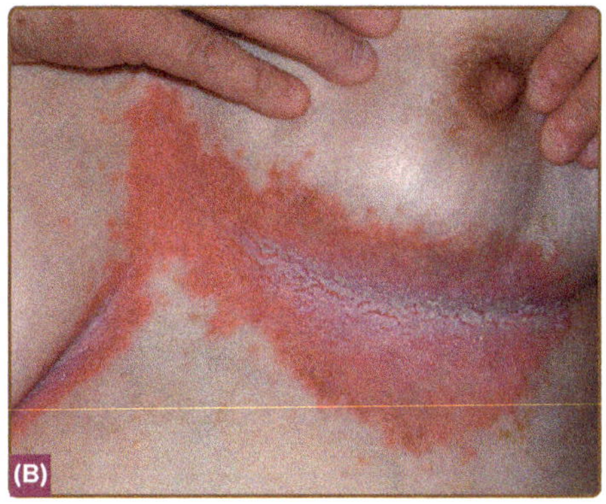

Reproduced, with permission, from Goldsmith LA, Katz SI, Gilchrest BA, Paller AS, Leffell DJ, Wolff K, eds. *Fitzpatrick's Dermatology in General Medicine*. 8th ed. New York, NY: McGraw-Hill Education; 2012.

A) There is prominent suprabasilar acantholysis forming large clefts between the basal and spinous layers.
B) Distinctive dyskeratotic keratinocytes are present in the upper spinous and granular layers with clumped keratohyaline granules and pyknotic nuclei, respectively.
C) Acantholysis is present throughout the entire epidermis, imparting a "dilapidated brick wall" appearance.
D) Immunohistochemical staining reveals diminished BCL-2 expression within the epidermis.
E) Acanthosis and hyperkeratosis may be present.

QUESTION 3-16.

A 45-year-old male patient presents with an eruption of pin-sized erythematous and slightly pruritic papules on the upper back, chest, and thighs that have persisted for several months. Biopsies are performed and the findings are illustrated below. The dermis contains scattered superficial lymphocytic infiltrates. Direct immunofluorescence reveals a nonspecific immunoreactant profile. There is no family history of similar findings. Which of the following diagnoses is CORRECT?

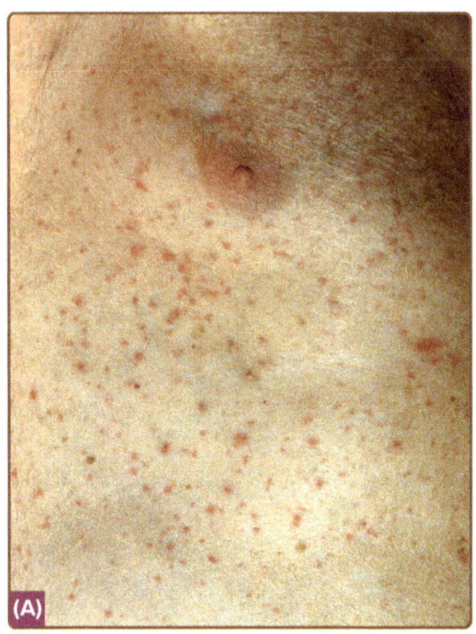

Reproduced, with permission, from Goldsmith LA, Katz SI, Gilchrest BA, Paller AS, Leffell DJ, Wolff K, eds. *Fitzpatrick's Dermatology in General Medicine*. 8th ed. New York, NY: McGraw-Hill Education; 2012.

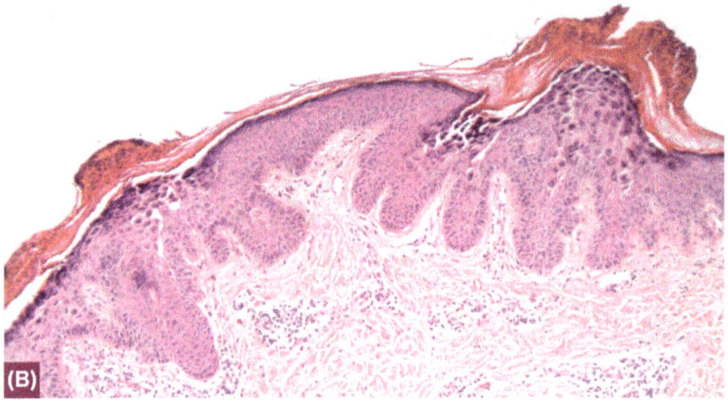

A) Keratosis follicularis
B) Benign familial pemphigus
C) Acantholytic dyskeratoma
D) Drug-induced pemphigus
E) Transient acantholytic dermatosis

QUESTION 3-17.

A 1-week-old infant presents with 2 to 3 cm, diffuse, blotchy erythematous macules and patches containing 1 to 4 mm, centrally located vesicles on the trunk, face, and limbs. There is sparing of the palms and soles. Biopsy is performed and the findings are illustrated below. Which of the following diagnoses is CORRECT?

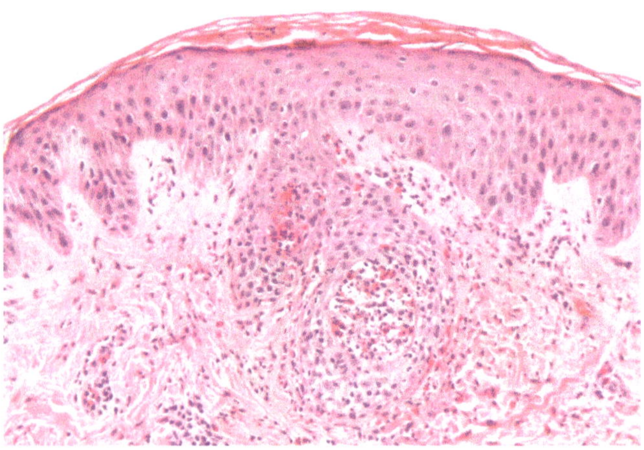

A) Erythema toxicum neonatorum
B) Incontinentia pigmenti
C) Transient neonatal pustular melanosis
D) Bullous impetigo
E) Herpes virus infection

QUESTION 3-18.

A healthy 2-day-old African American infant presented at birth with 1 to 3 mm individual pustules on a nonerythematous base localized to the head, neck, trunk, palms, and soles. Several of these pustules have ruptured, revealing a fine scale with hyperpigmentation. Serial blood cultures are negative for bacterial and fungal growth. Scrapings from the intact lesions are evaluated by KOH, Gram, and Tzanck smears and only reveal numerous neutrophils. A biopsy is performed. Microscopically, the epidermis is spongiotic with discrete pustules confined between the stratum corneum and upper spinous/granular layers. The pustules are predominantly composed of neutrophils with rare eosinophils. No acantholysis is identified. There are sparse papillary dermal neutrophilic infiltrates. The basal keratinocytes contain increased amounts of melanin pigment. Direct immunofluorescence reveals a nonspecific immunoreactant profile. Which of the following diagnoses is CORRECT?

A) Erythema toxicum neonatorum
B) Bullous impetigo
C) Transient neonatal pustular melanosis
D) Infantile acropustulosis
E) IgA pemphigus

QUESTION 3-19.

A 14-year-old ballerina presents with numerous clear blisters on the tips of the toes and interphalangeal joints. The patient reports no prior history of blistering and no known family history of blistering. A biopsy is performed and the findings are illustrated below. Direct immunofluorescence reveals a nonspecific immunoreactant profile. Which of the following diagnoses is CORRECT?

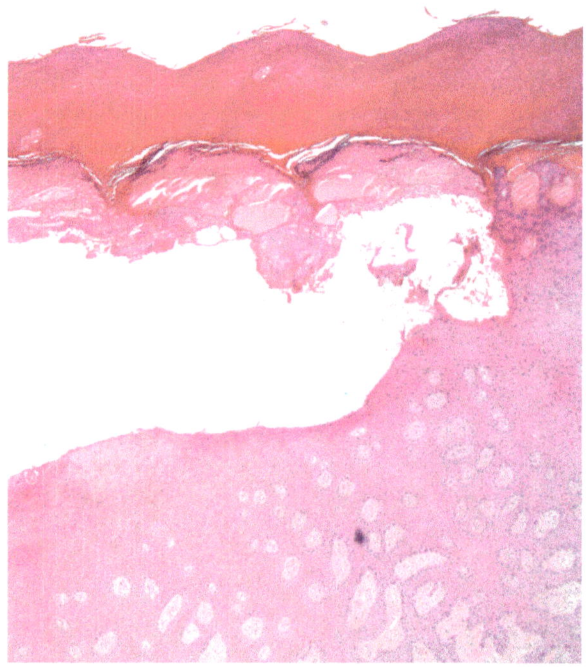

A) Talon noir
B) Epidermolysis bullosa simplex superficialis
C) Bullous tinea pedis
D) Friction blister
E) Suction blister

QUESTION 3-20.

A patient with chronic lymphocytic leukemia presents with painful vesicles and ulcerations on the lips. A scraping and smear are performed and the findings are illustrated below. Which of the following regarding these lesions is INCORRECT?

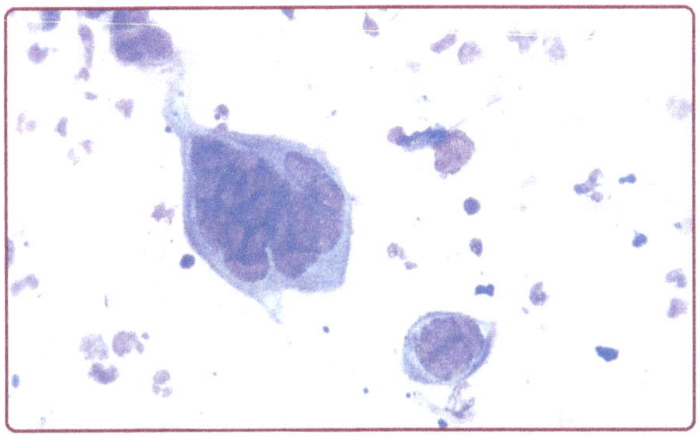

Reproduced, with permission, from Goldsmith LA, Katz SI, Gilchrest BA, Paller AS, Leffell DJ, Wolff K, eds. *Fitzpatrick's Dermatology in General Medicine*. 8th ed. New York, NY: McGraw-Hill Education; 2012.

- **A)** This condition most frequently arises within immunocompromised patients and may be associated with tissue eosinophilia in such instances.
- **B)** Indirect immunofluorescence studies of peripheral blood will most likely reveal a panoply of circulating autoantibodies directed against a number of epidermal antigens.
- **C)** Patients with HIV disease may exhibit follicular-based blisters with similar cytomorphologic features involving the outer root sheath epithelium.
- **D)** These lesions may follow a waxing and waning course.

QUESTION 3-21.

A 1-year-old boy visits your office for a second opinion about recurrent pruritic vesicles and pustules on his hands and feet. This is his third episode and in both previous episodes the physician thought the child had scabies. The child was treated with permethrin both times and within 2 to 3 weeks the skin cleared. No other family members have had lesions or symptoms. Several scrapings from the vesicles and pustules only reveal keratinous debris and scattered neutrophils. A biopsy is performed and reveals spongiosis and subcorneal and intraepidermal pustules containing neutrophils and a few eosinophils. Small multifocal areas of epidermal necrosis containing dyskeratotic keratinocytes are noted. Which of the following diagnoses is CORRECT?

- **A)** Infantile acropustulosis
- **B)** Erythema toxicum neonatorum
- **C)** Transient neonatal pustular melanosis
- **D)** Varicella
- **E)** Tinea pedis

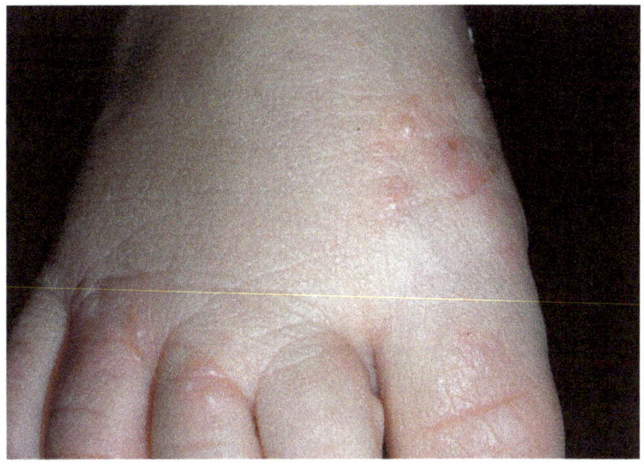

Reproduced, with permission, from Usatine RP, Smith MA, Mayeaux EJ Jr, Chumley HS, eds. *Color Atlas of Family Medicine*. 2nd ed. New York, NY: McGraw-Hill Education; 2012.

QUESTION 3-22.

Below is a diagram of the ultrastructural components of the cutaneous basement membrane. Using the numbered options below, correctly label these ultrastructural components.

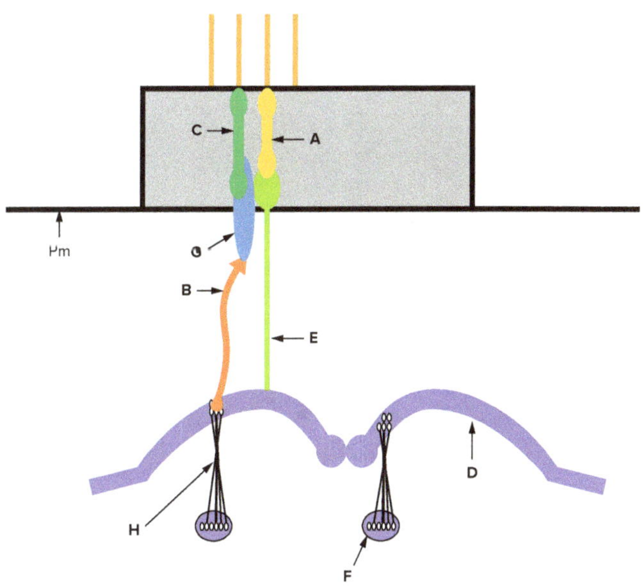

1) $\alpha_6\beta_4$ integrin
2) Bullous pemphigoid antigen 2
3) Plectin
4) Type VII collagen
5) Bullous pemphigoid antigen 1
6) Laminin 5
7) Lamina densa
8) Anchoring plaque

QUESTION 3-23.

A 69-year-old patient presents with tense serous blisters on slightly erythematous skin arising on the flexural surface of the forearms. The lesions are pruritic and are studded by tiny vesicles. Initially the lesions were raised, edematous papules and plaques surrounded by a zone of erythema without surface alteration. Rubbing of the skin does not produce blistering. A few of the ruptured lesions appear to have healed without scarring, leaving behind slight postinflammatory hyperpigmentation. Biopsies are performed and the findings are illustrated below. Immunohistochemical stain for type IV collagen reveals a linear band of staining along the floor of the blister cavity. Direct immunofluorescence of perilesional skin reveals linear deposition of IgG and C3 along the dermal epidermal junction. Which of the following statements regarding this condition is INCORRECT?

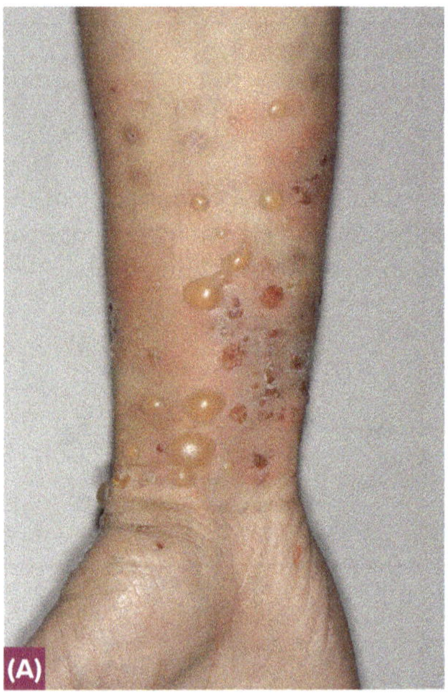

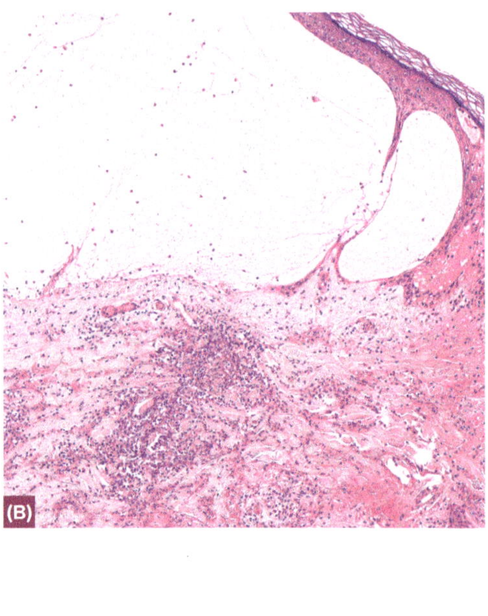

A) Certain medications have also been associated with the development of these lesions, including penicillamine, efalizumab, etanercept, and furosemide.
B) Direct immunofluorescence testing after incubating the sample in 1 M NaCl at 4°C for 72 hours reveals IgG deposition along the undersurface of the detached portion of epidermis. The separated portion of dermis exhibits no staining.
C) This condition is an immunobullous disease where patients have circulating autoantibodies directed against components of the lamina densa.
D) Early lesions are characterized microscopically by superficial perivascular and interstitial infiltrates of lymphocytes, numerous eosinophils, and variable neutrophils. The epidermis may be spongiotic with intraepidermal eosinophils.
E) Western blot and/or ELISA studies reveal antibodies against BPAG1 and/or BPAG2 in 90% and 50% of cases, respectively.

QUESTION 3-24.

A 27-year-old female admitted to the hospital for evacuation of a partial molar pregnancy presents postoperatively with an intensely pruritic, urticarial rash on the periumbilical region. The eruption gradually spreads peripherally to the flanks and a few small blisters develop. The patient reports waxing and waning of similar lesions within the past 9 weeks. Biopsies are performed and the findings are illustrated below. The dermal infiltrate is composed of scattered lymphocytes, eosinophils, and neutrophils. Eosinophils are present along the dermal-epidermal junction with vacuolar change. Which of the following statements regarding this condition is INCORRECT?

A) Direct immunofluorescence of perilesional skin using the salt-split technique will reveal linear deposition of IgG along the floor of the subepidermal cleft in 100% of cases.
B) Patients have circulating IgG antibodies of the IgG and IgG3 classes that have the ability to fix normal human complement to the basement membrane zone of normal human skin.
C) Patients have circulating antibodies mainly directed against BPAG2 and rarely BPAG1.
D) Patients most commonly experience this rare condition during normal pregnancies and experience exacerbation skin lesions immediately or shortly after delivery.
E) In the postpartum state, recurrence of lesions may occur with resumption of menstruation, on administration of oral contraceptives, or within subsequent pregnancies.

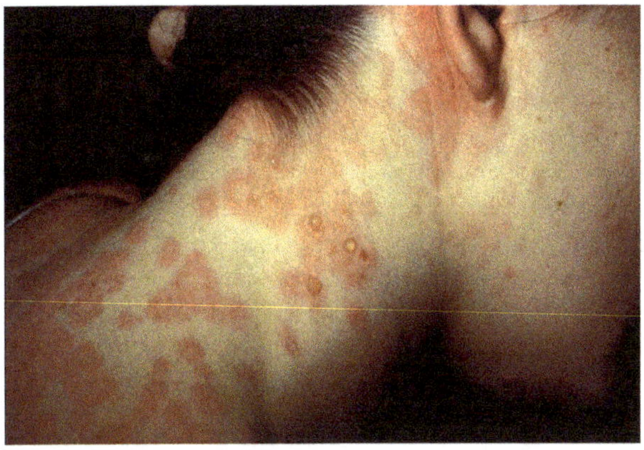

Courtesy of Dr. Amit Pandya.

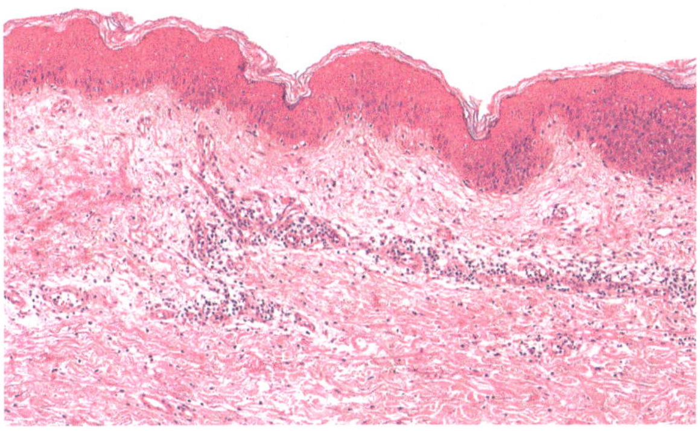

QUESTION 3-25.

Which of the following statements regarding lichen planus pemphigoides is INCORRECT?

A) Clinically, lesions present as flat-topped, purple, polygonal, pruritic, papules, and plaques surmounted by tense blisters on the extremities, trunk, and oral mucosa.
B) Microscopically, a band-like lymphocytic infiltrate with scattered eosinophils underlies a subepidermal blister.
C) Direct immunofluorescence on perilesional skin shows linear IgG deposits along the basement membrane zone with localization to the epidermal side on salt-split skin.
D) Immunohistochemical stain for type IV collagen will reveal linear deposition along the roof of the blister cavity.
E) Although patients have circulating antibodies against BPAG2, epitope mapping reveals that the sera of these patients react with different epitopes than bullous pemphigoid.

QUESTION 3-26.

An elderly female is referred to you by her dentist for evaluation of denuded and inflamed oral mucosa as well as sites of gingival recession and loss. The patient reports dysphagia and on clinical examination you notice the patient to also have vulvar erosions and conjunctivitis with shortened conjunctival fornices and symblepharon formation. Biopsies of the oral lesions are performed and the findings are illustrated below. Immunohistochemical staining of the de novo blister for type IV collagen reveals labeling at the floor of the blister cavity. Direct immunofluorescence (DIF) of perilesional clinically normal-appearing mucosa reveals linear homogenous deposition of IgG, IgA, and C3 along the basement membrane zone. Indirect immunofluorescence (IIF) using the patient's serum and monkey esophagus substrate fails to demonstrate circulating IgG antibodies to the basement membrane zone; however, a sample of salt-split skin reveals IgG deposition on both epidermal and dermal sides of the split. Western blotting using a panel of cell-derived and recombinant proteins reveals IgG and IgA autoantibodies directed against BPAG2; however, the target epitopes are both intra- and extracellular domains. Which of the following diagnoses is CORRECT?

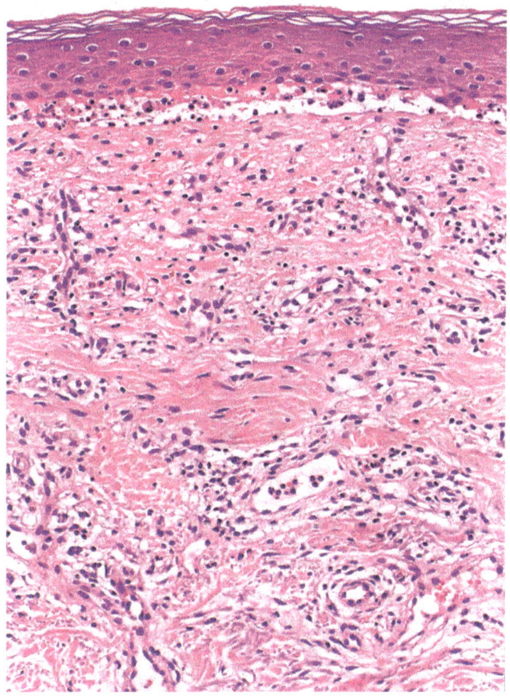

A) Linear IgA disease
B) Epidermolysis bullosa acquisita
C) Bullous systemic lupus
D) Bullous pemphigoid
E) Cicatricial pemphigoid

QUESTION 3-27.

Which of the following clinical presentations MOST likely reflects the biopsy findings illustrated below?

A) There are large, tense, pruritic, annular blisters on slightly erythematous skin involving the trunk, limbs, face, groin, and perineum. New blisters are present around resolving lesions, forming rosette or jewel-like clusters. Some of the blisters lie within erythematous areas in a linear distribution imparting a "string of pearls" appearance.

B) There are intensely pruritic, erythematous papules, urticarial plaques, papulovesicles, and vesicles in herpetiform groupings. The lesions are symmetrically distributed and appear mainly on elbows, knees, nape, scapular region, sacral region, and buttocks. Ruptured lesions heal with scar formation. Systemic symptoms include chronic gastrointestinal malabsorption with weight loss, bloating, and occasional diarrhea.

C) There are trauma-induced, tense, clear, and hemorrhagic blisters and erosions on the extensor surfaces of the limbs arising on normal-appearing skin. The lesions heal with scarring and milia formation.

D) There is a widespread eruption of tense blisters spontaneously forming on erythematous skin. These lesions occur on flexural and intertriginous areas and heal with scarring and milia formation.

E) There are well circumscribed, well demarcated, erythematous, scale-crusted papulovesicles involving the full circumference of a wrist only.

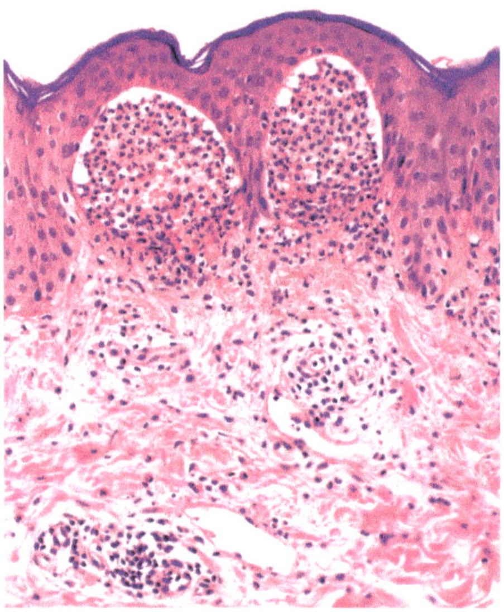

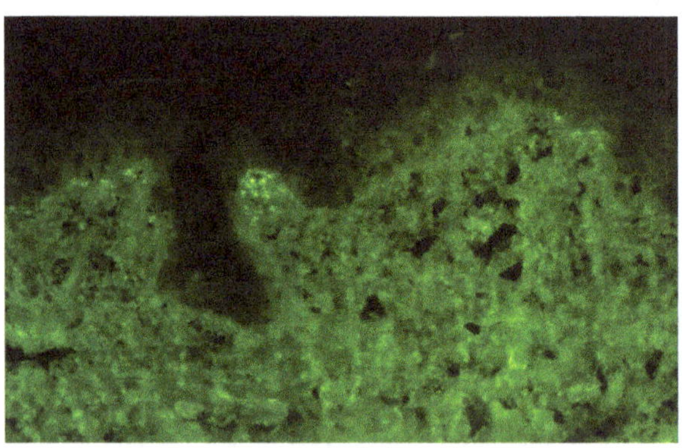

QUESTION 3-28.

A 5-year-old presents with extensive blistering on the upper extremities and trunk. The blisters are pruritic and both tense and flaccid. They are grouped with new blisters arising around resolving lesions, forming rosette or jewel-like clusters. Focally, blisters are arranged in a linear distribution imparting a "string of pearls" appearance. There is no notable inflammation. A few oral erosions are noted. Biopsies are performed and the findings are illustrated below. Direct immunofluorescence reveals homogenous linear deposition of IgA along the basement membrane zone. Other immunoreactants are either negative or nonspecific. Indirect immunofluorescence using salt-split skin reveals localization of the patient's IgA to the epidermal side of the split. Western blot analysis for the targeted antigen is pending. Serological studies are negative for antigliadin and antiendomysial antibodies. Which of the following diagnoses is CORRECT?

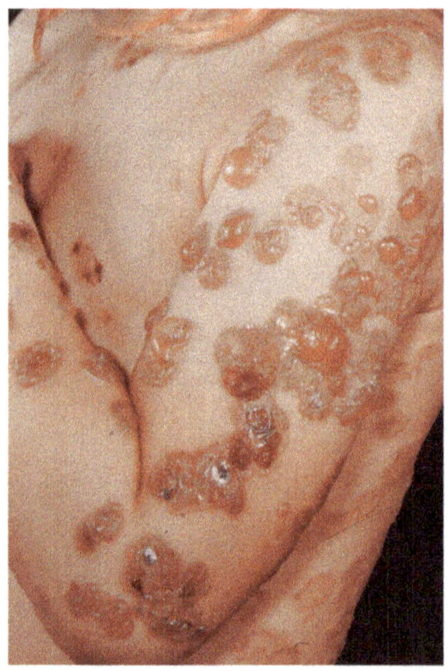

Reproduced, with permission, from Wolff K, Johnson RA, Saavedra AP. *Fitzpatrick's Color Atlas and Synopsis of Clinical Dermatology*. 7th ed. New York, NY: McGraw-Hill Education; 2013

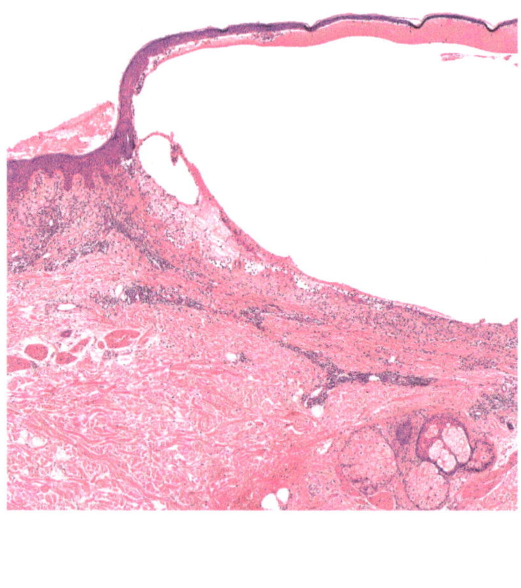

A) Chronic bullous disease of childhood
B) Bullous arthropod bite reaction
C) Bullous Sweet syndrome
D) Bullous systemic lupus erythematosus
E) Bullous pemphigoid

QUESTION 3-29.

An elderly patient presents with numerous erosions, tense blisters within noninflamed skin, and scars over trauma-prone surfaces such as the backs of the hands, knuckles, elbows, knees, sacral area, and toes. Some blisters are hemorrhagic and have developed scale crusts and erosions. The scarred areas are studded with pearl-like milia cysts. Biopsies are performed and the routine histopathological and salt-split immunofluorescent findings are illustrated below. Which of the following statements regarding this condition is CORRECT?

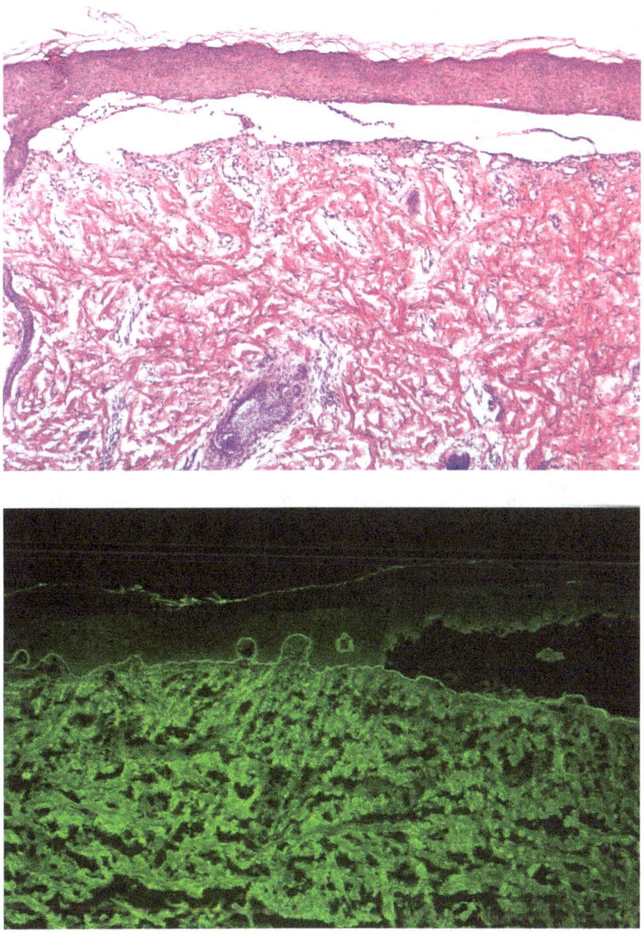

A) This condition is most commonly seen in patients on hemodialysis for chronic renal insufficiency or those taking drugs such as naproxen, furosemide, nalidixic acid, and tetracycline.
B) These patients typically have periorbital hypertrichosis and blisters preferentially affecting sun-exposed sites.
C) Immunohistochemical staining of the de novo blister for type IV collagen will reveal deposition along the base of the blister cavity.
D) Patients with this condition typically have circulating antinuclear antibodies.
E) This patient has circulating antibodies to type VII collagen.

QUESTION 3-30.

A 23-year-old female presents with tense blisters in a herpetiform arrangement on erythematous skin of the trunk and flexural surfaces. A few oral erosions are noted. The lesions are intensely pruritic. Some areas of scarring are noted. The patient has positive circulating antinuclear antibodies and low serum complement levels. Review of systems reveals arthritis and a history of proteinuria. A biopsy is performed and the findings are illustrated below. Which of the following microscopic descriptions of immunofluorescence performed on perilesional skin MOST closely supports the patient's condition?

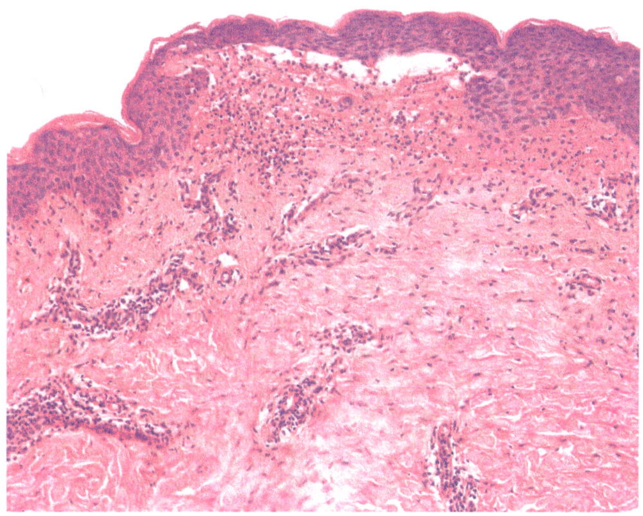

A) There are large chunky granular IgA deposits present within dermal papillae.
B) There is a linear band of deposition along the basement membrane zone of IgA only.
C) There is a linear band of IgG and granular deposits of IgM and C3 along the basement membrane zone.
D) Salt-split perilesional skin reveals deposits of IgG located on the epidermal side of the split.
E) There is a nonspecific immunoreactant profile with no immunoglobulin along the dermal-epidermal junction.

QUESTION 3-31.

A 34-year-old female presents with mottled pigmentation of sun-exposed areas and some areas exhibiting morphea-like changes. You notice hypertrichosis most pronounced on the zygomatic and malar skin. Numerous blisters containing clear fluid are present on the fingers and dorsal hands. The patient reports that these blisters frequently arise after minor trauma and heal with atrophic scars. You notice the scarred areas contain numerous scattered milia. A biopsy is performed and the findings are illustrated below. A PAS stain highlights markedly thickened superficial dermal blood vessels. Direct immunofluorescence reveals deposition of active complement components (ie, C3 and C5b-9) within superficial dermal vessels and along the dermal epidermal junction. Which of the following statements regarding this condition is CORRECT?

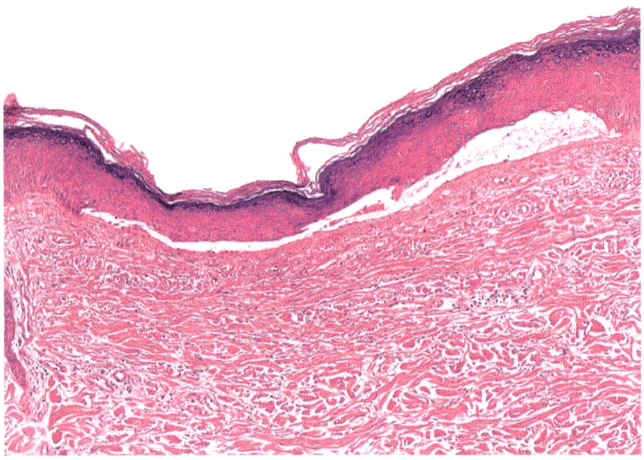

A) Clinical laboratory analysis will reveal reduced serum uroporphyrinogen decarboxylase activity and increased porphyrins in the serum, urine and stool.
B) Clinical laboratory analysis will reveal moderately increased plasma porphyrin levels and normal uroporphyrinogen decarboxylase activity.
C) Clinical laboratory analysis will reveal normal plasma porphyrin levels and normal uroporphyrinogen decarboxylase activity.
D) This patient's condition is most likely attributed to ingestion of certain drug such as furosemide, nalidixic acid, tetracycline, naproxen, pyridoxine, or isotretinoin.
E) Immunohistochemical staining of the de novo blister for type IV collagen will reveal deposition confined to the roof of the blister cavity.

QUESTION 3-32.

A hospitalized patient develops tense clear linear blisters on the sacrum and heels. A biopsy is performed and the findings are illustrated below. Direct immunofluorescence reveals a nonspecific immunoreactant profile. Which of the following diagnoses is CORRECT?

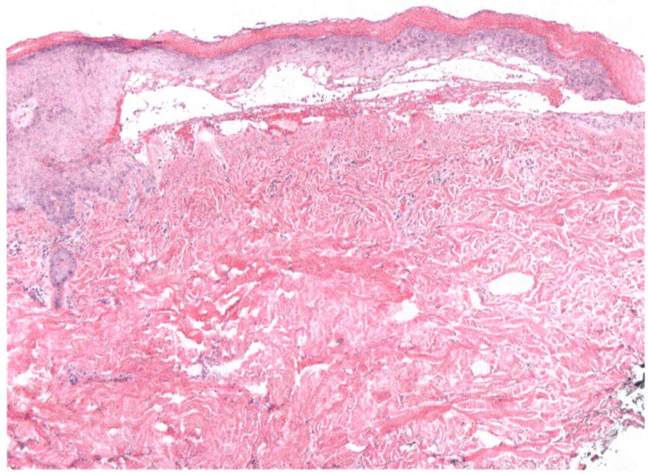

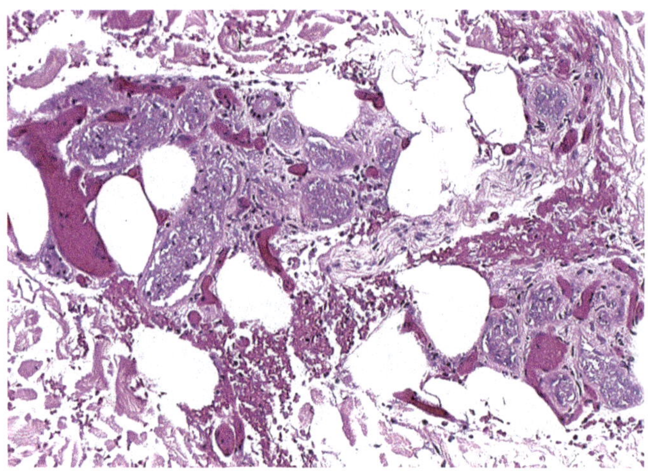

A) Thermal burn
B) Friction blister
C) Pseudoporphyria
D) Coma blister
E) Cell-poor bullous pemphigoid

ANSWERS

ANSWER 3-1:

1. D)
2. C)
3. B)
4. A)

Pemphigus foliaceus and fogo selvagem clinically and pathophysiologically represent two different entities. However, morphologic distinction may be impossible.

ANSWER 3-2: C.

The separation plane is relatively constant in each **vesiculobullous disease.** Each process tends to reliably produce blisters in either the subcorneal/granular, spinous, or suprabasal zones in the epidermis. Occasionally, blisters may extend from one plane to another. Pustules tend to form in the subcorneal or intracorneal zone but are not limited to those locations. Because of the relative consistency of this feature, the cleavage plane may be used to initially categorize the various forms of vesiculobullous disease. Vesiculobullous diseases are best classified as intraepidermal versus subepidermal on histopathology (Table 3-2A). Lesions can be further subclassified into immunobullous versus genodermatosis versus trauma-induced categories.

Another way to approach intraepidermal vesicular and pustular diseases is by evaluating the presence or absence of **acantholysis**, which must be differentiated from **spongiosis.** Spongiosis also contain vesicles and occasional bullae, but lacks or contains only small numbers of acantholytic cells. **Acantholysis** is characterized by the loss of intercellular bridges, resulting in dyscohesion between adjacent keratinocytes. These separated acantholytic keratinocytes exhibit a rounded shape and their cell membranes are usually rimmed by a bright eosinophilic band of keratin. In **spongiosis,** the intercellular bridges ("spines") are usually more prominent by the presence of extracellular intraepidermal edema. When the edema is severe, the intercellular bridges may rupture, destroying the keratinocytes in the process (**cytolysis**). Therefore, acantholytic keratinocytes are typically absent in spongiotic vesiculation. **Vesicles** may form in both acantholytic and spongiotic conditions and although they are filled predominantly with fluid, scattered inflammatory cells (ie, lymphocytes, Langerhans cells, eosinophils) are almost always present to some degree. **Pustules** are typically filled with abundant inflammatory cells, usually neutrophils.

A **blister** is a fluid-filled cavity within or beneath the epidermis containing tissue fluid, plasma, and a variable complement of inflammatory cells. **Vesicles** are blisters less than 0.5 cm in diameter, and **bullae** are blisters greater than 0.5 cm in diameter. A **vesicopustule** is a vesicle in which there are prominent neutrophils. Some diseases produce microscopic slit-like spaces within the epidermis that are known as **clefts**. Clefts characteristically occur in the group of diseases that have focal **acantholytic dyskeratosis** as their histopathologic reaction pattern and as a rule do not have clinically apparent blisters.

A **pustule** is a dense aggregate of neutrophils or eosinophils, viable or degenerated, with a small component of tissue fluid. A pustule is yellow-white clinically and resides intracorneally, within the stratum spinosum or at the dermal-epidermal junction. A **microabscess** is a small aggregate of neutrophils or eosinophils observed histopathologically. At times a microabscess may be predominated by mononuclear cells usually Langerhans cells and/or lymphocytes.

Spongiosis is the accumulation of extracellular fluid within the epidermis causing separation between adjacent keratinocytes. The keratinocytes often appear stellate with clear spaces separating them from their neighbors, producing a "spongy" appearance. As the degree of spongiosis increases, microscopic vesicles develop and may progress to macroscopic vesicles or bullae. In cases of severe spongiosis, **ballooning or hydropic degeneration** (intracellular edema) with subsequent rupture of the cell membranes (a form of cytolysis) may lead to a lace-like appearance (**reticular degeneration**). Spongiosis develops primarily due to transudation of serum from damaged or inflamed vessels within the superficial vascular plexus. Ballooning degeneration occurs when the keratinocytes lose osmotic control.

Acantholysis is the result of loss of appropriate keratinocyte-keratinocyte adherence. Tight junctions, adherens junctions, gap junctions, and desmosomes mediate this adherence. The role of desmosomes in keratinocytic adhesion is paramount, and they are the last structures to split when acantholysis occurs. Acantholytic disorders that have been well characterized develop as sequelae of desmosomal dysfunction or disruption of the desmosomal connections with the intracellular keratin structural matrix. Keratinocyte-keratinocyte adhesion is a dynamic process because the relationship of one keratinocyte to another must change during epidermal maturation. Thus acantholysis may be viewed as a loss of equilibrium between the formation and dissolution of junctions. This dysequilibrium may occur primarily when the adhesion junctions are impaired directly or secondarily when keratinocytic viability is affected. **Acantholytic keratinocytes** are rounded with condensed eosinophilic cytoplasm, large nuclei, peripherally marginated chromatin, and prominent nucleoli.

Cytolysis of keratinocytes, as well as apoptosis, may lead to blister formation. Although this phenomenon may occur in the setting of intraepidermal edema (spongiosis), the category of cytolytic vesiculobullous disease typically refers to conditions without spongiosis. Cytolysis may occur in the normal epidermis, when high levels of deleterious physical agents such as mechanical forces or heat overwhelm the structural matrix of the keratinocytes. Mechanical energy applied parallel to the epidermis (**friction**) may lead to shearing between

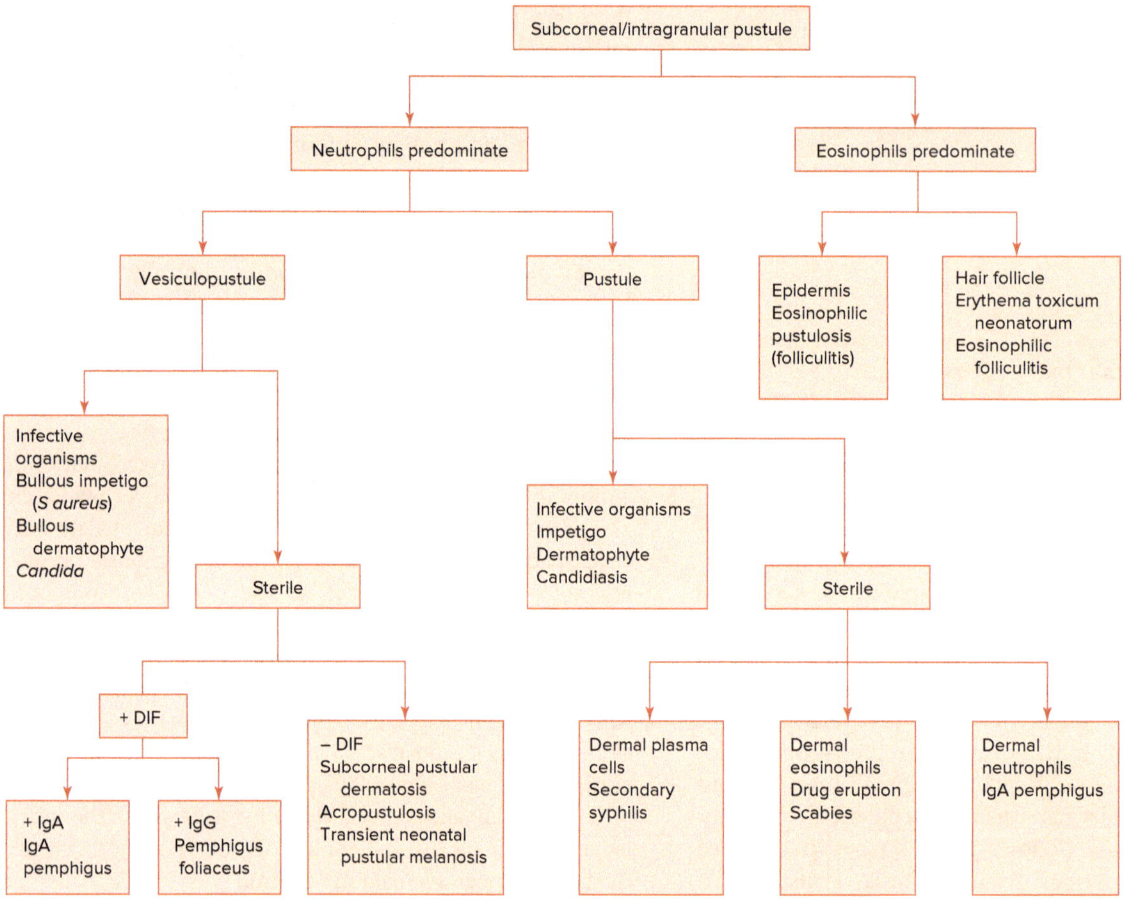
Subcorneal/intragranular pustule
Neutrophils predominate
Eosinophils predominate
Vesiculopustule
Pustule
Epidermis Eosinophilic pustulosis (folliculitis)
Hair follicle Erythema toxicum neonatorum Eosinophilic folliculitis
Infective organisms Bullous impetigo (S aureus) Bullous dermatophyte Candida
Sterile
Infective organisms Impetigo Dermatophyte Candidiasis
Sterile
+ DIF
– DIF Subcorneal pustular dermatosis Acropustulosis Transient neonatal pustular melanosis
Dermal plasma cells Secondary syphilis
Dermal eosinophils Drug eruption Scabies
Dermal neutrophils IgA pemphigus
+ IgA IgA pemphigus
+ IgG Pemphigus foliaceus

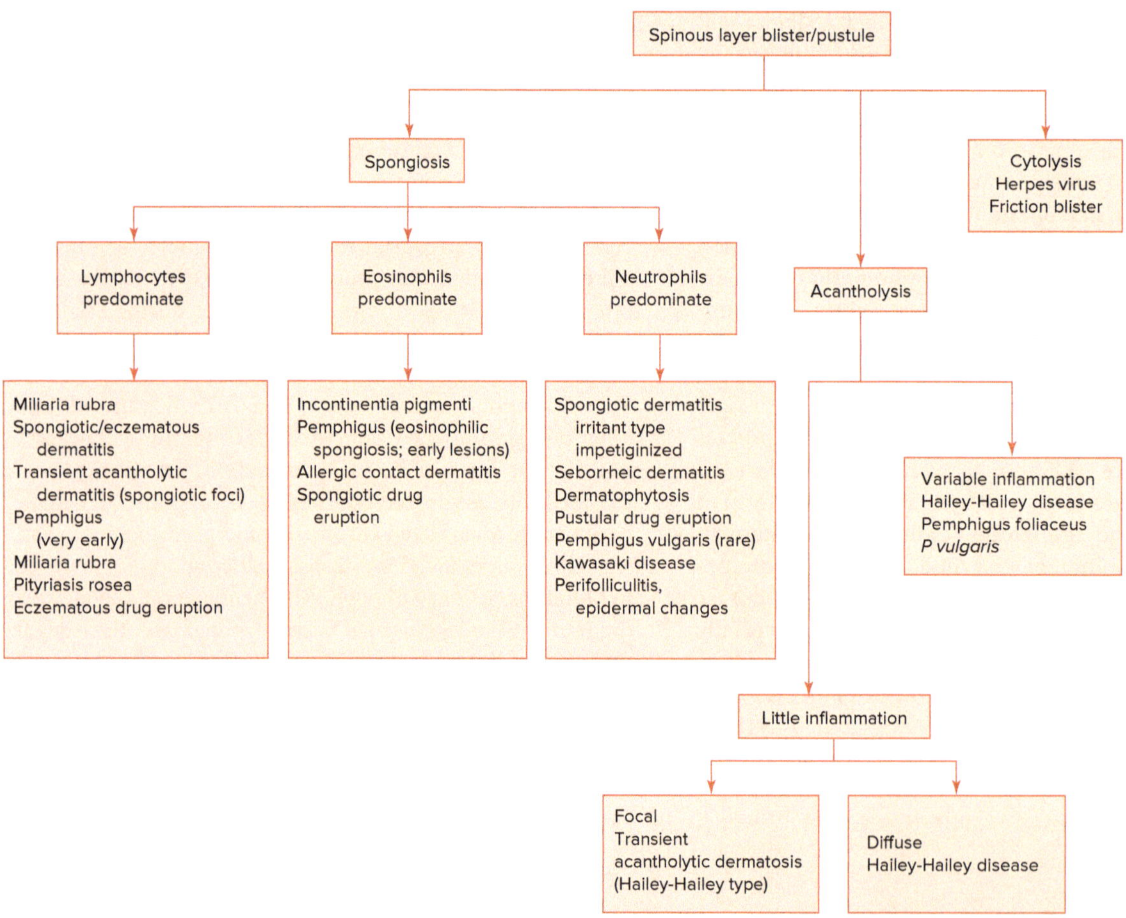
Spinous layer blister/pustule
Spongiosis
Cytolysis Herpes virus Friction blister
Lymphocytes predominate
Eosinophils predominate
Neutrophils predominate
Acantholysis
Miliaria rubra Spongiotic/eczematous dermatitis Transient acantholytic dermatitis (spongiotic foci) Pemphigus (very early) Miliaria rubra Pityriasis rosea Eczematous drug eruption
Incontinentia pigmenti Pemphigus (eosinophilic spongiosis; early lesions) Allergic contact dermatitis Spongiotic drug eruption
Spongiotic dermatitis irritant type impetiginized Seborrheic dermatitis Dermatophytosis Pustular drug eruption Pemphigus vulgaris (rare) Kawasaki disease Perifolliculitis, epidermal changes
Variable inflammation Hailey-Hailey disease Pemphigus foliaceus P vulgaris
Little inflammation
Focal Transient acantholytic dermatosis (Hailey-Hailey type)
Diffuse Hailey-Hailey disease

Table 3-2A. Intraepidermal Blistering and Pustular Diseases

SEPARATION PLANE	PATHOLOGIC PROCESS	INFLAMMATORY CELLS	DISEASE
Subcorneal/ intragranular	Spongiosis	Lymphocytes	Miliaria crystallina
	Acantholysis	—	Staphylococcal scalded skin syndrome Pemphigus foliaceus Transient acantholytic dermatosis (Pemphigus foliaceus–like foci)
	Pustules	Neutrophils	Impetigo Bullous impetigo Subcorneal pustular dermatosis IgA pemphigus Dermatophytosis Candidiasis Pustular secondary lues Pustular drug eruption Acropustulosis of infancy Transient neonatal pustular melanosis Pustular Id reaction Pemphigus vulgaris (rare) Pustular psoriasis
		Eosinophils	Scabies Erythema toxicum neonatorum
Spinous	Spongiosis	Lymphocytes	Miliaria rubra Spongiotic/eczematous dermatitis Transient acantholytic dermatitis (spongiotic foci) Pemphigus (very early) Miliaria rubra Pityriasis rosea Eczematous drug eruption
		Eosinophils	Incontinentia pigmenti Pemphigus (eosinophilic spongiosis; early lesions) Allergic contact dermatitis Spongiotic drug eruption
		Neutrophils	Spongiotic dermatitis irritant type impetiginized Seborrheic dermatitis Dermatophytosis Pustular drug eruption Pemphigus vulgaris (rare) Kawasaki disease Perifolliculitis, epidermal changes
	Acantholysis	Little inflammation	Hailey-Hailey disease Transient acantholytic dermatosis (Hailey-Hailey–like foci)
		Variable inflammation	Hailey-Hailey disease Pemphigus foliaceus and variants (extension from subcorneal plane) Pemphigus vulgaris and variants (extension from suprabasal plane) Irritant contact dermatitis (rare)

Table 3-2A. Intraepidermal Blistering and Pustular Diseases *(continued)*

SEPARATION PLANE	PATHOLOGIC PROCESS	INFLAMMATORY CELLS	DISEASE
	Cytolysis	Marked inflammation Little inflammation	Herpes virus infection Friction blister
Suprabasal	Cytolysis		Friction blister Epidermolytic hyperkeratosis Irritant contact dermatitis (rare)
	Acantholysis		Pemphigus vulgaris and variants Darier disease Transient acantholytic disease (Pemphigus vulgaris–like foci)

keratinocytes and within keratinocytes themselves, that is, cytolysis. Minimal friction may lead to cytolysis when keratinocytes have an abnormal structural matrix, as in **epidermolysis bullosa simplex**. Immune-mediated cell necrosis in the context of antibody-dependent cell-mediated immunity or a delayed-type hypersensitivity reaction may lead to blister formation, which most typically is subepidermal in nature. The morphologic hallmark of this pattern of **necrosis** is **karyolysis**, characterized by cellular disintegration. This is not to be confused with **apoptosis**, which is a unique form of cell death whereby individual, scattered single cells die without release of cellular contents. Such a pattern of programmed cell death usually does not lead to epidermal disruption. Both karyolysis and dyskeratosis (apoptosis) may eventuate in colloid body formation.

ANSWER 3-3: D.

The biopsy reveals an intraepidermal blister whose cleavage plane is above the basal layer (suprabasilar split). Numerous small rounded keratinocytes with dense eosinophilic cytoplasm are present, consistent with acantholytic keratinocytes. The acantholysis extends down into the hair follicle's outer root sheath epithelium. This is a classic example of **pemphigus vulgaris (PV)**, which is an autoimmune condition characterized by acantholysis of suprabasal keratinocytes. Antibodies are directed against **desmoglein 3** molecules of keratinocyte desmosomes; therefore, acantholysis is restricted between the lower spinous and upper spinous layers. Interestingly, it is not unusual for patients with cutaneous lesions to demonstrate circulating antibodies to both **desmoglein 1 desmoglein 3** via indirect immunofluorescence (IIF) using **monkey esophagus** as a substrate. Positive studies should be titrated to the weakest positive antibody titer, since this information is helpful in monitoring immunosuppressive therapy. The concentration of these anti-desmosomal cadherin antibodies generally correlates with disease severity. Direct immunofluorescence (DIF) studies must reveal intercellular deposition of IgG. The IgG consists predominantly of the IgG4 subclass. The pattern of intercellular space deposition of IgG may be identical in pemphigus vulgaris, pemphigus foliaceus (and their closely related variants pemphigus vegetans and erythematosus, respectively), and a percentage of patients with drug-induced pemphigus. The final diagnosis should be based on the level of cleavage observed by light microscopy and the clinical context. Intercellular deposition of C3d is usually present; however, its presence alone is not sufficient to warrant a diagnosis of PV. In addition to IgG, about 30% of cases will exhibit deposition of IgM and IgA.

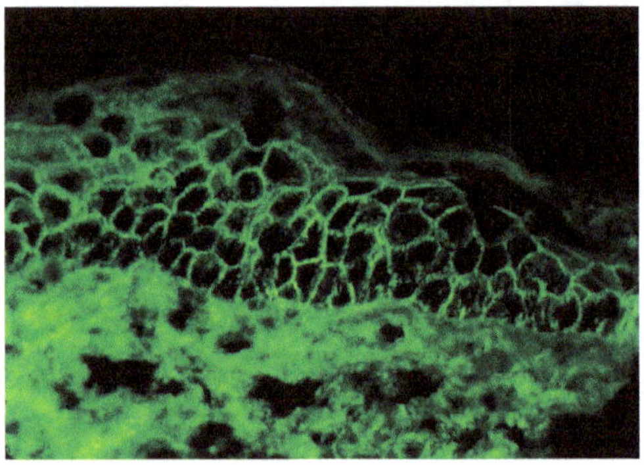

Direct immunofluorescence, pemphigus. There is intercellular IgG deposition in perilesional skin from a patient with pemphigus vulgaris. Note the staining throughout the epidermis. (Reproduced, with permission, from Goldsmith LA, Katz SI, Gilchrest BA, Paller AS, Leffell DJ, Wolff K, eds. *Fitzpatrick's Dermatology in General Medicine*. 8th ed. New York, NY: McGraw-Hill Education; 2012.)

If DIF is not readily available, immunohistochemical staining for C3d may be helpful in establishing a provisional diagnosis. Oral lesions are almost always present at some point during the evolution of PV, and may be the first manifestation in 10% to 15% of cases. The incorrect choice D describes the clinical presentation of **Grover disease**, which may exhibit histopathological features similar to pemphigus vulgaris (the so-called pemphigus vulgaris variant of Grover). The lesions of PV are large flaccid blisters and bullae, whereas Grover disease is characterized by small pin-sized papules. Additionally, mucosal (ie, oral) lesions are almost always present in PV and are not present in Grover disease. The histopathological clue separating PV from Grover disease is the presence of acantholysis extending down adnexal structures, which is not seen in Grover disease. Direct immunofluorescence of Grover disease is negative for intraepidermal immunoglobulin and complement deposition.

ANSWER 3-4: E.

This is a classic presentation of **pemphigus vulgaris (PV)** (Table 3-4A). Large and flaccid bullae develop on the oral mucosa, face, scalp, central chest, and intertriginous zones in older individuals (40-60 years of age). Oral lesions are the first manifestation in 10% to 15% of patients and almost invariably develop during the course of the disease. Since the blisters are fragile, they collapse rather quickly, giving place to erosions with few intact bullae typically present at clinical presentation. The surrounding skin of intact bullae is typically nonerythematous. The ability to extend blisters by external pressure has been referred to as **Nikolsky sign** and is helpful in distinguishing **pemphigus vulgaris** from **mucosal bullous pemphigoid**, where it is absent. A positive Nikolsky sign is also present in **Stevens-Johnson syndrome** and **toxic epidermal necrolysis.**

In PV, antibodies are directed against **desmoglein-3** molecules of keratinocyte desmosomes; therefore, acantholysis is restricted between the lower spinous and upper spinous layers. The basal keratinocytes remain attached to the basement membrane and protrude into the blister cavity, reminiscent of a **"row of tombstones."** The follicular outer root sheath epithelium is frequently involved. Early lesions are nonspecific and typically present as paucicellular spongiotic dermatitis with edema most prominent in the lower epidermis. Less commonly the early phase is characterized eosinophil-rich spongiotic vesicles (eosinophilic spongiosis). Older lesions may exhibit necrosis of the blister roof, with several regenerative layers of keratinocytes lining the base of the blister cavity. Additionally, epidermal rete ridges may elongate, giving rise

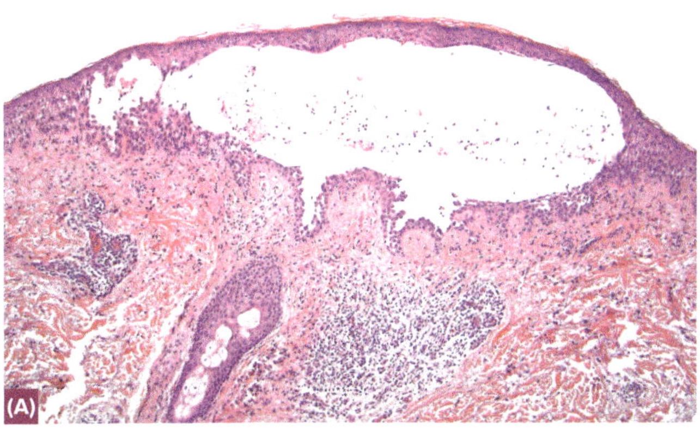

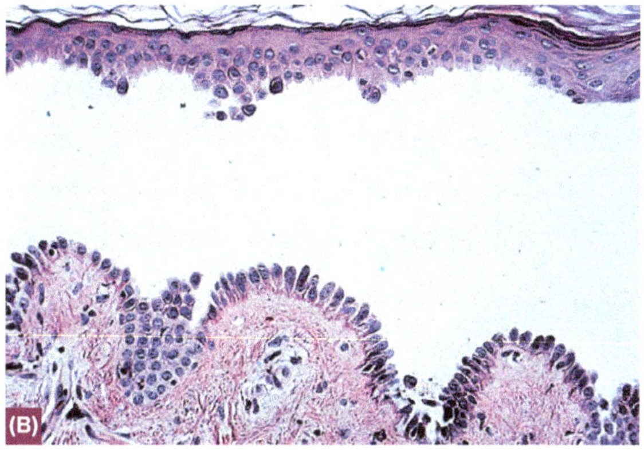

Pemphigus vulgaris. (A) Blister in suprabasilar location. In this well-developed lesion there is a suprabasilar cleft with acantholytic cells present in the blister cavity. **(B)** The row of intact basal cells protruding into the blister cavity imparts a "row tombstones" appearance. (Part **(B)** reproduced, with permission, from Goldsmith LA, Katz SI, Gilchrest BA, Paller AS, Leffell DJ, Wolff K, eds. *Fitzpatrick's Dermatology in General Medicine.*)

to the so-called villi. The dermal infiltrate characteristically contains perivascular lymphocytic infiltrates with scattered eosinophils and variable neutrophils.

The histopathological differential diagnosis includes **pemphigus foliaceus (PF), Darier disease, bullous pemphigoid (BP),** and **dermatitis herpetiformis (DH)** (choices A, B, C, and D, respectively). **Pemphigus foliaceus** may have a similar clinical presentation; however, the blisters are very superficial and are rarely intact at clinical presentation. Most importantly mucosal lesions are never present in PF, since antibodies directed against **desmoglein-1** cause this condition. The normal epidermis contains both desmoglein-1 (granular layer desmosomes) and desmoglein-3 (spinous layer desmosomes), whereas mucosal surfaces lack desmoglein-1 (as well as a granular layer). Histopathologically, the cleavage plane of acantholysis in PF is restricted to the granular cell layer where desmoglein-1 resides.

Darier disease is an autosomal dominant genodermatosis that presents within the first two decades of life as red-brown papules covered by tenacious scale, coalescing into large plaques of the chest, back, head, and groin. Warty papules are present at acral sites. Histopathologically, it is characterized by acantholysis accompanied by dyskeratosis (**corps ronds** and **corps grains**). Inflammation is generally absent since it is a genodermatosis. In **bullous pemphigoid,** there are large tense bullae characteristically presenting on erythematous skin. The tense nature of the bullae (negative Nikolsky sign) and rare mucosal involvement help to clinically distinguish BP from PV. **Dermatitis herpetiformis** presents as small groups papules and vesicles on elbows and flanks with extensive excoriations. The lesions are intensely pruritic and often heal with scarring. Histopathologically, both BP and DH are subepidermal bullous disorders, with the latter containing papillary dermal neutrophilic abscesses.

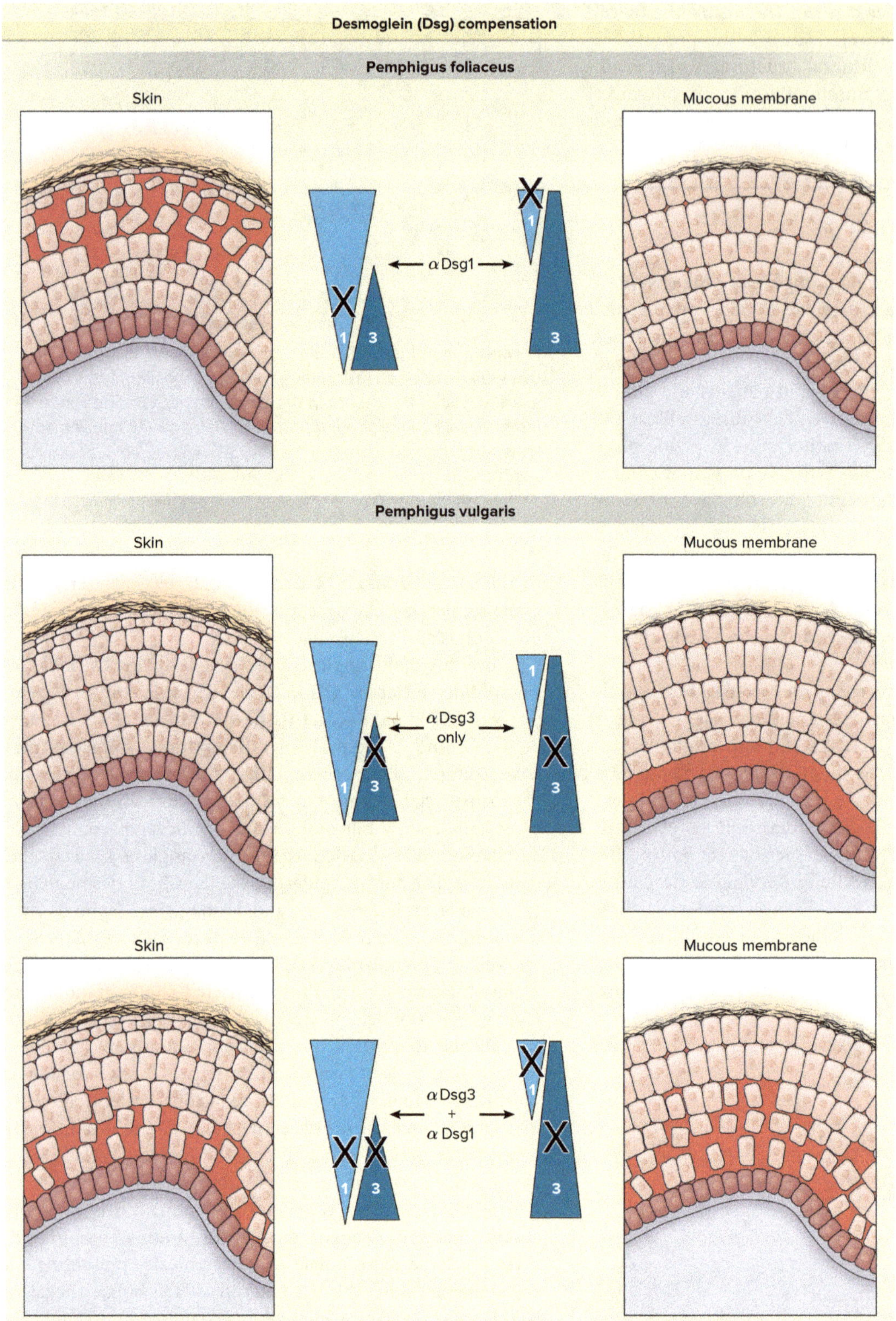

Desmoglein (Dsg) compensation. Triangles represent the distribution of Dsg1 and 3 in skin and mucous membranes. Anti-Dsg1 antibodies in pemphigus foliaceus cause acantholysis only in the superficial epidermis of skin. In the deep epidermis and in mucous membranes, Dsg3 compensates for antibody-induced loss of function of Dsg1. In early pemphigus vulgaris, antibodies are present only against Dsg3, which cause blisters only in the deep mucous membrane where Dsg3 is present without compensatory Dsg1. However, in mucocutaneous pemphigus, antibodies against both Dsg1 and Dsg3 are present, and blisters form in both mucous membrane and skin. The blister is deep probably because antibodies diffuse from the dermis and interfere first with the function of desmosomes at the base of the epidermis. (Reproduced, with permission, from Goldsmith LA, Katz SI, Gilchrest BA, Paller AS, Leffell DJ, Wolff K, eds. *Fitzpatrick's Dermatology in General Medicine*. 8th ed. New York, NY: McGraw-Hill Education; 2012.)

Table 3-4A. Pemphigus Vulgaris and Variants

Clinical Features
- Flaccid bullae on skin; face, scalp, chest, and intertriginous areas (especially pemphigus vegetans)
- Oral mucosa involved in 100% cases
- Older individuals

Histopathologic Features
- Suprabasal acantholysis with blister formation
- Involvement of hair follicles by acantholysis
- Spongiosis early
- Superficial perivascular mononuclear cell infiltrate
- Direct immunofluorescence: squamous epithelial intercellular deposition of IgG and possibly C3

Differential Diagnosis
- Other forms of pemphigus
- Benign familial pemphigus (Hailey-Hailey disease)
- Transient acantholytic dermatosis (Grover disease)
- Focal acantholytic dyskeratosis
- Acantholytic variants of actinic keratosis
- Herpesvirus infection

ANSWER 3-5: D.

This patient has **pemphigus vegetans**, which is a rare variant of **pemphigus vulgaris (PV)** that typically involves intertriginous areas and is seen in approximately 1% to 2% of cases. There are two subtypes: the **Hallopeau** and **Neumann types**. The differences between the two subsets are clinical presentation and course. The patient in this case has the **Hallopeau subtype**, which is a localized subtype of pemphigus vulgaris characterized by the transient formation of bullae breaking down into erythematous papules or vegetating plaques that are studded with pustules of varying sizes. The lesions usually arise on the flexural/intertriginous surfaces and the oral mucosa. The eroded areas do not heal like usual PV but instead form papillomatous growths and vegetations. This Hallopeau subtype typically exhibits a benign course with prolonged remission when treated with low-dose corticosteroids. In contrast, the **Neumann subtype** may develop extensive and widespread bullae similar to conventional pemphigus vulgaris with the formation of subsequent eroded plaques. Patients with the Neumann type have a course similar to pemphigus vulgaris, need higher doses of systemic corticosteroids, and have relapses and remissions.

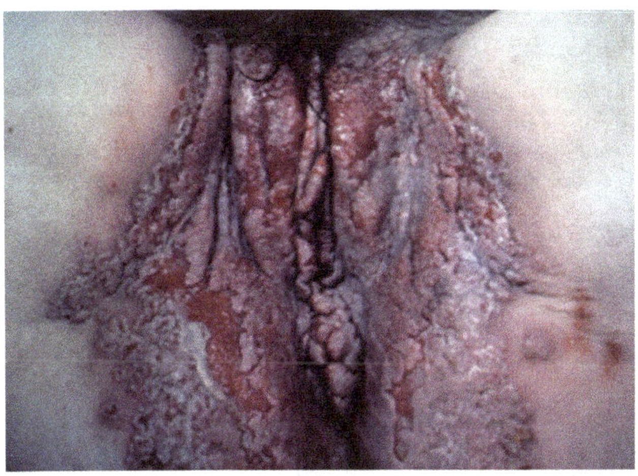

Pemphigus vegetans, Neumann subtype. Lesions become more extensive and widespread and may merge into extensive eroded vegetating plaques. Finally, with more severe disease, full-blown PV may appear. (Reproduced, with permission, from Usatine RP, Smith MA, Mayeaux EJ Jr, Chumley HS, eds. *Color Atlas of Family Medicine*. 2nd ed. New York, NY: McGraw-Hill Education; 2012.)

The histopathologic findings in these vegetating lesions are similar in both types. The direct immunofluorescence findings of both types are indistinguishable and similar to pemphigus vulgaris. Microscopically, early lesions exhibit acantholysis, most prominent in the suprabasal and lower spinous zones of the epidermis, just like conventional pemphigus vulgaris. In fact, initial lesions may be identical to pemphigus vulgaris. However, as the lesions age, verrucous epidermal hyperplasia develops with prominent eosinophilic spongiosis and eosinophilic pustules. Neutrophil-rich intraepidermal pustules may be present as well.

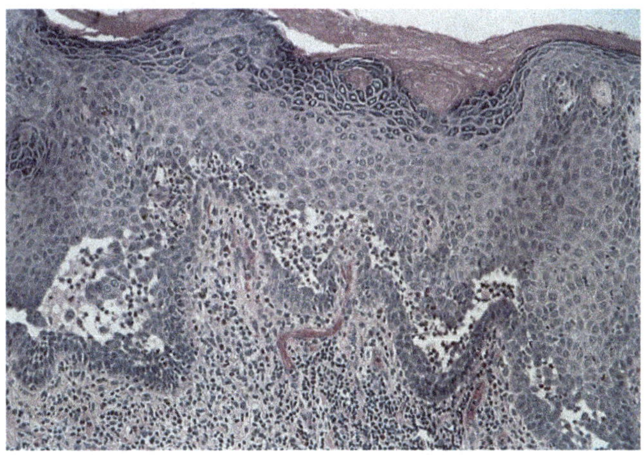

Lesion of pemphigus vegetans in mid-evolution.

This marked acanthosis is a unique feature of pemphigus vegetans. It is characterized by proliferation and downward expansion of the rete ridges within the papillary dermis separated by narrow elongated dermal papillae. The dermis is diffusely infiltrated by lymphocytes and eosinophils. Fully evolved lesions frequently exhibit a paucity of acantholytic cells, morphologically resembling reactive **pseudoepitheliomatous hyperplasia** (ie, fungal infections, halogenodermas, and perforating diseases). In these late stage lesions, clinical correlation and a diligent search for acantholytic keratinocytes may be required (ie, deeper levels). Direct immunofluorescence studies are confirmatory.

ANSWER 3-6: D.

The biopsy reveals interface dermatitis with scattered dyskeratotic keratinocytes. Additionally, there is a suprabasilar acantholytic blister containing rare acantholytic cells. The direct immunofluorescence reveals linear deposition of IgG in between basilar and suprabasilar keratinocytes (intercellular staining) and along the epidermal basement membrane zone. The combined findings are consistent with **paraneoplastic pemphigus (PNP)** (Table 3-6A). Paraneoplastic pemphigus is characterized by a generalized polymorphous eruption of blisters and lichenoid papules. Painful oral ulcerations are a prominent feature and have been present in

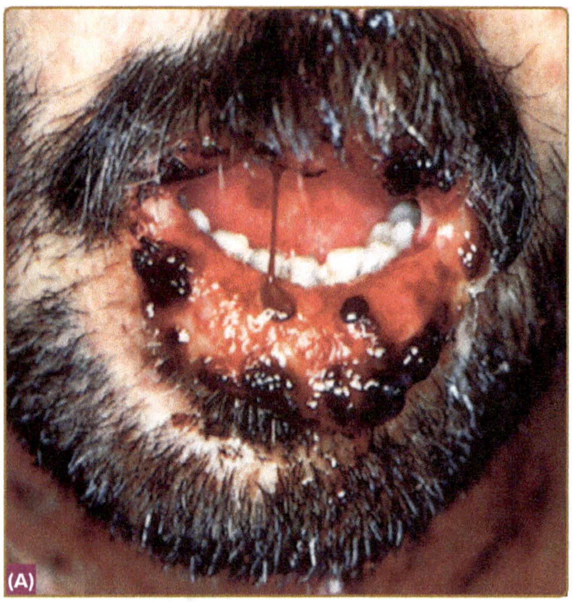

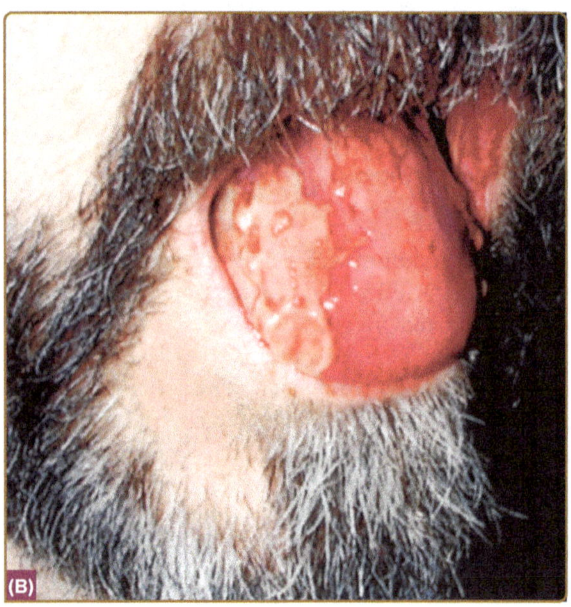

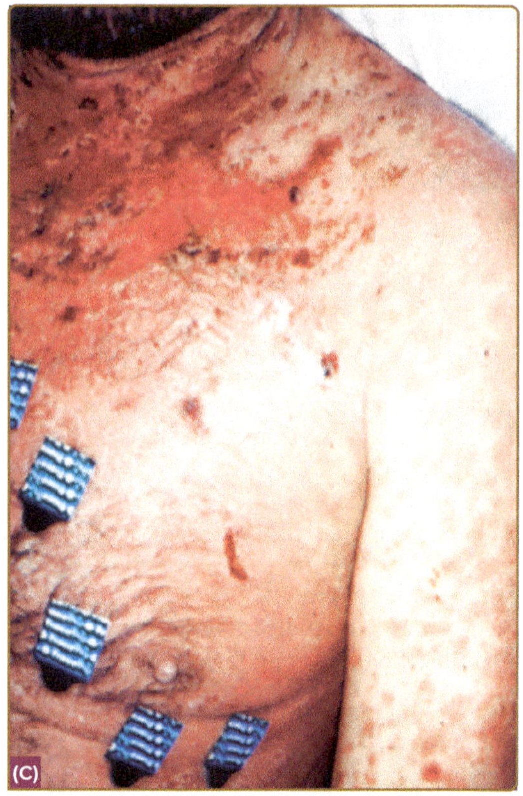

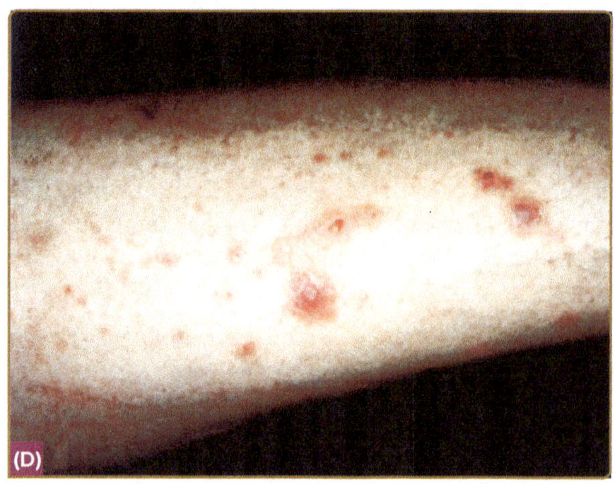

Paraneoplastic pemphigus. (A). Extensive erosions involving the vermillion of the lips in a patient presenting with paraneoplastic pemphigus and an occult lymphoma. The characteristic severe stomatitis, accompanied by polymorphous cutaneous lesions, is the most consistent feature of the disease. **(B).** Painful ulcerations tend to localize to the lateral border of the tongue. **(C).** Lesions of the trunk from the same patient pictured in **A.** Erythematous macules and papules coalesce and become erosive on the upper chest as the cutaneous lesions evolve. **(D).** Lesions from the forearm of the same patient. These lesions clinically resemble erythema multiforme, but biopsy shows a mix of individual cell necrosis, interface change, and acantholysis. (Reproduced, with permission, from Goldsmith LA, Katz SI, Gilchrest BA, Paller AS, Leffell DJ, Wolff K, eds. *Fitzpatrick's Dermatology in General Medicine*. 8th ed. New York, NY: McGraw-Hill Education; 2012.)

all cases. The ulcerations are often extensive over the lower lips, mimicking those of **Stevens-Johnson syndrome**. Any mucosal surface may be involved and pseudomembranous conjunctivitis is a common occurrence. Cutaneous involvement is characterized by lichenoid papules often involving the palms and the soles, which helps differentiate the disorder from pemphigus vulgaris. Associated neoplasms, in order of frequency, include non-Hodgkin lymphomas, chronic lymphocytic leukemia, Castleman disease, thymoma, sarcoma, and Waldenström macroglobulinemia. The disorder is aggressive and generally refractory to treatment. Successful treatment of the underlying malignancy may induce a remission of the pemphigus.

Microscopically, the hallmarks include suprabasal acantholysis with basal layer keratinocyte apoptosis (dyskeratotic keratinocytes) and variably dense interface dermatitis resembling **erythema multiforme** or **lichen planus**. Rarely, cases may appear identical to pemphigus vulgaris on H&E without interface dermatitis and dyskeratosis. It is important to note that acantholysis may be focal or not present at all in a single lesion. Thus the lesions may appear as either a purely erythema multiforme–like interface dermatitis or a cell-rich lichenoid interface dermatitis. Therefore, biopsies of more than one lesion or leveled sections of a biopsy specimen may be necessary to make the diagnosis. Severe refractory **chronic graft versus host disease** may also be histopathologically similar. **Bullous lichen planus** reveals a subepidermal cleavage plane, unlike the suprabasilar cleavage plane of PNP. Unlike **Stevens-Johnson syndrome, lichen planus,** or **lichenoid graft versus host disease**, direct immunofluorescence studies of PNP reveal intercellular IgG and C3 deposition as well as granular and linear areas of IgG and C3 along the dermal epidermal junction. Indirect immunofluorescence demonstrates intercellular IgG in all cases when using **rat bladder** as substrate. An impressive collection of autoantibodies is directed against a number of epidermal antigens and bind to simple, columnar, and transitional epithelia in addition to epidermis. PNP sera contain autoantibodies to plakin antigens (in the intercellular plaque of desmosomes), envoplakin and periplakin, and to desmoplakin I and II. Less commonly patient sera may also recognize bullous pemphigoid antigen (230 kDa), plectin, and plakoglobin, and an unidentified 170-kDa antigen. **Pemphigus erythematosus** shares features of both **pemphigus foliaceus** and **lupus erythematosus** with erythematous plaques of the nose and malar areas. Similar to PNP, these lesions usually exhibit basement membrane deposition of immunoglobulin and occasionally C3 (usually granular deposition c/w positive lupus band test) in addition to the intercellular immunoreactivity. However, unlike PNP, the most common immunoreactant is IgM. Further differentiating features from PNP include a subcorneal plane of cleavage and eosinophilic spongiosis and microabscesses/blisters confined to the subcorneal/granular layer accompanied by a few acantholytic keratinocytes and dyskeratotic granular cells.

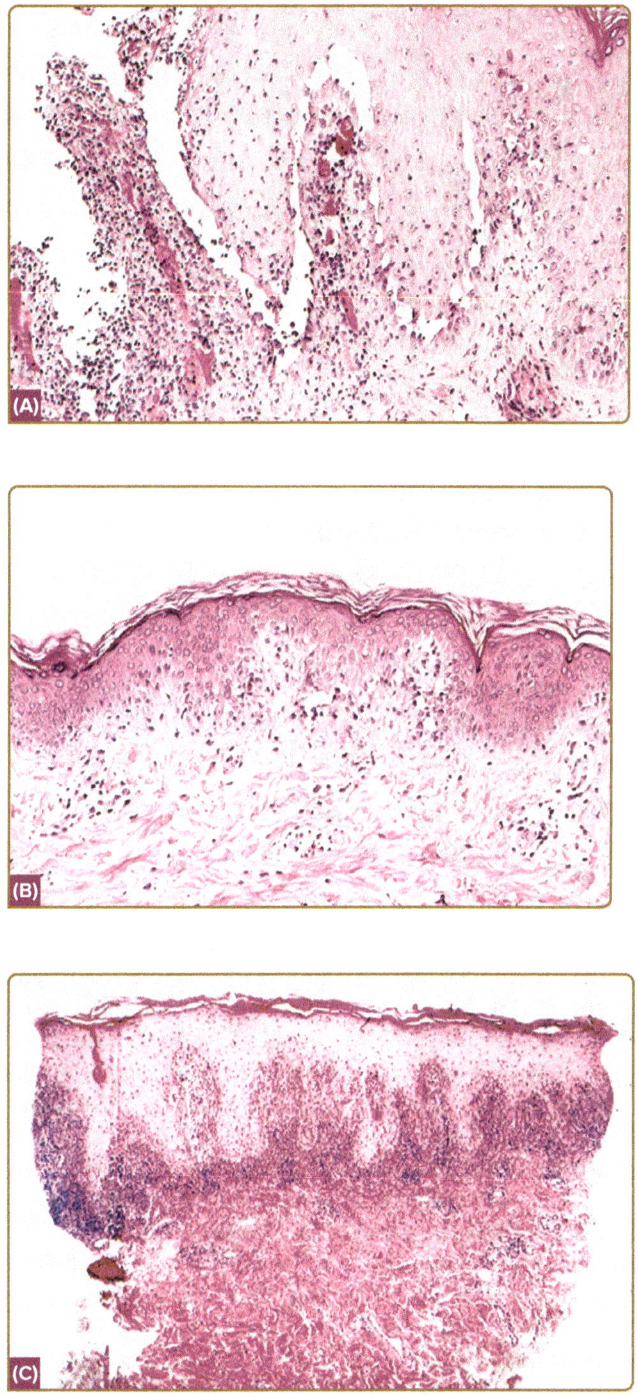

Paraneoplastic pemphigus. (A). Histopathology of a blistering cutaneous lesion in paraneoplastic pemphigus. This demonstrates the characteristic presence of vacuolar interface change and suprabasilar acantholysis. **(B).** Macular and papular lesions may show just vacuolar interface change. **(C).** Lichenoid lesions demonstrate lichenoid infiltrates on histopathologic examination. The presence of these varied histopathologic findings help differentiate paraneoplastic pemphigus from pemphigus vulgaris. (Reproduced, with permission, from Goldsmith LA, Katz SI, Gilchrest BA, Paller AS, Leffell DJ, Wolff K, eds. *Fitzpatrick's Dermatology in General Medicine*. 8th ed. New York, NY: McGraw-Hill Education; 2012.)

Table 3-6A. Paraneoplastic Pemphigus

Clinical Features
Polymorphous eruption of blisters and lichenoid papules
Painful oral ulcerations
Remission may be seen following successful treatment of underlying malignancy
Histopathologic Features
Suprabasal acantholysis
Interface dermatitis; either vacuolar or lichenoid type
Direct immunofluorescence: squamous epithelial intercellular deposition of IgG, or IgM, and possibly C3 usually shows linear or granular IgG, or IgM, and possibly C3 in epidermal basement membrane zone
Differential Diagnosis
Other forms of pemphigus
Benign familial pemphigus (Hailey-Hailey disease)
Transient acantholytic dermatosis (Grover disease)
Focal acantholytic dyskeratosis
Acantholytic variants of actinic keratosis
Lichen planus
Erythema multiforme

ANSWER 3-7: E.

This patient has **pemphigus foliaceus (PF),** which is an immunobullous disease where the plane of cleavage is restricted to within the granular layer or beneath the stratum corneum and is attributed to autoantibodies directed against **desmoglein-1** of granular layer desmosomes (Table 3-7A). As a consequence, these superficial blisters rarely remain intact and clinically manifest as shallow erythematous oozing and crusted erosions most commonly distributed on the face, scalp, chest, and back. Rare intact bullae may be identified with close inspection. Clinically these lesions may be confused with seborrheic dermatitis unless intact bullae are identified. The absence of mucosal lesions is an important diagnostic finding since **desmoglein-1** is not present in mucosal tissues. Since the superficial bullae are frequently ruptured, microscopic examination may only reveal small isolated foci of acantholytic keratinocytes on a superficially denuded epidermal surface. In those cases where the blister roof is absent, careful inspection of the hair follicles may reveal focal acantholysis. Typically there are diffuse dermal infiltrates of eosinophils and lymphocytes. Serum-imbued neutrophilic scale crusts with parakeratosis are common, making it difficult to distinguish from other subcorneal pustular disorders such as **impetigo, dermatophyte infection, candidiasis, pustular psoriasis, subcorneal pustular dermatosis (Sneddon-Wilkinson disease),** and **transient acantholytic dermatosis (Grover disease).** Unlike PF, these conditions lack intercellular deposition of IgG and C3d on direct immunofluorescence. **Impetigo** contains colonies of *Staphylococcus aureus* on the epidermal surface where an exotoxin cleaves **desmoglein-1**. While secondary impetiginization may occur in PF, it is not a characteristic feature.

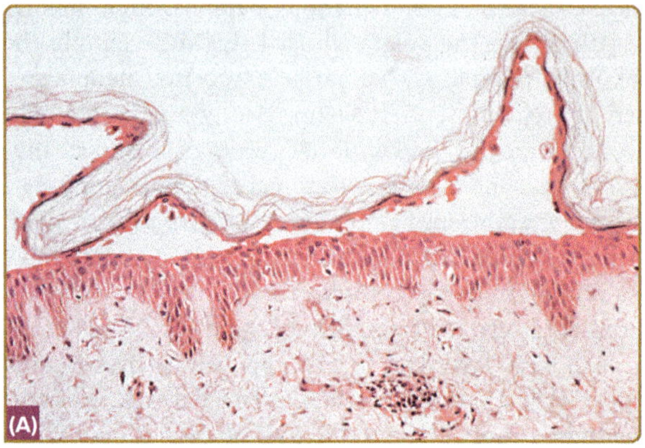

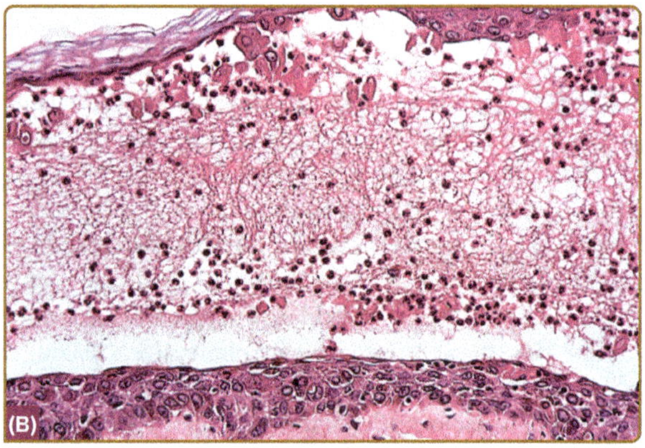

Histopathology of pemphigus foliaceus. (A). Acantholysis in the granular layer. **(B).** Subcorneal pustule with acantholysis. (Reproduced, with permission, from Goldsmith LA, Katz SI, Gilchrest BA, Paller AS, Leffell DJ, Wolff K, eds. *Fitzpatrick's Dermatology in General Medicine.* 8th ed. New York, NY: McGraw-Hill Education; 2012.)

In older evolved lesions, the granular cell layer may be thickened. Interestingly, patients treated with the drugs **penicillamine** and **captopril** have been noted to develop an illness identical to **pemphigus foliaceus** referred to as **drug-induced pemphigus. Fogo selvagem** is similar clinically but develops in people who live adjacent to rivers and streams in Brazil. An arthropod (*Simulium* sp) vector may mediate this disorder. It has been hypothesized that a component of the saliva within the arthropod vector triggers antibody development to **desmoglein-1**. Just like pemphigus foliaceus, fogo selvagem patients have circulating polyclonal IgG directed against desmoglein-1, which is found in greater concentrations in the upper epidermis. This distribution explains the subcorneal-granular layer cleavage plane of the blisters and lack of intraoral lesions. As with pemphigus vulgaris, the IgG in PF and fogo selvagem is of the IgG4 subclass. Definitive diagnosis requires careful consideration of the clinical information, and the results of bacterial culture and immunofluorescent studies.

Table 3-7A. Pemphigus Foliaceus and Variants

Clinical Features
Crusted erosions and patches
Very fragile flaccid bullae
Middle-aged and elderly
Trunk, head and neck, intertriginous areas, and proximal extremities
"Butterfly rash" mimicking lupus erythematosus seen in pemphigus erythematosus
Histopathologic Features
Subcorneal/granular blister with acantholytic keratinocytes or dyskeratotic granular cells
Variable eosinophilic spongiosis
Direct immunofluorescence: squamous epithelial intercellular deposition of IgG and possibly C3
Possible accentuation in superficial epidermis
Pemphigus erythematosus usually shows linear or granular IgG and possibly C3 at the epidermal basement membrane zone
Differential Diagnosis
Other forms of pemphigus
Impetigo
Staphylococcal scalded skin syndrome
Subcorneal pustular dermatosis

ANSWER 3-8: A.

The biopsy reveals a large subcorneal pustule with spongiform pustulation. The pustules are formed predominantly of neutrophils. This is a classic example of **IgA pemphigus** (aka **IgA pemphigus foliaceus**), which is a pruritic vesiculopustular eruption that develops in middle-aged to older individuals, often involving the axilla, trunk, and extremities (Table 3-8A). Flaccid vesicles, pustules, or bullae arise on erythematous bases similar to the lesions of **pemphigus foliaceus**. The pustules tend to coalesce and form an annular pattern. Mucous membrane involvement is very rare. Patients have been segregated into two groups: one resembling **subcorneal pustular dermatosis (Sneddon-Wilkinson disease like)** and the other resembling an **intraepidermal pustular eruption (pustular drug [AGEP] like)**. Many cases in the literature of subcorneal pustular dermatosis (Sneddon-Wilkinson disease), in which immunologic investigation was not undertaken, may represent IgA pemphigus.

Circulating IgA is directed against adhesion molecules within the epidermis. The antigens against which the antibodies are directed toward are neither **pemphigus foliaceus** nor **pemphigus vulgaris** antigens, but rather **desmocollins** and/or other **desmogleins.** The differing clinical presentation likely relates to the fact that the antibodies are directed against desmocollins in particular Dsc1 (subcorneal pustular type/Sneddon-Wilkinson type) and desmogleins (intraepidermal pustular type/pustular drug [AGEP] type) that have differing distributions within the epidermis.

Two histopathologic patterns, a subcorneal pustular pattern and an intraepidermal pustular pattern, are observed. In the former there are subcorneal vesiculopustules with minimal acantholysis. In the latter, there are intraepidermal pustules containing small to moderate numbers of neutrophils throughout the breadth of the epidermis. Suprabasal separation is not apparent. Minimal acantholysis is apparent such that the histopathologic reaction pattern is best considered an intraepidermal pustular dermatosis. The patient in the question exhibits the intraepidermal pustular pattern. Both variants of IgA pemphigus are defined by the presence of IgA intercellular deposition on immunofluorescence.

The differential diagnosis includes **pemphigus foliaceus (PF), subcorneal pustular dermatosis (Sneddon-Wilkinson disease), bacterial** and **fungal infection (particularly impetigo), pustular psoriasis,** and **pustular drug eruption (acute generalized exanthematous pustulosis [AGEP])**. Systematic evaluation with clinical history for evidence of psoriasis, drug ingestion, and so on; special stains and cultures for infective organisms; and immunofluorescence studies should facilitate making a specific diagnosis.

Table 3-8A. IgA Pemphigus

Clinical Features
Flaccid vesicles, pustules, and bullae arise on an erythematous base
Middle-aged to elderly patients
Histopathologic Features
Subcorneal or intraepidermal pustules
Direct immunofluorescence: intercellular IgA in epidermis
Differential Diagnosis
Other forms of pemphigus
Impetigo
Staphylococcal scalded skin syndrome
Subcorneal pustular dermatosis

ANSWER 3-9: C.

Drug-induced pemphigus usually begins as a nonspecific eruption of morbilliform, annular, or urticarial plaques without blisters (Table 3-9A). Patients with **penicillamine-induced pemphigus** have a characteristic generalized toxic erythema that has been labeled "a toxic pre-pemphigus rash." After a variable period of time, blisters develop on scaly, crusted patches, similar to those of pemphigus foliaceus in most cases. The most common causative drugs include **penicillamine** and **captopril**. Drug-induced pemphigus can be separated into two subsets. In the first group, representing 10% of cases, pemphigus antibodies are produced and cause acantholysis identical to that of classic "idiopathic" pemphigus (pemphigus foliaceus and pemphigus vulgaris). Direct binding of the drugs to the pemphigus antigens may render the antigens immunogenic in such cases. In the second group, the drugs or metabolites, rich in sulfhydryl groups, accumulate within the epidermis. They may cleave the disulfide bonds of keratin and incorporate into the keratin molecule itself because of their similarity to cystine, leading to acantholysis, which is nonimmunologically mediated. Another possible mechanism is the direct binding of the drugs to the pemphigus vulgaris and foliaceus antigens, disrupting their interchain disulfide bonds.

Microscopically, early eruptions exhibit an acute to subacute eczematous dermatitis. Eosinophils may be present, on occasion giving rise to eosinophilic spongiosis. The blister separation plane may either be in the subcorneal or suprabasal zones, such that in well-developed lesions, the histopathologic features are identical to pemphigus foliaceus or pemphigus vulgaris. The immunofluorescence findings may also be indistinguishable from other forms of pemphigus. However, in the majority of cases of drug-induced pemphigus where the acantholysis is not immunologically triggered, the direct immunofluorescence is characteristically negative.

Choice C describes the mechanism of action for **impetigo** and **staphylococcal scalded skin syndrome**. Cases of drug-induced pemphigus with secondary impetiginization may be difficult to distinguish from impetigo and staphylococcal scalded skin syndrome. Clinical correlation is required for definitive diagnosis in these situations.

Table 3-9A. Drug-Induced Pemphigus

Clinical Features
- Morbilliform, annular, or urticarial plaques progress to blisters
- Scaly crusted plaques
- Penicillamine and captopril are common causative agents

Histopathologic Features
- Plane of blister separation may occur in either subcorneal or suprabasal plane
- Subacute eczematous dermatitis seen in early lesions
- Direct immunofluorescence study: intercellular deposition of IgG and possibly C3 in epidermis in almost all active cases

Differential Diagnosis
- Other forms of pemphigus
- Benign familial pemphigus (Hailey-Hailey disease)
- Transient acantholytic dermatosis (Grover disease)
- Focal acantholytic dyskeratosis
- Acantholytic variants of actinic keratosis
- Herpesvirus infection
- Impetigo
- Staphylococcal scalded skin syndrome
- Subcorneal pustular dermatosis

ANSWER 3-10: E.

This patient has **pemphigus erythematosus (PE)**, which is a variant of **pemphigus foliaceus (PF)** that has features of both **pemphigus** and **lupus erythematosus.** It usually presents with erythematous plaques of the nose and malar areas. By definition, all cases demonstrate the direct immunofluorescence intercellular staining pattern classic for pemphigus, approximately 30% have positive antinuclear antibody titers, and 80% have concomitant positive lupus band tests. Nonlesional, non–sun-exposed skin reveals a positive lupus band test in only 20% to 40% of biopsies. In the vast majority of cases, indirect immunofluorescence is also positive. Most patients with PE do not develop systemic signs or symptoms of lupus, and some may progress from localized disease to generalized PF.

Three characteristic histopathologic patterns occur: eosinophilic spongiosis and abscesses, subcorneal/granular blisters with few acantholytic keratinocytes (identical to PF), and subcorneal/granular blisters with dyskeratotic granular layer cells. The latter pattern is considered diagnostic of this disorder. As in **pemphigus vulgaris**, the cleavage plane in most cases is not exact and may extend to the suprabasal zone, on occasion rendering histopathologic distinction of the two principal pemphigus variants difficult (PF vs PV). Rare cases exhibit interface dermatitis similar to that of **lupus erythematosus** and may resemble **paraneoplastic pemphigus (PNP)**. Just like PNP, PE demonstrates intercellular and granular basement zone deposition of immunoglobulin and complement. Unlike PNP, the immunoglobulin is typically IgM. In rare cases where IgG deposits in intercellular and BMZ patterns, discrimination between the two relies on other findings (clinical, histopathologic, and laboratory).

ANSWER 3-11: C.

This patient is presenting with **cephalic herpes zoster with facial palsy (Ramsay Hunt syndrome),** in which the eruption involves the facial and auditory nerves. In **herpes zoster** eruptions, or **"shingles,"** patients present with painful clusters of small vesicles with an erythematous base that frequently are eroded and crusted. Initial infection with the **varicella-zoster virus (VZV)** results in a disseminated vesiculopustular eruption (**chicken pox**). Secondary reactivated eruptions of varicella-zoster virus are clinically identical to the **HSV-1** and **HSV-2** eruptions, but arise in crops in a dermatome distribution corresponding to the infected sensory nerve. Clinically HSV-1 infections preferentially affect the oral mucosa and HSV-2 infections frequently infect the genital skin and mucosa. However, both strains of the virus may be recovered from either site. Microscopically, **herpes simplex virus 1 (HSV-1), herpes simplex 2 (HSV-2),** and **varicella-zoster virus (VZV)** are identical and cannot be distinguished. The infected keratinocytes are acantholytic, but have distinct viral cytopathic features of enlarged pale basophilic nuclei with effaced heterochromatin and peripheral beading of the nuclear membrane, imparting a "steel gray" appearance. Large multinucleated keratinocytes are frequently present. The multinucleated cells typically exhibit dense clusters of nuclei with molding and sharp contours. Frequently eosinophilic intranuclear inclusions are present which are pathognomonic.

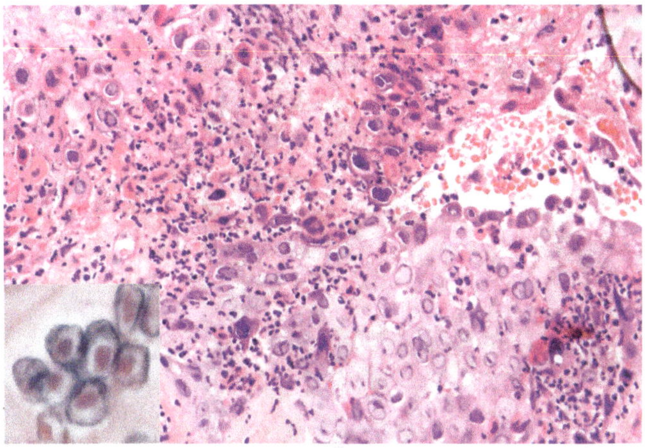

Herpes viral cytopathic changes. In this particular case of herpes there are striking cytopathic changes including an effaced heterochromatin, beading of the nuclear membrane, and multinucleation. The insert on the lower left reveals the eosinophilic nuclear inclusions that are pathognomonic for herpes infection.

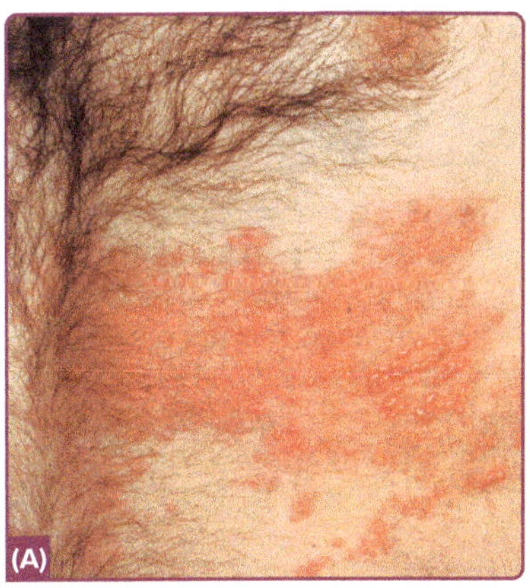

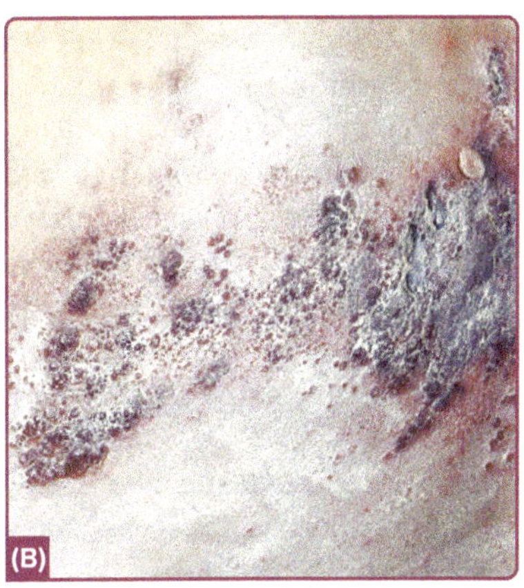

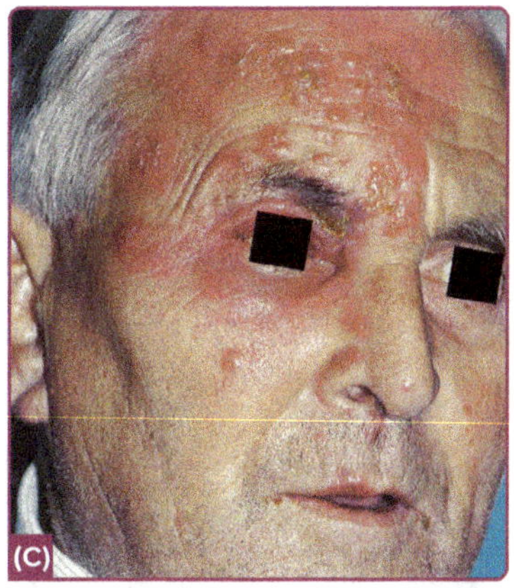

Herpes zoster. (A). Early involvement of a thoracic dermatome with erythema within the dermatome and areas of grouped vesicle formation. **(B).** Later involvement with crusted sites on the back, where the eruption first appeared, and many confluent hemorrhagic vesicles and bullae on the lateral chest wall, where the eruption appeared more recently; some vesicles are also seen outside the involved dermatome, representing hematogenous dissemination, a not uncommon occurrence. **(C).** Ophthalmic zoster. Note the involvement of the tip of the nose, which frequently signals involvement of the eye. (Reproduced, with permission, from Goldsmith LA, Katz SI, Gilchrest BA, Paller AS, Leffell DJ, Wolff K, eds. *Fitzpatrick's Dermatology in General Medicine*. 8th ed. New York, NY: McGraw-Hill Education; 2012.)

Additional features include marked acantholysis, leukocytoclastic vasculitis, and ulceration. Direct immunofluorescence studies reveal a nonspecific profile with immunoglobulin and complement deposition within vessels. The intercellular deposition of IgG and C3d consistent with pemphigus vulgaris is not present in herpes.

ANSWER 3-12: A.

The biopsy reveals a subcorneal blister containing only rare acantholytic cells. A sparse inflammatory infiltrate of rare lymphocytes and neutrophils is present. Gram stain reveals gram-positive cocci within the blister cavity. The findings are consistent with **bullous impetigo. Impetigo** refers to infections of the epidermis, which may extend into the dermis and are then referred to as **ecthyma. Bullous impetigo** is a contagious cutaneous infection by *Staphylococcus aureus*. Patients are typically young preschool-age children who develop pustules on an erythematous base at exposed sites. These large pustules are typically short-lived and rapidly breakdown into golden or honey-colored crusts. Self-inoculation is common. Patients with bullous impetigo frequently have a concomitant history of atopic dermatitis.

Ordinary **impetigo** (nonbullous) is characterized clinically by red papules that transform into vesicles and pustules developing at sites where abrasions, insect bites, or excoriations disrupt the cutaneous barrier. Honey-colored crusts also develop rapidly. Secondary impetiginization with bacteria

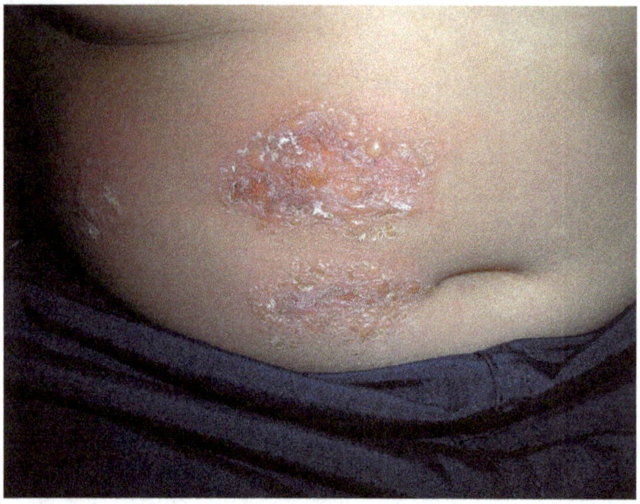

Bullous impetigo. This 8-year-old patient with atopic dermatitis demonstrates numerous bullae, some of which have ruptured forming honey crusted erosions. (Reproduced, with permission, from Usatine RP, Smith MA, Mayeaux EJ Jr, Chumley HS, eds. *Color Atlas of Family Medicine*. 2nd ed. New York, NY: McGraw-Hill Education; 2012.)

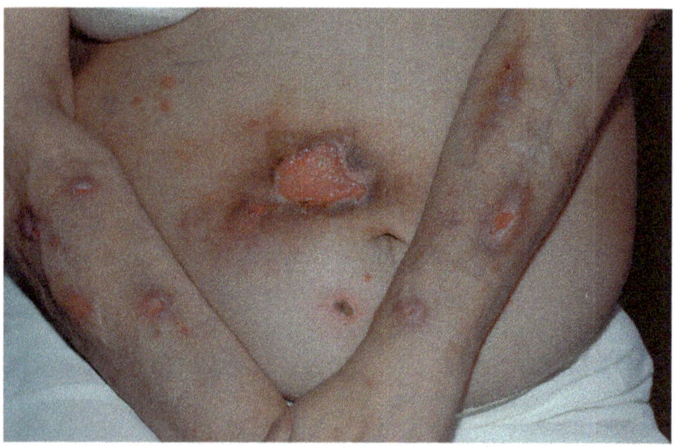

Secondary impetiginization of factitial ulcers: MRSA. 60-year-old female with end-stage renal disease (ESRD) and generalized pruritus has large self-induced excoriations and ulcers, which are secondarily infected. (Reproduced, with permission, from Wolff K, Johnson RA, Saavedra AP. *Fitzpatrick's Color Atlas and Synopsis of Clinical Dermatology.* 6th ed. New York, NY: McGraw-Hill Education; 2009)

may also develop in all varieties of eczematous dermatitis, particularly atopic eczema. Ordinary (nonbullous) impetigo is mostly caused by infection by group A *Streptococci*.

Bullous impetigo and **staphylococcal scaled skin syndrome (SSSS)** are almost exclusively associated with *Staphylococcus aureus*, primarily phage group 2, type 71. In fact, **bullous impetigo** may be viewed clinically as a localized form of **SSSS**. Patients with staphylococcal scalded skin syndrome (SSSS) are typically infants who develop fever and malaise followed by a painful, tender, orange-tinged erythematous rash associated with purulent conjunctivitis, otitis media, occult nasopharyngeal infection, or umbilical stump infection. Within 2 days, large, flaccid bullae develop in the axillae and groin and around body orifices and become generalized. The mucous membranes are not involved. Healing usually is complete within 5 to 7 days.

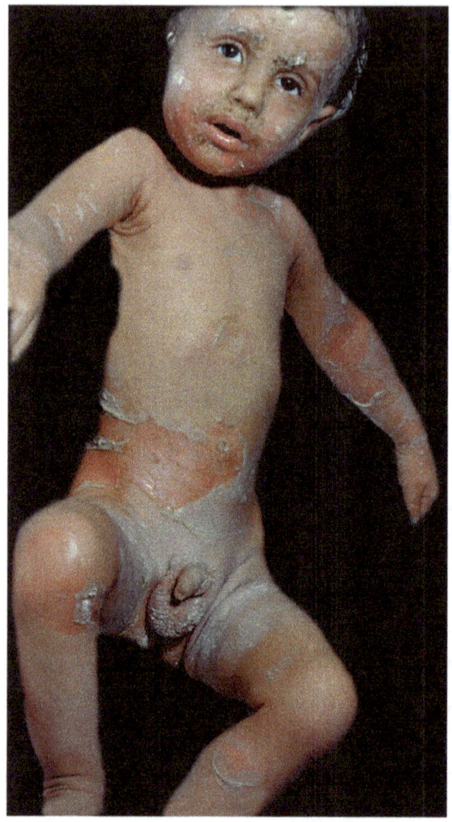

Staphylococcal scalded skin syndrome: desquamation. In this infant, painful, tender, diffuse erythema was followed by generalized epidermal sloughing and erosions. *S aureus* had colonized the nares with perioral impetigo, the site of exotoxin production. Extensive desquamation is seen on the face and anterior trunk. (Reproduced, with permission, from Wolff K, Johnson RA, Saavedra AP. *Fitzpatrick's Color Atlas and Synopsis of Clinical Dermatology.* 6th ed. New York, NY: McGraw-Hill Education; 2009.)

Bullous impetigo and **staphylococcal scalded skin syndrome** are both caused by a staphylococcal exotoxin called **exfoliatin** which targets **desmoglein-1**. The toxin is produced locally in bullous impetigo and systemically delivered in SSSS. Microscopically, both **bullous impetigo** and **staphylococcal scalded skin syndrome** are characterized by subcorneal and intragranular bullae with rare numbers of acantholytic keratinocytes. However, advanced lesions of bullous impetigo contain robust intraepidermal and superficial dermal neutrophilic infiltrates. Spongiosis and parakeratotic scale crusts are frequently identified. Gram stain reveals numerous gram-positive cocci in clusters within the stratum corneum. Staphylococcal scalded skin syndrome is characterized by a relative paucity of neutrophilic infiltrates and has complete necrosis of the upper granular layer keratinocytes. Bacteria are not identified on Gram stain in SSSS, since the condition is attributed to disseminated exotoxin. In the absence of immunofluorescence studies, the rarity of acantholytic keratinocytes combined with the presence of neutrophils differentiates **bullous impetigo** from **pemphigus foliaceus (PF).** PF only reveals bacteria within the stratum when secondarily infected. In these instances, clinical correlation and immunofluorescence are required to establish a definitive diagnosis. In ordinary **nonbullous impetigo**, neutrophils migrate singly throughout the epidermis to form small subcorneal pustules. The exocytosis of neutrophils as single cells and clusters into the hyperplastic and spongiotic epidermis resembles **psoriasis** or **lichen simplex chronicus.** There is usually prominent edema in the upper dermis and diapedesis of neutrophils from the superficial vessels. **Toxic epidermal necrolysis** may clinically resemble **SSSS** and can be distinguished microscopically from SSSS and bullous impetigo by the presence of necrotic keratinocytes throughout the full thickness of the epidermis and not just limited to the granular layer or higher.

The other major entities to be considered in the differential diagnosis include other infective processes such as **dermatophytosis, *Candida* infection, syphilis, IgA pemphigus, subcorneal pustular dermatosis, pustular psoriasis, pustular drug eruption, pustular bite reaction, pustular vasculitis, neutrophilic dermatoses** such as **pyoderma gangrenosum**, and a nutritional deficiency such as **migratory necrolytic erythema** and **acrodermatitis enteropathica**. Systematic evaluation with clinical history for evidence of psoriasis, drug ingestion, and so on; special stains and cultures for infective organisms; and immunofluorescence studies should facilitate making a specific diagnosis.

ANSWER 3-13: A.

The biopsy reveals a tense and intact subcorneal pustule containing robust neutrophilic infiltrates. The combined clinical, histopathological, and immunofluorescent findings are consistent with **subcorneal pustular dermatosis (Sneddon-Wilkinson disease [SW])**, in which patients present with several millimeter-sized tense subcorneal pustules in the groin and intertriginous areas (Table 3-13A). Clinically these lesions are distinctive by the tendency for pus to accumulate in the lower half of the pustules, referred to as a **hypopyon**. These pustules easily rupture and leave behind hyperpigmented serpiginous erosions with scaly crust. An important clinical finding is the absence of pruritus. There is an association with IgA paraproteinemias and IgA secreting myelomas, Crohn disease, rheumatoid arthritis, and Graves disease. It is presumed that the pustule containing neutrophils are responding to chemotactic factors present in the subcorneal zone, in particular TNF-α, which has been identified in the blister fluid.

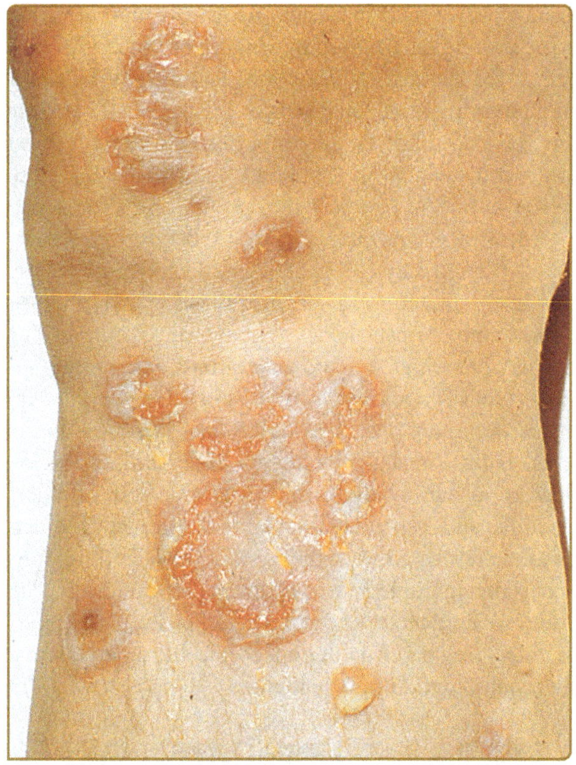

Subcorneal pustular dermatosis (Sneddon-Wilkinson disease). Close-up showing coalescence of pustules, which form annular and circinate patterns. Lesions of different developmental stages are seen side by side. At the lower right, newly formed pustule with characteristic hypopyon formation. (Reproduced, with permission, from Goldsmith LA, Katz SI, Gilchrest BA, Paller AS, Leffell DJ, Wolff K, eds. *Fitzpatrick's Dermatology in General Medicine.* 8th ed. New York, NY: McGraw-Hill Education; 2012.)

Microscopically, these lesions consist of well-contained, unilocular, neutrophilic pustules with rare eosinophils and rare acantholytic cells confined to subcorneal layer. The underlying granular layer is intact. The epidermal spinous layers are spongiotic with little to no neutrophilic permeation. There are sparse mixed perivascular and superficial papillary dermal neutrophilic and lymphocytic infiltrates. The differential diagnosis includes **pustular psoriasis, bullous impetigo, pemphigus foliaceus** + variants, and **pustular drug eruption (acute generalized exanthematous pustulosis).** There is epidermal hyperplasia in **pustular psoriasis** consisting of regular epidermal hyperplasia with elongation of the rete ridges and thinning of the suprapapillary plates and a uniform absence of the granular layer. In psoriasis, the smaller scattered intraepidermal neutrophilic pustules of Kogoj and Monro are located within the upper epidermis and stratum corneum, respectively. The pustules of Sneddon-Wilkinson disease are confined to the corneal layer and are much larger in size. The pustules of **bullous impetigo** are also subcorneal in location; however, they clinically present in young school-age children with a background history of atopic dermatitis. Histopathologically, these pustules are smaller and contain fewer inflammatory cells. Gram-positive cocci in clusters are usually present within or near the pustule on Gram stain. Culture of the lesions may be required for definitive distinction. **Pemphigus foliaceus (PF)** and **pemphigus erythematosus (PE)** typically present with abundant acantholytic keratinocytes and contain fewer neutrophils and eosinophils. Unlike PF and PE, direct immunofluorescence of SW reveals a nonspecific immunoreactant profile, and cases where intercellular IgA deposition is present are best classified as IgA pemphigus. In fact, many cases described in the literature as subcorneal pustular dermatosis where immunofluorescence was not performed may in fact represent IgA pemphigus. **Acute generalized exanthematous pustulosis (AGEP)**, also known as **pustular drug eruption**, most commonly occurs around 5 days postingestion of antibiotics. Diffuse macular erythema and multiple nonfollicular-based pustules characterize this eruption. In addition, malaise, chills, and low-grade fever may be present. The dermatitis rapidly resolves after withdrawal of the offending drug. Microscopically, multiple foci of neutrophilic spongiosis with or without subcorneal or intraepidermal pustules are seen. There is underlying papillary dermal edema and a perivascular infiltrate usually containing eosinophils.

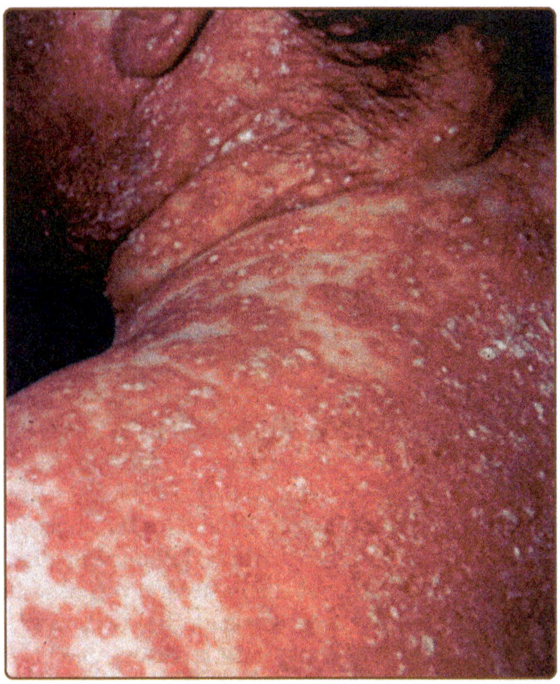

Acute generalized exanthematous pustulosis in a 48-year-old man who developed nonfollicular pustules and fever after 7 days of treatment with diltiazem. (Reproduced, with permission, from Goldsmith LA, Katz SI, Gilchrest BA, Paller AS, Leffell DJ, Wolff K, eds. *Fitzpatrick's Dermatology in General Medicine.* 8th ed. New York, NY: McGraw-Hill Education; 2012.)

Lastly, **dermatitis herpetiformis** is a chronic blistering disease associated with gluten intolerance **(Celiac disease)** and is characterized by tiny vesicles containing watery fluid usually distributed symmetrically on extensor surfaces. Unlike

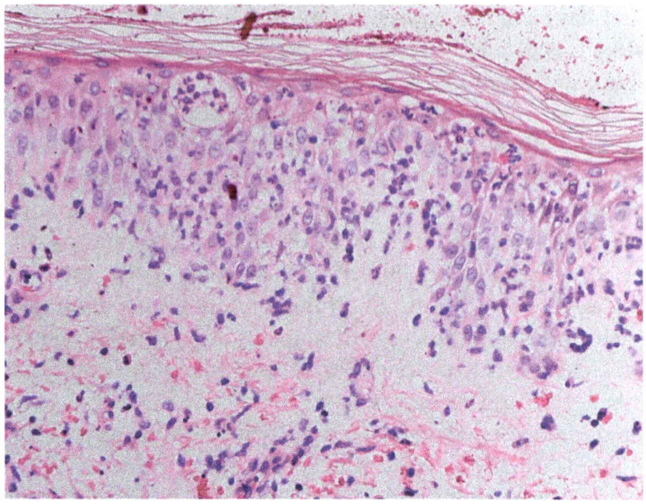

Acute generalized exanthematous pustulosis (AGEP). There are foci of neutrophilic spongiosis with subcorneal and intraepidermal pustules. There is underlying papillary dermal edema and a perivascular infiltrate usually containing eosinophils.

SW, these lesions are extremely pruritic. Microscopically, there are tiny microabscesses of neutrophils and rare eosinophils confined to the dermal papillae. Robust papillary dermal edema may lead to confluence and enlargement of the dermal papillae and the overlying epidermis may exhibit spongiotic vesiculation. Direct immunofluorescence of these lesions will reveal chunky granular IgA deposits confined to the dermal papillae.

Table 3-13A. Subcorneal Pustular Dermatosis (Sneddon-Wilkinson)

Clinical Features
Pustules develop in erythematous skin
Predilection for flexural skin, axillary and inguinal folds
Histopathologic Features
Subcorneal neutrophil-rich pustules
Superficial and deep perivascular mononuclear cell infiltrates
Direct immunofluorescence: negative
Differential Diagnosis
Impetigo
Candida
Dermatophytosis
Staphylococcal scalded skin syndrome
Psoriasis
Keratoderma blenorrhagicum (Reiter disease)
IgA pemphigus
Pemphigus foliaceus
Pustular drug eruption

ANSWER 3-14: E.

This patient has **benign familial pemphigus (Hailey-Hailey disease)** which is a benign autosomal dominant acantholytic condition in which acantholysis occurs throughout the full thickness of the epidermis, extending from the granular cell layer to the basal cell layer forming intraepidermal bullae (Table 3-14A). Morphologically the epidermis takes on the appearance of a **"dilapidated brick wall."** This condition is potentially disabling due to the fact that these circinate, pruritic, foul-smelling, oozing, and crusted plaques frequently become secondarily infected by bacteria and fungi. Therefore, the designation of **"benign familial pemphigus"** is actually misleading. Trauma has been implicated in the etiology of these lesions, as there is preferential localization to the flexural surfaces, axillae, and groin. Acantholysis is frequently incomplete with clusters of attached keratinocytes and single acantholytic keratinocytes present within the bullae. This nonimmunologically mediated form of acantholysis is due to mutations in the *ATP2C1* gene that codes for a P-type Ca^{2+} transport ATPase. Unlike immunologically mediated pemphigus, there is usually sparing of the follicular infundibula and dermis with absent or sparse dermal inflammatory infiltrates. Dyskeratotic keratinocytes are absent in this condition and when present one must consider **keratosis follicularis (Darier disease). Herpes virus infections** may also appear similarly due to acantholysis occurring throughout all the epidermal layers; however, **Hailey-Hailey disease** lacks the distinctive nuclear viral inclusions.

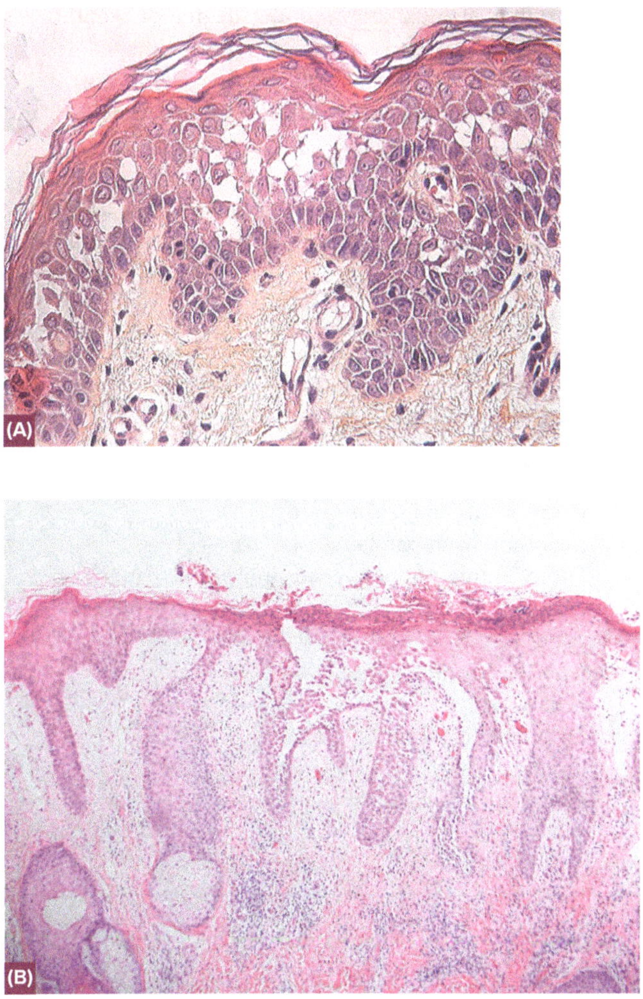

Hailey-Hailey disease. (A), (B) Extensive partial loss of intercellular contacts within the epidermis produces the appearance of a "dilapidated brick wall." (Part **(A)** reproduced, with permission, from Goldsmith LA, Katz SI, Gilchrest BA, Paller AS, Leffell DJ, Wolff K, eds. *Fitzpatrick's Dermatology in General Medicine*. 8th ed. New York, NY: McGraw-Hill Education; 2012.)

Table 3-14A. Hailey-Hailey Disease

Clinical Features
Fragile flaccid blisters give rise to scale crust
Intertriginous areas, neck, perianal, inframammary, and antecubital regions
Autosomal dominant
Histopathologic Features
Acantholysis giving rise to dilapidated brick wall appearance in at least half of epidermis
Acanthosis
Often slight dyskeratosis
Direct immunofluorescence: nonspecific pattern
Differential Diagnosis
Darier disease
Transient acantholytic dermatosis (Grover disease)
Pemphigus vulgaris

ANSWER 3-15: C.

The tiny coalescent brown papules are characteristic of **Darier disease**. The inflammatory plaques with fissures and maceration under the breasts simulate Hailey-Hailey disease; however, note the presence of dystrophic fingernails. **Keratosis follicularis (Darier disease),** an autosomal dominant condition, is characterized by multiple, brown, pruritic, and keratotic papules that frequently coalesce on the face, chest, and back (Table 3-15A). Lesions are exacerbated by sunlight, humidity, and heat exposure and frequently present in late childhood. The Darier disease gene has been localized to chromosome 12q23-q24.1. Mutations in the *ATP2A2* gene that encodes the sarco/endoplasmic reticulum Ca^{2+}-ATPase isoform 2 are found in patients with the disease. This is one of the proteins that catalyses the transport of calcium from the cytosol into the lumen of the endoplasmic reticulum, resulting in enhanced apoptosis. Not surprisingly, Bcl-2 expression (anti-apoptosis) is diminished in the lesional epidermis of patients with Darier disease. Microscopically, there is an acantholytic suprabasal cleft with an underlying intact basal cell layer. This acantholytic focus occurs over a broad zone within the epidermis. The rete may be elongated, giving rise to so-called villi, similar to what may be seen in **pemphigus vulgaris**. The distinguishing microscopic feature of Darier disease is the prominence of dyskeratotic keratinocytes, in addition to acantholytic keratinocytes, which may be found throughout all layers of the epidermis. Above the acantholytic cleft are compact and enlarged granular layer keratinocytes surmounted by a parakeratotic stratum corneum. These large upper spinous and granular layer keratinocytes contain clumped keratohyaline granules in an eosinophilic cytoplasm and have large nuclei with perinuclear chromatin clumping and halos about prominent nucleoli. These acantholytic cells are referred to as **corp ronds**. The parakeratotic stratum corneum contains small, seed-shaped cells with pyknotic, elongated nuclei and dense, eosinophilic cytoplasm. They are referred to as **corp grains**. Immunofluorescence studies do not detect any immunoreactants in Darier disease.

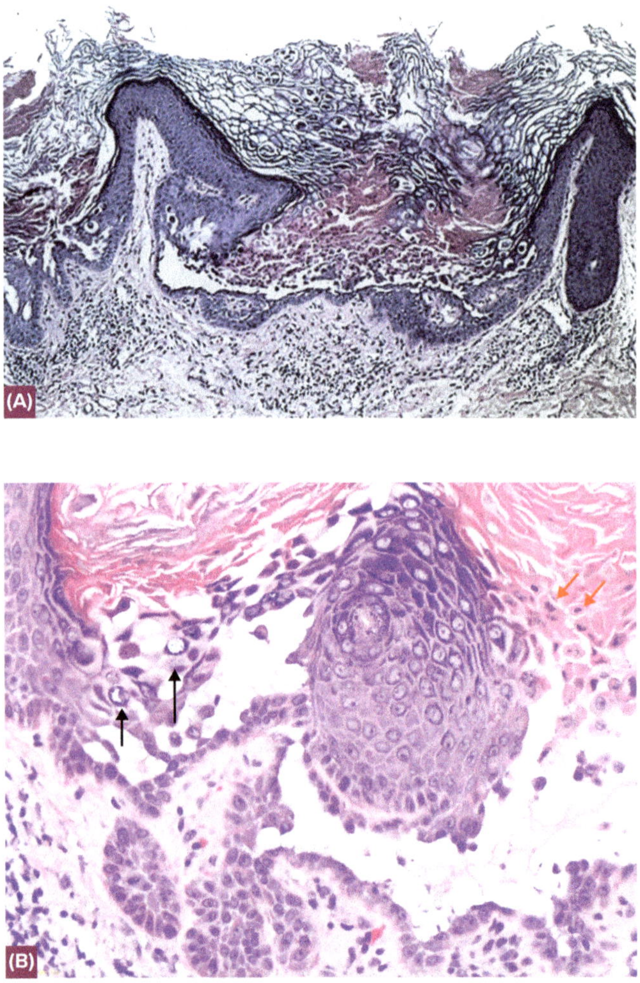

Darier disease. (A) There is an epidermal invagination filled with ortho- and parakeratotic debris. A suprabasilar lacuna with dyskeratotic acantholytic cells is present. **(B)** At higher power, the typical corps ronds (black arrows) and corps grains (red arrows) are noted.

In regard to the differential diagnosis, Darier disease can be distinguished from the other acantholytic diseases by the presence of extensive and distinctive dyskeratotic keratinocytes. The main histopathological similarity is **Grover disease**, which may be indistinguishable from Darier disease but usually shows additional histopathologic patterns resembling **pemphigus, Hailey-Hailey disease**, and **spongiotic dermatitis**. Like **Hailey-Hailey,** Darier disease is a nonimmunologically mediated genodermatosis and therefore typically lacks a dermal inflammatory infiltrate. However, Darier disease lacks the full-thickness acantholysis with a "dilapidated brick wall" appearance seen in Hailey-Hailey. **Warty dyskeratomas** also exhibit a similar degree of acantholysis with Darier-like dyskeratosis, but are cup-shaped lesions that are centered on the hair follicle. These lesions are easily distinguished from Darier disease since they are isolated and solitary lesions.

Table 3-15A. Darier Disease

Clinical Features
- Scaly papules and plaques of the head, back, chest, and groin
- Autosomal dominant

Histopathologic Features
- Acantholytic dyskeratosis with suprabasal split
- Corps ronds and corps grains
- Acanthosis and parakeratosis
- Direct immunofluorescence: nonspecific pattern of granular C3 at the epidermal basement membrane zone

Differential Diagnosis
- Hailey-Hailey disease
- Transient acantholytic dermatosis (Grover disease)
- Pemphigus vulgaris

ANSWER 3-16: E.

The biopsy reveals several, small, discrete foci of suprabasilar acantholysis with focal full-thickness acantholysis (dilapidated brick wall like) and prominent dyskeratotic keratinocytes within the granular layer. The dermis contains scattered inflammatory cells. This patient has **transient acantholytic dermatosis (Grover disease)** in which

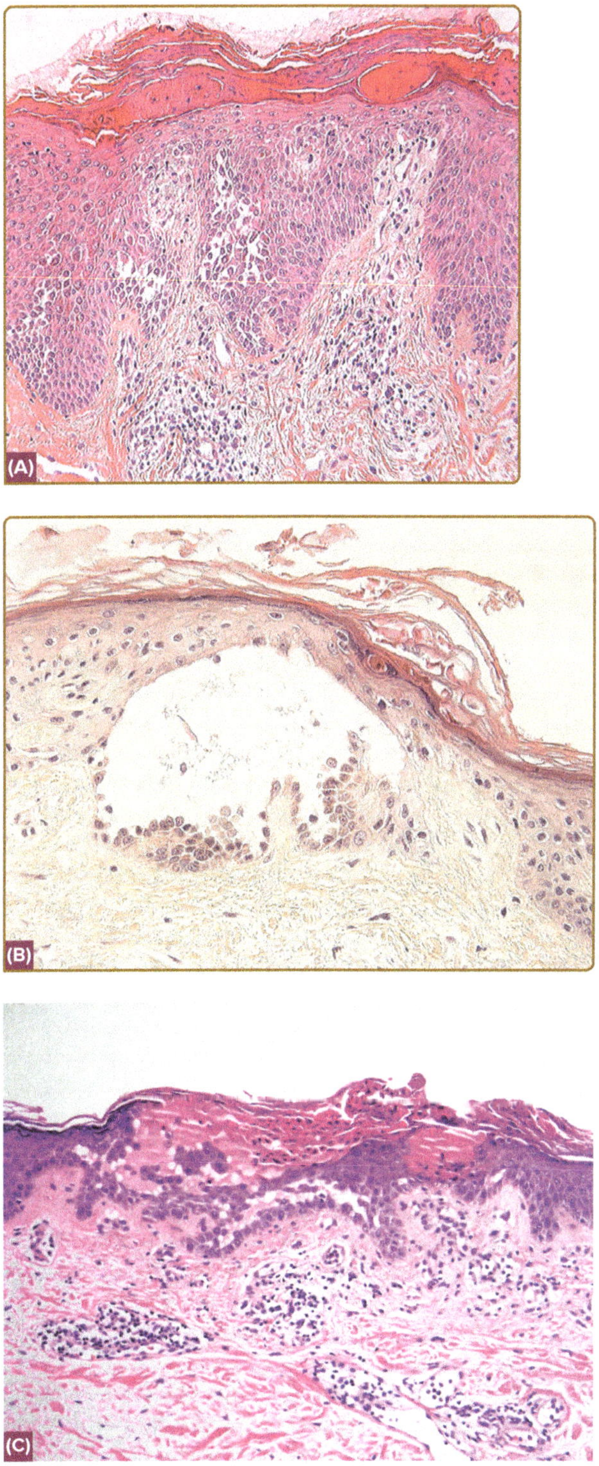

Grover disease. (A). Hailey-Hailey–like histological pattern in Grover disease with detached keratinocytes (acantholysis), focal spongiosis, and epidermal hyperplasia. **(B).** Pemphigus-like pattern in Grover disease with suprabasal acantholytic cleavage. (Reproduced, with permission, from Goldsmith LA, Katz SI, Gilchrest BA, Paller AS, Leffell DJ, Wolff K, eds. *Fitzpatrick's Dermatology in General Medicine*. 8th ed. New York, NY: McGraw-Hill Education; 2012.) **(C)** Darier's-like variant with spongiosis. Note the focal acantholysis with corp ronds and corp grains and overlying serum imbued crust. Grover's disease typically exhibits multiple "variant" patterns at once within individual lesions.

small pin-sized skin colored to erythematous and slightly pruritic papules arise on the upper back, chest, and thighs (Table 3-16A). Of clinical importance is the fact that these lesions are not transient, unlike how the name suggests, and may persist for several years. There are four histopathological subtypes of **Grover disease: pemphigus vulgaris pattern, Hailey-Hailey pattern, Darier pattern**, and a **spongiotic pattern**. The epidermal changes within these subtypes are identical to the condition for which they are named. The most distinguishing feature for Grover disease is the fact that acantholysis is focal, limited, and persistent. The Darier subtype is most frequently encountered, but lesions typically contain mixtures of any of these patterns. Unlike **Darier** and **Hailey-Hailey**, dermal lymphocytic infiltrates are usually present, but range from sparse to dense and diffuse. Direct immunofluorescence (DIF) examination is negative for intercellular IgG deposition in Grover disease, distinguishing this entity from pemphigus vulgaris and pemphigus foliaceus. Drug-induced pemphigus clinically manifests with larger clinical lesions. Both conditions typically exhibit nonspecific immunofluorescent findings and histopathological distinction from spongiotic variants of Grover disease may be difficult. Drug-induced pemphigus lacks the Darier-type dyskeratosis and Hailey-Hailey–like acantholysis that is frequently seen in Grover disease. Clinical correlation is essential.

Table 3-16A. Transient Acantholytic Dermatosis (Grover Disease)

Clinical Features
Pruritic papulovesicles on chest, back, and thighs
Middle-aged or elderly men
Histopathologic Features
Acantholytic dyskeratosis in small foci
Four histological patterns:
Focal acantholytic dyskeratosis as in Darier disease
Hailey-Hailey disease pattern
Pemphigus vulgaris or foliaceus pattern
Spongiotic dermatitis pattern
Any or all four patterns may be present in a single biopsy
Direct immunofluorescence: nonspecific pattern
Differential Diagnosis
Darier disease
Hailey-Hailey disease
Pemphigus vulgaris or foliaceus
Spongiotic dermatitis

Important Differential Diagnostic Features of Acantholytic Dermatoses

	PEMPHIGUS FOLIACEUS	SSSS	HAILEY-HAILEY DISEASE	PEMPHIGUS VULGARIS	PEMPHIGUS VEGETANS	DARIER DISEASE	GROVER DISEASE
Subcorneal cleavage	+++	+++	–	–	–	–	–
Intraspinous cleavage	0/+	–	+++	0/+	–	–	–
Suprabasal cleavage	–	–	0/+	+++	+++	+++	+ (small)
Cleft	–	–	–	–	–	++	++
Blister	+	+	+	+	+	–	–
Dyskeratosis	+ (some)	–	–	–	–	++	+ (some lesions)
Villi	–	–	+	+/+++	+++	+/+++	+
Tombstone basal keratinocyte	–	–	–	+++	+	–	–
Follicular involvement	+	–	–	++	+	+	–
Epidermal hyperplasia	–	–	+/++	0/+	+++	+	–
Spongiotic early change	+	–	–	+	+	–	+
Eosinophilic spongiosis	0/+	–	–	0/+ (some)	+++ (abscesses)	–	–

ANSWER 3-17: A.

This patient has **erythema toxicum neonatorum** (ETN), which is an idiopathic benign pustular eruption in healthy neonates that arises within the first week of life (Table 3-17A). Individual 1 to 3 mm pustules on an erythematous base erupt in crops on the trunk, face, and limbs. The palms and soles are characteristically spared. The lesions spontaneously resolve by 2 weeks of age without residual hyperpigmentation.

Histopathologically, these pustules are filled with eosinophils with a rare neutrophil component. In early lesions, the pustules are found in the lower epidermis adjacent to or within the intraepidermal portion of the hair follicle (acrotrichium). More evolved pustules are larger in size and may be found within the upper layers within the epidermis. Dermal inflammatory infiltrates range from superficial perivascular to diffuse and are composed of eosinophils and lymphocytes. The main histopathological differential diagnosis includes the initial phase of **incontinentia pigmenti, transient neonatal pustular melanosis** (**TNPM**), **disseminated candidiasis, impetigo,** and **herpes viral infection**. In **incontinentia pigmenti**, numerous scattered dyskeratotic keratinocytes are identified as well as diffusely distributed intraepidermal eosinophils. This patient's biopsy lacks dyskeratotic keratinocytes. **Transient neonatal pustular melanosis (TNPM)** presents at birth with numerous pustules on a nonerythematous base and resolves with basal layer hypermelanosis (increased pigment in basal keratinocytes). The pustules of TNPM are not follicular based but subcorneal and contain predominantly neutrophils. **Candidiasis, impetigo**, and **herpes viral infections** clinically all fall within the differential; however, they are also neutrophil rich and lack significant eosinophilia. Special stains (PAS and Gram) as well as culture are helpful in ruling out these infectious conditions. The presence of herpes viral infected keratinocytes must be investigated by either Tzanck smear or H&E (routine biopsy). Of note, there is a striking histopathological similarity between **follicular-based ETN** and **eosinophilic pustular folliculitis.**

Table 3-17A. Erythema Toxicum Neonatorum

Clinical Features
Pustules and macules arise in the first few days of life
Face, torso, and extremities
Histopathologic Features
Intraepidermal and subcorneal eosinophilic pustules in hair follicles
Differential Diagnosis
Scabies
Incontinentia pigmenti
Eosinophilic folliculitis

ANSWER 3-18: C.

Transient neonatal pustular melanosis (TNPM) is typically present at birth and in some instances babies are born with the tiny pigmented macules, suggesting in utero vesiculation. The condition is characterized by a transient eruption of 1 to 3 mm neutrophil-rich pustules without an erythematous base localized to the head, neck, trunk, palms, and soles. Infants with darkly pigmented skin are more commonly affected. The pustules arise in crops and rupture within about a week, leaving behind a fine scale with hyperpigmentation.

Histopathologically, the epidermis is spongiotic with numerous singly scattered intraepidermal neutrophils and neutrophilic subcorneal pustules. Acantholysis is absent. Rare eosinophils may be seen within the pustules. There are sparse papillary dermal neutrophilic infiltrates. The ruptured lesions will reveal increased melanin pigmentation within basal keratinocytes. The diagnosis is largely clinical and these lesions are rarely biopsied. Occasionally, microscopic examination of a smear from one of the vesicles is performed to document the presence of neutrophils.

The main differential diagnosis includes **erythema toxicum neonatorum, infantile acropustulosis, IgA pemphigus, bullous impetigo, candidal** and **bacterial sepsis,** and **herpesvirus viremia. Erythema toxicum neonatorum** (ETN) differs by the fact that the pustules are not present at birth but usually arise within the first week of life. These pustules arise on an erythematous base and do not resolve with basal hypermelanosis. In ETN, there are eosinophil-rich pustules found adjacent to the follicular ostia in the lower epidermis and larger progressive vesicles may be seen within the higher levels of the epidermis. Significant tissue neutrophilia is not a characteristic feature of erythema toxicum neonatorum. **Infantile acropustulosis (IAP)** is characterized by transient eruptions of intensively pruritic pustules in acral locations that may arise in infants that are several months old. The pustules are neutrophil-rich but may contain an admixture of eosinophils. In infantile acropustulosis, the pustules are found throughout all levels of the epidermis unlike transient neonatal pustular melanosis where the pustules are confined to the superficial epidermal or subcorneal layers. An association of scabetic infestation and IAP has been well documented. **IgA pemphigus** is a pruritic vesiculopustular eruption that develops in middle-aged to older individuals, often involving the axilla, trunk, and extremities. The pustules are flaccid and extremely pruritic. Microscopically these lesions can be similar to TNPM, but exhibit intercellular deposition IgA on direct immunofluorescence. Rare acantholytic cells may be seen within the blister in IgA pemphigus, a finding not present in TNPM. **Bullous impetigo** presents with multiple golden/honey-colored crusts and pustules with an erythematous base on the hands, fingers, mouth, and intertriginous sites. These subcorneal vesicles contain neutrophils but typically contain rare acantholytic cells. Additionally, bullous impetigo is caused by an exotoxin produced by *Staphylococcus aureus*, which are easily uncovered with swab culture and Gram stain. **Herpes virus infection** is unlikely since viral inclusions were not identified on Tzanck smear.

ANSWER 3-19: D.

The biopsy reveals an intraepidermal blister sharply confined to the mid-spinous layer without associated dermal inflammation or acantholytic keratinocytes. The blister roof is imbued with serum. This a classic example of **friction blisters**, which develop mainly on the soles and palms as a result of repetitive actions producing mechanical forces applied parallel to the cutaneous surface in normal individuals (Table 3-19A). Friction blisters are the result of shearing forces within the epidermis causing cytolysis of the spinous layer. They tend to occur where the epidermis is thick and firmly attached to the underlying tissues. There may be individual necrotic keratinocytes with cytoplasmic strands of disrupted keratinocytes. Pale, hydropic, degenerated keratinocytes, which have been sheared, are located on the superior and inferior aspects of the blister. There is typically an absence of inflammatory cells within the epidermis and dermis in early intact lesions. The blister fluid is usually clear due to transudation. When the shearing force extends into the dermis, hemorrhage into the blister cavity is common. **Talon noir** refers to hemorrhage entrapped in the stratum corneum following trauma. These lesions appear dark brown or black and clinically mimic melanocytic proliferations. They commonly occur on the toes and soles. In the mechanobullous genodermatoses (ie, epidermolysis bullosa simplex superficialis) only minimal friction will produce blisters due to a lack of appropriate structural integrity of the epidermis and dermis. **Epidermolysis bullosa simplex superficialis** is characterized by mutations in the collagen VII gene resulting numerous blisters, milia, and atrophic scarring, as well as involvement of oral and/or ocular surfaces with minimal surface trauma. These lesions tend to be apparent at an early age. This is unlikely in this patient since she has no prior history of blistering and no family history of a blistering condition. Additionally, the cleavage plane in these mechanobullous genodermatoses is subepidermal. **Suction blisters** typically produce subepidermal blisters with minimal inflammation. Distinction from mechanobullous genodermatoses may be difficult and requires clinical correlation. **Bullous tinea pedis** results from a dramatic inflammatory reaction to dermatophyte infection. The blisters are typically subepidermal and attributed to robust papillary dermal edema. PAS stain will reveal hyphae.

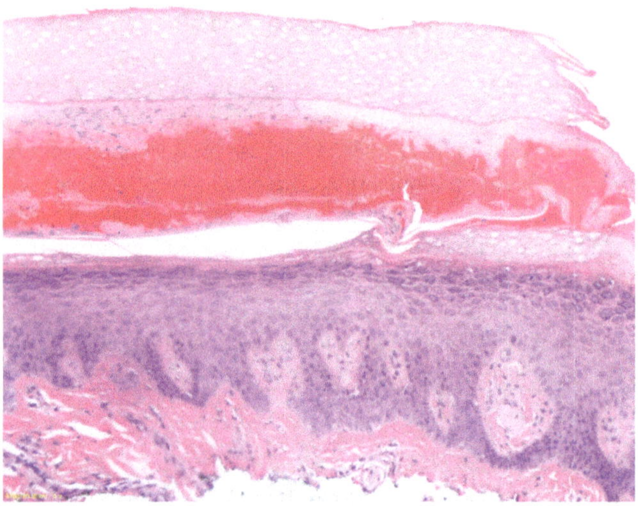

Talon noir. There is a large focus of intracorneal hemorrhage with little associated inflammation.

Table 3-19A. Friction Blister

Clinical Features
Palms and soles most common sites affected
History of mechanical injury at site affected
Histopathologic Features
Blister with intraepidermal cleavage
Individual necrotic keratinocytes
Hemorrhage is common
Differential Diagnosis
Epidermolysis bullosa simplex superficialis

ANSWER 3-20: B.

The Giemsa-stained smear reveals a giant, multinucleated keratinocyte. The nuclei are molded against one another and have a dispersed chromatin pattern. This is an example of a positive **Tzanck smear** and **herpes virus infection**. Regardless if samples are obtained via scraping or biopsy, the diagnosis depends on the viral cytopathic features of enlarged pale basophilic nuclei with effaced heterochromatin and peripheral beading of the nuclear membrane, imparting a "steel gray" appearance. Large multinucleated keratinocytes are characteristically present exhibiting dense clusters of nuclei with molding and sharp contours. Eosinophilic intranuclear inclusions, when present, are considered pathognomonic. A recurrent waxing and waning course is the characteristic of HSV-1 and HSV-2 infections and occasionally VZV infections. This risk is increased with immunosuppression. Patients with HIV disease or other forms of immune dysregulation are prone to developing follicular herpes, where the viral cytopathic changes involve the follicular outer root sheath epithelium. Additionally, the inflammatory infiltrates in these patients may contain large numbers of eosinophils. The cytomorphology of HSV-1, HSV-2, and VZV is identical and requires clinical correlation and viral typing for distinction.

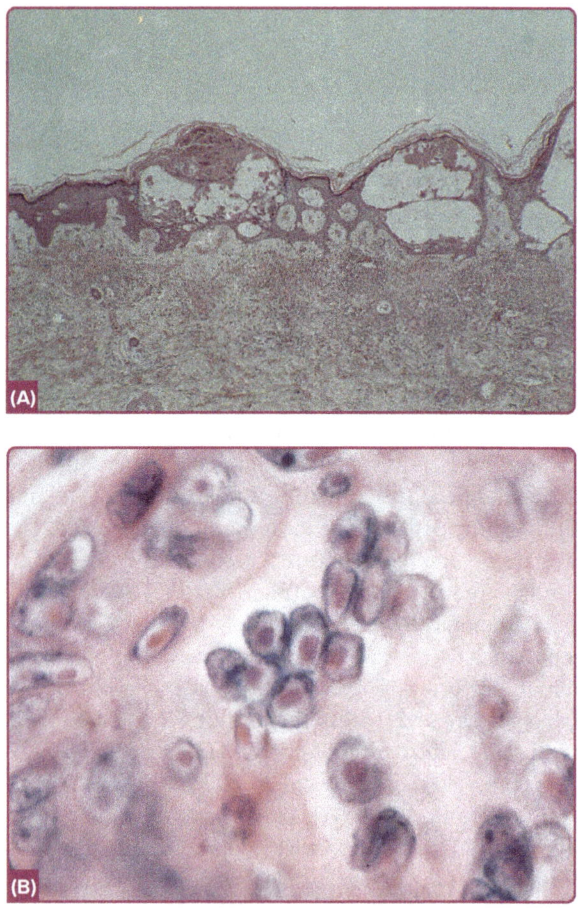

Herpes zoster, histopathology. (A). Intraepidermal vesicle, acantholysis, reticular degeneration; underlying dermis shows edema and vasculitis. **(B).** Multinucleated giant cells with characteristic nuclear changes including eosinophilic inclusions. (Reproduced, with permission, from Goldsmith LA, Katz SI, Gilchrest BA, Paller AS, Leffell DJ, Wolff K, eds. *Fitzpatrick's Dermatology in General Medicine.* 8th ed. New York, NY: McGraw-Hill Education; 2012.)

Choice C describes **paraneoplastic pemphigus (PNP).** Indirect immunofluorescence studies of peripheral blood from patients with PNP will reveal a panoply of circulating autoantibodies directed against a number of epidermal antigens (ie, BPAg 1, desmoplakin 1, and desmogleins 1 and 3). Immunofluorescence studies in cutaneous herpes reveal a nonspecific immunoreactant profile. **Cutaneous herpes** and **paraneoplastic pemphigus (PNP)** are both associated with immunosuppression and prominent painful mucosal ulcerations (lower lip especially in PNP). Microscopically, both conditions may exhibit multinucleation, varying degrees of interface dermatitis with dyskeratotic keratinocytes along the dermal-epidermal junction, and acantholysis involving the follicular outer root sheath epithelium, however, only herpes exhibits viral cytopathic features. PNP is associated with bronchogenic carcinomas, thymomas, retroperitoneal sarcomas, and various hematologic malignancies such as Hodgkin lymphoma and chronic lymphocytic leukemia. It is characterized by a generalized polymorphous eruption of blisters and lichenoid papules with painful mucocutaneous oral ulcerations. Clinical "lichenoid" papules and plaques are often present on the palms and soles, which may clinically resemble **erythema multiforme (EM)** and **Stevens-Johnson syndrome.** Remember that a majority of EM cases are associated with herpetic antigens. PNP generally follows an aggressive clinical course that is refractory to treatment, unlike the waxing and waning course of herpes. Direct immunofluorescence studies of PNP reveal a mixed pattern of intercellular IgG and possibly C3d along with linear and/or granular IgG, C3d, and possibly IgM deposition along the basement membrane zone.

ANSWER 3-21: A.

This patient has **infantile acropustulosis (IAP),** which is characterized by recurrent crops of intensely pruritic vesicles or pustules developing most commonly in black infants at birth or during the first year of life. Males are slightly affected more commonly than females. The lesions predominantly involve the distal extremities, particularly the palms and soles, dorsa of the hands and feet, and the sides of the fingers and toes. Individual lesions heal with hyperpigmentation, and the process resolves within 2 years in most cases. Some patients have a history of **atopic dermatitis,** and in several patients there has been associated **scabetic infestation.** The etiology is unknown. Some physicians speculate that IAP is a persistent reaction to scabies ("post-scabetic syndrome"). Suggestive of this infectious etiology is the occasional finding of concurrent scabetic infestation present among siblings. Also, patients diagnosed with this disorder frequently have received prior treatment for scabies, which may either provide evidence of an infectious etiology or demonstrate the frequent misdiagnosis, as in the patient above. Odom et al conclude that in some cases, this disease may represent a hypersensitivity reaction to *Sarcoptes scabiei.* Since mites or burrows within the stratum corneum are not present, a definitive diagnosis of scabies cannot be made.

Microscopically, early lesions reveal spongiosis and small foci of epidermal necrosis, apoptosis (dyskeratosis), and exocytosis of neutrophils and occasional eosinophils. Later lesions reveal subcorneal and intraepidermal vesiculopustules containing numerous neutrophils and admixed eosinophils. A few cases have shown a predominance of eosinophils. There is minimal papillary dermal edema and a sparse mixed-cell perivascular infiltration. **Erythema toxicum neonatorum** presents in neonates, 1 to 2 days after birth. This disease of unknown etiology causes 2 to 3 cm diffuse blotchy macules and patches with 1 to 4 mm central vesicles. The lesions, which spare the palms and soles, contain a predominance of eosinophils and resolve spontaneously by 2 weeks of age. **Transient neonatal pustular melanosis** is characterized by the presence at birth of 2 to 3 mm macules and pustules on a nonerythematous base. The lesions probably evolve prenatally and subsequently rupture postnatally in 1 to 2 days. They heal with hyperpigmented macules that fade by 3 months of age, with lighter-skinned patients experiencing less hyperpigmentation. Sometimes, the only evidence of the disease is the presence of small, brown macules with a rim of scale at birth. Microscopically, these lesions are composed of subcorneal pustules containing predominantly neutrophils and rare eosinophils. As in all intraepidermal pustular disorders, PAS stain and tissue Gram stain should be performed in order to exclude infection. **Varicella** is characterized clinically by "dew drops on a rose petal" that develop in childhood. The vesicles are uniformly distributed, pruritic, and most commonly associated with known exposure. Microscopically, viral cytopathic changes of herpes are diagnostic. This patient reveals no evidence of viral cytopathic changes or hyphae.

ANSWER 3-22:

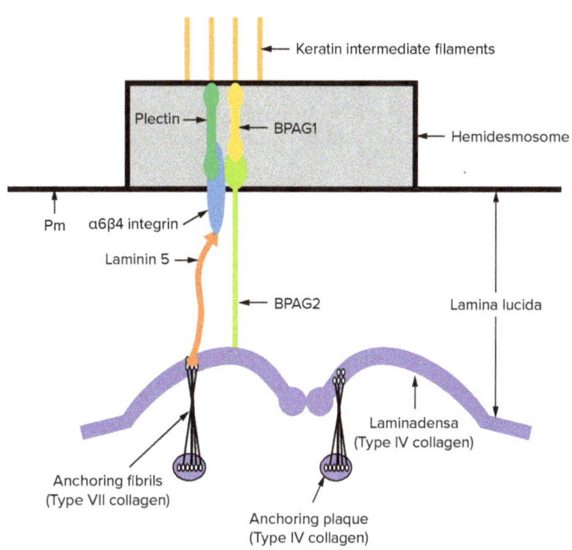

1) $\alpha_6\beta_4$ integrin (G)
2) Bullous pemphigoid antigen 2 (E)
3) Plectin (C)
4) Type VII collagen (H)
5) Bullous pemphigoid antigen 1 (A)
6) Laminin 5 (B)
7) Lamina densa (D)
8) Anchoring plaque (F)

ANSWER 3-23: C.

This is a classic example of **bullous pemphigoid (BP),** which is a subepidermal immunobullous disease caused by circulating autoantibodies against components of the basement membrane's lamina lucida, namely BPGA1 and BPAG2 (90% and 50%, respectively) (Table 3-23A). BP is considered the most common autoimmune blistering disease, with a reported incidence of 10 cases per 1 million. It affects mainly elderly patients (peak ago 70 years), but can also occur in any age, including infants and children. No ethnic or gender predominance has been found. BP is clinically characterized by large serous or hemorrhagic, tense blisters that arise on normal or erythematous skin. The sites of predilection are the inner and anterior thighs, groin, flexor surfaces of the upper extremities, and lower abdomen. Any skin region may, however, be involved. Erosions and crusts as a consequence of the blister rupture are usually present, and the lesions characteristically heal without scar formation. This regenerative capability without scarring is thought to be attributed to the plane of cleavage occurring above the lamina densa. A **Nikolsky sign** is characteristically absent. In the early stage of the disease, there are urticarial papules and plaques. Occasionally, pruritus is present and may range from mild to severe. Certain medications have also been associated with the development of these lesions including penicillamine, efalizumab, etanercept, and furosemide.

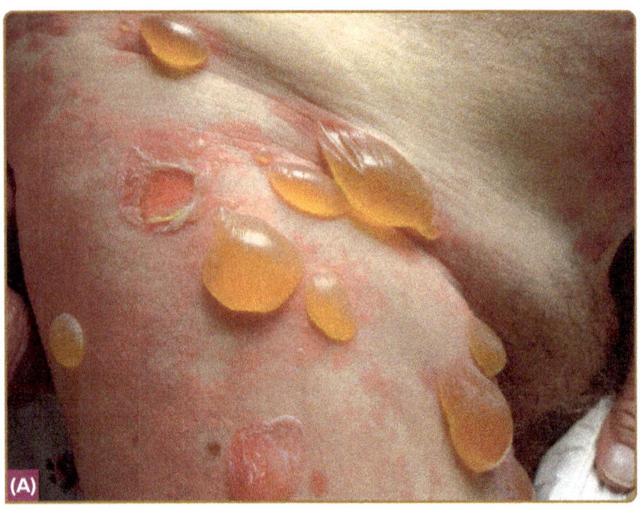

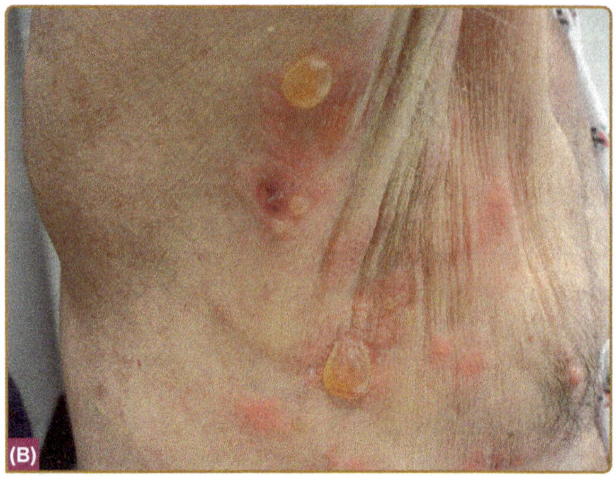

Bullous pemphigoid. (A) Large, tense bullae and erythematous patches studded of small vesicles on the thighs and lower legs. **(B)** Urticarial lesions of bullous pemphigoid with overlying tense vesicles and bullae in the axilla.

Microscopically, fully developed lesions of BP are characterized by the formation of subepidermal blisters. The blisters are usually accompanied by moderate to dense dermal infiltrates of lymphocytes, numerous eosinophils, and occasional neutrophils, referred toas **"cell rich" BP**. However, occasionally cases of **"cell poor" BP** with only sparse infiltrates may occur and are present clinically with little erythema, making distinction from **epidermolysis bullosa acquisita** very difficult.

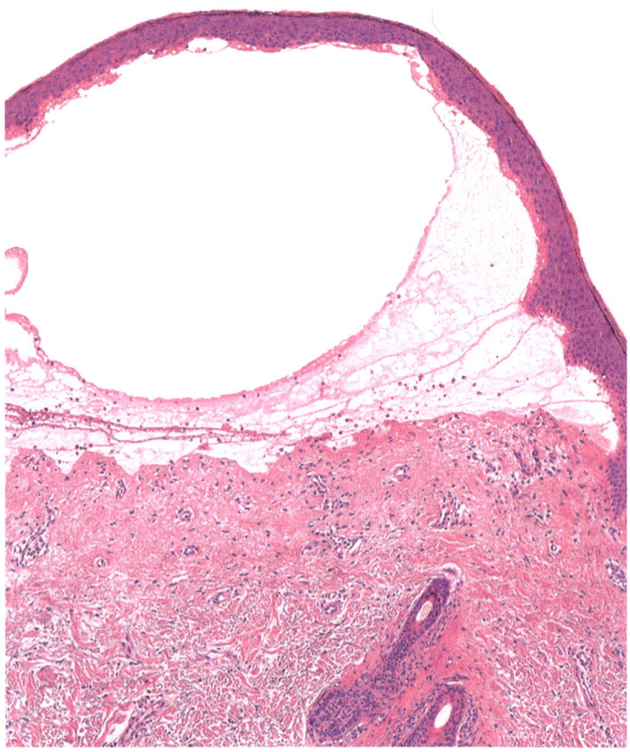

Cell-poor bullous pemphigoid displaying a subepidermal blister containing fibrin and few inflammatory cells.

Plasma, fibrin, and inflammatory cells are usually present within the blister cavity. The epidermis above the blister is flattened along its base and may be necrotic. In **cell-rich BP**, the infiltrate is usually present at the base and at the sides of the blister. Sometimes the infiltrate extends into the deep dermis. In some cases of cell-rich BP, neutrophils may dominate in the infiltrate and can be located along the dermal-epidermal junction, which usually shows vacuolar degeneration. The neutrophils may also collect in the dermal papillae, resulting in papillary neutrophilic abscesses similar to those seen in **dermatitis herpetiformis**. Early **urticarial lesions of BP** are characterized by a superficial perivascular and interstitial infiltrate of lymphocytes, numerous eosinophils, and variable neutrophils. Eosinophils and neutrophils may be observed in the epidermis and at the dermal-epidermal junction, which usually shows vacuolar degeneration. Eosinophilic or neutrophilic spongiosis, or a combination of both, may also be present. On immunomapping using antibodies to type IV collagen, the blister in BP is located within the lamina lucida.

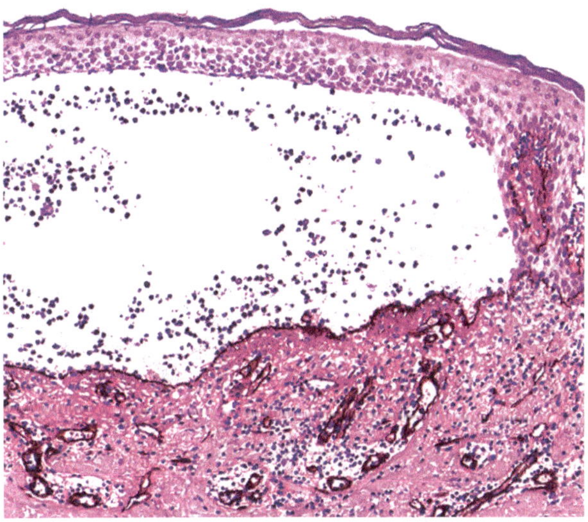

Epitope mapping (using antibodies against type IV collagen) in a cell-rich bullous lesion of bullous pemphigoid. There is staining along the floor of the blister cavity therefore the plane of cleavage is located within the lamina lucida region.

Direct immunofluorescence (DIF) on clinically normal appearing, perilesional skin characteristically shows linear deposits of IgG and C3 along the BM zone. Indirect immunofluorescence (IIF) examination with patients' sera applied to normal human skin as a substrate demonstrates circulating IgG antibodies to proteins of the BM zone in 65% to 80% of the cases with active disease. The **salt-split skin technique** may be applied to both direct and indirect immunofluorescence tests. This technique requires the incubation of skin with 1 M sodium chloride at 4°C for 72 hours, resulting in cleavage between the lamina lucida and the remainder of the epidermal basement membrane. In regard to DIF, this step is usually performed after IgG and C3 have been confirmed along the dermal-epidermal junction. In regard to IIF, patient serum may be applied to salt-treated normal control skin, and will reveal an identical localization of deposition. Both tests will reveal localization of the BP antigen to the roof of the artificially induced blister, whereas the **epidermolysis bullosa acquisita** antigen is located in its base. Although a properly done saline split-skin procedure is very valuable methodology, it is tedious, which explains why it is routinely used only in a few laboratories. However, on occasion, the IgG deposits may also be detected on the dermal side or even on the dermal and epidermal sides of the split. In such cases, Western blot and ELISA may be used to antibodies recognizing **BPAG1** and/or **BPAG2**.

In regard to the differential diagnosis, **epidermolysis bullosa acquisita (EBA)** may be indistinguishable from **bullous pemphigoid** on clinical and histologic grounds and on routine direct immunofluorescence of intact (nonbullous) skin. In the routine laboratory setting, the differential diagnosis hinges on direct immunofluorescence studies performed on salt-split skin. IgG is deposited on the floor of the blister in epidermolysis bullosa acquisita and localizes almost exclusively to the roof of the blister in bullous pemphigoid. The more specialized techniques that differentiate between the two entities, such as immunoblotting, immunoprecipitation, and immunoelectron microscopy, are limited to few facilities. The histopathologic alterations and direct immunofluorescence findings in **cicatricial pemphigoid** are the same as those seen in **bullous pemphigoid**. Clinical features usually differentiate the two diseases. The usual variant of cicatricial pemphigoid affects almost exclusively the mucous membranes as opposed to bullous pemphigoid that mainly involves the skin. Direct immunofluorescence performed on salt-split skin is of little help as cicatricial pemphigoid is a heterogeneous disease on the molecular level and the majority of antigens targeted by the autoantibody localize to the roof of the blister as in bullous pemphigoid.

The histopathological differential diagnosis also includes **herpes gestationis**. This entity is best distinguished by the clinical presentation. Direct immunofluorescence may be of some help: C3 is deposited in a linear fashion along the dermal-epidermal junction in nearly 100% of cases of **herpes gestationis and bullous pemphigoid**. IgG, in contrast, can be seen in 60% to 80% of cases of bullous pemphigoid but only in 30% of patients with herpes gestations. On histology, the presence of necrotic basal keratinocytes may also favor a diagnosis of herpes gestationis over bullous pemphigoid. Occasional cases of **dermatitis herpetiformis** and **linear IgA dermatosis** may have increased numbers of eosinophils. Conversely, occasional cases of bullous pemphigoid may display increased numbers of neutrophils. In these situations, direct immunofluorescence is probably the easiest way to distinguish these entities. Other conditions, which may give rise to a subepidermal blister with abundant eosinophils, include **bullous arthropod bite reaction** and **bullous drug eruption. Bullous arthropod bite reactions** tend to have an inflammatory infiltrate, which is more intense, extends deeper into the reticular dermis and subcutaneous fat, and may have eosinophils individually dispersed between collagen bundles. **Bullous drug eruptions** may also have a deeper infiltrate, but can be histopathologically indistinguishable from bullous pemphigoid. Bullous arthropod bite reactions and bullous drug eruptions will be negative, or demonstrate only nonspecific features of vascular leakage on direct immunofluorescence examination. Lesions of cell-poor bullous pemphigoid must be distinguished from each of the entities described as subepidermal blisters with minimal inflammation. These distinctions are best made on the basis of clinical and immunologic methods.

Table 3-23A. Bullous Pemphigoid

Clinical Features
- Usually elderly patients
- Tense blisters on erythematous base
- Blisters remain intact
- Predilection for extremities
- Mucosal surfaces can be involved

Histopathologic Features
- Subepidermal blister
- Scarce or moderate to dense infiltrate of lymphocytes, eosinophils, and/or neutrophils, or perivascular and interstitial infiltrate of lymphocytes, eosinophils, and sometimes neutrophils
- No necrosis of overlying epidermis

Laboratory Evaluation
- Blister mapping using antibodies against type IV collagen
- Intralamina lucida blister
- DIF examination
- Perilesional intact human skin:
- Linear deposits of IgG and C3 along the BM zone
- Perilesional salt-split skin:
- IgG deposits, along the epidermal, dermal, or both sides of the split
- IIF examination
- Linear deposits of IgG along the BM zone in most cases
- ELISA test
- Circulating IgG antibodies to BPAG1 and/or BPAG2
- Western blot
- Circulating IgG antibodies to 180- and/or 230-kDa protein bands

Differential Diagnosis

Cell-poor bullous pemphigoid
- Classical epidermolysis bullosa acquisita
- Toxic epidermal necrolysis
- Junctional epidermolysis bullosa
- Dystrophic epidermolysis bullosa
- Porphyria cutanea tarda
- Pseudoporphyria

Cell-rich bullous pemphigoid with numerous eosinophils
- Inflammatory epidermolysis bullosa acquisita
- Linear IgA disease
- Herpes gestationis
- Cicatricial pemphigoid
- Bullous drug eruption

Cell-rich bullous pemphigoid with numerous neutrophils
- Inflammatory epidermolysis bullosa acquisita
- Linear IgA disease
- Dermatitis herpetiformis
- Bullous systemic lupus erythematosus

Bullous pemphigoid, urticarial stage
- Urticarial stage of intraepidermal autoimmune bullous disease
- Urticarial stage of inflammatory EBA
- Linear IgA disease
- Herpes gestationis
- Drug reaction
- Insect bite

ANSWER 3-24: A.

Herpes gestationis (HG), also known as **pemphigoid gestationis**, is an acquired, autoimmune, subepidermal blistering disease that develops in association with pregnancy (Table 3-24A). It is estimated to occur in 1 of 3000 to 1 of 10000 pregnancies and usually begins in the second or third trimester. However, it may occur at any time during pregnancy or even in the postpartum period. In rare cases HG may develop in association with trophoblastic tumors such as molar pregnancies and choriocarcinoma. Clinically, patients present with severely pruritic, erythematous, urticarial papules and plaques. Occasionally, blisters develop and are usually arranged in a herpetiform pattern. Lesions of HG usually begin on the abdomen, with a predilection for the periumbilical region. As the disease evolves, the blisters spread peripherally and may become generalized. The lesions resolve within weeks or months and subside at the end of pregnancy; however, many patients may experience exacerbation of skin lesions immediately or shortly after delivery. Recurrence of HG may occur with resumption of menstruation, on administration of oral contraceptives, or within subsequent pregnancies.

Microscopically, lesions of HG are similar to **cell-rich bullous pemphigoid (BP)** with subepidermal blisters and dermal infiltrates of lymphocytes, numerous eosinophils, and occasional neutrophils. The blister usually contains plasma, fibrin, and inflammatory cells (lymphocytes, eosinophils, and sometimes also neutrophils). Urticarial lesions of HG are also histopathologically similar to those of BP.

Unlike BP, direct immunofluorescence of perilesional, clinically normal-appearing skin shows linear basement membrane zone deposits of C3 in 100% of the cases and IgG in only 27% of the cases. Salt-split skin assessment will reveal immunoreactant localization to the epidermal side of cleavage. Unlike BP, circulating antibodies in HG are mainly directed against **BPAG2** and, in rare cases, against **BPAG1**. These circulating autoantibodies can be detected by IIF testing in about 21% of the patients with normal human skin as a substrate. The circulating IgG antibodies in HG are of IgG1 and IgG3 classes and have the ability to fix normal human complement to the basement membrane zone of normal human skin. These circulating IgG antibodies are called HG factor and can be detected by the **complement fixation assay. Complement fixation assay** is more sensitive than conventional IIF and is performed by incubating the test serum with normal human skin, followed by normal human complement, and then a fluorescein-conjugated antibody specific for the complement. By complement fixation assay, circulating IgG antibodies are detected in 91% of HG patients. The circulating IgG antibodies in HG can also be detected by ELISA using recombinant proteins of BPAG1 and BPAG2.

Herpes Gestationis (Pemphigoid Gestationis)

Easy as "1, 2, 3, 4"

1. IgG**1** (fixes complement)
2. BPAG**2** (NC16A domain)
3. Linear C**3**; HLADR**3** association
4. HLADR**4** association

The histopathological differential diagnosis includes **bullous pemphigoid, bullous arthropod bite, bullous drug eruption,** and **pruritic urticarial papules and plaques of pregnancy (PUPPP).** On histologic sections, the presence of individually necrotic keratinocytes would favor **herpes gestationis** over **bullous pemphigoid**, but in most cases distinction relies on the clinical setting as well as differences in immunologic findings. **Bullous arthropod bite reactions** usually have a denser infiltrate, which extends deeper into the dermis. Direct immunofluorescence examinations are invariably negative for immune complexes in **bullous arthropod bite reactions** and **bullous drug eruptions.** Subepidermal blisters are not seen in **PUPPP**, but in some cases of **pemphigoid gestationis**, eosinophilic spongiosis without fully formed blisters may be present. In these cases, the histopathologic features of these two entities may be identical. The clinical features are most often different, and pruritic urticarial papules and plaques of pregnancy are always negative for linear C3 and IgG on direct immunofluorescence examination.

Table 3-24A. Herpes Gestationis

Clinical Features
Uncommon
Usually in second or third trimesters of pregnancy
Recurs with subsequent pregnancies
Most lesions on trunk and extremities
Newborn may have blisters
Mucosal lesions uncommon
Histopathologic Features
Subepidermal blister with sparse or moderate to dense infiltrate of lymphocytes, eosinophils, and/or neutrophils *or*
Perivascular and interstitial infiltrate of lymphocytes, eosinophils, and sometimes neutrophils
Papillary dermal edema
Rare necrotic keratinocytes
Laboratory Evaluation
Blister mapping using antibodies against type IV collagen
Intralamina lucida blister
DIF examination
Perilesional intact human skin:
Linear deposits of C3, IgG along the BM zone
Perilesional salt-split skin:
C3, IgG deposits on the epidermal sides of the split
Complement fixation assay
Detection of HG factor
ELISA test
Circulating IgG antibodies to BPAG1 or BPAG2
Western blot
Circulating IgG antibodies to 180- or 230-kDa protein bands
Differential Diagnosis
Blistering lesion of herpes gestationis
Cell-rich bullous pemphigoid with numerous eosinophils
Inflammatory epidermolysis bullosa acquisita
Linear IgA disease
Cicatricial pemphigoid
Bullous drug reaction
Bullous arthropod bite reaction
Urticarial lesion of herpes gestationis
Urticarial stage of intraepidermal autoimmune bullous diseases
Urticarial stage of inflammatory EBA, linear IgA disease, BP
Pruritic urticarial papules and plaques of pregnancy
Drug reaction
Arthropod bite reaction

ANSWER 3-25: D.

Lichen planus pemphigoides (LPPe) is a rare, acquired, autoimmune subepidermal blistering disease characterized by the simultaneous occurrence of lichen planus lesions and blisters (Table 3-25A). This form of blistering is different than the small **Max-Joseph spaces** seen microscopically in **classic lichen planus.** Circulating autoantibodies in sera from patients with LPPe recognize in most instances BPAG2 and in few cases a 200-kDa protein that remains uncharacterized. Epitope mapping using BPAG2 fusion proteins show that **LPPe** sera and **BP** sera react with different epitopes of **BPAG2.** These results suggest that LPPe is a distinct disease and not a coexistence of bullous pemphigoid (BP) and lichen planus, as previously suggested.

Clinically, there are typical lesions of lichen planus as well as tense blisters that surmount lesions of lichen planus or develop in clinically normal skin. Extremities, trunk, and oral mucosa are the sites of predilection. Like bullous pemphigoid, lesions are capable of regeneration without scar formation. The age of onset ranges between 9 and 85 years, with a mean age of 46 years. There is no race predominance.

The histopathological findings in LPPe are lesion dependent. Blisters on clinically normal skin will display a subepidermal blister with perivascular and interstitial infiltrate of lymphocytes and eosinophils, identical to cell-rich bullous pemphigoid. Occasionally, the accompanying infiltrate is sparse, as in cases of cell-poor bullous pemphigoid. A blister forming on lichen planus lesions will display a subepidermal vesicle as well as typical histopathological changes of lichen planus, namely compact stratum corneum, acanthosis, hypergranulosis, and a band-like infiltrate of lymphocytes. The blister of LPPe (with or without concurrent changes of lichen planus) immunohistochemically stained for type IV collagen will reveal localization of a linear band to the base of the blister cavity, confining that the plane of cleavage is within the lamina lucida. Immunofluorescence studies reveal findings identical to BP. Direct immunofluorescence (DIF) of perilesional skin shows in all patients with LPPe linear IgG deposits along the BM zone. On NaCl-split perilesional skin, the deposits are located on the epidermal side of the split. Indirect immunofluorescence (IIF) with sera of LPPe using human skin (intact or NaCl split) as a substrate shows, in about 64% of the reported cases, circulating IgG autoantibodies to proteins of the basement membrane zone. Via ELISA testing these autoantibodies predominantly recognize BPAG2.

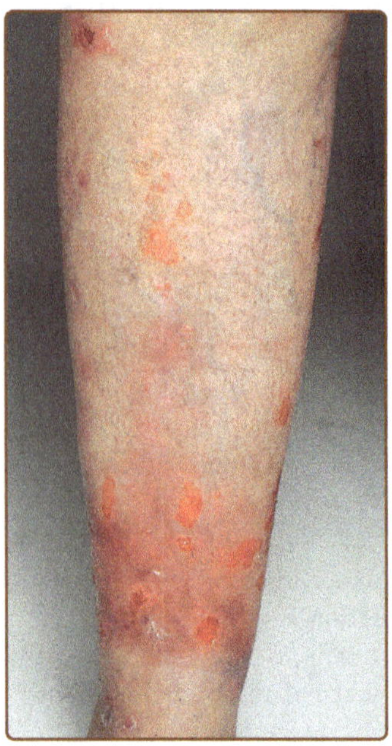

Lichen planus pemphigoides. Lichenoid maculopapular erythema, erosions, and bullae with direct immunofluorescence showing features of bullous pemphigoid. Indirect immunofluorescence was also positive. (Reproduced, with permission, from Goldsmith LA, Katz SI, Gilchrest BA, Paller AS, Leffell DJ, Wolff K, eds. *Fitzpatrick's Dermatology in General Medicine.* 8th ed. New York, NY: McGraw-Hill Education; 2012.)

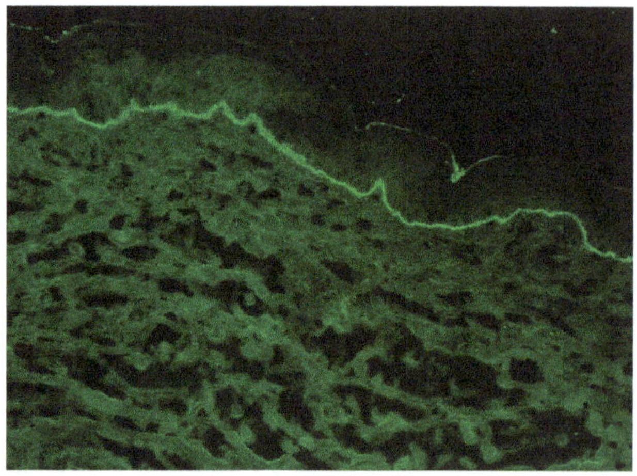

Lichen planus pemphigoides. DIF of perilesional clinically normal-appearing skin revealing linear homogenous deposition of IgG along the basement membrane zone.

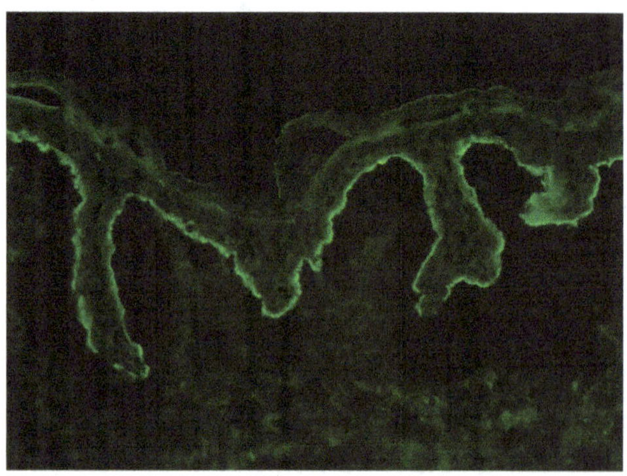

Lichen planus pemphigoides, Salt-split skin. DIF using salt-split, perilesional, clinically normal-appearing skin reveals linear homogenous IgG deposits along the epidermal side of the split, confirming a cleavage plane within the lamina lucida.

Table 3-25A. Lichen Planus Pemphigoides

Clinical Features
Adults, rarely in children
Lesions indistinguishable from lichen planus, ie, flat-topped violaceous papules with whitish scale
Tense blisters on normal-appearing skin or surmounting preexistent lesions of lichen planus
Histopathologic Features
Subepidermal blister with sparse or moderate to dense infiltrate of lymphocytes, eosinophils, and/or neutrophils or
Subepidermal as well as typical histopathological changes of lichen planus
Laboratory Evaluation
Blister mapping using antibodies against type IV collagen
Intralamina lucida blister
DIF examination
Perilesional intact human skin:
Linear deposits of IgG along the BM zone
Perilesional salt-split skin:
IgG deposits on the epidermal side of the split
ELISA test
Circulating IgG antibodies to BPAG2
Western blot
Circulating IgG antibodies to 180-kDa protein band
Differential Diagnosis
Lichenoid lesion
Lichen planus
Lichenoid drug eruption
Bullous lesion
Inflammatory epidermolysis bullosa acquisita
Linear IgA disease
Herpes gestationis
Cicatricial pemphigoid
Bullous drug eruption

ANSWER 3-26: E.

Cicatricial pemphigoid (CP) is a rare, heterogeneous, acquired, autoimmune, subepithelial blistering disease of mucous membranes and/or skin (Table 3-26B). A variety of different autoantigens have been recognized by autoantibodies from patients, suggesting that cicatricial pemphigoid is not a single nosologic entity but rather a disease phenotype. It affects mainly elderly persons and occurs in females more than in males.

No ethnical or geographic predominance is evident. The clinical spectrum of CP varies widely. It affects squamous mucosa, especially that of the oral cavity (85%), conjunctiva (65%), nasopharynx (20%), genitalia (20%), larynx (8%), esophagus (4%), and anus (3%). The skin is reportedly involved in 25% of the cases. The primary lesion of CP is a tense blister that on rupture heals slowly and usually with scar formation.

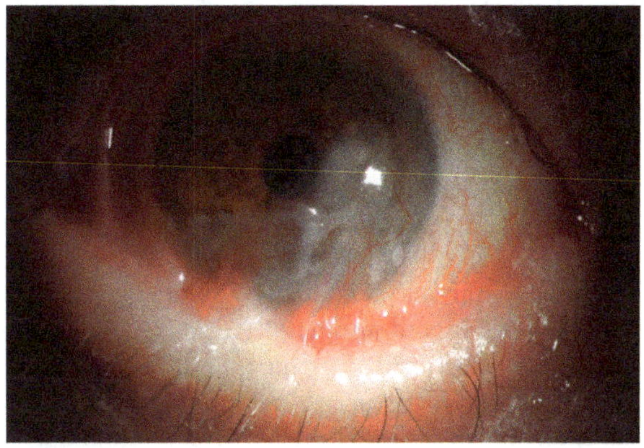

Advanced ocular cicatricial pemphigoid. There is symblepharon (adherence between the palpebral conjunctiva and the bulbar conjunctiva) and opacification and neovascularization of the inferior cornea. (Reproduced, with permission, from Imboden JB, Hellmann DB, Stone JH, eds. *Current Medical Diagnosis & Treatment: Rheumatology.* 3rd ed. New York, NY: McGraw-Hill Education; 2013.)

Microscopically, three histological patterns can be defined. In the first pattern, there is a subepidermal blister and a lymphocytic infiltrate at its base and sides. Eosinophils and occasionally neutrophils may be present. In oral and genital lesions, plasma cells are usually present. In the second pattern, there is a subepidermal blister, fibrosis, and lymphocytic infiltrates with eosinophils and sometimes also neutrophils. In the third pattern, the changes of the epithelium are similar to that seen in lichen planus. This histopathological pattern is observed only in oral and genital lesions.

DIF examination using perilesional clinically normal-appearing skin or mucosa shows linear IgG and/or C3 deposits along the basement membrane zone in 80% to 100% of cases. IgA, IgM, and/or fibrin are found in some patients. Patients with both IgG and IgA antibasement membrane autoantibodies appear to have a worse prognosis as defined by requirements for medications to control disease as well as overall clinical severity score. Indirect immunofluorescence (IIF) examination with CP patient sera demonstrates circulating IgG antibodies to the BM zone. These antibodies are usually present in a very low titer. The sensitivity of IIF on using conventional substrates (monkey esophagus, normal human skin) is reportedly very low (10%-36%). When using 1 M NaCl-split normal human skin, the sensitivity of IIF in CP markedly improves. The deposition of IgG in CP may be limited to the epidermal or dermal side of the split or even to both sides. In fact, this heterogeneity in autoantibody binding patterns was one of the first clues that cicatricial pemphigoid is a disease phenotype that is associated with different autoantigens. Western blot or immunoprecipitation examinations as well as ELISA-testing using recombinant fusion proteins

Table 3-26A. Antigenic Targets in Cicatricial Pemphigoid

The antigen (its molecular weight)
1. BPAG1 (230 kDa)
2. BPAG2 (180 kDa)
3. α_3 Chain of laminin 5 and laminin 6 (145 kDa)
4. β-Integrin subunit (205 kDa)
5. α-Integrin subunit (130 kDa)

of the basement membrane zone identify the target autoantigen. **Bullous pemphigoid antigen 2 (BPAG2)** appears to represent a major cicatricial pemphigoid autoantigen, and its location of cleavage appears to possibly affect whether lesions regenerate or heal with scarring. Other autoantigens of particular interest include **laminin 332, integrin subunit β_4, integrin subunit α_6,** and **bullous pemphigoid antigen 1 (BPAG1).** The best characterized IgA autoantigen linked to the cicatricial pemphigoid phenotype is the **ectodomain (FAD-1) of BPAG2** (Table 3-26A). While autoantibodies directed against some of these autoantigens have been shown to be pathogenic in vivo, it is conceivable that other mechanisms may contribute to the pathogenesis of cicatricial pemphigoid. For example, recent studies have demonstrated high stromal expression of IL-13 in $CD3^+$ T cells from patients with ocular cicatricial pemphigoid and that these cells may contribute both profibrotic and proinflammatory stimuli to conjunctival fibroblasts. Additionally, the IgG in CP is predominantly of the IgG4 subclass, which is a subclass associated with other fibrosing conditions.

The differential diagnosis includes **linear IgA disease (LAD), epidermolysis bullosa acquisita (EBA), bullous systemic lupus (BSLE),** and **bullous pemphigoid (BP). Linear IgA disease** and **mucosal epidermolysis bullosa acquisita** may occasionally present with mucosal involvement only and **bullous systemic lupus** may extensively involve the oral mucosa. Therefore, histopathology, immunofluorescence, and possibly Western blot and/or ELISA are needed to establish a definitive diagnosis. In regard to histopathology,lesions that are intensely inflammatory, the differential diagnosis would include linear **IgA bullous dermatosis,** which is not associated with dermal scarring. **Dermatitis herpetiformis** could also be in the differential diagnosis, but usually has neutrophils, which are more localized to dermal papillae than is seen in **cicatricial pemphigoid.**

Bullous lupus could appear quite similar to **cicatricial pemphigoid** on routine histology. The differences in direct immunofluorescence staining patterns are helpful in discriminating between these diseases. **Epidermolysis bullosa acquisita** would also be in the differential diagnosis and can also produce dermal scarring. Direct immunofluorescence on salt-split skin probably offers the most reliable method for distinguishing between these two entities.

Table 3-26B. Cicatricial Pemphigoid

Clinical Features
Elderly patients
More common in women
Vesiculobullous eruption primarily involves mucous membranes
Extensive scarring
Skin involvement in only 25% of cases
Histopathologic Features
Subepidermal blister
Moderate to dense infiltrate of lymphocytes, eosinophils, and/or neutrophils
With or without fibrosis *or*
Subepidermal blister
Band-like infiltrate of lymphocytes and eosinophils (occasionally also neutrophils and plasma cells)
Lichen planus–like changes of the epithelium
Fibrosis
Laboratory Evaluation
Epitope mapping using antibodies against type IV collagen
Intralamina lucida blister
DIF examination
Perilesional intact human skin:
Linear deposits of IgG, C3 along the BM zone
Perilesional salt-split skin:
IgG deposits, along the epidermal, dermal, or both sides of the split
ELISA test
Circulating IgG antibodies to BPAG1 and/or BPAG2; at present ELISA test for other proteins of the BMZ is not available
Western blot
Circulating IgG antibodies to 180-, 230-, 145-, 205-, or 130-kDa protein bands
Differential Diagnosis
Bullous pemphigoid
Linear IgA disease
Epidermolysis bullosa acquisita
Dystrophic epidermolysis bullosa
Bullous drug eruption
Dermatitis herpetiformis
Bullous lupus erythematosus
Epidermolysis bullosa acquisita
Sweet syndrome

ANSWER 3-27: B.

Dermatitis herpetiformis (DH) is an acquired, pruritic, autoimmune, subepidermal blistering disease characterized by IgA deposits in the dermal papillae (Table 3-27A). It occurs in males more than in females and usually begins in the second to fourth decade. It can, however, commence at any age. DH affects mainly Caucasians and is rarely seen in African Americans or Asians. The condition is clinically characterized by erythematous papules, urticarial plaques, papulovesicles, vesicles, and rarely bullae, either isolated or in herpetiform groupings. The lesions are intensely pruritic and often heal with scarring. The lesions are symmetrically distributed and appear mainly on elbows, knees, nape, scapular region, sacral region, and buttocks. All patients with DH have **gluten-sensitive enteropathy** indistinguishable from **celiac disease.** However, only 10% have clinical manifestations of intestinal disease. Choices A, C, D, and E describe the clinical presentations **of linear IgA disease, classic variant of epidermolysis bullosa acquisita (EBA), inflammatory variant of EBA,** and **allergic contact dermatitis,** respectively.

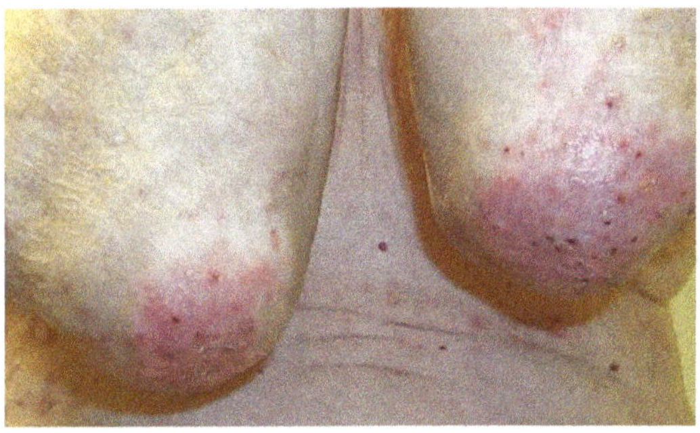

Dermatitis herpetiformis manifested by pruritic, grouped vesicles in a typical location. The vesicles are often excoriated and may occur on knees, buttocks, elbows, and posterior scalp. (Reproduced with permission from Kasper DL, Fauci A, Hauser SL et al: Harrison's Principles of Internal Medicine. 19th ed. New York, NY: McGraw-Hill Education; 2015.)

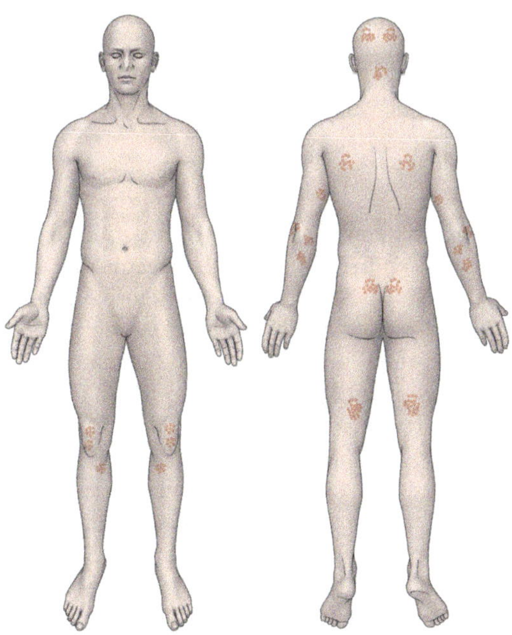

Dermatitis herpetiformis Pattern of distribution. (Reproduced, with permission, from Wolff K, Johnson RA, Saavedra AP. *Fitzpatrick's Color Atlas and Synopsis of Clinical Dermatology*. 7th ed. New York, NY: McGraw-Hill Education; 2013.)

In regard to the microscopic findings, early lesions exhibit superficial perivascular infiltrates of lymphocytes and neutrophils and an edematous papillary dermis. The neutrophils are also present in the epidermis and at the dermoepidermal junction, which usually shows vacuolar degeneration. With evolution of the lesions, neutrophils collect in some of the dermal papillae, and fibrin often appears at their tips. Eosinophils may also be present in the dermal infiltrate and in the papillary abscesses. With further lesional evolution, a subepidermal blister develops. The blister usually contains serum, fibrin, neutrophils, and eosinophils.

The dermis displays perivascular and interstitial infiltrates of lymphocytes, neutrophils, and eosinophils, the latter often numerous. The infiltrate may be dense and deep. At the sides of the blister, neutrophilic abscesses in the dermal papillae and subepidermal clefts are usually present. On immunomapping using antibodies to type IV collagen, the blister plane of DH is located in the lamina lucida.

Direct immunofluorescence (DIF) examination shows chunky granular IgA deposits in the dermal papillae. In some patients, linear IgA deposits occur concomitantly along the basement membrane zone. Indirect immunofluorescence (IIF) examination of DH patient sera reveals no evidence for circulating autoantibodies against proteins of keratinocytes or the basement membrane zone. However, patients with DH have IgA antibodies to **gliadin** (a component of gluten) and **endomysium** (connective tissue surrounding smooth muscles). The antiendomysial antibodies target **tissue transglutaminase,** which was recently identified as the autoantigen of celiac disease. IgA antibodies to tissue transglutaminase (detected via ELISA) serve nowadays as the serological diagnostic marker for DH and celiac disease.

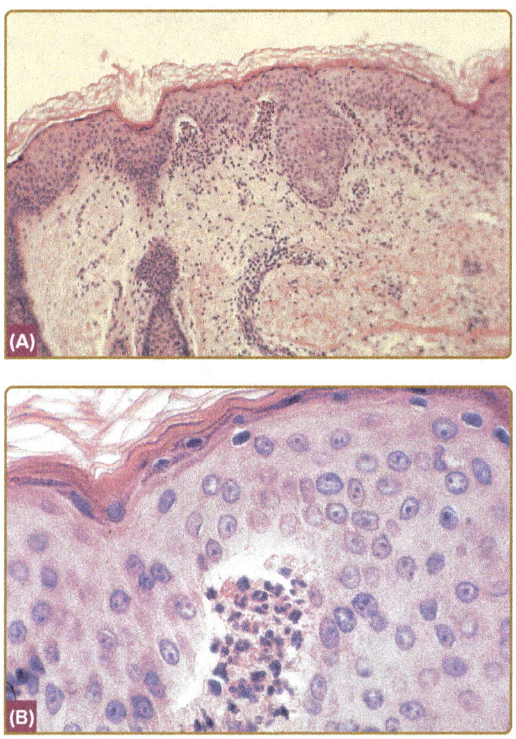

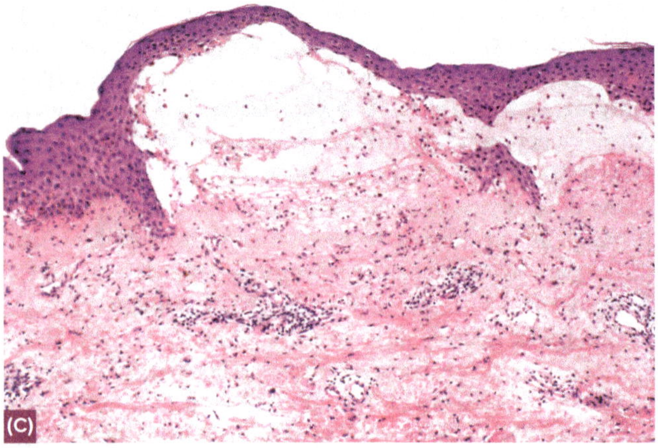

Dermatitis herpetiformis. Biopsy of an early lesion showing dermal papillary collections of neutrophils and eosinophils and subepidermal vesiculation at low **(A)** and high **(B)** magnification. **(C)** There is a subepidermal blister, which contains neutrophils, eosinophils, and fibrin. At the sides of the blister, there are papillary neutrophilic abscesses and subepidermal clefts. The dermis contains perivascular and interstitial infiltrates of lymphocytes, neutrophils, and eosinophils. (Parts **(A)** and **(B)** reproduced, with permission, from Goldsmith LA, Katz SI, Gilchrest BA, Paller AS, Leffell DJ, Wolff K, eds. *Fitzpatrick's Dermatology in General Medicine.* 8th ed. New York, NY: McGraw-Hill Education; 2012.)

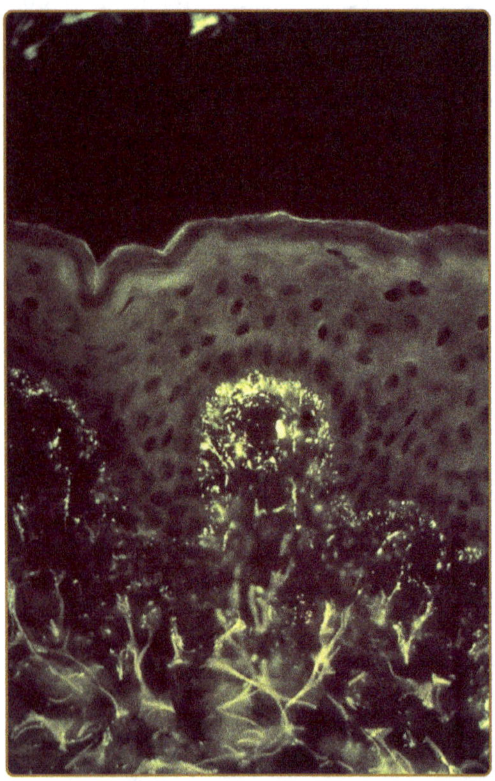

Dermatitis herpetiformis. Direct immunofluorescence showing granular dermal papillary deposits of immunoglobulin A (IgA). (Reproduced, with permission, from Goldsmith LA, Katz SI, Gilchrest BA, Paller AS, Leffell DJ, Wolff K, eds. *Fitzpatrick's Dermatology in General Medicine.* 8th ed. New York, NY: McGraw-Hill Education; 2012.)

Table 3-27A. Dermatitis Herpetiformis

Clinical Features
Intensely pruritic
Usual onset in early adulthood
Symmetrical vesicles on extensor surfaces of extremities
Mucous membrane involvement uncommon
Gluten-sensitive enteropathy associated with HLA-A1, HLA-B8, HLA-DR3
Histopathologic Features
Depends on the stage of the lesions
Subepidermal blister
Neutrophilic microabscesses in papillary dermal tips
Lymphocytic infiltrate around superficial vascular plexus
Laboratory Evaluation
Epitope mapping using antibodies against type IV collagen
Intralamina lucida blister
DIF examination (using perilesional, normal-appearing skin)
Granular IgA, C3 deposits in the dermal papillae *or*
Linear IgA deposits along the basement membrane zone, as well as granular IgA deposits in the dermal papillae
ELISA test
Circulating IgA antibodies to tissue transglutaminase
Differential Diagnosis
Linear IgA bullous dermatosis
Epidermolysis bullosa acquisita
Bullous lupus erythematosus
Cicatricial pemphigoid
Bullous pemphigoid
Pustular drug eruption

The histological differential diagnosis includes **linear IgA bullous dermatosis, epidermolysis bullosa acquisita, bullous lupus erythematosus, cicatricial pemphigoid, pustular drug eruptions (AGEP), subacute eczematous dermatitis,** and occasional cases of **bullous pemphigoid. Dermatitis herpetiformis** is the only one of these entities in which the neutrophils tend to aggregate within papillary dermal tips. The blister spaces tend to be smaller in dermatitis herpetiformis than in the other entities. **Epidermolysis bullosa acquisita** is less inflammatory in many cases, and **bullous pemphigoid** demonstrates a predominantly eosinophilic infiltrate in most cases. **Pustular drug eruptions** may exhibit papillary dermal collections of neutrophils similar to dermatitis herpetiformis, but in contrast to dermatitis herpetiformis also show intraepidermal microabscesses. The serological detection of antiendomysial antibodies should allow distinction of DH from the other entities and direct immunofluorescence staining patterns will be different for each of the disorders in this differential diagnosis and probably represent the most specific means of establishing a definitive diagnosis.

ANSWER 3-28: A.

Chronic bullous disease of childhood (**CBDC**) is a rare blistering disease that occurs predominantly in children younger than 5 years of age and has similar immunofluorescent and histopathological findings as **linear IgA bullous dermatosis (LAD)**. In fact, recent studies have demonstrated that some patients with CBDC and linear IgA dermatosis represent different presentations of the same disease process (Table 3-28B). Both CBDC and LAD are acquired, autoimmune, subepithelial blistering disease of the skin and/or mucous membranes characterized by the presence of linear IgA deposits along the basement membrane zone. CBDC presents with tense bullae, often in perineum and perioral regions, giving a "cluster of jewels" or "string of pearls" appearance. New lesions sometimes appear around the periphery of previous lesions with a collarette of blisters. The clinical picture of LAD is more heterogeneous and may clinically simulate **bullous pemphigoid, dermatitis herpetiformis, erythema multiforme, erythema annulare centrifugum,** or **Lyell syndrome (TEN).** In both conditions, early stages of the disease present with urticarial patches and plaques. Involvement of the mucous membranes, especially that of the oral cavity and conjunctiva, is not uncommon and may be the only presenting manifestations. A **drug-induced form of linear IgA disease** has been associated with the administration of vancomycin.

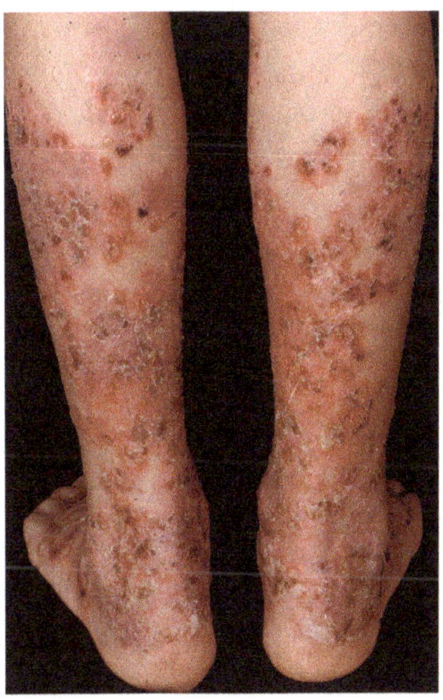

Linear IgA dermatosis. There are multiple grouped, confluent vesicles, bullae, and crusts on an urticarial and erythematous base. (Reproduced, with permission, from Wolff K, Johnson RA, Saavedra AP. *Fitzpatrick's Color Atlas and Synopsis of Clinical Dermatology.* 7th ed. New York, NY: McGraw-Hill Education; 2013.)

Microscopically, fully developed lesions reveal subepidermal blisters accompanied by infiltrates of lymphocytes, eosinophils, and neutrophils. The infiltrate is superficially situated at the sides and base of the blister. In most of the cases, neutrophils predominate over eosinophils. They are usually present along the basement membrane zone, which shows vacuolar degeneration. The neutrophils also accumulate in some of the dermal papillae as abscesses resembling those of dermatitis herpetiformis. Mucosal lesions may contain plasma cells. The ocular lesions of LAD are indistinguishable from those of **cicatricial pemphigoid**. Early lesions may demonstrate a dermal urticarial pattern with interstitial neutrophils and eosinophils accompanied by eosinophilic and neutrophilic spongiosis.

Direct immunofluorescence (DIF) examination of perilesional skin or mucosa displays linear IgA deposits along the basement membrane (BM) zone. Indirect immunofluorescence (IIF) examination with patients' sera demonstrates circulating IgA antibodies to proteins of the basement membrane zone. The sensitivity of IIF is 62% with normal human intact skin as substrate and 73% with NaCl-split normal human skin. With NaCl-split skin, the antibodies bind to the epidermal side of the split in most cases. In a few cases they bind to the dermal side, or both, of the split. Western blot or immunoprecipitation examinations, as well as ELISA-testing using recombinant fusion proteins of the basement membrane zone, may define the target autoantigen in LAD, which may include a variety of basement membrane antigens (Table 3-28A).

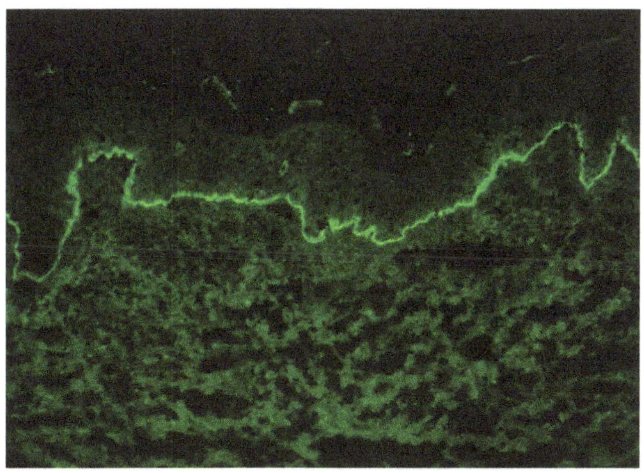

Linear IgA disease. DIF using perilesional, normal-appearing skin. IgA is deposited in a linear fashion along the basement membrane zone.

The major histologic differential diagnosis is **dermatitis herpetiformis.** In the classic situation, dermatitis herpetiformis has a less diffuse and more abscess-like distribution of neutrophils, confined to papillary dermal tips, whereas linear IgA dermatosis and chronic bullous disease of childhood display neutrophils in a more evenly distributed pattern along the dermal-epidermal junction. However, there is great

Table 3-28A. Autoantigens of Linear IgA Disease

ANTIGEN	MOLECULAR WEIGHT
1. BPAG1	230 kDa
2. BPAG2	180 kDa
3. LAD1 (LABD 97) (cleaved ectodomain of BPAG2)	120/97 kDa
4. Ladinin	95 kDa
5. LAD225 (still not characterized)	255 kDa
6. LAD285 (still not characterized)	285 kDa
7. Type VII collagen	290 kDa

Drug-Induced Linear IgA Disease

"SAD VIP CLIPS"

Sulfa
Amiodarone
Diclofenac

Vancomycin
IFN-γ
Penicillin, Phenytoin, Piroxicam

Captopril,
Lithium, Lasix
IL-2
PUVA
Somatostatin

Table 3-28B. Linear IgA Bullous Dermatosis

Clinical Features
- Childhood disease has onset within 5-6 years of birth
- Adult onset in sixth to eighth decades
- Often antecedent infection
- Annular erythematous patches with tense blisters at edges
- Trunk and extremities most commonly affected sites

Histopathologic Features
- Subepidermal blister
- Neutrophils linearly aligned along dermal-epidermal junction
- Papillary dermal edema
- Occasional eosinophils present

Laboratory Evaluation
- Epitope mapping using antibodies against type IV collagen
- Intralamina lucida blister (rarely sublamina densa blister)
- DIF examination
- Perilesional intact human skin:
- Linear deposits of IgA along the BM zone
- Perilesional salt-split skin:
- IgA deposits, along the epidermal, dermal, or both sides of the split
- ELISA test
- Circulating IgG antibodies to BPAG1 and/or BPAG2
- Western blot
- Circulating IgA antibodies to different protein bands

Differential Diagnosis
- Cell-rich bullous pemphigoid
- Inflammatory variant of epidermolysis bullosa acquisita
- Herpes gestationis
- Bullous drug eruption
- Cicatricial pemphigoid
- Dermatitis herpetiformis
- Bullous systemic lupus erythematosus
- Bullous arthropod bite reaction
- Sweet syndrome

overlap in these cases, and frequently, direct immunofluorescence demonstrating a linear versus granular staining pattern with IgA is the only way to distinguish these entities. Clinical parameters such as absent antigliadin and antiendomysial antibodies may further aid in the differential diagnosis. Occasional **arthropod bite reactions** can display neutrophil-predominant infiltrates, and these cases resemble linear IgA dermatosis. The presence of a punctum, or a deep component to the inflammatory infiltrate, as well as a negative or nonspecific direct immunofluorescence study would favor a bite reaction. The neutrophilic infiltrate in **Sweet syndrome** is usually far more florid and diffuse than that seen in linear IgA dermatosis or chronic bullous disease of childhood. In addition, Sweet syndrome is characterized by much more papillary dermal edema. **Bullous lupus erythematosus** can present with a histologic picture similar to linear IgA disease, most notably neutrophils along the dermal epidermal junction, vacuolar alteration of the basement membrane zone, and subepidermal blister formation. Patients with bullous lupus erythematosus have serologic findings of systemic lupus. On direct immunofluorescence, the staining pattern of lupus is granular and band like and is usually observed with several immunoglobulins and not just IgA. **Epidermolysis bullosa acquisita, cicatricial pemphigoid,** and **bullous pemphigoid** may have histologic features similar to linear IgA disease but can be discerned by direct immunofluorescence. Cases with neutrophilic blisters and with linear deposition of IgA and IgG along the dermal-epidermal junction are more problematic. One approach is to classify the disease according to the stronger staining immunoglobulin, that is, as linear IgA disease if

IgA is the predominant immunoglobulin or as bullous pemphigoid when IgG predominates. Some authors accept linear IgA disease as cases with exclusive staining with IgA and classify all others as **bullous pemphigoid** or **epidermolysis bullosa acquisita.**

ANSWER 3-29: E.

This patient has **epidermolysis bullosa acquisita (EBA),** which is an acquired subepidermal autoimmune blistering disease of the skin and/or mucous membranes, which is characterized by the presence of IgG deposits along the basement membrane zone and circulating IgG autoantibodies targeting type VII collagen (Table 3-29A). It affects mainly adults but can also occur in children and even infants. The mean age at onset is 47 years. EBA affects all races and is reported to be slightly more common in females. Clinically, EBA can be divided in three variants: classical, inflammatory, and mucosal. The **classical variant of EBA** is characterized by trauma-induced blisters and erosions on the extensor surface of the limbs. The blisters arise on normal-appearing skin, are tense, clear, or hemorrhagic, and heal with scarring and milia formation.

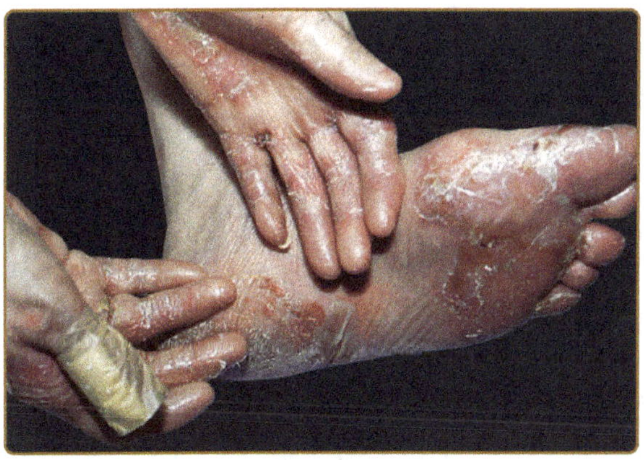

Patient with epidermolysis bullosa acquisita who has severe blistering, erosions, scarring, and milia formation on trauma-prone areas of her skin. This is the classic presentation. (Reproduced, with permission, from Goldsmith LA, Katz SI, Gilchrest BA, Paller AS, Leffell DJ, Wolff K, eds. *Fitzpatrick's Dermatology in General Medicine.* 8th ed. New York, NY: McGraw-Hill Education; 2012.)

The **inflammatory variant of EBA** displays widespread eruptions with tense blisters spontaneously forming on erythematous or nonerythematous skin. These lesions occur on flexural and/or intertriginous areas and tend to heal with less scarring and milia formation. The third variant is **mucosal EBA**, where the lesions are limited to the mucous membranes of the mouth, nose, pharynx, larynx, esophagus, eye, and genitourinary tract.

Histopathologically, lesions of EBA are characterized by formation of subepidermal blisters associated with no or sparse perivascular and interstitial infiltrates of lymphocytes in the upper dermis (**classic variant of EBA**). On occasion, a few

Table 3-29A. Epidermolysis Bullosa Acquisita

Clinical Features
Usually affects middle-aged to elderly adults
Blisters on noninflammatory skin
Scarring and milia
Predilection for trauma-prone sites
Nail dystrophy may be present
Histopathologic Features
Subepidermal blister
Sparse or moderate to dense infiltrates of lymphocytes, eosinophils, and/or neutrophils *or*
Eosinophilic and/or neutrophilic spongiosis
No keratinocyte necrosis
Dermal scarring may be present
Laboratory Evaluation
Epitope mapping using antibodies against type IV collagen
Sublamina densa blister
DIF examination
Perilesional intact human skin:
Linear deposits of IgG, C3 along the BM zone
Perilesional salt-split skin:
IgG deposits, along the dermal side of the split
ELISA test
Circulating IgG antibodies to collagen type VII
Western blot
Circulating IgG antibodies to a 290-kDa protein band
Differential Diagnosis
Classical epidermolysis bullosa acquisita
Cell-poor bullous pemphigoid
Bullous systemic lupus erythematosus
Toxic epidermal necrolysis
Junctional epidermolysis bullosa
Dystrophic epidermolysis bullosa
Porphyria cutanea tarda
Pseudoporphyria
Inflammatory epidermolysis bullosa acquisita
Cell-rich bullous pemphigoid
Linear IgA disease
Herpes gestationis
Cicatricial pemphigoid
Dermatitis herpetiformis
Bullous systemic lupus erythematosus
Bullous drug reaction
Epidermolysis bullosa acquisita (urticarial stage)
Urticarial stage of intraepidermal autoimmune bullous diseases
Urticarial stage of cell-rich bullous pemphigoid
Linear IgA disease
Herpes gestationis
Drug reaction
Arthropod bite reaction

eosinophils and/or neutrophils are present. In the **inflammatory variant of EBA**, the blister is associated with moderately dense lymphocytic infiltrates with eosinophils and neutrophils. Early urticarial lesions of the inflammatory variant are histopathologically indistinguishable from urticarial lesions of other autoimmune blistering diseases, showing perivascular and interstitial infiltrates of lymphocytes, neutrophils, and eosinophils. The eosinophils or the neutrophils may dominate the infiltrate and are present along the dermal-epidermal junction, which displays vacuolar degeneration. Eosinophilic and/or neutrophilic spongiosis may also be present. **Mucosal EBA** has findings similar to those of the inflammatory variant of EBA, although usually the infiltrate is denser and contains plasma cells. In all forms the blisters localize to the sublamina densa and fibrosis, with or without milia, may occur in relapsing lesions.

Direct immunofluorescence (DIF) using perilesional skin or perilesional mucosa displays in all active cases linear deposits of IgG along the basement membrane zone. Using NaCl-split perilesional skin or mucosa, the deposits segregate to the dermal side of the split. Circulating IgG antibodies to proteins of the basement membrane zone occur by IIF testing in about 25% to 50% of the patients with normal human skin or monkey esophagus as substrate. The sensitivity increases markedly with NaCl-split normal skin. The circulating antibodies react by Western blot or immunoprecipitation assay with a 290-kDa protein band which represents type VII collagen. These antibodies also react positively with recombinant fusion protein of type VII collagen by ELISA.

The histopathological differential diagnosis is dependent on the subtype of epidermolysis bullosa acquisita. In **classical EBA** (noninflammatory), the differential diagnosis includes **porphyria cutanea tarda, pseudoporphyria,** and **cell-poor bullous pemphigoid** (choices A, B, and C, respectively). These two conditions can be distinguished from epidermolysis bullosa acquisita on the basis of immunofluorescence staining patterns (requiring salt-split skin to differentiate bullous pemphigoid and epidermolysis bullosa acquisita). **Porphyria cutanea tarda** can be further distinguished with urine, fecal, and blood porphyrin studies.

In the **inflammatory variant of epidermolysis bullosa acquisita** with abundant dermal neutrophils, **bullous lupus erythematosus** is the major differential diagnostic possibility. Bullous lupus erythematosus may display other histologic features of lupus, such as a superficial and deep perivascular and periappendageal lymphocytic infiltrate, but these features are often absent. In fact, the histologic features of epidermolysis acquisita and bullous lupus erythematosus may be indistinguishable. Patients with the latter disease must meet the criteria of the American, Rheumatologic Association for systemic lupus erythematosus. Further, the granular nature of the immunoglobulin deposits seen in lupus erythematosus on direct immunofluorescence (positive lupus band test) often differentiates this entity from the homogenous linear deposits seen in epidermolysis bullosa acquisita.

ANSWER 3-30: C.

This patient has **bullous systemic lupus erythematosus (BSLE),** which is an acquired autoimmune disease characterized by the occurrence of vesiculobullous eruptions, often in a herpetiform arrangement, in patients diagnosed as having SLE by criteria of the American Rheumatism Association (ARA) (Table 3-30A). Similar to **epidermolysis bullosa acquisita**, the lesions are caused by antibodies directed toward type VII collagen of the sublamina densa. It affects mainly adults but may also occur in children. Clinically, there are tense blisters on normal or erythematous skin with a predilection to the trunk and flexural surfaces. Like all cicatricial subepidermal blistering diseases, there is a tendency to form milium cysts. Oral lesions have been frequently observed, and pruritus, which may be severe, has also been reported.

The histopathology of BSLE is similar to that of **dermatitis herpetiformis**, with subepidermal blisters and infiltrates of lymphocytes and numerous neutrophils. In contrast to dermatitis herpetiformis, the infiltrate in BSLE is also present around the hair follicles. Moreover, in BSLE there are interstitial mucin deposits and frequent evidence of **leukocytoclastic vasculitis**. Also in contrast to dermatitis herpetiformis, the blister in BSLE localizes to the sublamina densa region.

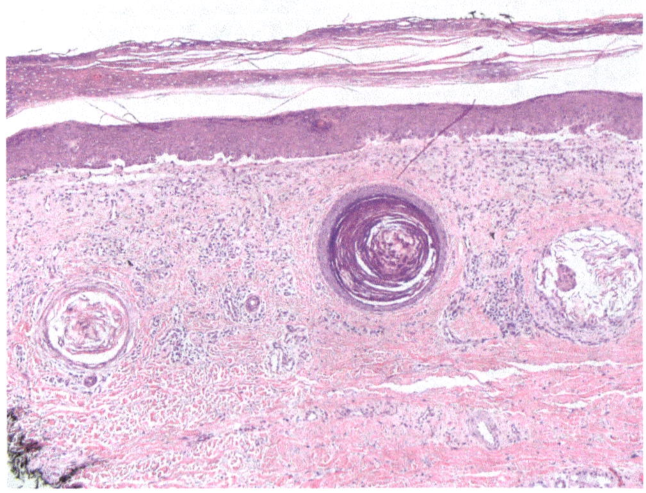

Bullous systemic lupus erythematosus, late stage lesion. There is a subepidermal blister with underlying dermal scar formation and numerous milium cysts.

Direct immunofluorescence (DIF) of perilesional skin displays linear and/or granular deposits of IgG and/or IgA, IgM, and C3 along the basement membrane zone. With NaCl-split perilesional skin, the deposits are located on the dermal side of the split. Patients' sera contain circulating IgG autoantibodies to the basement membrane zone by indirect immunofluorescence assay. These circulating IgG autoantibodies recognize in Western blot or by immunoprecipitation a 290-kDa protein band which represents type VII collagen.

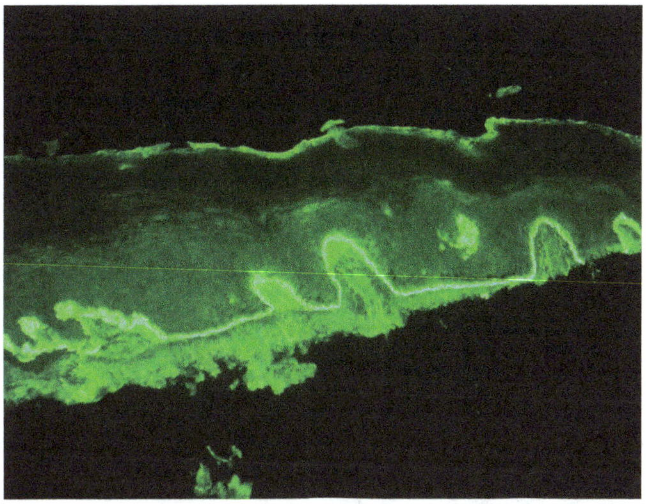

Bullous systemic lupus. Linear IgG deposition along the dermal epidermal junction, consistent with immunobullous disease.

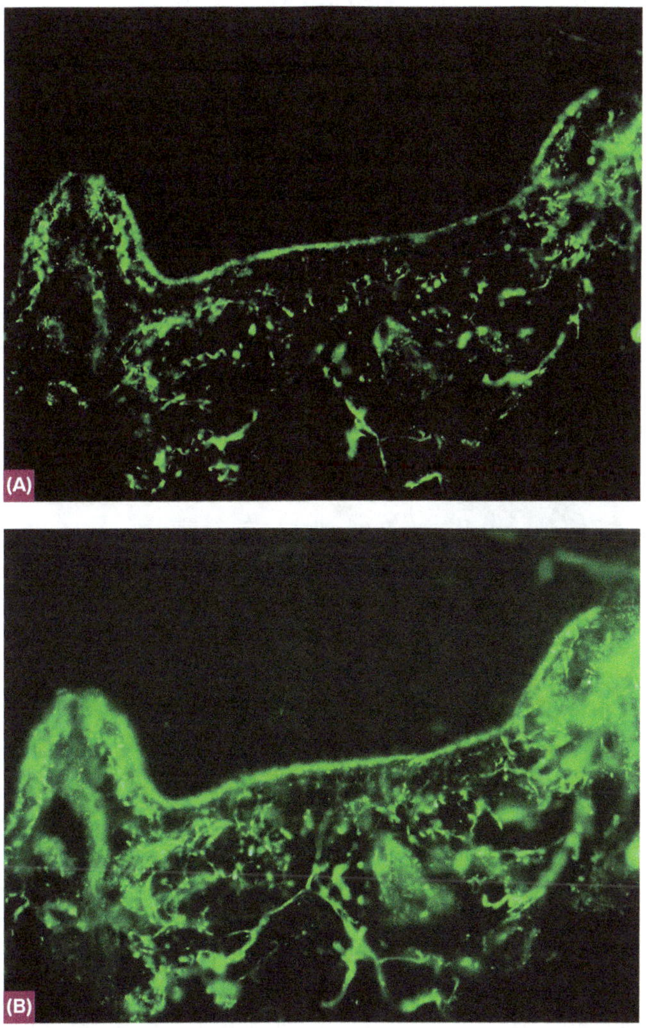

Bullous systemic lupus. Granular deposition of **(A)** IgA and **(B)** IgM along the dermal-epidermal junction, consistent with a positive lupus band test.

Table 3-30A. Bullous Systemic Lupus Erythematosus

Clinical Features
Young adults, women > men, particularly African American women
Widespread vesicles and bullae often on an erythematous base or plaques
Trunk and flexural surfaces most commonly involved
Predominately sun-exposed skin or any site
Four or more ARA criteria
Histopathologic Features
Subepidermal blister
Often numerous neutrophils in papillary dermis, often dermal papillae or in a more diffuse pattern
Usually prominent papillary dermal edema
Superficial and mid-dermal perivascular lymphoid infiltrates with occasional neutrophils and eosinophils
Uncommonly microvascular injury, rarely leukocytoclastic vasculitis
Extravasation of erythrocytes on occasion
Rarely typical features of lupus erythematosus: basal layer vacuolopathy, epidermal atrophy, thickened basement membrane, thickening
Laboratory Evaluation
Epitope mapping using antibodies against type IV collagen
Sublamina densa blister
DIF examination
Perilesional intact human skin:
Linear deposits of IgG along the BM zone
Perilesional salt-split skin:
IgG deposits along the dermal side of the split
ELISA test
Circulating IgG antibodies to collagen type VII
Western blot
Circulating IgG antibodies to a 290-kDa protein band
Differential Diagnosis
Dermatitis herpetiformis
Linear IgA bullous dermatosis
Epidermolysis bullosa acquisita
Cicatricial pemphigoid
Drug eruption
Neutrophilic dermatoses such as Sweet syndrome

The histopathological differential diagnosis includes **dermatitis herpetiformis, linear IgA bullous dermatosis, cicatricial pemphigoid,** and **Sweet syndrome** (choices A, B, D, and E, respectively). **Cicatricial pemphigoid** may reveal IgG deposition on the epidermal side, dermal side, or both by salt-split skin immunofluorescence. **Epidermolysis bullosa acquisita** will reveal linear deposition of IgG along the basement membrane zone, but lacks the granular deposition

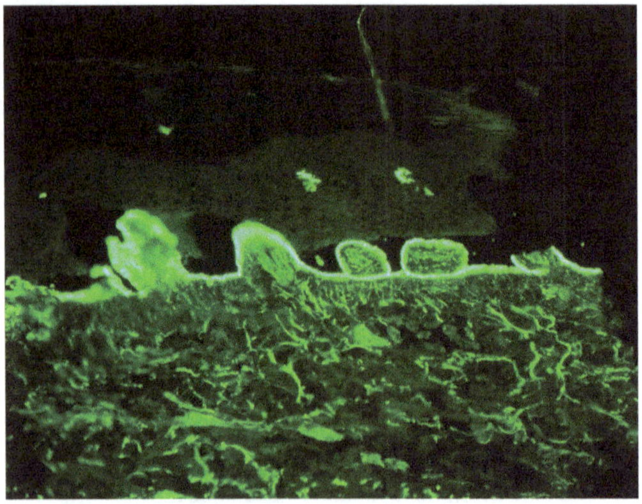

Bullous systemic lupus. Salt-split skin reveals linear homogenous IgG deposition along the base of the blister cleavage plane.

Subepidermal Blister with Neutrophils

"PLAID"

Pemphigoid (bullous, cicatricial)
Lupus, bullous systemic
Acquisita, epidermolysis bullosa
IgA, linear
Dermatitis herpetiformis

pattern (lupus band test) frequently encountered in BSLE. The presence of leukocytoclastic changes favors the diagnosis of lupus over the other entities listed. Other than the clinical information, the most compelling diagnostic information is found on direct immunofluorescence examination, which separates out each of these entities.

ANSWER 3-31: A.

The **porphyrias** comprise a group of disorders characterized by excessive accumulation of porphyrins or their precursors in tissues due to inherited or acquired deficiencies in any one of the enzymes that synthesize heme. There are several types of porphyrias. The patient in question has **porphyria cutanea tarda (PCT)**, which is the most common (Table 3-31A). It has an estimated incidence of 1:1000 to 1:30000. About 60% of the affected patients are males. PCT is due to reduced activity of the enzyme **uroporphyrinogen decarboxylase (UROD)**, which catalyzes several steps in heme synthesis. In PCT, this enzyme defect may occur spontaneously or through an autosomal dominant inheritance pattern. Age of onset is usually in the third to fourth decade of life. Clinically, blisters develop on

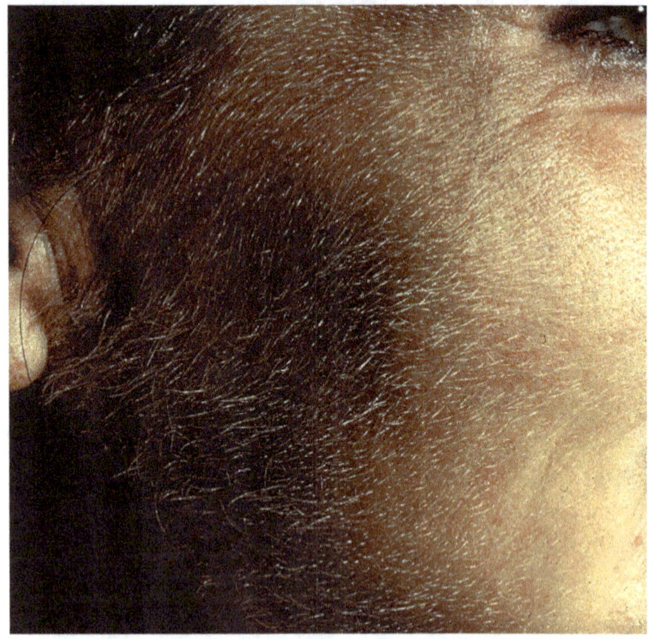

Porphyria cutanea tarda. Hypertrichosis in a woman who had been on a prolonged regimen with estrogens. (Reproduced, with permission, from Wolff K, Johnson RA, Saavedra AP. *Fitzpatrick's Color Atlas and Synopsis of Clinical Dermatology.* 7th ed. New York, NY: McGraw-Hill Education; 2013.)

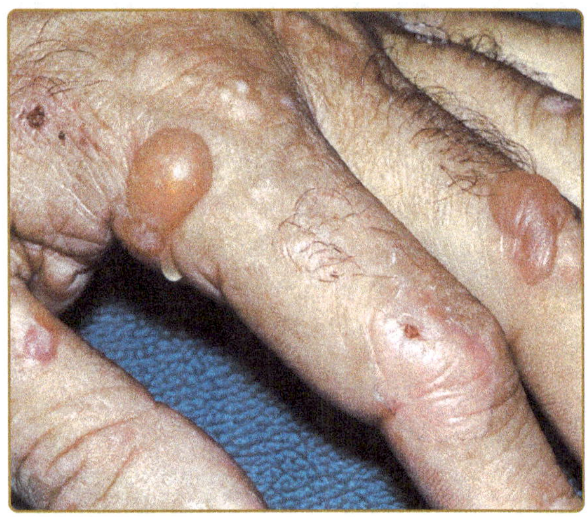

Porphyria cutanea tarda. This shows bullae filled with clear fluid. Elsewhere are remnants of blisters and over the second metacarpophalangeal joint are small milia. (Reproduced, with permission, from Goldsmith LA, Katz SI, Gilchrest BA, Paller AS, Leffell DJ, Wolff K, eds. *Fitzpatrick's Dermatology in General Medicine.* 8th ed. New York, NY: McGraw-Hill Education; 2012.)

the dorsal surfaces of the hands, in association with increased fragility of sun-exposed skin and hypertrichosis of the periorbital area. There is mottled pigmentation of sun-exposed areas and sometimes morphea-like changes. The blisters are usually induced by minor trauma and heal with atrophic scars and milia. **Pseudoporphyria** has an identical clinical presentation

Table 3-31A. Porphyria Cutanea Tarda

Clinical Features
Sporadic or familial
Blisters at sites of sun exposure and trauma
Scarring and milia
Facial hypertrichosis
Hyperpigmentation
Often associated with liver disease
Histopathologic Features
Subepidermal blister
Sparse perivascular and interstitial lymphoid infiltrates
Usually solar elastosis
Thick-walled blood vessels
Caterpillar bodies—basement membrane material (segment eosinophilic structures)
Laboratory Evaluation
Direct immunofluorescence
Linear dermal-epidermal and perivascular C3, and sometimes IgG, IgM, IgA
Epitope mapping using antibodies against type IV collagen
Intralamina lucida blister
Porphyrin laboratory tests
Elevated total porphyrin levels in urine
Isocoproporphyrin is demonstrable in feces
Differential Diagnosis
Cell-poor bullous pemphigoid
Epidermolysis bullosa (hereditary and acquired)
Thermal injury
Toxic epidermal necrolysis
Bullosis diabeticorum
Pseudoporphyria
Traumatic blisters

Table 3-31B. Pseudoporphyria

Clinical Features
Features often identical to porphyria cutanea tarda
Chronic renal failure with hemodialysis common
Secondary to particular medications:
Furosemide
Nalidixic acid
Tetracycline
Naproxen
Tense bullae in sun-exposed skin
Histopathologic Features
Subepidermal blister
In the dermis:
Sparse perivascular and interstitial infiltration by lymphocytes
Actinic elastosis and thick-walled blood vessels
Laboratory Evaluation
Blister mapping using antibodies against type IV collagen
Intralamina lucida split
Porphyrin laboratory tests
Dialysis-induced pseudoporphyria: elevated serum porphyrin levels, normal UROD activity
Drug-induced and UVA-induced pseudoporphyria: normal UROD activity and serum porphyrin levels
Differential Diagnosis
Porphyria cutanea tarda
Cell-poor bullous pemphigoid
Epidermolysis bullosa (hereditary and acquired)
Thermal injury
Toxic epidermal necrolysis
Bullosis diabeticorum
Traumatic blisters

Drugs Associated with Pseudoporphyria

"No Talking after Last Night's Party Dude"

Nalidixic acid
Tetracycline
Lasix
Naproxen
Pyridoxine
Dapsone

minus the facial hypertrichosis, which is frequently the initial chief complaint of patients with PCT (Table 3-31B).

Pseudoporphyria may occur in patients undergoing hemodialysis for chronic renal insufficiency (**dialysis-induced pseudoporphyria**) or in those taking drugs such as naproxen, furosemide, nalidixic acid, and tetracycline (**drug-induced pseudoporphyria**). Pseudoporphyria has also been attributed to PUVA therapy, excessive sun exposure, and tanning bed use (**UVA-induced pseudoporphyria**).

Microscopically, bullous lesions of PCT and pseudoporphyria are identical and are characterized by the formation of subepidermal blisters containing fibrin and a few inflammatory cells. The epidermis forming the blister roof is usually effaced and may be necrotic. In the dermis, there is solar elastosis and a sparse superficial perivascular and interstitial infiltration by lymphocytes. The blood vessels of the superficial dermal plexus usually have thickened walls that can be best demonstrated by PAS stain. On immunomapping with antibodies to type IV collagen, the blister in PCT is located in the lamina lucida.

Indirect immunofluorescence (IIF) examination of patients with PCT and pseudoporphyria are negative for immunoglobulin deposition. Direct immunofluorescence (DIF) usually reveals C3 and C5-9 deposits around the upper dermal vascular plexus and/or at the dermal-epidermal junction. Sometimes weak linear deposits of IgG and/or IgA may be seen at the dermal-epidermal junction and around vessels in pseudoporphyria.

Confirmation of the diagnosis of PCT requires porphyrin laboratory tests. In PCT, there is markedly reduced to absent serum uroporphyrinogen decarboxylase activity. Total porphyrin levels in urine are elevated (10-100 times than normal), with a predominance of **uroporphyrin** and **heptacarboxyporphyrin. Isocoproporphyrin** is demonstrable in feces. In pseudoporphyria serum uroporphyrinogen decarboxylase activity is normal. Porphyria levels in drug-induced pseudoporphyria and UVA drug-induced pseudoporphyria are also normal. In dialysis-induced pseudoporphyria, serum porphyrins are increased.

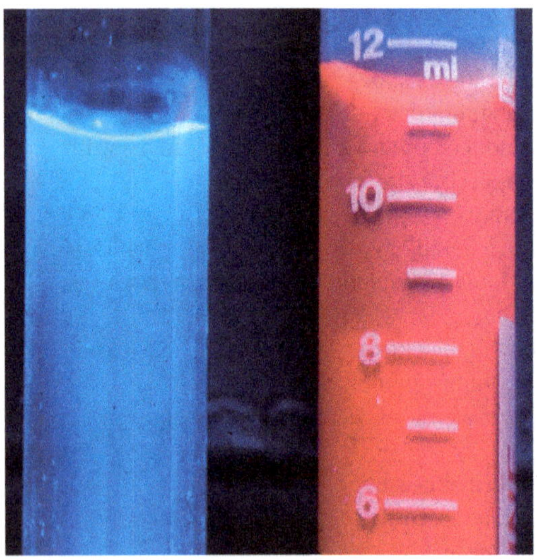

Porphyria cutanea tarda: Wood light. Coral-red fluorescence of the urine of a patient with PCT (right) as compared to that of a normal control (left).

ANSWER 3-32: D.

Coma blisters are bullae that appear at pressure sites in patients with drug-induced and nondrug-induced coma (Table 3-32A). Clinically the blisters are tense, usually clear, and occur at sites subjected to pressure, such as the hands, wrists, scapulae, sacrum, knees, legs, ankles, and heels. They appear on normal or erythematous skin, often in a linear distribution, and may reach substantial size.

Histopathologically, subepidermal blisters occur in association with necrosis of the eccrine sweat glands and ducts. Necrosis of pilosebaceous units may also be present. On immunomapping with antibodies against type IV collagen, the split localizes within the lamina lucida. DIF and IIF examinations in coma blisters are negative. The histology of coma blisters is diagnostic based on the necrosis of appendageal structures and in combination with the clinical picture allows definitive diagnosis.

Table 3-32A. Coma Blisters

Clinical Features
Blisters at sites of pressure in comatose patients: hands, wrists, scapulae, sacrum, knees, legs, ankles, heels
Often linear distribution
Tense clear blisters on normal-appearing or erythematous skin
Often quite large in size
Histopathologic Features
Subepidermal blister
Necrosis of eccrine sweat glands and ducts and less commonly pilosebaceous units
Sparse inflammation
Laboratory Evaluation
Direct immunofluorescence
Negative
Epitope mapping using antibodies against type IV collagen
Intralamina lucida blister
Differential Diagnosis
Cell-poor bullous pemphigoid
Epidermolysis bullosa (hereditary and acquired)
Thermal injury
Bullosis diabeticorum
Pseudoporphyria
Traumatic blisters

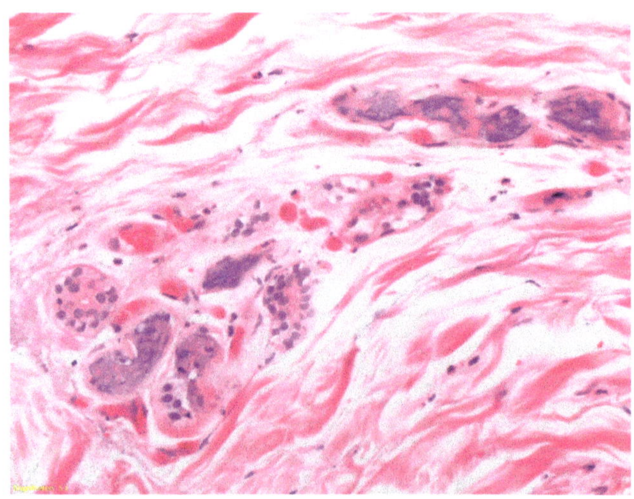

Coma blister. There is necrosis of the eccrine coil (pink-purple gritty appearance) underlying a denuded cutaneous surface.

BIBLIOGRAPHY

1. Anhalt GJ, Kim SC, Stanley JR, et al. Paraneoplastic pemphigus: an autoimmune disease associated with neoplasia. *N Engl J Med.* 1990;323:1729–1735.
2. Balding SD, Prost C, Diaz LA, et al. Cicatricial pemphigoid autoantibodies react with multiple sites on the BP l80 extracellular domain. *J Invest Dermatol.* 1996;106:141–146.
3. Briggaman RA, Yoshiike T, Cronce DJ. The epidermal-dermal junction and genetic disorders of this area. In: Goldsmith LA, ed. *Physiology, Biochemistry, and Molecular Biology of the Skin.* 2nd ed. New York, NY: Oxford University Press; 1991.
4. Burge SM, Wilkinson JD. Darier-White disease: a review of the clinical features in 163 patients. *J Am Acad Dermatol.* 1992;27:40.
5. Burgeson RE, Christiano AM. The dermal-epidermal junction. *Curr Opin Cell Biol.* 1997;5:651–658.
6. Cheng S, Edmonds E, Ben-Gashir M, et al. Subcorneal pustular dermatosis: 50 years on. *Clin Exp Dermatol.* 2008;33:229.
7. Chorzelski TP, Beutner EH, Sulej J, et al. IgA anti-endomysium antibody. A new immunological marker of dermatitis herpetiformis and coeliac disease. *Br J Dermatol.* 1984;111:395–402.
8. Crosby DL, Diaz LA. Endemic pemphigus foliaceus. Fogo selvagem. *Dermatol Clin.* 1993;11:453.
9. Davis MD, Dinneen AM, Landa N, et al. Grover's disease: clinicopathologic review of 72 cases. *Mayo Clin Proc.* 1999;74:229.
10. Devries DT, Warren SJ. Recent advances in intraepidermal blistering diseases. *Adv Dermatol.* 2002;18:203.
11. Dhitavat J, Fairclough RJ, Hovnanian A, et al. Calcium pumps and keratinocytes: lessons from Darier's disease and Hailey-Hailey disease. *Br J Dermatol.* 2004;150:821.
12. Dobson-Stone C, Fairclough R, Dunne E, et al. Hailey-Hailey disease: molecular and clinical characterization of novel mutations in the ATP2C1 gene. *J Invest Dermatol.* 2002;118:338.
13. Egan CA, Zone JJ. Linear IgA bullous dermatosis. *Int J Dermatol.* 1999;38(11):818–827.
14. Engineer L, Bhol K, Ahmed AR. Pemphigoid gestationis: a review. *Am J Obstet Gynecol.* 2000 Aug;183(2):483–491.
15. Fleming TE, Korman NJ. Cicatricial pemphigoid. *J Am Acad Dermatol.* 2000 Oct;43(4):571–591.
16. Florman AL, Holzman RS. Nosocomial scalded skin syndrome. Ritter's disease caused by phage group 3 *Staphylococcus aureus. Am J Dis Child.* 1980;134:1043.
17. Fritsch C, Lang K, von Schmiedeberg S, et al. Porphyria cutanea tarda. *Skin Pharmacol Appl Skin Physiol.* 1998 Nov–Dec;11(6):321–335.
18. Gammon WR, Fine JD, Forbes M, Briggaman RA. Immunofluorescence on split skin for the detection and differentiation of basement membrane zone autoantibodies. *J Am Acad Dermatol.* 1992 Jul;27(1):79–87.
19. Gammon WR, Woodley DT, Dole KC, Briggaman RA. Evidence that anti-basement membrane zone antibodies in bullous eruption of systemic lupus erythematosus recognize epidermolysis bullosa acquisita autoantigen. *J Invest Dermatol.* 1985;6:472–476.
20. Ghohestani R, Nicolas JF, Kanitakis J, Bedane C, Faure M, Claudy A. Pemphigoid gestationis with autoantibodies exclusively directed to the 230 kDa bullous pemphigoid antigen. *Br J Dermatol.* 1996;134:603–604.
21. Giancotti FG. Signal transduction by the alpha6beta4 integrin: charting the path between laminin binding and nuclear events. *J Cell Sci.* 1996;109:1165–1172.
22. Green JJ, Manders SM. Pseudoporphyria. *J Am Acad Dermatol.* 2001 Jan;44(1):100–108.
23. Guo L, Degenstein L, Dowling J, et al. Gene targeting of BPAG1: abnormalities in mechanical strength and cell migration in stratified epithelia and neurologic degeneration. *Cell.* 1995;81:233–243.
24. Hashimoto T, Yasumoto S, Nagata Y, et al. Clinical, histopathological and immunological distinction in two cases of IgA pemphigus. *Clin Exp Dermatol.* 2002;27:636.
25. Hopkinson SB, Riddelle KS, Jones JC. Cytoplasmic domain of the 180-kD bullous pemphigoid antigen, a hemidesmosomal component: molecular and cell biologic characterization. *J Invest Dermatol.* 1992;99:264–270.
26. Horn TD, Anhalt GJ. Histologic features of paraneoplastic pemphigus. *Arch Dermatol.* 1992;128:1091.
27. Hughes AP, Callen JP. Drug-induced linear IgA bullous dermatosis mimicking toxic epidermal necrolysis. *Dermatology.* 2001;202(2):138–139.
28. Korman NJ, Eyre RW, Zone J, et al. Drug-induced pemphigus: autoantibodies directed against the pemphigus antigen complexes are present in penicillamine and captopril-induced pemphigus. *J Invest Dermatol.* 1991;96:273.
29. Magro CM, Roberts-Barnes J, Crowson AN. Direct immunofluorescence testing in the diagnosis of immunobullous disease, collagen vascular disease, and vascular injury syndromes. *Dermatol Clin.* 2012 Oct;30(4):763–798.
30. Maynard B, Peters MS. Histologic and immunofluorescence study of cutaneous porphyrias. *J Cutan Pathol.* 1992 Feb;19(1):40–47.

31. Mehregan DR, Daoud M, Rogers RS III. Coma blisters in a patient with diabetic ketoacidosis. *J Am Acad Dermatol.* 1992 Aug;27(2 Pt 1):269–270.
32. Müller S, Klaus-Kovtun V, Stanley JR. A 230-kD basic protein is the major bullous pemphigoid antigen. *J Invest Dermatol.* 1989;92:33–38.
33. Ohnishi Y, Tajima S, Ishibashi A, Fujiwara SA. Vesicular bullous pemphigoid with an autoantibody against plectin. *Br J Dermatol.* 2000;142:813–815.
34. Ostezan LB, Fabre VC, Caughman SW, et al. Paraneoplastic pemphigus in the absence of a known neoplasm. *J Am Acad Dermatol.* 1995;33:312.
35. Pulkkinen L, Christiano AM, Airenne T, Haakana H, Tryggvason K, Uitto J. Mutations in the gamma-2 chain gene (LAMC2) of kalinin/laminin 5 in the junctional forms of epidermolysis bullosa. *Nat Genet.* 1994;6:293–298.
36. Resnick SD. Staphylococcal toxin-mediated syndromes in childhood. *Semin Dermatol.* 1992;11:11.
37. Reunala T. Dermatitis herpetiformis: coeliac disease of the skin. *Ann Med.* 1998;30:416–418.
38. Robinson ND, Hashimoto T, Amagai M, et al. The new pemphigus variants. *J Am Acad Dermatol.* 1999;40:649.
39. Sakuntabhai A, Ruiz-Perez V, Carter S, et al. Mutations in ATP2A2, encoding a Ca^{2+} pump, cause Darier disease. *Nat Genet.* 1999;21:271.
40. Sidoroff A, Halevy S, Bavinck JN, et al. Acute generalized exanthematous pustulosis (AGEP)—a clinical reaction pattern. *J Cutan Pathol.* 2001;28:113.
41. Sitaru C, Mihai S, Zillikens D. The relevance of the IgG subclass of autoantibodies for blister induction in autoimmune bullous skin diseases. *Arch Dermatol Res.* 2007 April;299(1):1–8.
42. Spencer JM, Silvers DN, Grossman ME. Pustular eruption after drug exposure: is it pustular psoriasis or a pustular drug eruption? *Br J Dermatol.* 1994;130:514.
43. Syder AJ, Yu QC, Paller AS, et al. Genetic mutations in the K1 and K10 genes of patients with epidermolytic hyperkeratosis. Correlation between location and disease severity. *J Clin Invest.* 1994;93:1533.
44. Tamada Y, Yokochi K, Nitta Y, Ikeya T, Hara K, Owaribe K. Lichen planus pemphigoides: identification of 180 kD hemidesmosome antigen. *J Am Acad Dermatol.* 1995;32:883–887.
45. Uitto J, Pulkkinen L. Molecular complexity of the cutaneous basement membrane zone. *Mol Biol Rep.* 1996;1:35–46.
46. Vainio E, Kalimo K, Reunala T, Viander M, Palosuo T. Circulating IgA- and IgG-class antigliadin antibodies in dermatitis herpetiformis detected by enzyme-linked immunosorbent assay. *Arch Dermatol Res.* 1983;275:15–18.
47. Warren SJ, Lin MS, Giudice GJ, et al. The prevalence of antibodies against desmoglein 1 in endemic pemphigus foliaceus in Brazil. Cooperative Group on Fogo Selvagem Research. *N Engl J Med.* 2000;343:23.
48. Wenzel FG, Horn TD. Nonneoplastic disorders of the eccrine glands. *J Am Acad Dermatol.* 1998 Jan;38(1):1–17.
49. Willsteed E, Bhogal BS, Black MM, McKee P, Wojnarowska F. Use of 1M NaCl split skin in the indirect immunofluorescence of the linear IgA bullous dermatoses. *J Cutan Pathol.* 1990 Jun;17(3):144–148.
50. Zambruno G, Kanitakis J. Linear IgA dermatosis with IgA antibodies to type VII collagen. *Br J Dermatol.* 1996;135:1004–1005.

CHAPTER 4

Vasculitis and Related Disorders

QUESTION 4-1.

Which of the following statements regarding vasculitis is INCORRECT?

A) Vasculitis is defined by clear-cut vascular damage, with or without a cellular inflammatory process.
B) The standardized nomenclature for the vasculitides is based primarily on the size of the involved vessels.
C) Clinically, medium vessel vasculitis results in ulcers, nodules, or reticulated purplish discoloration of the skin.
D) Clinically, small vessel vasculitis results in palpable purpura and petechiae.
E) The histopathologic criteria for recognizing microvascular injury are somewhat arbitrary, and the minimal criteria for vasculitis remain controversial.

QUESTION 4-2.

An otherwise healthy patient presents with erythematous and violaceous purpuric macules and papules involving the distal lower extremities. In addition, necrotic, eroded, and ulcerated lesions are present. The remainder of the skin exam is unremarkable. The patient recently was prescribed a course of antibiotics for a sore throat. Blood cultures are negative for growth of microorganisms. Serum analysis reveals normal complement levels. A biopsy is performed and the findings are illustrated below. Which of the following statements regarding this patient's condition is INCORRECT?

A) This is an example of an immune-complex mediated type III hypersensitivity reaction.
B) The presence of numerous eosinophils suggests a drug-based etiology.
C) Similar eruptions may occur in patients ingesting various foods and nondrug chemicals.
D) Similar eruptions may occur in patients with collagen vascular disease and certain malignancies.
E) This is an example of serum sickness.

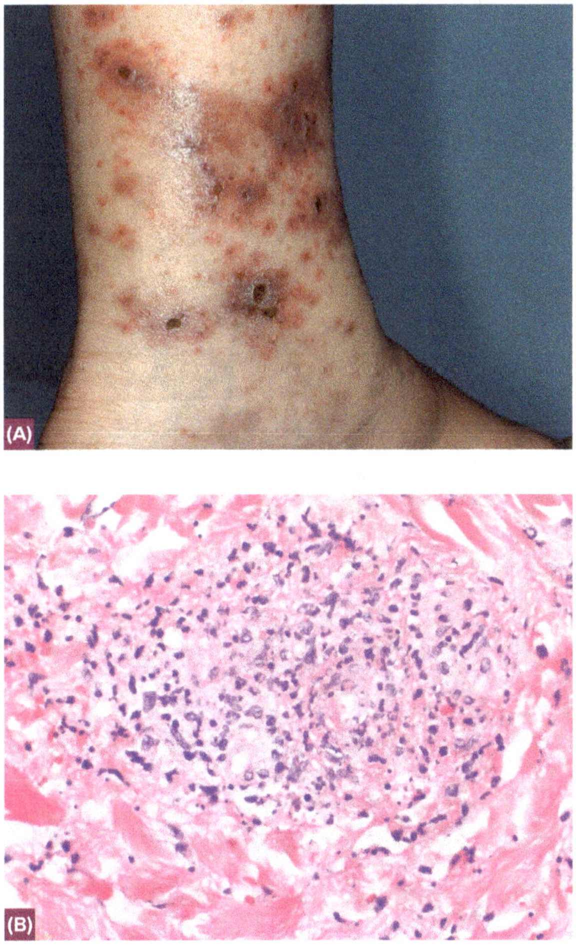

QUESTION 4-3.

An adult male presents with palpable purpura of the buttocks and lower extremities accompanied by abdominal pain, arthralgia, and hematuria. Focal retiform areas are noted. A few hemorrhagic bullae are present on the abdomen. Serum analysis reveals an elevated adenovirus antibody titer. A biopsy is performed and the findings are illustrated below. The dermatopathology report comes back with a diagnosis of pustular leukocytoclastic vasculitis containing large numbers of neutrophils. Direct immunofluorescence reveals granular IgA and C3 deposition within the dermal vessels. Which of the following statements regarding this condition is INCORRECT?

A) This patient has renal vasculitis that will most likely result in severe long-term renal impairment.
B) This condition most commonly occurs in children following Group A *Streptococcal* infections.
C) A similar condition without systemic involvement may occur in infants 4–24 months of age, characterized by initial purpuric annular plaques on the face, ears, and extremities followed by proximal spread.
D) Elderly patients with IgA-mediated leukocytoclastic vasculitis should be screened for malignancy.

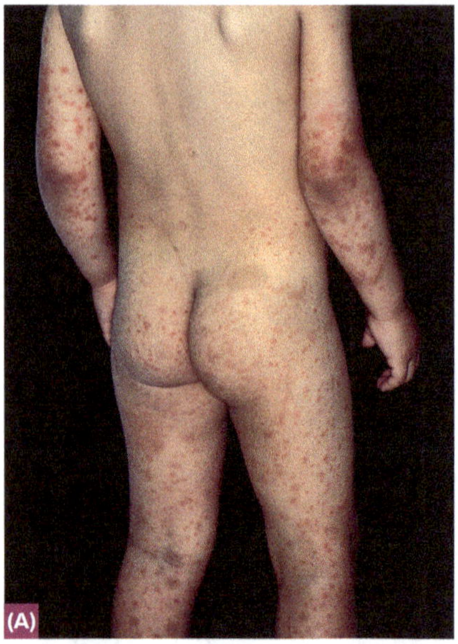

(A)

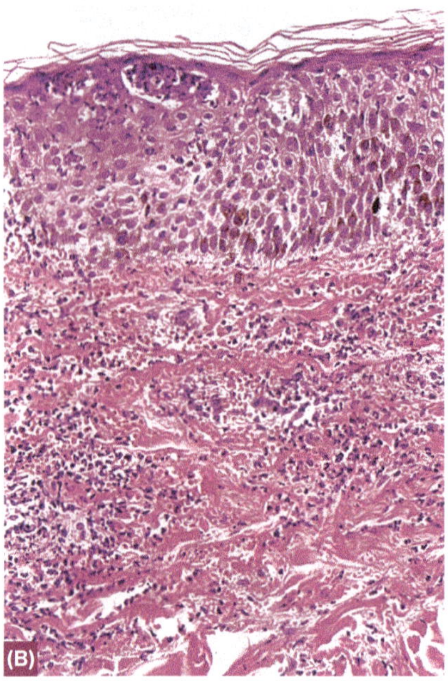

(B)

Reproduced, with permission, from Knoop KJ, Stack LB, Storrow AB, Thurman RJ. *The Atlas of Emergency Medicine*. 3rd ed. New York, NY: McGraw-Hill; 2010.

QUESTION 4-4.

A 30-year-old female patient, status-post tubal ligation, presents to the emergency department with acute pelvic inflammatory disease, fever, malaise, leukocytosis, and hypotension. Physical examination reveals a dermal nodule with hemorrhage and necrosis on the dorsum of a finger. Blood culture and serological studies are pending. A biopsy is performed and the H&E findings are illustrated below. The inflammatory infiltrate is composed mainly of neutrophils. Which of the following diagnoses is CORRECT?

A) Septic vasculitis
B) Henoch–Schönlein purpura
C) Hypersensitivity vasculitis attributed to medication
D) Urticarial vasculitis
E) Churg–Strauss syndrome

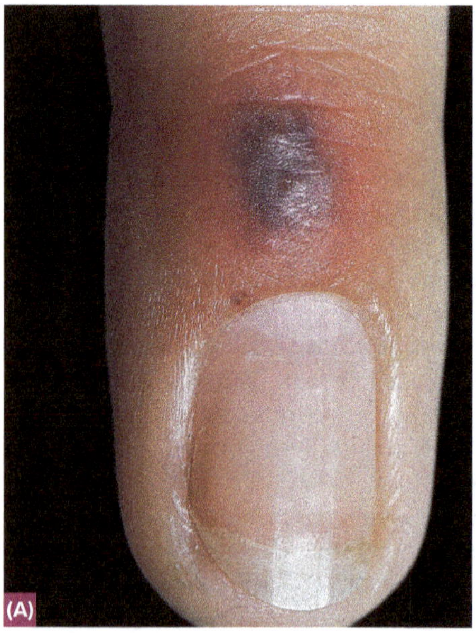

(A)

Reproduced, with permission, from Wolff K, Johnson RA, Saavedra AP. *Fitzpatrick's Color Atlas and Synopsis of Clinical Dermatology*. 7th ed. New York, NY: McGraw-Hill Education; 2013.

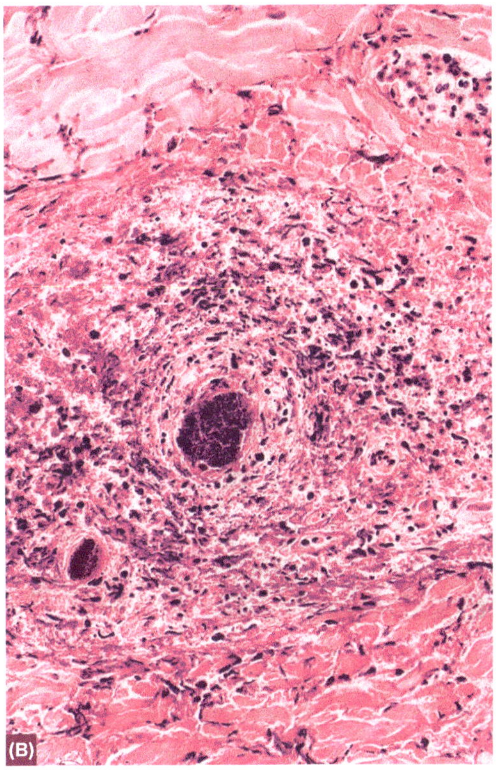
(B)

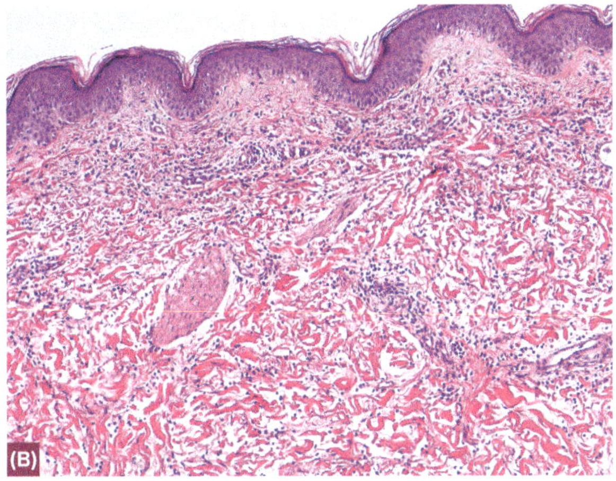
(B)

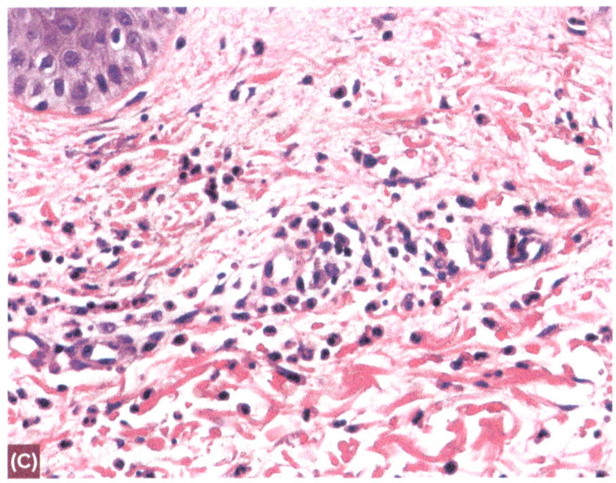
(C)

A) The condition frequently precedes the onset of lupus erythematosus.
B) Patients with this condition frequently have decreased serum complement levels.
C) This condition is vastly more common in women than men.
D) This condition is strongly associated with chronic urticaria.
E) This condition is characterized by true vascular damage with fibrinoid necrosis of vessel walls and luminal thrombosis.

QUESTION 4-5.

A 53-year-old female presents with erythematous plaques and wheals on the buttocks that, in part, do not blanch on diascopy. The lesions have been present for 2 days and the patient reports that they seem to have slightly changed in shape. A biopsy is performed and the findings are illustrated below. The cellular infiltrate is composed predominantly of neutrophils. Which of the following statements regarding this condition is INCORRECT?

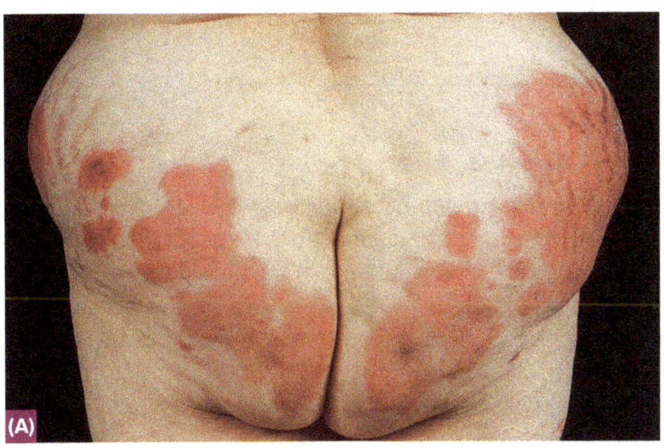
(A)

Reproduced, with permission, from Wolff K, Johnson RA, Saavedra AP. *Fitzpatrick's Color Atlas and Synopsis of Clinical Dermatology*. 7th ed. New York, NY: McGraw-Hill Education; 2013.

QUESTION 4-6.

A 45-year-old patient with tuberculosis, positive antinuclear antibody, and hepatitis C infection, returns from a skiing trip in Aspen with symmetrical purpuric papular lesions on toes and soles. Petechial macular lesions are present on the dorsal aspect of the foot. Similar lesions are present on the nose and fingertips. A variety of neurologic symptoms are also present, including blurred vision, headache, vertigo, nystagmus, dizziness, diplopia, ataxia, and confusion. Urine analysis reveals hematuria and proteinuria. A biopsy is performed revealing leukocytoclastic vasculitis. Direct immunofluorescence reveals IgG, IgM, and complement deposition within the vessels. Which of the following statements regarding this condition is INCORRECT?

A) A PAS stain may reveal bright eosinophilic material within vascular lumens.
B) Centrifugation of the patient's serum will reveal whitish precipitates when stored at 4°C (39.2°F) for 48 hours.
C) This condition is likely caused by monoclonal or polyclonal IgM that are complexed with a polyclonal IgG.
D) Nail-fold capillary abnormalities are common in this condition and include dilatation, altered orientation, capillary shortening, and neoangiogenesis.
E) The presence of leukocytoclastic vasculitis is a consistent finding in this condition.

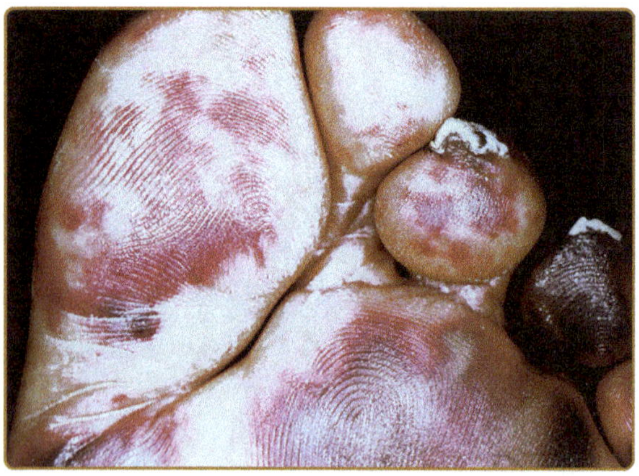

Reproduced, with permission, from Goldsmith LA, Katz SI, Gilchrest BA, Paller AS, Leffell DJ, Wolff K, eds. *Fitzpatrick's Dermatology in General Medicine*. 8th ed. New York, NY: McGraw-Hill Education; 2012.

QUESTION 4-7.

A patient with rheumatoid arthritis presents with multiple, persistent, symmetric, and erythematous to violaceous papules and plaques on the extensor surfaces of the hands, elbows, wrists, knees, ankles, fingers, toes, buttocks, face, ears, legs, forearms, and genitals. The trunk is spared. Some of the lesions are extremely firm when palpated and exhibit dyspigmentation. The patient reports that this condition is exacerbated by cold exposure. Additionally, the lesions become more raised, erythematous, and firm in the evening. A biopsy is performed and the findings are illustrated below. Which of the following diagnoses is CORRECT?

A) Granuloma annulare
B) Granuloma faciale
C) Rheumatoid nodule
D) Erythema elevatum diutinum
E) Rheumatoid neutrophilic dermatitis

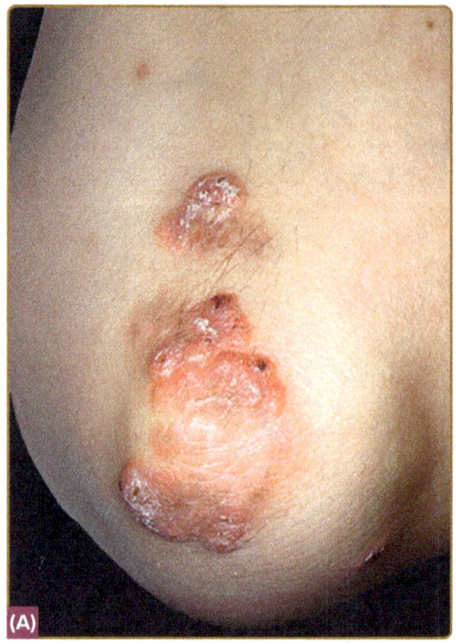

(A)

Reproduced, with permission, from Goldsmith LA, Katz SI, Gilchrest BA, Paller AS, Leffell DJ, Wolff K, eds. *Fitzpatrick's Dermatology in General Medicine*. 8th ed. New York, NY: McGraw-Hill Education; 2012.

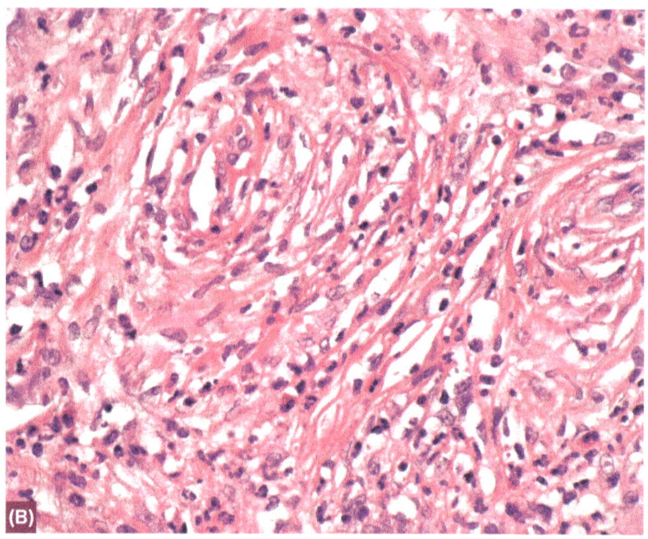

(B)

QUESTION 4-8.

A patient presents with raised edematous plaques on the cheek showing prominent follicular ostia. A biopsy is performed and the findings are illustrated below. The inflammatory infiltrate is mixed and contains lymphocytes, histiocytes, eosinophils, neutrophils, and plasma cells. Which of the following diagnoses is CORRECT?

A) Angiolymphoid hyperplasia with eosinophilia
B) Erythema elevatum diutinum
C) Papular rosacea
D) Sweet syndrome
E) Granuloma faciale

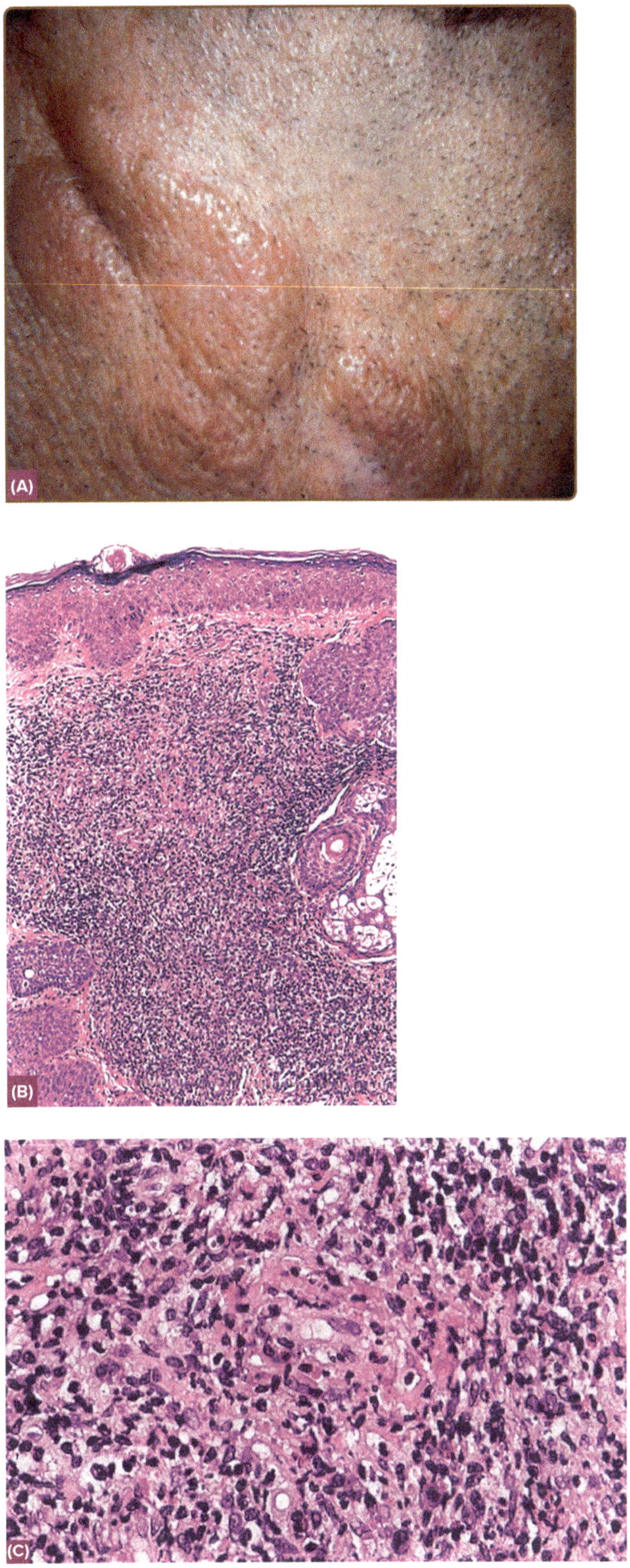

Part **(A)** reproduced, with permission, from Goldsmith LA, Katz SI, Gilchrest BA, Paller AS, Leffell DJ, Wolff K, eds. *Fitzpatrick's Dermatology in General Medicine*. 8th ed. New York, NY: McGraw-Hill Education; 2012.

QUESTION 4-9.

A 45-year-old male with myelodysplastic syndrome presents with the acute onset of fever, leukocytosis, and painful erythematous and edematous plaques on the face and neck. Some of the plaques exhibit central yellowish discoloration and tend to coalesce, forming well circumscribed, irregularly bordered plaques. A biopsy is performed and the findings are illustrated below. The infiltrate is composed mainly of neutrophils. Which of the following statements regarding this condition is INCORRECT?

A) The pathogenesis of this condition involves aberrant neutrophil chemotaxis into the involved tissues with minimal leukocytoclasia and usually with minimal or no vascular damage.
B) Extensive involvement of the subcutis is associated with hematologic malignancy.
C) This condition classically occurs in middle-aged women after a nonspecific infection of the respiratory or gastrointestinal tract.
D) Direct immunofluorescence typically demonstrates immunoglobulin deposition within the dermal vessels.
E) Tissue culture and special stains are consistently negative and are required for definitive diagnosis.

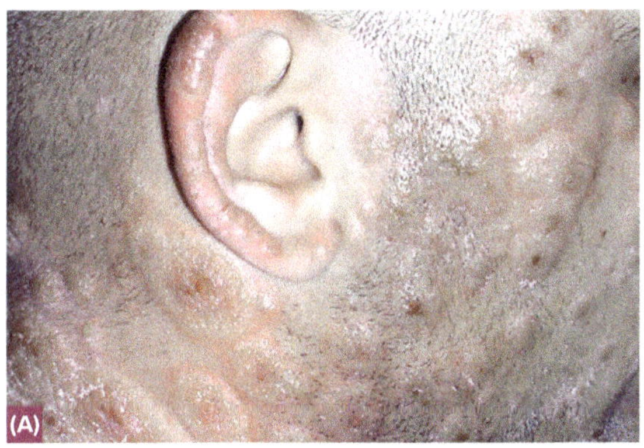

Reproduced, with permission, from Kaushansky K, Lichtman MA, Beutler E, Kipps TJ, Seligsohn U, Prchal JT, eds. *Williams Hematology*. 8th ed. New York, NY: McGraw-Hill Education; 2010.

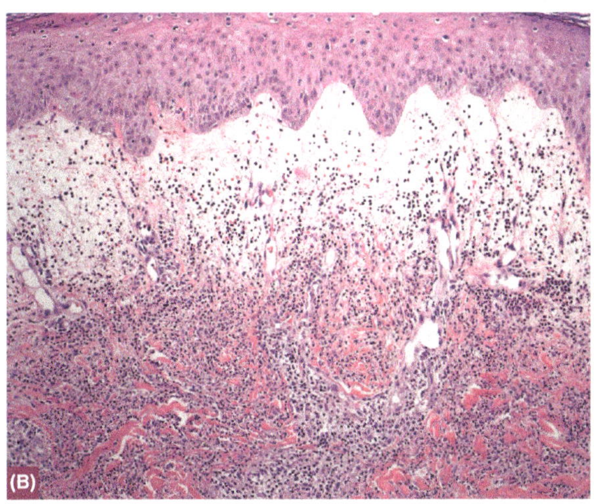

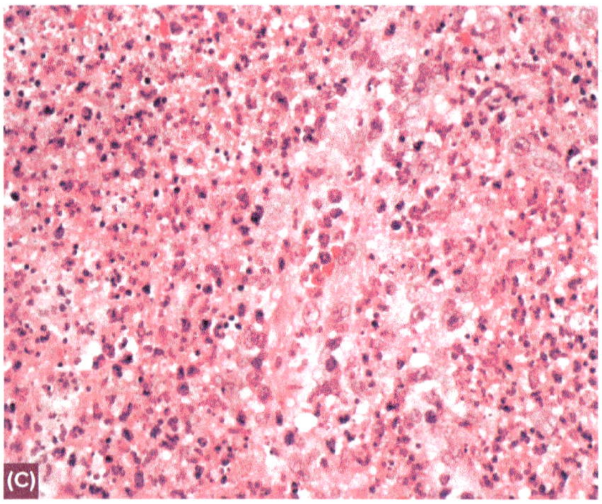

QUESTION 4-10.

A 32-year-old man with Crohn disease presents with two chronic ulcers of the lower extremity. The lesions were preceded by minor trauma and have progressively enlarged despite continuous wound management from his podiatrist. Which of the following statements regarding this condition is INCORRECT?

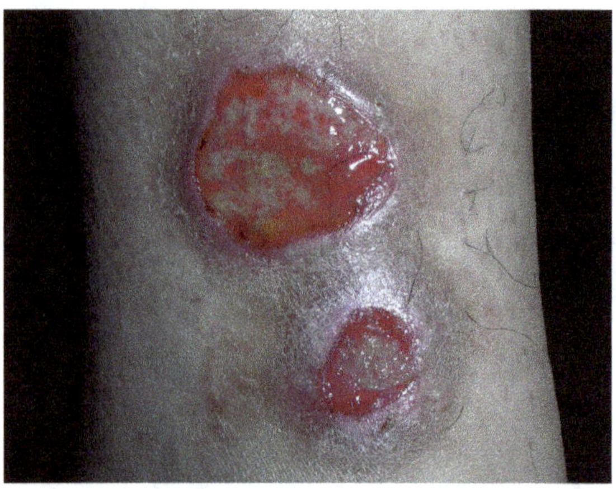

Reproduced, with permission, from Usatine RP, Smith MA, Mayeaux EJ Jr, Chumley HS, eds. *Color Atlas of Family Medicine*. 2nd ed. New York, NY: McGraw-Hill Education; 2012.

A) This is a multisystem disease characterized by oral aphthous lesions, genital aphthae, synovitis, posterior uveitis, superficial thrombophlebitis (STP), cutaneous pustular vasculitis, and meningoencephalitis.
B) This condition has several different clinical presentations, including ulceration with undermined borders, discrete and painful pustules, painful bullae with progression to superficial ulceration, and vegetative painless ulcers with an ostraceous scale and nonundermined exophytic borders.
C) Tissue culture and special stains are consistently negative and are required for definitive diagnosis.
D) The typical lesion is histopathologically characterized by robust neutrophilic infiltrates with minimal edema, significant leukocytoclasia, focal true vascular damage, and ulceration with dermal necrosis.
E) Surgical debridement of these ulcers should be immediately stopped and the lesions should be gently treated with topical immunosuppressive agents.

QUESTION 4-11.

Which of the following conditions does NOT exhibit the vascular reaction pattern illustrated below?

A) Perniosis
B) Pigmented purpuric dermatitis
C) Viral exanthem
D) Pityriasis lichenoides
E) Henoch–Schönlein purpura

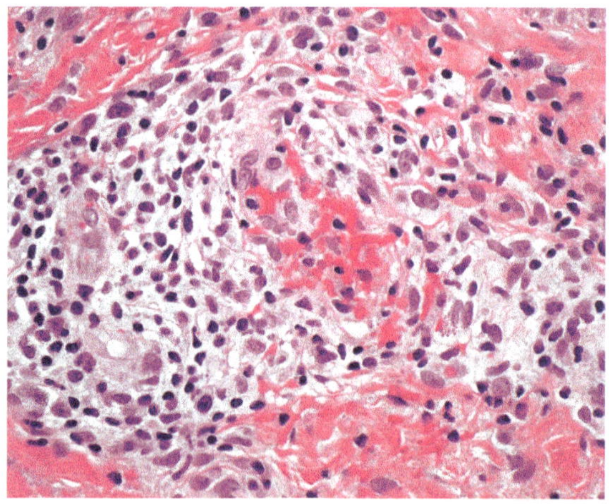

QUESTION 4-12.

You receive an outside case for consultation without clinical history. The histopathological findings are significant for leukocytoclastic vasculitis involving both superficial and deep dermal vessels. Scattered eosinophils are noted. Indirect immunofluorescence using the patient's serum and normal circulating neutrophils as a substrate is performed and the findings are illustrated below. A repeat biopsy and direct immunofluorescence are pending. Which of the following statements regarding this case is INCORRECT?

A) This patient has circulating antibodies directed against myeloperoxidase.
B) Direct immunofluorescence is characteristically negative for immunoglobulin deposition within vessels.
C) Based on the histopathological and serological findings, the differential diagnosis includes Churg–Strauss syndrome and microscopic polyarteritis.
D) Rare drug-associated cases may demonstrate immunoglobulin deposition within vessels via direct immunofluorescence.

E) Although this patient's biopsy revealed leukocytoclastic vasculitis, cutaneous biopsies most commonly exhibit granulomatous vasculitis.

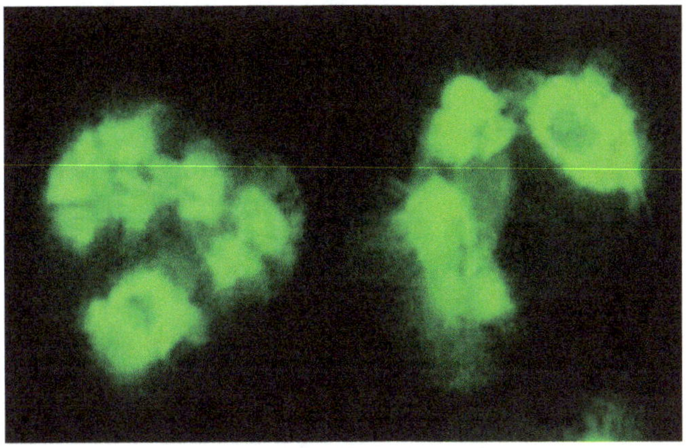

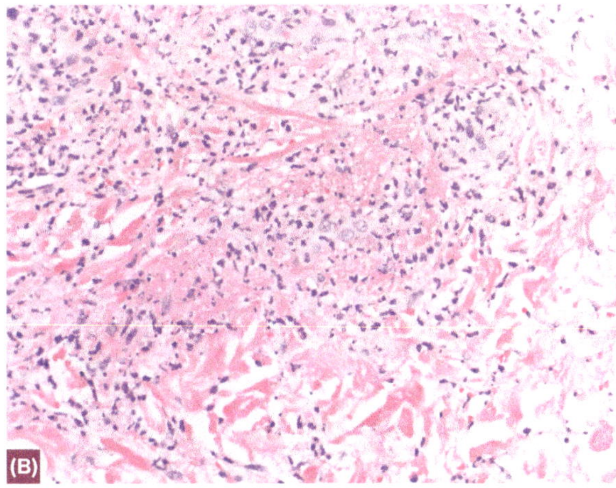

(B)

QUESTION 4-13.

A 56-year-old male presents with microhematuria, proteinuria, and acute oliguric renal failure, as well as livedo reticularis and palpable purpura. He reports prodromal symptoms of fever, myalgias, arthralgias, and a sore throat. A biopsy is performed and the findings are illustrated below. Direct immunofluorescence is negative for immunoglobulin deposition within vessels. Indirect immunofluorescence using normal peripheral blood neutrophils as a substrate reveals perinuclear staining. Which of the following diagnoses is CORRECT?

A) Microscopic polyarteritis nodosa
B) Polyarteritis nodosa
C) Wegener granulomatosis
D) Churg–Strauss syndrome
E) Drug-induced ANCA-positive vasculitis

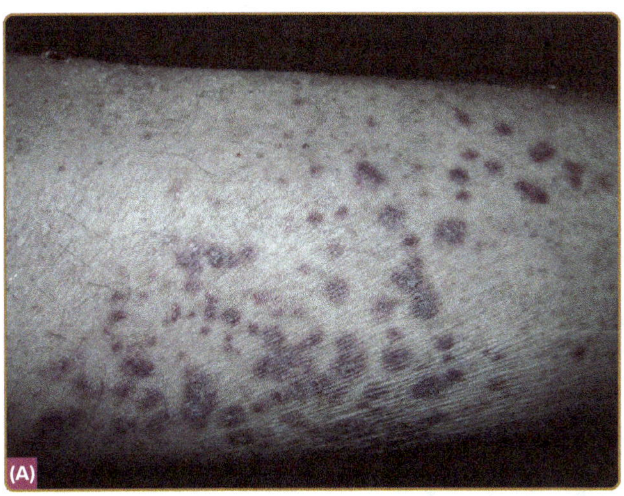

(A)

Reproduced, with permission, from Goldsmith LA, Katz SI, Gilchrest BA, Paller AS, Leffell DJ, Wolff K, eds. *Fitzpatrick's Dermatology in General Medicine*. 8th ed. New York, NY: McGraw-Hill Education; 2012.

QUESTION 4-14.

A 40-year-old patient with asthma presents with fever, dyspnea, gastroenteritis, and peripheral eosinophilia. Cutaneous findings are remarkable for livedo reticularis and a cutaneous ulcer just superior to the medial malleolus. The patient's foot is held in extension because of a left foot drop. Bronchoalveolar lavage produces large numbers of eosinophils. Urinalysis, BUN, and creatinine are normal. A skin biopsy lateral to the ulcer is performed and the findings are illustrated below. Direct immunofluorescence is negative for immunoglobulin deposition within vessels. Indirect immunofluorescence using the patient's serum and normal circulating neutrophils as a substrate reveals a perinuclear pattern of staining. Which of the following statements regarding this condition is INCORRECT?

A) Levels of anti-MPOs immunoglobulins have been found to correlate with disease activity.
B) Distinct extravascular granulomas characterized by radially arranged histiocytes and multinucleated giant cells centered around degenerated collagen fibers and numerous eosinophils are occasionally present in this condition.
C) The absence of renal failure is an important diagnostic finding.
D) This condition is most likely attributed to a medication.

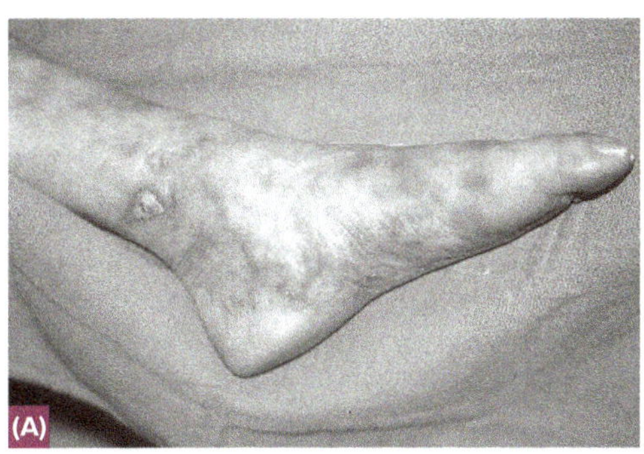

(A)

Reproduced, with permission, from Imboden JB, Hellmann DB, Stone JH, eds. *Current Medical Diagnosis & Treatment: Rheumatology*. 3rd ed. New York, NY: McGraw-Hill Education; 2013.

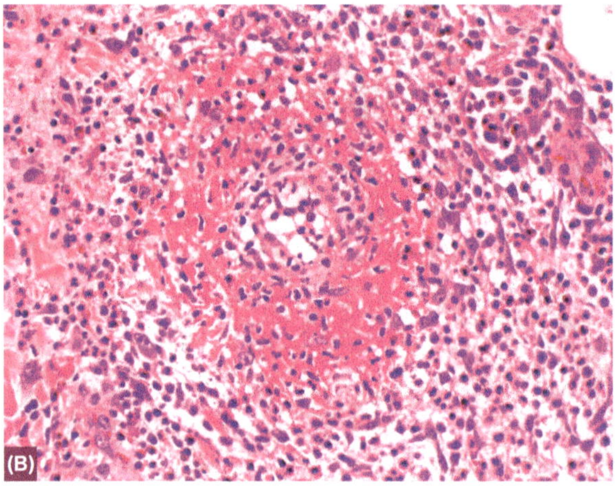

(B)

QUESTION 4-15.

Which of the following conditions is LEAST likely to exhibit the histopathological findings illustrated below?

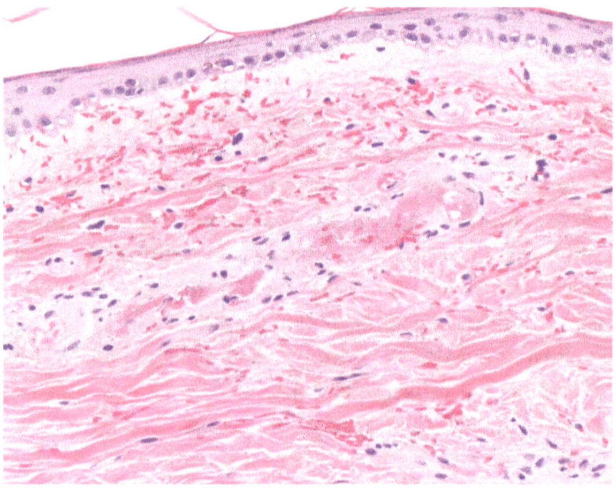

A) Antiphospholipid antibody syndrome
B) Protein C and S deficiencies
C) Heparin-induced skin necrosis
D) Type II cryoglobulinemia
E) Cocaine/levamisole-induced retiform purpura

QUESTION 4-16.

A 56-year-old female presents with porcelain-white atrophic areas with telangiectases over the medial malleolus. A biopsy is performed and the findings are illustrated below. Which of the following diagnoses is CORRECT?

A) Livedo reticularis
B) Livedo racemosa
C) Atrophie blanche
D) Purpura fulminans
E) Retiform purpura

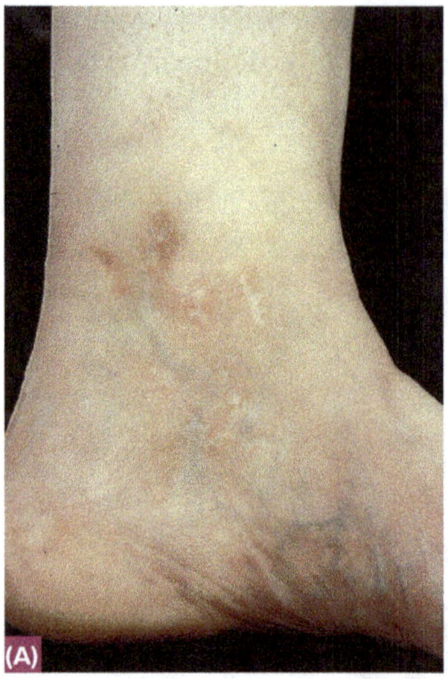

(A)

Reproduced, with permission, from Goldsmith LA, Katz SI, Gilchrest BA, Paller AS, Leffell DJ, Wolff K, eds. *Fitzpatrick's Dermatology in General Medicine*. 8th ed. New York, NY: McGraw-Hill Education; 2012.

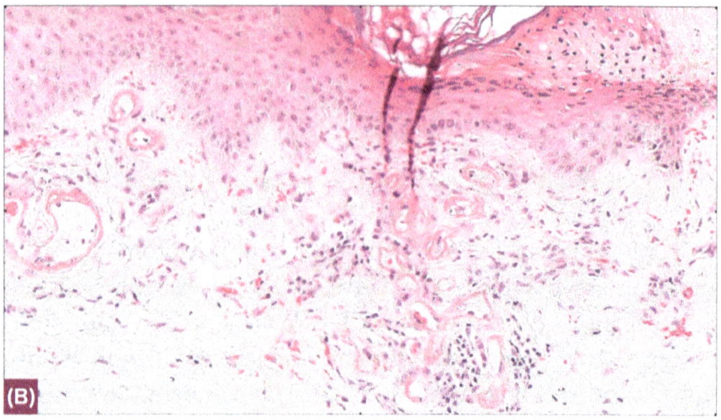

(B)

QUESTION 4-17.

An 82-year-old male develops painful purpura on the tips of the toes shortly following cardiac catheterization. A biopsy is performed and the findings within the deep dermis are illustrated below. Which of the following diagnoses is CORRECT?

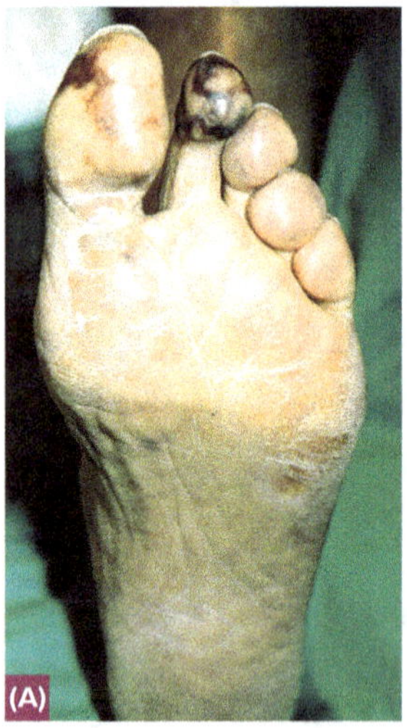

(A)

Reproduced, with permission, from Kaushansky K, Lichtman MA, Beutler E, Kipps TJ, Seligsohn U, Prchal JT, eds. *Williams Hematology*. 8th ed. New York, NY: McGraw-Hill Education; 2010.

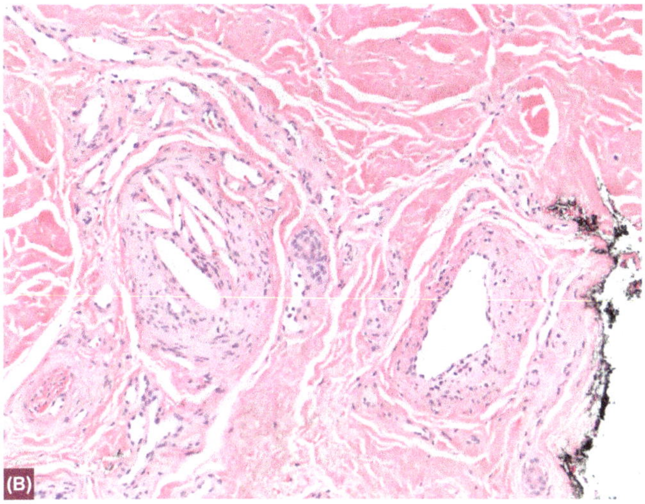

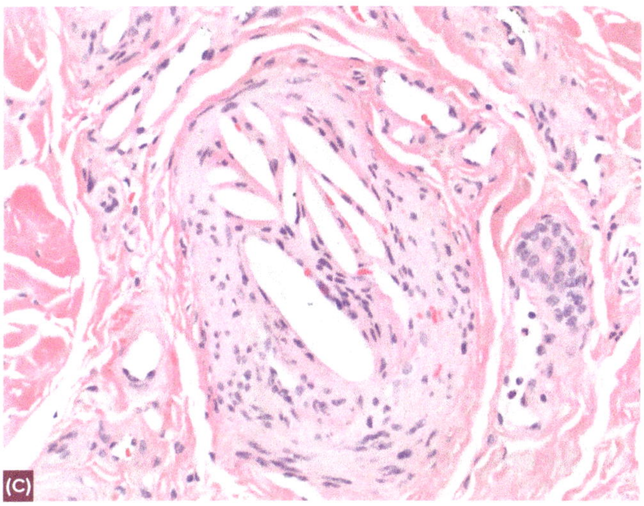

A) Septic vasculitis
B) Perniosis
C) Cryoglobulinemia
D) Cholesterol embolism
E) Calciphylaxis

QUESTION 4-18.

A patient presents to the emergency room with severe acute abdominal pain and mental status changes. Physical examination reveals numerous scattered asymptomatic papules with porcelain-white centers and erythematous raised borders on the trunk and extremities. A skin biopsy is performed and the findings are illustrated below. Alcian blue stain reveals increased dermal mucin. Which of the following diagnoses is CORRECT?

A) Tumid lupus erythematosus
B) Malignant atrophic papulosis
C) Henoch–Schönlein purpura
D) Microscopic polyarteritis
E) Lichen sclerosus

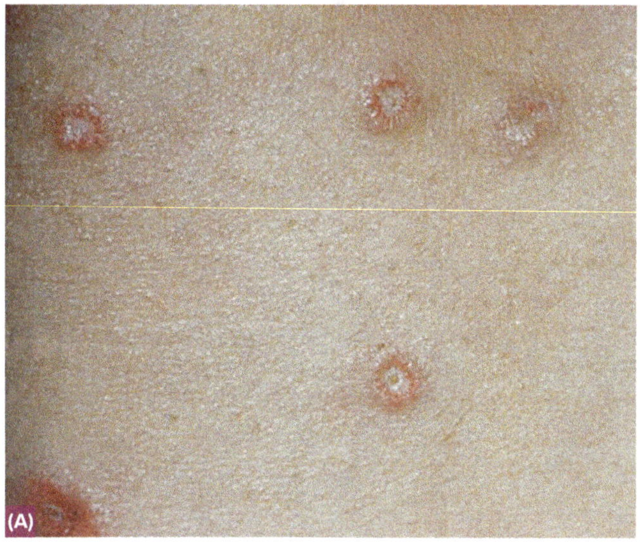

Reproduced, with permission, from Goldsmith LA, Katz SI, Gilchrest BA, Paller AS, Leffell DJ, Wolff K, eds. *Fitzpatrick's Dermatology in General Medicine*. 8th ed. New York, NY: McGraw-Hill Education; 2012.

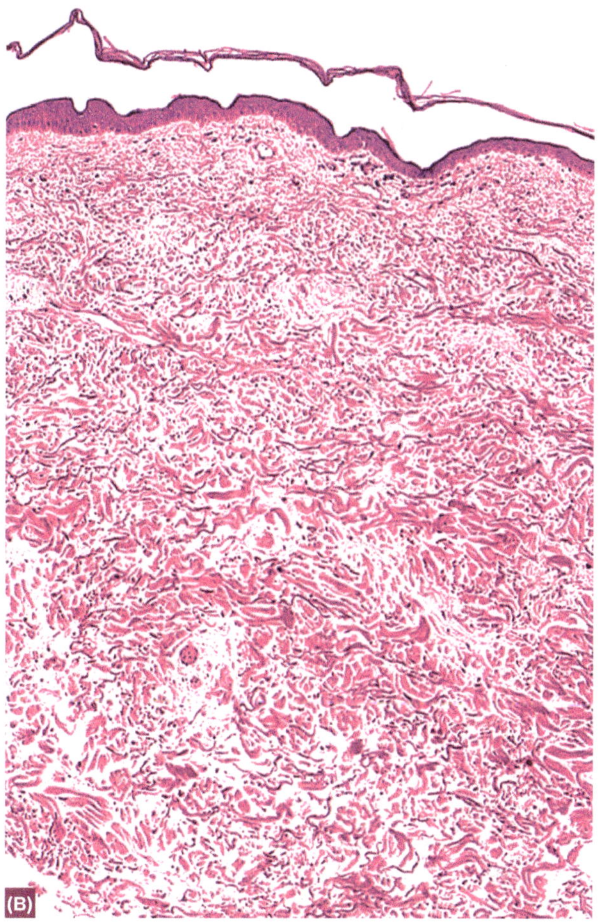

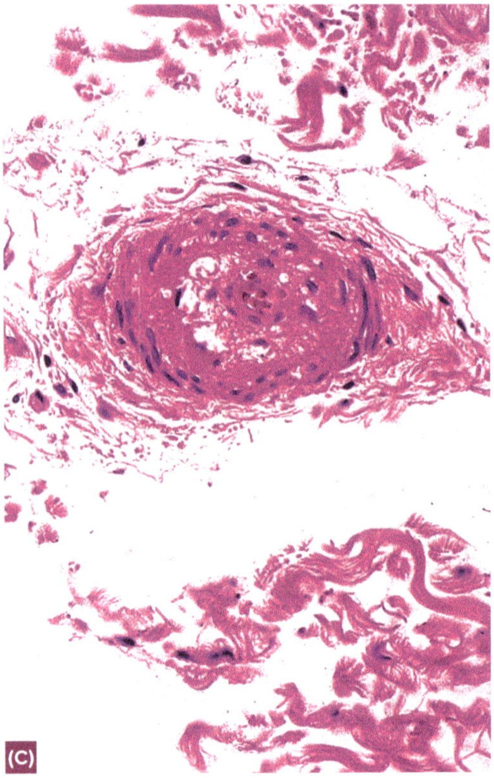

(C)

QUESTION 4-19.

Which of the following conditions is MOST likely to exhibit the histopathological findings illustrated below?

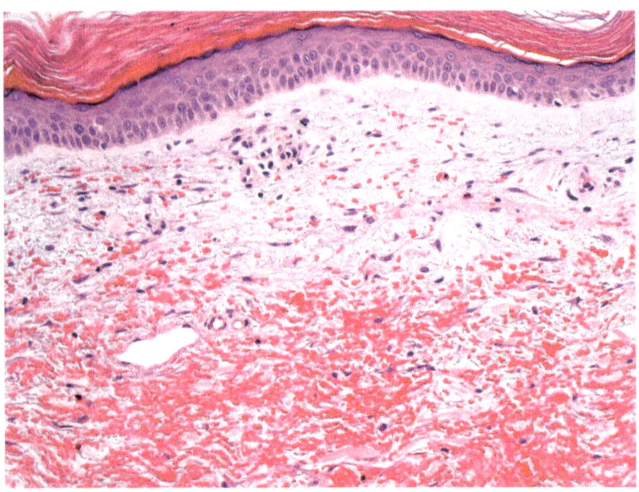

A) Disseminated intravascular coagulation
B) Senile purpura
C) Traumatic ecchymosis
D) Thrombotic thrombocytopenic purpura
E) Antiphospholipid antibody syndrome

QUESTION 4-20.

A 43-year-old Caucasian male presents dyspnea as well as palpable purpura and a deep ulcer of the soft palate. Urinalysis reveals hematuria and proteinuria. Two skin biopsies are performed. The first biopsy reveals leukocytoclastic vasculitis, whereas the findings of the second biopsy are illustrated below. Direct immunofluorescence is negative for immunoglobulin deposition within vessels. Indirect immunofluorescence using the patient's serum and normal circulating neutrophils as a substrate reveals a diffuse cytoplasmic staining pattern. Which of the following diagnoses is CORRECT?

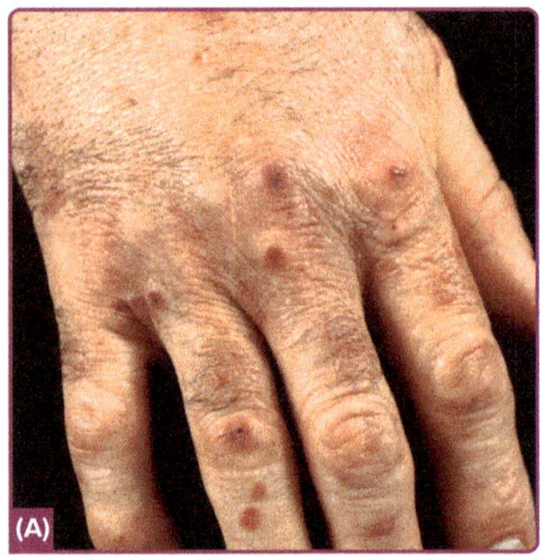

(A)

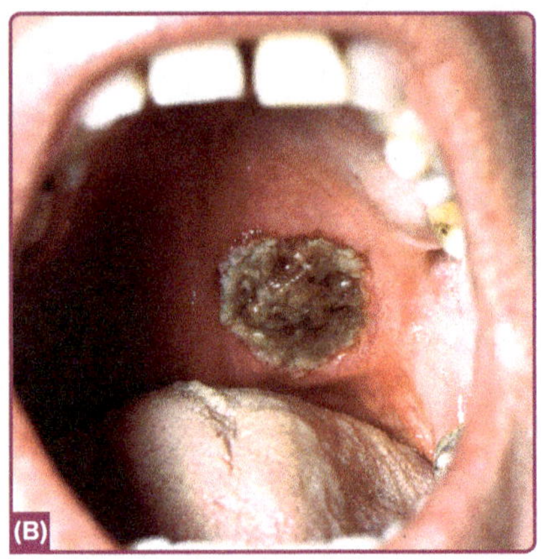

(B)

Reproduced, with permission, from Goldsmith LA, Katz SI, Gilchrest BA, Paller AS, Leffell DJ, Wolff K, eds. *Fitzpatrick's Dermatology in General Medicine*. 8th ed. New York, NY: McGraw-Hill Education; 2012.

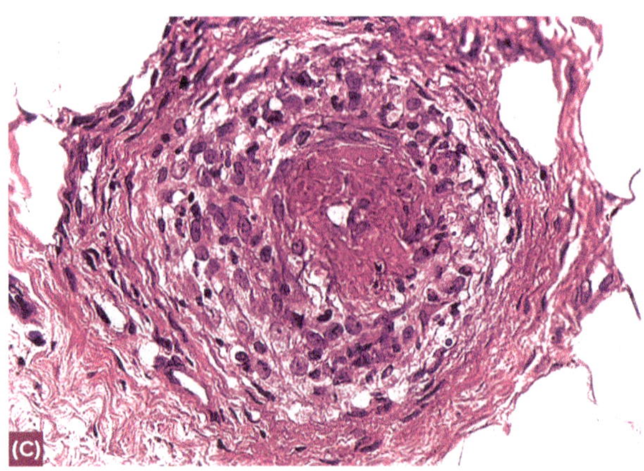

(C)

A) Henoch–Schönlein purpura
B) Churg–Strauss syndrome
C) Microscopic polyarteritis
D) Wegener granulomatosis
E) Septic vasculitis

QUESTION 4-21.

A 40-year-old male heroine abuser with cirrhosis presents with fever, malaise, weight loss, weakness, myalgias, arthralgias, anorexia, and abdominal pain. Additional findings include hematuria, proteinuria, hypertension, and azotemia. Physical examination reveals subcutaneous nodules that pulsate as well gangrene of fingers and toes. An incisional biopsy is performed on one the posterior calf nodules and the findings involving a lobular subcutaneous vessel are illustrated below. Direct immunofluorescence reveals immunoglobulin deposition within the involved vessel. Indirect immunofluorescence is negative for anti-neutrophil cytoplasmic antibodies. Which of the following diagnoses is CORRECT?

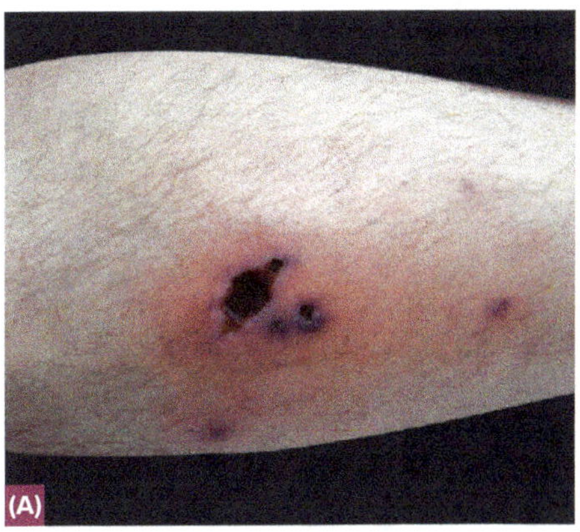

(A)

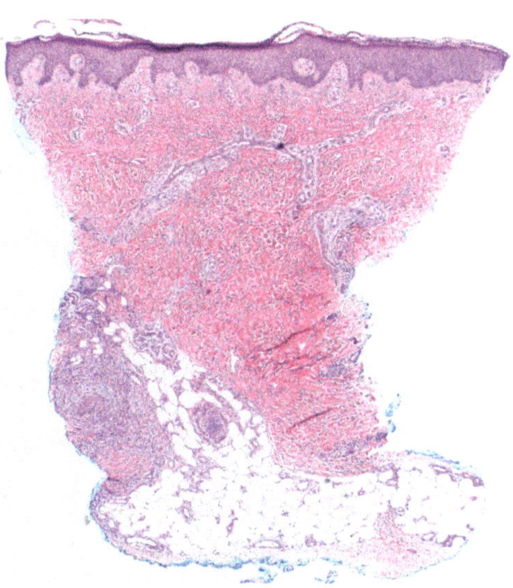

(B)

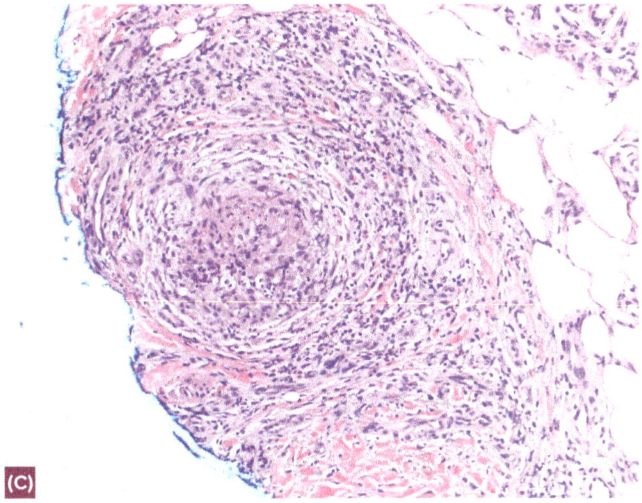

(C)

A) Microscopic polyarteritis
B) Superficial thrombophlebitis
C) Polyarteritis nodosa
D) Henoch–Schönlein purpura
E) Nodular vasculitis

ANSWERS

ANSWER 4-1: A.

Vascular injury can occur in forms limited to the skin. However, in many instances vascular injury occurs in the context of a systemic disease (Table 4-1A). Vascular damage may be the principal event of a disease process, such as in **polyarteritis nodosa (PAN)**; a significant component of a complex disease, as in connective tissue disease or hypercoagulable states; or simply a secondary effect to a localized injury, such as an **arthropod bite** or **traumatic ulcer**. **Vasculitis** is defined as an inflammatory process resulting in clear-cut vascular damage. Histopathologic recognition of vasculitis relies on the recognition of two components: (1) an inflammatory cell infiltrate and (2) evidence of vascular injury. The composition and cellularity of the inflammatory infiltrate of a vasculitis may correlate with the chronology of the process, but not always. Early on, neutrophils and/or eosinophils may predominate. In the late healing stage, the inflammatory cell infiltration may be minimal with an excess of lymphocytes and macrophages.

The histopathologic criteria for recognizing microvascular injury are somewhat arbitrary, and the minimal criteria for vasculitis remain controversial. Various histopathologic features are considered to be indicative of vascular injury. Certain changes, including edema, extravasation of erythrocytes, infiltration of vessel walls by inflammatory cells, leukocytoclasia, and thrombosis, may occur without actual damage to the structural integrity of the vessel. Vessels become leaky for physiologic reasons, leading to edema or even extravasation

Table 4-1A. Definitions of Vascular Injury

Primary Vascular Injury
- Vasculitis
  - Inflammatory cell infiltrate
  - Clear-cut vascular damage (ie, fibrinoid necrosis of vessel wall)
- Inflammatory vascular reaction
  - Inflammatory cell infiltrate
  - Limited vascular damage (insufficient for vasculitis)
- Vasculopathy
  - Lack of inflammation
  - Vascular damage of any degree

Secondary Vascular Injury
- May present as vasculitis, inflammatory vascular reaction, or vasculopathy
- Secondary to another insult such as external trauma, ulceration
  - Variable vascular alterations with sparing of some vessels
  - Peripheral perivascular fibrinoid deposition

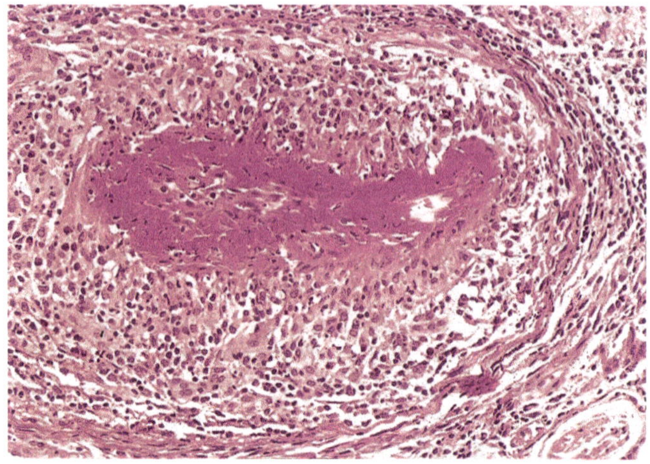

Fibrinoid degeneration. Bright pink fibrinoid material is deposited within a vessel. There is also a polymorphonuclear (neutrophilic) infiltrate.

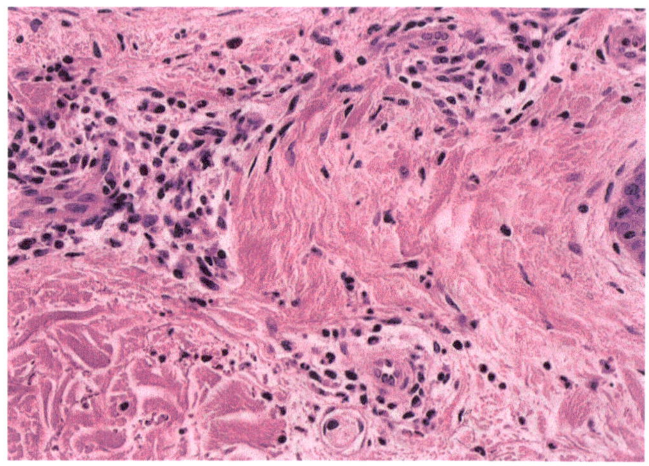

Inflammatory vascular reaction. Occasional perivascular karyorrhectic debris (leukocytoclasia), extravasated red blood cells, and endothelial cell swelling are noted. However, no fibrinoid necrosis is present.

of erythrocytes and leukocytes. **Leukocytoclasia** may result from the breakdown of a perivascular neutrophilic infiltrate during the resolution of an inflammatory process unrelated to vasculitis. Similarly, fibrin thrombi may be present in essentially uninjured vessels in the setting of a hypercoagulable state. Unequivocal injury to the vascular wall is manifested by deposition of fibrinoid material and/or necrosis (**fibrinoid necrosis**). In other words, a diagnosis of vasculitis is established histopathologically if vascular inflammation is accompanied by fibrinoid alterations of the vessel wall. Is the presence of fibrinoid necrosis an absolute prerequisite for the pathologist to render a diagnosis of vasculitis? For didactic purposes, it is tempting to answer the question with an unambiguous "yes." Yet in some cases other features of vascular damage, such as leukocytoclasia or intraluminal thrombi, are developed to such a degree that the constellation of findings favors vasculitis despite the lack of clear-cut fibrinoid necrosis. As a general rule, however, we advise the application of strict criteria for the diagnosis of vasculitis and caution in diagnosing vasculitis in the absence of fibrinoid necrosis.

Many vascular diseases exist in which inflammation is present, but the extent of vascular injury usually is limited and appears insufficient for vasculitis. This group of disorders encompasses a great number of heterogeneous inflammatory conditions, which may regularly or occasionally manifest vascular injury. In fact, many of these conditions are referred to as "vasculitis" (ie, **lymphocytic vasculitis, urticarial vasculitis**). We have included those diseases whose histopathologic or clinical presentation warrants distinction from "true" vasculitis. Since the only common denominator for these disorders is the presence of an inflammatory infiltrate and some limited vascular damage, it is best to designate these conditions as "**inflammatory vascular reactions.**" This term is an adaptation and generalization of the more established term "**neutrophilic vascular reactions,**" which was coined to define a group of inflammatory disorders that showed histological overlap with neutrophilic small-vessel vasculitis.

The term **vasculopathy** (aka **pseudovasculitis**) is used to describe evidence of vascular damage in the absence of inflammation. The degree of vascular damage is variable. The spectrum of clinical settings in which noninflammatory vascular injury commonly occurs includes mainly **coagulopathies** and other vascular occlusive conditions. Hemorrhage, intraluminal thrombi, or emboli are histopathologic findings in these disorders.

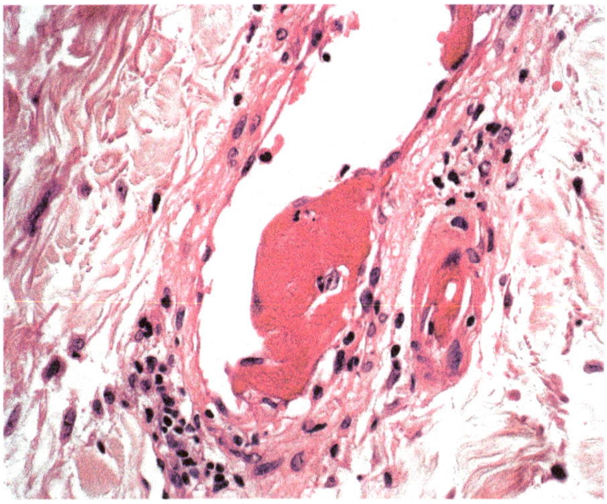

Vasculopathy. Fibrin thrombi in small dermal vessels are seen with a minimal inflammatory cell infiltrate.

The classification of **vasculitis** is difficult for a number of reasons. The various vasculitic disease entities do not have specific histological features, and the same disease process may show a spectrum of histological changes depending on the stage of the disease, the level of activity, and whether or not treatment has modified its course. Moreover, advances in research have redefined or expanded the definitions of certain disease processes with subsequent loss of histopathologic criteria previously thought to be specific. Considerable overlap between vasculitis syndromes exists with many case reports describing patients with hybrid disease states. In an attempt to standardize nomenclature for the vasculitides, an international conference has proposed a system based primarily on the size of the involved vessels (Table 4-1B).

Classification based on vessel size is helpful because there is some correlation with the clinical presentation. **Petechiae, purpura, palpable purpura, urticaria, vesicles** and **bullae**, and **splinter hemorrhages** typically reflect small-vessel injury. Cutaneous **nodules, ulcers, livedo reticularis,** and **racemosa** and **digital gangrene** suggest the involvement of medium-sized arteries. If vascular damage is severe, vascular occlusion may lead to ischemic injury resulting in necrosis, gangrene, and/or ulceration. However, classification based on vessel size alone is of limited value in dermatopathology because most cutaneous vasculitides affect primarily small dermal vessels. In addition,

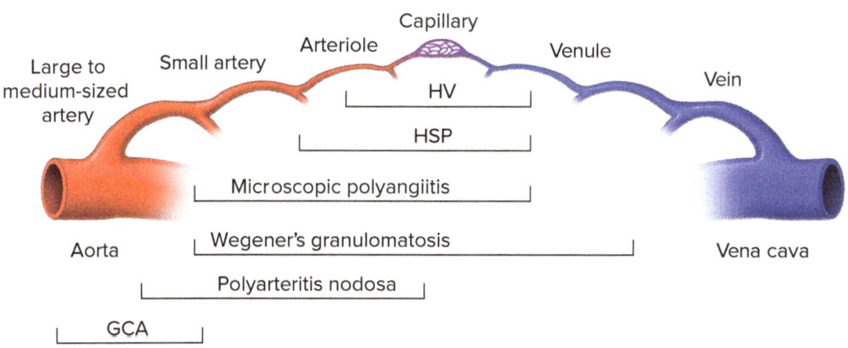

Classification scheme for the primary vasculitides. HV, hypersensitivity vasculitis; HSP, Henoch–Schönlein purpura; GCA, giant cell arteritis. (Adapted, with permission, from Jennette JC et al. Nomenclature of systemic vasculitides. Proposal of an international consensus conference. *Arthritis Rheum*. 1994;37:187.)

Table 4-1B. Names and Definitions of Vasculitis Adopted by the Chapel Hill (NC) Consensus Conference on the Nomenclature of Systemic Vasculitis[a]

CONDITION	DEFINITION
	Large-Vessel Vasculitis[b] (>10 mm in diameter)
Giant cell (temporal) arteritis	Granulomatous arteritis of the aorta and its major branches, with a predilection for the extracranial branches of the carotid artery; often involves the temporal artery; usually occurs in patients older than 50 years and often is associated with polymyalgia rheumatica
Takayasu arteritis	Granulomatous inflammation of the aorta and its major branches; usually occurs in patients younger than 50 years
	Medium-Sized Vessel Vasculitis[b] (about 0.3-10 mm)
Polyarteritis nodosa (classic polyarteritis nodosa)	Necrotizing inflammation of medium-sized or small arteries without glomerulonephritis or vasculitis in arterioles, capillaries, or venules

Table 4-1B. Names and Definitions of Vasculitis Adopted by the Chapel Hill (NC) Consensus Conference on the Nomenclature of Systemic Vasculitis *(continued)*

CONDITION	DEFINITION
Kawasaki disease	Arteritis involving large, medium-sized, and small arteries, and associated with mucocutaneous lymph node syndrome; coronary arteries are often involved; aorta and veins may be involved; usually occurs in children
	Small-Vessel Vasculitis[b] *(10-20 μm to 300 μm)*
Wegener granulomatosis[c,d]	Granulomatous inflammation involving the respiratory tract, and necrotizing vasculitis affecting small- to medium-sized vessels, eg, capillaries, venules, arterioles, and arteries; necrotizing glomerulonephritis is common
Churg–Strauss syndrome[c,d]	Eosinophil-rich and granulomatous inflammation involving the respiratory tract and necrotizing vasculitis affecting small- to medium-sized vessels, and associated with asthma and blood eosinophilia
Microscopic polyangiitis (microscopic polyarteritis)[c,d]	Necrotizing vasculitis with few or no immune deposits affecting small vessels, ie, capillaries, venules, or arterioles; necrotizing arteritis involving small- and medium-sized arteries may be present; necrotizing glomerulonephritis is very common; pulmonary capillaritis often occurs
Henoch–Schönlein purpura[d]	Vasculitis with IgA-dominant immune deposits affecting small vessels, ie, capillaries, venules, or arterioles; typically involves skin, gut, and glomeruli, and is associated with arthralgias or arthritis
Essential cryoglobulinemic vasculitis[d]	Vasculitis with cryoglobulin immune deposits affecting small vessels, ie, capillaries, venules, or arterioles, and associated with cryoglobulins in serum; skin and glomeruli are often involved
Cutaneous leukocytoclastic angiitis	Isolated cutaneous leukocytoclastic angiitis without systemic vasculitis or glomerulonephritis

[a]Modified from Jennette et al.[1]

[b]Larger artery refers to the aorta and the largest branches directed toward major body regions (eg, to the extremities and the head and neck); medium-sized artery refers to the main visceral arteries (eg, renal, hepatic, coronary, and mesenteric arteries), and small artery refers to the distal arterial radicals that connect with arterioles (eg, renal arcuate and interlobular arteries). Note that some small- and large-vessel vasculitides may involve medium-sized arteries; but large- and medium-sized vessel vasculitides do not involve vessels smaller than arteries.

[c]Strongly associated with antineutrophil cytoplasmic autoantibodies.

[d]May be accompanied by glomerulonephritis and can manifest as nephritis or pulmonary-renal vasculitis syndrome.

medium-sized vessel vasculitis frequently will show some degree of small-vessel involvement and vice versa. Classification by etiology or pathogenetic mechanism is difficult because much remains to be learned about the causes of vasculitis. Therefore, in the absence of clinical and serological information, the most important information to communicate in the pathology report is whether or not "true vasculitis" is present, accompanied by the type of cellular inflammatory infiltrate (neutrophilic vs granulomatous) and vessel size involved (typically based on anatomic cutaneous compartment; smallest being papillary dermal vessels and the largest being subcutaneous vessels).

[1] Reproduced with permission from Jennette JC, Falk RJ, Andrassy K, et al: Nomenclature of systemic vasculitides. Proposal of an international consensus conference, *Arthritis Rheum.* 1994 Feb;37(2):187-192.

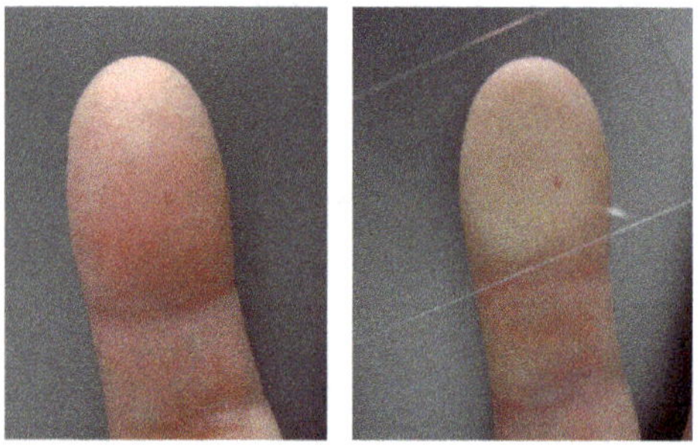

Petechia. Confirmed by diascopy. Several red vascular markings are seen on the index fingertip. Diascopy discloses that the lesions do not blanch and are therefore extravasated blood. By definition, hemorrhagic lesions less than 3 mm in diameter are called *petechiae*. (Reproduced, with permission, from LeBlond RF, Brown DD, DeGowin RL. *DeGowin's Diagnostic Examination*. 9th ed. New York, NY: McGraw-Hill; 2009.)

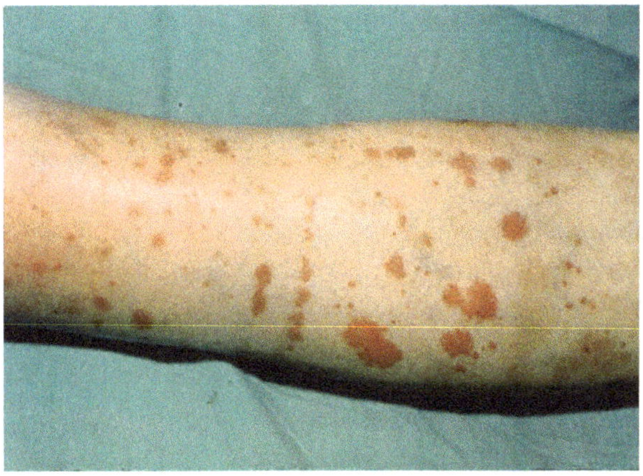

Palpable purpura (leukocytoclastic vasculitis). Erythematous to violaceous plaques on the lower extremity, which do not blanch with pressure. The palpable quality indicates an inflammatory component is present. By definition, purpura measure between 0.3 and 1 cm. (Reproduced, with permission, from Hall JB, Schmidt GA, Wood LDH, eds. *Principles of Critical Care*. 3rd ed. New York, NY: McGraw-Hill; 2005: Courtesy of Denise Rubenstein Collection)

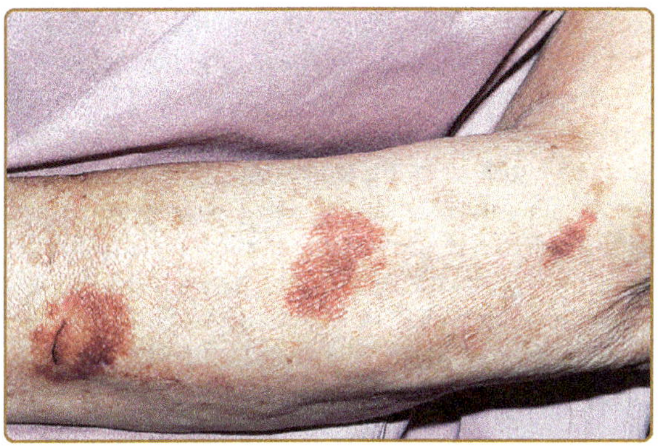

Nonpalpable ecchymoses in a patient on chronic oral glucocorticoid therapy. Note the rectangular and linear lesions that suggest the minor trauma component; the distal lesion shows that the ecchymosis surrounds a linear traumatic injury. By definition, ecchymoses measure greater than 1 cm. (Reproduced, with permission, from Goldsmith LA, Katz SI, Gilchrest BA, Paller AS, Leffell DJ, Wolff K, eds. *Fitzpatrick's Dermatology in General Medicine*. 8th ed. New York, NY: McGraw-Hill Education; 2012.)

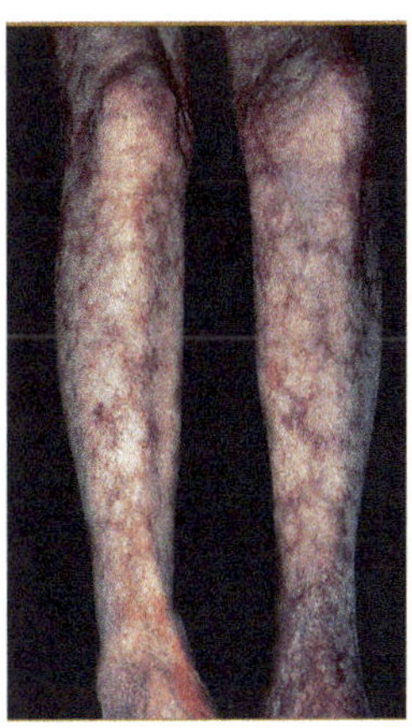

Livedo reticularis/racemosa. This is a lacy pattern of cutaneous vascular injury on the legs. These manifestations reflect vasculitis of "medium-sized" arteries in the subcutis, which are frequently too deep to be sampled in a routine punch biopsy. (Reproduced, with permission, from Goldsmith LA, Katz SI, Gilchrest BA, Paller AS, Leffell DJ, Wolff K, eds. *Fitzpatrick's Dermatology in General Medicine*. 8th ed. New York, NY: McGraw-Hill Education; 2012.)

An important step in evaluating vascular injury is to determine whether the vascular damage is a primary or secondary process (**primary vasculitis** vs **secondary vasculitis**). Primary vascular injury implies that the vascular insult is the predominant disease process. Secondary vascular injury indicates that another disease process outside the vessels is the primary pathologic process. An example of the latter would include vessels engulfed by the necrotizing inflammation around an ulcer initiated by external trauma or infection. Usually, the primary disease process is evident microscopically. Unlike primary vascular injury, secondary vascular injury often is variable, with sparing of some vessels in the zone of tissue injury. Other indications of secondary vascular injury include vascular injury and inflammation confined to areas near ulceration or tissue destruction (ie, abscess), deposition of fibrinoid material at the periphery of the vessel wall, focal thrombosis without significant infiltration by inflammatory cells, and extensive inflammation or granulation tissue between blood vessels (robust interstitial infiltrates) (Table 4-1C).

Table 4-1C. Approach to Vasculitis

Determine if vasculitis or vasculopathy is present or absent
Determine if primary or secondary vascular injury, if possible
Size of vessel and type
Large
Medium
Small
Composition of infiltrate
Neutrophilic/leukocytoclastic
Lymphocytic
Histiocytic/granulomatous
Evaluation for infection (special stains for microorganisms and cultures)
Additional histologic clues:
Intravascular PAS-positive bright red material (suspicious for cryoprecipitates)
Viral cytopathic changes (eg, HSV-associated vascular damage)
Plasma cells (spirochetes)
Presence of eosinophils (r/o drug, hypersensitivity reaction)
Changes suggestive of connective tissue disease (eg, interface dermatitis; dermal mucin)
Edema (urticarial reaction)
Serologic and immunopathologic evaluation
antineutrophil cytoplasmic antibody (ANCA), antinuclear antibody (ANA), rheumatoid factor, cryoglobulins
immunofluorescence, and other studies for the detection of immune complexes, eg, IgA fibronectin aggregates
Clinical context
Cutaneous involvement only
Extent of systemic involvement

Abbreviation: HSV, herpes simplex virus.

ANSWER 4-2: E.

The biopsy reveals a perivascular neutrophilic infiltrate with extensive leukocytoclasia (degenerating/degranulating neutrophils) accompanied by obliteration of the vessel wall and lumen. There is focal residual bright eosinophilic fibrinoid material and extravasated red blood cells. This is an example of **leukocytoclastic vasculitis (LCV)**, which is a **hypersensitivity vasculitis,** referring to type III hypersensitivity most likely attributed to the antibiotic (Table 4-2A). The single most common clinical manifestation of this form of vasculitis is **palpable purpura**, that is, small papules associated with purpura. The distal lower extremities are the most common location, although any site may be involved. The pathophysiology involves circulating antibody–antigen complexes (immune-complexes) that become embedded in the small vessels (usually post-capillary venules). Once embedded, regional complement activation occurs and recruits neutrophils to the site. Additionally, the exposed Fc portion of the antibodies may bind to the Fc-receptor of neutrophils resulting in degranulation and localized destruction of the vessel walls. Implicated antigens include medications (most commonly), foods, nondrug chemicals, microorganisms, and host antigens (ie, tumors, antibodies [rheumatoid factor], phospholipids). **Rheumatoid arthritis, lupus erythematosus, dermatomyositis,** and other diseases in the spectrum of **connective tissue disease** may develop **leukocytoclastic vasculitis (LCV)**. LCV may also occur in patients with **antiphospholipid antibody syndrome.** Clinical and serologic information is critical to arrive at the correct interpretation of the cutaneous findings in these clinical settings. Primary **Sjögren syndrome** not associated with connective tissue disease may present with purpura in addition to ocular and glandular involvement. Skin biopsy commonly shows an **LCV** or **lymphocytic vasculitis.** A wide spectrum of vasculitic processes has been associated with neoplastic disorders. The most common associations include **polyarteritis nodosa** with **hairy cell leukemia** and **cutaneous small-vessel vasculitis** with **lymphoproliferative** or **myeloproliferative disorders.** Solid tumors are less commonly implicated. Occasional cases of **Wegener granulomatosis, microscopic polyarteritis nodosa (aka microscopic polyangiitis),** and **Henoch–Schönlein purpura** have been reported.

Table 4-2A. Common Examples of Drugs Associated with Vasculitis[a]

Allopurinol
Penicillin and aminopenicillins
Sulfonamides
Thiazide diuretics
Pyrazolones
Hydantoins
Propylthiouracil

[a]Data from Wolkenstein and Revuz (1995).[2]

The histopathological findings are referred to as **leukocytoclastic vasculitis (LCV)**. Depending on its severity, this process can be subtle and limited to the superficial dermis or pandermal and florid and associated with necrosis and ulceration. If edema is prominent, a subepidermal blister may form. In a typical case of LCV, the dermal vessels show swelling of the endothelial cells and deposits of strongly eosinophilic strands of fibrin within and around their walls. The deposits of fibrin and the marked edema together give

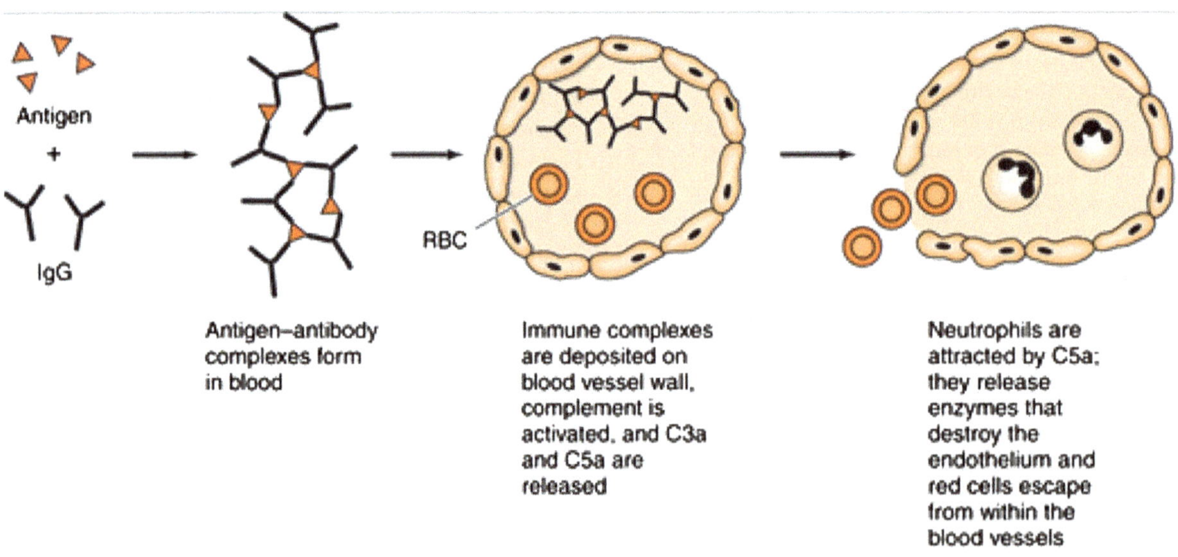

Immune complex (type III) hypersensitivity. (Reproduced, with permission, from Levinson W, ed. *Review of Medical Microbiology and Immunology.* 13th ed. New York, NY: McGraw-Hill Education; 2012.)

[2] Wolkenstein P, Revuz J. Drug-induced severe skin reactions. *Pharmacoepidemiology.* 1995;13:56-68.

the walls of the vessels a "smudgy" appearance referred to as **fibrinoid degeneration.** Actual necrosis of the perivascular collagen, however, is seen primarily in conjunction with lesions of vasculitis showing ulceration. Luminal occlusion of vessels by an expanded, inflamed, edematous vessel wall or by microthrombi may be observed. The cellular infiltrate is present predominantly around or within dermal blood vessel wall, blurring the vascular outlines. Neutrophils and varying numbers of eosinophils and mononuclear cells are found in the infiltrate. Karyorrhectic nuclear debris, or **leukocytoclasia**, gives these infiltrates a dirty appearance and is reflective of neutrophil activation and degranulation. Increased tissue eosinophil counts (5.2 vs 1.05 per 10 high-power fields) have recently been shown to correlate with drug-induced versus nondrug-induced LCV.

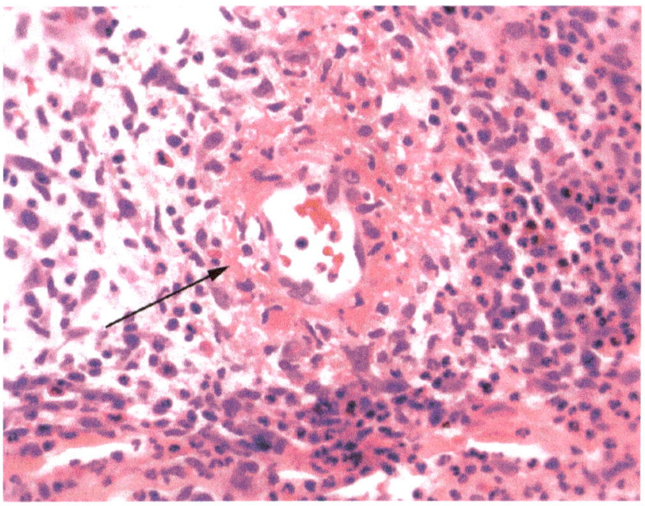

Leukocytoclastic vasculitis. Vascular damage with fibrinoid necrosis (red material at arrow head) and a perivascular neutrophilic infiltrate and nuclear debris are seen.

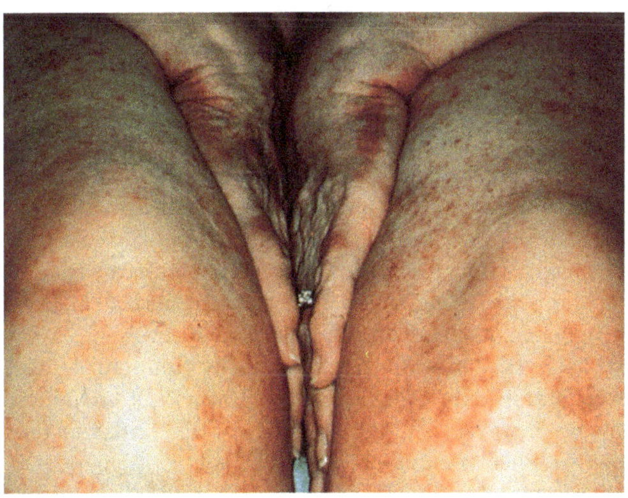

Serum sickness caused by antithymocyte globulin. (Reproduced, with permission, from Kaushansky K, Lichtman MA, Beutler E, Kipps TJ, Seligsohn U, Prchal JT, eds. *Williams Hematology.* 8th ed. New York, NY: McGraw-Hill Education; 2010.)

Arthus reaction is the name given to the inflammation caused by the deposition of immune complexes at a localized site. In contrast, **serum sickness** is a systemic inflammatory response to the presence of circulating immune complexes deposited in many areas of the body. This self-limited syndrome is characterized by a morbilliform-urticarial eruption, fever, arthralgias-myalgias, and lymphadenopathy occurring 7-10 days after a primary antigen exposure, or 2-4 days after a repeat exposure. The offending antigen may be a drug, arthropod sting, antecedent infection, or therapeutic serum immuoglobulins (Table 4-2B). The LCV of serum sickness is not distinctive.

Table 4-2B. Drugs and Sera Associated with Serum-Sickness Reactions[a]

Cefaclor
Minocycline
Penicillins
Propranolol
Streptokinase
Horse serum diphtheria antitoxin
Horse serum antithymocyte globulins
Human diploid cell rabies vaccine

[a]Data from Wolkenstein and Revuz (1995).[3]

ANSWER 4-3: A.

The biopsy reveals a perivascular inflammatory cell infiltrate composed of neutrophils with leukocytoclasia and fibrinoid necrosis of the vessel walls. Extravasated red blood cells are present. Additionally, the infiltrate is diffusely present in the dermis and forms pustules in the epidermis accompanied by spongiosis. The combined clinical, histopathological, and immunofluorescent findings are consistent with **Henoch-Schönlein purpura (HSP).** HSP is characterized clinically by palpable purpura of the buttocks and lower extremities, abdominal pain, and hematuria. Retiform or patterned purpura is considered characteristic of HSP. Occasionally, hemorrhagic bullae may be seen. Typically, but not exclusively, children are affected after a *Streptococcal* upper respiratory tract infection or other infection. However, the clinical picture of HSP is often incomplete. A diagnostic skin biopsy can clarify such cases before significant renal injury occurs. In adults, HSP is less common and histologic confirmation is also important to exclude mimics including serious underlying illnesses such as malignancy. **Acute infantile hemorrhagic edema (AHE)** is an uncommon benign form of cutaneous vasculitis occurring in children less than 2 years of age and is considered by some to be a variant of HSP. AHE often presents with

[3] Wolkenstein P, Revuz J. Drug-induced severe skin reactions. *Pharmacoepidemiology*. 1995;13:56-68.

striking inflammatory edema and ecchymotic purpura with a targetoid or cockade appearance. Recently rotavirus infection has been implicated in one case. Theoretically, abnormalities in the production of IgA follow stimulation of the mucosal immune system. A self-limited syndrome results and usually resolves within 6-16 weeks after onset. Complications generally arise from renal involvement that may even necessitate kidney transplantation. Although renal vasculitis is common, long-term renal impairment occurs in only 2% of patients. Risk factors for severe renal impairment include adult onset, more pronounced systemic symptoms (fever, arthralgias), and lesions above the waist. Various genetic polymorphisms may lead to a predisposition to or protection from these complications. IgA myeloma also has resulted in HSP-like manifestations. Familial Mediterranean fever is also associated with HSP, and occult cases of this genetic disease may be uncovered in patients presenting with HSP.

Microscopically, HSP cannot be distinguished from other forms of leukocytoclastic vasculitis (LCV). In general, conditions involving IgA deposition (ie, **dermatitis herpetiformis, IgA pemphigus**) tend to recruit robust infiltrates of neutrophils. When the leukocytoclastic vasculitis is accompanied by robust neutrophilic infiltrates and intraepidermal pustulation, the term **pustular vasculitis** is sometimes used to describe the process. The histopathological differential diagnosis in these cases includes secondary vasculitis attributed to infection due to the epidermal inflammation. However, in HSP, immunofluorescence studies typically demonstrate deposition of IgA in capillaries. IgA-associated vasculitis may occur outside the symptom complex of HSP, but serologic detection of IgA-fibronectin aggregates tend to be associated with greater likelihood of renal or systemic disease in patients with cutaneous LCV.

ANSWER 4-4: A.

An infectious process needs to be ruled out early in the evaluation of **leukocytoclastic vasculitis (LCV)**. The patient in question has **septic vasculitis**, most likely secondary to *Staphylococcal* infection from the prior surgery. The biopsy in question contains intraluminal and scattered basophilic smudgy debris indicative of bacteria. Clinically, the spectrum of findings ranges from small macules to papules, pustules, and purpura. Septic vasculitis characteristically involves the distal extremities due to emboli containing microorganisms; however diffuse infiltration of vessels by microorganisms may result in widespread purpura. Histopathologically, localized or embolic infection-related vasculitis probably shows a greater frequency of the following changes: subcorneal, intraepidermal, and subepidermal neutrophilic pustules and abscesses (**pustular vasculitis**); dermal infiltrates with more neutrophils relative to other cell types; and intravascular fibrin thrombi, some of which will occasionally contain microorganisms. On the other hand, diffuse infection-related vasculitis may show a lesser degree of vascular damage compared with noninfectious vasculitides. Microorganisms may invade vessels directly or damage them by an immune-mediated mechanism. In septic vasculitis, emboli containing microorganisms frequently become lodged within the microvasculature of the distal extremities. Gram, PAS, and AFB (Fite) stains should always be ordered in patients with any clinical suspicion for infection.

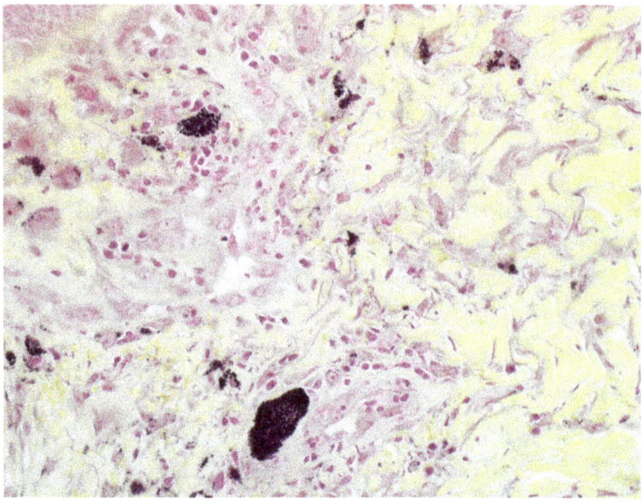

Septic vasculitis, gram stain. There are numerous gram-positive cocci occluding the vessel lumens.

Neisseria meningitidis is a common cause of infectious cutaneous leukocytoclastic vasculitis. Meningococci may be found within endothelial cells and neutrophils at sites of vascular inflammation. However, other gram-positive or gram-negative bacteria and fungi also may cause cutaneous small-vessel vasculitis. ***Staphylococcal* sepsis** can lead to neutrophilic vasculitis with purpura or nodular lesions that may contain microabscesses.

Acid-fast organisms also cause vasculitis. **Lucio phenomenon (erythema necroticans)** and **erythema nodosum leprosum (ENL)** are syndromes that may arise during the course of **lepromatous leprosy.** In both cases, biopsies show vascular damage, including LCV. Histologically, Lucio phenomenon shows necrotizing small-vessel vasculitis, and Fite-Faraco staining reveals large aggregates of acid-fast bacilli within the vascular walls and endothelium and throughout the dermis. Ischemia and necrosis of the epidermis, dermis, and adnexal structures often with ulceration are seen. Some researchers have suggested that the massive endothelial mycobacterial burden in Lucio phenomenon may lead directly to vascular damage.

Rickettsial infections, such as **Rocky Mountain spotted fever (RMSF),** are characterized by invasion of endothelial cells by organisms causing vascular damage. Inflammation, however, often is minimal in RMSF. The Brown-Hopps stain and direct immunofluorescence microscopy may demonstrate the organism.

Many viral organisms such as **hepatitis C, herpesvirus,** and **parvovirus B19** may result in LCV on occasion.

ANSWER 4-5: E.

Urticarial vasculitis is not a specific disease but is a pattern of minimal vasculitis associated with increased vascular permeability. Microscopically, the vessels are lined by swollen endothelial cells and are infiltrated and surrounded by neutrophilic infiltrates with mild leukocytoclasia and red blood cell extravasation. Luminal thrombosis and fibrinoid necrosis of vessel walls are characteristically absent (distinguishing it from **leukocytoclastic vasculitis**). Scattered eosinophils may also be present. Similar to its clinical presentation, the histopathological findings are somewhere in between **urticaria** and **leukocytoclastic vasculitis (LCV)**. Approximately 70% of affected individuals are women. The prevalence of this disorder remains unknown. Clinically, persistent wheals (lasting more than 24 hours by convention) with faint purpura are a typical finding. Often, residual purpura is seen after resolution of the urticarial lesions. Similar to **urticaria**, the lesions are not static and tend to slightly change in size and shape over their evolutionary course. The clinical course generally is benign and episodic, lasting several months. There is a strong association with **chronic urticaria**. Additionally, urticarial vasculitis occurs with some frequency in **lupus erythematosus** and may be the initial clinical manifestation of the disease. Approximately one-third of patients with vasculitic urticaria have decreased complement levels (**hypocomplementemic vasculitis**). These patients may have systemic findings, such as arthralgias and adenopathy, and may be more likely to have underlying systemic lupus erythematosus. Low complement levels and positive anti-C1q antibodies may indicate greater likelihood of more severe systemic disease. Direct immunofluorescence frequently reveals immunoglobulin and complement (occasionally C1q) within the vessels walls.

ANSWER 4-6: E.

Small-vessel vasculitis may be associated with **paraproteins,** that is, abnormal serum proteins, including **cryoglobulins, cryofibrinogens, macroglobulins,** and **gamma heavy chains.** Purpuric lesions tend to form in the microvasculature of the distal extremities and occasionally the nose, which are sites vulnerable to cold temperatures (Table 4-6A).

Type I cryoglobulinemia most commonly leads to an occlusive vasculopathy without inflammation (**thrombogenic vasculopathy**), but also can be associated with **leukocytoclastic vasculitis (LCV)**. Examples include the hyperglobulinemic purpura of **Waldenström hyperglobulinemia** and **Schnitzler syndrome,** which manifests as chronic urticaria with macroglobulinemia (usually monoclonal IgM) and other paraproteinemias.

Types II and III or mixed cryoglobulinemia frequently are associated with connective tissue disorders or infection, in particular, **hepatitis C (HCV) infection**. Idiopathic cases are referred to as **essential cryoglobulinemia.** The cryoprecipitates in **mixed cryoglobulinemias** are typically a composite of polyclonal IgG and an IgM rheumatoid factor that may be monoclonal. Rheumatoid factor is an antibody directed against another antibody, forming an immune complex. Clonal expansion of the rheumatoid factor-synthesizing B-lymphocytes is

Table 4-6A. Types of Cryoglobulins, Composition of Cryoprecipitates, and Disease Associations

TYPE OF CRYOGLOBULINEMIA (ESTIMATED FREQUENCY)	COMPOSITION OF CRYOPRECIPITATES	DISEASE ASSOCIATIONS
Type I (25%)	Monoclonal IgM (sometimes IgG, IgA), immunoglobulin light chain, complexed to other proteins	Hematological disorders • Multiple myeloma • Waldenström macroglobulinemia • Plasma cell dyscrasias, monoclonal gammopathy of undetermined significance (MGUS) • Other lymphoproliferative diseases with M components
Type II (25%)	Combination of monoclonal (usually IgM with rheumatoid factor activity) and polyclonal (usually IgG)	Chronic infection • Viral (HCV) Autoimmune diseases • Sjögren syndrome • Cold agglutinin disease Hematological disorders • Waldenström macroglobulinemia • Chronic lymphocytic leukemia • B-cell non-Hodgkin lymphoma

Table 4-6A. Types of Cryoglobulins, Composition of Cryoprecipitates, and Disease Associations *(continued)*

TYPE OF CRYOGLOBULINEMIA (ESTIMATED FREQUENCY)	COMPOSITION OF CRYOPRECIPITATES	DISEASE ASSOCIATIONS
Type III (50%)	Polyclonal Igs	Chronic infection • Viral (eg, HCV, HIV, HBV) • Bacterial (eg, subacute bacterial endocarditis, leprosy, spirochetal) • Fungal, parasitic Autoimmune diseases • Systemic lupus erythematosus • Rheumatoid arthritis • Dermatomyositis/polymyositis • Inflammatory bowel diseases • Biliary cirrhosis
Type II–III (frequency unknown)	Oligoclonal IgM, intermediate state between the entirely polyclonal type III and the monoclonal, polyclonal type II	Chronic infection (eg, HCV) Autoimmune diseases Lymphoproliferative diseases Chronic liver disease Proliferative glomerulonephritis

Reproduced, with permission, from Goldsmith LA, Katz SI, Gilchrest BA, Paller AS, Leffell DJ, Wolff K, eds. Fitzpatrick's Dermatology in General Medicine. 8th ed. New York, NY: McGraw-Hill Education; 2012. Data from Crowson AN et al. Cutaneous vasculitis: a review. *J Cutan Pathol.* 2003;30:161-173; and Kallemuchikkal U, Gorevic PD. Evaluation of cryoglobulins. *Arch Pathol Lab Med.* 1999;123:119-125.

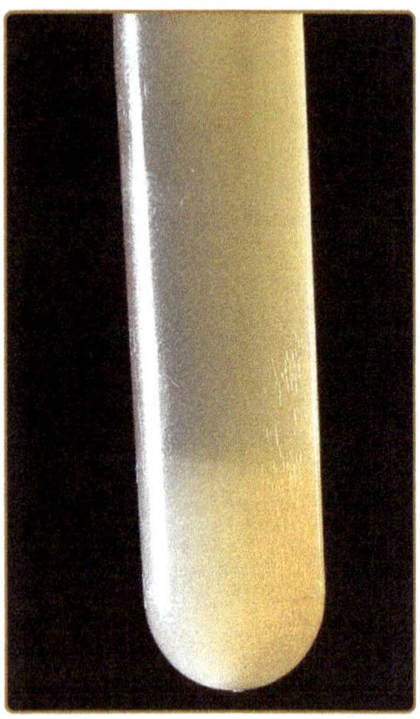

Whitish cryoprecipitates after keeping tube at 4°C (39.2°F) for 48 hours and centrifugation. (Reproduced, with permission, from Goldsmith LA, Katz SI, Gilchrest BA, Paller AS, Leffell DJ, Wolff K, eds. *Fitzpatrick's Dermatology in General Medicine.* 8th ed. New York, NY: McGraw-Hill Education; 2012.)

fundamental to the development of mixed cryoglobulinemia. In cases of cryoglobulinemia associated with HCV, HCV particles and nonenveloped nucleocapsid protein participate in the formation of immune complexes. The rheumatoid factor B-cell clonal expansion primarily takes place in the liver and correlates directly with intrahepatic HCV viral load, indicating the critical role of HCV in the pathogenesis of such B-cell clonality.

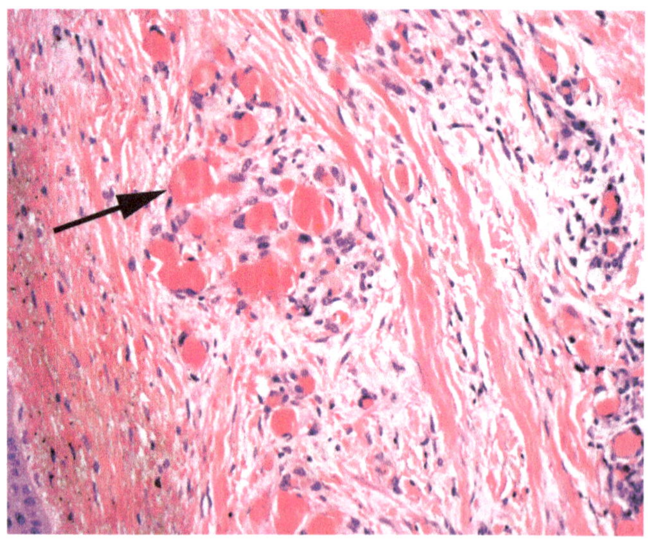

Type I cryoglobulinemia. PAS-positive bright red cryoprecipitates (arrow) are seen in small superficial dermal vessels. In this type of cryoglobulinemia there is typically no inflammation. Types II and III cryoglobulinemia result in immune complex formation and classic leukocytoclastic vasculitis. PAS stain may also occasionally reveal eosinophilic material within the vessels.

In any case, mixed cryoprecipitates commonly trigger a cutaneous LCV but occasionally may form periodic acid-Schiff (PAS)-positive intramural and intravascular deposits.

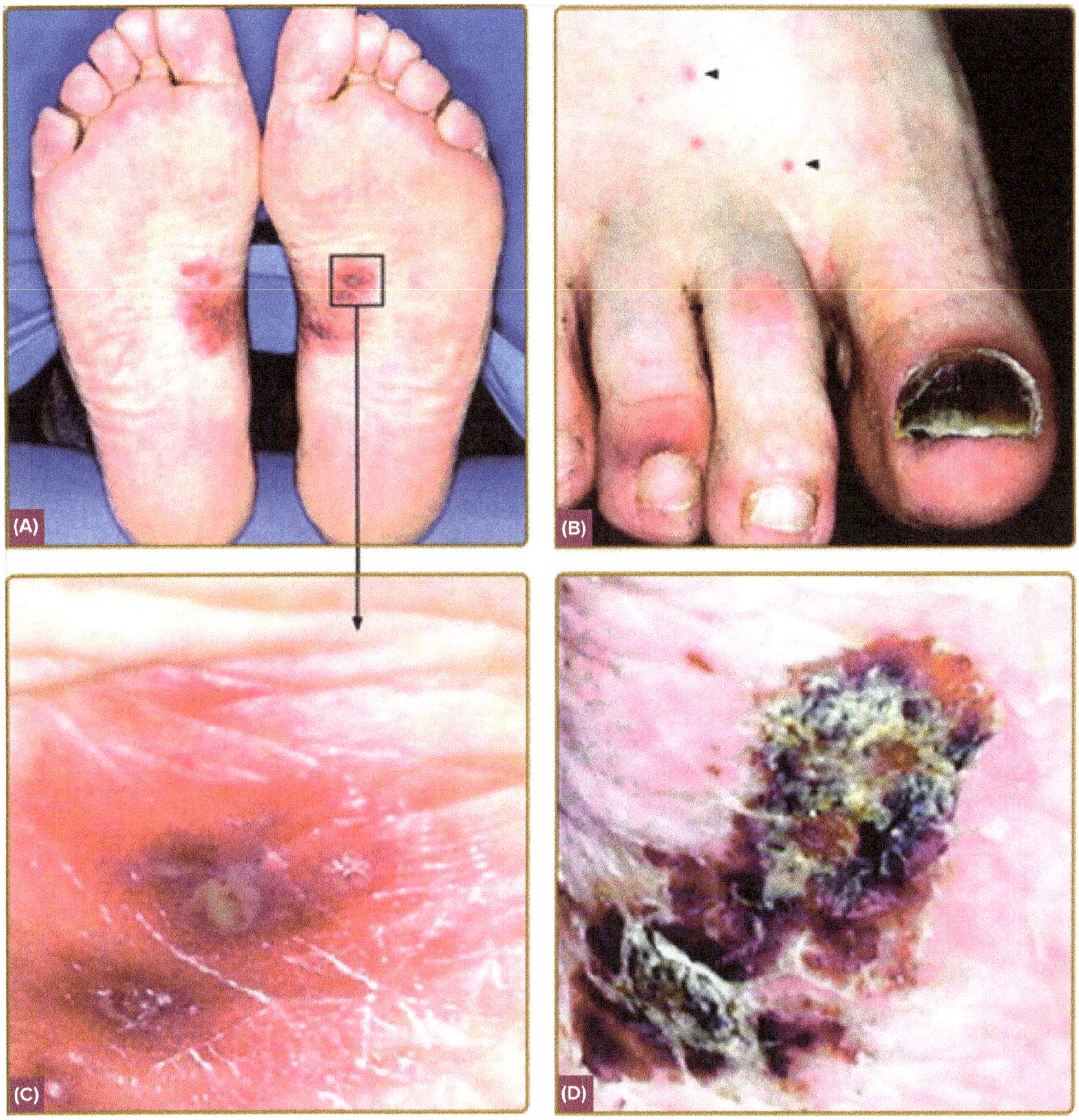

Dermal findings in a patient with type II/III cryoglobulinemia associated with chronic alcoholic liver disease in the absence of viral hepatitis. **(A)** Symmetrical purpuric papular lesions on the medial aspect of the foot soles. **(B)** Petechial macular lesions on the dorsal aspect of the foot on presentation. **(C)** Magnification of the boxed area from panel **A**. **(D)** Partial healing of the foot sole lesion after 8 weeks of oral steroid treatment. Presence of type II/III cryoglobulin in the absence of other pathologic immune serologies or evidence for neoplasm or internal organ involvement confirmed the diagnosis of isolated dermal cryoglobulinemic vasculitis in this patient. (Reproduced, with permission, from Braun GS et al. Cryoglobulinaemic vasculitis: classification and clinical and therapeutic aspects. *Postgrad Med J*. 2007;83:87-94.)

ANSWER 4-7: D.

Erythema elevatum diutinum (EED) is rare condition characterized by persistent, initially red-to-violaceous and later brown-to-yellow papules, nodules, and plaques (Table 4-7A). The lesions, typically distributed symmetrically on the extensor surfaces of the extremities, initially are soft and then evolve into fibrous nodules. EED probably is not a distinct disease entity but rather a clinicopathologic reaction pattern most often developing in association with either a monoclonal or polyclonal gammopathy and in particular IgA hyperglobulinemia. **Inflammatory bowel disease**, **rheumatoid arthritis**, and **systemic lupus erythematosus** also may be associated with EED. HIV-infected patients also develop EED, which can mimic Kaposi sarcoma clinically.

Microscopically, the condition is characterized by ongoing **leukocytoclastic vasculitis** (LCV) with subsequent fibrosis (scar formation). In the early stages, nonspecific LCV is observed. In later stages, granulation tissue and fibrosis develop with a diffuse

Table 4-7A. Erythema Elevatum Diutinum

Clinical Features
Red to violaceous, soft papules
Nodules and plaques evolving into brown-to-yellow fibrous nodules primarily on the extensor surfaces of the extremities
Histopathologic Features
Early: LCV
Mature:
Granulation tissue
Fibrosis with vertical vessels
A diffuse mixed-cell infiltrate with neutrophils
Capillaries with fibrinoid necrosis or fibrous thickening
Late:
Fibrosis
Lipid material may also be present as cholesterol clefts
Active vasculitis may still be observed
Differential Diagnosis
Early:
Sweet syndrome
Other causes of LCV
Rheumatoid neutrophilic dermatitis
Bowel bypass–associated dermatosis
Neutrophilic drug reaction
Behçet syndrome
Mature:
Granuloma faciale
Late:
Kaposi sarcoma
Dermatofibroma
Granuloma annulare

mixed-cell infiltrate showing a predominance of neutrophils. The capillaries may still show deposits of fibrinoid material or merely fibrous thickening. Vertically oriented vessels, as noted in scars, suggest EED. In the late fibrotic stage, lipid material also may be present as well as cholesterol clefts. Serial sections may be required to demonstrate vascular damage in late lesions.

In regards to the differential diagnosis, early lesions of EED show nonspecific LCV. Fully developed lesions of EED may be difficult to distinguish from **Sweet syndrome, rheumatoid neutrophilic dermatitis, bowel bypass-associated dermatosis, neutrophilic drug reaction** (AGEP), **and Behçet syndrome**; however these conditions lack the fibroplasia of EED. **Granuloma faciale (GF)** also may resemble EED but is distinguished by clinical localization to the face, and prominence of eosinophils and plasma cells in addition to neutrophils. Occasional cases of EED may show neutrophilic microabscesses in the tips of dermal papillae that might suggest **dermatitis herpetiformis**. Older lesions of EED must be differentiated from **Kaposi sarcoma, dermatofibroma**, or **granuloma annulare**. In old, fibrotic lesions of EED there is an orderly array of spindle cells and collagen bundles often parallel to the skin surface with vertically arranged capillaries similar to a scar. Many of the spindle cells have the immunohistochemical and electron microscopic features of macrophages. Neutrophils, nuclear dust, and fibrin owing to persistent vascular damage may be present, helping to distinguish these lesions from dermatofibromas or scars. The irregularly arranged, jagged vascular spaces of Kaposi sarcoma are absent. EED is negative for HHV8. Focal areas of basophilic collagen caused by nuclear dust in EED can resemble the mucin seen in granuloma annulare but this material does not stain with alcian blue. **Rheumatoid nodules** are well circumscribed and arise in the deep dermis and subcutis; however they are composed of palisading granulomas with marked fibrosis, which may otherwise resemble EED.

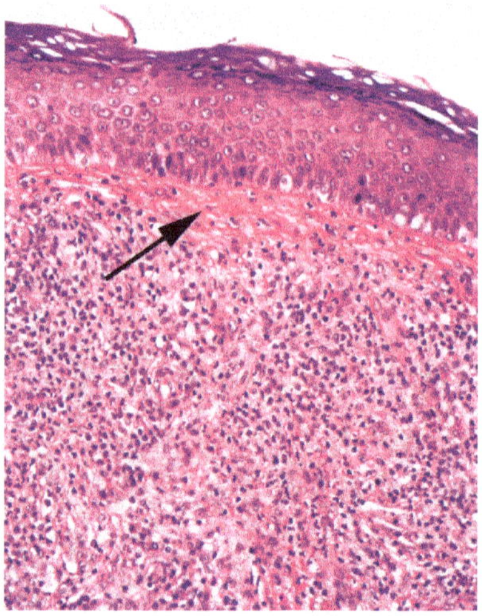

Erythema elevatum diutinum. A mixed infiltrate is noted in the dermis with a grenz zone (arrow). Higher magnification would reveal leukocytoclastic vasculitis, neutrophilic infiltrates, and fibroplasia.

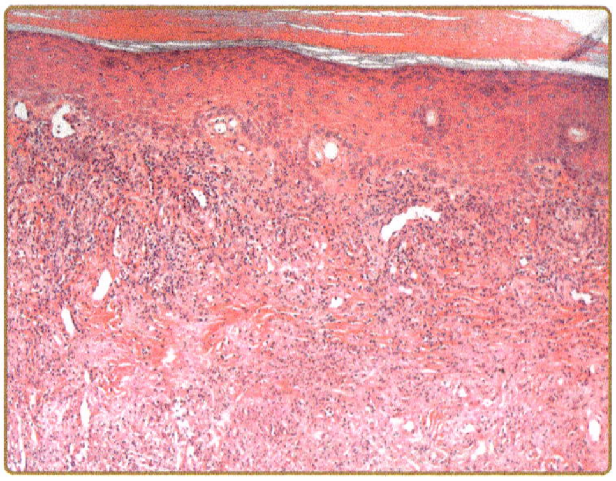

Early stage lesion of erythema elevatum diutinum. Focal leukocytoclastic vasculitis with a fairly dense perivascular and interstitial infiltrate composed of neutrophils, lymphocytes, histiocytes, and leukocytoclastic debris. Mild capillary proliferation is also evident. (Reproduced, with permission, from Goldsmith LA, Katz SI, Gilchrest BA, Paller AS, Leffell DJ, Wolff K, eds. *Fitzpatrick's Dermatology in General Medicine*. 8th ed. New York, NY: McGraw-Hill Education; 2012.)

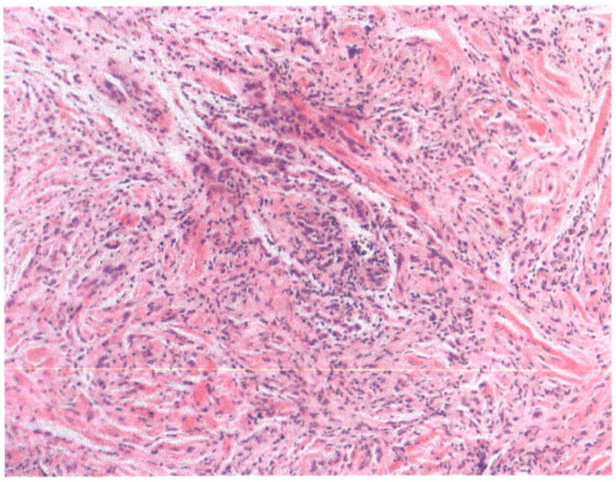

Early stage lesion of erythema elevatum diutinum. Higher magnification highlighting the early granulation tissue-like response. (Reproduced, with permission, from Goldsmith LA, Katz SI, Gilchrest BA, Paller AS, Leffell DJ, Wolff K, eds. *Fitzpatrick's Dermatology in General Medicine*. 8th ed. New York, NY: McGraw-Hill Education; 2012.)

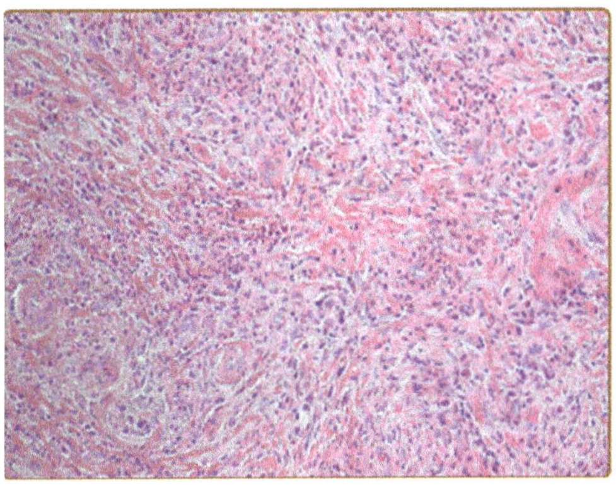

Later-stage lesion of erythema elevatum diutinum. Prominent perivascular and interstitial fibrosis with scattered lymphocytes and histiocytes. Marked stromal fibrosis. (Reproduced, with permission, from Goldsmith LA, Katz SI, Gilchrest BA, Paller AS, Leffell DJ, Wolff K, eds. *Fitzpatrick's Dermatology in General Medicine*. 8th ed. New York, NY: McGraw-Hill Education; 2012.)

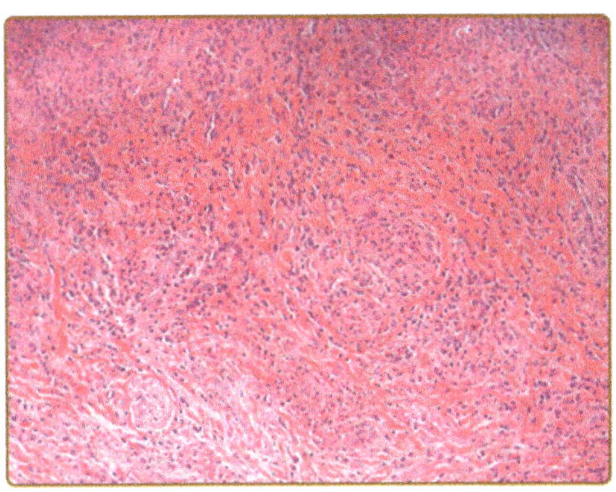

End-stage lesion of erythema elevatum diutinum. Concentric perivascular fibrosis and interstitial fibrosis with lymphocytes and histiocytes. (Reproduced, with permission, from Goldsmith LA, Katz SI, Gilchrest BA, Paller AS, Leffell DJ, Wolff K, eds. *Fitzpatrick's Dermatology in General Medicine*. 8th ed. New York, NY: McGraw-Hill Education; 2012.)

ANSWER 4-8: E.

Granuloma faciale (GF) is characterized by solitary papules, plaques, or nodules most commonly involving the face (Table 4-8A). The lesions are typically asymptomatic red, brown, or violaceous plaques that are soft, smooth, and well circumscribed, often showing follicular accentuation and telangiectasias. Ulceration is rare. Sites of predilection include the nose, preauricular area, cheeks, forehead, eyelids, and ears. Lesions may be present for weeks or months and tend to follow a chronic course. Lesions are typically asymptomatic; however, patients may complain of tenderness, burning, or pruritus. Photoexacerbation of lesions has been reported. Rare upper respiratory tract forms have been described.

Microscopically, a dense polymorphous infiltrate is present mainly in the upper half of the dermis, but it may extend into the lower dermis and occasionally even into the subcutaneous tissue. Quite characteristically, the infiltrate does not invade the epidermis or the pilosebaceous appendages but is separated from them by a narrow **grenz zone** of normal collagen. The pilosebaceous structures tend to remain intact. The polymorphous infiltrate consists primarily of neutrophils and eosinophils, but mononuclear cells, plasma cells, and mast cells are also present. Vascular damage in GF is seen but often is limited, and thus perhaps GF is best termed a **neutrophilic vascular reaction**. However, vascular damage may be important to the pathogenesis of this lesion because direct immunofluorescence data suggest an immune complex–mediated event with deposition of mainly IgG in and around vessels. Frequently, the nuclei of some of the neutrophils are fragmented, especially in the vicinity of the capillaries, thus forming nuclear dust. Often there

Table 4-8A. Granuloma Faciale

Clinical Features
Asymptomatic, soft, brown-red, slowly enlarging papules or plaques usually on the face
Histopathologic Features
Dense polymorphous dermal infiltrate primarily of neutrophils but also eosinophils, plasma cells
Grenz zone beneath epidermis and around pilosebaceous appendages
Intact pilosebaceous structures
Subtle evidence of vascular damage
Nuclear dust
Fibrinoid material within and around vessels
Foam cells and fibrosis in older lesions
Differential Diagnosis
Infections
Erythema elevatum diutinum
Acne vulgaris or rosacea
Acute folliculitis
Other neutrophilic dermatoses
Sweet syndrome

is some evidence of vasculitis with deposition of fibrinoid material within and around vessel walls. Occasionally, some hemorrhage is noted. Foam cells and fibrosis are observed frequently in older lesions.

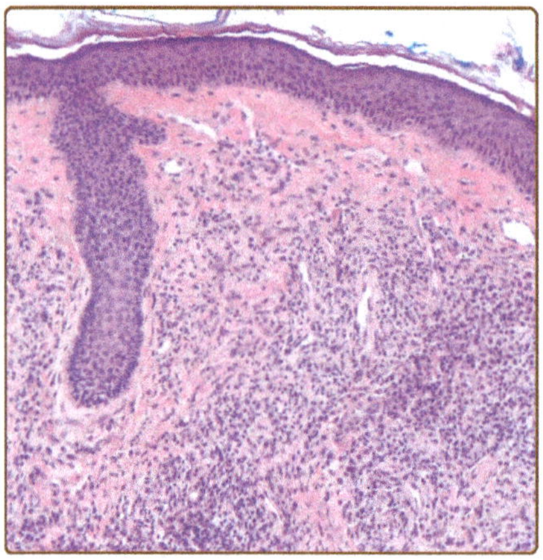

Granuloma faciale. This low-power histologic section shows a mixed infiltrate of lymphocytes, histiocytes, neutrophils, plasma cells, and eosinophils. There is sparing of a narrow grenz zone between the inflammatory infiltrate and the overlying epidermis. (Reproduced, with permission, from Goldsmith LA, Katz SI, Gilchrest BA, Paller AS, Leffell DJ, Wolff K, eds. *Fitzpatrick's Dermatology in General Medicine.* 8th ed. New York, NY: McGraw-Hill Education; 2012.)

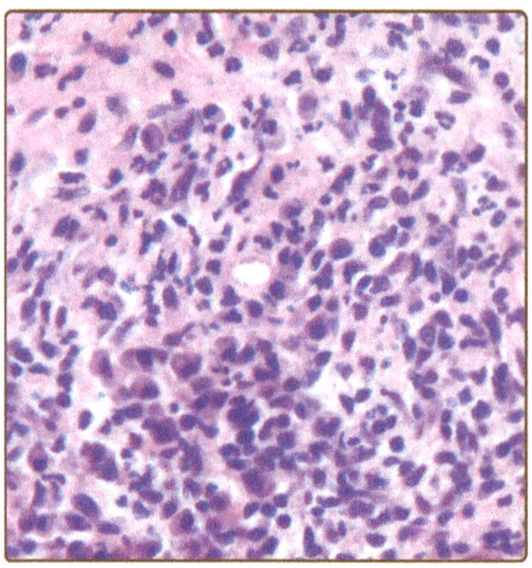

Granuloma faciale. This histologic section shows perivascular deposition of fibrin and a mixed infiltrate of lymphocytes, neutrophils, plasma cells, and eosinophils. (Reproduced, with permission, from Goldsmith LA, Katz SI, Gilchrest BA, Paller AS, Leffell DJ, Wolff K, eds. *Fitzpatrick's Dermatology in General Medicine.* 8th ed. New York, NY: McGraw-Hill Education; 2012.)

In regards to the differential diagnosis, GF can appear similar to **erythema elevatum diutinum (EED)**, although the prevalence of eosinophils and plasma cells favor GF. Other neutrophilic dermatoses can be distinguished from GF by the lack of a grenz zone and clinical features. **Sweet syndrome** contains marked papillary dermal edema and characteristically lacks vascular damage. Frank **leukocytoclastic vasculitis** should not be seen in GF. In acneiform lesions and folliculitides (ie, **rosacea**), pilosebaceous units are invaded by inflammatory cells and may be destroyed or disrupted. **Angiolymphoid hyperplasia with eosinophilia (epithelioid hemangioma)** also commonly presents as papules on the face, preauricular areas, and ears. Additionally, they also contain robust lymphocytic and eosinophilic infiltrates; however GF contains large numbers of plasma cells and lacks the brightly eosinophilic plump epithelioid endothelial cells seen in angiolymphoid hyperplasia with eosinophilia.

ANSWER 4-9: D.

This is a classic example of **Sweet syndrome** (Table 4-9A). In many clinical conditions there are reactions characterized by a neutrophilic infiltrate with variable leukocytoclasis and some vascular damage. However, the extent of vascular damage is insufficient for necrotizing vasculitis; that is, fibrinoid necrosis is lacking. This histologic pattern needs to be distinguished from necrotizing vasculitis. However, occasionally a

Table 4-9A. Sweet Syndrome

Clinical Features
- Women greater than men
- Adults, but patients of any size
- Fever
- Leukocytosis
- Elevated erythrocyte sedimentation rate
- Erythematous plaques
- Vesicles and pustules of the face or extremities, rarely trunk
- Response to systemic steroids or potassium iodide
- Involvement of noncutaneous sites: eye, joints, oral mucosa, visceral sites
- Associations:
  - Gastrointestinal or upper respiratory tract infection (classic Sweet syndrome)
  - Malignancy, especially myeloproliferative disorders
  - Sjögren syndrome
  - Pustular psoriasis
  - Rheumatoid arthritis
  - Subacute lupus erythematous
  - Subacute thyroiditis
  - Pregnancy

Histopathologic Features
- Superficial dermal neutrophilic infiltrate with some leukocytoclasis
- Vascular alterations, including vasodilation and swelling of endothelium
- Erythrocyte extravasation
- Prominent edema with subepidermal blister formation

Table 4-9A. Sweet Syndrome *(continued)*

Differential Diagnosis
Infection
Vasculitis
Other neutrophilic dermatoses
Dermatitis herpetiformis or linear IgA disease
Neutrophilic drug reaction
Leukemia cutis
Suppurative panniculitides
Neutrophilic arthropod bite
Secondary syphilis

neutrophilic vascular reaction may be a precursor to or associated with full-blown necrotizing vasculitis. Conditions with a neutrophilic vascular reaction that rarely develop necrotizing vasculitis generally are categorized as **neutrophilic dermatoses** (Table 4-9B). The term "**neutrophilic dermatosis**" includes a number of conditions characterized (1) histopathologically by a neutrophilic infiltrate, which may be clonal even if unassociated with myelodysplasia, (2) by the lack of microorganisms on special stains and cultures, and (3) by clinical improvement with systemic steroid treatment. The lesions are most commonly associated with hematologic, gastrointestinal, or rheumatologic diseases. A relationship between these entities is suggested by their occasional co-occurrence in patients with predisposing conditions. The stimulus for the aggregation of neutrophils is unclear. However, as more is understood about the inherited disorders associated with neutrophilic aggregates, termed autoinflammatory disorders, revelations regarding the etiology of acquired neutrophilic dermatoses may be around the corner. Vascular damage has been observed in these conditions, but is likely secondary to the dense neutrophilic infiltrate.

Table 4-9B. Differential Diagnosis of Neutrophilic Dermatoses

Neutrophilic dermatoses
Granuloma faciale
Sweet syndrome
Inherited autoinflammatory syndromes
Bowel-associated neutrophilic dermatosis
Pyoderma gangrenosum
Infection
Neutrophilic vesicular dermatoses
Linear IgA disease
Dermatitis herpetiformis
Leukocytoclastic vasculitis
Leukemia cutis
Neutrophilic drug reaction

In 1964, Sweet described a disease process that he termed "**acute febrile neutrophilic dermatosis**" that was characterized by acute onset of fever, leukocytosis, and erythematous plaques infiltrated by neutrophils. This condition classically occurs in middle-aged women after a nonspecific infection of the respiratory or gastrointestinal tract. Abrupt onset of painful or tender erythematous plaques, nodules, vesicles, and pustules on the face, extremities, and rarely, the trunk is characteristic. Occasional cases are limited to the hands. Involvement of noncutaneous sites, such as the eyes, joints, and oral mucosa, as well as visceral sites (ie, lung, liver, brain, and kidney), has been reported. A number of disorders have been associated with neutrophilic dermatoses similar to those seen in Sweet syndrome. About 20% of cases are associated with malignancy, especially those involving the subcutis (**subcutaneous Sweet syndrome**). The etiology of Sweet syndrome is unknown. Current hypotheses include altered T-cell activation and altered function of neutrophils. The neutrophils within the lesions may be clonal whether or not associated with myelodysplasia. The vascular alterations seen in Sweet syndrome may be secondary to the massive extravasation of activated neutrophils. Direct immunofluorescence studies generally are negative in Sweet syndrome.

Microscopically, a dense, band-like, and perivascular infiltrate composed largely of neutrophils occupies the superficial dermis. Some of the neutrophils may show leukocytoclasis; however it is typically minimal. Lymphocytes, histiocytes, and occasionally eosinophils may be included in the infiltrate. Cases associated with myelodysplastic syndrome may exhibit perivascular infiltrates of atypical mononuclear cells. This finding may herald the transformation into acute myelogenous leukemia. The density of the neutrophilic infiltrate varies and may be limited in a small proportion of patients. Although extensive vascular damage is not a feature of Sweet syndrome, common vascular alterations include vasodilation, swelling of endothelium, erythrocyte extravasation, and occasional karyorrhectic debris. Frank fibrinoid

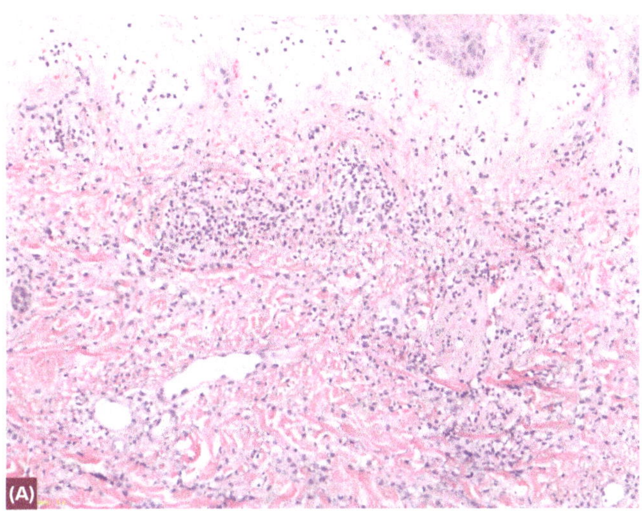

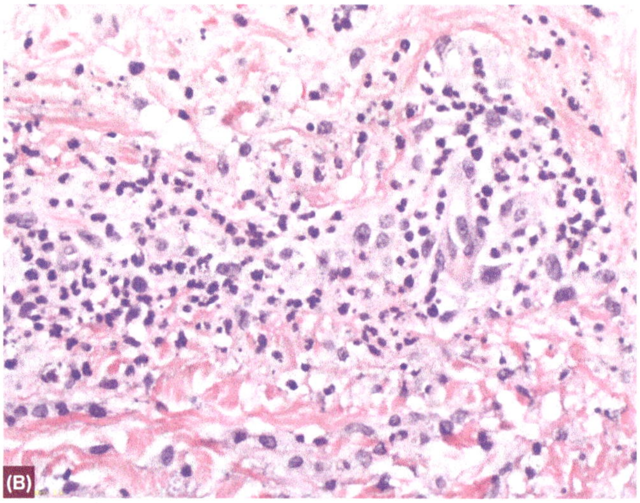

Sweet syndrome. (A) There is striking papillary dermal edema accompanied by perivascular and interstitial inflammatory infiltrates. **(B)** High magnification reveals numerous neutrophils without significant leukocytoclasia and no vascular damage.

necrosis may occur but is rare and most commonly is seen in vessels underlying areas of ulceration (**localized secondary vasculitis**). A striking feature is the presence of prominent superficial dermal edema, which may result in subepidermal blister formation (**bullous Sweet syndrome**). As expected, the histologic appearance varies depending on the stage of the process. In later stages, lymphocytes and histiocytes may predominate.

In regards to the differential diagnosis, **infection** (bacterial or fungal especially) must be excluded by special stains and tissue culture. **Vasculitis** should be considered, but necrotizing vasculitis, with fibrinoid necrosis, should not be observed in Sweet or Sweet-like lesions. The findings overlap with other neutrophilic dermatoses such as early or **bullous pyoderma gangrenosum, bowel-associated dermatosis-arthritis, periodic fever syndromes**, and **erythema elevatum diutinum (EED)**. Clinical features should distinguish these entities. **Bowel-associated dermatosis–arthritis syndrome (BADAS)** was initially described in patients after jejunoileal bypass surgery. This syndrome has been expanded to include neutrophilic cutaneous lesions associated with many bowel diseases. Patients may have inflammatory bowel disease or a blind loop after peptic ulcer surgery. The cutaneous lesions are characterized by initial small macules that develop through a papular phase into pustules on a purpuric base. This evolution usually occurs within a 2-day period. The lesions commonly reach a size of 0.5-1.5 cm. They are typically distributed on the upper part of the body, especially the arms, rather than the dependent sites of the legs, and often occur in episodic, recurrent crops. Fever, myalgias, and arthralgias may accompany the disease process. An immune complex–mediated reaction triggered by intestinal bacteria-derived antigens may lead to the initiating vascular insult. Microscopically, BADAS is

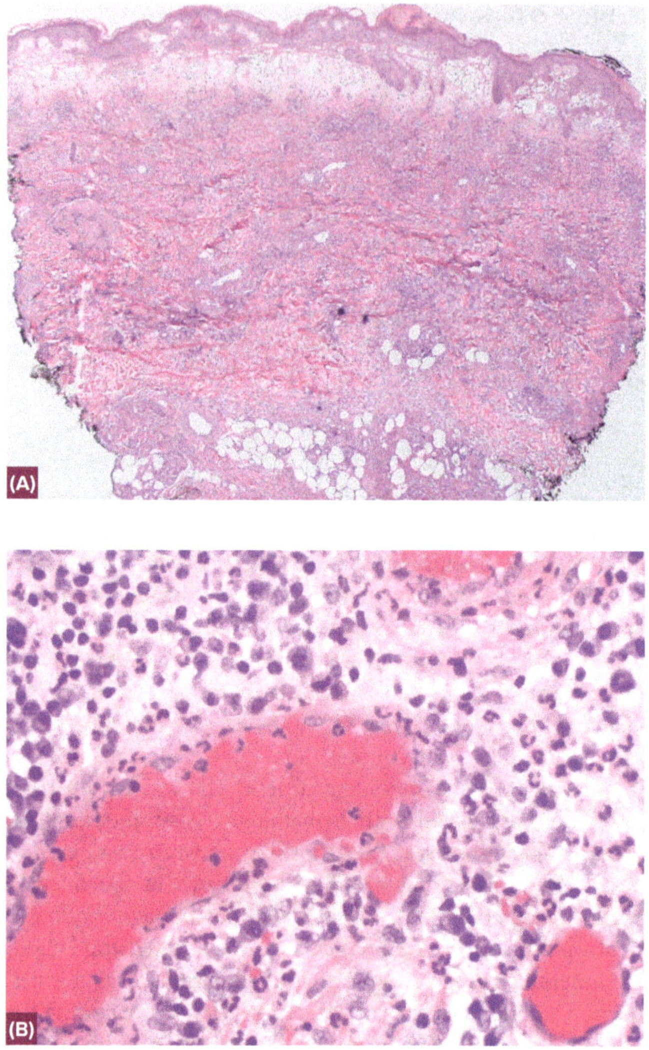

Sweet syndrome involving the subcutis. (A) There is prominent papillary dermal edema and a diffuse inflammatory infiltrate extending into the subcutaneous fat. **(B)** High magnification reveals numerous perivascular atypical (dysplastic) mononuclear cells and mature neutrophils. The vessel walls contain emigrating neutrophils without significant vascular injury (no thrombi or fibrinoid necrosis). This case arose in association with myelodysplastic syndrome and preceded the onset of acute myelogenous leukemia.

similar to Sweet syndrome; however unlike Sweet syndrome, frank leukocytoclastic vasculitis with intraepidermal pustulation may be seen.

Neutrophilic vesicular diseases such as **dermatitis herpetiformis** or **linear IgA disease** may be suspected in cases of Sweet syndrome with vesicle formation. In addition, some cases of **lupus erythematosus** or **polymorphous light eruption** with an unusual robust neutrophilic component may resemble Sweet syndrome. Clinicopathologic and immunofluorescence studies should distinguish these entities. **Secondary**

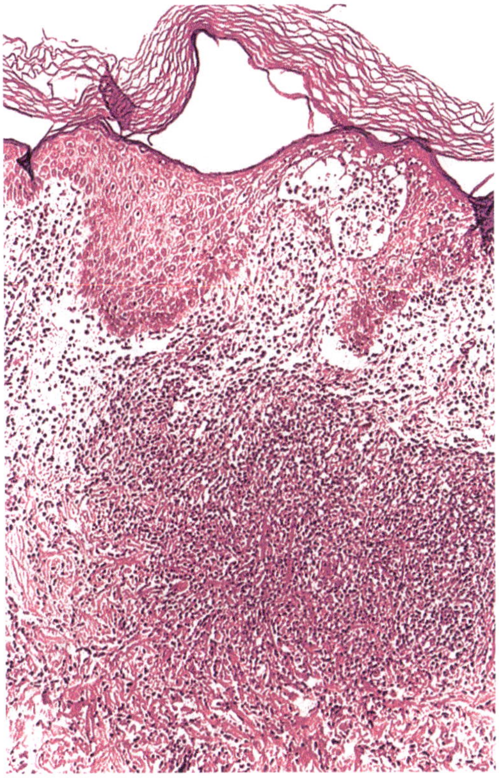

Bowel-associated dermatosis–arthritis syndrome (BADAS). In addition to edema and dense superficial dermal neutrophilic infiltrates accompanied by mild vascular damage, there is an intraepidermal neutrophilic pustule.

syphilis also may mimic Sweet syndrome. Other considerations include a neutrophilic drug reaction (**pustular drug eruption**). Leukemia cutis must be excluded in the appropriate clinical setting.

ANSWER 4-10: A.

This is a classic clinical presentation of **ulcerative pyoderma gangrenosum (PG)**. As with other **neutrophilic dermatoses**, an infection must be excluded to arrive at the correct diagnosis. Several clinical types have been described: **ulcerative PG** with an undermined border; **pustular PG** with discrete, painful pustules; painful **bullous PG** with progression to a superficial ulceration; and **vegetative PG** with a painless ulcer and a nonundermined exophytic border (Table 4-10A). Classically, lesions begin as tender papulopustules or folliculitis that eventually ulcerate. Again, as with other neutrophilic dermatoses, **pyoderma gangrenosum**, especially the vegetative form, may occur as an isolated cutaneous phenomenon or may be a cutaneous manifestation associated with a number of systemic disease processes, such as inflammatory bowel disease, connective tissue disease, or a lymphoproliferative disorder. **Bullous PG**, when associated with **leukemia**, is an

Table 4-10A. Pyoderma Gangrenosum

Clinical Features
Tender papulopustules or folliculitis
Ulcerated lesions with bluish borders
Vegetating lesions
Associated diseases:
Inflammatory bowel disease
Malignancy (especially leukemia)
Connective tissue disease
Immunologic abnormalities
Monoclonal gammopathy (hypogammaglobulinemia, hyperimmunoglobulin E, iatrogenic immunosuppression)
Histopathologic Evaluation
Possible lymphocytic infiltrates early
Extensive neutrophilic infiltrates often involving follicular structures
Neutrophilic vascular reaction with variable vascular damage
Pustular vasculitis
Ulceration
Necrosis
Occasional granulomatous inflammation
Differential Diagnosis
Deep fungal infection
Mycobacterial lesions
Traumatic deep ulceration (factitial diseases)
Sweet and Sweet-like dermatosis
Subcorneal pustular dermatosis
Erythema elevatum diutinum
Bowel-associated dermatosis
Spider bite
Pustular drug reactions
Blastomycosis-like pyoderma (from vegetative PG)

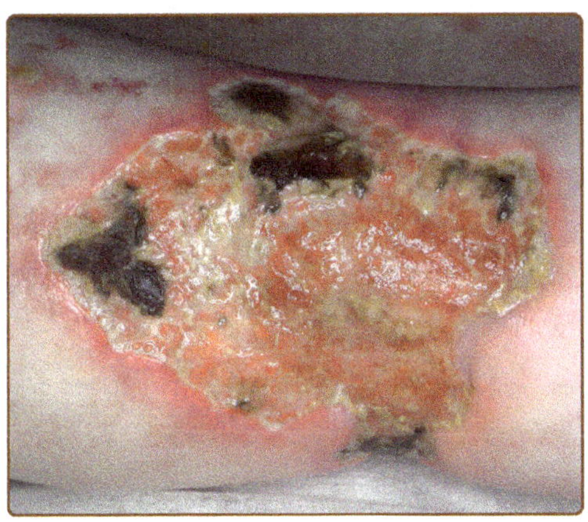

Established lesion of ulcerative pyoderma gangrenosum showing well-defined ulceration with surrounding zone of erythema. (Reproduced, with permission, from Goldsmith LA, Katz SI, Gilchrest BA, Paller AS, Leffell DJ, Wolff K, eds. *Fitzpatrick's Dermatology in General Medicine*. 8th ed. New York, NY: McGraw-Hill Education; 2012.)

indicator of poor prognosis. A uniting feature for this condition is **pathergy**, in which mild trauma or inflammation of any cause results in the aberrant influx of neutrophils and the eventual tissue break down and ulceration. The classic clinical presentation is that of a small wound, such as a cut, bug bite, or ruptured hair follicle, transforming into a large ulcer. Surgical management via debridement worsens in the condition and may result in significant tissue destruction and eventual scar formation.

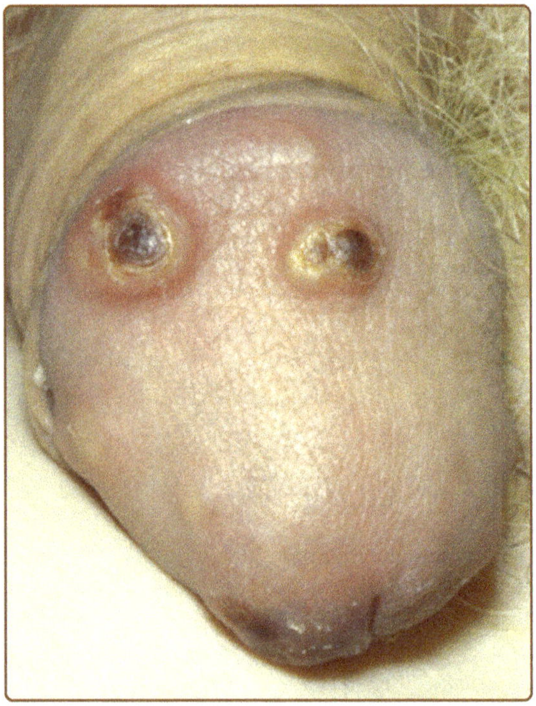

Pustular pyoderma gangrenosum lesions of the penis in a patient who also had ulcerative pyoderma gangrenosum. (Reproduced, with permission, from Goldsmith LA, Katz SI, Gilchrest BA, Paller AS, Leffell DJ, Wolff K, eds. *Fitzpatrick's Dermatology in General Medicine*. 8th ed. New York, NY: McGraw-Hill Education; 2012.)

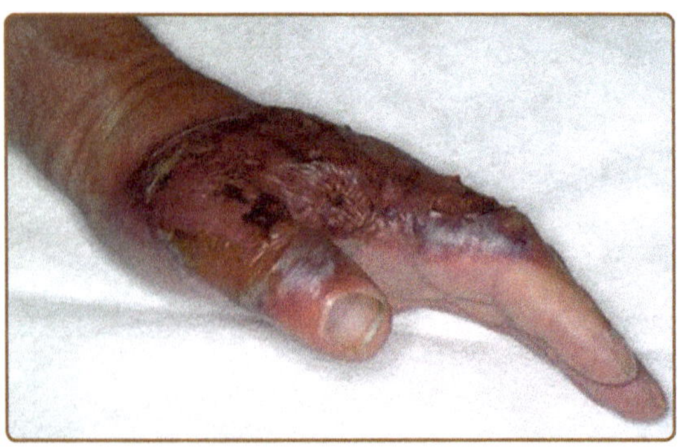

Bullous pyoderma gangrenosum lesion showing collapsed roof of blister and superficial erosive quality of the subsequent ulceration. (Reproduced, with permission, from Goldsmith LA, Katz SI, Gilchrest BA, Paller AS, Leffell DJ, Wolff K, eds. *Fitzpatrick's Dermatology in General Medicine*. 8th ed. New York, NY: McGraw-Hill Education; 2012.)

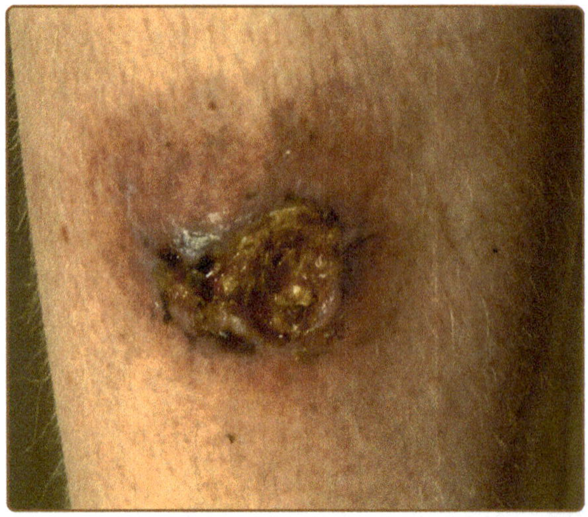

Vegetative pyoderma gangrenosum. An indolent area of chronic inflammation and ulceration that was present for months. (Reproduced, with permission, from Goldsmith LA, Katz SI, Gilchrest BA, Paller AS, Leffell DJ, Wolff K, eds. *Fitzpatrick's Dermatology in General Medicine*. 8th ed. New York, NY: McGraw-Hill Education; 2012.)

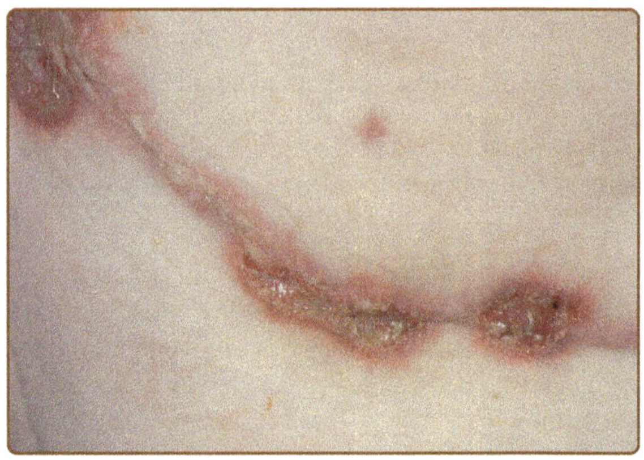

Several pathergic pyoderma gangrenosum lesions occurring along a thoracotomy scar site. Note central ulceration, violaceous borders, and peripheral rim of erythema. (Reproduced, with permission, from Goldsmith LA, Katz SI, Gilchrest BA, Paller AS, Leffell DJ, Wolff K, eds. *Fitzpatrick's Dermatology in General Medicine*. 8th ed. New York, NY: McGraw-Hill Education; 2012.)

The histopathological findings are nonspecific and depend on the type of lesion and timing of the biopsy. The diagnosis primarily is clinical. Most authors studying early lesions have reported a primarily neutrophilic infiltrate that frequently involves follicular structures. Other authors, however, have stated that the lesions begin with a lymphocytic reaction. Degrees of vessel involvement range from none to fibrinoid necrosis. In the majority of biopsied lesions, a neutrophilic vascular reaction is present with limited vascular damage. The infiltrate tends to be deeper and more extensive than in **classic Sweet syndrome**. Additionally, PG does not exhibit the extensive papillary dermal edema seen in Sweet.

A pattern of pustular vasculitis may be present. Fully developed lesions show ulceration, necrosis, and a mixed inflammatory cell infiltrate. Involvement of the deep reticular dermis and subcutis may exhibit primarily mononuclear cell and granulomatous inflammatory reactions.

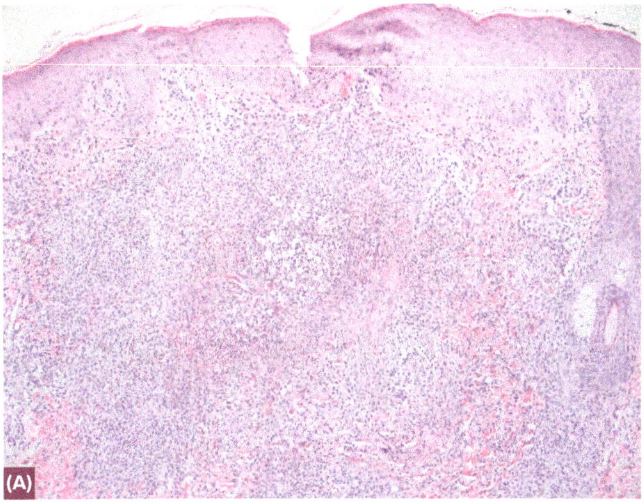

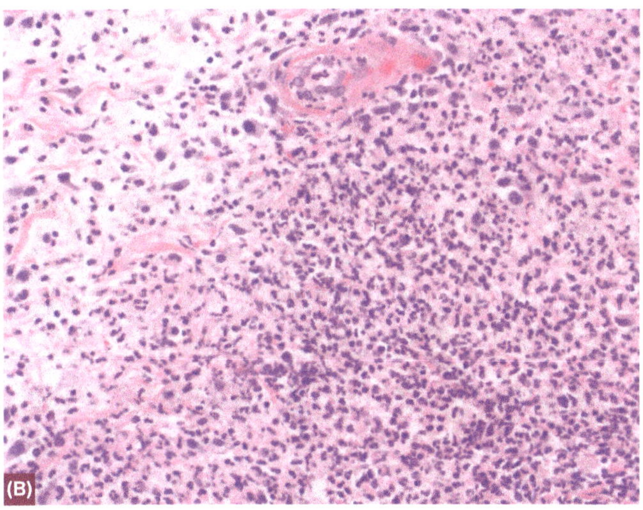

Pyoderma gangrenosum. (A) There are diffuse inflammatory infiltrates without prominent superficial dermal edema. **(B)** High magnification reveals predominantly neutrophils and necrosis of the dermal collagen. A small vessel with peripheral fibrinoid change is present.

Answer choice A describes **Behçet disease**, which is a multisystem disease characterized by oral **aphthous ulcers** and at least two of the following criteria: genital aphthae, synovitis, posterior uveitis, superficial thrombophlebitis (STP), cutaneous pustular vasculitis, and meningoencephalitis (Table 4-10B). Exacerbations and remissions are unpredictable. Just like PG, Behçet also exhibits **pathergy** and the skin pathergy test, which elicits a nonspecific hyperreactive lesion in response to a needle-prick, has been used in the diagnosis of Behçet disease. This reaction is similar to the erythematous papules or pustules that appear spontaneously in these patients. Behçet disease is most common from the Middle East through Asia, but is rare in northern Europe and the United States. An association with HLA-B51 has been reported. The clinical presentation is extremely variable and so is the vascular involvement. Vascular lesions include not only active inflammatory lesions but also aneurysms, arterial or venous occlusions, and varices. The etiology of Behçet disease remains unknown. Enhanced inflammatory response to minor stimuli and the possibility of a genetic susceptibility suggest that Behçet disease may be an autoinflammatory disorder, similar to familial Mediterranean fever.

Table 4-10B. Behçet Syndrome

Clinical Features
- Oral and genital aphthae
- Synovitis
- Posterior uveitis
- Meningoencephalitis
- Vascular lesions: cutaneous pustular vasculitis, aneurysms, arterial or venous occlusions, varices
- Middle East and Japan, rare in Northern Europe and the United States
- HLA-B51 associated

Histopathologic Features
- Early: neutrophilic, fully developed necrotizing leukocytoclastic vasculitis or pustular vasculitis
- Late: lymphocytic and granulomatous vascular reactions

Differential Diagnosis
- Infection and infectious vasculitis
- Vasculitis in connective tissue disease
- Paraneoplastic vasculitis
- Neutrophilic vascular reactions
  - Sweet syndrome
  - Pyoderma gangrenosum
- Inflammatory bowel disease
- Other pustular vasculitides
- Bowel bypass–associated process

The histopathologic spectrum of mucocutaneous inflammatory vascular lesions in **Behçet disease**, depending on the stage and activity of the lesion, includes neutrophilic, lymphocytic, and granulomatous vascular reactions. Biopsy specimens of early lesions typically show a neutrophilic vascular reaction, and Behçet disease is sometimes classified as a **neutrophilic dermatosis/neutrophilic vascular reaction**. However, unlike in the neutrophilic dermatoses, fully developed **necrotizing leukocytoclastic vasculitis, pustular**

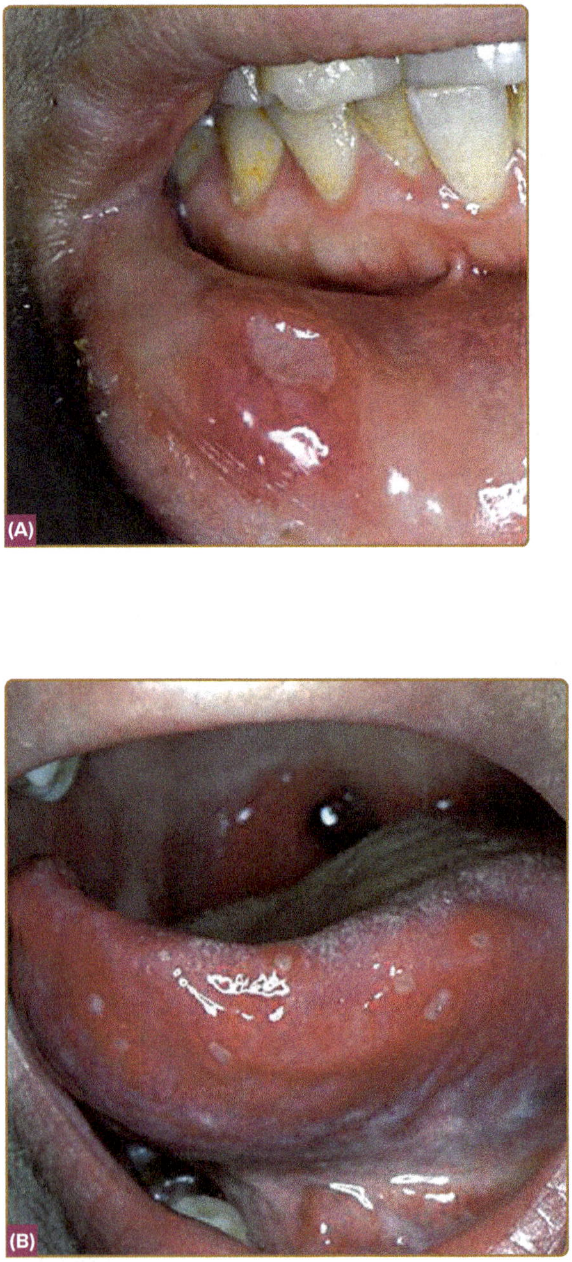

Behçet disease. Single **(A)** and multiple **(B)** oral aphthous ulcers. (Part **A** reproduced, with permission, from Altenburg A et al. Epidemiology and clinical manifestations of Adamantiades-Behçet disease in Germany—current pathogenetic concepts and therapeutic possibilities. *J Dtsch Dermatol Ges.* 2006;4:49; part **B** from Goldsmith LA, Katz SI, Gilchrest BA, Paller AS, Leffell DJ, Wolff K, eds. *Fitzpatrick's Dermatology in General Medicine*. 8th ed. New York, NY: McGraw-Hill Education; 2012.)

vasculitis, or **lymphocytic vasculitis** may develop. Fully developed lesions typically contain large numbers of mononuclear cells admixed with neutrophils and occasional plasma cells. Unlike the neutrophilic vascular reactions, Behçet is associated with phlebothrombosis of medium-sized vessels in the subcutis.

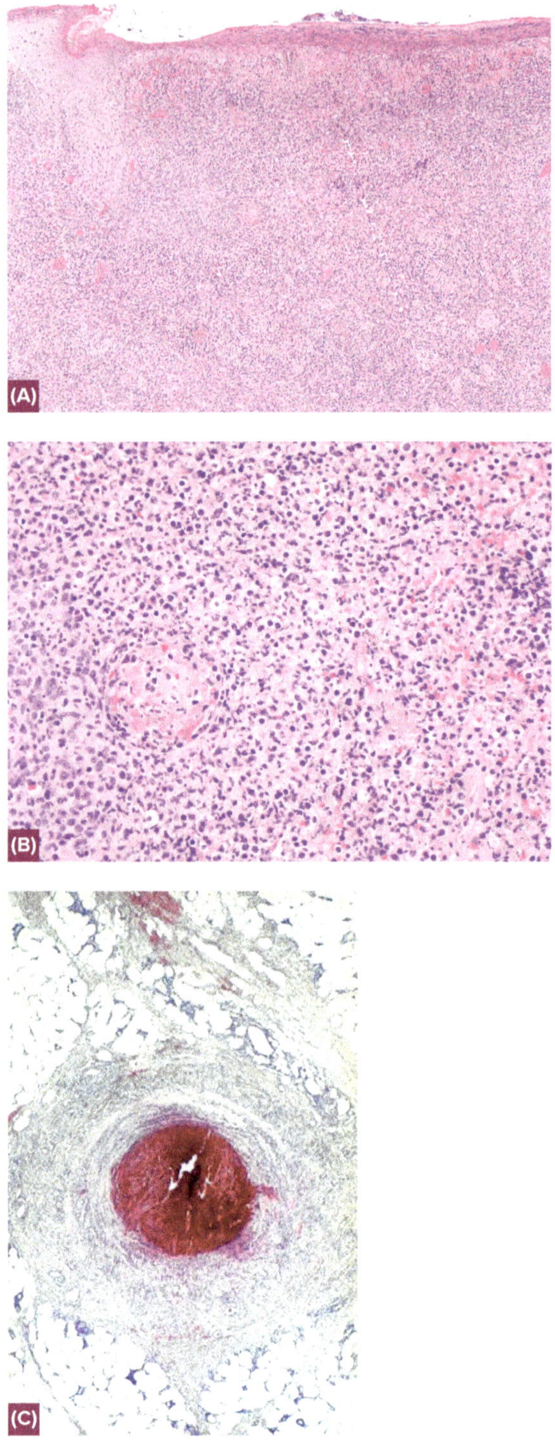

Behçet disease, fully evolved lesion. (A) The epidermis is ulcerated and there are robust and diffuse infiltrates composed of neutrophils and mononuclear cells (lymphocytes and macrophages). **(B)** Neutrophils are seen within vessel walls producing focal areas of fibrinoid degeneration. Vessel lumens are occluded by fibrin thrombi. **(C)** Medium-sized vessel thrombosis in the subcutis. (Part **C** reproduced, with permission, from Goldsmith LA, Katz SI, Gilchrest BA, Paller AS, Leffell DJ, Wolff K, eds. *Fitzpatrick's Dermatology in General Medicine.* 8th ed. New York, NY: McGraw-Hill Education; 2012.)

ANSWER 4-11: E.

The image in question reveals so-called **"lymphocytic vasculitis"** characterized by a perivascular lymphocytic infiltrate with lymphocytes permeating the vessels walls and concomitant red blood cell extravasation (Table 4-11A). Fibrinoid necrosis of the vessel walls is absent. **Henoch–Schönlein purpura** is characterized by true necrotizing **leukocytoclastic vasculitis** with neutrophilic infiltrates. A histologic diagnosis of a lymphocytic vasculitis may be made if there is sufficient evidence of vascular damage and the inflammatory infiltrate is predominantly lymphocytic. Often the vascular damage is subtle, and in many cases there may be disagreement among dermatopathologists on whether the term **"vasculitis"** is warranted or not. Clear-cut evidence of vasculitis again is indisputable if an inflammatory infiltrate is present together with fibrinoid necrosis of the vascular wall. A diagnosis of lymphocytic vasculitis may still be rendered in the absence of fibrinoid necrosis if the constellation of findings suggests clear-cut vascular damage. Features indicative of vascular damage include lamination of the adventitia of venules by concentrically arranged pericytes and basement membrane material, lymphocytic nuclear fragmentation, and subendothelial or intramural infiltration of arterioles by lymphocytes. Lymphocytic vasculitis, if rigidly defined as here, is rare. However, in the majority of conditions to manifest lymphocytic vasculitis, "true vasculitis" is the exception rather than the rule. In instances one might use the term **"lymphocytic vascular reaction"** to indicate that a lymphocytic infiltrate is accompanied by some, albeit limited, vascular injury. The disease processes in which lymphocytic vasculitis is seen commonly include a variety of hypersensitivities and reactive processes, autoimmune and connective tissue diseases, infections, and idiopathic conditions. Again, Henoch–Schönlein purpura is characterized by true necrotizing leukocytoclastic vasculitis with neutrophilic infiltrates.

Table 4-11A. Differential Diagnosis of Lymphocytic Vasculitis and Lymphocytic Vascular Reactions

Pernio (chilblains)
Arthropod bites
Drug-induced or other hypersensitivity reactions
Infection-associated reactions (eg, viral)
Connective tissue diseases
Behçet disease
Pigmented purpuric dermatitides
Pityriasis lichenoides (acute and chronic)
Lymphomatoid papulosis
Cutaneous lymphoma
Autoimmune diseases
Polymorphous light eruption
Atrophie blanche
Malignant atrophic papulosis (Degos disease)
Infestations (eg, scabies)

The histologic picture of **lymphocytic vasculitis** or **lymphocytic vascular reaction** also may occur in other situations. Leukocytoclastic vasculitides (eg, drug reactions), neutrophilic vascular reactions (eg, Sweet syndrome and pyoderma gangrenosum), or usually noninflammatory vasculopathies (eg, atrophie blanche) may show a lymphocytic vasculitis-like picture at some stages. Clinical information and other histologic features are needed to determine the significance of lymphocytic vasculitis. The most common conditions to exhibit **lymphocytic vasculitis** include **perniosis, pigmented purpuric dermatitis, viral exanthems, pityriasis rosea,** and **pityriasis lichenoides.**

Pernio (chilblains) is perhaps the most commonly biopsied condition in which lymphocytic vasculitis is observed. Most patients are young or middle-aged women. The acral surfaces and less commonly the thighs and buttocks are involved. Erythematous to purpuric lesions develop in response to cold damp air or cold water. Histologically, a biopsy typically shows a superficial and possibly deep dermal perivascular and perieccrine lymphocytic infiltrate accompanied by variable degrees of vascular damage, most commonly in the form of fibrin in the walls of venules. There may be associated papillary dermal edema or interface dermatitis. Alcian blue stain typically reveals an increase in dermal mucin.

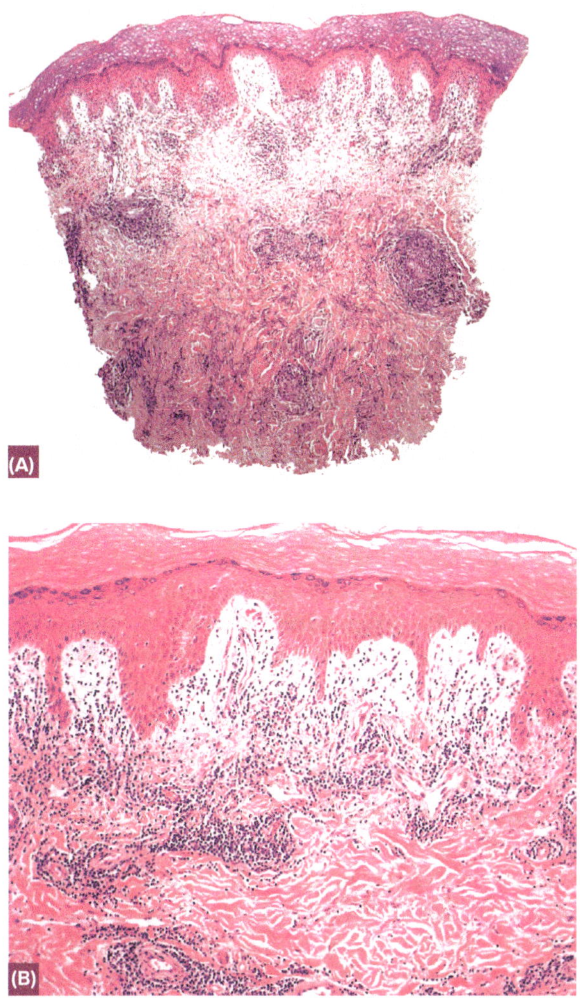

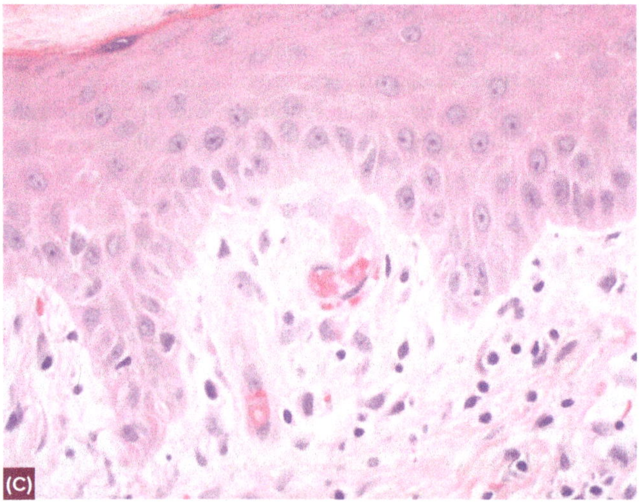

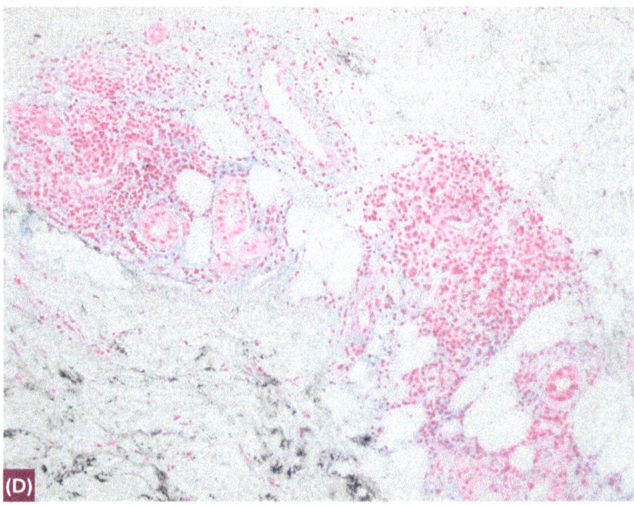

Pernio. **(A)** A superficial and deep, mostly perivascular lymphocytic infiltrate is present with **(B)** superficial edema. **(C)** There is focal vascular thrombosis of a papillary dermal vessel. **(D)** Alcian blue stain reveals abundant dermal mucin surrounding the eccrine coil which is also surrounded by lymphocytic infiltrates.

In regards to **pigmented purpuric dermatitis (PPD)**, four clinical presentations of these entities have been described and named: **purpura annularis telangiectoides of Majocchi (Majocchi disease), progressive pigmentary dermatosis of Schamberg (Schamberg disease), pigmented purpuric dermatitis of Gougerot and Blum, and eczematid-like purpura of Doucas and Kapetanakis.** However, they are closely related and often cannot be reliably distinguished on clinical and histologic grounds. Precise subclassification may not be necessary in dermatopathologic practice, but some knowledge of the spectrum of their various appearances is helpful. **Lichen aureus** is a closely related entity because the clinical lesion has a purpuric component and the histologic findings are similar to the other four variants of **pigmented purpuric dermatitis (PPD).** The etiology of PPD is essentially unknown, and there are probably a number of different factors involved. Some degree of venous insufficiency or stasis is present in most or many patients with PPD. In some instances PPD also may be related to drug or contact hypersensitivity. Eruptions with the clinical and histologic appearance of a PPD have also been associated with subsequent development of a T-cell lymphoproliferative disorder. Thus it is possible that some PPD may be the initial manifestation of T-cell lymphoproliferative disease. Clinically, the primary lesion consists of persistent, bilateral, discrete puncta and pigmentation. Telangiectatic puncta may appear as a result of capillary dilatation and pigmentation as a result of hemosiderin deposits. In some cases, telangiectasia predominates **(Majocchi disease)**, and in others, pigmentation **(Schamberg disease)**. In Majocchi disease, the lesions usually are irregular in shape and occur predominantly on the lower legs. In some cases the findings may mimic those of stasis. Frequently, clinical signs of inflammation are present, such as erythema, papules, and scaling **(Gougerot–Blum disease)** or papules, scaling, and lichenification **(eczematid-like purpura)**. The disorder often is limited to the lower extremities and is bilateral.

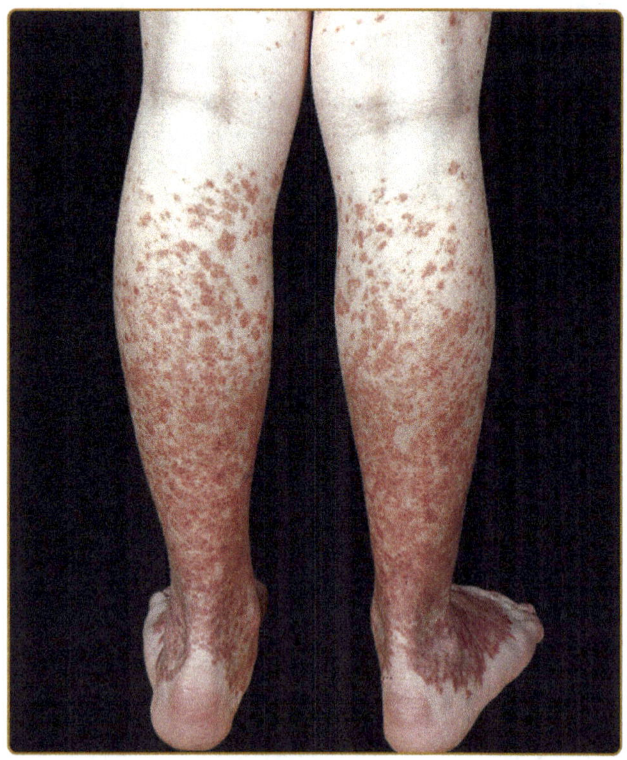

Pigmented purpuric dermatosis: Schamberg disease. Multiple, discrete, and confluent nonpalpable, nonblanching purpuric lesions of many months' duration on the legs. Acute microhemorrhages resolve with deposition of hemosiderin, creating a disfiguring dark-brown peppered stain. (Reproduced, with permission, from Goldsmith LA, Katz SI, Gilchrest BA, Paller AS, Leffell DJ, Wolff K, eds. *Fitzpatrick's Dermatology in General Medicine.* 8th ed. New York, NY: McGraw-Hill Education; 2012.)

In rare cases it may be extensive and involve other sites. Mild pruritus may be present, but usually there are no systemic symptoms. **Lichen aureus** is a localized, unilateral variant of PPD, and most commonly involves the lower extremities but may occur anywhere. One or a few patches are composed of closely set, flat papules of rust, copper, or orange color. In some cases petechiae are present within the patches. Lichen aureus shows a male predilection, and its peak incidence is in the fourth decade.

The principal histopathologic finding of PPD is a lymphocytic perivascular infiltrate limited to the papillary dermis. The pattern of the infiltrate often is not strictly confined to the perivascular area and may infiltrate the adjacent papillary dermis between vessels. In some instances the infiltrate may assume a band-like or lichenoid pattern, particularly in the **lichenoid variant of Gougerot–Blum**, and may involve the reticular dermis in a perivascular distribution. Epidermal alterations are variable and include parakeratosis, slight acanthosis, spongiosis, exocytosis, and basal layer vascuolopathy. Evidence of vascular damage may be present, and the reaction pattern then may be termed **lymphocytic vasculopathy** or **lymphocytic vasculitis**. However, the extent of vascular injury usually is mild and often insufficient to justify the term vasculitis.

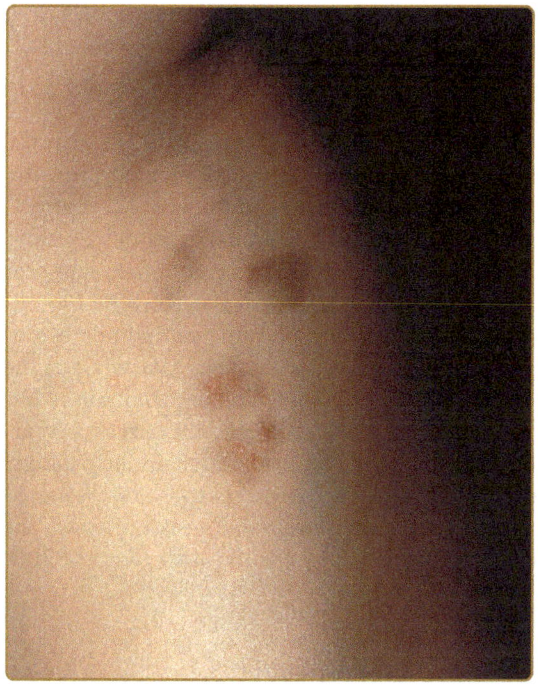

Pigmented purpuric dermatosis: lichenoid dermatosis of Gougerot and Blum. Note the reddish-brown polygonal or round lichenoid papule, in association with purpura or telangiectasia. (Reproduced, with permission, from Goldsmith LA, Katz SI, Gilchrest BA, Paller AS, Leffell DJ, Wolff K, eds. *Fitzpatrick's Dermatology in General Medicine*. 8th ed. New York, NY: McGraw-Hill Education; 2012.)

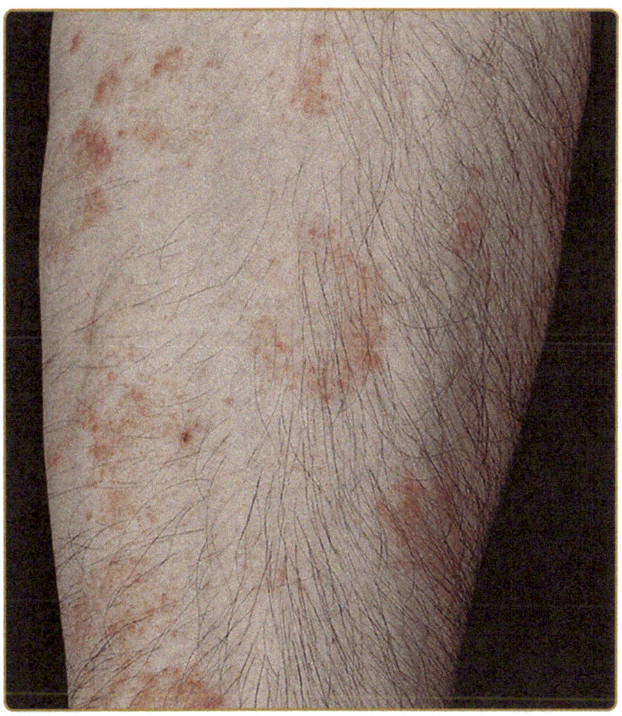

Pigmented purpuric dermatosis: Majocchi disease. Multiple nonpalpable, nonblanching purpuric lesions arranged in annular configurations and associated with tiny telangiectasias. Note brownish discoloration of older lesions. (Reproduced, with permission, from Goldsmith LA, Katz SI, Gilchrest BA, Paller AS, Leffell DJ, Wolff K, eds. *Fitzpatrick's Dermatology in General Medicine*. 8th ed. New York, NY: McGraw-Hill Education; 2012.)

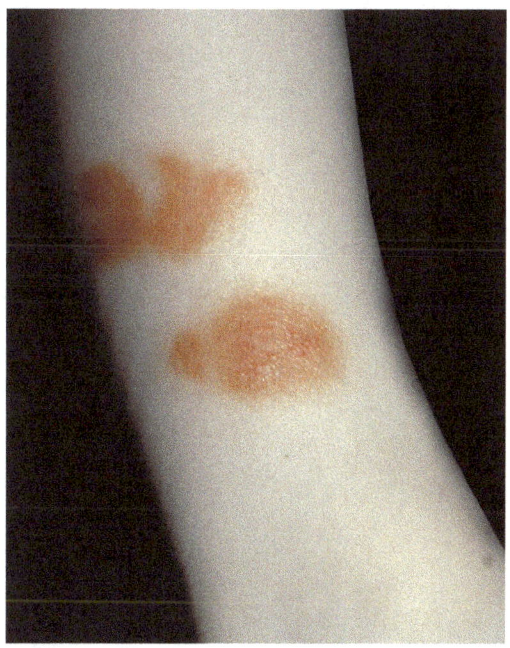

Lichen aureus. Typically unilateral, circumscribed areas of confluent gold to copper-orange to, less commonly, purple macules or papules. (Reproduced, with permission, from Goldsmith LA, Katz SI, Gilchrest BA, Paller AS, Leffell DJ, Wolff K, eds. *Fitzpatrick's Dermatology in General Medicine*. 8th ed. New York, NY: McGraw-Hill Education; 2012.)

Vascular damage commonly consists only of endothelial cell swelling and dermal hemorrhage. Extravasated red blood cells and often-subtle hemosiderin deposits usually are found in the vicinity of the capillaries. However, less commonly one may observe deposition of fibrinoid material in vessel walls. This may be observed particularly in **pigmented purpuric lichenoid dermatitis of Gougerot and Blum** and **eczematid-like purpura of Doucas and Kapetanakis**. In older lesions the capillaries often show dilatation of their lumen and proliferation of their endothelium. Extravasated red blood cells may no longer be present, but one frequently finds hemosiderin deposition. An iron stain (Perl's stain) may aid in the diagnosis in these cases. The inflammatory infiltrate is less pronounced than in the early stage. **Lichen aureus** is characterized by a dense granulomatous infiltrate in the papillary dermis, typically distributed in a band-like fashion. Scattered within the infiltrate are hemosiderin-laden macrophages. The epidermal changes are variable, as in the other forms of PPD.

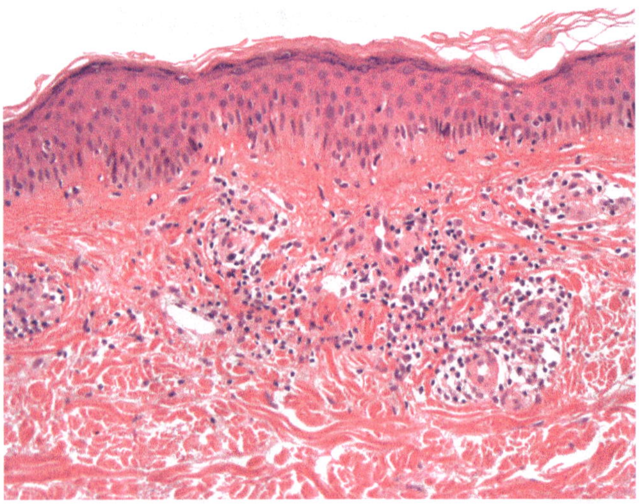

Pigmented purpuric dermatitis. There is a papillary dermal lymphocytic perivascular infiltrate and extravasation of red blood cells.

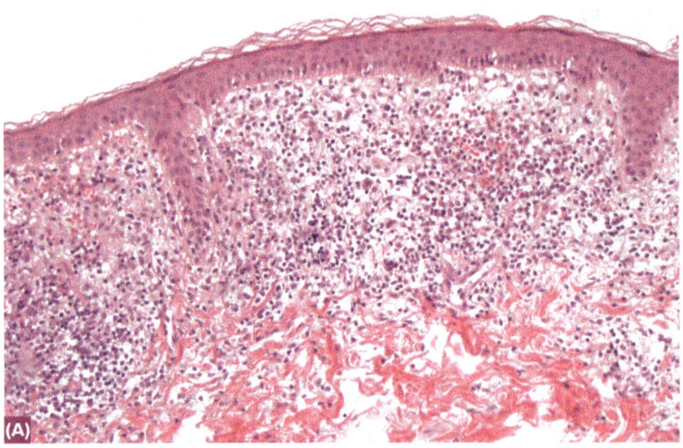

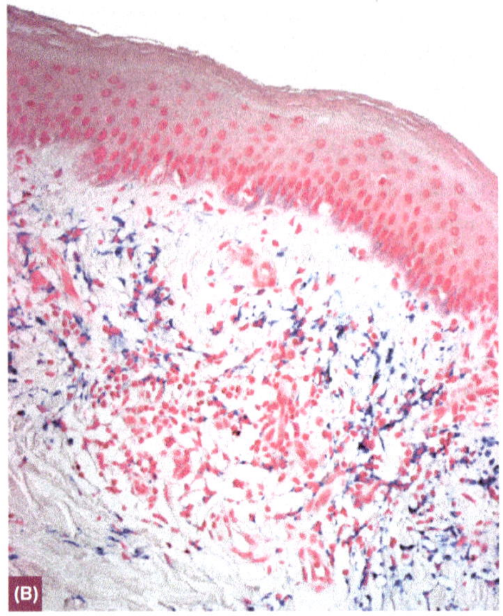

Pigmented purpuric dermatitis. (A) A lichenoid infiltrate of lymphocytes and hemorrhage are seen. **(B)** Iron stain shows positivity (blue) in the superficial dermis.

ANSWER 4-12: E.

Antineutrophil cytoplasmic antibodies (ANCAs) are important serologic markers of certain vasculitides (Table 4-12A). ANCAs may be demonstrated by a combination of indirect immunofluorescence of normal peripheral blood neutrophils followed by enzyme-linked immunosorbent assay (ELISA) to detect specific autoantibodies. Indirect immunofluorescence assays reveal two staining patterns: cytoplasmic **(c-ANCAs)** and perinuclear **(p-ANCAs)**. The patient in this case exhibits a circumferential perinuclear pattern of immunoglobulin localization **(p-ANCA)**. ELISAs show that the majority of c-ANCAs are autoantibodies to **proteinase 3**, and most p-ANCAs are specific for **myeloperoxidase (MPO)**. Combined with clinical features, these antibodies are especially helpful in the differential diagnosis of three primarily small-vessel vasculitides:

Table 4-12A. ANCA-Positive Vasculitides

DISEASE PROCESS	ANTI-MYELOPEROXIDASE (p-ANCA)	ANTI-SERINE PROTEINASE (c-ANCA)
Wegener granulomatosis	Rare (5%)	Common (80%)
Microscopic polyarteritis	Common (50–60%)	Common (45%)
Churg–Strauss syndrome	Common (70%)	Rare (7%)

Wegener granulomatosis (WG), Churg–Strauss syndrome (CSS), and **microscopic polyarteritis (MPA).** WG is usually associated with c-ANCAs, MPA with either p- or c-ANCAs, and CSS with p-ANCAs. However, these syndromes cannot be discriminated by ANCA subtype alone as exceptional cases and population differences are seen.

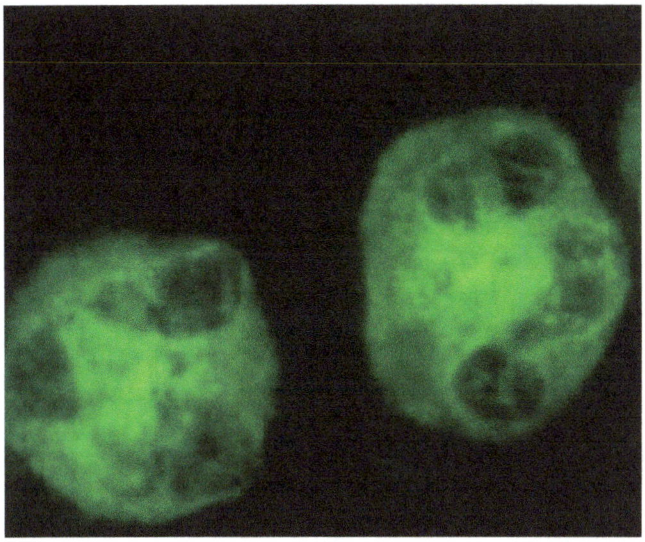

c-ANCA. Note the diffuse cytoplasmic deposition of immunoglobulin. The antigenic target is proteinase 3 in the vast majority of cases.

These three syndromes are termed **pauci-immune vasculitides** because vascular injury is not associated with immunoglobulin deposition in vessel walls, in contrast to the immune-complex–mediated small-vessel injury seen in entities such as **Henoch–Schönlein purpura** and **hypersensitivity vasculitis.** The pathogenesis of the vascular injury and the role of ANCAs in these disease processes are still unclear although there is evidence for a direct role.

ANCAs may play a role in inducing vasculitis by activating circulating neutrophils and monocytes, causing them to adhere to vessels, degranulate, and release toxic metabolites, thereby causing vascular injury. Another possibility is that immune deposits are present at an early stage of vasculitis but are degraded rapidly, resulting in pauci-immune lesions.

Both environmental insult and genetic predisposition have been implicated in the pathogenesis of WG. A recessive genetic defect completely unrelated to ANCAs has been shown to lead to a vasculitis/granulomatosis syndrome similar to WG. This inherited syndrome differs from WG, though, showing familial clustering and not responding to immunosuppression. Recurrent bacterial infection is also a feature. A mutation in the transporter associated with antigen processing (TAP) leads to a decreased cell surface expression of HLA class I molecules and possibly increased self-reactivity. Novel immunologic defects may await detection in patients with systemic vasculitis. A number of cases of ANCA-associated vasculitis have been reported in patients with **Graves disease** receiving treatment, most commonly with **propylthiouracil.** Other medications that may induce ANCA-positive vasculitis include **hydralazine, penicillamine,** and **minocycline.** Unlike the classic ANCA-positive vasculitides, drug-associated ANCA-positive vasculitis frequently demonstrates immunoglobulin deposition within the vessels.

CSS and WG most often are classified as granulomatous vasculitides in textbooks. However, the most common cutaneous histopathologic finding in both diseases is **leukocytoclastic vasculitis.** The granulomatous inflammation seen in the skin usually is not angiodestructive. Although MPA does not have a significant cutaneous granulomatous component, it is discussed here because there is significant overlap, histologically and clinically, with WG and CSS patients who show an extensive vasculitic diathesis. In fact, significant overlap between these three syndromes as well as **microscopic polyarteritis nodosa** is well recognized. Over time, particular patients may shift from one disease category to another.

ANSWER 4-13: A.

Microscopic polyarteritis nodosa (MPA; aka microscopic polyangiitis) is a systemic small-vessel vasculitis that is typically associated with focal necrotizing glomerulonephritis with crescents and serum **myeloperoxidase-antineutrophil cytoplasmic autoantibodies (p-ANCA)** (Table 4-13A). Involvement of the small vessels of the kidneys, lungs, and skin gives MPA a particular clinical picture and separates MPA from "classic" polyarteritis nodosa, which is to a greater degree a disease of medium-sized vessels. Clinically, most patients with MPA are male and over 50 years of age. Prodromal

Table 4-13A. Microscopic Polyarteritis Nodosa (MPA)

Clinical Features
Males over 50 years of age
Viral-like prodrome
Renal disease:
Microhematuria, proteinuria, or acute oliguric renal failure
Cutaneous symptoms:
Palpable purpura, splinter hemorrhages, and ulcerations
Pulmonary involvement without granulomas
Histopathologic Features
LCV
Differential Diagnosis
Wegener granulomatosus
Churg–Strauss syndrome
PAN
Other causes of LCV

symptoms include fever, myalgias, arthralgias, and sore throat. The most common clinical feature is renal disease, manifesting as microhematuria, proteinuria, or acute oliguric renal failure. Although cutaneous involvement is rare in classic PAN, at least 30-40% of patients with MPA have skin changes. These include erythematous macules (100% in one study), livedo reticularis, palpable purpura, splinter hemorrhages, and ulcerations. Tender erythematous nodules typical of classic PAN are exceedingly rare in MPA. Pulmonary involvement without granulomatous tissue reaction occurs in approximately one-third of patients. Other organ systems (ie, gastrointestinal tract, central nervous system, serosal and articular surfaces) also may be affected, but this is less common. Serious clinical complications usually arise from renal and pulmonary disease.

Microscopcially, a **leukocytoclastic vasculitis (LCV)** primarily affecting arterioles, venules, and capillaries is observed. Necrotizing vasculitis of medium-sized arteries typical of classic PAN is also present on occasion. Cutaneous granulomatous inflammation is only rarely seen in MPA.

In regards to the differential diagnosis, **MPA** and **classic polyarteritis nodosa (PAN)** may not be distinguishable in every case, practically speaking. Glomerulonephritis, typical skin signs, ANCA positivity, and lack of arteriographic findings (aneurysms and stenoses reflecting medium-sized vessel involvement) favor MPA over classic PAN. MPA also tends not to be associated with viral hepatitis in contradistinction to some cases of classic PAN. Biopsy findings are less useful in distinguishing between these two syndromes because the size of diseased vessels detected is highly dependent on biopsy site, size of specimens, and number of tissue samples. Thus lack of medium-sized vessel involvement by no means excludes classic PAN. Detection of small-vessel involvement also does not exclude classic PAN, which may show small-vessel disease. A number of cases of vasculitis show overlapping features, leading to introduction of the term **overlapping syndrome of vasculitis** to encompass vasculitis affecting both small- and medium-sized arteries. The differential diagnosis also includes **Wegener vasculitis (WG)** and other small-vessel vasculitides that are occasionally ANCA-positive, such as certain drug reactions. The granulomatous inflammation of WG should be lacking in MPA; however, these two entities share many features, and some physicians are of the opinion that the distinction between MPA and WG is largely artificial. Although **Churg–Strauss syndrome (CSS)** is also typically positive for p-ANCA, renal involvement is characteristically absent. Additionally, the LCV of CSS typically contains increased numbers of eosinophils.

ANSWER 4-14: D.

The biopsy reveals small-vessel leukocytoclastic vasculitis with scattered eosinophils. This is a classic example of **Churg–Strauss syndrome (CSS)**, also known as **allergic granulomatosis** (Table 4-14A). This clinicopathologic syndrome is characterized by asthma, fever, hypereosinophilia, eosinophilic tissue infiltrates, necrotizing vasculitis, and extravascular granuloma formation. Short of an autopsy, the classic pathologic triad of necrotizing vasculitis, eosinophilic tissue infiltration, and extravascular granulomas is extremely difficult to demonstrate because of the focality of the process. A broader definition of CSS requiring asthma, hypereosinophilia greater than 1.5×10^9/L, and systemic vasculitis involving two or more extrapulmonary organs has been suggested. Considerable overlap with other systemic vasculitides and with other inflammatory disorders associated with eosinophils, such as **eosinophilic pneumonitis**, has brought the legitimacy of the CSS into question.

Table 4-14A. Churg–Strauss Syndrome

Clinical Features
Men and women equally affected, 20-40 years of age
Asthma
Allergic rhinitis
Eosinophilia
Petechiae, extensive ecchymoses
Necrotic ulcers
Cutaneous-subcutaneous nodules
Histopathologic Features
Leukocytoclastic vasculitis
Tissue eosinophilia
Churg–Strauss granulomata (extravascular granulomas with numerous eosinophils)
Differential Diagnosis
Infection
Connective tissue disease
Wegener granulomatous
Microscopic polyarteritis nodosa

Clinically, despite multiple reports, CSS appears to be rare. Between 1950 and 1995, only 120 cases were identified at the Mayo Clinic. The incidence of CSS is similar in males and females. It typically presents in the third and fourth decades of life. Patients tend to move through several phases of disease development from nonspecific signs and symptoms such as asthma and allergic rhinitis (prodromal phase), to a phase of hypereosinophilia with eosinophilic pneumonitis or gastroenteritis (second phase), and finally, to systemic vasculitis (third phase). The three disease phases are not always sequential and on occasion may occur simultaneously. The internal organs most commonly involved are the lungs, the gastrointestinal tract, and less commonly, the peripheral nerves and heart. In contrast to **polyarteritis nodosa**, renal failure in CSS is extremely rare. A limited form of allergic granulomatosis is characterized by preexisting asthma and lesions confined to the conjunctiva, skin, and subcutaneous tissue. Two types of cutaneous lesions occur in about two-thirds of patients: (1) hemorrhagic lesions varying from petechiae to palpable purpura to extensive ecchymoses, sometimes accompanied by necrotic ulcers and often associated with areas of erythema (similar to Henoch–Schönlein purpura) and (2) cutaneous-subcutaneous nodules. The most common sites of skin lesions are the extremities, followed by the trunk. In some instances the petechiae and ecchymoses are generalized. Other skin manifestations include urticaria, erythematous macules, and livedo reticularis.

Diagnostically helpful laboratory findings include an elevated peripheral eosinophil count. Patients with active CSS have anti-MPOs (p-ANCAs) in most cases. The levels of anti-MPOs have been found to correlate with disease activity. Anti-MPOs are found less often in patients with limited forms of the disease. Anti-serine proteinase antibodies (c-ANCAs) are uncommon in patients with CSS.

Microscopically, the areas of cutaneous hemorrhage typically show **small-vessel leukocytoclastic vasculitis (LCV)** often with numerous eosinophils. **Granulomatous arteritis** may also be occasionally observed. In some instances the dermis shows a distinctive granuloma typified by radially arranged histiocytes and multinucleated giant cells centered around degenerated collagen fibers. The central portion of these so-called **"red" palisading granulomas** contains not only degenerated collagen fibers but also disintegrated cells, particularly eosinophils, in great numbers. These granulomas initially were thought to be characteristic and were referred to as **Churg–Strauss granulomas**. However, they are not always present and are not a prerequisite for the diagnosis. Therefore, although a "red-flag" for introducing CSS into the histopathological differential diagnosis, these granulomas are neither sensitive nor specific for the diagnosis. The **"Churg–Strauss granuloma"** can also be observed in other disease processes, such as connective tissue disease (rheumatoid arthritis and lupus erythematosus), WG, PAN, lymphoproliferative disorders, subacute bacterial endocarditis, chronic active hepatitis, and inflammatory bowel disease (Crohn disease and ulcerative colitis). The extravascular granulomas may involve subcutaneous fat, where they may attain considerable size through expansion and confluence, thus giving rise to the clinically apparent cutaneous-subcutaneous nodules. These palisading granulomas are embedded in a diffuse inflammatory exudate rich in eosinophils. Erythematous plaques, sometimes annular or bullous lesions can show the histopathology of **eosinophilic cellulitis (Wells syndrome)** with an intense dermal eosinophilic infiltrate encrusting collagen bundles with eosinophilic granules **(flame figures)**.

In regards to the differential diagnosis, CSS is a clinicopathologic entity whose diagnosis depends on the presence of respiratory disease, in particular a history of asthma, p-ANCA positivity, and particular histologic features such as extravascular granulomas described earlier, necrotizing vasculitis, and eosinophilia. The differential diagnosis includes all varieties of **small-vessel leukocytoclastic vasculitis (LCV)** but in particular, **polyarteritis (PAN)**, **microscopic polyarteritis (MPA)**, and **Wegener granulomatosis (WG)**, and the conditions mentioned earlier that might show extravascular necrotizing granulomas. Although Churg and Strauss initially characterized allergic granulomatosis as a "strikingly uniform clinical picture," there is less clarity today about its distinction from other vasculitic processes, particularly WG and PAN. **Medication-associated hypersensitivity leukocytoclastic vasculitis** also typically contains eosinophils, but systemic involvement is rare. Additionally, these lesions typically exhibit immunoglobulin deposition within vessels via direct immunofluorescence and negative peripheral blood analysis for p-ANCA and c-ANCA antibodies. A drug-associated ANCA-positive vasculitis typically exhibits immunoglobulin deposition within vessels via direct immunofluorescence.

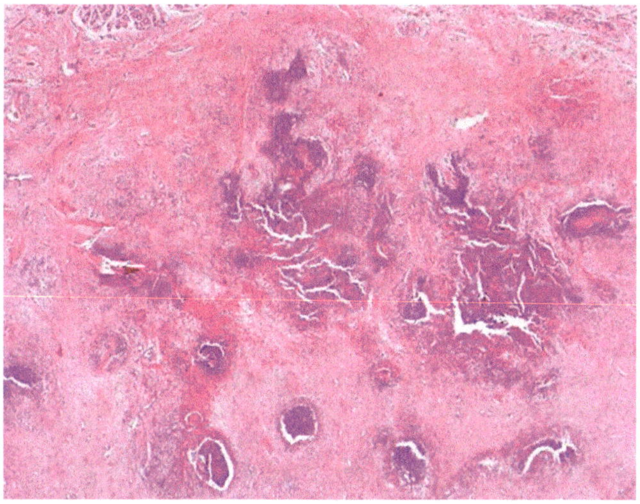

Palisading necrotizing granuloma (Churg–Strauss granuloma). Eosinophilic necrobiotic collagen is surrounded by epithelioid histiocytes. High power examination would reveal numerous eosinophils.

ANSWER 4-15: D.

A **vasculopathic reaction** refers to vascular damage without inflammation. The term **pseudovasculitis** has been used to describe a closely related group of conditions in which fibrin thrombi and vascular damage are associated with a sparse (minimal) inflammatory cell infiltrate (Table 4-15A). The microscopic image in question reveals dilated superficial vessels occluded by fibrin thrombi with peripheral eosinophilic hyalinization of the vessel walls, indicative of damage. There is also extensive red blood cell extravasation. Note the absence of inflammation. Vasculopathies or pseudovasculitis may be associated with vascular occlusive phenomena, including thrombi or emboli, pathologic alterations of the vessel wall or structural deficiencies of the perivascular connective tissue, and miscellaneous other disease processes including drug-induced vasospasm and repetitive vascular injury. The clinical presentation associated with vasculopathies correlates with the size of vessels involved, extent of vascular injury, and whether or not the vessels are partially versus completed occluded.

In **vascular occlusive** conditions, thrombi are present in blood vessels of the dermis and/or subcutis. Extensive infarctions and necrosis may be associated and are more characteristic of some **coagulopathies** (ie, **antiphospholipid antibody syndrome, protein C deficiency,** etc), **cryoglobulinemias, atrophie blanche, cholesterol emboli,** and **calciphylaxis. Livedo reticularis** and **late atrophie blanche** present a more fibrotic chronic picture. Usually, the various conditions can be histopathologically distinguished by additional distinctive findings such as calcification in **calciphylaxis**, needle-shaped crystals in **cholesterol emboli**, or the wedge-shaped dermal alteration of **Degos syndrome**. Characteristic clinical findings or serologic tests (eg, cryoglobulinemia, cryofibrinogenemia, coagulopathy) further narrow the differential diagnosis. **Cryoglobulins** are serum immunoglobulins that precipitate when the serum is cooled and redissolve with rewarming. There are three major types of cryoglobulinemia. In **type I cryoglobulinemia,** monoclonal IgG or IgM cryoglobulins are found (Table 4-15B). This type of cryoglobulinemia may be idiopathic but often is associated with lymphoma, leukemia, Waldenström macroglobulinemia, or multiple myeloma. **Types II and III cryoglobulinemia** form immune complexes resulting in **leukocytoclastic vasculitis** (Table 4-15C). Cutaneous lesions in patients with cryoglobulinemia may manifest as chronic palpable purpura, urticaria-like lesions, livedo reticularis, Raynaud phenomenon, acrocyanosis, digital gangrene, and leg ulcers. Systemic manifestations may include arthralgia, hepatosplenomegaly, lymphadenopathy, and glomerulonephritis. Any coagulopathy may be accompanied by vasculopathic changes, although the extent of vascular damage is variable. Vascular damage may occur in the setting of altered platelet counts, such as in

Table 4-15A. Vasculopathic Reactions and Pseudovasculitis

MECHANISM	CONDITION
Coagulopathies	Idiopathic thrombocytopenic purpura Coagulation factor deficiencies (eg, protein C and S deficiencies) Antiphospholipid antibody syndrome Thrombotic thrombocytopenic purpura Coumadin/warfarin-induced skin necrosis Heparin-induced skin necrosis Calciphylaxis Purpura fulminans Disseminated intravascular coagulation Monoclonal gammopathy Sickle cell disease Livedo vasculopathy
Pathological alterations of the vessel wall	Calciphylaxis Primary hyperoxaluria Diabetes mellitus Amyloidosis Porphyria Radiation vasculopathy
Embolic phenomena	Cholesterol embolism Atrial myxoma
Structural deficiencies of the perivascular connective tissue	Solar/senile purpura Scurvy
Vasospasm	Ergot derivatives Cocaine Methamphetamines
Repetitive vascular trauma	Hypothenar hammer syndrome

Table 4-15B. Type I Cryoglobulinemia

Clinical Features
Cutaneous:
Palpable purpura
Urticaria-like lesions
Livedo reticularis
Acrocyanosis
Digital gangrene
Leg ulcers
Raynaud phenomenon
Systemic:
Arthralgia
Hepatosplenomegaly
Lymphadenopathy
Glomerulonephritis
Histopathologic Evaluation
Amorphous, PAS-positive thrombi
Cracking of thrombi
Extensive extravasation of erythrocytes
Differential Diagnosis
Coagulopathies

Table 4-15C. Clinical-Pathologic Associations of Cryoglobulinemias

	IMMUNOGLOBULIN	ASSOCIATIONS	SITE	CLINICAL FINDINGS HISTOPATHOLOGY	CHARACTERISTIC
Type I	Monoclonal IgG or IgM	Lymphoma, leukemia, Waldenström macroglobulinemia, or multiple myeloma	Head, neck, oral, or nasal mucosa	Hemorrhagic crusts, skin ulcerations	Noninflammatory hyaline thrombosis Cutaneous infarction
Type II	Monoclonal and polyclonal immune complexes	Connective tissue disorders idiopathic (essential) Infection Autoimmune diseases	Legs	Erythematous to purpuric macules or papules	Leukocytoclastic vasculitis

idiopathic thrombocytopenic purpura, in coagulation factor deficiencies (ie, **inherited or acquired protein C and S deficiencies**), coagulopathies associated with connective tissue disease (ie, **lupus anticoagulant, antiphospholipid antibody syndrome**), and platelet thrombosis (**heparin-induced skin necrosis and cocaine/levamisole ingestion**). Extensive vascular damage and hemorrhage with luminal occlusion by thrombotic material may develop in **coumarin/warfarin-induced skin necrosis, thrombotic thrombocytopenic purpura,** and **disseminated intravascular coagulation,** in particular in the setting of **purpura fulminans.**

The histopathology illustrated in this question may be seen in all of the answer choices, as well as **type I cryoglobulinemia. Mixed cryoglobulinemias (types II and III)** typically show a leukocytoclastic vasculitis, as previously discussed.

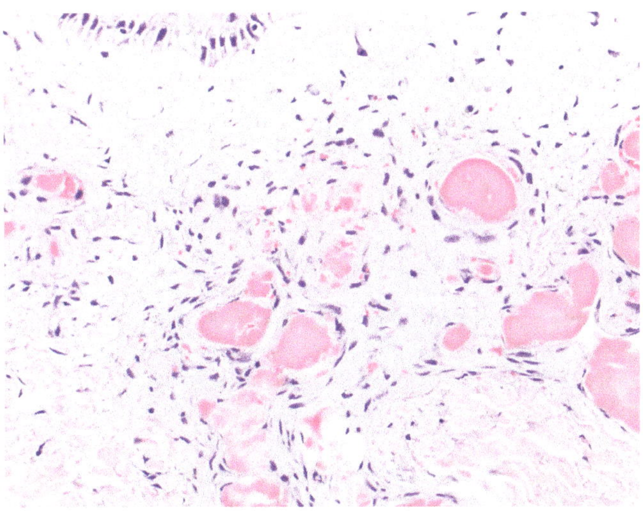

Type I cryoglobulinemia, PAS stain. Superficial dermal vessels are dilated and occluded by bright pink-red cryoprecipitate.

Additional specific features of type I cryoglobulinemia include amorphous material (**precipitated cryoglobulins**) deposited subjacent to endothelium, throughout the vessel wall, and within the vessel lumen, resulting in a thrombus-like appearance. These precipitates stain pink with hematoxylin and eosin and bright red-pink with PAS stain, as opposed to less intense staining of fibrinoid material. Cracking of the precipitate may be a prominent feature. Some capillaries are filled with red blood cells, and extensive extravasation of erythrocytes may be present. PAS-positive intramural and intravascular cryoprecipitate also may be found in mixed cryoglobulinemia, but less frequently than in type I cryoglobulinemia.

ANSWER 4-16: C.

All of the answer choices represent different clinical presentations associated with vascular damage, most commonly without inflammation (**vasculopathy**). **Atrophie blanche** is a common condition that may be seasonal, with greatest disease activity in the summer and winter months (Table 4-16A). Usually middle-aged or elderly females are affected. Initially, purpuric macules and papules develop into small, painful ulcers with a tendency to recur. Healing of the ulcers results in the classic white atrophic areas that have given the disease its name. Typically lesions are located on the lower portions of the legs, particularly on the ankles and the dorsa of the feet. In the fully developed state, there are irregularly outlined, whitish atrophic areas with peripheral hyperpigmentation and telangiectasia. Many of the patients may also have associated livedo reticularis. The etiology of atrophie blanche is unknown. Immune-complex deposits that have been observed in late lesions are likely secondary changes. A primary disturbance of fibrinolysis in the endothelium of affected microvessels has been postulated.

Table 4-16A. Atrophie Blanche

Clinical Features
- Seasonal
- Middle-aged or elderly females
- Lower portions of the legs ankles and the dorsa of the feet
- Purpuric macules and papules develop into small, painful ulcers followed by irregularly outlined atrophic scars with peripheral hyperpigmentation and telangiectasia

Histopathologic Features
- Early:
  - Fibrinoid material in vessel walls or lumina
  - Infarction with hemorrhage and an inflammatory infiltrate
- Late:
  - Thinning of epithelium
  - Dermal sclerosis with little cellular thickening and intimal hyalinization of dermal vessel walls
  - Occlusion of vessel lumina by intimal proliferation and/or fibrinoid recanalized vessels

Differential Diagnosis
- Stasis
- Coagulopathy
- Lymphocytic vasculitis, not otherwise specified

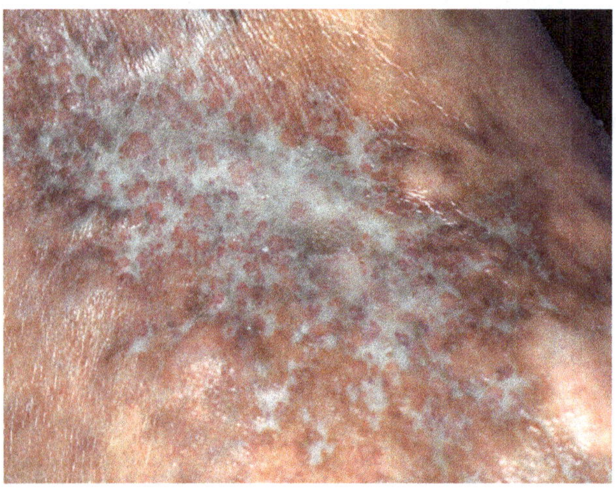

Atrophie blanche associated with chronic venous insufficiency. An area of diffuse and mottled pigmentation due to hemosiderin and ivory-white patches of atrophie blanche. Such lesions are both itchy and painful. (Reproduced, with permission, from Wolff K, Johnson RA, Saavedra AP. *Fitzpatrick's Color Atlas and Synopsis of Clinical Dermatology.* 7th ed. New York, NY: McGraw-Hill Education; 2013.)

The histopathologic findings of **atrophie blanche** are nonspecific and vary with the stage of the lesion. However, in all stages, vascular changes are present. In early lesions, fibrinoid material may be noted in vessel walls or vessel lumina. Infarction with hemorrhage and an inflammatory infiltrate may be present as well. In late atrophic lesions, the epithelium is thinned, and the dermis is sclerotic with little, if any, cellular infiltrate. The walls of the dermal vessels may show thickening and intimal hyalinization. Occlusion of vessel lumina by intimal proliferation and/or fibrinoid material and sometimes-recanalized thrombotic vessels may be seen. In some cases the vessels in the superficial dermis are predominantly affected; in others, the vessels in the middle and even deep dermis are mostly affected. **Cutaneous polyarteritis nodosa** can show atrophie blanche-like histology in superficial biopsies and can look similar to atrophie blanche clinically. A deep biopsy may aid in distinguishing these two conditions.

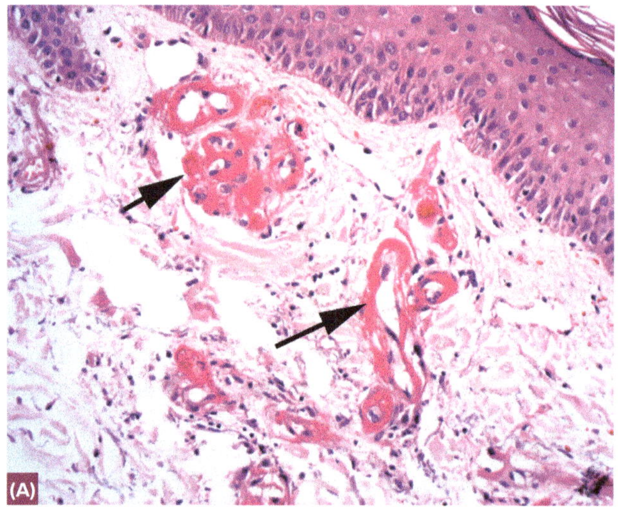

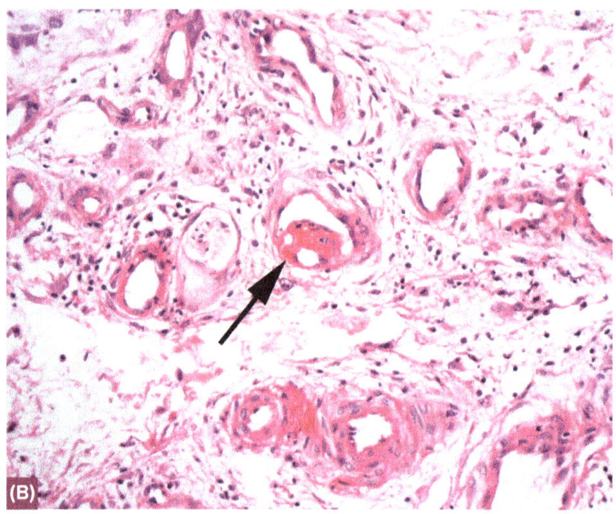

Atrophie blanche. (A) The microvessels show deposition of fibrinoid material in their walls (arrow) and an associated sparse lymphoid infiltrate. **(B)** Fibrin thrombi (arrow) may be found in other vessels. (Used with permission of Dr. Charles Palmer.)

Livedo reticularis is red-blue mottling of the skin in a netlike pattern. This nonspecific physical sign indicates sluggish blood flow, which may result from a number of causes (Table 4-16B). The vessels involved are typically deep dermal or subcutaneous and are **partially occluded**. Physiologic livedo (**cutis marmorata**), commonly seen in young women, is mottling of the skin that subsides with warming. An idiopathic form, that is persistent and does not respond to warming, is limited to the lower extremities, may be associated with subtle coagulation abnormalities, and autoimmune phenomena. Drug-induced livedo has been seen with interferon-alpha therapy for melanoma and amantadine therapy for Parkinson disease.

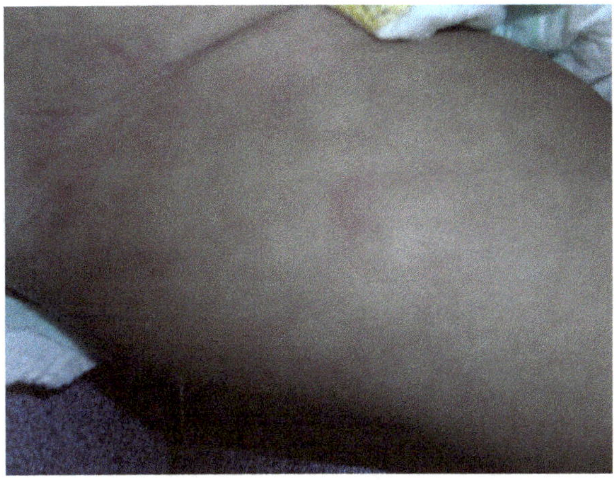

Cutis marmorata in a 4-month-old infant in a cold exam room. Notice the reticular pattern. This resolved when the infant was warmed. (Reproduced, with permission, from Usatine RP, Smith MA, Mayeaux EJ Jr, Chumley HS, eds. *Color Atlas of Family Medicine*. 2nd ed. New York, NY: McGraw-Hill Education; 2012. Used with permission of Richard P. Usatine, MD.)

Livedo racemosa is also a violaceous mottling of the skin similar to livedo reticularis, but more generalized and widespread, and showing irregularities and breaks in the network patterning.

Table 4-16B. Livedo Reticularis/Racemosa

Clinical Features
Persistent red-blue mottling of the skin in a netlike pattern
Histopathologic Features
Erythematous areas: no distinct findings
White areas: thick vessel walls, thrombi, arterioles obliteration, red blood cell slugging
Associations
Vasculitis or a vasculopathies due to infection
Atrophie blanche
Cholesterol emboli
Connective tissue disease
Calciphylaxis and oxalosis
Idiopathic
Sneddon syndrome

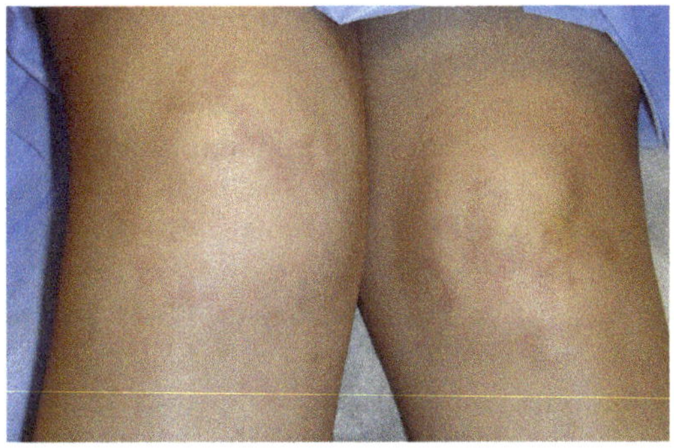

Livedo racemosa. Violaceous mottling of the skin similar to livedo reticularis, but with irregularity and breaks in the network pattern. (Reproduced, with permission, from Imboden JB, Hellmann DB, Stone JH, eds. *Current Medical Diagnosis & Treatment: Rheumatology*. 3rd ed. New York, NY: McGraw-Hill Education; 2013.)

Persistent **livedo reticularis** and **livedo racemosa** may be associated with vasoocclusive disorders, vasculitides (usually ANCA+ or polyarteritis nodosa), or connective tissue diseases including the antiphospholipid antibody syndrome. Lupus patients with livedo reticularis are more likely to suffer cerebral vascular accidents. Generalized livedo reticularis and livedo racemosa are also part of a potentially severe arterio-occlusive syndrome (**Sneddon syndrome**) that often is complicated by cerebrovascular disease.

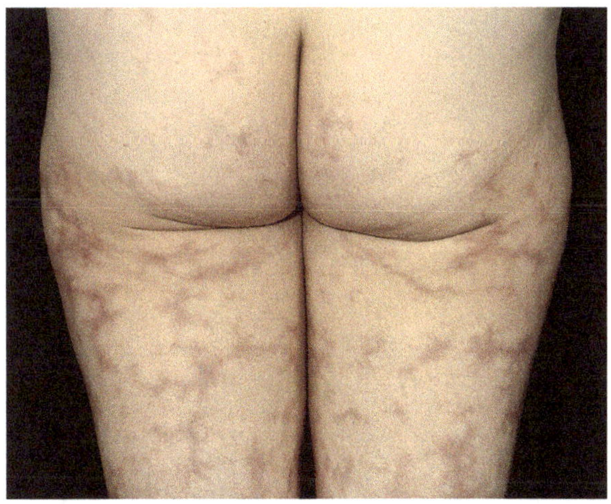

Symptomatic livedo reticularis. A netlike, arborizing pattern on the posterior thighs and buttocks defined by violaceous, erythematous streaks resembling lightning. The skin within the erythematous areas is normally pale. This occurred in a patient with labile hypertension and multiple cerebrovascular attacks and was thus pathognomonic for Sneddon syndrome. (Reproduced, with permission, from Wolff K, Johnson RA, Saavedra AP. *Fitzpatrick's Color Atlas and Synopsis of Clinical Dermatology*. 7th ed. New York, NY: McGraw-Hill Education; 2013.)

Microscopically, the changes of **livedo reticularis/racemosa** may only be detected in punch biopsies sampling the dermis–subcutis boundry, since the small vessels are typically not involved. Multiple areas from different areas of the livedo may need to be sampled, especially the seemingly uninvolved white skin at the center. Initially, blood vessels may show attachment of lymphohistiocytic cells and detachment of endothelial cells. Later, **partial occlusion** of the lumen by a plug of lymphohistiocytic cells and fibrin may be seen, which is replaced by proliferating subendothelial cells accompanied by dilated capillaries in the adventitia of the **partially occluded vessel**. Late-stage vessels may show fibrosis and shrinkage, similar to that of **atrophie blanche**. Intravascular aggregates of red blood cells suggest a low-flow state.

Retiform purpura is a netlike (livedoid) pattern of cutaneous hemorrhage representing severe damage to both medium and small vessels. These palpable plaques are characteristic of **antiphospholipid antibody syndrome, heparin-induced skin necrosis, coumadin/warfarin-induced skin necrosis, cocaine/levamisole-induced retiform purpura,** and **calciphylaxis**. Among inflammatory causes of hemorrhage (i.e. **vasculitis**), only **benign cutaneous polyarteritis nodosa** is likely to cause such large necrotic thick plaques with early inflammation.

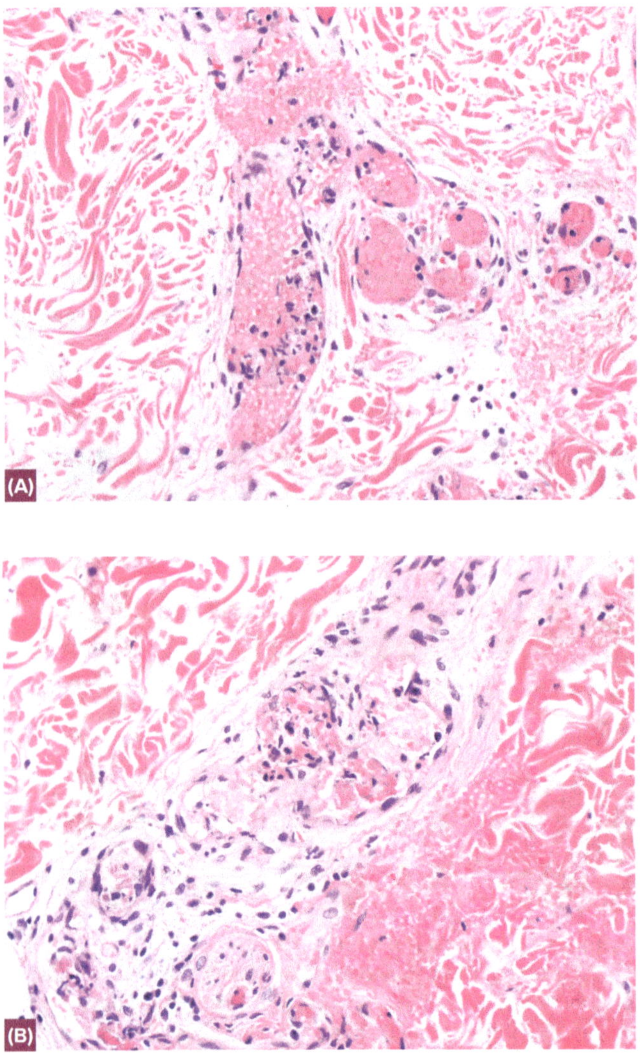

Pauci-inflammatory thrombogenic vasculopathy associated livedo reticularis. (A) Note the vascular congestion (dilatation filled with red blood cells) and fibrin thrombi (solid pink foci) partially occluding the vessels. **(B)** Rare entrapped inflammatory cells are present within the thrombi.

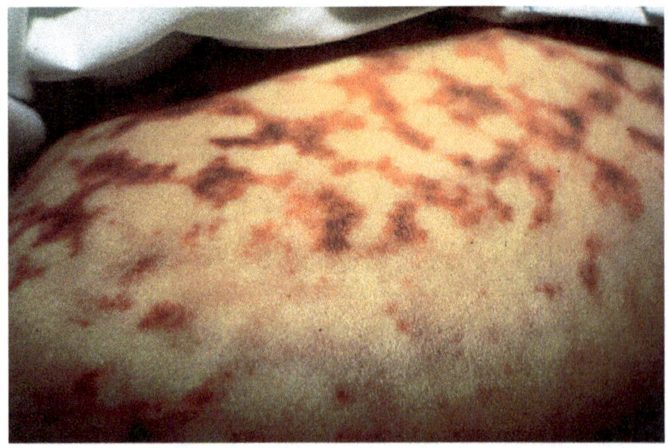

Noninflammatory retiform purpura on the thigh in a patient with disseminated intravascular coagulation secondary to sepsis, and sepsis-associated protein C depletion eventually leading to purpura fulminans. None of the lesional color faded on compression. The biopsy showed multiple dermal vessels completely occluded by clot without inflammation. (Reproduced, with permission, from Goldsmith LA, Katz SI, Gilchrest BA, Paller AS, Leffell DJ, Wolff K, eds. *Fitzpatrick's Dermatology in General Medicine.* 8th ed. New York, NY: McGraw-Hill Education; 2012.)

Purpura fulminans is a severe form of coagulopathy characterized by palpable purpura and large areas of ecchymoses, often on the extremities. Large hemorrhagic bullae may overlie the ecchymoses, and in some instances, necrosis may supervene. The condition is most commonly associated with **catastrophic antiphospholipid antibody syndrome, disseminated intravascular coagulation,** or **protein C depletion** (septic [Meningococcemia], acquired [vitamin K deficiency, cirrhosis], or congenital).

The histopathologic findings include **complete thrombotic vascular occlusion** leading to hemorrhagic infarcts, epidermal and dermal necrosis, or subepidermal bullae formation. Systemic intravascular coagulation with widespread thrombosis of the small vessels of internal organs leading to hemorrhagic necrosis may also develop.

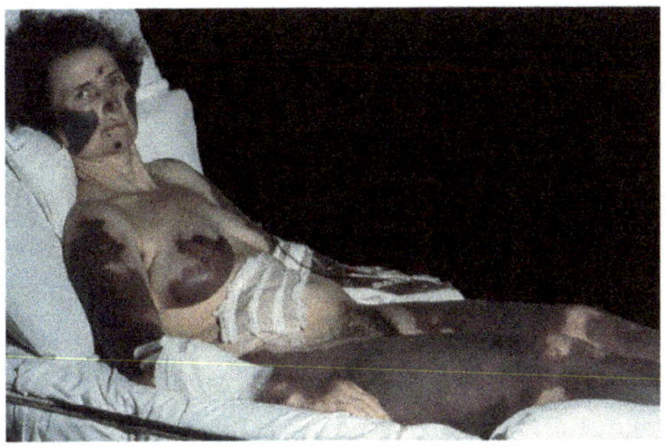

Purpura fulminans. Disseminated intravascular coagulation and sepsis, with presumed sepsis-associated protein C depletion leading to purpura fulminans. Extensive geographic areas of cutaneous infarction with hemorrhage involving the face, breast, and extremities; although the patient looked alert, she died within several days. This catastrophic event followed sepsis after abdominal surgery. (Reproduced, with permission, from Goldsmith LA, Katz SI, Gilchrest BA, Paller AS, Leffell DJ, Wolff K, eds. *Fitzpatrick's Dermatology in General Medicine.* 8th ed. New York, NY: McGraw-Hill Education; 2012.)

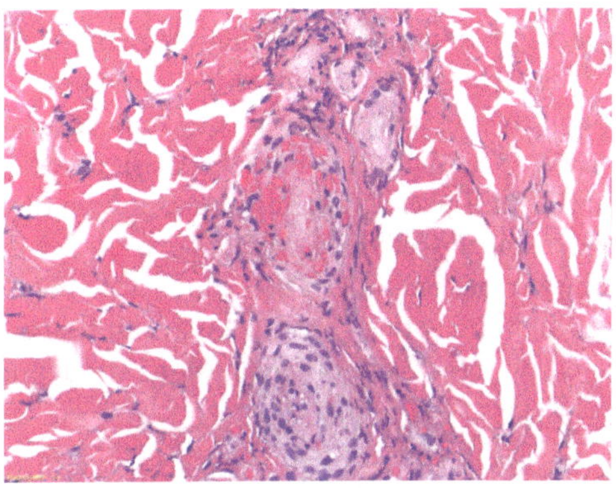

Pauci-inflammatory thrombogenic vasculopathy with complete vascular occlusion associated with purpura fulminans. There is complete thrombotic occlusion of the vessels.

ANSWER 4-17: D.

Cholesterol crystal embolization (aka **atheroembolism**) is usually a disease of the elderly with significant atherosclerosis (Table 4-17A). Atheromatous plaque material may detach spontaneously or, more commonly, may follow an invasive procedure, such as arterial catheterization. Microemboli, composed of cholesterol crystals and/or other components of atheromatous plaque, often result in ischemic changes, most commonly involving the lower extremities. The cutaneous manifestations include livedo reticularis (purple netlike discoloration) or, like the patient in question, small, painful nodules or indurated plaques of the distal extremities (toes most common) often resulting in gangrene. In regards to the other answer choices, the former clinical presentation (livedo reticularis) may mimic **calciphylaxis** and the latter presentation (distal extremities) closely mimics **septic vasculitis, cryoglobulinemia**, and

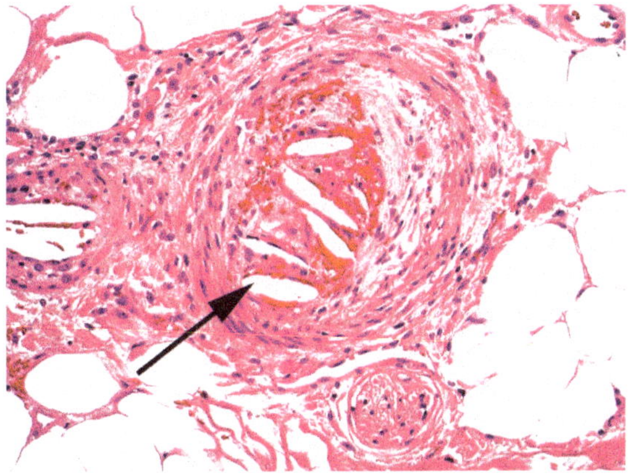

Cholesterol emboli. Needle-shaped clefts (arrow) are present within the lumen of a small vessel.

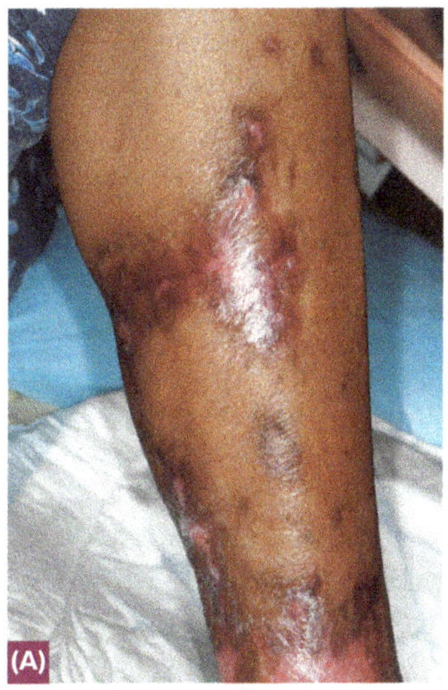

Calciphylaxis. **(A)** Hyperpigmented and purpuric plaques with vaguely livedoid, reticulate, and arciform patterns showing coalescence on the lower extremity. Large atheroemboli may rarely manifest with a similar presentation. **(B)** High power image revealing purple vascular calcification of a small blood vessel in the panniculus. (Used with permission of Dr. Charles Palmer.)

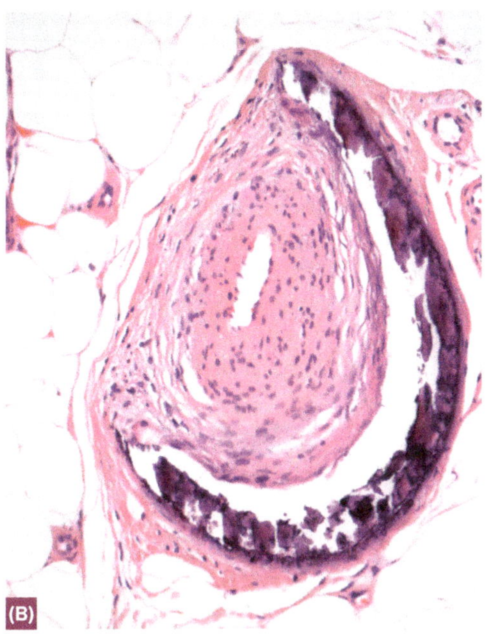

Table 4-17A. Cutaneous Cholesterol Embolism (Atheroembolism)

Clinical Features
- Elderly patient with significant atherosclerosis
- Often status post-arterial catheterization
- Often lower extremities effected
- Extremity with adequate pulsation
- Livedo reticularis, purple discoloration, gangrene of toes, and small, painful ulcerations on the legs, nodules, or indurated plaques

Histopathologic Features
- Emboli with needle-shaped clefts in the lumina of small vessels associated with amorphous eosinophilic material
- Macrophages
- Foreign body giant cell reaction
- Intimal fibrosis
- Obliteration of lumina
- Fibrin thrombi

perniosis (chilblains). A helpful feature is the presence of intact arterial pulses on examination of the affected extremity, indicating that the ischemia is secondary to small-vessel involvement rather than major arteries.

Microscopically, **cholesterol emboli** may be found as needle-shaped clefts within the lumina of small vessels. The intravascular clefts, that are actually dissolved crystals, may be single or multiple and commonly are associated with amorphous eosinophilic material, macrophages, or a foreign body giant cell reaction. Vascular walls exhibit intimal fibrosis and often obliteration of lumina in older lesions. In many instances only fibrin thrombi are observed. Often a deep biopsy is needed to reveal such emboli, which are distributed focally and therefore difficult to find. **Calciphylaxis** is a condition of systemic vascular calcification associated with chronic renal failure and is microscopically characterized by small-vessel wall calcification in the subcutis with subsequent thrombus formation (Table 4-17B). The calcification has a dark purple color and is refractile.

Table 4-17B. Calciphylaxis

Clinical Features
- Renal failure with secondary hyperparathyroidism
- Primary hyperparathyroidism
- Hypercalcemia of malignancy
- Livedo reticularis
- Firm, indurated, painful, violaceous lesions
- Progression to bullae, ulcers, eschars, and gangrene
- Trunk and extremities involved

Histopathologic Features
- Calcium deposition in soft tissue and small blood vessels
- Intimal proliferation and luminal occlusion
- Thrombi in uncalcified, noninflamed small vessels of the subcutis
- Full-thickness ischemic necrosis of skin

Differential Diagnosis
- Coagulopathies
- Calcinosis cutis
- Panniculitis with calcification

ANSWER 4-18: B.

The biopsy reveals a strikingly pauci-cellular dermis with increased dermal mucin. The epidermis is unremarkable (the cleft is artifactual separation of the stratum corneum). The small vessels in the papillary dermis are obliterated by thrombus and are surrounded by thick eosinophilic hyaline material. This patient has **malignant atrophic papulosis (MAP)**, also known as **Degos disease** (Table 4-18A). Degos initially described a cutaneointestinal syndrome in which distinct skin findings (**"drops of porcelain"**) were associated with recurrent attacks of abdominal pain that often ended in death from intestinal perforations. He chose the name **malignant atrophic papulosis** to emphasize the serious clinical course of the disease. Originally, the cutaneous lesions were thought to be specific and pathognomonic for a unique disease entity (Degos disease). Currently, MAP is considered to be a clinicopathologic reaction pattern that can be associated with a number of conditions other than the cutaneointestinal syndrome described by Degos and others. Lesions similar, if

Table 4-18A. Degos Syndrome

Clinical Features
- Crops of asymptomatic, slightly raised, yellowish-red or pale rose papules which umbilicate and develop an atrophic porcelain-white center with a livid red, telangiectatic surrounding
- Trunk and proximal extremities commonly affected
- Acute abdominal crisis
- Cerebral infarction

Histopathologic Features
- Atrophic epidermis with hyperkeratosis
- Wedge-shaped area of altered dermis
- Necrosis or edema
- Mucin deposition and slight sclerosis
- Vascular damage at the base of the wedge
- Fibrin thrombi common

Differential Diagnosis
- Coagulopathies
- Cryoglobulinemia
- Atrophie blanche
- Pityriasis lichenoides

not identical, to MAP have been noted in particular in **connective tissue diseases** such as **lupus erythematosus, dermatomyositis**, and **progressive systemic sclerosis**; in **atrophie blanche**; and in **Creutzfeldt–Jakob disease**. A "benign" form, involving only the skin, has been reported. The etiology of Degos syndrome is unclear. The findings have been ascribed to a coagulopathy, vasculitis, or mucinosis. However, convincing evidence to support any single causal factor is lacking. Recently, a case with intense C5b-9 deposition within the dermal microvasculature and absent immunoglobulins has been reported. This patient was successfully treated with eculizumab (terminal complement inhibitor).

The cutaneous manifestations of Degos syndrome include crops of asymptomatic, slightly raised, yellowish red or pale-rose papules. Gradually the papules become umbilicated and develop an atrophic porcelain white center with a livid red, telangiectatic margin (**"porcelain papules"**). These papules tend to affect the trunk and proximal extremities. Symptoms of an acute abdomen or, less commonly, of a cerebral infarction may supervene.

The histopathology observed varies with the evolution of the lesions. Early papular lesions may show a superficial and deep perivascular, periadnexal, and perineural chronic inflammatory cell infiltrate associated with interstitial mucin deposition and an overlying mild vacuolar interface reaction mimicking **tumid lupus**. More evolved lesions with the porcelain white scale show a wedge-shaped area of altered dermis covered by atrophic epidermis with slight hyperkeratosis. Dermal alterations may include frank necrosis. However, more commonly, edema, extensive mucin deposition (which may mimic tumid lupus), and slight sclerosis or a **lichen sclerosis-like** appearance is seen. Typically, vascular damage is noted in the vessels at the base of the "**cone of necrobiosis.**"

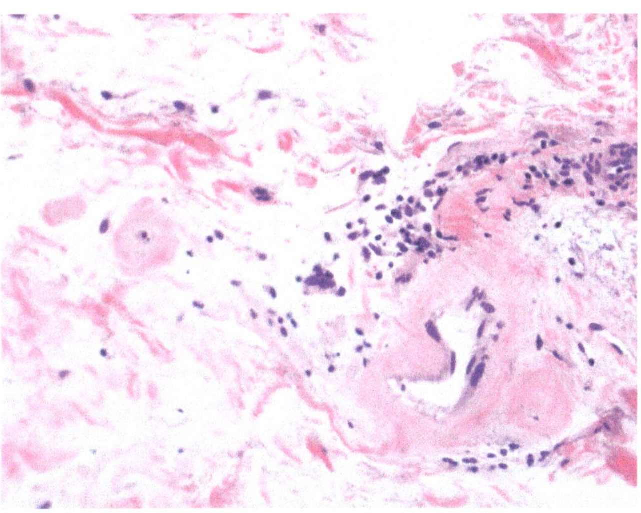

Degos disease. Note the sparse lymphocytic infiltrate and small vessels surrounded by eosinophilic hyaline material. The vessel of the left is almost completely obliterated. The endothelial lining exhibits degenerative changes.

Vascular alterations may be subtle and manifest as endothelial swelling only. However, more characteristically, intravascular fibrin thrombi may be noted. Their presence suggests that the dermal and epidermal changes result from ischemia. Altered vessels usually lack an inflammatory infiltrate.

In regards to the other answer choices, **Henoch–Schönlein pupura** and **microscopic polyarteritis** may manifest systemic symptoms in addition to cutaneous lesions; however these conditions are histopathologically characterized by leukocytoclastic vasculitis, which is not present in MAP. As previously discussed, **tumid lupus** may histopathologically mimic MAP; however tumid lupus typically lacks significant vasculopathic changes and contains robust lymphocytic infiltrates. Clinically, tumid lupus lacks systemic involvement and presents with indurated plaques, rather than ulcerated papules. **Lichen sclerosus** may exhibit similar microvascular damage, but is accompanied by papillary dermal sclerosis and also lacks systemic findings. Clinical correlation may be required to establish the correct diagnosis.

ANSWER 4-19: E.

The biopsy reveals extravasated red cells within an elastotic dermis. There is no evidence of vasculitis (inflammation, fibrinoid necrosis, or thrombosis). This is an example of a vasculopathy owing to a deficiency of vascular connective tissue support. Structural deficiencies of the perivascular connective tissue may contribute to vascular fragility and the attendant extravasation of erythrocytes. Such alterations underlie the hemorrhage in **senile purpura** and **scurvy**. This group of conditions can be described as **noninflammatory purpura**.

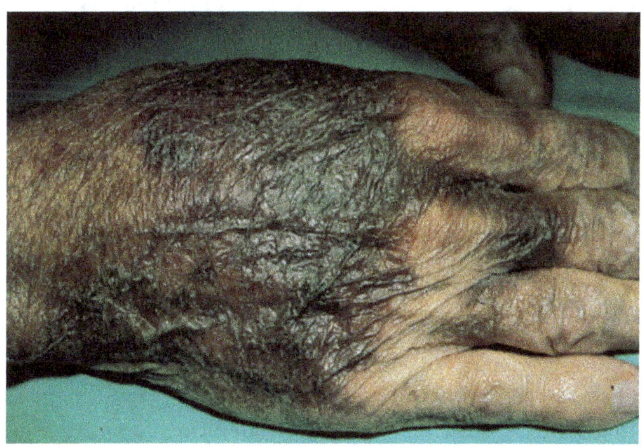

Senile purpura. Note accompanying skin atrophy. (Reproduced, with permission, from Kaushansky K, Lichtman MA, Beutler E, Kipps TJ, Seligsohn U, Prchal JT, eds. *Williams Hematology*. 8th ed. New York, NY: McGraw-Hill Education; 2010.)

In **senile purpura**, extravasation of red blood cells occurs in atrophic skin with severe solar elastosis and normal-appearing capillaries. Such lesions may simulate melanoma

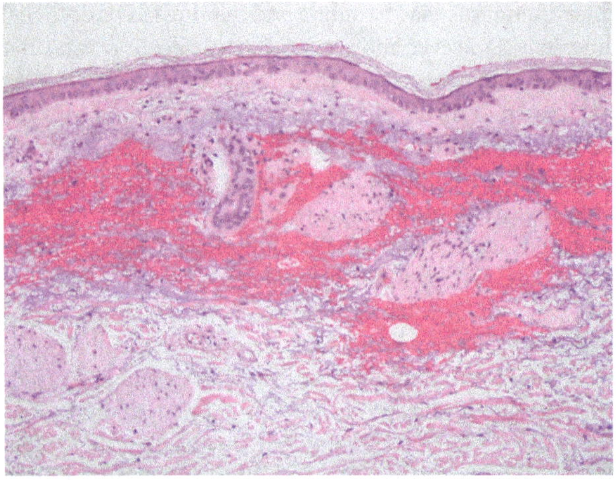

Non-inflammatory purpura, consistent with "senile purpura". There is extensive red blood cell extravasation without obvious vascular injury. Note the background of severe solar elastosis.

or angiosarcoma clinically. **Scurvy** is characterized by dermal hemorrhage predominantly in the vicinity of hair follicles without evidence of vascular damage. Hemosiderin-laden macrophages, follicular keratotic plugs, and coiled hair are also seen.

In regards to the other answer choices, they may also exhibit extensive dermal hemorrhage, but are typically accompanied by vascular thrombosis, at least focally.

ANSWER 4-20: D.

The second skin biopsy reveals a small- to medium-sized vessel with thrombosis and infiltration of its walls by macrophages and lymphocytes, consistent with **granulomatous vasculitis** (Table 4-20A). **Wegener granulomatosis (WG)** was first recognized as a distinct clinicopathologic disease process in 1936, when Wegener reported three patients with a "peculiar rhinogenic granulomatosis." Godman and Churg summarized postmortem studies in 1954, from which the classic triad of this clinicopathologic complex evolved: (1) necrotizing and granulomatous inflammation of the upper and lower respiratory tracts, (2) glomerulonephritis, and (3) systemic vasculitis. Limited variants of the disease involving only the respiratory tract have been described. In the protracted superficial variant, ulcerated, necrotizing lesions remain localized to the mucosa and skin for many years, with pulmonary and renal involvement eventually developing in some of these patients. With the recognition of an association between ANCAs and WG, the concept of WG has been modified, and the need for demonstrating granulomatous inflammation as a prerequisite for the diagnosis of WG has been challenged. A less restrictive definition has been proposed: Wegener vasculitis. Subsumed under this less restrictive category are ANCA-positive patients with clinical presentations of WG, such as sinusitis, pulmonary infiltrates, and nephritis, and documented necrotizing vasculitis

Table 4-20A. Wegener Granulomatosis

Clinical Features
- Sinusitis
- Recurrent pneumonitis
- Glomerulonephritis
- Myalgia, arthralgia, fever
- Palpable purpura, nodules, and ulcers

Histopathologic Features
- LCV
- Granulomatous inflammation with suppuration and necrosis
- Cutaneous extravascular necrotizing granuloma
- Erythema elevatum diutinum, granuloma annulare, or erythema nodosum
- Nonspecific acute or chronic inflammatory lesions and ulcerations

Differential Diagnosis
- Vasculitic component
  - MPA, CSS, other causes of LCV
  - Metastatic Crohn disease
- Granulomatous component
  - Granulomatous infections
  - CSS
  - Sarcoidosis
  - Granulomatous rosacea
  - Foreign body reactions
  - Ruptured cysts

but without biopsy-proven granulomatous inflammation. **Wegener syndrome**, a more generic term can include both classic WG and Wegener vasculitis.

Clinically, two-thirds of patients with WG are male, and the mean age of diagnosis is 35-54 years. The vast majority of patients are Caucasians. The clinical presentation is extremely variable, ranging from an insidious course with a prolonged period of nonspecific constitutional symptoms and upper respiratory tract findings to abrupt onset of severe pulmonary and renal disease. The most commonly involved anatomic sites include the upper respiratory tract, lower respiratory tract, and kidney. Other organ systems that are commonly affected include the joints and skin. Migratory polyarticular arthralgia of large and small joints is found in up to 85% of patients with WG.

Cutaneous involvement is extremely variable in different series, ranging from less than 20% to over 50% of patients. The most common presentation is palpable purpura. Other cutaneous manifestations include macular erythematous eruptions, papulonecrotic lesions, subcutaneous nodules with and without ulceration, and pyoderma gangrenosum. Occasionally, cutaneous lesions are the first indication of WG. However, because of their nonspecific appearance, they are infrequently recognized as presentations of WG.

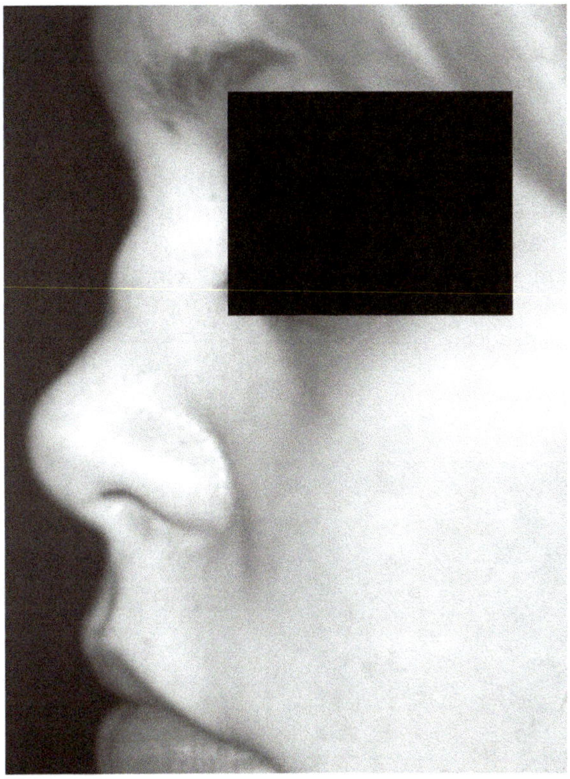

Saddle-nose deformity of Wegener granulomatosis. Cartilaginous inflammation of the nose in granulomatosis with polyangiitis (Wegener granulomatosis) may lead to nasal septal perforation and ultimately to collapse of the nasal bridge ("saddle-nose" deformity). (Reproduced, with permission, from Imboden JB, Hellmann DB, Stone JH, eds. *Current Medical Diagnosis & Treatment: Rheumatology*. 3rd ed. New York, NY: McGraw-Hill Education; 2013.)

Microscopically, the majority of skin biopsies in patients with WG are nonspecific, such as perivascular lymphocytic infiltrates. However, in about 25%-50% of patients the histopathologic findings are fairly characteristic. The most frequent reaction patterns that are distinctive include **necrotizing leukocytoclastic small-vessel vasculitis** and **granulomatous inflammation**. The small-vessel vasculitis is characterized by neutrophilic infiltrates and is indistinguishable from the LCV of many other processes. Eosinophils can be as numerous in LCV lesions from patients with WG, as in those with **Churg-Strauss syndrome (CSS)**. The granulomatous reactions contain histiocytes, lymphocytes, and giant cells and show suppurative necrosis. Microgranulomas, minute foci of tissue necrosis surrounded by histiocytes, are characteristic and are similar to lesions described in open lung biopsies from WG patients. True **granulomatous vasculitis**, acneiform perifollicular granulomatous inflammation, **erythema elevatum diutinum (EED),** and **erythema nodosum-like reaction** patterns have been described. The granulomatous vasculitis is characterized by a perivascular histiocytic infiltrate, few neutrophils, and focal vascular damage. The **palisading granulomas** of WG resemble those of CSS, except that the center of the WG granuloma contains necrobiotic collagen and basophilic fibrillar necrotic debris admixed with neutrophils, the so-called "**blue**" **palisading granuloma**. Tissue eosinophilia and eosinophilic debris are observed less frequently in the granulomata of WG. These lesions, also referred to as **cutaneous extravascular necrotizing granuloma**, are not specific for WG and may be associated with systemic vasculitis, connective tissue disease, or lymphoproliferative disease. Cutaneous ulcerations in WG may show granulomatous inflammation and necrotizing vasculitis and also secondary nonspecific vascular damage.

The histopathologic differential diagnosis of WG includes numerous entities causing LCV and palisading granulomas. Infective processes causing granulomatous inflammation and possibly vasculitis should be excluded; the list of such agents is large and includes mycobacteria, deep fungi, viruses, and syphilis, among others. **Septic vasculitis and Henoch-Schönlein purpura** demonstrate immunoglobulin deposition within vessels via direct immunofluorescence. Other conditions causing LCV and granulomatous reactions include **CSS, metastatic Crohn disease, rheumatoid arthritis**, and sarcoidosis. Granulomatous vascular reactions may also be a manifestation of T-cell lymphomas such as **angiocentric T-cell lymphoma** or **panniculitis-like T-cell lymphoma**. Tightly packed, nonnecrotizing granulomas characteristic of sarcoid are not typical of WG. The distinction between WG and these other diseases relies primarily on clinical findings. In contrast to WG, CSS is associated with asthma, lacks lesions in the upper respiratory tract, rarely shows severe renal involvement, and typically is accompanied by peripheral eosinophilia or eosinophilic infiltrates and p-ANCA positivity.

ANSWER 4-21: C.

The biopsy reveals leukocytoclastic vasculitis involving a medium-sized vessel. The combined clinical and histopathological findings are consistent with **polyarteritis nodosa (PAN)** (Table 4-21A). The first report of polyarteritis nodosa (PAN) in 1885 describes a 27-year-old man with fever, abdominal pain, muscle weakness, peripheral neuropathy, and renal disease. The fatal illness was termed "periarteritis nodosa," referring to nodular protuberances along the course of medium-sized muscular arteries. Ferrari in 1903 emphasized the characteristic presence of inflammatory cells within all levels of the affected vessels (panarteritis) and suggested the term "polyarteritis" instead of periarteritis.

The term PAN now subsumes three entities: (1) **classic systemic PAN**, (2) **cutaneous PAN**, and (3) **microscopic polyarteritis**. Classic PAN is a multisystem disorder characterized by inflammatory vasculitis involving arterioles and small- and medium-sized arteries. **Cutaneous PAN** according to some authors is the only variety of PAN consistently involving the deep dermis and subcutaneous fat with diagnostic

Table 4-21A. Polyarteritis Nodosa

Clinical Features
Fever, malaise, weight loss, weakness myalgias, arthralgias, and anorexia
Hematuria, proteinuria, hypertension, and azotemia
Acute abdominal crises, strokes, myocardial infarction, and mononeuritis multiplex
Subcutaneous nodules which may pulsate or ulcerate
Ecchymoses and gangrene of fingers and toes
Livedo reticularis, bullae, papules, scarlatiniform lesions, and urticaria
Histopathologic Features
Early: leukocytoclastic vasculitis of small- to medium-sized arteries
Late: intimal proliferation and thrombosis, chronic inflammatory infiltrate, fibrosis
Differential Diagnosis
Infection (bacterial, eg, pseudomonas; viral, eg, hepatitis B or HIV)
Connective tissue disease (lupus erythematosus, rheumatoid arthritis)
Vasculitides with granulomatosis
Wegener granulomatosis
Churg–Strauss syndrome

features of arteritis. Some authors maintain that if there is no evidence of systemic involvement by (skin-limited) PAN at the time of initial diagnosis, then the condition will remain confined to the skin despite a potentially prolonged clinical course with multiple recurrences. The pathogenesis of PAN is poorly understood. Direct immunofluorescence testing of skin lesions of PAN shows some immune deposits in dermal vessels. However, these deposits may reflect a secondary event after vascular injury from another cause. There is some clinical overlap with microscopic PAN, although ANCAs generally are absent in classic systemic and cutaneous PAN. PAN is more common in men than in women, usually occurring between the ages of 20 and 60 years. Clinical manifestations may be dramatic and protean. Fever, malaise, weight loss, weakness, myalgias, arthralgias, and anorexia are common symptoms reflecting the systemic nature of the disease. Other findings may reflect infarction of specific organs. Renal involvement, present in about 75% of patients, is the most common cause of death. Hematuria, proteinuria, hypertension, and azotemia may result from both infarction owing to disease of renal arteries or focal, segmental necrotizing glomerular lesions suggesting involvement of small vessels. Acute abdominal crises, strokes, myocardial infarction, and mononeuritis multiplex result from involvement of the relevant arteries. Arteriography of visceral arteries often shows multiple aneurysms that are highly suggestive of PAN. Symptoms such as asthma, Löffler syndrome, and rashes may be related to the hypereosinophilia sometimes seen in these patients. Cutaneous manifestations include subcutaneous nodules that may pulsate or ulcerate, ecchymoses, and gangrene of fingers and toes. Livedo reticularis, bullae, papules, scarlatiniform lesions, and urticaria occur in some patients. A limited form of PAN without visceral involvement may exist (cutaneous PAN), but this concept is controversial and patients must be closely monitored. So-called cutaneous PAN actually may show skin, muscle, peripheral nerve, and joint involvement. The course of disease is benign but protracted and shows steroid dependence.

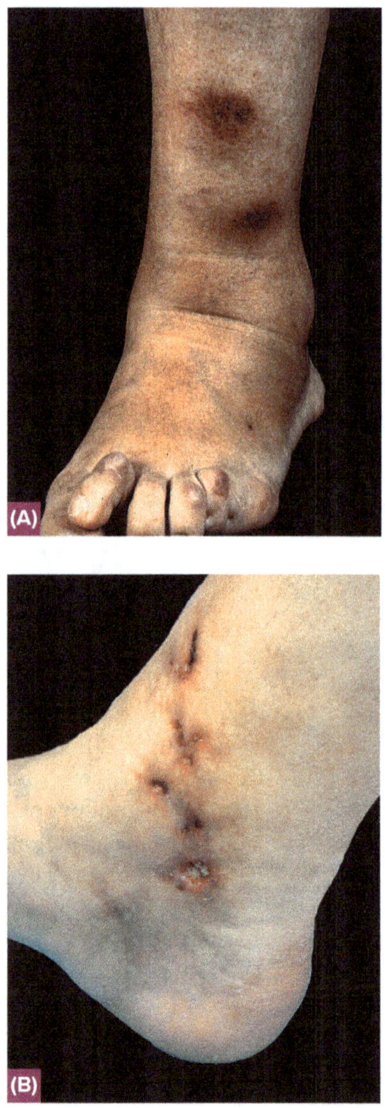

Polyarteritis nodosa. (A) Two dermal and subcutaneous nodules occurring on the pretibial aspects of the lower leg. **(B)** A starburst pattern can be seen in the supra- and retromalleolar region of the right leg in another patient. These lesions represent cutaneous infarction with ulceration. (Reproduced with permission from Kemp WL, Burns DK, Travis Brown TG. *Pathology: The Big Picture*. 1st ed. New York, NY: McGraw-Hill Education; 2008.)

Microscopically, although affected skin often shows only a small-vessel necrotizing vasculitis, the characteristic lesion of classic PAN is a panarteritis involving medium-sized and small arteries in visceral sites. A panarteritis of the larger arteries in deeper dermis or subcutis is observed most commonly in patients presenting with cutaneous nodules. Lesions typically are in different stages of development. Early lesions show degeneration of the arterial wall with deposition of fibrinoid material. There is partial to complete destruction of the external and internal elastic laminae. An infiltrate present within and around the arterial wall is composed largely of neutrophils showing evidence of leukocytoclasis, although eosinophils often are admixed. At a later stage, intimal proliferation and thrombosis lead to complete occlusion of the

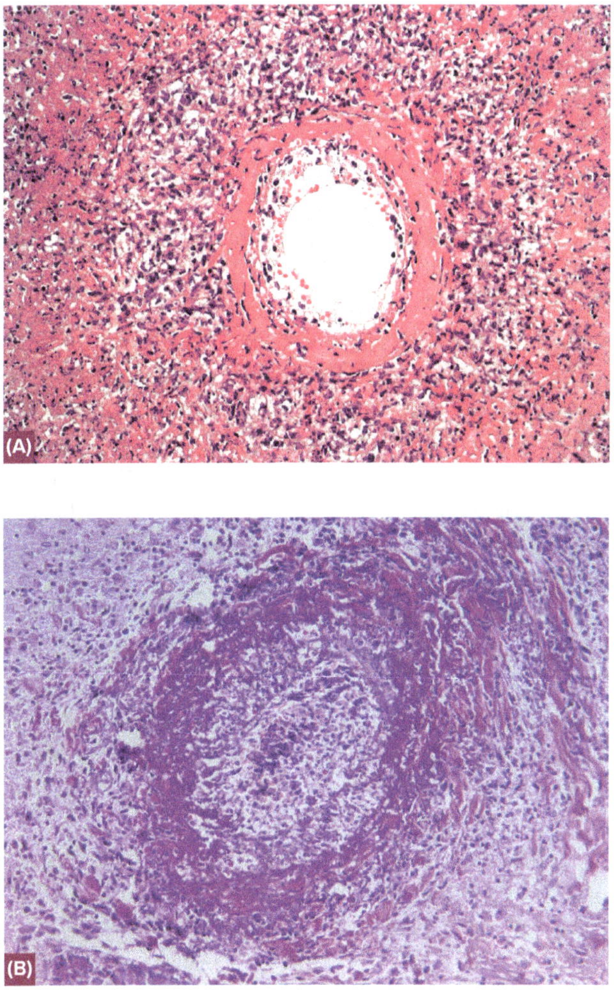

Polyarteritis nodosa. (A), (B) Note the prominent fibrinoid necrosis (smudgy eosinophilic changes) of the wall of this vessel and the accompanying inflammatory infiltrate. Polyarteritis nodosa can affect many different medium-sized vessels (with the exception of the pulmonary vasculature) and, thus, patients can present with a wide variety of signs and symptoms. Hematoxylin and eosin, 200×. (Reproduced, with permission, from Kemp WL, Burns DK, Travis Brown TG. *Pathology: The Big Picture*. 8th ed. New York, NY: McGraw-Hill Education; 2008.)

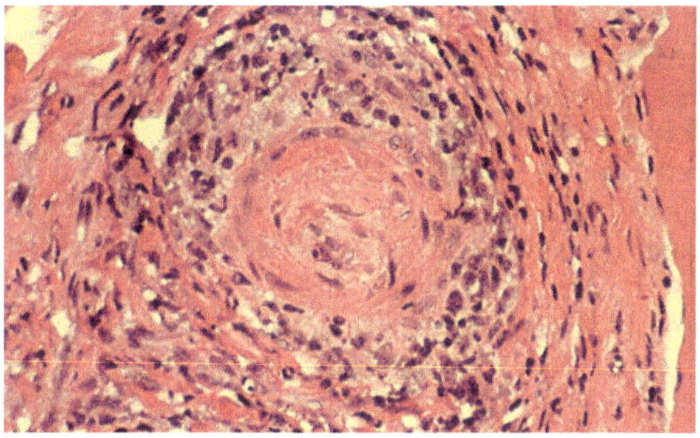

Sural nerve biopsy in polyarteritis nodosa. This sural nerve biopsy was performed in a patient with polyarteritis nodosa, who had presented with a mononeuritis multiplex. Neutrophils are seen infiltrating all layers of this medium-sized vessel, which resulted in vessel occlusion and nerve infraction. (Reproduced with permission from Kasper DL, Fauci A, Hauser SL et al: Harrison's *Principles of Internal Medicine*. 19th ed. New York, NY: McGraw-Hill Education; 2015.)

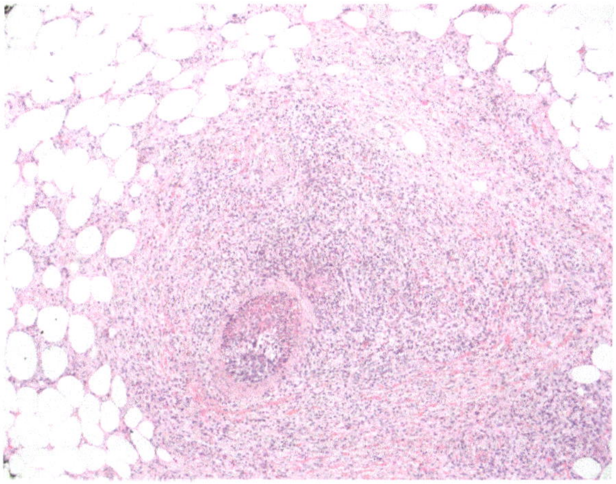

Erythema induratum/Nodular vasculitis. Note the medium vessel vasculitis with extensive lobular inflammation and fibrosis. Polyarteritis nodosa lacks significant inflammation of the fat lobules.

lumen with subsequent ischemia and possibly ulceration. The subacute infiltrate often contains lymphocytes, histiocytes, and some plasma cells. The healing stage is distinguished by a fibroblastic proliferation extending into the perivascular area. The small vessels of the middle and upper dermis often show a nonspecific lymphocytic perivascular infiltrate.

In regards to the differential diagnosis, vasculitides indistinguishable from idiopathic PAN may be observed in **infection** (bacterial, eg, *Streptococcus* and *Pseudomonas*; viral, eg, hepatitis B or HIV), **connective tissue disease** (lupus erythematosus, rheumatoid arthritis), **Wegener granulomatosis, Churg–Strauss syndrome**, and other settings without explanation, for example, acute myelogenous leukemia. Some cases of **erythema induratum/nodular vasculitis** with limited septolobular panniculitis can mimic PAN histologically. In general, any panniculitis accompanying PAN should be limited to the area directly adjacent to the affected vessel. Widespread inflammation of the fat suggests panniculitis as the primary disease category. Additionally, erythema induratum/nodular vasculitis lacks the systemic findings and is typically confined as nodules on the posterior lower legs. These conditions present with nodules on the posterior calves and are associated with mycobacteria id (erythema induratum) and other infectious id reactions (nodular vasculitis).

As with all vasculitides, the disease process should be defined by ruling out infection, searching for underlying systemic diseases, and then documenting the extent of systemic involvement and associated findings. **Superficial thrombophlebitis (STP)** of small- to medium-sized veins may be seen at many anatomic sites but especially the lower extremities. The usual presentation is a tender, erythematous cordlike structure or nodule, similar to PAN. Affected individuals often have predisposing factors such as varicose veins, a hypercoagulable state, ingestion of oral contraceptives, or an underlying malignancy. **Superficial septic thrombophlebitis** is usually secondary to peripheral venous infusion. **Mondor disease** is a thrombophlebitis of the subcutaneous veins of the chest region and is also often manifested clinically by a cordlike induration. It usually is not accompanied by general symptoms and tends to resolve within weeks. In most cases the etiology remains unknown; however, local interference with venous flow may be a factor as associations include trauma and surgical procedures. PAN affects medium-sized arteries rather than veins, is more inflammatory and less thrombogenic than STP. Finally, PAN shows conspicuous fibrinoid necrosis whereas STP usually does not. An elastic tissue stain to demonstrate the presence of an internal elastic lamina in an arterial vessel versus its usual absence (not always) in a vein may facilitate the differentiation of PAN and STP.

BIBLIOGRAPHY

1. Abdul-Ghaffar S, Chan SK, Burrows NP. Haemorrhagic bullae in a child with Henoch-Schonlein purpura. *Br J Dermatol.* 2007;156(6):1408.
2. Bahrami S, Malone JC, Webb KG, Callen JP. Tissue eosinophilia as an indicator of drug-induced cutaneous small-vessel vasculitis. *Arch Dermatol.* 2006;142(2):155–161.
3. Bansal PJ, Tobin MC. Neonatal microscopic polyangiitis secondary to transfer of maternal myeloperoxidase-antineutrophil cytoplasmic antibody resulting in neonatal pulmonary hemorrhage and renal involvement. *Ann Allergy Asthma Immunol.* 2004;93:398–401.
4. Barnhill RL, Bravermann IM. Progression of pigmented purpura-like eruptions to mycosis fungoides: report of 3 cases. *J Am Acad Dermatol.* 1988;19:25–31.
5. Bonaci-Nikolic B, Nikolic MM, Andrejevic S, Zoric S, Bukilica M. Antineutrophil cytoplasmic antibody (ANCA)-associated autoimmune diseases induced by antithyroid drugs: comparison with idiopathic ANCA vasculitides. *Arthritis Res Ther.* 2005;7(5):R1072–R1081.
6. Burns BV, Roberts PF, De Carpentier J, Zarod AP. Eosinophilic angiocentric fibrosis affecting the nasal cavity: a mucosal variant of the skin lesion granuloma faciale. *J Laryngol Otol.* 2001;115:223–226.
7. Callen JP. Cutaneous vasculitis: relationship to systemic disease and therapy. *Curr Probl Dermatol.* 1993;5:45–80.
8. Caputo R, Marzano AV, Vezzoli P, Lunardon L. Wells syndrome in adults and children: a report of 19 cases. *Arch Dermatol.* 2006;142(9):1157–1161.
9. Carlson JA, LeBoit PE. Localized chronic fibrosing vasculitis of the skin: an inflammatory reaction that occurs in settings other than erythema elevatum diutinum and granuloma faciale. *Am J Surg Pathol.* 1997;21:698–705.
10. Chen KR, Kawahara Y, Miyakawa S, Nishikawa T. Cutaneous vasculitis in Behçet's disease: a clinical and histopathologic study of 20 patients. *J Am Acad Dermatol.* 1997;36:689–696.
11. Chen KR, Sakamoto M, Ikemoto K, Abe R, Shimizu H. Granulomatous arteritis in cutaneous lesions of Churg-Strauss syndrome. *J Cutan Pathol.* 2007;34(4):330–337.
12. Churg J, Strauss L. Allergic granulomatosis, allergic angiitis, and periarteritis nodosa. *Am J Pathol.* 1951;27:277–301.
13. Cohen SJ, Pittelkow MR, Su WPD. Cutaneous manifestations of cryoglobulinemia: clinical and histopathologic study of 72 patients. *J Am Acad Dermatol.* 1992;26:38–44.
14. Comfere NI, Macaron NC, Gibson LE. Cutaneous manifestations of Wegener's granulomatosis: a clinicopathologic study of 17 patients and correlation to antineutrophil cytoplasmic antibody status. *J Cutan Pathol.* 2007;34(10):739–747.
15. Cribier B, Djeridi N, Peltre B, Grosshans E. A histologic and immunohistochemical study of chilblains. *J Am Acad Dermatol.* 2001;45:924–929.
16. Davis MDP, Daoud MS, Kirby B, et al. Clinicopathologic correlation of hypo-complementemic and normocomplementemic urticarial vasculitits. *J Am Acad Dermatol.* 1998;38:899–905.

17. Díaz-Pérez JL, De Lagrán ZM, Díaz-Ramón JL, Winkelmann RK. Cutaneous polyarteritis nodosa. *Semin Cutan Med Surg.* 2007 Jun;26(2):77–86.
18. Dillon MJ, Ozen S. A new international classification of childhood vasculitis. *Pediatr Nephrol.* 2006;21(9):1219–1222.
19. Dillon MJ. Henoch-Schonlein purpura: recent advances. *Clin Exp Rheumatol.* 2007;25(1 Suppl 44):S66–S68.
20. Edsall L, English JC III, Patterson JW. Calciphylaxis and metastatic calcification associated with nephrogenic fibrosing dermopathy. *J Cutan Pathol.* 2004;31(3):247–253.
21. Faclieru D, Bergman R, Lanir N, et al. A study of coagulation and anti-endothelial antibodies in idiopathic livedo reticularis. *Acta Derm Venereol (Stockh).* 1997;77:181–183.
22. Fain O, Hamidou M, Cacoub P, et al. Vasculitides associated with malignancies: analysis of sixty patients. *Arthritis Rheum.* Dec 15, 2007;57(8):1473–1480.
23. Falanga V, Fine MJ, Kapoor WN. The cutaneous manifestations of cholesterol crystal embolization. *Arch Dermatol.* 1986;122:1194–1198.
24. Fernandes SRM, Singsen BH, Hoffman GS. Sarcoidosis and systemic vasculitits. *Semin Arthritis Rheum.* 2000;30:33–46.
25. Ferreres JR, Marcoval J, Bordas X, et al. Calciphylaxis associated with alcoholic cirrhosis. *J Eur Acad Dermatol Venereol.* 2006;20(5):599–601.
26. Francès C, Niang S, Laffitte E, le Pelletier F, Costedoat N, Piette JC. Dermatologic manifestations of the antiphospholipid syndrome: two hundred consecutive cases. *Arthritis Rheum.* 2005;52(6):1785–1793.
27. Greer KE, Cooper PH, Campbell R, Westervelt FB. Primary oxalosis with livedo reticularis. *Arch Dermatol.* 1980;116:213–214.
28. Guillevin L, Lhote F, Amouroux J, et al. Antineutrophil cytoplasmic antibodies, abnormal angiograms, and pathological findings in polyarteritits nodosa and Churg-Strauss syndrome: indications for the classification of vasculitides of the polyarteritits nodosa group. *Br J Rheumatol.* 1996;35:958–964.
29. Hoffman GS, Specks U. Antineutrophil cytoplasmic antibodies. *Arthritis Rheum.* 1998;41:1521–1537.
30. Ikeda E, Uchigasaki S, Baba S, Suzuki H. Multiple rheumatoid papules characteristic of the early stage of rheumatoid vasculitis. *Eur J Dermatol.* 1999;4:313–316.
31. Jennette JC, Falk RJ, Andrassy K, et al. Nomenclature of systemic vasculitides: proposal of an international consensus conference. *Arthritis Rheum.* 1994;37: 187–192.
32. Jennette JC, Falk RJ. Diagnostic classification of antineutrophil cytoplasmic autoantibody-associated vasculitides. *Am J Kidney Dis.* 1991;16:184–187.
33. Jones A, Walling H. Retiform purpura in plaques: a morphological approach to diagnosis. *Clin Exp Dermatol.* 2007;32(5):596–602.
34. 1. Jorizzo JL, Solomon AR, Zanolli MD, et al. Neutrophilic vascular reactions. *Arch Dermatol.* 1988;19:983–1005.
35. Kanazawa N, Furukawa F. Autoinflammatory syndromes with a dermatological perspective. *J Dermatol.* 2007;34(9):601–618.
36. Kawakami T, Soma Y, Mizoguchi M. Initial cutaneous manifestations associated with histopathological leukocytoclastic vasculitis in two patients with antiphospholipid antibody syndrome. *J Dermatol.* 2005;32(12):1032–1037.
37. Kumar B, Narang T, Radotra BD, Gupta S. Mondor's disease of penis: a forgotten disease. *Sex Transm Infect.* 2005;81(6):480–482.
38. Landing BH, Larson EJ. Pathologic features of Kawasaki disease (mucocutaneous lymph node syndrome). *Am J Cardiovasc Pathol.* 1987;4:75–84.
39. Lynch JM, Barrett TL. Collagenolytic (necrobiotic) granulomas: part 1—the 'blue' granulomas. *J Cutan Pathol.* 2004;31(5):353–361.
40. Magro CM, Crowson AN. A clinical and histologic study of 37 cases of immunoglobulin A-associated vasculitis. *Am J Dermatopathol.* 1999;21:234–240.
41. Magro CM, Kiani B, Li J, Crowson AN. Clonality in the setting of Sweet's syndrome and pyoderma gangrenosum is not limited to underlying myeloproliferative disease. *J Cutan Pathol.* 2007;34(7):526–534.
42. Magro CM, Poe JC, Kim C, et al. Degos disease: a C5b-9/interferon-α-mediated endotheliopathy syndrome. *Am J Clin Pathol.* 2011 Apr;135(4):599–610.
43. Mehregan DR, Hall MJ, Gibson LE. Urticarial vasculitis: a histopathologic and clinical review of 72 cases. *J Am Acad Dermatol.* 1992;26:441–448.
44. Mehta RL, Scott G, Sloand JA, Francis CW. Skin necrosis associated with acquired protein C deficiency in patients with renal failure and calciphylaxis. *Am J Med.* 1990;88:252–257.
45. Mimouni D, Ng PP, Rencic A, Nikolskaia OV, Bernstein BD, Nousari HC. Cutaneous polyarteritis nodosa in patients presenting with atrophie blanche. *Brit J Dermatol.* 2003;148(4):789–794.
46. Patel A, Prussick R, Buchanan WW, Sauder DN. Serum sickness-like illness and leukocytoclastic vasculitis

after intravenous streptolinase. *J Am Acad Dermatol.* 1991;24:652–653.

47. Perniciaro CV, Winkelmann RK, Hunder GG. Cutaneous manifestations of Takayasu's arteritis. *J Am Acad Dermatol.* 1987;17:998–1005.
48. Price RD, Murdoch DR. Perniosis (chillblains) of the thigh: report of five cases, including four following river crossings. *High Alt Med Biol.* 2001;2:535–538.
49. Ramelet AA. Exercise-induced purpura. *Dermatology.* 2004;208(4):293–296.
50. Ruiz-Genao D, García-F-Villalta MJ, Hernández-Núñez A, Ríos-Buceta L, Fernández-Herrera J, García-Díez A. Livedo reticularis associated with interferon-a therapy in two melanoma patients. *J Eur Acad Dermatol Venereol.* 2005;19(2):252–254.
51. Sanchez-Guerro J, Gutierrez-Urena S, Vidaller A, et al. Vasculitis as a paraneoplastic syndrome: report of 11 cases and review of the literature. *J Rheumatol.* 1990;17:1458–1462.
52. Sansonno D, Dammacco F. Hepatitis C virus, cryoglobulinaemia, and vasculitis: immune complex relations. *Lancet Infect Dis.* 2005;5(4):227–236.
53. Schneider JW, Jordaan HF. The histologic spectrum of erythema induratum of Bazin. *Am J Dermatopathol.* 1997;19(4):323–333.
54. Stiefler RE, Bergfeld WF. Atrophie blanche (review). *Int J Dermatol.* 1982;21:1–7.
55. Stinco G, Di Gaetano L, Rizzi C, Patrone P. Leukocytoclastic vasculitis in urticaria induced by sun exposure. *Photodermatol Photoimmunol Photomed.* 2007;23(1):39–41.
56. Uthman IW, Khamashta MA. Livedo racemosa: a striking dermatological sign for the antiphospholipid syndrome. *J Rheumatol.* 2006;33(12):2379–2382.
57. Wallach D, Vignon-Pennamen MD. From acute febrile neutrophilic dermatosis to neutrophilic disease: forty years of clinical research. *J Am Acad Dermatol.* 2006;55(6):1066–1071.
58. Weenig RH, Bruce AJ, McEvoy MT, Gibson LE, Davis Mark DP. Neutrophilic dermatosis of the hands: four new cases and review of the literature. *Int J Dermatol.* 2004;43(2):95–102.

CHAPTER 5

Inflammatory Diseases of Adnexal Structures and Subcutis

QUESTION 5-1.

The microanatomy of the subcutaneous layer is supplied by arteries and arterioles in the ______ portion and venules and veins in the _______ portion.

A) Centrilobular, Septal
B) Septal, Centrilobular
C) Septal, Septal
D) Centrilobular, Centrilobular

QUESTION 5-2.

A 27-year-old female presents with abdominal pain, arthralgias, diarrhea, fever, headache, and rapid onset of symmetric crops of exquisitely tender, bright-red nodules on the ankles, knees, and anterior shins. One of the nodules is biopsied to reveal a mixed inflammatory infiltrate involving the fibrous trabeculae of the subcutis composed of neutrophils, lymphocytes, and eosinophils. Extravasated red blood cells are noted. The infiltrates extend to the peripheries of the fat lobules with little infiltration into the fat. Over a period of 6 weeks the nodules resolve with a bruise-like appearance. No ulcers ever appeared. Which of the following regarding this patient's disease is INCORRECT?

A) In regard to pathogenesis, this is a nonspecific hypersensitivity reaction that in children is most commonly preceded by streptococcal infections and in adults is associated with drugs, sarcoidosis, tuberculosis, and inflammatory bowel disease.
B) Late stage lesions of this condition reveal widened fibrotic septae with clusters of mononuclear cells arranged in radial arrays with multinucleation.
C) In late stage lesions, gradual obliteration of fat lobules by septal fibrosis is commonly seen.
D) Fat necrosis with saponification is a characteristic feature of this disease.
E) Although vasculitis is not a major feature, low-grade vascular injury and thrombophlebitis may be encountered in these lesions.

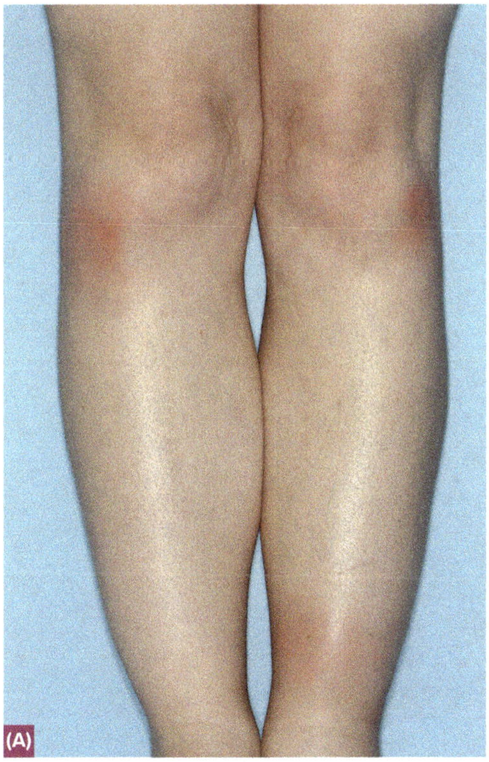

(A)

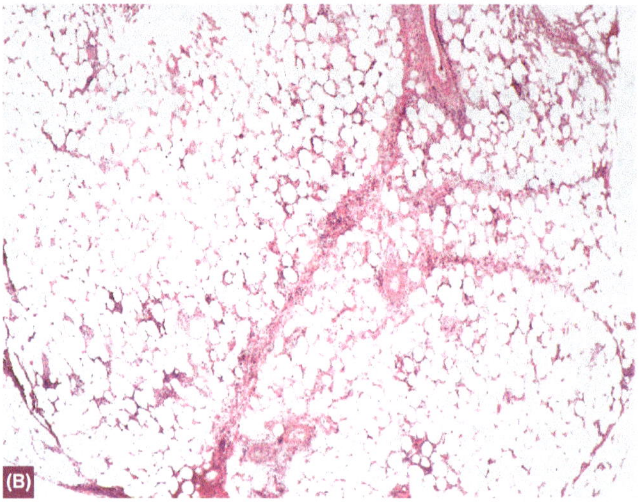

(B)

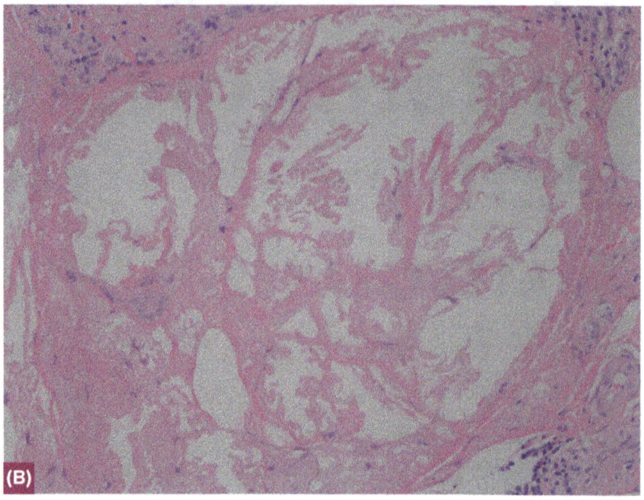

(B)

QUESTION 5-3.

A 67-year-old hypertensive female with a history of venous stasis presents with striking induration of the lower third portions of both legs. The areas are circumferential, erythematous, and wood-like in consistency. A biopsy is performed and reveals marked septal fibrosis with encroachment on the fat lobules. Septal lymphocytic infiltrates admixed with pigmented macrophages are present. A section from the center of the fat lobule is illustrated below. Which of the following regarding this disease is INCORRECT?

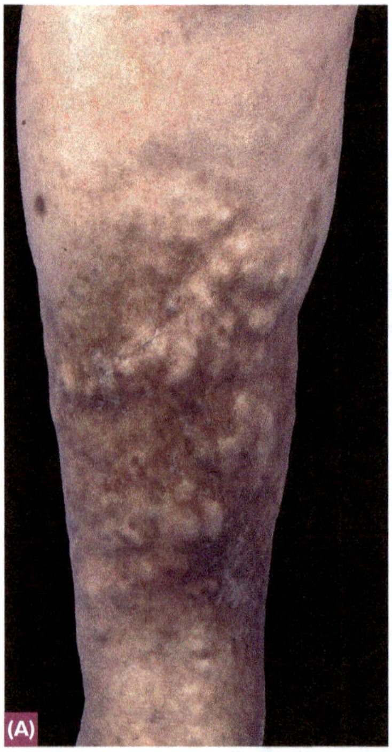

(A)

Reproduced, with permission, from Wolff K, Johnson RA, Saavedra AP. *Fitzpatrick's Color Atlas and Synopsis of Clinical Dermatology*. 7th ed. New York, NY: McGraw-Hill Education; 2013.

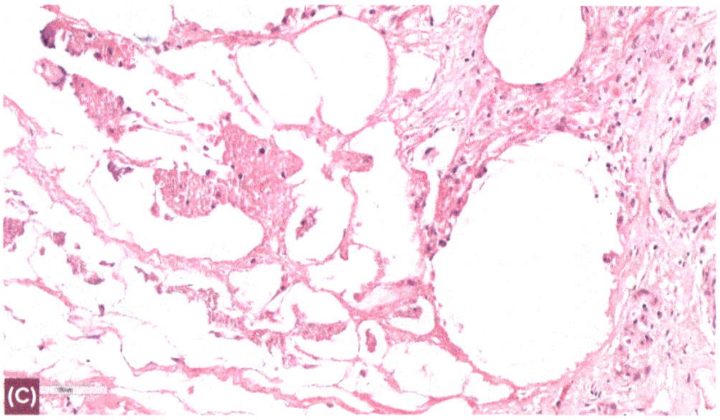

(C)

A) The most specific finding for this condition is lipomembranous fat necrosis since these lesions are attributed to ischemia.
B) Matrix metalloproteinase-2 is elevated in the affected tissues.
C) PAS-D stain will highlight degenerated adipocyte membranes.
D) Pigment present within macrophages will appear bright blue on Prussian blue stain.
E) The most common association is with venous incompetence and chronic stasis.

QUESTION 5-4.

A 67-year-old male with hepatorenal syndrome presents with painful erythematous dusky lesions in a livedo-like pattern on the trunk and extremities. A few of the lesions are ulcerated. Radiographic examination reveals calcification of the vessel walls. Which of the following regarding this disease is INCORRECT?

A) Microscopically, purple appearing calcification of the small vessels (<0.5 mm) and endovascular fibrosis are the most specific findings for this diagnosis.
B) The mortality rate has been reported to be as high as 80%.

C) The vessel walls contain calcium oxalate, which is birefringent under polarized light.
D) Fibrin thrombi within calcified vessels, septal fibrosis, intralobular calcification of fat, and ischemic lobular fat necrosis are regular findings.
E) Osteopontin, thrombospondins, and matrix glutamic acid protein have been found to be upregulated in the lesional blood vessels in this condition.

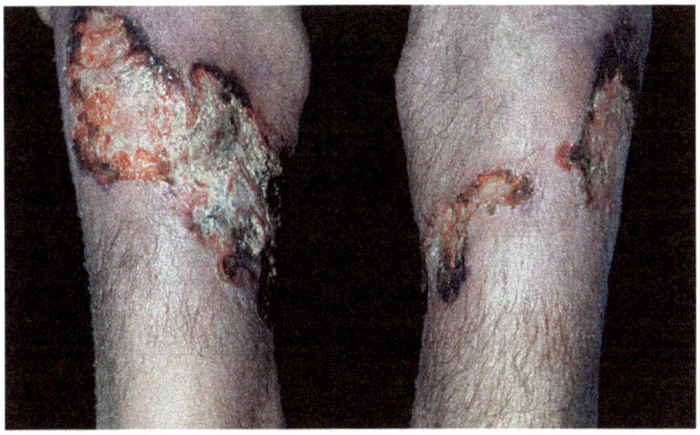

Reproduced, with permission, from Wolff K, Johnson RA, Saavedra AP. *Fitzpatrick's Color Atlas and Synopsis of Clinical Dermatology*. 7th ed. New York, NY: McGraw-Hill Education; 2013.

QUESTION 5-5.

A 42-year-old male with a recent diagnosis of myelodysplastic syndrome develops pitting edema followed by extensive symmetrical sleeve-like circumferential induration with dimpling of the arms and legs. There is sparing of the hands and feet. The onset occurred shortly after an intensive hiking trip in the Catskill Mountains. He has peripheral blood eosinophilia. A deep incisional biopsy is performed and the findings within the deep subcutis and fascia are illustrated below. The reticular dermis, papillary dermis, and epidermis are unremarkable. The inflammatory infiltrate is composed of lymphocytes and rare eosinophils and plasma cells. Which of the following about this disease is INCORRECT?

A) This condition has been associated with drugs, vigorous exercise, *Borrelia* infection, and malignancy.
B) Tissue eosinophils are a requisite finding for the diagnosis.
C) The sclerosis present in this lesion is generally felt to develop in the fascia and extend upward into the subcutaneous tissue and reticular dermis.
D) The sclerosis gradually resolves in most patients over a period of months to years.
E) A similar condition has been reported in association with the ingestion of herbal supplements containing L-tryptophan.

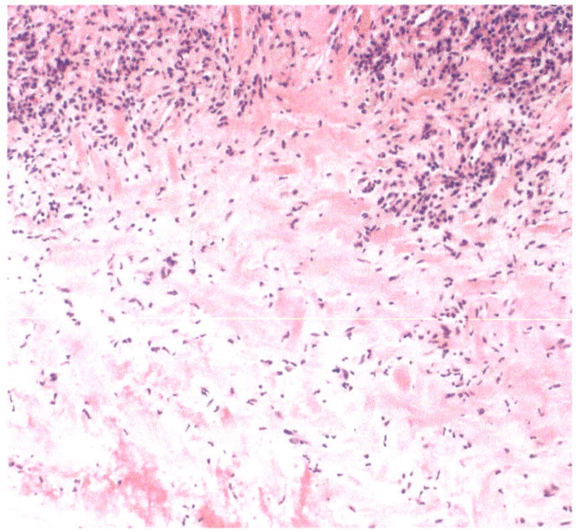

QUESTION 5-6.

A 47-year-old patient presents with multiple large erythematous nodules involving the trunk and upper extremities. One nodule is ulcerated and ecchymotic. Review of systems reveals constitutional symptoms including pyrexia, malaise, weight loss, fatigue, and myalgia. A deep punch biopsy is performed and the findings are illustrated below. T-cell rearrangement analysis reveals a clonal infiltrate. Immunohistochemistry for BF-1 reveals diffusely positive expression within the lymphocytic infiltrate. Which of the following regarding this disease is INCORRECT?

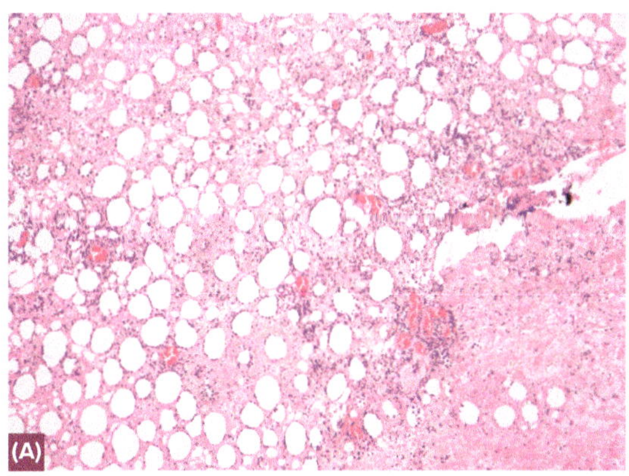

(A)

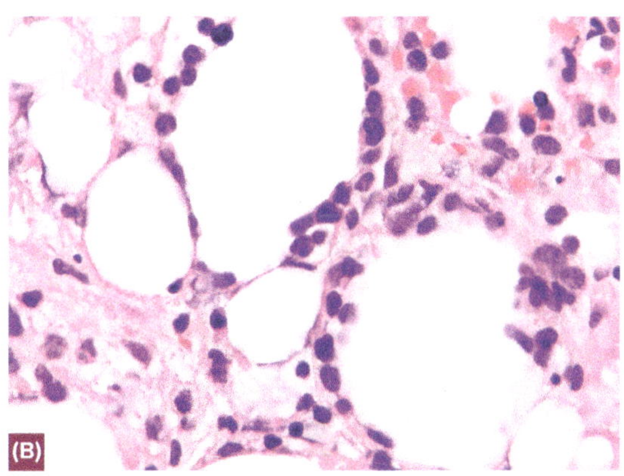

(B)

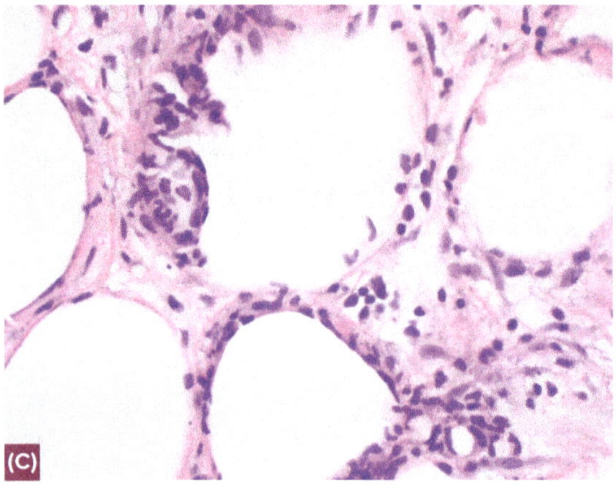

Parts **(A)** and **(B)** reproduced, with permission, from Kantarjian HM, Wolff RA, Koller CA. *The MD Anderson Manual of Medical Oncology.* 2nd ed. New York, NY: McGraw-Hill Education; 2011.

- **A)** Phagocytosis of erythrocytes and leukocytes by macrophages in the fat lobule is a poor prognostic finding.
- **B)** A precursor form of this lesion exists that is frequently clonal and presents with waxing and waning indurated plaque-like lesions.
- **C)** Approximately one-third of patients present with pancytopenia, fever, and hepatosplenomegaly.
- **D)** The lymphocytes, especially those involving the inner rim of adipocyte membranes, express CD3, CD4, and TIA-1.
- **E)** The clonal population identified by T-cell-receptor rearrangement analysis will most likely be of the alpha/beta type.

QUESTION 5-7.

A 40-year-old alcoholic male presents with severe epigastric pain that radiates to the back and several tender erythematous nodules on the anterior shins and trunk. One of the lesions is ulcerated draining a creamy oily substance. He is febrile with complaints of arthralgias and arthritis. A biopsy at the edge of the ulcerated nodule is performed and the findings are illustrated below. Which of the following regarding this condition is INCORRECT?

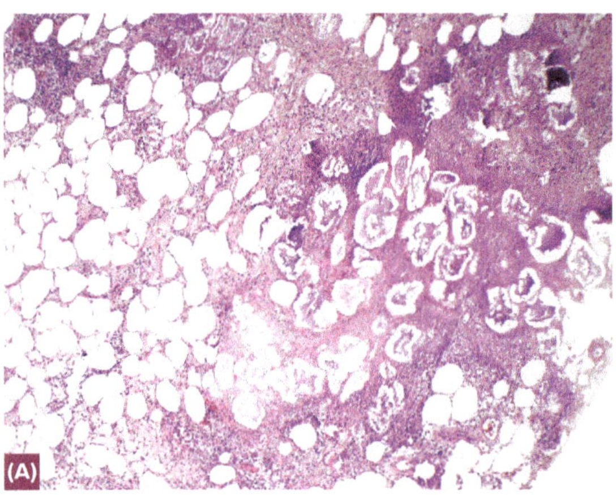

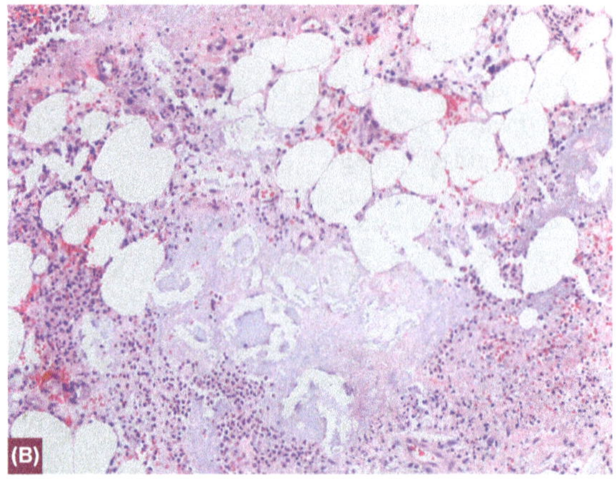

- **A)** This syndrome may also include pancreatic disease, arthritis, lytic bone lesions, and polyserositis.
- **B)** This syndrome is associated with pancreatitis, cholelithiasis, pancreatic cysts and pseudocysts, acinar cell carcinoma, pancreatic ductal carcinoma, pancreatic divisum, and ingestion of sulindac.
- **C)** Patients typically have elevated lipase and amylase levels.
- **D)** The changes characteristic of this condition are limited to the subcutaneous fat.
- **E)** The basophilic discoloration of the adipocytes is attributed to calcification.

QUESTION 5-8.

A healthy full-term infant develops variably sized, red to violaceous, indurated nodules on the back. The nodules are well circumscribed and freely mobile with palpation. The lesions developed 11 days following delivery. No steroids have been

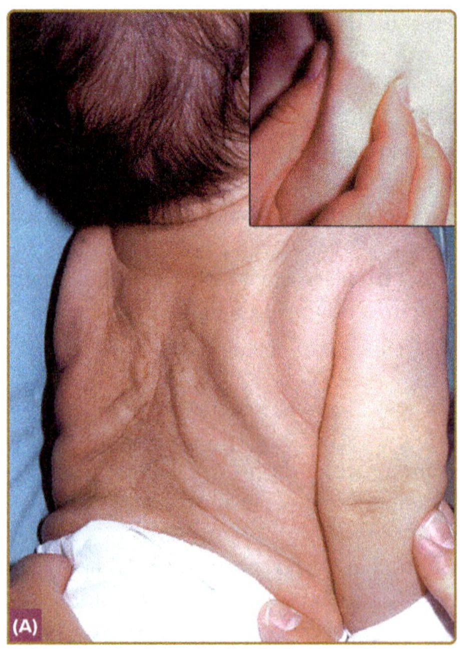

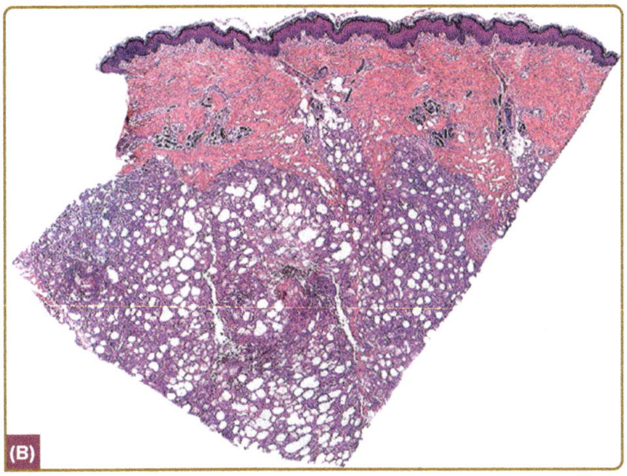

(B)

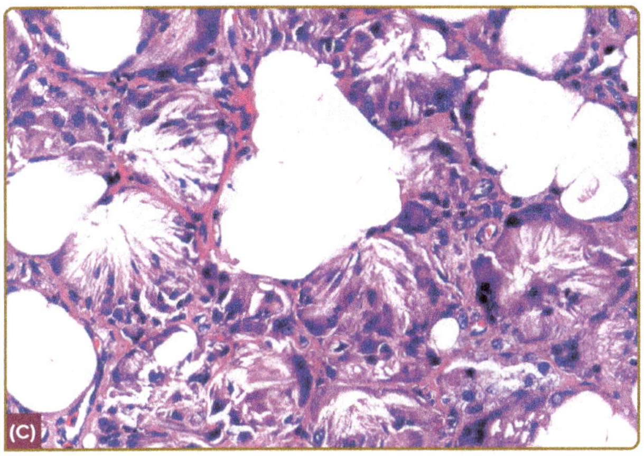

(C)

Reproduced, with permission, from Goldsmith LA, Katz SI, Gilchrest BA, Paller AS, Leffell DJ, Wolff K, eds. *Fitzpatrick's Dermatology in General Medicine*. 8th ed. New York, NY: McGraw-Hill Education; 2012.

administered to this patient. Which of the following regarding this disease is INCORRECT?

A) This condition is partially attributed to the greater proportion of saturated fats in children and their higher melting point compared to unsaturated fats.

B) Associated conditions include prematurity, hypothermia, and stress.

C) This condition is associated with dehydration, undernourishment, and a high mortality rate.

D) Occasionally these infants can develop hypercalcemia and extensive calcification.

E) The presence of granulomatous inflammation within the fat lobules is an important diagnostic finding.

QUESTION 5-9.

A 23-year-old type I diabetic male was admitted to the emergency room for ketoacidosis. He later becomes febrile and develops painful erythematous and dusky lesions in a livedo-like distribution. Blood cultures grow *Klebsiella pneumoniae.* A punch biopsy is performed and is illustrated below. Which of the following is INCORRECT about this condition?

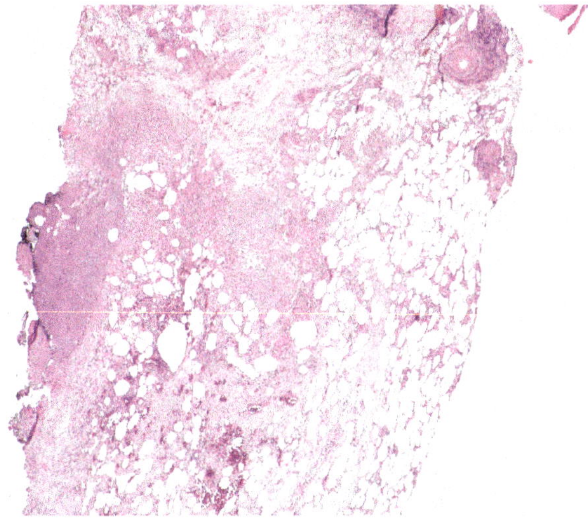

A) Special stains such as PAS, GMS, Gram, and AFB (Fite) are required to investigate an infectious etiology.

B) This category of panniculitis most frequently exhibits additional epidermal and dermal inflammatory changes.

C) High-power microscopic examination will most likely reveal lobular involvement by granulomatous inflammation.

D) In this category of panniculitis, both small- and medium-sized vessel vasculitis with thrombosis are common.

E) Despite the positive blood culture, a tissue sample should be submitted for culture.

QUESTION 5-10.

A 40-year-old female presents with multiple indurated, deep-seated nodules involving the upper extremities, trunk, and buttocks. A few areas exhibit ulceration. A biopsy is performed and the findings are illustrated below. The inflammatory infiltrate is composed predominantly of lymphocytes and plasma cells. The lesions eventually heal with lipoatrophy and depressed scars. Which of the following regarding this disease is INCORRECT?

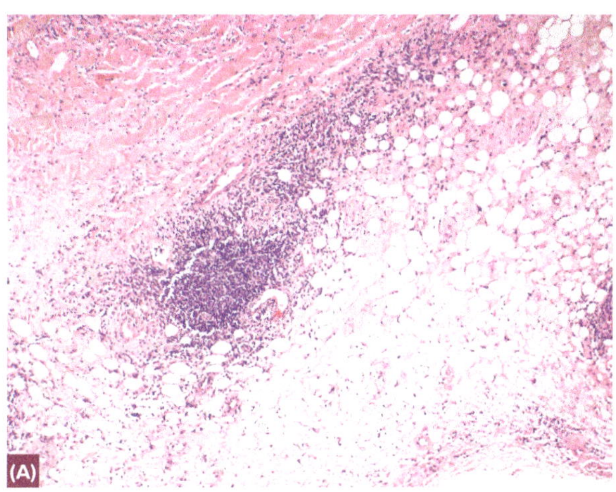

(A)

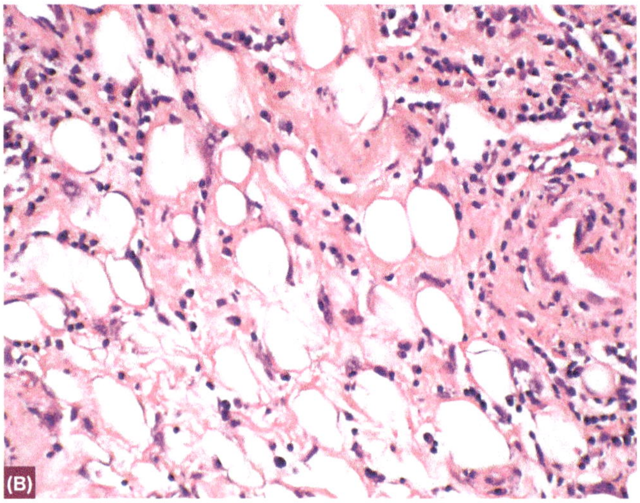

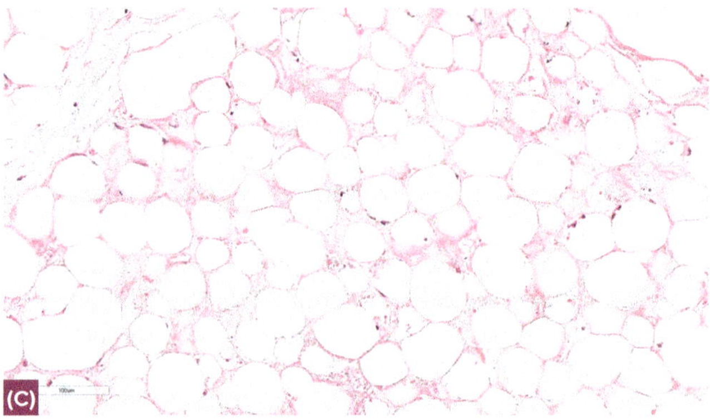

Used with permission of Claudia Vidal, MD, PhD, St. Louis University School of Medicine

A) Approximately half of patients with this condition have concomitant collagen vascular disease.
B) Lesions tend to arise at sites of prior trauma, such as injection or prior biopsy sites.
C) By definition, this condition lacks epidermal and dermal inflammatory components.
D) Alcian blue stain will reveal increased mucin in the vast majority of cases.
E) Special stains are needed to rule out an infectious process.

QUESTION 5-11.

A 30-year-old obese female ice skating instructor presents with bilateral, tender, dusky, bluish nodules on the posterior calves with ulceration. She reports to experiencing a similar but milder eruption several years ago that healed very slowly resulting in atrophic scars. A punch biopsy is performed and the findings are illustrated below. Which of the following statements regarding this condition is INCORRECT?

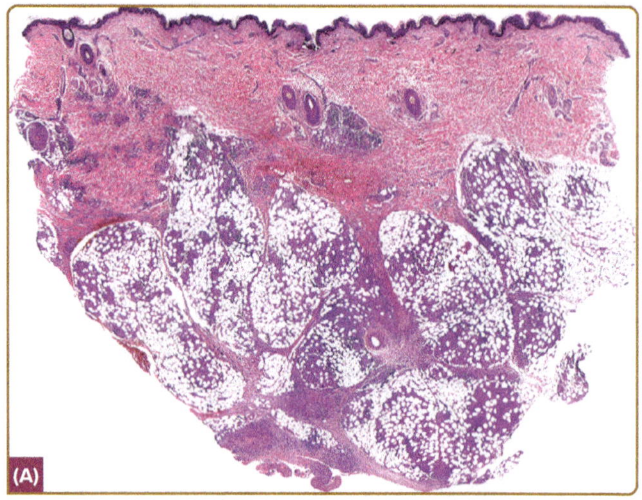

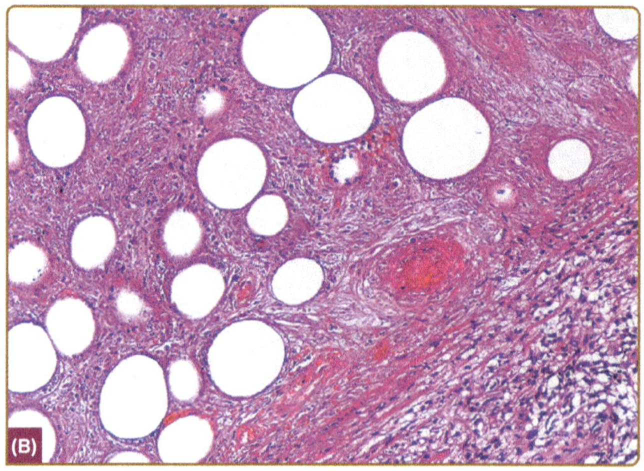

Reproduced, with permission, from Goldsmith LA, Katz SI, Gilchrest BA, Paller AS, Leffell DJ, Wolff K, eds. *Fitzpatrick's Dermatology in General Medicine*. 8th ed. New York, NY: McGraw-Hill Education; 2012.

A) This condition is frequently associated with erythrocyanosis.
B) Although special stains are negative for microorganisms, tissue culture using Löwenstein-Jensen agar frequently grows microorganisms.
C) A subset of patients with this condition exhibits invariable hypersensitivity to intradermal injection of purified protein derivative and a complete clearing of all skin lesions following treatment with isoniazid, rifampin, pyrazinamide, or ethambutol.
D) There is an association with acute myeloid leukemia, chronic hepatitis C infection, and various medications such as propylthiouracil.
E) An atypical variant of this condition occurs in men, in which lesions are unilateral and commonly involve the shins and thighs.

QUESTION 5-12.

A woman who recently survived a car crash presents to your office 3 months later with brawny, discolored, indurated plaques and nodules with a *peau d'orange* appearance on the breasts. A punch biopsy is performed and the findings are illustrated below. Which of the following diagnoses is MOST accurate?

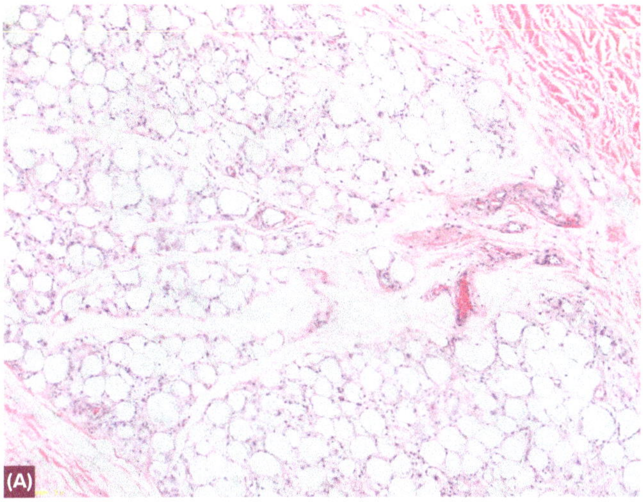

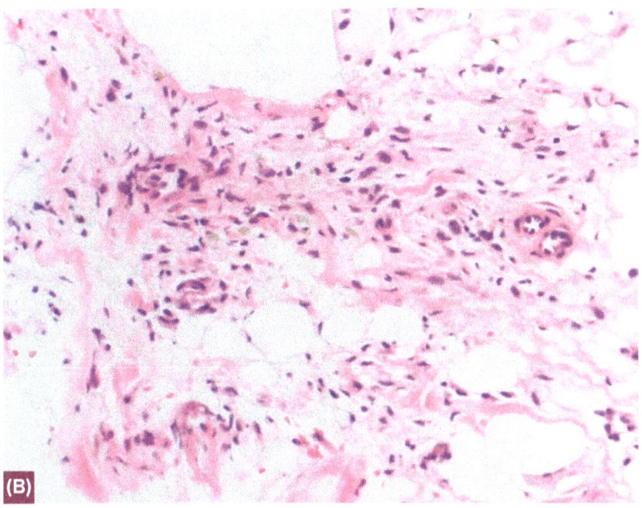

A) Traumatic fat necrosis
B) Lipoatrophia semicircularis
C) Benign symmetric lipomatosis
D) Secrétan syndrome
E) Encapsulated lipoma

QUESTION 5-13.

A 37-year-old social worker with a history of depression and anxiety presents with multiple erythematous nodules with disparate appearance and location. Several lesions contain round and angulated foci of ulceration. A biopsy is performed on one of the lesions and the findings are illustrated below. Which of the following diagnoses is CORRECT?

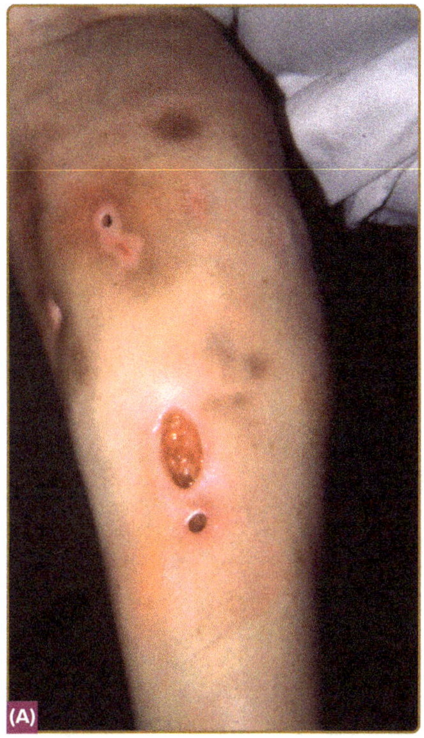

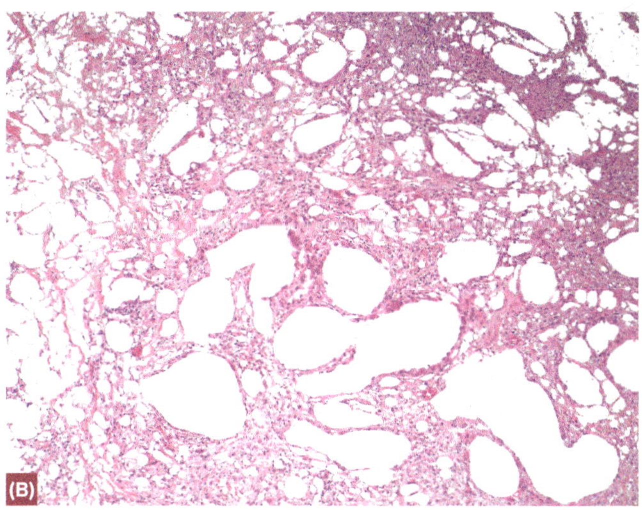

Part **(A)** reproduced, with permission, from Goldsmith LA, Katz SI, Gilchrest BA, Paller AS, Leffell DJ, Wolff K, eds. *Fitzpatrick's Dermatology in General Medicine*. 8th ed. New York, NY: McGraw-Hill Education; 2012.

A) Subcutaneous panniculitis-like T-cell lymphoma
B) Lupus profundus
C) Erythema nodosum
D) Factitial panniculitis
E) Pancreatic panniculitis

QUESTION 5-14.

A 38-year-old female with insulin-dependent diabetes mellitus presents with numerous indented areas in the fatty regions of the thighs and buttocks. A biopsy is performed and the findings are illustrated below. Which of the following diagnoses is CORRECT?

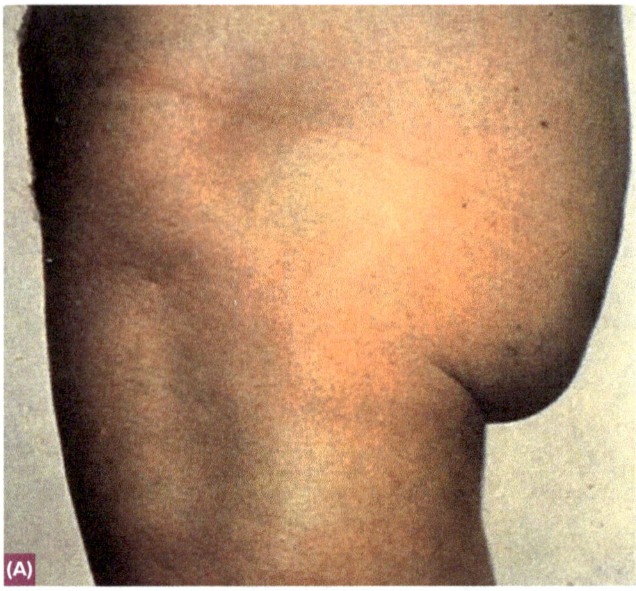

Courtesy of Joslin Diabetes Center, Boston, MA

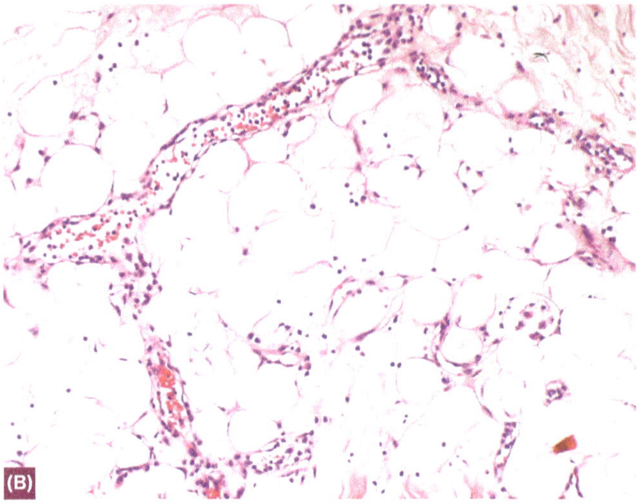

A) Lipoatrophy
B) Lipodystrophy
C) Lupus profundus
D) Infectious panniculitis
E) Erythema nodosum

QUESTION 5-15.

A 57-year-old patient with restrictive lung disease presents with several nodules of the left arm. A biopsy is performed and the findings are illustrated below. The inflammatory process involves the dermis as well as the subcutaneous lobules and septae. Special stains are negative for microorganisms. Alcian blue stain is negative for mucin. Which of the following diagnoses is CORRECT?

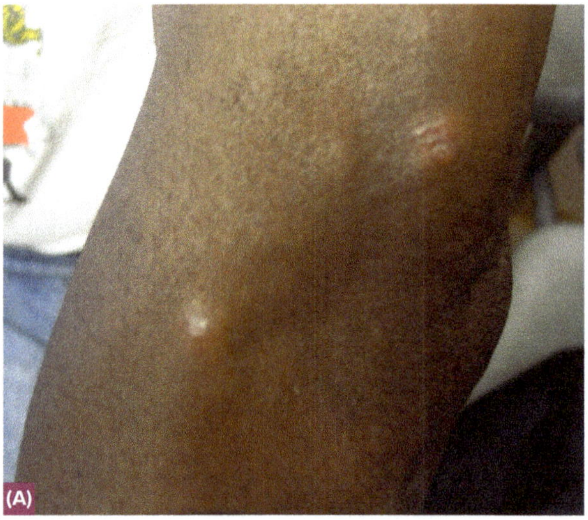

Reproduced, with permission, from Usatine RP, Smith MA, Mayeaux EJ Jr, Chumley HS, eds. *Color Atlas of Family Medicine*. 2nd ed. New York, NY: McGraw-Hill Education; 2012.

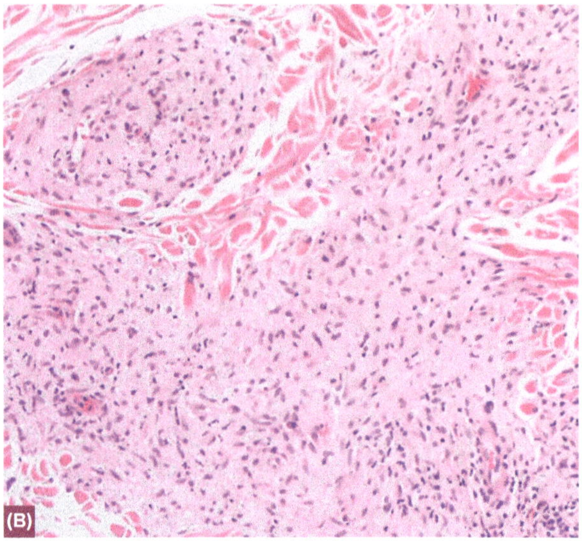

A) Granulomatous reaction secondary to arthropod bites
B) Metastatic Crohn disease
C) Sarcoidosis
D) Wells syndrome
E) Subcutaneous granuloma annulare

QUESTION 5-16.

A 45-year-old patient with chronic obstructive lung disease and idiopathic hepatitis presents with recurrent, tender, erythematous, subcutaneous nodules with ulceration involving the face, trunk, buttocks, and proximal extremities. The nodules are localized with well-demarcated peripheral edges. The patient reports that the nodules commonly follow trauma and occasionally drain clear or serosanguineous material. There is a sibling with a similar condition. A biopsy is performed and the findings are illustrated below. In addition to panniculitis, there is liquefactive necrosis of the dermis. Special stains and tissue culture are negative for infection. Which of the following diagnoses is most likely CORRECT?

A) Alpha-1-antitrypsin deficiency
B) Weber-Christian disease
C) Factitial panniculitis
D) Pancreatic panniculitis
E) Erythema induratum of Bazin/nodular vasculitis

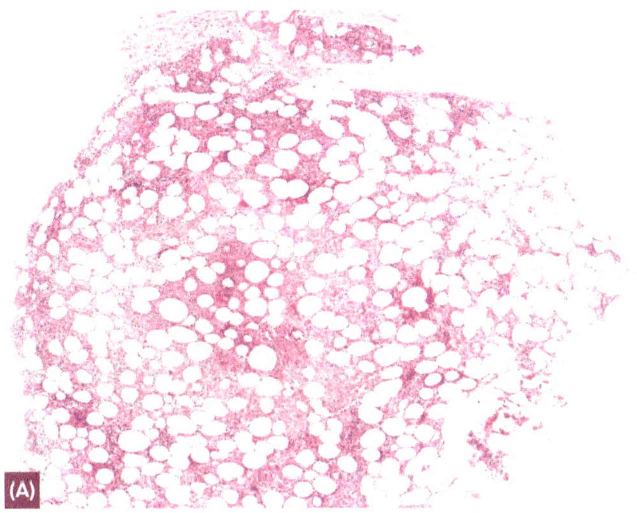

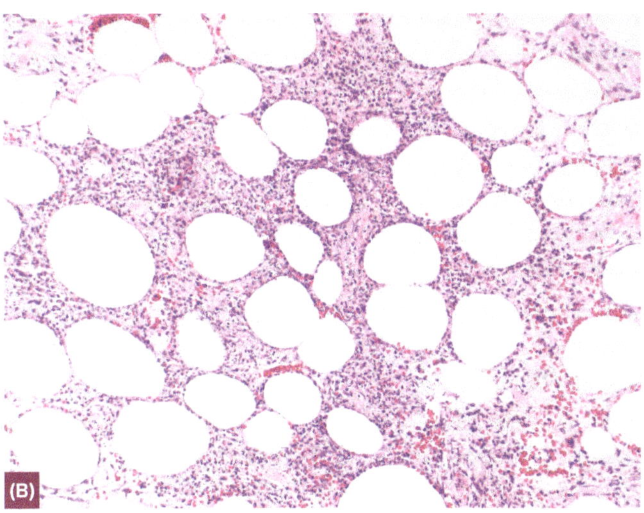

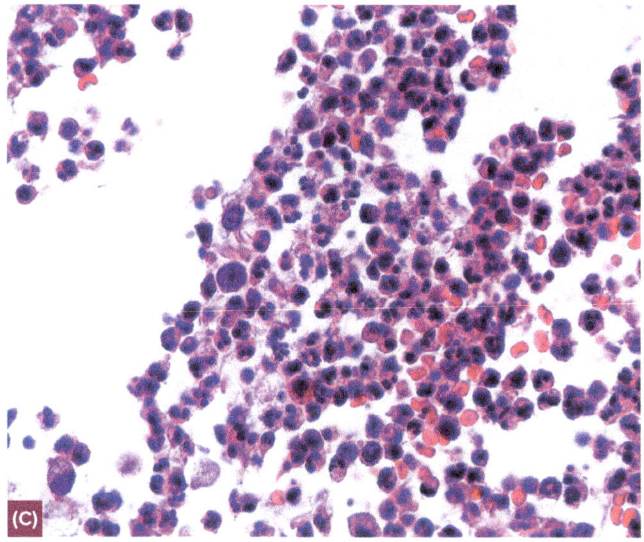

Part **(C)** reproduced, with permission, from Goldsmith LA, Katz SI, Gilchrest BA, Paller AS, Leffell DJ, Wolff K, eds. *Fitzpatrick's Dermatology in General Medicine*. 8th ed. New York, NY: McGraw-Hill Education; 2012.

QUESTION 5-17.

The interpretation of scalp biopsies from patients with hair loss can be difficult. Traditionally, alopecias have been divided into scarring and nonscarring categories based on their ability to regrow hair at the affected site. While scarring alopecias are typically defined by the type and pattern of inflammatory infiltrate, nonscarring alopecias are typically determined by assessing the ratios of hair sizes and growing and involuting hairs. Therefore, understanding the normal hair microanatomy is critical to understanding both scarring and nonscarring alopecia. Below is a diagram of a terminal hair. Please MATCH the following structures with their appropriate designations.

A) Infundibulum
B) Bulb
C) Isthmus
D) Suprabulbar region
E) Bulge area
F) Subcutaneous fat
G) Hair matrix
H) Sebaceous gland
I) Arrector pili muscle
J) Medulla of hair shaft
K) Cortex of hair shaft
L) Fibrous root sheath
M) Outer root sheath
N) Inner root sheath
O) Dermal papilla

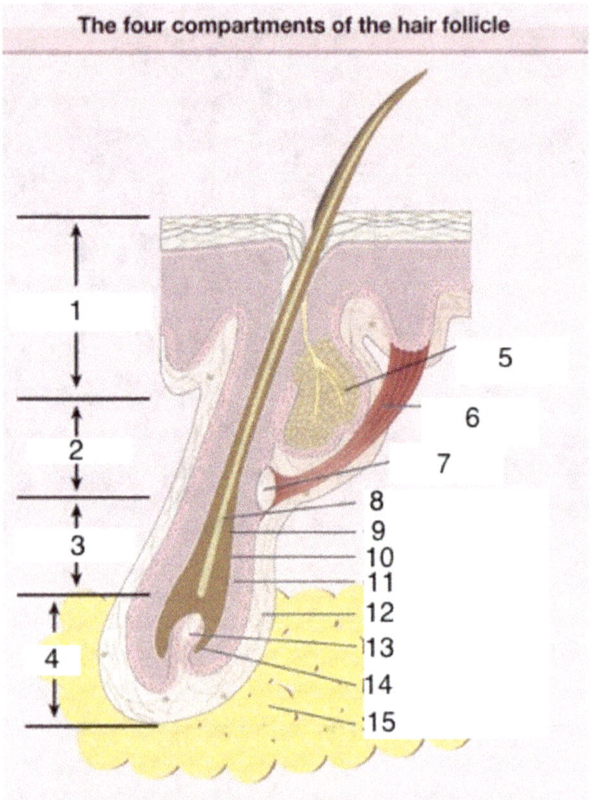

Reproduced, with permission, from Goldsmith LA, Katz SI, Gilchrest BA, Paller AS, Leffell DJ, Wolff K, eds. *Fitzpatrick's Dermatology in General Medicine*. 8th ed. New York, NY: McGraw-Hill Education; 2012.

QUESTION 5-18.

Two separate processing techniques have been applied to biopsies of alopecia: vertical and transverse (horizontal). Which of the following statements regarding these techniques is INCORRECT?

A) Transverse processing is more commonly performed and is superior in identifying the various patterns of inflammation seen in scarring alopecias.
B) Transverse processing provides larger numbers of hairs for evaluation and therefore improves assessment of anagen-telogen and terminal-vellus hair ratios.
C) Vertical sections provide a better and easier assessment of the dermal-epidermal interface.
D) Transverse sections require familiarity with the scalp microanatomy in different planes of sectioning.
E) Vertical sections do not require special training of the histology laboratory staff.

QUESTION 5-19.

A 46-year-old male presents with alopecia involving the temporal areas. Additionally, he reports an overall thinning of the scalp over the past several years. Two biopsies are performed. Both vertical and transverse sections are illustrated below. Which of the following diagnoses is CORRECT?

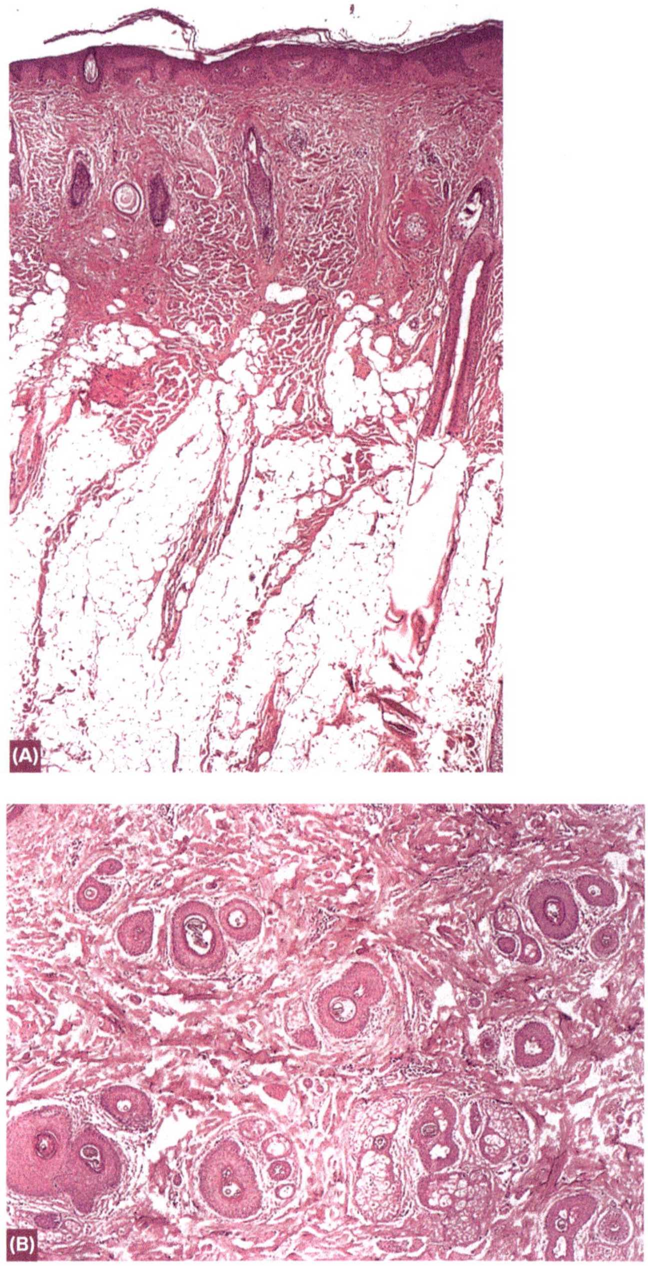

A) Telogen effluvium
B) Androgenetic alopecia
C) Alopecia areata
D) Frontal fibrosing alopecia
E) Trichotillomania

QUESTION 5-20.

A 21-year-old female patient presents with diffuse alopecia. She provides you with a bag of "falling out" hair and she reports that the hair loss abruptly began approximately 3 months ago following a miscarriage and breakup with her boyfriend. As you examine the scalp you notice a large number of shedding hairs. A hair "pull test" yields seven hairs. Although the hair loss appears to be diffuse, there is considerable hair loss in the temporal regions. A biopsy is performed and processed using vertical sections. Which of the following microscopic descriptions MOST accurately characterizes this condition?

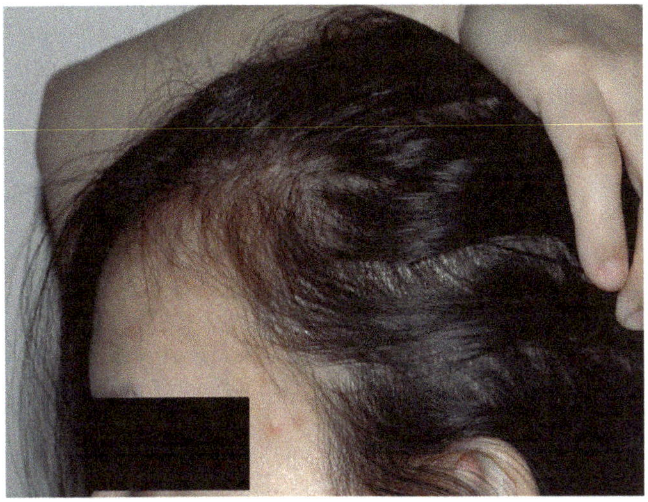

Reproduced, with permission, from Goldsmith LA, Katz SI, Gilchrest BA, Paller AS, Leffell DJ, Wolff K, eds. *Fitzpatrick's Dermatology in General Medicine*. 8th ed. New York, NY: McGraw-Hill Education; 2012.

A) The terminal-to-vellus hair ratio is 5:1 and the anagen-to-catagen/telogen ratio is 6:1. The hairs are normal in shape and miniaturization of hairs is not appreciated. A sparse perifollicular lymphocytic infiltrate is present. There is no evidence of trichomalacia.

B) The terminal-to-vellus hair ratio is 2:1 and the anagen-to-catagen/telogen ratio is 9:1. The hairs are normal in shape but range in size. Several hairs of intermediate size have hair bulbs residing in the deep dermis. A sparse perifollicular lymphocytic infiltrate is present. There is no evidence of trichomalacia.

C) The terminal-to-vellus hair ratio is 2:1 and the anagen-to-catagen/telogen ratio is 4:1. The hairs are normal in shape and miniaturization of hairs is not appreciated. A peribulbar lymphocytic infiltrate is present with scattered melanophages in the surrounding deep dermis and subcutaneous fat. There is no evidence of trichomalacia.

D) The terminal-to-vellus hair ratio is 3:1 and the anagen-to-catagen/telogen ratio is 4:1. The hairs are normal in size; however, there is considerable architectural disorder with empty anagen follicles and pigment casts in hair canals. A sparse perifollicular lymphocytic infiltrate is present. Trichomalacia is present.

QUESTION 5-21.

A 26-year-old patient presents with an area of alopecia on the occipital scalp without scaling, erythema, atrophy, or scarring. Short, broken-off hair shafts appear as very short stubs emerging from the bald scalp. A biopsy is performed and the findings are illustrated below. Although an elastic stain reveals clumps of elastic fiber aggregates at the sites of antecedent follicular papillae, the overall dermal elastic fiber network is intact. Which of the following diagnoses is CORRECT?

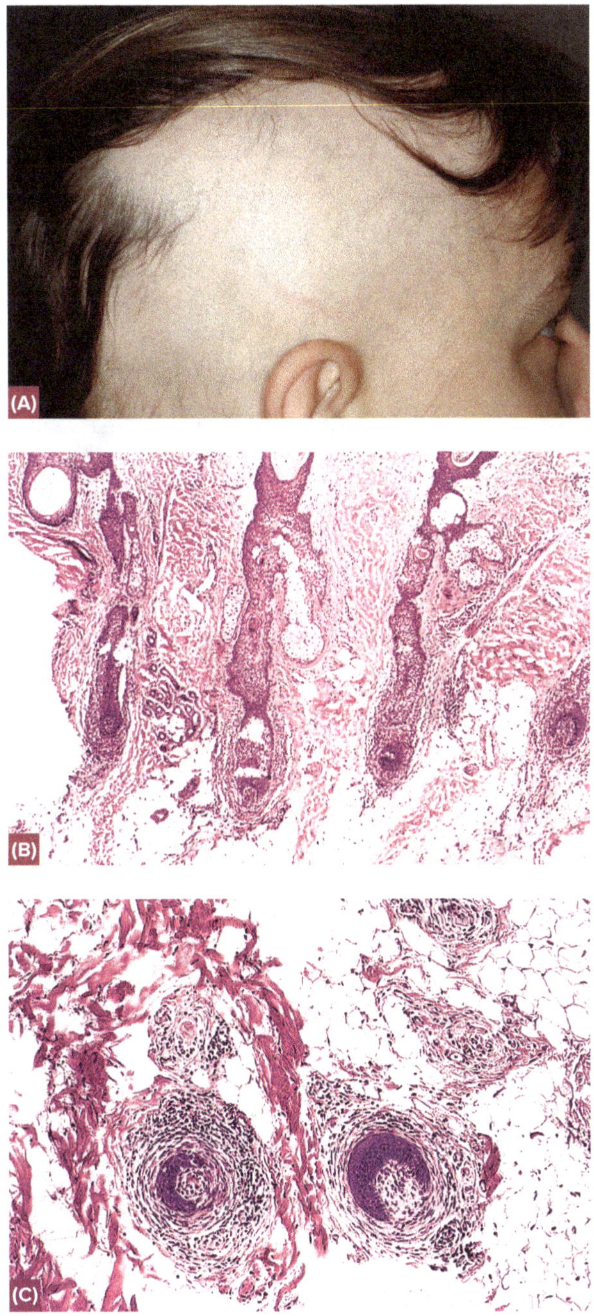

A) Telogen effluvium
B) Androgenetic alopecia
C) Trichotillomania
D) Lichen planopilaris
E) Alopecia areata

QUESTION 5-22.

An 11-year-old boy presents with incomplete hair loss in an unusual geometric pattern. He is recently experiencing a lot of stress due to the recent divorce of his parents. A biopsy is performed and the findings are illustrated below. An elastic stain reveals an intact elastic fiber network within the dermis. Which of the following diagnoses is CORRECT?

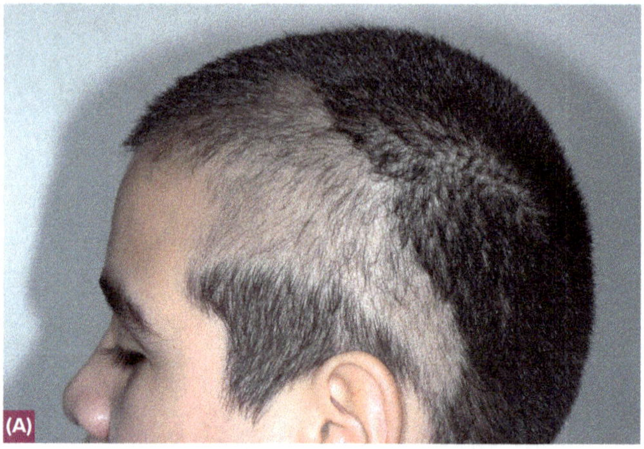

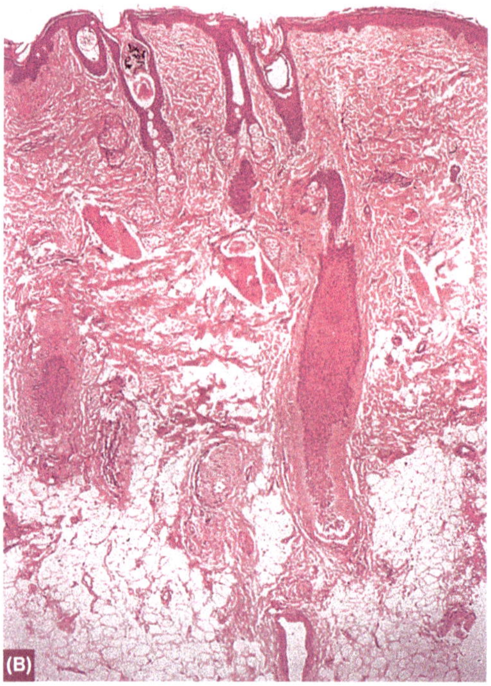

Part **(A)** reproduced, with permission, from Usatine RP, Smith MA, Mayeaux EJ Jr, Chumley HS, eds. *Color Atlas of Family Medicine*. 2nd ed. New York, NY: McGraw-Hill Education; 2012.

A) Alopecia areata
B) Traction alopecia
C) Tinea capitis
D) Trichotillomania
E) Pseudopelade of Brocq

QUESTION 5-23.

Which of the following statements regarding scarring alopecia is INCORRECT?

A) Biopsies of end-stage scarring alopecia rarely reveal the precise pathophysiology of the condition; however, they are still valuable since scarring alopecias usually will progress to permanent hair loss unless therapeutic intervention is successful, whereas nonscarring alopecias are less predictable.
B) Scarring alopecias are classified based on the type of cellular inflammatory infiltrate and whether or not the process results in the preferential destruction of the hair follicle.
C) Elastic stains will typically reveal disruption of the elastic fiber network in the surrounding dermis.
D) Examination of vertical sections in primary scarring alopecia provides an advantage in assessing the relationship of the inflammatory infiltrate with the hair follicle.
E) The presence of postinflammatory alteration characterized by dermal melanophages is considered pathognomonic for scarring alopecia.

QUESTION 5-24.

A 38-year-old patient presents with a localized area of alopecia with skin depigmentation and scaling at the peripheral edges of the lesion. A biopsy is performed and the findings are illustrated below. PAS stain reveals thickened basement membranes. Alcian blue stain reveals a diffuse accumulation of dermal mucin. Which of the following diagnoses is CORRECT?

A) Lichen planopilaris
B) Central centrifugal cicatricial alopecia
C) Discoid lupus erythematosus
D) Alopecia areata
E) Alopecia mucinosa

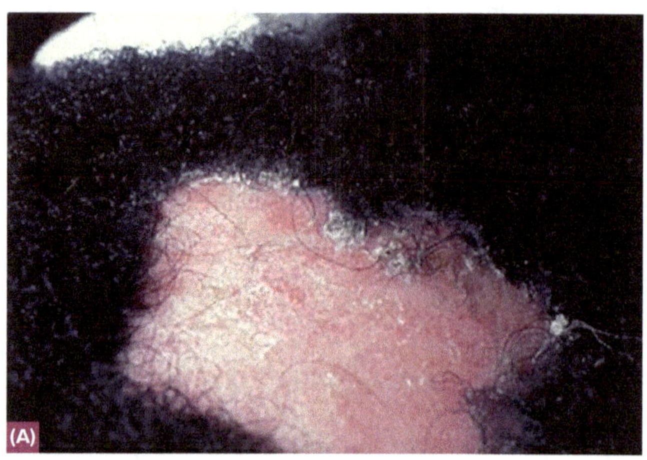

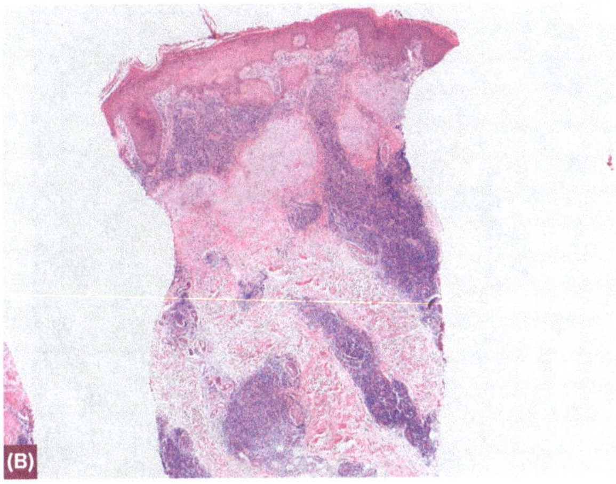

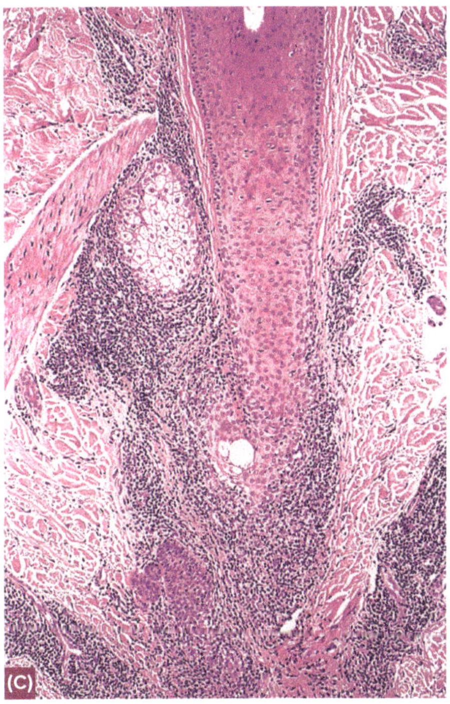

Part **(A)** Reproduced, with permission, from Papadakis MA, McPhee SJ, eds. *Current Medical Diagnosis & Treatment 2016*. 55th ed. New York, NY: McGraw-Hill Education; 2016: Courtesy S. Goldstein

QUESTION 5-25.

A 68-year-old female presents with a gradually receding hairline along the frontal scalp. The areas of alopecia are hypopigmented. Additionally, you notice that both eyebrows have no hair. The eyelashes appear normal. A biopsy is performed and the findings are illustrated below. Which of the following diagnoses is CORRECT?

A) Androgenetic alopecia
B) Discoid lupus erythematosus
C) Central centrifugal cicatricial alopecia
D) Frontal fibrosing alopecia
E) Alopecia areata

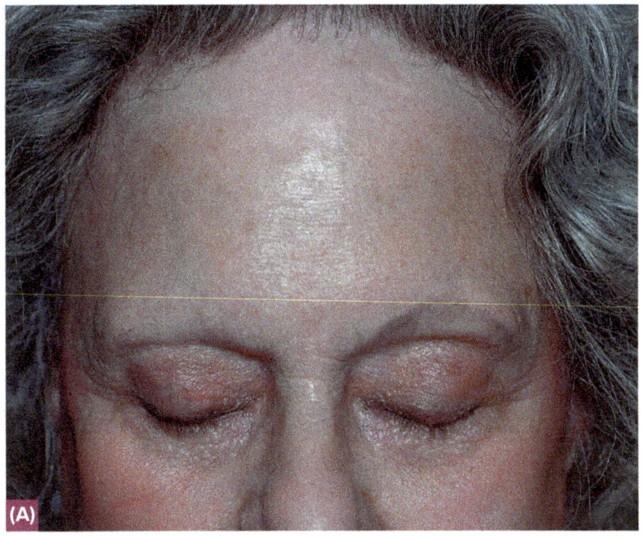

Reproduced, with permission, from Wolff K, Johnson RA, Saavedra AP. *Fitzpatrick's Color Atlas and Synopsis of Clinical Dermatology*. 7th ed. New York, NY: McGraw-Hill Education; 2013.

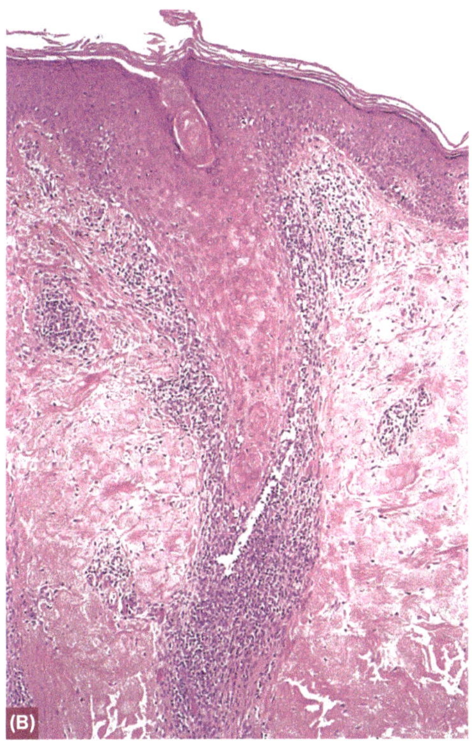

QUESTION 5-26.

A patient presents with extensive scarring alopecia of the vertex of the scalp. There are residual islands where several residual hair follicles emerge in groups. Erythema, scale, and crusting are absent. The patient reports the condition has been progressive over the past year. A biopsy is performed and the findings are illustrated below. Which of the following diagnoses is CORRECT?

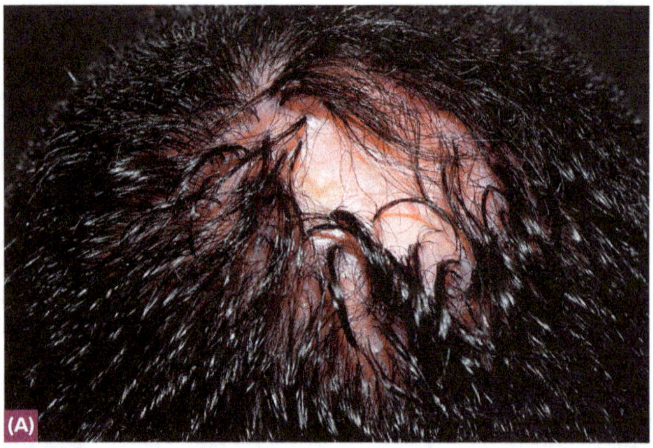

Reproduced, with permission, from Wolff K, Johnson RA, Saavedra AP. *Fitzpatrick's Color Atlas and Synopsis of Clinical Dermatology*. 7th ed. New York, NY: McGraw-Hill Education; 2013.

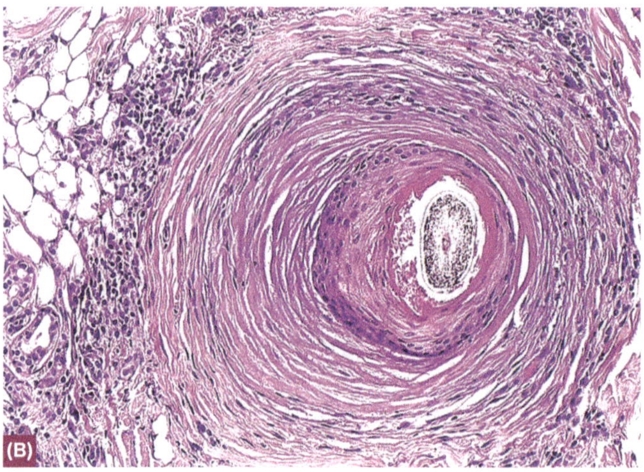

A) Discoid lupus erythematosus
B) Lichen planopilaris
C) Folliculitis decalvans
D) Central centrifugal cicatricial alopecia
E) Alopecia areata

QUESTION 5-27.

A 19-year-old male patient presents with fluctuant scalp nodules that coalesce progressively to form complex, interconnected, crusted abscesses and sinus tracts that drain spontaneously or with slight pressure. The lesions are painful and are associated with alopecia. One of the abscesses is aspirated and sent for culture; however, it is negative for bacterial and fungal growth. A biopsy is performed and the findings are illustrated below. The inflammatory infiltrate is mixed and contains neutrophils, lymphocytes, macrophages, and rare plasma cells. Which of the following diagnoses is CORRECT?

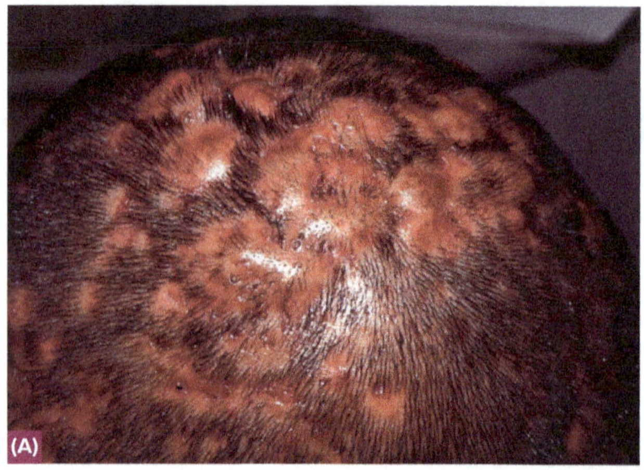

Reproduced, with permission, from Goldsmith LA, Katz SI, Gilchrest BA, Paller AS, Leffell DJ, Wolff K, eds. *Fitzpatrick's Dermatology in General Medicine*. 8th ed. New York, NY: McGraw-Hill Education; 2012.

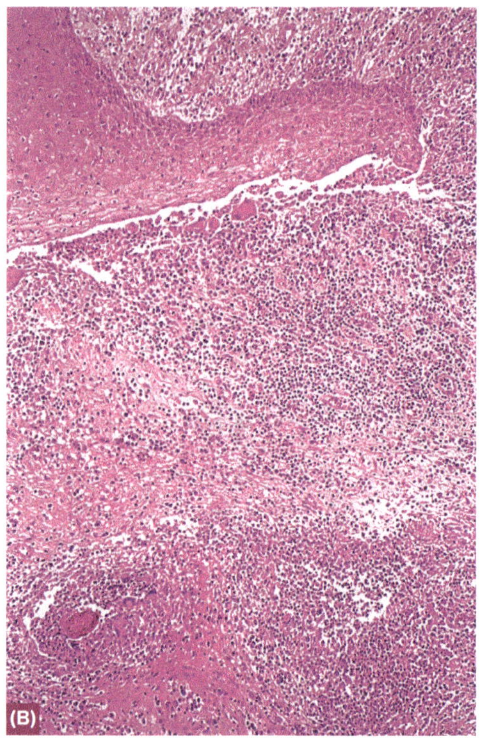

A) Folliculitis decalvans
B) Acne keloidalis nuchae
C) Erosive pustular dermatosis of the scalp
D) Lipedematous alopecia
E) Dissecting cellulitis

QUESTION 5-28.

A 32-year-old male presents with irregular erythematous patches of alopecia involving the vertex of the scalp. There are numerous follicular pustules and areas of follicular hyperkeratosis. Tufted folliculitis is noted where several hair shafts emerge from a common follicular ostium. A biopsy is performed and the findings are illustrated below. The inflammatory infiltrate is composed of neutrophils, lymphocytes, macrophages, and occasional plasma cells. Special stains are negative for microorganisms. Which of the following diagnoses is CORRECT?

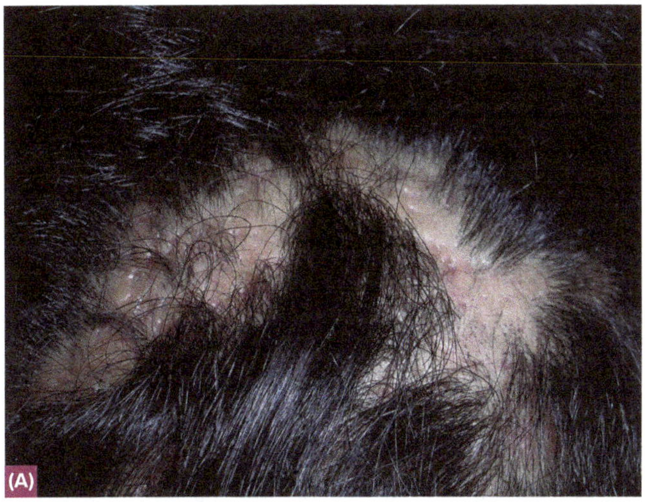

Reproduced, with permission, from Usatine RP, Smith MA, Mayeaux EJ Jr, Chumley HS, eds. *Color Atlas of Family Medicine*. 2nd ed. New York, NY: McGraw-Hill Education; 2012.

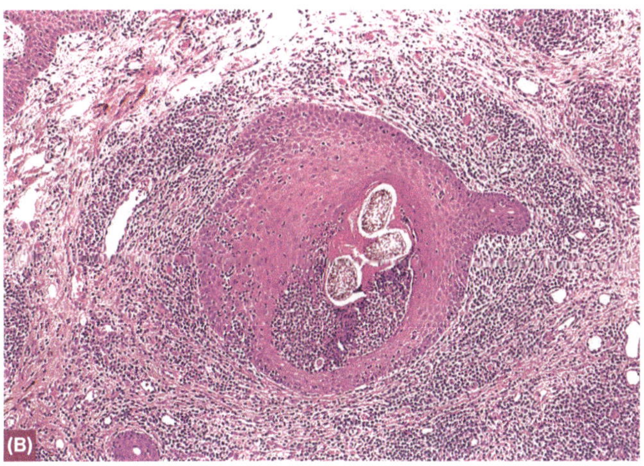

A) Folliculitis decalvans
B) Acne keloidalis nuchae
C) Erosive pustular dermatosis of the scalp
D) Lipedematous alopecia
E) Dissecting cellulitis

QUESTION 5-29.

An African American male presents with numerous follicular-based pustules on the occipital scalp with alopecia. Focal areas of scarring are present. Similar areas are also present within the beard area. A biopsy of the scalp is performed and the findings are illustrated below. Which of the following diagnoses is CORRECT?

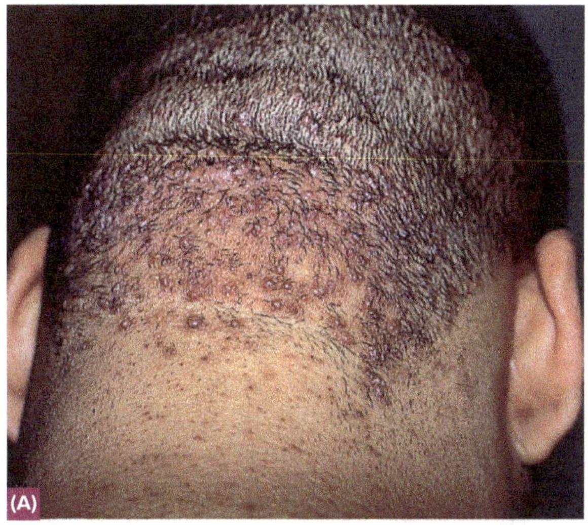

Reproduced, with permission, from Goldsmith LA, Katz SI, Gilchrest BA, Paller AS, Leffell DJ, Wolff K, eds. *Fitzpatrick's Dermatology in General Medicine*. 8th ed. New York, NY: McGraw-Hill Education; 2012.

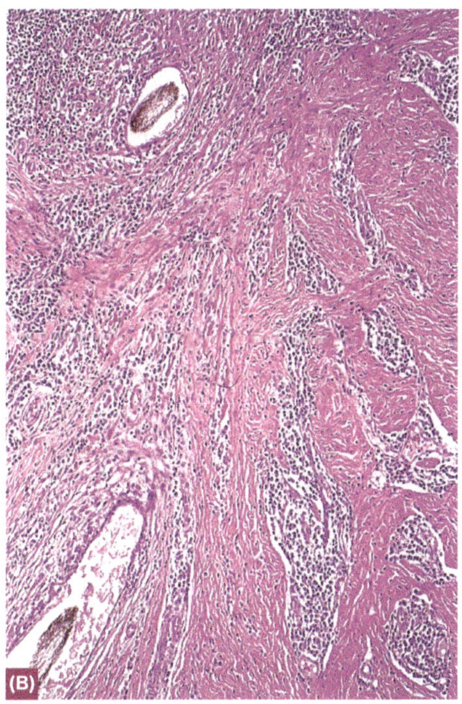

A) Folliculitis decalvans
B) Acne keloidalis nuchae
C) Erosive pustular dermatosis of the scalp
D) Lipedematous alopecia
E) Dissecting cellulitis

QUESTION 5-30.

A 5-year-old African American boy presents with an inflammatory mass on the scalp. There is overlying alopecia and boggy swelling with multiple pustules accompanied by postauricular lymphadenopathy. The condition has worsened since another physician prescribed him topical corticosteroids. A biopsy is performed and the findings are illustrated below. Which of the following diagnoses is CORRECT?

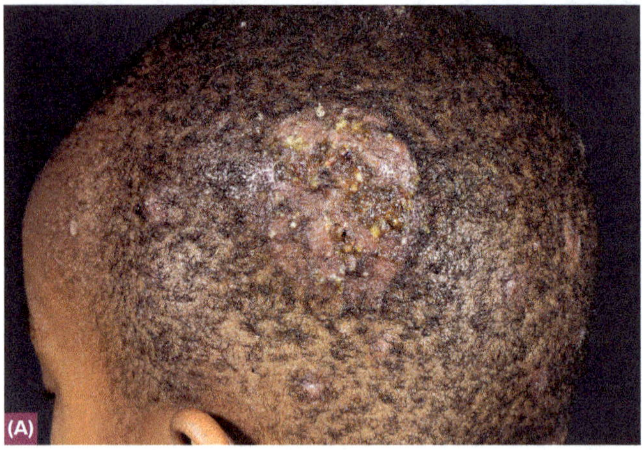

(A)

Reproduced, with permission, from Wolff K, Johnson RA, Saavedra AP. *Fitzpatrick's Color Atlas and Synopsis of Clinical Dermatology*. 7th ed. New York, NY: McGraw-Hill Education; 2013.

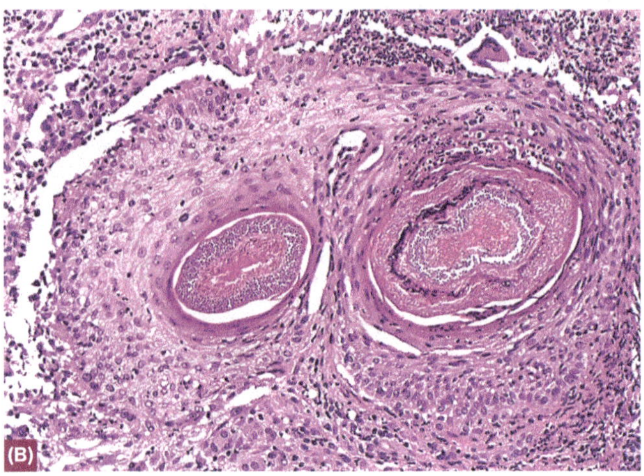

(B)

A) Favus
B) Folliculitis decalvans
C) Kerion
D) Hot tub folliculitis
E) Majocchi granuloma

QUESTION 5-31.

Which of the following is NOT a cause of secondary scarring alopecia?

A) Keratosis pilaris
B) Basal cell carcinoma
C) Lichen sclerosus et atrophicus
D) Radiation dermatitis
E) Necrobiosis lipoidica

QUESTION 5-32.

A 17-year-old male bodybuilder presents with the sudden worsening of his "skin condition", characterized by numerous nodules and cysts on his chest and back covered by hemorrhagic crusts. He also reports polymyalgia and arthralgia. He is currently taking several topical and oral medications for the condition that were prescribed by another physician. He cannot recall the names of these medications; however, the dosage of one of his oral medications has been recently increased. Palpable lymphadenopathy is appreciated on physical examination. A biopsy is performed and reveals an abscess cavity within the superficial and deep dermis filled with neutrophils and liquefactive necrosis. Which of the following statements regarding this patient's condition is INCORRECT?

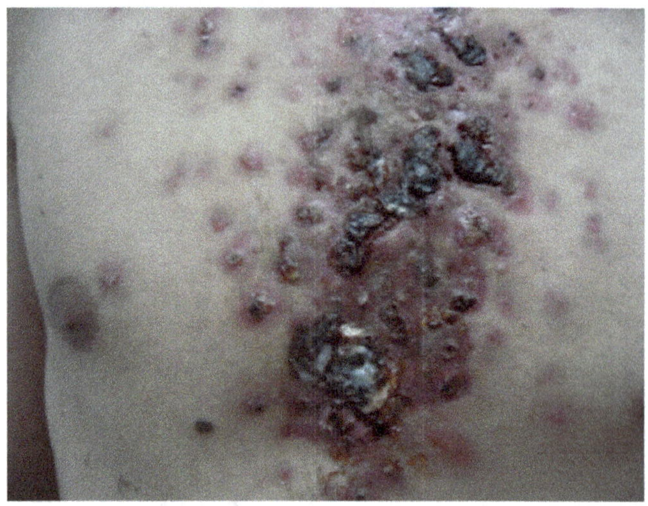

Reproduced, with permission, from Usatine RP, Smith MA, Mayeaux EJ Jr, Chumley HS, eds. *Color Atlas of Family Medicine*. 2nd ed. New York, NY: McGraw-Hill Education; 2012.

A) This patient's underlying condition is one of a triad of follicular occlusion diseases.
B) This condition is attributed to the regrowth of recently shaved hairs reentering the skin and eliciting a granulomatous inflammatory response.
C) This recent flare is likely attributed to an increased dose of oral isotretinoin.
D) This patient is at risk for developing deep abscesses in the axilla, groin, and possibly the scalp.
E) A biopsy is rarely, if ever, required for making this diagnosis.

QUESTION 5-33.

A 34-year-old woman presents with extensive papulopustular facial lesions. She has a history of easy facial flushing since her teen years. Her face has been persistently redder in the past 5 years and thus she is seeking your medical attention. She acknowledges that her mom has similar redness in her face and that she is of northern European heritage. In the last 6 months, since her daughter was born, she has developed many "pimples." Physical examination reveals papules, pustules, and telangiectasias. No comedones are seen. She knows that the sun makes it worse but finds that many sunscreens are irritating to her skin. The patient is started on oral tetracycline daily and 0.75% metronidazole cream to use once daily. She agrees to wear a hat and stay out of the sun during the middle of the day. She will continue to look for a sunscreen she can tolerate. She knows that precipitating factors for her include hot and humid weather, alcohol, hot beverages, and spicy foods. She will do her best to avoid those factors. Two biopsies are performed and the findings are illustrated below. Which of the following statements regarding this patient's condition is INCORRECT?

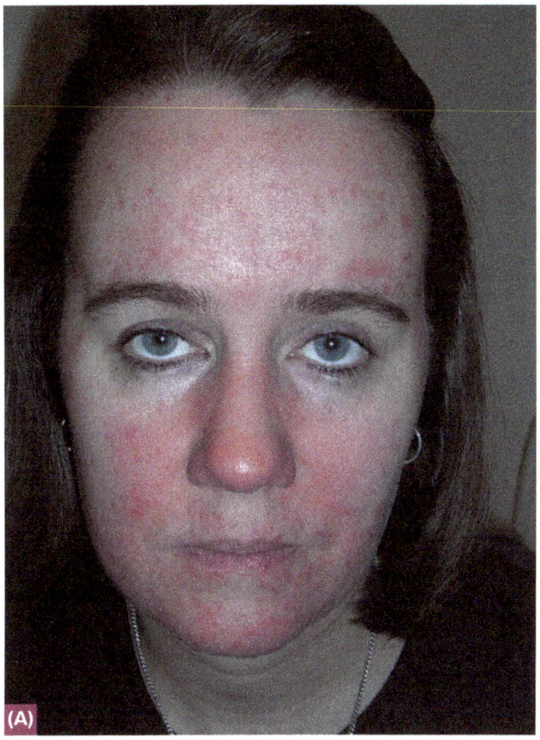

(A)

Reproduced, with permission, from Usatine RP, Smith MA, Mayeaux EJ Jr, Chumley HS, eds. *Color Atlas of Family Medicine*. 2nd ed. New York, NY: McGraw-Hill Education; 2012.

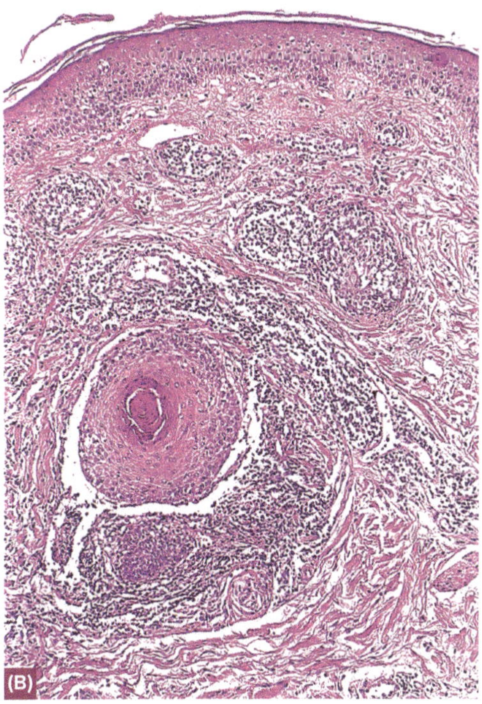

(B)

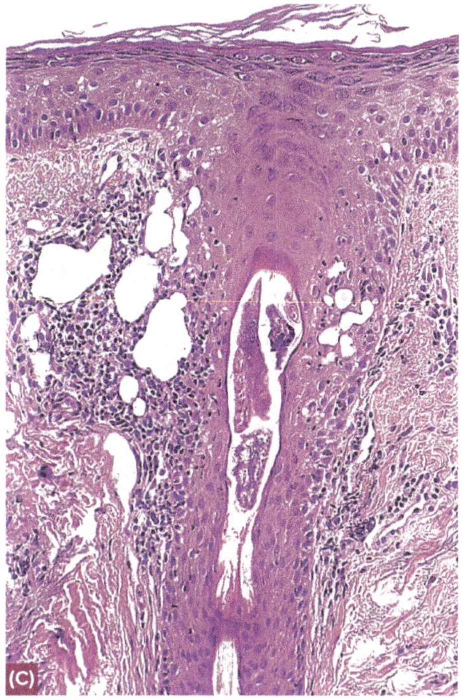

(C)

A) Patients with chronic untreated disease may eventually develop enlargement of the nose, especially the nasal tip, due to sebaceous gland hypertrophy.
B) The findings in this patient's biopsies are incidental and are not associated with the clinical presentation.
C) The use of topical steroids in some patients may elicit a similar presentation around the mouth.
D) This condition is strongly associated with Pityrosporum, HIV, and neurological diseases such as Parkinson disease.
E) The histopathology for this disease is rather non-specific and correlates best with the clinical stage at presentation.

QUESTION 5-34.

A 9-month-old male infant presents with persistent, pruritic, indurated, and erythematous plaques with pustules on the scalp and forehead. There is a history of atopic dermatitis. A biopsy is performed and the findings are illustrated below. Which of the following statements regarding this condition is INCORRECT?

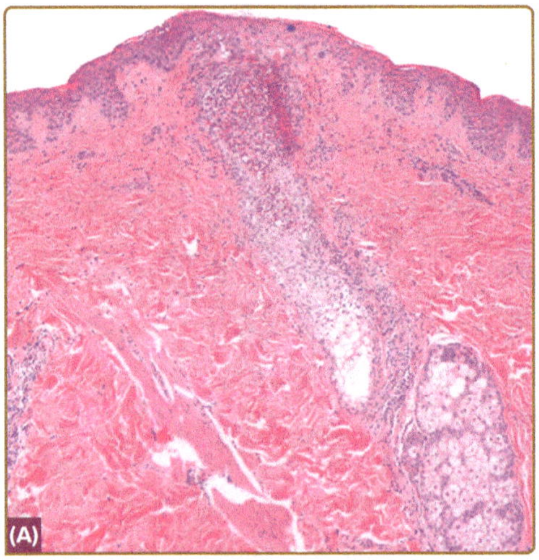

(A)

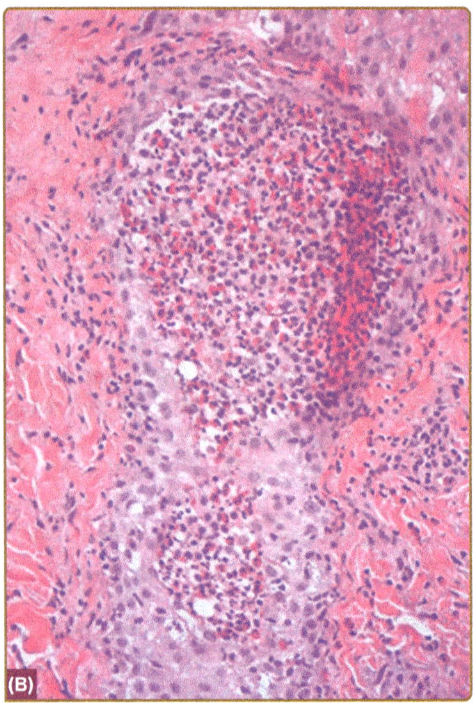

(B)

Courtesy of Scott R. Florell, MD.

A) This condition is strongly associated with *Pityrosporum* colonization of affected hair follicles.
B) This condition commonly affects immunocompromised patients.
C) This condition may be seen in healthy Japanese patients accompanied by peripheral leukocytosis and eosinophilia.
D) This condition may be associated with follicular mucinosis.
E) In healthy patients, this condition is most commonly associated with atopy.

QUESTION 5-35.

A patient with acute myelogenous leukemia recently treated with cytarabine presents with a polymorphous cutaneous eruption affecting the neck, trunk, and extremities. The lesions consist of tender erythematous macules, papules, and plaques. A biopsy of the palm is performed and the findings are illustrated below. The inflammatory infiltrate is composed mainly of neutrophils. Focal areas of squamous metaplasia of the eccrine ducts are noted. Which of the following diagnoses is CORRECT?

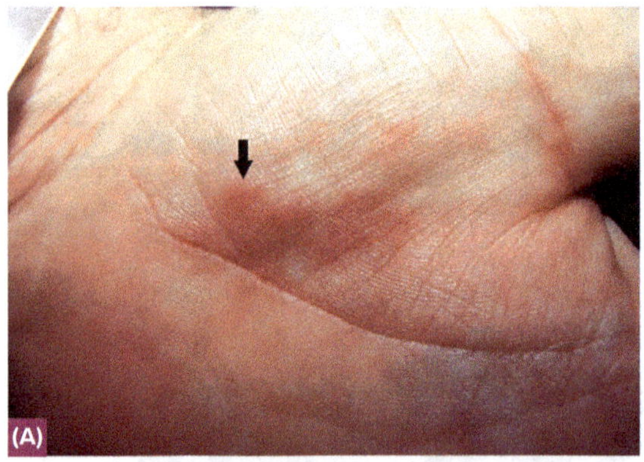

(A)

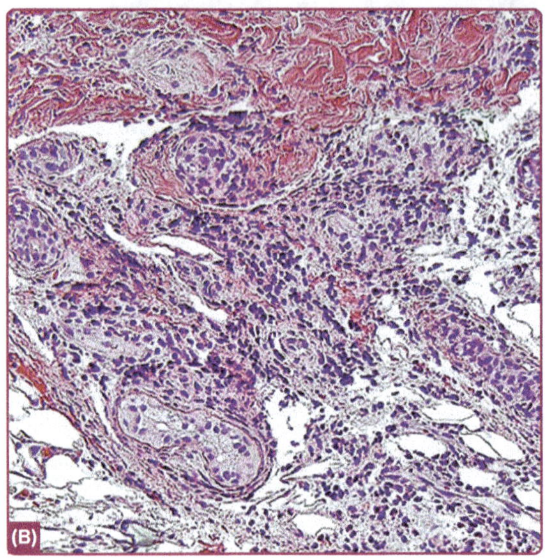

(B)

Reproduced, with permission, from Goldsmith LA, Katz SI, Gilchrest BA, Paller AS, Leffell DJ, Wolff K, eds. *Fitzpatrick's Dermatology in General Medicine*. 8th ed. New York, NY: McGraw-Hill Education; 2012.

A) Coma blister
B) Idiopathic palmoplantar eccrine hidradenitis
C) Neutrophilic eccrine hidradenitis
D) Sweet syndrome
E) Leukocytoclastic vasculitis

ANSWERS

ANSWER 5-1: A.

The subcutaneous tissue consists of depot fat sandwiched between the reticular dermis above and the superficial fascia beneath. Adipose tissue is organized into two compartments: (1) discrete round or ovoid lobules composed of confluent aggregates of the clear-appearing fat cells and (2) fibrous trabeculae (or *septa*) that form a meshwork separating the individual fat lobules. The fibrous septa are continuous with collagen of the reticular dermis and the superficial fascia and contain all the blood vessels, lymphatics, and nerves of the subcutaneous fat. In one sense, the fibrous septa simply serve as scaffolding for vascular and nerve plexi traversing the subcutis from deeper tissue to supply the skin (Table 5-1A). Thus, inflammatory conditions affecting the fat often involve the reticular dermis and fascia, and vice versa. Arterial vessels in the fat are small to medium in size and are categorized as muscular arteries. Thus, it is not possible to develop large-vessel arteritis in the subcutaneous fat but rather an arteritis affecting vessels of the caliber noted in polyarteritis nodosa.

Each fat lobule is vascularized by a single arteriole and, in effect, is an end organ with no collateral blood supply. There are no lymphatics within the lobules. Any interruption to this arterial supply will eventuate in ischemia or infarction of the fat lobule depending on the speed with which vascular compromise develops (Table 5-1B). The individual fat cells are supplied by arterial capillaries, which drain to venous capillaries and venules at the peripheries of the fat lobules. Based on these vascular patterns, in very general terms pathologic processes affecting arterial vessels may result in a **"lobular"** pattern of panniculitis versus a **"septal"** pattern associated with venular or venous inflammatory disorders (Table 5-1C).

Table 5-1A. Evaluation of Panniculitis

1. Excisional wedge biopsy is necessary for adequate sampling.
2. Punch biopsies are to be discouraged and may be misleading.
3. Biopsy is an active rather than a late-stage lesion.
4. Special stains for infectious organisms include Gram, acid-fast, fungal, Warthin-Starry, Fite-Faraco.
5. Examine specimen under polarized light for foreign material.
6. Laboratory investigation includes cultures and other techniques, such as immunostaining and polymerase chain reaction, for infection; serologic testing for syphilis, borreliosis, connective tissue disease, vasculitis, alpha-antitrypsin deficiency, calcium, phosphorus, oxalate, coagulopathy, lipase, and amylase.
7. Directed clinical history for isolated lesion (eg, ruptured cyst), trauma, factitial causes, psychiatric illness, drug abuse, cold exposure, recent medications, systemic disease, eg, vasculitis, connective tissue disease, sarcoidosis, infections, and malignancy.

Table 5-1B. Manifestations of Fat Necrosis

Lipophages—macrophages containing phagocytosed lipid following necrosis of adipocytes
Microcysts—coalesced tissue spaces in fat following fat necrosis
Liquefactive alterations—granular cellular debris
Hyalinizing (sclerosing) alterations—intact mummified lipocytes with a grainy and, at late stages, glassy amorphous appearance
Membranous (lipomembranous) microcyst formation—microcysts lined by feathery, almost ciliated membranes
Ischemic alterations—pallor of adipocytes with loss of nuclei and microvessels, hemorrhage, hemosiderin deposits, karyorrhexis

Table 5-1C. Predominant Patterns of the Panniculitides

CONDITION	PATTERN OF PANNICULITIS
Hypersensitivity reactions	
Short duration (erythema nodosum reactions)	Septal → lobular
Longer duration (chronic EN)	Septal → lobular
Vasculitis	
Small-vessel vasculitis	Septal → lobular
Medium- to large-vessel vasculitis	Septal and lobular
Lipodermatosclerosis	Septal and lobular Septal early
Calciphylaxis	Septal and lobular
Oxalosis	Septal and lobular
Morphea profunda, scleroderma, eosinophilic fasciitis	Septal → lobular Septal early
Palisading granulomas	Septal → lobular

(*continued*)

Table 5-1C. Predominant Patterns of the Panniculitides *(continued)*

CONDITION	PATTERN OF PANNICULITIS
Alpha-antitrypsin deficiency	Septal and lobular
Cytophagic histiocytic panniculitis	Lobular → septal
Pancreatic panniculitis	Lobular → septal
Subcutaneous fat necrosis	Lobular → septal
Sclerema neonatorum	Lobular → septal
Post-steroid panniculitis	Lobular → septal
Infection-related panniculitis	Septal and lobular
Physical panniculitis	
Cold panniculitis	Septal and lobular
Trauma related	Lobular → septal
Chemical and factitial	Lobular → septal
Connective tissue disease	
Lupus panniculitis	Septal and lobular
Dermatomyositis	Septal and lobular
Connective tissue panniculitis	Septal and lobular
Eosinophilic panniculitis	Septal and lobular
Noninfectious granulomatous panniculitis	
Sarcoidosis	Septal and lobular
Metastatic Crohn disease	Septal and lobular
Lymphoma and leukemia	Lobular → septal

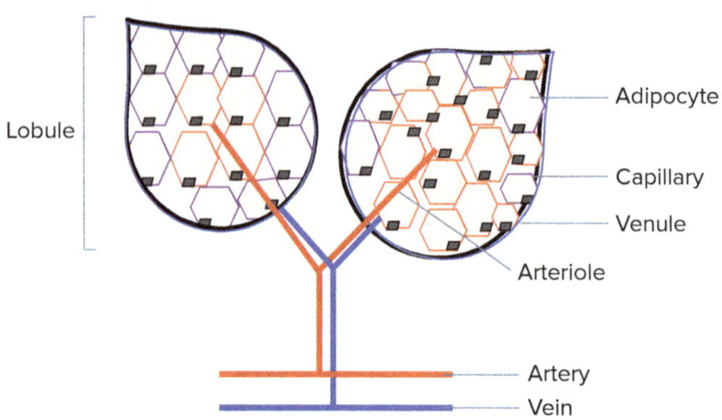

ANSWER 5-2: D.

This is a classic example of **acute erythema nodosum (EN)**, a septal panniculitis. Although believed by many clinicians to be a rather distinctive clinicopathologic entity, EN is in fact a relatively nonspecific hypersensitivity reaction associated with a wide variety of causes eventuating in fairly short-lived tender red nodules and raised plaques most often located on the extensor aspects of the legs.

Causes of Erythema Nodosum
"SORE SHINS"

1. **S**treptococci
2. **O**ral contraceptive pills
3. **R**ickettsia
4. **E**ponymous (Bechet)
5. **S**ulfonamides
6. **H**ansen's Disease (Leprosy), Histoplasmosis
7. **I**nflammatory bowel disease
8. **N**on-Hodgkins lymphoma
9. **S**arcoidosis

Typical EN lesions last 3 to 6 weeks and often resolve with a bruise-like appearance **(erythema contusiformis),** but always without ulceration. Lesions are usually accompanied by systemic symptoms such as abdominal pain, arthralgias, cough, diarrhea, fever, headache, malaise, and vomiting. Women are afflicted three to six times more often than men. **Chronic erythema nodosum (EN)** and **erythema nodosum migrans (EN)** appear to represent hypersensitivity reactions of longer duration, often 1 to 4 years or more. Some authors maintain that **chronic EN** is characterized by fairly discrete persistent nodules that are symmetric and not migratory, whereas **EN migrans** tends to show nodules that coalesce into spreading plaques that are commonly unilateral. Microscopically, early or acute lesions commonly show changes primarily confined to the fibrous trabeculae (septae): edema, hemorrhage, and variable inflammatory cell infiltrates composed primarily of neutrophils, possibly with some admixture of lymphocytes and eosinophils. This infiltrate often extends into the peripheries of the fat lobules. Otherwise, the fat lobules are largely unaffected. Older lesions often exhibit some thickening of the septa and a predominance of mononuclear cells, lymphocytes in particular. There may be greater encroachment into the fat lobules by the inflammatory cell infiltrates. Often at this stage, one begins to encounter in the thickened fibrotic septa, radial arrays of mononuclear and multinucleate histiocytic giant cells (the so-called **Miescher granulomas**). This latter feature is considered by some authors to be diagnostic or supportive of EN. Although some fat necrosis is observed occasionally, this is not a prominent feature in EN. To the extent that fat necrosis does occur, lipophages and granulomatous inflammation are present. By definition, vasculitis is not a major feature of EN. However, low-grade vascular injury and thrombophlebitis have been emphasized as findings commonly encountered in the EN reaction pattern. One must determine whether septal panniculitis or thrombophlebitis is the predominant finding and also consider the clinical features in order to arrive at a final interpretation of their significance.

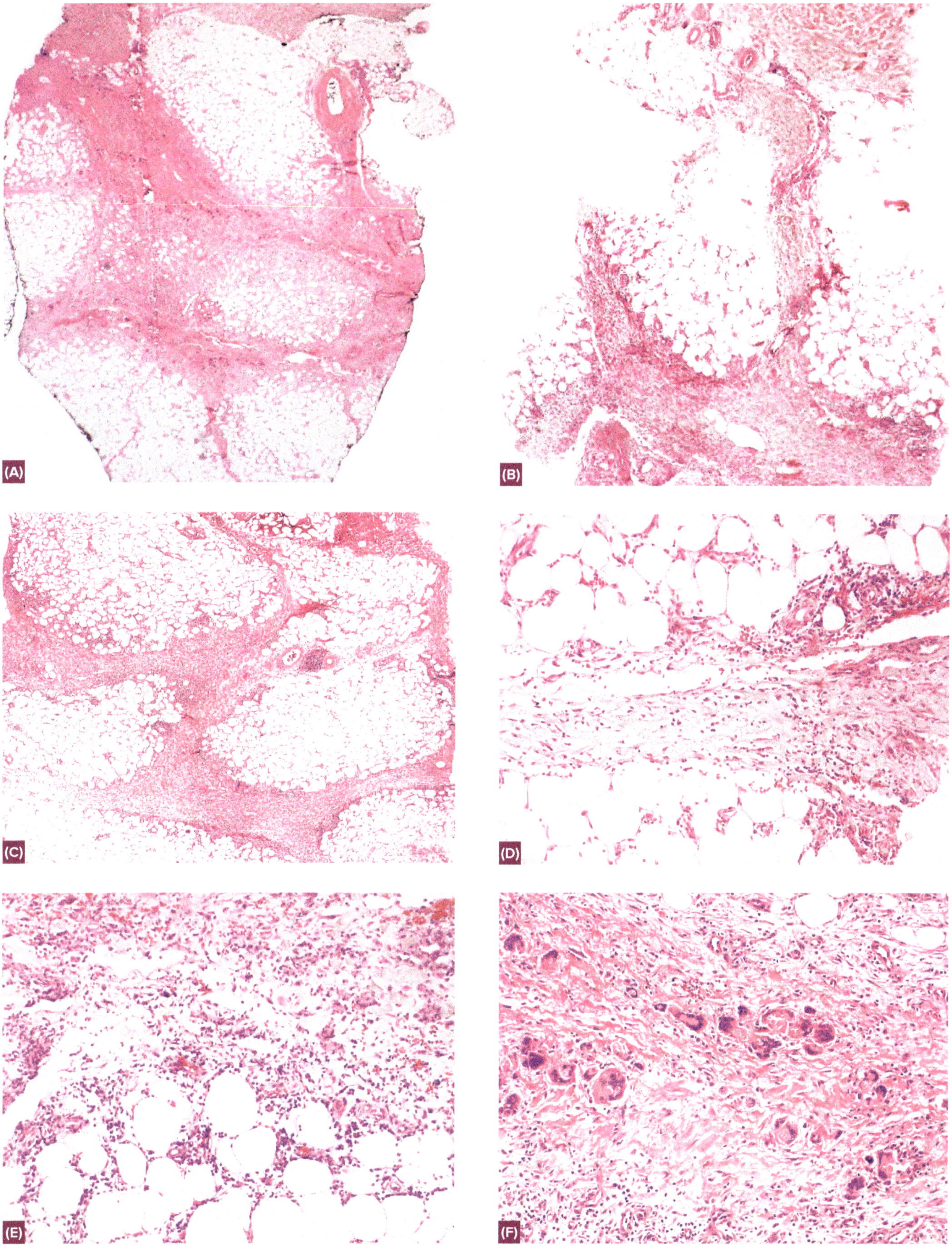
(A)
(B)
(C)
(D)
(E)
(F)

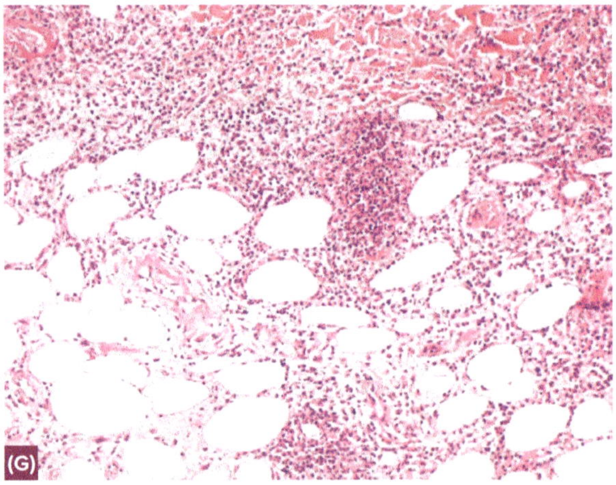

Erythema nodosum reaction pattern. (A), (B), (C) Well-developed erythema nodosum. The fibrous trabeculae are thickened by fibroplasia. **(D)** Higher magnification showing thickened fibrous trabeculum. **(E)** Inflammatory cell infiltrates are present at the periphery of fat lobules. **(F)** A thickened fibrous septum contains Miescher granulomas. **(G)** Acute neutrophilic lobular panniculitis associated with clinical presentation of erythema nodosum.

ANSWER 5-3: A.

This is a classic example of **lipodermatosclerosis** (aka **sclerosing panniculitis),** which is a distinctive clinicopathologic entity characterized by striking induration of the distal third of the lower extremity and ischemic fat necrosis (Table 5-3A). An **"inverted bottle"** appearance resulting from atrophy of the subcutaneum secondary to deep fibrosis is the prototypic presentation. Therefore, lipodermatosclerosis represents a circumferential process rather than an isolated nodule. Clinical correlation is needed to discriminate from focal ischemic conditions such as trauma. One or both of the lower extremities may be affected, often resulting from superficial or deep thromboses, thrombophlebitis, arterial ischemia, or varicosities. Elevated expression of urokinase-type plasminogen activator and its receptor (CD87) has been reported as a possible early step in lipodermatosclerosis and other venous stasis disorders through activation of **matrix metalloproteinase-2** (MMP2). MMP2 is an interstitial collagenase thought to contribute to the development of the ulcers found in advanced lipodermatosclerosis.

Microscopically, the epidermis and dermis commonly show **stasis dermatitis** with variable acanthosis, spongiosis, lobular ("glomeruloid") vascular proliferation, fibroplasia, dermal atrophy, and hemosiderin deposition. The panniculitis, compared to erythema nodosum, is relatively pauci-inflammatory. In early lesions, there is a septal mixed inflammatory infiltrate of lymphocytes, macrophages (some lipidized), and plasma cells that may spill over to affect the periphery of the fat lobules. The central portions of the fat lobules exhibit characteristic features related to ischemia, with adipocyte infarction, vascular congestion/hemorrhage, and hemosiderin deposition. Although vascular thrombosis may be present, features of true

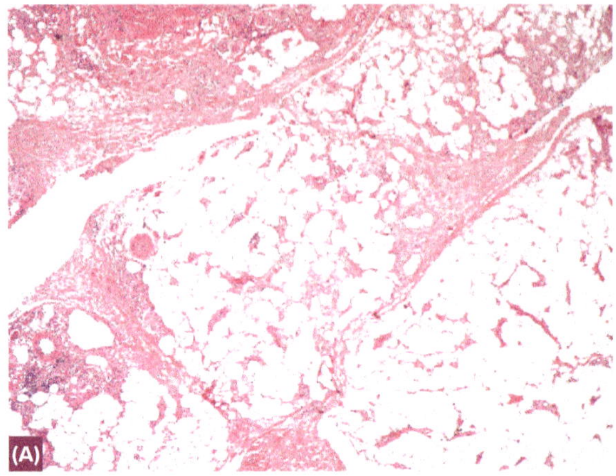

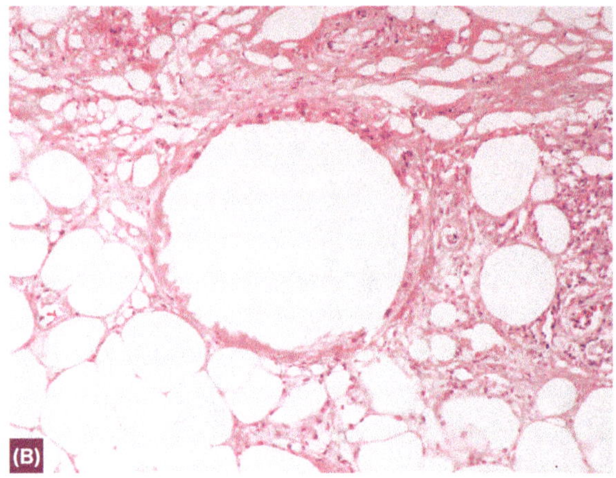

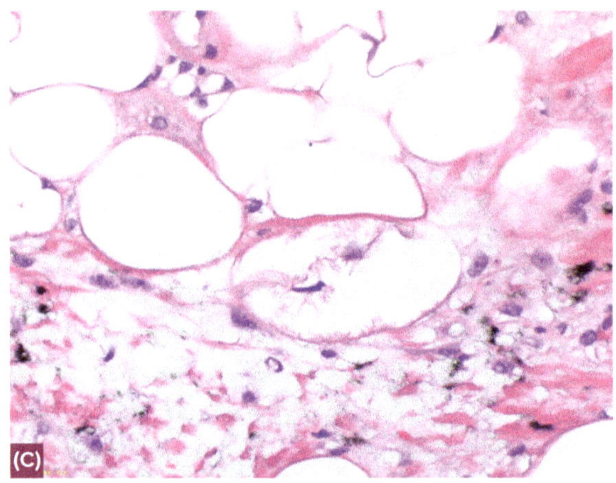

Lipodermatosclerosis. (A) There is obliteration of fat lobules by hyalinized fibrous tissue. There is relatively little inflammation at this late stage. **(B)** There is prominent lipomembranous alteration resulting in a feathery membrane in this fat lobule. The latter changes are nonspecific. **(C)** Note the scattered hemosiderin pigment surrounding the lipomembranous fat necrosis.

vasculitis (inflammatory-mediated necrosis) are not present. As the ischemia progresses, increased septal scarring and gradual obliteration of fat lobules ensues. These later stages show marked septal sclerosis with little or no inflammation. Centrilobular cystic fat necrosis with lipomembranous change **(lipomembranous fat necrosis)** is a highly sensitive finding but is not

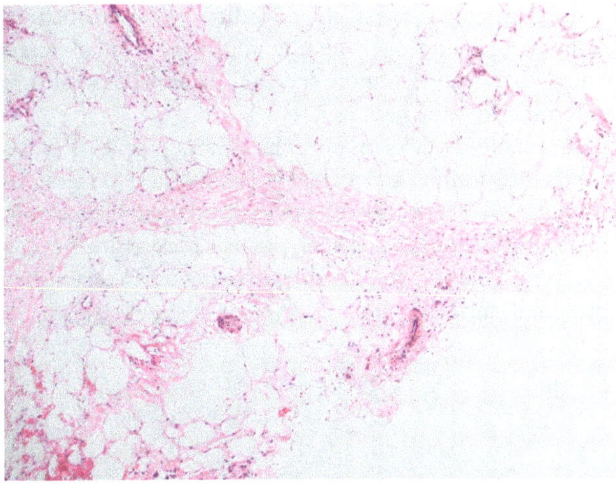

Lipodermatosclerosis. There is dense septal fibrosis with only mild inflammatory infiltrates. The fat lobules are tightly encased in the fibrosis and exhibit varying degrees of atrophy and lipomembranous fat necrosis.

specific and corresponds with any form of ischemic injury to fat. Lipomembranous change is characterized by cystic spaces lined by eosinophilic, feathery, crenulated membranous structures. These membranes stain with periodic acid–Schiff (PAS)-diastase and the lipid stains with Sudan black and Luxol fast blue.

Table 5-3A. Lipodermatosclerosis

Clinical Features
Adult women > men
Venous insufficiency
Stasis
Thromboses
Erythematous, edematous indurated plaques with "inverted bottle" appearance, distal lower extremities above ankles
Histopathologic Features
Stasis dermatitis
Septal and lobular involvement
Perivascular lymphocytic infiltrates
Ischemic fat necrosis
Pallor of adipocytes, loss of nuclei
Karyorrhexis, hemorrhage, hemosiderin deposition
Progressive fibrosis, obliteration of fat lobules and vessels
Lipomembranous fat necrosis
Fat microcysts
Differential Diagnosis
Septal panniculitides (erythema nodosum)
Other fibrosing panniculitides
Lupus panniculitis
Morphea profunda, fasciitis
Physical panniculitis

In regard to the differential diagnosis, more developed lesions may be difficult to distinguish from **lupus profundus** and other fibrosing panniculitides (Table 5-3B). **Lipodermatosclerosis** shows ischemic fat necrosis, whereas lupus profundus is notable for prominent lymphoplasmacytic infiltrates and hyalinizing fat necrosis. **Morphea** and related conditions should not show stasis changes, dermal atrophy, and ischemic necrosis to the degree observed in lipodermatosclerosis. An elastic stain will reveal a disrupted elastic fiber network in the scarred septa of lipodermatosclerosis, but a preserved elastic network sandwiched in between thickened collagen bundles is seen in morphea. The clinical manifestations should easily allow distinction of even late-stage sclerosing panniculitis from collagen-vascular disease.

Table 5-3B.

Lipodermatosclerosis DDX
1. Lupus profundus
1. Lymphoplasmacytic infiltrates
2. Hyalinizing fat necrosis
2. Morphea
1. No stasis change
2. No dermal atrophy
3. Lipophages not prominent
4. Lipodystrophy not prominent

ANSWER 5-4: C.

This is a classic presentation of **calciphylaxis**, which is a rare syndrome of vascular calcification and ischemic necrosis with a poorly understood pathophysiology (Table 5-4A). Patients

Table 5-4A. Calciphylaxis

Clinical Features
Abnormalities of calcium and/or phosphorus metabolism
Chronic renal failure
Primary or secondary hyperparathyroidism
Protein C deficiency
Livedo reticularis
Painful inflammatory nodules that ulcerate
Vascular calcification
Histopathologic Features
Small vessels (30-600 μm) show:
Mural calcification
Intimal proliferation
Soft-tissue calcification
Fibrin thrombi, variable
Ischemic fat necrosis
Mixed inflammatory cell infiltrates involving panniculus with neutrophils and mononuclear cells

(continued)

Table 5-4A. Calciphylaxis *(continued)*

Differential Diagnosis
- Other calcifying panniculitides (dystrophic and metastatic calcification)
- Connective tissue disease
- Peripheral vascular disease, sclerosing panniculitis
- Cholesterol emboli
- Marantic and septic emboli
- Oxalosis
- Intravascular thrombotic and occlusive vasculopathies
- Vasculitis
- Infection
- Pyoderma gangrenosum

presenting with this dramatic condition often have a systemic disease commonly associated with perturbation of calcium and/or phosphorus metabolism, such as chronic renal failure and/or renal transplant, primary or secondary hyperparathyroidism, idiopathic hypercalcemia, or hypervitaminosis D. However, rare patients without any of the latter conditions and normal calcium and phosphorus levels have been reported. Possible etiologic factors include (1) endovascular fibrosis and calcification of small vessels, (2) a hypercoagulable state, and (3) luminal narrowing by calcification (Table 5-4B).

Table 5-4B. Risk Factors for Calciphylaxis

Calciphylaxis Risk Factors
1. AIDS
2. Arterial hypertension
3. Calcium/phosphate imbalance
4. Caucasian race
5. Chronic dialysis
6. Corticosteroid use
7. Crohn disease
8. Type I diabetes mellitus
9. Female gender
10. Hypotension
11. Liver disease (hypoalbuminemia)
12. Malnutrition, morbid obesity
13. Iron overload
14. Peripheral vascular disease
15. Polycythemia
16. Posthemodialysis
17. Metabolic alkalosis
18. Protein C or S deficiency
19. Recent weight loss
20. Localized trauma
21. Warfarin use

The clinical manifestations of calciphylaxis are distinctive. Radiographic examination commonly reveals vascular calcification of large vessels, the so-called pipe-stem pattern of calcific medial stenosis, which is nonspecific. Small-vessel (<0.5 mm) calcification is more specific. The mortality rate has been reported to be as high as 80%.

Microscopically, calcium phosphate (dark purple) deposits are found in the intimal and medial layers of small- to medium-sized blood vessels of the subcutaneous fat and reticular dermis. The vascular calcification and endovascular fibrosis are thought to be the precipitating factors leading to ischemia. In established lesions, mural calcification of small vessels is observed.

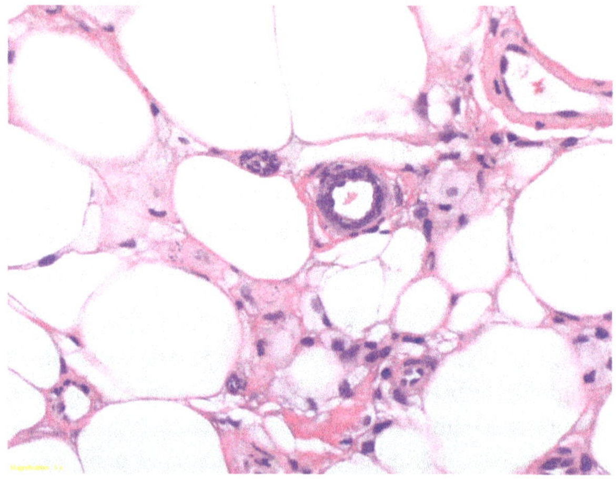

Calciphylaxis. Note the central small arterioles with mural calcification (gritty dark purple material).

A regular finding is the presence of fibrin thrombi in vessels. The adipose tissue generally shows foci of intralobular calcification and ischemic lobular fat necrosis **(lipomembranous fat necrosis)**, as well as variable mixed inflammatory cell infiltrates containing neutrophils and mononuclear cells.

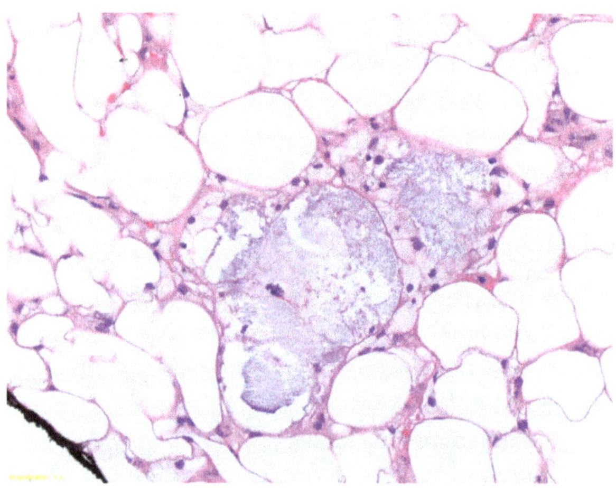

Calciphylaxis. There is focal ischemic lobular fat necrosis with calcification.

Recently, osteopontin (OPN), thrombospondins (TSPs), and matrix glutamic acid protein (MGP) have been found to be upregulated in calciphylactic blood vessels. These three proteins are not normally expressed in blood vessels, but in addition to being localized in calciphylactic vessels, they have also been found in atherosclerotic vessels, suggesting a possible common mechanism.

In regard to the differential diagnosis, the clinical presentation and the presence of small-vessel calcification with endovascular proliferation and fat necrosis should allow distinction from other entities. **Monckeberg medial calcific sclerosis** is a form of arteriosclerosis where dystrophic calcification occurs in the muscular middle layer of the walls of arteries (the tunica media). **Benign nodular calcification** is also in the differential diagnosis, but lesions will disappear with resolution of the abnormal serum calcium and phosphate levels. **Oxalosis** is an extremely rare form of panniculitis associated with deposition of the crystalline calcium oxalate in vessels and may closely resemble calciphylaxis, except that the calcifications are clear birefringent oxalate crystals instead of purple calcium phosphate within the walls of small blood vessels situated in the deep dermis and subcutaneous fat. It may occur as a primary inherited autosomal recessive metabolic enzyme defect or as a secondary metabolic condition resulting from excessive ingestion of oxalate and other substances, such as glycolic acid and ethylene glycol (antifreeze).

ANSWER 5-5: B.

This is a classic presentation of **eosinophilic fasciitis (EF)**. **Morphea profunda, scleroderma,** and **eosinophilic fasciitis** may all show prominent involvement of subcutaneous fat, dermis, and fascia, and although there are clinical and histopathologic features shared by these entities, there are also substantial differences. There is still no consensus as to whether EF is simply a deep variant of morphea/scleroderma or a distinct entity. EF has been associated with drugs, vigorous exercise, Borrelia infection, and a rare paraneoplastic phenomenon most often associated with hematopoietic malignancies. **Tryptophan-related fasciitis** (the **eosinophilia-myalgia syndrome**) refers to a disorder with features of morphea, scleroderma, and eosinophilic fasciitis occurring after ingestion of L-tryptophan. In the case of **morphea**, the lesions are generally well-circumscribed guttate (<10 mm in diameter) or oval plaques most commonly found on the trunk or occasionally linear processes (**coup de sabre**) that commonly involve the lower limbs. The plaques often have an ivory appearance with an erythematous or purple border. **Scleroderma** is characterized by diffuse cutaneous induration principally involving the trunk and upper limbs that leaves atrophic, hyperpigmented areas when healed. EF is distinctive and usually typified by a sudden onset following stress or intense exercise. The extremities are involved most frequently and demonstrate an extensive sleeve-like circumferential, symmetric induration with dimpling of the skin and have a **peau d'orange** appearance (Table 5-5A).

A peripheral eosinophilia is present in up to 60% of patients. The face, fingers, and feet are usually spared. Unlike morphea or scleroderma, patients with EF usually improve

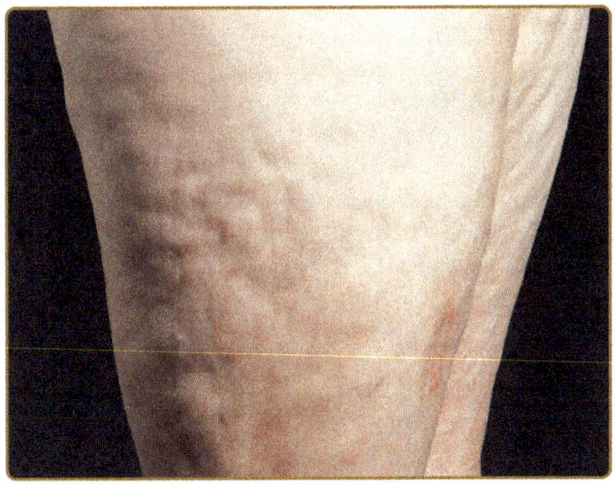

Eosinophilic fasciitis. Puckered skin of the thighs in a diffuse circumferential distribution. (Reproduced, with permission, from Goldsmith LA, Katz SI, Gilchrest BA, Paller AS, Leffell DJ, Wolff K, eds. *Fitzpatrick's Dermatology in General Medicine.* 8th ed. New York, NY: McGraw-Hill Education; 2012.)

gradually with or without treatment. Many recover completely over a period of a few years, yet others may develop hematologic or myelodysplastic disorders or other associated complications.

Quick Fact

- Circumferential panniculitis = lipodermatosclerosis, eosinophilic fasciitis

Microscopically, the involvement of the panniculus by these disorders is characterized by two principal features: (1) inflammatory infiltrates localized to the fibrous trabeculae composed principally of lymphocytes and plasma cells with a variable admixture of eosinophils, neutrophils, and mucinous edema and (2) a progressive sclerosis of the fibrous trabeculae resulting in the obliteration of the fat lobules in the final stages. The septal sclerosis is often continuous, with sclerosis involving the reticular dermis, fascia, and perimysium. The septa and fascia show progressive hypertrophy and hyalinization of the collagen fibers as in the dermis. Collagen is also deposited in place of the normal fat surrounding the eccrine glands, which causes them to incorrectly appear as though they are located in the dermis. Edema and inflammatory infiltrates generally are most prominent in the initial stages and have a perivascular and septal localization with involvement of the peripheries of the fat lobules. The lymphoplasmacytic infiltrates also vary in density from sparse infiltrates to large nodules with germinal centers. While the "center of gravity" for the disease activity in **morphea** and **scleroderma** is frequently the interface of the reticular dermis and subcutis, the focus of **eosinophilic fasciitis** is the fascia and immediately contiguous deep adipose tissue. Morphea and scleroderma often show progressive involvement of the entire panniculus (including blood vessels, nerves, and other adnexae except arrector pilae muscles) and occasionally the fascia (termed **morphea profunda**). Features that distinguish morphea/scleroderma from other forms of

Table 5-5A.

	MORPHEA/ SCLERODERMA	EOSINOPHILIC FASCIITIS
Gender predilection	F > M	M > F
Lesion morphology	Morphea: well-circumscribed, guttate or oval ivory-appearing plaques with purple border Scleroderma: diffuse cutaneous induration; heals with atrophy and hyperpigmentation	*peau de orange* appearance; "groove sign"
Lesion distribution	Morphea: trunk; extremities (linear) Scleroderma: trunk, upper limbs	Extremities; spares the face, fingers, and feet
"Center of gravity"	Interface of the reticular dermis and subcutis "Top-down"	Fascia and contiguous deep adipose tissue "Bottom-up"
Involvement of subcutis	Progress to entire panniculus (including blood vessels, nerves, other adnexae excluding the arrector pilae muscle); occasionally fascia (*morphea profunda*)	Progress to upper subcutaneous fat and reticular dermis

sclerosing panniculitis (ie, **lipodermatosclerosis**) include a variable loss of CD34+ proliferating dermal fibroblasts and preservation of elastic fibers on Elastic van Gieson stain. Straightening of fibers with parallel orientation and compression between thickened collagen bundles is frequently present. The extent of elastic fiber alteration correlates with the degree of sclerosis. Conversely, **eosinophilic fasciitis** commonly progresses to involve the upper subcutaneous fat and overlying reticular dermis. It may also show occasional lymphoid follicles in the septa and eosinophils in the fascia. Tissue eosinophilic infiltrates range from none to marked in EF. Other distinguishing features include frequent edema, hemorrhage, and variable mucin deposition. Vascular damage is observed commonly as fibrinoid deposition, thrombosis, lymphocytic vasculitis, or uncommonly as a necrotizing vasculitis. On occasion, spirochetes consistent with *Borrelia* can be demonstrated with silver stains, such as the Warthin-Starry reaction.

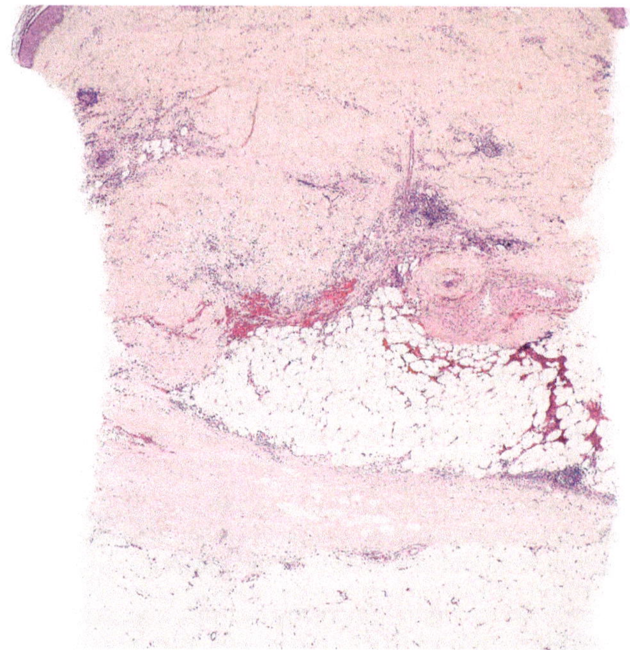

Morphea profunda. The fibrous septa are markedly thickened and sclerotic with inflammation at the periphery of the fat lobules. The process is concentrated in the dermis and extends into the subcutis ("top-down").

ANSWER 5-6: D.

This patient has **subcutaneous panniculitis-like T-cell lymphoma (SPTCL)**, and although is presenting with clinical findings of panniculitis, does not truly suffer from an actual panniculitis. Patients are usually adults who present with multiple subcutaneous nodules that may occasionally ulcerate. Approximately, one-third of patients present with **hemophagocytic syndrome** causing systemic symptoms, pancytopenia, fever, and hepatosplenomegaly. Originally this condition was classified as having either alpha/beta or gamma/delta lineages. Subcutaneous lymphomas with a gamma/delta phenotype of T-cell-receptor (TCR) rearrangement **(subcutaneous gamma-delta T-cell lymphoma)** show a much more aggressive course and are nowadays classified separately. Although earlier literature suggests that SPTCL is an aggressive disease with a high mortality, this is largely due to the inclusion of gamma-delta-positive cases. Cases ending in death are usually a result of hemophagocytic syndrome.

Microscopically, SPTCLs involve subcutaneous tissue, with minimal involvement of overlying dermis. There is lobular infiltration of the subcutaneous fat by T lymphocytes and benign macrophages (histiocytes) with a "beanbag" appearance. Marked **hyaline necrosis** and fat necrosis are common, resembling panniculitis. A characteristic finding is the rimming of malignant lymphocytes along the inner aspects of the adipocyte cell membranes. The tumor cells are cytologically atypical and may be a mixture of small and large cells or predominantly large cells. Large cells typically accrue over time. Karyorrhexis is often prominent and mitotic figures are easily identified. Although the "rimming" pattern of lymphocyte infiltration is sensitive for SPTCL, it is not specific and other conditions such as **lupus profundus** may occasionally exhibit this finding. **Lupus profundus** also exhibits hyaline fat necrosis. It has been proposed that there is a spectrum of disease encompassing **lupus profundus, SPTCL**, and a T-cell dyscrasia referred to as **"atypical" lymphocytic lobular panniculitis**. **Cytophagic histiocytic panniculitis (CHP)** is characterized by phagocytosis of erythrocytes and leukocytes by macrophages in the fat lobule **(hemophagocytic syndrome in the subcutis)**. This process may extend into the bone marrow. CHP is similar to the infection-activated reaction associated with perforin mutations found **in familial hemophagocytic lymphohistiocytosis (HLH)**. Causes of CHP are varied and include **subcutaneous panniculitis-like T-cell lymphomas, infections, connective tissue diseases,** and **other malignancies.**

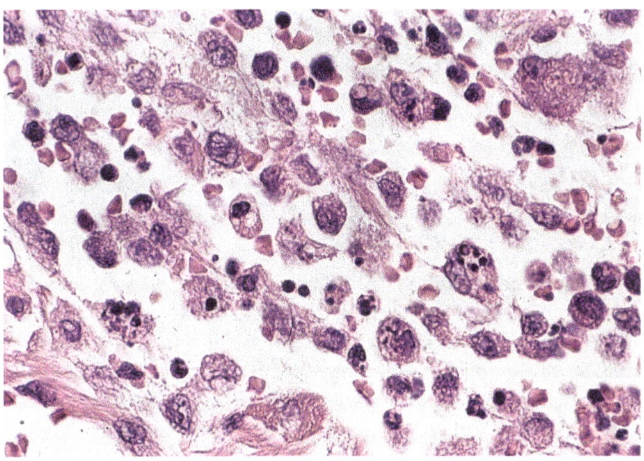

Cytophagic histiocytic panniculitis. High magnification shows phagocytosis of erythrocytes and leukocytes by macrophages in a fat lobule.

The lymphocytes that rim the inner adipocyte cell membranes are T cells (CD3+) with a cytotoxic phenotype (CD8 and cytotoxic proteins TIA-1 and granzyme). They are also BF1-positive reflective of alpha/beta TCR rearrangement. The cells are characteristically negative for CD4 and CD56. A cytokine phagocytosis-inducing factor (PIF) secreted by other T lymphocytes, which are CD4-positive, may be responsible for the prominent phagocytic properties of monocytes/macrophages in **hemophagocytic syndrome**. **Gamma/delta lymphomas** are CD3 and CD56 positive and typically negative for both CD4 and CD8. They are also negative for BF1 since they lack alpha/beta TCR restriction.

Quick Fact

Cytophagic Histiocytic Panniculitis

Key Histologic Findings

- Monocyte-macrophage infiltration
- "Beanbag" cells
- RBC extravasation
- Infiltration by other cell types
- Most often lobular
- Occasionally septal

ANSWER 5-7: D.

This is a classic example of **pancreatic panniculitis** (Table 5-7A). A syndrome including pancreatic disease, subcutaneous fat necrosis, arthritis, lytic bone lesions, eosinophilia, and polyserositis has been recognized for over a century. This syndrome is associated most commonly with alcohol-related acute pancreatitis but also has been associated with chronic pancreatitis, cholelithiasis, pancreatic cysts and pseudocysts, acinar cell carcinoma, pancreatic ductal carcinoma, pancreatic divisum, and ingestion of sulindac. Intramedullary fat of the bone marrow may also be affected and intestinal involvement has been documented. The pathogenesis of these lesions, including those in the panniculus, is poorly understood but thought secondary to lipolytic enzymes released into the systemic circulation from the diseased pancreas. In particular, elevations of serum lipase and, to a lesser extent, amylase have been reported. Subcutaneous lesions associated with cancer tend to be more chronic, recurrent, and ulcerative and may spread beyond the usual location of the lower extremities. Skin manifestations may precede the diagnosis of a pancreatic disease by several months, and with correction of the underlying pancreatic disorder the skin lesions fade away.

Pancreatic panniculitis is more common in men than in women (3:1) and generally presents as a tender, erythematous nodule or nodules on the lower extremities clinically resembling **erythema nodosum (EN)**. The nodules often measure about 1 to 2 cm and commonly involve the anterior shins. Unlike EN, these lesions may also break down and drain a creamy, oily substance resulting from liquefactive necrosis of the fat. Patients commonly exhibit systemic involvement with fever, arthralgias, arthritis, and occasionally, widespread necrosis of fat, including the bone marrow.

In the fully developed state, the histologic findings in **pancreatic panniculitis** are diagnostic. The fat lobules show a characteristic form of necrosis with formation of "ghost cells." The latter finding refers to necrotic adipocytes with intact but thickened eosinophilic cell walls and absence of nuclei. At the peripheries of necrotic foci with ghost cells, there is variable calcification, resulting in a basophilic lamellation that constitutes saponification, that is, formation of calcium soaps from the reaction of free fatty acids with ionizable calcium. Neutrophilic infiltration of fat lobules accompanies the fat necrosis and later gives place to mononuclear cells and granulomatous inflammation.

Table 5-7A. Pancreatic Panniculitis

Clinical Features
Men > women
Age 30-50 years
Alcohol-related pancreatitis
Pancreatic carcinoma
Traumatic pancreatitis
Fluctuant tender erythematous nodules
Extremities, especially pretibial
Buttocks
Arthritis
Polyserositis
Histopathologic Features
Early septal panniculitis with perivascular lymphocytic infiltrates
Fat necrosis with ghost cells
Basophilic alteration (saponification)
Calcification
Neutrophilic infiltration of fat lobules
Mononuclear cells later
Laboratory Evaluation
Elevated lipase, amylase levels
Differential Diagnosis
Early septal panniculitides
Infection

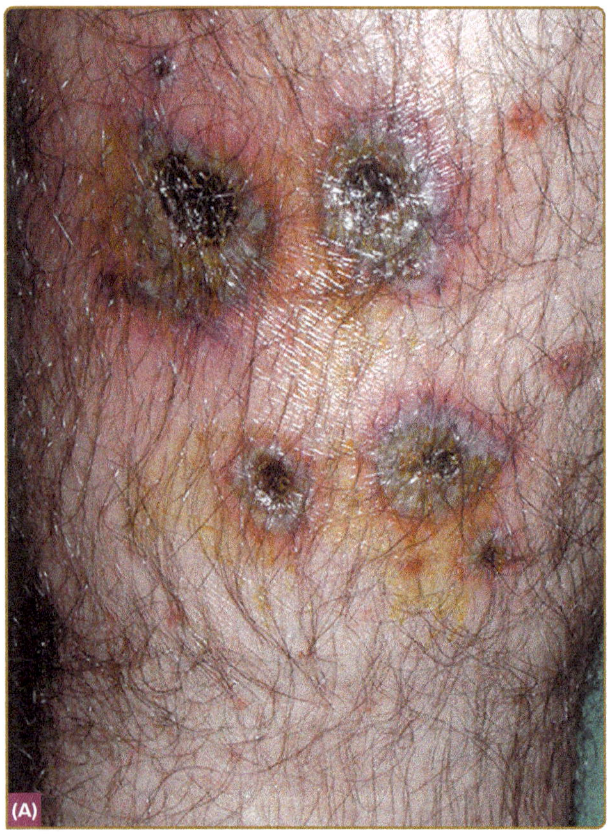

(A)

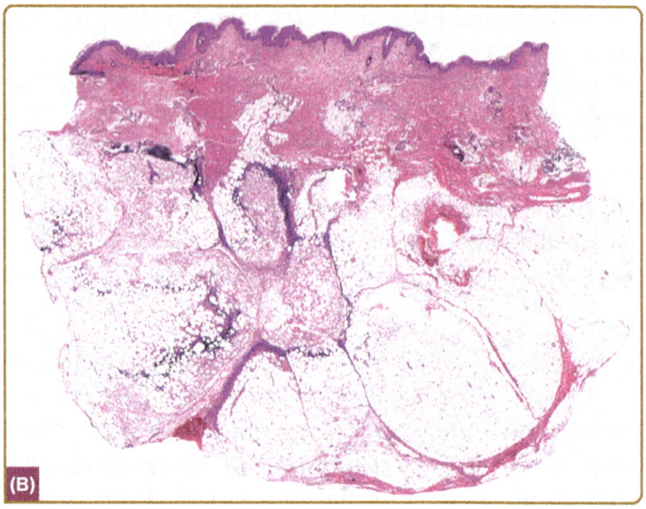

(B)

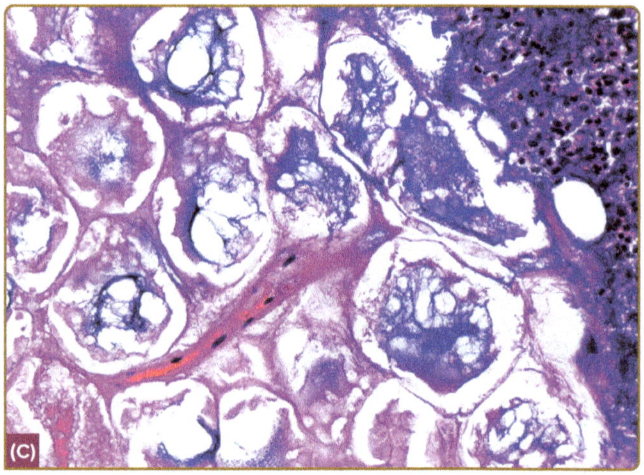

(C)

Pancreatic panniculitis. (A) Clinical features: erythematous subcutaneous nodules that ulcerate and exude an oily material. **(B)** Scanning power shows a mostly lobular panniculitis with adipocyte necrosis at the center of the fat lobule. **(C)** Higher magnification shows ghost adipocytes, necrotic adipocytes without nuclei and with cytoplasmic fine granular basophilic material due to calcification. (Reproduced, with permission, from Goldsmith LA, Katz SI, Gilchrest BA, Paller AS, Leffell DJ, Wolff K, eds. *Fitzpatrick's Dermatology in General Medicine*. 8th ed. New York, NY: McGraw-Hill Education; 2012.)

ANSWER 5-8: C.

The biopsy reveals a mostly lobular panniculitis. Higher magnification shows narrow needle-shaped clefts within adipocytes, histiocytes, and multinucleated giant cells. This is a classic presentation of **subcutaneous fat necrosis of the newborn** (SFN). **SFN, sclerema neonatorum** (SN), and **post-steroid panniculitis** (PSP) are three forms of panniculitis occurring in either neonates or children and showing crystallization of subcutaneous fat (Table 5-8A).

The pathogenesis of this crystal formation remains poorly understood, but certain factors may contribute to its development. At least with respect to SFN and SN, the composition of the subcutaneous fat in infants differs from that in older individuals. In this age group, hydrolases that break down unsaturated fatty acids are released in unusual events, such as mild trauma. The large ratio of body surface area to weight combined with a higher ratio of saturated to unsaturated fatty acids compared with adults favors this release. Since saturated fatty acids have a higher melting point than unsaturated fatty acids, solidification of fat (**crystallized fat necrosis**) may occur at lower temperatures. Additional factors that have some bearing on this phenomenon include prematurity, trauma, infection, fetal asphyxia, hypothermia, and other stresses. It should be pointed out that none of the latter factors have been consistently implicated in precipitating these diseases.

In SFN, full-term or postmature infants develop variably sized red to violaceous-indurated nodules that are reasonably well circumscribed and not bound down to deep tissue. The lesions are localized primarily to the cheeks, shoulders, back, buttocks, and thighs. The lesions usually develop in the first few days or weeks of life and generally resolve over 3 to 5 months with an excellent outcome in most newborns. Occasional infants develop an associated hypercalcemia that potentially can result in extensive calcification. **Sclerema neonatorum (SN)** presents in premature infants and develops within 1 week of birth. These newborns are usually seriously ill at the onset of disease, and many are dehydrated or undernourished. In general, a widespread yellow-white board-like induration involves the entire cutaneous surface except the palms, soles, and scrotum. In contrast to **SFN**, there is a high mortality rate associated with **SN**, often resulting from sepsis. **Post-steroid panniculitis** is a rare form of panniculitis, thus far only observed in young children 1 to 13 days after the rapid discontinuation of high doses of oral corticosteroids. Subcutaneous nodules develop particularly in areas of fat accumulation, especially the cheeks. The lesions generally are asymptomatic and resolve without scarring over a period of weeks to months.

Microscopically, in **subcutaneous fat necrosis of the newborn (SFN)** the epidermis and dermis generally are uninvolved. The most characteristic findings are patchy fat necrosis with crystallization of fat. Typically, macrophages and, to a lesser extent, adipocytes contain radially oriented needle-shaped clefts that correspond to triglyceride crystals dissolved during tissue processing. In addition to macrophages and foreign-body giant cells, other inflammatory cells, including neutrophils, lymphocytes, and plasma cells, may be observed. **Post-steroid panniculitis** is histopathologically indistinguishable from SFN. In **sclerema neonatorum** the characteristic needle-shaped clefts are present predominantly in adipocytes instead of macrophages and inflammation is absent. Clinical correlation may be required for definitive diagnosis.

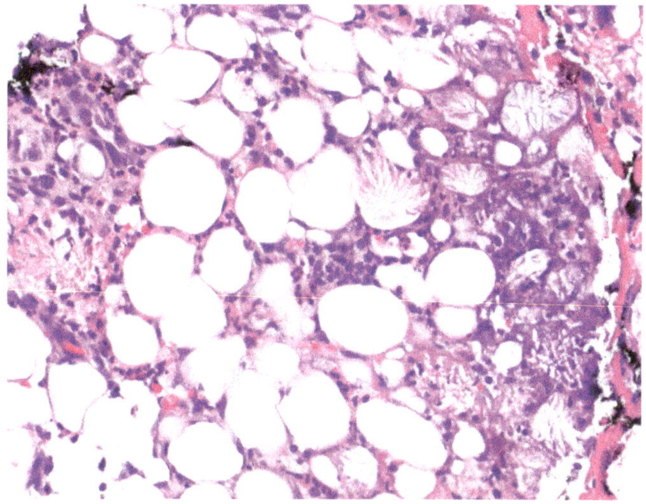

Subcutaneous fat necrosis of the newborn. There is a prominent lobular panniculitis with scattered lymphohistiocytic infiltrates. The characteristic stellate clefting from triglyceride crystals is evident in the center of the field.

Table 5-8A. Crystal-Related Panniculitis

SUBCUTANEOUS FAT NECROSIS (SFN) OF THE NEWBORN	SCLEREMA NEONATORUM	POST-STEROID PANNICULITIS
Clinical Features		
Full- or post-term Healthy Onset first few days or weeks	Often premature Seriously ill Onset within 1 week of birth Widespread board-like induration	Young children Healthy Onset days after stopping high-dose steroids
Reddish indurated nodules Cheeks, shoulder, back, buttocks Good prognosis	Often fatal	
Histopathologic Features		
Inflammation	Little or no inflammation	Similar to SFN
Needle-shaped clefts in macrophages and lipocytes Variable fat necrosis	Crystals mainly in adipocytes	

ANSWER 5-9: C.

Infection is a relatively frequent cause of panniculitis (**infectious panniculitis**), which has a mixed septal and lobular pattern of inflammation (Table 5-9A). Bacterial organisms are probably the most common agents, including *Staphylococcus*, *Streptococcus*, and both conventional and atypical mycobacteria. They are followed in incidence by fungi, *Nocardia*, and recently, *Acanthamoeba*. A particularly important predisposing factor to infection-related panniculitis is immunosuppression, such as organ transplantation, diabetes mellitus, AIDS, cancer, and connective tissue disease. Lesions may be primary (sites of inoculation) or secondary (sites of direct or hematogenous spread). The most common route of infectious entry is via the respiratory tract. Microscopically, epidermal and dermal changes are more frequent in infection-related panniculitis than in the other panniculitides (with the exception of lupus profundus). Often there are overlying changes of spongiosis combined with dermal edema and neutrophil-rich inflammatory infiltrates. A predominantly septal panniculitis with infiltration of fibrous trabeculae and extension into the peripheries of fat lobules may be noted with bacterial infection. Other notable features include a prominent neutrophilic infiltrate with occasional abscess formation, hemorrhage, basophilic liquefactive necrosis, and associated necrosis of sweat glands. Bacterial panniculitis as a general rule does not exhibit granulomatous inflammation. However, granulomatous inflammation is a common finding in other forms of infection-related panniculitis, particularly those with mycobacterial infection. Granulomas may or may not exhibit caseous necrosis.

Table 5-9A. Infection-Related Panniculitis

Clinical Features
- Immunosuppression
  - Organ transplantation
  - Corticosteroid and cytotoxic therapy
  - Cancer
  - Connective tissue disease
- Diabetes mellitus
- Inflammatory nodules—lower extremities most common

Histopathologic Features
- Epidermal and dermal changes common
  - Neutrophil-rich infiltrate
  - Edema
- Septal and lobular panniculitis often
  - Septal changes frequent with bacterial infection
  - Neutrophilic infiltrates
  - Abscess formation
  - Basophilic necrosis
  - Hemorrhage
  - Granulomatous inflammation in nonbacterial panniculitis
  - Vascular damage and vasculitis

Differential Diagnosis
- Acute neutrophilic panniculitis (erythema nodosum syndromes)
- Neutrophilic dermatoses
  - Sweet syndrome
  - Pyoderma gangrenosum
- Inflammatory bowel disease—metastatic Crohn disease
- Physical and factitial panniculitis

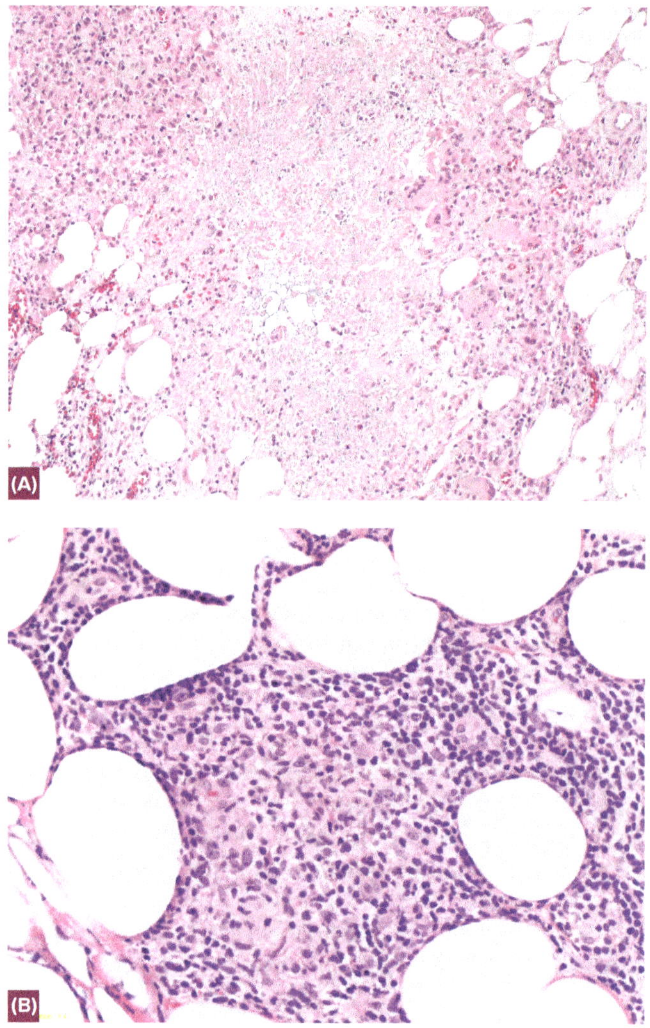

Infection-related panniculitis. (A) Bacterial panniculitis. There is granular and basophilic liquefactive necrosis of fat. **(B)** Septal and lobular granulomatous panniculitis with caseation necrosis. These changes are nonspecific but may be associated with infectious agents such as mycobacteria or fungi.

Both small- and medium-sized vessel vasculitis may be observed. In primary lesions, the superficial dermis is the center of the inflammation, whereas secondary lesions are deeper and involve the reticular dermis and subcutaneum. Blood vessels are thrombosed and are expanded with large numbers of the infective organism, especially in disseminated fungal and bacterial panniculitis. Clinical correlation and identification of microorganisms (on special stains or culture) is required for definitive diagnosis.

ANSWER 5-10: C.

The biopsy reveals a septal and lobular panniculitis composed predominantly of lymphocytes. Lymphoid aggregates are present in the septum and the inflammation spills over to diffusely involve the fat lobule. The individual adipocytes are separated from one another by inflammation and eosinophilic hyaline material. Large areas of completely necrotic fat admixed with eosinophilic material are present. This is a classic example of **lupus profundus,** which is a rare form of septal and lobular lymphocytic panniculitis (Table 5-10A). Approximately 50% of cases arise in association with autoimmune conditions such as **systemic lupus erythematosus** (1%-30%). Patients with systemic lupus erythematosus (SLE) and lupus profundus seem to have a milder course, often exhibiting only arthralgias, polyserositis, and Raynaud phenomenon. Trauma to the subcutaneum often occurs to sites where lesions later arise, for example, injection, biopsy, or excision sites. Women are afflicted two to four times as often as men. Patients commonly present with multiple indurated, deep-seated subcutaneous nodules or plaques involving the proximal extremities, particularly the upper extremities, as well as the shoulders, breasts **(lupus mastitis)**, buttocks, trunk, or face. Ulceration may develop, and the lesions often heal with lipoatrophy and depressed scars. Cutaneous manifestations overlying the panniculitis most commonly show changes consistent with **discoid lupus erythematosus (DLE)**, including epidermal atrophy, increased thickness of the basement membrane, vacuolar change within the junction of the dermis and epidermis, mucin among bundles of collagen in the dermis, and a lymphocytic perivascular dermal inflammatory infiltrate that may be superficial and/or deep. The remaining cases are characterized by poikiloderma, atrophy, telangiectasia, dyspigmentation, or changes confined to the subcutaneous fat only.

Table 5-10A. Lupus Panniculitis

Clinical Features
Women > men
Age 20-60 years
Multiple indurated subcutaneous nodules or plaques—proximal extremities, buttocks, breasts, trunk, or face
Ulceration
Overlying discoid lupus erythematosus, poikiloderma
Lipoatrophy, depressed scars late
Histopathologic Features
Epidermis and dermis may or may not show features of lupus erythematosus
Septal and lobular panniculitis
Hyaline necrosis of fat lobules
Hyalinization of adipocytes, connective tissue, blood vessels ("onion-skin" pattern)
Karyorrhectic material
Lymphocytic infiltrates and nodules at peripheries of fat lobules
Plasma cells often
Lymphocytic vasculopathy and vasculitis
Occasional fibrin thrombi
Mucin deposition
Variable fibrous thickening of septa
Differential Diagnosis
Septal panniculitis
Panniculitis in connective tissue disease
Morphea/scleroderma
Eosinophilic fasciitis
Dermatomyositis
Lipoatrophy, not otherwise specified
Borreliosis
Necrobiosis lipoidica

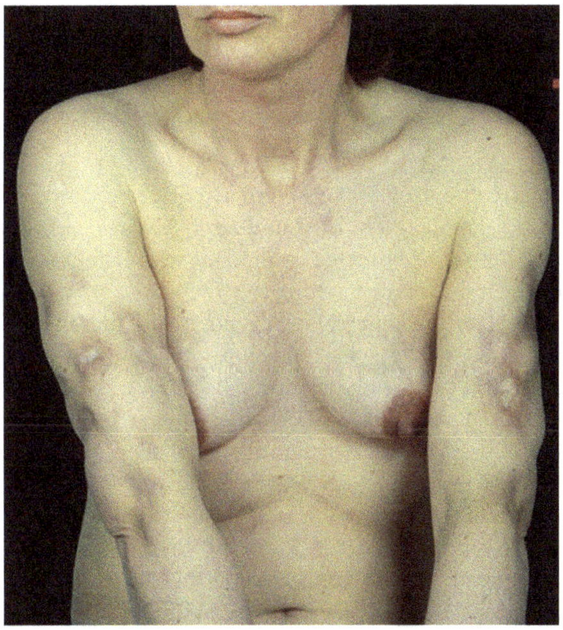

Lupus profundus. Chronic panniculitis with atrophy of the subcutaneous tissue, resulting in large sunken areas of overlying skin, representing resolving lesions. Where erythema is still visible, palpation reveals firm subcutaneous nodules and plaques. Also, some lesions reveal scarring in the center. (Reproduced, with permission, from Wolff K, Johnson RA, Saavedra AP. *Fitzpatrick's Color Atlas and Synopsis of Clinical Dermatology.* 7th ed. New York, NY: McGraw-Hill Education; 2013.)

Microscopically, there are distinctive changes involving septal and lobular areas characterized by lymphocytic infiltrates at the septal-lobular interface often-forming nodules with occasional germinal centers, scattered nuclear dust (karyorrhectic debris), and hyaline fat necrosis. The **hyaline fat necrosis** refers to the degeneration of fat lobules and connective tissue with development of a progressive glassy eosinophilic appearance. This alteration is often accompanied by mucin deposition. The fat lobules are commonly characterized by the formation of hyalinized microcysts and onion skin–like concentric layering of involved blood vessels.

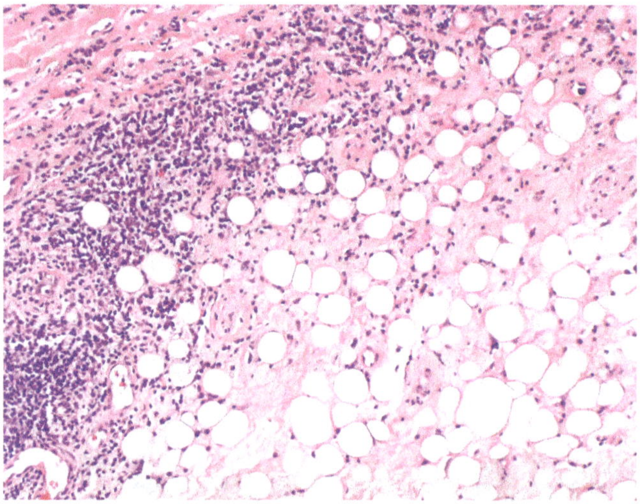

Lupus profundus (lupus panniculitis). Higher magnification shows hyalinizing necrosis of fat with mononuclear infiltrates.

Almost without exception, plasma cells are an integral part of the infiltrate, often surrounding it. Variable degrees of vascular injury are observed commonly, with lymphocytic vasculitis the most frequent finding.

In regard to the differential diagnosis, the presence of lymphoid follicles in the subcutaneum is highly suggestive of lupus profundus but not diagnostic because of their presence in other panniculitides such as **erythema induratum of Bazin**, **panniculitis in dermatomyositis, deep morphea**, and **erythema nodosum (EN).** Early lesions of lupus panniculitis may be confused with septal patterns of panniculitis (the EN reaction pattern). However, the major entities to be considered include connective tissue disease–related panniculitis, that is, **morphea, eosinophilic fasciitis**, and allied conditions; **dermatomyositis; necrobiosis lipoidica; lipoatrophy**; and **borreliosis**. The greatest difficulty may be distinguishing lupus panniculitis from morphea profunda/eosinophilic fasciitis. Both may present as clinically indurated plaques or nodules, and both exhibit prominent lymphoplasmacytic infiltrates, thickening of fibrous septa, lymphocytic vasculitis, and mucinosis. **Morphea profunda, scleroderma,** and **eosinophilic fasciitis** lack the epidermal changes of lupus erythematosus such as hyperkeratosis, atrophy, basal layer vacuolar degeneration, basement membrane thickening, and prominent dermal mucin. Additionally morphea profunda and eosinophilic fasciitis exhibit prominent sclerosis of the subcutis and dermis and lack the hyalinizing necrosis of adipose tissue of lupus profundus. **Subcutaneous panniculitis-like T-cell lymphoma** may contain hyaline fat necrosis but the adipocytes contain internalized atypical lymphocytes rimming the cell membranes as well as clonality. Recent evidence suggests a close relationship of lupus panniculitis to subcutaneous lymphoma, an observation that requires further study and clarification.

ANSWER 5-11: B.

The biopsy reveals an extensive lobular and partially septal panniculitis with extensive fat necrosis. Additionally, there is necrotizing vasculitis involving medium-sized vessels. **Erythema induratum of Bazin** and **nodular vasculitis** should be used interchangeably when discussing this most frequent form of lobular panniculitis associated with vasculitis. In regard to erythema induratum, some authors have provided convincing evidence for a relationship to ***mycobacterium tuberculosis*** **(MTB)** based on documentation of tuberculosis at other sites, positive Mantoux (tuberculin-purified protein derivative) tests, and response to antituberculous therapy. By definition, special histochemical stains and tissue culture are consistently negative for microorganisms; however, recent studies using molecular diagnostic techniques (PCR) have isolated MTB DNA from 25% to 77% of lesions. Taken together, there is increasing evidence that many cases of **erythema induratum** are likely to be a form of florid hypersensitivity reaction directed against components of MTB organisms. Others have disavowed any relationship, proposing the term **"nodular vasculitis"** to describe nodules not having any clear association with MTB. Some cases of **"nodular vasculitis"** have been associated with acute myeloid leukemia, chronic hepatitis C infection, and various medications such as propylthiouracil. Nonetheless, many clinicians maintain that erythema induratum/nodular vasculitis is a distinctive clinical entity characterized by bilateral, tender, dusky, bluish nodules, principally localized to the posterior calves of obese adult women.

These nodules seem to have some relationship to **cold exposure, cutis marmorata, erythrocyanosis,** and column-like weighty calves. Lesions frequently ulcerate with slow healing and eventual atrophic scars. An atypical variant occurs in men, in whom the lesions are unilateral involving the shins and thighs most commonly.

The histopathologic features described in these lesions are entirely nonspecific and often are related to the age of the lesion biopsied. In general, there is a robust lobular panniculitis with vasculitis involving small- and medium-sized lobular vessels. Early lesions primarily contain neutrophils with extensive ischemic necrosis, whereas evolved lesions contain infiltrates of lymphocytes, foamy macrophages, and multinucleated giant cells with caseous necrosis. The caseous process may extend to the dermis and epidermis, causing ulceration and exudation of the necrotic, liquefied fat. Vasculitis is not

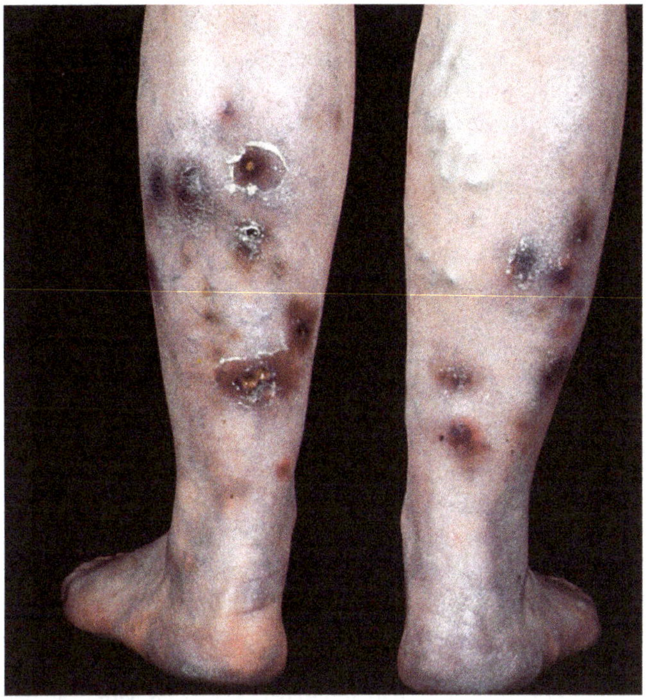

Erythema induratum. Erythematous to brown and bluish nodules with ulceration on the posterior calves. (Reproduced, with permission, from Goldsmith LA, Katz SI, Gilchrest BA, Paller AS, Leffell DJ, Wolff K, eds. *Fitzpatrick's Dermatology in General Medicine*. 8th ed. New York, NY: McGraw-Hill Education; 2012.)

always identified but is accepted as one of the major histopathologic criteria. This may be attributed to sampling error.

Many dermatopathologists recommend that the terms erythema induratum and nodular vasculitis be abandoned in favor of more objective morphologic descriptions. For example, such panniculitides are best designated as "granulomatous panniculitis associated with MTB detection," "granulomatous panniculitis without specific cause" (failure to detect an infective agent), or "panniculitis associated with small- or medium-sized vessel vasculitis." Patients should have a thorough evaluation for a local or systemic cause of their panniculitis.

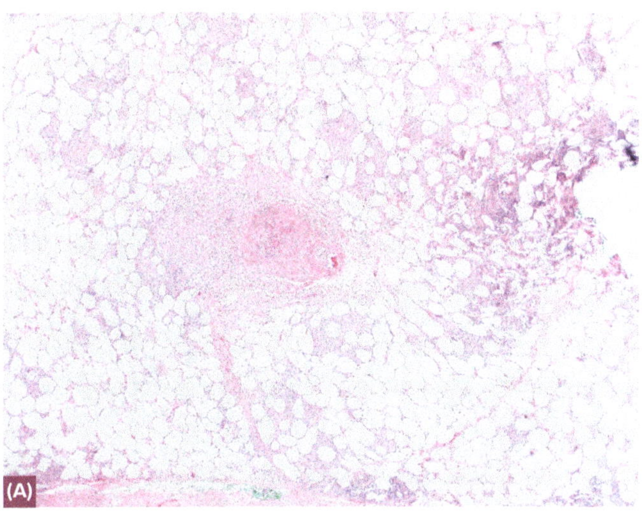

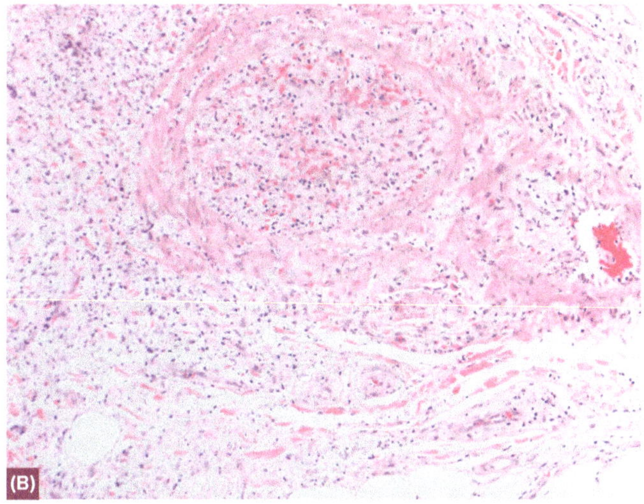

Erythema induratum/nodular vasculitis. (A) Histopathology: scanning power shows a mostly lobular panniculitis. **(B)** Higher magnification: extensive adipocyte necrosis and vascular damage-necrotizing vasculitis of small-medium vessels in the fat lobule.

ANSWER 5-12: A.

The biopsy reveals a shrunken fat lobule surrounded by dense fibrosis. A few of the vessels feeding into the lobule may be occluded by thrombi. There is a lobular panniculitis characterized by infiltrates of lymphocytes and lipophages. Additionally, there is interstitial fibrosis between adipocytes and scattered hemosiderin pigment. The findings are consistent with **traumatic fat necrosis.** Physical trauma, whether self-inflicted (factitial) or otherwise, is a major cause of injury to fat. Common locations include the breasts of women and accessible sites, such as the extremities. This is a classic scenario for traumatic fat necrosis of the breast after impact with the steering wheel during a car accident. Clinically, one observes traumatic edema and hemorrhage, often resulting in purpuric, discolored, indurated plaques or nodules that may have a ***peau d'orange*** appearance, especially when located on the breast. Scarring usually occurs, but it may resolve with **lipoatrophy**. **Secrétan syndrome** and ***l'oedeme bleu*** are clinical forms of **factitial panniculitis** resulting from blunt trauma to the dorsal hand and forearm and upper arm, respectively, or any site. **Lipoatrophia semicircularis** is possibly another clinical variant of trauma-related panniculitis that occurs when individuals, particularly women, bump one of their thighs on a hard object. It manifests as a semicircular ring of atrophic subcutaneous fat around half the anterolateral thigh. Nodular-cystic fat necrosis, also known as **encapsulated fat necrosis** (aka **encapsulated lipoma**), is also another possible variant of trauma-related panniculitis. These subcutaneous, well-circumscribed, movable nodules are induced by trauma and are located on the elbows, lower extremities, and hips.

Histopathologically, the subcutaneous nodules of traumatic fat necrosis show organizing hematoma, granulation tissue, fibrosis and hemosiderin often in the late stage, and focal fat necrosis accompanied by hemorrhage. Degenerating adipocytes are typically of various shapes and sizes. They are bordered by foamy histiocytes and lymphocytes. Mobile **encapsulated fat necrosis (encapsulated lipoma)** differs from normal lipoma in that they are bordered by anucleated, necrotic adipocytes (coagulative necrosis). Their thin, fibrous capsule completely or almost completely surrounds normal-appearing adipocytes.

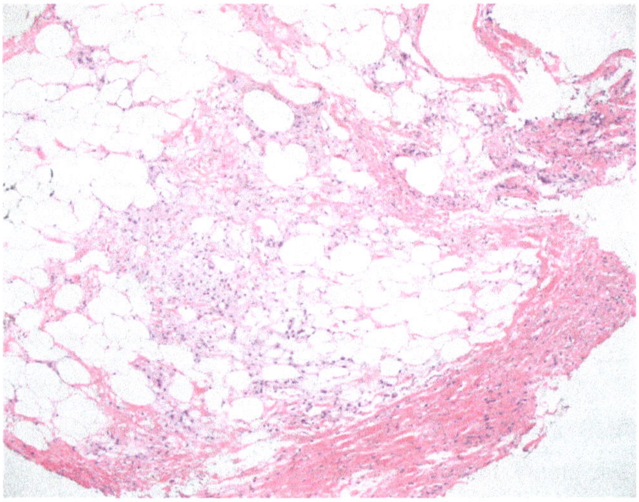

Traumatic fat necrosis. The architecture of the fat lobule is significantly distorted by dense scar tissue. The fat is infiltrated by numerous lipophages.

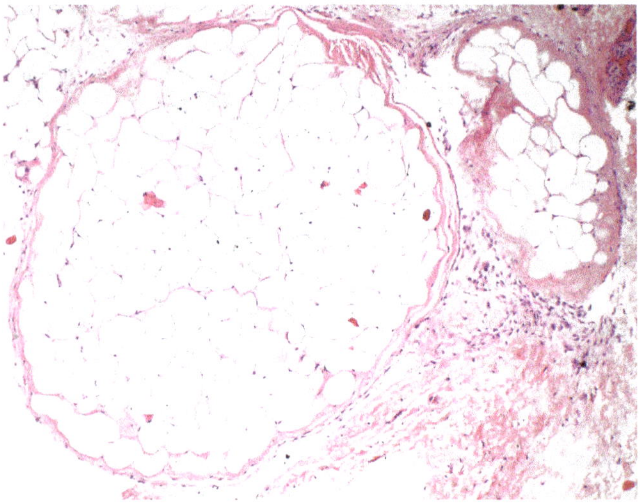

Encapsulated fat necrosis/encapsulated lipoma. Small nodule of necrotic adipose tissue compartmentalized by fibrous tissue capsule. Note that the adipocytes lack viable nuclei.

ANSWER 5-13: D.

The biopsy reveals extensive lobular panniculitis where cystic spaces of varying size and shape are present imparting a "Swiss cheese" appearance. The combined clinical and histopathological findings are consistent with **factitial panniculitis** (Table 5-13A). Injection of various foreign or organic substances and medications is also a common cause of panniculitis. **Sclerosing lipogranuloma** is a term used to describe the reaction of adipose tissue to various mineral, animal, and vegetable oils, silicone, and other hydrocarbons injected into the subcutaneous fat for cosmetic and other reasons. Almost every conceivable substance, including milk, feces, and blood, has been injected into the subcutis. Many injectable medications have been associated with panniculitis, including meperidine, pentazocine, povidone-iodine, morphine, corticosteroids, vitamin K, tetanus toxoid, and augmentation substances such as paraffin, silicone, PMMA microspheres, and polymethylsiloxane.

The injection or implantation of various oils, paraffin, and other hydrocarbons may involve any site. However, particularly common locations include the male genitalia, face and scalp, female breasts, and hands (**"greasegun granuloma"**). Such lesions are often indurated and may break down with drainage of oily material. Many such patients have health profession backgrounds and psychiatric histories and exhibit unusual or bizarre manifestations. There may be systemic signs, such as fever and, in some instance, a liquefying panniculitis.

Table 5-13A. Chemical and Factitial Panniculitis

Clinical Features
- Injection of foreign or organic substances, oils, paraffin, silicone, medications
- Psychiatric history
- Health care professionals
- Unusual or bizarre manifestations
- Indurated lesions—drainage

Histopathologic Features
- Sclerosing lipogranuloma
  - Variable-size vacuoles ("Swiss cheese" pattern)
  - Foreign body reaction
  - Dense hyalinized fibrous tissue
  - Variable inflammation
- Fat necrosis
- Microcyst formation
- Mixed and granulomatous inflammation
- Fibrosis
- Calcification
- Birefringent material, often

Differential Diagnosis
- Infection
- Alpha-antitrypsin deficiency
- Pancreatic panniculitis

Microscopically, **sclerosing lipogranuloma** shows a rather characteristic constellation of findings involving fat lobules: the so-called **"Swiss cheese"** pattern, with variably sized vacuoles corresponding to lipid removed with tissue processing, variable foreign-body giant cell reaction associated with vacuolated spaces, dense hyalinized fibrous tissue, and variable inflammatory cell infiltrates. The histopathologic features associated with injection or implantation of other substances is in general nonspecific but varies with the particular agent. Commonly, there is patchy, sometimes focal fat necrosis accompanied by microcyst formation and inflammatory infiltrates composed of neutrophils, especially early lesions; mononuclear cells; and granulomatous elements, more specifically in late-stage lesions. Birefringent material may be demonstrated with polarized light. Some agents such as meperidine may result in exuberant fibrotic reactions. Various methods can be used to identify the offending material, such as slide polarization or special staining techniques.

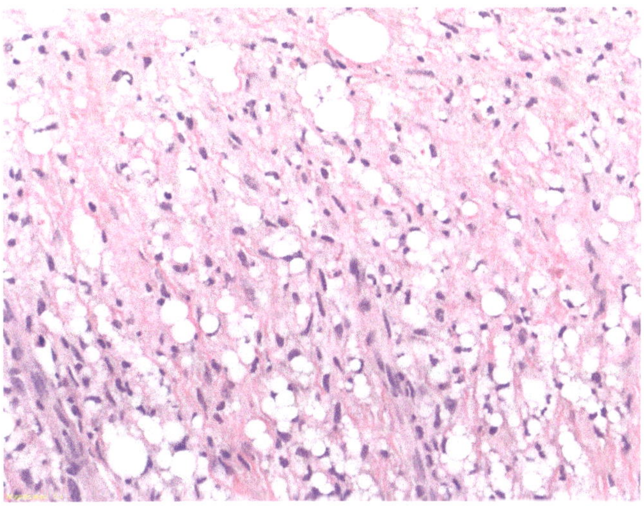

Silicone granuloma. Note the fibrosis and scattered inflammatory cells surrounding clear "Swiss cheese–like" spaces.

In regard to the differential diagnosis, in many instances the cause of physical panniculitis is obvious. Unusual forms of panniculitis, particularly persistent or recurrent, should raise suspicion for factitial etiologies. Evaluation for birefringent material and calcification may provide evidence for self-administered local injections. **Lupus profundus** and **subcutaneous panniculitis-like T-cell lymphoma** exhibit hyaline fat necrosis and may contain focal individual **lipogranulomas**, but lack the irregular "Swiss cheese" vacuolization of factitial panniculitis attributed to injected oils, silicone, or paraffin. **Subcutaneous panniculitis-like T-cell lymphoma** contains atypical lymphocytes that rim the inner cell membranes of adipocytes. The nodules of **erythema nodosum** do not ulcerate and the inflammation is characteristically septal. **Pancreatic fat necrosis** contains the characteristic basophilic saponification.

ANSWER 5-14: A.

This patient has **lipoatrophy** associated with chronic insulin injections. The patient's biopsy reveals prominent microvessels associated with diminished overall size of the fat lobule. This category includes a highly heterogeneous and confusing group of conditions perhaps only related by the clinical finding of loss of subcutaneous fat. This atrophy or disappearance of fat may be localized, partial, or generalized (total). Specifically, **lipoatrophy** is the loss of a previously inflamed subcutaneum, whereas **lipodystrophy** is a similar condition but lacks a preceding inflammatory episode of the panniculus (Table 5-14A). Much more work is needed to characterize the pathogenesis of these various disorders. Various classifications have been proposed, but until a more definitive nosology is devised, this text will continue with the current classification: localized, partial, and generalized or total lipoatrophy. Recent studies in this area have shown mutations in several genes in patients with **inherited lipodystrophies.** In patients with partial lipodystrophies, mutations in LMNA, PPARG, and ZMP-STE24 and in total lipodystrophy BSCL2 and AGPAT2 have been noticed. The **localized lipoatrophies** probably encompass the most heterogeneous grouping of conditions. One well-recognized outcome of panniculitis occurring in connective tissue disease, (i.e. **lupus panniculitis** and **morphea profunda**), is localized lipoatrophy, which has been designated as **atrophic connective tissue panniculitis.** However, other autoimmune diseases such as diabetes mellitus, Hashimoto thyroiditis, and juvenile rheumatoid arthritis may result in localized lipoatrophic panniculitis. Localized lipoatrophy may be secondary to a variety of local insults to fat, such as injections of depot corticosteroids, antibiotics, vasopressin, human growth hormone, and insulin, and factitial disease. Other unusual and poorly understood variants include centrifugal lipodystrophy and the annular and semicircular lipoatrophies. **Centrifugal lipodystrophy** is characterized by round, depressed lesions having a raised erythematous border, often involving the trunk and groin areas of children. The annular and semicircular variants show circumscribed bands of lipoatrophy involving the upper extremities and thighs, respectively, of adult patients. **Annular lipoatrophy** of the ankles is typified by a broad (~10 cm) annulus of lipoatrophy involving the distal leg above the ankle. It is often induced secondarily by compression of tightly fitted clothing on the abdomen, sacrum, and extremities, especially the thighs and ankles. The **partial lipodystrophies** most commonly show progressive loss of facial fat that may extend gradually to the upper trunk and arms (cephalothoracobrachial lipodystrophy). They are more common in female than male children. Many patients have reduced serum complement (C3) levels, a circulating immunoglobulin that activates C3 (the C3 nephritic factor), membranoproliferative glomerulonephritis, SLE, scleroderma, Sjögren syndrome, sicca syndrome, dermatomyositis, recurrent infections, high thyroid autoantibody titers, hypertriglyceridemia, insulin resistance, and diabetes. The generalized or **total lipodystrophies** may

Table 5-14A. Lipoatrophies and Lipodystrophies

CONDITION	CLINICAL FEATURES
Localized lipoatrophies	
Atrophic connective tissue panniculitis; lipoatrophic panniculitis	Children or adults with connective tissue and autoimmune diseases
Secondary localized lipoatrophies	Localized lipoatrophy secondary to local processes such as injections, factitial disease
Centrifugal lipodystrophy (lipodystrophia centrifugalis, abdominalis infantilis)	Annular erythematous lesions involving abdomen and other sites of children, possibly related to Kawasaki disease
Annular lipoatrophy, semicircular lipoatrophy, annular lipoatrophy of the ankle	Circumferential band of lipoatrophy affecting circumscribed areas of the extremities
Localized lipoatrophy	Localized lipoatrophy without evidence of inflammation
Partial lipoatrophies, dystrophies; cephalothoracic lipodystrophy	Progressive loss of fat from the face and upper trunk; relationship to hypocomplementemia, C3 nephritic factor, glomerulonephritis, and diabetes; often inherited
Generalized lipodystrophies	Congenital or acquired; generalized loss of fat; diabetes and other endocrine abnormalities; often inherited

present at birth or develop later in life. They are more common in females and show a number of cutaneous signs, including acanthosis nigricans, hypertrichosis, and hyperpigmentation. Endocrine abnormalities, including diabetes and hypothalamic dysfunction, often are present. Patients with human immunodeficiency virus 1 (HIV-1) infection have been reported with lipodystrophy while undergoing combination antiretroviral therapy that has specifically included protease inhibitors. The most commonly areas affected are the gluteal region, face, and extremities.

Microscopically, all forms of lipoatrophy are characterized by loss of subcutaneous fat in their established or fully developed stages; that is, fat lobules are greatly diminished in size and associated with prominent microvessels and myxoid alteration. Mostly, small fat lobules are surrounded by lipophagic granulomas and perilobular fibrosis. Early lesions, particularly those associated with inflammation and autoimmune or connective tissue disease in localized lipoatrophy, have been reported to show infiltration of fat lobules by lymphocytes, plasma cells, and macrophages with little change to the surrounding adipocytes or blood vessels. Direct immunofluorescence highlights the walls of blood vessels or the basement membrane at the junction of the dermis and epidermis. An involutional phase of localized lipoatrophy has been described and may or may not have a relationship to antecedent inflammation. This stage is characterized by diminished sizes of fat lobules, variation in the sizes of adipocytes, prominent vascularity, and a hyaline or myxoid stromal alteration. The latter findings greatly resemble fetal adipose tissue.

Part of the clinical differential diagnosis consists of **SHORT syndrome** (*s*hort height, *h*yperextensability of limbs, *o*cular depression, *R*eiger anomaly, and *t*eething delay), Werner syndrome, Wiedemann Rautenstrauch syndrome, leprechaunism, and Cushing syndrome. In regard to the histopathological differential diagnosis, the absence of hyaline fat necrosis and dermal mucin excludes **lupus profundus**. The minimal inflammatory infiltrate makes an infectious process unlikely. Although sparse septal inflammation may be seen in **erythema nodosum**, the clinical presentation does not fit.

ANSWER 5-15: C.

This is a classic example of **cutaneous sarcoidosis**. The patient's biopsy reveals numerous granulomas composed of epithelioid histiocytes with a scanty rim of lymphocytes. A number of (presumed) noninfectious processes may involve the subcutaneous fat, eventuating in varying degrees of septal and/or lobular panniculitis, in addition to the palisading/necrobiotic granulomatous disorders. These conditions include **metastatic Crohn disease, sarcoidosis,** granulomatous reactions secondary to **arthropod bites, rupture folliculitis, ruptured cysts, and granulomatous angiopanniculitis (GAP). Subcutaneous granuloma annulare** contains palisading granulomas with central necrobiosis of collagen and increased dermal mucin. In **Crohn disease**, the lesions may resemble **erythema nodosum (EN)** clinically and usually are located on the lower extremities. Histopathologically, they may show noncaseating granulomas in the subcutaneous septa or within the fat lobules accompanied by a lymphocytic vasculitis in the medium-sized vessels at the dermal-subcutis junction. In **sarcoidosis,** deep subcutaneous nodules are present on the lower extremities, but there are usually no visible indications of an inflammatory process except for pink to tan coloration. Microscopically, these small noncaseating granulomas are associated with the subcutaneous septa and fat lobules but show only a few lymphocytes around their perimeter (**"naked" granulomas**). Occasionally, these sarcoid granulomas will undergo necrosis in their centers, and calcification may develop. **GAP** may appear microscopically similar to carcinoma, as in GAP of the breast, but close inspection will reveal granulomas lacking involvement of breast lobules and ducts. Because a possible infectious etiology still exists in patients with panniculitis and Crohn disease or sarcoidosis, noninfectious granulomatous panniculitis must be a diagnosis of exclusion. Granulomatous reactions secondary to **arthropod bites** generally contain robust eosinophilic infiltrates and form **eosinophilic panniculitis. Eosinophilic panniculitis** is a nonspecific form of lobular panniculitis containing large numbers of eosinophils that may be associated with drug injections, arthropod bites, and parasitic infections (Table 5-15A). **Wells syndrome (eosinophilic cellulitis)** is recurrent granulomatous dermatitis with eosinophilia that presents as mildly pruritic or tender papules, plaques, and nodules. A characteristic but nonspecific finding is the presence of flame figures, where degranulated eosinophilic granules are admixed with degenerative collagen. The condition may be familial or associated with arthropod bites. Cases where inflammation extends into the subcutis may also produce an eosinophilic panniculitis.

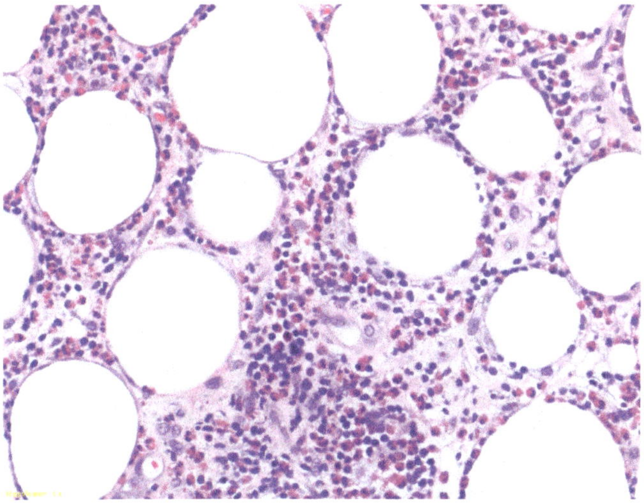

Eosinophilic panniculitis. There is a lobular inflammatory infiltrate composed of robust eosinophilic and lymphocytic infiltrates.

Table 5-15A. Eosinophilic Panniculitis

Clinical Features
Many etiologies
Atopy
Local injections
Cancer (especially lymphoma)
Vasculitis
Borrelial infection
Inflammatory subcutaneous nodules
Vesicles, pustules, urticarias
Histopathologic Features
Infiltration of fat lobules by eosinophils
Other inflammatory cells to variable extent
Occasional "flame figures"
Occasional eosinophilic cellulitis and fasciitis
Laboratory Evaluation
Special stains and serologic evaluation for Borrelial infection
Differential Diagnosis
Lymphoma

ANSWER 5-16: A.

The biopsy reveals a lobular panniculitis with robust neutrophilic infiltrates. Liquefactive necrosis is present in the subcutis and the dermis. The combined clinical and histopathological findings are most consistent with **alpha-1-antitrypsin deficiency–associated panniculitis**. Severe homozygous deficiency of the protease inhibitor alpha-1-antitrypsin may result in a recurrent ulcerating lobular panniculitis thought in the past to be **Weber-Christian disease**. **Alpha-1-antitrypsin**, which is synthesized in the liver, is the major inhibitor of serine proteases circulating in the blood. The deficiency of alpha-1-antitrypsin is thought to result in unopposed proteolytic activity and the promotion of inflammatory reactions. There is often a history of tender, recurrent, erythematous, subcutaneous nodules associated with ulceration that involves the face, trunk, buttocks, and proximal extremities. The nodules commonly follow trauma and exhibit drainage of clear or serosanguineous material. There may also be an exudate similar to necrotic adipocytes. In some instances, particularly early in the disease, the clinical picture is similar to cellulitis. Patients may have other manifestations of the protease inhibitor deficiency such as emphysema, hepatitis, and acquired angioedema. Laboratory evaluation usually discloses a reduction in level of the serum alpha-1-antitrypsin activity, although too few cases have been reported to make a definitive correlation. Resolution of the lesions results in atrophic scarring.

Microscopically, two patterns of panniculitis have been described: (1) a lobular panniculitis with fat necrosis and (2) a septal panniculitis with proteolysis of collagen and necrosis of the fibrous trabeculae. The first pattern, seen in our patient, is commonly characterized by neutrophilic infiltration of fat lobules that may be focal, but often is indistinguishable from other forms of lobular panniculitis. The entire fat lobule may be destroyed. The septal pattern of panniculitis also shows neutrophilic infiltration of fibrous septa of the reticular dermis but usually is accompanied by prominent numbers of macrophages. Concomitant lobular involvement with fat necrosis may or may not be present. An important feature is the presence of liquefactive necrosis of the dermis, which, along with a similar pattern in the fibrous septa, is thought to be characteristic of alpha-1-antitrypsin deficiency panniculitis. As the necrosis progresses and scar formation ensues, the number of neutrophils and macrophages found on biopsy decreases. Having well-demarcated edges and being well localized are other unique features of alpha-1-antitrypsin deficiency. Vasculitis usually is not present on biopsy except in the necrotic areas surrounding the panniculitis.

In regard to the differential diagnoses, the lobular form of **alpha-1-antitrypsin deficiency** may be indistinguishable from other lobular panniculitides, particularly those associated with **infection** and **physical** or **factitial agents**. Cultures, special stains, polaroscopy, clinical history, and laboratory evaluation of serum alpha-1-antitrypsin activity are needed to sort out these possibilities. **Marshall syndrome** is considered part of the clinical spectrum of alpha-1-antitrypsin deficiency. Just like alpha-1-antitrypsin deficiency, many other disease processes may eventuate in a predominately lobular panniculitis. These panniculitides may also be septal initially, remain septal, or display both septal and lobular patterns. In a large proportion of cases, the lobular panniculitis is entirely nonspecific. However, the particular features observed in any given biopsy, while nonspecific, may be influenced by when the biopsy was taken in the natural history of the panniculitis and the severity of the insult to the fat. Early lesions tend to show predominately neutrophilic infiltrates, and older lesions, mononuclear cell infiltrates with lymphocytes, lipid-laden macrophages, granulomatous elements, and finally, fibrosis. It is incumbent on the histopathologist to look for certain histopathologic features that are clues to diagnosis. Historically, **Weber-Christian disease (WCD)** refers to recurrent crops of erythematous nodules on the lower limbs or trunk accompanied by fever, malaise, arthralgias, and fatigue. It has been called "**idiopathic lobular panniculitis, nodular panniculitis, idiopathic nodular panniculitis,** and **relapsing febrile nonsuppurative nodular panniculitis.**" These nodules occasionally discharge oily material and hence have been termed **liquefying panniculitis**. Women aged 30 to 60 years have been affected most commonly. Histopathologically, **Weber-Christian disease** has been reported to show a predominately lobular panniculitis, and the presence of numerous lipophages has been considered diagnostic. Like most forms of lobular panniculitis, it is likely that WCD is entirely a nonspecific reaction pattern whose histologic picture varies according to the age of the lesion biopsied, for example, neutrophils early > mononuclear cells/lipophages > granulomas > fibrosis. Over the years, specific causes of WCD have been recognized and probably will continue to be identified. For example, when revisited, cases of WCD have been reclassified as **alpha-1-antitrypsin deficiency panniculitis, cytophagic histiocytic panniculitis (CHP), erythema induratum of Bazin/nodular vasculitis, erythema nodosum, factitial panniculitis, pancreatic panniculitis, subcutaneous panniculitic lymphoma, superficial thrombophlebitis,** and **traumatic panniculitis**. Many believe that the entity is only of historical significance and most likely does not exist. However, recently WCD-like symptoms and findings were found in patients with detected mutations in the TNFRSF 1A gene, coding for the p55 TNF receptor. Mutations in this gene are the cause of tumor necrosis factor (TNF) receptor–associated periodic syndrome (TRAPS), with an unbalanced TNF-alpha action. Beyond acknowledging WCD as a historical entity, the term should probably be abandoned. If no cause of a particular panniculitis can be established, the process should be designated as **lobular panniculitis of unknown etiology,** and the patient should continue to be evaluated.

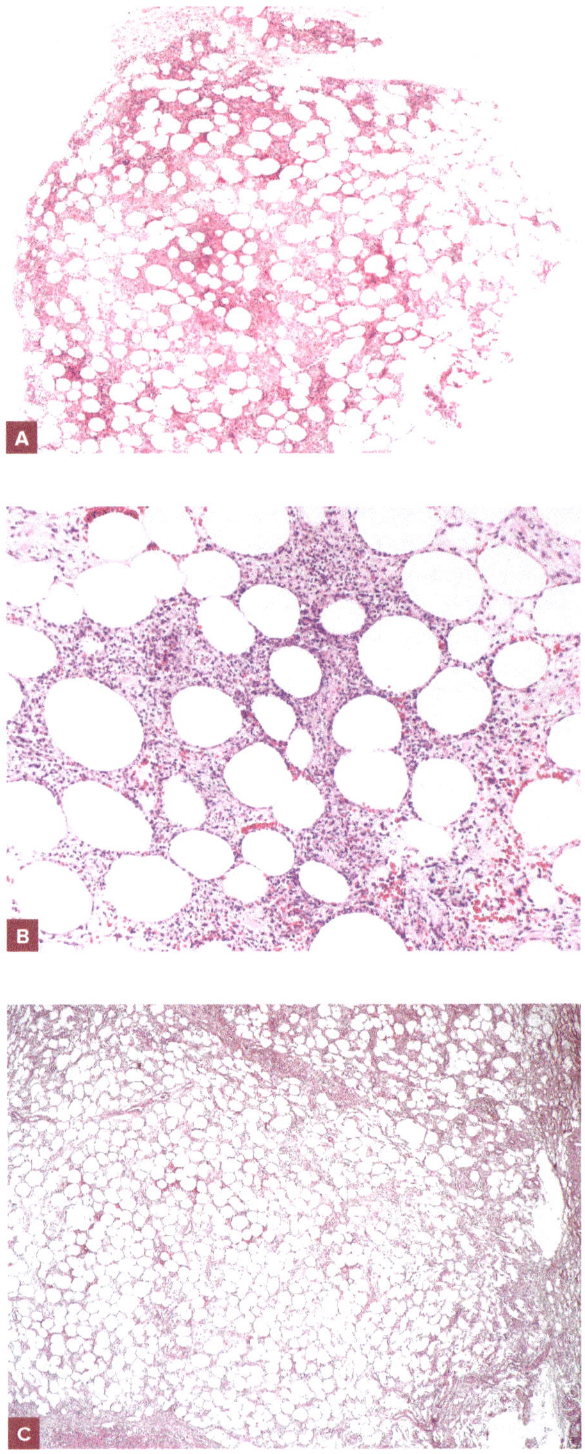

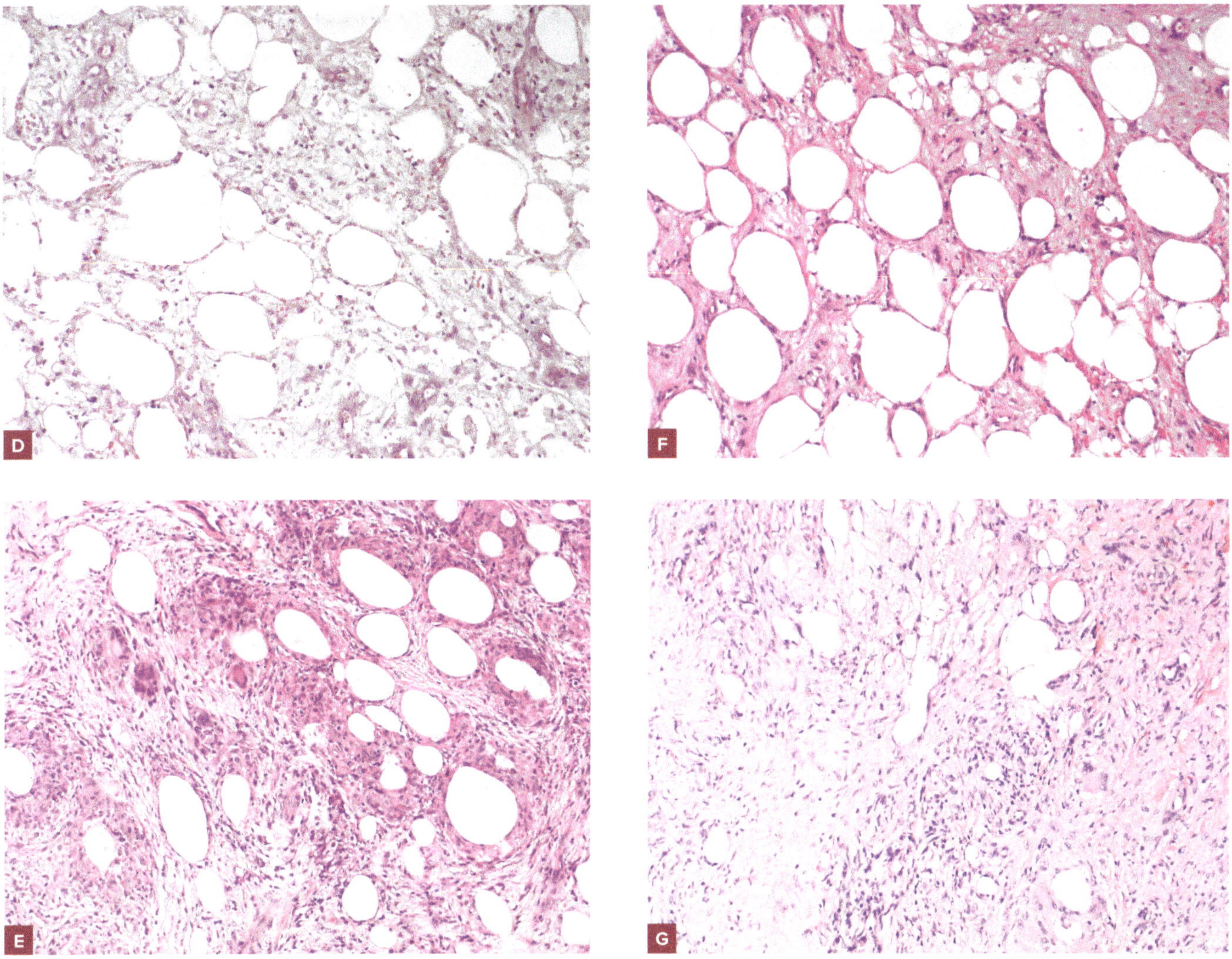

Lobular panniculitis. (A) Acute lobular panniculitis. The fat lobule shows prominent infiltration by neutrophils. These changes are nonspecific and may be associated with a wide variety of etiologies. **(B)** Acute lobular panniculitis. The adipocytes are separated by sheets of neutrophils. **(C)** Lobular panniculitis at a later stage of evolution and characterized by predominance of mononuclear cells infiltrating fat lobule. These changes represent the typical sequence of inflammation irrespective of etiology. **(D)** Lipidized macrophages diffusely infiltrate fat lobule. **(E)** Granulomatous inflammation involving fat lobules. **(F)** Later fibrosing stage of lobular panniculitis. Mononuclear and granulomatous infiltrates progressively subside and the fat lobule gradually undergoes fibrosis. **(G)** End-stage lobular panniculitis. The fat lobules are obliterated by fibrosis.

ANSWER 5-17:

1-A; 2-C; 3-D; 4-B; 5-H; 6-I; 7-E; 8-J; 9-K; 10-K; 11-N; 12-M; 13-L; 14-O; 15-G; 16-F

A basic understanding of the hair follicle and the hair cycle is needed to interpret scalp biopsies (Table 5-17A). The human hair follicle consists of a permanent upper segment, comprised of **infundibulum** and **isthmus**, and an impermanent lower segment, comprised of lower follicle (suprabulbar region) and **hair root** (hair bulb). The **infundibulum** is lined with keratinized skin surface epithelium (contains a granular layer) and ends at the entry of the sebaceous duct into the follicle. Many believe this portion of the hair follicle to simply be an invagination of the epidermis. The **isthmus** extends down from the sebaceous duct and ends at the **bulge** where the **arrector pili muscle** inserts into the follicle. It is lined by trichilemmal (**external root sheath**) and trichilemmal keratin (no granular layer). The lower segment surrounds a growing hair with **internal and external root sheaths**, hyaline membrane, and fibrous sheath, which are layers providing structural support of the hair shaft. The **hair bulb** consists of the **dermal papilla** surrounded by **hair matrix cells**. The **dermal papilla** is a stromal (spindle cell) structure that provides anchorage and signaling to the matrical cells to generate the growing hair. The dermal papilla and fibrous sheath are

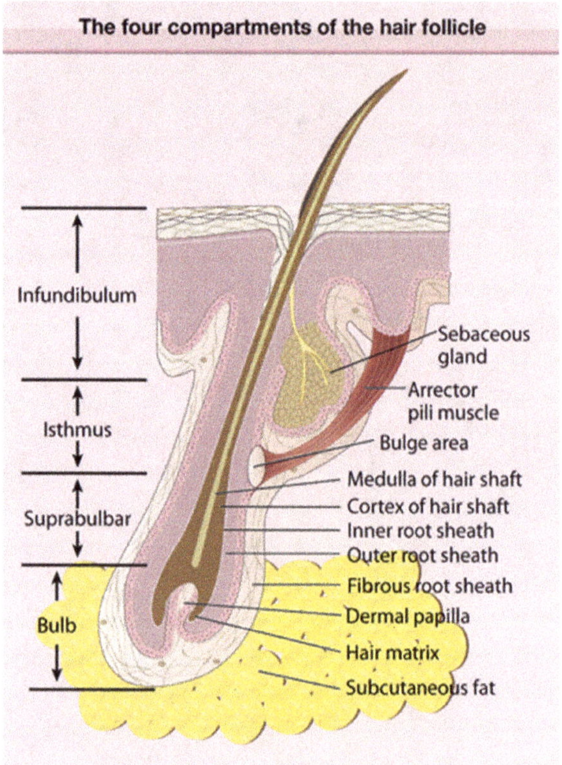

The hair follicle can be divided into four compartments: the infundibulum, isthmus, suprabulbar, and bulb regions. (Reproduced, with permission, from Goldsmith LA, Katz SI, Gilchrest BA, Paller AS, Leffell DJ, Wolff K, eds. *Fitzpatrick's Dermatology in General Medicine*. 8th ed. New York, NY: McGraw-Hill Education; 2012.)

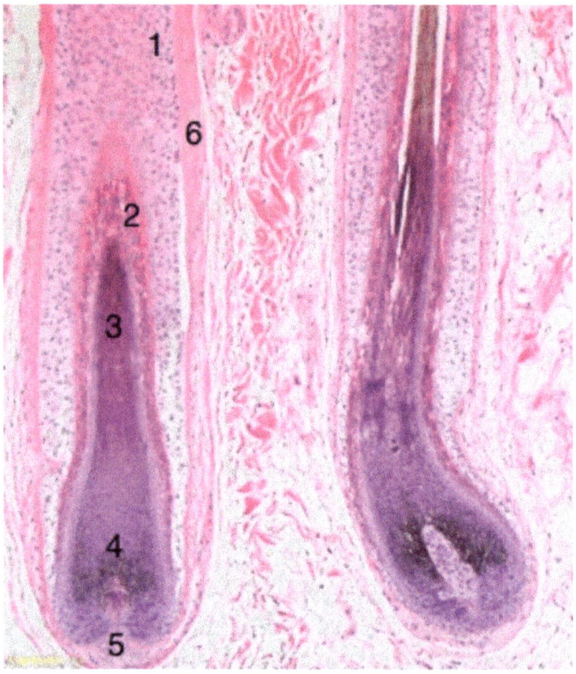

Normal hair microanatomy in anagen phase. (1) Outer root sheath epithelium. (2) Inner root sheath epithelium. (3) Hair shaft. (4) Hair matrix epithelium. (5) Dermal papilla. (6) Fibrous root sheath.

Table 5-17A. Description of Follicular Structures

Terminal (big hair)	Shaft diameter exceeds 0.03 mm and is thicker than its inner root sheath. A medullary cavity and/or pigment may be present. This definition includes "intermediate" hair shafts of diameter 0.03-0.06 mm.
Vellus (small)	Shaft diameter equals 0.03 mm or less and is thinner than its inner root sheath. Shaft lacks pigment and medullary cavity, and arrector pili muscle is usually not found. All hairs of this size are counted as *vellus* hairs, whether true vellus hairs or vellus-like hairs secondary to miniaturization from any cause.
Hair bulb	The hair bulb consists of root sheath, hair matrix, and dermal papilla.
Anagen hairs	Hair bulbs or hair shafts surrounded by inner and outer root sheaths. Only identifiable in lower follicle below bulge area.
Telogen hairs	Catagen hairs with trichilemmal apoptosis and thickened, corrugated, vitreous membrane, telogen hairs containing trichilemmal keratin, and telogen germinal units (resting telogen follicles containing basaloid cells). Only identifiable in lower follicle below bulge area.
Follicular stelae	Residual fibrous tracts or streamers representing the impermanent lower third of the hair follicle below the bulge area. Not counted as extra hair-forming structures because they are either downward prolongations of follicular structures that are counted in horizontal sections of the papillary dermis anyway or are permanently fibrosed follicles.
Follicular units	Hexagonal areas seen in horizontal sections at sebaceous duct level, surrounded by collagen and containing terminal and vellus hairs, sebaceous glands and ducts, and arrector pili muscles. Not counted as follicular structures, but if fibrosed, represent severe cicatricial alopecia.

Source: Data from Whiting DA: Chronic telogen effluvium: increased scalp hair shedding in middle-aged women, J Am Acad Dermatol. 1996 Dec;35(6):899-906 continuous. Human scalp hair follicles cycle continuously through periods of growth and rest. Asynchronous follicular growth produces an ever-changing mosaic pattern of growing follicles on the scalp. The growth or **anagen phase** lasts 2 to 7 years (1000 days on average) and the resting or **telogen phase** lasts 2 to 4 months (an average of 100 days). The appearance of a new anagen hair and the shedding of the telogen hair signal the end of telogen. Assuming an average of 100,000 hairs on the human scalp, with 5% to 10% in telogen at any one time, then up to 10,000 hairs are shed every 100 days, an average loss of 100 hairs per day.

Quick Fact

Terminal-to-Vellus Hair Ratios

- Normal terminal-vellus hair ratio is 7:1.
- Terminal-to-vellus hair ratio <4:1 suggests pathology.

Large hairs with a diameter exceeding 0.03 mm, growing more than 1 cm in length, often pigmented and medullated, are classified as ***terminal* hairs.** Small hairs with a diameter of less than 0.03 mm, growing less than 1 cm in length, and with no pigment or medullary cavity, are classified as ***vellus* hairs** (downy hairs or peach fuzz). Depigmented hairs less than 0.03 mm in diameter that have been miniaturized by **androgenetic alopecia, alopecia areata**, or any other cause can be classified as ***vellus-like* hairs**. The designation ***vellus hairs*** used in this chapter includes true vellus hairs and vellus-like hairs. Terminal hairs are rooted in the subcutaneous tissue, but vellus hairs are rooted in the dermis. **Terminal-to-vellus ratios** therefore denote the proportions of large hairs to small hairs, and a normal scalp averages **seven terminal hairs per vellus hair.** Less than four terminal hairs to one vellus denotes a relative increase in vellus hairs, perhaps indicating a miniaturization process.

Quick Fact

Anagen vs Telogen

- Normal anagen-to-telogen hair ratio should be in excess of 10:1.
- An anagen-to-telogen ratio of less than 9:1 suggests pathology.

The termination of **anagen** is signaled by the onset of **catagen**. **Catagen** is the short, 10- to 14-day intermediate phase between anagen and telogen that indicates the onset of **telogen**, since it irrevocably commits the growing follicle to a resting phase. In **catagen**, the hair shaft retracts upward, the hyaline basement membrane thickens and corrugates, and individual cell necrosis or apoptosis occurs in the outer root

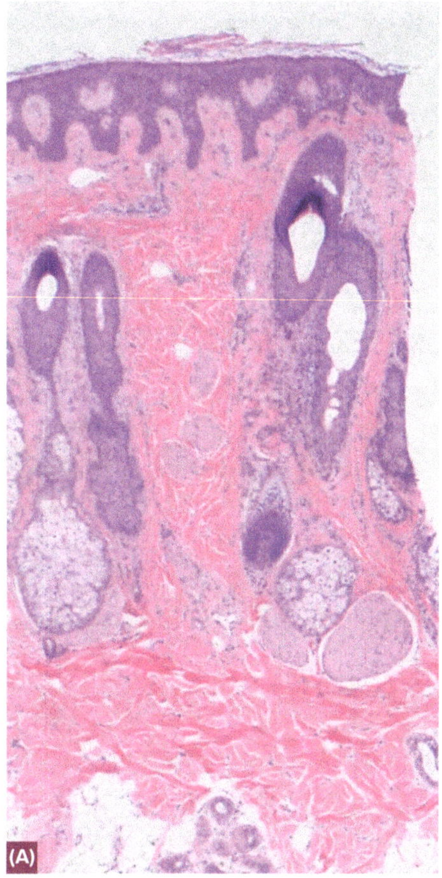

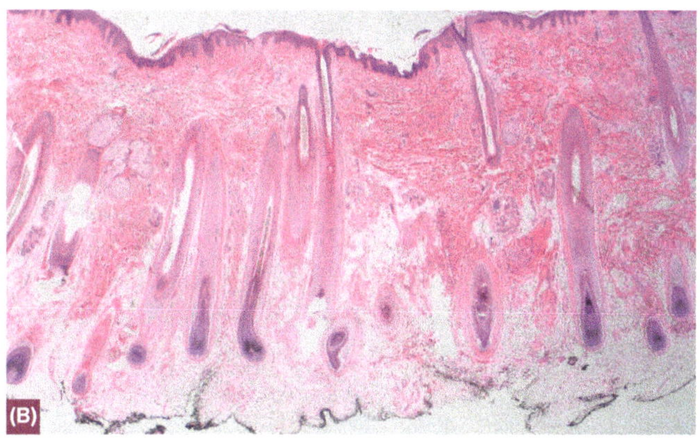

Normal hair microanatomy. (A) Vellus hairs, two of which are in involution. Note the overall small size and the hair bulb located within the dermis. **(B)** Terminal hairs. Note how the hairs are large and the bulbs are anchored in either the deep dermis or subcutis.

sheath. Involuting hairs exhibit a wrinkled outer root sheath with an undulating appearance. The hair displacement and volumetric reduction of root sheath lead to the progressive disappearance of the lower or impermanent part of the hair follicle so that in **telogen** the resting hair root is seen near the insertion of the arrector pili muscle, where the permanent follicle begins. A **telogen bulb** lacks pigment and structurally supportive internal root sheaths and is surrounded by outer

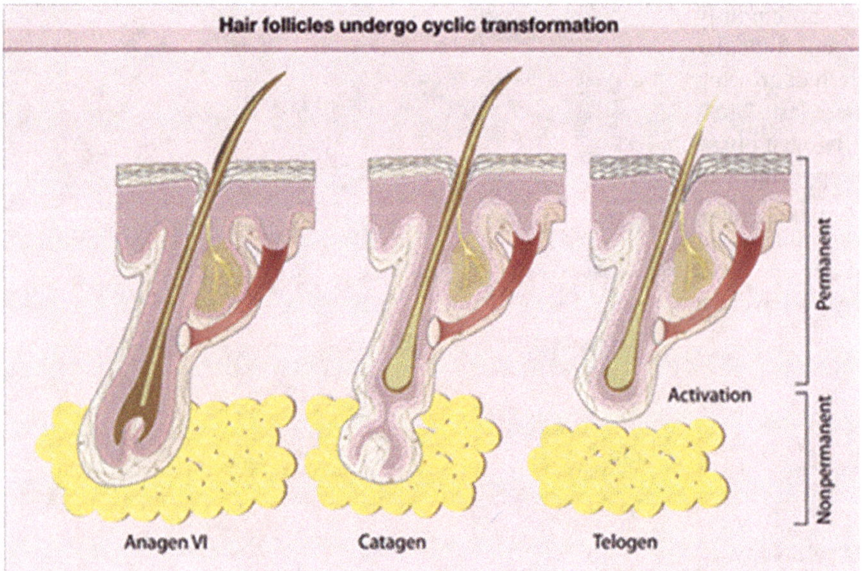

Hair follicles undergo cyclic transformation. Rapid growth (anagen) is followed by apoptosis-driven regression (catagen) and eventual resting period where the hair shaft is unanchored and easily falls out (telogen). (Reproduced, with permission, from Goldsmith LA, Katz SI, Gilchrest BA, Paller AS, Leffell DJ, Wolff K, eds. *Fitzpatrick's Dermatology in General Medicine*. 8th ed. New York, NY: McGraw-Hill Education; 2012.)

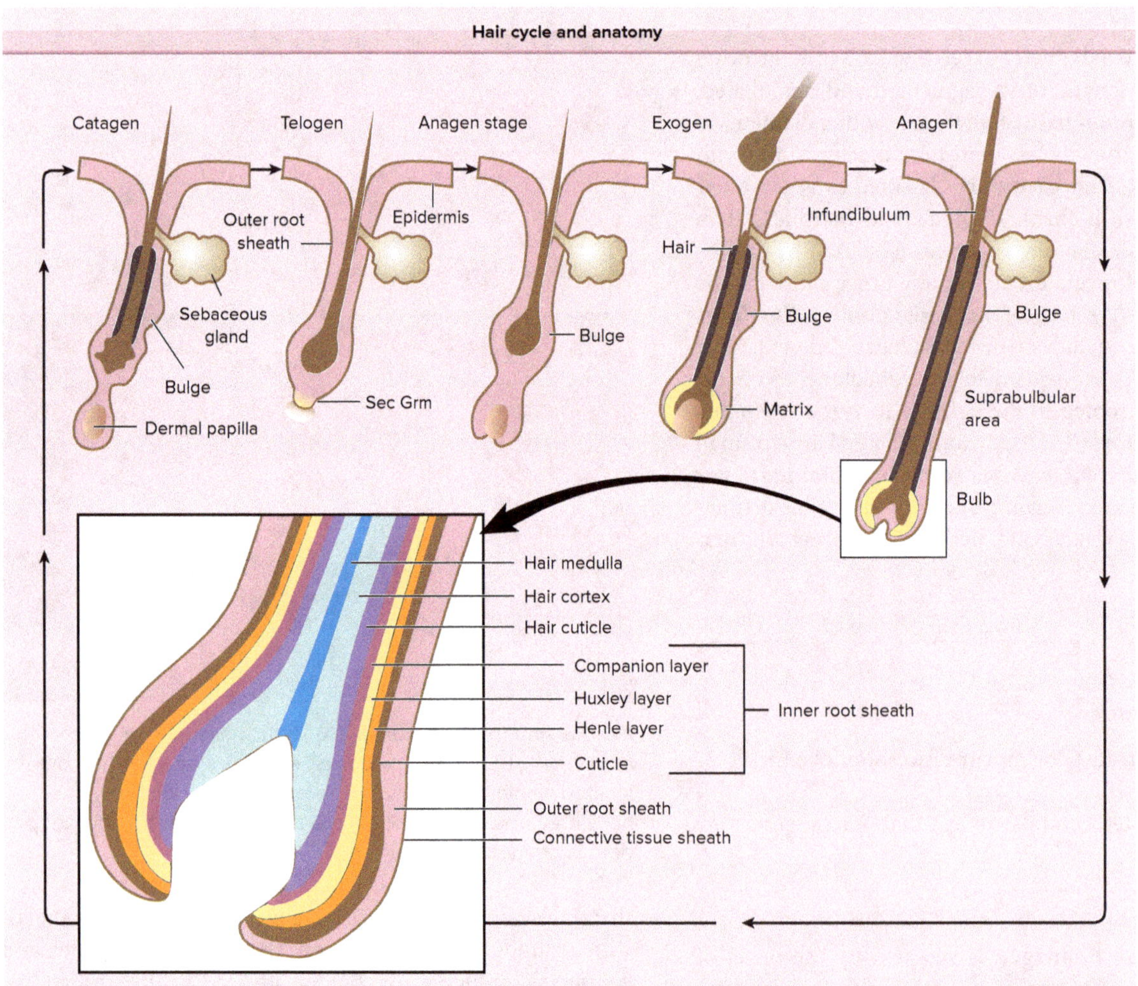

Hair cycle and anatomy. The hair follicle cycle consists of stages of rest (telogen), hair growth (anagen), follicle regression (catagen), and hair shedding (exogen). The entire lower epithelial structure is formed during anagen and regresses during catagen. The transient portion of the follicle consists of matrix cells in the bulb that generate seven different cell lineages, three in the hair shaft and four in the inner root sheath. B = bulge; E = epidermis; DP = dermal papilla; H = hair shaft; M = matrix; ORS = outer root sheath; S = sebaceous gland; Sec Grm = secondary germ. (Reproduced, with permission, from Goldsmith LA, Katz SI, Gilchrest BA, Paller AS, Leffell DJ, Wolff K, eds. *Fitzpatrick's Dermatology in General Medicine.* 8th ed. New York, NY: McGraw-Hill Education; 2012.)

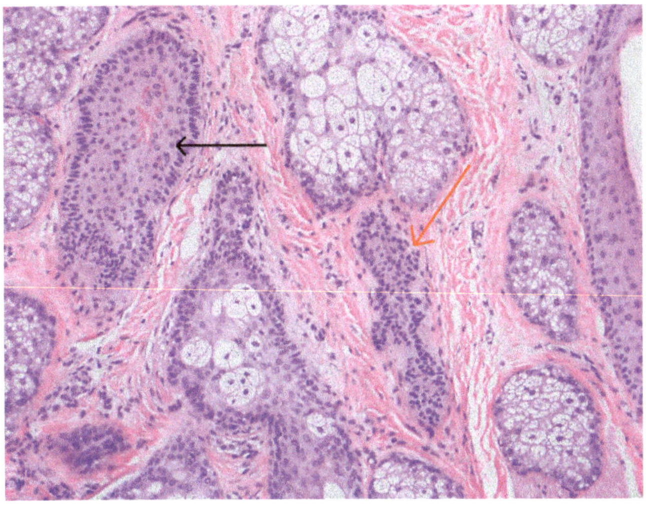

Involuting hairs. Late catagen hair (black arrow) and telogen hair (red arrow).

root sheath only. An angiofibrotic strand extending down from the permanent follicle, known variously as a ***fibrous tract, streamer***, or ***stela***, indicates the former position of the retracted follicle.

ANSWER 5-18: A.

Histopathologic examination is helpful for diagnostic purposes and for evaluating the capacity for future hair regrowth (**scarring alopecia vs nonscarring alopecia**). If possible, the biopsy should be taken from an area of active alopecia. For predictive purposes, an area of maximal hair loss can be sampled. Punch biopsies of the scalp are adequate substitutes for excisional biopsies. A sharp trephine of at least 4 mm diameter is used. The biopsy is angled in the direction of any emerging hairs and taken deep enough to include subcutaneous tissue and therefore hair bulbs. For additional information, two 4-mm punch biopsies are taken from comparable sites. One biopsy is bisected vertically parallel to the direction of any hairs, and both halves are placed in a cassette for formalin fixation and standard staining with hematoxylin and eosin (H&E). If necessary, one-half of the vertical biopsy can be reserved for immunofluorescence or any other purpose that requires different processing. The other 4-mm punch is carefully bisected horizontally (transversely) parallel to the epidermis and 1 to 1.5 mm below it. Both segments are embedded in paraffin side by side with the cut surfaces face down in the block. Sectioning will progress down toward the subcutaneous tissue in one-half and up toward the epidermis in the other. The pathologist who uses this technique and is familiar with the transverse anatomy of the hair follicle can then count the hair bulbs; terminal anagen, catagen, and telogen hairs; telogen germinal units; and stelae (fibrous tracts or streamers) in sections through reticular dermis. Terminal hairs, vellus hairs (which include true vellus hairs and miniaturized or vellus-like hairs), and **follicular units** can be counted in sections of the papillary dermis (Table 5-18A).

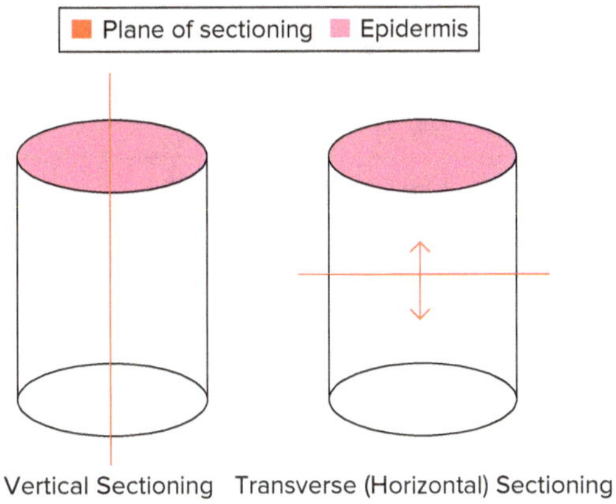

Biopsy processing techniques in the assessment of alopecia.

Table 5-18A. Normal Transverse Section Microanatomy: 4-mm Punch Biopsy

Follicular unit[a] composition	2-4 terminal follicles 2-4 vellus follicles Sebaceous lobules Arrector pili muscles
Follicular unit density	10-14 follicular units
Hair follicle[a] density	20-40 terminal follicles
Anagen follicles	90%±
Telogen follicles	10%±

[a]Follicular units include terminal and vellus hairs, sebaceous glands and ducts, and arrector pili muscles; hair follicle refers to terminal follicular units.

From these data, total follicular counts are derived with **anagen-telogen ratios, terminal-vellus hair ratios**, and **follicular concentration per square millimeter**. Comparative data for controls versus androgenetic alopecia, chronic telogen effluvium, alopecia areata, and trichotillomania are shown in Table 5-18B. For pathologists who rely only on vertical sections, multiple sections may be required to estimate the total follicular counts and the terminal-vellus and anagen-telogen ratios, which are helpful in the diagnosis of nonscarring alopecia. The presence or absence of inflammatory changes and fibrosis is also important in establishing the diagnosis.

The advantages of **transverse sections** in evaluating alopecia are many; however, familiarity with follicular microanatomy is essential for proper interpretation. **Transverse sections** allow for rapid detection of pathologic alteration of this normal follicular microanatomy, especially follicular density,

Table 5-18B. Horizontal Sections of 4-mm Scalp Biopsies Mean Follicular Counts in Differential Diagnosis of Alopecia: 1987-2007

DIAGNOSIS	NO. OF PATIENTS	AGE, YEARS	SEX (M:F)	TERMINAL (T) HAIRS	+	VELLUS (V) HAIRS	=	TOTAL HAIRS	T:V RATIO	ANAG: TELO %
Controls	22	43	1.4:1	35	+	5	=	40	7:1	93.5:6.5
Male pattern alopecia	305	34.4	M	20.9	+	14.7	=	35.6	1.4:1	80:20
Female pattern alopecia	1338	46.2	F	21.6	+	11.1	=	32.6	1.9:1	86:14
Diffuse alopecia	1061	48.4	1:36	32.8	+	4.4	=	37.2	7.4:1	89:11
Alopecia areata	834	31.9	1:2	16.4	+	12.9	=	29.3	1.3:1	56:44
Trichotillomania	85	20.2	1:5.5	27.5	+	6.6	=	34.1	4.2:1	65:35

Table 5-18C. Advantages and Disadvantages of Transverse Sections

Advantages
- More follicles per section
- Rapid, accurate assessment of follicle density, the number of terminal follicles, and the preservation or loss of normal follicular unit morphology
- Easy assessment of follicle and shaft diameters
- Most accurate anagen-telogen ratios

Disadvantages
- Must be familiar with scalp microanatomy in a different plane of sectioning
- Gross tissue specimen processing requires a different protocol
- The epidermis and dermal-epidermal interface are not easily evaluated in transverse sections

Limitations of Both Methods
- The 4- to 6-mm scalp biopsy is a small sample compared with the total scalp area
- Biopsy site selection is critical
- The specificity of the histopathologic diagnosis decreases with the duration and extent of follicular destruction

and provides for either quantitative or semiquantitative evaluation of numerous follicles and follicular units in one section. Evaluation of follicular density is more difficult using traditional **vertical sections** because multiple serial sections must be examined. However, gross tissue specimen processing for **transverse sections** requires a different protocol and many labs are not properly trained in this technique. Additionally, follicular unit morphology and its relation to inflammation are better assessed with **vertical sections**, especially since the dermal-epidermal junction cannot be readily visualized with **transverse sections**. In general, **transverse sections** are better in **nonscarring alopecias** where hair counts and various ratios are needed for diagnosis, whereas **vertical sections** are better for evaluating **scarring alopecias** and their associated inflammatory patterns (Table 5-18C).

ANSWER 5-19: B.

The biopsies in this case are processed using both vertical and transverse sections. The **vertical sections** reveal approximately five hairs in total. There are a strikingly increased number of small vellus-like hairs (four out of five). All of the hairs appear to be in anagen phase. There is essentially no inflammation within the dermis. A prominent follicular stela is present (fibrous streak/column extending from the subcutis into the dermis). The **transverse sections** confirm this increased vellus-to-terminal hair ratio. Additionally, the transverse sections reveal several hairs with sizes in between those of terminal and vellus hairs, known as miniaturization. This is a classic example of **androgenetic alopecia**. Androgenetic alopecia is the most common form of nonscarring alopecia (Table 5-19A). The terms ***scarring*** and ***nonscarring*** are firmly entrenched in the dermatologic lexicon and are helpful for classification and prognosis in many cases of alopecia. However, some of the traditionally designated nonscarring alopecias may eventuate in permanent follicular atrophy and hair loss. **Androgenetic alopecia, alopecia areata, traction alopecia,** and **trichotillomania** are examples of **nonscarring alopecia** that may progress to complete, permanent hair loss. Thus the terms ***scarring*** and ***nonscarring*** as they have been used historically do not always correlate with prognosis for hair regrowth. **Androgenetic alopecia,** or common baldness, affects at least 50% of the population by age 50 years in males and a decade later in females. The familiar pattern of fronto-parietal hair loss is due to a genetically determined end-organ sensitivity of the hairs on the crown to androgens.

Finer and shorter hairs replace the affected terminal hairs progressively. Androgenetic alopecia predominantly affects the top of the scalp in both sexes, with relative sparing of the back and sides. It is of dominant inheritance with variable penetrance. Hair thinning occurs in males at any time after puberty. It often begins with bitemporal hair recession followed by a circular patch of hair loss over the vertex and then thinning of the frontal hairline. In females, hair thinning also can begin after puberty, but an onset at between 25 and 35 years of age is more common, and many patients only present around menopause. Female-pattern alopecia causes diffuse thinning over the top of the scalp with an intact frontal hair margin and without total baldness. In females, severe bitemporal recession, vertex baldness, acne, hirsutism, and abnormal menses reflect significant hyperandrogenism, which needs investigation.

The histopathologic changes in **androgenetic alopecia** are similar in males and females and reflect the pathogenesis of the condition. The pathognomonic finding for androgenetic alopecia is **miniaturization** of **terminal hairs** to become **vellus hairs**; hence with shorter hair cycles, terminal hairs progressively become vellus-like. The hair roots retreat upward toward the epidermis so that many of the miniaturized hair bulbs are found in mid- or papillary dermis. Residual **follicular stelae** (fibrous tracts or streamers) extending from the subcutaneous tissue up the old follicular tract to the miniaturized hair mark the former position of the original terminal follicle. Thus the expected findings in **androgenetic alopecia** are decreased terminal hairs, increased follicular stelae, and increased vellus hairs. A varying number of intermediate hairs, with a shaft diameter less than the average 0.06-mm terminal hair diameter but more than the 0.03-mm vellus hair diameter, may be present; for simplicity, these intermediate hairs are classified as terminal hairs in follicular counts quoted in this chapter. The progressive reduction in duration of anagen, but not telogen, causes a relative increase in telogen hairs.

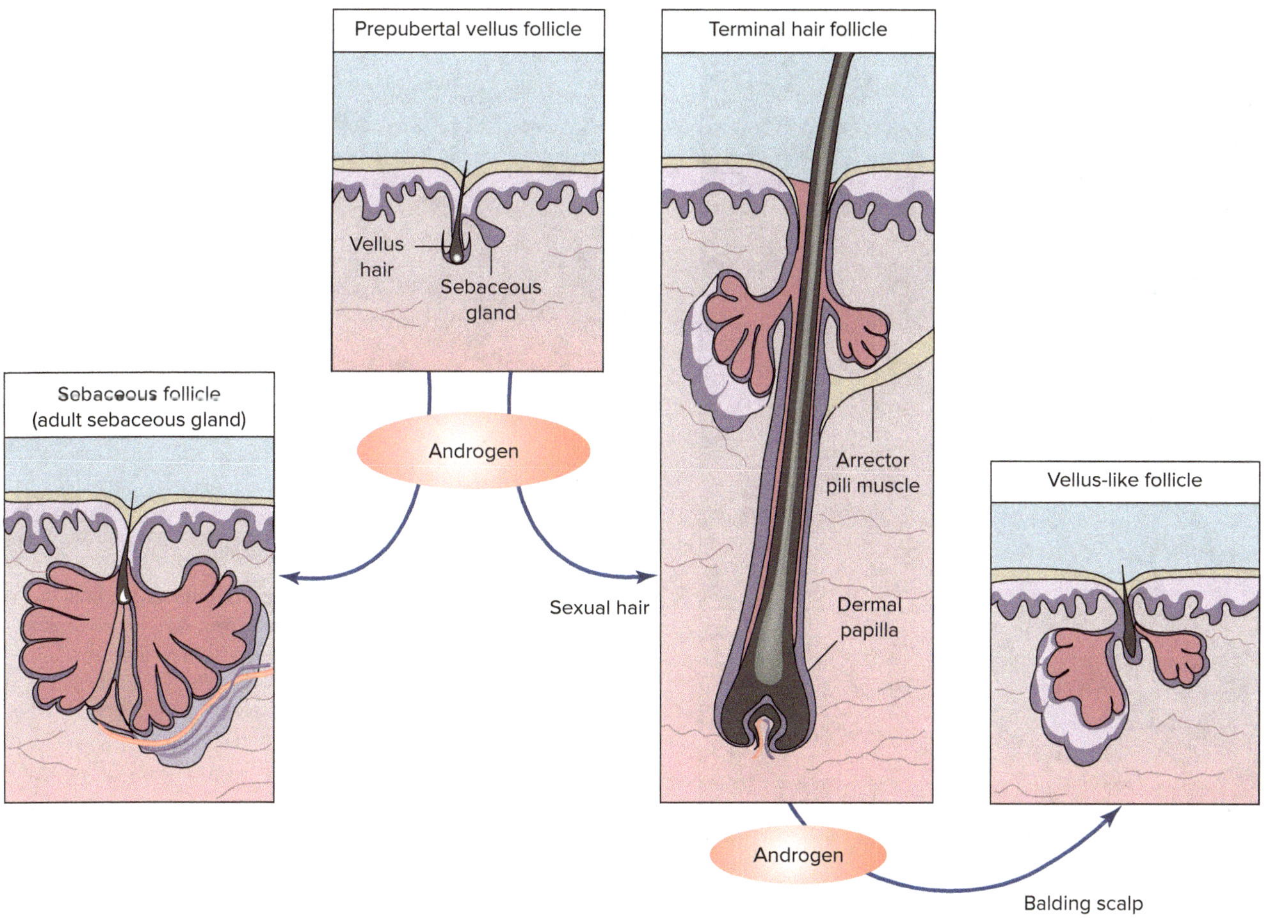

Androgenic effects on the pilosebaceous unit. In some hair-bearing areas, androgens stimulate sebaceous glands, and increased sebum may lead to acne. In other areas, vellus follicles respond to androgens and are converted to terminal follicles, leading to hirsutism. Under the influence of androgens, terminal hairs that were not previously dependent on androgens revert to a vellus form and balding results. (Reproduced with permission from Rosenfield RL: Clinical practice. Hirsutism, N Engl J Med. 2005 Dec 15;353(24):2578-2588.)

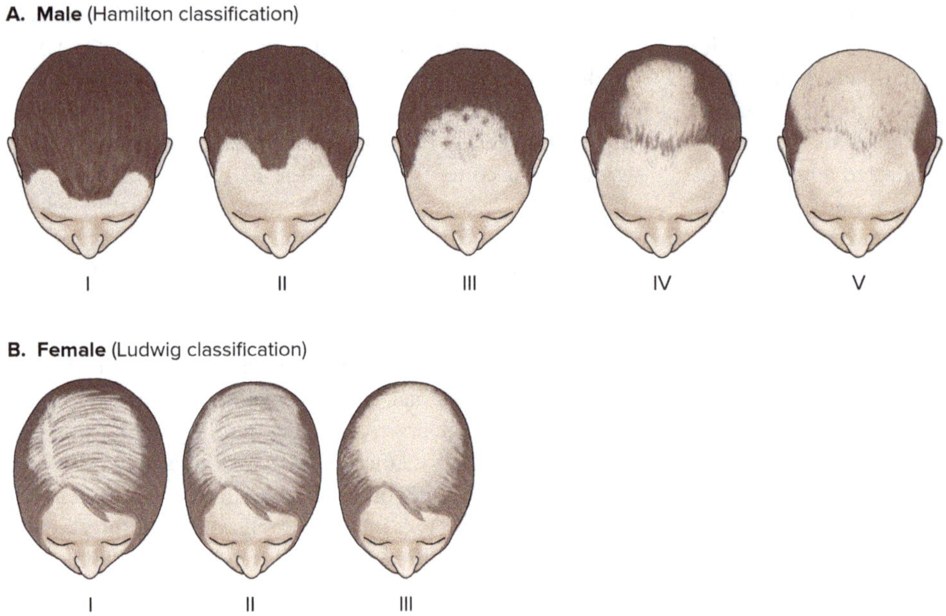

Androgenetic alopecia: patterns in men and women. (A) Hamilton classified the severity and pattern of hair loss in men into types I to V. **(B)** Ludwig classified hair loss in women into types I to III. (Reproduced, with permission, from Wolff K, Johnson RA, Saavedra AP. *Fitzpatrick's Color Atlas and Synopsis of Clinical Dermatology*. 7th ed. New York, NY: McGraw-Hill Education; 2013.)

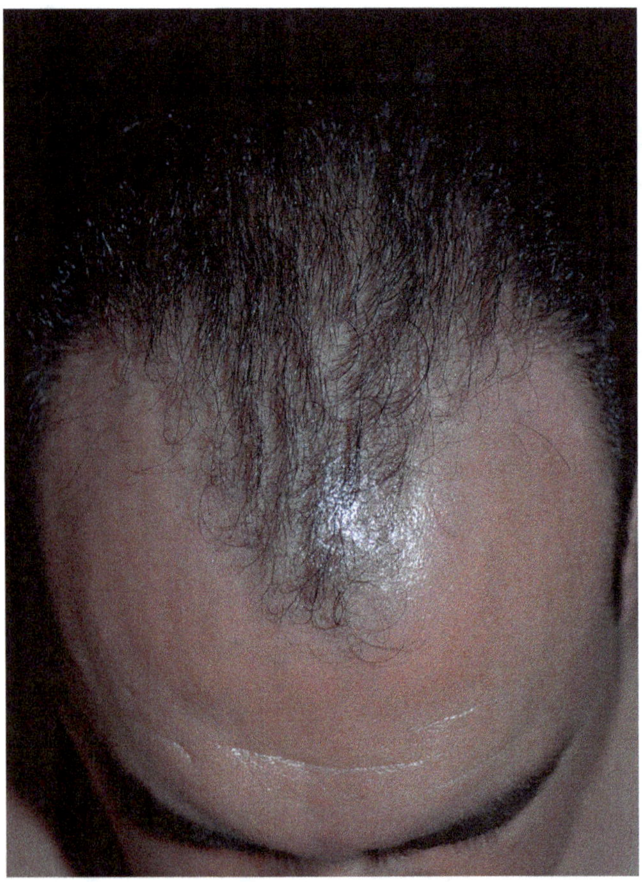

Pattern hair loss: male, Hamilton type III. A 46-year-old male with bitemporal recession of hairline and frontal thinning of hair. (Reproduced, with permission, from Wolff K, Johnson RA, Saavedra AP. *Fitzpatrick's Color Atlas and Synopsis of Clinical Dermatology*. 7th ed. New York, NY: McGraw-Hill Education; 2013.)

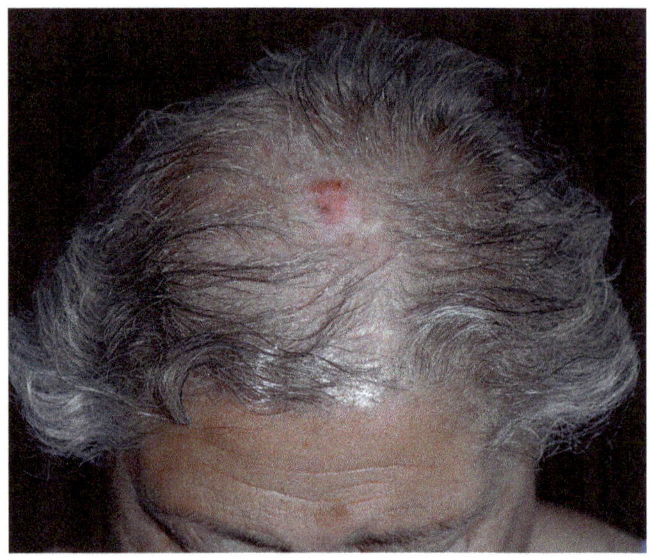

Pattern hair loss: female, Ludwig type III with basal cell carcinoma (BCC). A 67-year-old Greek female with advanced alopecia of the crown with BCC arising within it. (Reproduced, with permission, from Wolff K, Johnson RA, Saavedra AP. *Fitzpatrick's Color Atlas and Synopsis of Clinical Dermatology*. 7th ed. New York, NY: McGraw-Hill Education; 2013.)

Using **transverse sectioning**, the average follicular counts of a 4-mm punch biopsy of male pattern alopecia are 20.9 terminal hairs + 14.7 vellus hairs + 35.6 total hairs, with a terminal-vellus ratio of 1.4:1 and a ratio of 80% anagen to 20% telogen. The follicular counts in female pattern alopecia are 21.6 terminal hairs + 11.1 vellus hairs = 32.6 total hairs, with a terminal-vellus ratio of 1.9:1, and 86% anagen hairs and 14% telogen hairs. These counts contrast with those in normal controls, which are 35 terminal hairs + 5 vellus hairs + 40 total hairs, with a terminal-vellus ratio of 7:1 and a ratio of 93.5% anagen to 6.5% telogen.

In **vertical sections**, a terminal-vellus ratio of less than 4:1 indicates increased follicular miniaturization. A significant reduction in the total follicular count is seen in 10% of cases of androgenetic alopecia, indicating a decreased capacity for follicular regrowth in these cases. A mild perifollicular lymphohistiocytic infiltrate, usually around upper follicles, is present in one-third of cases of androgenetic alopecia, as it is in one-third of normal controls. A moderate perifollicular lymphohistiocytic infiltrate, perhaps with concentric layers of collagen deposition, is present in 40% of cases of androgenetic alopecia but only in 10% of normal controls. Occasional mast cells and even eosinophils are seen. Despite the inflammatory changes, sebaceous glands remain intact in androgenetic alopecia. Routine stains are adequate to evaluate androgenetic alopecia, but periodic acid–Schiff (PAS) stains apoptotic cells and vitreous layer to highlight catagen, and elastic stains highlight **Arao-Perkins bodies** (ie, elastin aggregates at the site of an antecedent follicular papilla) in **follicular stelae**; however, the elastic fiber network throughout the dermis will be intact, consistent with a nonscarring alopecia.

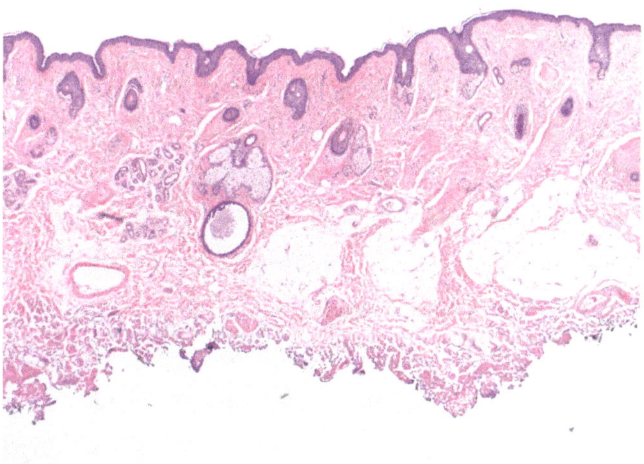

Androgenetic alopecia, vertical section. There is a marked predominance of small vellus hairs whose hair bulbs reside in the superficial to mid-dermis. The anagen to catagen/telogen ratio is within normal limits. Note the large (normal) sized sebaceous glands in relation to the small miniaturized hairs.

In regard to the differential diagnosis, **androgenetic alopecia** must be distinguished from **diffuse alopecia, alopecia areata,** and **trichotillomania.** Hair miniaturization does not occur in diffuse alopecia or in trichotillomania but is present in alopecia areata, often with a peribulbar lymphocytic infiltrate. Increased catagen hairs are present in trichotillomania and alopecia areata. **Trichomalacia** is characteristic of **traction alopecia** and **trichotillomania,** but can also occasionally occur in alopecia areata. It is absent in androgenetic alopecia.

Table 5-19A. Androgenetic Alopecia

Clinical Features
- Progressive miniaturization of hairs on crown, with relative sparing of hair on back and sides of scalp
- Male: onset from puberty to 50 years; marked bitemporal recession with balding of vertex
- Female: onset often one decade later than males; intact frontal hairline with diffuse thinning over crown

Histopathologic Features
- Increased miniaturized, vellus hairs
- Increased follicular stelae
- Decreased terminal hairs
- Increased telogen hairs
- Mild to moderate perifollicular lymphohistiocytic inflammation in 70% of cases
- Intact sebaceous glands

Differential Diagnosis
- Diffuse alopecia, especially telogen effluvium
- Diffuse alopecia areata
- Diffuse trichotillomania

ANSWER 5-20: A.

Diffuse alopecia implies generalized hair loss or shedding involving the back, sides, and top of the scalp (Table 5-20A). The underlying mechanism is often a **telogen effluvium.** Answer choices B, C, and D describe **androgenetic alopecia, alopecia areata,** and **trichotillomania,** respectively.

Headington has described five functional types of **telogen effluvium** based on changes occurring in different phases of the hair cycle. These consist of **immediate anagen release**

Table 5-20A. Causes of Diffuse Alopecia

Classic acute telogen effluvium	Nutritional causes
Chronic telogen effluvium	Malabsorption
Anagen effluvium	Renal failure
Drugs	Hepatic failure
Other chemicals	Systemic disease
Thyroid disorders	Miscellaneous causes
Iron deficiency	Idiopathic

Source: Data from Simpson NB: Diffuse alopecia: endocrine, metabolic, and chemical influences on the follicular cycle. In: Rook A, Dawber R, eds. *Diseases of the Hair and Scalp*. 2nd ed. Oxford: Blackwell Scientific; 1991: Chap 5, 136-166.

(postfebrile), **delayed anagen release** (postpartum), **short anagen cycle** (inability to grow long hair), **immediate telogen release** (minoxidil), and **delayed telogen release** (molting). Basically, an abnormal number of hairs go into the telogen phase and only fall out 1 to 3 months later when new anagen hairs grow in. The classic presentation of **acute telogen effluvium** occurs after childbirth, severe illness, operations, stress, crash diets, or various drugs (Table 5-20B). In **chronic telogen effluvium**, the trigger factor may be obscure, and any one of Headington's functional types can be implicated, although short anagen cycle may be the most common. **Anagen effluvium** is a severe condition, often resulting from antimitotic drugs (chemotherapy), in which large amounts of hair fall out within a few weeks of impaired DNA synthesis.

In an **acute phase of diffuse alopecia**, **hair pull tests** are positive from all over the scalp. In **telogen effluvium**, the extracted hairs show depigmented club roots and no root sheaths, reflective of telogen hairs. In **anagen effluvium**, extracted hairs show a proximal taper with a fracture (broken anagen hairs). When the antimitotic influence is removed, hairs grow back promptly with a distal taper due to reversal of the pencil-pointing process. A **hair pluck test** involves using forceps and forcibly removes a small bundle of hairs. The hairs should include both anagen and involuting (catagen and telogen) hairs. **Classic acute telogen effluvium** affecting any age group has an abrupt onset and a short course of 3 to 6 months. **Chronic telogen effluvium** can last from 6 months to 7 years or more, with an abrupt or gradual onset and a cyclic course. It is often idiopathic, usually affects middle-aged women, and usually does not cause severe baldness.

The histopathology of **telogen effluvium** is often similar to that seen in a normal scalp, except for the definite increase in telogen hairs seen during an active phase of hair loss. In vertical sections the terminal to vellus hair ratio is within normal limits (at least 4:1); however, the anagen to catagen/telogen ratio is less than 9:1. Follicular stelae may be seen in normal numbers.

Due to the smaller number of hairs present in vertical sections, transverse sections are beneficial in providing a better assessment hair counts and ratios. Follicular counts in

Table 5-20B. Drugs Causing Diffuse Alopecia

Allopurinol	Alpha receptor blockers	Amiodarone
Amoxapine	Amphetamine^{TE}	Androgens
ACE inhibitors^{TE}	Anticancer drugs^{AE}	Anticoagulants^{TE}
Anticonvulsants^{TE}	Antithyroid drugs^{TE}	Arsenicals^{TE}
Aspirin^{TE}	Azathioprine	Azulfidine
Beta-blockers^{TE}	Birth control drugs^{TE}	Bismuth^{AE}
Boric acid^{AE}	Bromocriptine^{TE}	Calcium channel blockers^{TE}
Carbamazepine	Cholesterol reducers^{TE}	Cimetidine^{TE}
Clomiphene	Clonidine	Colchicine^{AE}
Danazol^{TE}	Estrogen	Ethambutol
Ethionamide	Fluoxetine	Gentamycin
Gold^{AE}	Haloperidol	Histamine 2 blockers
Levodopa^{TE}	Lithium^{TE}	Mercury
Methyldopa	Methysergide^{TE}	Methyrapone^{TE}
Nitrofurantoin^{TE}	NSAIDs^{TE}	Omerprazole
Para amino salicylic acid	Penicillamine	Prazosin
Probenecid	Pyridostigimine bromidet^{TE}	Retinoids^{TE}
Retinol^{TE}	Salicylates^{TE}	Sulfasalazine
Terfenadine	Thallium salts^{AE}	Tricyclic antidepressants

^{AE}Cause of anagen effluvium.
^{TE}Cause of telogen effluvium.

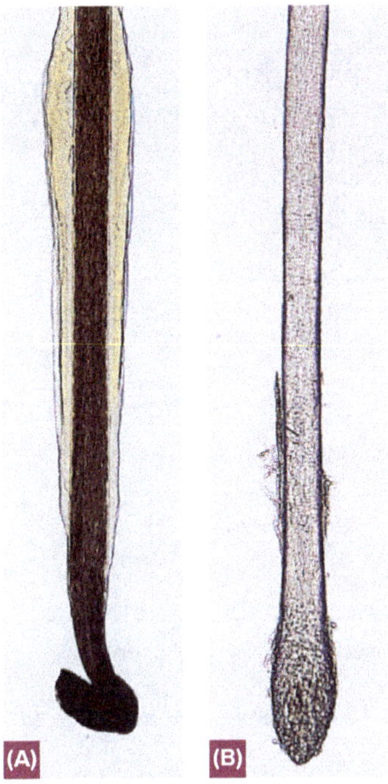

Hair mount from a pluck test. (A) Anagen: note the malleable proximal ends and retained inner root sheath surrounding the hair central shaft. **(B)** Telogen: club hairs without inner root sheath. (Reproduced, with permission, from Wolff K, Johnson RA, Saavedra AP. *Fitzpatrick's Color Atlas and Synopsis of Clinical Dermatology.* 7th ed. New York, NY: McGraw-Hill Education; 2013.)

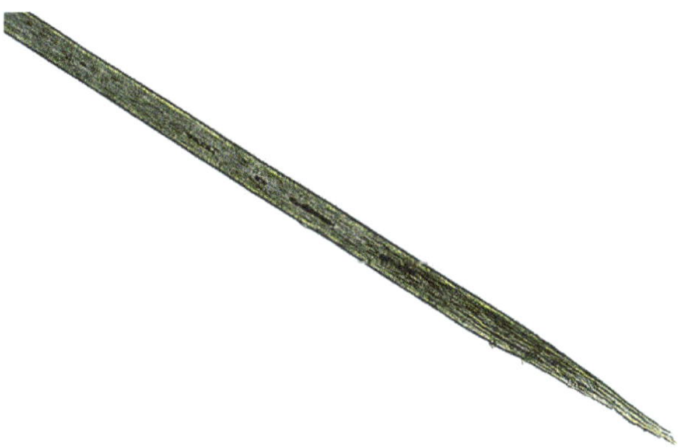

Anagen effluvium, pluck test. The broken-off hair shaft shows proximal tapering adjacent to the fracture.

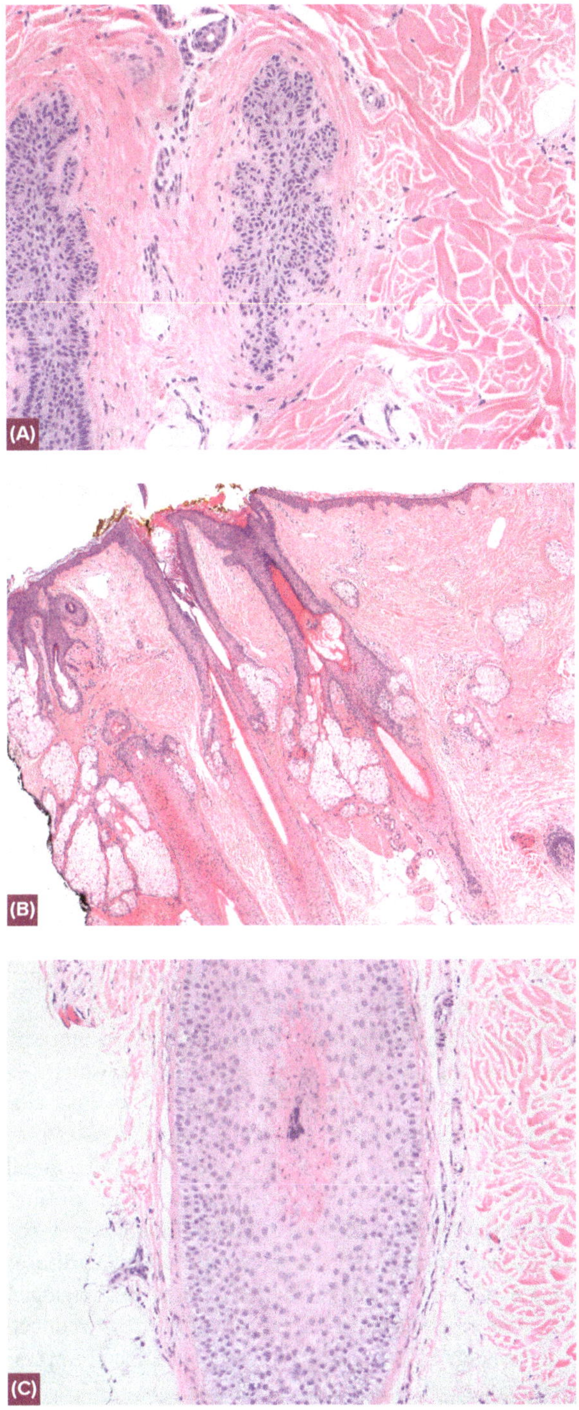

Acute telogen effluvium, vertical section. (A) Note the two telogen hairs with wrinkled outer root sheath epithelium. **(B)(C)** Catagen hair with disintegration of the inner root sheath and apoptosis of the outer root sheath keratinocytes.

transverse (horizontal) sections of a 4-mm punch biopsy of the crown in chronic telogen effluvium average 32.8 terminal hairs + 4.4 vellus hairs = 37.2 total hairs, with a terminal-vellus ratio of 7:1 and a ratio of 89% anagen to 11% telogen. These findings are the same as in normal controls, except that the 11% telogen hairs exceed the 6.5% telogen hairs found in normal individuals. The telogen count can increase to 20% to 30% or higher in active phases of telogen effluvium. Inflammatory changes are similar to controls in that mild perifollicular lymphohistiocytic infiltration occurs in one-third and moderate infiltration in 10% of cases of telogen effluvium. Normal numbers of follicular stelae are found.

The diffuse alopecia caused by hypothyroidism, other systemic diseases, and many drugs and chemicals results from a **telogen effluvium** and shows a similar histology. **Anagen effluvium** involves 90% of scalp hairs in anagen. The diagnosis is usually simple, since there is a clear history of the drug or influence that interferes with DNA synthesis. Examination

Table 5-20C. Histopathologic Features of Nonscarring Alopecias

	FOLLICULAR LOSS	TERMINAL-VELLUS RATIO	ANAGEN-TELOGEN RATIO	PERIFOLLICULAR LYMPHOID INFILTRATES	PERIBULBAR LYMPHOID INFILTRATES	TRICHOMALACIA
Congenital hypotrichosis	Moderate	NA	Large decrease	Usually absent	Absent	Absent
Congenital triangular alopecia	Moderate	Decreased	Large decrease	Usually absent	Absent	Absent
Androgenetic alopecia	Mild	Decreased	Slight decrease	70%	Absent	Absent
Alopecia areata	Mild	Decreased	Moderate decrease	Usually absent	Present	Absent
Diffuse alopecia (telogen effluvium)	None	Normal	Slight decrease	40%	Absent	Absent
Trichotillomania	None	Normal	Large decrease	Usually absent	Absent	Often present
Traction alopecia	None	Normal	Large decrease	Usually absent	Absent	Often absent

of plucked hairs is diagnostic, so biopsies are usually not indicated, except in cases of persistent hair loss following chemotherapy. The proximal tapering of a plucked hair in anagen effluvium is characteristic.

In regard to the differential diagnosis, diffuse alopecia usually can be diagnosed on clinical grounds but sometimes is confused with female **androgenetic alopecia, diffuse alopecia areata,** or **congenital hypotrichosis**, and biopsies may be necessary (Table 5-20C). There is no reduction in terminal hair numbers in diffuse alopecia (telogen effluvium or anagen effluvium). However, there is a definite reduction in the terminal-to-vellus hair ratio in androgenetic alopecia, diffuses alopecia areata, and congenital hypotrichosis. Both telogen effluvium and alopecia areata are characterized by reduced anagen-to-telogen hair ratios; however, peribulbar lymphocytes are typically present in alopecia areata.

ANSWER 5-21: E.

The biopsy reveals an increased number of involuting hairs with wrinkled outer root sheath epithelium and lymphocytic infiltrates surrounding the hair bulbs. Lymphocytic infiltrates are also present within follicular stelae (upper right corner). The findings are consistent with **alopecia areata (AA)** (Table 5-21A). **Alopecia areata** typically presents with patchy hair loss; however, rare diffuse presentations can occur. It is not

Table 5-21A. Alopecia Areata

Clinical Features
- Periodic attacks of circumscribed patches of hair loss
- Unpredictable course: patches may regrow or progress to confluent patches, alopecia totalis, or alopecia universalis

Histopathologic Features
- Peribulbar and intrabulbar mononuclear cell infiltrate
- Degenerative changes in hair matrix
- Decreased numbers of terminal anagen hairs
- Increased numbers of terminal catagen and telogen hairs
- Increased numbers of follicular stelae
- Increased numbers of miniaturized vellus hairs
- Pigment incontinence of hair bulbs and follicular stelae

Differential Diagnosis
- Other causes of patchy alopecia include tinea capitis, trichotillomania, traction and pressure alopecia, loose anagen syndrome, secondary syphilis, congenital triangular alopecia, familial focal alopecia, aplasia cutis, pseudopelade, tick-bite alopecia, etc.

uncommon and may affect 1.7% of Americans by age 50. The etiology of alopecia areata is unknown, and many believe it to be an autoimmune disease. Helper T cells are consistently found in the predominately lymphocytic infiltrate around affected hair bulbs. A family history is present in 20% of cases. Recent studies have shown the importance of the HLA class II antigen DQ3, DR4, and DR11 genes in susceptibility to alopecia areata and of DRW52A in resistance to the condition. Longstanding **alopecia totalis** or **alopecia universalis** patients have unique associations with HLA antigens DR4, DR11, and DQ7. Trigger factors include seasonal variation, emotional stress, and infections. Clinically, the initial patch of alopecia areata on the scalp is often barely noticeable, but it may enlarge, and further patches may appear. "Exclamation point" hairs at the spreading margin of lesions indicate disease activity.

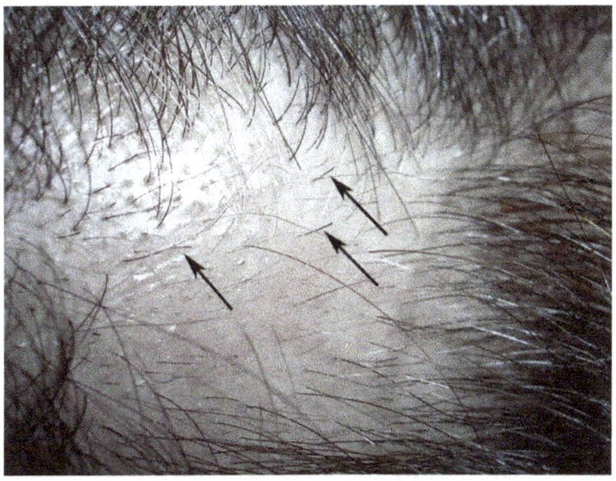

Exclamation point hairs (*arrows*) can be seen in this case of alopecia areata. The hair is narrow at the base, short and wide at the end. (Reproduced, with permission, from Usatine RP, Smith MA, Mayeaux EJ Jr, Chumley HS, eds. *Color Atlas of Family Medicine*. 2nd ed. New York, NY: McGraw-Hill Education; 2012.)

Specific forms of alopecia areata include **ophiasis**, a persistent band-like loss of hair; diffuse alopecia areata including an acute form labeled alopecia areata incognito; and reticular alopecia areata with multiple patches of hair loss. In some cases the alopecia primarily involves beard, eyebrow, eyelash, and rarely, body hair. In the most severe cases all scalp (**alopecia totalis**) and body (**alopecia universalis**) hair is lost. Alopecia areata is more common in females, except in children. Its course is unpredictable.

Microscopically, in the active stage of **alopecia areata** there is a characteristic cluster of mononuclear cells around follicular bulbs that has been likened to a **"swarm of bees."** The infiltrate in alopecia areata consists primarily of CD4 lymphocytes and Langerhans cells, but some eosinophils and plasma cells may be seen. This lymphocytic infiltrate can invade the hair bulb and cause pigment incontinence. The infiltrate can also surround the adjacent suprabulbar portion of the hair shaft. Inflammatory cells invading bulbar epithelium can cause inter- and intracellular edema; nuclear pyknosis; apoptosis of matrix and outer sheath keratinocytes, melanocytes, Langerhans cells, and

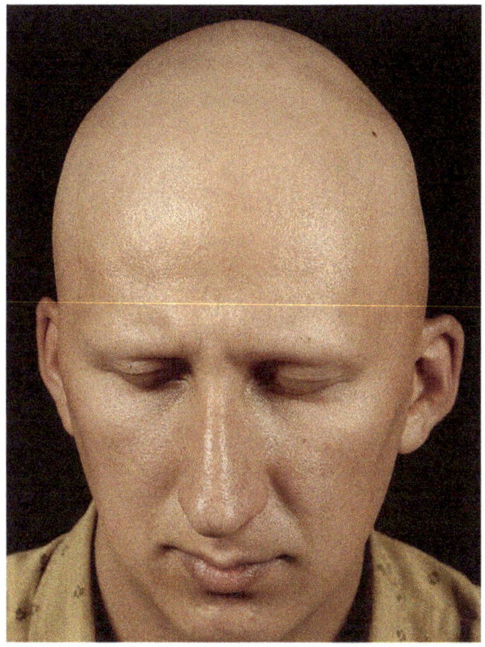

Alopecia areata universalis (AAU). This patient has lost all scalp hair (alopecia totalis), eyebrows, eyelashes, beard, and all body hair (alopecia universalis) and has dystrophic ("hammered brass") nails. (Reproduced, with permission, from Wolff K, Johnson RA, Saavedra AP. *Fitzpatrick's Color Atlas and Synopsis of Clinical Dermatology.* 7th ed. New York, NY: McGraw-Hill Education; 2013.)

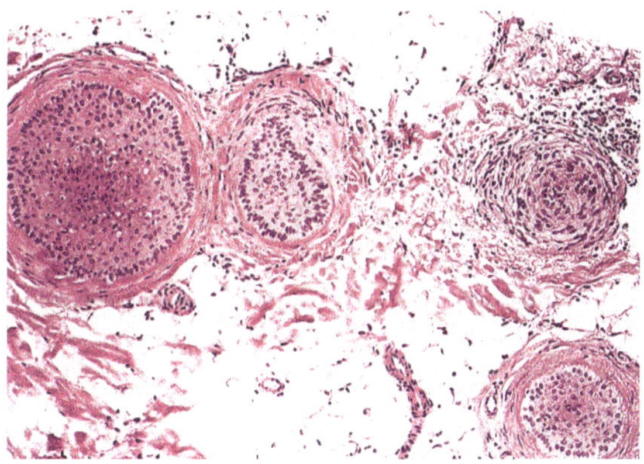

Alopecia areata. Transverse section, reticular dermis. One catagen hair (left lateral margin), one follicular stela infiltrated by lymphocytes (right lateral margin), and one telogen hair with wrinkled outer root sheath epithelium is visible.

dermal dendritic cells; and necrosis and microvesicle formation in the upper bulb above the dermal papilla.

In the initial stages the disease usually involves terminal hairs, but later on miniaturized vellus-like hairs are also involved. As the disease progresses, follicular stelae infiltrated with lymphocytes and melanin pigment are common. The inflammatory process involves anagen hairs that become either tapered or dystrophic, sometimes progressing to **trichomalacia**. More commonly the lymphocytic infiltrate converts the anagen hair into catagen and telogen phases. The increased

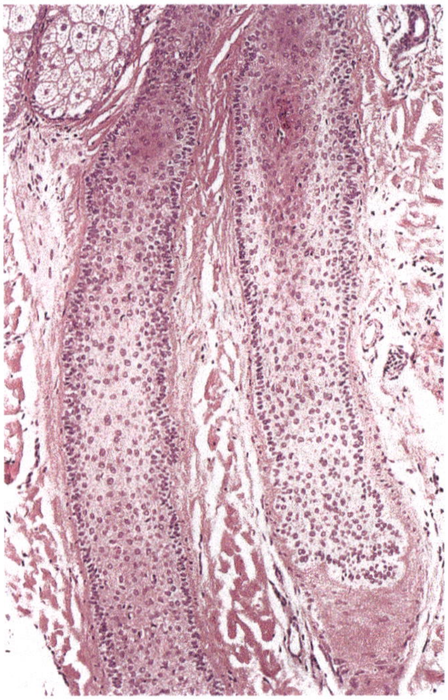

Alopecia areata. Vertical section. Two catagen hairs are present showing a thickened vitreous membrane (fibrous sheath) and central apoptotic cells. Note how no inflammation is present in the more superficial portions of the hair follicle.

number of catagen hairs that results is equaled or exceeded only by the number of catagen hairs found in **trichotillomania.**

Persistent disease results in **miniaturization** of hairs with decreased terminal hairs and increased vellus hairs and follicular stelae. The average follicular count found in transverse (horizontal) sections of a 4-mm punch biopsy consists of 16.4 terminal hairs + 12.9 vellus hairs = 29.3 total hairs, a terminal-vellus ratio of 1.3:1, and 56% of terminal hairs in anagen and 44% in telogen. The reduction in total hairs and the increase in vellus and telogen hairs contrast with normal controls.

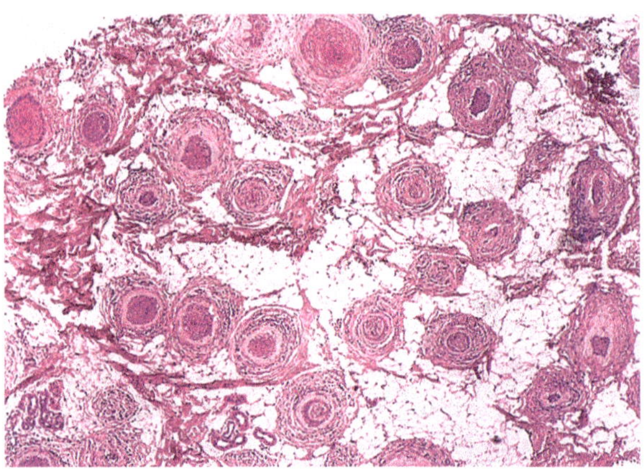

Alopecia areata. Transverse section, reticular dermis. Several hair bulbs surrounded by lymphocytes, a large number of catagen hairs surrounded by thickened vitreous membranes and lymphocytes, several telogen germinal units, and some follicular stelae infiltrated by lymphocytes are visible.

Contrary to general belief, there is a definite follicular dropout with fibrosis in about 10% of patients with a long history of attacks of alopecia areata. Peribulbar lymphocytic infiltration may not be prominent between acute attacks. Additionally, many dermatologists initially treat these areas of alopecia with injections of steroids before performing a biopsy. Therefore, the inflammatory **"swarm of bees"** infiltrate may be absent in the sections. In these cases, the most helpful findings are decreased terminal-to-vellus hair and anagen-to-catagen/telogen ratios, combined with postinflammatory melanophages within follicular stelae and adjacent hair bulb stroma. The presence of **trichomalacia** and foreign-body tissue reaction may be further diagnostic pointers.

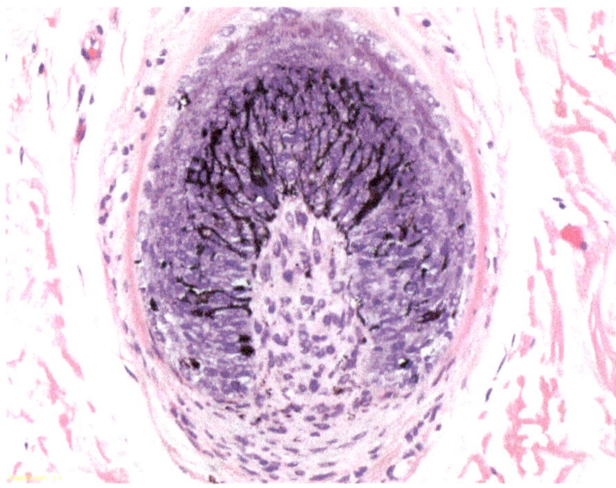

Alopecia areata treated with steroid injection. Note the absence of inflammation; however, scattered melanophages are present within the dermal papilla and adjacent peribulbar stroma.

Quick Fact

Alopecia Areata

- Peribulbar lymphocytic infiltrates
- Decreased anagen-to-telogen ratio
- Decreased terminal-to-vellus hair ratio
- Trichomalacia
- Pigmentary incontinence in deep dermis or subcutis

In regard to the differential diagnosis, causes of patchy alopecia that may be confused with alopecia areata include **tinea capitis, trichotillomania, traction alopecia, pressure alopecia, congenital triangular alopecia, loose anagen syndrome, familial focal alopecia, secondary syphilis, tick-bite alopecia,** and **scarring alopecia** such as **lichen planopilaris, aplasia cutis**, and **pseudopelade**. These usually can be distinguished by the history and clinical appearance, but biopsies may be necessary. **Tinea capitis** shows chronic folliculitis, often granulomatous, with intrafollicular neutrophils; fungal spores and hyphae may still be present. Inflammation and miniaturized hairs are lacking in

trichotillomania and other forms of traumatic alopecia, but involuting catagen/telogen hairs occur. Inflammation is absent in **congenital triangular alopecia** and **loose anagen syndrome** and in **familial focal alopecia**, in which a marked increase of telogen germinal units with no scarring indicates telogen arrest; terminal hairs are reduced in **congenital triangular alopecia** but not in **loose anagen syndrome.** Plasma cells may be sparse or plentiful in the diffuse inflammation of **secondary syphilis. Cicatricial (scarring) alopecia** is characterized by permanent destruction of hair follicles with replacement by fibrosis with result disrupted elastic fiber networks. Follicles are undamaged in **tick-bite alopecia**, which is a localized **telogen effluvium** caused by an anticoagulant in tick saliva.

ANSWER 5-22: D.

The vertical section of this patient's biopsy demonstrates one terminal hair (left), one telogen hair (right), and two follicular stelae projecting into the subcutaneous tissue. Another telogen hair is seen in the middle dermis and one follicular infundibulum shows trichomalacia with a pigment cast (upper left corner). There is an absence of inflammatory cells. **Trichotillomania** is an abnormal compulsion to pull out hair (Table 5-22A). It affects more children than adults and after age 6 years is more common in females. Two polar forms of **trichotillomania** occur: The **juvenile type** peaks between 2 and 6 years of age, and the **adult type** peaks between 11 and 17 years of age. In children, the habit may develop subconsciously and replace thumb sucking or represent an effort to gain attention. Mental retardation or severe psychological disturbances are more common in adults. Clinically, trichotillomania presents with one or more patches of hair thinning contrasted with complete hair loss seen in alopecia areata, etc. The patches are characterized by irregular stubble due to hair breakage at different times. In severe patches, only newly growing anagen hairs remain. The underlying scalp is usually normal. Trichotillomania can involve eyebrows and lashes. The onset is often sudden, and the course is fluctuating and prolonged.

Table 5-22A. Trichotillomania

Clinical Features
Recurrent attacks of patchy hair loss—chronic course
Affected hairs broken off at different lengths
Underlying scalp usually normal
Histopathologic Features
Normal follicular counts with normal terminal:vellus ratio
Marked increase in catagen and telogen hairs
Follicular damage may be present
Follicles may contain pigmented casts
Trichomalacia can occur
Inflammatory changes usually absent
Differential Diagnosis
Other causes of patchy alopecia include alopecia areata, tinea capitis, loose anagen syndrome, traction and pressure alopecia, secondary syphilis, tick-bite alopecia, aplasia cutis, congenital triangular alopecia, familial focal alopecia, pseudopelade, etc.

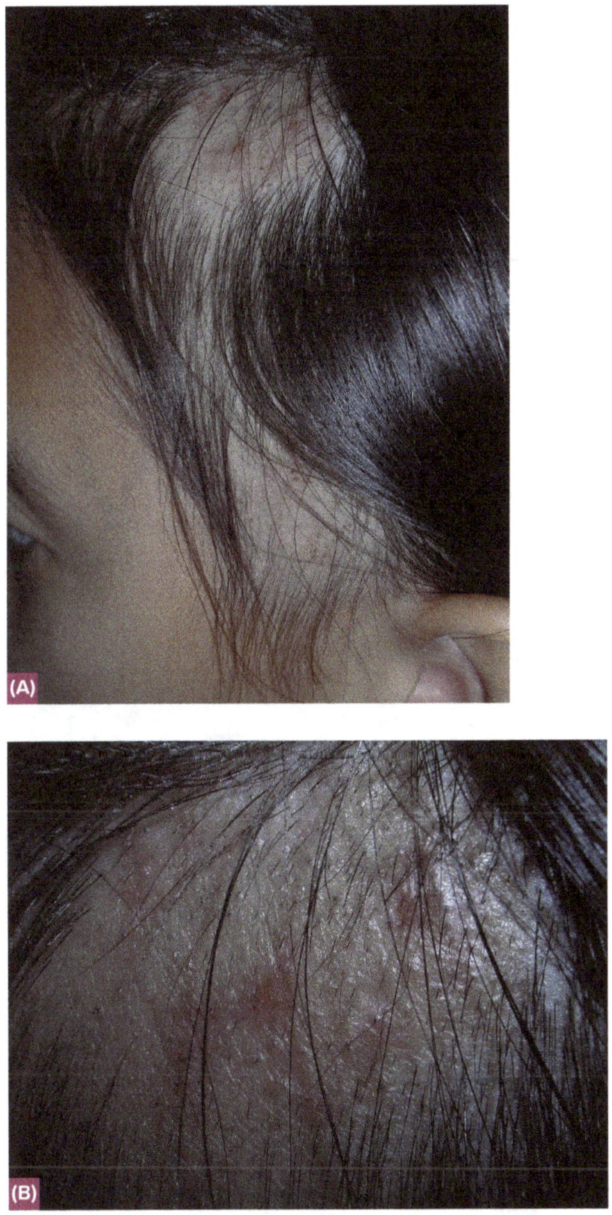

Trichotillomania. (A) 12-year-old girl undergoing much stress because of conflict in her family. **(B)** Close-up of trichotillomania showing broken hairs, black dots, and excoriations. (Reproduced, with permission, from Usatine RP, Smith MA, Mayeaux EJ Jr, Chumley HS, eds. *Color Atlas of Family Medicine.* 2nd ed. New York, NY: McGraw-Hill Education; 2012.)

Microscopically, normal numbers of hair follicles are present, although some may be distorted by hair shaft avulsion and show perifollicular shearing and hemorrhages. Follicular plugging and pigment casts are common, but true **trichomalacia**, or softened, twisted hair, is less frequent. Hair plucking/trauma

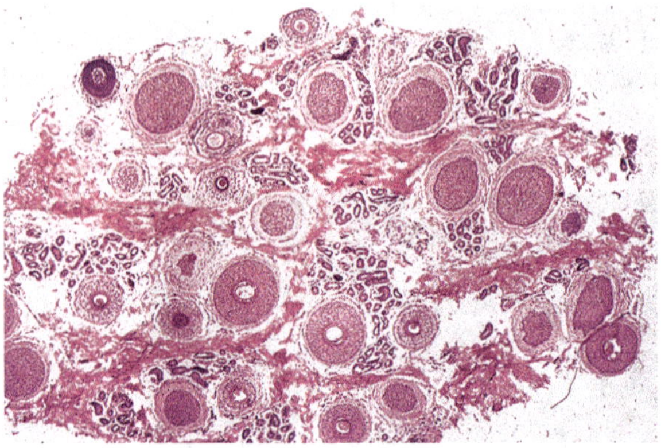

Trichotillomania. Transverse section, reticular dermis. One hair bulb, some terminal hairs, many catagen hairs, a telogen hair, and a telogen germinal unit are visible.

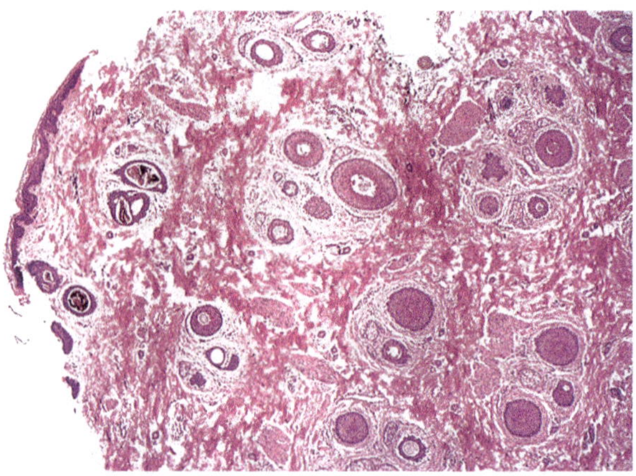

Trichotillomania. Transverse section, papillary dermis. Terminal hairs, telogen hairs, telogen germinal units, and vellus hairs are visible. Several follicular infundibula show pigment casts or trichomalacia (left). There is no inflammation.

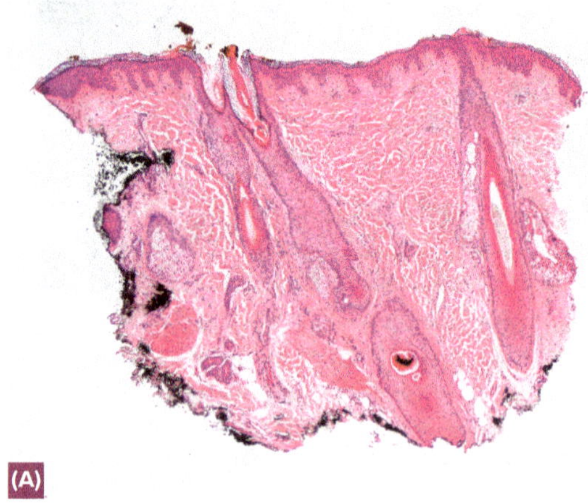

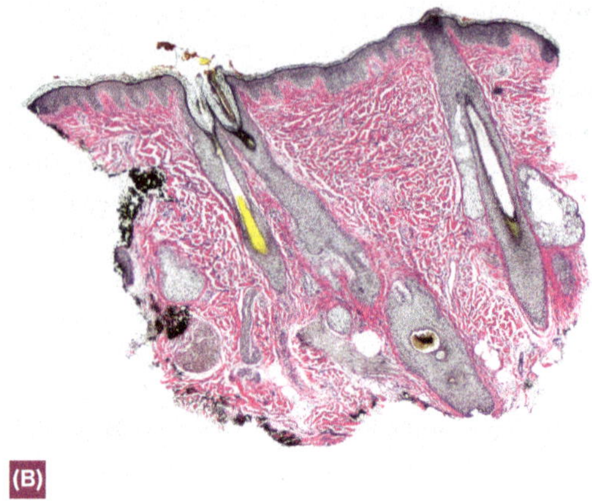

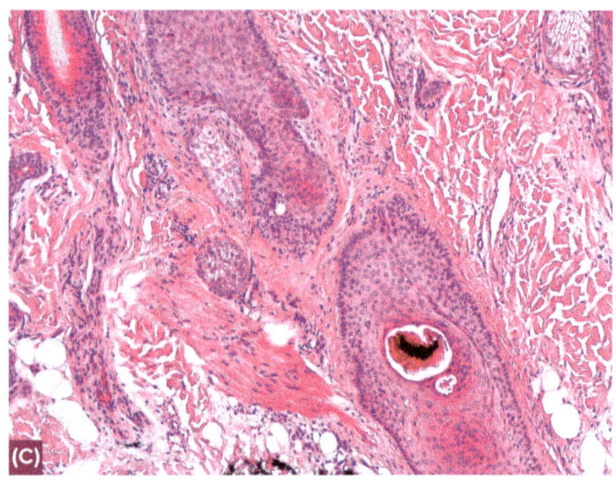

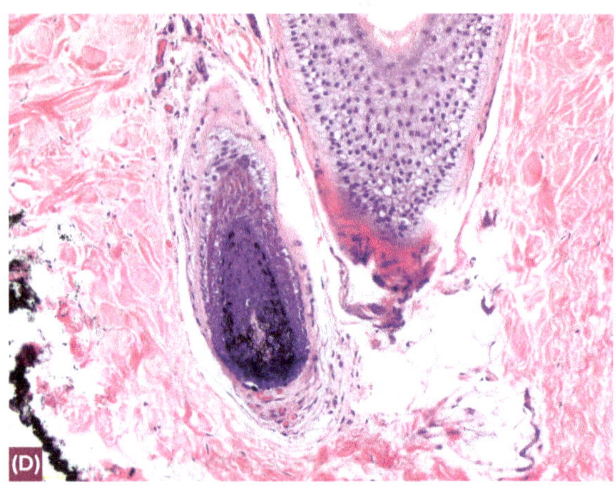

Trichotillomania. Vertical section. (A) There is a marked increase in involuting hairs, many of which exhibit distorted size and shape. Also note a slight reduction in terminal hairs. **(B)** EVG (elastic) stain reveals an intact elastic fiber network, consistent with a nonscarring process. **(C)** A dark brown pigment cast is present within a follicular lumen. **(D)** Note the hemorrhage surrounding the fibrous sheath and the congested vessels. These findings are consistent with trauma.

induces hair involution (**conversion to telogen**), accounting for the high catagen and telogen counts seen in trichotillomania. **Miniaturized** hairs are not typically seen, although true vellus hairs persist, because they are too small to grasp, thereby reducing the terminal-to-vellus ratio. Inflammatory changes are not a feature of **trichotillomania**, unless excoriations are complicated by secondary bacterial infection with infiltration of neutrophils, lymphocytes, and histiocytes.

The average follicular count in horizontal sections of a 4-mm punch biopsy of trichotillomania consists of 27.5 terminal hairs + 6.6 vellus hairs = 34.1 total hairs, with a terminal-vellus ratio of 4.2:1, just within normal limits; however, a ratio of 65% anagen to 35% telogen and an average of 5 catagen hairs are strikingly abnormal. Catagen hairs are rare in normal controls.

In regard to the differential diagnosis, other causes of patchy alopecia must be excluded. **Trichotillomania** is often misdiagnosed as **tinea capitis, alopecia areata,** or even **loose anagen syndrome**. **Secondary syphilis, congenital triangular alopecia, tick-bite alopecia,** and subtle forms of **scarring alopecia** such as **pseudopelade** and **congenital aplasia cutis** may also fall into the differential diagnosis. The history and appearance are often diagnostic, but in some cases scalp biopsies are necessary. The lack of inflammation, fungal elements, and scarring and the presence of terminal hairs, catagen hairs, and trichomalacia exclude most other conditions. The major histopathological differential diagnosis includes **traction alopecia** and **pressure alopecia**, which in many cases requires correlation with the clinical history and presentation for diagnostic distinction (Table 5-22B).

Acute traction alopecia results from sudden, painful avulsion in accidental or intentional hair pulling or domestic or industrial accidents. **Chronic traction alopecia** is more common and insidious and results from hair weaves, other hair additions glued or clipped in place, excessive brushing, backcombing, braiding, or tight ponytails. Prolonged pressure on the scalp from prolonged immobility can cause alopecia. Clinically, band-like traction alopecia involving frontal, temporal, and occipital scalp hair margins is usually due to ponytails with the maximum pull on peripheral hairs. **Traction alopecia** from hair weaves and other hair additions occurs at the point of attachment. **Traction alopecia** can occur between tight braids and in areas where hair is wound too tightly on rollers. Sustained traction usually induces telogen in affected hairs, which eventually fall out.

Pressure alopecia can occur in the newborn and in patients of any age who are severely injured, very ill, or anesthetized or who have sustained blunt trauma to the scalp. It usually results from prolonged immobilization of the patient on a hard operating table, bed, or floor. The soft-tissue compression over underlying skull causes ischemia. A patch of alopecia develops over the compressed scalp within 2 to 4 weeks but regrows within a few months, unless permanent scarring has resulted from necrosis and ulceration.

The histopathology of **traction alopecia** is similar to **trichotillomania.** Due to the sustained traction, many catagen and telogen hairs are seen, which reduces the anagen-telogen ratio. There is usually a lack of inflammation. Total follicular counts on horizontal section are identical to normal controls. Unlike **trichotillomania**, **pigment casts** and **trichomalacia**

Table 5-22B. Traction and Pressure Alopecia

Clinical Features

Acute traction alopecia from avulsion: easily diagnosable from history and clinical findings
Obvious linear alopecia at scalp hair margins, caused by chronic traction from ponytails
Chronic traction alopecia under points of attachment of hair weaves or other hair additions more subtle
Pressure alopecia: localized to the area of pressure and usually transient

Histopathologic Features

Normal follicular counts with normal terminal: vellus ratio
Marked increase in catagen and telogen hairs
Occasional pigmented casts; trichomalacia uncommon
Inflammatory changes usually absent
In late cases of marginal alopecia, terminal hairs decreased due to follicular fibrosis
Catagen and telogen hairs increased from pressure alopecia

Differential Diagnosis

Common causes of patchy alopecia to be differentiated from traumatic alopecia include trichotillomania, alopecia areata—especially ophiasis, tinea capitis, loose anagen syndrome, and other causes of localized alopecia

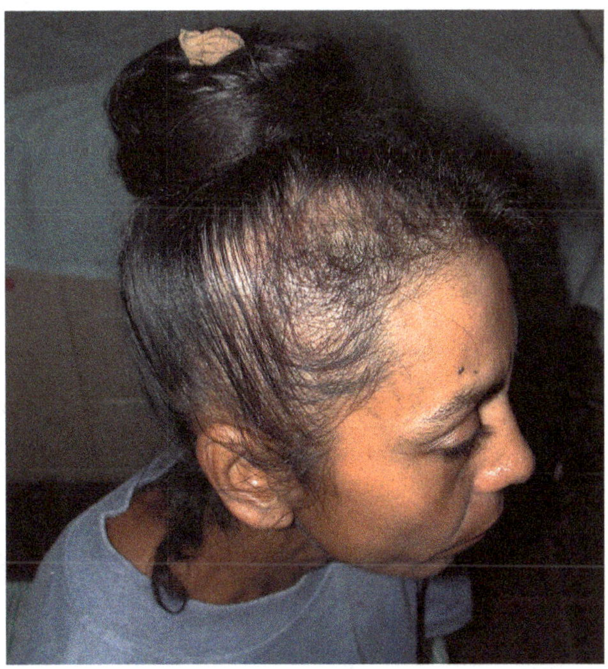

Traction alopecia from pulling the hair up in a tight bun. (Reproduced, with permission, from Usatine RP, Smith MA, Mayeaux EJ Jr, Chumley HS, eds. *Color Atlas of Family Medicine*. 2nd ed. New York, NY: McGraw-Hill Education; 2012.)

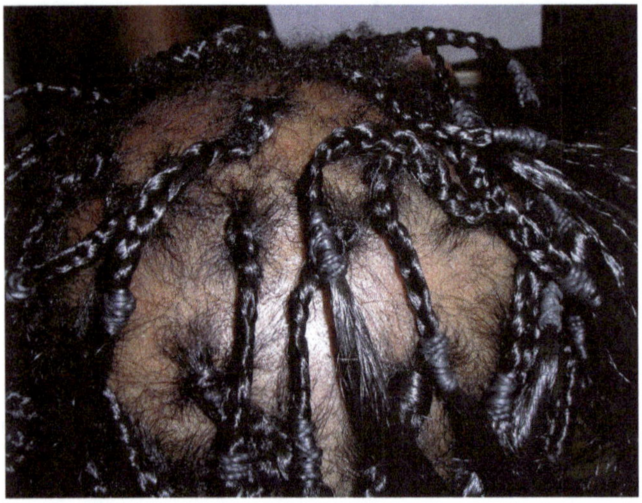

Traction alopecia in a young African American girl whose mom braids her hair tightly.

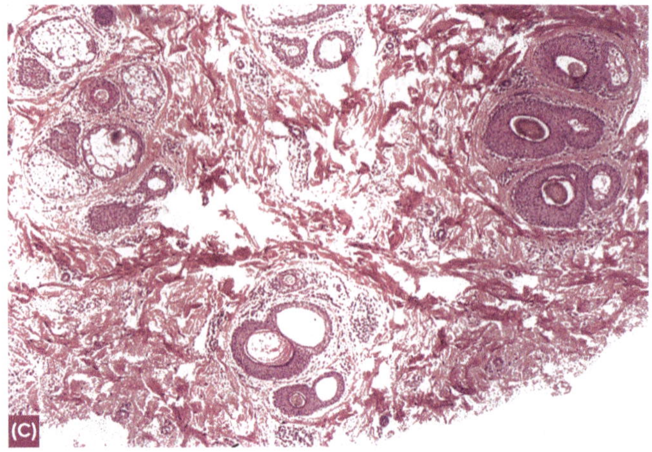

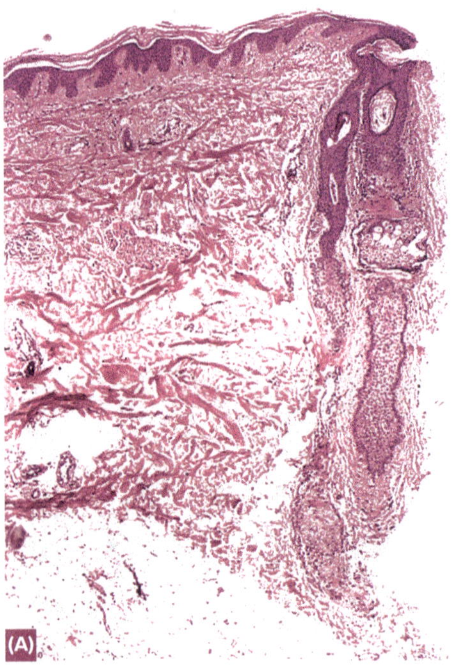

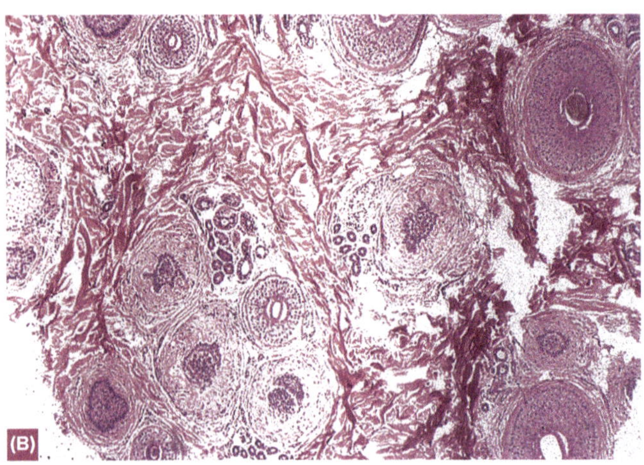

Traction alopecia. (A) Vertical section: One terminal catagen hair and one terminal telogen hair are seen. A mild lymphohistiocytic infiltrate is present around one follicular infundibulum. **(B)** Horizontal section, reticular dermis: Three terminal hairs, three vellus hairs, and seven telogen germinal units are visible. There is no inflammation. This is a striking increase in involuting hairs, outside the spectrum typically seen in telogen effluvium. The clinical presentations of traction alopecia and telogen effluvium are strikingly different (diffuse thinning vs localized hair loss). **(C)** Horizontal section, papillary dermis: Terminal and vellus hairs are seen. Several follicular infundibula are empty. No trichomalacia is present. There is a mild lymphohistiocytic infiltrate around a few follicular infundibula.

are rare. In chronic traction alopecia affecting hair margins, dense fibrosis may be present around upper and lower follicles.

In the early stages of **pressure alopecia**, vascular thrombosis and tissue necrosis, with a mild lymphohistiocytic infiltrate, may be present. Most of the terminal hairs are then projected into a catagen or telogen phase. Fat necrosis with foamy macrophages and varied degrees of dermal fibrosis may eventuate.

ANSWER 5-23: E.

Clinically, **scarring alopecia (cicatricial alopecia)** is characterized by loss of follicular orifices. Distinguishing characteristics that aid in diagnosis include the pattern of alopecia, pigmentary alteration, follicular prominence, keratinous plugs, and follicular pustules. While postinflammatory alteration with scattered melanophages is more typical in scarring alopecias, they are also helpful in establishing a diagnosis of **alopecia areata**, where they are present within follicular stelae and around the hair bulbs at the deep dermal and subcutaneous interface. **Pigment casts** and rare scattered dermal melanophages may be present in **trichotillomania**. Histopathologic evaluation of progressive, "active" alopecia is often very helpful for diagnosis of specific scarring alopecias. However, biopsies from patients with end-stage, "burned-out" scarring alopecia frequently yield a nonspecific diagnosis, but these specimens still may be

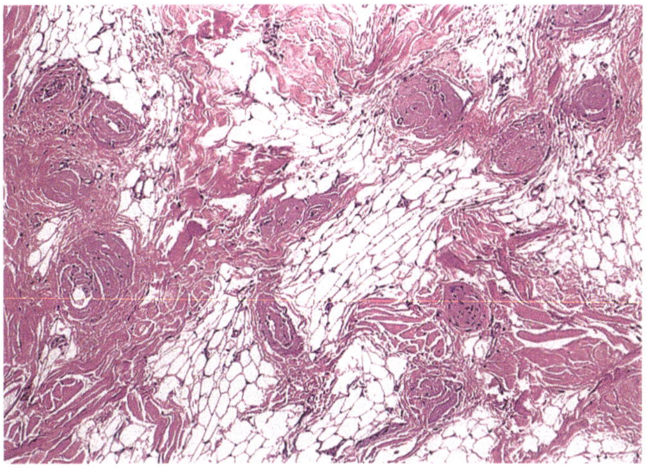

End-stage scarring alopecia. Horizontal sections: Complete follicular dropout with numerous residual fibrous tracts. These end-stage features occur in many primary scarring alopecias and are not diagnostic of a specific entity.

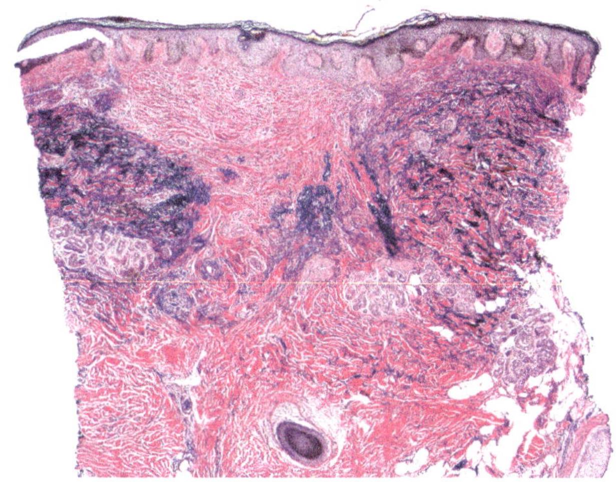

Scarring alopecia, elastic stain. There is a focal fibrosis and disruption of the elastic fiber network (absent black staining fibers) in the superficial dermis. This is reflective of a completely destroyed follicular infundibulum.

useful in assessment of the extent of follicular destruction and regrowth potential.

The traditional separation of alopecia into either **"scarring"** or **"nonscarring"** is not very helpful from a patient's perspective because he or she is concerned with only one issue—whether or not the hair loss is potentially reversible or permanent. If a patch of alopecia areata never regrows, the patient will not be comforted by the fact that he or she has **"*nonscarring*" alopecia**. Nevertheless, histopathologic differentiation of scarring from nonscarring alopecia remains of value because the former usually will progress to permanent hair loss unless therapeutic intervention is successful, whereas the latter is less predictable. While examination of **transverse sections** is advantageous for **nonscarring alopecias** since they provide increased numbers of follicular units for assessment, they are of limited value when assessing the relationship of an inflammatory infiltrate with various portions of the hair follicle. Although **vertical sections** reveal fewer numbers of hair follicles per section, they adequately demonstrate the relationship of inflammation with the hair follicle; therefore, they are the preferred method for interpreting **scarring alopecias**. Elastic stains in scarring alopecias typically reveal an absent or disrupted elastic fiber network within the dermis. Many classification systems of scarring alopecia have been proposed according to clinical, histologic, and pathogenic factors. We endorse the concept of primary and secondary scarring alopecia based on the pattern of follicular destruction. **Primary scarring alopecia** occurs as the result of preferential destruction of follicular epithelium and/or its associated adventitial dermis, with relative sparing of the intervening reticular dermis. In primary scarring alopecia, the hair follicle is the primary target of destruction. Although the interfollicular epidermis may be affected, as in **lupus erythematosus** and **lichen planopilaris (LPP),** the epidermal changes in and of themselves do not result in follicular destruction. Primary scarring alopecias are a diverse group of diseases with differing or uncertain etiologies. The unifying feature of these varied disorders is destruction of sufficient follicles to yield permanent alopecia. Microscopically, **primary scarring alopecia** can be further categorized into two groups according to the predominant inflammatory cell type: (1) lymphocyte-associated scarring alopecia and (2) neutrophil-associated (pustulofollicular) scarring alopecia. **Secondary scarring alopecia** occurs as the result of nonfollicular events that impinge on and eventually destroy the follicle. Follicular destruction and subsequent permanent scarring alopecia are not the primary pathologic process, but they occur secondarily due to the close anatomic location of follicles to the primary pathologic event (ie, dermal sclerosis in coup de sabre linear morphea).

ANSWER 5-24: C.

The biopsy reveals a band-like lymphocytic infiltrate along the dermal-epidermal junction with vacuolar alteration of the basal layer and modest premature terminal differentiation. The infiltrate also involves adnexal structures and extends into the deep dermis. Increased dermal mucin is present throughout the dermis and is not just confined to the areas of inflammation. This is a classic example of **discoid lupus erythematosus (DLE)**. Scalp involvement in DLE is common, and 30% to 50% of patients develop scarring alopecia. DLE typically occurs in young to middle-aged females (2:1 female predominance), and lesions occur on sun-exposed sites, especially the face, scalp, and conchal bowl of the ear. Early lesions are scaly erythematous papules, whereas late lesions are sclerotic plaques with follicular plugging, telangiectasia, and pigmentary alteration. Patients with DLE uncommonly progress to **systemic lupus erythematosus**. Diffuse, **nonscarring alopecia** may occur in patients with **systemic lupus erythematosus** but is best categorized as **nonscarring inflammatory telogen effluvium**.

Microscopically, vacuolar interface alteration at the level of the epidermis and hair follicle is the primary feature of DLE. Epidermal and follicular dyskeratosis are also present but less so than in **lichen planopilaris (LPP)**. The epidermis is often atrophic with overlying orthokeratotic hyperkeratosis, but the hypertrophic variant of DLE is characterized by marked acanthosis and hyperkeratosis. Focal parakeratosis may be seen in some lesions. Laminated keratin fills dilated follicular ostia corresponding to the clinical follicular plugs. The basement membrane zone of the epidermis and/or follicle may be thickened with a corrugated appearance. This finding is best seen with the PAS stain and ultrastructurally represents a multilayered basal lamina. Superficial and deep perivascular and periadnexal lymphocytic infiltrates of variable density are present. Occasional admixed plasma cells can be found. Lymphocyte exocytosis into the epidermis and follicular epithelium may be present but usually is not prominent. Pigment incontinence with melanophagocytosis is seen commonly in the papillary dermis. Increased dermal mucin (hyaluronic acid) is present both superficially and deep and is best detected in colloidal iron or Alcian blue stained sections. Dermal sclerosis and complete follicular dropout with disrupted elastic fiber networks occurs in advanced lesions and is similar to end-stage microscopic findings of other primary scarring alopecias. Biopsies of well-established clinical lesions for immunofluorescence usually show granular immunoglobulin and complement at the dermal-epidermal junction (positive lupus band test). IgM deposits are more common but less specific for DLE than IgG deposits. The incidence of lesional immunoglobulin deposition in DLE is about 75%, with older, sun-exposed lesions more likely to be positive.

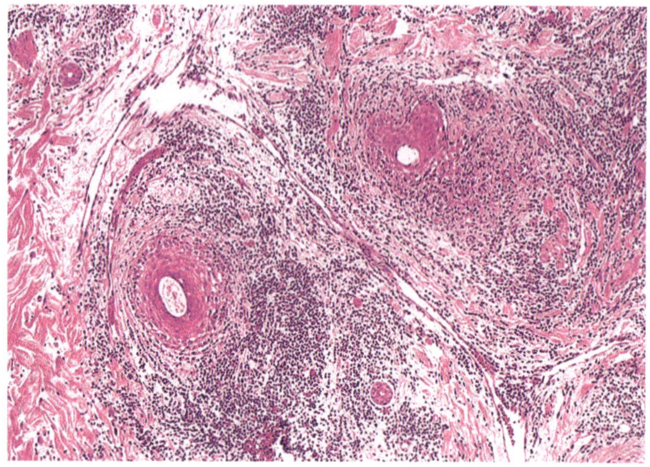

Discoid lupus erythematosus. Transverse sections. Perifollicular lymphocytic infiltrate with vacuolar interface alteration of the follicular epithelium.

Lichen planopilaris (LPP), central centrifugal cicatricial (follicular degeneration syndrome; FDS), and **alopecia mucinosa (follicular mucinosis)** are the primary differential diagnostic considerations. All of these entities are **lymphocyte-associated scarring alopecias**, and end-stage biopsies from all these entities can be identical (Table 5-24A).

Table 5-24A. Lymphocyte-Associated Primary Scarring Alopecia

	DISCOID LUPUS ERYTHEMATOSUS	LICHEN PLANOPILARIS	CENTRAL CENTRIFUGAL SCARRING ALOPECIA/ FOLLICULAR DEGENERATION SYNDROME	FOLLICULAR MUCINOSIS
Clinical Features				
	Young to middle-aged Women > men Erythematous papules to sclerotic plaques Follicular plugging, telangiectasia, dyspigmentation	Adults Women > men Acuminate, spinous hyperkeratotic follicular papules Perifollicular erythema Smooth atrophic polygonal patches of alopecia	Young to middle-aged African American Women >> men Slowly progressive, irregularly shaped alopecic patches ("footprints in the snow") Confluence of patches Noninflammatory	All ages Head and neck > trunk, extremities Erythematous infiltrate Sometimes boggy plaques with scaling, expression of mucin Adults have lymphoproliferative disorder in about 30% of cases

Table 5-24A. Lymphocyte-Associated Primary Scarring Alopecia *(continued)*

	DISCOID LUPUS ERYTHEMATOSUS	LICHEN PLANOPILARIS	CENTRAL CENTRIFUGAL SCARRING ALOPECIA/ FOLLICULAR DEGENERATION SYNDROME	FOLLICULAR MUCINOSIS
Histopathological Features				
Interface alteration				
at DEJ	Primarily vacuolar	Primarily lichenoid if present	Absent	Absent
at follicle	Primarily vacuolar	Primarily lichenoid	Absent	Absent
Dyskeratosis	Minimal to moderate	Moderate to prominent	Absent	Absent
Inflammation type	Lymphocytic	Lymphocytic	Lymphocytic	Lymphocytic
Perivascular pattern	Superficial and deep	Minimal superficial perivascular, primarily perifollicular	Mostly superficial	May be superficial and deep in lymphoma
Perifollicular infiltrates	Present, prominent	Present, prominent	Present, sparse	Present, variable
Perieccrine infiltrates	Present	Absent	Absent	Absent
Intrafollicular mucin	Minimal	Absent	Absent	Prominent
Dermal mucin	Moderate to prominent	Absent	Absent	Minimal
Concentric lamellar fibrosis	End-stage finding	Yes in advanced lesions	Prominent	No
Pigment incontinence	Yes	Yes	Minimal	No

However, in "active" clinical lesions, interface alteration in **DLE** is primarily vacuolar rather than lichenoid, as in **LPP**. The superficial and deep infiltrates are both perivascular and periadnexal in DLE as opposed to tightly perifollicular in LPP. **FDS** lacks interface alteration around follicles. The presence of increased dermal mucin distributed throughout the dermis is an important finding that points toward **DLE** rather than **LPP** or **FDS. Alopecia mucinosa** contains mucin within the outer root sheath epithelium only, unlike DLE which contains mucin in the dermis. Alopecia mucinosa typically contains lymphocytes with nuclear contour irregularity. The inflammatory infiltrate of nonscarring **alopecia areata** is confined to the bulbar and suprabulbar regions.

ANSWER 5-25: D.

This is a classic example of **frontal fibrosing alopecia (FFA),** which is considered a unique clinical presentation of **lichen planopilaris (LPP).** LPP is an uncommon scarring alopecia. First described in 1895 by Pringle, LPP presents as acuminate, spinous, and hyperkeratotic follicular papules with perifollicular erythema. LPP is more common in women, and onset ranges from young adulthood to elderly age. As follicles are destroyed, smooth, atrophic, polygonal-shaped patches of complete alopecia result. Typical **lichen planus** papules and plaques are present elsewhere on the body in 50% to 70% of patients. The clinical triad of typical lichen planus, spinous or acuminate lesions, and alopecia of the scalp or other nonglabrous skin is known as the ***Graham-Little syndrome***.

In 1994, Kossard described a distinctive form of cicatricial alopecia that he termed postmenopausal **frontal fibrosing alopecia (FFA).** The patients presented with a band-like progressive zone of alopecia that ultimately spanned the entire frontal hairline from temple to temple. The frontal alopecia is usually accompanied by alopecia of the eyebrows and perifollicular erythema. FFA has subsequently been reported to also occur in premenopausal women and men. FFA may develop in association with other findings of the **Graham-Little syndrome** (follicular papules and alopecia in sites remote from the scalp).

Microscopically, lichenoid interface alteration of follicular epithelium is the primary microscopic feature of **LPP** and **FFA**. Although not always completely distinct from vacuolar interface alteration, lichenoid interface alteration of the follicle is characterized by disruption of the epithelial-adventitial dermal junction with angular, glassy, basal keratinocytes and a tight perifollicular lymphocytic infiltrate that is largely confined to the follicular adventitial dermis. Exocytosis into the follicular epithelium and dyskeratosis are more prominent in **LPP** than **DLE**. Artifactual clefting similar to that seen at the dermal-epidermal junction in **lichen planus (Max Joseph space)** can also occur around hair follicles in LPP. In a minority of cases, lichenoid interface alteration typical of lichen planus may affect the intervening epidermis. Superficial and deep perivascular lymphocytic infiltrates and dermal mucin typical of **DLE** are lacking in **LPP**.

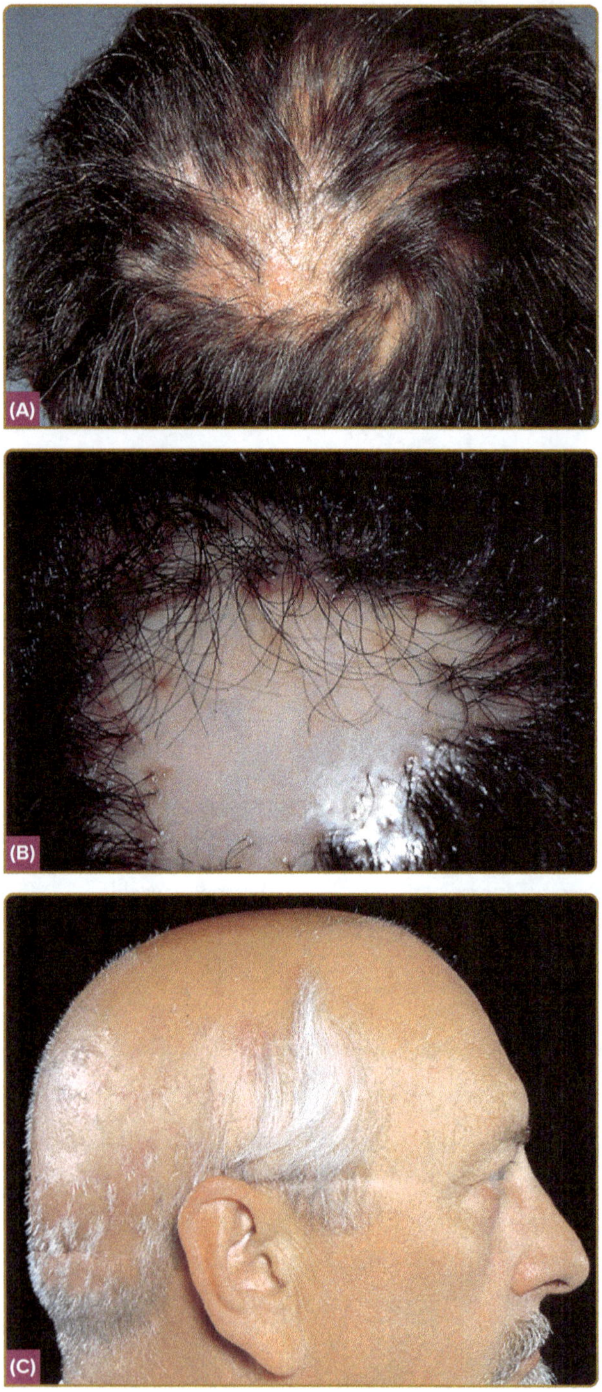

Lichen planopilaris. (A) Irregular patches of alopecia with violaceous papules and coalescing plaque of lichen planus within scalp. **(B)** Lichen planopilaris resulting in atrophic, scarred, porcelain-colored area centrally with bordering follicular involvement consisting of dusky erythema, perifollicular hyperkeratosis and scale, and follicular convergence resulting in doll's hair formation. **(C)** Extensive hair loss leading to pseudopelade of Brocq appearance. Several remaining tufts of hair showing violaceous erythema and disease activity. (Reproduced, with permission, from Goldsmith LA, Katz SI, Gilchrest BA, Paller AS, Leffell DJ, Wolff K, eds. *Fitzpatrick's Dermatology in General Medicine.* 8th ed. New York, NY: McGraw-Hill Education; 2012.)

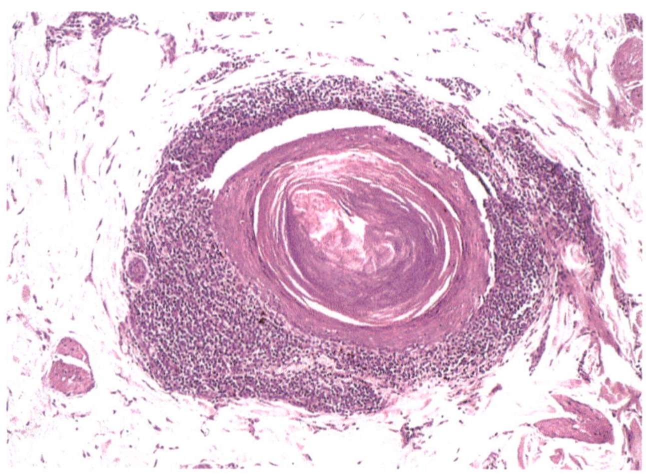

Lichen planopilaris. Transverse sections. Dense perifollicular lichenoid infiltrates with artifactual clefting.

Complete follicular dropout with scattered unsheathed hair shafts surrounded by sparse histiocytic and granulomatous infiltrates occurs in late lesions. These end-stage features are not specific for LPP but may occur in all scarring alopecias. Lesional biopsy for direct immunofluorescence reveals globular IgM deposits on cytoid (colloid) bodies and fibrin at the dermal-epidermal junction and infundibular-adventitial dermal junction. However, these immunofluorescent findings are not specific for LPP and may be seen in other dermatoses with interface dermatitis. The histopathologic findings in **FFA** are reported to be identical to those of **LPP**. Abbas and coauthors reported a greater number of apoptotic (dyskeratotic) cells and less dense lymphocytic infiltrates in FFA along with complete sparring of the interfollicular epidermis, although these findings may be difficult to apply to individual cases.

Discoid lupus and **central centrifugal cicatricial alopecia (follicular degeneration syndrome)** are the primary entities considered in the differential diagnosis. In practice, it can be very difficult to distinguish between vacuolar and lichenoid interface change at the level of infundibulum, so that the presence or absence of other findings is extremely helpful, for example, increased dermal mucin in **DLE**. Another common cause of confusion is artifactual clefting that simulates true interface change between remnants of the infundibulum and the encompassing lymphocytes in advanced lesions of **central centrifugal cicatricial alopecia**. Although sparse peri-isthmic lymphocytic infiltrates may be present in **androgenetic alopecia**, there is miniaturization of hairs with decreased terminal-to-vellus hair ratios. The sebaceous glands are spared in **androgenetic alopecia,** while they are frequently destroyed in LPP/FFA. Additionally, the lymphocytic infiltrate of androgenetic alopecia does not have interface activity. Lastly, androgenetic alopecia results in nonscarring frontal alopecia in males but is diffuse in females. In regard to **alopecia areata**, the inflammatory infiltrate is confined to the bulbar and suprabulbar regions, whereas LPP involves the infundibular and isthmic regions.

ANSWER 5-26: D.

The biopsy reveals concentric perifollicular fibrosis accompanied by a moderate lymphocytic infiltrate. The outer root sheath epithelium exhibits degenerative changes in an eccentric fashion. Active interface dermatitis involving the hair follicle is absent and dyskeratotic keratinocytes are not present. The inner root sheath epithelium reveals degeneration. This is a classic example of **central centrifugal scarring alopecia (CCSA).** A century after it was coined, controversy still surrounds the term ***pseudopelade***. Brocq first described this form of alopecia in 1885 as a clinically noninflammatory, progressive, idiopathic scarring alopecia. Since then, conflicting opinions have arisen as to whether **pseudopelade of Brocq (PPOB)** is a disease *sui generis* or the end-stage lesion of various types of scarring alopecia. Support for the concept of pseudopelade as a unique clinicopathologic entity appears to be dwindling, given the substantial overlap in the clinical and histopathologic features with other forms of scarring alopecia. The main argument for elimination of the term ***pseudopelade*** is that it has never been defined as a unique clinicopathologic entity. In other words, if defined clinically, there is no specific histopathology. If defined microscopically, there is no specific clinical presentation. To address the pseudopelade issue and the problem of overlap in the clinical and histopathologic findings of several types of scarring alopecia, Sperling and coauthors introduced the concept of ***central centrifugal scarring alopecia***. As described, this term is meant to be a unifying concept with the goal of more rational clinical and microscopic diagnosis and eventually better therapeutic approaches. **Central centrifugal scarring alopecia (CCSA)** denotes alopecia with the following common clinical features: (1) primary involvement of the crown and vertex, (2) relentless progression to broad areas of scalp devoid of follicular orifices, and (3) symmetric expansion with an active, inflammatory border. These clinical features are common to several subtypes of scarring alopecia, such as the **follicular degeneration syndrome (hot comb alopecia), folliculitis decalvans**, and **tufted folliculitis**. Other well-defined types of scarring alopecia, including **LPP** and **DLE**, may also present as **CCSA.** These subtypes of scarring alopecia usually can be defined by the clinical presentation and histopathologic features, but there may be significant overlap in both, especially in chronic lesions with extensive follicular destruction. The concept of **CCSA** is most useful in addressing the late-stage lesions because attempts to make a specific clinicopathologic diagnosis are frequently futile. Therefore, some would argue that **CCSA** represents a "waste basket" diagnosis encompassing a number of end-stage scarring alopecia. Others contend that it represents a unique clinicopathologic entity. It should be noted that **pseudopelade** was included in the construct for conceptual reasons, but we conclude that it should be abolished. In this discussion, **follicular degeneration syndrome (FDS)** will be discussed as an early discrete entity within **CCSA** in order to highlight the important clinical findings. The **follicular degeneration syndrome**, described by Sperling and Sau, usually can be recognized both clinically and microscopically in early-stage lesions. The condition was first described in association with the hot oil used in the cosmetic practices of African American women and was referred to as **"hot comb" alopecia**. Since then, poor correlation has been noted between the usage of a hot comb and the onset and progression of disease. It remains unclear whether the use of any of a variety of hair care products and techniques plays a role in the pathogenesis of this condition; hence the term has been replaced by FDS. The central scalp (crown) is by far the most frequent location. The alopecia progressively expands centrifugally to involve the entire crown and vertex, leaving a smooth skin surface devoid of follicular orifices. Variable perifollicular erythema and scale are present. Only isolated hair fibers remain in

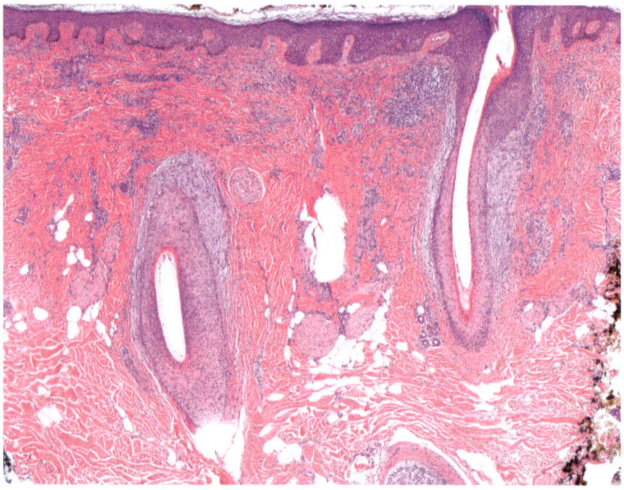

Follicular degeneration syndrome/early central centrifugal cicatricial alopecia, vertical section. There is eccentric thinning of the outer root sheaths with premature disintegration of the inner root sheath. The follicles are surrounded by lymphocytic infiltrates embedded within a loose fibromyxoid stroma. No interface activity and dyskeratotic outer root sheath keratinocytes are not present. Note the absence of sebaceous glands.

the alopecic regions. Polytrichia may be present, resulting in a **"doll's hair"** appearance. It is the most common form of scarring alopecia in African American women. It occurs occasionally in Caucasian women and African American men as well.

Microscopically, the earliest findings of **FDS** are perifollicular lymphocytic infiltrates and perifollicular fibroplasia without interface alteration. The infiltrate is more dense in these early lesions and present from the level of the follicular infundibulum to the midsegment of the follicle. Sparse adjacent perivascular lymphocytic infiltrates may also be present. Follicular density is diminished, and follicular unit morphology is disrupted. Scattered residual fibrous tracks indicating the site of destroyed follicles are present. In more advanced lesions **(evolved CCSA)**, the predominant finding is concentric lamellar fibroplasia and follicular epithelial atrophy. Frequently, the follicular canal is eccentrically located, and premature disintegration of the inner root sheath is emphasized. Finally, the residual follicular epithelium ruptures, and a foreign-body giant cell reaction ensues. In end-stage CCSA, only rare, viable though somewhat miniaturized follicles and numerous residual fibrous tracts are present. Direct immunofluorescence usually is negative, but occasional, minimal, nonspecific IgM deposits may be seen around the follicular infundibulum.

In regard to the differential diagnosis, **DLE, LPP**, and end-stage **folliculitis decalvans (FD)** may be considered. The lack of follicular interface dermatitis in FDS is the primary distinguishing microscopic feature from DLE and LPP.

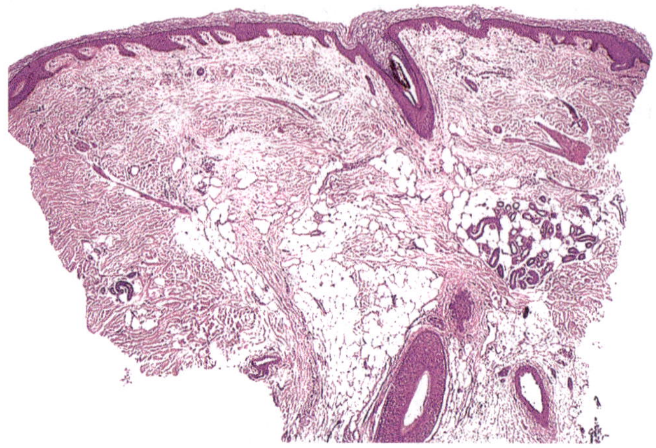

End-stage scarring alopecia. Vertical sections. Diminished follicular density with vertically oriented residual fibrous tracts and sparse lymphocytic infiltrates.

Although robust perifollicular lymphocytic infiltrates may be present in CCSA, interface activity with dyskeratotic outer root sheath keratinocytes is absent. The neutrophil is the predominant inflammatory cell in **active folliculitis decalvans**. End-stage lesions of **FDS, DLE, LPP**, and **folliculitis decalvans** are indistinguishable from each other, forming the basis for the concept of **CCSA.**

ANSWER 5-27: E.

This patient has **dissecting cellulitis of the scalp**. Vertical sections reveal a fibroinflammatory process that destroys the hair follicle. A partially squamous-lined abscess with unsheathed hair shaft (lower left) is present. The **pustulofollicular neutrophil-associated primary scarring alopecias** are **dissecting cellulitis of the scalp (DCS), folliculitis decalvans, acne keloidalis nuchae (AKN), erosive pustular dermatosis of the scalp (EPDS),** and **tinea capitis** (TC) (Table 5-27A). Common features include early follicular dilatation and predominately neutrophilic infiltrates within and around the affected follicles. Early lesions have overlapping clinical and microscopic features, but well-developed cases usually are distinct both clinically and microscopically.

Dissecting cellulitis of the scalp (DCS) is most common in young black men and begins as fluctuant scalp nodules that coalesce progressively to form complex, interconnected, crusted abscesses, and sinus tracts that drain spontaneously or with slight pressure. Well-developed lesions are painful and result in extensive scarring of the scalp. Some patients with **DCS** also have **acne conglobata** and **hidradenitis suppurativa** and are said to have the ***follicular occlusion triad***.

Microscopically, the initial finding is acneiform follicular dilatation with neutrophilic infiltrates. Biopsies from fluctuant nodules and sinuses reveal large dermal and subcutaneous abscesses. Well-developed lesions are abscesses and sinus

Table 5-27A. Pustulofollicular, Neutrophil-Associated Primary Scarring Alopecia

	DISSECTING CELLULITIS	FOLLICULITIS DECALVANS	ACNE KELOIDALIS	TINEA KERION AND FAVUS
Clinical Features				
	African American men	Adults of either sex	African American men	Children, adolescents
	Fluctuant scalp nodules Progression to extensive interconnected abscesses, sinus tracts Spontaneous drainage Painful, prominent scarring Associated follicular occlusion triad	Round or irregularly shaped patches of alopecia with follicular pustules Other sites may be affected	Occipital scalp, neck Follicular papules, pustules progress to large, exophytic, keloidal alopecic plaques	Boggy, erythematous, crusted, scaling nodules and plaques with variable alopecia Zoophilic and geophilic forms of dermatophyte Yellow, cup-shaped crusts (scutula) with favus
Histopathologic Features				
Acneiform follicular dilatation	Early finding, persists	Early finding, persists	Early finding, persists	Early finding, persists
Follicular rupture	Present	Present	Present	Present
Abscess formation	Extensive dermal and subcutaneous	Present in dermis	Less prominent in dermis	Variable, may be prominent
Sinus tract formation	Yes, partially squamous lined	Absent	Largely absent	Absent
Location of fibrosis	Dense fibrotic scar around sinus tracts in dermis and subcutis	Less dense perifollicular fibrosis in dermis	Dense dermal hypertrophic scar and/or keloid	Perifollicular dermal scar, may be extensive in favus
Infectious agents	Occasional staph within follicular infundibulum	Occasional staph within follicular infundibulum	Occasional propionibacteria acnes	Endothrix and ectothrix
Inflammation type	Neutrophilic initially, later mixed granulomatous with plasma cells	Neutrophilic initially, later mixed granulomatous with plasma cells	Neutrophilic initially, later mixed with lymphocytes and prominent plasma cells	Neutrophilic initially, later mixed granulomatous with plasma cells
Location	Initially peri-infundibular, progresses to involve entire follicle and subcutis	Primarily peri-infundibular, may extend to involve entire follicle	Primarily peri-infundibular, may extend to involve entire follicle	Primarily peri-infundibular, may extend to involve entire follicle

tracts partially lined with squamous epithelium derived from the overlying epidermis or follicular epithelium. Bacteria may be seen superficially in follicular infundibula but not in abscesses, and the pathogenic significance is unclear. Dense dermal and subcutaneous fibrosis eventually surrounds the sinus tracts, and the hair follicles are eventually destroyed by the fibroinflammatory process. The infiltrate in older, more scarred lesions is primarily lymphoplasmacytic and histiocytic with few neutrophils.

In regard to the differential diagnosis, other pustulofollicular scarring alopecias need to be considered. The microscopic features of **DCS** are very similar to those in **hidradenitis suppurativa**. PAS and Gram stains should be done to rule out fungal and bacterial infection. Where the inflammatory process of **DCS** typically involves the dermis and subcutis, the pustular inflammation of **folliculitis decalvans** is confined to the dermis and does not produce draining sinus tracts. **Acne keloidalis** characteristically involves the occipital portion of the scalp and results in extensive scar tissue formation with bundles of keloidal collagen. **Erosive pustular dermatosis** of the scalp is an uncommon erosive and pustular process that may lead to permanent alopecia. It is strongly associated with chronic sun exposure and generally begins on the crown as a localized area of crusted erosion with occasional pustules. It occurs most commonly in elderly Caucasian women. The histopathology is not specific and consists of neutrophilic pustules, ulcers, and erosions with subjacent-mixed inflammatory infiltrates and abscesses. **Lipedematous alopecia** (**LA**) is the term used to describe alopecia associated with boggy thickening of the subcutaneous adipose tissue of the scalp. This rare form of alopecia has been described primarily in African American females, but has also been reported in Caucasian women and a Japanese man. The defining clinical feature is the compressible bogginess of the thickened scalp. The latter may occur without associated alopecia (lipedematous scalp). When present, the associated alopecia ranges from extensive and diffuse to limited and patchy. Some patients with this condition state their hair will not grow beyond a short length. Histopathologic studies have found the primary abnormality to be an increase in the thickness of the subcutaneous adipose tissue of the scalp. In some cases, the latter structure is nearly 1 cm thick, as opposed to the reported 3 mm in normal scalp. In addition, the thickened adipose tissue shows other abnormalities including edema and dilated lymphatics, but neither inflammation nor mucin is increased. Peculiarly, characteristic and reproducible follicular changes in lipedematous scalp have not yet been documented.

ANSWER 5-28: A.

This is a classic early example of **folliculitis decalvans** (**FD**). Transverse sectioning of the patient's biopsy reveals pustular folliculitis with incipient rupture and adjacent mixed dermal infiltrates. Several hair shafts converge into a single follicular ostium, referred to as **polytrichia. Folliculitis decalvans** (**FD**)

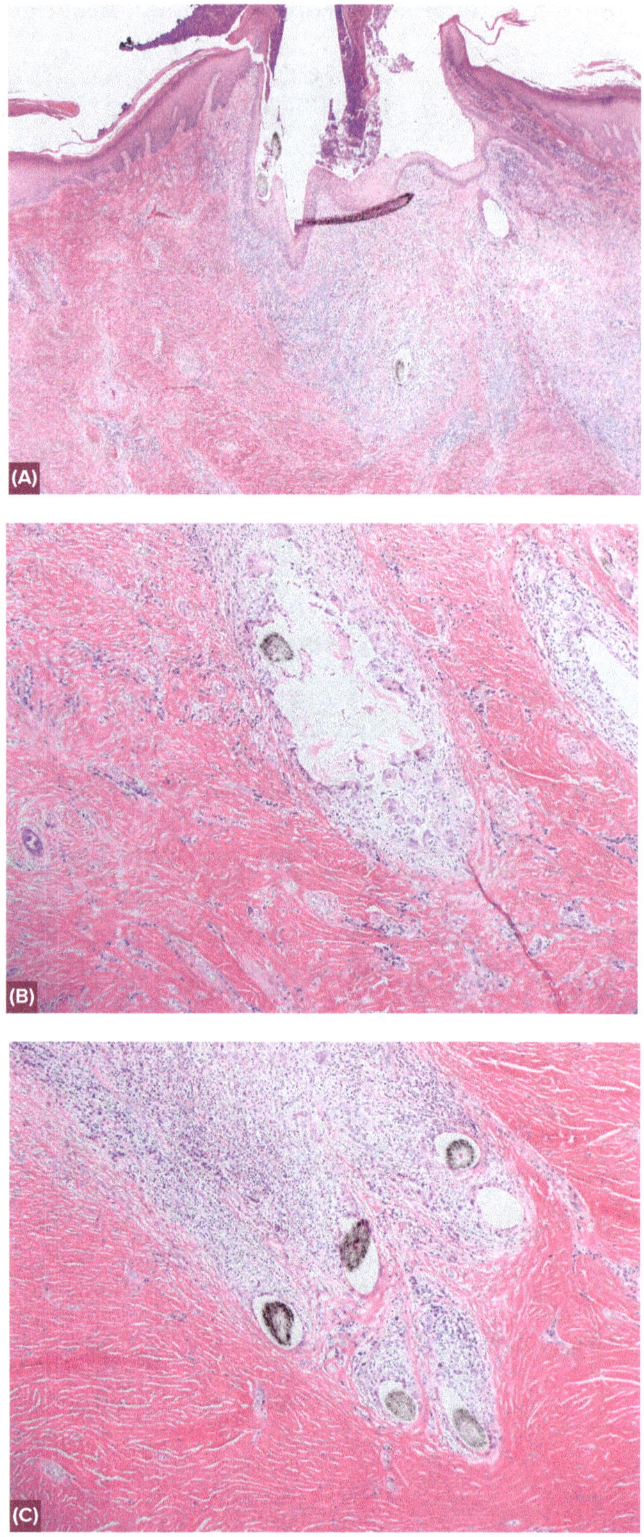

Folliculitis decalvans, late stage. (A) There is a superficial fibroinflammatory process localized at a markedly dilated follicular ostium. Numerous hair shafts appear to converge on this opening. **(B)** The follicular epithelium has been destroyed, resulting in a foreign body giant cell reaction toward naked hair shafts. **(C)** Numerous naked hair shafts are embedded within dense scar tissue admixed with mixed inflammatory infiltrates.

is a rare pustulofollicular alopecia that presents as round to irregular-shaped patches of alopecia with follicular pustules at the peripheral, advancing edge. Microscopic polytrichia corresponds clinically with **tufted folliculitis**, where clustered tufts of hair shafts arise from a common opening resulting in a "doll's hair" appearance. This finding is common in FD, but is nonspecific and may be seen in other forms of scarring alopecia. FD occurs in both sexes and primarily affects the scalp, but involvement of the beard, axillae, pubic area, arms, and legs may also occur. End-stage FD without pustules is included within central centrifugal cicatricial alopecia **(CCSA)** by some, but not all, authors.

Microscopically, the initial finding is comedonal dilatation with intra- and perifollicular neutrophilic infiltrates. Follicular rupture ensues with resulting perifollicular fibrosis and eventual permanent follicular destruction. Localized perifollicular dermal abscesses are often present but are not as extensive or deep as seen in **dissecting cellulitis of the scalp (DCS)**. Sinus tracts are not seen in FD. In later stages, the infiltrate is mixed with lymphocytes, plasma cells, and neutrophils. Unsheathed hair shafts surrounded by foreign-body giant cells are present after the follicular epithelium has been destroyed, and as in all primary scarring alopecias, numerous residual fibrous tracts mark sites of destroyed follicles. Special stains are necessary to rule out fungal and bacterial folliculitis.

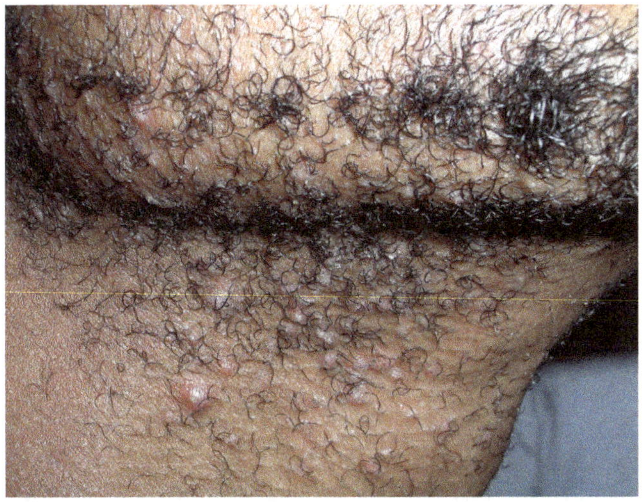

Pseudofolliculitis barbae in a Dominican man. Note the active pustules on the neck. The painful nodules become worse every time he shaves. (Reproduced, with permission, from Usatine RP, Smith MA, Mayeaux EJ Jr, Chumley HS, eds. *Color Atlas of Family Medicine.* 2nd ed. New York, NY: McGraw-Hill Education; 2012.)

ANSWER 5-29: B.

Acne keloidalis nuchae (AKN) is a destructive pustulofollicular process that primarily affects the occipital scalp and neck of young black men. Lesions begin as discrete follicular papules or pustules and may progress to large exophytic keloidal plaques devoid of hair. Similar lesions may occur in the beard region in patients with **pseudofolliculitis barbae**. The pathophysiology is not completely understood; however, most believe the condition involves the reentry of the free end of tightly coiled hairs back into the skin, causing a foreign-body-like inflammatory reaction. Shaving produces a sharp free end below the skin surface. Tightly curled hair has a greater tendency for the tip to pierce the surface of the skin and form ingrown hairs. This explains the relative predominance of this condition in patients of African ethnicity. The hair eventually forms a loop and if the embedded tip is pulled out, there may be spontaneous resolution of symptoms. As such, multiple hairs can be seen growing from a single follicle (hair tufts) in the midst of the keloidal scarring.

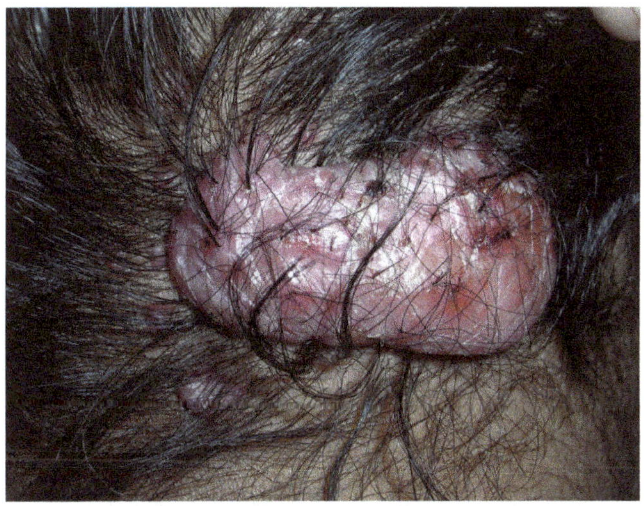

Acne keloidalis nuchae with large keloidal scar in a Hispanic man. Note multiple hairs can be seen growing from single follicles (hair tufts). Surgery is the only treatment that can remove this keloidal mass. (Reproduced, with permission, from Usatine RP, Smith MA, Mayeaux EJ Jr, Chumley HS, eds. *Color Atlas of Family Medicine.* 2nd ed. New York, NY: McGraw-Hill Education; 2012.)

Microscopically, early lesions display comedonal dilatation and pustular folliculitis as in other **pustulofollicular alopecias**. Follicular rupture with subsequent mixed neutrophilic infiltrates occurs. Well-developed lesions are characterized by dense dermal scar with many entrapped unsheathed hair shafts surrounded by lymphohistiocytic infiltrates with admixed neutrophils and abundant plasma cells. Variable numbers of broad eosinophilic hyalinized keloidal collagen bundles may be present but are not essential for diagnosis. Special stains are necessary to rule out bacterial and fungal infections. The extensive dermal fibrosis typical of keloidal scar is the most distinctive microscopic feature of AKN.

ANSWER 5-30: C.

Kerion and **favus** are subtypes of **tinea capitis** (TC) that can result in permanent alopecia and are seen most commonly in children. The transverse sectioning of the patient's biopsy reveals hyphae extensively permeating **(endothrix)** and surrounding **(ectothrix)** hair shafts. Numerous neutrophils are seen. Fungal infections are notorious for rapidly progressing following topical steroid therapy for various forms of dermatitis. **Kerion** is inflammatory TC caused by a zoophilic or geophilic follicular dermatophyte infection and presents as boggy, erythematous, scaling, crusted, partially alopecic plaques with regional adenopathy. **Favus** is an uncommon follicular dermatophyte infection of the scalp seen in rural regions and associated with poor nutrition and poor hygiene. Yellow, cup-shaped crusts termed ***"scutula"*** are present on the scalp and often result in permanent alopecia.

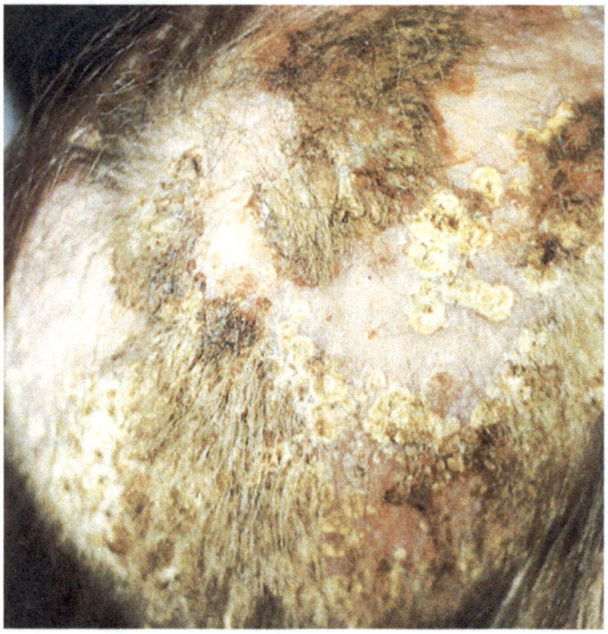

Favus caused by *Trichophyton schoenleinii*. There is extensive hair loss with atrophy, scarring, and so-called scutula (yellowish adherent crusts present on the scalp). The remaining hairs pierce the scutula. (Reproduced, with permission, from Goldsmith LA, Katz SI, Gilchrest BA, Paller AS, Leffell DJ, Wolff K, eds. *Fitzpatrick's Dermatology in General Medicine*. 8th ed. New York, NY: McGraw-Hill Education; 2012.)

The causative organism for both **kerion** and **favus** is *Trichophyton schoenleinii*. In adults, noninflammatory **endothrix dermatophyte infections,** usually *T tonsurans*, occasionally can cause a more diffuse alopecia without clinically appreciable inflammation mimicking **female-pattern androgenetic alopecia** or **follicular degeneration syndrome**.

Microscopically, the follicular infundibula generally are dilated and often hyperkeratotic. Pustular folliculitis with incipient or complete rupture is seen commonly in kerion. Dense, mixed inflammatory infiltrates including many neutrophils surround the affected follicles. ***Endothrix*** (hyphae within hair shafts) and ***ectothrix*** (hyphae around hair shafts) patterns of **follicular dermatophytosis** may be seen. In the skin, PAS

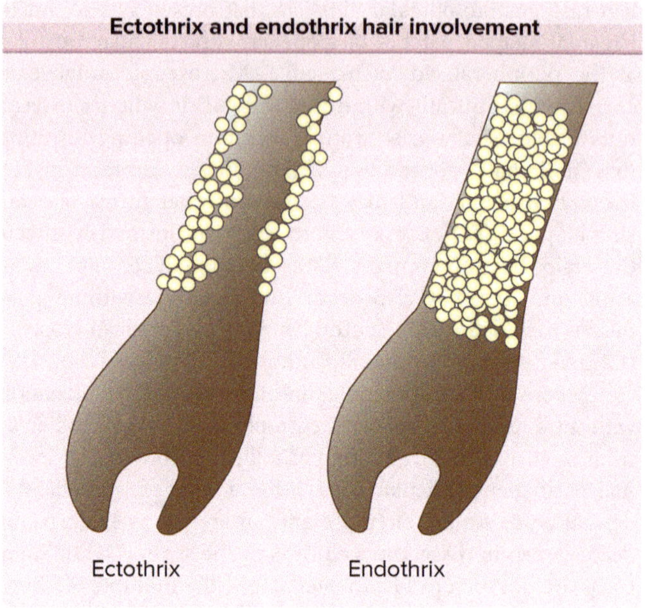

Ectothrix and endothrix hair involvement. (Reproduced, with permission, from Goldsmith LA, Katz SI, Gilchrest BA, Paller AS, Leffell DJ, Wolff K, eds. *Fitzpatrick's Dermatology in General Medicine*. 8th ed. New York, NY: McGraw-Hill Education; 2012.)

stain with diastase (dissolves glycogen) is preferred over silver stains (GMS; Gomori methenamine silver stain) since the latter stains dermal elastic fibers and is difficult to interpret.

Hyphae usually are not seen in the overlying epidermis. Some **endothrix infections** do not elicit a brisk inflammatory response but result in a relatively noninflammatory diffuse

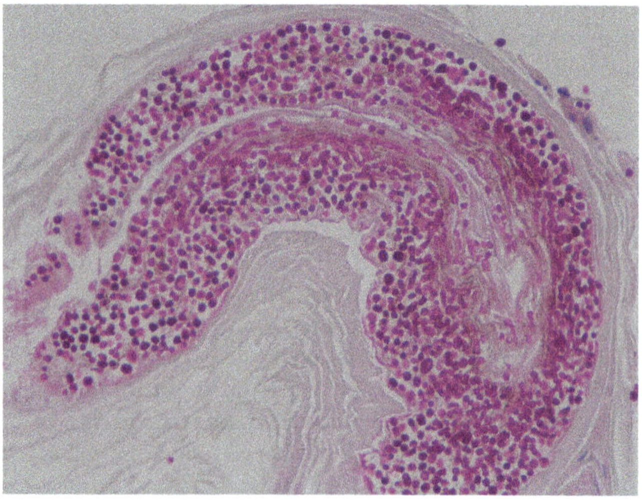

Kerion with endothrix; PAS stain. Note the numerous hyphae within the hair shaft. There is little inflammation surrounding the hair follicle.

alopecia with broken shafts and perifollicular fibroplasia. Thick parakeratotic and orthokeratotic hyperkeratosis overlying an atrophic dermis with lymphoplasmacytic and granulomatous dermal infiltrates and follicular dermatophytosis are seen in **favus**.

In regard to the differential diagnosis, diagnostic distinction from **folliculitis decalvans** and **dissecting cellulitis of the scalp** requires demonstration of the fungal organisms in either routine or special stains. Several different clinical entities involve fungal infection of hair follicles. Fungal folliculitis is typically caused by *Malassezia furfur,* formerly termed *Pityrosporum ovale* (***Pityrosporum*** **folliculitis**) or dermatophytes (**Majocchi granuloma** and **tinea capitis** [already discussed]). ***Pityrosporum*** **folliculitis** occurs on the trunk as pruritic acneiform papules and pustules most commonly in young adults. Microscopically, acneiform dilatation with budding yeast and follicular hyperkeratosis is seen in ***Pityrosporum*** **folliculitis.**

Majocchi granuloma is a form of follicular dermatophytosis that occurs on nonglabrous skin, most commonly on extremities. The lesions present as grouped, somewhat annular inflammatory papulopustules or as deep furuncle-like nodules. Topical corticosteroid usage prior to a correct diagnosis is common in **Majocchi granuloma** and may allow for more extensive infection of hair shafts. The histopathology of **Majocchi granuloma** is similar to **tinea capitis/kerion** with follicular rupture, abscess, and dermatophyte-infected hair shafts.

Both bacterial and fungal folliculitis share similar microscopic features and show intra- and perifollicular, predominantly neutrophilic inflammatory infiltrates. Follicular rupture with adjacent dense, mixed inflammatory infiltrates, abscess formation, and granulation tissue is common. **Bacterial**

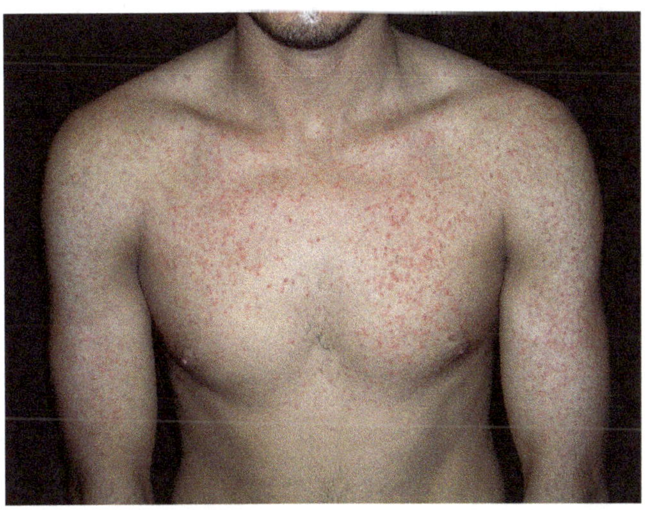

Pityrosporum **folliculitis** on the chest, shoulders, and arms of a young man. KOH preparation showed *Pityrosporum* looking like ziti and meatballs. (Reproduced, with permission, from Usatine RP, Smith MA, Mayeaux EJ Jr, Chumley HS, eds. *Color Atlas of Family Medicine.* 2nd ed. New York, NY: McGraw-Hill Education; 2012.)

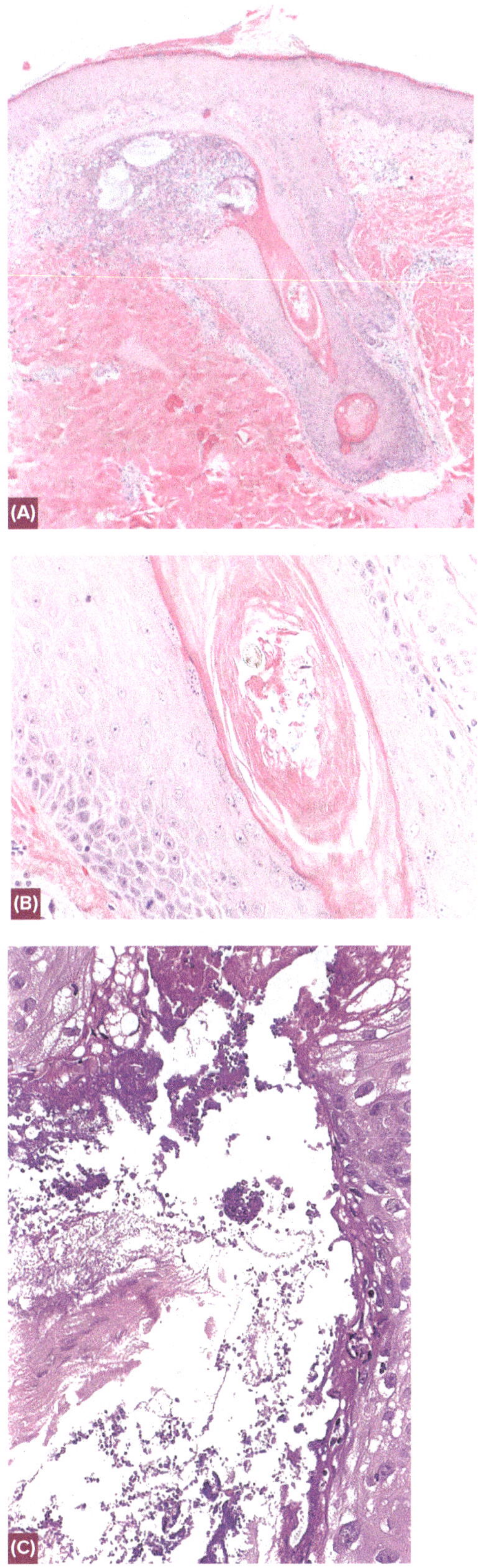

Pityrosporum **folliculitis. (A)** Note the ruptured follicular infundibulum associated with pustular inflammation. There is overlying follicular hyperkeratosis. **(B, C)** Numerous *Pityrosporum* yeasts are present within the follicular canal.

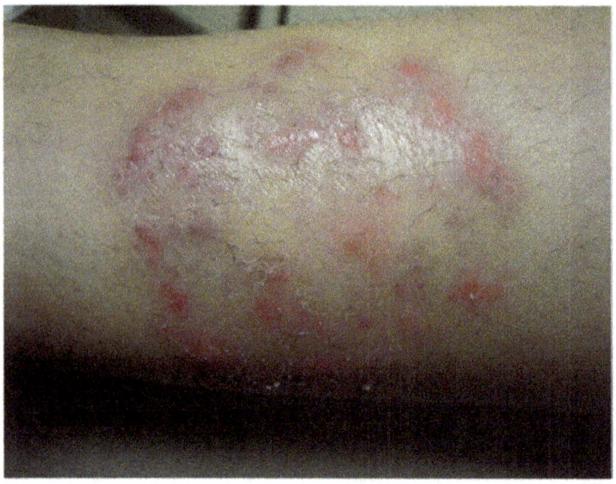

Majocchi granuloma. Follicular papules and nodules with scale coalescing to form an annular-shaped plaque on the leg of a woman applying topical corticosteroids to the area. (Reproduced, with permission, from Goldsmith LA, Katz SI, Gilchrest BA, Paller AS, Leffell DJ, Wolff K, eds. *Fitzpatrick's Dermatology in General Medicine*. 8th ed. New York, NY: McGraw-Hill Education; 2012.)

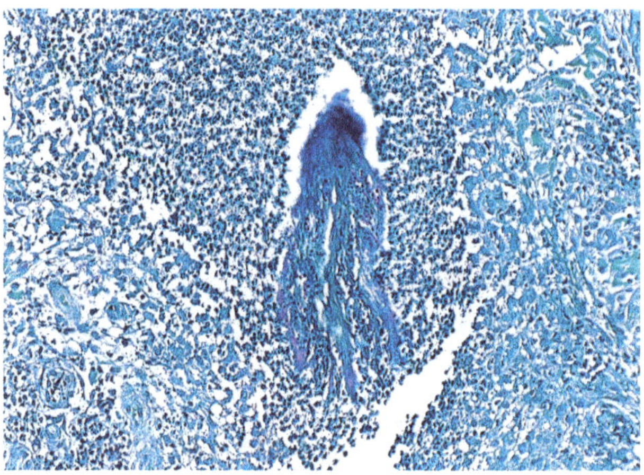

Majocchi granuloma; GMS stain. A disintegrating hair shaft with numerous endothrix and ectothrix dermatophyte hyphae is present in a dermal abscess.

folliculitis may affect the superficial portion of the hair follicle and present clinically as a pustule or the deep portion of the hair follicle and present as indurated, erythematous nodules or plaques. Superficial bacterial folliculitis, also known as ***Bockhart impetigo***, is usually caused by *Staphylococcus aureus*. **Furuncles**, or deep folliculitis, are larger, tender, warm, erythematous nodules and plaques with central pustules, generally caused by *S aureus*. Furuncles may occur on any nonglabrous skin but are more common on the legs, buttocks, posterior neck, and axillae. **Carbuncles**, composed of two or more coalescing furuncles, are more common in diabetics. Gram-negative folliculitis may occur as a complication of long-term oral antibiotic treatment for acne and presents clinically as worsening acneiform papules and pustules around the nose, mouth, and cheeks. Culture of these lesions usually grows a species of *Enterobacter, Klebsiella*, or *Escherichia coli*. **Hot-tub folliculitis** is a less common gram-negative folliculitis usually caused by *Pseudomonas aeruginosa* and acquired

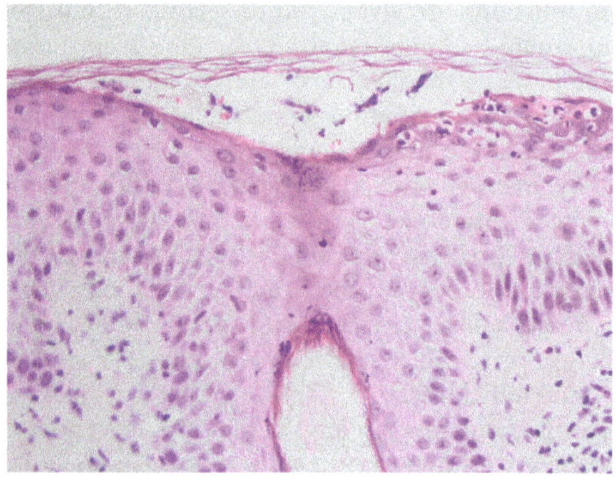

Bockhart impetigo. There is a subcorneal pustule localized within the follicular ostium. Scattered neutrophils are present. Gram stain revealed rare gram-positive cocci in clusters.

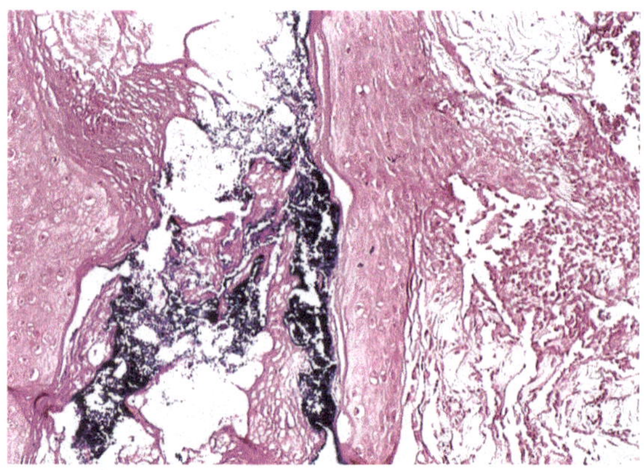

Bacterial folliculitis. Numerous intrafollicular bacteria are seen as well as early follicular rupture.

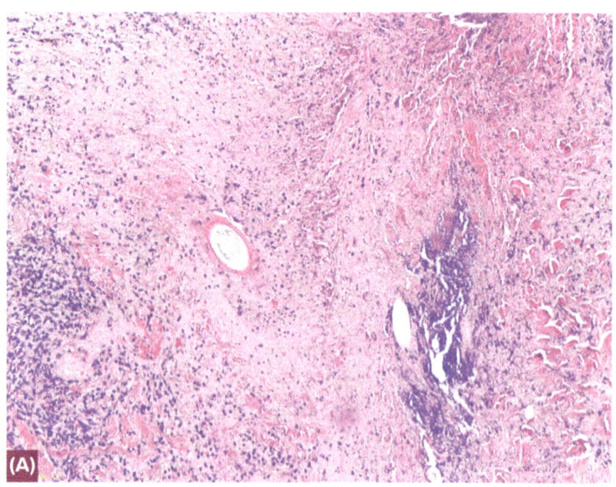

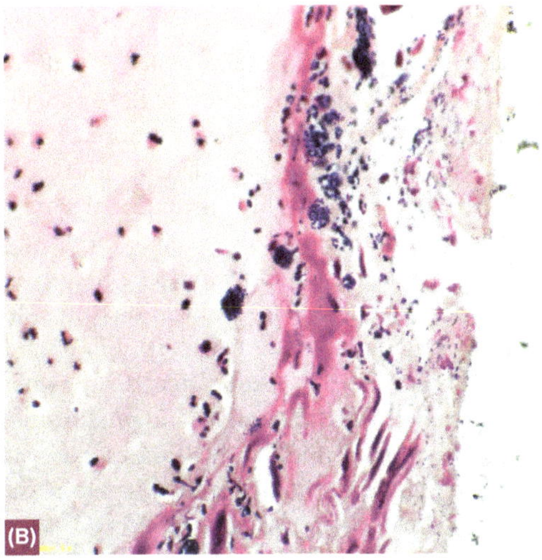

Furuncle. (A) There is an abscess characterized by extensive liquefactive dermal necrosis accompanied by mixed inflammatory infiltrates. A naked hair shaft is present. The blue "smokey" material represents bacteria. **(B)** Gram stain reveals numerous gram-positive cocci.

through exposure to inadequately chlorinated water in swimming pools and hot tubs. Lesions generally are distributed over areas covered by the bathing suit. **Mud-wrestling folliculitis** caused by soil bacteria, Enterobacteriaceae, also occurs on covered skin in individuals participating in this activity.

ANSWER 5-31: A.

Hair loss in **secondary scarring alopecias** is the result of non-folliculocentric skin disease (Table 5-31A). The pilosebaceous apparatus is not the focus of disease but is collateral damage. The clinical and microscopic features of **secondary scarring alopecia** are characteristic for the specific disease involved. Some examples include hair loss produced by **neoplasms, sarcoidal granulomas, sclerodermoid porphyria cutanea tarda, necrobiosis lipoidica,** and dermal sclerosis from **morphea, lichen sclerosus et atrophicus,** and **external trauma**.

Keratosis pilaris (KP) is a common follicular dermatosis often associated with **ichthyosis** and **atopic dermatitis**. Onset occurs in the first and second decades of life with persistence into adulthood. Lesions consist of patches of follicular hyperkeratosis with variable perifollicular erythema commonly affecting the upper outer arms, thighs, and buttocks. **Scarring alopecia** is typically not associated with **classic KP. Lichen spinulosus (LS)** is a closely related follicular hyperkeratotic condition presenting in children as patches of minute horny follicular spines. Patients with vitamin A deficiency develop numerous follicular hyperkeratotic lesions termed ***phrynoderma*** that begin on the thighs and posterolateral arms with subsequent involvement of extensor surfaces. Night blindness, xerophthalmia, keratomalacia, diarrhea, weakness, and generalized wasting may occur in hypovitaminosis A. Several genetically determined syndromes

Table 5-31A. Secondary Scarring Alopecia

Sclerosing disorders
Morphea
Sclerodermoid porphyria cutanea tarda
Lichen sclerosus et atrophicus
Parry-Romberg syndrome
Physical/chemical agents
Mechanical trauma, laceration
Thermal burns
Chemical burns
Radiation dermatitis
Dermal infiltrative processes
Tumors
Basal cell carcinoma
Squamous cell carcinoma
Metastatic carcinoma
Lymphoma
Adnexal tumors
Dermatofibrosarcoma protuberans
Others
Granulomatous conditions
Sarcoidosis
Necrobiosis lipoidica
Miescher
Actinic granuloma
Infections
Syphilis (tertiary)
Tuberculosis
Viral infections
Protozoal infections
Other
Amyloidosis

characterized by KP, follicular destruction, and typical clinical findings have been described. This group of disorders is often termed ***scarring follicular keratosis***. Three major variants include **keratosis pilaris spinulosa decalvans (KPSD), keratosis pilaris atrophicans (KPA),** and **atrophoderma vermiculata (AV)**. Scarring alopecia with KP-like lesions occurs in **KPSD** with onset during the teenage years. Loss of eyebrow hair with atrophy and follicular hyperkeratosis is characteristic of **KPA. AV** is characterized by reticulate, "ice-pick" scarring of the cheeks with follicular hyperkeratosis. Overlapping clinical findings may be seen in these three clinical subtypes of scarring follicular keratosis.

Microscopically, follicular dilatation with compact follicular hyperkeratosis, at times tightly adherent to the hair shaft, is present in KP and LS. Follicular infundibular atrophy with slight perifollicular lymphocytic infiltrates is also present. Follicular rupture with subsequent inflammatory folliculitis may occur.

Similar findings are seen in the **scarring follicular keratosis**. Early lesions display typical KP-like features but may have more prominent infundibular hypergranulosis.

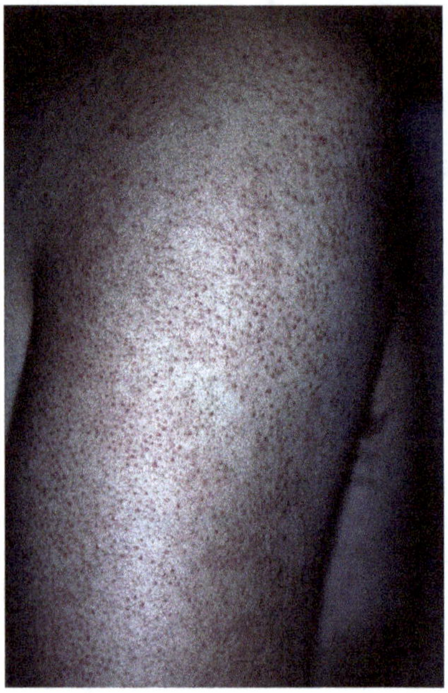

Classic keratosis pilaris on the lateral upper arm. Note how the papules can vary in color from pink to brown to white depending on the skin color of the person. (Reproduced, with permission, from Usatine RP, Smith MA, Mayeaux EJ Jr, Chumley HS, eds. *Color Atlas of Family Medicine.* 2nd ed. New York, NY: McGraw-Hill Education; 2012.)

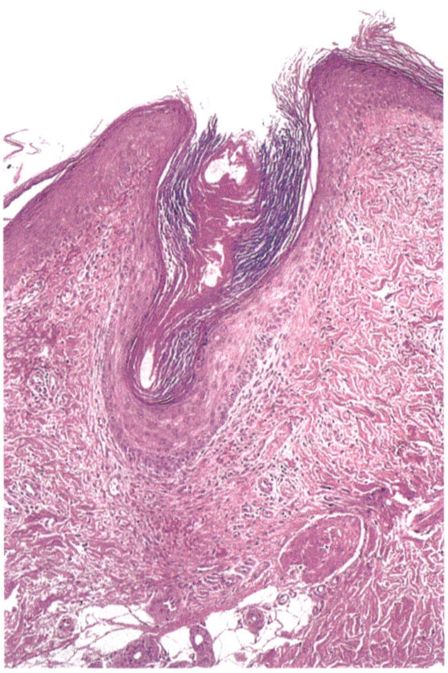

Keratosis pilaris. Follicular hyperkeratosis with slight perifollicular fibroplasia and sparse lymphocytic infiltrates are seen.

Inflammatory and pustular lesions show follicular rupture and folliculitis. Late lesions are no different from other end-stage scarring alopecias, with complete follicular dropout, numerous residual fibrous tracts, and scattered "naked" hair shafts.

ANSWER 5-32: B.

This is a classic example of **acne fulminans**, which is a clinical diagnosis characterized by the sudden severe flare of acne (usually **acne conglobata**) following an elevated dose of oral retinoids. The condition is typically preceded by myalgias, arthralgias, lymphadenopathy, and mild constitutional symptoms. It is believed to be immunologically mediated resulting in increased follicular colonization of *Propionibacterium acnes* (Gram+ rod). The most frequent flare associations include testosterone and increased doses of oral isotretinoin. **Acne vulgaris**, other acne subtypes, **pseudofolliculitis barbae** (answer choice B), **hidradenitis suppurativa**, and **pustulofollicular scarring alopecias** (ie, dissecting cellulitis, etc) are all examples of acneiform folliculitis. Some forms of rosacea are also included in this group of diseases (Table 5-32A).

Acne can be comedonal, papular, pustular, nodular, or cystic. The face, chest, and back are involved, and this disorder primarily affects adolescents and young adults. Comedonal, papular, and pustular acnes are the most common variants and are termed ***acne vulgaris*** (Table 5-32B). **Comedones** are either open (blackheads) or closed (whiteheads). **Acne conglobata** is a severe form of nodulocystic acne that usually involves the back, chest, and posterior neck and consists of numerous coalescing large comedones, acne cysts, and nodules. Extensive irregularly shaped scars and epidermoid cysts occur in the later stages, and association with the follicular occlusion triad is common. This condition, along with **hidradenitis suppurativa** and **dissecting cellulitis of the scalp**, forms the follicular occlusion triad (Table 5-32C). **Chloracne** is a rare acne variant occurring after exposure to halogenated aromatic compounds, especially dioxin. Patients using systemic and topical corticosteroids may develop a monomorphic acneiform follicular eruption termed ***steroid acne***. A number of other drugs, including anticonvulsants,

Table 5-32A. Folliculitis Subtypes

Infectious folliculitis
Bacterial—*Staphylococcus, Pseudomonas,* other
Fungal folliculitis—Majocchi granuloma,
Pityrosporum folliculitis
Demodex folliculitis
Herpesvirus folliculitis
Acneiform folliculitis
Acne variants
Hidradenitis suppurativa
Pseudofolliculitis barbae
Pustulofollicular scarring alopecias
Rosacea
Perioral dermatitis
Eosinophilic folliculitis
Neonatal and adult
HIV associated

Table 5-32B. Acne Vulgaris

Clinical Features
Adolescence, early adulthood
Men ≥ women
Face >> back, chest, shoulder
Comedones
Erythematous papules, pustules, nodules, cysts
Occasional scarring
Association with hidradenitis suppurativa and dissecting cellulitis
Histopathologic Features
Comedone: dilated follicular infundibulum with keratinous plug, open to surface or closed
Follicular pustule with or without rupture into surrounding dermis
Neutrophilic and foreign-body granulomatous reaction to keratin and follicular contents in dermis
Epithelial cyst and sinus tract formation
Dermal scarring
Differential Diagnosis
Keratosis, pilaris, and related conditions
Other forms of folliculitis, eg, bacterial, fungal, viral

Table 5-32C. Hidradenitis Suppurativa

Clinical Features
Onset after puberty
Axillae, inguinal, and perineal areas, other sites
Erythematous nodules followed by draining abscesses, sinus tracts, prominent scarring
Association with severe acne, dissecting cellulitis of scalp
Histopathologic Features
Early lesions
Follicular plugging, folliculitis
Chronic lesions
Features of chronic folliculitis
Abscesses within apocrine glands and in the dermis and subcutis
Prominent foreign body granulomatous reaction
Dermal scarring often extensive
Sinus tract and cyst formation
Differential Diagnosis
Other chronic active deep folliculitides, infectious and noninfectious
Pyoderma gangrenosum
Crohn disease

anabolic steroids, lithium, isoniazid, azathioprine, cyclosporine A, etretinate, and epidermal growth factor inhibitors, may also cause acneiform eruptions. **Acne cosmetica (pomade acne)** is more common in women and occurs on the face as the result of persistent follicular occlusion by cosmetics and applied hair oils. Noninflammatory comedones and cysts associated with nodular solar elastosis are termed the ***Favre-Racouchot syndrome*** and generally occur on the upper to lateral cheeks and temples near the eyes.

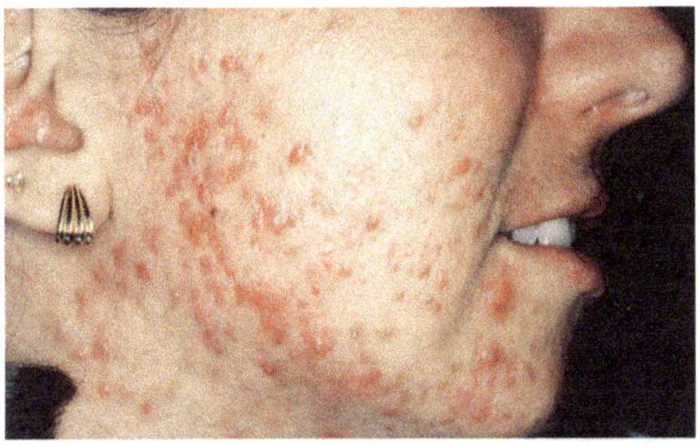

Acne vulgaris. An example of acne vulgaris with inflammatory papules, pustules, and comedones. (Reproduced, with permission, from Longo DL, Fauci AS, Kasper DL, Hauser SL, Jameson JL, Loscalzo J, eds. *Harrison's Principles of Internal Medicine.* 18th ed. New York, NY: McGraw-Hill Education; 2011.)

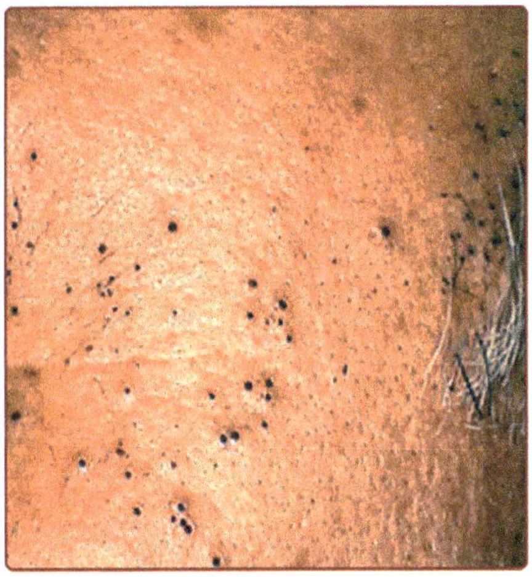

Open comedones in the temporal region are called Favre-Racouchot disease. (Reproduced, with permission, from Goldsmith LA, Katz SI, Gilchrest BA, Paller AS, Leffell DJ, Wolff K, eds. *Fitzpatrick's Dermatology in General Medicine.* 8th ed. New York, NY: McGraw-Hill Education; 2012.)

Microscopically, the follicular infundibulum is thinned, dilated, and filled with compact hyperkeratosis in acne comedones. Inflammatory comedones, papules, and pustules show mixed infiltrates of increasing density within and around dilated follicles. Follicular rupture with dermal abscess is seen in nodulocystic acne lesions, and subsequent scarring is common. Extensive abscesses and partially squamous-lined sinuses with prominent scarring are seen in **acne conglobata**. Focal dystrophic calcification may occur in old, scarred acne lesions.

Extensive solar elastosis, open comedones, and small epidermoid cysts are seen in the **Favre-Racouchot syndrome**. Typically there is little to no inflammation in this latter condition.

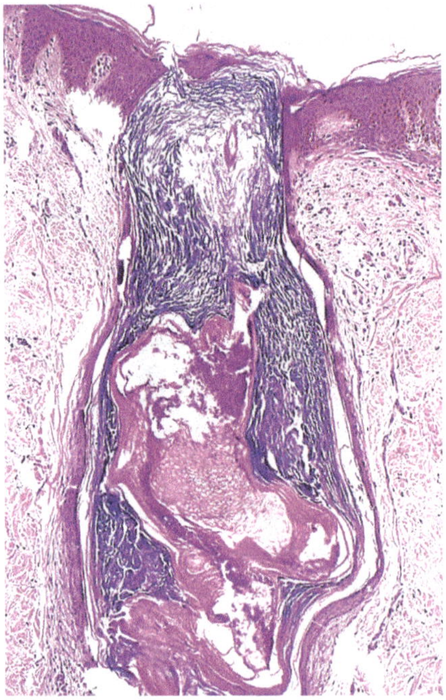

Large closed comedone displays a keratin-filled dilated follicle with atrophy of infundibular epithelium.

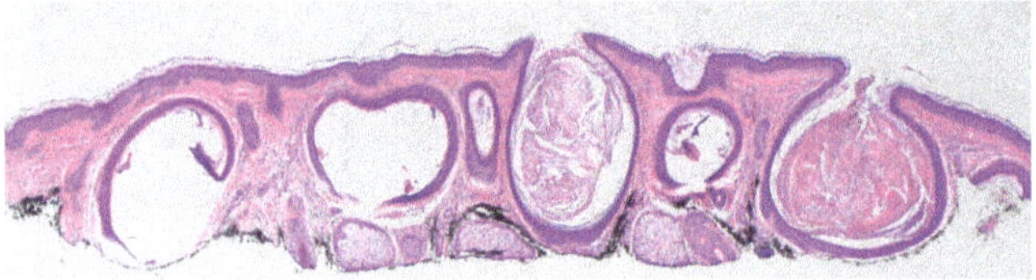

Favre-Racouchot disease. Numerous open comedones containing keratinous debris. There is a background of solar elastosis and inflammation is absent.

Answer choice B describes the pathophysiology of **pseudofolliculitis barbae**, which is an acneiform eruption of the bearded area most common in men with thick, tightly curled hair. This condition is related to **acne keloidalis**, and not surprisingly concomitant **acne keloidalis** often occurs in these patients. **Pseudofolliculitis barbae** results from close shaving in individuals with thick, tightly curled hair. The hair shafts either penetrate their own follicular infundibulum or curl back and penetrate the adjacent epidermis after exiting the acrotrichium. The histopathologic features show a follicular and perifollicular mixed inflammatory infiltrate with an associated foreign-body histiocytic giant cell response and variable fibrosis and naked hair shafts.

The histopathological differential diagnosis also includes **hidradenitis suppurativa** and **dissecting cellulitis of the scalp,** both of which share a very similar histomorphology to **acne conglobata**. The clinical presentations for these conditions are obviously different and are required for the correct diagnosis. In fact, these three conditions form the **follicular occlusion triad**. **Hidradenitis suppurativa** is a painful, deep, scarring folliculitis of the axillae and groin often associated with nodulocystic acne. **Dissecting cellulitis of the scalp** consists of numerous fluctuant abscesses that converge via draining sinus tracts and overlying scarring alopecia.

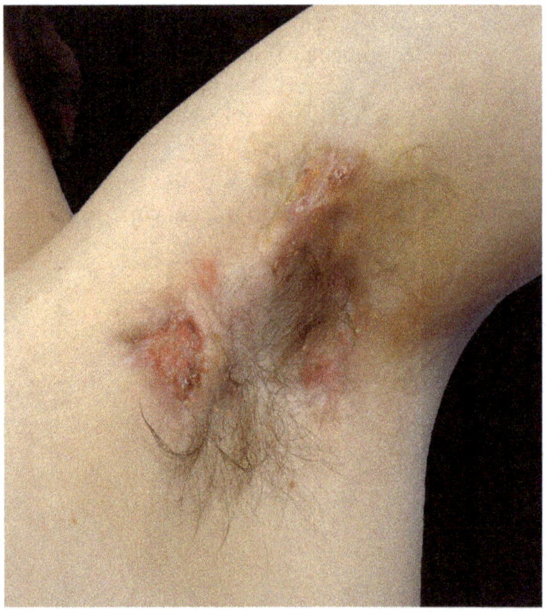

Hidradenitis suppurativa. Multiple bulging and depressed scars, draining sinuses and larger ulcer in the axilla of a 24-year-old male. (Reproduced, with permission, from Wolff K, Johnson RA, Saavedra AP. *Fitzpatrick's Color Atlas and Synopsis of Clinical Dermatology*. 7th ed. New York, NY: McGraw-Hill Education; 2013.)

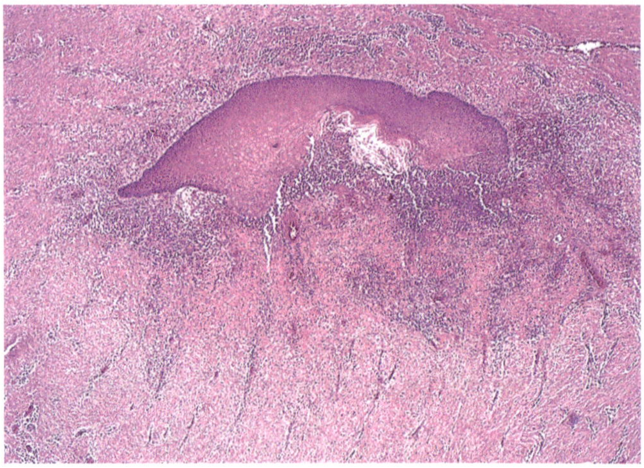

Hidradenitis suppurativa. Extensive dermal scarring is present with a partially squamous-lined sinus tract and associated suppurative infiltrates.

Microscopically, all three conditions consist of extensive scarring of the dermis and subcutis with deep dermal and subcutaneous abscesses and sinuses tracts partially lined with squamous epithelium. Follicular occlusion occurs initially with subsequent superficial and deep folliculitis and abscess formation. A persistent fibroinflammatory response occurs as the result of continuous keratin production by ruptured squamous-lined sinuses. Abundant granulation tissue is seen in some patients. Suppurative inflammation of apocrine glands occurs secondarily and only in a minority of patients with hidradenitis suppurativa. In one study, secondary apocrine gland involvement was found in 12% of specimens, and secondary involvement of eccrine glands was found in 25%.

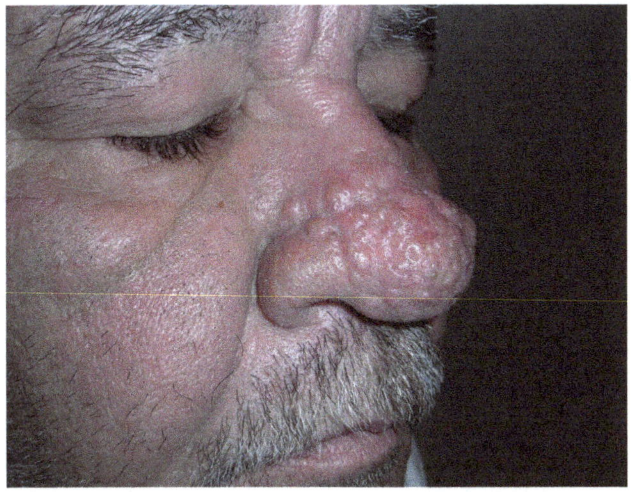

Rhinophymatous rosacea with hypertrophy of the skin of the nose of a 51-year-old Hispanic man. The patient acknowledges previous heavy alcohol intake. (Reproduced, with permission, from Usatine RP, Smith MA, Mayeaux EJ Jr, Chumley HS, eds. *Color Atlas of Family Medicine*. 2nd ed. New York, NY: McGraw-Hill Education; 2012.)

ANSWER 5-33: D.

This is a classic example of **papulopustular rosacea**. The patient's biopsies show nonspecific perifollicular and perivascular lymphohistiocytic infiltrates and elongated *Demodex folliculorum* mites present within in a follicular infundibulum with perifollicular infiltrates (**Demodex folliculitis**). **Rosacea** is an acneiform disorder that most commonly affects the middle-aged and elderly (Table 5-33A). **Telangiectatic, papulopustular, granulomatous,** and **rhinophyma** variants occur. The nose, cheeks, and chin typically are affected, but extrafacial involvement can occur rarely. Transient and persistent flushing of the face is common and may be aggravated by external and psychological factors. Inflammatory papular and granulomatous lesions can mimic **basal cell carcinoma** clinically and therefore often are biopsied. Although once considered a tuberculid, **lupus miliaris disseminatus faciei** is now considered a variant of granulomatous rosacea and consists of discrete red-brown papules distributed over the face and eyelids. **Rhinophyma** is an end-stage variant of rosacea that results in enlargement of the nose, especially the nasal tip, due to sebaceous gland hypertrophy. On occasion, other areas of the face or ears may be involved by rhinophyma.

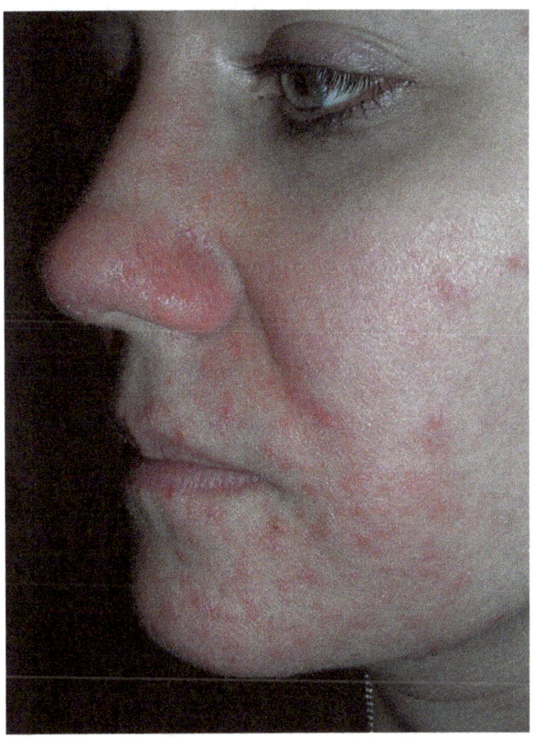

Papulopustular rosacea. Close-up showing telangiectasias on the nose and papules around the mouth and chin. Note the absence of comedones. This is not acne. (Reproduced, with permission, from Usatine RP, Smith MA, Mayeaux EJ Jr, Chumley HS, eds. *Color Atlas of Family Medicine*. 2nd ed. New York, NY: McGraw-Hill Education; 2012.)

The pathogenesis is poorly understood, but the vascular flushing reaction is one of the earliest stages in the development of rosacea and recent evidence suggests angiogenesis is an important factor in the pathogenesis of rosacea. Aggravating factors include hot, spicy foods and liquids, alcohol, certain vasodilatory drugs, and sunlight. Ocular rosacea is relatively common, with symptoms of stinging, burning, tearing, photophobia, scratchiness, and feelings of foreign material in the eye. Answer choice D describes associations with **seborrheic dermatitis. Perioral dermatitis** is a relatively common related facial eruption consisting of acneiform papules and pustules distributed around the mouth of young women. Use of topical fluorinated corticosteroids on the face is often the inciting cause, but idiopathic cases occur. Clinically, **perioral dermatitis** has features of **acne rosacea** and **seborrheic dermatitis**. Granulomatous variants of perioral dermatitis occur, especially in children, and in these cases involvement of the eyelids and neck is common.

Table 5-33A. Rosacea and Rhinophyma

Clinical Features
Age 20-50 years common
Women > men
Fair-skinned individuals
Central face: nose, cheek, chin, glabella, forehead; rarely neck, upper trunk
Blushing, flushing
Erythema, telangiectasia, edema
Papules, pustules
Rhinophyma, other phymas involving forehead, chin
Histopathologic Features
Variable degrees of the following:
Vascular ectasia
Perivascular and perifollicular lymphoid infiltrates
Folliculitis
Solar elastosis
Edema
Granulomatous inflammation
Epithelioid granulomas, especially perifollicular
Sebaceous hyperplasia
Rhinophyma and other phymas show variable degrees of the following:
Florid sebaceous gland hyperplasia
Diffuse fibroplasia
Ectatic venular vessels
Nodular solar elastosis
Differential Diagnosis
Lupus erythematosus
Perioral dermatitis
Acne vulgaris
Sarcoidosis
Other granulomatous dermatitides

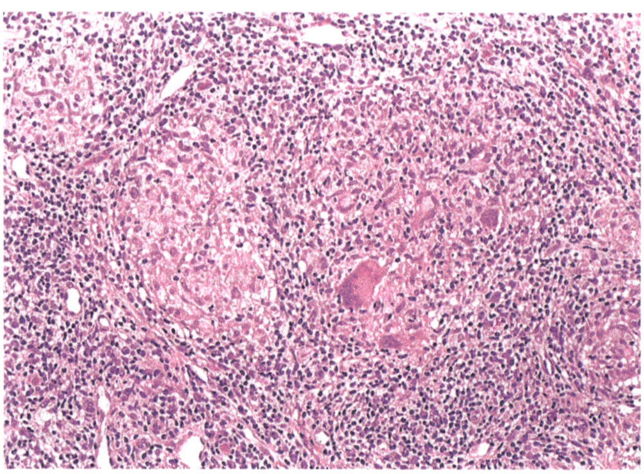

Granulomatous rosacea. Loose to well-formed granulomas comprised of histiocytes and multinucleate giant cells are seen. Granulomas may or may not be perifollicular.

Microscopically, the features of **rosacea** are nonspecific and vary according to clinical subtype. In **telangiectatic rosacea**, increased numbers of ectatic venules with sparse perivascular lymphocytic infiltrates are seen. Solar elastosis is common. **Papular rosacea** lesions have perivascular and perifollicular lymphohistiocytic infiltrates involving the superficial to middle dermis. Admixed multinucleate histiocytes and loose granulomas are seen in **papular rosacea** and **granulomatous rosacea**. Nonfollicular epithelioid granulomas that occasionally exhibit caseation necrosis occur less frequently.

The inflammatory infiltrate in papular rosacea may have a perivascular to nodular pattern rather than a strictly perifollicular distribution. Suppurative folliculitis with admixed lymphohistiocytic infiltrates, including foreign-body giant cells, is characteristic of **pustular rosacea**. Extensive hypertrophy of mature sebaceous glands, follicular dilatation, and hyperkeratosis with variable inflammation are seen in **rhinophyma.** In contrast to discrete lesions of sebaceous hyperplasia, in which sebaceous lobules radiate around a central dilated sebaceous duct, **rhinophyma** exhibits more extensive and diffuse sebaceous gland hypertrophy, fibroplasia, fibrovascular hypertrophy (fibroplasia with prominent vascular ectasia), and nodular accumulation of solar elastotic material. The histopathology of **perioral dermatitis** is similar to that of papular, pustular, and granulomatous variants of rosacea. The ectoparasites *Demodex folliculorum* and *D brevis* are hair follicle mites found frequently in normal adult skin. The pathogenicity of the mites in folliculitis, especially acne rosacea, is controversial. However, in some cases, facial rosacea-like papules and pustules respond to topical acaricidal therapy, suggesting that *Demodex* mites may play a role in some instances. In addition, the mean mite count in a facial biopsy was significantly higher in patients with rosacea than in matched control patients in one study. *Demodex* mites are elongated eosinophilic ectoparasites and are more numerous on the head and neck. One or more mites may be found in normal follicular infundibula. Mites may also be seen within the sebaceous duct. Follicular spongiosis with perifollicular lymphohistiocytic infiltrates can occur in rosacea-like lesions, especially on the face.

ANSWER 5-34: A.

This is a classic example of **eosinophilic folliculitis (eosinophilic pustular folliculitis),** characterized by a dilated follicular infundibulum containing numerous eosinophils (Table 5-34A). The infiltrate involves the entire pilosebaceous unit. **Eosinophilic folliculitis (EF)** is a histopathologically distinct group of diseases that occur in several patient populations: (1) adult males, usually Japanese **(classic EF/Ofuji disease),** (2) neonates and young children, (3) HIV-infected and other immunocompromised patients, and (4) a miscellaneous group of patients, including those with atopic dermatitis. The etiology of EF has not been determined. Classic EF was first

Table 5-34A. Eosinophilic Folliculitis

Clinical Features
Adult young to middle-aged men, mainly Japanese
Neonates and young children
HIV-infected patients
Face, trunk, upper extremities
Erythematous follicular pustules
Polycyclic plaques often with centripetal extension, central clearing
Urticarial follicular papules often in HIV patients
Low CD4 counts (usually <200 cells/mm^3)
Histopathologic Features
Peri and intrafollicular eosinophilic infiltration
Occasional subcorneal eosinophilic pustules
Follicular spongiosis often
Perivascular and interstitial lymphocytic infiltrates
Flame figures rare
Differential Diagnosis
Other folliculitides, especially infectious
Arthropod bite reaction
Papular urticaria
Papular eruption of HIV

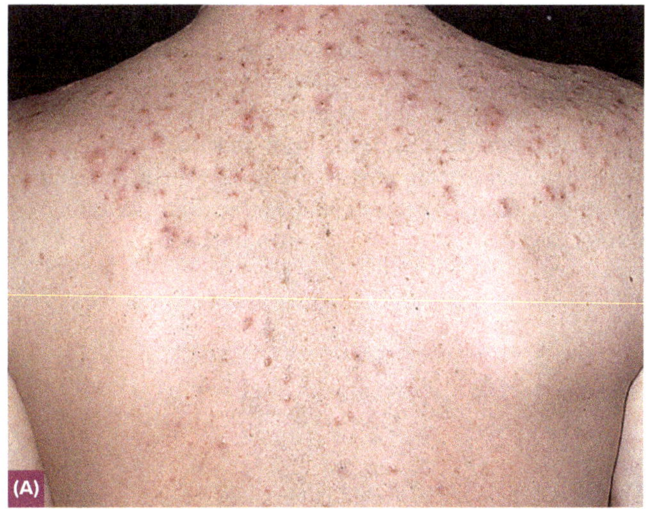

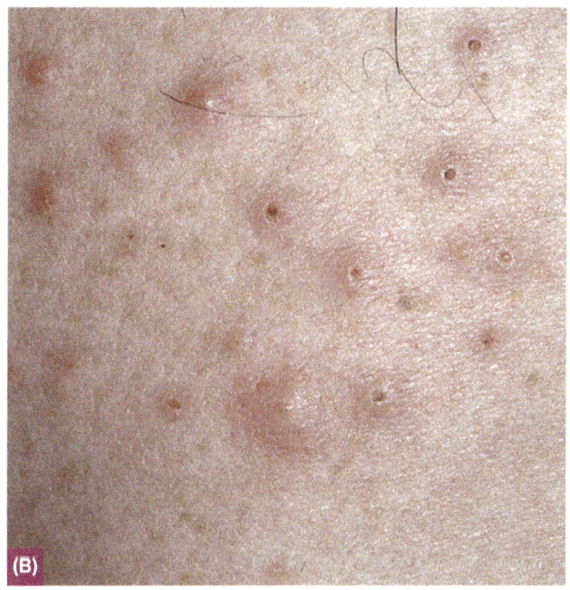

Eosinophilic folliculitis. (A) Multiple erythematous pruritic papules and a few pustules in an individual with a CD4 cell count of 50/μL. **(B)** Close-up showing urticaria papules, pustules, and crusted erosions secondary to rubbing. (Reproduced, with permission, from Goldsmith LA, Katz SI, Gilchrest BA, Paller AS, Leffell DJ, Wolff K, eds. *Fitzpatrick's Dermatology in General Medicine*. 8th ed. New York, NY: McGraw-Hill Education; 2012.)

described in Japanese men by Ofuji and colleagues in 1970 but has since been reported in non-Japanese patients.

Clinically, patients present with erythematous follicular papules and pustules that coalesce to form polycyclic plaques with centrifugal extension and central clearing. Postinflammatory hyperpigmentation occurs frequently. The lesions typically affect the face, trunk, and proximal extremities and can be pruritic. Peripheral leukocytosis and eosinophilia are often present. The pediatric variant occurs predominately in males younger than 1 year of age and generally affects the scalp and forehead as pruritic indurated erythematous plaques with pustules. Lesions can also occur on the face, trunk, and extremities. The lesions typically lack the polycyclic morphology and centrifugal extension seen in the adult form. Peripheral leukocytosis and eosinophilia are often present. HIV-associated EF was described initially by Soeprono and authors in 1986. In contrast to classic EF, **HIV-associated EF** is associated with severe pruritus, rare pustules, and the absence of polycyclic plaques. Discrete follicular urticarial papules, which are often excoriated, occur on the head, neck, and trunk with sparing of the lower extremities. Females may show predominantly facial involvement. CD4 counts typically are below 200 cells/mm^3, and the presence of EF suggests more advanced disease. Serum IgE levels frequently are elevated. **Follicular mucinosis** has been coexistent in two reported cases; however, lymphocytic atypia and progression to follicular mycosis fungoides has never been documented. Therefore, this follicular mucinosis represents merely a reaction pattern and should not be confused with **alopecia mucinosa**. EF has also been reported in immunocompromised patients secondary to bone marrow transplantation. A **necrotizing variant of EF** has been described in nine patients with an **atopic diathesis**. The cases in atopic patients differed from the presentation of **classic EF** clinically by ulceration and nodule formation and microscopically by follicular necrosis and eosinophilic vasculitis.

Microscopically, the various subtypes of **EF** share similar microscopic features. Intra- and perifollicular mixed inflammatory infiltrates with numerous eosinophils and associated follicular spongiosis are characteristic of EF. Spongiosis of the sebaceous lobules is commonly present. Subcorneal eosinophilic pustules may also be seen. In many cases, variably dense, perivascular and interstitial lymphocytic infiltrates are present in both the superficial and deep reticular dermis. Flame figures are rare. In the variant reported in atopic patients, follicular necrosis and eosinophilic vasculitis are present in addition to follicular inflammation.

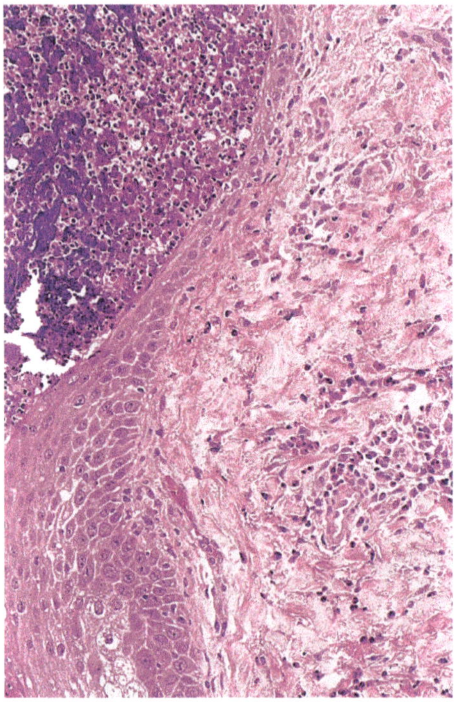

Eosinophilic folliculitis. Both intrafollicular and perifollicular eosinophils are seen in this case of eosinophilic folliculitis.

In regard to the differential diagnosis, lesions that may present with a similar eosinophilic infiltrate include **papular urticaria, arthropod bite reactions, papular eruption of HIV, scabies infestation, dermatophyte infection, drug reactions,** and **erythema toxicum neonatorum.** A PAS and/or silver stain should be performed to exclude an infectious etiology. The inflammatory infiltrate in **papular urticaria, arthropod bite reactions,** and **drug reactions** generally lacks the folliculocentric distribution of EF. The neonatal presentation and rapid resolution of **erythema toxicum neonatorum** should allow clinical distinction from EF.

ANSWER 5-35: C.

Neutrophilic eccrine hidradenitis (NEH) was described initially by Harrist and colleagues in 1982 as a complication of cytarabine chemotherapy in patients with acute myelogenous

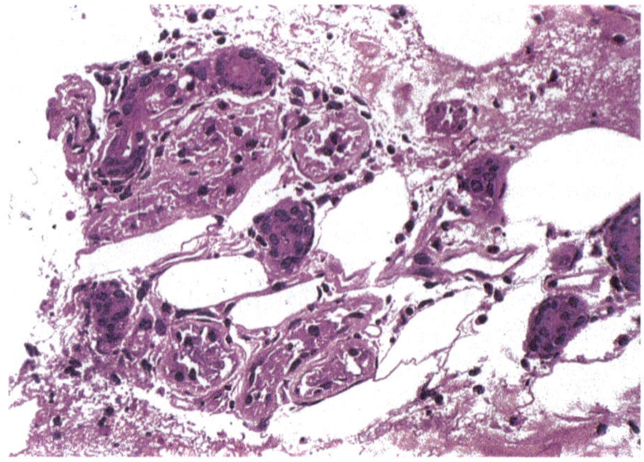

Neutrophilic eccrine hidradenitis. An eccrine sweat coil is infiltrated by neutrophils. The epithelial tubular structures show degenerative changes.

leukemia. It has since been reported in association with other chemotherapeutic agents, particularly bleomycin, nonmyeloid malignancies, and granulocyte colony-stimulating factor (Table 5-35A). It also has occurred in HIV-infected patients and in patients with myeloid leukemia prior to induction chemotherapy. **NEH** is a polymorphous cutaneous eruption affecting the neck, trunk, and extremities. Lesions consist of tender erythematous macules, papules, and plaques. Spontaneous resolution of the lesions may occur.

The predominant microscopic finding in **classic NEH** is a sparse to dense neutrophilic infiltrate surrounding eccrine units. Secretory coils in the superficial subcutis generally show more extensive involvement by the neutrophilic infiltrate, and eccrine epithelial vacuolization and necrosis are commonly present. Focal degenerative mucinous changes often are evident in the adjacent subcutis. Squamous

Table 5-35A. Cytotoxic Agents Associated With Adnexal Toxicity

Neutrophilic Eccrine Hidradenitis	Eccrine Syringosquamous Metaplasia
Bleomycin	Bleomycin
Chlorambucil	Cytarabine (common)
Cytarabine (common)	
Daunorubicin	Daunorubicin
Doxorubicin (common)	Doxorubicin
Mitoxantrone	Mitoxantrone
Vincristine	Suramin

Table 5-35B. Neutrophilic Eccrine Hidradenitis

Clinical Features
Onset a few days after administration of chemotherapeutic agents such as cytarabine, bleomycin
Neck, trunk, extremities
Tenderness
Erythematous macules, papules, plaques
Spontaneous resolution
Histopathologic Features
Neutrophilic infiltrates associated with eccrine sweat coil
Eccrine epithelial cells show vacuolar degeneration and necrosis
Mucin deposition in perieccrine adipose tissue
Dermal edema
Sparse dermal infiltrates composed of lymphocytes and neutrophils
Differential Diagnosis
Infectious hidradenitis and pyoderma
Other neutrophilic dermatitides

metaplasia and variable dyskeratosis can affect part or the entire eccrine unit in chemotherapy and has been termed ***eccrine squamous syringometaplasia***. In association with chemotherapy, it is considered in the histopathologic spectrum of NEH (Table 5-35B).

The clinical differential diagnosis includes **idiopathic palmoplantar eccrine hidradenitis (IPEH). IPEH** shares clinical and microscopic features with **NEH**. It presents as an abrupt onset of tender, erythematous papules and nodules on the plantar and less commonly palmar surfaces. The lesions resolve spontaneously in most cases. The disease affects children and young adults of both sexes. There is no disease or chemotherapy association, and no specific etiology has been identified. Squamous metaplasia of the eccrine apparatus is characteristically absent in **IPEH**. The other entities in the microscopic differential diagnosis include **infectious hidradenitis, neutrophilic dermatoses (Sweet syndrome), leukocytoclastic vasculitis**, and **coma blister** or **pressure-induced eccrine necrosis**. Special stains and/or tissue culture should be used to exclude an infectious hidradenitis. **NEH** has been hypothesized to be in the spectrum of neutrophilic dermatoses; however, in contrast to **Sweet syndrome**, the neutrophilic infiltrate is confined to the eccrine unit. Although the pattern of the infiltrate in NEH may mimic vasculitis at low magnification, vessels typically are not affected. Patients in a comatose state due to carbon monoxide poisoning, drug overdose (especially barbiturates), severe illness, or trauma may develop bullae with sweat gland necrosis at pressure sites **(coma blister)**. The cause of these blisters is thought to be related to pressure-induced ischemia and possible toxic effect of offending drugs. Intra- and subepidermal vesiculation with variable dyskeratosis and necrosis is present in the epidermis. Eosinophilic coagulative necrosis of the eccrine secretory coils with minimal inflammation is the most characteristic finding in this entity. Similar necrotic changes can be observed in adjacent hair follicles and sebaceous lobules. The dermis may be acellular or contain degenerating fibroblasts. Generally, the inflammatory infiltrate is minimal, but sparse neutrophils can be present around necrotic adnexal structures.

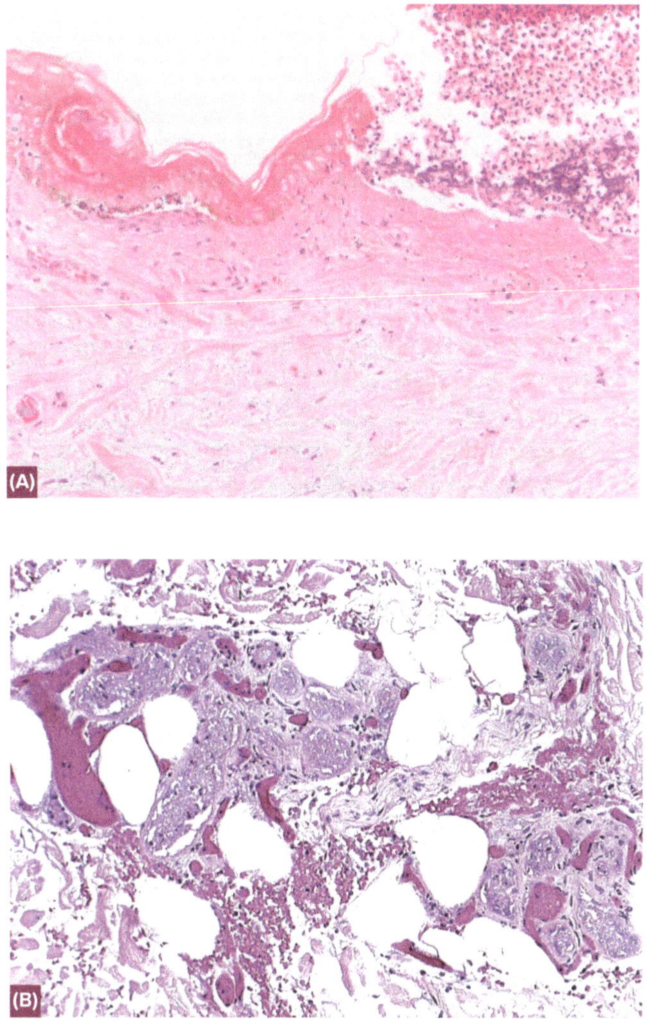

Coma blister. (A) There is a subepidermal blister with necrotic epidermis. Although the epidermal surface is crusted secondary to ulceration, the dermis exhibits a striking absence of inflammatory cells. **(B)** Evaluation of the subcutis reveals extensive noninflammatory necrosis of the eccrine sweat units.

BIBLIOGRAPHY

1. Abbas O, Chedraoui A, Ghosn S. Frontal fibrosing alopecia presenting with components of Piccardi-Lassueur-Graham-Little syndrome. *J Am Acad Dermatol.* 2007;57:S15–S18.
2. Aimes RT, Quigley JP. Matrix metalloproteinase-2 is an interstitial collagenase: inhibitor-free enzyme catalyses the cleavage of collagen fibrils and soluble native type I collagen generating the specific 3/4-and 1/4-length fragments. *J Biol Chem.* 1995;270:5872.
3. Amato L, Mei S, Massi D, et al. Cicatricial alopecia: a dermatopathologic and immunopathologic study of 33 patients (pseudopelade of Brocq is not a specific clinico-pathologic entity). *Int J Dermatol.* 2002;41:8–15.
4. Annessi G, Lombardo G, Gobello T, et al. A clinicopathologic study of scarring alopecia due to lichen planus: comparison with scarring alopecia in discoid lupus erythematosus and pseudopelade. *Am J Dermatopathol.* 1999;21:324–331.
5. Anshu, Gangane N, Vagha S, Samal N. Cytodiagnosis of erythema nodosum leprosum: a case report. *Acta Cytol.* 2002;46(2):386–388.
6. Aroni K, Tsagroni E, Kavantzas N, et al. A study of the pathogenesis of rosacea: how angiogenesis and mast cells may participate in a complex multifactorial process. *Arch Dermatol Res.* 2008;300:125–131.
7. Attanoos R, Appleton M, Douglas-Jones A. The pathogenesis of hidradenitis suppurativa: a closer look at apocrine and apoeccrine glands. *Br J Dermatol.* 1995;133:254–258.
8. Attie, Alan D. The adipocyte comes of age. *J Lipid Res.* 2007;48:1251–1252.
9. Au S, Crawford RI. Three-dimensional analysis of a calciphylaxis plaque: clues to pathogenesis. *J Am Acad Dermatol.* 2002;47(1):53–57.
10. Bachmeyer C, Aractingi S. Neutrophilic eccrine hidradenitis. *Clin Dermatol.* 2000;18:319–330.
11. Baden H, Byers H. Clinical findings, cutaneous pathology, and response to therapy in 21 patients with keratosis pilaris atrophicans. *Arch Dermatol.* 1994;130:469–475.
12. Benedek TG, Rodnan GP. The early history and nomenclature of scleroderma and of its differentiation from sclerema neonatorum and scleredema. *Semin Arthritis Rheum.* 1982;12:52–67.
13. Blume-Peytavi U, Chen W, Djemadji N, et al. Eosinophilic pustular folliculitis (Ofuji's disease). *J Am Acad Dermatol.* 1997;37:259–262.
14. Brooke R, Griffiths C. Folliculitis decalvans. *Clin Exp Dermatol.* 2001;26:120–122.
15. Bruce AJ, Bennett DD, Lohse CM, et al. Lipodermatosclerosis: review of cases evaluated at Mayo clinic. *J Am Acad Dermatol.* 2002;46(2):187–192.
16. Buezo G, Fraga J, Abajo P, et al. HIV-associated eosinophilic folliculitis and follicular mucinosis. *Dermatology.* 1998;197:178–180.
17. Canfield AE, Farrington C, Dziobon MD, et al. The involvement of matrix glycoproteins in vascular calcification and fibrosis: an immunohistochemical study. *J Pathol.* 2002;196(2):228–234.
18. Chapalain V, Winter H, Langbein L. Is the loose anagen hair syndrome a keratin disorder? *Arch Dermatol.* 2002;138:501–506.
19. Chuang SD, Chiu HC, Chang CC. Subcutaneous fat necrosis of the newborn complicating hypothermic cardiac surgery. *Br J Dermatol.* 1995;132:805–810.
20. Connolly SM, Quimby SR, Griffing WL, Winkelmann RK. Scleroderma and L-tryptophan: a possible explanation of the eosinophilia-myalgia syndrome. *J Am Acad Dermatol.* 1990;23:451–457.
21. Dawber R, Simpson N, Barth J. Diffuse alopecia: endocrine, metabolic and chemical influences on the follicular cycle. In: Dawber R, ed. *Diseases of the Hair and Scalp.* 3rd ed. Oxford: Blackwell Scientific Publication; 1997.
22. DeBerker D, Sinclair R. Defects of the hair shaft. In: Dawber R, ed. *Diseases of the Hair and Scalp.* 3rd ed. Oxford: Blackwell Scientific; 1997.
23. Degitz K. Detection of mycobacterial DNA in the skin: etiologic insights and diagnostic perspectives. *Arch Dermatol.* 1996;132:71–75.
24. DeVillez R, Jacobs J, Szpunar C, et al. Androgenetic alopecia in the female: treatment with 2 percent minoxidil solution. *Arch Dermatol.* 1994;130:303–307.
25. Diaz-Cascajo C, Borghi S. Subcutaneous pseudomembranous fat necrosis: new observations. *J Cutan Pathol.* 2002;29(1):5–10.
26. Dyer J, Guitart J, Klein-Gitelman M, Mancini A. Neutrophilic panniculitis in infancy: a cutaneous manifestation of juvenile rheumatoid arthritis. *JAAD.* 2007;57(5):S65–S68.
27. Elmer K, George R. Congenital triangular alopecia: a case report and review. *Pediatr Dermatol.* 2002;69:255–262.
28. Elston D, McCollough M, Angeloni V. Vertical and transverse sections of alopecia biopsy specimens: combining the two to maximize diagnostic yield. *J Am Acad Dermatol.* 1995;32:454–457.
29. Elston D, McCollough M, Bergfeld W. Eosinophils in fibrous tracts and near hair bulbs: a helpful diagnostic feature of alopecia areata. *J Am Acad Dermatol.* 1997;37:101–106.

30. Erbagci Z, Ozgoztasi O. The significance of Demodex folliculorum density in rosacea. *Int J Dermatol.* 1998;37:421–425.
31. Faulkner C, Wilson N, Jones S. Frontal fibrosing alopecia associated with cutaneous lichen planus in a premenopausal woman. *Aust J Dermatol.* 2002;43:65–67.
32. Fiedler V, Gray A. Diffuse alopecia: telogen hair loss. In: Olsen E, ed. *Disorders of Hair Growth: Diagnosis and Treatment.* 2nd ed. New York, NY: McGraw-Hill; 2003.
33. Förström L, Winkelmann RK. Factitial panniculitis. *Arch Dermatol.* 1974;110:747–750.
34. Friedman SJ, Winkelmann RK. Subcutaneous fat necrosis of the newborn: light, ultrastructural and histochemical microscopic studies. *J Cutan Pathol.* 1989;16:99–105.
35. Galende J, Vasquez ML, Almeida J, et al. Case report. Histiocytic cytophagic panniculitis: a rare late complication of allogeneic bone marrow transplantation. *Bone Marrow Transplant* 1994;14:637–639.
36. Gilaberte Y, Coscojuela C, Vazquez C, et al. Perforating folliculitis associated with tumour necrosis factor-alpha inhibitors administered for rheumatoid arthritis. *Br J Dermatol.* 2007;156:368–371.
37. Grossberg E, Scherschun L, Fivenson DP. Lupus profundus: not a benign disease. *Lupus.* 2001;10(7):514–516.
38. Hanly A. Post operative pressure induced alopecia: a report of a case and discussion of the rate of apoptosis in nonscarring alopecia. *J Cutan Pathol.* 1999;26:357–361.
39. Harrist TJ, Fine JD, Berman RS, et al. Neutrophilic eccrine hidradenitis. A distinctive type of neutrophilic dermatosis associated with myelogenous leukemia and chemotherapy. *Arch Dermatol.* 1982;118:263–266.
40. Headington J. Telogen effluvium: new concepts and review. *Arch Dermatol.* 1993;129:356–363.
41. Herouy Y, Aizpurua J, Stetter C, et al. The role of the urokinase-type plasminogen activator (uPA) and its receptor (CD87) in lipodermatosclerosis. *J Cutan Pathol.* 2001;28(6):291–297.
42. Hogan D. Perioral dermatitis. *Curr Probl Dermatol.* 1995;22:98–104.
43. Hordinsky M. Alopecia areata. In: Olsen E, ed. *Disorders of Hair Growth: Diagnosis and Treatment.* 2nd ed. New York, NY: McGraw-Hill; 2003.
44. Hoss D, Grant-Kels J. Diagnosis: alopecia areata or not? *Semin Cutan Med Surg.* 1999;18:84–90.
45. Jaap J, Van der Velden J, van Marion A, et al. Erythema nodosum as an early sign of Crohn's disease. *Int J Dermatol.* 2007;46:27–29.
46. Jansen T, Plewig G. Rosacea: classification and treatment. *J R Soc Med.* 1997;90:144–150.
47. Jordaan H, Louw M. The moth-eaten alopecia of secondary syphilis: a histopathological study of 12 patients. *Am J Dermatopathol.* 1995;17:158–162.
48. Kirsner RS, Pardes JB, Eaglstein WH, Falanga V. The clinical spectrum of lipodermatosclerosis. *J Am Acad Dermatol.* 1993;28:623–627.
49. Kligman A. Ocular rosacea. Current concepts and therapy. *Arch Dermatol.* 1997;133:89–90.
50. Kossard S, Lee MS, Wilkinson B. Postmenopausal frontal fibrosing alopecia: a frontal variant of lichen planopilaris. *J Am Acad Dermatol.* 1997;36:59–66.
51. Kossard S. Diffuse alopecia with stem cell folliculitis: chronic diffuse alopecia areata or a distinct entity? *Am J Dermatopathol.* 1999;21:46–50.
52. Krauser RE, Tuthill RJ. Eosinophilic fasciitis. *Arch Dermatol.* 1977;113:1092–1093.
53. Magro CM, Crowson AN, Kovatich AJ, Burns F. Lupus profundus, indeterminate lymphocytic lobular panniculitis and subcutaneous T-cell lymphoma: a spectrum of subcuticular T-cell lymphoid dyscrasia. *J Cutan Pathol.* 2001;28(5):235–247.
54. Mehregan D, Gibson L, Muller S. Follicular mucinosis: histopathologic review of 33 cases. *Mayo Clin Proc.* 1991;66:387–390.
55. Mirmirani P, Willey A, Headington JT, et al. Primary cicatricial alopecia: histopathologic findings do not distinguish clinical variants. *J Am Acad Dermatol.* 2005;52:637–643.
56. Mori Y, Kahari VM, Varga J. Scleroderma-like cutaneous syndromes. *Curr Rheumatol Rep.* 2002;4(2):113–122.
57. Muller S. Trichotillomania: a histopathologic study of sixty-six patients. *J Am Acad Dermatol.* 1990;23:50–62.
58. Naylor E, Hu S, Robinson-Bostom L. Nephrogenic systemic fibrosis with septal panniculitis mimicking erythema nodosum. *JAAD.* 2008;58(1):149–150.
59. Olsen E, Hordinsky M, Roberts J, et al. Female pattern hair loss. *J Am Acad Dermatol.* 2002;47:795.
60. Olsen E, Messenger A, Shapiro J, et al. Evaluation and treatment of male and female pattern hair loss. *J Am Acad Dermatol.* 2005;52:301–311.
61. Olsen E. Pattern hair loss in men and women. In: Olsen E, ed. *Disorders of Hair Growth: Diagnosis and Treatment.* 2nd ed. New York, NY: McGraw-Hill; 2003.
62. Oranje AP, van Osch LD, Oosterwijk JC. Keratosis pilaris atrophicans. One heterogeneous disease or a symptom in different clinical entities? *Arch Dermatol.* 1994;130:500–502.
63. Pantanowitz L, Harton A, Beckwith B. Cutaneous gangrene in a renal dialysis patient. *Postgrad Med J.* 2001;77(913):735, 741–742.
64. Parker SRS, Parker DC, McCall CO. Eosinophilic folliculitis in HIV-infected women: case series and review. *Am J Clin Dermatol.* 2006;7:193–200.
65. Patton D, Lynch PJ, Fung MA, et al. Chronic atrophic erosive dermatosis of the scalp and extremities: a

recharacterization of erosive pustular dermatosis. *J Am Acad Dermatol.* 2007;57:421–427.

66. Perry P, Cook-Bolden F, Rahman Z, et al. Defining pseudofolliculitis barbae in 2001: a review of the literature and current trends. *J Am Acad Dermatol.* 2002;46:S113–S119.
67. Phelps RG, Shoji T. Update on panniculitis. *Mt Sinai J Med.* 2001;68(4–5):262–267.
68. Philpott H, Hissaria P, Warren L, et al. Eosinophilic fasciitis as a paraneoplastic phenomenon associated with metastatic colorectal carcinoma. *Australas J Dermatol.* 2008;49:27–29.
69. Poelman SM, Nguyen K. Pancreatic panniculitis associated with acinar cell pancreatic carcinoma. *J Cutan Med Surg.* 2008;12(1):38–42.
70. Poskitt L, Wilkinson JD. Natural history of keratosis pilaris. *Br J Dermatol.* 1994;130:711–713.
71. Powell J, Dawber RP. Folliculitis decalvans and tufted folliculitis are specific infective diseases that may lead to scarring, but are not a subset of central centrifugal scarring alopecia. *Arch Dermatol.* 2001;137:373–374.
72. Price V. Structural anomalies of the hair shaft. In: Orfanos C, Happle R, eds. *Hair and Hair Diseases.* Berlin: Springer-Verlag; 1990.
73. Requen L, Sanchez Yus E. Panniculitis. I. Mostly septal panniculitis. *J Am Acad Dermatol.* 2001;45(2):163–183.
74. Requen L, Sanchez Yus E. Panniculitis: II. Mostly lobular panniculitis. *J Am Acad Dermatol.* 2001;45(3):325–361.
75. Roustan G, Salas C, Cabrera R, et al. Neutrophilic eccrine hidradenitis unassociated with chemotherapy in a patient with acute myelogenous leukemia. *Int J Dermatol.* 2001;40:144–147.
76. Sehgal V, Jain S, Thappa D, et al. Perforating dermatoses: a review and report of four cases. *J Dermatol.* 1993;20:329–340.
77. Sinclair R, Grossman K, Kvedar J. Anagen hair loss. In: Olsen E, ed. *Disorders of Hair Growth: Diagnosis and Treatment.* 2nd ed. New York, NY: McGraw-Hill; 2003.
78. Sinclair R, Jolley D, Mallari R, et al. The reliability of horizontally sectioned scalp biopsies in the diagnosis of chronic diffuse telogen hair loss in women. *J Am Acad Dermatol.* 2004;51:189–199.
79. Smith KJ, Neafie R, Skelton H, et al. Majocchi's granuloma. *J Cutan Pathol.* 1991;18:28–35.
80. Snow JL, Su WPD. Lipomembranous (membranocystic) fat necrosis: clinicopathologic correlation of 38 cases. *Am J Dermatopathol.* 1996;18:151–155.
81. Solomon A. The transversely sectioned scalp biopsy specimen: the technique and an algorithm for its use in the diagnosis of alopecia. *Adv Dermatol.* 1994;9: 127–157, discussion 158.
82. Sperling L, Heimer W. Androgen biology as a basis for the diagnosis and treatment of androgenic disorders in women. *J Am Acad Dermatol.* 1993;28:669–683.
83. Sperling L, Lupton G. Histopathology of non-scarring alopecia. *J Cutan Pathol.* 1995;22:97–114.
84. Sperling L, Winton G. The transverse anatomy of androgenetic alopecia. *J Dermatol Surg Oncol.* 1990;16:1127–1133.
85. Sperling L. Hair anatomy for the clinician. *J Am Acad Dermatol.* 1991;25:1–17.
86. Sperling L. Transverse anatomy of telogen effluvium. *J Assoc Mil Med.* 1990;16:3–12.
87. Sperling LC, Homoky C, Pratt L, et al. Acne keloidalis is a form of primary scarring alopecia. *Arch Dermatol.* 2000;136:479–484.
88. Sperling LC, Sau P. The follicular degeneration syndrome in black patients. 'Hot comb alopecia' revisited and revised. *Arch Dermatol.* 1992;128:68–74.
89. Sperling LC. Scarring alopecia and the dermatopathologist. *J Cutan Pathol.* 2001;28:333–342.
90. Su WPD, Person JR. Morphea profunda: a new concept and a histopathologic study of 23 cases. *Am J Dermatopathol.* 1981;3:251–260.
91. Su WPD, Smith KC, Pittelkow MR, Winkelmann RK. Alpha-1-antitrypsin deficiency panniculitis: a histopathologic and immunopathologic study of four cases. *Am J Dermatopathol.* 1987;9(6):483–490.
92. Suwattee P, Cham P, Pope E, Ho N. Pancreatic panniculitis in a 4 year old child with nephritic syndrome. *Pediatr Dermatol.* 2007;24(6):659–660.
93. Tausche A-K, Hansel S, Tausche K, Unger S, Scroder HE. Case number 31: nodular panniculitis as expression of Munchausen's syndrome (panniculitis artefacta). *Ann Rheum Dis.* 2004;63(1):1195–1196.
94. Templeton SF, Solomon AR. Scarring alopecia: a classification based on microscopic criteria. *J Cutan Pathol.* 1994;21:97–109.
95. Ter Poorten JC, Hebert AA, Ilkiw R. Cold panniculitis in a neonate. *J Am Acad Dermatol.* 1995;33(2):383–385.
96. Ter Poorten MA, Theirs BH. Systemic Weber-Christian disease. *J Cutan Med Surg.* 2000;4(2):110–112.
97. Tobin D, Fenton D, Kendall M. Ultrastructural observations on the hair bulb melanocytes and melanosomes in acute alopecia areata. *J Invest Dermatol.* 1990;94:803–807.
98. Tope W, Sangueza O. Rhinophyma's fibrous variant. Histopathology and immunohistochemistry. *Am J Dermatopathol.* 1994;16:307–310.
99. Tosti A. Loose anagen hair syndrome and loose anagen hair. *Arch Dermatol.* 2002;138:521–522.

100. Trent JT, Kirsner RS. Unusual wounds: calciphylaxis: diagnosis and treatment. *Adv Skin Wound Care.* 2001;14(6):309–312.

101. Van Exel CE, English JC III. Erosive pustular dermatosis of the scalp and nonscalp. *J Am Acad Dermatol.* 2007;57:S11–S14.

102. Wang TC, Tzen CY, Su HY. Erythema induratum associated with tuberculous lymphadenitis: analysis of a case using polymerase chain reactions with different primer pairs to differentiate Bacilli Calmette-Guérin (BCG) from virulent strains of *Mycobacterium tuberculosis* complex. *J Dermatol.* 2000;27(11):717–723.

103. Whiting D. Chronic telogen effluvium. *Dermatol Clin.* 1996;14:723–731.

104. Whiting D. Dermatopathology of common hair problems. *J Cutan Med Surg.* 1999;S2–S13.

105. Whiting D. Diagnostic and predictive value of horizontal sections of scalp biopsy specimens in male pattern androgenetic alopecia. *J Am Acad Dermatol.* 1993;28:755–763.

106. Whiting D. Hair and nail histology: histology of normal hair. In: Hordinsky M, Sawaya M, Scher R, eds. *Atlas of Hair and Nails.* Philadelphia, PA: Churchill-Livingstone; 2000.

107. Whiting D. Histopathologic features of alopecia areata. *Arch Dermatol.* 2003;139:1555–1559.

108. Whiting D. Horizontal sections of scalp biopsies. In: Burgdorf W, Katz S, eds. *Dermatology: Progress and Perspectives. The Proceedings of the 18th World Congress of Dermatology, New York, June 12–18, 1992.* New York, NY: Parthenon; 1993.

109. Whiting D. Possible mechanisms of miniaturization during androgenetic alopecia or pattern hair loss. *J Am Acad Dermatol.* 2001;45:S81–S86.

110. Whiting D. Scalp biopsy as a diagnostic and prognostic tool in androgenetic alopecia. *Dermatol Ther.* 1998;8:24–33.

111. Whiting D. *The Structure of the Human Hair Follicle: Light Microscopy of Vertical and Horizontal Sections of Scalp Biopsies.* Fairfield, NJ: Canfield Publishing; 2004.

112. Whiting D. The value of horizontal sections of scalp biopsies. *J Cut Aging Cosm Dermatol.* 1990;1:165–173.

113. Whiting DA. Traumatic alopecia. *Int J Dermatol.* 1999;38:34–44.

114. Wilson CL, Burge SM, Dean D, et al. Scarring alopecia in discoid lupus erythematosus. *Br J Dermatol.* 1992;126:307–314.

115. Winkelmann RK, Barker SM. Factitial traumatic panniculitis. *J Am Acad Dermatol.* 1985;13:988–994.

116. Winkelmann RK, Frigas E. Eosinophilic panniculitis: a clinicopathologic study. *J Cutan Pathol.* 1986;13:1–12.

117. Won et al. Erythema nodosum: clinicopathologic correlations and their use in differential diagnosis. *Yonsei Med J.* 2007;48(4):601–608.

118. Yasar S, Mansur AT, Goktay F, et al. Lipedematous scalp and lipedematous alopecia: report of three cases in white adults. *J Dermatol.* 2007;34:124–130.

CHAPTER 6

Alterations to Components of the Epidermis and Dermis

QUESTION 6-1.

An 8-year-old girl presents to her dermatologist with hypopigmented patches on the trunk. A biopsy of one of the lesions is performed. Immunohistochemical staining with Melan-A is illustrated below. Which entity on the clinician's differential diagnosis is NOT supported by the biopsy findings?

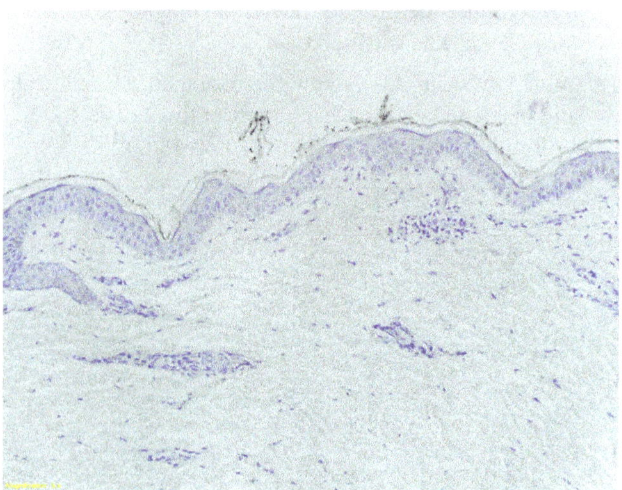

A) Piebaldism
B) Vitiligo
C) Hypopigmented burn scar
D) Ash leaf spots of tuberous sclerosis
E) Waardenburg syndrome

QUESTION 6-2.

A child presents with white hair, milky white skin, and blue-gray eyes. The condition has been present since birth. A plucked hair bulb does not become darker after incubation in DOPA solution. Which of the following statements is MOST accurate regarding this patient's condition?

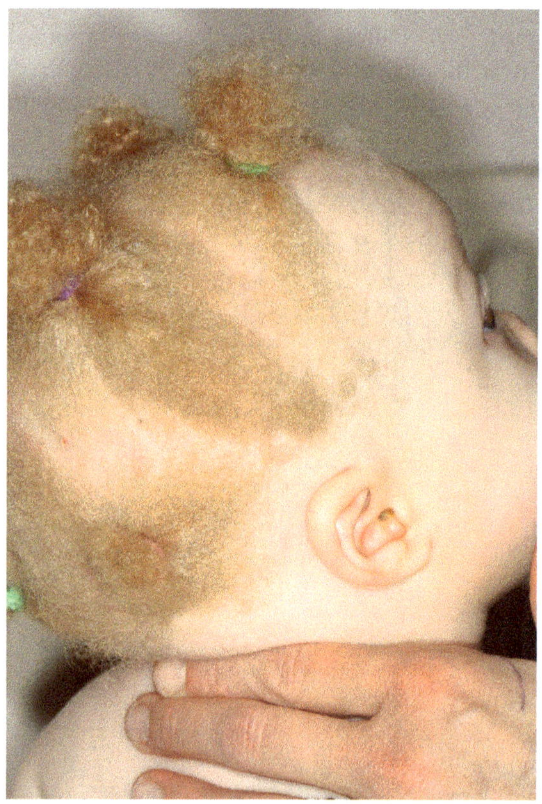

Reproduced, with permission, from Wolff K, Johnson RA, Saavedra AP. *Fitzpatrick's Color Atlas and Synopsis of Clinical Dermatology*. 7th ed. New York, NY: McGraw-Hill Education; 2013.

A) Biopsy of the skin will reveal a paucity of melanocytes.
B) This patient may develop freckles and pigmented nevi later in life.

C) This condition is associated with alterations in the optic systems that will manifest as decreased visual acuity, nystagmus, and photophobia.
D) The mutated gene in this disorder normally encodes a protein thought to play a role in regulating organelle pH and vacuolar accumulation of glutathione.
E) Sunburns are unusual.

QUESTION 6-3.

A 27-year-old female with long-standing discoid lupus presents with concerns regarding the appearance of some lesions on her cheeks, nose, and forehead. On physical exam there are several atrophic depigmented plaques and patches surrounded by hyperpigmentation and erythema associated with alopecia. The patient's medication list includes hydroxychloroquine and naproxen. Which of the following statements is MOST accurate regarding this patient's leukoderma?

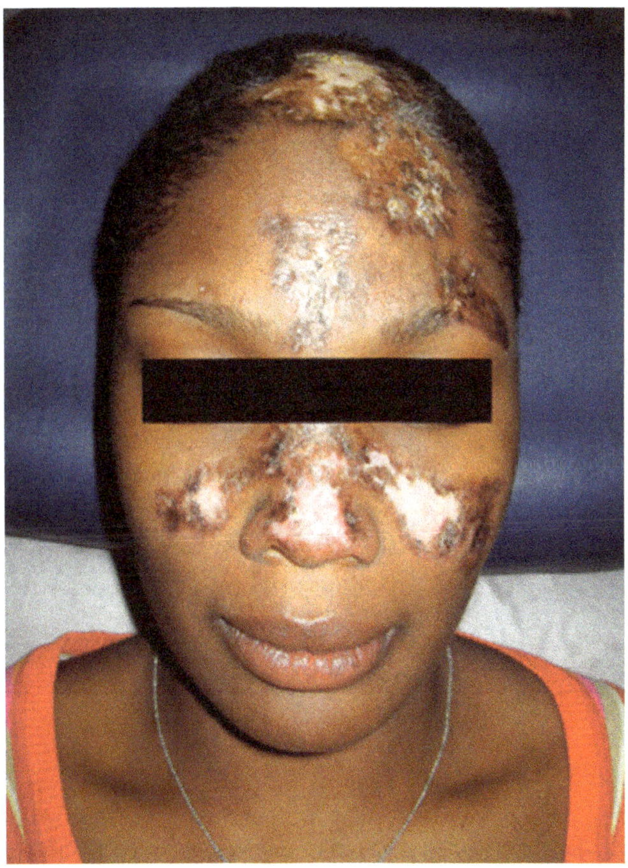

Reproduced with permission from Kasper DL, Fauci A, Hauser SL et al: *Harrison's Principles of Internal Medicine*. 19th ed. New York, NY: McGraw-Hill Education; 2015

A) The depigmentation is most likely attributed to an acquired defect in tyrosinase.
B) This patient's depigmentation is completely reversible with regeneration of basilar melanocytes and keratinocyte melanin pigment.
C) This patient likely has a lichenoid drug eruption that is resolving with post-inflammatory hypopigmentation. She should stop her medications, and the lesions will completely repigment slowly after cessation of the offending medication.
D) This patient's condition is best described as post-inflammatory hypopigmentation, where the epidermis contains normal concentrations of hypopigmented melanocytes and keratinocytes.
E) While destroyed melanocytes may recover in these depigmented lesions, fibrosis and a paucity of blood vessels will most likely contribute to a persistent white color.

QUESTION 6-4.

A 12-year-old patient presents with a congenital white patch on the chest with an irregular border. Rubbing the border makes the normal surrounding skin erythematous while the lesion remains white. The border and extent of the lesion become imperceptible when the pressure of diascopy is applied, whereas the application of heat or ice will accentuate the lesion. A biopsy of the hypopigmented area reveals normal numbers of epidermal melanocytes, normal basal layer melanization, and dermal blood vessels of normal size and number. Which of the following regarding this condition is INCORRECT?

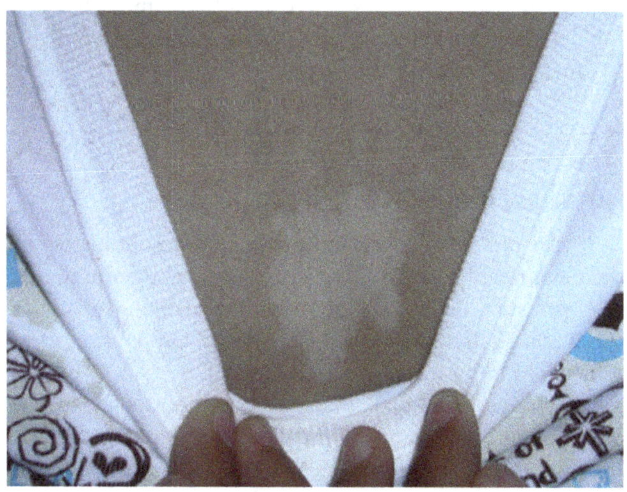

Reproduced, with permission, from Usatine RP, Smith MA, Mayeaux EJ Jr, Chumley HS, eds. *Color Atlas of Family Medicine*. 2nd ed. New York, NY: McGraw-Hill Education; 2012.

A) This condition is considered a vascular malformation in which the abnormality of the involved vessels is functional rather than anatomic.

B) This condition is linked with certain genodermatoses, including neurofibromatosis and phakomatosis pigmentovascularis.
C) The condition is possibly mediated by an abnormality in endothelial E-selectin expression.
D) The hypopigmentation is due to increased dermal fibrosis.
E) Intralesional injection of α-adrenergic blockers may induce erythema; however, vasodilators such as histamine and acetylcholine do not induce erythema.

QUESTION 6-5.

In regards to clinical melanotic hyperpigmentation disorders, which of the following is INCORRECT?

A) Epidermal melanocytes may manifest an increase in function, in number, or both.
B) Vacuolar degeneration of basal cells releases melanin granules into the upper dermis, which are concentrated in macrophages (melanophages).
C) Disorders of hyperpigmentation may be classified histopathologically according to the predominant patterns: epidermal, dermal, or mixed epidermal and dermal.
D) The predominant location of the excess melanin correlates with the color of the hyperpigmentation: blue-gray (epidermal), brown (dermal), and gray-brown (mixed epidermal and dermal).
E) Chronic irritation frequently induces hyperpigmentation of keratinocytes with concentrated melanin deposits within the stratum corneum and scattered melanophages in the dermis.

QUESTION 6-6.

A 76-year-old female presents with a 3-month history of weakness, fatigue, nausea, low blood sugar and sodium, low blood pressure, daily bouts of abdominal pain and diarrhea, as well as a 20 lb unintentional weight loss. On physical exam she is noted to have sparse pubic and axillary hair, hyperpigmentation over the knuckles, as well as the nipples, axillae, perineum, and within the skin creases of the palms. She has no prior surgical history. Which of the following additional findings is MOST commonly associated with this patient's disease?

A) Pituitary adenoma
B) Type II diabetes mellitus
C) Elevated serum ferritin
D) Elevated ACTH
E) Small, round, black granules surrounding sweat glands

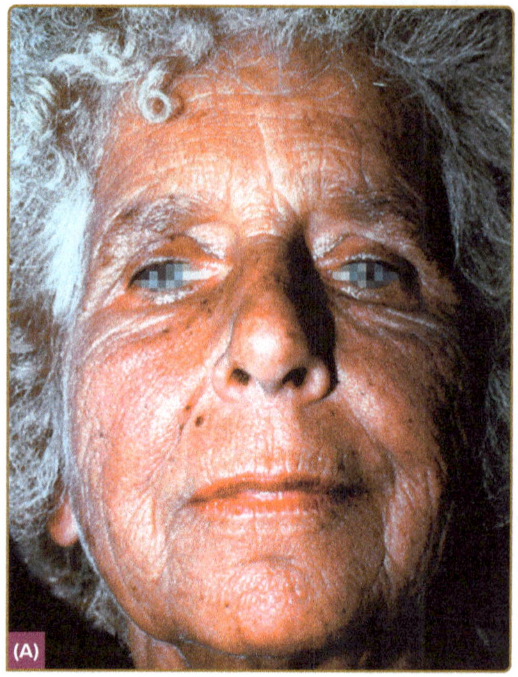

(A)

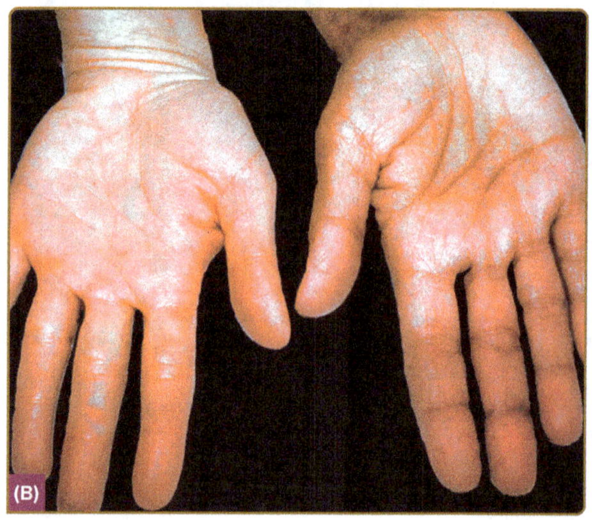

(B)

Reproduced, with permission, from Goldsmith LA, Katz SI, Gilchrest BA, Paller AS, Leffell DJ, Wolff K, eds. *Fitzpatrick's Dermatology in General Medicine*. 8th ed. New York, NY: McGraw-Hill Education; 2012.

QUESTION 6-7.

A 37-year-old patient presents with numerous dark-brown to gray-blue pigmented macules on the lips, around the mouth, buccal mucosa, and on the fingers. These lesions developed in early childhood. Some lesions have disappeared over time; however, the intraoral lesions have remained constant. Additional complaints include abdominal symptoms such as pain, GI bleeding, and anemia. A recent colonoscopy revealed several polyps within the small intestine. A biopsy of one of the pigmented lip lesions reveals heavily pigmented basal cells, but no increase in the number of melanocytes. Which of the following diagnoses is CORRECT?

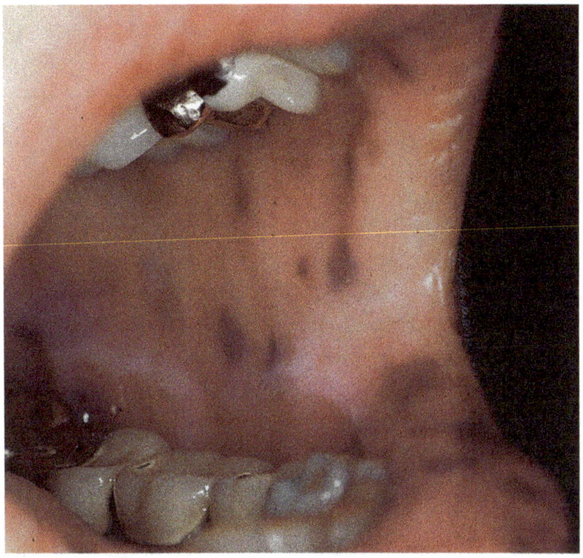

Reproduced, with permission, from Wolff K, Johnson RA, Saavedra AP. *Fitzpatrick's Color Atlas and Synopsis of Clinical Dermatology*. 7th ed. New York, NY: McGraw-Hill Education; 2013.

A) Generalized lentignosis
B) Peutz–Jeghers syndrome
C) LEOPARD syndrome
D) Carney syndrome
E) Laugier–Hunziker syndrome

QUESTION 6-8.

A 32-year-old patient presents with slowly spreading areas of reticular hyperpigmentation involving the axillae, neck, groin, and inframammary folds. Perioral comedo-like follicular keratosis and pitted scars are present. The hair, nails, and teeth are unremarkable. A biopsy of one of the hyperpigmented lesions is illustrated below. Which of the following diagnoses is CORRECT?

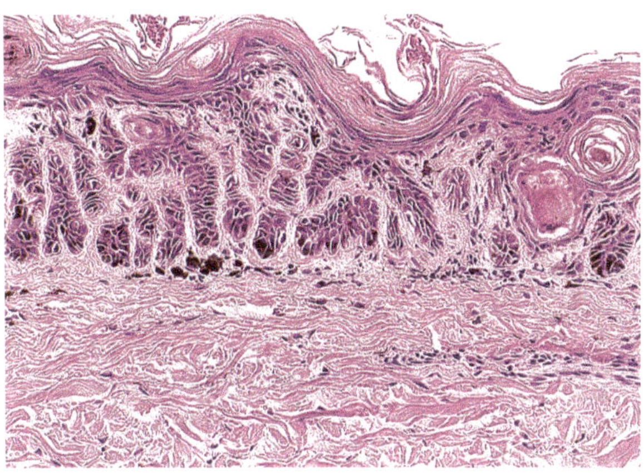

A) Dowling–Degos disease
B) Dermatopathia pigmentosa reticularis
C) Naegli–Franceschetti–Jadassohn syndrome
D) Cantu syndrome
E) Acanthosis nigricans

QUESTION 6-9.

A 23-year-old female presents with spotty centrofacial pigmentation involving the vermillion border of the lips, the lacrimal caruncle, the conjunctival semilunar fold, and the sclera. Additionally, she has darkly pigmented lentigines on the vulva. You notice in the medical chart that the patient has a history of neuromas and atrial fibrillation. A biopsy of the lip was performed and the findings are illustrated below. Which of the following additional clinical findings is MOST consistent with this patient's disorder?

A) Punctate palmoplantar keratoderma
B) Epithelioid blue nevi
C) Increased distance between the eyes
D) Multiple polyps in the small intestine

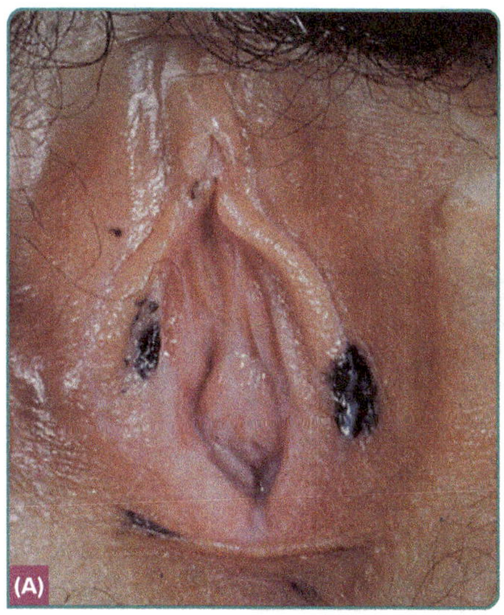

(A)

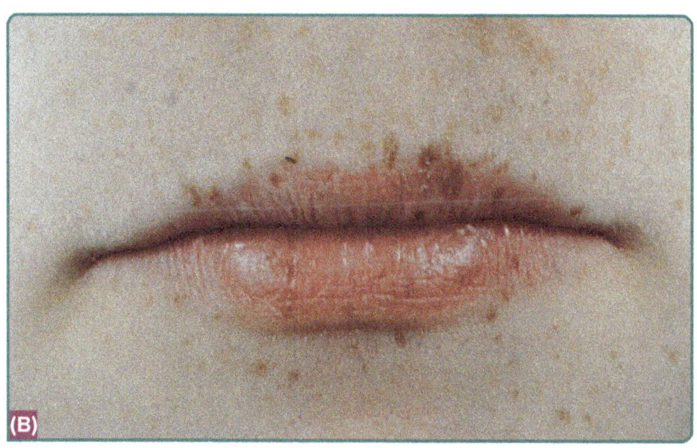

(B)

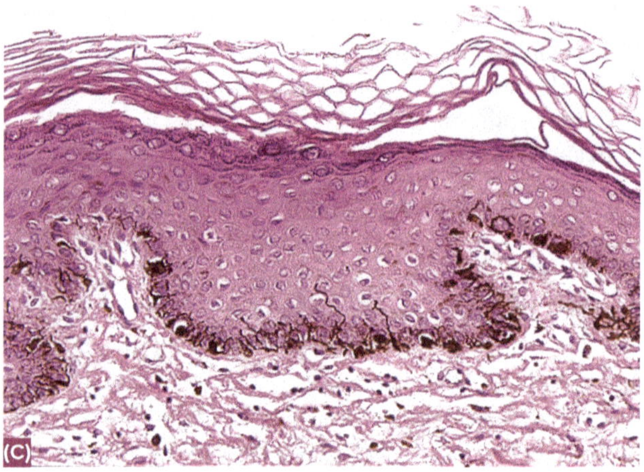

Parts **(A)** and **(B)** reproduced, with permission, from Goldsmith LA, Katz SI, Gilchrest BA, Paller AS, Leffell DJ, Wolff K, eds. *Fitzpatrick's Dermatology in General Medicine*. 8th ed. New York, NY: McGraw-Hill Education; 2012.

QUESTION 6-10.

A 31-year-old pregnant Puerto Rican female presents with symmetrical centrofacial hyperpigmentation involving the forehead, nose, cheeks, upper lip, and chin. A biopsy reveals an increased number of enlarged hyperpigmented epidermal melanocytes with prominent dendritic processes. No areas of confluent growth are noted. Numerous scattered melanophages are present. Which of the following diagnoses is CORRECT?

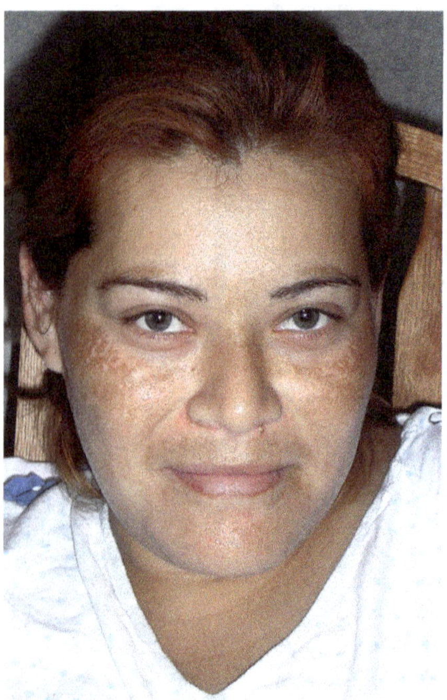

Reproduced, with permission, from Usatine RP, Smith MA, Mayeaux EJ Jr, Chumley HS, eds. *Color Atlas of Family Medicine*. 2nd ed. New York, NY: McGraw-Hill Education; 2012.

A) Erythema dyschromicum perstans
B) Cholasma
C) Hermansky–Pudlak syndrome
D) Riehl melanosis
E) Exogenous ochronosis

QUESTION 6-11.

A young female patient presents with diffuse pigmented macules outlined by smooth and rounded borders, reminiscent of "the coastline of California." These macules are located primarily on the trunk, axillae, inguinal region, and under the breasts. You identify at least six patches that measure greater than 1.5 cm in diameter. The pigmentation of these lesions is not altered by sun exposure. Additionally, there are several flesh-colored to hyperpigmented soft papules and nodules scattered on the back, extremities, and face. The patient describes a "buttonholing" sensation when a finger is rubbed gently over the surface of one of the smaller lesions. A biopsy is performed on one of the larger pigmented patches. Which of the following microscopic descriptions BEST describes this lesion?

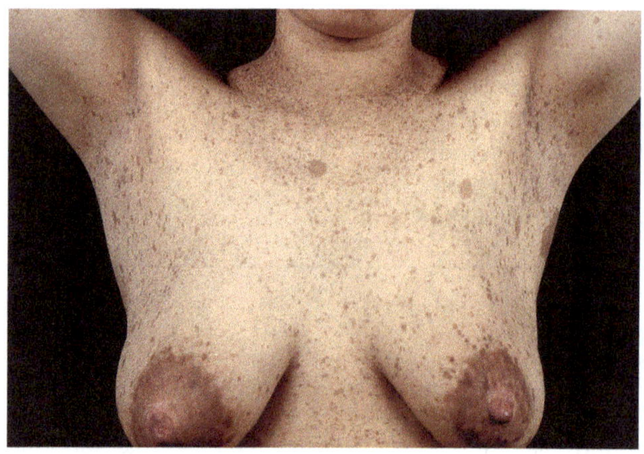

Reproduced, with permission, from Wolff K, Johnson RA, Saavedra AP. *Fitzpatrick's Color Atlas and Synopsis of Clinical Dermatology*. 7th ed. New York, NY: McGraw-Hill Education; 2013.

A) Basal layer hypermelanization and a normal number of melanocytes containing large melanin globules. Electron microscopy reveals giant melanosomes within melanocytes.
B) Basal cell hypermelanization concentrated at the tips of elongated rete ridges and increased numbers of melanocytes containing large melanin globules. Electron microscopy reveals giant melanosomes within melanocytes. No solar elastosis is present.
C) A normal to slightly attenuated epidermis with diffuse basal cell hypermelanization and slightly decreased numbers of melanocytes with prominent elongated dendrites. Electron microscopy reveals normal melanosomes.

D) An epidermis with basal cell hypermelanization concentrated at the tips of elongated "club-shaped" rete ridges, hyperkeratosis, and normal numbers of melanocytes. There is a background of solar elastosis.

E) A hyperplastic epidermis with acanthosis and papillomatosis, diffuse basal cell hypermelanization, and slightly increased numbers of normal melanocytes. Smooth muscle bundles are present in the dermis without associated hair follicles.

F) An epidermis with discontinuous foci of basal cell hypermelanization and occasional small nests of melanocytes at the tips of elongated rete ridges.

G) An attenuated epidermis with basal cell hypermelanization, partial thickness keratinocytic atypia, hypogranulosis, parakeratosis, and marked solar elastosis. There is a normal number of melanocytes.

QUESTION 6-12.

An elderly Asian female presents with the rapid onset of a reticular gray-bro wn to almost black hyperpigmentation of the lateral face and neck. She works as a cosmetic chemist and has applied, over years, most of the scented products she was involved in producing to her own skin. She currently lives in Hawaii. One of the hyperpigmented lesions is biopsied. Which of the following statements is MOST accurate regarding with these lesions?

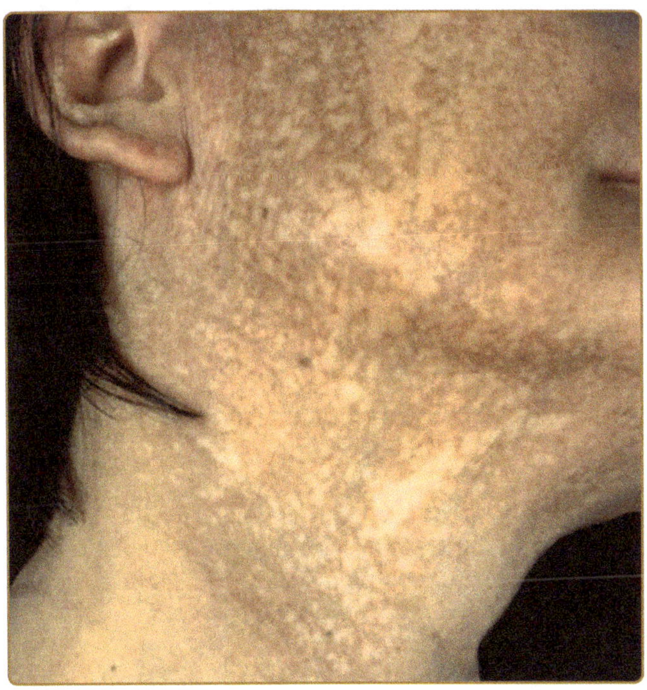

Reproduced, with permission, from Goldsmith LA, Katz SI, Gilchrest BA, Paller AS, Leffell DJ, Wolff K, eds. *Fitzpatrick's Dermatology in General Medicine*. 8th ed. New York, NY: McGraw-Hill Education; 2012.

A) The upper dermis contains small, refractile, brown-black mercury granules, either free or in macrophages.

B) There are increased numbers of melanocytes along the basal layer.

C) Pigment is found exclusively in the epidermis.

D) Dark-skinned individuals are protected from these pigmentary changes because individual melanosomes are more heavily melanized than fairer-skin types.

E) Interface dermatitis may be visible in early lesions.

QUESTION 6-13.

A patient presents with generalized slate-blue discoloration of the skin, mucous membranes, and conjunctivae. The patient has a history of a deeply invasive malignant melanoma. Which of the following statements regarding this form of generalized melanosis is INCORRECT?

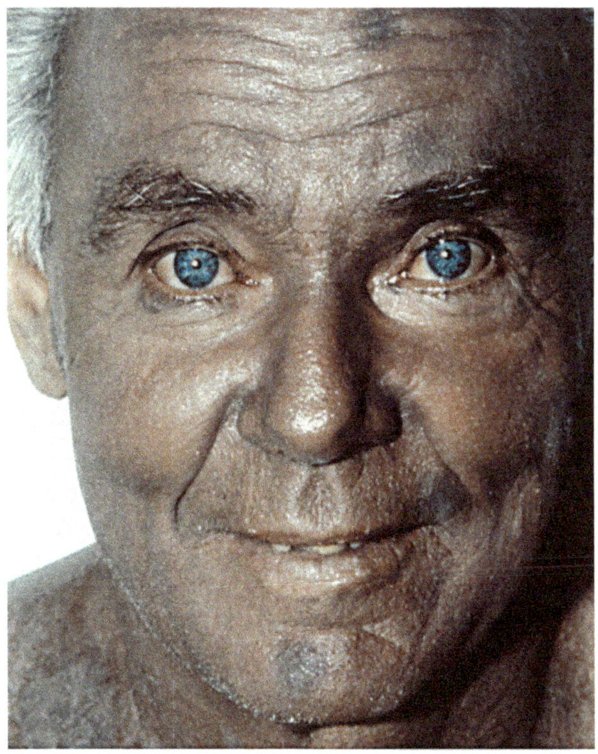

Reproduced, with permission, from Wolff K, Johnson RA, Saavedra AP. *Fitzpatrick's Color Atlas and Synopsis of Clinical Dermatology*. 7th ed. New York, NY: McGraw-Hill Education; 2013.

A) Tumor-derived factors seem to drive the hyperproliferation of normal melanocytes.

B) Neutrophils in this patient's circulation may contain melanin, and the intima of arteries and many visceral organs may also appear black.

C) Perivascular macrophages may contain melanin granules that are DOPA positive, indicating active melanin synthesis within phagocytosed melanosomes.

D) The pigmented macrophages will be positive on both Fontana-Masson and Prussian blue stains.
E) The urine of these patients frequently has a dark-brown to black color.

QUESTION 6-14.

A 48-year-old patient with facial discoid lupus presents with blue-black pigmentation most prominently of the cheeks, forehead, nose, and chin. The patient has been using topical cream for the discoid lesions. Physical exam reveals no other pertinent findings. A biopsy is performed and the findings are illustrated below. Which of the following statements regarding this patient's condition is CORRECT?

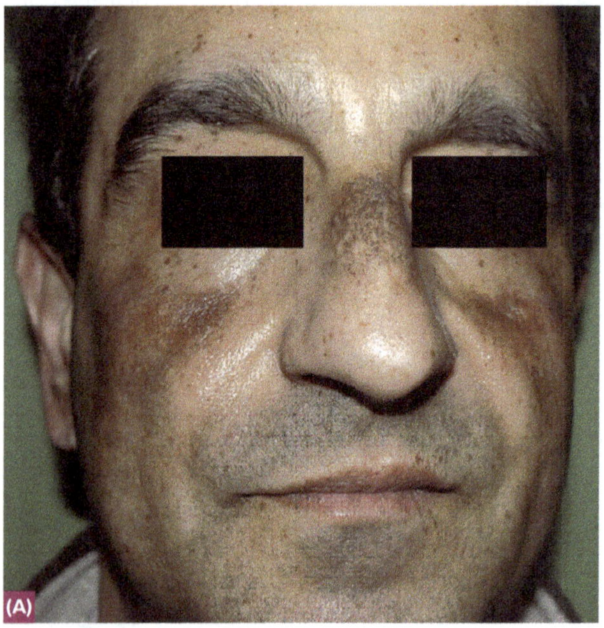

Reproduced, with permission, from Goldsmith LA, Katz SI, Gilchrest BA, Paller AS, Leffell DJ, Wolff K, eds. *Fitzpatrick's Dermatology in General Medicine*. 8th ed. New York, NY: McGraw-Hill Education; 2012.

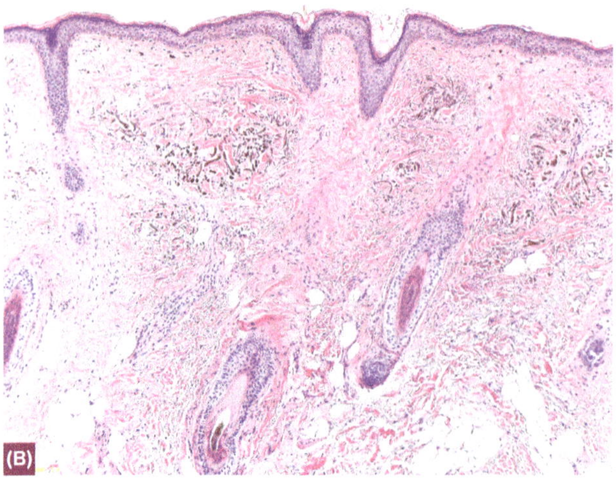

A) The discoloration will fade with discontinuation of the topical cream.
B) The hyperpigmentation is due to chronic topical use of high-concentration (6%-8%) hydroquinone, resorcinol, phenol, quinine injection, systemic antimalarial therapy, or exposure to benzene.
C) This patient has an autosomal recessive disease of homogentisic decarboxylase deficiency, which causes pigmentation of cartilage and eventually the skin.
D) The patient's urine will turn pink to brown if exposed to the air or an alkalizing agent.
E) The pigment will stain positively with both Prussian blue and Fontana-Masson stains.

QUESTION 6-15.

A 65-year-old coal miner presents with an irregular blue-black linear papule adjacent to an old scar. There is a family history of melanoma. A biopsy is performed and the findings are illustrated below. Which of the following diagnoses is CORRECT?

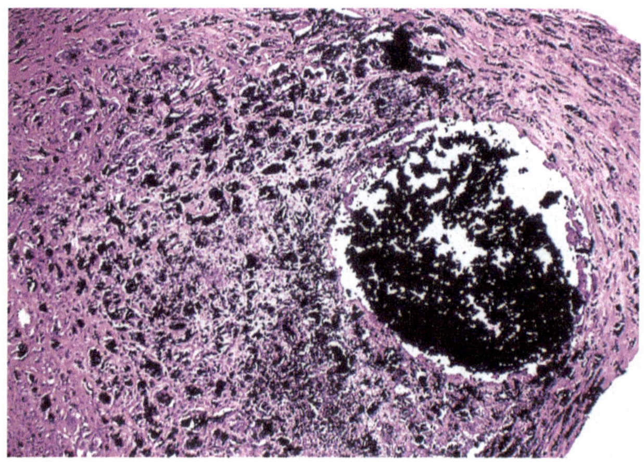

A) Blue nevus
B) Calcinosis cutis
C) Carbon tattoo
D) Hemochromatosis
E) Tumoral melanosis

QUESTION 6-16.

A patient presents with raised areas inside a tattoo. A biopsy of the raised area reveals nodular lymphoid infiltrates admixed with foreign-body giant cells. Which of the following pigments is most likely responsible for this complication?

A) Cinnabar
B) Chromic oxide
C) Cobaltous albuminate
D) Cadmium sulfide
E) Iron oxide

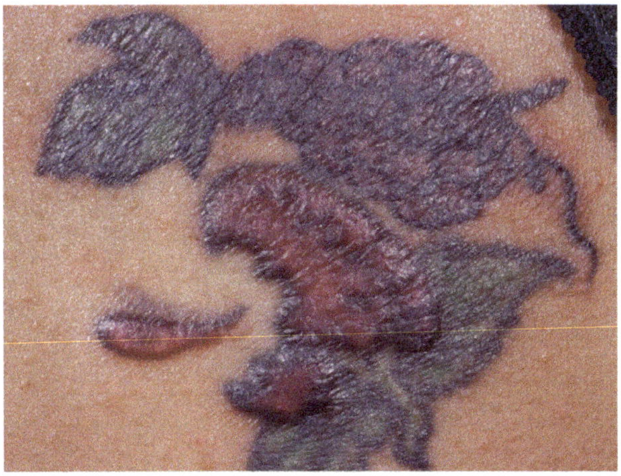

Reproduced, with permission, from Goldsmith LA, Katz SI, Gilchrest BA, Paller AS, Leffell DJ, Wolff K, eds. *Fitzpatrick's Dermatology in General Medicine*. 8th ed. New York, NY: McGraw-Hill Education; 2012.

QUESTION 6-17.

A patient has taken 100 mg PO BID minocycline for the last 3 years for acne. Over the last year blue-black pigmentation has formed at sites of old acne scars; however, recently bluish macules have developed on previously normal skin of the anterior lower legs and around the eyes. Additionally, a generalized gray-brown discoloration (ie, "muddy skin syndrome") has started to develop, particularly in sun-exposed areas, the gingiva, the hard palate, the teeth, and the nails. Biopsies of the acne, lower leg, and muddy brown hyperpigmentation are performed. Which of the following statements regarding these different forms of pigmentation is INCORRECT?

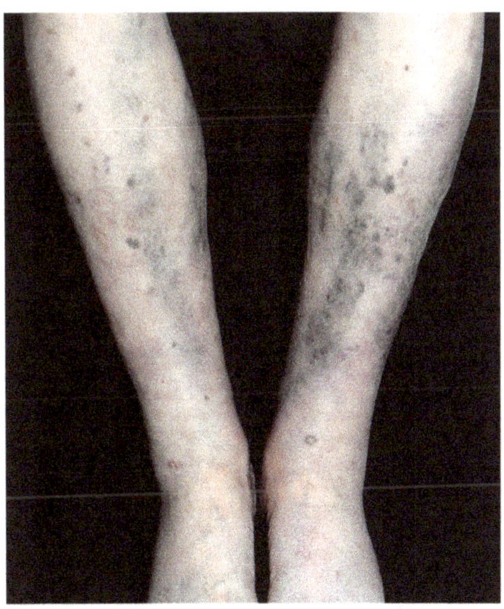

Reproduced, with permission, from Wolff K, Johnson RA, Saavedra AP. *Fitzpatrick's Color Atlas and Synopsis of Clinical Dermatology*. 7th ed. New York, NY: McGraw-Hill Education; 2013.

A) The acne scar biopsy reveals pigmented macrophages distributed mainly around the vasculature and sweat gland coils that are positive for iron with Prussian blue stain and negative for melanin with Fontana-Masson stain.
B) The macular lesion on the leg contains pigmented macrophages distributed mainly around the vasculature and sweat gland coils that are positive on both Prussian blue and Fontana-Masson stains, but fails to bleach with potassium permanganate, indicating that melanin is not present.
C) The generalized muddy brown skin sample shows increased epidermal basal layer melanization and melanophages in the upper dermis, but negative staining for iron.
D) The pigment of the macular leg lesion fluoresces yellow under ultraviolet light.
E) The acne and macular leg lesions contain pigmented macrophages that are distributed mainly around the vasculature and sweat gland coils and appear bright pink on PAS stain.

QUESTION 6-18.

Which of the following medications is NOT associated with cutaneous hyperpigmentation?
A) Hydroxychloroquine
B) Quinacrine
C) Amiodarone
D) Clofazimine
E) Imipramine
F) Phenothiazine
G) Tetracycline
H) Azithromycin
I) Bleomycin
J) Busulfan
K) Cyclophosphamide
L) Doxorubicin
M) 5-fluorouracil
N) Topical carmustine

QUESTION 6-19.

Which of the following leukodermas is characterized by an absence of melanocytes within hypopigmented lesions?
A) Albinism
B) Ash leaf spots of tuberous sclerosis
C) Hypomelanosis of Ito
D) Hermansky–Pudlak syndrome
E) Nevus depigmentosus
F) Pityriasis alba
G) Idiopathic guttate hypomelanosis
H) Piebaldism

QUESTION 6-20.

A 7-year-old girl presents with chronic diffuse fine scales on the trunk and extremities. There is sparing of the popliteal fossae, antecubital fossae, and sides of the lateral neck. There are numerous rough, hyperpigmented bumps on the lateral arms. Hyperlinearity and chafing of the palms and soles are also present. The patient's father and brother have a similar condition. A biopsy of the leg is performed and the findings are illustrated below. Which of the following diagnoses is CORRECT?

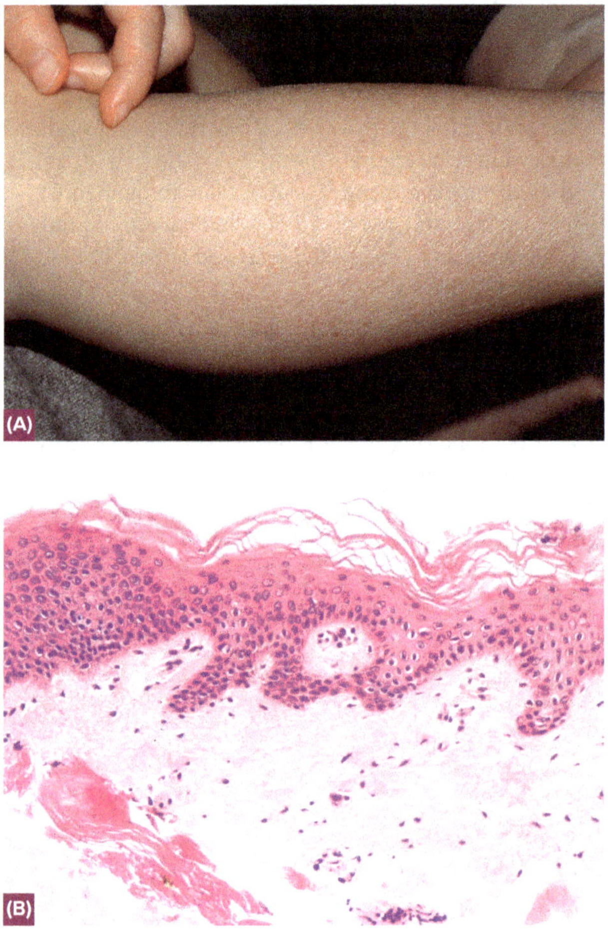

A) Lamellar ichthyosis
B) X-linked recessive ichthyosis
C) Ichthyosis vulgaris
D) Acquired ichthyosis
E) Harlequin ichthyosis

QUESTION 6-21.

A patient presents with erythematous to brown keratotic papules and plaques in the axilla. The lesions are pruritic. The patient is otherwise healthy. A biopsy is performed and the findings are illustrated below. Which of the following diagnoses is CORRECT?

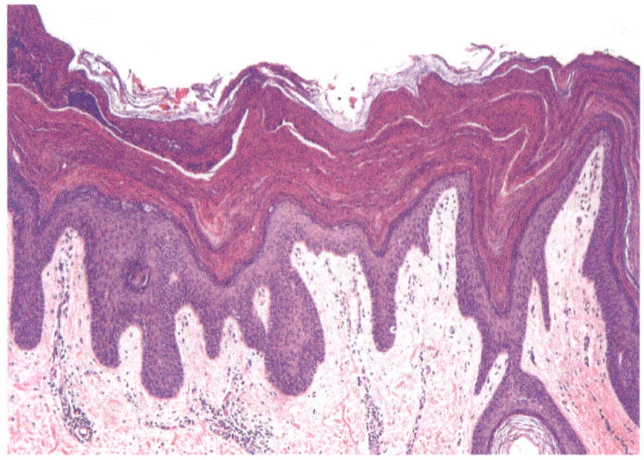

A) Acanthosis nigricans
B) Pityriasis rubra pilaris
C) Inverse psoriasis
D) Seborrheic dermatitis
E) Axillary granular parakeratosis

QUESTION 6-22.

Which of the following statements regarding the biopsy findings illustrated below is INCORRECT?

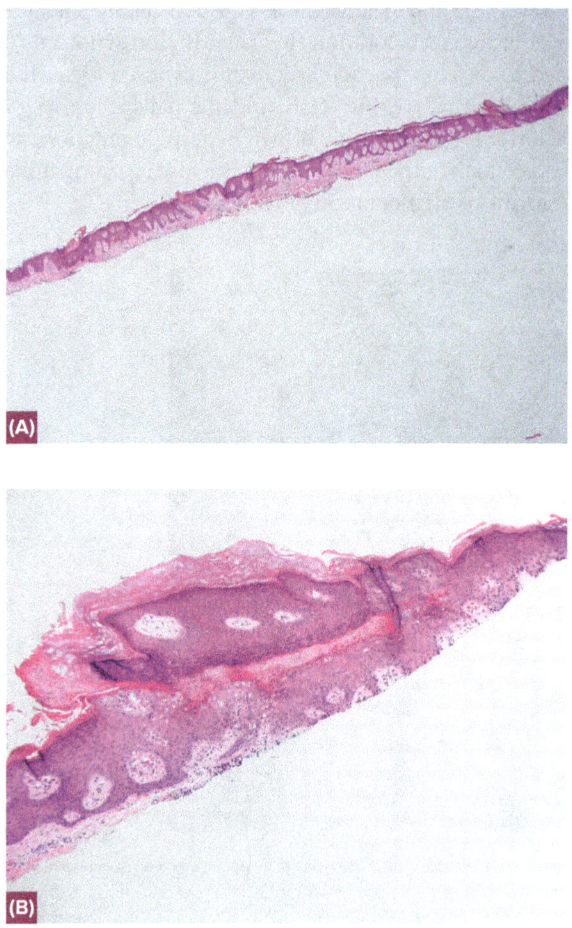

A) These lesions may clinically present as small annular lesions preferentially arising on sun-exposed extremities.
B) This condition may clinically present as a unilateral lesion confined to an extremity following Blaschko lines.
C) This condition is strongly associated with HPV infection.
D) These lesions may be associated with an autosomal dominant inheritance pattern.
E) These lesions may be associated with point mutations in the *SART3* gene and an increased incidence of squamous cell carcinoma.

QUESTION 6-23.

Which of the following conditions is NOT characterized by the histopathological findings illustrated below?

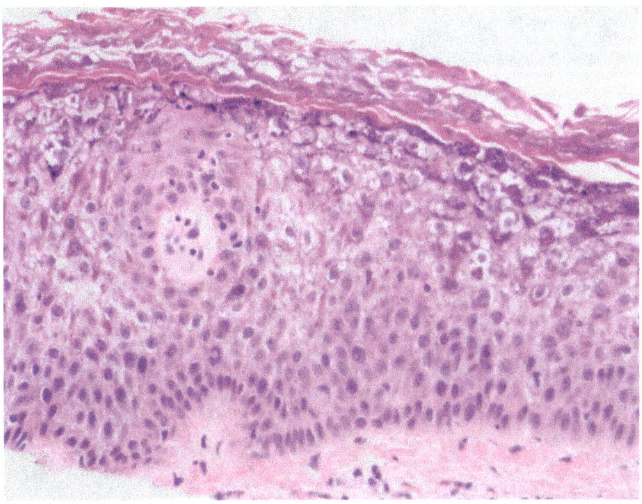

A) Epidermolytic acanthoma
B) Bullous congenital ichthyosiform erythroderma
C) Epidermal nevus
D) Palmoplantar keratoderma, Voerner-type
E) Benign familial pemphigus

QUESTION 6-24.

A 64-year-old female presents with hyperkeratotic, crusted, and erythematous papules coalescing into plaques on the axillae and inframammary regions. Additionally, there are keratotic papules on the palms and soles and red and white longitudinal streaks on the fingernails with V-nicking in the distal portions of plates. She reports that her father had similar lesions. A biopsy is performed and the findings are illustrated below. Which of the following diagnoses is CORRECT?

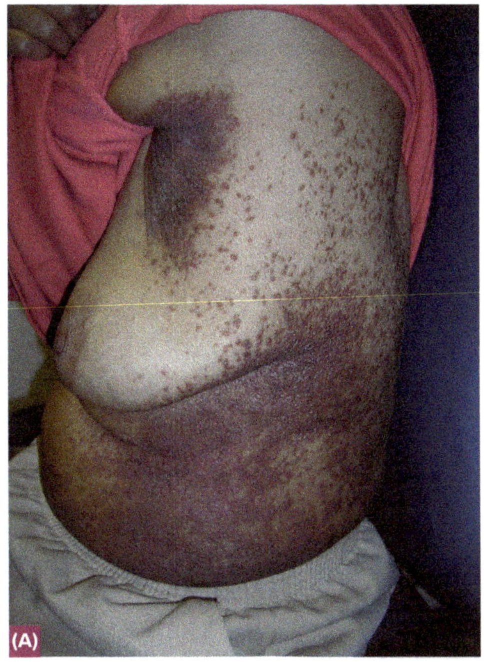

(A)

Reproduced, with permission, from Usatine RP, Smith MA, Mayeaux EJ Jr, Chumley HS, eds. *Color Atlas of Family Medicine*. 2nd ed. New York, NY: McGraw-Hill Education; 2012.

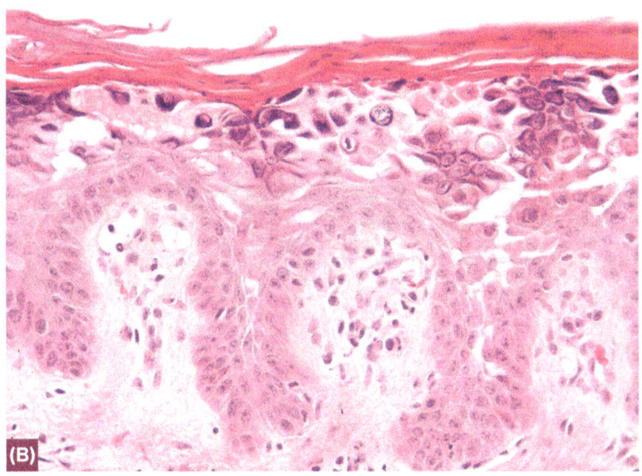

(B)

A) Hailey–Hailey disease
B) Grover disease
C) Warty dyskeratoma
D) Acantholytic dyskeratoma
E) Darier disease

QUESTION 6-25.

A 27-year-old patient presents with oozing lesions on both armpits and groin. He reports that occasionally lesions form in the popliteal fossae and on the nape of the neck. The lesions become worse during summer months. His father and sister have similar lesions. The lesions wax and wane, are painful, and show cracks and fissures within a partially erosive erythematous plaque. A biopsy is performed and the findings are illustrated below. Direct immunofluorescence reveals a nonspecific immunoreactant profile. Tissue swab culture grows *Staphylococcus aureus*. Which of the following diagnoses is CORRECT?

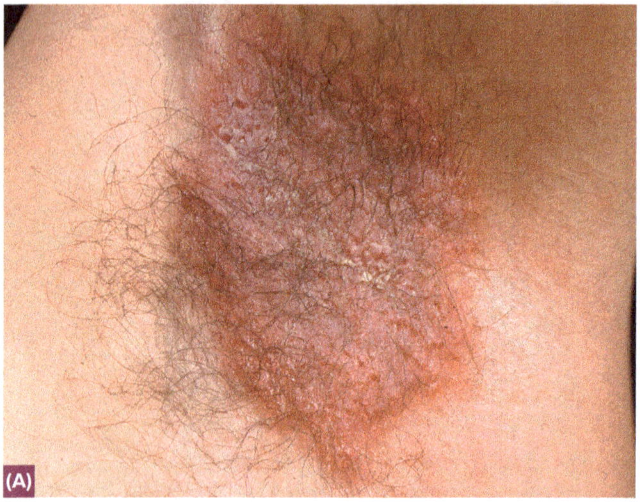

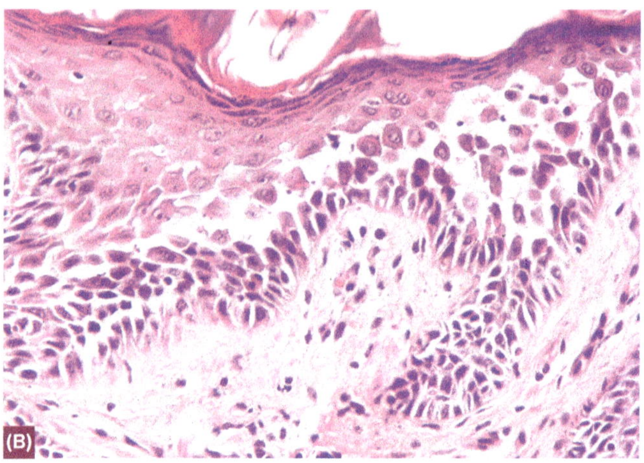

Part **(A)** reproduced, with permission, from Wolff K, Johnson RA, Saavedra AP. *Fitzpatrick's Color Atlas and Synopsis of Clinical Dermatology*. 7th ed. New York, NY: McGraw-Hill Education; 2013.

A) Keratosis follicularis
B) Benign familial pemphigus
C) Transient acantholytic dermatosis
D) Pemphigus vulgaris
E) Bullous impetigo

QUESTION 6-26.

An infant presents at birth with extensively denuded skin and generalized blistering accompanied by severe periorificial granulation, loss of nails, and involvement of most mucosal surfaces. Biopsies are performed and the findings are illustrated below. Direct immunofluorescence reveals a nonspecific immunoreactant profile without immunoglobulin deposition along the dermal epidermal junction. Indirect immunofluorescence is negative for circulating antibodies against basement membrane antigens. Immunohistochemical staining for type IV collagen reveals deposition along the floor of the blister cavity. Despite aggressive supportive therapy, the infant dies after 2 months. Which of the following statements regarding this condition is most likely CORRECT?

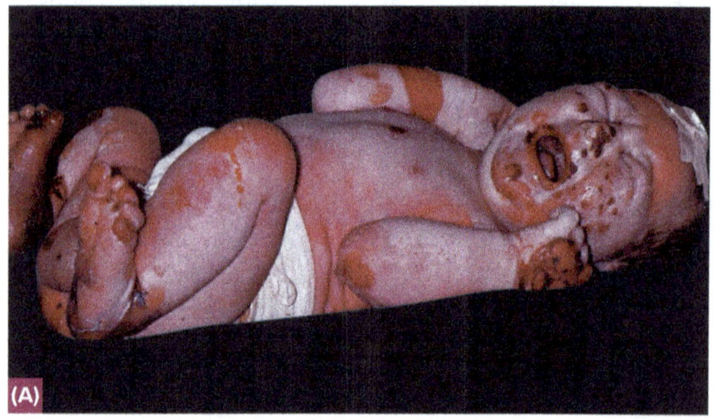

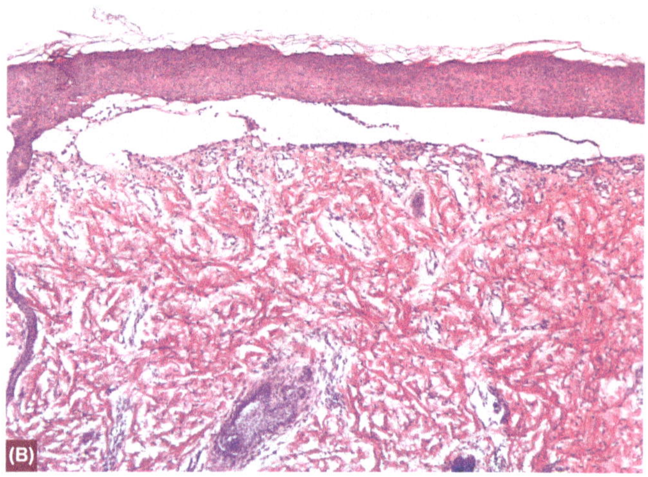

Part **(A)** reproduced, with permission, from Wolff K, Johnson RA, Saavedra AP. *Fitzpatrick's Color Atlas and Synopsis of Clinical Dermatology*. 7th ed. New York, NY: McGraw-Hill Education; 2013.

A) Epitope mapping using antibodies to type IV collagen reveals the plane of cleavage localized to the sublamina densa.
B) Gene analysis reveals mutations in the gene encoding $\alpha 3$, $\beta 3$, and/or the $\chi 2$ polypeptide chains of laminin 5.
C) Gene analysis reveals mutations in the gene encoding type VII collagen.
D) A subset of patients with this condition will have defects in porphyrin metabolism.
E) This condition demonstrates an autosomal dominant mode of inheritance.

QUESTION 6-27.

A 13-year-old girl presents with a cluster of bullae on the thigh following minor trauma. Her father and brother also have a history of forming blisters following minor trauma. A biopsy of the skin adjacent to the blister is performed and the findings are illustrated below. Which of the following statements regarding this condition is INCORRECT?

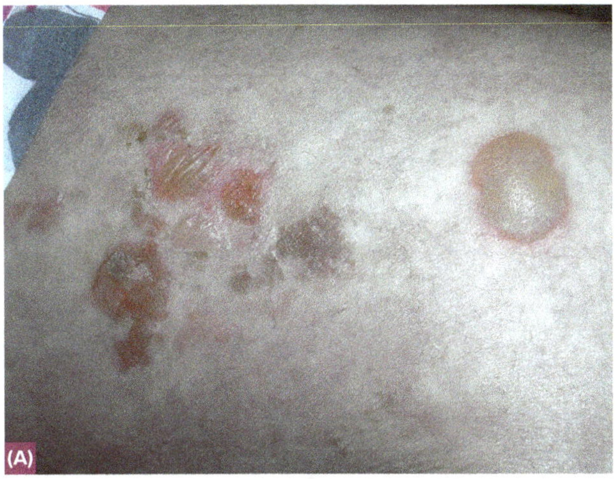

Reproduced, with permission, from Usatine RP, Smith MA, Mayeaux EJ Jr, Chumley HS, eds. *Color Atlas of Family Medicine*. 2nd ed. New York, NY: McGraw-Hill Education; 2012.

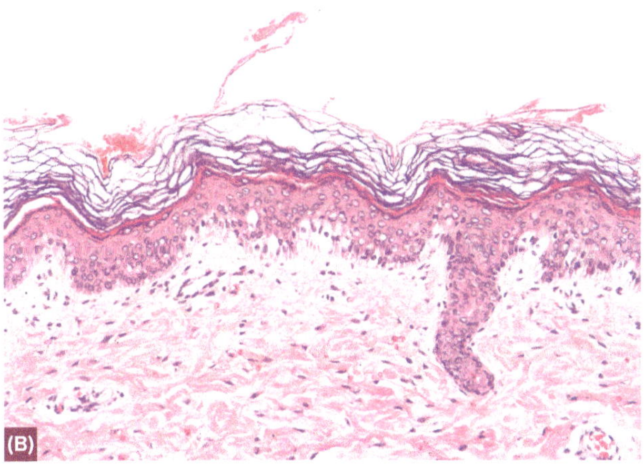

A) This condition is attributed to point mutations in the genes for either keratin 5 or keratin 14 (*K5* or *K14*).
B) This condition is associated with an autosomal dominant mode of inheritance.
C) There are three clinical variants of this condition: generalized blisters, herpetiform clustering of blisters, and localized acral blisters.
D) Immunohistochemical staining for type IV collagen of the blister will reveal staining along the roof of the blister cavity.
E) These blisters will most likely heal without scarring.

QUESTION 6-28.

A 10-year-old girl presents to the emergency room with fever and sepsis. She has a long-standing history of blisters that lead to erosions and eventually evolve into ulcers that have a low tendency to heal. When healing does occur, it results in scarring with scattered milium cysts. You notice that she has enamel defects with numerous caries and considerable growth retardation. Imaging reveals strictures of the esophagus. She also has severe anemia. It is obvious that these large wounds are portal entries for systemic infection. A biopsy of one of the intact blisters reveals a pauci-inflammatory subepidermal blister. Immunohistochemical stain for type IV collagen reveals deposition confined to the roof of the blister cavity. Immunofluorescence is negative for antibodies directed against basement membrane antigens. Gene analysis reveals a mutation in the gene that encodes type VII collagen. Which of the following diagnoses is CORRECT?

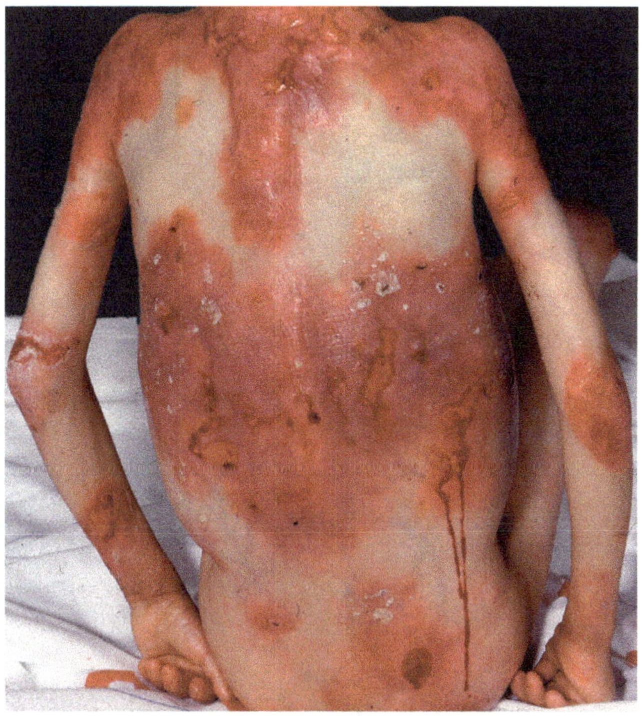

Reproduced, with permission, from Wolff K, Johnson RA, Saavedra AP. *Fitzpatrick's Color Atlas and Synopsis of Clinical Dermatology*. 7th ed. New York, NY: McGraw-Hill Education; 2013.

A) Epidermolysis bullosa simplex
B) Junctional epidermolysis bullosa
C) Kindler syndrome
D) Dystrophic epidermolysis bullosa, Hallopeau–Siemens variant
E) Epidermolysis bullosa acquisita

QUESTION 6-29.

A 73-year-old patient with a history of a pancreatic mass develops multiple perioral, perineal, and acral pustules and vesicles, some of which are ruptured revealing weeping scaling erythematous plaques and erosions. The patient reports multiple crops of these lesions arising and resolving over the last several months. The patient's nails are also brittle. A biopsy reveals sharp zonal necrosis of the upper half of the epidermis with markedly hydropic keratinocytes. The underlying lower layers of the epidermis are spared. A few subcorneal bullae with cytolysis are identified. Multiple pyknotic keratinocytes with pale cytoplasm are identified. There is spongiosis and sparse intraepidermal and dermal neutrophilic infiltrates. Interface activity is not identified. Which of the following diagnoses is CORRECT?

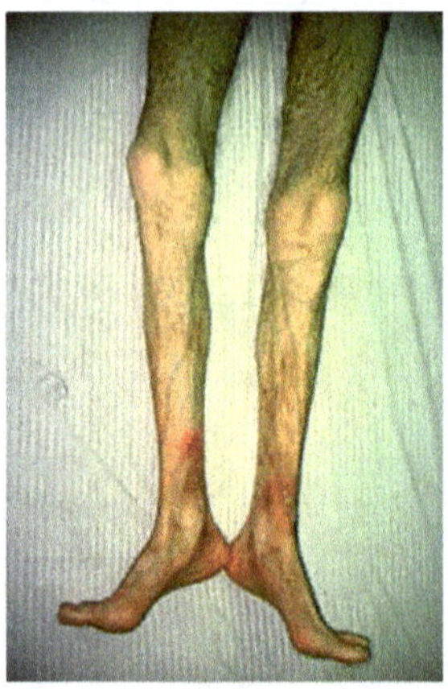

Courtesy of C Grunfeld

A) Necrolytic acral erythema
B) Migratory necrolytic erythema
C) Hand foot and mouth disease
D) Pellagra
E) Acrodermatitis enteropathica

QUESTION 6-30.

Which of the following clinical presentations is LEAST likely to be associated with the histopathological findings illustrated below?

A) A 5-year-old patient presents with numerous small, keratotic papules on the extremities and face following minor trauma. The lesions have an adherent keratinous plug. The patient's mother reports that the lesions start as pin-sized lesions that eventually grow into larger papules/nodules over a course of several weeks. There is a tendency for them to form on sun-exposed skin, and in some areas the papules exhibit a linear configuration, corresponding with scratching. The lesions heal with only minor scarring. The patient's brother has a similar condition.
B) A 30-year-old patient with diabetes mellitus and renal failure presents with numerous, round, hyperpigmented papules, each with a central keratotic plug, distributed on the extensor aspects of extremities, trunk, head, and neck.
C) A 76-year-old male with dermatomyositis presents with a solitary, extremely painful, dome-shaped papule on the helix of the right ear. A central, small, crusted umbilication is present.
D) A Down syndrome patient with rheumatoid arthritis currently being treated with penicillamine presents with an annular array of erythematous keratotic papules with central invagination on the nape of the neck.
E) A 30-year-old patient with HIV and tinea versicolor presents with discrete, erythematous follicular papules, 2-8 mm in diameter, each containing a small central white keratotic core. The lesions are present on the hair-bearing skin of the extremities.

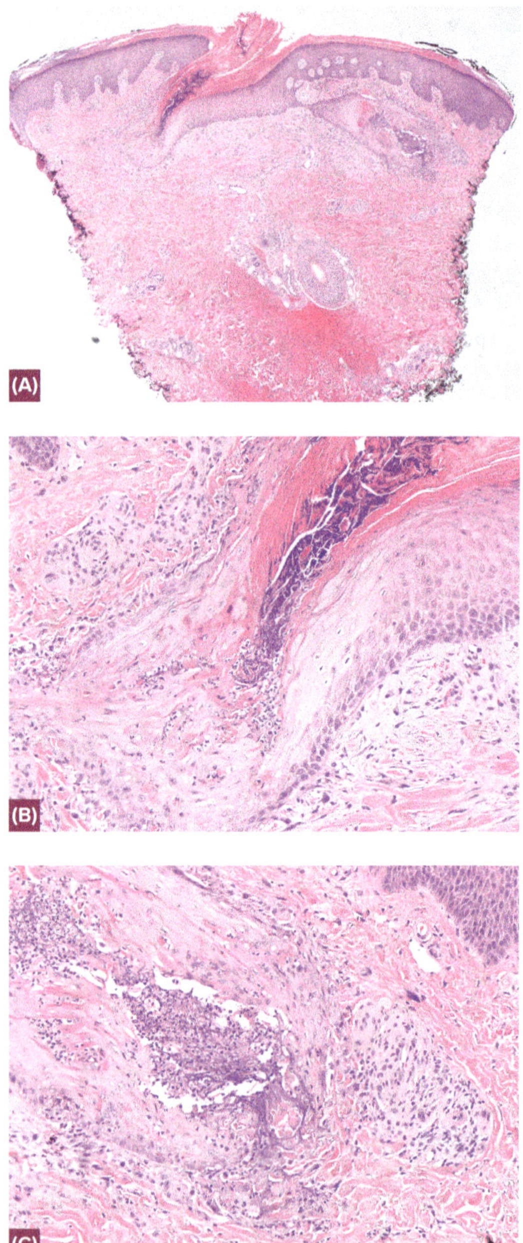

QUESTION 6-31.

Which of the following microscopic descriptions regarding dermal depositional substances is INCORRECT?

A) PAS stain reveals dense bright pink material in the dermis, consistent with hyaline.
B) Congo red stain examined under light microscopy reveals apple green amorphous material in the dermis, consistent with amyloid.
C) Colloidal iron stain reveals bright blue material in the dermis, consistent with dermal mucin.
D) Alcian blue stain reveals bright blue material in the dermis, consistent with dermal mucin.
E) Crystal violet stain reveals dark purple amorphous material in the dermis, consistent with amyloid.

QUESTION 6-32.

An elderly woman presents with elevated, knobby plaques and dome-shaped nodules on the anterior shins and dorsal feet. The cutaneous surface is waxy with peau d'orange follicular openings and follicular plugs. The skin appears edematous, but prolonged compression fails to produce an indentation. Serum analysis reveals normal TSH, T3, and T4 levels. The patient's medications include propylthiouracil and methimazole. A biopsy of the leg is performed and the findings of the H&E and Alcian blue stained sections are illustrate below. Which of the following diagnoses is CORRECT?

A) Generalized myxedema
B) Pretibial myxedema
C) Lymphedematous mucinosis
D) Lipodermatosclerosis
E) Focal cutaneous mucinosis

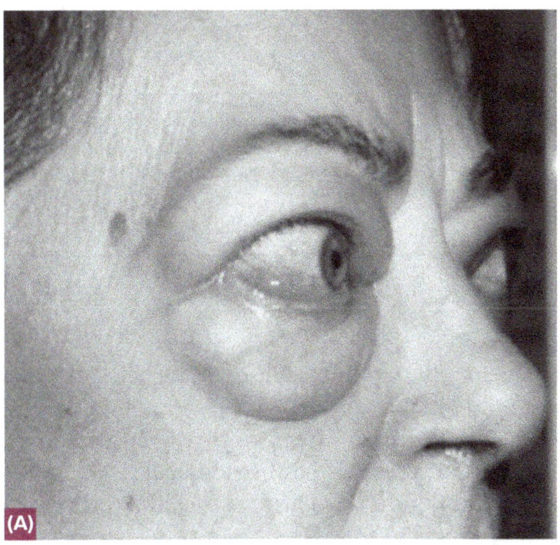
(A)

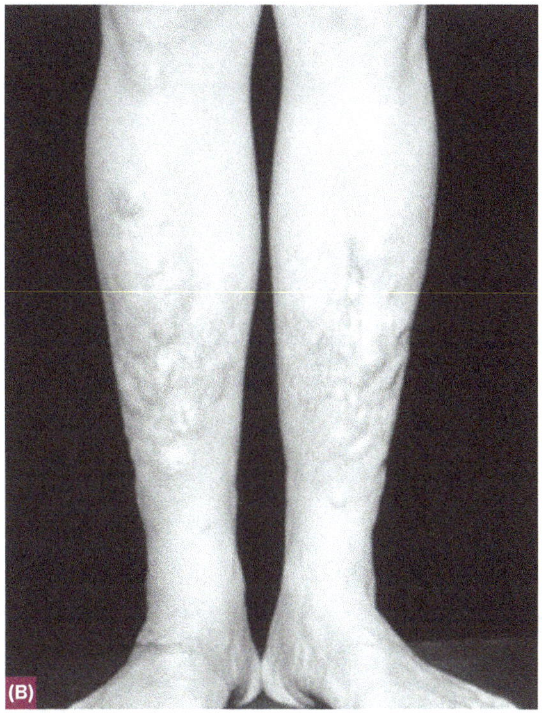
(B)

Reproduced, with permission, from Brunicardi FC et al, eds. *Schwartz's Principles of Surgery*. 9th ed. New York, NY: McGraw-Hill Education; 2010.

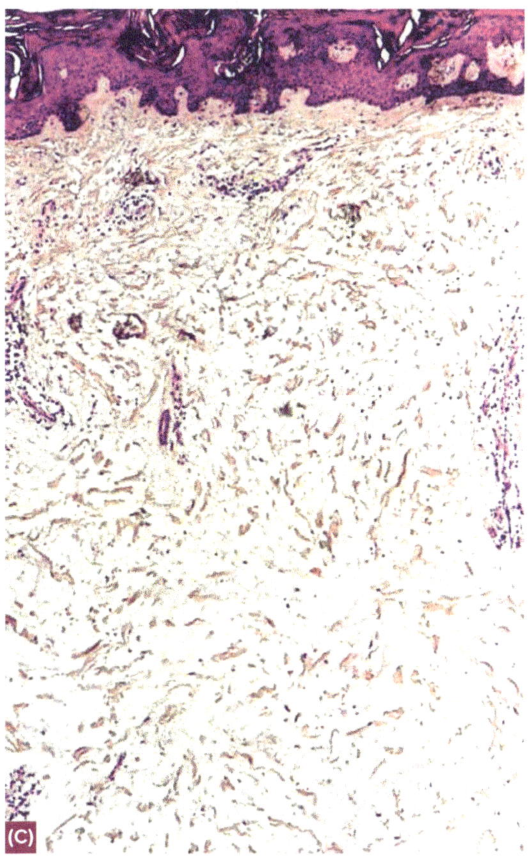
(C)

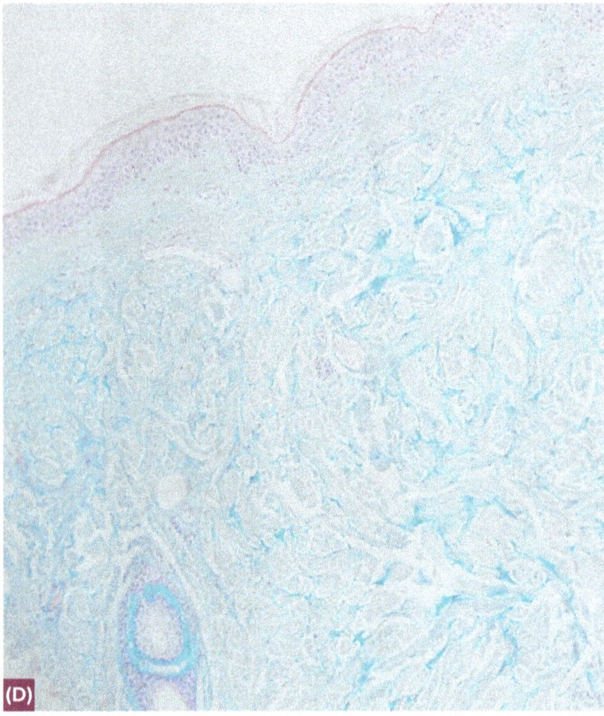

QUESTION 6-33.

A patient presents with a widespread symmetric eruption of small closely set papules accompanied by thickened bound-down skin. The eruption involves the face, upper trunk, and peripheral extremities. Serum analysis reveals a monoclonal gammopathy. A biopsy is performed and the findings are illustrated below. Which of the following diagnoses is CORRECT?

A) Nodular lichen myxedema
B) Scleromyxedema
C) Nephrogenic systemic fibrosis
D) Acral persistent papular mucinosis
E) Self-healing juvenile mucinosis

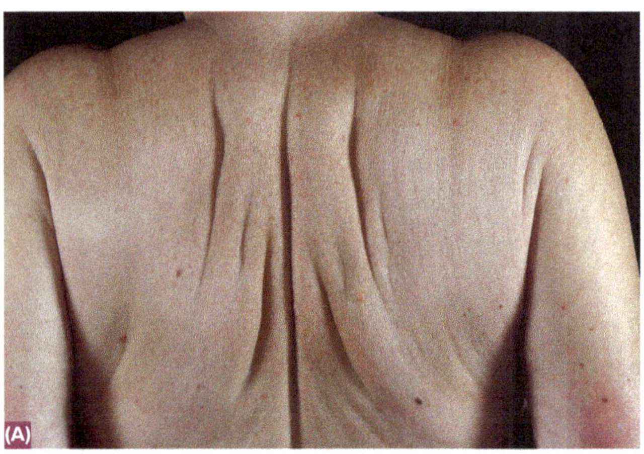

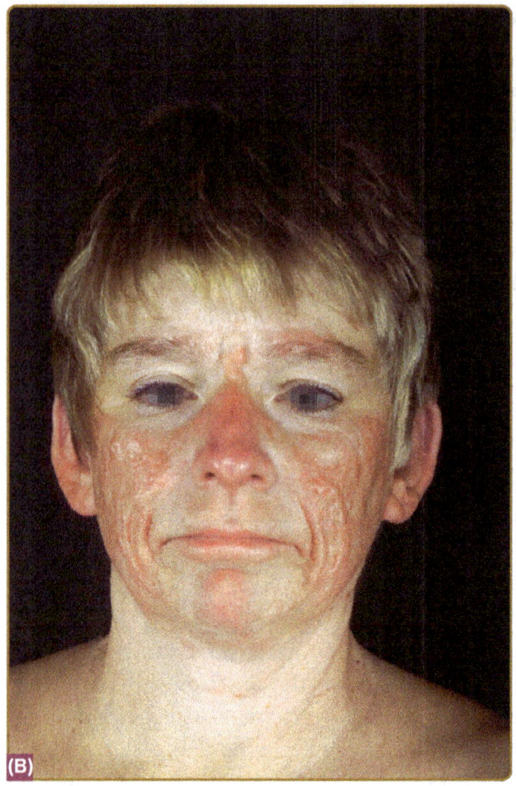

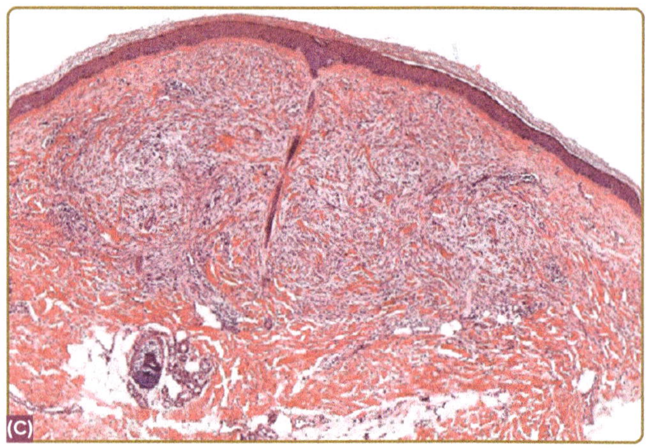

Parts **(A)–(C)** reproduced, with permission, from Goldsmith LA, Katz SI, Gilchrest BA, Paller AS, Leffell DJ, Wolff K, eds. *Fitzpatrick's Dermatology in General Medicine*. 8th ed. New York, NY: McGraw-Hill Education; 2012.

QUESTION 6-34.

An adult patient with chronic adult-onset diabetes presents with non-pitting indurated edema elevating the skin of the shoulder blade area with deep associated vertebral folds. He reports that the condition has been gradual. A biopsy is performed and the findings are illustrated below. Which of the following diagnoses is CORRECT?

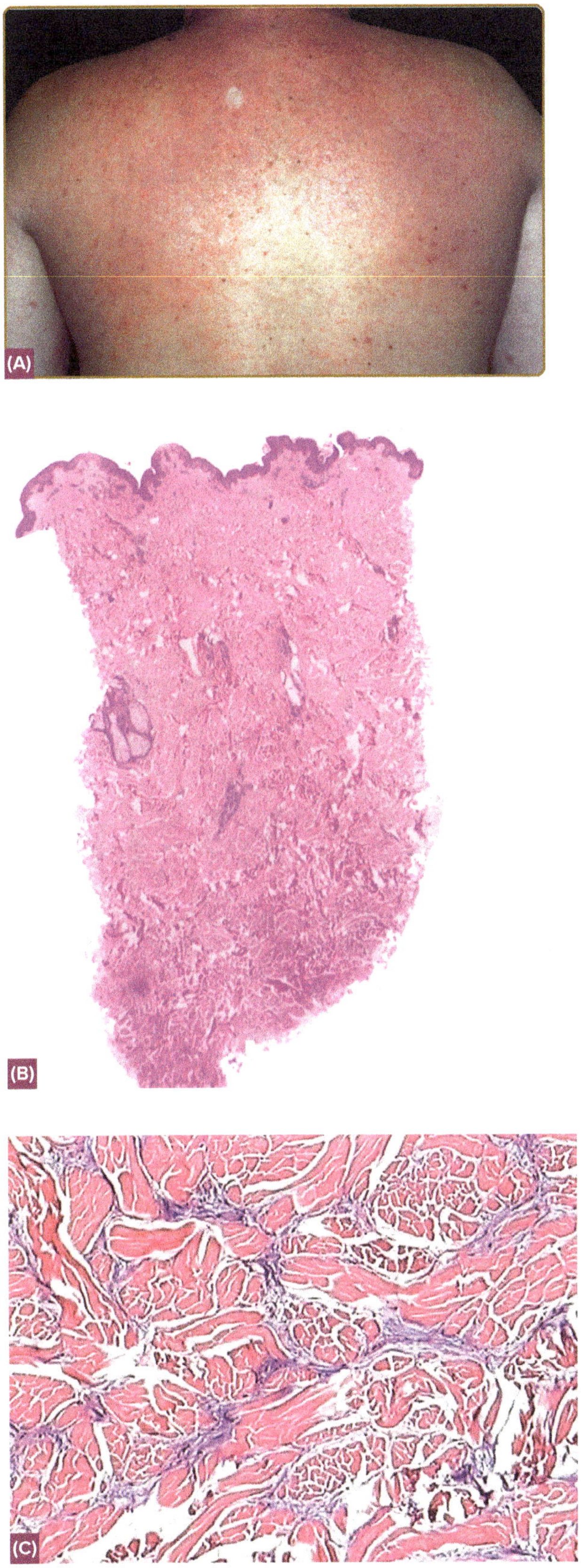

Part **(A)** reproduced, with permission, from Goldsmith LA, Katz SI, Gilchrest BA, Paller AS, Leffell DJ, Wolff K, eds. *Fitzpatrick's Dermatology in General Medicine*. 8th ed. New York, NY: McGraw-Hill Education; 2012.

A) Scleredema
B) Morphea
C) Scleromyxedema
D) Scleroderma
E) Follicular mucinosis

QUESTION 6-35.

The histopathological findings illustrated below represent a solitary lesion. Which of the following diagnoses is CORRECT?

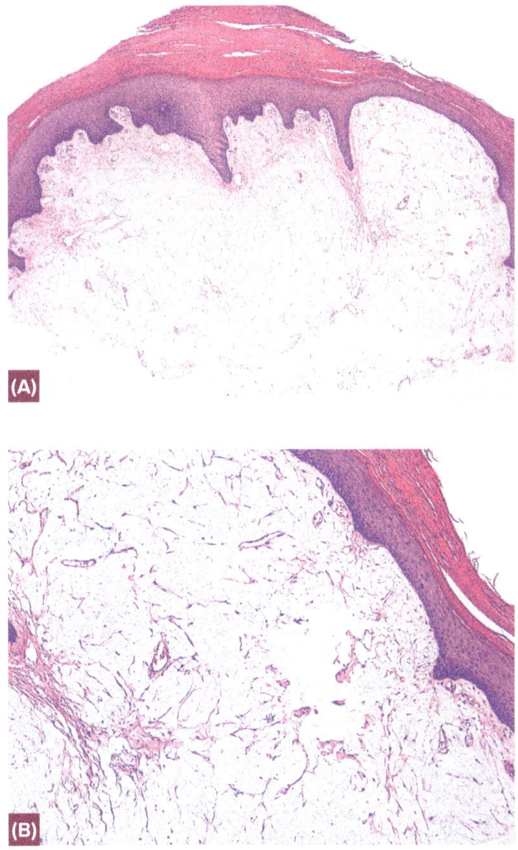

A) Focal cutaneous mucinosis
B) Digital mucous cyst
C) Mucocele of the lip
D) Cutaneous myxoma
E) Mucinous nevus

QUESTION 6-36.

An elderly patient presents with numerous firm waxy papules in the upper and lower palpebrae, as well as the tongue and oral mucosa. A biopsy is performed and the findings are illustrated below. Congo red stain reveals bright red amorphous material in the dermis, even after treatment with potassium permanganate. A bone marrow biopsy reveals a similar substance. Which of the following diagnoses is CORRECT?

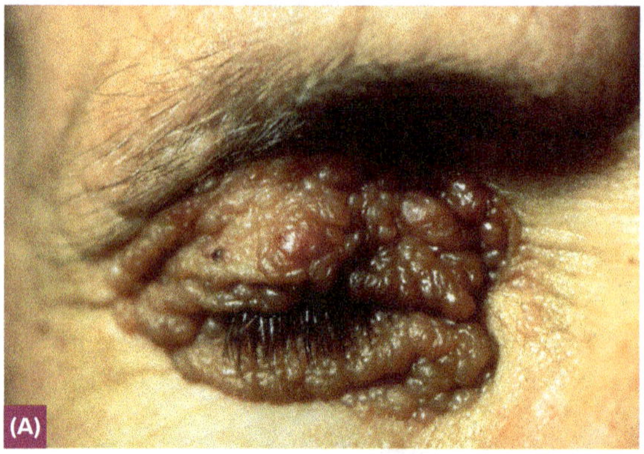

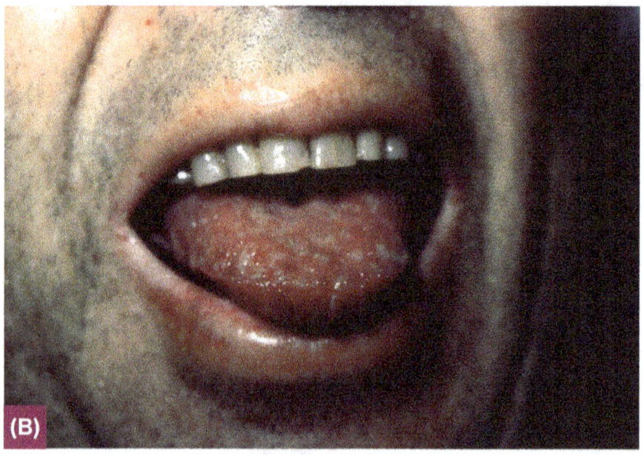

Reproduced, with permission, from Kaushansky K, Lichtman MA, Beutler E, Kipps TJ, Seligsohn U, Prchal JT, eds. *Williams Hematology*. 8th ed. New York, NY: McGraw-Hill Education; 2010.

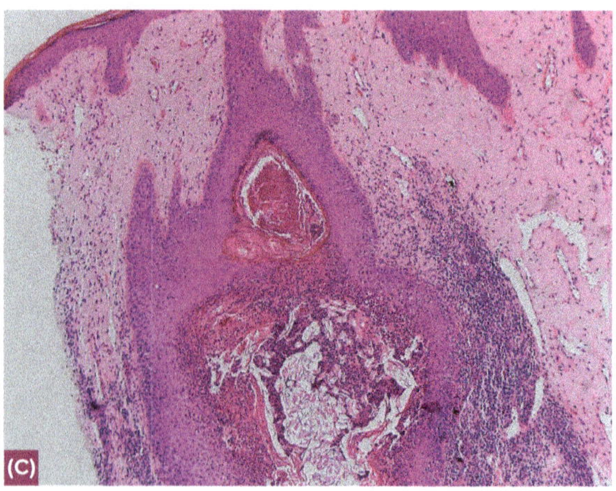

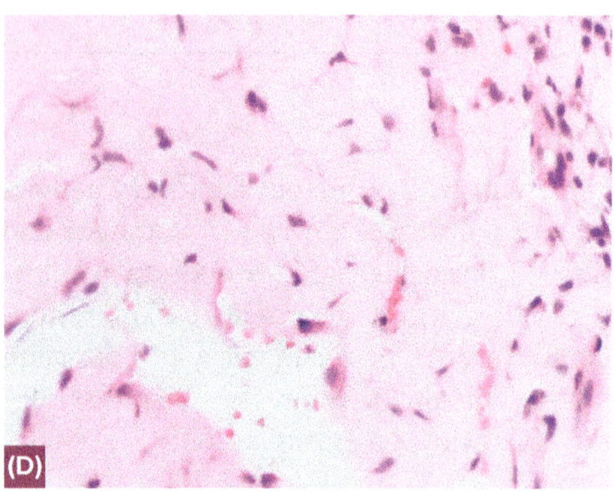

A) Systemic AL amyloidosis
B) Systemic AA amyloidosis
C) Familial amyloidotic polyneuropathy
D) β2-Microglobulin amyloid
E) Hyalinosis cutis et mucosae

QUESTION 6-37.

A patient presents with numerous hyperkeratotic papules on the shins. The lesions are extremely pruritic. A biopsy is performed and the findings are illustrated below. Thioflavine T fluorescence reveals deposition within the dermis. Which of the following diagnoses is CORRECT?

A) Macular amyloidosis
B) Lichen amyloidosis
C) Actinic amyloidosis
D) Nodular amyloidosis
E) Adult colloid milium

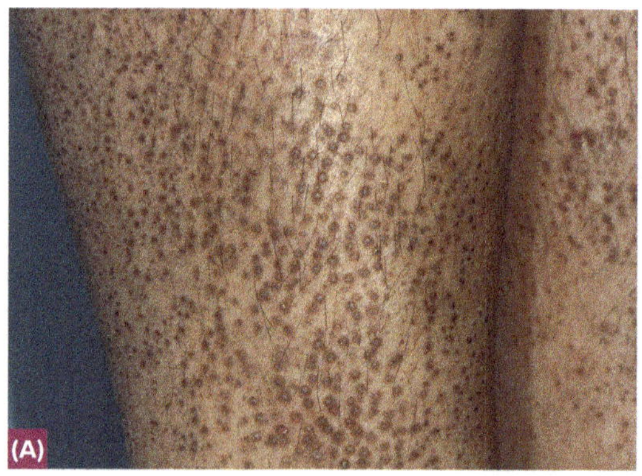

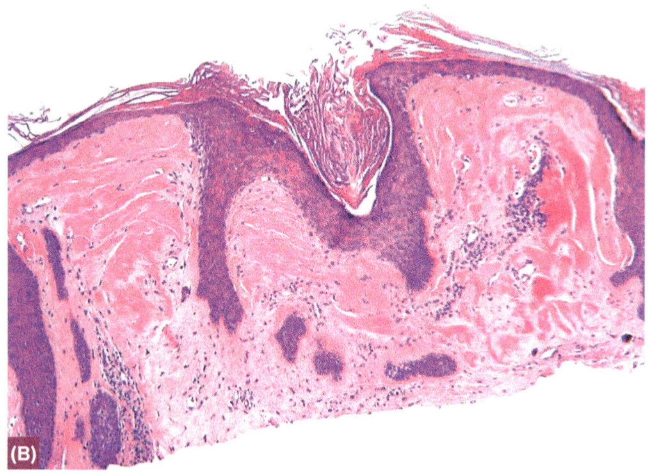

QUESTION 6-38.

A male patient presents with a hard yellow nodule on the auricle. A biopsy is performed and the findings are illustrated below. Which of the following statements regarding this condition is INCORRECT?

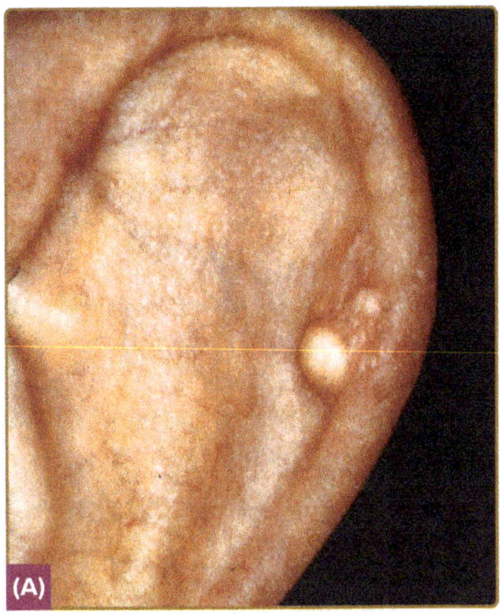

Reproduced, with permission, from Goldsmith LA, Katz SI, Gilchrest BA, Paller AS, Leffell DJ, Wolff K, eds. *Fitzpatrick's Dermatology in General Medicine*. 8th ed. New York, NY: McGraw-Hill Education; 2012.

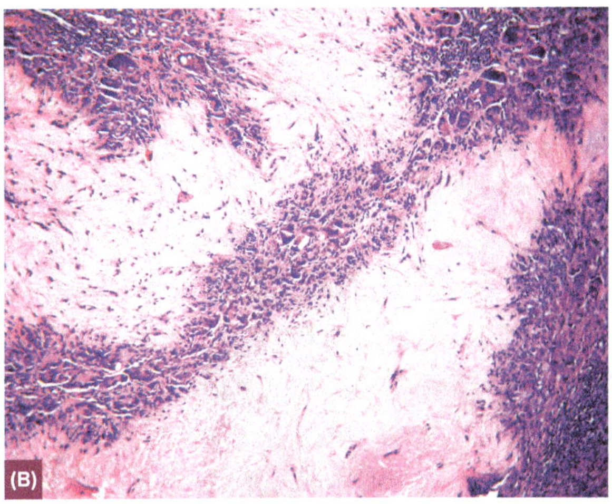

A) This condition tends to exhibit an autosomal dominant pattern of inheritance.
B) This condition may occur secondary to decreased renal function, diuretic therapy, and myeloproliferative syndromes.
C) Specimens fixed in alcohol exhibit multicolor birefringence under polarized light.
D) This condition is an episodic inflammatory process involving auricular cartilage that may also result in polyarthritis, nasal chondritis, ocular inflammation, and respiratory tract chondritis.
E) De Galantha stain, will stain the deposited material brown-black.

QUESTION 6-39.

A female patient presents with loose, thickened skin on the neck with a distinct yellowish hue. Review of systems reveals melena, hypertension, stable angina, and claudication. A biopsy of the neck is performed and the findings are illustrated below. Which of the following diagnoses is CORRECT?

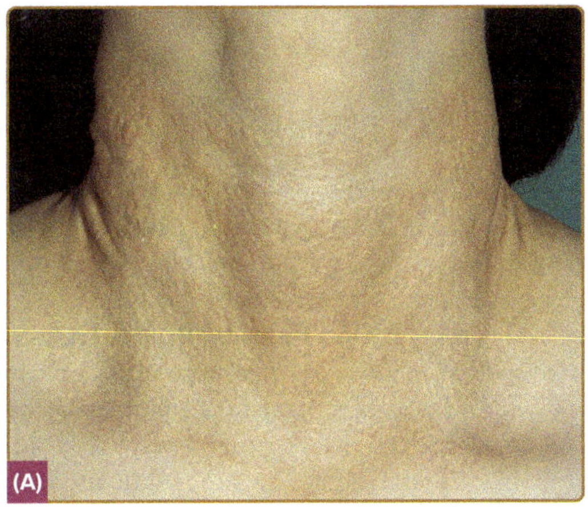

Reproduced, with permission, from Goldsmith LA, Katz SI, Gilchrest BA, Paller AS, Leffell DJ, Wolff K, eds. *Fitzpatrick's Dermatology in General Medicine*. 8th ed. New York, NY: McGraw-Hill Education; 2012.

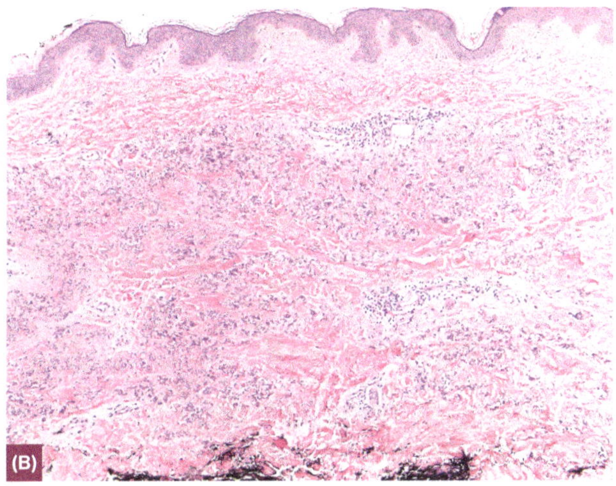

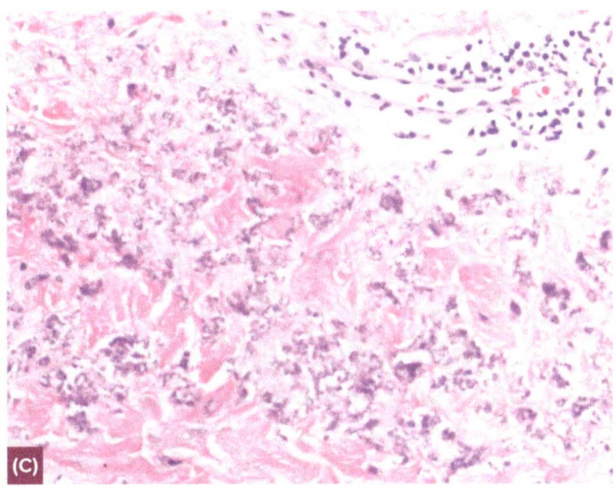

A) Macular atrophy (anetoderma)
B) Mid-dermal elastolysis
C) Pseudoxanthoma elasticum
D) Perifollicular elastolysis
E) Cutis laxa

ANSWERS

ANSWER 6-1: D.

Leukoderma is a clinical term that designates disorders characterized by skin lightening. The term does not reflect the cause of **hypopigmentation**, which may be the result of decreased epidermal melanin content or secondary to a decreased blood supply to the skin. **Hypomelanosis** denotes reduced melanin pigment within the skin, whereas **amelanosis** refers to the total absence of melanin pigment. **Depigmentation** implies total loss of skin color, whereas **pigmentary dilution** describes a generalized partial lightening of the skin and hair.

> **Quick Fact**
>
> **Disorders of Hypopigmentation**
>
> **Melanocytopenic hypomelanosis**
> Established vitiligo
> Piebaldism, Waardenberg syndrome, Woolf syndrome
> Physical leukoderma
> Onchocerciasis
> Pinta
> Scleroderma
> Halo nevus
> Melanoma-associated leukoderma
>
> **Melanopenic hypomelanosis**
> Early vitiligo/margin of vitiligo
> Albinism
> Idiopathic guttate hypomelanosis
> Pityriasis alba
> Post-inflammatory hypomelanosis
> Pityriasis alba
> Tinea versicolor
> Tuberous sclerosis
> Chediak–Higashi syndrome
> Hypomelanosis of Ito
> Nevus depigmentosus
> Malnutrition

Hypomelanosis can be classified into two histopathological categories: **melanocytopenic** or **melanopenic**. **Melanocytopenic hypomelanosis** is due to partial loss or total absence of epidermal and/or follicular melanocytes. The normal ratio of melanocytes to keratinocytes within the epidermis is approximately 1:10, with the exception of facial and genital skin, where it is about 1:4. This Melan-A stained biopsy exhibits a striking absence of melanocytes. **Melanopenic hypomelanosis**, on the other hand, is characterized by a normal number of epidermal and/or follicular melanocytes, but they either fail to synthesize normal amounts of melanin pigment or fail to transfer it to surrounding keratinocytes. All of the listed choices are examples of **melanocytopenic hypomelanosis**, with the exception of the **ash leaf spots of tuberous sclerosis**, which represent melanopenic hypomelanosis.

Piebaldism is an autosomal dominant condition characterized by congenital circumscribed patches of **leukoderma** and a white forelock, termed **poliosis**. Melanocytes are absent within involved sites. There are scattered areas of **hyperpigmentation** that contain a normal number of melanocytes. The condition results from mutations in the *KIT* proto-oncogene, which encodes a cell surface receptor tyrosine kinase important for the production of embryonic growth factors. Functional KIT receptor is required for melanocyte development both before melanoblast migration from the neural crest as well as postnatally.

Waardenburg syndrome (WS) is an autosomal dominant or less frequently autosomal recessive disorder characterized by various combinations of the following features: a white forelock, congenital patches of leukoderma, congenital deafness, synophrys, a broad nasal root, and dystopia canthorum. There are four clinical subtypes of WS. WS1 and WS3 are due to autosomal dominant mutations in PAX3, with WS3 demonstrating limb defects. WS2 is due to AD mutation in MITF, has an increased risk of deafness, but no dystopia canthorum. WS4 is due to AR mutation in SOX10, endothelin-3 ligand, and endothelin-3 receptor genes and has **Hirschsprung disease**.

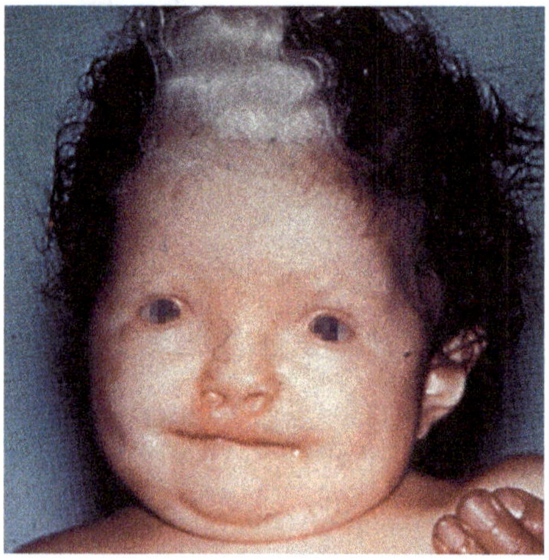

Waardenburg syndrome type 1. Note poliosis (white forelock) and dystopia canthorum (lateral displacement of the medial canthi of the eyes). (Reproduced, with permission, from Goldsmith LA, Katz SI, Gilchrest BA, Paller AS, Leffell DJ, Wolff K, eds. *Fitzpatrick's Dermatology in General Medicine*. 8th ed. New York, NY: McGraw-Hill Education; 2012.)

Vitiligo is acquired patchy pigment loss of the skin and rarely **leukotrichia**. Individuals may present at any age with a focal isolated macule, segmental unilateral lesions, or generalized symmetric lesions. It has a predilection for sites that are normally relatively hyperpigmented and/or subjected to repeated trauma or friction, including the face, dorsal hands, nipples, axillae, umbilicus, sacral, inguinal, and anogenital areas. The borders are usually convex and lesions enlarge centrifugally, as if the **depigmenting** process were "invading" normally pigmented skin. Rarely universal involvement may be seen. Microscopically, scattered lymphocytes are frequently seen along the dermal epidermal junction with minimal interface change and rare scattered papillary dermal melanophages. Melanocytes are markedly reduced or absent within involved skin.

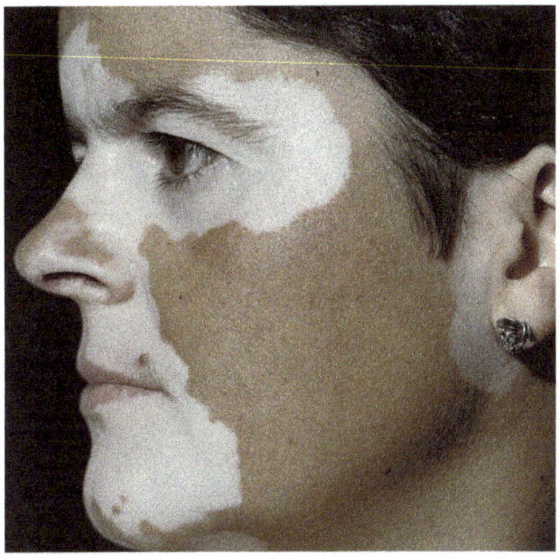

Vitiligo: face. Extensive depigmentation of the central face. Involved vitiliginous skin has convex borders, extending into the normal pigmented skin. Note the chalk-white color and sharp margination. Note also that the dermal nevomelanocytic nevus on the upper lip has retained its pigmentation. (Reproduced, with permission, from Wolff K, Johnson RA, Saavedra AP. *Fitzpatrick's Color Atlas and Synopsis of Clinical Dermatology*. 7th ed. New York, NY: McGraw-Hill Education; 2013.)

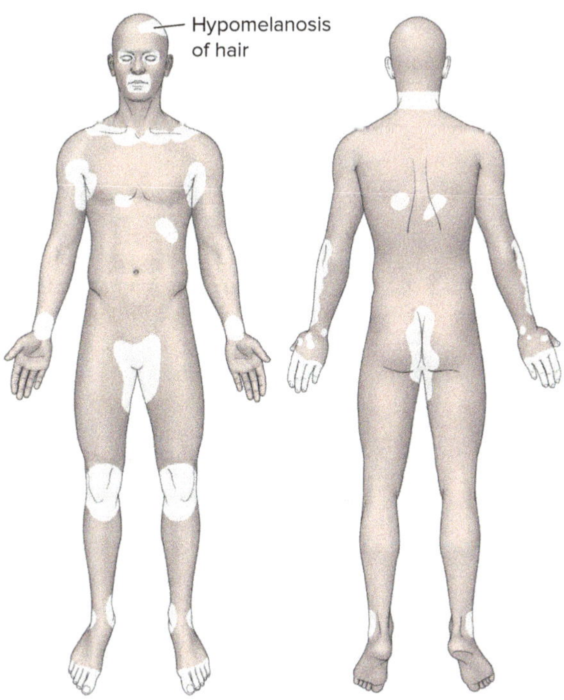

Vitiligo: predilection sites. (Reproduced, with permission, from Wolff K, Johnson RA, Saavedra AP. *Fitzpatrick's Color Atlas and Synopsis of Clinical Dermatology*. 7th ed. New York, NY: McGraw-Hill Education; 2013.)

Trauma, chemical burns, and **thermal burns** frequently result in scarring with loss of all epidermal melanocytes. These **depigmented** areas may be permanent. Dermal fibrosis and loss of vessels in the resultant scar may further contribute to the pallor seen clinically.

Tuberous sclerosis (TS), the incorrect choice, is an autosomal dominant disorder characterized by hamartomas in multiple organs, including the skin, brain, eye, heart, and kidney. The classic findings of **facial angiofibromas**, seizures, and mental deficits are preceded by white macules. These **hypomelanotic** macules are often evident at birth, and can have a lance-ovate configuration, which resembles an ash leaf (ie, **ash leaf spots**). These macules are a dull white color (**hypomelanotic**) and not the bone white color of **vitiligo (amelanotic)**. This **melanopenic hypomelanosis** is microscopically characterized by a normal to slightly reduced number of intraepidermal melanocytes and markedly reduced keratinocyte melanin pigment content. In the **ash leaf spots of TS**, the DOPA reaction is weak compared with the surrounding normal skin, thus indicating an impaired ability to produce melanin pigment. By electron microscopy, the size of melanosomes and degree of melanization are less than the normal counterparts, and their dendrites are less well developed.

ANSWER 6-2: C.

This patient has **oculocutaneous albinism** type 1 (OCA1), an autosomal recessive melanopenic condition due to mutations in the *TYR* gene, which encodes for tyrosinase. There are tyrosinase negative and tyrosinase positive subtypes of OCA. OCA 1 is tyrosinase negative and is further subclassified into OCA-1A, in which there is no tyrosinase activity; OCA-IB and OCA 1MP, in which some tyrosinase activity is present; and OCA-2TS, which is temperature sensitive. These patients are extremely sensitive to UV light and have a strong predisposition for skin cancer. The tyrosinase-positive subtypes are OCA2, OCA3, and OCA4. The OCA2 subtype is caused by a mutation in the *OCA2* gene (formerly P-gene) responsible for regulating organelle pH and vacuolar accumulation of glutathione. OCA3 is due to a mutated tyrosinase-related protein (TYRP 1), which leads to early degradation of tyrosinase. OCA4 is characterized by mutations of the membrane-associated transporter protein gene (*MATP*, also known as *SLC45A2*). In all disease subtypes, basal melanocytes are observed, but the epidermal melanin content is greatly diminished or absent (Table 6-2A).

A DOPA stain can be used to highlight intact DOPA oxidase (tyrosinase) activity and will result in the formation of brownish black pigment. A positive **DOPA reaction** indicates an intact and complete metabolic pathway to melanin synthesis. In **tyrosinase positive albinism**, a plucked hair bulb becomes dark after incubation in DOPA solution.

Table 6-2A. Oculocutaneous Albinism

TYPE	GENE	FUNCTION OF PROTEIN	PHENOTYPE
OCA1A	*TYR*	• Melanin synthesis	Tyrosinase negative OCA • No pigment from birth • No pigment over time • Decreased visual acuity, nystagmus, photophobia
OCA1B	*TYR*	• Melanin synthesis	Yellow mutant OCA • No pigment at birth • Some improvement with time • Milder eye findings
OCA2	*OCA2*	• Vacuolar glutathione accumulation • Organelle pH regulation tyrosinase processing and trafficking	Tyrosinase-positive OCA • Minimal pigment at birth • Skin darkens over time • White/yellow/red hair • Moderate nystagmus and visual impairment
OCA3	*TYRP1*	• Stabilizes tyrosinase	Brown OCA • Minimal to tan pigment from birth • White/red/light brown hair • Nystagmus with light retinal pigment
OCA4	*SLC45A2*	• Tyrosinase processing • Trafficking of proteins to the melanosome	• Most common among individuals with albinism from Japan, China, and India • White/yellow-brown hair

These patients may develop freckles and pigmented nevi later in life. In **tyrosinase negative albinism**, the hair bulb does not become dark after incubation in DOPA solution, and patients never become pigmented.

Reduction of melanin within eye structures and misrouting of optic nerve fibers during development are responsible for the ocular manifestations seen in all forms of OCA. These include a translucent iris that transmits light upon globe transillumination, a hypopigmented retina and fovea that result in photophobia and decreased visual acuity, nystagmus, and a lack of binocular vision. The severity of these findings is proportional to the amount of reduction in melanin pigment.

Electron microscopy proves the presence of normal melanocytes. In the **tyrosinase-positive type**, some melanosomes mature to stages III and IV, but in the **tyrosinase-negative type**, the melanosomes are not pigmented, even after incubation with DOPA. Microscopically, the skin of both forms exhibits reduced or absent melanin pigment within basal keratinocytes. This reduction can be highlighted using on Fontana-Masson stain. Melan-A stain will reveal normal numbers of intraepidermal melanocytes.

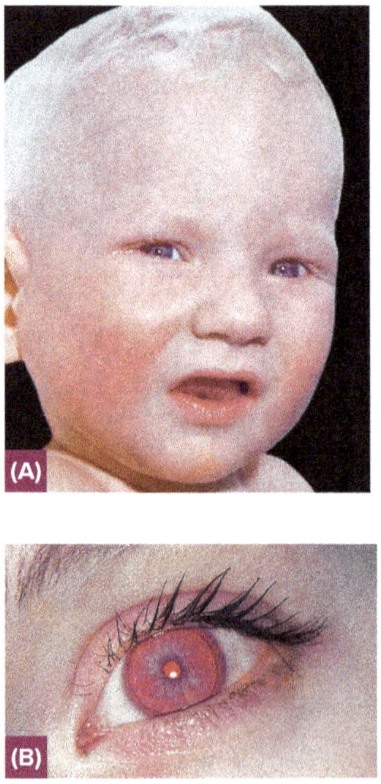

Oculocutaneous albinism. **(A)** White skin, white eyelashes, eyebrows, and scalp hair. The irises appear translucent. Heme pigment gives the face a pinkish hue. There is squinting due to photophobia and nystagmus. **(B)** Iris translucency is a sine qua non in all types of oculocutaneous albinism, even in those patients in whom the iris is brown. The iris is rarely pink except in infants, and the diagnosis of albinism depends on the detection of iris translucency. This is best done in a dark room with a flashlight pointed at the sclera.

ANSWER 6-3: E.

This patient has extensive cutaneous involvement by **discoid lupus erythematosus** with areas of porcelain-white scar formation. Inflammatory skin diseases, as well as various physical, chemical, thermal, and other pathologic injuries, can result in **leukoderma** (Table 6-3A). Inflammatory dermatitides can result in hypomelanotic macular lesions and are referred to as **post-inflammatory hypomelanosis (post-inflammatory leukoderma)**. Associated condition include **eczematous dermatitis, seborrheic dermatitis, psoriasis, drug eruptions, pityriasis lichenoides chronica, lupus erythematosus, lichen planus, alopecia mucinosa, sarcoidosis**, and **mycosis fungoides**. Clinically, the lesions of **post-inflammatory hypomelanosis** are off-white (not fully depigmented), have indistinct margins, and may show gradual repigmentation with a restoration of normal numbers of basilar melanocytes and keratinocyte melanin pigment. Scattered dermal melanophages may be present. Repigmentation may occur rapidly on sun-exposed sites and in less severely damaged areas. The repigmentation is irregular and often shows a mottled appearance.

Table 6-3A. Leukoderma

	POST-INFLAMMATORY LEUKODERMA	PHYSICAL LEUKODERMA
Clinical features	Hypopigmented, off-white (not fully depigmented) Widespread or localized Ill-defined margins Repigmentation usually occurs	Depigmented Macular lesions at sites of exposure/injury Repigmentation rarely occurs
Causes	Eczematous dermatitis Psoriasis Pityriasis lichenoides Lichen planus Lupus erythematosus Seborrheic dermatitis Mycosis fungoides Drug eruption	Physical injury Thermal injury Radiation Chemical exposure: phenols, catechols, sulfhydrl compounds Infections: Onchocerciasis Pinta
Histopathologic features	Reduced or absent basilar melanocytes Reduced melanin in epidermis (often blocked transfer to keratinocytes) Evidence of antecedent inflammatory process may be present in early lesions Reparative changes (depending on condition)	Absence of melanocytes and melanin pigment Reparative changes (depending on agent)

Less commonly, the leukoderma is permanent and characterized by an absence of intraepidermal melanocytes and melanin. Various physical, chemical, thermal, and other pathologic injuries can severely damage melanocytes, resulting in a **permanent leukoderma (physical leukoderma)**. Total destruction of melanocytes in burns, exposure to certain chemicals, infectious diseases such as **pinta** or **onchocerciasis, discoid lupus erythematosus, scleroderma, halo nevi**, and so on are associated with **physical leukoderma**. In old scars, even if the melanocytes have recovered, the fibrosis and the relative paucity of blood vessels will contribute to a persistent white color; examples include **atrophie blanche, discoid lupus, lichen sclerosis**, and **nevus anemicus**. Pigmentary side effects of hydroxychloroquine and NSAIDs are characterized by **hyperpigmentation**. The patient in question has areas of complete pigment loss (**depigmentation**) associated with extensive scar formation. The peripheral areas of hyperpigmentation and erythema most likely represent post-inflammatory pigmentary alteration and melanophage accumulation. While cases of cutaneous lupus most frequently result in **post-inflammatory leukoderma** with subsequent repigmentation, the severe nature of this patient's condition with porcelain-white **depigmentation** and scarring is indicative of **permanent leukoderma**. Even if these lesions were to regain a basilar melanocyte population, the underlying scar tissue will result in a persistent white color.

ANSWER 6-4: D.

This is a classic example of **nevus anemicus**, which is characterized by a congenital white patch with an irregular border and is found most commonly on the trunk, particularly the chest. Familial cases have been reported. Rubbing the border makes the normal skin erythematous while the lesion remains white. It is a vascular malformation in which the abnormality of the involved vessels is functional rather than anatomic. The abnormality seems to be a focal hypersensitivity of blood vessels to catecholamines, possibly mediated by an abnormality in endothelial adhesion molecule induction (E-selectin expression), resulting in vasoconstriction. An intralesional injection of α-adrenergic blockers, unlike vasodilators such as histamine and acetylcholine, may induce erythema. **Nevus anemicus** may be linked with certain genodermatoses, including **neurofibromatosis** and **phakomatosis pigmentovascularis**. Microscopically,

Quick Fact

✓ Nevus anemicus is catecholamine-related
✓ Nevus depigmentosus is melanin-related
✓ Vitiligo is melanocyte loss

the epidermal melanocytes and dermal blood vessels are normal in number and size. Other dermal components are likewise normal. Dermal fibrosis is not present in this condition.

ANSWER 6-5: D.

Melanotic hyperpigmentation disorders may be classified histopathologically according to the predominant pattern as epidermal, dermal (pigment incontinence), or mixed epidermal and dermal. In the epidermal pattern of hyperpigmentation, there is increased melanin production and/or transfer of melanin to keratinocytes. Inflammatory and mechanical mediators may play a role in this process by enhancing pigment production and transfer. In the dermal pattern, damage to the basement membrane causes melanin to "fall into" the dermis where it is phagocytosed and concentrated within dermal macrophages (referred to as melanophages). Melanin within dermal melanophages tends to persist for long periods of time. The color of the hyperpigmentation corresponds to the location of the pigment: brown (epidermal), blue-gray (dermal), and brown-gray (mixed epidermal and dermal). Attempting to classify these disorders may sometime be difficult because many patients have varying degrees of both epidermal and dermal hyperpigmentation. These disorders are also classified by clinical distribution as generalized or diffuse and patterned or circumscribed.

Quick Fact

Melanotic Hyperpigmentation

✓ Epidermal = brown
  - ↑melanocyte function
  - ↑melanocyte number
✓ Dermal = blue-gray
  - melanophages
✓ Mixed = brown-gray

ANSWER 6-6: D.

Addison disease is a primary disorder of adrenocortical insufficiency, marked by decreased levels of plasma cortisol, urinary 17-hydorxy-corticosteroids, and 17-ketosteroids. Adrenocorticotropic hormone (ACTH) levels are typically elevated due to a lack of feedback inhibition from the adrenal glands. Patients present with hyperpigmentation pronounced in sun-exposed areas that normally exhibit dark skin, sites of trauma, the palmar creases, axillae, perineum, nipples, tongue, and mucous membranes. There can be darkening of existing melanocytic nevi, hair, and nails. Calcification of the auricular cartilages may occur in long-standing primary or secondary adrenal insufficiency, a finding that occurs exclusively in men. This finding is thought to result from chronic cortisol deficiency, and does not improve with glucocorticoid replacement. Patients exhibit fatigue, nausea, loss of appetite, weight loss, hypoglycemia, hyponatremia, and low blood pressure. Loss of ambisexual hair occurs in postpubertal women, in whom androgen production occurs primarily in the adrenal gland. Most cases are an autoimmune disorder, with autoantibodies targeting steroid 21-hydroxylase and causing adrenocoritcal atrophy or hypofunction. Non-autoimmune causes include **metastatic tumors**, bilateral adrenal hemorrhage due to **anticoagulant therapy**, adrenal gland infarction in the setting of **antiphospholipid antibody syndrome** or **factor V Leiden**, **infections (TB, CMV, histoplasmosis)**, and infiltrative diseases (**sarcoidosis, amyloidosis**).

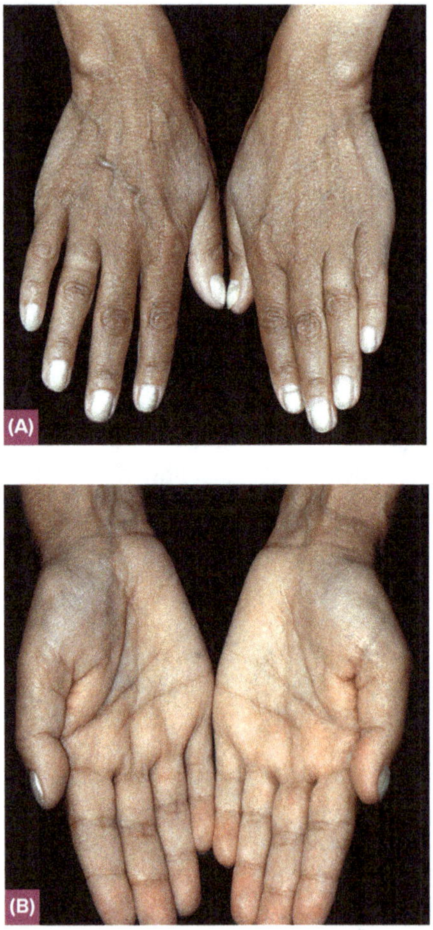

Addison disease. (A) Hyperpigmentation representing an accentuation of normal pigmentation of the hand of a patient with Addison disease. **(B)** Note accentuated pigmentation in the palmar creases. (Reproduced, with permission, from Wolff K, Johnson RA, Saavedra AP. *Fitzpatrick's Color Atlas and Synopsis of Clinical Dermatology*. 7th ed. New York, NY: McGraw-Hill Education; 2013.)

Choice A would suggest **Nelson syndrome**, and is incorrect given the negative surgical history. Nelson syndrome occurs in patients who have had bilateral adrenalectomy for **Cushing disease** who then develop secondary **ACTH-producing pituitary adenomas**. Remember, **Cushing disease** is when hypersecretion of ACTH is attributed to a primary anterior pituitary defect, most commonly a pituitary adenoma. **Cushing syndrome** is characterized by any condition resulting in elevated cortisol levels. **Nelson syndrome** occurs in 10%-47% of patients who undergo bilateral adrenalectomy for Cushing disease. **Hyperpigmentation** is similar to that in **Addison disease** and consists of generalized darkening of the skin and hair by hyperactive melanocytes in normal numbers. In addition, **multiple lentigines** and pigmented bands involving the nails may be seen. In both **Addison disease** and **Nelson syndrome**, ACTH and MSH are increased with MSH stimulating melanin synthesis. Because the **pituitary adenoma** in **Nelson syndrome** may be slow growing and because tumor volume and plasma ACTH levels correlate, it may take decades for symptoms to occur after adrenalectomy.

Cushing syndrome (choice B) may be associated with either high plasma ACTH levels (pituitary hyperproduction and "ectopic ACTH syndrome") or a nearly complete lack of ACTH (**adrenal primary nodular hyperplasia, adrenal adenoma, carcinoma**, or iatrogenic). Regardless, all patients have an increase in plasma cortisol, unlike **Addison disease**. Clinical features include central obesity, moon facies, "buffalo hump," purple striae, ecchymoses, hypertension, insulin resistance, and hyperglycemia. Like **Addison disease**, **Cushing syndrome** is due to increased ACTH and can cause hyperpigmentation. This is due to melanocyte-stimulating hormone production as a byproduct of ACTH synthesis from pro-opiomelanocortin. Other than hyperpigmentation, the patient in question does not exhibit any of the other clinical signs of **Cushing syndrome**.

Skin pigmentation, liver cirrhosis, cardiac failure, and diabetes mellitus make up the clinical tetrad of **hemochromatosis** (choice C). **Hereditary hemochromatosis** is a spectrum of autosomal recessive diseases characterized by hyper-absorption of dietary iron, with elevated serum ferritin. **Secondary hemochromatosis** is caused by disorders of erythropoiesis and treatment with blood transfusions. Iron freed from the heme that is released from damaged or transfused red blood cells accumulates in the body. In white skin, discoloration varies from bronze (bronze diabetes) to blue-gray, whereas in pigmented individuals it is brown to black. Pigmentation is most pronounced in the sun-exposed areas, skin creases and folds, and the nipples. It often precedes other symptoms, and is an important sign because treatment with phlebotomy and chelating agents improves the prognosis if serum ferritin levels are kept at 100 ng/mL or lower. Hemosiderin deposition is seen later in the cytoplasm of eccrine secretory cells, periglandular connective tissue, and perivascular macrophages, best highlighted with a Prussian blue stain.

Argyria (choice E) refers to silver deposition that results from prolonged contact with or ingestion of silver salts. It is characterized by gray to gray-black staining of the skin on sun-exposed sites and the azure lunula of nails. Absorption from mucous membranes may cause local as well as **systemic argyria**. In some patients the entire skin acquires a slate blue-gray color. Visceral organs accumulate silver and show blue discoloration. Silver particles have a dark brown to black granular appearance and are scattered extracellularly in the

Table 6-6A. Metal Deposition and Dyspigmentation

DISORDER	EPIDERMAL HYPERMELANOSIS	DERMAL ALTERATION	OTHER FINDINGS
Hemochromatosis	Present	Hemosiderin	
Argyria (silver deposition)	Present, sun-exposed skin	Silver particles, basement membranes of sweat glands, elastic fibers	Refractile granules on dark-field examination
Chrysiasis (gold deposition)	May be present	Gold particles in macrophages and endothelium	Refractile granules on dark-field microscopy
Mercury	May be present	Brown-black mercury granules either free or in macrophages	
Arsenic	Present	Arsenic particles	
Lead		Lead particles	
Bismuth		Bismuth granules in papillary and reticular dermis	

dermis. They are concentrated in the basement membranes of eccrine sweat glands, perifollicular sheath, nerves, capillary walls, and elastic fibers. Silver particles are best demonstrated by polarized light microscopy as refractile particles. Silver particles are absent in the epidermis, but **hypermelanosis** of the epidermis, particularly in exposed areas, is also evident. The accumulation of other metals in the skin can result in dyspigmentation (Table 6-6A).

ANSWER 6-7: B.

Peutz–Jeghers syndrome is an autosomal dominant disorder associated with mutations of the serine threonine kinase gene *STK11/LKB1*. Patients have **mucocutaneous melanotic macules**, which are present at birth or appear during childhood. Skin lesions have an acrofacial distribution pattern and favor the perioral region. Mucosal lesions may affect the palate, tongue, buccal mucosa, and conjunctivae. Macules on the lips may disappear over time, but not the pigmentation of the mouth; therefore the mouth pigmentation is the sine qua non for diagnosis. In the majority of cases, multiple **hamartomatous polyps** develop in the small intestines, which if not resected may become malignant in 2%-3% of patients. Additionally, there is an increased incidence of **breast, ovarian**, and **pancreatic cancer**. These pigmented lesions are best characterized as **melanotic macules** (vs **lentigines**) since the pigmentation is located within basal cells and there is no increase in the number of melanocytes. There may be some disturbance of pigment transfer to basal keratinocytes.

> **Quick Fact**
>
> Melanotic macules=basal keratinocyte pigment and normal number of melanocytes.
>
> Lentigines=basal keratinocyte pigment and increased number of melanocytes.

Generalized lentiginosis is an autosomal dominant condition in which patients have many lentigines that appear at birth in a generalized dense distribution yet sparing mucous membranes and without associated abnormalities. The histopathological findings include increased basal cell melanization and increased intraepidermal melanocytes.

LEOPARD syndrome is an autosomal dominant disease typified by multiple lentigines affecting any part of the body from the scalp to the feet. Most cases are associated with mutations of protein-tyrosine phosphatase, nonreceptor type 11 (PTPN11). In addition to lentigines, electrocardiographic abnormalities, ocular hypertelorism, pulmonic stenosis, abnormal genitalia, growth retardation, and deafness are present. The histopathological findings are largely nonspecific and consist of elongation of rete ridges, increased melanocytes, and increased melanization of the epidermis. On electron microscopy, giant melanosomes and complex melanosomes are seen.

Carney complex is an autosomal dominant syndrome characterized by inactivating mutations in the *PRKAAR1A* gene coding for the cyclic AMP-dependent protein kinase A regulatory subunit type 1A. **Mucous membrane lentiginosis** and associated cardiac, cutaneous, and/or mammary **myxomas**, as well as endocrine abnormalities, primary **pigmented nodular adrenocortical disease**, and **psammomatous melanotic schwannomas (neuromas)** can occur. Microscopically, the findings are identical to those of generalized lentiginosis.

Laugier–Hunziker syndrome is a rare acquired condition characterized by diffuse oral hyperpigmentation and longitudinal pigmented streaks of the nails. The pathogenesis is unknown, but no systemic involvement or malignant predisposition has been described. Microscopically, the basal layer keratinocytes contain increased melanin pigment and there are slightly increased numbers of normal melanocytes. Scattered melanophages may be present.

ANSWER 6-8: A.

Dowling–Degos disease is a rare dominantly inherited condition that manifests as slowly spreading areas of reticular hyperpigmentation involving flexural or frictional surfaces such as the axillae, neck, groin, and in women the inframammary folds. Perioral comedo-like follicular keratosis and pitted scars may be present. The age of onset is typically in the third to fourth decades of life. The distribution of hyperpigmentation is similar to that in **acanthosis nigricans**, but the lesions of **acanthosis nigricans** manifest a velvety texture. The age of onset is usually in the third and fourth decades of life. **Haber syndrome** consists of rosacea-like facial erythema and telangiectasia associated with black keratotic papules of the axillae, neck, and occasionally trunk; it may be the same as **Dowling–Degos disease. Dowling–Degos disease** and **Haber syndrome** both manifest elongated, tapered, heavily melanized retia with small horn cysts or follicular plugs generating an appearance similar to **reticulated seborrheic keratosis.**

Dermatopathia pigmentosa reticularis is a heterogeneous autosomal dominant condition that involves reticulated pigmentation over the trunk and extremities. Loss of the fingernails and toenails; hypohidrosis; and atrophy of the skin of the elbows and knees and extremities may occur.

Naegli–Franceschetti–Jadassohn syndrome is a rare autosomal dominant disease of childhood onset in which punctate pigmentation involves the axillae, neck, and trunk. Mutations in *KRT14* may render keratinocytes more susceptible to TNFα-induced apoptosis. Hypohidrosis, palmoplantar hyperkeratosis, and abnormalities of the teeth and nails may be present. Increased epidermal melanization of melanophages in the upper dermis may be detected.

Cantu syndrome is an autosomal dominant disorder characterized by hypertrichosis, osteodysplasia, and cardiomegaly

Quick Fact

Genodermatoses: Reticulated Hyperpigmentation

- Dowling–Degos (DDD)
- Galli-galli (acantholytic DDD)
- Haber syndrome (Rosacea + DDD)
- Pigmentatio reticularis facei et colli (DDD face + epidermoid cysts)
- Dyskeratosis congenita
- Fanconi anemia
- X-linked reticulate pigmentary disorder
- Epidermolysis bullosa simplex herpetiformis (Dowling–Meara)
- Epidermolysis bullosa simplex with mottled pigmentation
- Mendes de Costa disease
- Dermatopathia pigmentosa reticularis
- Naegeli–Fraceschetti–Jadassohn syndrome
- Reticulate acropigmentation of Kitamura
- Cantu syndrome
- Mitochondrial disorders
- ANOTHER syndrome

with onset in adolescence. Small, punctate, hyperpigmented macules that often have a reticular pattern involve the face, forearms, and feet. Hyperkeratosis of the palms and soles may be associated with this disorder.

Acanthosis nigricans is not a disease per se, but a condition reflective of underlying malignancy, reaction to medications, or various systemic conditions such as glucose intolerance. Clinically, the lesions are ill-defined hyperpigmented plaques that most commonly also arise in the axillae and on the posterior neck. However, the surface has a velvety texture and may be surfaced by papillomatous projections. Acanthosis nigricans is not associated with perioral comedo-like follicular keratosis and pitted scars. Microscopically, there is an acanthotic epidermis with hyperorthokeratosis and slight hyperpigmentation of basal keratinocytes. Horn cysts and a reticulated distribution of rete ridges are typically absent.

ANSWER 6-9: B.

This patient most likely has **Carney complex,** which is an autosomal dominant disorder characterized by myxomas, lentiginosis, and endocrine hyperactivity. Historically, it was referred to as two syndromes: **NAME syndrome** and **LAMB syndrome**. Nonmyxoid tumors associated with Carney complex are primarily of endocrine differentiation and include **primary pigmented nodular adrenal disease** (Cushing syndrome), **testicular large-cell calcifying Sertoli cell tumor** (sexual precocity), **pituitary adenoma** (acromegaly), **thyroid tumors**, and **ovarian cysts**. Multiple types of

Quick Fact

NAME SYNDROME

Nevi (epithelioid blue nevi)
Atrial myxomas
Myxomas (skin, breast, neuroma/neurofibroma)
Ephelides

LAMB SYNDROME

Lentigines
Atrial myxomas
Mucocutaneous myxomas

hyperpigmentation such as **lentigines, ephelides, blue nevi, junctional, dermal** and **compound nevi**, and **café-au-lait** spots have been described. Diagnostic criteria for Carney complex have been recently published. The typical lesions consist of spotty centrofacial pigmentation involving the vermillion border of the lips, the lacrimal caruncle, the conjunctival semilunar fold, and sometimes the sclera. Intraoral-pigmented spots are present in a limited number of cases. In at least half of the patients with **Carney complex**, a mutation in the gene encoding protein kinase A regulatory subunit 1A (*PRKAR1A*) mapped to 17q22–24 has been identified.

Cantu syndrome (choice A) is an autosomal dominant disorder characterized by hypertrichosis, osteodysplasia, and cardiomegaly with onset in adolescence. Small, punctate, hyperpigmented macules that often have a reticular pattern involve the face, forearms, and feet. Hyperkeratosis of the palms and soles may be associated with this disorder. The histopathology of the lentigines is identical to common acquired lentigines and those of Carney complex.

LEOPARD syndrome (choice C) is an autosomal dominant disorder with multiple lentigines affecting any part of the body from the scalp to the feet. Most cases are associated with mutations of protein-tyrosine phosphatase, nonreceptor type 11 (*PTPN11*). In addition to lentigines, electrocardiographic abnormalities, ocular hypertelorism (increased distance between the eyes), pulmonic stenosis, abnormal genitalia, growth retardation, and deafness are present. Myxoid tumors are not a feature of **LEOPARD syndrome**. The lentigines are characterized by elongation of rete ridges, increased melanocytes, and increased melanization of the epidermis. On electron microscopy, giant melanosomes and complex melanosomes are seen.

Peutz-Jeghers syndrome (choice D) is an autosomal dominant disorder associated with mutations of the serine threonine kinase gene *STK11/LKB1*. Patients have small, irregularly contoured **melanotic macules** localized on the oral mucosa, lips, perioral skin, and dorsal skin of the fingers. In the majority of cases, multiple polyps develop in the small intestines that may become malignant in 2%-3% of patients. The **melanotic macules** are characterized by heavily pigmented

Quick Fact

Disorders with Multiple Lentigines

Generalized

- LEOPARD (*PTPN11*)
- Generalized lentiginosis
- Carney complex; NAME/LAMB (*PRKARI1A*)
- Arterial dissection plus lentiginosis
- Gastrocutaneous syndrome
- Tay syndrome
- Pipkin syndrome

Localized

- Peutz–Jeghers (*STK11*)
- Bandler syndrome
- Laugier–Hunzinker
- Cantu; hyperkeratosis-hyperpigmentation syndrome
- Cowden disease (*PTEN*)
- Centrofacial lentiginosis
- Inherited patterned lentiginosis
- Cronkhite–Canada syndrome

Genital

- Bannayan–Riley–Ruvalcaba (*PTEN*)
- Lentiginosis perigenito-axillaris

Photodistributed

Xeroderma pigmentosum

Segmental

Partial unilateral lentiginosis

basal cells with a number of melanocytes. There may be some disturbance of pigment transfer to keratinocytes.

ANSWER 6-10: B.

Melasma is observed most commonly on the faces of dark-skinned women living in tropical or subtropical locations where UV irradiation is intense. Increased estrogen and progesterone levels seem to be causative in susceptible women; pregnancy, contraceptive use, estrogen replacement therapy, and ovarian tumors are often linked to the onset. **Cholasma** is a synonym and refers to the "**mask of pregnancy**." The face is symmetrically involved in one of three patterns: a centrofacial pattern involving the forehead, nose, cheeks, upper lip, and chin; a malar pattern; and a mandibular pattern. The hyperpigmentation may be predominantly epidermal and consequently brown, dermal, and therefore bluish, or both epidermal and dermal and thus both brown and blue. Microscopically, epidermal melanocytes are usually slightly increased in number and activity. Corresponding to the clinical patterns, increased melanin may be localized primarily to the epidermis, upper dermis, or both. Immunohistochemical stains highlight enlarged, intensely stained melanocytes with prominent dendritic processes. Melanocytes may demonstrate increased numbers of melanosomes on electron microscopy.

Quick Fact

Melasma Clinical DDX

- Drug-induced (eg, doxycyline, amiodarone)
- Post-inflammatory hyperpigmentation
- Actinic lichen planus
- Lichen planus pigmentosus
- Pigmented contact dermatitis (Riehl melanosis)
- Exogenous ochronosis
- Acquired bilateral nevus of Ota-like macules (Hori nevus)
- Erythema dyschormicum perstans
- Poikiolderma of Civatte
- Erythromelanosis follicularis faciei et colli
- Cutaneous mercury deposits

The major entities to be considered in the histopathological differential diagnosis include **post-inflammatory hyperpigmentation, café-au-lait macules (CALMs), solar lentigo**, and **lentigo maligna**. **Melasma** may be histopathologically indistinguishable from **café-au-lait macules** (cases with epidermal pigmentation) and **post-inflammatory hyperpigmentation** (cases with dermal pigmentation), but the clinical presentation should readily allow its discrimination. **Solar lentigo** reveals elongated slender rete ridges with increased epidermal melanization and only a slightly increased concentration of melanocytes. There is also a background of solar elastosis. **Lentigo maligna (melanoma in situ)** presents as a confluent lentiginous growth of enlarged and atypical melanocytes along the basal layer of the epidermis and possible pagetoid ascent.

Post-inflammatory hyperpigmentation is extremely common in individuals with more darkly pigmented skin. However, it develops after inflammation or injury to the skin, such as cutaneous lupus erythematosus or photosensitivity reactions, rather than during pregnancy. Primary lesions with active inflammation may be found elsewhere on the body. **Erythema dyschromicum perstans** or "**ashy dermatosis**" is essentially a specific clinical presentation of **post-inflammatory hyperpigmentation**. It is most frequently seen in patients from Latin America, and consists of oval, circular, or irregularly shaped slate-gray to blue-brown macules and patches. Lesions initially can have an erythematous rim, and their distribution includes sun-protected areas. Microscopically, the findings are identical to **post-inflammatory hyperpigmentation** with abundant superficial dermal melanophages. Sparse vacuolar interface dermatitis with rare scattered dyskeratotic keratinocytes along the dermal–epidermal junction may be seen.

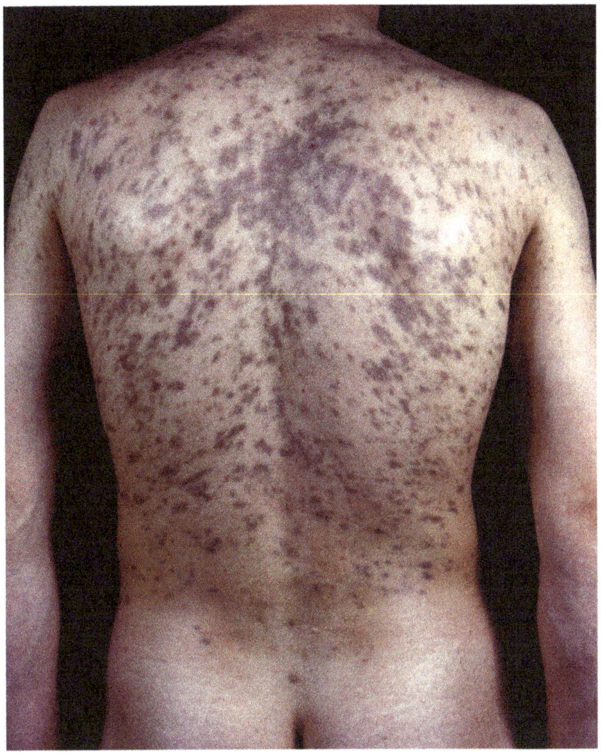

Erythema dyschromicum perstans (Ashy dermatosis). This form of post-inflammatory hyperpigmentation exhibits dark gray-black discoloration due to a dermal-based localization of the pigment. It is most common in skin phototypes V and VI. (Reproduced, with permission, from Wolff K, Johnson RA, Saavedra AP. *Fitzpatrick's Color Atlas and Synopsis of Clinical Dermatology*. 7th ed. New York, NY: McGraw-Hill Education; 2013.)

Hermansky–Pudlak syndrome (HPS) is a rare autosomal recessive disorder with the highest prevalence within Puerto Rico. The condition is characterized by oculocutaneous albinism, bleeding problems due to a platelet abnormality (platelet storage pool defect), and lysosomal storage disease (accumulation of lipofuscin).

Riehl melanosis, also referred to as **pigmented contact dermatitis**, favors sites of application of contactants, especially cosmetics. It may be reticulated, and the coloration is usually brown-gray due to dermal melanin deposits. Histopathologically, it is an unusual form of contact dermatitis characterized by vacuolar degeneration of the basal layer as well as a band-like lichenoid inflammatory infiltrate in early lesions. Numerous scattered melanophages are present.

Exogenous ochronosis is caused by the chronic topical use of high-concentration (6%-8%) hydroquinone, resorcinol, phenol, quinine injection, systemic antimalarial therapy, or exposure to benzene. In hydroquinone-induced ochronosis, blue-black pigmentation is seen most obviously on parts of the face suggesting photoinduction. The discoloration is usually permanent despite discontinuation of the hydroquinone. Annular lesions similar to actinic granuloma may occur.

ANSWER 6-11: A.

These are **café-au-lait macules (CALMs)**, which are one of the hallmarks of **von Recklinghausen multiple neurofibromatosis (NF1)**. **NF1** is associated with mutations in the *NF1* gene, resulting in abnormal expression of neurofibromin, an inhibitor of the Ras growth-promoting pathway. These patients present with numerous neurofibromas, which may rarely transform into malignant peripheral nerve sheath tumors. If an individual has six **CALMs** of 1.5 cm or larger, the development or presence of **NF1** is 100% certain. Microscopically, **CALMs** reveal a normal to slightly attenuated epidermis (flattened rete ridges) with diffuse basal cell hypermelanization and normal numbers of melanocytes. Electron microscopy reveals giant melanosomes.

Quick Fact

NF-1 DX, 2/7 ("NFL ROCS")

- **N**eurofibromas (>1 or 1 plexiform NF)
- **F**reckling, axillary/inguinal (Crowe sign)
- **L**isch nodules (>1) = iris hamartomas
- **R**elative with NF1—1st degree
- **O**ptic glioma
- **C**ALMs (>6 lesions, >5 mm prepuberty, >15 mm postpuberty)
- **S**phenoid wing dysplasia

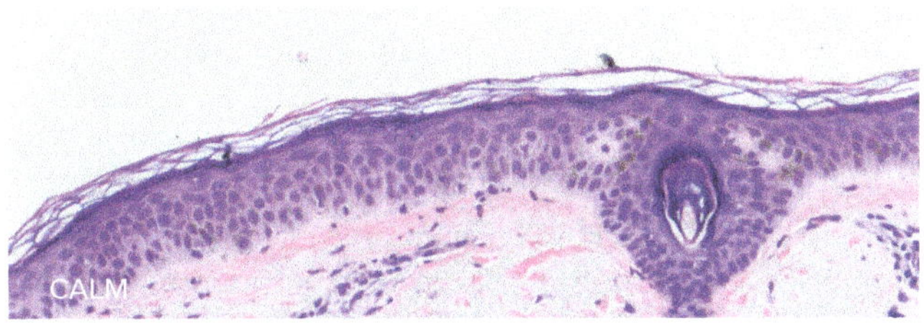

Café-au-lait macule.

McCune–Albright syndrome is a disorder due to sporadic somatic mutations of the *GNAS1* gene that encodes a subunit of a signal transducing guanine nucleotide-binding (G) protein and the mosaic distribution of cells that express that mutation. Patients present with polyostotic fibrous dysplasia, melanotic macules, and hyperfunctional endocrinopathies (ie, precocious puberty). **CALMs** in this disorder have an identical microscopic appearance; however, in contrast to the **CALMs** of **NF1**, they are usually unilateral and manifest irregular borders that have been likened to the coastline of Maine.

Ephelides (freckles) (choice C) are light-brown macules that predominately affect light-skinned individuals and occur on sun-exposed areas, such as the face, upper back, shoulders, and dorsa of the hands and forearms. Lesions are almost always smaller than 4 mm in diameter, with irregular borders and uniform pigmentation. An **ephelide** can be difficult to distinguish from a **simple lentigo** (choice B) both clinically and histopathologically. In general, they are lighter in color and are confined to sun-exposed skin. Most importantly, these lesions fade without sun exposure. In contrast, **simple lentigines (lentigo simplex)** may occur on any site and are persistent. A freckle reflects increased melanization of the epidermis attributed to increased melanin production within melanocytes and transfer to basal keratinocytes unaccompanied by elongation of the rete ridges. The number of melanocytes is not increased; in fact, melanocytes may even be decreased relative to uninvolved skin. With silver preparations, melanocytes with prominent dendritic processes may be identified, a finding associated with a photoadaptive effect. Electron microscopy reveals normal melanosomes. **Ephelides** and **CALMs** are essentially identical via histopathology and distinction requires clinical correlation. A distinguishing feature is the presence of giant melanosome in **CALMs** on electron microscopy, which are normal in **ephelides**. Unlike the sun-associated facial **freckles** common to light-skinned individuals, **CALMs** and the axillary, inguinal, and inframammary **"freckles"** of **NF1** do not darken by sun exposure and are persistent.

Lentigo simplex, solar lentigo, and **spreading pigmented actinic keratosis (SPAK)** (choices B, D, and G, respectively) are lesions in which hyperpigmentation is typically accentuated at the tips of elongated rete ridges (Table 6-11A). Melanocyte hyperplasia is characteristic in **lentigo simplex. Solar lentigo** and **SPAK** contain a normal number of melanocytes, but may exhibit a markedly increased number of melanocytes when arising in severely sun-damaged skin. Electron microscopy reveals giant melanosomes in **lentigo simplex. Solar lentigo** and **SPAK** arise in sun-damaged skin and contain a background of solar elastosis. **Spreading pigmented actinic keratosis (SPAK)** exhibits partial thickness keratinocytic atypia, hypogranulosis, and thick parakeratosis.

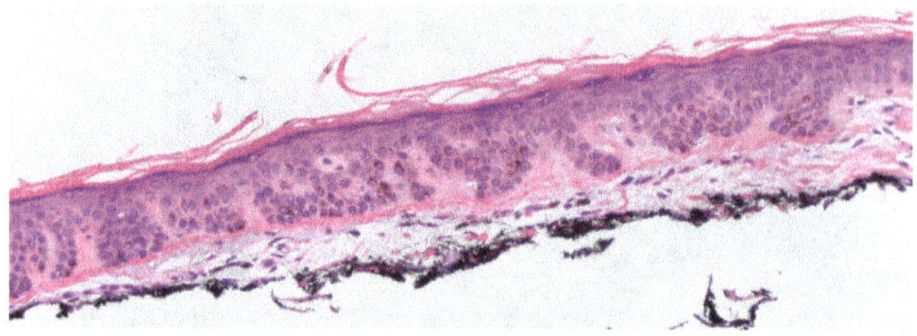

Solar lentigo. There are elongated club-shaped rete ridges with keratinocyte hyperpigmentation. Significant keratinocytic atypia is absent. There is a background of solar elastosis.

Table 6-11A. Circumscribed Hypermelanosis

LESION	CLINICAL FEATURES	EPIDERMIS	BASILAR MELANOCYTES	OTHER FEATURES
Freckle	Transient, sunlight responsive, 1-3 mm macules Light to medium brown	Normal	Reduced, normal, increased	Melanocytes are larger with increased development of dendrites
Lentigo simplex	Persistent 1-5 mm macule	Elongated, club-shaped epidermal rete ridges	Increased	Melanin macroglobules Electron microscopy reveals giant melanosomes
Solar lentigo	Persistent on sun-exposed skin, 5-15 mm macules	Elongated, club-shaped epidermal rete ridges Solar elastosis	Increased	
Café-au-lait macule	Persistent 2-5 cm oval macule, uniform tan to dark brown	Normal	Normal or slightly increased	Association with neurofibromatosis Melanin macroglobules Electron microscopy reveals giant melanosomes
Melasma	Patterned macular pigmentation on face	Normal	Normal or slightly increased	Pigment incontinence may be prominent
Becker melanosis	Persistent macular or raised lesion, a few to several centimeters Tan to dark brown, often hypertrichoic	Elongated rete ridges to frank acanthosis and papillomatous	Normal or slightly increased	Often with a smooth muscle hamartoma in dermis

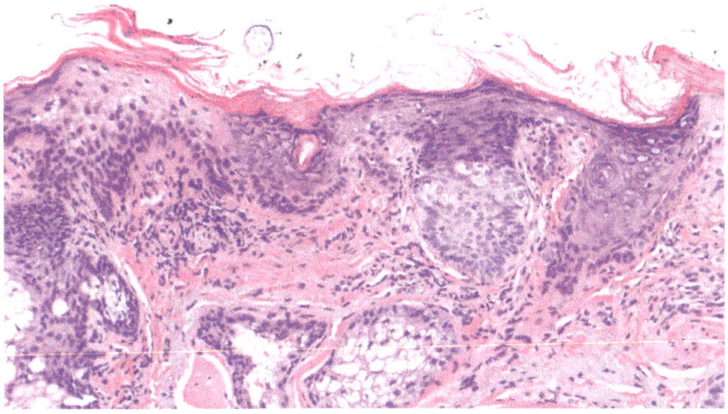

Spreading pigmented actinic keratosis (SPAK). There are focal areas of partial thickness keratinocytic atypia characterized by hypogranulosis and parakeratosis. Pigment is present within the basal keratinocytes. There is a background of solar elastosis.

Becker nevus (choice E) is a hamartoma that appears in childhood or early adolescence and is characterized by macular hyperpigmentation with irregular borders, usually located on the upper lateral trunk. The pigmentation typically develops during the first decade of life, and hypertrichosis can appear in the second decade. The epidermal changes vary from almost normal to showing acanthosis, papillomatosis, elongation of rete ridges, and hyperpigmentation of the basal layer. Melanocytes may be slightly increased in number in the epidermis. Dermal melanophages are often present and increased bundles of smooth muscle are usually present in the reticular dermis.

Nevus spilus (speckled lentiginous nevus) (choice F) is a slightly hyperpigmented (tan) macular lesion that contains hyperpigmented foci or speckles that may be either flat or raised. The **nevus spilus** may be congenital or acquired and often becomes more prominent after solar exposure. The tan macular area commonly varies from less than 1 cm to 10 or 20 cm in greatest diameter. The hyperpigmented speckles are approximately 1-6 mm in greatest diameter and may be macular or papular. Large **nevi spili** may be unilateral, segmental, or zosteriform (**speckled zosteriform lentiginous nevus**). Microscopically, the tan macule or patch exhibits lentiginous melanocytic hyperplasia associated with elongated epidermal rete ridges. Whereas the hyperpigmented macular foci show lentiginous melanocytic hyperplasia, or junctional nevus, the papular foci contain junctional or compound nevus elements. Varying degrees of architectural disorder or cytologic atypia may be observed in nevus spilus.

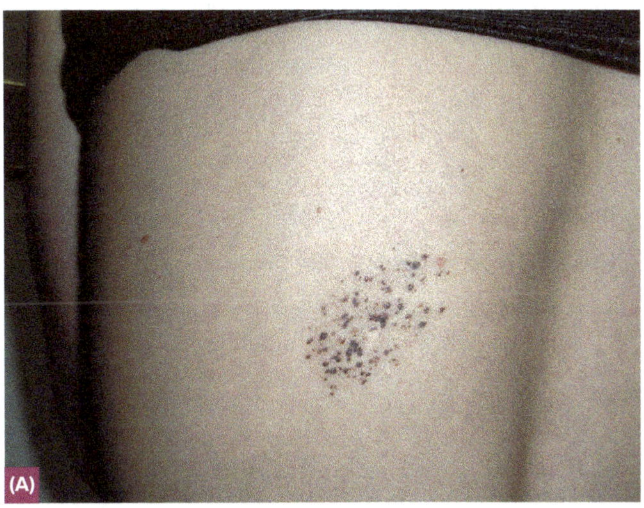

(A)

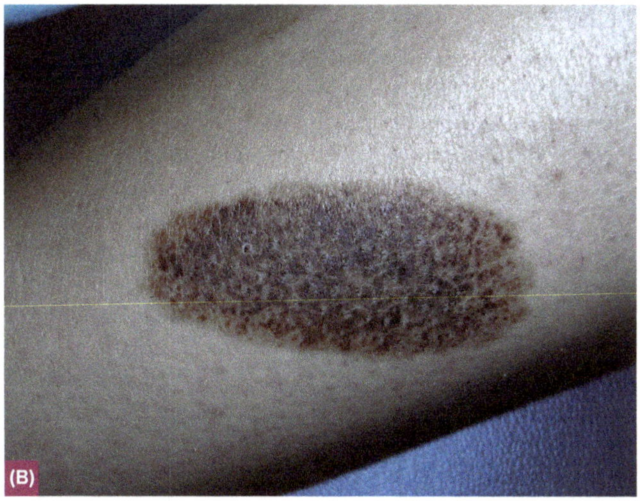

(B)

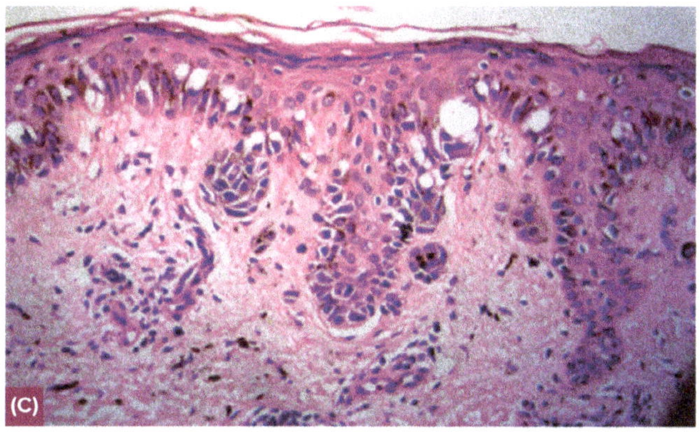

(C)

Nevus spilus. (A) There is a cluster of pigmented macules and papules. **(B)** A large pigmented patch studded with areas of hyperpigmentation. **(C)** There is basal layer hypermelanization accompanied by a lentiginous proliferation of melanocytes along the basal layer and occasional nests at the tips of rete ridges. (Parts **(A)** and **(B)** reproduced, with permission, from Usatine RP, Smith MA, Mayeaux EJ Jr, Chumley HS, eds. *Color Atlas of Family Medicine*. 2nd ed. New York, NY: McGraw-Hill Education; 2012; part **(C)** reproduced, with permission, from Goldsmith LA, Katz SI, Gilchrest BA, Paller AS, Leffell DJ, Wolff K, eds. *Fitzpatrick's Dermatology in General Medicine*. 8th ed. New York, NY: McGraw-Hill Education; 2012.)

ANSWER 6-12: E.

This is an example of **post-inflammatory hyperpigmentation**, in which inflammation of the epidermis results in melanin incontinence of basal keratinocytes and sometimes melanocytes (Table 6-12A). Variable epidermal inflammatory changes, such as **interface dermatitis**, are often visible in early lesions together with melanin deposition in the upper dermis, either free or in melanophages. Epidermal melanization may be increased. Long-standing lesions typically show pigment incontinence without active inflammation. The changes are typically more pronounced in patients with heavily pigmented skin. The pigmentary alteration alone is entirely nonspecific and an etiologic diagnosis depends on identification of the antecedent inciting injury. Clinical correlation should exclude other causes such as regression of a pigmented lesion.

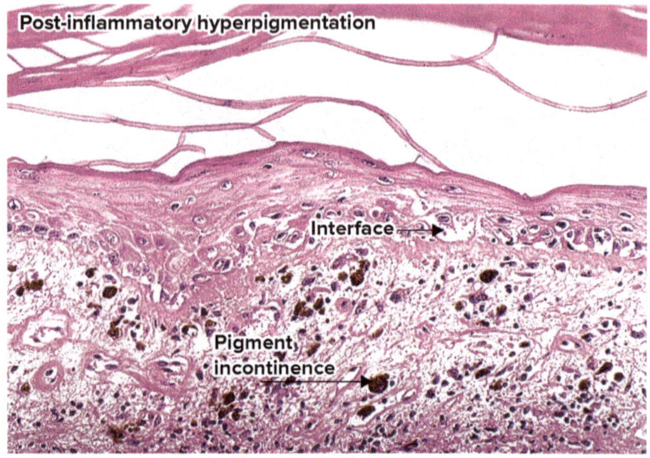

Lupus erythematosus. Vacuolization of the basal cells and incontinence of the released melanin into upper dermis are seen. These melanin granules are tattooed in the dermis semi-permanently. A thin epidermis makes these pigment granules more readily visible.

Table 6-12A. Post-inflammatory Hypermelanosis

Clinical Features
- Usually follows inflammatory processes
- Localized or widespread
- Common dermatoses = lichen planus, lupus erythematosus, eczematous dermatitis, psoriasis, phytophotodermatitis, drug eruptions
- Gradual loss of pigmentation, but may be permanent

Histopathologic Features
- Variable degrees of epidermal hypermelanosis and pigment incontinence

Differential Diagnosis
- Melasma
- Addison disease
- Malnutrition

In **fixed drug eruption** and **erythema dyschromicum perstans ("ashy dermatosis")**, repeated episodes of interface dermatitis eventuate in a gray-blue dyspigmentation as the incontinent melanin accumulates in large amounts in a deeper location in the dermis. Trauma or chronic irritation may also cause **post-inflammatory hyperpigmentation.**

Mercury-containing cream (choice A) was once used extensively by dermatologists to treat bacterial and fungal infections and to bleach hyperpigmented skin. The chronic use of such cream caused slate-gray pigmentation, with small, refractile, brown-black mercury granules in the upper dermis, either free or in macrophages.

This patient's condition is most consistent with **melanodermatitis toxica (Riehl melanosis)**, which is believed to be a type IV cytotoxic hypersensitivity contact dermatitis. Some believe **phototoxicity** is an important component to this eruption. Chemicals, such as cosmetics, are most frequently implicated. The face (especially the forehead, zygomatic area, and temples) and the neck are principally involved, but the hands, forearms, and trunk can also be affected. Inflammatory findings such as erythema and pruritus are usually absent. Other causative dermatoses frequently ending with **post-inflammatory pigmentary alteration** include **lichen planus, lichenoid drug eruption, discoid lupus erythematosus, dermatomyositis, notalgia paresthetica**, and **mycosis fungoides**.

ANSWER 6-13: D.

This patient is presenting with a rare form of **generalized melanosis** secondary to **metastatic melanoma**. These patients frequently present with **melanouria**, and at autopsy have black hyperpigmented visceral organs. The exact mechanism is unknown; however, it is believed that tumor-derived factors seem to drive the hyperproliferation of normal melanocytes.

Quick Fact

Helpful Stains for Pigmentary Disorders

- Fontana-Masson (silver stain) = melanin granules, seen especially in dendritic melanocytes
- DOPA reaction (specific for tyrosinase) = melanocytes producing pigment
- Melan-A, MITF, or HMB-45 antibodies = melanocytes
- Prussian blue = iron, hemosiderin

Perivascular melanophages contain melanin granules that are often DOPA positive, indicating that melanin synthesis is still active in the phagocytosed melanosomes, which most likely are derived from blood-borne melanoma cells carried to the skin. The dermal blood vessels may be occluded with DOPA-positive pigment granules. In some cases, only melanophages are present; in other cases, both melanoma cells and melanophages are admixed in the dermis. The pigment will stain black (positive) on Fontana-Masson stain, but will be negative for iron on Prussian blue stain.

ANSWER 6-14: B.

Ochronosis is the accumulation of yellow-brown pigment created by the inhibition of the enzyme homogentisic oxidase. It may be acquired (**exogenous ochronosis** or **pseudo-ochronosis**) or inherited (**endogenous ochronosis**). This patient is presenting with **exogenous ochronosis**.

Endogenous ochronosis is an autosomal recessive disease of homogentisic acid oxidase deficiency (not decarboxylase, as in choice C). A slow accumulation of homogentisic acid, which is an intermediate product of metabolism of phenylalanine to tyrosine, causes pigmentation of cartilages and eventually the skin. An affected child's urine, if exposed to the air or an alkalizing agent for a few hours, turns pink to brown (**alkaptonuria**), and staining of the diaper is the first sign of the disease in 50% of cases. Cutaneous signs usually do not develop until 30 years of age. This is a rare disease in the United States. Because the cartilage of the ear is covered with thin skin, a bluish gray to dark brown color is readily noticed. A butterfly pattern of pigmentation of the face, including the nose, may suggest photosensitivity. Axillary sweat may be variously colored from greenish blue to greenish yellow-brown. The sclera and teeth may also be pigmented. **Alkaptonuria** is diagnosed by gas chromatography–mass spectrometry analysis or a colorimetric assay of a 24-hour urine specimen.

Exogenous ochronosis or **pseudo-ochronosis** is caused by the chronic topical use of high-concentration (6%-8%) hydroquinone, resorcinol, phenol, quinine injection, systemic antimalarial therapy, or exposure to benzene. In **hydroquinone-induced ochronosis**, blue-black pigmentation is seen most obviously on prominent parts of the face (ie, the cheeks, forehead, nose, and in some cases, the chin), suggesting photoinduction. The discoloration is usually permanent despite discontinuation of hydroquinone. Annular lesions similar to actinic granuloma may occur.

Microscopically, both forms exhibit yellow-brown or ochre-colored pigment in the dermis, hence the designation **ochronosis**. A blue-gray-brown color is produced by scattering of light from the deep-seated ochre-colored pigment (**Tyndall effect**). The pigment is also observed in the endothelial cells of the blood vessels, basement membranes, secretory cells of eccrine glands, and dermal macrophages. However, the most diagnostic form of deposition is the banana-shaped dermal collagen fibers that become swollen, rigid, and fragmented with jagged ends. The same pigment is deposited on elastic fibers, which also degenerate. The epidermis is normally pigmented. **Sarcoidal granulomas** may occasionally be present, as may transepidermal elimination of degenerated collagen. The pigment does not contain iron or melanin, and therefore stains negatively with respective Prussian blue and Fontana-Masson stains.

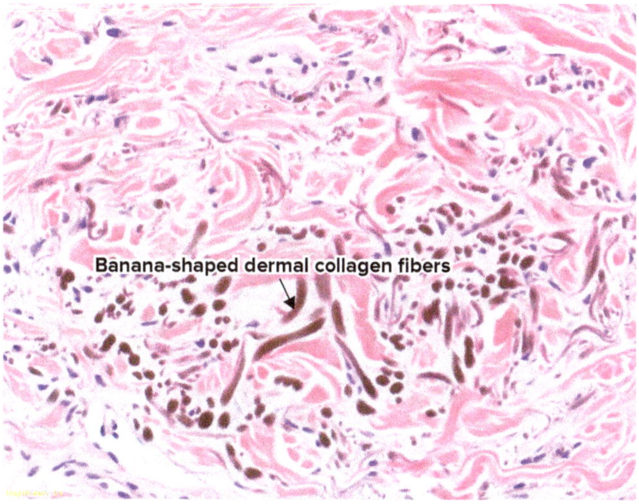

Exogenous ochronosis. There are swollen collagen and elastic fibers with a brown discoloration. The collagen bundles have been referred to as having the appearance of "rotten bananas."

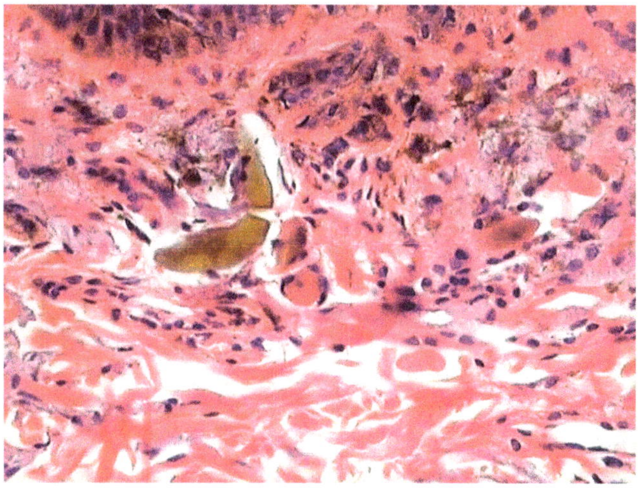

Alkaptonuric ochronosis. Yellow-brown, ochre-colored, bizarre (banana-shaped) masses deposited in the upper dermis with solar elastosis and a granulomatous reaction.

ANSWER 6-15: C.

This is a classic example of a **carbon tattoo**. Coal miners frequently develop these characteristic tattoos owing to coal dust getting into wounds. Graphite of lead pencils may also produce identical lesions when purposely or accidentally introduced to the skin. The biopsy reveals black pigment particles scattered from the main body of inoculated carbon accompanied by a granulomatous reaction. The usual microscopic appearance for the common carbon tattoo is that of a jet-black material rather than the granular-brown character of melanin in dermal melanocytic lesions.

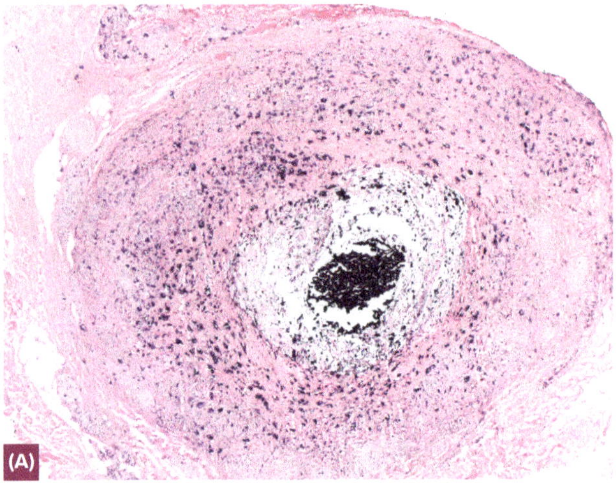

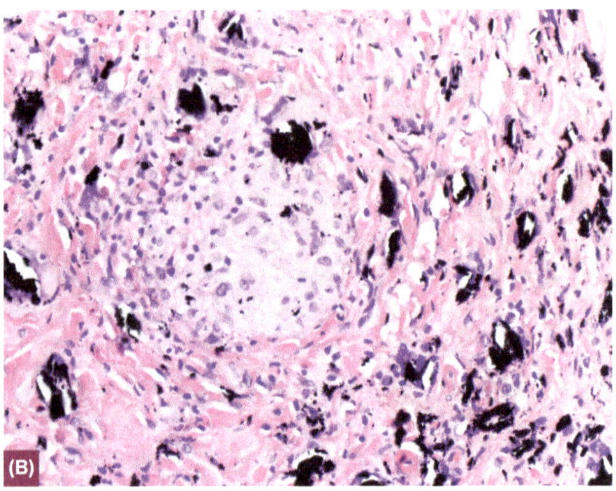

Carbon tattoo. (A) There is a nodular focus composed of scattered clusters of black pigmented and dense fibrosis. **(B)** The pigment is black and associated with focal granulomatous inflammation.

Blue nevi may have pigmented melanophages, but also contain scattered pigmented spindle melanocytes. The pigment is not black but rather dark brown. They do not normally contain granulomatous infiltrates. **Tumoral melanosis** represents nodular clusters of melanophages without viable melanocytes. The condition most commonly represents a completely regressed melanocytic proliferation, possibly **malignant melanoma**. **Calcinosis cutis (tumor calcinosis)** may complicate epithelial cysts or neoplasms and presents as scattered fragments of purple dystrophic calcification (H&E stain) accompanied by a granulomatous reaction. Clinically these lesions are not pigmented. **Hemochromatosis** may be a primary autosomal recessive condition of system iron accumulation or secondary to exogenous iron overload (ie, multiple blood transfusions). The condition is not localized but generalized with yellow-brown discoloration of skin and internal organs. In addition to the skin pigmentation, liver cirrhosis, cardiac failure, and diabetes mellitus make up the clinical tetrad. Microscopically, large chunky yellow-brown hemosiderin is seen in the cytoplasm of eccrine secretory cells, periglandular connective tissue, and perivascular macrophages. Focal resolving hematomas secondary to trauma may produce a similar clinical picture as this patient. Microscopically, free hemosiderin pigment and hemosiderin-laden macrophages surround blood vessels and are frequently accompanied by scattered red blood cells. Hemosiderin is bright blue on Prussian blue stain.

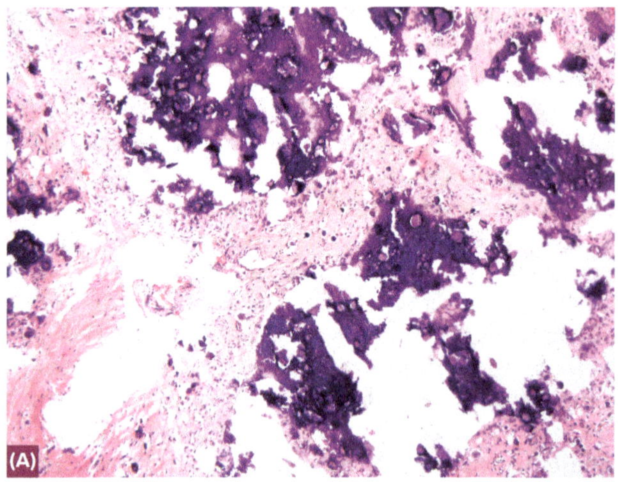

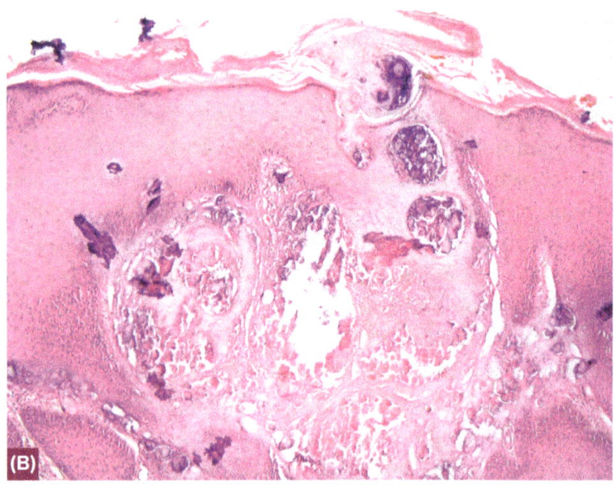

Tumoral calcinosis (calcinosis cutis). (A) There are nodular foci of calcification with associated fibrosis and foreign-body reaction compatible with tumoral calcinosis. The calcification appears dark purple on routine H&E staining. **(B)** In this child, a biopsy of a hard cheek nodule revealed nodular collections of calcium in the dermis with associated transepidermal elimination of calcium through the epidermis.

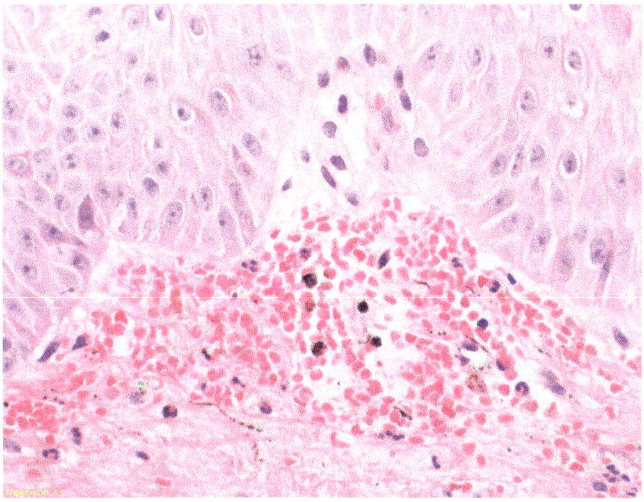

Traumatic purpura. There is dermal hemorrhage admixed with scattered pigmented macrophages containing golden-brown hemosiderin pigment.

ANSWER 6-16: A.

Note that the elevated area is confined to the red portion of the tattoo. Many, but not all, of the pigment-based reactions are in response to **cinnabar** or **mercuric sulfide (red)**. Other pigment-color combinations include: chromic oxide (green), cobaltous albuminate (light blue), cadmium sulfide (yellow), and iron oxide or ochre (brown) (Table 6-16A).

Table 6-16A. Tattoo Pigments

Tattoo Pigments
• **Traumatic**: lead, dirt, gunpowder • **Amateur black**: India ink, carbon • **Professional black**: carbon, iron oxide, logwood extract • **Blue**: cobalt aluminate (azure blue) • **Green**: chromium oxide (casalis green), hydrated chromium sesquioxide (guignet green), malachite green, curcumin green, phthalocyanine dyes (copper salts with yellow coal tar dyes) • **Red**: mercury sulfide (cinnabar), cadmium selenide (cadmium red), sieena (red ochre; ferric hydrate and ferric sulfate), azo dyes • **Yellow**: cadmium sulfide (cadmium yellow), ochre, curcumin yellow • **Brown**: ochre • **Violet**: manganese violet • **White**: titanium dioxide, zinc oxide • **Skin colored**: iron oxides

Reactions may be photosensitive and histology may be pseudolymphomatous, lichenoid, or granulomatous (foreign body and sarcoidal types). **Lymphomatoid reactions** (resembling lymphoma) are most commonly seen with cinnabar tattoos. Several patients have developed hilar lymphadenopathy together with **sarcoidal reactions** at tattoo sites; patients with underlying sarcoidosis manifest exaggerated reactions to injected dyes.

ANSWER 6-17: E.

Minocycline is notorious for generating skin discoloration. Three clinical variants of cutaneous **minocycline pigmentation** are generally recognized:

- Type I: blue-black macules localized to areas of scarring and inflammation (eg, facial acne scars).
- Type II (most common): blue-black, brown or slate-gray pigmentation on the shins, ankles, and arms. This pigment usually fluoresces yellow under ultraviolet light.
- Type III: generalized muddy-brown pigmentation, which may be exacerbated on sunlight-exposed areas.

The histological features of minocycline pigmentation are variable depending on clinical type.

- Type I: macrophages containing golden-brown to brown-black granules are distributed mainly around the vasculature and sweat gland coils that are Prussian blue positive (iron+) and negative for melanin by Fontana-Masson stain. It is believed to represent minocycline or its breakdown product chelated with hemosiderin, ferritin, or iron. Other elements such as calcium, sulfur, and chlorine are also present but melanin is absent. Melanocytes and the epidermis show no increase in melanin pigmentation.
- Type II: macrophages containing golden-brown to brown–black granules are distributed mainly around the vasculature and sweat gland coils that are positive on iron and Fontana-Masson stains, but fails to bleach with potassium permanganate, indicating that melanin is actually not present. Melanocytes and the epidermis show no increase in melanin pigmentation.
- Type III: hyperpigmentation is characterized by an increase in epidermal basal cell melanin pigmentation, best highlighted with a Fontana-Masson stain. Prussian blue stain is negative for iron.

A recent case report found pigmented lipomembranous changes in the subcutis of two patients with pretibial minocycline pigmentation (type II). These different types of pigmentation may manifest individually or in combination. The pigments are PAS negative in all three forms. Types I and II are usually reversible with cessation of the medication (Table 6-17A).

Table 6-17A. Minocycline Pigmentation

TYPE	APPEARANCE	LOCATION	DURATION OF TREATMENT AND DOSE	HISTOPATHOLOGIC CHARACTERISTICS
I	Blue-black	Areas of inflammation and scar	Not related to duration	Pigment in macrophages; Prussian blue stain (+), Fontana-Masson stain (−)
II	Blue-gray (mistake for bruise)	Otherwise normal skin (arms, legs, face)	11-35 mo; 22-104 g total dose	Prussian blue stain (+), Fontana-Masson stain (+)
III	Muddy-brown	Diffuse or generalized (exposed areas, gingival, hard palate, teeth, nails)	Depends on total dose and duration; about 3 years' duration; about 130-144 g total dose	Increased basilar melanin; brown-black pigment in macrophages is Prussian blue stain (−), Fontana-Masson stain (+)

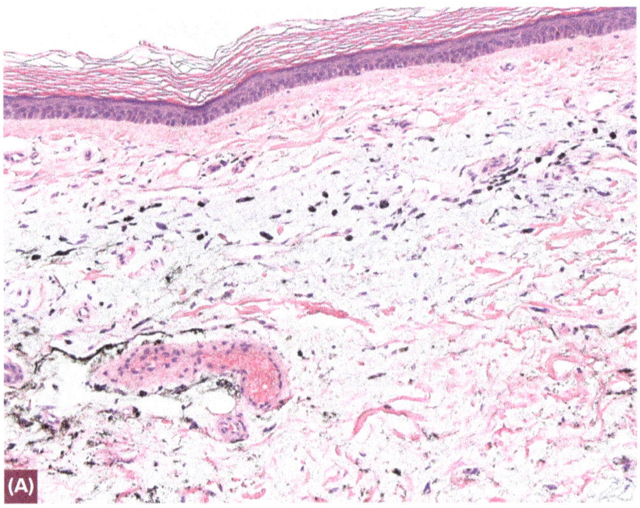
(A)

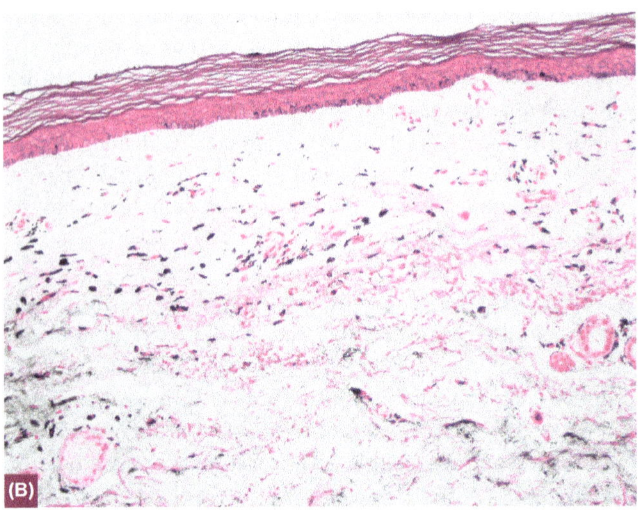
(B)

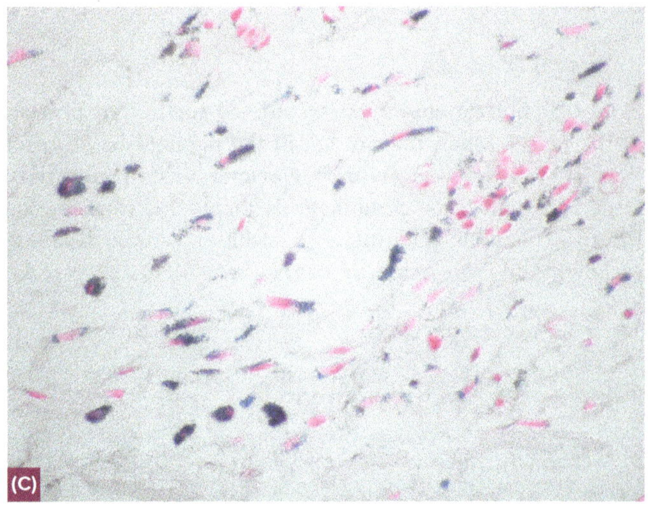
(C)

Minocycline hyperpigmentation, type II. (A) There are scattered dermal macrophages containing brown-black pigment. **(B)** The granules appear dark black with Fontana-Masson stain. **(C)** The granules are both black and bright blue with Prussian blue stain.

ANSWER 6-18: H.

Numerous classes of medications may result in cutaneous dyspigmentation (Table 6-18A).

Antimalarials (Hydroxychloroquine, Chloroquine, and Quinacrine)

Quinacrine produces a diffuse lemon-yellow color if taken for a long period, particularly in fair-skinned patients. The yellow color is probably the direct stain of **quinacrine** itself. **Hydroxychloroquine** has been reported to cause widespread

Table 6-18A. Drug-Related Dyspigmentation

DRUG	EPIDERMAL HYPERMELANOSIS	DERMAL ALTERATION	OTHER
Minocycline			
Type I	Usually not present	Drug metabolite–protein complex in macrophages that stains for iron but not melanin	
Type II	Usually not present	Drug metabolite–protein complex that stains for iron and is positive by the Fontana reaction but fails to bleach (thus is not melanin)	
Type III	Present	Melanin, negative iron stain	
Antimalarials			
Chloroquine		Drug–melanin complex, hemosiderin	
Quinacrine		Quinacrine	
Amiodarone		Drug metabolite in endothelium, macrophages	Drug metabolite pigment granules in phagolysosomes
Clofazimine	Present	Melanin, ceroid-like material	
Psychotropic drugs	Present	Drug metabolite bound to melanin in macrophages, endothelial cells	
Chemotherapeutic drugs	Present	Melanin	

slate-gray or bluish-gray macular hyperpigmentation. **Chloroquine** may cause irregular grayish macules on the shins and diffuse pigmentation of the face. Hard palate and nail discoloration may occur after chronic ingestion. The pigment is found in the dermis as a drug–melanin complex. Hemosiderin is deposited around capillaries.

Amiodarone

Chronic use of **amiodarone**, an antiarrhythmic drug, may cause a blue-gray discoloration in sun-exposed areas such as the face and hands; at least 20 months of continuous medication totaling about 250 g seems to be necessary to cause this discoloration. In addition to basilar melanization and melanocyte photoactivation, endothelia and dermal macrophages may accumulate pigment demonstrable ultrastructurally in phagolysosomes in the form of lipid membranous structures, likely undigested drug metabolites stored as residual bodies.

Clofazimine

Used in the treatment of atypical mycobacterial infection and leprosy, **clofazimine** may induce a reddish discoloration that represents the color of the drug and occurs in the conjunctivae and skin within 4 weeks of beginning the medication in 49%-65% of patients. After 2-3 months of therapy, the infective lesions and occasionally even normal skin turn a brown or violaceous hue. This color may be due to a combination of epidermal and dermal melanin and a ceroid-like substance in the dermis.

Psychotropic Drugs (Phenothiazine and Imipramine)

Prolonged use of **phenothiazine** and the **tricyclic antidepressant imipramine** may cause blue-gray to slate-gray discoloration, mainly in sun-exposed locations. The dark granules associated with **chlorpromazine** discoloration and scattered golden pigments in **imipramine** pigmentation are noted in the upper dermis and perivascular spaces. Both melanosomes and electron-dense substances representing drug metabolites are found in dermal macrophages, fibroblasts, vascular endothelial cells, and dermal dendrocytes. The epidermis is hyperpigmented.

Chemotherapeutic Drugs (Bleomycin, Busulfan, Cyclophosphamide, Doxorubicin, and 5-Fluorouracil and Topical Carmustine)

The ingestion of agents such as **bleomycin, busulfan, cyclophosphamide, doxorubicin**, and **5-fluorouracil** or topical application of **nitrogen mustard (mechlorethamine)** and **carmustine** (BCNU) may result in diffuse hypermelanosis or, in the case of **bleomycin**, so-called "flagellate streaks" after long-term ingestion. **Sunitinib**, a multi-kinase inhibitor, has

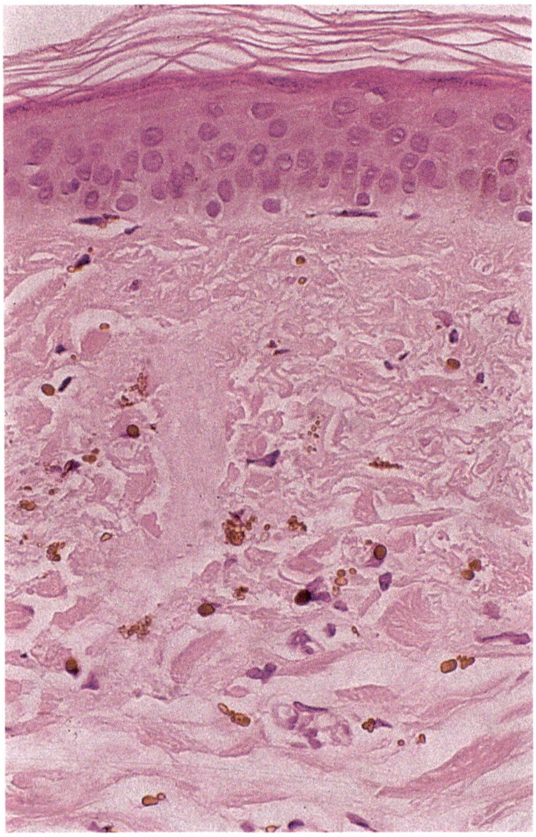

Imipramine pigmentation. Yellow granules are scattered in the upper and mid-dermis.

been reported to cause transient yellow discoloration of the skin. **Capecitabine** is a prodrug of **5-fluorouracil** that causes marked hyperpigmentation. The epidermis shows increased melanin, usually with some pigment incontinence.

Various antibiotics, such as **minocycline** and **tetracycline**, may produce hyperpigmentation; however, **azithromycin** has not been reported to be associated with hyperpigmentation.

ANSWER 6-19: H.

The histopathological findings of all of the listed conditions, with the exception of **piebaldism**, are consistent with **melanopenic hypomelanosis**, characterized by reduced or absent melanin pigment within keratinocytes and normal to only slightly reduced numbers of intraepidermal melanocytes with a dysfunctional ability to synthesize and/or transfer melanin pigment. Melan-A immunohistochemical staining is very helpful for assessing intraepidermal melanocyte concentrations and Fontana-Masson histochemical staining is helpful for assessing melanin pigment within keratinocytes.

Piebaldism is an autosomal dominant melanocytopenic condition characterized by congenital patches of **depigmentation**, **poliosis**, and scattered areas of hyperpigmentation. Skin biopsy will reveal a striking absence of melanocytes within the hypopigmented areas. The distinction between the remaining choices diagnoses relies on clinical findings.

Oculocutaneous albinism is a congenital and recessively inherited condition in which patients are unable to produce melanin pigment. The two subtypes are **tyrosinase positive** and **tyrosinase negative**. In the former, a plucked hair bulb becomes dark after incubation in DOPA solution. These patients may develop freckles and pigmented nevi. In the latter, the hair bulb does not become dark after incubation in DOPA solution, and patients never become pigmented. Due to a lack of melanin pigment in the developing eye, optical findings, such as foveal hypoplasia, misrouting of optic nerve to the brain, and reduced visual acuity, are universal for all types of albinism.

Tuberous sclerosis (TS) is an autosomal dominant condition in which hypopigmented macules (ie, **ash leaf spots**) are the earliest and most frequent cutaneous finding. **Poliosis** and depigmented spots on the iris and retina are also seen. Additionally, numerous, small, "guttate" hypopigmented macules may be seen on the extremities, referred to as

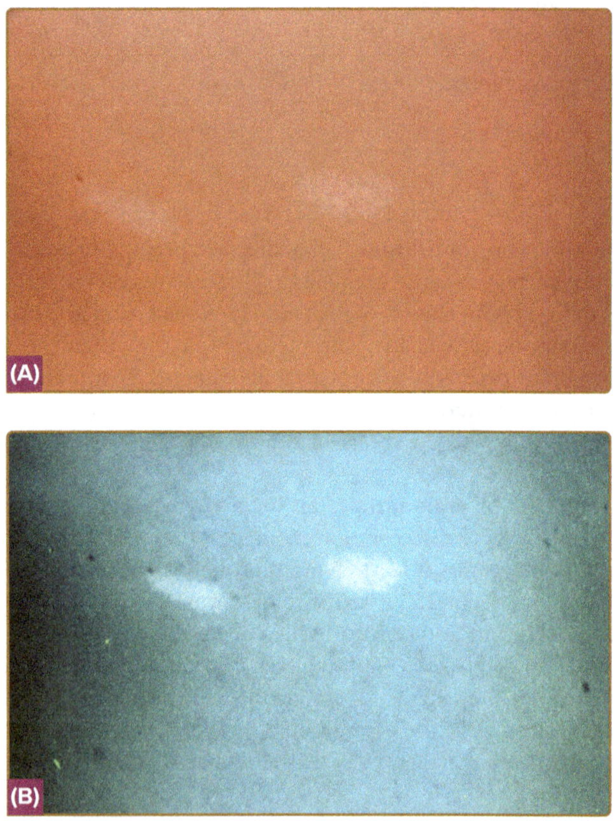

Ash leaf spot of tuberous sclerosis. (A) Hypomelanotic macules on the lateral chest of an adult with tuberous sclerosis complex. The macules may be easily overlooked. **(B)** Wood lamp accentuates the macules. (Reproduced, with permission, from Goldsmith LA, Katz SI, Gilchrest BA, Paller AS, Leffell DJ, Wolff K, eds. *Fitzpatrick's Dermatology in General Medicine*. 8th ed. New York, NY: McGraw-Hill Education; 2012.)

"**confetti macules.**" Other findings include numerous facial **angiofibromas** that spare the upper lip, **shagreen patches**, and **periungual fibromas**. Multiple organ systems may have hamartomatous involvement, including the CNS, kidneys, heart, and other viscera. When there is pulmonary involvement, the condition is known as **pulmonary lymphangioleiomyomatosis (LAM)**. The combination of three or more **congenital hypopigmented lesions** with seizures and mental retardation strongly suggests a diagnosis of TS. The gene for TS has been mapped to chromosomes 9q(33−) 34.3 (*TS1*) and 16p13.3 (*TS2*), which encode **hamartin** and **tuberin** respectively. Hamartin interacts with tuberin and negatively regulates signaling by the small GTPases Rab and Rheb. This complex inhibits the mammalian target of rapamycin (mTOR), which results in abnormal cell differentiation and proliferation. Mutations in *TS2* are seen in the majority of de novo cases and 50% of familial cases and usually portend a more severe clinical phenotype. Hypomelanosis in TS does not result from a reduction in melanocytes but rather from decreased size and poor melanization of melanosomes. Microscopically, there is a normal to slightly reduced density of melanocytes with a weak DOPA reaction compared with the surrounding normal skin. By electron microscopy, the size of melanosomes and degree of melanization are less than the normal counterparts, and their dendrites are less well developed.

Hypomelanosis of Ito (HI) refers to hypopigmentation in a distribution following Blaschko lines due to a clone of skin cells with decreased ability to produce pigment. It presents at birth or during the first year of life. Repigmentation may occur in some cases. Structural hair shaft abnormalities are often associated. Extracutaneous manifestations can occur and include CNS, eye, and musculoskeletal system defects. HI can be caused by mosaicism for a wide variety of abnormalities in the structure or number of autosomes and X chromosomes, and approximately 90% of the chromosomal aberrations reported in patients with HI overlap with genes known to be involved in pigmentation. Microscopically, the hypopigmented areas have fewer and smaller melanocytes than the normal skin; electron microscopy demonstrates decreased numbers of melanosomes in the melanocytes and basal keratinocytes, with some melanocytes showing degenerative changes and containing no melanosomes.

Hermansky–Pudlak syndrome (HPS) includes a group of genetically distinct disorders characterized by **tyrosinase-positive oculocutaneous albinism**, a platelet storage pool deficiency that results in a **bleeding diathesis**, and impaired formation or trafficking of intracellular vesicles (**lysosomal storage disease**). It is an autosomal recessive disorder that affects mainly persons of Puerto Rican origin. Additionally, these patients exhibit **inflammatory bowel disease** and **pulmonary fibrosis**. The skin of these patients contains normal numbers of melanocytes that manifest shortened dendritic processes with a reduced number of melanosomes. Electron microscopy reveals that the melanosomes mature to only stages I–III.

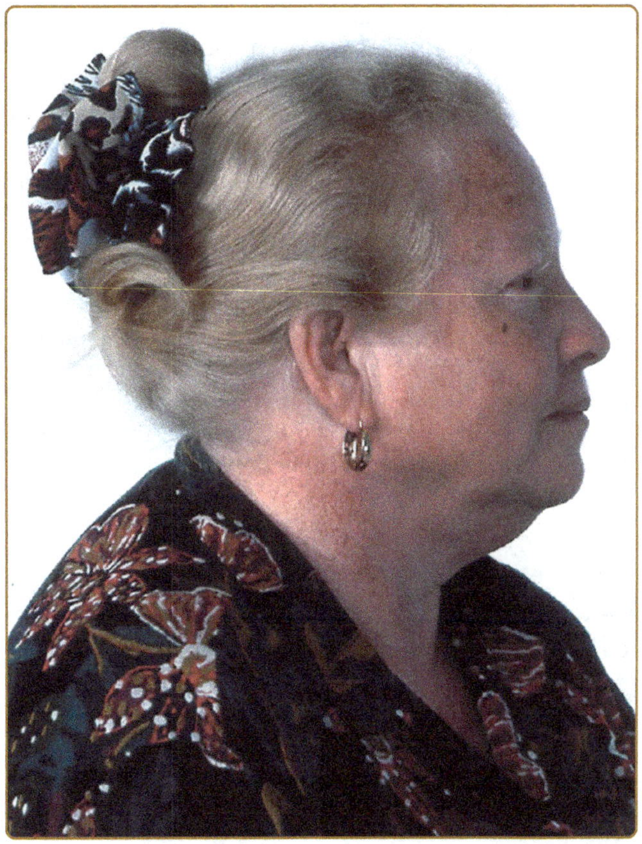

Puerto Rican with Hermansky–Pudlak syndrome. The patient died of pulmonary fibrosis. (Reproduced, with permission, from Goldsmith LA, Katz SI, Gilchrest BA, Paller AS, Leffell DJ, Wolff K, eds. *Fitzpatrick's Dermatology in General Medicine*. 8th ed. New York, NY: McGraw-Hill Education; 2012.)

Nevus depigmentosus manifests at birth as a solitary congenital patch of hypopigmentation on the trunk, neck, and other locations. The name is a misnomer because it represents **congenital hypomelanosis** rather than **acquired depigmentation**. Such a lesion may be localized, segmental, or less often systematized. Lesions may be circumscribed, irregular, oval or round, or a unilateral band or streak that may be arranged along one or more lines of Blaschko. A block-like variant referred to as the hypopigmented form of "segmental pigmentation disorder" typically features midline demarcation and less distinct lateral borders. When systematized, the lesion is indistinguishable from **hypomelanosis of Ito**. In contrast to **vitiligo** or **piebaldism**, depigmentation is not complete, and the contour is usually not smooth as in **vitiligo** but is rather ragged. **Nevus depigmentosus** may be associated with either ipsilateral or contralateral segmental lentiginosis or with the acquired onset of multiple pigmented nevi within the hypopigmented region.

Pityriasis alba is a common condition of slightly scaly, round to oval, ill-defined macules and patches with mild-to-moderate hypopigmentation around the nose, cheeks, and eyebrow areas of children. It is more noticeable in darkly pigmented individuals and is often misdiagnosed as **tinea faciae** because fine scales may cover the lesion. The condition is probably a variant of **seborrheic dermatitis** or **atopic dermatitis**, with *Pityrosporum* infection a contributing factor. Microscopically, there is hyperkeratosis with patchy parakeratosis, slight acanthosis with spongiosis, follicular spongiosis, and a superficial perivascular lymphocytic infiltrate. There is decreased basal layer melanin, best highlighted with a Fontana-Masson stain. The number of basilar melanocytes is normal or only slightly decreased, and these cells produce fewer and smaller melanosomes. Transfer of melanosomes to the keratinocytes is normal. The clinical depigmentation may reflect **post-inflammatory alterations**, but it is possible that *Pityrosporum* species are involved in the etiology because the tyrosinase inhibitor azelaic acid is produced by these lipophilic yeasts.

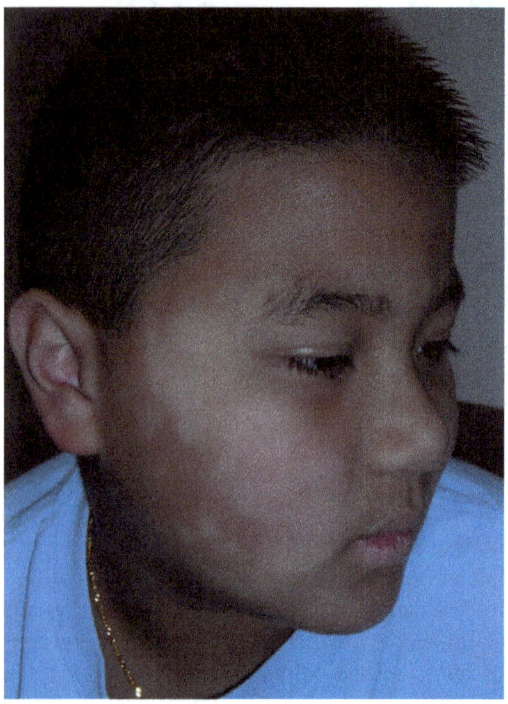

Pityriasis alba on the face of a young boy. (Reproduced, with permission, from Usatine RP, Smith MA, Mayeaux EJ Jr, Chumley HS, eds. *Color Atlas of Family Medicine*. 2nd ed. New York, NY: McGraw-Hill Education; 2012. Used with permission of Richard P. Usatine, MD.)

Idiopathic guttate hypomelanosis is common among older (>50 years) African American men and women and may be equally frequent in whites but is not as noticeable. Numerous well-demarcated hypopigmented (pigmentary dilution) and depigmented (porcelain white) macules 2-10 mm in diameter are seen on the shins and, less frequently, on the extensor aspects of the arms. The pathogenesis is uncertain, but given the distribution, a link to chronic UV exposure has been proposed. Microscopically, the epidermis is atrophic with flattened rete ridges and shows decreased melanin content. Biopsies taken at the interface between normal and hypopigmented skin show an abrupt loss of basal layer melanization. Basilar melanocytes are present but are slightly reduced in number. Ultrastructurally, most melanosomes are immature (stages I and II), and their dendrites are underdeveloped. Normal melanocytes may be intermingled with these less active ones.

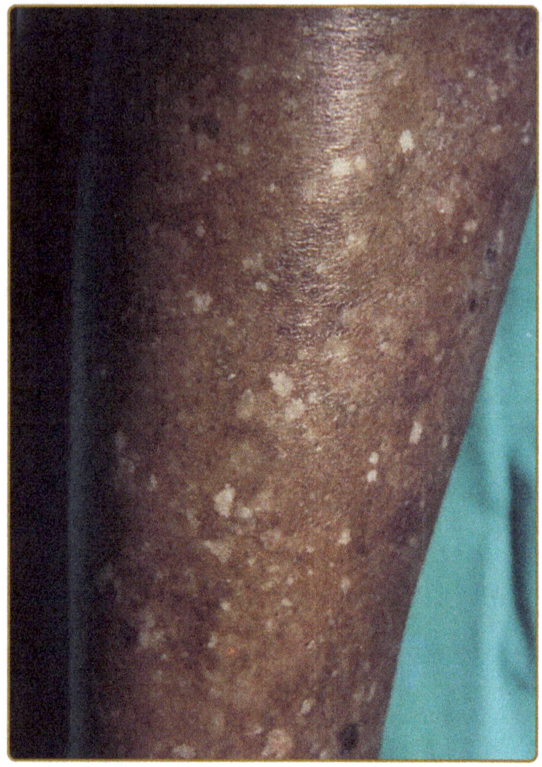

Idiopathic guttate hypomelanosis. Lesions on the leg of an African American individual. (Reproduced, with permission, from Goldsmith LA, Katz SI, Gilchrest BA, Paller AS, Leffell DJ, Wolff K, eds. *Fitzpatrick's Dermatology in General Medicine*. 8th ed. New York, NY: McGraw-Hill Education; 2012.)

ANSWER 6-20: C.

The biopsy reveals moderate hyper-orthokeratosis of the stratum corneum overlying a mildly acanthotic epidermis with hypogranulosis, consistent with **ichthyosis vulgaris**. The designation "**ichthyosis**" is fundamentally a descriptive term covering a variety of keratinization disorders that are usually genetic in nature. Although their genetic bases are heterogeneous, all of them share the common clinical feature of scaling skin, which is usually generalized, but as in the instances of the **palmoplantar keratodermas** and the **erythrokeratodermas**, they may also be localized. The organization of these hyperkeratotic disorders, which has been adapted from the work of Traupe, follows the diagnostic algorithm presented in the table below. This scheme focuses initial attention on whether the predominant mode of keratinization is ortho- or parakeratotic and secondarily on the morphologic status of the stratum granulosum.

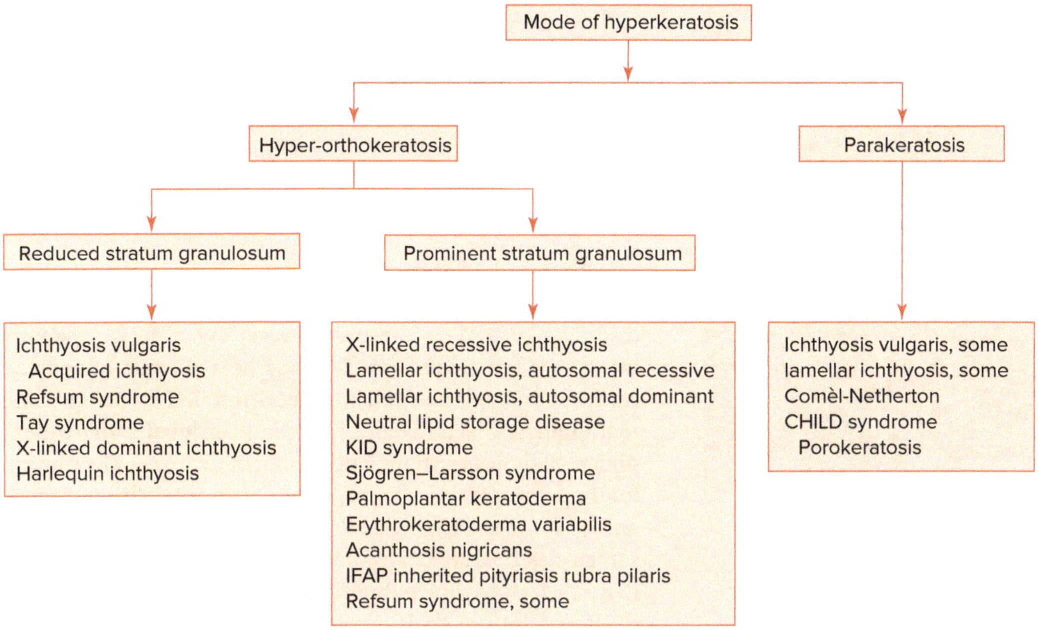

Hyperkeratosis without epidermolytic change: diagnostic algorithm for the non-bullous ichthyoses and related disorders. The pathway for differential diagnosis is dichotomized on the preponderant mode of hyperkeratosis, whether ortho- or parakeratotic, and if the former, whether the stratum granulosum is reduced or retained. CHILD = congenital hemidysplasia, ichthyosiform erythroderma, limb defects; IFAP = ichthyosis follicularis with atrichia and photophobia; KID = keratitis, ichthyosis-like hyperkeratosis, and deafness.

Ichthyosis vulgaris is the most common ichthyosis, and is a retention hyperkeratosis disorder inherited as an autosomal dominant trait (Table 6-20A). The markedly reduced granular cell layer in this condition has led to investigations of the role of **profilaggrin** (the predominant keratohyaline protein in the human epidermis) in **ichthyosis vulgaris**. **Profilaggrin** expression in the affected epidermis is decreased or absent, depending on the disease severity. A subset of individuals with the clinical findings of **ichthyosis vulgaris** and no granular layer has been identified. Keratinocytes cultured from such individuals have very little detectable **profilaggrin** protein, and the **profilaggrin** mRNA level is reduced by approximately 50% in these cells. A mouse model, known as flaky tail, presents a clinical phenotype resembling that of the human condition, and at the histologic level, keratohyaline granules are absent from the epidermis; molecular analysis has suggested a defect in the processing of **profilaggrin** to **filaggrin** as the potential basis for the phenotype. Following from the animal models and genetic linkage analyses, subsequent mutational analyses have identified specific mutations in the **profilaggrin** gene that cause **ichthyosis vulgaris** and predispose individuals to **atopic dermatitis**, presumably mediated by defects in barrier function.

Table 6-20A. Ichthyosis Vulgaris

Clinical Features
Onset within the first year of life
Fine, white scales on the trunk and extensor extremities, sparing the sides of the neck
Hyperlinearity and chafing of the palms and soles
Associated with atopy and keratosis pilaris
Histopathology
Mild-to-moderated compact hyper-orthokeratosis
Generally no parakeratosis
Diminished to absent stratum granulosum
Follicular dilatation and hyperkeratosis
Epidermis usually of normal thickness
Differential Diagnosis
Acquired ichthyosis
Xerosis
Syndromes with associated ichthyosis: Refsum syndrome, ichthyosis, and trichothiodystrophy,
X-linked dominant ichthyosis with chondrodysplasia punctata

Clinically, **ichthyosis vulgaris** presents early in life, usually within the first year, but is rarely present at birth. Fine, white scales are found on the trunk and extensor surfaces of the extremities in association with superficial fissuring in severe cases. The central face and cheeks may be involved. The popliteal fossae, antecubital fossae, and sides of the neck are almost always spared. The condition is associated with **atopy** and **keratosis pilaris**. Hyperlinearity and chafing of the palms and soles are often present, but whether this is linked to the **atopy** or the **ichthyosis** is disputed.

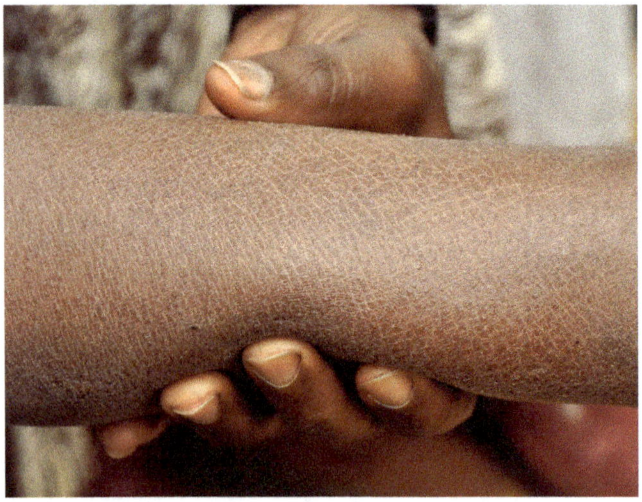

Ichthyosis vulgaris starts in childhood and has a fine scale. (Reproduced, with permission, from Usatine RP, Smith MA, Mayeaux EJ Jr, Chumley HS, eds. *Color Atlas of Family Medicine*. 2nd ed. New York, NY: McGraw-Hill Education; 2012. Used with permission of Richard P. Usatine, MD.)

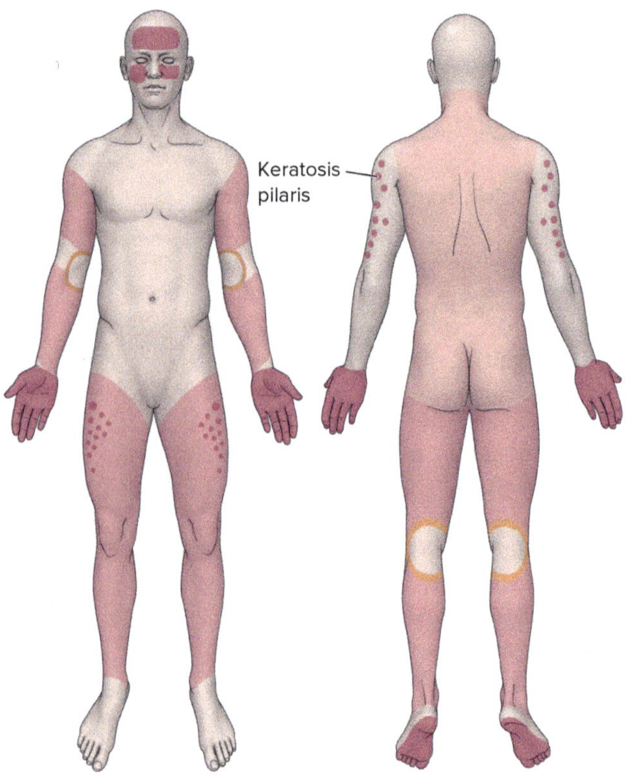

Distribution of ichthyosis vulgaris. Dots indicate keratosis pilaris. (Reproduced, with permission, from Wolff K, Johnson RA, Saavedra AP. *Fitzpatrick's Color Atlas and Synopsis of Clinical Dermatology*. 7th ed. New York, NY: McGraw-Hill Education; 2013.)

Microscopic examination of the stratum corneum in patients with **ichthyosis vulgaris** reveals compact hyper-orthokeratosis. The degree of hyperkeratosis varies from mild to moderate. This alteration is associated with a uniformly reduced granular layer that is absent in at least some foci. Parakeratosis is generally not observed. Follicular dilatation and hyperkeratosis are regularly present, consistent with **keratosis pilaris**. The epidermis is usually of normal thickness, but on occasion, acanthosis or even atrophy may be present. The rete ridge pattern is not accentuated. The sebaceous glands are atrophic. Minimal perivascular inflammation is found in the papillary dermis.

Acquired ichthyosis, which usually presents in adults, has been described in association with a number of systemic disorders (including **thyroid disease, sarcoidosis, systemic lupus erythematosus, graft versus host disease after bone marrow transplantation, malnutrition, HIV**), **drugs**, and **malignancies**. Nearly half of people with **insulin-dependent diabetes** clinically show ichthyosiform changes. The clinical findings are reported to resemble those of **ichthyosis vulgaris**, although large platelike or hyperpigmented scales are sometimes observed. Hyperlinearity of the palms and soles is not a feature, but **palmar-plantar keratoderma** has been described. Microscopically, in **acquired ichthyosis**, there is less hypogranulosis than that seen in **ichthyosis vulgaris** and immunohistochemical staining for anti-profilaggrin or filaggrin antibodies demonstrates the presence of **profilaggrin** or **filaggrin**, respectively.

Because of the overlap in clinical phenotype, **ichthyosis vulgaris** and **X-linked recessive ichthyosis** are often confused clinically (Table 6-20B). The usual mistake in diagnosis is labeling **X-linked recessive ichthyosis** as **ichthyosis vulgaris**. A careful examination of the family history will reveal the inheritance pattern. Mutations (deletions) in the **steroid sulfatase** gene are responsible for the defect in **X-linked recessive ichthyosis**. The resulting accumulation of cholesterol sulfate in keratinocytes (as well as in other tissues such as leukocytes) is thought to result in retention hyperkeratosis and scaling, and the increased cholesterol sulfate in combination with decreased cholesterol within the stratum corneum contributes to a deficiency in barrier function. Assay for reduced levels of

Table 6-20B. X-Linked Recessive Ichthyosis

Clinical Features
- Present at birth or shortly thereafter
- Generalized fine scaling, especially at flexural sites
- Progresses over the first 6 months to large, pigmented, platelike scales

Histopathologic Features
- Marked hyper-orthokeratosis with occasional parakeratotic foci
- Granular layer usually thickened
- Variable acanthosis and papillomatosis

Differential Diagnosis
- Ichthyosis vulgaris
- Autosomal recessive lamellar ichthyosis

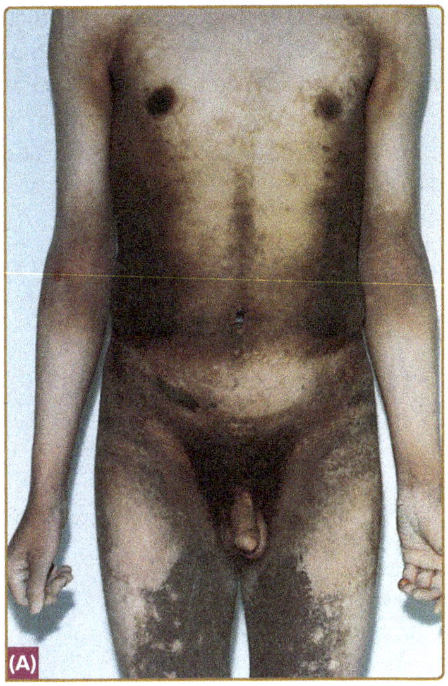

X-linked recessive ichthyosis. The scales are large and dark and most evident on the flexural areas in this patient. (Reproduced, with permission, from Goldsmith LA, Katz SI, Gilchrest BA, Paller AS, Leffell DJ, Wolff K, eds. *Fitzpatrick's Dermatology in General Medicine.* 8th ed. New York, NY: McGraw-Hill Education; 2012.)

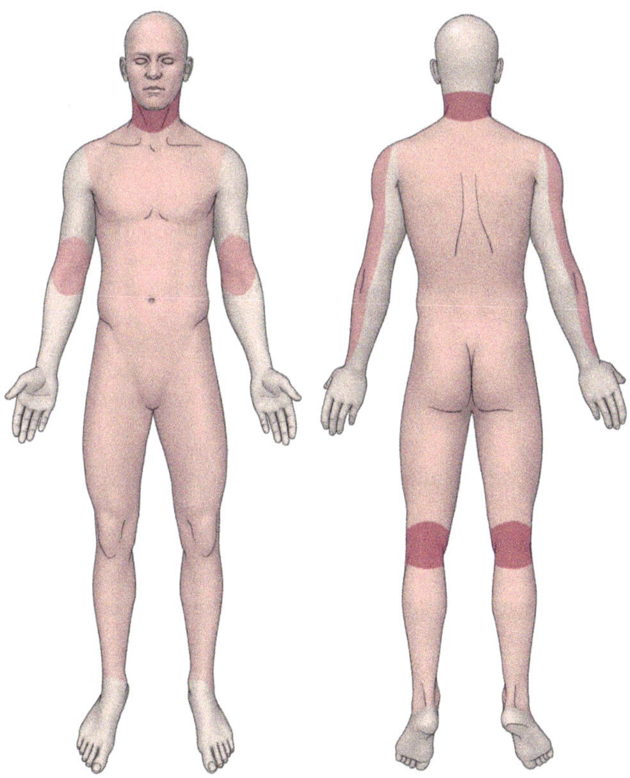

Distribution of X-linked ichthyosis. Dark pink areas represent severe involvement. (Reproduced, with permission, from Wolff K, Johnson RA, Saavedra AP. *Fitzpatrick's Color Atlas and Synopsis of Clinical Dermatology.* 7th ed. New York, NY: McGraw-Hill Education; 2013.)

steroid sulfatase activity can be used to confirm the diagnosis of **X-linked recessive ichthyosis**. Individuals with **X-linked recessive ichthyosis** present at birth or soon thereafter. A collodion membrane is seen infrequently, but affected infants more commonly manifest fine, relatively mild scaling at birth. The scaling worsens or generalizes in the first 2-6 months as larger, pigmented scales that appear on the trunk, extremities, axillae, sides of the neck, and the popliteal and antecubital fossae, although the volar epidermis is spared. The brownish scales tend to be large polygonal plates that are adherent. Associated findings may include cryptorchidism and asymptomatic corneal opacities. Obstetric complications, such as a late-for-dates pregnancy, weak labor, and prolonged delivery, occur in as many as 30% of affected pregnancies because of blocked placental estrogen synthesis.

Microscopically, patients have marked hyper-orthokeratosis with occasional foci of parakeratosis. The granular layer is usually thickened, although this can vary, and it may be thinned in some sections. The spinous layer is variably acanthotic and papillomatous. Perivascular lymphoid infiltrates within the papillary dermis range from mild to marked. Follicular dilatation and plugging are usually absent but may occasionally be observed.

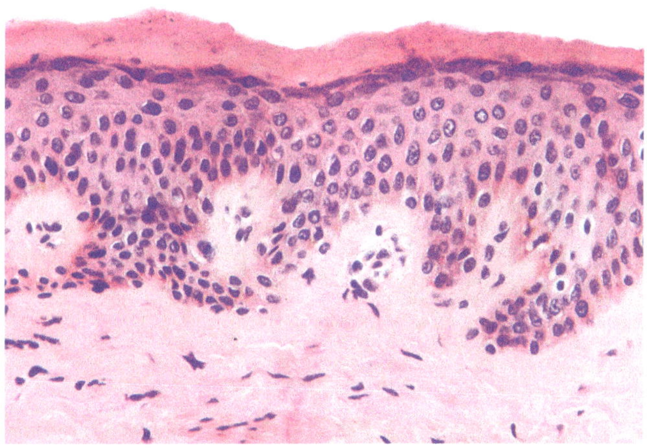

X-linked recessive ichthyosis. A continuous granular layer of normal to slightly increased thickness separates the densely compact orthokeratotic corneum from the histopathologically unremarkable stratum spinosum.

Lamellar ichthyosis is a genetically heterogeneous disease. Most cases are transmitted as an autosomal recessive trait, but cases with dominant transmission have also been described. The recessively inherited form is a severe and often generalized dermatosis, usually presenting at birth and accounting for the majority of cases of **collodion baby syndrome** (Table 6-20C). There are erythrodermic and non-erythrodermic clinical variants. Patients with the most severe phenotype show large, brown, platelike scales and pronounced ectropion. Those with milder phenotypes may have involvement of only the flexural sites and the palms and soles.

Table 6-20C. Autosomal Recessive Lamellar Ichthyosis

Clinical Features
Present at birth with generalized involvement, often with a collodion membrane
Erythrodermic and non-erythrodermic variants
Large platelike scales, ectropion
Histopathology
Mild to marked compact hyper-orthokeratosis
Normal to widened stratum granulosum
Often acanthosis and papillomatosis
Differential Diagnosis
X-linked recessive ichthyosis

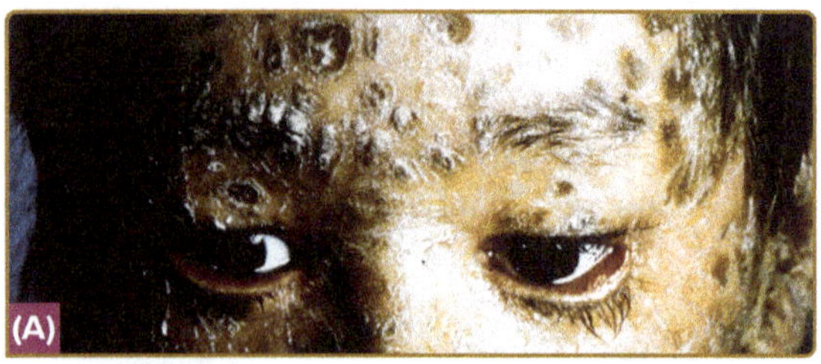

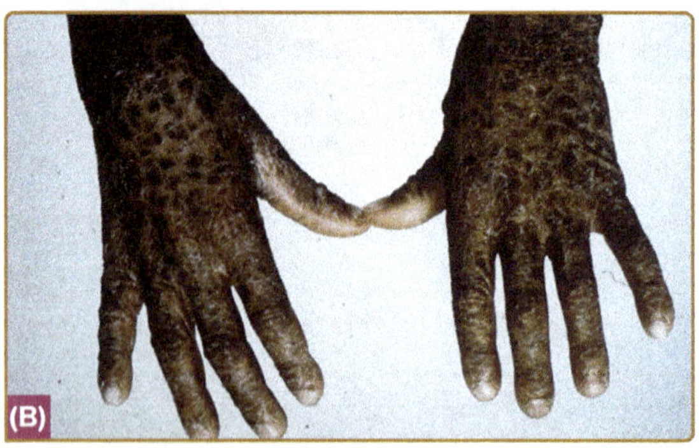

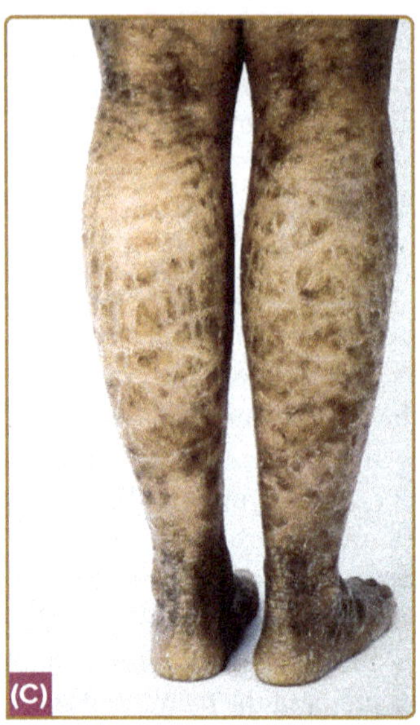

Classic lamellar ichthyosis phenotype. (A) Ectropion (lower eyelids turn outwards). **(B)**, **(C)** Large, brown, platelike scales. (Reproduced, with permission, from Russell LJ et al. Linkage of autosomal recessive lamellar ichthyosis to chromosome 14q. *Am J Hum Genet.* 1994;55:1146.)

Mutations in **keratinocyte (type I) transglutaminase**, which cross-links the cornified envelopes of terminally differentiating keratinocytes, are associated with most cases of **lamellar ichthyosis**. Defective **transglutaminase** activity results in incomplete cross-linking of substrates such as **loricrin** and **involucrin**, disrupted assembly of cornified envelopes, and defective barrier function.

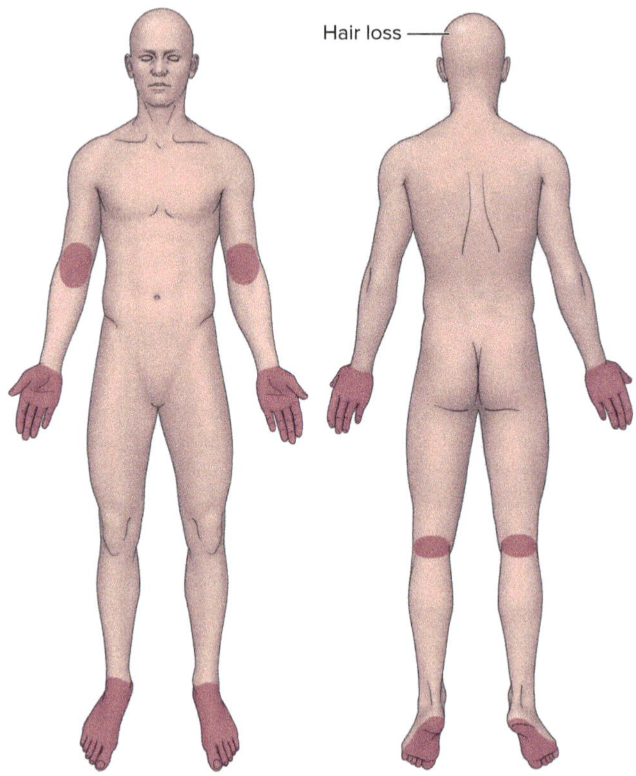

Lamellar ichthyosis. Shoulder tessellated (tile-like) hyperkeratosis gives the appearance of reptilian scales on the shoulder and back. The entire body is involved, and ectropium is present. Dark pink areas represent severe involvement. (Reproduced, with permission, from Wolff K, Johnson RA, Saavedra AP. *Fitzpatrick's Color Atlas and Synopsis of Clinical Dermatology*. 7th ed. New York, NY: McGraw-Hill Education; 2013.)

The histopathologic patterns are indistinguishable across all erythrodermic and non-erythrodermic clinical variants of **lamellar ichthyosis** of autosomal recessive type, as well as cases with autosomal dominant transmission. Mild to marked compact hyper-orthokeratosis and a normal to increased stratum granulosum are observed in these patients. Often acanthosis and occasionally papillomatosis are seen. Parakeratotic foci associated with a focally thinned granular layer are occasionally observed. The papillary dermis may contain a perivascular lymphocytic infiltrate of variable intensity.

Harlequin ichthyosis is a rare, severe keratinizing disorder thought to be inherited as an autosomal recessive trait or a new dominant mutation. The disorder is phenotypically heterogeneous. Abnormal or absent **lamellar granules** within

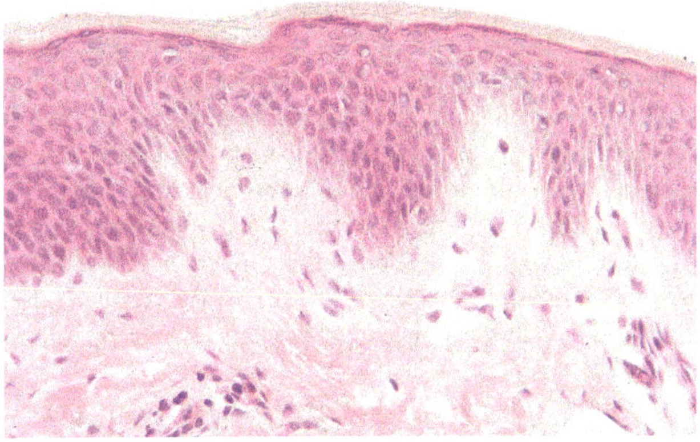

Lamellar ichthyosis. The compact and mildly thickened orthokeratotic stratum corneum is separated from the slightly acanthotic stratum spinosum by a continuous granular layer of normal thickness.

keratinocytes are observed by electron microscopy in all forms. **Lamellar granules** function in lipid transport. A member of the ATP-binding cassette transporter family designated ABCA12 ultrastructurally localizes to **lamellar granules** and functions in lipid secretion in and out of the cells via these granules. Mutational analyses of *ABCA12* as a candidate gene for **Harlequin ichthyosis** and complementary single nucleotide polymorphism mapping strategies have shown that missense and nonsense mutations in highly conserved regions of the gene are etiologic for the condition; the phenotype is thus mediated by deleterious effects on skin barrier function resulting from defective lipid transport.

Clinically, the condition is the most severe of the congenital ichthyoses. Newborns are incarcerated in a massively thick, platelike scale affecting the entire integument, which produces **ectropion** and **eclabium**; restricts respiration and feeding; and alters development of the ears, nose, eyes, and mouth. The cuirass cracks soon after birth, resulting in deep fissures in geometric patterns. Death usually ensues. If the affected infant survives beyond the newborn period, the phenotype evolves into that of a severe non-bullous congenital erythroderma.

The histologic pattern in **Harlequin ichthyosis** varies between reports. Across all categories, however, there is massive compact hyper-orthokeratosis, creating a stratum corneum that is much thicker than the spinous layer. Changes in the granular layer are variable. This zone is usually thinned, with keratohyaline granules either reduced in density or totally absent, but it may be normal. The follicles are dilated and hyperkeratotic. Inconstant and less striking changes include mild acanthosis and papillomatosis. Pronounced parakeratosis may be observed in patients who completely lack keratohyaline granules. A superficial perivascular lymphocytic infiltrate is an inconstant feature.

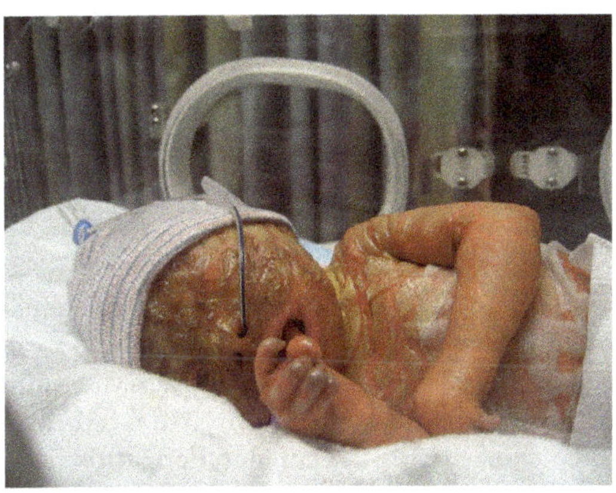

Harlequin fetus. Stratum corneum consists of thick plates separated by deep cracks. (Reproduced, with permission, from Wolff K, Johnson RA, Saavedra AP. *Fitzpatrick's Color Atlas and Synopsis of Clinical Dermatology*. 7th ed. New York, NY: McGraw-Hill Education; 2013. Used with permission of Benjamin Solky, MD.)

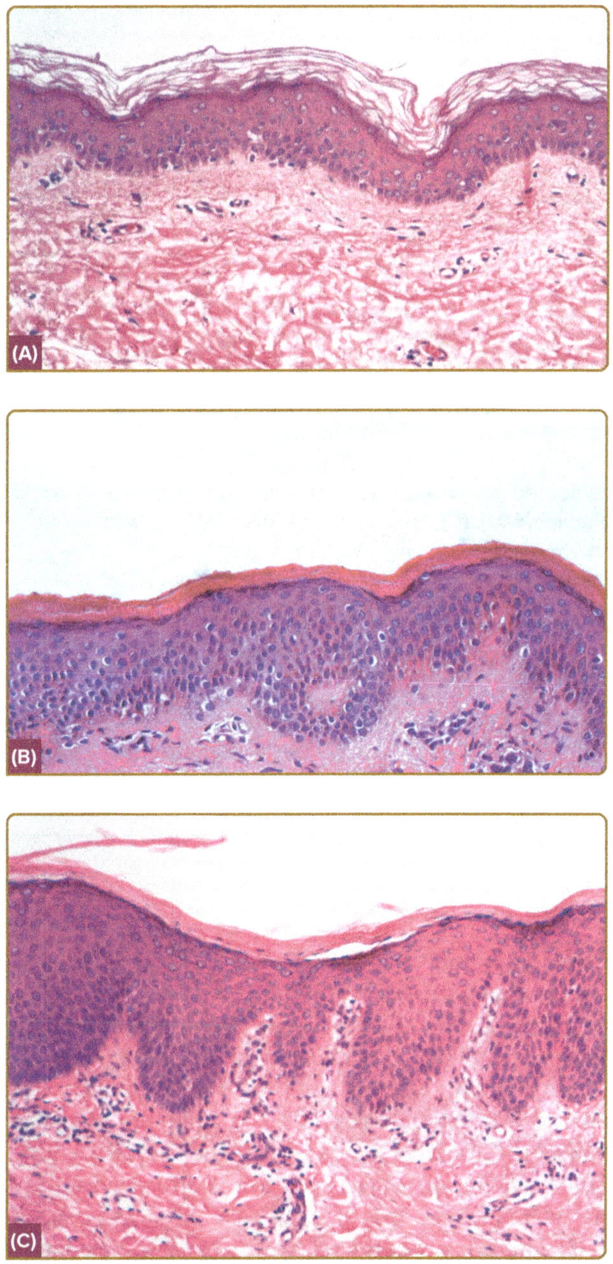

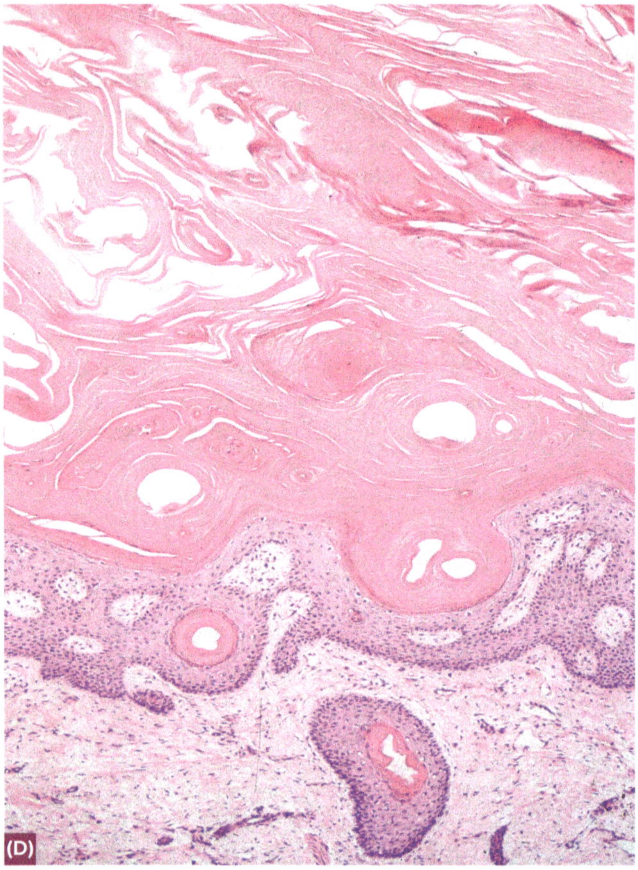

Histopathology of ichthyosis (retention hyperkeratoses). **(A)** Ichthyosis vulgaris. Note absent granular layer. **(B)** X-linked recessive ichthyosis. Note compact hyperkeratosis and accentuated granular layer. (Used with permission from Rob McFarlane, MD). **(C)** Autosomal recessive lamellar ichthyosis. Thickened stratum corneum composed of compact hyperkeratosis with foci of parakeratosis. **(D)** Harlequin ichthyosis. Massive orthokeratotic thickening of the stratum corneum is seen in association with a thinned stratum granulosum and a spinous layer that is mildly acanthotic and papillomatous. The follicular ostia are dilated and plugged with keratin. (Reproduced, with permission, from Goldsmith LA, Katz SI, Gilchrest BA, Paller AS, Leffell DJ, Wolff K, eds. *Fitzpatrick's Dermatology in General Medicine*. 8th ed. New York, NY: McGraw-Hill Education; 2012.)

ANSWER 6-21: E.

The stratum corneum is dramatically thickened with compact parakeratosis, psoriasiform epidermal hyperplasia, slight papillomatosis, and a perivascular lymphocytic infiltrate. Keratohyaline granules are diffusely present within the parakeratotic stratum corneum, and the retained granular layer manifests focal vacuolization. The findings are consistent with **axillary granular parakeratosis**. There are few entities in which prominent parakeratosis is a clue to the diagnosis. More often, parakeratosis is found as a transient or inconstant feature in a disorder with hyperkeratosis developing in an orthokeratotic fashion. **Granular parakeratosis** is a rare acquired condition thought to be a disorder of keratinization. Although an irritant contact reaction appears operative, other forms of mechanical irritation may also figure into the pathogenesis of these lesions. Recent studies on this entity suggest a basic defect in the processing of **profilaggrin** to **filaggrin**, resulting in a failure to degrade keratohyaline granules and to aggregate keratin filaments during cornification. Associated abnormalities of the cell surface structures and dysregulation of cornified envelope components may account for the retention hyperkeratosis.

Clinically, individuals of all ages ranging from younger than 1 year of age to the elderly present with intertriginous (most commonly axillary), erythematous, brown or red, scaly or keratotic papules and plaques that are often pruritic. Other sites, including the face, trunk, and buttocks, may also be involved.

Characteristic microscopic features include a conspicuously thickened stratum corneum with compact parakeratosis, slight epidermal hyperplasia (psoriasiform, papillomatous, or both), and a sparse perivascular lymphohistiocytic infiltrate. Keratohyaline granules are diffusely present within the parakeratotic stratum corneum, and the retained granular layer manifests focal vacuolization.

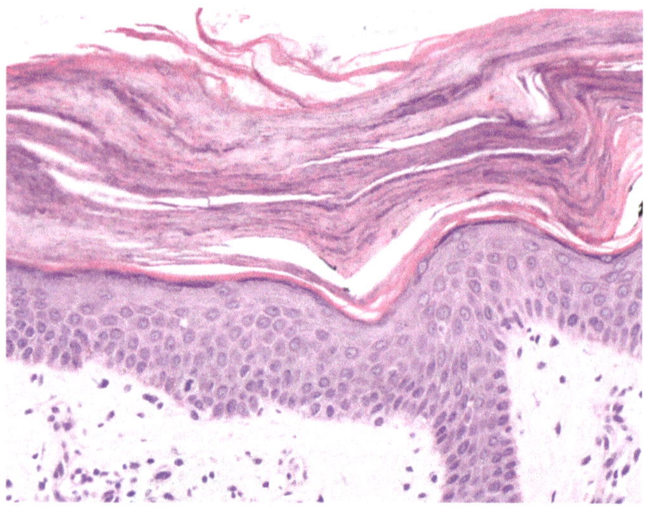

Granular parakeratosis. Note the thick parakeratosis with retained keratohyaline granules. The epidermis is slightly acanthotic with hypergranulosis.

In regards to the differential diagnosis, **granular parakeratosis** must be distinguished from a number of inflammatory and noninflammatory conditions. Various psoriasiform dermatitides to be considered are **psoriasis, pityriasis rubra pilaris, seborrheic dermatitis, allergic or irritant contact dermatitis, atopic dermatitis, nummular dermatitis, dyshidrotic eczema**, nodules secondary to **scabetic infestation**, and **dermatophyte** and **candidal infection**. **Psoriasis** typically demonstrates a diminished granular layer and fairly regular psoriasiform hyperplasia. **Pityriasis rubra pilaris** shows alternating ortho- and parakeratosis. Additionally, the parakeratosis does not contain prominent keratohyaline granules. **Seborrheic dermatitis** frequently displays spongiosis and parafollicular parakeratosis. The various other dermatitides usually exhibit a spongiotic reaction pattern. The fungal infections are easily ruled out by stains for fungi. Noninflammatory processes, such as **acanthosis nigricans, confluent and reticulated papillomatosis, seborrheic keratoses**, and **epidermal nevi**, are excluded by their lack of basophilic granules within the parakeratotic layer.

ANSWER 6-22: C.

Porokeratosis is a morphologically distinct disorder of keratinization, characterized clinically by hyperkeratotic papules or plaques surrounded by a thread-like elevated border that expands centrifugally. Histopathologically, a thin column of parakeratotic cells extends throughout the stratum corneum and is seen in all variants. This distinctive histopathologic feature, known as the **cornoid lamella**, corresponds to the raised hyperkeratotic border evident clinically.

At least six clinical variants of **porokeratosis** are recognized; however, the clinical distinction between these morphological variants may not be justified. Reports of one type of porokeratosis coexisting with other forms and different types developing in multiple members of an affected family suggest more similarities than disparities, particularly in the disseminated forms.

Classic **porokeratosis of Mibelli** begins during infancy or childhood as asymptomatic small brown to skin-colored annular papules with a characteristic annular border. The well-demarcated hyperkeratotic border is usually more than 1 mm in height, with a characteristic longitudinal furrow. The center of the lesion may be hyperpigmented, hypopigmented, depressed, atrophic, or anhidrotic. Lesions range in diameter from millimeters to several centimeters, but giant lesions measuring up to 20 cm may occur. Such giant **porokeratoses** are rare and occur predominantly on the lower leg and foot. Large lesions are associated with a higher malignant potential. Multiple lesions may arise; however, they are usually regionally localized and unilateral. The condition may be familial and inherited as an autosomal dominant trait. Lesions persist indefinitely.

Disseminated superficial actinic porokeratosis (DSAP) is the most common of the **porokeratoses**. Lesions are characteristically uniformly small, annular, asymptomatic, or mildly pruritic papules ranging from 2 to 5 mm in diameter, distributed symmetrically on the extremities. Lesions are more generalized than other forms of **porokeratosis**, with typically in excess of 50 lesions located predominantly in sun-exposed sites. Although widespread, lesions typically spare palms, soles, and mucous membranes. Compared with **porokeratosis of Mibelli**, the hyperkeratotic border is characteristically subtler. As the lesions progress, the older, central area becomes atrophic and anhidrotic. **DSAP** tends to be inherited as an autosomal dominant disorder, with the earliest reported age of onset at 7 years, and is usually fully penetrant by the third or fourth decade of life. Point mutations in the *SART3* gene on chromosome 12q have been identified in kindreds affected with **disseminated superficial actinic porokeratosis (DSAP)**. **Porokeratosis** is associated with immunosuppression, and malignancies such as **Bowen disease** arise within these lesions, but the relative risk of malignant degeneration is unknown.

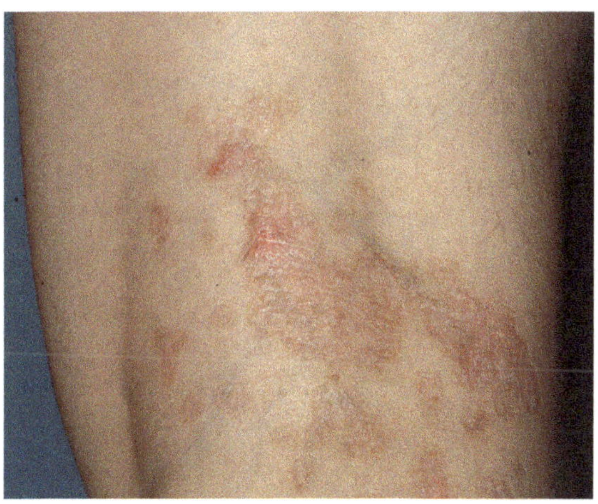

Porokeratosis of Mibelli. Coalescent erythematous papules and plaques with distinctive raised, fine, threadlike annulus at the periphery of each lesion corresponding to histologic cornoid lamella.

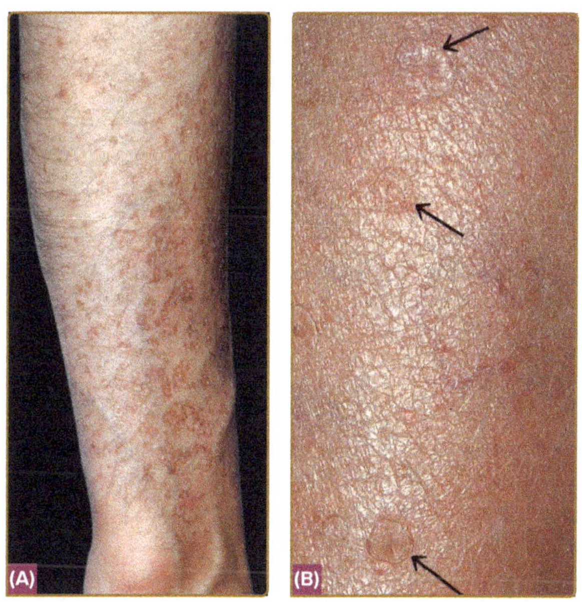

Disseminated superficial actinic porokeratosis. (A) Multiple lesions on the forearm in this severely affected individual. **(B)** The characteristic furrowing (*arrows*) is clearly demonstrated on the forearm of this patient. (Reproduced, with permission, from Goldsmith LA, Katz SI, Gilchrest BA, Paller AS, Leffell DJ, Wolff K, eds. *Fitzpatrick's Dermatology in General Medicine*. 8th ed. New York, NY: McGraw-Hill Education; 2012.)

Linear porokeratosis is an uncommon variant, traditionally categorized as a separate entity, but is increasingly recognized as mosaic manifestation of one of the other types of **porokeratosis**. Typically, it presents in early childhood, although congenital presentations have been reported. Two distinct clinical variants have been described. The more common presentation consists of a unilateral lesion confined to an extremity following Blaschko lines. In the rare generalized form, multiple lesions affect several extremities and may involve the trunk. **Linear porokeratoses** have the highest potential for malignant degeneration of all the **porokeratoses**. It has been postulated that this association can be attributed to allelic loss due to a postzygotic mutation. The proband in Mibelli's original publication most likely had coexistent **linear porokeratosis** and **DSAP**, with several subsequent reports confirming this phenomenon. These findings may be explained by the loss of heterozygosity for the **DSAP** allele and provide an example of the type 2 segmental manifestations of an autosomal dominant disorder.

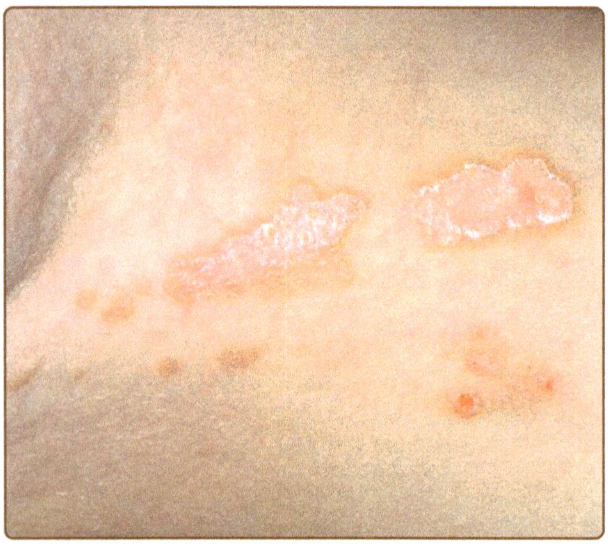

Linear porokeratosis showing the characteristic distribution along Blaschko lines. (Reproduced, with permission, from Goldsmith LA, Katz SI, Gilchrest BA, Paller AS, Leffell DJ, Wolff K, eds. *Fitzpatrick's Dermatology in General Medicine*. 8th ed. New York, NY: McGraw-Hill Education; 2012.)

Porokeratosis palmaris et plantaris disseminata (porokeratosis punctata palmaris et plantaris) is a genodermatosis with an autosomal dominant inheritance pattern characterized by small, relatively uniform lesions that initially appear on the palms and soles. Subsequently, lesions spread to involve other parts of the body, including the mucous membranes and non-sun-exposed sites. The palmar and plantar lesions are generally more hyperkeratotic, and the characteristic longitudinal furrow along this ridge may be quite pronounced. Typically, the lesions appear during adolescence or early adulthood and are bilateral and distributed symmetrically. **Porokeratosis palmaris et plantaris disseminata** affects males twice as often as females.

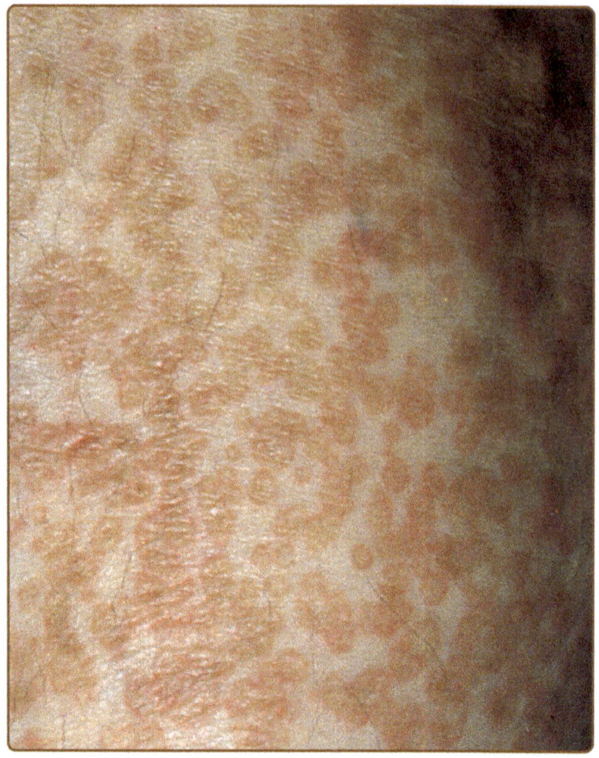

Porokeratosis palmaris et plantaris disseminata showing multiple superficial lesions on the calf. Note the clinical similarity to DSAP. (Reproduced, with permission, from Goldsmith LA, Katz SI, Gilchrest BA, Paller AS, Leffell DJ, Wolff K, eds. *Fitzpatrick's Dermatology in General Medicine*. 8th ed. New York, NY: McGraw-Hill Education; 2012.)

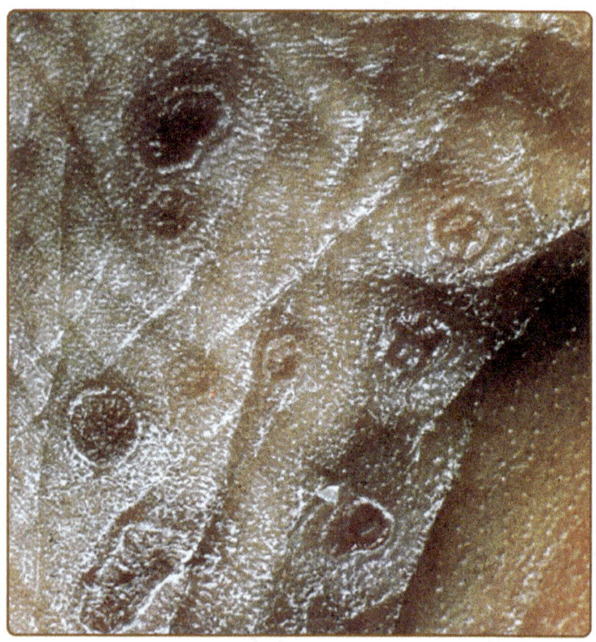

Porokeratosis palmaris et plantaris disseminata. Sole of the foot. The ridge and furrow are clearly seen. (Reproduced, with permission, from Goldsmith LA, Katz SI, Gilchrest BA, Paller AS, Leffell DJ, Wolff K, eds. *Fitzpatrick's Dermatology in General Medicine*. 8th ed. New York, NY: McGraw-Hill Education; 2012.)

Punctate porokeratosis usually appears during adolescence or adulthood and may be seen concomitantly with other types of **porokeratosis**. Multiple minute and discrete punctate, hyperkeratotic lesions surrounded by a thin, raised margin are present on the palms and soles. Lesions may occur in a linear arrangement, or they may aggregate to form plaques. **Punctate porokeratosis** must be differentiated clinically and histopathologically from **punctate keratoderma**, also referred to as **punctate porokeratotic keratoderma** or as **porokeratosis punctata palmaris et plantaris**.

CDAGS syndrome (*c*raniosynostosis and clavicular hypoplasia, *d*elayed closure of the fontanel, *a*nal anomalies, *g*enitourinary malformations, *s*kin eruption), also referred to as ***CAP* syndrome** (*c*raniosynostosis, *a*nal anomalies, and *p*orokeratosis), is a rare genodermatosis reported in four ethnically diverse families to date. The main phenotypic features consist of craniosynostosis and clavicular hypoplasia, anal anomalies, and porokeratosis. It appears to segregate as an autosomal recessive trait, with possible linkage to chromosome band 22q12–13. The cutaneous manifestations are strikingly consistent, with the development of small, widespread porokeratotic papules from 1 month of age in affected individuals, predominantly affecting the face and extremities, with reported photoaggravation of lesions.

The histopathologic hallmark of all clinical varieties of **porokeratosis** is the **cornoid lamella**, which is sometimes distributed to both sides of a biopsy sample, delimiting a central zone of either acanthokeratosis or atrophy. It consists of a thin, layered column within the corneum created by parakeratotic corneocytes. This tier of cells is often obliquely oriented to the epidermal surface and appears to arise from a dell in the upper viable layers of the epidermis in association with a focal absence of the stratum granulosum. Dyskeratotic cells are frequently observed in the subjacent upper spinous layer. Edema and patchy, band-like infiltrates with scattered apoptotic bodies may be a feature within the papillary dermis subjacent to the inner zone of a porokeratotic lesion, particularly in the **DSAP** variant, in which the pattern may be lichenoid in quality.

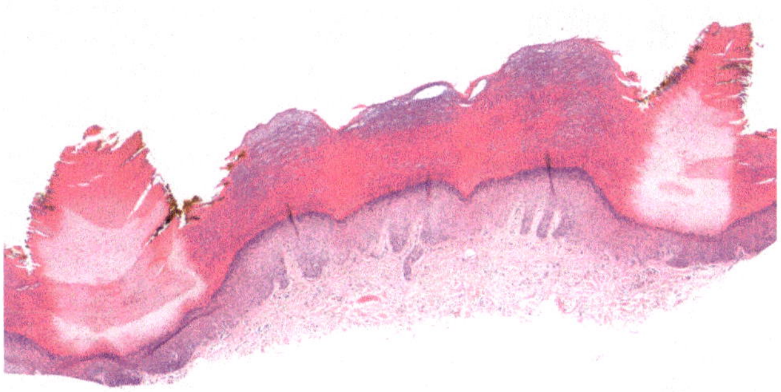

Punctate keratoderma (porokeratosis). Multiple minute and discrete punctate columns of hyperkeratosis occurring on acral skin.

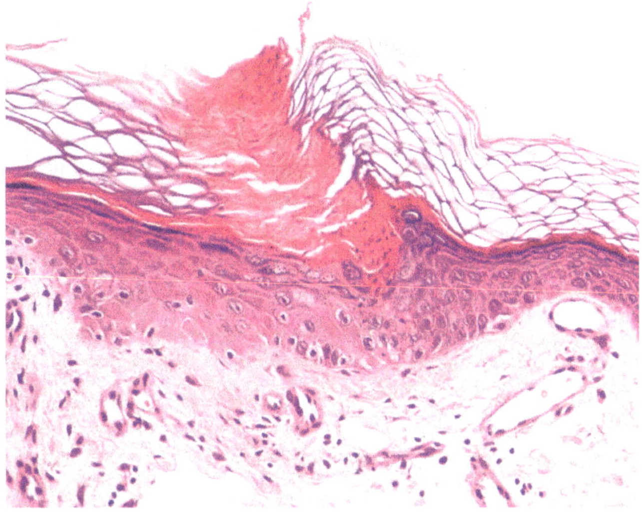

Porokeratosis. The obliquely oriented cornoid lamella containing parakeratotic corneocytes has arisen from a superficial dell, the base of which contains several dyskeratotic cells.

> **Quick Fact**
>
> **Porokeratosis**
>
> Cornoid lamella must have:
> 1) Parakeratotic column
> 2) Dyskeratotic keratinocytes at the base

In regards to the differential diagnosis, the **cornoid lamella** is a distinctive structure that is not usually confused with other processes, although its presence in tissue sections may be subtle and easily overlooked. Although it is the characteristic finding in **porokeratosis**, it is not completely specific to the diagnosis. A **cornoid lamella** may occasionally be found in a variety of other conditions, such as **warts, actinic keratosis, seborrheic keratosis, squamous cell carcinoma**, and **basal cell carcinoma**. Clinicopathologic correlations or observation of other pathologic processes in the tissues are necessary to resolve the differential diagnosis in instances associated with incidental **cornoid lamellae**.

ANSWER 6-23: E.

The biopsy reveals a markedly acanthotic and hyperkeratotic epidermis with a widened stratum granulosum containing coarsely clumped keratohyaline granules. There is mild cytolysis (clear spaces) at the levels of the mid- to upper spinous and granular cell layers. The findings are consistent with **epidermolytic hyperkeratosis**, which is a morphologic manifestation of congenital or acquired disorders of keratinocytic maturation that may be focal or diffuse. It is defined by hyperkeratosis and suprabasilar vacuolar and reticular degeneration (cytolysis) of the strata spinosum and granulosum. **Epidermolytic hyperkeratosis** is the hallmark feature of generalized ichthyosis known as **bullous congenital ichthyosiform erythroderma** and of related but more anatomically restricted disorders of either the glabrous or volar skin, such as **ichthyosis bullosa of Siemens, ichthyosis hystrix of Curth and Macklin**, some **epidermal nevi (hamartomas)**, and **palmoplantar keratoderma of Voerner type**. **Epidermolytic hyperkeratosis** is also found rather commonly as a focal histologic phenomenon due to spontaneous mutations in unrelated lesions, including **melanocytic nevi, seborrheic keratoses, actinic keratoses, acrochordons**, and **inflammatory dermatoses**, or in morphologically normal skin. A solitary lesion of **epidermolytic hyperkeratosis** presenting as a wart-like papule is designated **epidermolytic acanthoma**. **Benign familial pemphigus** (aka **Hailey–Hailey disease)** is an autosomal dominant condition in which there is extensive suprabasilar to mid-spinous layer acantholysis resulting in a "dilapidated brick wall" appearance. **Cytolysis** (cell rupture) and clumped hypergranulosis are not features of **benign familial pemphigus**.

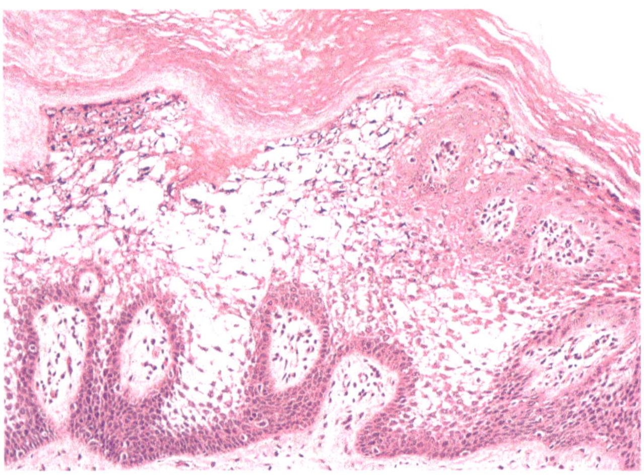

Epidermolytic hyperkeratosis in bullous ichthyosiform erythroderma. The markedly acanthotic and hyperkeratotic epidermis exhibits prominent epidermolysis at the levels of the mid- to upper spinous and granular cell layers. The widened stratum granulosum contains coarsely clumped keratohyaline granules.

Bullous congenital ichthyosiform erythroderma (aka **epidermolytic hyperkeratosis and bullous ichthyosis)** is an uncommon autosomal dominant dermatosis presenting with generalized erythroderma, severe scaling, and blistering (Table 6-23A). Cornrow-like scaling accumulates in the antecubital fossae, axillae, and over the knees and dorsal ankles.

Table 6-23A. Bullous Congenital Ichthyosiform Erythroderma

Clinical Features
Onset at birth or early childhood
Erythema, blistering, and verrucous plaques, usually widespread
Flexural accentuation
Abatement of blistering with age
Histopathologic Features
Massive hyper-orthokeratosis
Thickened granular layer with coarse keratohyaline granules
Acanthotic spinous layer with epidermolytic changes
Differential Diagnosis
Ichthyosis bullosa of Siemens
Palmoplantar keratoderma, Voerner type
Incidental finding in hyperproliferative epidermal disorders

Original ultrastructural studies of **ichthyosiform erythroderma** indicated clumping and aggregation of suprabasal keratin filaments (tonofilaments) at the cell periphery, suggesting molecular defects in keratin genes. Genetic linkage studies have shown point mutations in the critical rod domains of both suprabasal keratins 1 and 10 associated with the phenotype. The etiologic role of the keratin mutations has been established experimentally by expression of mutant keratin alleles in transgenic mice that reproduce the phenotype. In some families, somatic mutations with associated **epidermal nevi** exhibiting the histologic changes of **epidermolytic hyperkeratosis** have resulted in **generalized bullous congenital ichthyosiform**

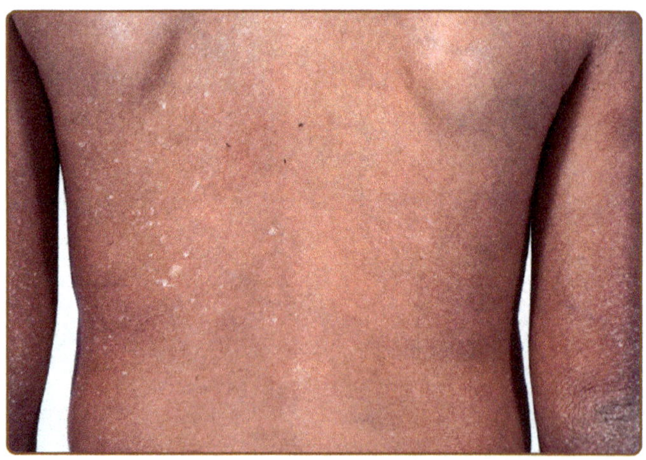

Congenital ichthyosiform erythroderma. Bright, red erythroderma with fine, white scale. (Reproduced, with permission, from Goldsmith LA, Katz SI, Gilchrest BA, Paller AS, Leffell DJ, Wolff K, eds. *Fitzpatrick's Dermatology in General Medicine*. 8th ed. New York, NY: McGraw-Hill Education; 2012.)

erythroderma in subsequent generations as a result of gonadal mosaicism. **Epidermolytic hyperkeratosis** is clinically heterogeneous, but the phenotype is relatively uniform within affected kindreds. In most cases, widespread erythema, blistering, and hyperkeratotic verrucous plaques are noted at birth or during childhood, frequently with accentuation in the flexures. Clinical blistering often abates after the first few years of life. The presence or absence of **palmoplantar keratoderma** distinguishes some pedigrees.

Palmoplantar keratoderma of Voerner (aka **epidermolytic palmoplantar keratoderma**) is an autosomal dominant form of diffuse **palmoplantar keratoderma** showing **epidermolytic hyperkeratosis** on biopsy of the affected skin, to which the designation *Voerner* is eponymously assigned. The condition has been linked to mutations in the 1A domain of the keratin 9 gene, the expression of which is restricted to the suprabasal zone of the palms and soles. Some kindreds with mild **epidermolytic palmoplantar keratodermas** harbor mutations in keratin 1. The clinical presentation of diffuse **palmoplantar keratoderma** does not allow distinction of the epidermolytic variant of Voerner from the ostensibly **non-epidermolytic palmoplantar keratoderma of Unna and Thost**. The volar lesions typically are sharply demarcated with erythematous borders. The lesions may be associated with knuckle-pad–like changes and nail clubbing.

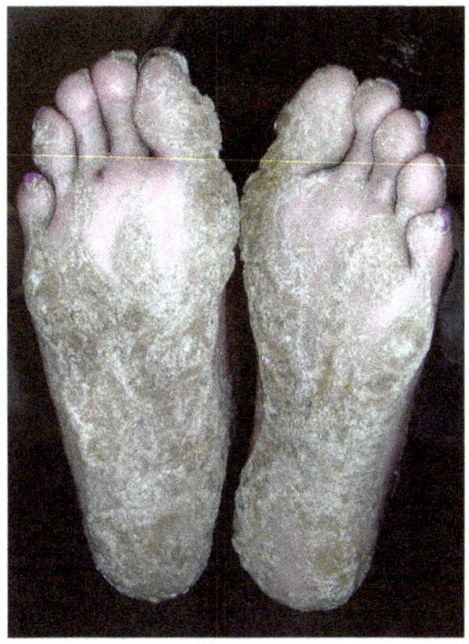

Diffuse palmoplantar keratoderma of the soles in an 11-year-old girl. This is an inherited genodermatosis with severe functional consequences. Biopsy revealed epidermolytic hyperkeratosis. (Reproduced, with permission, from Usatine RP, Smith MA, Mayeaux EJ Jr, Chumley HS, eds. *Color Atlas of Family Medicine*. 2nd ed. New York, NY: McGraw-Hill Education; 2012. Used with permission of Richard P. Usatine, MD.)

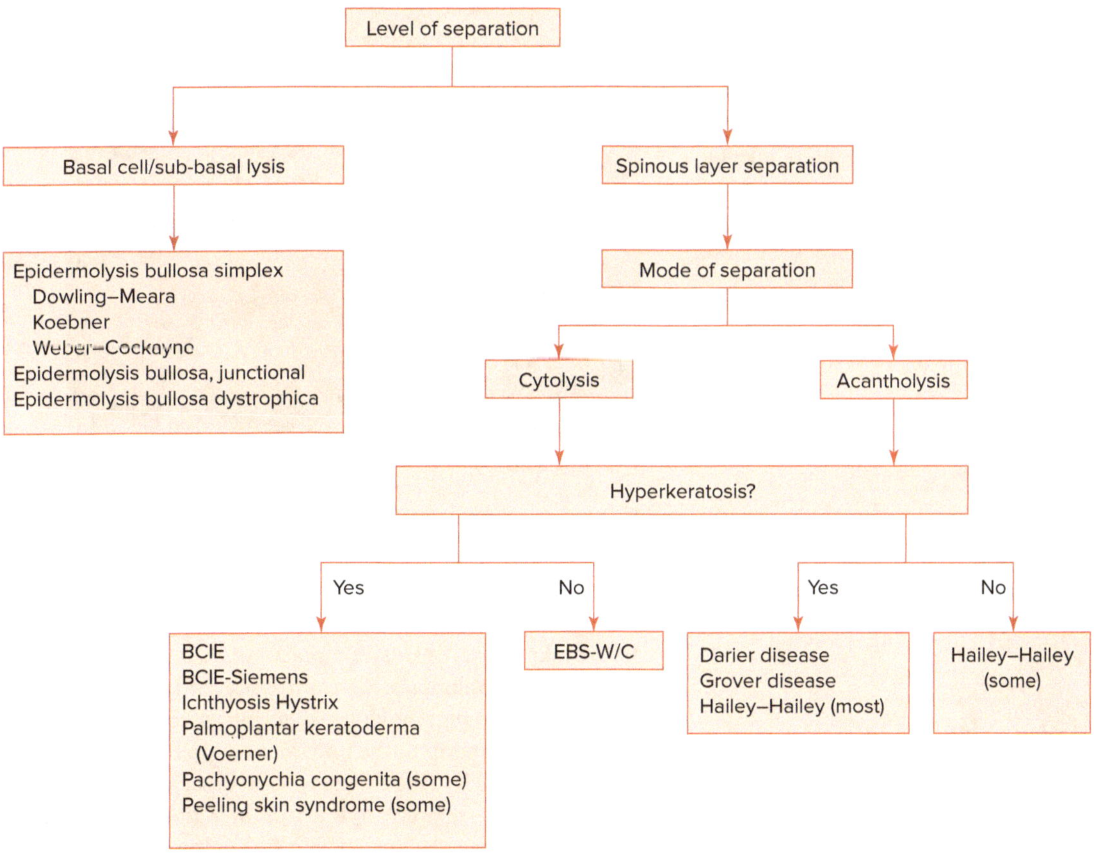

Diagnostic algorithm for the epidermolytic disorders. The hierarchy for differential diagnosis follows primarily from the level of separation within the epidermis or basement membrane zone and secondarily from the mode of separation, whether cytolysis or acantholysis. BCIE = bullous congenital ichthyosiform erythroderma; EBS = epidermolysis bullosa simplex; W/C = Weber/Cockayne.

ANSWER 6-24: E.

The biopsy reveals prominent suprabasal acantholysis in association with dyskeratotic cells (**corp ronds** [large purple cells] and **corp grains** [small eosinophilic cells]), hypergranulosis, and hyperkeratosis. **Darier disease** (aka **keratosis follicularis**) is an uncommon dominantly inherited dermatosis, which manifests as focal keratinocyte defects in intercellular adhesions that are restricted to the sites of the clinical lesions. Fine structure studies have suggested that the initial event in the lesions is separation of the paired desmosomal plaques, followed by retraction of the tonofilaments from their attachment sites in the plaques and redistribution to a perinuclear pattern; dyskeratosis occurs after the initiating acantholytic event. The mutant genetic locus responsible for Darier disease is highly penetrant and has been mapped to chromosome 12q, but genes for keratins and other known epidermal proteins were excluded as candidate loci. The gene *ATP2A2*, which encodes the endosarcoplasmic reticulum calcium ATPase isoform 2, is now established as the locus for **Darier disease**. Spontaneous mutations account for some cases.

The clinical onset of **Darier disease** ranges from childhood to the early adult years. The lesions are hyperkeratotic, crusted, erythematous papules coalescing as plaques, often with a follicular localization, that are predisposed to seborrheic areas, especially the presternal skin; however, flexural, volar, and oral mucosal lesions also occur occasionally. Clinical variants include hypertrophic, vesicular, and linear lesions. Distinctive nail changes are present in most patients and are often associated with palmar pits and keratoses. Neuropsychiatric disorders, including mental retardation, cosegregate in some families. **Darier disease** confers an infection-prone diathesis to a range of fungal, bacterial, and viral pathogens, which in turn exacerbate the clinical condition. The disorder typically has an unremitting course.

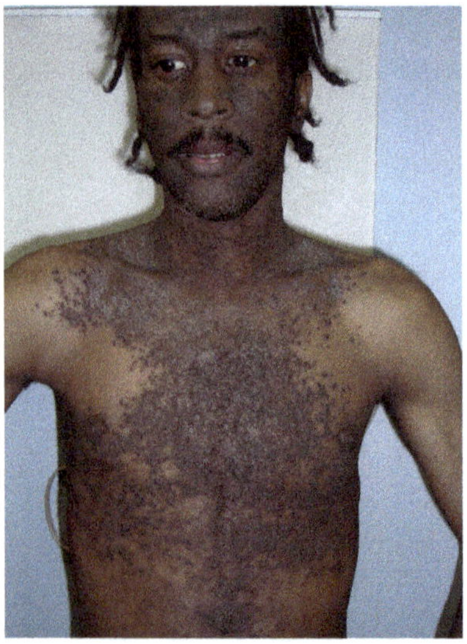

Darier disease with greasy scales, hyperkeratotic and hyperpigmented papules and plaques in a seborrheic distribution involving the face, neck, and chest. (Reproduced, with permission, from Usatine RP, Smith MA, Mayeaux EJ Jr, Chumley HS, eds. *Color Atlas of Family Medicine*. 2nd ed. New York, NY: McGraw-Hill Education; 2012.)

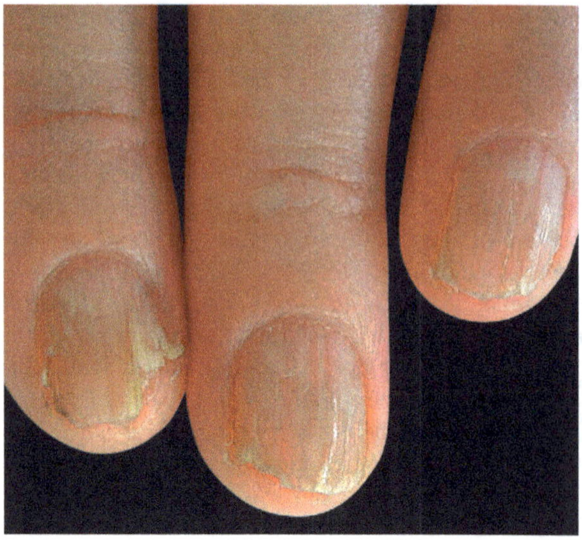

Darier disease. Red and white longitudinal streaks on the fingernails with V-nicking in distal portion of plate. (Reproduced with pemission of Goldsmith LA, Katz SI, Gilchrest BA, Paller AS, Leffell DJ, Wolff K, eds. *Fitzpatrick's Dermatology in General Medicine*. 8th ed. New York, NY: McGraw-Hill Education, 2012.)

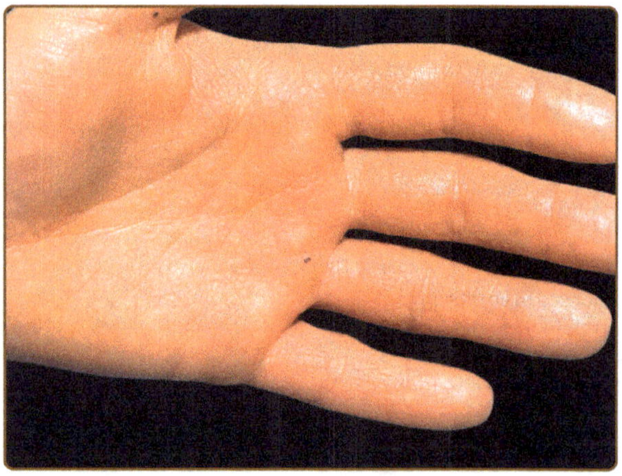

Darier disease. Keratotic papules of the palms. (Reproduced with pemission of Goldsmith LA, Katz SI, Gilchrest BA, Paller AS, Leffell DJ, Wolff K, eds. *Fitzpatrick's Dermatology in General Medicine*. 8th ed. New York, NY: McGraw-Hill Education, 2013.)

Microscopically, the characteristic pattern of **acantholytic dyskeratosis** in **Darier disease** occurs in association with epidermal papillomatosis, acanthosis, and hyperkeratosis. Acantholytic changes giving rise to microscopic lacunae and dyskeratosis develop in the immediate suprabasal zone. Villus structures lined by single cell layers of basal keratinocytes are created by the apparent upward proliferation of the dermal papillae into these lacunae. Lying free within the lacunae are dyskeratotic spinous keratinocytes, which have lost their intercellular bridges and may have prematurely keratinized. In the upper epidermis, the acantholytic cells take the morphologic forms of **corp ronds** and **corp grains**. **Corp ronds** reside in the upper spinous and granular layers and consist of acantholytic cells with homogeneously pyknotic nuclei; a clear pericellular halo; and refractile, basophilic cytoplasms. **Corp grains** are smaller counterparts within the stratum granulosum or higher, displaying pericellular halos and sparse cytoplasms and resembling (but more plump than) parakeratotic corneocytes. The folliculosebaceous elements may have infundibular dilatation and plugging. A perivascular mixed lymphocytic infiltrate occurs in the superficial dermis, which is typically sparse. Variants of **Darier disease** include vesiculobullous lesions, created by large lacunae, and hypertrophic lesions, with accentuation of downward proliferation by the rete.

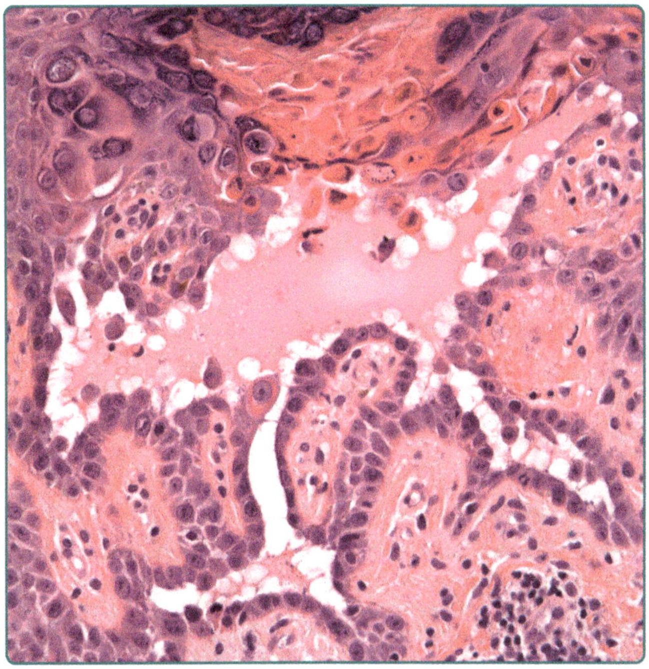

Darier disease. The association of dyskeratosis and acantholysis is seen in this high-power view, which also demonstrates the intraepidermal cleft formation resulting from these phenomena. Note the corp rounds (purple cells) and corp grains (small eosinophilic cells) in the upper strata spinosum/granulosum and stratum corneum. (Reproduced, with permission, from Goldsmith LA, Katz SI, Gilchrest BA, Paller AS, Leffell DJ, Wolff K, eds. *Fitzpatrick's Dermatology in General Medicine*. 8th ed. New York, NY: McGraw-Hill Education; 2012.)

In regards to the differential diagnosis, the pattern of **acantholytic dyskeratosis** is not specific to **Darier disease** because it is often found in **warty dyskeratoma, Grover disease**, and **focal acantholytic dyskeratoma** and may reside as an incidental finding in diverse lesions, such as **verrucae, basal cell carcinoma, keratoacanthoma, psoriasis**, and **angiomata**. **Warty dyskeratoma** is a solitary cup-shaped tumor with central endophytic acantholytic dyskeratosis. **Grover disease** frequently exhibits numerous small foci with combined features of suprabasilar acantholysis (pemphigus-like), acantholytic dyskeratosis (Darier-like), and superficial mixed perivascular inflammatory infiltrates. **Acantholytic dyskeratoma** is a solitary lesion often found incidentally on excision specimens. Although **acantholytic dyskeratosis** may be evident on rare occasion in **Hailey–Hailey disease**, the latter disorder usually exhibits few corp ronds or grains and more widespread acantholysis.

ANSWER 6-25: B.

Hailey–Hailey disease (aka **benign familial pemphigus**) represents a widespread subclinical abnormality of cell adhesion mediated by dissolution of desmosomal plaques (Table 6-25A). Its clinical manifestations, however, are usually restricted to intertriginous anatomic regions that are subject to friction, maceration, and opportunistic infection. This uncommon disorder is genetic, segregating as an autosomal dominant trait linked to chromosome 3q21, and the responsible locus is *ATP2C1*, which encodes a calcium transport ATPase; regulation of cytoplasmic calcium is defective in cultured keratinocytes from patients with the disease.

Clinically, the disease often presents in the second to fourth decades of life with vesicles, bullae, and chronic erosive plaques on the neck and in flexural sites, especially the axillae, inframammary folds, and groin, that are well demarcated, often arcuate, and spread centrifugally. They are subject to exacerbation by perspiration, secondary infection, friction, and heat and confer a burning sensation or mild itch. Uncommon morphologic variants include dermatitic, verrucoid, and papular lesions. Although the condition is chronic, remissions occur, and spontaneous improvement may occur later in the adult years. With rare exceptions, the mucous membranes are unaffected. The erosions are often secondarily infected. Longitudinal white bands may be found in the nail beds.

Table 6-25A. Hailey–Hailey Disease

Clinical Features
Onset in the second to fourth decades of life
Bullae and erosions at flexural sites that are exacerbated by friction and heat
Dermatitic, verrucoid, and papular variants
Histopathologic Features
Widespread acantholysis affecting more than half of the spinous layer
"Dilapidated brick wall" appearance
Infrequent dyskeratotic cells
Villi projecting into lacunae
Acanthosis
Differential Diagnosis
Grover disease
Darier disease
Pemphigus vulgaris

Microscopically, the most typical finding in patients with **Hailey–Hailey disease** is widespread acantholysis of the spinous layer, which characteristically involves at least half the thickness of the epidermis. Acanthosis is usually present. Whereas numerous completely acantholytic cells may be situated free within the resulting intraspinous vesicles, other regions of contiguously affected cells are not completely separated but rather remain partially tethered to each other. When fully developed, this suprabasal change gives an appearance that has been aptly likened to a "dilapidated brick wall." As in **Darier disease**, villus projections of elongated papillae lined by a single row of basal cells often project into the lacunae and bullae. The acantholytic cells generally retain an otherwise normal appearance without morphologically apparent dyskeratosis, but focally, the latter may develop and resemble the corp ronds and grains of **Darier disease**.

In regards to the differential diagnosis, **Hailey–Hailey** and **Darier diseases** share common features of suprabasal acantholysis and formation of villus structures that protrude into separations created by acantholytic keratinocytes. In **Darier disease** (aka **keratosis follicularis**), however, the separations take the form of small lacunae, contrasted with larger vesicles and bullae resulting from more widespread acantholysis in **Hailey–Hailey disease**. Moreover, dyskeratosis is typically a feature of **Darier disease** and is associated with the development of corp ronds and grains. The discrimination of **Hailey–Hailey disease** from **pemphigus vulgaris** may be difficult because the initial pathologic process in each disorder is suprabasal acantholysis. In **pemphigus vulgaris**, however, less acantholysis is present overall, and the separations are often strikingly restricted to the cell layer immediately superficial to the basal keratinocytes, lacking the "dilapidated brick wall" effect of **Hailey–Hailey disease**. When present, the finding of intralesional eosinophils supports the diagnosis of **pemphigus vulgaris**. Definitive resolution of the differential diagnosis requires direct immunofluorescence assay for display of the characteristic intercellular autoantibody deposition in **pemphigus** but not in **Hailey–Hailey disease**. **Bullous impetigo** results in superficial acantholysis restricted to the subcorneal and granular layers due to *Staphylococcus aureus* exotoxin mediated cleavage of desmoglein-1. Full thickness acantholysis, as is seen in **Hailey–Hailey**, is not a feature of **bullous impetigo. Grover disease** (aka **transient acantholytic dermatosis**) is a common, acquired abnormality, which is a nonimmune-mediated, non-congenital acantholytic disorder of the epidermis that affects middle-aged or elderly men most often. The onset is often acute, and the duration may be transient or persistent for several years. Although resembling **Darier** and **Hailey–Hailey diseases**, **Grover disease** does not share an abnormality in the *ATP2A2* or *ATP2C1* genes, respectively. Clinically, **Grover disease** presents with small intensely pruritic papules, and occasionally papulovesicles occurring predominantly on the trunk and less often on the buttocks and thighs. The principal microscopic finding of **Grover disease** consists of small foci of spinous layer acantholysis accompanied by dermal inflammatory infiltrates. The spectrum of acantholysis in **Grover disease** includes both superficial and deep variants, which respectively mimic **pemphigus foliaceus** and **pemphigus vulgaris**. Most often, however, the acantholytic changes are accompanied by prominent **Darier-type dyskeratosis**. Robust inflammatory infiltrates are generally not a feature of **Darier** or **Hailey–Hailey diseases**, unless superimposed infection is present.

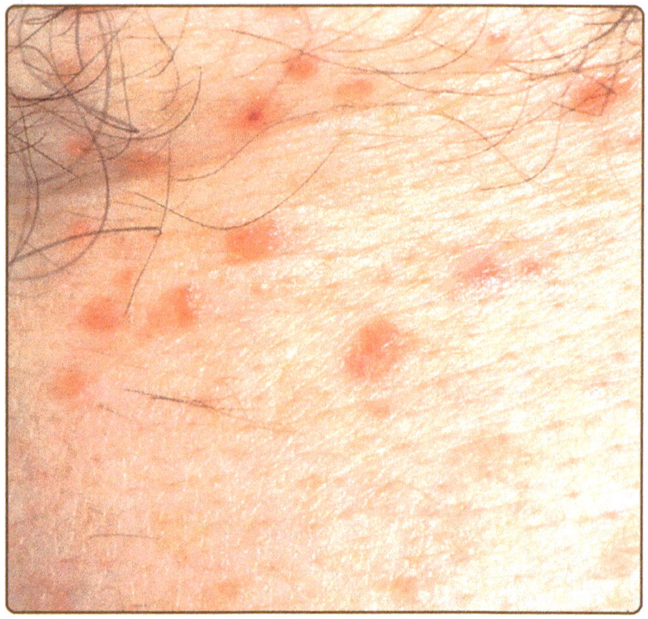

Grover disease. Discrete papulovesicular lesions with crusts in a 53-year-old man. (Reproduced, with permission, from Goldsmith LA, Katz SI, Gilchrest BA, Paller AS, Leffell DJ, Wolff K, eds. *Fitzpatrick's Dermatology in General Medicine.* 8th ed. New York, NY: McGraw-Hill Education; 2012.)

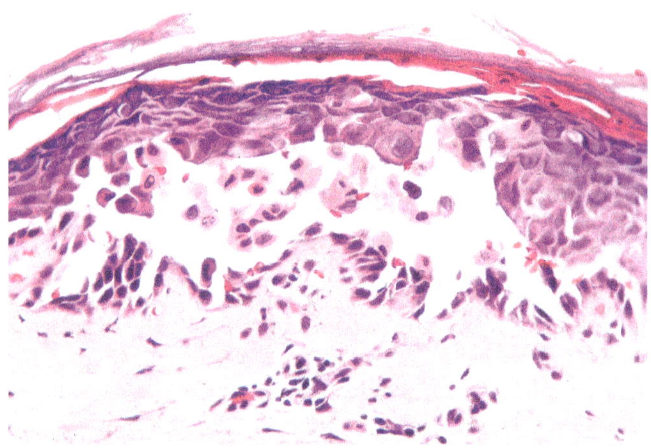

Grover disease. This microscopic lacuna, which has been created by acantholysis restricted to the suprabasal keratinocytes, contains dyskeratotic cells and is lined at the base by cells anchored to the basement membrane. Corp ronds and grains are situated in the upper epidermal strata.

ANSWER 6-26: B.

This patient unfortunately has the **Herlitz type of junctional epidermolysis bullosa (JEB)**, also referred to as **lethal junctional epidermolysis bullosa. Junctional epidermolysis bullosa** includes several genetically heterogeneous diseases that, although phenotypically variable, share autosomal recessive transmission and subepidermal separation through the lamina lucida of the basement membrane zone due to reduced numbers of hemidesmosomes. All forms of **JEB** share the pathologic feature of trauma-induced bullae formation within the lamina lucida of the basement membrane. **JEB** can be classified into three main subgroups distinguished by their clinical and genotypic characteristics: **junctional epidermolysis bullosa of the Herlitz type, junctional epidermolysis bullosa of the non-Herlitz type**, and **junctional epidermolysis bullosa with pyloric atresia**. Patients with the **Herlitz type** often do not survive infancy with a mortality rate reaching 40% during the first year of life. There is generalized blistering at birth or shortly thereafter and clinically distinctive and severe periorificial granulation, loss of nails, and involvement of most mucosal surfaces. The skin of these children may be completely denuded, representing oozing painful erosion. Associated findings include all symptoms resulting from generalized epithelial blistering with respiratory, gastrointestinal, and genitourinary organ system involvement. The **non-Herlitz type** characteristically presents at birth with a similar yet milder eruption to the **Herlitz type**, at a later age (4-10 years) with lesions involving the scalp, nails, and periorificial non-healing erosions, or with a condition characterized by blisters that heal with scarring. **Junctional epidermolysis bullosa with pyloric atresia** presents at birth with severe mucocutaneous fragility and gastric outlet obstruction. Gene analysis will reveal mutations in genes that encode the α3, the β3, and χ2 polypeptide chains of laminin 5 in the **Herlitz type**, BPAG2 (BP180) in the **non-Herlitz type**, and the α6 and β4 integrin subunits in the **pyloric stenosis type**. More severe phenotypes (**Herlitz type**) are linked to premature termination codon mutations in both alleles of one of the three laminin 5 subunit genes, *LAMB3*, but the less severe variants are associated with slice junction or missense mutations of one allele in trans to a premature termination codon mutation of the other (Table 6-26B).

Histopathologically, all variants of **JEB** are characterized by the formation of subepidermal blisters associated with sparse inflammatory infiltrates in the dermis. On immunomapping using antibodies to type IV collagen, the split localizes to the lamina lucida. Immunohistochemical staining for type IV collagen (lamina densa) will reveal staining along the base of the blister cavity. Direct and indirect immunofluorescence examinations are negative. Mutation analysis demonstrating the gene defect confirms the diagnosis (Table 6-26A).

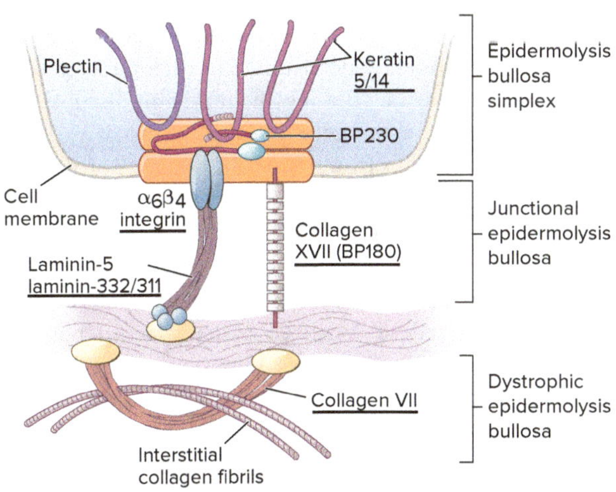

Schematic of the components of dermal–epidermal basement membrane (underlined items in the left panel) and levels of dermal-epidermal separation in hereditary bullous diseases with dermal-epidermal cleavage. (Reproduced, with permission, from Wolff K, Johnson RA, Saavedra AP. *Fitzpatrick's Color Atlas and Synopsis of Clinical Dermatology.* 7th ed. New York, NY: McGraw-Hill Education; 2013.)

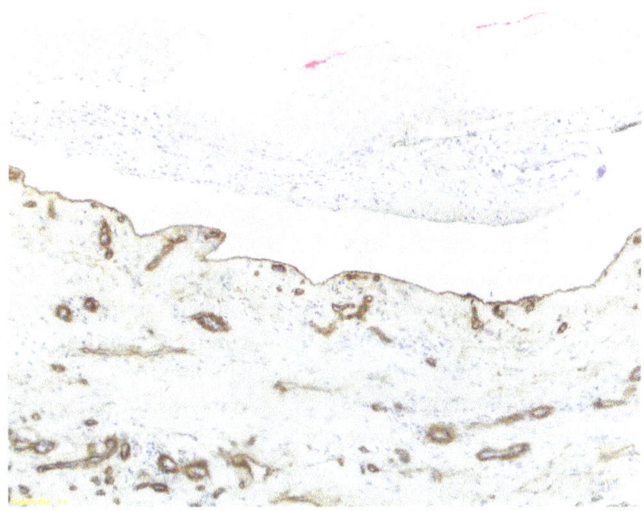

Type IV collagen immunohistochemistry in JEB. There is linear staining along the base of the blister cavity, indicating that the defect and plane of cleavage to be within the lamina lucida.

Table 6-26A. Diagnostic Criteria of Junctional Epidermolysis Bullosa

1. Histology: Subepidermal blister with sparse infiltrates in the dermis
2. Epitope mapping using antibodies against type IV collagen: Intra-lamina lucida split
3. Mutation analysis:
   - Mutations of the genes coding for the α3, β3, or χ2 polypeptide chains of laminin 5
   - Mutations of the gene encoding for the α6 or the β4 integrin subunits
   - Mutations of the gene encoding for BPAG2 (BP180)

Table 6-26B. Variants of Junctional Epidermolysis Bullosa and Their Molecular Defects

	MOLECULAR DEFECT	MODE OF INHERITANCE	ONSET	BLISTERS	OTHER CHANGES
Junctional epidermolysis bullosa of Herlitz type (JEB-H)	Mutations of the genes coding for the α3, the β3, and the χ2 polypeptide chains of laminin 5	Autosomal recessive	Birth or shortly thereafter	Generalized	Dystrophic nails, dysplastic teeth, growth retardation, anemia, mucous membrane lesions
Junctional epidermolysis bullosa of the non-Herlitz type (JEB-nH)	Mutations of the genes encoding for BPAG2 or any of the three polypeptide chains of laminin 5	Autosomal recessive	Birth, shortly thereafter or in early childhood	Localized or generalized	There may be pigmentary changes, dystrophic nails, and dysplastic teeth
Junctional epidermolysis bullosa with pyloric atresia (JEB-PA)	Mutations of the genes encoding for α6 or the β4 integrin subunits	Autosomal recessive	Birth or shortly thereafter	Generalized	Congenital esophageal, pyloric or duodenal atresia, aplasia cutis congenital, renal abnormalities

In regards to the histopathological differential diagnosis, the microscopic findings of **JEB** are nonspecific and can be seen in other diseases as **cell-poor bullous pemphigoid, epidermolysis bullosa acquisita, porphyria cutanea tarda, pseudoporphyria, dystrophic epidermolysis bullosa**, and **epidermolysis bullosa simplex.** By light microscopy, **junctional epidermolysis bullosa** may be simulated by **dystrophic epidermolysis bullosa** or by subepidermal autoimmune vesiculobullous disorders such as **bullous pemphigoid.** The clinical context will direct the histopathologic interpretations along the appropriate pathways. Resolution of the differential diagnosis for the mechanobullous disorders is usually obtained by immunolabeling for markers of basement membrane components, such as type IV collagen and laminin, to localize the plane of separation or by electron microscopy. The autoimmune disorders are confirmed diagnostically by the characteristic patterns of autoantibody deposition as shown by direct immunofluorescence methods.

ANSWER 6-27: D.

The biopsy reveals prominent cytolytic degeneration of basal and suprabasal keratinocytes. **Epidermolysis bullosa** represents a group of **mechanobullous diseases** that have in common heritable lesions in genes coding for structural proteins of basal keratinocytes or for components of the basement membrane zone. **Epidermolysis bullosa simplex** is a genetically heterogeneous disease that shares an autosomal dominant inheritance, pathophysiologic changes of minor trauma–induced cytolysis within the basal or suprabasal keratinocytes, and the tendency for lesions to heal without scarring. Tonofilament clumps within basal and suprabasal keratinocytes are observed by electron microscopy in the **Dowling–Meara variant of epidermolysis bullosa simplex**; these structures contain the keratin pair 5 and 14 by immunolabeling. Point mutations occur in either gene (*K5* or *K14*) in all clinical variants of **epidermolysis bullosa simplex**. The clinical severity is evidently determined in each affected kindred by the extent to which the specific mutation disrupts the functional properties of the gene product. Unusual variants of the disorder may result from mutations in other structural genes, such as the cell-linker protein plectin. The clinical phenotypes include the **generalized Koebner variant**; the **Dowling–Meara variant**, which is characterized by herpetiform clustering of blisters; and the **Weber–Cockayne variant**, which is characterized by localized (usually acral) blisters. The **Weber–Cockayne variant** may represent a mild variant of the **Koebner variant**. Whereas the **Dowling–Meara** and **Koebner variants** usually present early in infancy with blisters and erosions induced by minor trauma, the onset of the **Weber–Cockayne** variant is often delayed. Mucosal lesions, minor scarring, nail shedding, and widespread erosions with a risk of secondary pyogenic infection occur in severely affected patients. Spontaneous improvement is sometimes seen in later childhood and adulthood.

Microscopically, in all variants of **epidermolysis bullosa simplex**, vesicles form by cytolysis within the basal or lower

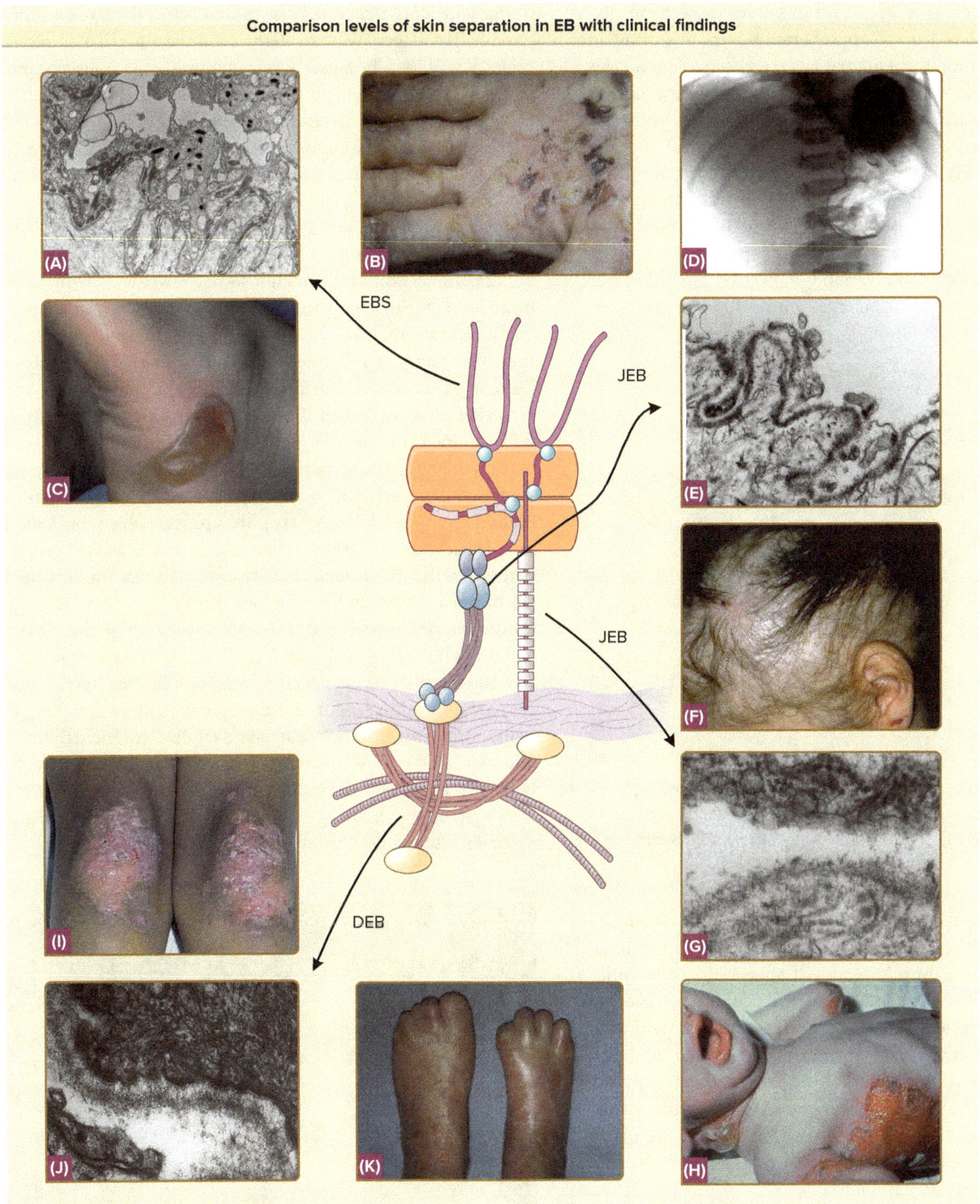

Comparison of levels of skin separation in epidermolysis bullosa with clinical findings. **(A)** Transmission electron micrograph showing typical intraepidermal separation in epidermolysis bullosa simplex (EBS). **(B)** Palmar hyperkeratosis and herpetiform erosions in EBS (Dowling–Meara variant). **(C)** Localized blister on heel in EBS (Weber–Cockayne variant). **(D)** Radiograph showing pyloric atresia associated with junctional epidermolysis bullosa (JEB). **(E)** Transmission electron micrograph showing typical separation at level of hemidesmosome in JEB with pyloric atresia, alternatively classified as EBS or JEB. **(F)** Nonscarring diffuse alopecia and scalp erosions in generalized atrophic benign junctional epidermolysis bullosa (non-Herlitz type). **(G)** Transmission electron microscopy showing typical intralamina lucida separation in JEB. **(H)** Generalized blistering in Herlitz JEB. **(I)** Localized dystrophic changes with milia in dominant dystrophic epidermolysis bullosa (JEB). **(J)** Transmission electron microscopy showing typical sublamina densa separation in DEB. **(K)** Pseudosyndactly in recessive DEB. EBS = epidermolysis bullosa simplex; DEB = dystrophic epidermolysis bullosa; JEB = junctional epidermolysis bullosa. (Reproduced, with permission, from Goldsmith LA, Katz SI, Gilchrest BA, Paller AS, Leffell DJ, Wolff K, eds. *Fitzpatrick's Dermatology in General Medicine*. 8th ed. New York, NY: McGraw-Hill Education; 2012.)

spinous cell layers. Histologic sections thus show focal dissolution of the basal or spinous keratinocytes, resulting in epidermal separation through that layer. Dyskeratotic changes may manifest histopathologically within the cells, especially in the **Dowling–Meara variant**. The cleavage plane occurs above the lamina densa; therefore, immunohistochemical staining for type IV collagen will reveal deposition along the floor of the blister cavity. On occasion, the **Dowling–Meara** and **Koebner variants** have been associated with **palmoplantar keratoderma** in which the histologic sections exhibit compact hyper-orthokeratosis and a variably thickened granular layer in addition to the cytolytic changes within the keratinocytes. Lesions typically heal without significant scarring.

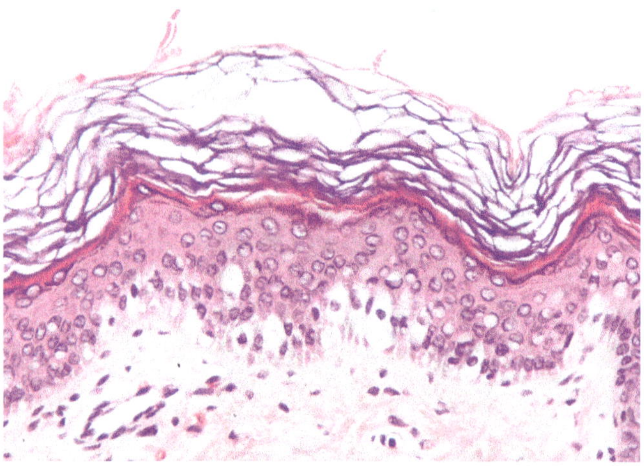

Epidermolysis bullosa simplex, Dowling–Meara variant. Basal and suprabasal keratinocytes display prominent cytolytic degeneration. The more superficial epidermal layers appear normal.

In regards to the differential diagnosis, in the **Dowling-Meara subtype**, the separation may occur deep in the basal layer such that by light microscopy it appears that the entire epidermis has formed the roof of the blister; this may simulate the findings in **junctional epidermolysis bullosa** and may require electron microscopy or immunomapping of basement membrane components for resolution of the level of the separation. The **Dowling–Meara variant** is distinguished from the other two varieties by herpetiform clustering of the clinical lesions and by keratin filament clumping on electron microscopy of lesional skin samples.

ANSWER 6-28: D.

Dystrophic epidermolysis bullosa (DEB) is characterized by trauma-induced blisters that heal with scarring and milia. **DEB** is genetically heterogeneous, with either autosomal dominant or recessive inheritance (Table 6-28A). Cases of **dystrophic epidermolysis bullosa** have long been known to demonstrate morphologic abnormalities of the anchoring fibrils, which are structures distributed below the basal lamina. Type VII collagen was an early candidate for the etiologic molecular defect because it is a major collagenous component of the anchoring fibrils. Immunolabeling for type VII collagen demonstrates either reduced content or disarrayed organization of this component. Genetic studies confirmed linkage between markers for the collagen VII locus on chromosome 3 and both the dominantly and recessively inherited clinical phenotype; mutational analyses subsequently confirmed mutations in the *COL7A1* gene. Clinically, **DEB** may be autosomal dominant or autosomal recessive. **Autosomal dominant DEB** comprises four subtypes: (1) dystrophic epidermolysis bullosa with congenital, localized absence of the skin (**Bart syndrome**); (2) **dystrophic epidermolysis bullosa—Cockayne-Touraine variant**; (3) **albopapuloid dystrophic epidermolysis bullosa**, or **dystrophic epidermolysis bullosa, Pasini type**; and (4) **transient bullous dermatolysis of new-born**. **Autosomal recessive DEB** encompasses two subtypes: (1) **dystrophic epidermolysis bullosa—Hallopeau-Siemens type** and (2) **dystrophic epidermolysis bullosa—non-Hallopeau-Siemens type**. As a reflection of genetic heterogeneity, the clinical severity of **dystrophic epidermolysis bullosa** varies widely. On one hand, the recessive form (**Hallopeau–Siemens syndrome**) presents in infancy with extensive blistering and scarring of the entire cutaneous and squamous mucosal surfaces of the oropharynx, anus, and esophagus, eventuating in mutilating deformities, shedding of nails, joint contractures, pseudosyndactylies, enteric strictures, and increased risk of squamous cell carcinoma, which may be clinically aggressive. The phenotype of the dominant form, although also exhibiting mechanically induced blisters and secondary scarring, is usually much less severe.

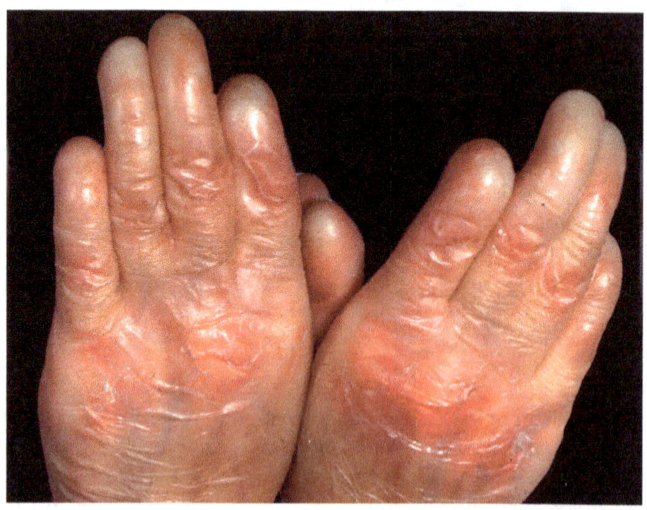

Generalized recessive dystrophic epidermolysis bullosa (Hallopeau–Siemens type). Loss of all fingernails, syndactyly, and severe atrophic scarring on the dorsa of hands. (Reproduced, with permission, from Wolff K, Johnson RA, Saavedra AP. *Fitzpatrick's Color Atlas and Synopsis of Clinical Dermatology*. 7th ed. New York, NY: McGraw-Hill Education; 2013.)

Table 6-28A. Variants of Dystrophic Epidermolysis Bullosa: Features and Molecular Defects

	MOLECULAR DEFECT	MODE OF INHERITANCE	ONSET	BLISTERS	OTHER CHANGES
1. Bart syndrome	Mutations of the gene coding for type VII collagen	Autosomal dominant	Birth	Affects skin and mucous membranes	Congenital absence the skin, dystrophic or absent nails
2. Dystrophic epidermolysis Cockayne-Touraine (DEB-CT)	Mutations of the gene coding for type VII collagen	Autosomal dominant	Birth, infancy, early childhood	Localized mainly to extremities	Dystrophic nails
3. Dystrophic epidermolysis bullosa, albopapulodea	Mutations of the gene coding for type VII collagen	Autosomal dominant	Blisters: birth, infancy, early childhood: adolescence	Localized mainly to extremities	Albopapuloid papules, dystrophic nails
4. Transient bullous dermatolysis of newborn	Mutations of the gene coding for type VII collagen	Autosomal dominant	Birth	Generalized, disappear spontaneously in the first few months of life	
5. Dystrophic epidermolysis bullosa-Hallopeau-Siemens	Mutations of the gene coding for type VII collagen	Autosomal recessive	Birth or shortly thereafter	Generalized and heal with marked scarring	Contracture, mittenlike deformities, scarring alopecia, dysplastic teeth, dystrophic nails, mucosal strictures, ocular involvement
6. Dystrophic epidermolysis bullosa-non-Hallopeau-Siemens	Mutations of the gene coding for type VII	Autosomal recessive	Birth or shortly thereafter	Generalized	Dysplastic teeth, dystrophic nails

Histopathologically, all variants of **DEB** are characterized by the formation of a subepidermal blister with sparse lymphocytic infiltration in the upper dermis (Table 6-28B). In recurrent lesions, fibrosis and/or milia may be present. On immunomapping using antibodies to type IV collagen, the blister localizes to the sublamina densa region. DIF and IF examinations are negative. Mutation analysis confirms the diagnosis by showing the gene defect.

In regards to the differential diagnosis, the histopathology of **DEB** is not diagnostic and can be seen in such other diseases as **cell-poor bullous pemphigoid, epidermolysis bullosa acquisita, porphyria cutanea tarda, pseudoporphyria**, and **junctional epidermolysis bullosa**. It should therefore be correlated with the clinical findings, the results of immunofluorescence, and immunomapping with antibodies to type VII collagen. Immunostaining for type IV collagen will reveal deposition along the roof of the blister cavity, confirming that the basal lamina remains attached to the epidermis. Immunostaining also demonstrates reduced labeling for collagen type VII in the anchoring fibril zone.

Table 6-28B. Diagnostic Criteria of Dystrophic Epidermolysis Bullosa

Histology: Subepidermal blister with sparse infiltrates in the dermis
Epitope mapping using antibodies against type IV collagen: Sublamina densa blister
Mutation analysis: Mutations of the gene coding for type VII collagen

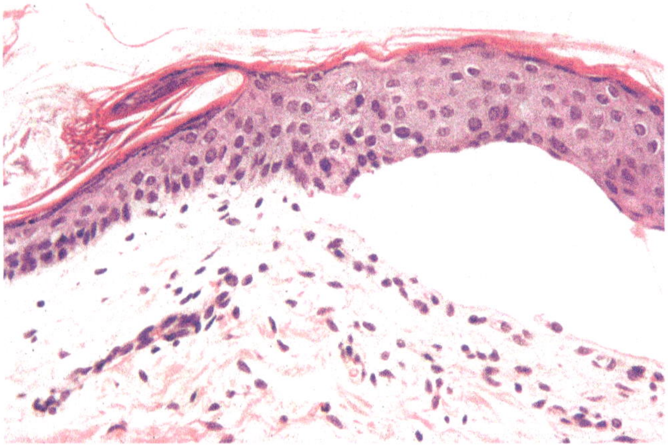

Dystrophic epidermolysis bullosa. There is a subepidermal blister with minimal inflammation. Dermal fibrosis is present.

ANSWER 6-29: B.

This patient has **migratory necrolytic erythema (glucagonoma syndrome)**, in which patients develop multiple cyclical perioral, perineal, and acral vesicles and pustules that rupture to form weeping and scaling circinate erythematous plaques and erosions. These lesions arise in the setting of systemic amino acid degradation and negative nitrogen balance due to elevated levels of serum glucagon, resulting in sustained gluconeogenesis. This patient's pancreatic mass is an alpha islet cell tumor that secretes high levels of glucagon. Noncutaneous manifestations of **glucagonoma syndrome** include glucose intolerance, weight loss, and anemia. Microscopically these cutaneous lesions are characterized by zonal necrosis of the upper half of the epidermis with an unremarkable or slightly psoriasiform hyperplastic underlying epidermis. The necrotic layer is formed by hydropic pale keratinocytes with pyknotic nuclei, extravasated plasma, neutrophils, and parakeratotic scale crust. The zonal necrosis may separate from the underlying viable epidermis, resulting in vesiculation or neutrophilic pustulation. The subcorneal bullae can be distinguished from **pemphigus foliaceus** and **pemphigus erythematosus** by the absence of acantholytic cells which are characterized by separated keratinocytes, rounded in shape with a brightly eosinophilic band of keratin beneath the cell membrane. The cells of **necrolytic migratory erythema** are true necrotic keratinocytes via cytolysis. Resolving nonbullous lesions may closely resemble psoriasis with acanthosis, hypogranulosis, and broad parakeratosis.

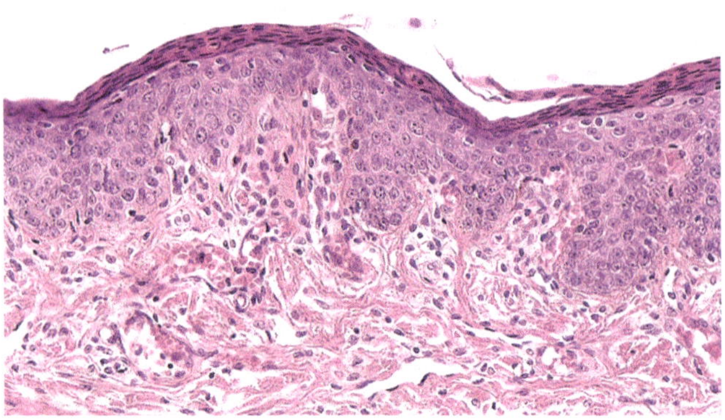

Resolving well-developed lesion of migratory necrolytic erythema. This well-developed lesion displays confluent parakeratosis, absence of the granular layer, and psoriasiform epidermal hyperplasia.

The histopathological differential diagnosis includes exogenous **trauma** (ie, excoriation), **pellagra, acrodermatitis enteropathica, necrolytic acral erythema**, and **hand, foot, and mouth disease**. Rarely are the effects of physical trauma limited exclusively to the upper layers of the epidermis. The histopathologic findings of the latter entities are strikingly similar, except that **necrolytic acral erythema** exhibits concomitant cytotoxic interface dermatitis. **Pellagra, acrodermatitis enteropathica, necrolytic acral erythema**, and **hand, foot, and mouth disease** are associated with niacin deficiency, zinc deficiency, HCV infection, and Coxsackie virus infection, respectively. Clinical correlation is essential.

ANSWER 6-30: C.

The biopsy demonstrates epidermal invagination surfaced by thick hyperkeratosis. At the base of the invagination, the epidermal keratinocytes exhibit reactive eosinophilic cytoplasm and abrupt keratinization. There is basophilic karyorrhectic debris admixed with inflammatory cells. Eosinophilic and basophilic (degenerated) collagen fibers, elastic fibers, and fibrin are seen penetrating through the epidermis. This histopathology may be seen in any of the four primary perforating dermatoses: **reactive perforating collagenosis, Kyrle disease, elastosis perforans serpiginosa**, and **perforating folliculitis** (answer choices A, B, D, and E, respectively). These conditions have traditionally been defined among the conditions displaying transepidermal elimination of stromal elements (Table 6-30A). In addition, numerous reports have discussed secondary transepidermal elimination in association with a clearly identifiable primary cutaneous process. The prototype for the primary perforating diseases is **Kyrle disease**, as described early in the early 1900s. With further studies, however, it became evident that there are more clinicopathologic similarities than there are differences between **Kyrle disease** and the other entities, which has obscured the criteria that were originally advanced for their recognition. Kyrle disease itself may not be a distinct entity but rather the extreme phenotype of a more common pathophysiologic process. **Perforating folliculitis** and **reactive/acquired perforating collagenosis**, according to the current trend for unification, may be phenotypic variants of a disease spectrum or merely different stages in lesional development. The term **reactive perforating collagenosis** has been used to represent an inherited form

Table 6-30A. Primary Perforating Dermatoses

	KYRLE DISEASE/ ACQUIRED PERFORATING COLLAGENOSIS	REACTIVE PERFORATING COLLAGENOSIS	PERFORATING FOLLICULITIS	ELASTOSIS PERFORANS SERPIGINOSA
Age of onset	4th decade (avg.)	Childhood	3rd decade (avg.)	2nd decade (avg.)
Site	Extensor lower and upper extremities; head, neck, and trunk	Upper and lower extremities; face	Hair-bearing portions of extremities	Nape of neck; upper extremities; face; lower extremities
Disease associations	Renal failure, hemodialysis, diabetes mellitus, hepatic insufficiency	None	Idiopathic, minor association with renal failure, hemodialysis, diabetes mellitus	Down syndrome; Ehlers–Danlos syndrome; osteogenesis imperfecta; pseudoxanthoma elasticum
Koebner phenomenon	Occasionally	Positive	Negative	Occasionally
Mode of inheritance		Autosomal recessive and autosomal dominant		Occasionally autosomal dominant

that manifests in childhood, whereas **acquired perforating collagenosis** has been used for the sporadic form that occurs in adulthood. It is still debated whether **perforating folliculitis** represents a true primary perforating disease since ruptured follicles are a feature of many infective conditions, such as *Pityrosporum* folliculitis. Given these considerations and in view of their common clinical association with renal disease and diabetes mellitus, **Kyrle disease, adult onset acquired perforating collagenosis**, and **perforating folliculitis** have been incorporated for the present purposes under the general "umbrella" designation of **acquired perforating dermatosis**. Many also incorporate **elastosis perforans serpiginosa** under this designation since there is strikingly similar histopathology. **Elastosis perforans serpiginosa** has a distinctive clinical presentation, which will be discussed below. Answer choice C describes the clinical presentation of **chondrodermatitis nodularis helicis.**

Acquired perforating dermatosis (including Kyrle disease, perforating folliculitis, and adult onset acquired perforating collagenosis) is commonly associated with chronic renal failure, hemodialysis, and diabetes mellitus. Its pathogenesis is poorly understood and has been the subject of wide-ranging conjecture, which includes theories of alterations in vitamin A metabolism, accumulation of nondialyzable metabolic products recognized as foreign by the skin, disordered keratinocyte maturation (ie, keratinization occurring at the expense of proliferation), and an unusual effect of humoral and cell-mediated immunity. The pathophysiologic mechanism may not be the same for all cases of **acquired perforating dermatosis**; rather, the mechanism may represent a common response pathway to a variety of epidermal and dermal alterations acting alone or in combination. The common association with uremia during the early phases of hemodialysis tends to support the theory of dermal deposition of a nondialyzable toxic metabolite. Autosomal recessive inheritance patterns in some kindreds diagnosed with **childhood onset reactive perforating collagenosis** have raised the possibility of a genetic diathesis in those instances. The pathogenesis of **elastosis perforans serpiginosa** remains unclear, but some cases are familial, with an autosomal dominant pattern of inheritance, indicating a genetic substrate. The frequent association in approximately 25% of patients with either **Down syndrome** or an inborn disorder of connective tissue metabolism, such as **Ehlers–Danlos syndrome, osteogenesis imperfecta, pseudoxanthoma elasticum**, or **Marfan syndrome**, suggests that the pathophysiology is based on a molecular defect in the connective tissues. Some cases have been coincident with penicillamine therapy. From these associations, hyperplastic connective tissue fibers may act as local irritants, provoking epidermal hyperplasia that envelops the altered material, which is then carried upward by the process of keratinocyte differentiation for transepidermal elimination.

Quick Fact

Primary Perforating Disease

Reactive perforating collagenosis (childhood onset)

Acquired perforating collagenosis

- Kyrle disease
- Adult onset acquired perforating collagenosis
- Perforating folliculitis

Elastosis perforans serpiginosa*

*Degenerated elastic fibers are predominantly extruded over collagen fibers, but both are typically present.

In regards to the clinical presentation of **acquired perforating dermatosis**, the florid (Kyrle disease–like) presentation is rare, but the milder phenotype is rather common in the setting of chronic renal failure, diabetes, or (less commonly) liver disease. At clinical presentation, which may occur at any age, there may be few to many lesions, which are often localized to the legs, or the onset may be more generalized to all extremities and the torso, with a predilection for the extensor surfaces. The mucous membranes and volar surfaces are spared. The condition is characteristically pruritic but not invariably so. The early lesions are pinhead-sized follicular and extrafollicular papules that resemble **keratosis pilaris**. With progression, the lesions evolve into larger, red-brown or purplish papules and nodules or occasionally plaques and tend to remain non-confluent. Mature lesions display a central cuplike depression containing a conical, keratinous plug. An isomorphic (Koebner) response is frequent, especially in the inherited form (**reactive perforating collagenosis**). It is uncommon for the condition to remit spontaneously, but improvement may occur after renal transplantation. The lesions of **elastosis perforans serpiginosa**, which are often asymptomatic, occur in arcuate to annular arrays that are characteristically localized to one region of the body, most often the nape but on occasion the face or upper extremities. The lesions are coalescent flesh-colored or erythematous, keratotic papules with central invaginations. There may be clinical resemblance to **granuloma annulare** or **porokeratosis of Mibelli**. Spontaneous remissions occur.

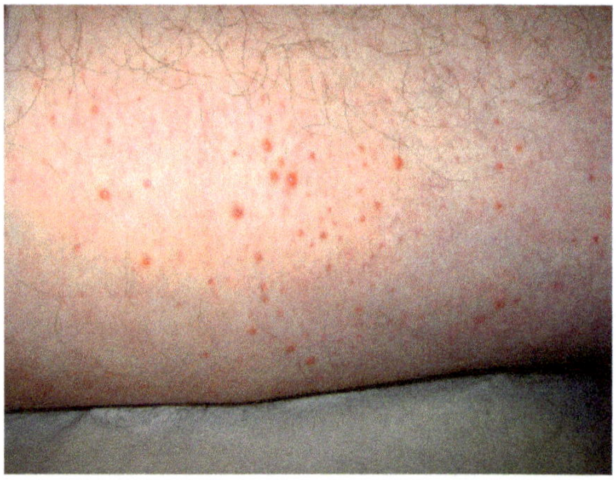

Perforating folliculitis. Multiple follicular, erythematous, firm papules with variable central crusting. (Reproduced, with permission, from Goldsmith LA, Katz SI, Gilchrest BA, Paller AS, Leffell DJ, Wolff K, eds. *Fitzpatrick's Dermatology in General Medicine*. 8th ed. New York, NY: McGraw-Hill Education; 2012.)

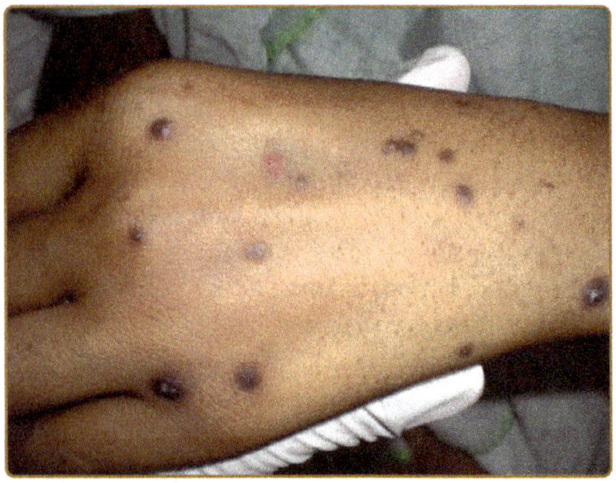

Acquired perforating collagenosis, adult onset. Multiple, round, hyperpigmented papules, each with a central keratotic plug, distributed on the extensor aspects of the hand and wrist in a patient with chronic kidney disease. (Reproduced, with permission, from Goldsmith LA, Katz SI, Gilchrest BA, Paller AS, Leffell DJ, Wolff K, eds. *Fitzpatrick's Dermatology in General Medicine*. 8th ed. New York, NY: McGraw-Hill Education; 2012.)

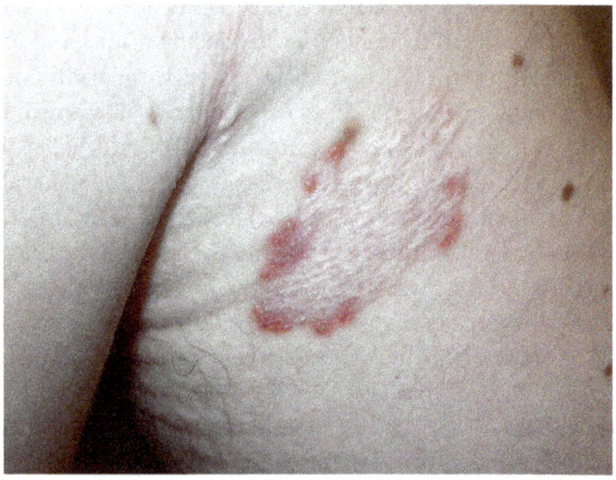

Acquired elastosis perforans serpiginosa in a patient taking penicillamine for Wilson disease. Annular plaque with variably crusted erythematous papules at the periphery and central cribriform scarring. (Reproduced, with permission, from Goldsmith LA, Katz SI, Gilchrest BA, Paller AS, Leffell DJ, Wolff K, eds. *Fitzpatrick's Dermatology in General Medicine*. 8th ed. New York, NY: McGraw-Hill Education; 2012.)

Microscopically, early lesions of **acquired perforating dermatosis** are associated with variable acanthosis, follicular and perifollicular hyperkeratosis, neutrophils in the subjacent dermis, and (variably) tinctorial changes in the connective tissue fibers. Some foci are clearly follicular, and others are perifollicular. The central cuplike keratotic plug within the epidermal invagination overlies the locus of epithelial perforation, with its apex oriented downward. Some reports describe vacuolar changes in the keratinocytes at the base of the plug and breaks in the basement membrane before channelization. The basophilic material undergoing transepidermal elimination is composed of a mixture of inflammatory cells and karyorrhectic debris, a parakeratotic column of keratinous material, and fragments of basophilic collagen or eosinophilic elastin. At the base may be a foreign-body granulomatous reaction, with or without a suppurative inflammatory component, occurring after the epithelium has been breached. The walls of the channels are bordered by flattened, anucleate, and variably glycogenated keratinocytes, which suggest premature keratinization. These altered keratinocytes follow the outflow of material through the epidermis. Extracellular lysosomal enzymes derived from the neutrophils may play an initiating role by altering elastin and collagen (with its basophilic degeneration) and possibly opening up the channel. Under this model, however, the mechanism initiating the chemoattraction of the neutrophils is undefined. The findings of **elastosis perforans serpiginosa** are strikingly similar, except that transepidermal elimination of altered elastin occurs through a central, narrow channel with a funnel-like or corkscrew configuration.

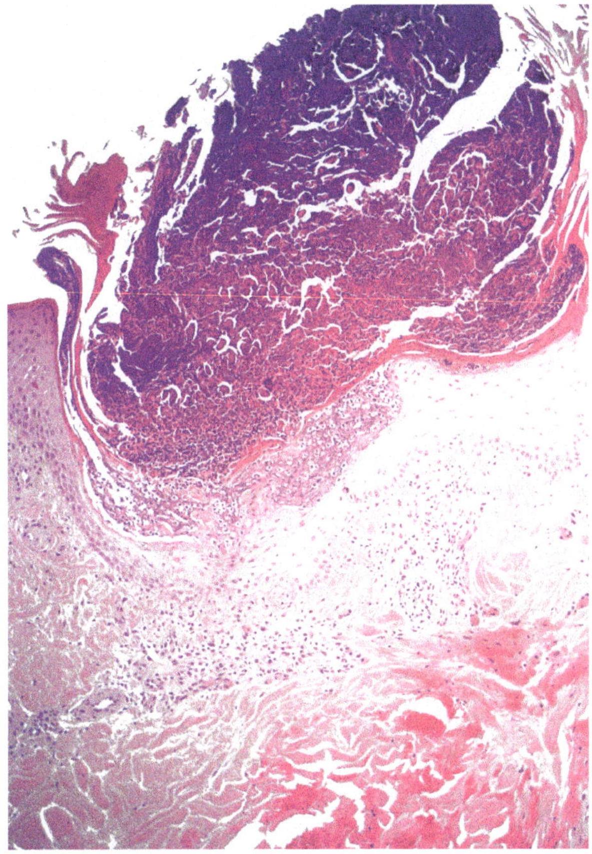

Acquired perforating dermatosis. The perforation is situated at an extrafollicular site.

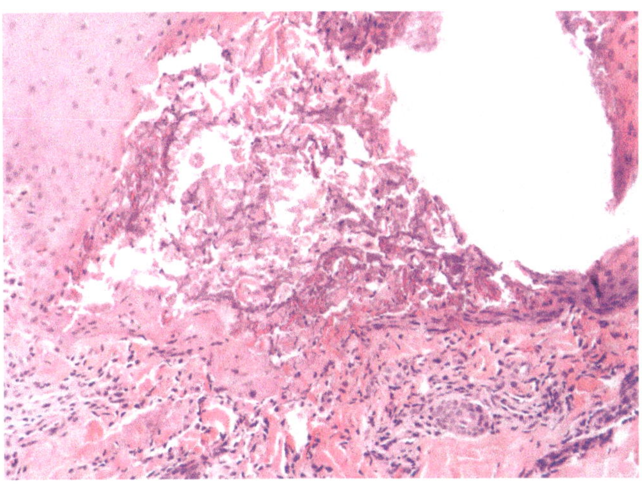

Acquired perforating dermatosis. The perforation in this follicular lesion has occurred through the infundibulum. Brightly eosinophilic elastin fibers are seen within the basophilic collagenous debris filling the transepithelial channel. The adjacent stroma contains a sparse, mixed mononuclear infiltrate.

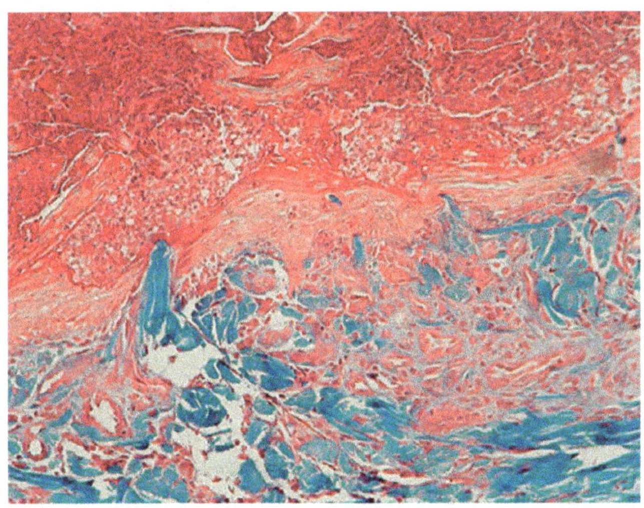

Acquired perforating dermatosis, trichrome stain (stains collagen blue). Collagen bundles can be seen crossing from the reticular dermis through the epidermis into an epidermal depression containing necrotic debris. (Reproduced, with permission, from Goldsmith LA, Katz SI, Gilchrest BA, Paller AS, Leffell DJ, Wolff K, eds. *Fitzpatrick's Dermatology in General Medicine*. 8th ed. New York, NY: McGraw-Hill Education; 2012.)

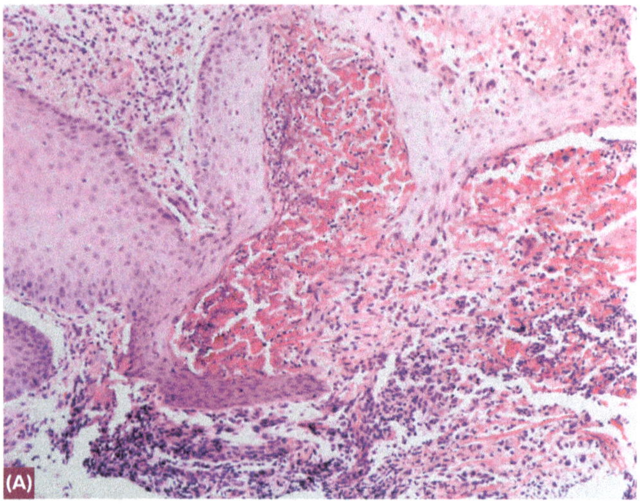

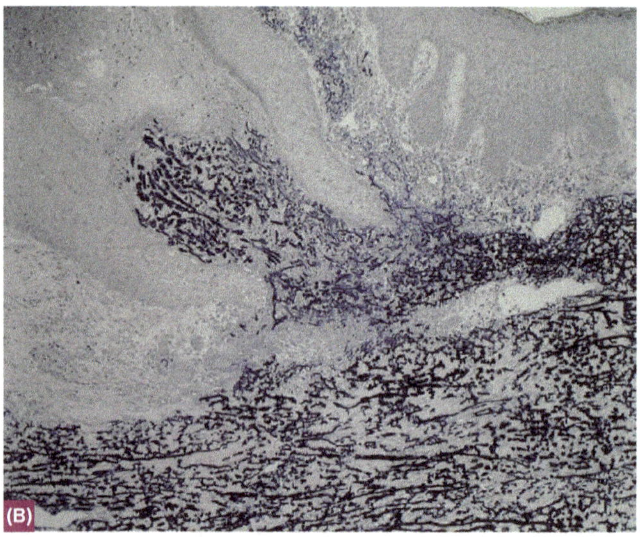

Acquired elastosis perforans serpiginosa. (A) Dilated follicular structure with transepidermal elimination of densely eosinophilic elongated bundles (Hematoxylin and eosin stain). **(B)** Transepidermally eliminated elongated bundles are elastin fibers (elastin stain). (Reproduced, with permission, from Goldsmith LA, Katz SI, Gilchrest BA, Paller AS, Leffell DJ, Wolff K, eds. *Fitzpatrick's Dermatology in General Medicine*. 8th ed. New York, NY: McGraw-Hill Education; 2012.)

In regards to the differential diagnosis, no absolute criteria discriminate the classic perforating dermatoses of **Kyrle disease, perforating folliculitis**, and **reactive/acquired perforating collagenosis** because transepidermal elimination of altered collagen, elastin, or both via a central, cuplike invagination may occur in each. The locus of the elimination may be follicular, extrafollicular, or both. Moreover, each condition may be associated with chronic renal failure or diabetes mellitus. Observation of an infundibular locus with hair material destined for transepidermal elimination, as defined for perforating folliculitis, may depend on the stage of disease or the extent of the histologic sampling of the biopsy specimen. For these reasons, it seems arbitrary to separate them. **Elastosis perforans serpiginosa** also exhibits histologic similarities, but this condition is distinctive clinically, and it exhibits microscopically a definite increase in the number and thickness of the papillary dermal elastic fibers on elastin stains. A cuplike invagination plugged with keratinous material is a feature of **keratosis pilaris**, but there should be no epithelial breach nor elimination of degenerated collagen or elastin in the condition.

Chondrodermatitis nodularis chronica helicis (CNH) (answer choice C) is a unique form of perforating disease that presents as one or two and rarely several, at times bilateral, small 2- to 3-mm dome-shaped papules, usually at the apex of the helix or antihelix. The nodules are remarkably tender for their bland clinical appearance, and attempts to examine them are frequently met with a prominent withdrawal response by the patient. A central, small, crusted or plugged umbilication is usually present. Patients are classically elderly males. The exact pathogenesis is unknown; however, the condition is most likely attributed to impaired blood supply to the ear. Associations include prolonged and excessive pressure, collagen vascular disease (ie, dermatomyositis), diabetes mellitus, and solar elastosis. Microscopically, within the center of a lesion of **CNH** is usually a dilated, horn-filled follicular infundibulum, often with perforation of the infundibular epithelium at its base. Scale crust may also overlie an epidermal ulceration, adjacent to which are features simulating **prurigo nodularis** or **lichen simplex chronicus**, including hyperkeratosis, hypergranulosis, irregular epidermal hyperplasia, and dense fibrosis of the papillary dermis. At the base of the ulceration or perforation is prominent fibrin deposition. At times, the dermis has a chondroid appearance with fibroblasts simulating chondrocytes, and there is adjacent fibrosing granulation tissue. Ear cartilage at the base of the lesion is often uninvolved.

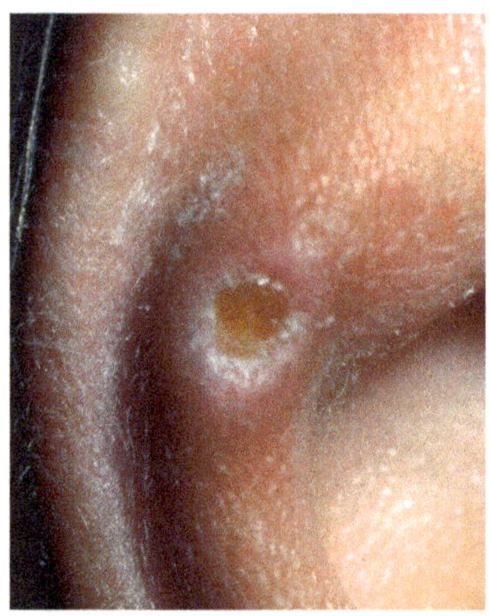

Chondrodermatitis nodularis helicis. An extremely painful nodule with central ulceration on the antihelix of a 60-year-old female. The central ulcer is covered with a crust and can be mistaken for a basal cell carcinoma. (Reproduced, with permission, from Wolff K, Johnson RA, Saavedra AP. *Fitzpatrick's Color Atlas and Synopsis of Clinical Dermatology*. 7th ed. New York, NY: McGraw-Hill Education; 2013.)

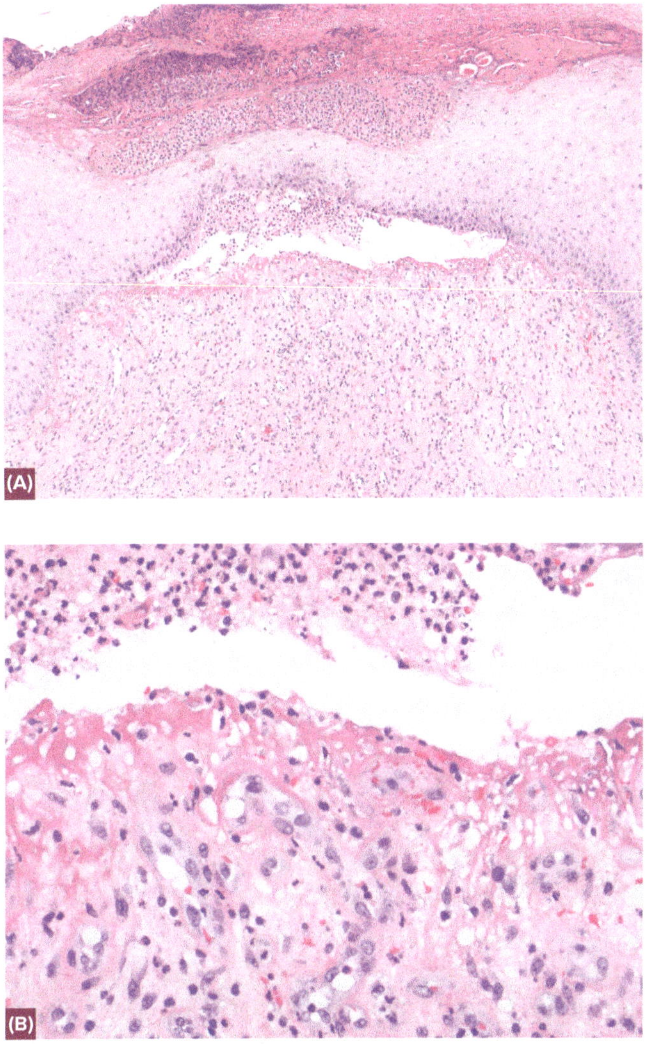

Chondrodermatitis nodularis helicis. **(A)** There is an ulcerated epidermal surface with adjacent hyperplastic changes. The underlying dermis contains granulation tissue. **(B)** There is a thick band of fibrinoid material at the ulcer base that is being eliminated transepidermally.

ANSWER 6-31: B.

Various substances may form deposits in the skin. They may be classified as endogenous and exogenous. Endogenous substances include substances that are normal constituents of the skin but are abnormally deposited (ie, increased deposition of mucin) and substances that are not normal constituents of the skin (ie, amyloid). Abnormal deposition of endogenous substances exhibits particular histochemical staining properties. However, different substances may show similar staining by the hematoxylin and eosin (H&E) stain. These deposits with similar staining properties are often grouped together and were once considered to be the same chemical substances. Examples are **amyloid, hyaline**, and **colloid**. In fact, these terms are frequently used interchangeably in microscopic descriptions of H&E-stained tissue sections that contain eosinophilic amorphous material. The dermatopathologist then focuses on the subset of conditions that manifests these particular characteristics. Special stains, immunostains, electron microscopy, and clinical information provide further aid in the differential diagnosis. In many instances, clinical knowledge is essential in the final synthesis of all data to reach a reasonable conclusion. This process is always at work in the experienced pathologist's mind. An algorithmic approach to differential diagnosis is presented in the figure below.

"**Hyaline**" is not a single substance. Traditionally, this term has included a variety of skin deposits that appeared eosinophilic and somewhat glassy because of the refraction of light. **Hyaline** stains bright pink on PAS stain and is diastase resistant. Therefore, the recognition of **hyaline** invokes the differential diagnosis of a limited yet diverse group of conditions. **Hyaline** is therefore a nonspecific "umbrella term" and includes **basement membrane material, colloid**, and **amyloid**. Additional stains may be used to further decipher the precise nature of the material.

Amyloid was once considered to be a single substance regardless of the differences in clinical presentations. It is now known that the origin and chemical nature of amyloid are quite diverse. Why then do we still use the term "**amyloid**"? The answer is that so-called "**amyloid**" defined by Virchow as a starch-like, iodine-stainable substance shares several common characteristics, including an eosinophilic amorphous appearance with the H&E stain. Congo red staining results in a red appearance under normal light microscopy, and a doubly refractile apple green color under polarized light. Thioflavine T fluorescence also produces a green color under UV-light. **Amyloid** reveals straight, nonbranching filaments (6-10 nm in diameter) are seen on electron microscopy. **Amyloid** stains dark purple with crystal violet stain. Keratin, immunoglobulin, insulin, thyrocalcitonin, and other chemical substances can produce β-pleated anti-parallel polypeptide sheets and therefore are amyloidogenic. All **amyloid** deposits, irrespective of their chemical nature and the clinical type of **amyloidosis**, have a common **amyloid P** component, which is a nonfibrillar protein derived from a serum precursor, known as serum **amyloid P (SAP)**. **Amyloid** can be detected by immunohistochemical stains on paraffin-embedded sections using antibodies against human component P (**anti-SAP**); however, the specificity of this reaction is limited because **amyloid P** is also present in elastic tissue. The current classification of **amyloidoses** is based on the chemical nature of the **amyloids** with significant consideration of the conventional clinical subclassification.

"**Colloid**" refers to globular pale eosinophilic material. In many cases, this material represents **keratin-derived amyloid** (ie, **juvenile colloid milium, colloid bodies** of interface dermatitis) or **degenerated elastic tissue** (ie, **adult colloid milium**). The material is PAS positive-diastase resistant and variably positive for Congo red stain.

Dermal mucin or **protein–hyaluronic acid complex** is a normal component of the dermal connective tissue produced by

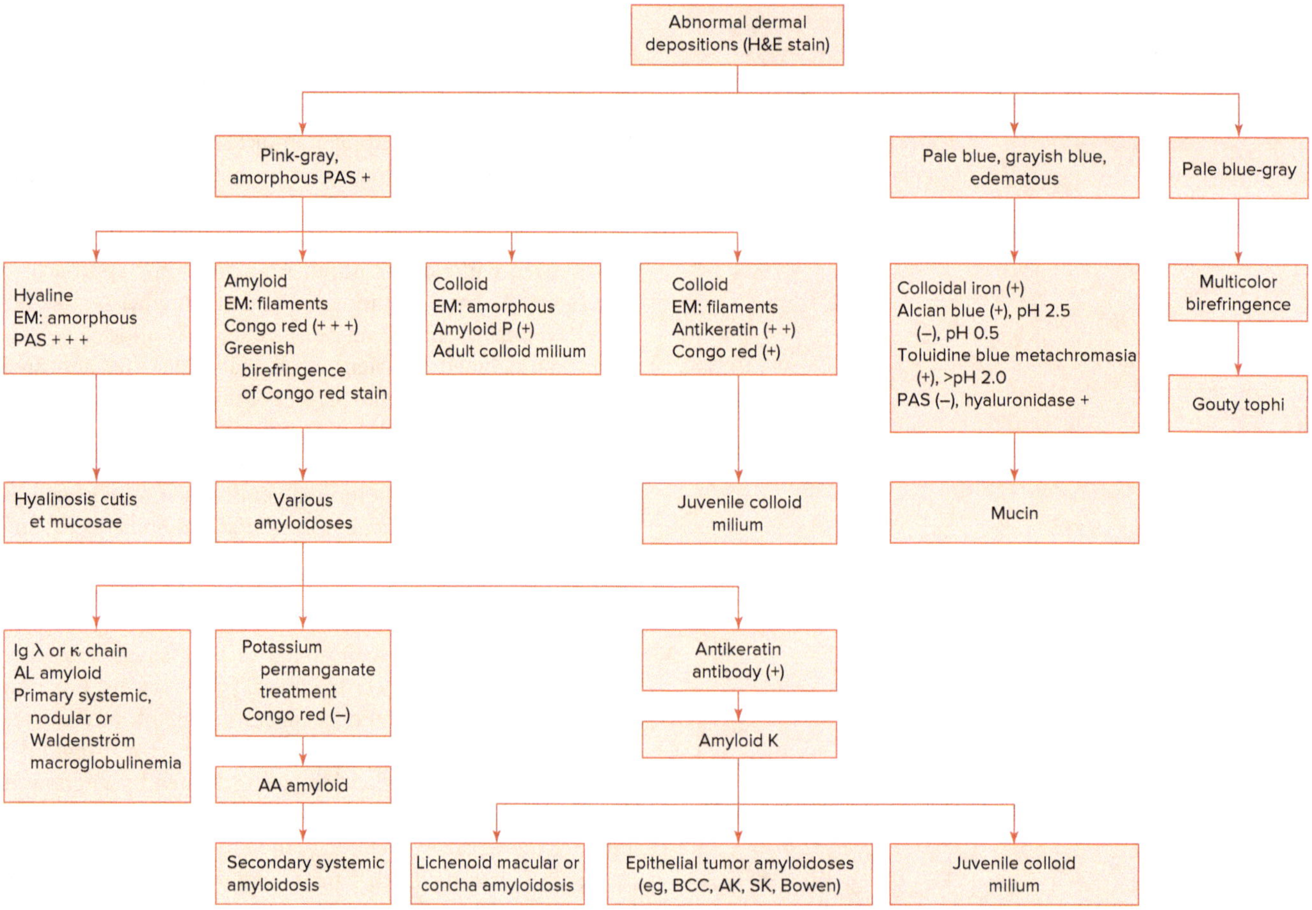

fibroblasts and mast cells. In disease conditions, it is increased, and because **hyaluronic acid** holds water (hygroscopic), the dermal connective tissue is swollen (**myxedema**). If this condition persists, the dermis and sometimes the subcutaneous connective tissues react with production of excessive collagen, leading to scleroderma-like fibrosis (**scleromyxedema**). **Mucin** is usually present in early lesions and may diminish or even disappear in late stages. Also, during tissue processing, **mucin** may largely be washed out. If one suspects **mucin** deposition because of light blue staining between widely separated collagen bundles or empty spaces, special stains should be used such as Alcian blue at a pH of 2.5 (negative at 0.5), toluidine blue

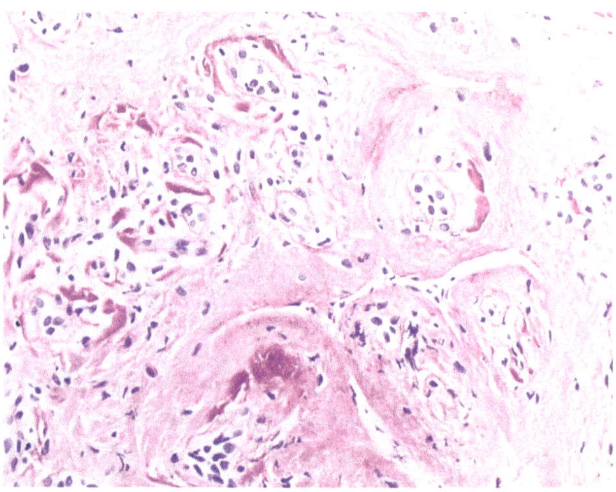

PAS stain with diastase reveals bright pink hyaline material deposited around vessels in a case of porphyria. This material represents excessive accumulations of basement membrane material.

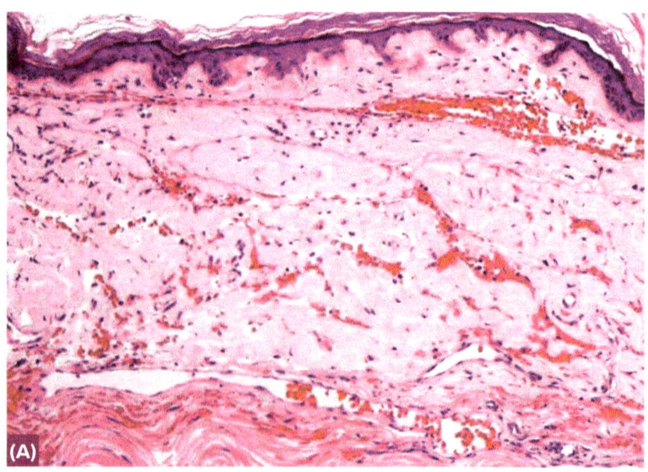

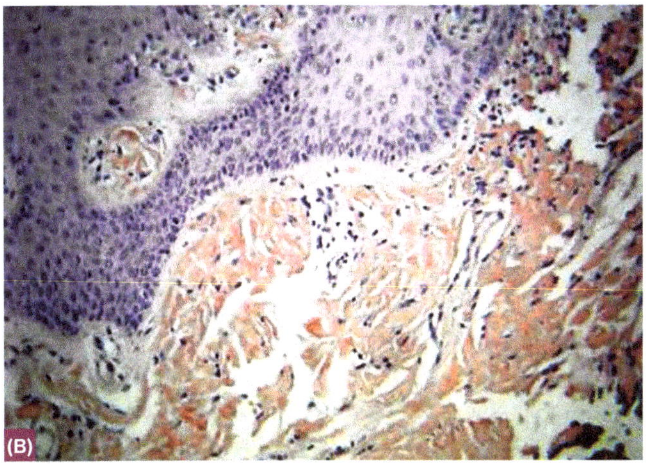

Systemic amyloid light chain amyloidosis. (A) A hyaline substance (ie, amyloid) occupies the entire dermis. There are some fissures and hemorrhages with vascular ectasia. **(B)** Congo red stain highlights the red material in the dermis, consistent with amyloid.

with metachromasia at a pH of 4.0 and 7.0 (negative below 2), and colloidal iron. The **mucin** stains bright blue. Furthermore, **mucin** is hyaluronidase sensitive and periodic acid Schiff (PAS) negative. Fixation in absolute alcohol may improve detection. Monoclonal antibodies to hyaluronan, although not routinely indicated, have been used.

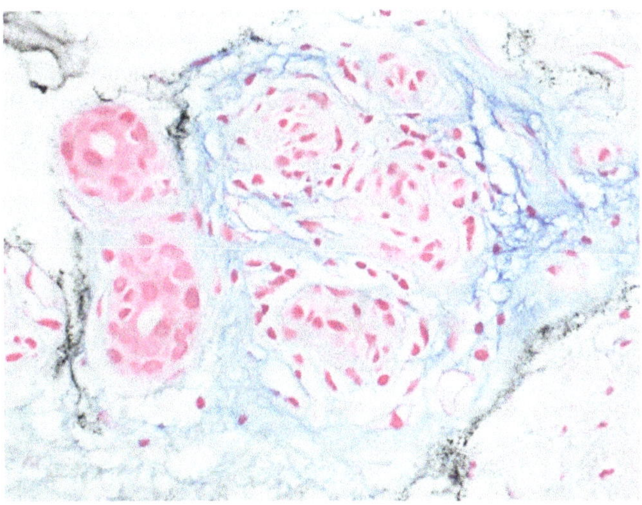

Alcian blue stain. The bright blue material in between the collagen bundles is dermal mucin.

ANSWER 6-32: B.

The **cutaneous mucinoses** are a heterogeneous group of disorders in which an abnormal amount of mucin deposits in the skin. The cutaneous mucinoses are categorized into two groups: **primary cutaneous mucinoses**, in which the mucin deposit is the main histologic feature resulting in clinically distinctive lesions, and **secondary mucinoses**, in which the mucin deposition is only an additional histologic finding. A typical example of **secondary mucinosis** is **granuloma annulare**, in which mucin deposition is associated with necrobiotic-palisaded granulomas, which is the diagnostic hallmark. **Primary cutaneous mucinoses** are further categorized into degenerative and inflammatory forms, which may be dermal, follicular, hamartomatous, and neoplastic forms. Diagnosing a **primary dermal mucinosis** on histologic grounds alone is a difficult task and always requires clinicopathologic correlation. Three histopathologic clues should be considered: the pattern of mucin distribution, the level of mucin deposition in the dermis, and some additional findings such as the numbers of fibroblasts and collagen deposition. The microscopic pattern of mucin distribution may be diffuse or focal. In the former, it is interstitial and poorly circumscribed (**generalized myxedema, pretibial myxedema, lymphedematous mucinosis**, and **scleromyxedema**); in the latter, mucin is localized and well circumscribed (ie, **focal cutaneous mucinosis**).

Pretibial myxedema is most commonly observed in patients with established **hyperthyroidism** (usually due to **Graves' disease**) that has been treated. These patients are usually euthyroid by the time they develop this condition, although they may still exhibit exophthalmos. With regard to pathophysiology, a serum factor (unrelated to long-acting thyroid-stimulating factor or hormone) seems to stimulate fibroblasts to produce mucin. Fibroblasts from the dermis of the lower extremities have been found to be more sensitive to this factor than are fibroblasts from other areas of the body. An insulin-like growth factor, trauma, and lymphatic obstruction due to mucin may be involved. The anterior shins and occasionally dorsal feet demonstrate elevated, knobby plaques or dome-shaped nodules. The cutaneous surface is shiny or waxy, and peau d'orange follicular openings with follicular plugging are noted in new lesions. In severe cases, marked edema and verrucoid surface changes, possibly resembling elephantiasis nostras verrucosa, may be seen. Rarely, the condition affects the shoulder, arms, and abdomen. After biopsy, transparent, viscous fluid continues to ooze.

Microscopically, the typical features consist of conspicuous, diffuse deposition of mucin (glycosaminoglycans) throughout the reticular dermis with attenuation of collagen fibers. With extensive deposition of mucin, the collagen fibers are frayed, fragmented, and widely separated. Spindle-shaped and large stellate fibroblasts appear to float in the edematous areas, but the number of fibroblasts is not increased. Lymphatic dilated vessels can be seen. In chronic lesions, increased collagen production occurs in the deep dermis and subcutaneous fat, resulting in the replacement of fat lobules by fibrosis. Alcian blue stain is strongly positive and differentiates mucin from conventional **lymphedema**. Hyperkeratosis and follicular plugging, the presence of mast cells, and sparse lymphoid infiltrates with occasional eosinophils are additional findings.

Generalized myxedema is associated with a severe form of **chronic hypothyroidism.** The face, particularly the eyelids and lips, are prominently swollen, and the entire skin is dry, pale, waxy, and edematous but not pitted with pressure.

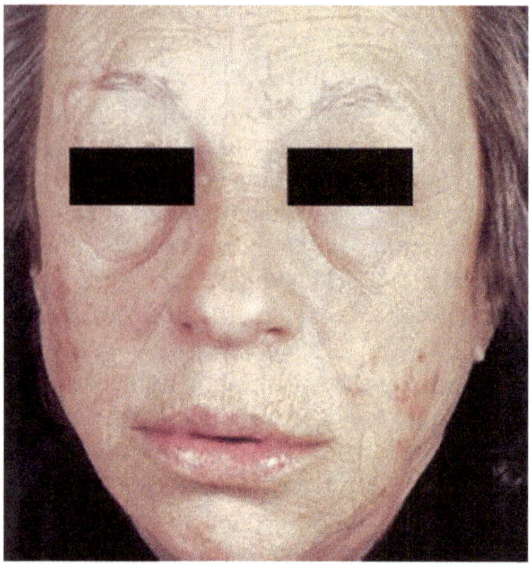

Typical features of severe hypothyroidism (generalized myxedema), including dry doughy skin, coarse hair, periorbital puffiness, lateral thinning of the eyebrows, and a dull and apathetic facial expression. (Reproduced with permission from Wolff K, Goldsmith LA, Katz SI, et al. *Fitzpatrick's Dermatology in General Medicine*. 7th ed. New York, NY: McGraw-Hill; 2008.)

Microscopic features of **generalized myxedema** include hyperkeratosis, occasional keratinous cysts **(epidermoid cysts)**, and only slight mucin accumulation within the dermis in most cases; usually requiring mucin stains for confirmation. The mucin is frequently deposited around the blood vessels and hair follicles of the upper and mid-dermis only. In some instances, there is massive accumulation of mucin, resulting in the disruption of collagen bundles, similar to **pretibial myxedema**. Usually, fibroblasts are not increased. Elastic fibers are fragmented and reduced. In the late stages, fibrosis in the deep dermis and subcutis may simulate **scleroderma**. The diagnosis is mainly clinical, and histopathologic findings are only confirmatory.

In regards to the differential diagnosis, **pretibial myxedema** should be distinguished from **lymphedematous mucinosis** associated with chronic obesity without thyroid disease. In the latter, vesicles and bullae, semitranslucent papules, or woody plaques are found on the shins in the setting of morbid obesity and bilateral pitting edema of the distal lower extremities. Histopathologically, epidermal atrophy with effacement of the rete ridge pattern, mucin deposition within the superficial papillary dermis, perivascular glomeruloid neovascularization, and hemosiderin deposition are seen. **Lipodermatosclerosis** also occurs on the lower extremities, but is associated with deep dense sclerosis and does not contain increased mucin.

ANSWER 6-33: B.

Myxedematosus is a chronic idiopathic disorder characterized by lichenoid papules, nodules, or plaques in the absence of thyroid disease, which includes two clinicopathologic subsets: (1) a generalized and sclerodermoid form (also called **scleromyxedema**) associated with a monoclonal gammopathy and systemic, even lethal, manifestations and (2) a localized form (**lichen myxedema**) that does not run a disabling course (Table 6-33A). The terms **lichen myxedematosus, scleromyxedema**, and **papular mucinosis** are often used interchangeably; however, an attempt to identify the clinicopathologic subset should be pursued. Occasional patients have overlapping or atypical features and fall between having **scleromyxedema** and **localized lichen myxedematosus**. In **scleromyxedema**, a widespread symmetric eruption of closely set papules, often arranged in a linear array and accompanied by skin thickening, involves the face, upper trunk, and peripheral extremities. Involvement of the glabella gives rise to leonine facies. The localized form, in which the papules are confined to only a few sites (usually the limbs and trunk) in the absence of paraproteinemia and systemic features, include four subtypes: a **discrete papular mucinosis, acral persistent papular mucinosis, cutaneous mucinosis of infancy**, and **nodular lichen myxedematosus**. An association of **discrete lichen myxedematosus** with HIV infection, toxic oil syndrome, eosinophilia myalgia syndrome, and hepatitis C virus (HCV) infection has been reported. **Self-healing papular mucinosis**, both of the juvenile and adult types, previously considered as a subtype of localized lichen myxedematosus, is probably a mucinosis suis generis.

Microscopically, in **scleromyxedema**, patients have a characteristic triad that includes diffuse mucin deposition in the upper and mid-reticular dermis, increased collagen deposition, and a marked proliferation of irregularly arranged fibroblasts. The epidermis is usually normal, but in old

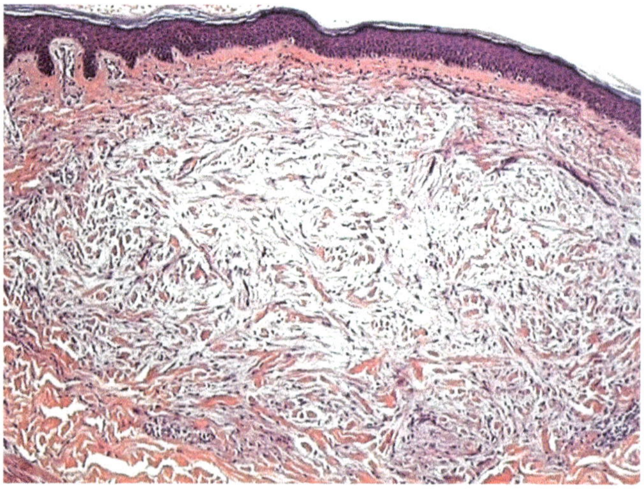

Scleromyxedema. The characteristic triad of mucin deposition, fibroblast proliferation, and fibrosis in the upper and mid-dermis.

Table 6-33A. The Cutaneous Mucinoses

DERMAL AND FOLLICULAR DEGENERATIVE/ INFLAMMATORY MUCINOSES	DISTRIBUTION, CHARACTERIZATION	ASSOCIATED DISORDERS	HISTOPATHOLOGIC FEATURES
Generalized myxedema	Generalized waxiness, non pitting, waxy facial edema	Hypothyroidism	Scant mucin, upper dermis around blood vessels, hair follicles
Pretibial myxedema	Shin, dorsal feet	Thyrotoxicosis, treated	Prominent mucin, lower two-thirds of dermis, hyperkeratosis, follicular plugging, mast cells
Myxedematosus (papular mucinosis)			
– Scleromyxedema	Generalized papules, including face, sclerodermoid features	Monoclonal gammopathy, systemic involvement	Diffuse mucin, upper dermis, increased collagen and fibroblasts
Localized forms (lichen myxedematosus)			
– Discrete type	Papules on trunk and extremities	Sometimes HIV	Focal or diffuse mucin, upper dermis, variable increased numbers of fibroblasts
– Acral persistent papular mucinosis	Papules on dorsa of hands and forearms		Focal mucin, upper dermis, grenz zone, normal fibroblast number
– Self-healing juvenile mucinosis	Children, linear infiltrated plaques, head, trunk, thighs; deep periarticular nodules	Sometimes rheumatologic symptoms	Mucin, upper dermis, increased fibroblasts, mast cells
– Cutaneous mucinosis of infancy	Firm papules on extremities		Focal mucin, papillary dermis
Scleredema	Induration of upper back, nape	Diabetes, acute infection, monoclonal gammopathy	Thickened dermis, fenestrated collagen, mucin may be absent on H&E stain, normal fibroblast number
Focal mucinosis	Solitary papulo-nodule		Focal mucin in dermis, clefts
Digital mucous cyst	Distal interphalangeal joint, posterior nail fold	Arthrosis	Focal mucin in dermis, collagen pseudocapsule
Mucocele of the lip, oral mucous cyst	Mucosal side of lower lip		Sialomucin (PAS+) with inflammatory reaction
Papular and nodular mucinosis associated with lupus erythematosus	Lumpy papulonodules, trunk and extremities	LE (mainly SLE)	Diffuse mucin in reticular dermis, normal epidermis, lymphocytic infiltrate
Follicular mucinosis	Tumid plaques with follicular papules, alopecia, face and scalp	Mycosis fungoides	Mucin within pilosebaceous units, lymphocytes, eosinophils

lesions, it may be thinned by the pressure of the underlying mucin and fibrosis; the follicles may be atrophic; and a slight perivascular, superficial lymphoplasmacytic infiltrate is often present. Rarely, eosinophils are found. The elastic fibers are fragmented and decreased in number. Reactive sweat gland proliferation is an occasional finding.

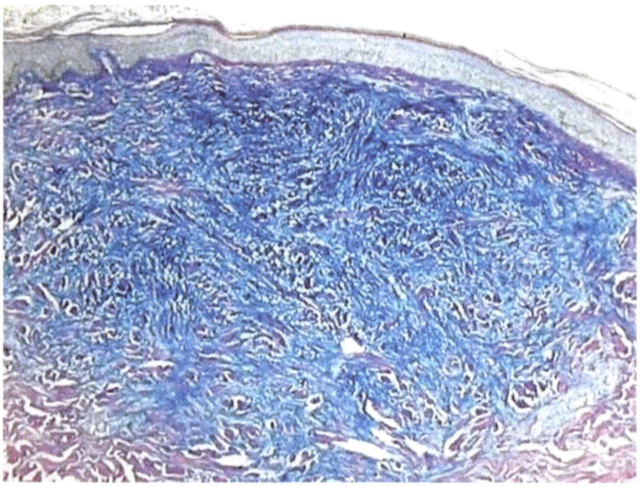

Scleromyxedema. Colloidal iron stain confirms increased mucin deposition in the upper dermis.

The changes in **localized lichen myxedema** are not as characteristic as in **scleromyxedema** but are still recognizable. The pattern of mucin distribution may be diffuse or focal, involving the upper and mid-reticular dermis. Fibroblast proliferation is variable. Fibrosis is not marked and may even be absent. In **acral persistent papular mucinosis**, a large, focal, well-circumscribed amount of mucin sparing a subepidermal zone is seen. Fibroblast proliferation is lacking. In **cutaneous mucinosis of infancy**, sometimes the mucin deposition in the papillary dermis is pronounced as to appear "hugged" by the epidermis.

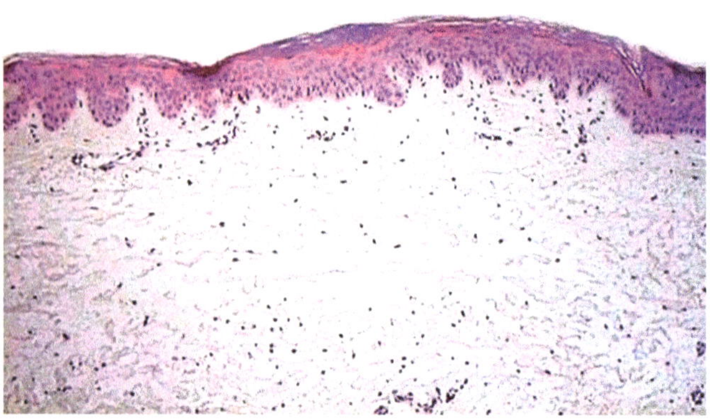

Localized lichen myxedematosus (papular mucinosis) of the discrete type. Increased mucin deposition splitting collagen fibers in the upper dermis with slight fibroblast proliferation and absence of fibrosis.

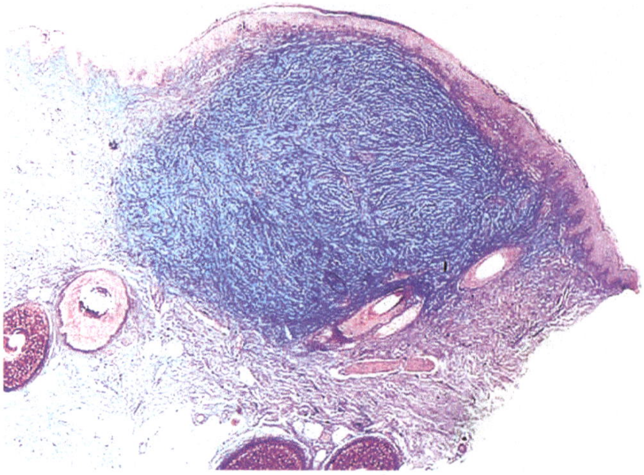

Acral persistent papular mucinosis. Pattern of focal dermal deposition of mucin. Alcian blue stain; pH, 2.5.

In regards to the differential diagnosis, **scleromyxedema** can only be distinguished from the other mucinoses by clinical features and dermal fibrosis, which is not observed in the other mucinoses until the late stages. Outside of **myxedematosus**, the differential diagnosis includes **nephrogenic systemic fibrosis (nephrogenic fibrosing dermopathy)** and **granuloma annulare**. Nephrogenic systemic fibrosis is observed in patients with renal disease and more recently liver failure and a history of exposure to gadolinium-containing contrast agents. This entity is microscopically similar to **scleromyxedema**.

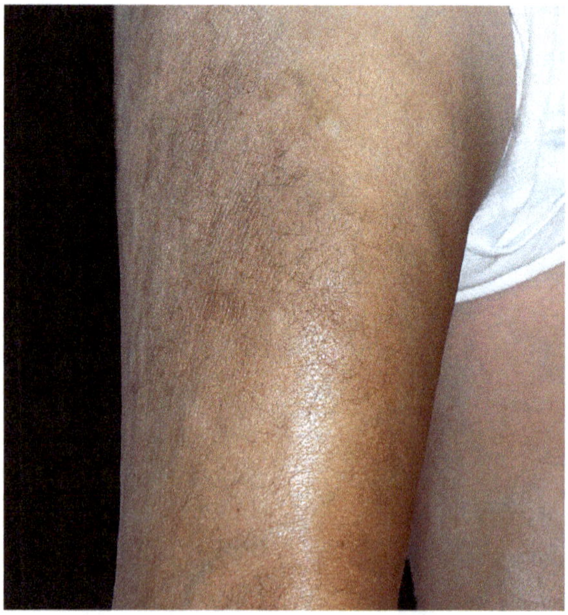

Nephrogenic systemic fibrosis. A brawny platelike induration bound down upon palpation, with an uneven surface on the legs. This patient had end-stage chronic renal failure and was on hemodialysis. (Reproduced, with permission, from Wolff K, Johnson RA, Saavedra AP. *Fitzpatrick's Color Atlas and Synopsis of Clinical Dermatology*. 7th ed. New York, NY: McGraw-Hill Education; 2013.)

Although the initial manifestations of this disorder may be a cutaneous, fibrosing reaction, it may involve extracutaneous sites such as the lungs, heart, and muscle, hence the more recent and preferred name **nephrogenic systemic fibrosis**. Infection at the time of gadolinium administration and the nature of the gadolinium used (ie, ionic vs nonionic preparations and linear vs macrocyclic chelates) define potential risk factors associated with the development of **nephrogenic systemic fibrosis**. Fibrosis and mucin deposition of the deep dermis and septa of the subcutis in concert with an increase of CD34+ stromal spindle cells that coexpress procollagen-I and CD45RO are typical. **Granuloma annulare** may resemble early **papular mucinosis**; however, in the former, the cells accompanying the deposit of mucin are histiocytes arranged in palisaded or interstitial pattern.

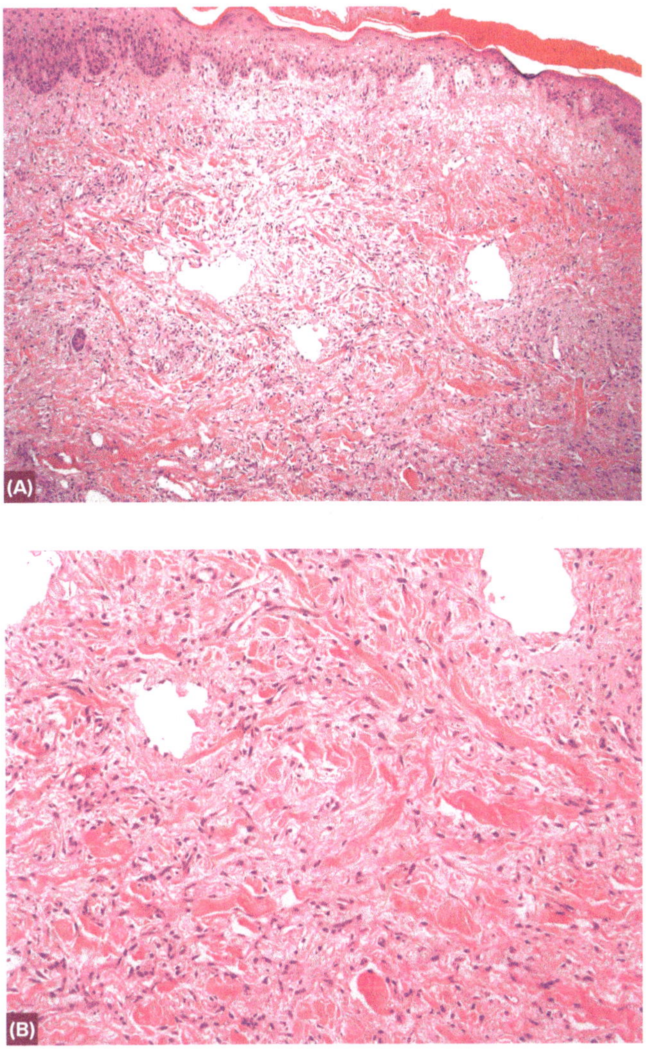

Nephrogenic systemic fibrosis. (A), (B) Nodular foci of fibrosis are seen. The collagen bundles exhibit a haphazard pattern, and the fibrocytes are increased in number, manifesting an activated appearance. Increased dermal mucin is present.

ANSWER 6-34: A.

The biopsy reveals a thickened superficial and deep reticular dermis with sclerotic collagen bundles that are separated from one another (fenestration). These fenestrations contain abundant interstitial mucin deposits, recognizable even with H&E staining. Although the collagen bundles are thickened, the number of dermal fibroblasts is normal. The combined clinical and histopathological findings are consistent with **scleredema adultorum**. The most common cause of this disorder is chronic adult-onset diabetes. Other associated conditions are monoclonal gammopathies and acute streptococcal

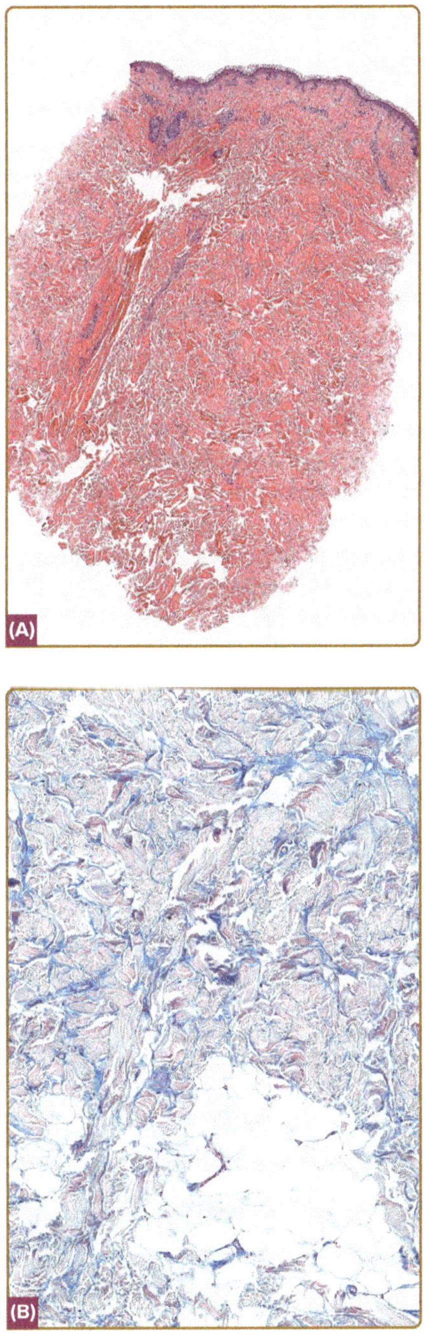

Scleredema. (A) Thickened dermis characterized by enlarged collagen bundles separated by clear spaces (15× original magnification). **(B)** Mucin deposition identified in clear spaces by acid mucopolysaccharide stain (80× original magnification). (Reproduced, with permission, from Goldsmith LA, Katz SI, Gilchrest BA, Paller AS, Leffell DJ, Wolff K, eds. *Fitzpatrick's Dermatology in General Medicine*. 8th ed. New York, NY: McGraw-Hill Education; 2012.)

respiratory infections. The onset of the type related to diabetes is insidious, and it often begins on the upper back with subsequent extension to the neck and occipital scalp. In advanced cases, non-pitting indurated edema elevates the skin of the shoulder blade area with deep associated vertebral folds. Such patients are usually obese, and the mobility of the neck and head may be severely restricted. The skin is shiny and often uneven. The clinical course is usually chronic. **Scleredema** after a respiratory infection is typically acute and resolves rapidly. Very rarely, the tongue, skeletal muscle, pleura, or pericardium is involved.

Microscopically, the dermis is significantly thickened, sometimes up to two to three times normal, by increased collagen, which sometimes replaces subcutaneous fat. In general, the patient has thick, hyalinized collagen bundles that are widely separated (resulting in so-called "fenestrations") by abundant interstitial deposits of mucin. After the early stage of disease, mucin stains may become negative. However, frozen sections may be stained with Alcian blue at a pH of 2.5 or toluidine blue at a pH of 7.0. Sometimes multiple biopsies and cetylpyridinium chloride fixation are needed to demonstrate mucin in the dermis. No increase in the number of fibroblasts and no prominent inflammatory infiltrates are present, and the elastic fibers are reduced in number.

In regards to the differential diagnosis, **scleredema** differs from other forms of **mucinosis** by showing marked thickening of the dermis, hypertrophied collagen bundles, and the fenestrations between collagen bundles filled with mucin. **Scleromyxedema** is distinguished by more superficial deposits of mucin in the dermis and a fibroblastic proliferation. In contrast to **scleredema**, **morphea** and **scleroderma** tend to exhibit tightly packed hypertrophied collagen bundles without fenestrations or abundant mucin deposition and the presence of a superficial and deep perivascular lymphoplasmacytic infiltrate. **Follicular mucinosis** results in the accumulation of mucin within follicular outer root sheath epithelium accompanied by lymphocytic infiltrates.

ANSWER 6-35: D.

A **cutaneous myxoma** is a benign acquired neoplasm. It may be solitary without systemic abnormalities or multiple. In the latter scenario, **myxomas** may represent a manifestation of **Carney complex** (cutaneous myxomas, cardiac myxoma, spotty pigmentation, and endocrine hyperactivity). **Cardiac myxoma** may be fatal, and **cutaneous myxoma** may be an important first indication of this serious condition. **Cutaneous myxomas** and **superficial angiomyxomas** are very similar clinically and histopathologically. **Acral fibromyxoma** is a distinct acral-based neoplasm that has many overlapping features with **superficial acral angiomyxoma**. Microscopically, **cutaneous myxoma** is a lobulated lesion characterized by a mucinous matrix involving the dermis and subcutis, with variably shaped fibroblasts, mast cells, and a few collagen and reticulin fibers. Bizarre multinucleated cells and regular mitotic figures can be seen. Prominent dilated capillaries are a typical finding. An epithelial component consisting of keratinous cysts or epithelial strands with trichoblastic features is often entrapped in the lesion. Stromal cells are vimentin positive and smooth muscle α-actin positive, supporting myofibroblastic differentiation. The discriminating features for **acral fibromyxoma** include greater collagen deposition, and the stromal fibroblasts are typically CD34 and CD99 positive.

In regards to the differential diagnosis, the major process to be distinguished from **cutaneous myxoma** is **focal cutaneous mucinosis**, in which mucin involves only the dermis and spares the subcutis in the absence of increased vascularity. This localized form of mucinosis is characterized by a benign, solitary, symptomless, skin-colored papule or nodule occurring anywhere on the body, except on the skin overlying the joints of the hands and feet, in adults and more rarely in children. Mucin deposition replaces the dermal collagen focally and spares the subcutaneous fat. Spindle-shaped or stellate, vimentin-positive fibroblasts are noted in such mucinous materials. Cleft-like spaces, but no cysts, are seen. A minor population of dermal dendrocytes that are partially factor XIIIa positive and partially CD34 positive is also found. The elastic and reticulum fibers are absent in the mucinous area, and the capillaries are normal in number. The differentiation is important because **myxoma** is a true neoplasm, although benign, which may recur after incomplete excision. Moreover, **cutaneous myxoma** may be a marker of **Carney complex**.

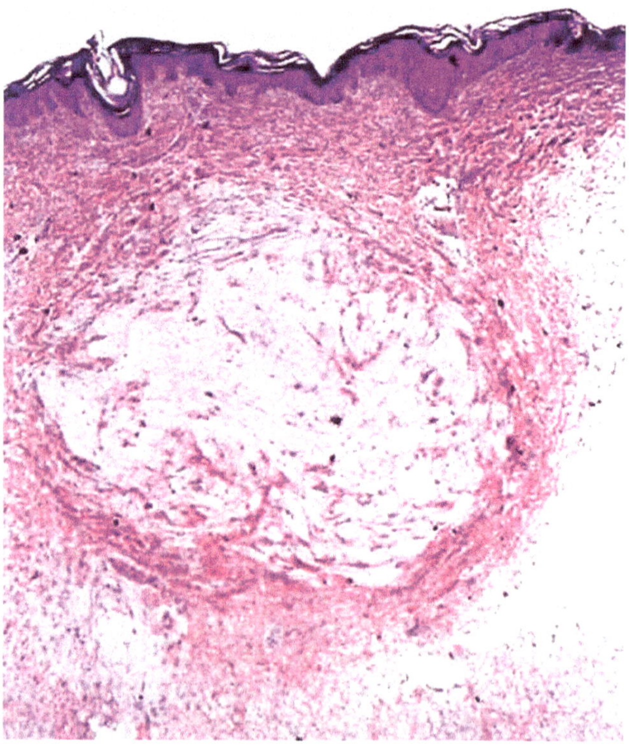

Focal cutaneous mucinosis. Large, focal deposit of mucin in the dermis with some fibroblasts floating in the mucinous material.

Digital mucous (myxoid) cyst is a dome-shaped elevation with or without visible semitransparent contents that forms on the dorsal skin on or near the distal interphalangeal joint of the finger. It may present near the nail. Subungual and eruptive variants have been reported. There are two principal variants. One subtype is derived from synovial cells (**ganglion cyst**) and is almost always localized to the surfaces of the interphalangeal joints, and the other major variant is derived from dermal-based fibroblasts and is usually present between the interphalangeal joints. Puncture or biopsy results in the drainage of viscous, stringy mucin from the cyst. Microscopically, the lesion is not a true cyst. The variety that originates in the dermis shows a large deposit of mucin-containing stellate fibroblasts, some vascular spaces, and multiple clefts. The less frequent variant of synovial origin is characterized by a large dermal cavity surrounded by a collagenous pseudocapsule. The overlying epidermis may be acanthotic at the peripheries of the cyst, sometimes forming a "collarette," and effaced over the central part of the cyst. Transepidermal elimination of mucinous material may be seen.

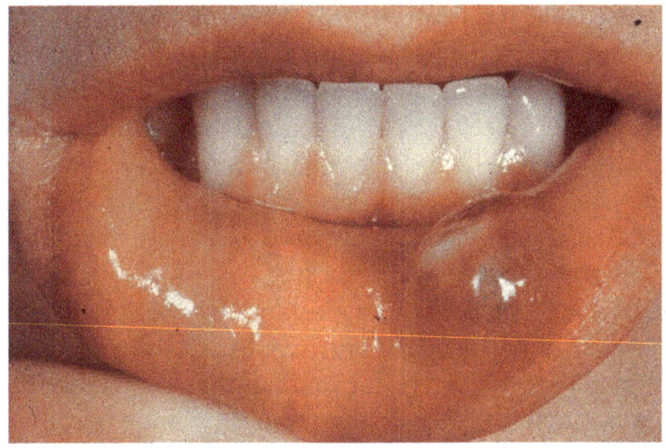

Mucocele. A well-defined, soft bluish submucosal fluctuant nodule on the lip. Thick clear mucus drained when the lesion was incised. (Reproduced, with permission, from Wolff K, Johnson RA, Saavedra AP. *Fitzpatrick's Color Atlas and Synopsis of Clinical Dermatology*. 7th ed. New York, NY: McGraw-Hill Education; 2013.)

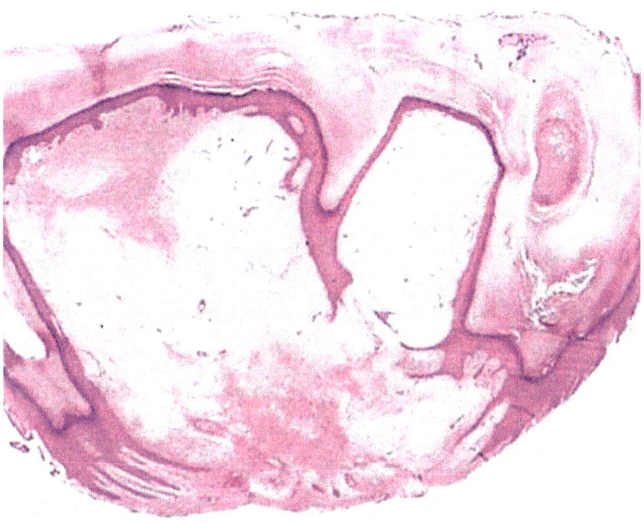

Digital mucous cyst. This is a pseudocyst with a large pool of mucin in the dermis and some vascular spaces and clefts. The epidermis is laterally acanthotic, forming a peripheral "collarette," and centrally more atrophic.

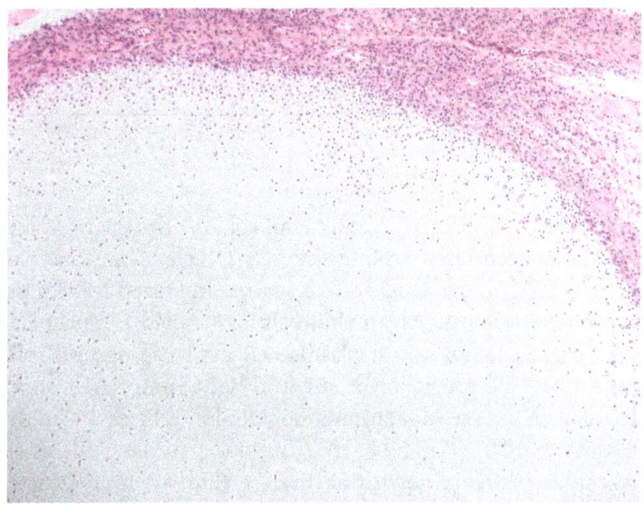

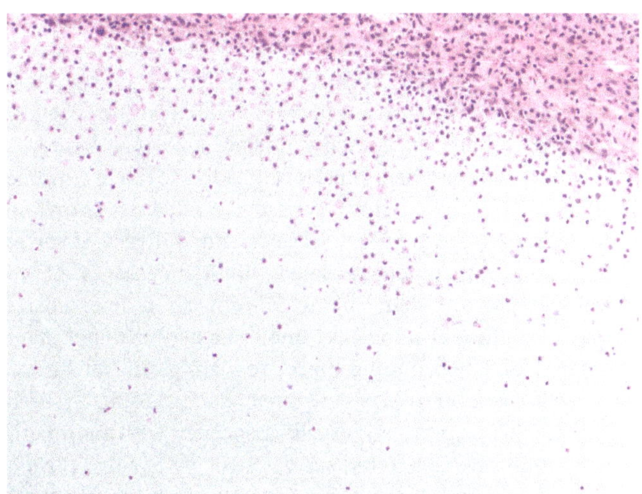

Mucocele of the lip. A cavity contains pale blue mucinous material and numerous mucin-containing macrophages. There is no true cyst lining, but instead a granulomatous inflammatory infiltrate and fibrosis.

The ordinary **oral mucous cyst** develops on areas prone to traumatic insult such as the lower lip, tongue, and bottom of the oral cavity. The superficial variant (called "**superficial mucocele**") usually develops on the soft palate and buccal mucosa. Microscopically, the **oral mucous cyst** forms below the basal membrane or in connective tissue and clinically appears as a submucosal nodule. The superficial mucocele forms in the mucous epithelium or immediately below the subepithelium and appears clinically as a vesicle or bulla. The mucin deposits are composed of **sialomucin** (neutral glycosaminoglycans) rather than acid glycosaminoglycans. **Sialomucin** is an epithelial-derived mucin (secreted by salivary glands) that is

PAS positive and diastase resistant. Alcian blue stain is also positive, but hyaluronidase does not abolish this staining. In ordinary **oral mucous cysts**, multiple edematous pockets of sialomucin are present in the submucosa. An inflammatory cell reaction surrounds these foci. Frequently large numbers of mucin-containing macrophages (muciphages) are present within the cavity. In an old lesion, one large cavity filled with faintly eosinophilic material is observed.

Although stromal mucin deposition may be found in a large number of cutaneous tumors (eg, basal cell carcinoma, neurofibroma) as an incidental finding, the mucin deposition is a distinctive histologic feature in **mucinous nevus**. A **mucinous nevus** is a benign hamartoma that may be either congenital or acquired. It consists of a cobblestoned plaque, usually in a unilateral nevoid pattern. Microscopically, a diffuse deposition of mucin is seen in the upper dermis, and collagen and elastic fibers are diminished or absent in the mucinous area. The epidermis may be normal or may be hyperplastic with elongation of the rete ridges and hyperkeratosis, as in an epidermal nevus. In the latter case, a **mucinous nevus** may be considered a combined hamartoma.

ANSWER 6-36: A.

The biopsy reveals pale pink amorphous material in the dermis concentrated around the hair follicles. The material contains numerous cracked-like spaces. Ruptured folliculitis is present. **Systemic AL amyloidosis** is classified as a primary type caused by an occult plasma cell dyscrasia or **multiple myeloma**. The precursor of **amyloid light chain** (AL) **amyloidosis** is a monoclonal immunoglobulin light chain, more frequently of the lambda type. This form of amyloidosis is mainly a systemic deposition disease (kidney, liver, heart), but cutaneous lesions are observed in 30%-40% of patients. Pinch hemorrhages, periorbital waxy papules and plaques with hemorrhage, enlargement of the tongue (macroglossia), and hardening of the oral mucous membranes are the most common signs. Microscopically, amyloid deposition begins in the perivascular and periappendageal areas (surrounding the sweat glands and hair follicles) and adipose tissue with the formation of "amyloid rings" (about the fat cells). Amyloid eventually fills the papillary dermis and diffusely involves the entire dermis, often associated with hemorrhages due to blood vessel involvement by amyloid infiltration. In extensive infiltrates, diffuse or nodular eosinophilic deposits often have a fissured or cracked appearance, rendering smaller aggregates with facets. Fibroblasts are often attached to the fissured edges. The deposits are not usually associated with an inflammatory infiltrate. Congo red stain is strongly positive (bright red) in dermal amyloid and reveals apple green birefringence under polarized light. Amyloid deposits are reactive with the antibodies against immunoglobulin light chains. In a rare subtype called **amyloid elastosis**, which is seen in the setting of systemic amyloidosis, the amyloid deposits surround individual elastic fibers. These elastic fibers appear shortened and fragmented and show no evidence of elastorrhexis and calcification. Abdominal subcutaneous fat and gingival biopsies may be useful in the absence of specific mucocutaneous lesions.

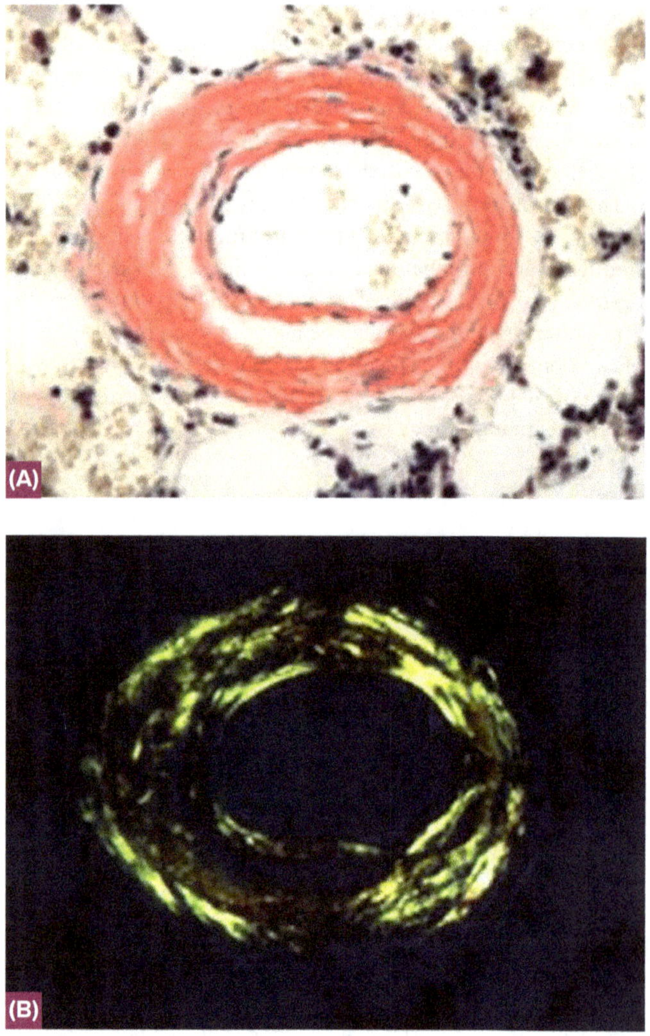

Patient with AL amyloidosis. (A) Small vessel stained with Congo red. Bright red amyloid infiltration of vascular wall. **(B)** Same image as in (A) viewed under polarized light with the polarizing filters set at 90-degree angles. The Congo red-stained material shows birefringence with transmission of apple-green colored light. This is due to the characteristic β-pleated sheet structure of the abnormal amyloid proteins deposited in tissue. (Reproduced, with permission, from Kaushansky K, Lichtman MA, Beutler E, Kipps TJ, Seligsohn U, Prchal JT, eds. *Williams Hematology*. 8th ed. New York, NY: McGraw-Hill Education; 2010.)

Systemic AA Amyloidosis (secondary systemic amyloidosis) is a disorder that occurs in association with a variety of chronic inflammatory and infectious diseases such as **rheumatoid arthritis, familial Mediterranean fever, lepromatous leprosy, hidradenitis suppurativa**, and **generalized arthropathic psoriasis.** Visible skin lesions are rare, except in

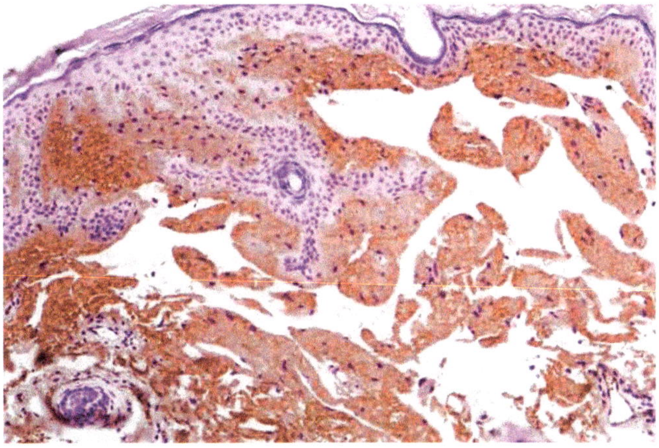

AL amyloidosis. The deposited material is monoclonal immunoglobulin light chains. The brown color is a corresponding immunohistochemical stain for λ light chains confirming the presence of a monoclonal plasma cell population in this patient's marrow sample. The light chains may also be of the κ-type, thus both immunostains should be performed.

Muckle–Wells syndrome, in which geographic skin lesions are seen (probably not containing amyloid). The major sites of **amyloid A (AA) deposition** are not the skin but rather the parenchymatous organs such as the kidneys, liver (speckled or wax liver), and spleen (sago spleen). **AA** is not immunoglobulin but instead is derived from **α-globulin called serum amyloid A (SAA)**, which is split into **AA amyloid** in chronic febrile conditions. Microscopically, deep-needle biopsy of the lower abdomen may show amyloid deposition around the subcutaneous fat cells (amyloid rings) and eccrine glands in about 66% of cases. As the amount of amyloid increases, the dermis may be diffusely infiltrated. Rectal biopsy usually shows amyloid deposition in the submucosa. After treatment with potassium permanganate, **AA amyloid** becomes nonreactive for alkaline Congo red stain; **AL amyloid** is not affected by this treatment.

Familial amyloidotic polyneuropathy constitutes a group of autosomal dominant diseases in which a mutant protein forms amyloid fibrils. The most common form is caused by mutant **transthyretin**. Skin changes consist of trophic leg ulcers and atrophic scars due to the accumulation of **transthyretin-derived amyloid** in peripheral nerves. This variety has long been confused with **leprosy** because of nerve involvement and the deformity of the joints. There are Portuguese, Japanese, and Swedish subtypes. Microscopically, in the skin, blood vessels, arrector pili muscles, and elastic fibers are infiltrated by amyloid, similar to that seen in **AL amyloidosis**. Large accumulations of amyloid are present around cutaneous nerves in **familial amyloidotic polyneuropathy**. The pancreas and testes may be affected, but the liver and spleen are usually spared.

β2-microglobulin amyloidosis presents as small, shiny lichenoid papules on the arms and trunk of patients who have had long-term hemodialysis. Dermal deposition of amyloid is similar to that in patients with **AL amyloidosis**.

Hyalinosis cutis et mucosae (lipoid proteinosis) may have a similar clinical presentation to **systemic AL amyloidosis**, but is not attributed to amyloid deposition. It is a rare autosomal recessive (OMIM 247100) or sporadic (new mutation) disease. In the hereditary form, which is caused by mutations in the **extracellular matrix protein 1 gene**, the initial symptom is hoarseness due to hyaline infiltration of the vocal cords. A diffuse infiltration of hyaline into the pharynx, larynx, and oral mucosa (including the tongue) produces extensive induration of the mouth. Early lesions consist of bullae and varicelliform scars on the face and arms, which are similar to those of **erythropoietic protoporphyria**. The free edges of the eyelids and nostrils show small, waxy, semitransparent papulonodules resembling a "string of beads." Large plaque-type infiltration may occur on the face and over the joints. The nonfamilial type occurs in an older age group and is typified by similar lesions except bullae and scars on the face are present. Microscopically, hyaline deposition begins around the dermal blood vessels and eccrine glands where PAS-positive diastase-resistant hyaline is demonstrated in concentric rings (onion-skin pattern). This material also stains with Alcian blue at a pH of 2.5, but only stains very weakly or negatively with Congo red. The material may be seen around pilosebaceous units and in arrector pili muscles. Hyaline deposits oriented perpendicularly to the dermal–epidermal junction gradually fill the entire dermis. Small lipid droplets may be demonstrated with the scarlet red stain, particularly around the blood vessels in late lesions. The epidermis may show hyperkeratosis and papillomatosis

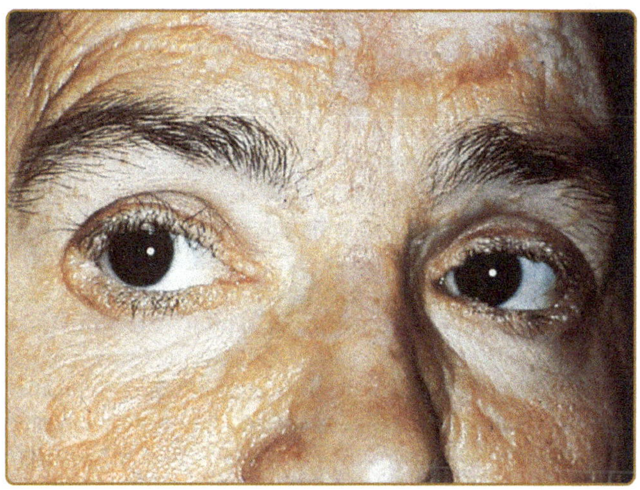

Lipoid proteinosis. Beaded papules along margin of the eyelids (moniliform blepharosis). Note increased severity of yellowish, waxy lesions in sun-exposed areas. (Reproduced, with permission, from Goldsmith LA, Katz SI, Gilchrest BA, Paller AS, Leffell DJ, Wolff K, eds. *Fitzpatrick's Dermatology in General Medicine*. 8th ed. New York, NY: McGraw-Hill Education; 2012. Courtesy of O. Braun-Falco, Munich.)

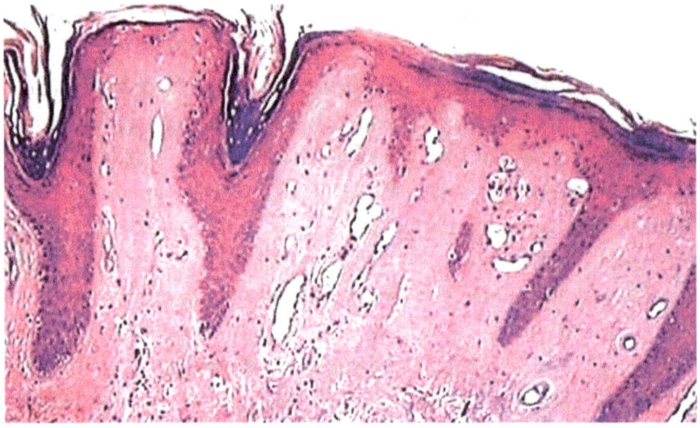

Hyalinosis cutis et mucosae. A widened dermal papilla is entirely occupied by vertically oriented hyaline material. Several dilated blood vessels are seen. The tissue reaction against this massive deposition is minimal. (Used with permission of A. Amantea, MD and P. Donati, MD.)

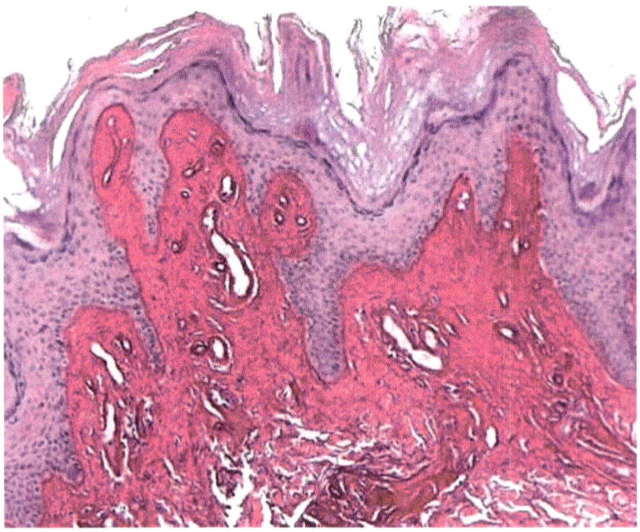

Hyalinosis cutis et mucosae. Periodic acid Schiff stain is strongly positive in the hyaline deposition in the upper dermis.

in verrucous lesions. Calcified foci and a failure of mucocutaneous lymphangiogenesis have also been described. Electron microscopy demonstrates multiplication of lamina densa (basal lamina) in perivascular and periglandular spaces. The hyaline substance is mainly homogeneous, but some filament components are also admixed. Significant degeneration of collagen fibers is seen as longitudinal splitting or fragmentation of fibers. The dermal deposits contain type IV collagen, laminin, neutral mucopolysaccharides, hyaluronic acid, and ceramide or more complex lipids, but the precise pathogenesis of the disease remains unknown. PAS-positive material in **lipoid proteinosis** is differentiated from **amyloidosis** by its negative or weak staining on Congo red stain. In **erythropoietic protoporphyria**, the deposits are more limited in distribution, being perivascular only, and the sweat glands are not involved.

ANSWER 6-37: B.

All skin-limited (skin only) amyloid depositions are of the keratin type, except **nodular amyloidosis**, which is derived from the light chain of immunoglobulins. The source of keratins is either epidermal or from tumors of epidermal or hair follicle origin. Individuals of color, such as African Americans, Asians, Latin Americans, and those of Middle Eastern origin, are more frequently affected than whites. **Macular, lichenoid, and biphasic amyloidosis** are the three most common variants (Table 3-37A).

The typical lesions of **lichen amyloidosis** are hyperkeratotic papules and plaques involving the shins and, in severe cases, the extensor surface of the arms, including the shoulders. Severe pruritus is a characteristic feature, and some authors have proposed that **lichen amyloidosis** is almost always a consequence of scratching in the setting of an underlying pruritic condition. Familial cases of **lichen amyloidosis** and cases associated with genetic diseases (ie, **multiple endocrine neoplasia syndrome type 2A**) have been reported.

In **macular amyloidosis** the upper back and scapular areas of middle-aged, dark-skinned women are most commonly affected by pruritic macules showing irregular pigmentation with a "rippled" pattern. The constant use of a nylon brush or towel is sometimes involved as a causal factor (**frictional amyloidosis**).

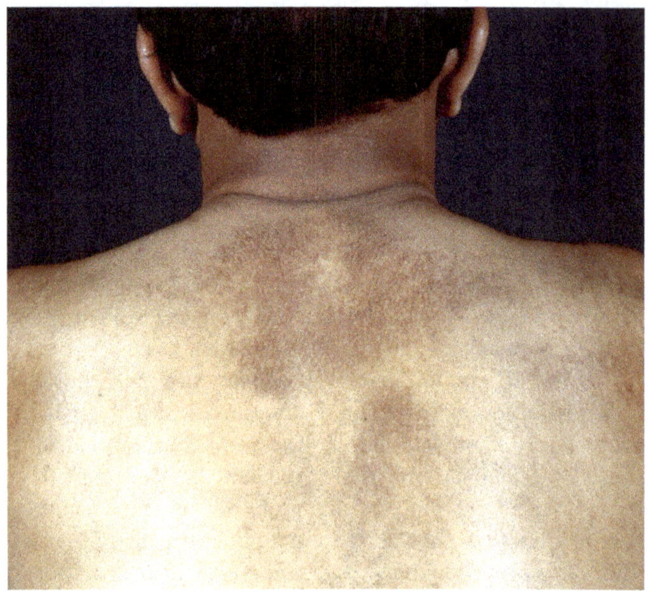

Macular amyloidosis. Gray-brown, reticulated pigmentation on the back of a 56-year-old Arab. (Reproduced, with permission, from Wolff K, Johnson RA, Saavedra AP. *Fitzpatrick's Color Atlas and Synopsis of Clinical Dermatology*. 7th ed. New York, NY: McGraw-Hill Education; 2013.)

In **biphasic amyloidosis,** both **lichenoid** and **macular amyloidoses** are present in the same area or separate locations in the same patient. The lichenoid lesions are commonly pruritic.

Table 6-37A. Skin-Limited Amyloidoses

	CLINICAL FEATURES	HISTOPATHOLOGIC FEATURES	DIFFERENTIAL DIAGNOSIS
Keratin-derived amyloidoses			
- Macular amyloidosis	Rippled pigmentation on the upper back, scapular areas, often middle-aged women of color, often with pruritus	Scant eosinophilic globules in the papillary dermis, pigment incontinence, occasional dyskeratotic cells	Post-inflammatory hypermelanosis
- Lichen amyloidosis	Hyperkeratotic papules or plaques on the shins, extensor surfaces, pruritus	Hyperkeratosis, papillomatous epidermal hyperplasia, aggregates of eosinophilic globules in the papillary dermis	Colloid milium, lipoid proteinosis
- Biphasic amyloidosis (macular and lichen amyloidosis)			
- Friction amyloidosis (see macular amyloidosis)			
- Epithelioma-associated keratin amyloidosis	Various cutaneous neoplasms: basal cell carcinoma, Bowen disease, actinic keratosis, seborrheic keratosis	Deposition of eosinophilic globules in both the parenchyma and stroma	
Actinic amyloidosis - Juvenile colloid milium	Waxy or pearly papules or nodules on sun-exposed skin	Large aggregates of pink eosinophilic material	
Insulin-derived amyloidosis			
Insulin amyloidosis	Sites of repeated insulin injection	Eosinophilic globules, reparative changes	
Immunoglobulin-derived amyloidosis			
Nodular amyloidosis	Single or multiple nodules on the face, scalp, and legs of middle-aged women	Massive accumulation of pink amorphous material in the dermis and occasionally the subcutis, plasma cells	Primary amyloidosis, **Waldenström** macroglobulinemia

Microscopically, small numbers of eosinophilic globular deposits of amyloid, barely distinguishable from collagen, accumulate initially in the papillary dermis in **macular amyloidosis**, resembling **the cytoid (colloid) bodies** of **lichen planus**. Although **cytoid bodies** or other evidence of keratinocyte degeneration are not routinely observed in the epidermis, a careful search may identify such cells. These epidermal cytoid bodies are considered to be the source of amyloid in these varieties of amyloidoses, breaking through the basement membrane and dropping into the dermis. In **lichen amyloidosis**, large clumps of amyloid expand dermal papillae, pressing the rete ridges into thin septae.

Lichen amyloidosis may be distinguished from **macular amyloidosis** by hyperkeratosis, acanthosis with hyperpigmentation of the basal layer, and larger deposits of amyloid. In the later stages, diffuse homogeneous eosinophilic amyloid fills the papillary dermis and infiltrates the upper reticular dermis. Adnexal structures and blood vessels are not involved. Some degree of pigment incontinence and hemorrhage is usually present in both forms of cutaneous amyloidosis. Definitive diagnostic distinction requires clinical correlation. A characteristic feature of **familial lichen amyloidosis** is the transepidermal elimination of amyloid. **Keratin amyloids (amyloid K)** are strongly stained with polyclonal anti-keratin antibodies that contain combinations of antibodies against basal cell keratins (K5, K14) and upper epidermal keratins (K1, K10). **Amyloid P** component is always positive. Maturation of degenerated keratin proteins into amyloid may require a digestion process in the lysosomes of dermal macrophages.

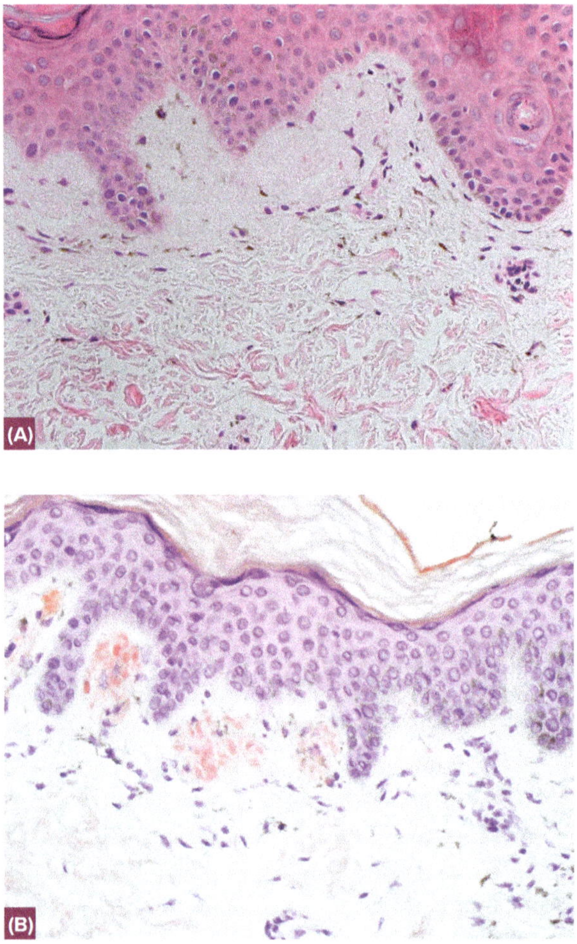

Macular amyloidosis. (A) There are small globules of pale eosinophilic material in the papillary dermis. **(B)** The material stains bright red with Congo red staining.

Routine Congo red, Dylon, thioflavine T, toluidine blue, and Crystal violet stains are positive, but they are not always reliable in formalin or alcohol fixed-tissue sections. These stains are more reliable in fresh-frozen sections. Electron microscopic demonstration of 6- to 10-nm straight filaments is the most specific and reliable diagnostic method.

The differential diagnosis of **lichen amyloidosis** also includes **nodular amyloidosis, actinic amyloidosis, adult colloid milium, lipoid proteinosis**, and **Waldenström macroglobulinemia.** A major condition confused with **macular amyloidosis** is **post-inflammatory pigmentary alteration** (PIPA). However, **post-inflammatory pigmentary alteration** does not exhibit amyloid and is clinically distinctive.

Nodular amyloidosis usually shows much more extensive amyloid accumulation in the dermis (and possibly the subcutis) and waxy or translucent nodules of the head and neck compared with **lichen amyloidosis** which typically forms papules on the extremities. In addition, immunoglobulin light chains can be demonstrated via immunohistochemistry (kappa or lambda) in **nodular amyloidosis.** Single and sometimes multiple nodules may occur anywhere on the cutaneous surface, but the face, scalp, and leg of middle-aged women are the most common sites. Individual nodules are firm, waxy and tumor-like, or appear semitransparent, amber colored, or hemorrhagic. About 7% of these patients develop **multiple myeloma. Nodular amyloidosis** may be associated with **Sjögren syndrome** and **subacute cutaneous lupus erythematosus.** In such cases, serum autoantibodies Sjögren syndrome antigen A/Sjögren syndrome antigen B (SSA/SSB) are positive. Microscopically, a massive deposition of weakly eosinophilic amorphous amyloid substance is noted throughout the entire dermis, often extending into the subcutis and around the blood vessels and the dermal appendages. Greenish birefringence of Congo red stain makes contrast with white birefringence of collagen fibers. Numerous plasma cells, some with large Russell bodies, are often seen, but they are sparse or absent in nodular lesions of **systemic primary AL amyloidosis (myeloma-associated).**

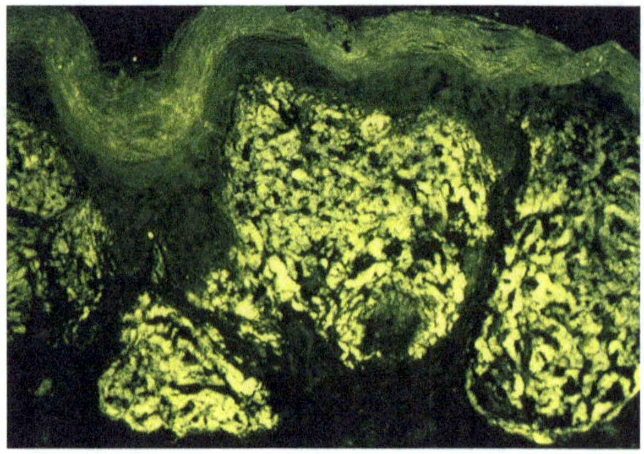

Lichen amyloidosis. Thioflavine T fluorescence is seen in amyloid deposition in the papillary dermis.

Quick Fact

- Nodular amyloidosis = Cutaneous AL amyloid without systemic paraproteinemia
- Systemic amyloidosis = Cutaneous and visceral AL amyloid with systemic paraproteinemia

Monoclonality of infiltrating plasma cells by polymerase chain reaction has been detected. Giant cells and focal calcification may be found. Contrary to the other localized cutaneous amyloidoses, the amyloid deposits are **AL type**, derived from immunoglobulin light chains. In all types of amyloid, immunoglobulins are present, probably passively trapped in the meshwork of amyloid filaments. These immunoglobulins can be eluted in acidic buffer without disrupting the filamentous nature of amyloid or altering the standard amyloid stains. In **nodular amyloidosis**, the same elution procedure abolishes amyloid staining, suggesting that this amyloid is immunoglobulin itself. However, the origin of immunoglobulin is not always elucidated.

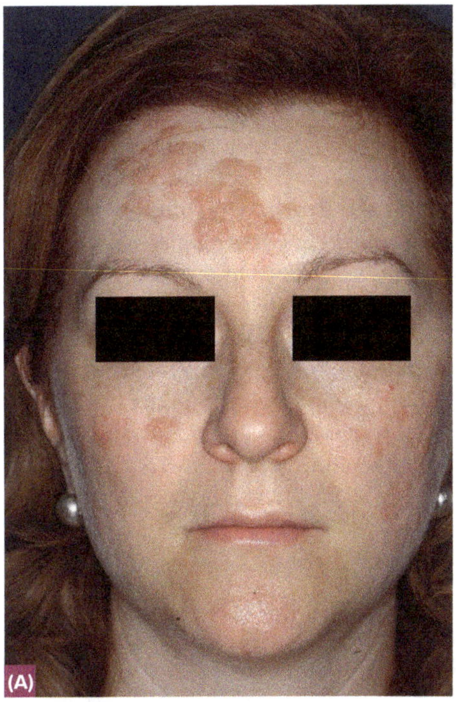

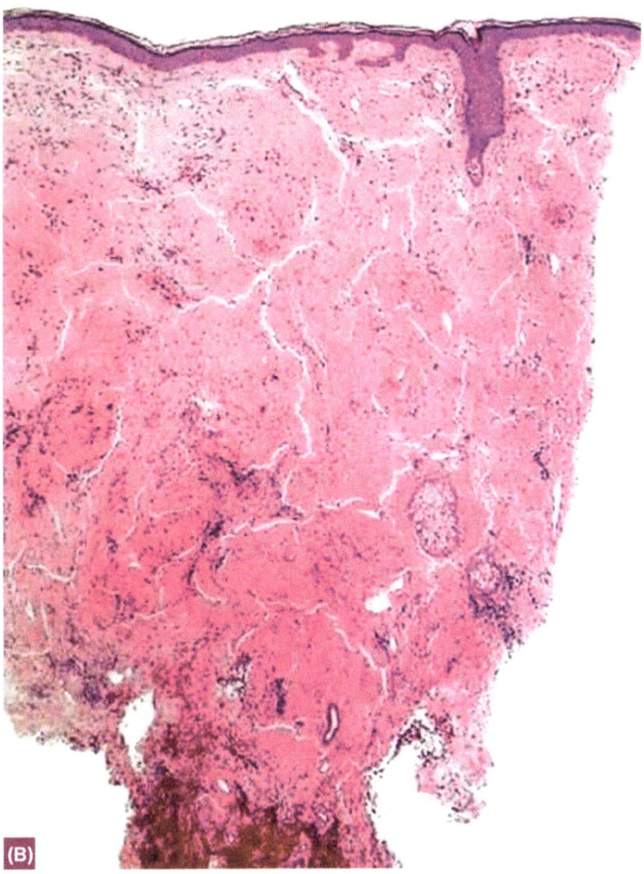

Nodular amyloidosis. (A) Characteristic infiltrative firm, waxy nodules on the face. **(B)** A massive deposition of amorphous amyloid substance throughout the entire dermis. There are many fissures and cracks caused by processing artifact due to the lack of elasticity in amyloid.

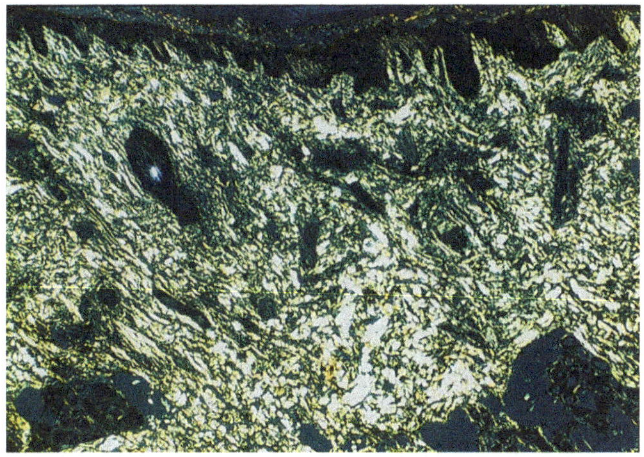

Nodular amyloidosis. Congo red stain observed under polarized light. Greenish birefringence of Congo red–stained amyloid makes contrast with white birefringence of collagen fibers.

Actinic amyloidosis includes **juvenile colloid milium** and **amyloidosis of the auricular concha**. Ultraviolet rays have a severe injurious effect on keratinocytes, as evidenced by sunburn cells. Chronic sun exposure of the skin leads to the amyloidal degeneration of the epidermal keratinocytes. For example, **actinic keratosis** is often associated with the deposition of keratin amyloid. **Concha amyloidosis** of the inner auricle or helix of the ear is clinically an aggregation of cobblestone-like waxy or pearly papulonodules. Severe keratinocyte degeneration into cytoid bodies is present in the epidermis. Microscopically, in **juvenile colloid milium**, subepidermal, eosinophilic, fissured colloid masses abut the epidermis without a grenz zone. Colloid-like material appears to develop in basal keratinocytes and drop off into the papillary dermis. Histiocytes and melanophages are noted within the colloid material. Epidermal cytoid bodies and dermal amyloid can be stained with polyclonal anti-keratin antibodies in addition

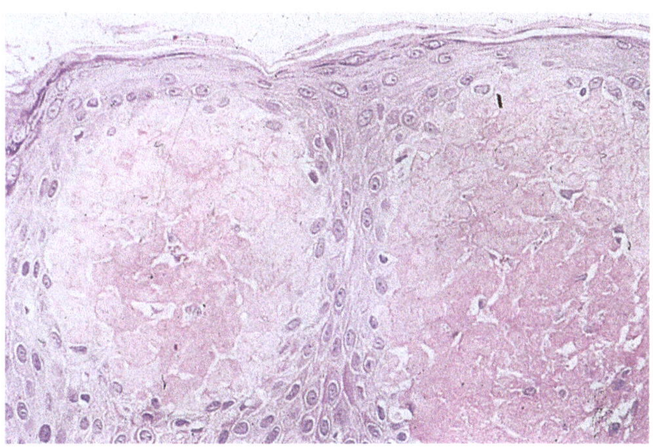

Juvenile colloid milium. Pink-stained hyaline substance (ie, amyloid) occupies widened dermal papillae. Round cytoid body–like amyloid globules can be recognized at the periphery.

to standard amyloid stains. The filaments derived from these cytoid bodies meet the ultrastructural criteria for amyloid filaments. **Juvenile colloid milium** may be histopathologically indistinguishable from **lichen amyloidosis** except by distribution and clinical features.

Whereas the "colloid" substance in **juvenile colloid milium** is actually keratin amyloid, **adult-type colloid milium** contains severely degenerated elastic fibers (Table 6-37B). Yellowish semitransparent papules and plaques occur on the face and dorsum of the hands. Interestingly, the left side of the face and left hand are more frequently and severely affected because of more sun exposure on that side while driving. The condition usually occurs in older men with fair skin, particularly farmers and other outdoor workers, sportsmen, and truck drivers. The lesions are soft, and a small incision and pressure allow the expression of the gelatinous substance. Hemorrhage is common in large lesions. Microscopically, colloid in **adult colloid milium** is the final degeneration product of elastic fibers. H&E-stained sections show a pink hyaline substance in large sheets occupying the papillary and upper reticular dermis. Many cracks and fissures within the colloid material and fibroblasts are commonly seen along the lines of fissuring. Inflammation is lacking. Solar elastosis is always present. A narrow grenz zone of normal collagen separates the atrophic epidermis from the colloid substance. Histochemical studies have shown that the material is PAS positive and only weakly positive or negative with Congo red or thioflavine T. The disparity in the results of Congo red stain could be due to the different technical procedures performed. An elastic fiber stain is largely negative in the main body of colloid and positive in the grenz zone and at the periphery of the colloid deposition (**solar elastosis**). **Amyloid P component**, which is present in normal elastic fibers, is strongly stained in the lesion with immunohistochemistry. On electron microscopy the colloid substance is a moderately electron-dense amorphous substance with some granules and fine filaments. These findings are in contrast to the colloid of **juvenile colloid milium**, despite the clinical and histologic similarity of the juvenile and adult types. As already discussed, **juvenile colloid milium** contains typical keratin-derived amyloid filaments.

Table 6-37B. Comparison of Lichen Amyloidosis and Colloid Milium of Adults

LICHEN AMYLOIDOSIS	COLLOID MILIUM OF THE ADULT
Small deposits within broadened dermal papillae	Large deposits within the upper half of the dermis
Amyloid in small globules	Colloid in large, nodular accumulations
Amyloid is amphophilic or eosinophilic in sections stained with H&E	Colloid is amphophilic or basophilic in sections stained with H&E
Stellate fibroblasts and melanophages intimately associated with globules of amyloid	A few fibroblasts associated with colloid, but no macrophages
No clefts within the globules of amyloid	Clefts within the nodules of colloid
Vascular proliferation associated with amyloid	No vascular proliferation associated with colloid
Papillary epidermal hyperplasia usually with hyperkeratosis overlies amyloid	Thin epidermis with loss of the rete pattern and grenz zone overlies colloid
Solar elastosis not usually seen	Solar elastosis always present

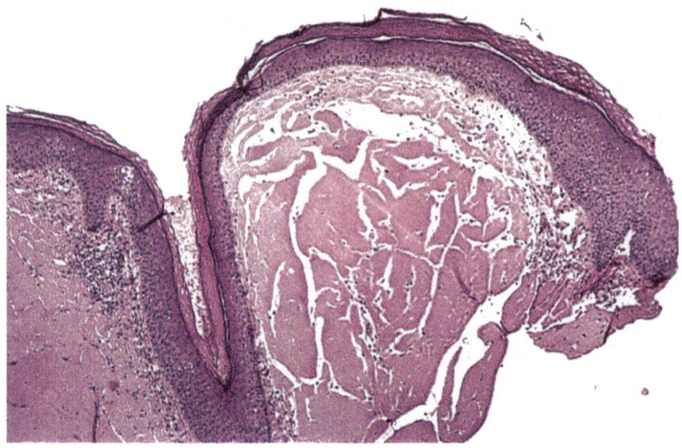

Adult colloid milium. Hyaline substance (ie, colloid) occupies dilated dermal papillae. There are many fissures in these masses.

Lipoid proteinosis (and **erythropoietic porphyria**) shows a perivascular pattern of accumulation of amorphous pink material that is PAS+D and weakly positive or negative on Congo red stain. The storage papules of **Waldenström macroglobulinemia** may closely resemble **adult colloid milium** and **lichen amyloidosis** because of the presence of clefts and fissures. The hyaline material in such storage papules is PAS+D positive and Congo red negative and reacts with antibodies against IgM.

ANSWER 6-38: D.

The biopsy reveals gray-pink amorphous material surrounded by robust granulomatous inflammatory infiltrates with foreign body giant cells, consistent with **gout**. **Gout** is a dominantly inherited abnormality of purine metabolism resulting in high levels of serum uric acid, which deposits as monosodium urate crystals in small joints, typically those of the great toe. Increased serum purine levels may be secondary to decreased renal function, diuretic therapy, or an increased purine synthesis in myeloproliferative diseases. Skin deposition of uric acid (called "**gouty tophi**") occurs most frequently on the auricle. The elbow and finger joints are also commonly affected.

Microscopically, **gouty tophi** are characterized by palisading granulomas surrounding grayish amorphous material with needlelike clefts in the dermis. The nuclei in macrophages may be altered by crystals and appear atypical. If fixed in alcohol, uric acid crystals are preserved and yield characteristic multicolor birefringence under polarized light. Upon examination with a red condenser, these crystals assume a yellow color when parallel to the condenser and blue when perpendicular to the plane of projected light. In formalin-fixed tissues, the crystals are less obvious, and no birefringence is observed. With the De Galantha stain, the crystals appear brown to black. Secondary calcification or even ossification is common. Late-stage **gouty tophi** are surrounded by a fibrous pseudocapsule and contain mucopolysaccharides.

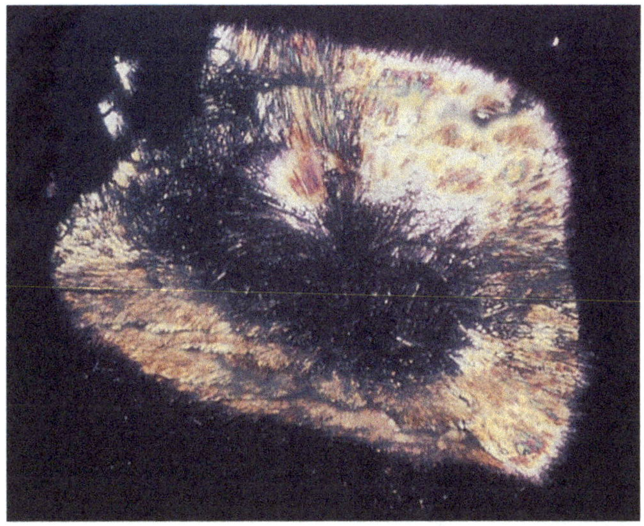

Gouty tophus. Under polarized light, urate crystals give rise to multicolored birefringence. (Used with permission of Min W. Lee, MD.)

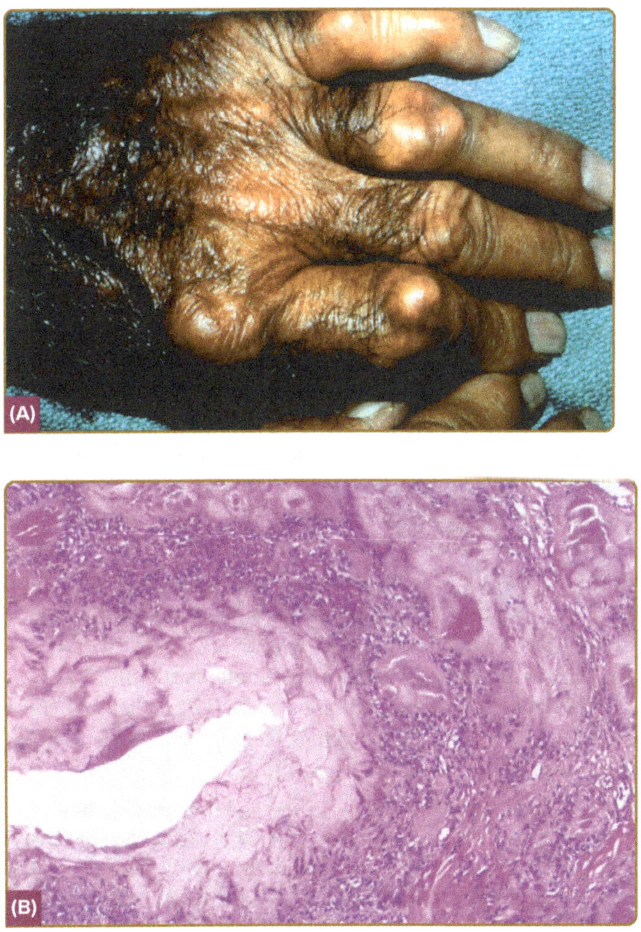

Gouty tophi. (A) Tender nodules overlying joints and tendons, which may drain chalky white material. **(B)** Histopathology shows granulomatous "fluffy" appearing infiltrate surrounding radially arranged needlelike spaces. (Reproduced, with permission, from Goldsmith LA, Katz SI, Gilchrest BA, Paller AS, Leffell DJ, Wolff K, eds. *Fitzpatrick's Dermatology in General Medicine*. 8th ed. New York, NY: McGraw-Hill Education; 2012.)

Answer choice D describes **relapsing polychondritis**, which is typically a progressive, episodic inflammatory process involving most commonly auricular cartilage in up to 90% of patients who also have polyarthritis, nasal chondritis, ocular inflammation, and respiratory tract chondritis. Deposition of crystalline material is not present. Mortality may be up to 25%, usually the result of respiratory tract involvement or from cardiac valvular chondritis. Clinically, painful erythema and edema involving both the ears and nose develop intermittently, ultimately leading to soft and flabby ears and saddle-nose deformity due to cartilage degeneration. Cutaneous lesions occur rarely and are described as purpuric or erythema nodosum–like.

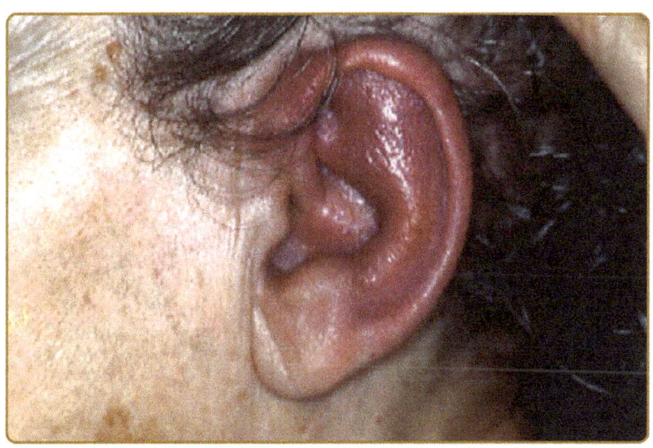

Relapsing polychondritis. Painful inflammation of the cartilaginous portion of ear. (Reproduced, with permission, from Goldsmith LA, Katz SI, Gilchrest BA, Paller AS, Leffell DJ, Wolff K, eds. *Fitzpatrick's Dermatology in General Medicine*. 8th ed. New York, NY: McGraw-Hill Education; 2012.)

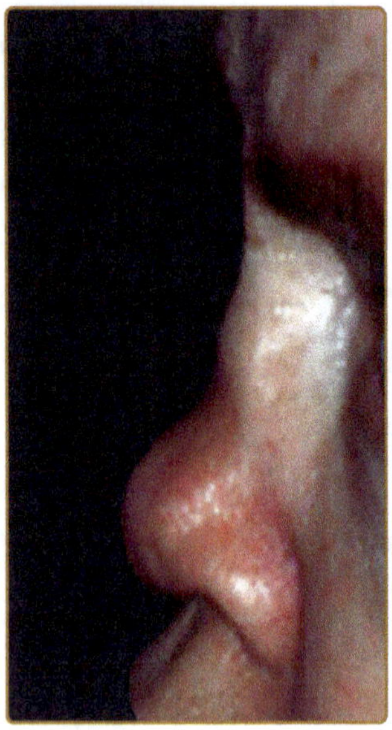

Relapsing polychondritis. Saddle nose deformity. (Reproduced, with permission, from Goldsmith LA, Katz SI, Gilchrest BA, Paller AS, Leffell DJ, Wolff K, eds. *Fitzpatrick's Dermatology in General Medicine*. 8th ed. New York, NY: McGraw-Hill Education; 2012.)

Microscopically, **relapsing polychondritis** is characterized by a mixed inflammatory infiltrate of lymphocytes, neutrophils, and plasma cells surrounding deeper cartilage structures. Cartilage changes include vacuolization and pyknosis of chondrocytes with eventual loss of cartilage basophilia. Elastic stains reveal destruction of elastic fibers within cartilage. With each succeeding attack, more chondrocytes are destroyed and replaced by fibrous tissue. Cutaneous lesions have shown vasculitis with fibrin deposition involving vessels that are surrounded by lymphocytes and eosinophils.

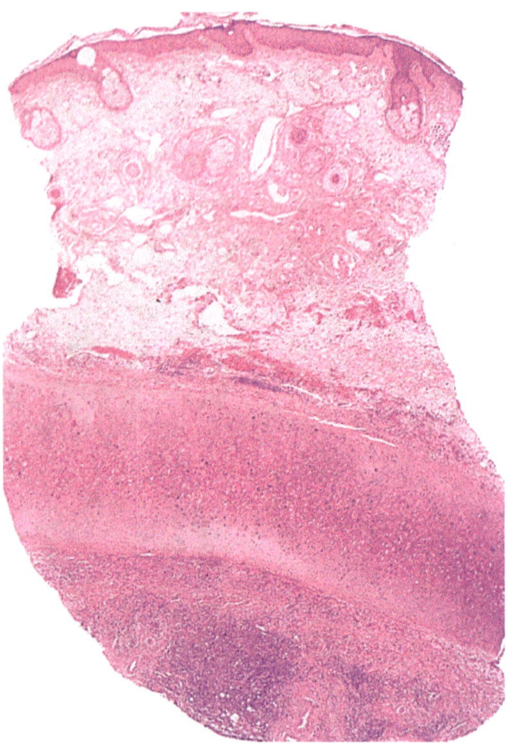

Relapsing polychondritis. At low power, a mixed inflammatory infiltrate is seen in the perichondrial connective tissue.

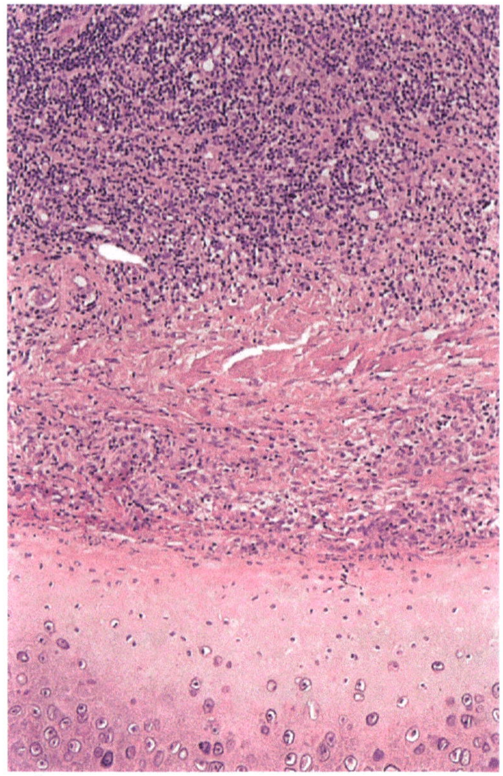

Relapsing polychondritis. At higher power, a mixed inflammatory infiltrate of neutrophils, lymphocytes, plasma cells, and eosinophils is seen adjacent to the auricular cartilage with some loss of normal staining (devitalization) of the cartilage.

ANSWER 6-39: C.

The biopsy reveals numerous fragmented and calcified (basophilic material) elastic fibers in the mid and deep dermis. The epidermis is unremarkable. The findings are consistent with **pseudoxanthoma elasticum (PXE)**. **Pseudoxanthoma elasticum** may be inherited as an autosomal recessive or dominant trait, with the inheritance pattern and disease severity varying widely from patient to patient. Apparently, two recessive and two dominant forms of pseudoxanthoma elasticum exist. It is reported to be caused by mutations in the ***ABC66*** gene on chromosome 16p13.1. In **PXE**, genetically abnormal elastic fibers develop prominent calcium deposition and are present in the skin, retina, and arterial walls, including those supplying gastric mucosa and myocardium, as well as larger peripheral arteries. Rupture of Bruch membrane results in angioid streaks of the ocular fundus, and calcification and degeneration of elastic tissue fibers in internal organs lead to gastrointestinal bleeding, renal hypertension, angina pectoris, and intermittent claudication of the extremities. Clinically, patients with **PXE** develop yellowish plaques with pebbly surfaces ("chicken skin") primarily involving the flexures, such as the antecubital fossae, groin, axillae, and especially the lateral neck. In white skin, the cutaneous lesions may be mistaken for **solar elastosis** or **xanthomas**.

Microscopically, with H&E stain, the middle third of the reticular dermis is filled with numerous short, wavy, fragmented, irregularly shaped, granular elastic fibers that are frequently deeply basophilic due to prominent calcium deposition. Consequently, the fibers stain deeply black with both elastic (orcein or Verhoef) and calcium (von Kossa) stains. Some cases with marked elastic fiber calcification result in a granulomatous infiltrate. Electron microscopy shows abnormalities of small elastic fibers, even those spared calcification, and most of the larger fibers show dense calcium deposition.

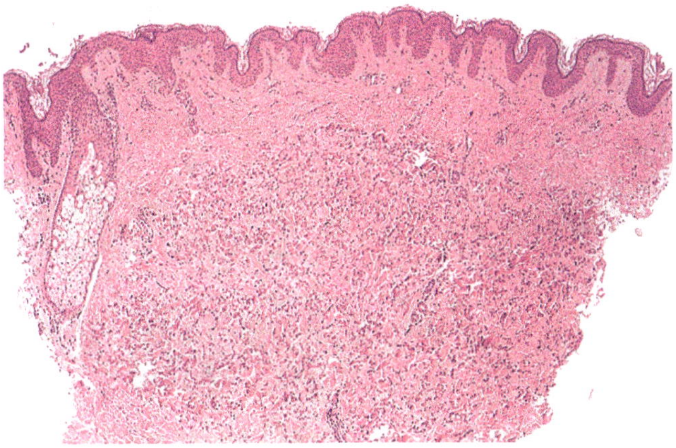

Pseudoxanthoma elasticum. Within the middle third of the dermis, numerous small, fragmented, distorted elastic fibers are seen.

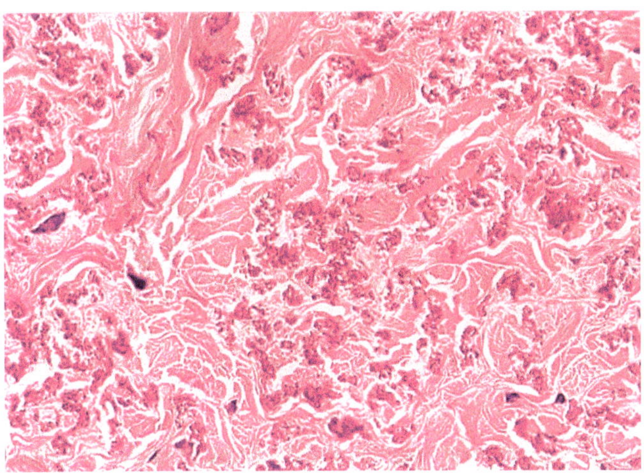

Pseudoxanthoma elasticum. Higher magnification shows the characteristic fragmented elastic fibers with calcium deposition.

In regards to the differential diagnosis, **solar elastosis** also demonstrates abnormal elastic tissue located in the upper third of the dermis, usually beneath a small zone of spared papillary dermis, rather than the mid-reticular dermal location characteristic of the abnormal elastic fibers of **pseudoxanthoma elasticum**. Calcium deposition does not occur in **solar elastosis**.

Mid-dermal elastolysis is a rare acquired disorder of elastic tissue degradation first described in 1977 by Shelly and Wood. To date less than 100 cases have been described in the literature, and there is growing evidence that the entity represents a rather characteristic histological reaction pattern to a wide variety of (predominately inflammatory) pathological processes. As the term implies the cardinal feature marking this entity is the well-defined obliteration of elastic fibers in the mid-dermis. Clinically, affected individuals, usually adult women aged approximately 30-50 years, present with asymptomatic and generally symmetrical skin lesions in one of three, sometimes concurrent, patterns: (1) well-defined or diffuse

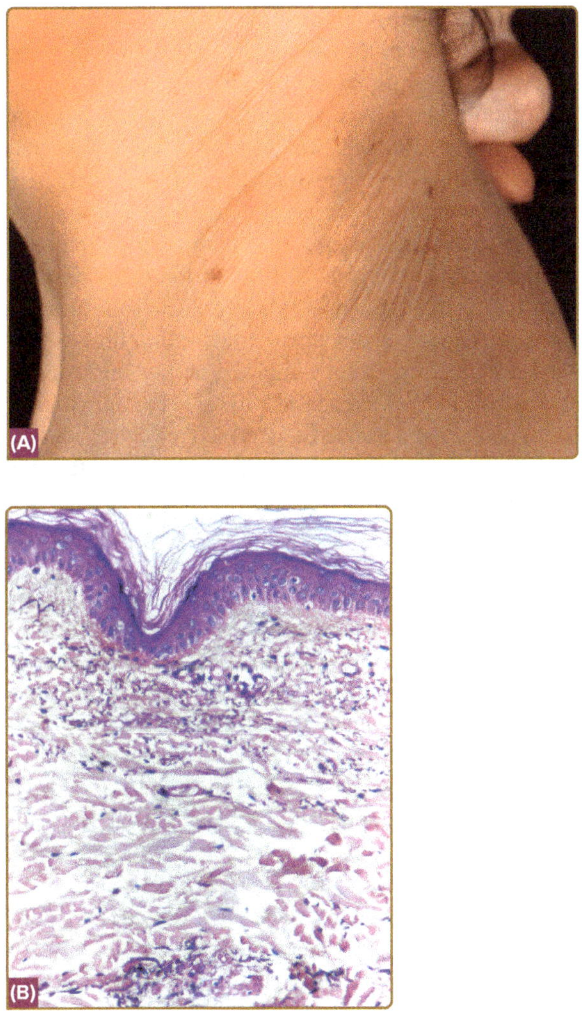

Mid-dermal elastolysis. (A) Well-circumscribed area of fine wrinkling on the neck of a middle-aged woman. **(B)** Histology of mid-dermal elastolysis. Note selective loss of elastic fibers in the mid-dermis. Normal elastic tissue is preserved in the superficial papillary dermis and in the reticular dermis (Weigert stain). (Reproduced, with permission, from Goldsmith LA, Katz SI, Gilchrest BA, Paller AS, Leffell DJ, Wolff K, eds. *Fitzpatrick's Dermatology in General Medicine*. 8th ed. New York, NY: McGraw-Hill Education; 2012. Part A courtesy of Richard Dubuc, MD; part B courtesy of Danielle Bouffard, MD.)

patches characterized by fine-wrinkling of skin, (2) discrete perifollicular papules, and (3) reticular and annular patches with central atrophy. Sites of predilection include the neck, trunk, and extremities. The pathogenesis of the condition has not been clearly delineated but has been linked to ultraviolet light exposure and a wide variety of inflammatory and autoimmune processes including connective tissue disease, **HIV, urticaria, neutrophilic dermatoses**, and granulomatous reactions such as **granuloma annulare** and **actinic granuloma (annular elastolytic giant cell granuloma)**. Microscopically, the essential histological criterion needed for recognition of this entity is a well-demarcated band-like absence of elastic fibers in the mid-dermis. Loss of elastic fibers is verified by elastic tissue staining (ie, Orcein stain, or potentially immunohistochemical staining for elastin). Characteristically, the elastic fibers are intact in the overlying papillary and underlying deep reticular dermis in lesional skin.

Perifollicular elastolysis is characterized by tiny pinpoint lesions with finely wrinkled perifollicular atrophy that may bulge outward with lateral pressure. Most likely, perifollicular elastolysis results from preceding follicular inflammation, explaining its common occurrence in patients with follicular diseases such as acne vulgaris and its anatomic distribution involving the face and upper back. Microscopically, as the name implies, elastic stains demonstrate a markedly diminished number to absence of elastic fibers within the dermis immediately surrounding hair follicles associated with little inflammation.

Cutis laxa (aka **generalized elastolysis**) may be congenital or acquired, affecting people of both genders, with autosomal dominant, recessive, and linked forms described. **Cutis laxa** is characterized by degenerative changes in elastic fibers. Some patients show normal microfibrils and a deficiency of elastin; in other patients elastin is preserved and microfibrils are absent. **Cutis laxa** may be preceded by an inflammatory rash or may develop spontaneously. Clinically, **cutis laxa** is characterized by loose, pendulous skin imparting a prematurely aged appearance. In both the congenital and acquired types, systemic involvement is seen frequently, involving the lungs (pulmonary emphysema), bladder, and GI tract (diverticula and rectal prolapse) with inguinal, umbilical, and hiatal hernias. In some congenital cases, growth retardation and multiple joint dislocations involving the hip joints may also be present.

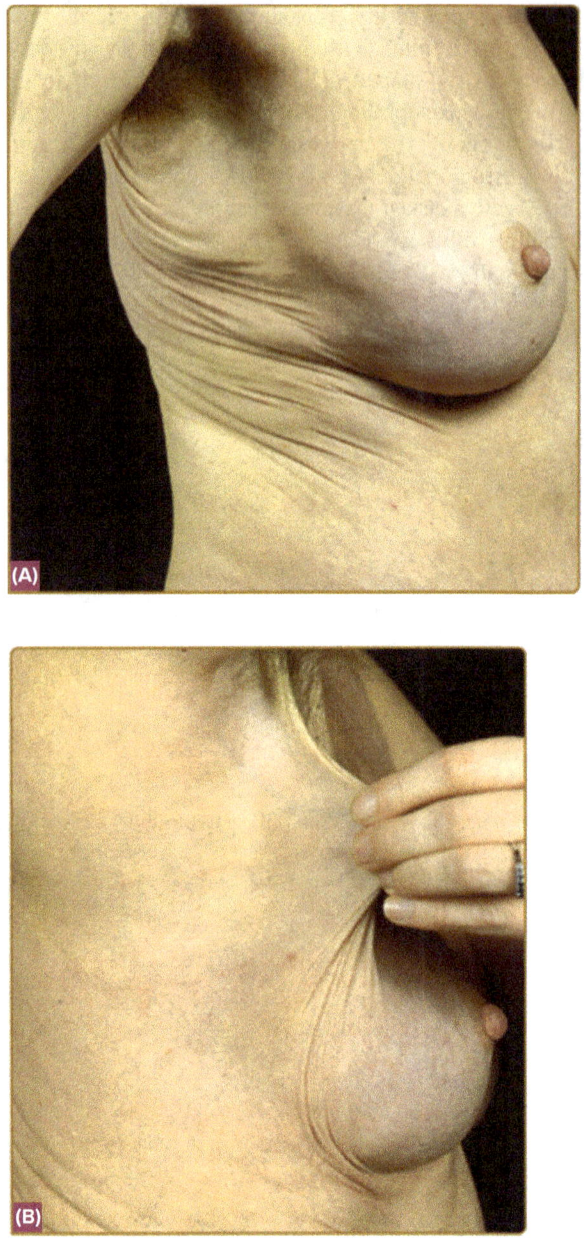

Cutis laxa. (A) The skin sags if it were too wide for the patient. **(B)** Skin can be picked up like a loose sheet. When released, it will return only slowly to the original position.

Microscopically, the elastic fiber abnormalities in **cutis laxa** vary depending on the stage and severity of the disease, either with elastic fibers diminished throughout the dermis or the decrease in elastic tissue confined to the upper or the lower dermis. The remaining elastic fibers may be shortened, fragmented, and strikingly variable in diameter. Elastic tissue stains may be used to demonstrate the abnormalities. In severe examples, no elastic fibers may be present, and only fine, dust-like or dot-like particles are scattered through the dermis. In cases preceded by an inflammatory eruption such as **urticaria**, erythematous plaques, or vesicles, the inflammatory infiltrate may be mononuclear (lymphocytes and histiocytes) or mixed, containing neutrophils. When vesicles are present, they are subepidermal, with papillary collections of neutrophils and eosinophils mimicking **dermatitis herpetiformis**. Involved internal organs show granular changes in elastic fibers similar to those seen in the skin. Collagen abnormalities have also been described but are ultrastructurally nonspecific.

Macular Atrophy (anetoderma) may be classified as primary, where it may either be preceded by inflammation (**Jadassohn–Pellizzari type**) in which the atrophic cutaneous lesions appear initially red and demonstrate an inflammatory infiltrate on histologic examination, or the lesions may lack clinical and histologic evidence of inflammation (**Schweninger–Buzzi type**). **Primary anetoderma** has been

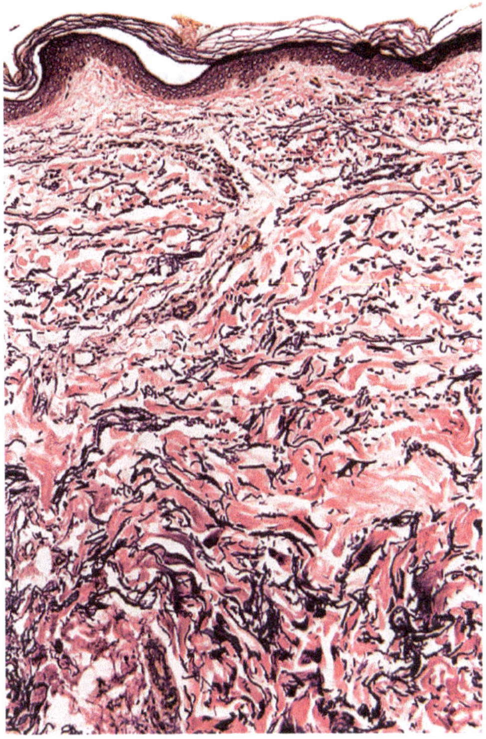

Cutis laxa. Elastic tissue stain of normal skin from a patient with cutis laxa showing the expected pattern of elastic tissue (elastic stain).

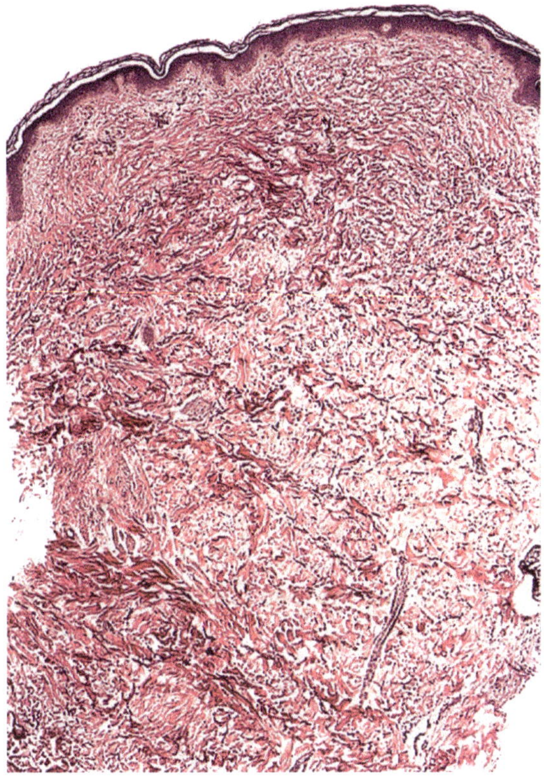

Anetoderma (macular atrophy). Elastic tissue stain shows loss of normal elastic tissue throughout the papillary and upper reticular dermis that allows the skin to bulge (elastic stain).

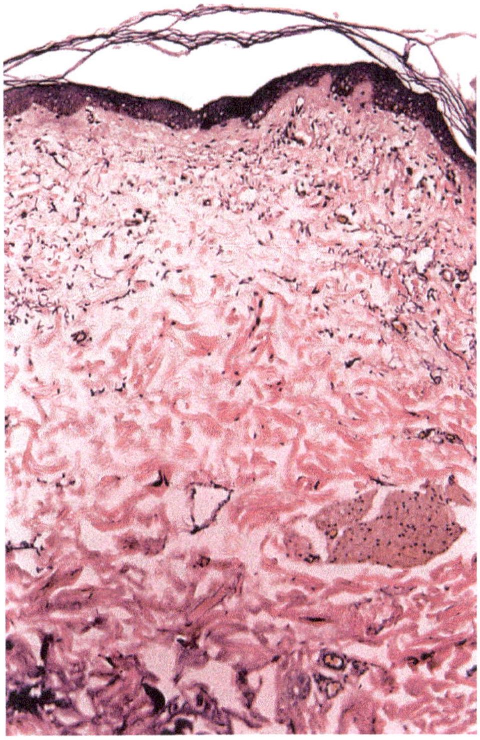

Cutis laxa. Elastic tissue stain from the involved skin of a patient with cutis laxa shows virtually no elastic tissue remaining with little evidence of an inflammatory infiltrate (elastic stain).

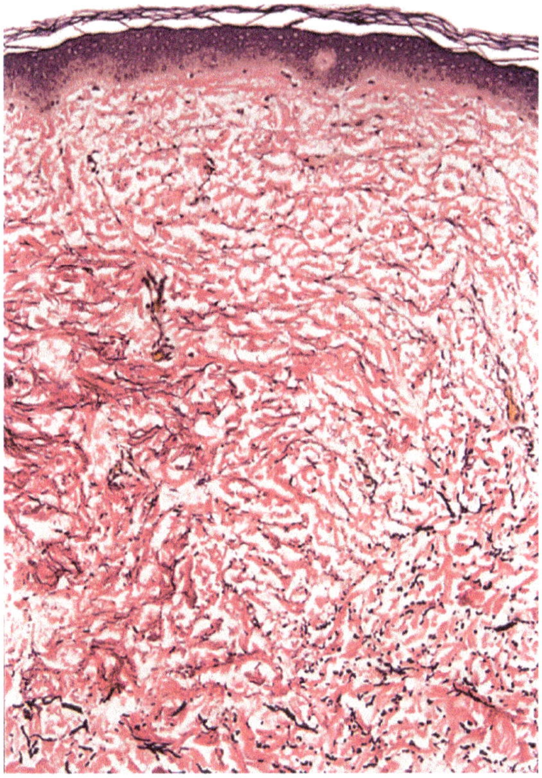

Anetoderma (macular atrophy). A higher power view shows markedly reduced elastic tissue (elastic stain).

Table 6-39A. Elastolytic Disorders of the Skin

ELASTOLYSIS IN DERMIS	DISORDER	CLINICAL FEATURES	HISTOPATHOLOGICAL FEATURES
Total	Cutis laxa	Coarsely wrinkled, loose redundant skin folds	Loss of elastic fibers throughout dermis and fragmentation of remaining fibers
	Blepharochalasis	Recurrent eyelid edema leading to atrophy of periorbital skin	Almost complete loss of elastic fibers in dermis, epidermal atrophy, and thinned collagen fibers
	Anetoderma	Small papules and cobblestone plaques	Absent elastic fibers in the dermis; elastophagocytosis may be present; perivascular inflammatory infiltrate may be present in clinically inflammatory lesions
Zonal	Papillary elastolysis	Small papules and cobblestone plaques	Complete loss of elastic fibers in the papillary dermis; almost complete loss of elastic fibers from papillary dermis and atrophic epidermis
	Papillary pseudoxanthoma-like elastolysis	Multiple small yellow nonfollicular papules that coalesce to form plaques resembling pseudoxanthoma elasticum	
	Mid-dermal elastolysis	Type I: fine wrinkling arranged parallel to skin cleavage lines; type II: papular perifollicular protrusions	Focal loss of elastic fibers in the reticular dermis
Focal	Perifollicular elastolysis	Small finely wrinkled macules in association with hair follicle associated with acne vulgaris	Almost complete loss of elastic fibers confined to the immediate vicinity of hair follicle; no inflammation
	Striae	Linear atrophic depression along skin cleavage lines, initially violaceous then fade	Reduction of elastic tissue in early lesions and thickened elastic fibers in older lesions; epidermis flattened, atrophic blunted rete ridges, dermal thickness decreased, collagen bundles thinned and parallel to epidermis, and absent subepidermal appendages
	Scars		Elastic fibers initially absent; thinned elastic fibers present at 3 months; absent subepidermal appendages

associated with a number of conditions; the most significant of which is antiphospholipid antibodies. **Secondary anetoderma** has been reported after numerous cutaneous conditions. No hereditary forms of macular atrophy have been established. The cause of **anetoderma** is controversial, but elastolysis is a likely candidate. In all forms of **macular atrophy (anetoderma)**, round to oval atrophic patches primarily involving the upper trunk develop and are characterized by thin skin that bulges with movement. Palpation of **macular atrophy** transmits the sensation of a soft depression suggesting an orifice. Microscopically, in **inflammatory anetoderma (Jadassohn–Pellizzari type)**, early lesions show a moderately dense perivascular, predominately lymphocytic infiltrate. Occasionally, plasma cells and eosinophils predominate, and rarely, neutrophils and epithelioid histiocytes may be present. In chronic **noninflammatory anetoderma (Schweninger-Buzzi type)**, elastic tissue stains show a virtually complete loss of elastic tissue either in the upper reticular and papillary dermis or confined to the upper reticular dermis. Inflammatory cells may surround degenerated elastic fibers. A summary of these elastolytic conditions is provided in Table 6-39A.

BIBLIOGRAPHY

1. Ajoka RS, Kushner JP. Hereditary hemochromatosis. *Semin Hematol.* 2002;39:235–241.
2. Akiyama M, Sugiyama-Nakagiri Y, Sakai K, et al. Mutations in lipid transporter ABCA12 in harlequin ichthyosis and functional recovery by corrective gene transfer. *J Clin Invest.* 2005;115:1777–1784.
3. Al-Aboosi M, Abalkhail A, Kasim O, et al. Friction melanosis: a clinical, histologic, and ultrastructural study in Jordanian patients. *Int J Dermatol.* 2004;43(4):261–264.
4. Amichai B, Gat A, Grunwald MH. Cutaneous hyperpigmentation during therapy with hydroxychloroquine. *J Clin Rheumatol.* 2007;13(2):113.
5. Aretz S, Stienen D, Uhlhaas S, et al. High proportion of large genomic STK11 deletions in Peutz-Jeghers syndrome. *Hum Mutat.* 2005;26(6):513–519.
6. Banasiak MJ, Malek AR. Nelson syndrome: comprehensive review of pathophysiology, diagnosis, and management. *Neurosurg Focus.* 2007;23(3):E13.
7. Beers W, Ince A, Moore T. Scleredema adultorum of Buschke: a case report and review of the literature. *Semin Arthritis Rheum.* 2006;35:355.
8. Bittar M, Happle R, Grzeschik KH, et al. CHILD syndrome in 3 generations: the importance of mild or minimal skin lesions. *Arch Dermatol.* 2006;142:348–351.
9. Bowen AR, McCalmont TH. The histopathology of subcutaneous minocycline pigmentation. *J Am Acad Dermatol.* 2007;57(5):836–839.
10. Butler D, Davis G, Greene J. Multiple mucinous (myxoid) cysts of a single finger. *J Am Acad Dermatol.* 2005;53:914.
11. Chan H, Liu FT, Naguwa S. A review of pityriasis rubra pilaris and rheumatologic associations. *Clin Dev Immunol.* 2004;11:57–60.
12. Charlín R, Barcaui CB, Kac BK, et al. Hydroquinone-induced exogenous ochronosis: a report of four cases and usefulness of dermoscopy. *Int J Dermatol.* 2008;47(1):19–23.
13. Choi JC, Yang JH, Lee UH, et al. Progressive cribriform and zosteriform hyperpigmentation—the late onset linear and whorled nevoid hypermelanosis. *J Eur Acad Dermatol Venereol.* 2005;19(5):638–639.
14. Chowdhury MM, Blackford S, Williams S. Juvenile colloid milium associated with ligneous conjunctivitis: report of a case and review of the literature. *Clin Exp Dermatol.* 2000;25:138.
15. Common JE, O'Toole EA, Leigh IM, et al. Clinical and genetic heterogeneity of erythrokeratoderma variabilis. *J Invest Dermatol.* 2005;125:920–927.
16. Conlin PA, Jimenez-Quintero LP, Rapini RP. Osteomas of the skin revisited: a clinicopathologic review of 74 cases. *Am J Dermatopathol.* 2002;24:479.
17. Dale BA, Kam E. Harlequin ichthyosis. Variability in expression and hypothesis for disease mechanism. *Arch Dermatol.* 1993;129:1471–1477.
18. Danarti R, König A, Salhi A, et al. Becker's nevus syndrome revisited. *J Am Acad Dermatol.* 2004;51(6):965–969.
19. Davis MD, Pittelkow MR, Lindor NM, et al. Progressive extensive osteoma cutis associated with dystrophic features: a new syndrome? Case report and review of the literature. *Br J Dermatol.* 2002;146:1075.
20. de Sanctis L, Delmastro L, Russo MC, et al. Genetics of McCune-Albright syndrome. *J Pediatr Endocrinol Metab.* 2006;19(Suppl 2):577–582.
21. De Schepper S, Boucneau JM, Westbroek W, et al. Neurofibromatosis type 1 protein and amyloid precursor protein interact in normal human melanocytes and colocalize with melanosomes. *J Invest Dermatol.* 2006;126(3):653–659.
22. Desai AM, Pielop JA, Smith-Zagone MJ, Hsu S. Colloid milium: a histopathologic mimicker of nodular amyloidosis. *Arch Dermatol.* 2006;142:784.
23. Di Lernia V. Segmental nevus depigmentosus: analysis of 20 patients. *Pediatr Dermatol.* 1999;16: 349–321.
24. DiGiovanna JJ, Robinson-Bostom L. Ichthyosis: etiology, diagnosis, and management. *Am J Clin Dermatol.* 2003;4:81–95.
25. Du-Thanh A, Cave H, Bessis D, et al. A novel PTPN11 gene mutation in a patient with LEOPARD syndrome. *Arch Dermatol.* 2007;143(9):1210–1211.
26. Ferreira M, Sanches M, Lobo I, Selores M. Alkaptonuric ochronosis. *Eur J Dermatol.* 2007;17:336.
27. Fulk CS. Primary disorders of hyperpigmentation. *J Am Acad Dermatol.* 1984;10:1–16.
28. Fusco F, Bardaro T, Fimiani G, et al. Molecular analysis of the genetic defect in a large cohort of IP patients and identification of novel NEMO mutations interfering with NF-kappaB activation. *Hum Mol Genet.* 2004;13(16):1763–1773.
29. Garg A, Mahalingam M, Alavian C. Pruritic patches on the back and papules on the legs. Primary localized cutaneous amyloidosis (PLCA) (cutaneous lichen amyloidosis and macular amyloidosis). *Arch Dermatol* 2007;143:255.
30. Geist DE, Phillips TJ. Development of chrysiasis after Q-switched ruby laser treatment of solar lentigines. *J Am Acad Dermatol.* 2006;55(Suppl 2):S59–S60.

31. Gilhar A, Zelickson B, Ulman Y, Etzioni A. In vivo destruction of melanocytes by the IgG fraction of serum from patients with vitiligo. *J Invest Dermatol.* 1995;105:683–686.
32. Goldstein N. IV. Complications from tattoos. *J Dermatol Surg Oncol.* 1979;5:869–878.
33. Grange DK, Lorch SM, Cole PL, et al. Cantu syndrome in a woman and her two daughters: further confirmation of autosomal dominant inheritance and review of the cardiac manifestations. *Am J Med Genet A.* 2006;140(15):1673–1680.
34. Grimes P, Yamada N, Bhawan J, et al. Light microscopic, immunohistochemical, and ultrastructural alterations in patients with melasma. *Am J Dermatopathol.* 2005;27(2):96.
35. Grønskov K, Ek J, Brondum-Nielsen K. Oculocutaneous albinism. *Orphanet J Rare Dis.* 2007;2:43.
36. Hamada T. Lipoid proteinosis. *Clin Exp Dermatol.* 2002;27:624.
37. Harrison C, Khair K, Baxter B, et al. Hermansky-Pudlak syndrome: infrequent bleeding and the first report of Turkish and Pakistani kindreds. *Arch Dis Child.* 2002;86:297–301.
38. Hatchwell E. Hypomelanosis of Ito and X; autosome translocations: a unifying hypothesis. *J Med Genet.* 1996;33:177–183.
39. Hatsell SJ, Eady RA, Wennerstrand L, et al. Novel splice site mutation in keratin 1 underlies mild epidermolytic palmoplantar keratoderma in three kindreds. *J Invest Dermatol.* 2001;116:606–609.
40. Heidary N, Naik H, Burgin S. Chemotherapeutic agents and the skin: an update. *J Am Acad Dermatol.* 2008;58(4):545–570.
41. Hernandez-Martin A, Gonzalez-Sarmiento R, De Unamuno P. X-linked ichthyosis: an update. *Br J Dermatol.* 1999;141:617–627.
42. Horn HM, Tidman MJ. The clinical spectrum of dystrophic epidermolysis bullosa. *Br J Dermatol.* 2002;146:267–274.
43. Horn HM, Tidman MJ. The clinical spectrum of epidermolysis bullosa simplex. *Br J Dermatol.* 2000;142:468–472.
44. Horvath A, Bossis I, Giatzakis C, et al. Large deletions of the PRKAR1A gene in Carney complex. *Clin Cancer Res.* 2008;14(2):388–395.
45. Hu Z, Bonifas JM, Beech J, et al. Mutations in ATP2C1, encoding a calcium pump, cause Hailey-Hailey disease. *Nat Genet.* 2000;24:61–65.
46. Hutton SM, Spritz RA. Comprehensive analysis of oculocutaneous albinism among non-Hispanic Caucasians shows that OCA1 is the most prevalent OCA type. *J Invest Dermatol.* 2008;128(10):2442–2250.
47. Introcaso CE, Hivnor C, Cowper S, Werth VP. Nephrogenic fibrosing dermopathy/nephrogenic systemic fibrosis: a case series of nine patients and review of the literature. *Int J Dermatol.* 2007;46:447.
48. Ito M, Fujiwara H, Maruyama T, et al. Morphogenesis of the cornoid lamella: histochemical, immunohistochemical, and ultrastructural study of porokeratosis. *J Cutan Pathol.* 1991;18:247–256.
49. Jambrosic J, From L, Hanna W. Lichen amyloidosus: ultrastructure and pathogenesis. *Am J Dermatopathol.* 1984;6:151–158.
50. Jonas L, Bloch C, Zimmermann R, et al. Detection of silver sulfide deposits in the skin of patients with argyria after long-term use of silver-containing drugs. *Ultrastruct Pathol.* 2007;31(6):379–384.
51. Kalajian AH, Waldman M, Knable AL. Nodular primary localized cutaneous amyloidosis after trauma: a case report and discussion of the rate of progression to systemic amyloidosis. *J Am Acad Dermatol.* 2007 Aug;57(Suppl 2):S26–S29.
52. Kaya TI, Yazici AC, Tursen U, et al. Idiopathic guttate hypomelanosis: idiopathic or ultraviolet induced? *Photodermatol Photoimmunol Photomed.* 2005;21(5):270–271.
53. Kelsell DP, Norgett EE, Unsworth H, et al. Mutations in ABCA12 underlie the severe congenital skin disease harlequin ichthyosis. *Am J Hum Genet.* 2005;76:794–803.
54. Kemp E, Gavalas N, Gawkrodger D, et al. Autoantibody responses to melanocytes in the depigmenting skin disease vitiligo. *Autoimmun Rev.* 2007;6(3):138–142.
55. Kemp E, Waterman E, Hawes B, et al. The melanin-concentrating hormone receptor 1, a novel target of autoantibody responses in vitiligo. *J Clin Invest.* 2002;109(7):923–930.
56. Kim SK, Kang HY, Lee ES, et al. Clinical and histopathologic characteristics of nevus depigmentosus. *J Am Acad Dermatol.* 2006;55(3):423–428.
57. Komatsu N, Saijoh K, Jayakumar A, et al. Correlation between SPINK5 gene mutations and clinical manifestations in Netherton syndrome patients. *J Invest Dermatol.* 2007;128(5):1148–1159.
58. Konrad K, Woolf K. Pathogenesis of diffuse melanosis secondary to malignant melanoma. *Br J Dermatol.* 1974;91:635–655.
59. Lacz NL, Vafaie J, Kihiczak NI, et al. Postinflammatory hyperpigmentation: a common but troubling condition. *Int J Dermatol.* 2004;43(5):362–365.
60. Landau M, Krafchik BR. The diagnostic value of café-au-lait macules. *J Am Acad Dermatol.* 1999;40:877–890.

61. Langer K, Konrad K, Wolff K. Keratitis, ichthyosis and deafness (KID)-syndrome: report of three cases and a review of the literature. *Br J Dermatol.* 1990;122: 689–697.
62. Langeveld-Wildschut EG, Toonstra J, van Vloten WA, et al. Familial elastosis perforans serpiginosa. *Arch Dermatol.* 1993;129:205–207.
63. Lee HS, Chun YS, Hann SK. Nevus depigmentosus: clinical features and histopathologic characteristics in 67 patients. *J Am Acad Dermatol.* 1999;40:21–26.
64. Lesesky EB, Pelle MT, O'Grady TC. Diffuse nodules in a woman with renal failure: chronic tophaceous gout. *Arch Dermatol.* 2007;143:1201.
65. Libow LF, Mawhinney JP, Bessinger GT. Cutaneous Waldenstrom's macroglobulinemia: report of a case and overview of the spectrum of cutaneous disease. *J Am Acad Dermatol.* 2001;45(Suppl):S202.
66. Lin RL, Janniger CK. Pityriasis alba. *Cutis.* 2005;76(1): 21–24.
67. Lugassy J, McGrath JA, Itin P, et al. KRT14 haploinsufficiency results in increased susceptibility of keratinocytes to TNF-alpha-induced apoptosis and causes Naegeli-Franceschetti-Jadassohn syndrome. *J Invest Dermatol.* 2008;128(6):1517–1524.
68. Mahalingam M, Palko M, Steinberg-Benjes L, Goldberg LJ. Amyloidosis of the auricular concha: an uncommon variant of localized cutaneous amyloidosis. *Am J Dermatopathol.* 2002;24:447.
69. Mancini AJ, Lawley LP, Uzel G. X-linked ectodermal dysplasia with immunodeficiency caused by NEMO mutation: early recognition and diagnosis. *Arch Dermatol.* 2008;144(3):342–346.
70. Maruyama H, Ohbayashi C, Hino O, et al. Pathogenesis of multifocal micronodular pneumocyte hyperplasia and lymphangioleiomyomatosis in tuberous sclerosis and association with tuberous sclerosis genes TSC1 and TSC2. *Pathol Int.* 2001;51:585–594.
71. McClelland M, VanLock JS, Patterson JW, Greer KE. Radiation-induced morphea
72. McCormack CJ, Cowen P. Haber's syndrome. *Australas J Dermatol.* 1997;38(2):82–84.
73. Mevorah B, Krayenbuhl A, Bovey EH, et al. Autosomal dominant ichthyosis and X-linked ichthyosis. Comparison of their clinical and histological phenotypes. *Acta Derm Venereol.* 1991;71:431–434.
74. Moon AO, Calamia KT, Walsh JS. Nodular amyloidosis: review and long-term follow-up of 16 cases. *Arch Dermatol.* 2003;139:1157.
75. Moretti S, Spallanzani A, Amato L, et al. New insights into the pathogenesis of vitiligo: imbalance of epidermal cytokines at sites of lesions. *Pigment Cell Res.* 2002;15:87–92.
76. Mukherji M, Chien W, Kershaw NJ, et al. Structure-function analysis of phytanoyl-CoA 2-hydroxylase mutations causing Refsum's disease. *Hum Mol Genet.* 2001;10:1971–1982.
77. Murakami T, Hosomi N, Oiso N, et al. Analysis of KIT, SCF, and initial screening of SLUG in patients with piebaldism. *J Invest Dermatol.* 2005;124(3):670–672.
78. Nakano A, Chao SC, Pulkkinen L, et al. Laminin 5 mutations in junctional epidermolysis bullosa: molecular basis of Herlitz vs. non-Herlitz phenotypes. *Hum Genet.* 2002;110:41–51.
79. Oji V, Traupe H. Ichthyoses: differential diagnosis and molecular genetics. *Eur J Dermatol.* 2006;16:349–359.
80. Oriba HA, Lo JS, Dijkstra JWE, Bergfeld WF. Reticulate nonmelanocytic hyperpigmentation anomaly: a probable variant of Dowling-Degos disease. *Int J Dermatol.* 1991;30:39–42.
81. Pasternak S, Wright B, Walsh N. Soft tissue amyloidoma of the extremities: report of a case and review of the literature. *Am J Dermatopathol.* 2007;29:152–155.
82. Patel N, Spencer LA, English JC III, et al. Acquired ichthyosis. *J Am Acad Dermatol.* 2006;55:647–656.
83. Patel S, Zirwas M, English JC III. Acquired palmoplantar keratoderma. *Am J Clin Dermatol.* 2007;8:1–11.
84. Pinto FJ, Bolognia JL. Disorders of hypopigmentation in children. *Pediatr Clin North Am.* 1991;38:991–1017.
85. Pourrabbani S, Marra DE, Iwasaki J, et al. Colloid milium: a review and update. *J Drugs Dermatol.* 2007;6:293.
86. Ramesh V, Sood N, Kubba A, et al. Familial reactive perforating collagenosis: a clinical, histopathological study of 10 cases. *J Eur Acad Dermatol Venereol* 2007;21:766–770.
87. Requena L, Sangueza OP. Cutaneous vascular anomalies: I. Hamartomas, malformations, and dilation of preexisting vessels. *J Am Acad Dermatol.* 1997;37:523–549.
88. Rhodes AR, Albert LS, Barnhill RL, Weinstock MA. Sun-induced freckles in children and young adults: a correlation of clinical and histopathologic features. *Cancer.* 1991;67:1990–2001.
89. Riccardi VM. Neurofibromatosis: past, present, and future. *New Engl J Med.* 1991;324:1283–1285.
90. Rieger E, Kofler R, Borkenstein M, et al. Melanotic macules following Blaschko's lines in McCune-Albright syndrome. *Br J Dermatol.* 1994;130:215–220.
91. Rongioletti F, Rebora A. Cutaneous mucinoses: microscopic criteria for diagnosis. *Am J Dermatopathol.* 2001;123:257.

92. Rongioletti F, Rebora A. Updated classification of papular mucinosis, lichen myxedematosus, and scleromyxedema. *J Am Acad Dermatol.* 2001;44:273.
93. Rousseau K, Kauser S, Pritchard LE, et al. Proopiomelanocortin (POMC), the ACTH/melanocortin precursor, is secreted by human epidermal keratinocytes and melanocytes and stimulates melanogenesis. *FASEB J.* 2007;21(8):1844–1856.
94. Rugg EL, Common JE, Wilgoss A, et al. Diagnosis and confirmation of epidermolytic palmoplantar keratoderma by the identification of mutations in keratin 9 using denaturing high-performance liquid chromatography. *Br J Dermatol.* 2002;146:952–957.
95. Rugg EL, Horn HM, Smith FJ, et al. Epidermolysis bullosa simplex in Scotland caused by a spectrum of keratin mutations. *J Invest Dermatol.* 2007;127:574–580.
96. Sakuntabhai A, Dhitavat J, Burge S, et al. Mosaicism for ATP2A2 mutations causes segmental Darier's disease. *J Invest Dermatol.* 2000;115:1144–1147.
97. Salvini C, Fabroni C, Francalanci S, et al. Generalized nevus anaemicus in an adult. *J Eur Acad Dermatol Venereol.* 2007;21(8):1142–1144.
98. Sandilands A, O'Regan GM, Liao H, et al. Prevalent and rare mutations in the gene encoding filaggrin cause ichthyosis vulgaris and predispose individuals to atopic dermatitis. *J Invest Dermatol.* 2006;126:1770–1775.
99. Saray Y, Seckin D, Bilezikci B. Acquired perforating dermatosis: clinicopathological features in twenty-two cases. J *Eur Acad Dermatol Venereol.* 2006;20:679–688.
100. Savage SA, Giri N, Baerlocher GM, et al. TINF2, a component of the shelterin telomere protection complex, is mutated in dyskeratosis congenita. *Am J Hum Genet.* 2008;82(2):501–509.
101. Schamroth JM, Zlotogorski A, Gilead L. Porokeratosis of Mibelli. Overview and review of the literature. *Acta Derm Venereol.* 1997;77:207–213.
102. Scheinfeld NS, Mones J. Granular parakeratosis: pathologic and clinical correlation of 18 cases of granular parakeratosis. *J Am Acad Dermatol.* 2005;52(5):863–867.
103. Schwartz RA, Fernández G, Kotulska K, et al. Tuberous sclerosis complex: advances in diagnosis, genetics, and management. *J Am Acad Dermatol.* 2007;57(2):189–202.
104. Siragusa M, Ferri R, Cavallari V, Schepis C. Friction melanosis, friction amyloidosis, macular amyloidosis, towel melanosis: many names for the same clinical entity. *Eur J Dermatol.* 2001;11:545–548.
105. Smahi A, Courtois G, Rabia SH, et al. The NF-κB signaling pathway in human diseases: from incontinentia pigmenti to ectodermal dysplasia and immunodeficiency syndromes. *Hum Mol Genet.* 2002;11:2371–2375.
106. Smoller BR, Horn TH. Endocrine abnormalities and the skin. In: Smoller BR, Horn TH, eds. *Dermatopathology in Systemic Diseases.* New York, NY: Oxford University Press; 2001:179.
107. Spenny ML, Suwannarat P, Gahl WA, et al. Blue pigmentation and arthritis in an elderly man. *J Am Acad Dermatol.* 2005;52(1):122–124.
108. Spritz RA, Ho L, Strunk KM. Inhibition of proliferation of human melanocytes by KIT antisense oligodeoxynucleotide: implications for human piebaldism and mouse dominant white spotting (W). *J Invest Dermatol.* 1994;103:148–150.
109. Syrris P, Heathcote K, Carrozzo R, et al. Human piebaldism: six novel mutations of the protooncogene KIT. *Hum Mutat.* 2002;20:234.
110. Tee AR, Manning BD, Roux PP, et al. Tuberous sclerosis complex gene products, tuberin and hamartin, control mTOR signaling by acting as a GTPase-activating protein complex toward Rheb. *Curr Biol.* 2003;13:1259–1268.
111. Terrinoni A, Cocuroccia B, Gubinelli E, et al. Identification of the keratin K9 R162W mutation in patients of Italian origin with epidermolytic palmoplantar keratoderma. *Eur J Dermatol.* 2004;14:375–378.
112. Tokuda Y, Kawachi S, Murata H, Saida T. Chronic obesity lymphoedematous mucinosis: three cases of pretibial mucinosis in obese patients with pitting oedema. *Br J Dermatol.* 2006;154:157.
113. Tominaga A, Tajima S, Ishibashi A, et al. Reticular erythematous mucinosis syndrome with an infiltration of factor XIIIa+ and hyaluronan synthase 2+ dermal dendrocytes. *Br J Dermatol.* 2001;145:141.
114. Torley D, Bellus GA, Munro CS. Genes, growth factors and acanthosis nigricans. *Br J Dermatol.* 2002;147:1096–1101.
115. Touart DM, Sau P. Cutaneous deposition diseases, part II. *J Am Acad Dermatol.* 1998;39:527–544.
116. Uchida T, Hayashi H, Inaoki M, et al. A failure of mucocutaneous lymphangiogenesis may underlie the clinical features of lipoid proteinosis. *Br J Dermatol.* 2007;156:152–157.
117. Uhle P, Norvell SS. Generalized lentiginosis. *J Am Acad Dermatol.* 1988;18:444–447.
118. van Geel M, van Steensel MA, Kuster W, et al. HID and KID syndromes are associated with the same connexin 26 mutation. *Br J Dermatol.* 2002;146:938–942.
119. Varki R, Sadowski S, Pfendner E, et al. Epidermolysis bullosa. I. Molecular genetics of the junctional

and hemidesmosomal variants. *J Med Genet.* 2006;43:641–652.

120. Varki R, Sadowski S, Uitto J, et al. Epidermolysis bullosa. II. Type VII collagen mutations and phenotype-genotype correlations in the dystrophic subtypes. *J Med Genet.* 2007;44:181–192.

121. Wallace ML, Grichnik JM, Prieto VG, Shea CR. Numbers and differentiation status of melanocytes in idiopathic guttate hypomelanosis. *J Cutan Pathol.* 1998;25:375–379.

122. Ward DM, Shiflett SL, Kaplan J. Chédiak-Higashi syndrome: a clinical and molecular view of a rare lysosomal storage disorder. *Curr Mol Med.* 2002;2:469–477.

123. Wei M. Hermansky-Pudlak syndrome: a disease of protein trafficking and organelle function. *Pigment Cell Res.* 2006;19(1):19–42.

124. Wu YH, Lin YC. Generalized Dowling-Degos disease. *J Am Acad Dermatol.* 2007;57(2):327–334.

125. Yang JM, Ahn KS, Cho MO, et al. Novel mutations of the transglutaminase 1 gene in lamellar ichthyosis. *J Invest Dermatol.* 2001;117:214–218.

126. Zhang ZH, Niu ZM, Yuan WT, et al. A mutation in SART3 gene in a Chinese pedigree with disseminated superficial actinic porokeratosis. *Br J Dermatol.* 2005;152:658–663.

CHAPTER 7

Infectious Diseases of the Skin

QUESTION 7-1.

A 31-year-old HIV-positive veterinary assistant presents with an erythematous smooth nodule on the shin with focal ulceration. There is regional lymphadenopathy. You forget to include the pertinent clinical history on the specimen requisition form and a diagnosis of "pyogenic granuloma" is rendered. Which of the following statements regarding this lesion is INCORRECT?

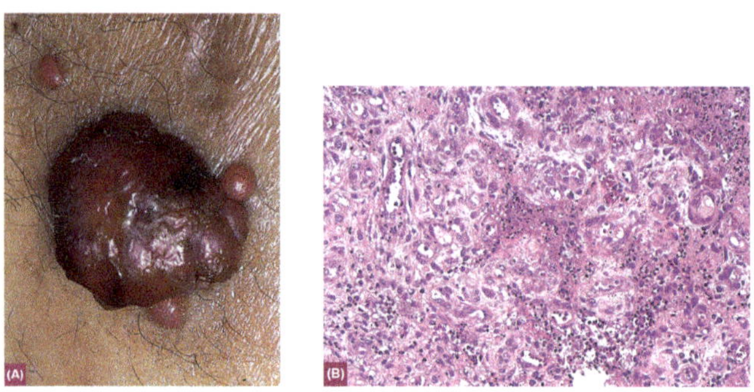

Part **(A)** reproduced, with permission, from Wolff K, Johnson RA, Saavedra AP. *Fitzpatrick's Color Atlas and Synopsis of Clinical Dermatology*. 7th ed. New York, NY: McGraw-Hill Education; 2013.

A) The causative microorganisms are best highlighted with a Warthin-Starry stain, revealing granular clusters of bacilli within endothelial cells, macrophages, and within the dermis.
B) This condition is associated with exposure to cats and cat fleas.
C) Low-power microscopic examination will reveal a well-circumscribed pedunculated proliferation of small vessels with an overlying epidermal collarette.
D) These lesions typically respond to a course of antibiotics.
E) The endothelial cells will stain positive for HHV8 via immunohistochemistry.

QUESTION 7-2.

In the clinic during your summer externship to South Africa, you encounter a 21-year-old male with a painful ulcerated erythematous ulcer on the coronal sulcus of the penis with suppuration. The ulcer edge is ragged, undermined, and its base is formed by granulation tissue covered by a necrotic, yellowish-gray exudate. Gram stain of a scraping reveals short gram-negative bacilli that form parallel chains resembling a "school of fish." His last sexual encounter was 7 days ago. There is associated regional lymphadenopathy with an overlying draining sinus tract producing copious amount of suppurative material. Which of the following statements regarding this condition is CORRECT?

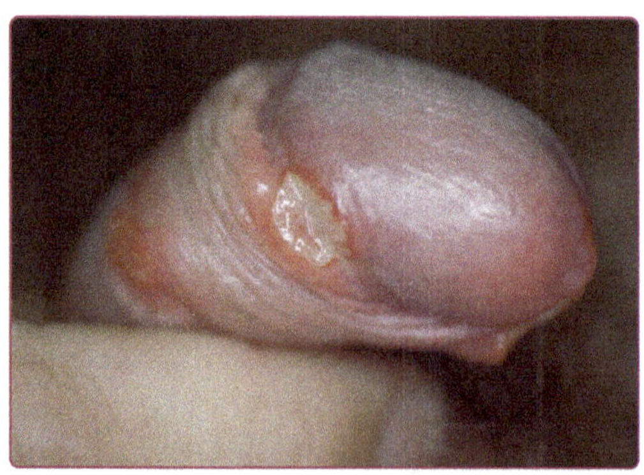

Reproduced, with permission, from Goldsmith LA, Katz SI, Gilchrest BA, Paller AS, Leffell DJ, Wolff K, eds. *Fitzpatrick's Dermatology in General Medicine*. 8th ed. New York, NY: McGraw-Hill Education; 2012.

A) The causative microorganism is *Haemophilus ducreyi.*
B) The ulcer is histopathologically characterized by two distinct layers: necrosis and granulation tissue.
C) Tissue cultures consistently fail to grow the causative microorganisms.
D) Smears from the ulcer examined under dark field microscopy consistently reveal organisms.
E) Clumped collections of the microorganisms form structures referred to as Donovan bodies.

QUESTION 7-3.

Three weeks after having unprotected intercourse, a 22-year-old Jamaican male presents with serpiginous painless ulcers with central red friable centers on the penis, perianal, and pubic regions. Regional lymphadenopathy is absent. A scraping of the ulcer is stained with Giemsa and illustrated below. A biopsy of the ulcer reveals peripheral pseudoepitheliomatous hyperplasia and an ulcer bed composed of granulation tissue with numerous large macrophages. Which of the following diagnoses is CORRECT?

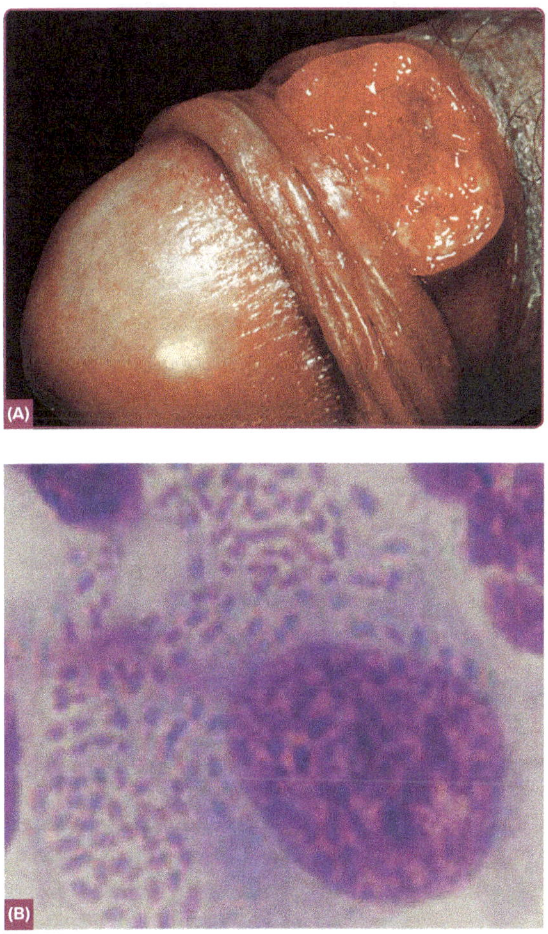

Reproduced, with permission, from Goldsmith LA, Katz SI, Gilchrest BA, Paller AS, Leffell DJ, Wolff K, eds. *Fitzpatrick's Dermatology in General Medicine.* 8th ed. New York, NY: McGraw-Hill Education; 2012.

A) Leishmaniasis
B) Histoplasmosis
C) Leprosy
D) Donovanosis
E) Chancroid

QUESTION 7-4.

A 4-year-old child presents with multiple golden/honey-colored crusts and blisters with an erythematous base on the hands, fingers, and face. The patient has a history of asthma, eczematous dermatitis, and allergic rhinitis. A biopsy of the face is performed and the findings are illustrated below. A PAS stain is negative for pseudohyphae and yeasts. Culture of the bullous fluid is positive for *Staphylococcus aureus.* The mother reports that several other children in the child's preschool class have developed similar lesions. Which of the following diagnoses is CORRECT?

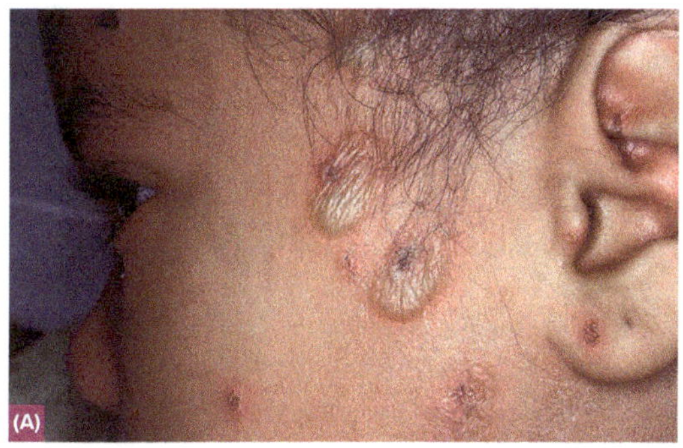

Reproduced, with permission, from Knoop KJ, Stack LB, Storrow AB, Thurman RJ. *The Atlas of Emergency Medicine.* 3rd ed. New York, NY: McGraw-Hill; 2010.

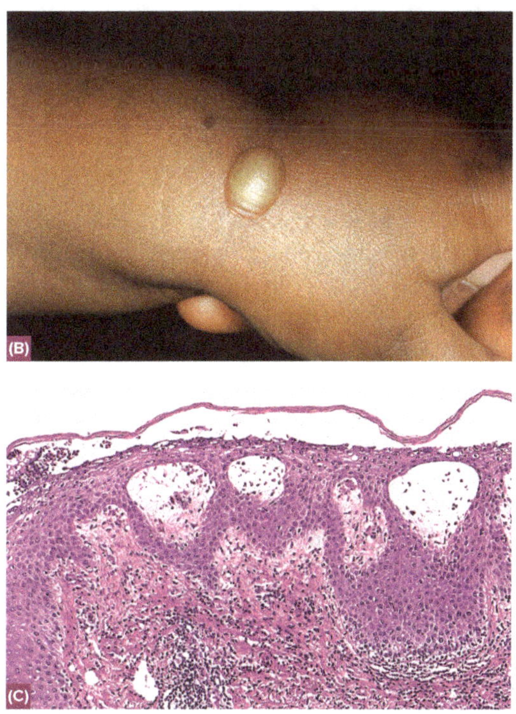

A) Impetigo
B) Bullous impetigo
C) Staphylococcal scalded skin syndrome
D) Ecthyma
E) Pemphigus foliaceus

QUESTION 7-5.

A 5-year-old child presents with several small erythematous papulopustules surrounding a bite wound on the hand from his pet cat. One of the small papulopustules is biopsied and submitted for tissue culture and routine H&E processing. The biopsy findings are illustrated below. You thoroughly cleanse and dress the wound and give the patient a course of broad-spectrum antibiotics. Two weeks after the visit, the mother reports that the bite wound has healed; however, she is concerned since the surrounding lesions have resolved with considerable scar formation. Which of the following regarding this condition is INCORRECT?

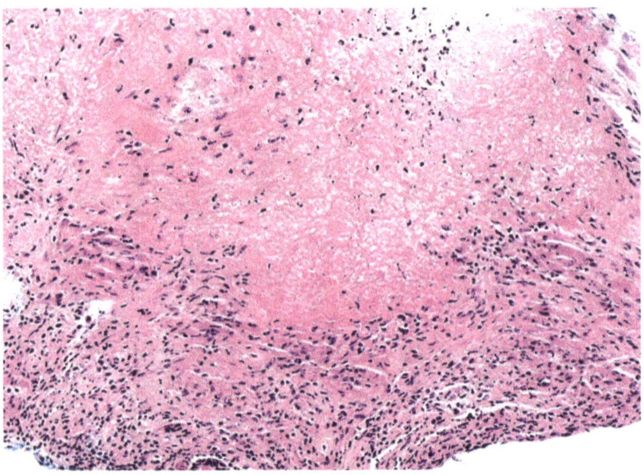

A) Tissue culture will yield gram-negative bacilli and the patient's infection will respond to the prescribed course of antibiotics.
B) The patient may present several weeks later with massive axillary lymphadenopathy.
C) GMS or Warthin-Starry stains of the skin biopsy should be examined for clumps of bacilli.
D) A Hanger-Rose test will be positive when done within the first week of infection.
E) The causative microorganism of this condition is also implicated in the pathogenesis of cutaneous nodules composed of lobular vessels with robust inflammatory infiltrates seen almost exclusively in immunocompromised patients.

QUESTION 7-6.

A 65-year-old diabetic patient with a history of stasis dermatitis presents with erythema and swelling of the left lower extremity accompanied by constitutional symptoms of fever and chills. Tissue culture grows *Staphylococcus aureus*. A biopsy is performed and reveals diffuse superficial and deep dermal as well as subcutaneous inflammatory infiltrates composed of neutrophils and lymphocytes. The epidermis is slightly spongiotic. Which of the following diagnoses is CORRECT?

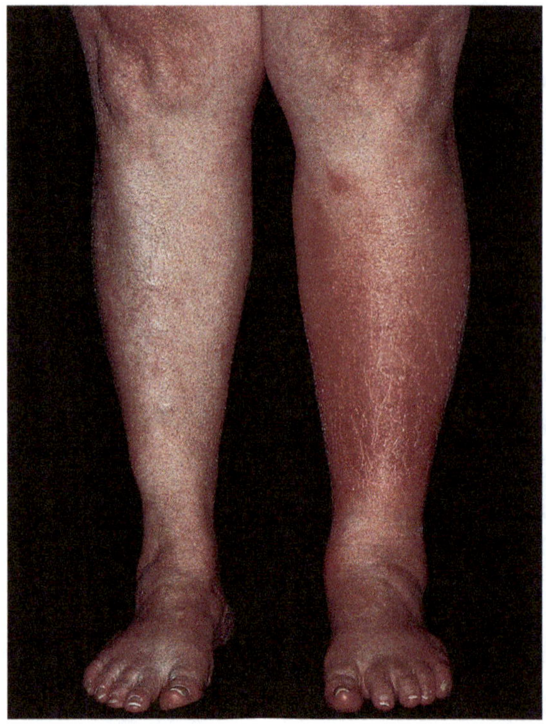

Reproduced, with permission, from Knoop KJ, Stack LB, Storrow AB, Thurman RJ. *The Atlas of Emergency Medicine*. 3rd ed. New York, NY: McGraw-Hill; 2010.

A) Urticaria
B) Cellulitis
C) Erysipeloid
D) Erysipelas
E) Sweet syndrome

QUESTION 7-7.

A 32-year-old man with HIV infection presents with the onset of a very tender plaque on the right buttock associated with fever and malaise. He claims that the lesion has been present for 5 days (image A). Biopsies are performed for tissue culture and routine H&E processing. The biopsy findings are illustrated below (image C) and the tissue culture grows gram-negative rods. The patient is lost to follow-up and presents 5 weeks later with a large necrotic ulcer (image B) and bacteremia. Which of the following diagnoses is CORRECT?

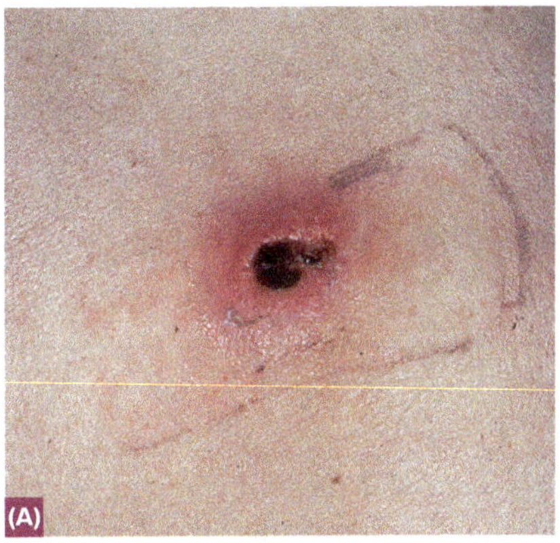

(A)

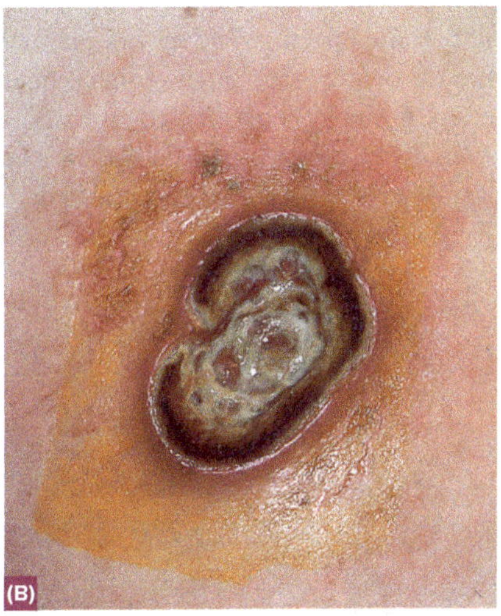

(B)

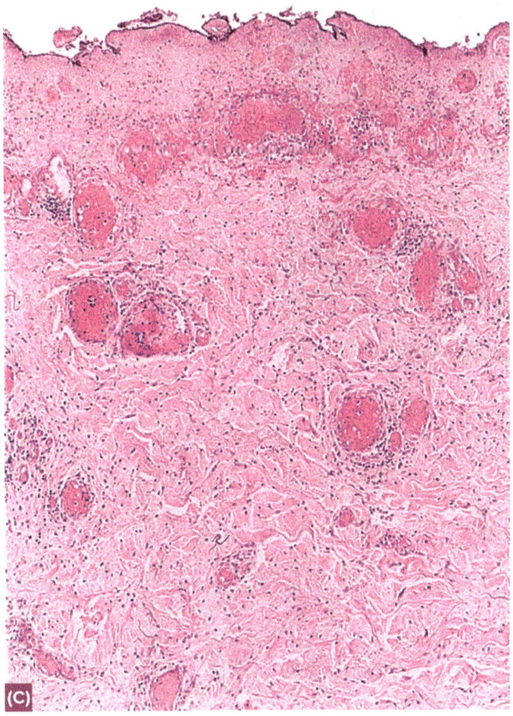

(C)

Part **(A)** reproduced, with permission, from Wolff K, Johnson RA, Saavedra AP. *Fitzpatrick's Color Atlas and Synopsis of Clinical Dermatology*. 7th ed. New York, NY: McGraw-Hill Education; 2013.

A) Cellulitis
B) Ecthyma
C) Ecthyma gangrenosum
D) Pyoderma gangrenosum
E) Toxic epidermal necrolysis

QUESTION 7-8.

A 56-year-old male presents with rapidly advancing indurated erythema on the lower extremity surfaced by a large bulla and focal areas of necrosis. The patient has a high fever and reports extreme pain out of proportion to the cutaneous findings. Palpation reveals an edematous, wooden consistency of the subcutaneous tissues extending beyond the margin of erythema. The patient reports to recently stepping on a nail in his garage for which he self-treated with a course of left over antibiotics. An incisional biopsy is performed and the findings are illustrated below. Tissue culture is pending. Which of the following statements regarding this condition is INCORRECT?

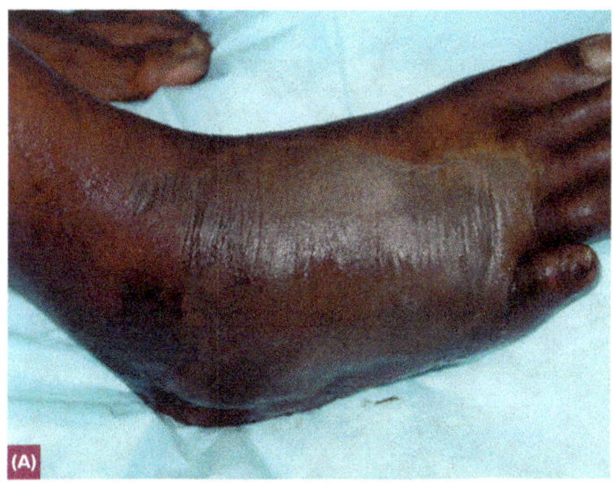

(A)

Reproduced, with permission, from Usatine RP, Smith MA, Mayeaux EJ Jr, Chumley H, Tysinger J. *The Color Atlas of Family Medicine*. McGraw-Hill, 2009; Courtesy of Ramesh Subramaniam, MD.

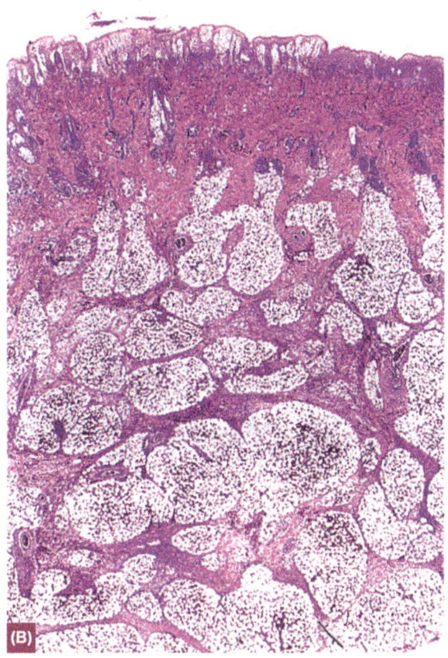

(B)

A) This condition is more common in children than adults.
B) When this condition is caused by mixed bacterial infection in surgical wounds, it is referred to as Meleney synergistic gangrene.
C) When this condition is caused by mixed bacterial infection in the genitalia, it is referred to as Fournier gangrene.
D) This condition is classically caused by infection with group A streptococci.
E) With appropriate antibiotic therapy, this condition is associated with a low mortality rate.

QUESTION 7-9.

A 55-year-old obese diabetic patient presents with slightly pruritic, raised, ill-defined, red/brown patches located in the axillae and groin. The patient is examined with a Wood lamp and the findings are illustrated below. Which of the following statements regarding this condition is INCORRECT?

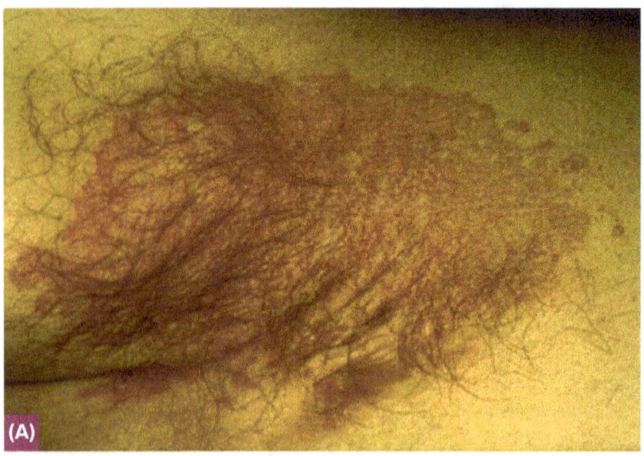
(A)

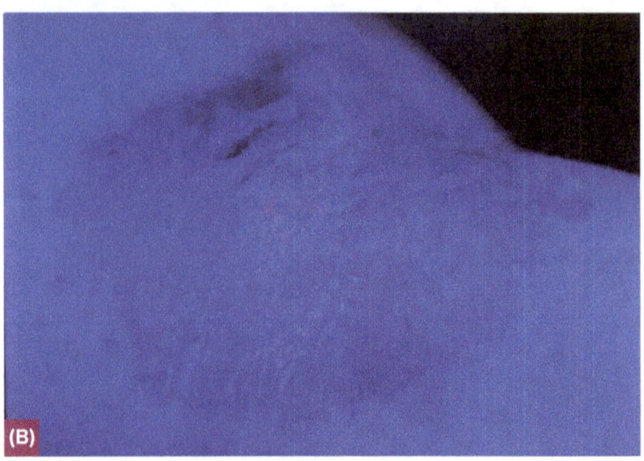
(B)

(A) and **(B)** Courtesy of K Zipperstein.

A) This patient has trichomycosis axillaris.
B) The causative organism is a gram-positive rod called *Corynebacterium minutissimum.*
C) The coral-red color seen under the Wood lamp is due to porphyrins produced by a microorganism.
D) The microscopic findings that characterize this condition include mild acanthosis and hyperkeratosis with cleft-like spaces within the stratum corneum.
E) PAS stain will highlight thin filamentous organisms within the stratum corneum.

QUESTION 7-10.

A 48-year-old female presents with painful swelling of the right middle finger for 4 months. She recalled cleaning a fish tank several weeks before the distal finger became red and tender. The finger and hand became progressively more inflamed and red nodules appeared on the forearm. Slight enlargement of axillary nodes is detected. A biopsy is performed and H&E- and Fite-stained sections are illustrated below. Which of the following infectious organisms is MOST likely implicated in this condition?

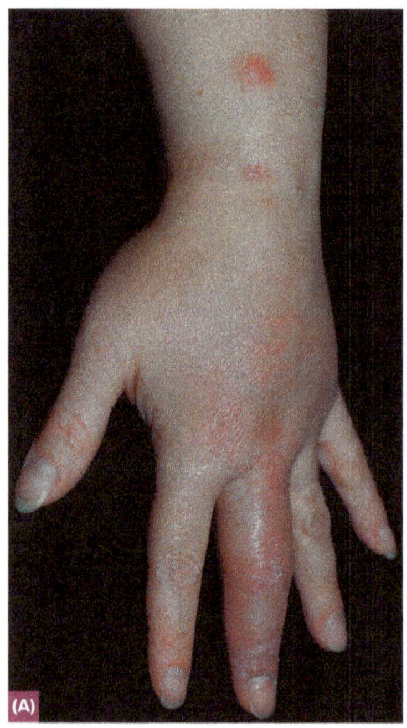
(A)

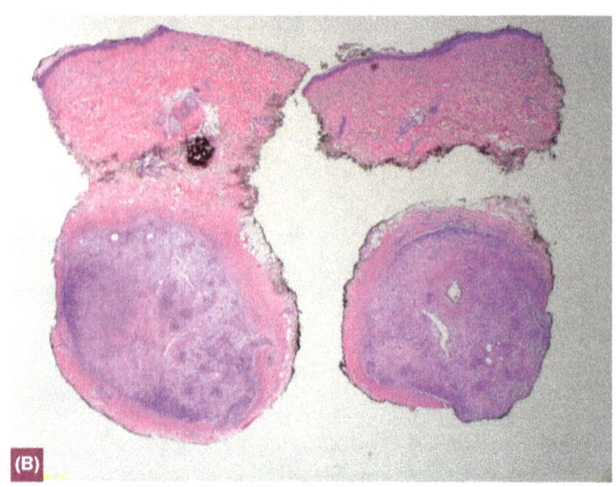
(B)

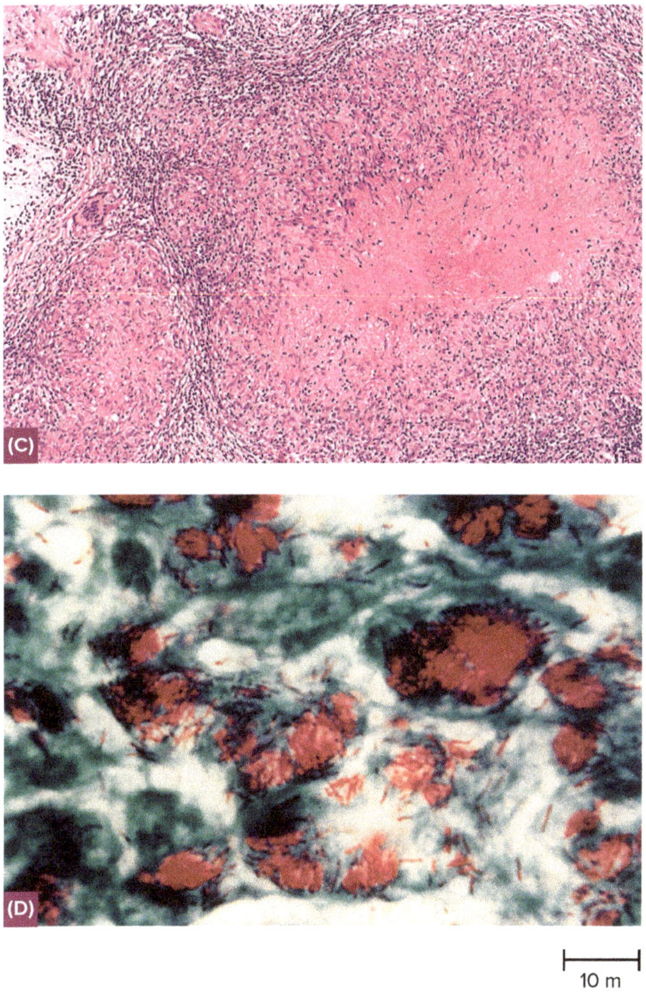

Part **(A)** reproduced, with permission, from Wolff K, Johnson RA, Saavedra AP. *Fitzpatrick's Color Atlas and Synopsis of Clinical Dermatology*. 7th ed. New York, NY: McGraw-Hill Education; 2013; part **(D)** reproduced, with permission, from Nester FW. *Microbiology: A Human Perspective*. 6th ed. New York: McGraw-Hill; 2009.

A) *Sporothrix schenckii*
B) *Mycobacterium marinum*
C) *Leishmania braziliensis*
D) *Nocardia brasiliensis*
E) *Mycobacterium ulcerans*

QUESTION 7-11.

A patient who recently emigrated from Brazil presents with scattered erythematous plaques and nodules with concomitant alopecia on the abdomen, face, nose, arms, and backs of the hands. There is sparing of the axillae, groins, and perineum. The lesions are anesthetic and the patient reports frequent epistaxis. There is no fever or other constitutional symptoms. A biopsy of the arm is performed and the findings are illustrated below. Which of the following statements regarding this condition is INCORRECT?

A) Fite stain will reveal numerous acid-fast–positive bacilli in clusters.
B) This patient has poor cell-mediated immunity against the causative infectious microorganism, but will have high levels of circulating antibodies.
C) Patients with this condition may occasionally develop new tender red plaques and nodules on normal skin, accompanied by constitutional symptoms. This type of reaction involves immune complexes and is frequently associated with leukocytoclastic vasculitis.
D) The causative infectious microorganism is *Mycobacterium chelonae.*
E) Patients treated with antibiotics for this condition may develop enhanced cellular immunity with swelling of preexisting cutaneous and neural lesions, accompanied by constitutional symptoms.

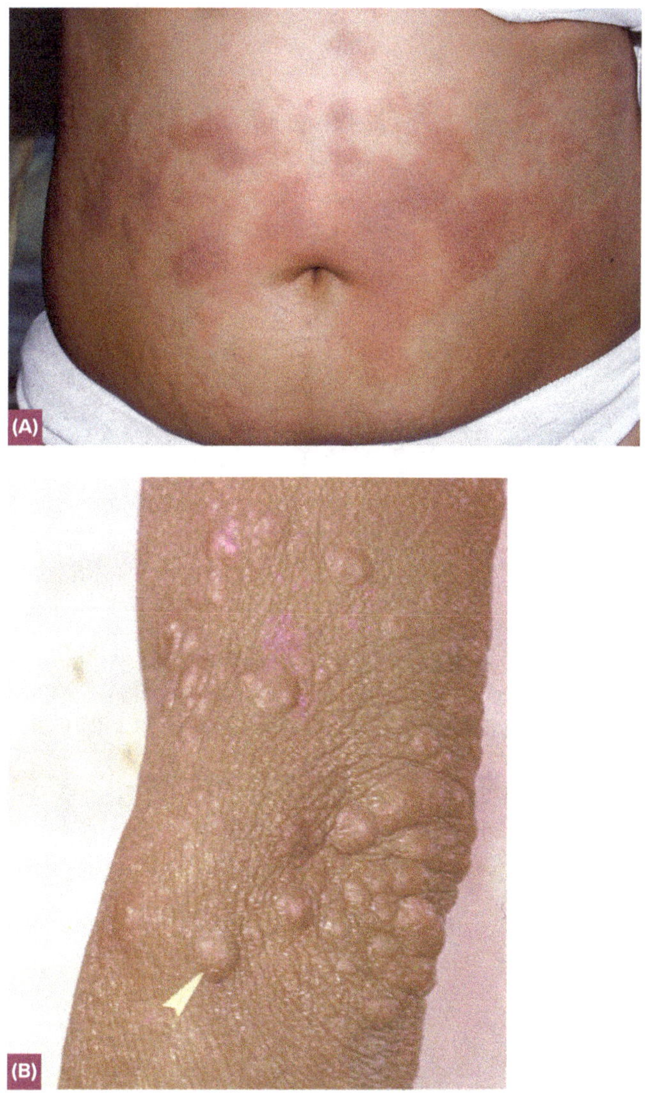

Reproduced, with permission, from Longo DL, Fauci AS, Kasper DL, Hauser SL, Jameson JL, Loscalzo J, eds. *Harrison's Principles of Internal Medicine*. 19th ed. New York, NY: McGraw-Hill Education; 2015

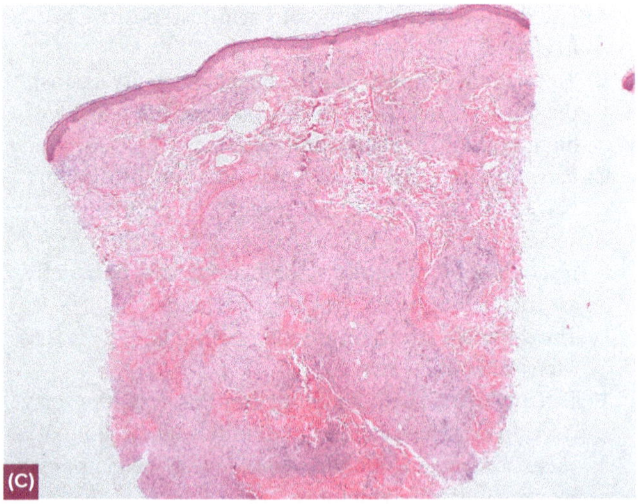

(C)

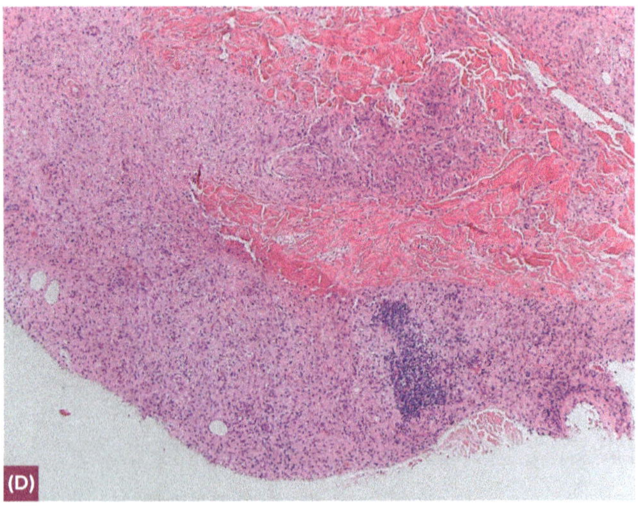

(D)

QUESTION 7-12.

A young male patient presents with an annular scaly patch with a raised erythematous margin on the chest. A biopsy is performed and the findings of the PAS stained sections are illustrated below. Which of the following diagnoses is CORRECT?

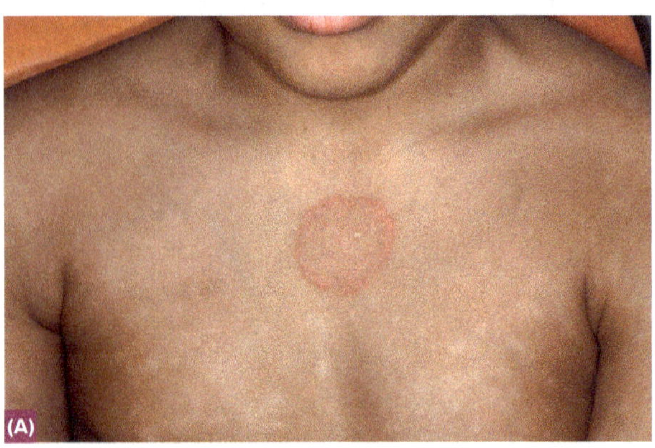

(A)

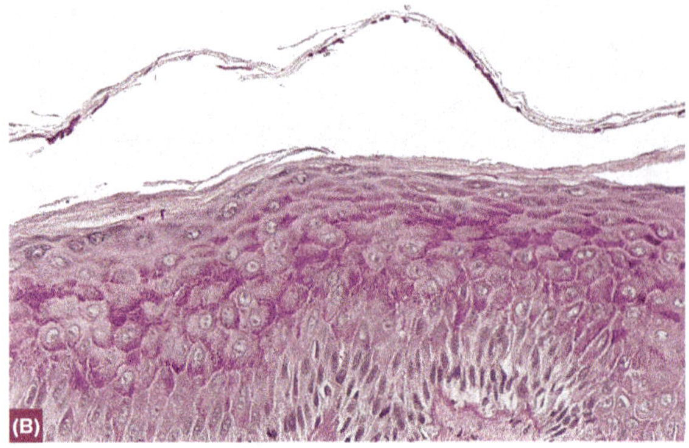

(B)

A) Allergic contact dermatitis
B) Seborrheic dermatitis
C) Tinea Corporis
D) Nummular eczema
E) Pityriasis rosea

QUESTION 7-13.

An adult patient presents with alopecia involving the scalp. Close examination reveals hairs that are broken off at the level of the scalp. Grouped black dots are identified within these patches of polygonal alopecia. Normal hairs also remain adjacent to the broken hairs. Minimal erythema is appreciated. Wood lamp examination is negative for fluorescence. Which of the following microorganisms is MOST likely implicated in this patient's alopecia?

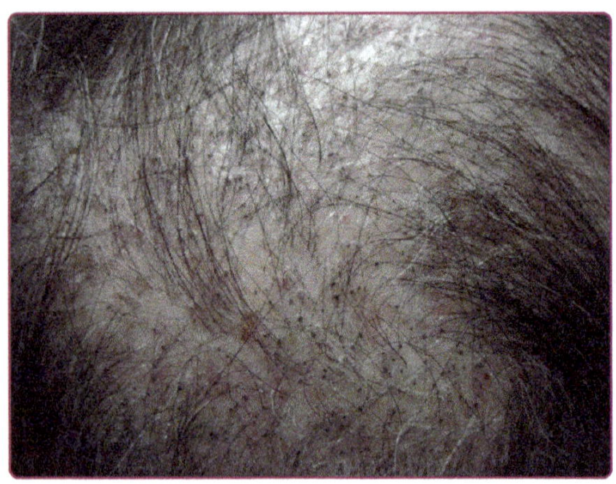

Reproduced, with permission, from Goldsmith LA, Katz SI, Gilchrest BA, Paller AS, Leffell DJ, Wolff K, eds. *Fitzpatrick's Dermatology in General Medicine*. 8th ed. New York, NY: McGraw-Hill Education; 2012.

A) *Microsporum canis*
B) *Trichophyton tonsurans*
C) *Trichophyton schoenleinii*
D) *Microsporum audouinii*
E) *Microsporum ferrugineum*

QUESTION 7-14.

An infant presents with erythematous moist and macerated macules with erosions, irregular edges, peripheral scaling, and satellite papules and pustules. A biopsy is performed and the findings are illustrated below. Which of the following infectious microorganisms is MOST likely implicated?

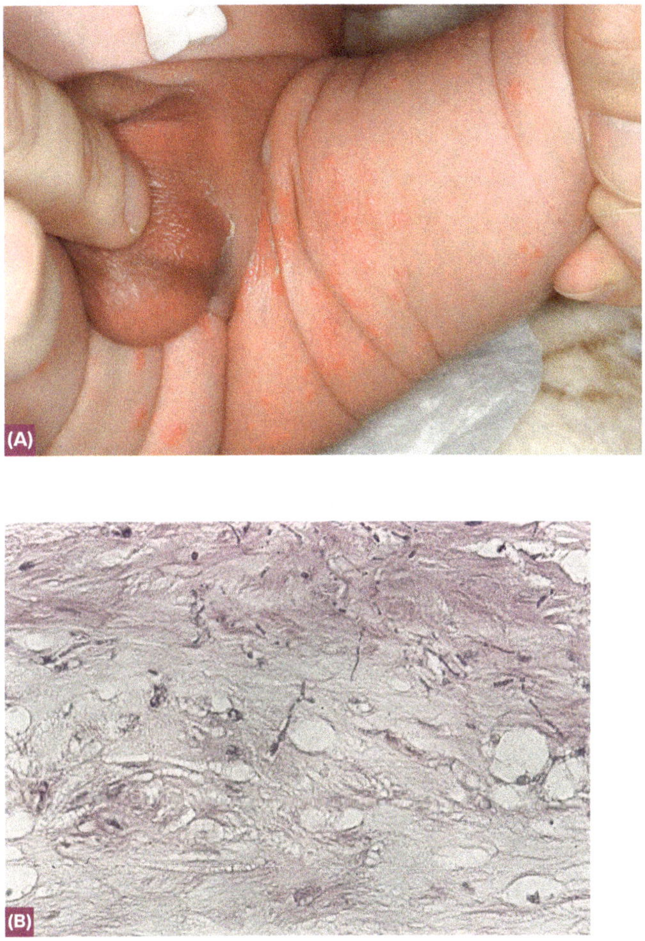

A) *Pseudomonas aeruginosa*
B) *Histoplasma capsulatum*
C) *Candida albicans*
D) *Aspergillus fumigatus*
E) *Corynebacterium minutissimum*

QUESTION 7-15.

Below is a skin scraping stained with Swartz-Lamkins stain. Which of the following clinical presentations is LEAST likely to be associated with this microorganism?

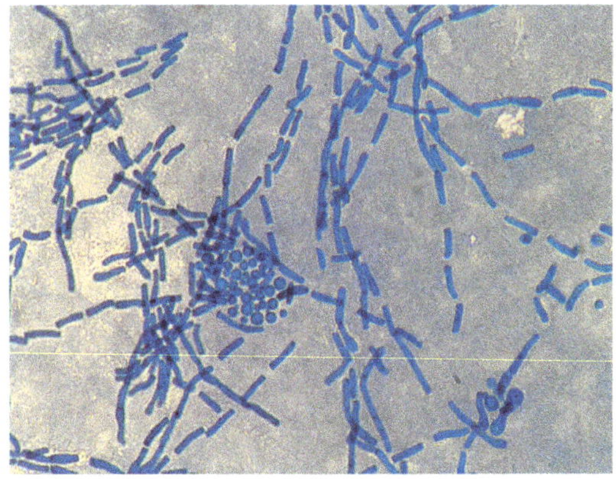

Reproduced, with permission, from Usatine RP, Smith MA, Mayeaux EJ Jr, Chumley HS, eds. *Color Atlas of Family Medicine*. 2nd ed. New York, NY: McGraw-Hill Education; 2012.

A)

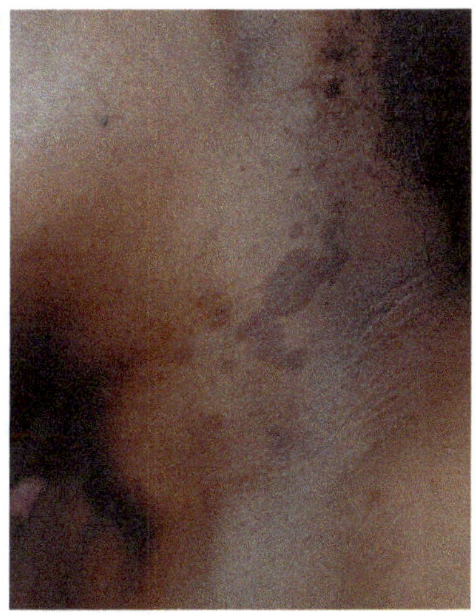

Reproduced, with permission, from Wolff K, Johnson RA, Saavedra AP. *Fitzpatrick's Color Atlas and Synopsis of Clinical Dermatology*. 7th ed. New York, NY: McGraw-Hill Education; 2013.

B)

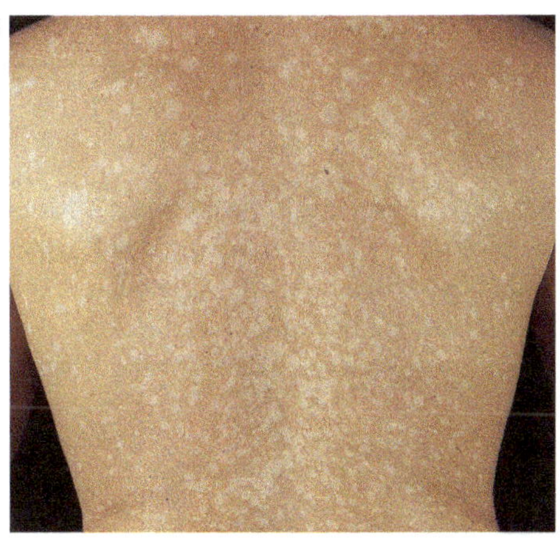

Reproduced, with permission, from Wolff K, Johnson RA, Saavedra AP. *Fitzpatrick's Color Atlas and Synopsis of Clinical Dermatology*. 7th ed. New York, NY: McGraw-Hill Education; 2013.

C) 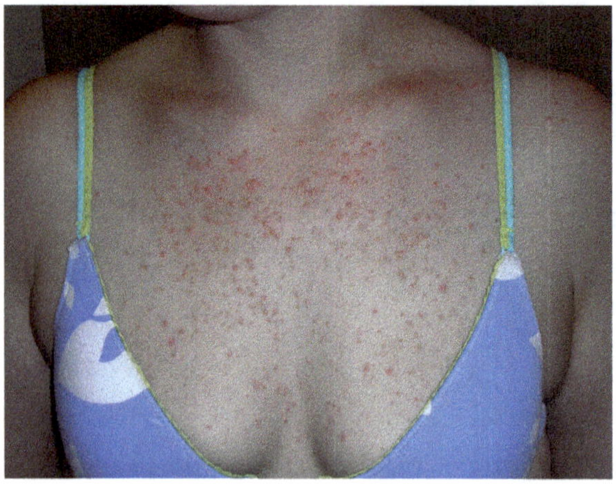

Reproduced, with permission, from Usatine RP, Smith MA, Mayeaux EJ Jr, Chumley HS, eds. *Color Atlas of Family Medicine*. 2nd ed. New York, NY: McGraw-Hill Education; 2012.

D) 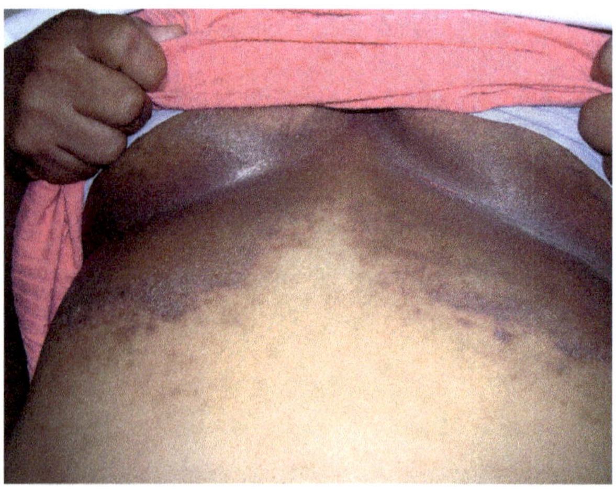

Reproduced, with permission, from Usatine RP, Smith MA, Mayeaux EJ Jr, Chumley HS, eds. *Color Atlas of Family Medicine*. 2nd ed. New York, NY: McGraw-Hill Education; 2012.

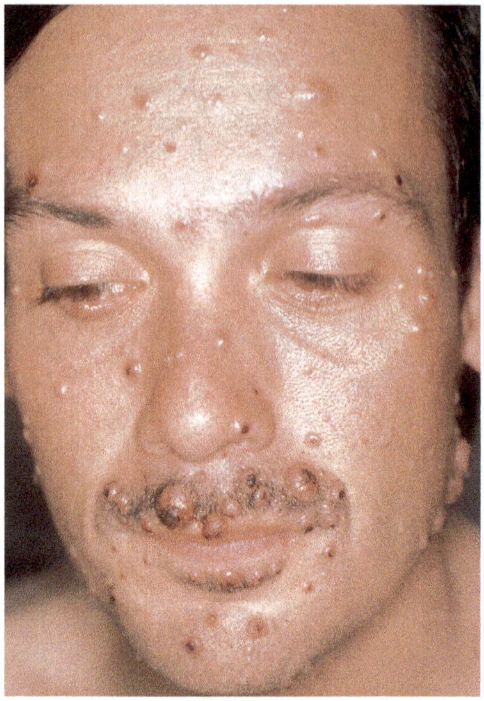

Reproduced, with permission, from Wolff K, Johnson RA, Saavedra AP. *Fitzpatrick's Color Atlas and Synopsis of Clinical Dermatology*. 7th ed. New York, NY: McGraw-Hill Education; 2013.

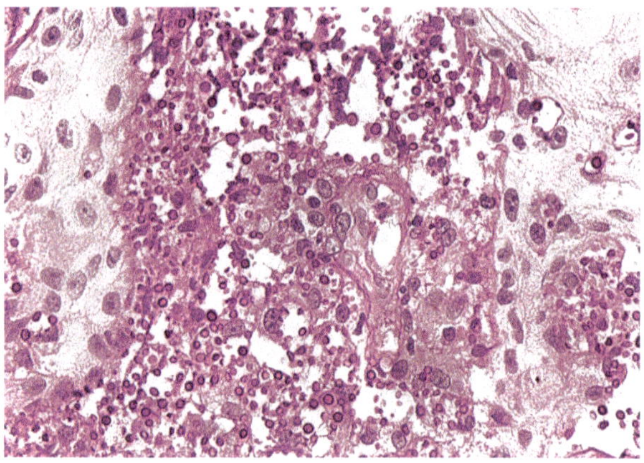

QUESTION 7-16.

An HIV-positive patient presents with multiple, skin-colored papules and nodules on the face. A biopsy is performed and the findings of the PAS stained sections are illustrated below. Fontana-Masson stain reveals numerous black yeasts with narrow-based budding. Which of the following diagnoses is CORRECT?

A) *Blastomyces dermatitidis*
B) *Histoplasma capsulatum*
C) *Lacazia loboi*
D) *Cryptococcus neoformans*
E) *Molluscum contagiosum*

QUESTION 7-17.

A veterinary assistant from Arkansas presents with dyspnea and an ulcerated, inflammatory plaque with surrounding erythema, edema, and fibrosis on the elbow. A biopsy is performed and the PAS-stained sections are illustrated below. Which of the following diagnoses is CORRECT?

A) Pyoderma gangrenosum
B) Coccidioidomycosis
C) Paracoccidioidomycosis
D) Chromoblastomycosis
E) Blastomycosis

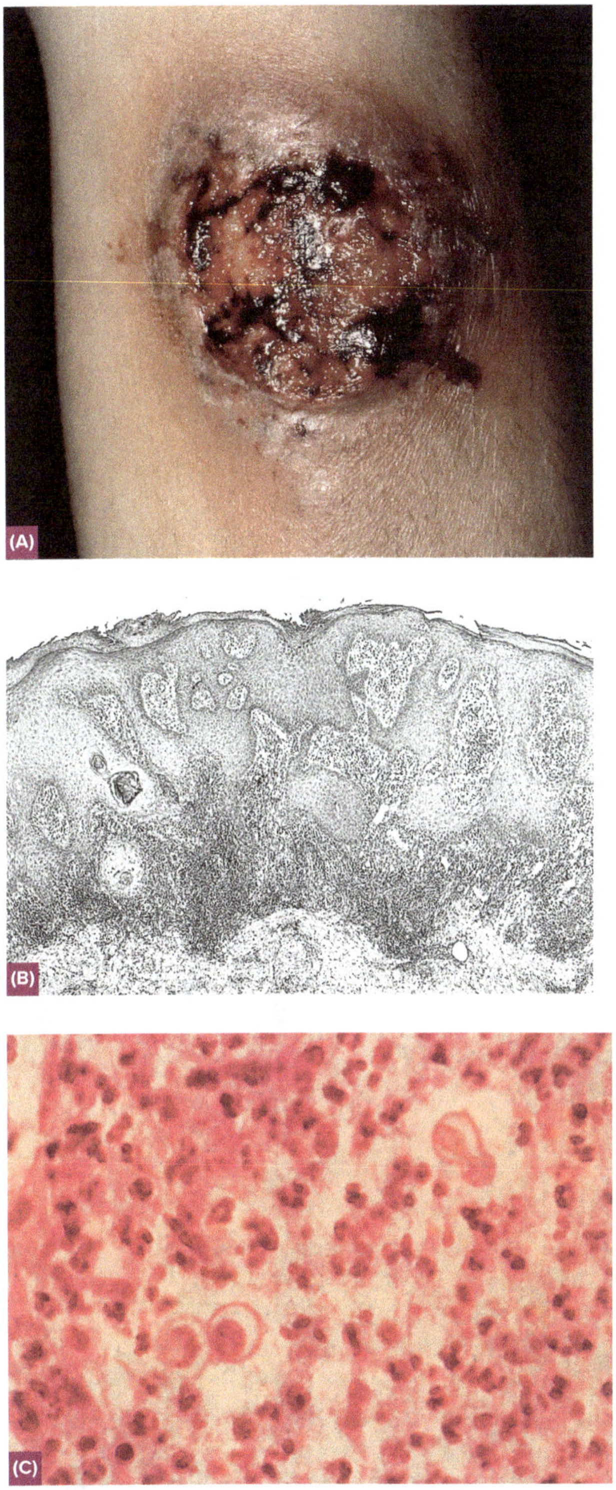

Part **(A)** reproduced, with permission, from Wolff K, Johnson RA, Saavedra AP. *Fitzpatrick's Color Atlas and Synopsis of Clinical Dermatology*. 7th ed. New York, NY: McGraw-Hill Education; 2013; part **(C)** reproduced, with permission, from Carroll KC et al, eds. *Jawetz, Melnick & Adelberg's Medical Microbiology*. 26th ed. New York, NY: McGraw-Hill Education; 2013.

QUESTION 7-18.

A male patient who recently emigrated from Colombia presents with progressive, painful, ulcerated, crusted plaques with well-defined, raised borders involving the gingivae, tongue, lips, palate, and nasal septum. The patient reports that the lesions began as acne-like papules that slowly evolved into their current state. Palpable cervical and submandibular lymphadenopathy is appreciated. A biopsy is performed and the findings are illustrated below. Which of the following diagnoses is CORRECT?

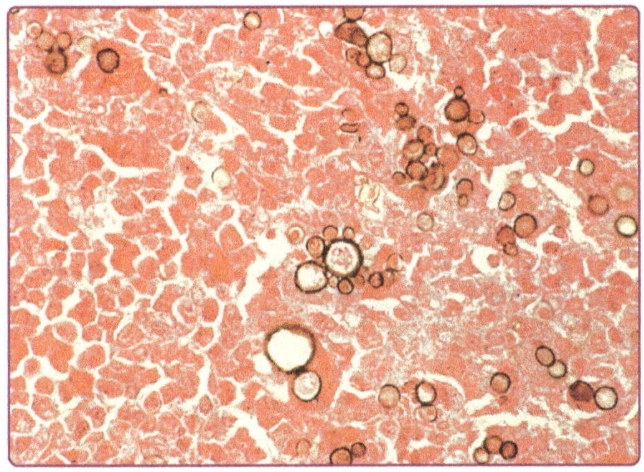

Reproduced, with permission, from Goldsmith LA, Katz SI, Gilchrest BA, Paller AS, Leffell DJ, Wolff K, eds. *Fitzpatrick's Dermatology in General Medicine*. 8th ed. New York, NY: McGraw-Hill Education; 2012.

A) North American blastomycosis
B) Coccidioidomycosis
C) Histoplasmosis
D) Paracoccidioidomycosis
E) Lobomycosis

QUESTION 7-19.

A Filipino College Professor of Agricultural and Environmental Sciences at UC San Diego presents to the emergency department in acute respiratory distress. You are called in for consultation and notice several ulcerated and crusted nodules on the cheek and nose. His past medical history is significant for systemic lupus for which he underwent kidney transplantation last year. He reports that he developed fever, chest pain, headache, and cough approximately 2 months ago followed by the onset of painful erythematous nodules on the anterior shins. The cutaneous lesions of the face began as acne-like pustules that gradually progressed to their current state. A biopsy of one of the facial lesions is performed and the findings are illustrated below. Which of the following diagnoses is CORRECT?

A) North American blastomycosis
B) Lobomycosis
C) Histoplasmosis
D) Coccidioidomycosis
E) Rhinosporidiosis

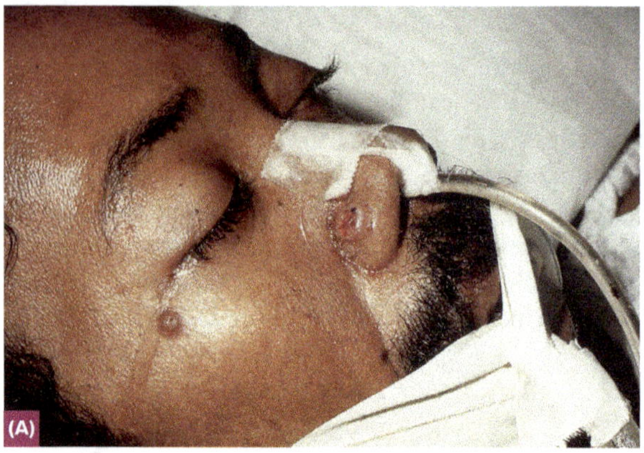

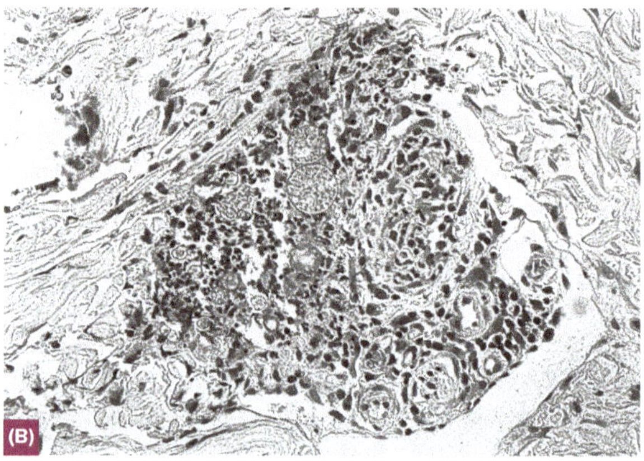

Part **(A)** reproduced, with permission, from Wolff K, Johnson RA, Saavedra AP. *Fitzpatrick's Color Atlas and Synopsis of Clinical Dermatology*. 7th ed. New York, NY: McGraw-Hill Education; 2013.

QUESTION 7-20.

A 35-year-old HIV-positive male from Cincinnati presents in January with a subacute febrile illness, dry cough, and multiple erythematous keratotic papules and small plaques resembling guttate psoriasis on the chest and arms. Oral and genital mucosal ulcerations are also present. Despite the cold weather, the patient appears to have a diffuse tan and denies any recent travel. Hepatosplenomegaly, anemia, and fever are present. A biopsy is performed and the high power findings of the H&E- and GMS-stained sections are illustrated below (images A & B, respectively). Gram and Fontana-Masson stains are negative. Low-power examination reveals an ulcerated epidermis and a neutrophilic and granulomatous dermatitis. A peripheral blood smear stained with Giemsa stain is also provided (image C). The patient dies before tissue culture and biopsy results are received. Which of the following microorganisms is MOST likely responsible for this patient's condition?

- **A)** *Histoplasma capsulatum* var *capsulatum*
- **B)** *Candida glabrata*
- **C)** *Cryptococcus neoformans*
- **D)** *Leishmania donovani*
- **E)** *Cryptococcus neoformans*

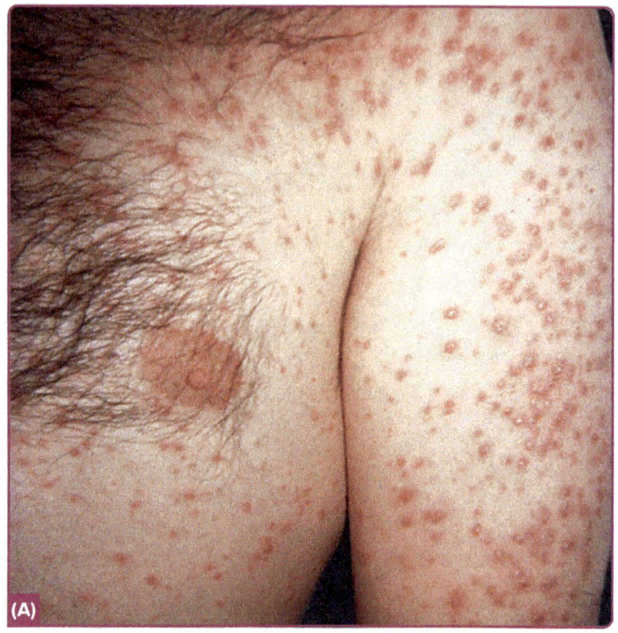

Reproduced, with permission, from Goldsmith LA, Katz SI, Gilchrest BA, Paller AS, Leffell DJ, Wolff K, eds. *Fitzpatrick's Dermatology in General Medicine*. 8th ed. New York, NY: McGraw-Hill Education; 2012.

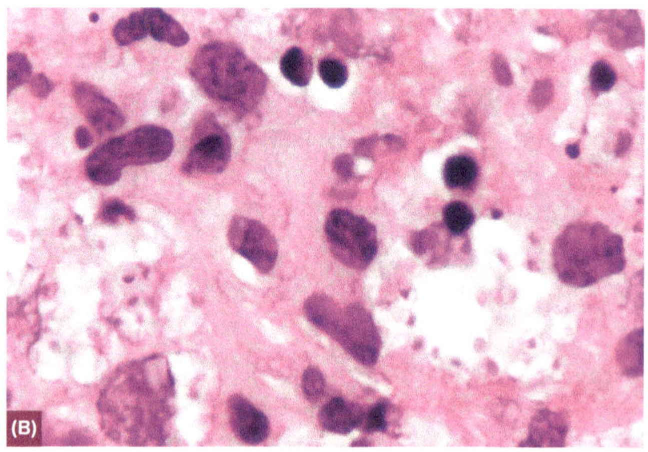

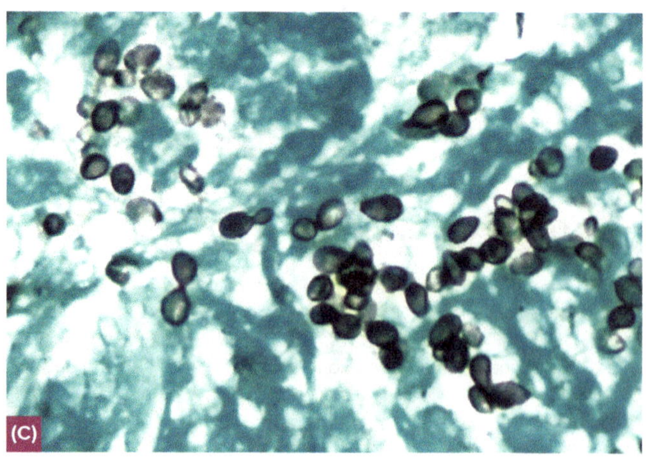

Reproduced, with permission, from Brunicardi FC et al, eds. *Schwartz's Principles of Surgery*. 9th ed. New York, NY: McGraw-Hill; 2010.

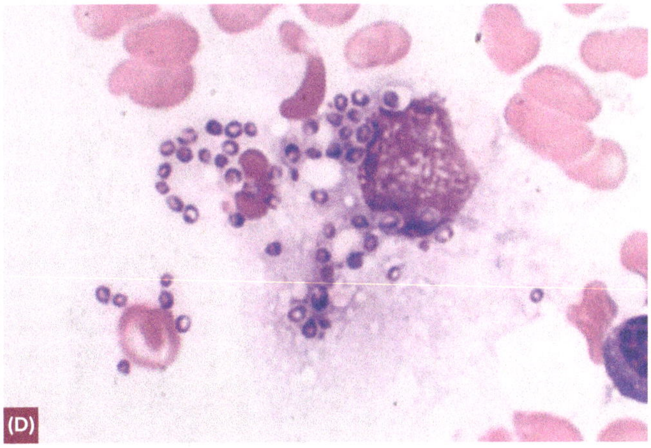

Reproduced, with permission, from McKean SC et al, eds. *Principles and Practice of Hospital Medicine*. New York, NY: McGraw-Hill; 2012.

QUESTION 7-21.

A carpenter from Peru presents with a solitary, large, verrucous plaque on the shin surrounded by a halo of erythema. Close-up view reveals hyperkeratosis with focal areas of pigmentation within the scale. A biopsy is performed and the findings are illustrated below. Which of the following microorganisms is LEAST likely to be implicated in this infection?

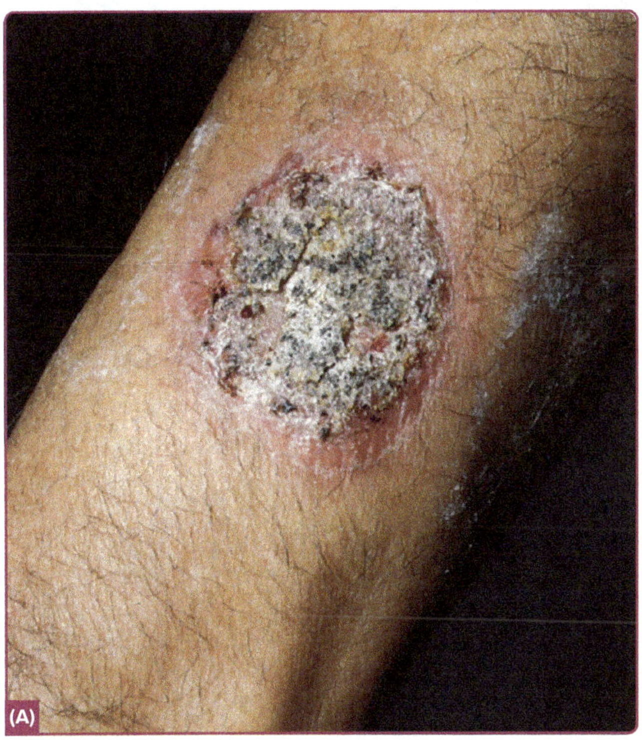

Reproduced, with permission, from Goldsmith LA, Katz SI, Gilchrest BA, Paller AS, Leffell DJ, Wolff K, eds. *Fitzpatrick's Dermatology in General Medicine*. 8th ed. New York, NY: McGraw-Hill Education; 2012.

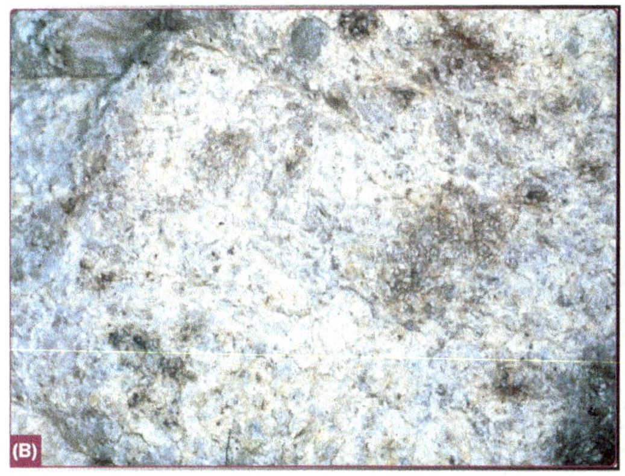

Reproduced, with permission, from Goldsmith LA, Katz SI, Gilchrest BA, Paller AS, Leffell DJ, Wolff K, eds. *Fitzpatrick's Dermatology in General Medicine*. 8th ed. New York, NY: McGraw-Hill Education; 2012.

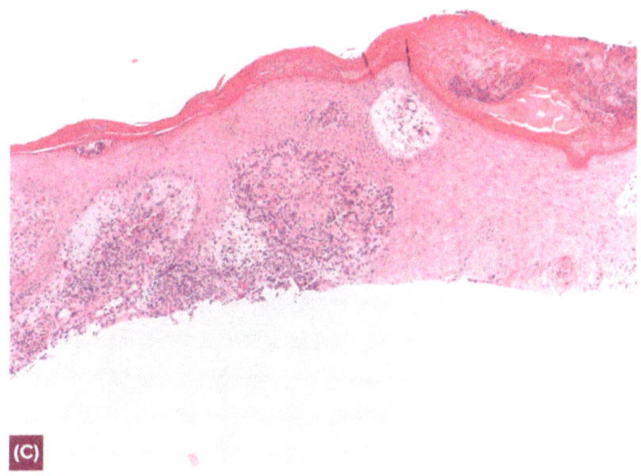

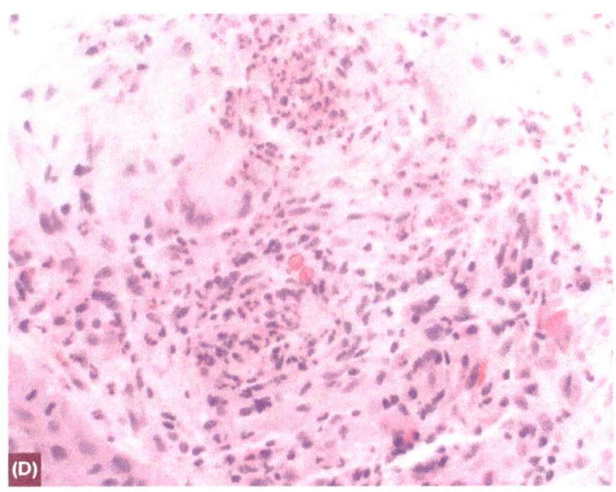

A) *Fonsecaea pedrosoi*
B) *Exophiala jeanselmei*
C) *Cladophialophora carrionii*
D) *Fonsecaea compacta*
E) *Rhinocladiella aquaspersa*

QUESTION 7-22.

An East Indian patient presents with painless swelling of the foot with a draining sinus tract over the lateral surface of the foot. The area is hyperpigmented and significant structural and function distortion of the foot is appreciated. The patient reports that dark brown/black gritty material is occasionally extruded from the sinus tract. A biopsy is performed and the findings are illustrated below. Which of the following diagnoses is CORRECT?

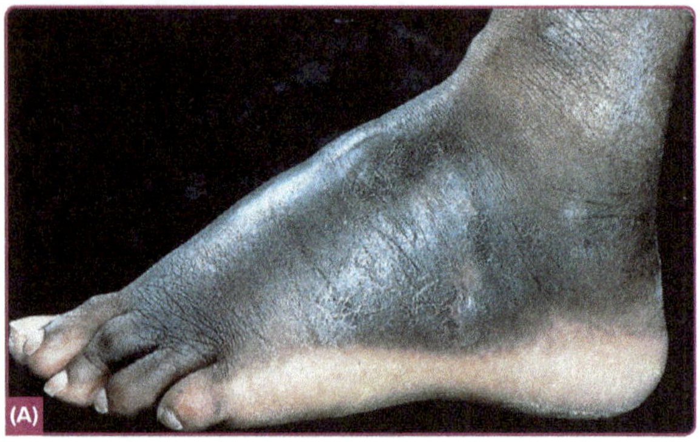

(A)

Reproduced, with permission, from Goldsmith LA, Katz SI, Gilchrest BA, Paller AS, Leffell DJ, Wolff K, eds. *Fitzpatrick's Dermatology in General Medicine*. 8th ed. New York, NY: McGraw-Hill Education; 2012.

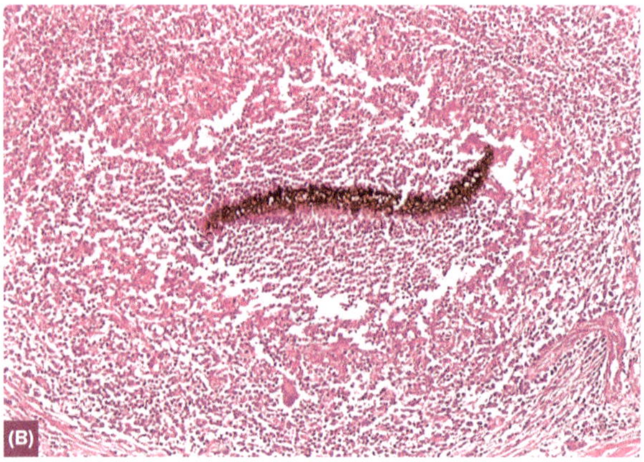

(B)

A) Botryomycosis
B) Eumycetoma
C) Actinomycetoma
D) Tinea versicolor

QUESTION 7-23.

A young woman with diabetes mellitus presents to the emergency department with proptosis, unilateral facial edema, and a right-sided facial palsy. Inspection of the nasopharynx reveals black nasal discharge. There is also an ulcer on the leg that has been self-treated with gauze and store-purchased medical tape. A biopsy of the nasopharynx is performed and the findings of the PAS-stained sections are illustrated below. Which of the following diagnoses is CORRECT?

A) Aspergillosis
B) Fusarium infection
C) Lobomycosis
D) Mucormycosis
E) Paracoccidioidomycosis

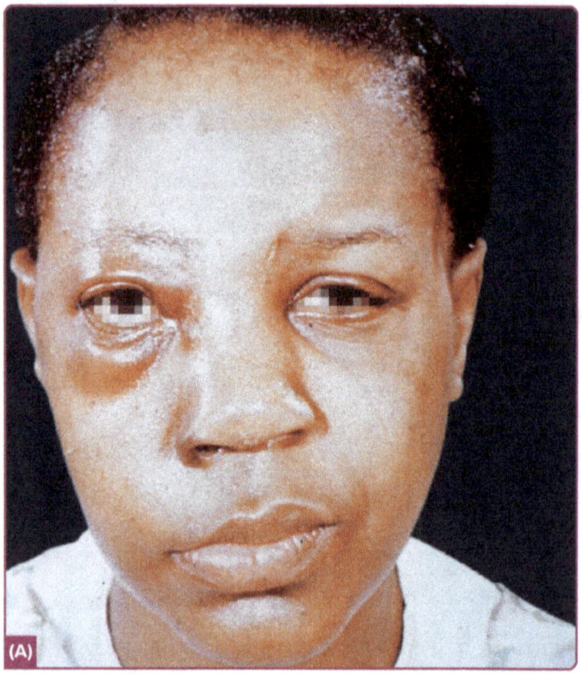

(A)

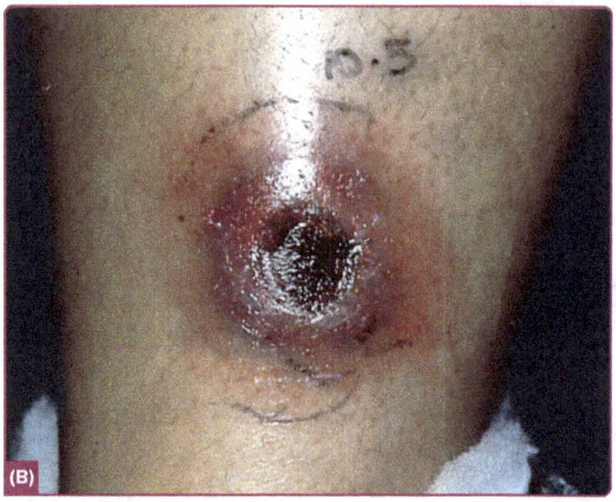

(B)

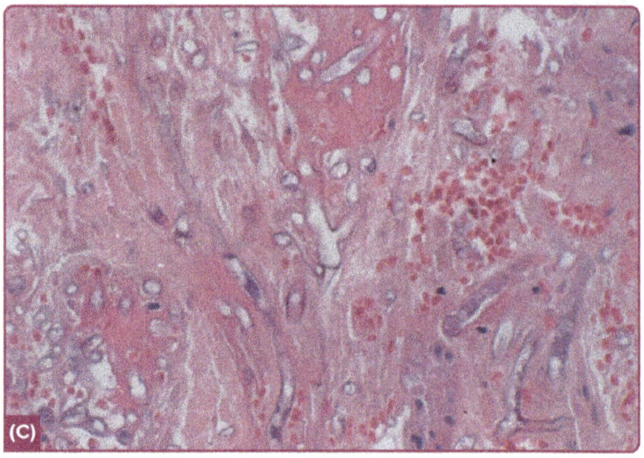

(C)

Reproduced, with permission, from Goldsmith LA, Katz SI, Gilchrest BA, Paller AS, Leffell DJ, Wolff K, eds. *Fitzpatrick's Dermatology in General Medicine*. 8th ed. New York, NY: McGraw-Hill Education; 2012.

QUESTION 7-24.

A young male patient presents with fever (101°F/38.6°C), malaise, sore throat and mouth, and refusal to eat. The mother reports that the patient has recently had a cough and diarrhea. Physical examination reveals multiple small discrete vesicles on the fingers, palms, soles, and oral mucosa. A biopsy of one of the vesicles of the palm is performed and the findings are illustrated below. Which of the following regarding this entity is INCORRECT?

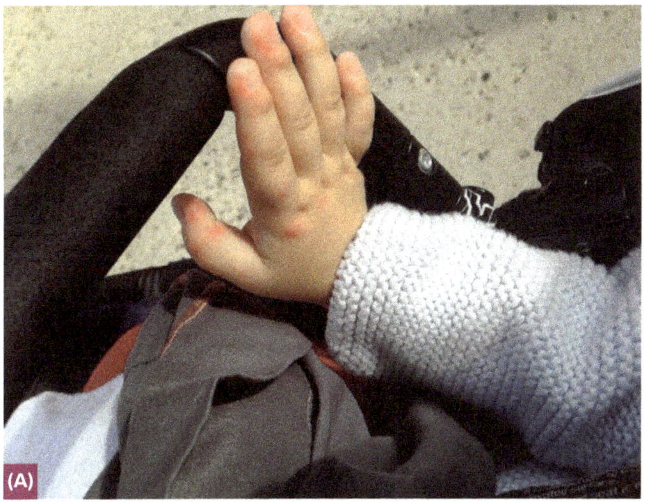

(A)

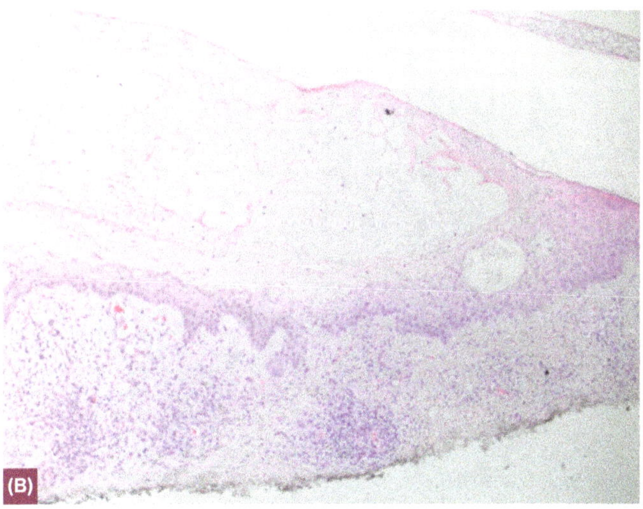

(B)

A) This lesion most likely represents the cutaneous manifestations of Coxsackievirus infection.
B) Viral cytopathic changes are characteristically absent in this condition.
C) This patient has virus-associated erythema multiforme.
D) Most outbreaks of this condition occur between June and October.
E) Serum analysis will reveal normal zinc and niacin levels.

QUESTION 7-25.

Which of the following clinical presentations is LEAST likely to be associated with the histopathology illustrated below?

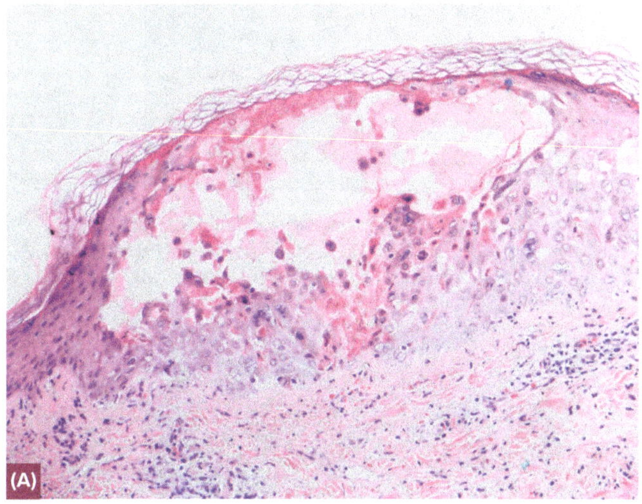

(A)

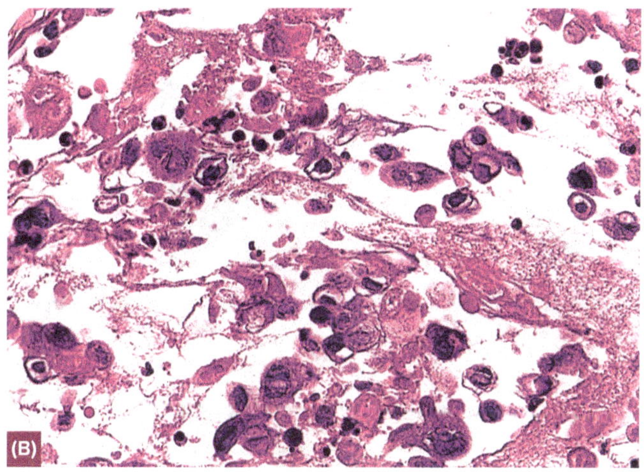

(B)

A)

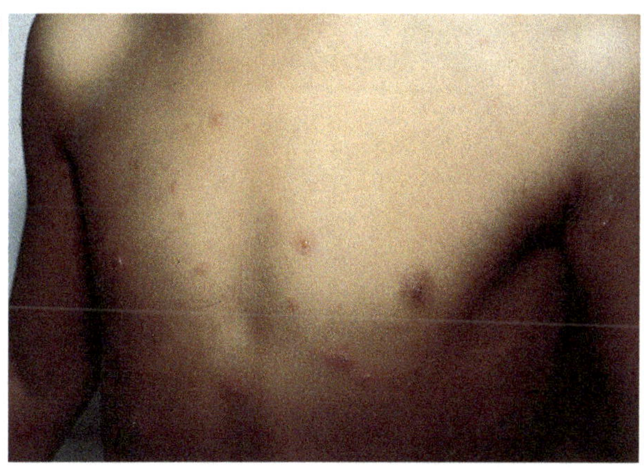

Reproduced, with permission, from Knoop KJ, Stack LB, Storrow AB, Thurman RJ. *The Atlas of Emergency Medicine*. 3rd ed. New York, NY: McGraw-Hill; 2010.

B)

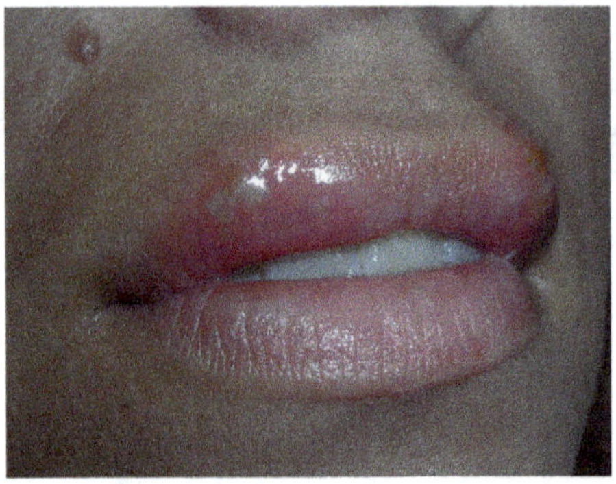

Reproduced, with permission, from Usatine RP, Smith MA, Mayeaux EJ Jr, Chumley HS, eds. *Color Atlas of Family Medicine*. 2nd ed. New York, NY: McGraw-Hill Education; 2012.

C)

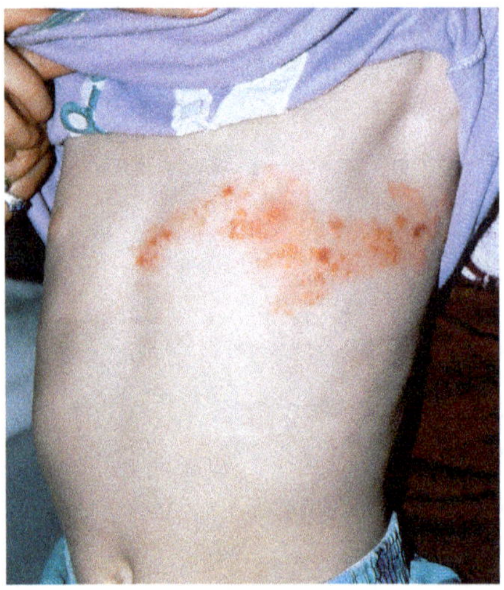

Reproduced, with permission, from Knoop KJ, Stack LB, Storrow AB, Thurman RJ. *The Atlas of Emergency Medicine*. 3rd ed. New York, NY: McGraw-Hill; 2010.

D)

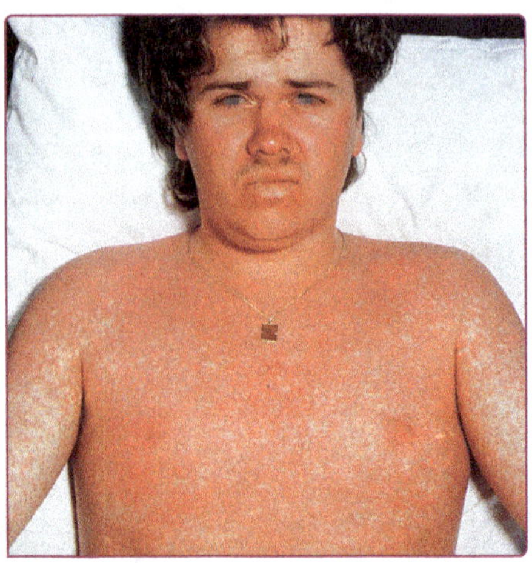

Reproduced, with permission, from Goldsmith LA, Katz SI, Gilchrest BA, Paller AS, Leffell DJ, Wolff K, eds. *Fitzpatrick's Dermatology in General Medicine*. 8th ed. New York, NY: McGraw-Hill Education; 2012.

QUESTION 7-26.

A 44-year-old male with HIV disease presents with extensive flat papules on face, neck, trunk, and abdomen. A biopsy is performed and the findings are illustrated below. Which of the following statements regarding this condition is INCORRECT?

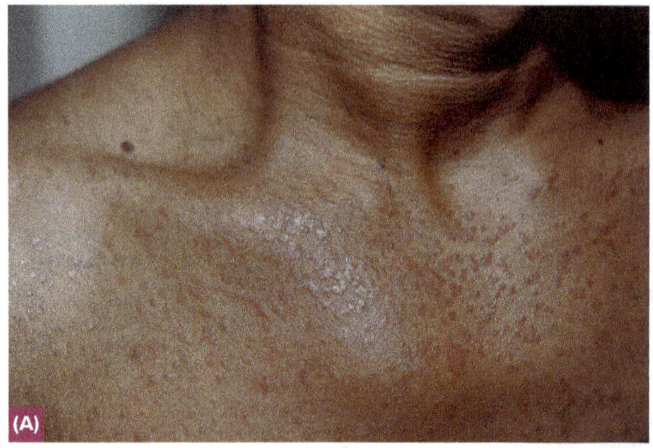

(A)

Reproduced, with permission, from Wolff K, Johnson RA, Saavedra AP. *Fitzpatrick's Color Atlas and Synopsis of Clinical Dermatology*. 7th ed. New York, NY: McGraw-Hill Education; 2013.

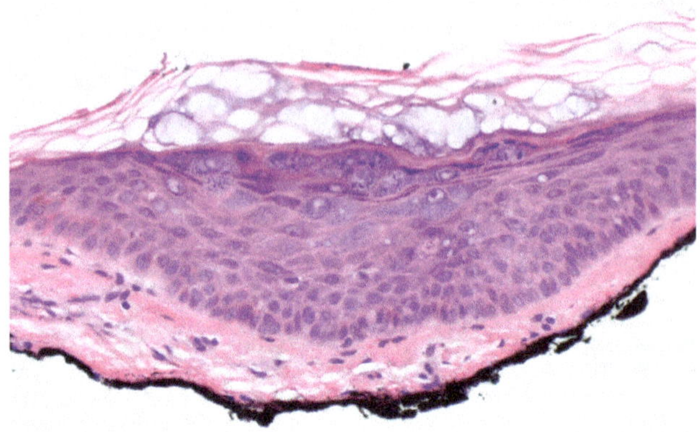

(B)

A) This condition is attributed to infection with HPV types 3, 5, 8, and 10.

B) This condition may be familial with autosomal recessive and x-linked patterns of inheritance.

C) Patients with this condition have an abnormal propensity for developing squamous cell carcinomas.

D) This condition is linked to defective cell–mediated immunity, with elucidation of mutations in *EVER1* and *EVER2* genes (band 17q25).

E) This condition is associated with mucous membrane hyperplasia of the lips, tongue, buccal mucosa, floor of the mouth, and palate.

QUESTION 7-27.

A 65-year-old male patient presents with multiple 3 to 5 mm well-demarcated erythematous plaques with mild scaling on the penis. A biopsy is performed and the findings are illustrated below? Which of the following HPV types is MOST likely associated with these hyperproliferative lesions?

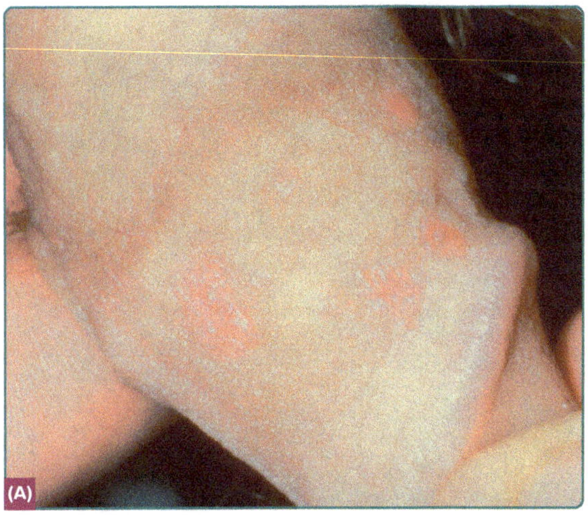

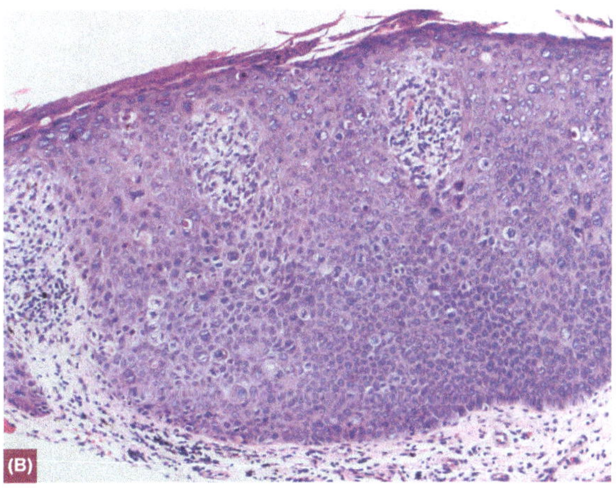

Reproduced, with permission, from Goldsmith LA, Katz SI, Gilchrest BA, Paller AS, Leffell DJ, Wolff K, eds. *Fitzpatrick's Dermatology in General Medicine*. 8th ed. New York, NY: McGraw-Hill Education; 2012.

- A) HPV types 6, 8, and 11
- B) HPV types 2 and 4
- C) HPV types 1 and 2
- D) HPV type 3
- E) HPV 61
- F) HPV 16 and 18

QUESTION 7-28.

A 27-year-old large-animal veterinarian from Montana presents with a large, firm, red, crusted nodule. A biopsy is performed and the findings are illustrated below. Which of the following diagnoses is CORRECT?

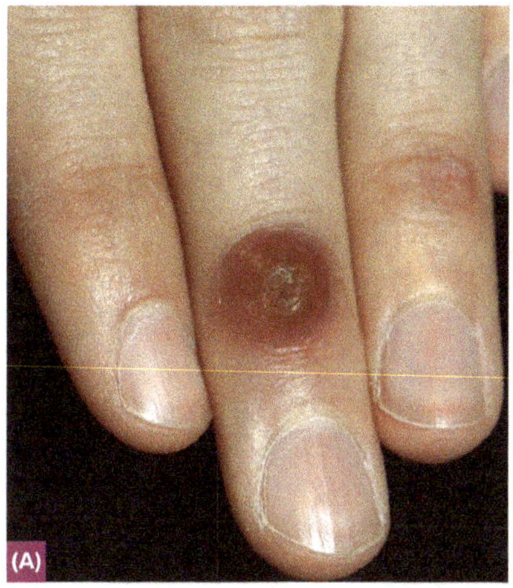

Reproduced, with permission, from Wolff K, Johnson RA, Saavedra AP. *Fitzpatrick's Color Atlas and Synopsis of Clinical Dermatology*. 7th ed. New York, NY: McGraw-Hill Education; 2013.

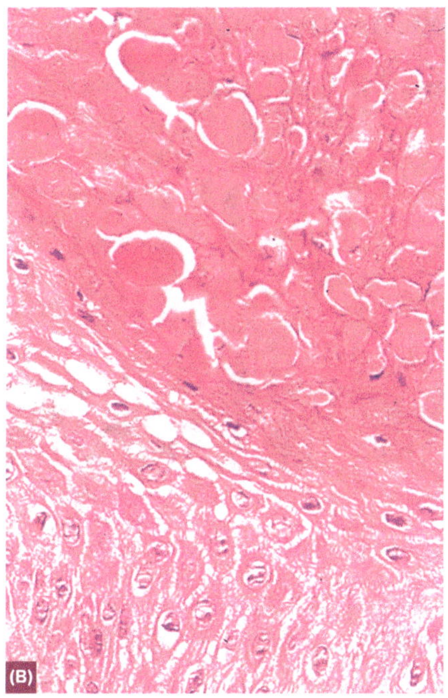

- A) Molluscum contagiosum
- B) Milker's nodule
- C) Orf
- D) Small pox
- E) Cytomegalovirus infection

QUESTION 7-29.

A young child from Bolivia presents with multiple facial ulcers with raised edges. A biopsy is performed and the findings are illustrated below. Which of the following diagnoses is CORRECT?

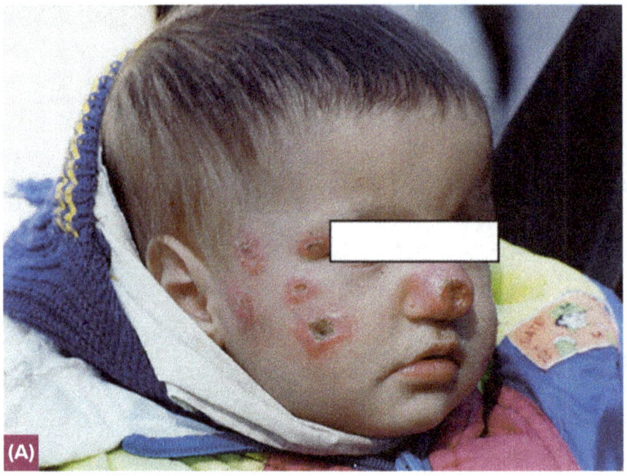

Reproduced, with permission, from Longo DL, Fauci AS, Kasper DL, Hauser SL, Jameson JL, Loscalzo J, eds. *Harrison's Principles of Internal Medicine*. 18th ed. New York, NY: McGraw-Hill Education; 2011.

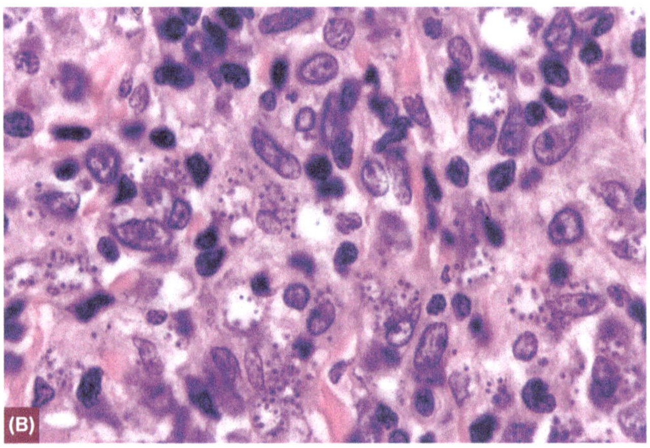

A) Chagas disease
B) Leishmaniasis
C) Histoplasmosis
D) Rhinoscleroma
E) Lepromatous leprosy

QUESTION 7-30.

An HIV-positive patient with chronic diarrhea presents with rapidly progressive, foul smelling, and painful punched-out perianal ulcers with glairy, hemopurulent, raw beef-like bases. The ulcers are necrotic with undermined borders. A biopsy is performed and the findings are illustrated below. Which of the following diagnoses is CORRECT?

A) Cutaneous herpes infection
B) Primary syphilis
C) Chancroid
D) Amebiasis
E) Condyloma acuminatum

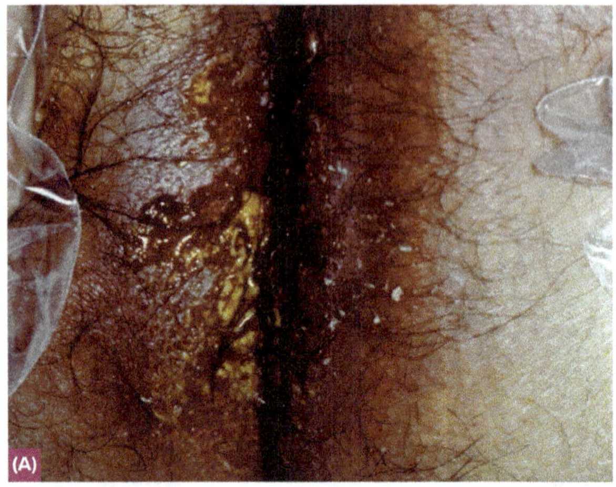

Reproduced, with permission, from Usatine RP, Smith MA, Mayeaux EJ Jr, Chumley HS, eds. *Color Atlas of Family Medicine*. 2nd ed. New York, NY: McGraw-Hill Education; 2012.

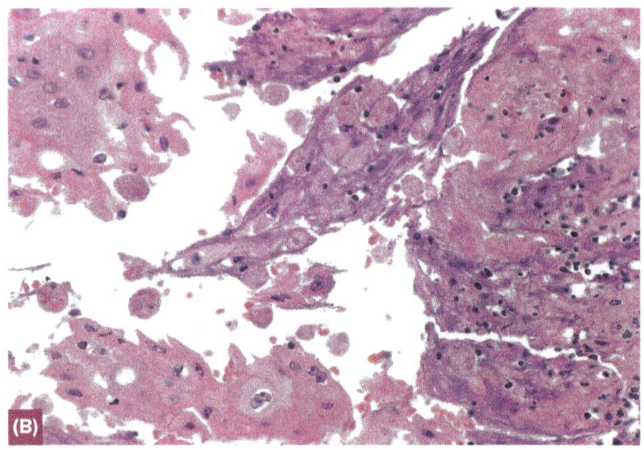

QUESTION 7-31.

A 31-year-old scuba diving instructor with chronic eczematous dermatitis presents with a swollen olecranon bursa 3 weeks after an injury to the elbow. A biopsy is performed and the findings of the GMS-stained sections are illustrated below. Which of the following diagnoses is CORRECT?

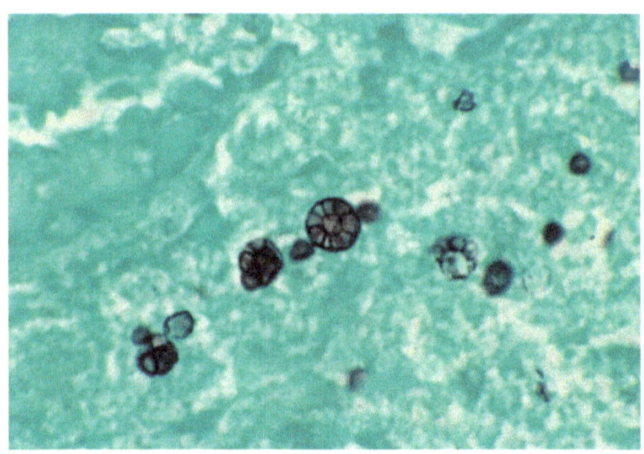

A) Cryptococcosis
B) Blastomycosis
C) Coccidioidomycosis
D) Chromoblastomycosis
E) Protothecosis

QUESTION 7-32.

A 23-year-old man is the next patient you see in the clinic. Under chief complaint, the nurse has written, "Wants a general checkup." You enter the room and greet a generally healthy-appearing young, white man, who seems nervous. He finally admits that he has been worried about a lesion on his penis. He denies pain or dysuria. He has never had any sexually transmitted diseases (STDs) and has an otherwise unremarkable medical history. He is afebrile, and his examination is notable for a shallow clean ulcer without exudates or erythema on the shaft of his penis, which is nontender to palpation, and has a cartilaginous consistency. There are some small, nontender, inguinal lymph nodes bilaterally. A biopsy is performed and the findings are illustrated below. The infiltrate is composed of lymphocytes, neutrophils, and plasma cells. Additionally, a Warthin-Starry stain is performed and the findings are illustrated below (image D). Which of the following diagnoses is CORRECT?

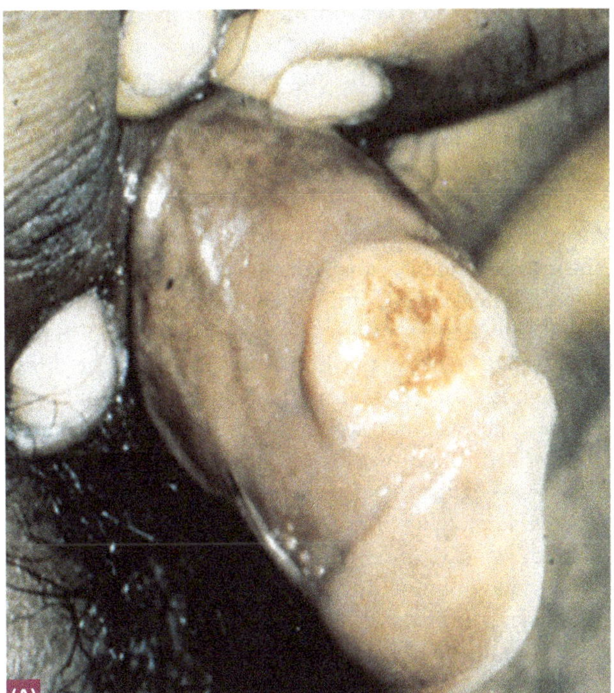

(A)

Courtesy of Gregory Cox, MD.

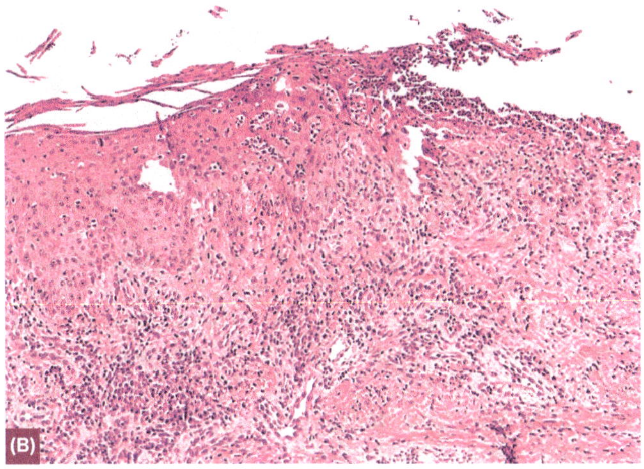

(B)

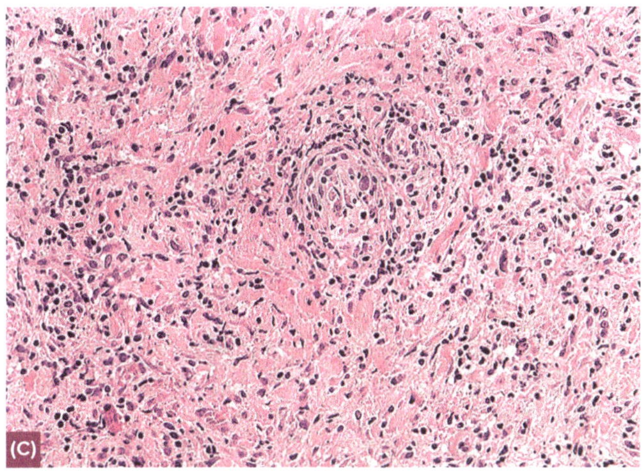

(C)

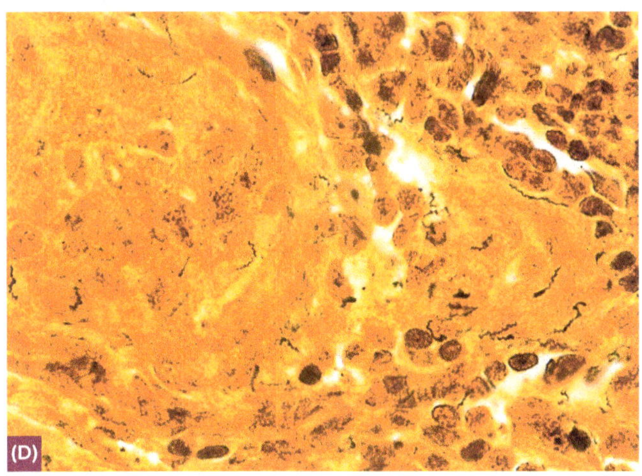

(D)

A) Chancre
B) Yaws
C) Chancroid
D) Zoon balanitis
E) Granuloma inguinale

ANSWERS

ANSWER 7-1: E.

This patient has **bacillary angiomatosis**. This condition is a multiorgan infection caused by gram-negative *Bartonella henselae* bacilli. Cats and cat fleas classically transmit these organisms to immunocompromised patients. Clinically, the lesions may be solitary or multiple, depending on the immune status of the patient and the extent of the infection. Mucosal lesions may occur. Typically there is associated regional lymphadenopathy. These erythematous papules or nodules are smooth with frequent ulceration. Microscopically, there is a raised pedunculated proliferation of well-circumscribed small vessels surfaced by an epidermal collarette. The proliferation may be superficial, deep, or both, and is accompanied by a robust mixed inflammatory infiltrate composed of neutrophils, lymphocytes, plasma cells, macrophages, and leukocytoclastic debris. Vessels in the deep portions of the lesion may be collapsed without obvious lumina. On H&E, the bacilli appear as purple or amphophilic granular clusters within endothelial cells, macrophages, or within the dermis. Warthin-Starry or GMS stains should be ordered to better highlight the organisms.

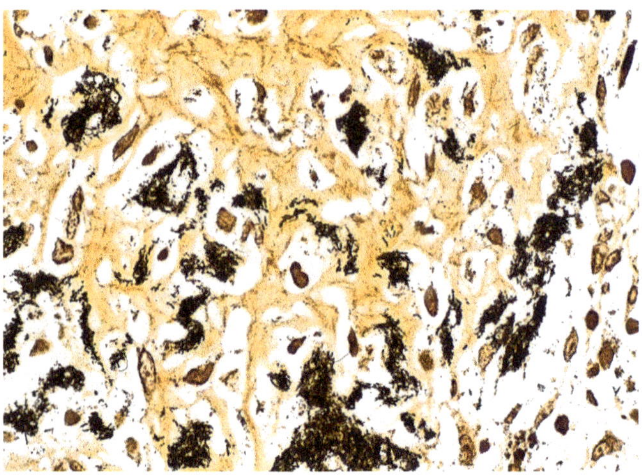

Bacillary angiomatosis. Warthin-Starry stain reveals numerous black, clumped bacilli.

Immunohistochemical stains and PCR are also commercially available to confirm infection. *B henselae* is the causative organism of both **bacillary angiomatosis** and **catscratch disease**; however, unlike **catscratch disease**, these lesions do respond to antibiotic therapy. The differential diagnosis includes **pyogenic granuloma, angiolymphoid hyperplasia with eosinophilia (epithelioid hemangioma), Kaposi sarcoma,** and **erythema elevatum diutinum. Pyogenic granuloma** can appear very similar to **bacillary angiomatosis**. Lesions of **pyogenic granuloma** often have less of a neutrophilic infiltration and lack the clusters of bacilli. All severely immunocompromised patients that present with pyogenic granuloma–like lesions should have GMS or Warthin-Starry stains performed to confirm the presence or absence of clusters of *B henselae* bacilli. **Angiolymphoid hyperplasia with eosinophilia (epithelioid hemangioma)** may present as solitary or clustered erythematous papules, typically on the head and neck, and may also have associated regional lymphadenopathy. However, microscopically, these lesions are poorly circumscribed with abundant eosinophils and only rare to absent neutrophils. The endothelial cells of **angiolymphoid hyperplasia with eosinophilia** are enlarged ("histiocytoid") with abundant eosinophilic cytoplasm devoid of organisms. **Kaposi sarcoma (KS)** is also frequently seen in HIV+ and immunocompromised patients; however, the vessels in **Kaposi sarcoma** are jagged and not round like those seen in **bacillary angiomatosis**. Additionally, the endothelial cells of **KS** will stain positive for HHV8 (LANA) via immunohistochemistry.

ANSWER 7-2: A.

This patient has **Chancroid**, which is a sexually transmitted disease that is most frequently seen in young African or South American males. The lesions begin to develop on the penis after 3 to 7 days postinoculation and form painful erythematous ulcerated papules/nodules with a ragged base and a yellow/green suppurative center. There is frequent regional lymphadenopathy, which may be bilateral. The skin overlying the regional lymph nodes may ulcerate and form draining sinus tracts. The causative organism is *Haemophilus ducreyi*, a gram-negative coccobacillus. The gold standard for diagnosis is tissue culture; however, organisms may be identified by Gram or Giemsa staining of ulcer scrapings or in the superficial portions of a biopsy. The organisms form parallel chains resembling a "school of fish" or "railroad tracks." The literature has stressed that the microscopic examination of these lesions contains three distinct layers; however, this is not as specific as often implied. Classically, the ulcers have a superficial layer of fibrin, neutrophils, and red blood cells admixed with the organisms. The middle zone consists of granulation tissue, swollen endothelial cells, and vessels that may contain fibrin thrombi. The deepest layer is composed of a deep dermal dense infiltrate of plasma cells and lymphocytes. The differential diagnosis includes **syphilitic chancre** and **granuloma inguinale**. The histomorphology of the ulcer in **chancroid** is distinct from these two entities, which generally lack the three layers. A diagnosis of **primary syphilis (chancre)** rests on positive serology (RPR or VDRL) and will reveal multiple spirochetes on dark field microscopy. Warthin-Starry stain and spirochete immunohistochemical stain will also identify the organisms in biopsied tissue. Microscopically, **granuloma inguinale** reveals numerous macrophages containing gram-negative, Warthin-Starry-positive, and Giemsa-positive clusters of bacilli of *Klebsiella granulomatis* clumped into collections of 10 to 20 organisms **(Donovan bodies)**.

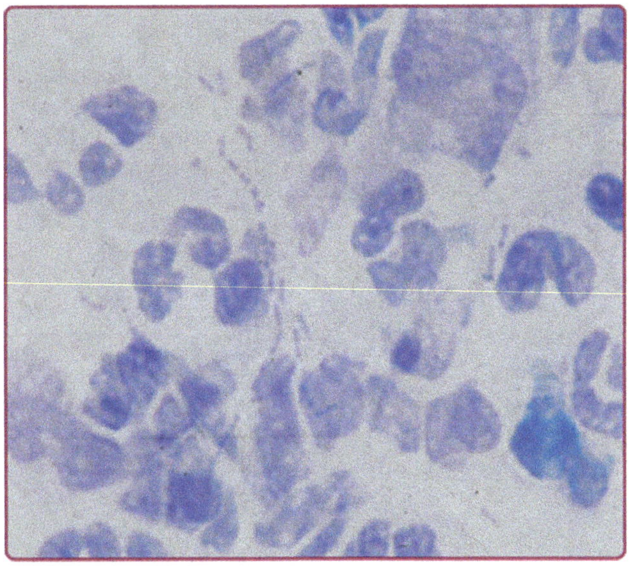

Chancroid. Giemsa-stained smear from a soft ulcer demonstrates the "school-of-fish" pattern of *Haemophilus ducreyi* (coccobacilli). (Reproduced, with permission, from Goldsmith LA, Katz SI, Gilchrest BA, Paller AS, Leffell DJ, Wolff K, eds. *Fitzpatrick's Dermatology in General Medicine*. 8th ed. New York, NY: McGraw-Hill Education; 2012.)

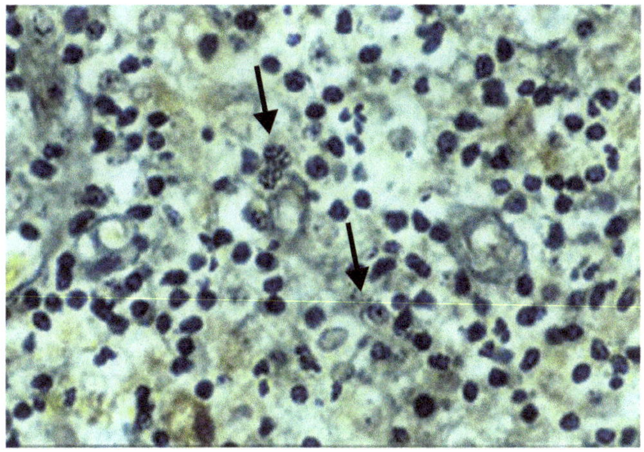

Granuloma inguinale. Donovan bodies ("safety pin") are readily stained with Giemsa stain. (Reproduced, with permission, from Goldsmith LA, Katz SI, Gilchrest BA, Paller AS, Leffell DJ, Wolff K, eds. *Fitzpatrick's Dermatology in General Medicine*. 8th ed. New York, NY: McGraw-Hill Education; 2012.)

ANSWER 7-3: D.

This patient has **granuloma inguinale** (aka **Donovanosis**), which is a sexually transmitted disease most frequently seen in patients living in tropical regions. The lesions are caused by infection with gram-negative bacilli called **Klebsiella granulomatis**. The lesions typically present as rapidly enlarging firm papules/nodules in the genitalia, perianal, and pubic regions approximately 15 days after inoculation. The nodules rapidly ulcerate to form irregular serpiginous ulcers with central red friable granulation tissue. Lymphadenopathy is characteristically absent. Development of squamous cell carcinoma and lymphatic obstruction leading to elephantiasis of the external genitalia has been described. Microscopically, there is reactive pseudoepitheliomatous hyperplasia adjacent to the ulcer bed characterized by diffuse neutrophilic, plasmacytic, and histiocytic infiltrates admixed with granulation tissue extending deep into the dermis and subcutaneous tissue. Intraepidermal and subepidermal neutrophilic microabscesses are common. Vacuolated macrophages contain encapsulated structures known as **Donovan bodies** which are composed of intracellular accumulations of bacilli best highlighted with GMS, Warthin-Starry, or Giemsa stains. The bacilli have a characteristic "safety pin" appearance once stained with Giemsa.

The clinical differential diagnosis includes **chancroid,** which is clinically associated with massive lymphadenopathy and overlying draining sinus tracts. **Granuloma inguinale** is not typically associated with lymphadenopathy. Ulcers of **chancroid** are composed of three distinct layers: superficial necrotic and fibrinous suppurative inflammation, mid-dermal granulation tissue with neutrophilia, and deep plasmacytosis. **Chancroid** is caused by *Haemophilus ducreyi,* characterized by extracellular coccobacilli lining up in a "school of fish" or "railroad track" pattern. This is in contrast to the intracellular bacilli in **granuloma inguinale (Donovanosis).**

The histopathological differential diagnosis includes **American trypanosomiasis, leishmaniasis, histoplasmosis, penicilliosis, rhinoscleroma, leprosy**, and **atypical mycobacteriosis.** Each of these entities is characterized by an infiltrate of parasitized histiocytes (intracellular organisms) admixed

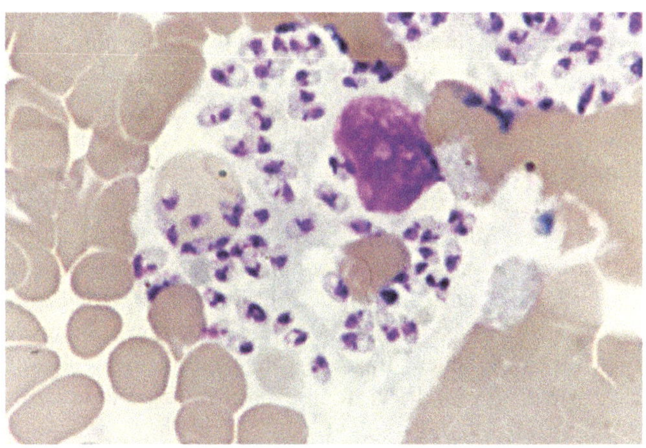

Leishmaniasis. Macrophage engorged with the amastigotes of *Leishmania donovani.* Note that these round-oval organisms contain a nucleus and a separate dot-like kinetoplast. (Reproduced, with permission, from Lichtman MA, Shafer JA, Felgar RE, Wang N. *Lichtman's Atlas of Hematology*. New York, NY: McGraw-Hill; 2007.)

Table 7-3A. Infectious Causes of Diffuse Histiocytic Infiltrates (Parasitized Histiocytosis)

	ORGANISM	TISSUE MORPHOLOGY	HISTOPATHOLOGICAL FEATURES
Lepromatous leprosy	*M leprae*	Fite-positive AFB	Foamy lepra cells; grenz zone; globi Organisms within and outside of macrophages
Histoid leprosy and atypical mycobacteria in HIV	*M leprae* and atypical mycobacteria	Fite-positive AFB, Ziehl-Neelsen-positive AFB	Spindle cell pseudotumor confused with neoplasm Organisms within and outside of macrophages
Donovanosis (granuloma inguinale)	*Klebsiella granulomatis*	GMS, Warthin-Starry, or Giemsa stains reveal "safety pin" bacilli	Reactive pseudoepitheliomatous hyperplasia and neutrophilic, plasmacytic, and histiocytic infiltrates admixed with granulation tissue. Organisms within macrophages
Histoplasmosis	*H capsulatum*	2-4 μm intracellular yeasts with clear halo; no hyphae	Organisms within macrophages
Leishmaniasis	*L tropica* *L mexicana* *L brasiliensis* *L donovani*	2-4 μm round-oval protozoa with nucleus and kinetoplast (Giemsa-positive)	Organisms within macrophages; nucleus and kinetoplast stain red with Giemsa

with chronic inflammatory cells (Table 7-3A). Although clinical correlation may be the easiest means of diagnostic distinction, the causative intracellular organisms have distinguishing features. ***Leishmania*** amastigotes generally can be differentiated histopathologically from the *Klebsiella granulomatis* of **granuloma inguinale** since they contain a kinetoplast, which is a small round basophilic structure located adjacent to the nucleus of the organism. ***Trypanosoma*** species are similar to **Leishmania**, but unlike the other conditions in the differential diagnosis, they are able to invade mesenchymal cells and are often seen in myocytes.

Cutaneous histoplasmosis is typically a systemic mycosis (primary cutaneous inoculation is rare) presenting in immunocompromised patients as scattered erythematous papules and plaques. Microscopically, macrophages contain multiple round-oval intracellular yeasts, unlike the rod-shaped bacteria *Klebsiella*. The yeasts of *Penicillium marneffei* in **penicilliosis** are elongated ovals that divide by transverse septae. Spores of both fungi are better visualized with Gomori methenamine silver stain (GMS). They are also positive to periodic acid-Schiff (PAS).

The histologic spectrum seen in **leprosy** varies with the type of disease. Histiocytes have abundant foamy or vacuolated cytoplasm, may be epithelioid, and are often separated from the epidermis by a narrow grenz zone. The histiocytes may be scattered among other inflammatory cells in the dermis or form granulomas. The granulomas tend to be elongated and course along nerves. Organisms stain poorly with Ziehl-Neelsen stain and are best seen with a Fite-Faraco acid-fast stain. They appear as red-staining bacilli measuring approximately 0.5 by 5.0 μm, primarily within histiocytes. **Atypical mycobacteriosis** also has a varied histologic

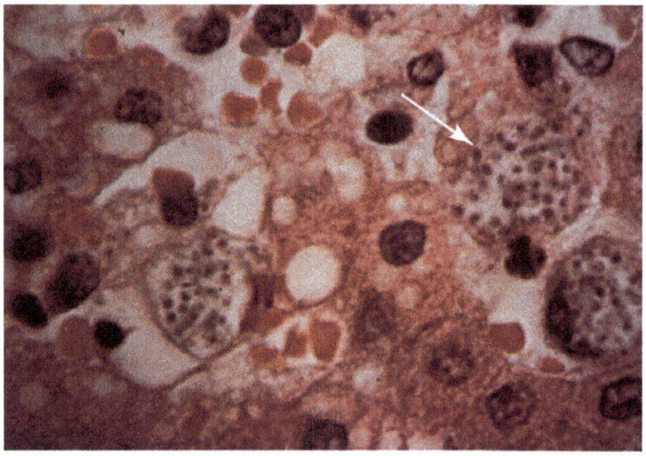

Histoplasmosis, disseminated. Lesional biopsy specimen shows dermal macrophages packed with dozens of tiny yeast forms of *Histoplasma capsulatum* (*arrow*). These round yeasts lack a kinetoplast. (Reproduced, with permission, from Goldsmith LA, Katz SI, Gilchrest BA, Paller AS, Leffell DJ, Wolff K, eds. *Fitzpatrick's Dermatology in General Medicine*. 8th ed. New York, NY: McGraw-Hill Education; 2012.)

appearance. Earlier lesions show dermal infiltrates of histiocytes, lymphocytes, and neutrophils with occasional microabscess formation. As the lesions age, epithelioid and tuberculoid type granulomas as well as **Langhans giant cells** are noted. Epithelial hyperplasia and hyperkeratosis may also be present. Variable numbers of bacilli primarily within histiocytes are seen in acid-fast–stained sections.

DDX for Parasitized Histiocytes (Intracellular Microorganisms)

Lizzie Grubman Loves To ReHeat Nasty Microwave Pizza:

Lepromatous leprosy
Granuloma Inguinale (Donovan bodies—does not stain with GMS)
Leishmania (Kinetoplasts)
Toxoplasmosis (not TB)
Rhinoscleroma (not *Rhinosporidium*)—Mikulicz cells
Histoplasmosis (stains with GMS)
Nocardia
Malakoplakia (Michaelis-Gutman bodies)
Penicillium marneffei

ANSWER 7-4: B.

The biopsy reveals a subcorneal blister containing neutrophils, acantholytic keratinocytes, and prominent papillary dermal edema consistent with **bullous impetigo. Bullous impetigo** is an infectious acantholytic dermatosis. These patients frequently have a concomitant history of **atopic dermatitis**. It is caused by phage group II, Type 71 *Staphylococcus aureus*. Gram stain frequently reveals gram-positive cocci in clusters within the stratum corneum. **Bullous impetigo** is clinically characterized by flaccid blisters in nontraumatized skin or moist erosions with surrounding erythema. Lesions are distributed on the face, buttocks, trunk, and perineum. It occurs mainly in newborns, infants, and young children, but only occasionally in adults. **Bullous impetigo** is pathogenically distinct from **nonbullous impetigo**. **Nonbullous impetigo** (or simply **"impetigo"**) is more common and begins on the skin of the face and extremities following minor trauma. Chicken pox, arthropod bite, abrasion, laceration, and burns are common predisposing factors. **Nonbullous impetigo** can also occur as a complication of systemic diseases such as diabetes mellitus, acquired immunodeficiency syndrome, and other skin diseases that cause a break in the skin barrier (ie, scabies, atopic dermatitis, and Darier disease). The skin lesions begin as small vesicles or pustules that progress into honey-colored crusted plaques, usually less than 2 cm in diameter. Lymphadenopathy is common. Lesions normally resolve in 2 to 3 weeks without scarring. Infection may spread rapidly by direct contact, especially in conditions such as crowding, poor hygiene, and contact sports, or through fomites. In the past, *Streptococcus pyogenes* (group A beta-hemolytic streptococcus) was the organism most frequently implicated. Recently, however, *Staphylococcus aureus* has been increasingly isolated. Non-Group A (Groups B, C, and G) streptococci may be responsible for rare cases of impetigo. Group B streptococci are associated with impetigo in the newborn. Microscopically, numerous subcorneal and intragranular pustules with extensive intraepidermal and superficial dermal neutrophilic infiltrates characterize nonbullous impetigo. Spongiosis and parakeratotic scale crusts are frequently identified, especially after the pustules have ruptured and crusted over. Acantholytic cells are absent in nonbullous impetigo.

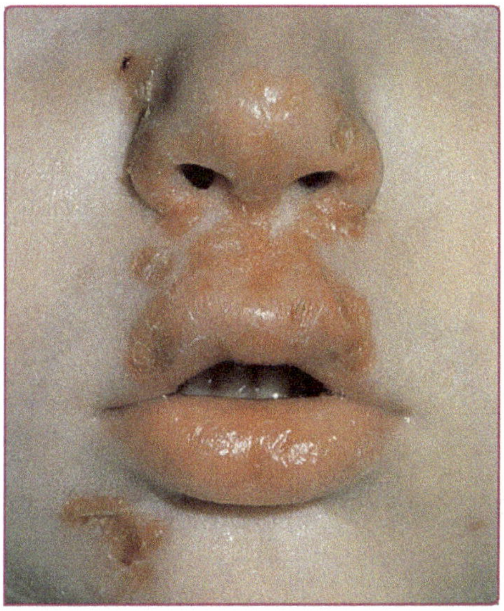

Nonbullous impetigo. There are honey-colored crusts, pustules, and erythematous weeping erosions on the nose, mouth, and chin. (Reproduced, with permission, from Goldsmith LA, Katz SI, Gilchrest BA, Paller AS, Leffell DJ, Wolff K, eds. *Fitzpatrick's Dermatology in General Medicine*. 8th ed. New York, NY: McGraw-Hill Education; 2012.)

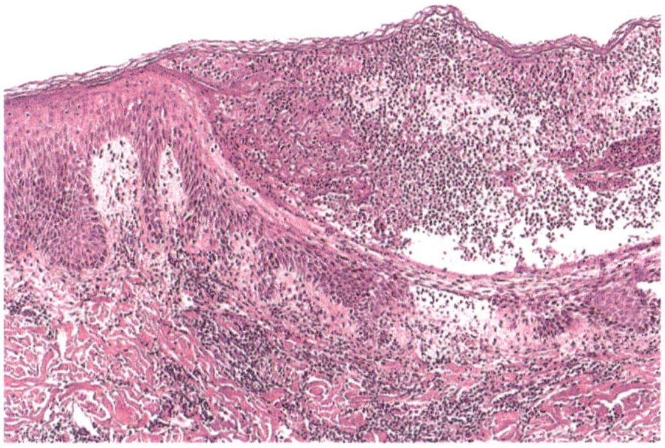

Nonbullous impetigo. Subcorneal pustule containing neutrophils.

The differential diagnosis for **bullous impetigo** also includes **staphylococcal scalded skin syndrome**, **ecthyma, candidiasis,** and **pemphigus foliaceus**. **Bullous impetigo** and **Staphylococcal scalded skin syndrome** are both caused by a staphylococcal exotoxin called **exfoliatin**, which cleaves **desmoglein 1.** Whereas **bullous impetigo** presents with localized lesions, **staphylococcal scalded skin syndrome** is attributed to systemic dissemination of **exfoliatin** and presents with large flaccid bullae, which may coalesce and form exfoliative sheets accompanied by fever (Table 7-4A). Both **bullous impetigo** and **staphylococcal scalded skin syndrome** are characterized by subcorneal and intragranular bullae; however, **staphylococcal scalded skin syndrome** is characterized by a relative paucity of neutrophilic infiltrates and complete necrosis of the upper granular layer keratinocytes. Additionally, Gram stain will be negative for bacteria in the lesions of **staphylococcal scalded skin syndrome.**

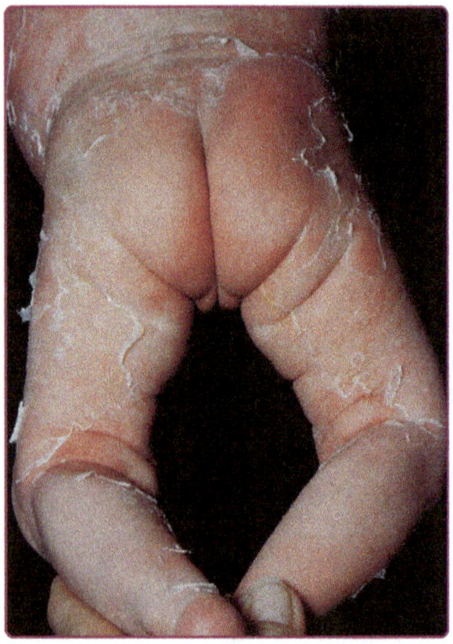

Late stage of staphylococcal scalded skin syndrome. Generalized desquamation with large sheets. (Reproduced, with permission, from Goldsmith LA, Katz SI, Gilchrest BA, Paller AS, Leffell DJ, Wolff K, eds. *Fitzpatrick's Dermatology in General Medicine*. 8th ed. New York, NY: McGraw-Hill Education; 2012.)

Table 7-4A. Staphylococcal Scalded Skin Syndrome

Clinical Features
Superficial peeling of bright red skin
Head and neck most common
Children usually
Constitutional symptoms, usually of acute onset
Occult source of staphylococci in nonlesional sites (eg, conjunctiva, nares, groin, blood)
Histopathologic Features
Pauci-inflammatory subcorneal blister that may contain few acantholytic keratinocytes
Minimal perivascular inflammatory infiltrate
Bacteria not present in lesional skin
Differential Diagnosis
Pemphigus erythematosus or foliaceus
Toxic epidermal necrolysis (clinical)
Kawasaki disease

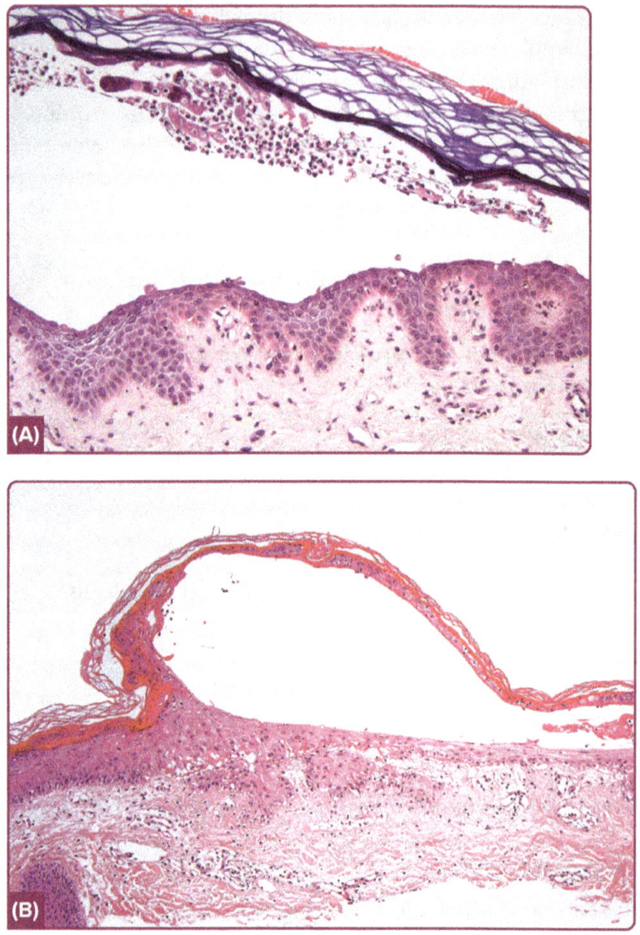

(A) Bullous impetigo vs (B) Staphylococcal scalded skin syndrome. In both conditions, the intraepidermal cleavage induced by the epidermolytic toxin occurs within or just below the stratum granulosum. Note paucity of cells in generalized disease (staphylococcal scalded skin syndrome) in image **(B)**, compared to the large numbers of neutrophils found in the localized form (bullous impetigo) in image **(A)**. In both, cleavage occurs in the granular layer and is due to acantholysis. Note: free-floating acantholytic cells in **(A)** and compacted acantholytic cells in the blister roof of **(B)**. Gram-positive cocci will only be found in bullous impetigo **(A)**, unless the lesions of Staphylococcal scalded skin syndrome are secondarily infected. (Reproduced, with permission, from Goldsmith LA, Katz SI, Gilchrest BA, Paller AS, Leffell DJ, Wolff K, eds. *Fitzpatrick's Dermatology in General Medicine*. 8th ed. New York, NY: McGraw-Hill Education; 2012.)

Ecthyma is an ulcer caused by Group A streptococci, and is essentially an ulcerated **impetigo** (Table 7-4B). It occurs most commonly on the lower extremity of children or in elderly patients following minor trauma. The lesion begins as vesicle or vesiculopustule with an erythematous base and a surrounding halo. The lesion undergoes ulceration and becomes crusted. The ulcer has a punched-out appearance with an indurated, raised, and violaceous border. The lesion heals slowly. Microscopically, a crust is present within the ulceration. Gram-positive cocci may be present in the ulcer bed. Neutrophils are usually found diffusely throughout the dermis.

Table 7-4B. Impetigo and Ecthyma

Clinical Features
"Honey-colored" crusted lesions, usually of acute onset
Bullae in "bullous impetigo"
Ulceration in "ecthyma"
Children are more commonly affected
Paranasal, axilla, groin are common sites
Histopathologic Features
Subcorneal pustule filled with neutrophils and sometimes occasional acantholytic cells
Subcorneal bullae in bullous impetigo, with acantholytic cells and few inflammatory cells
Ulceration in ecthyma
Sometime gram-positive cocci found in the pustule or on the surface of crusts or ulcers
Variable dermal infiltrate (usually sparse)
Differential Diagnosis
Other diseases with subcorneal pustules
Pemphigus foliaceus and erythematosus

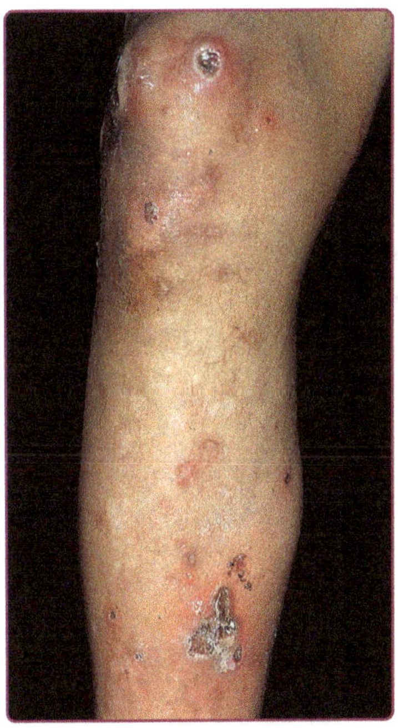

Ecthyma. Multiple thickly crusted ulcers on the leg of a patient with diabetes and renal failure. Ecthymatous lesions were also present on the other leg, the arms, and the hands. (Reproduced, with permission, from Goldsmith LA, Katz SI, Gilchrest BA, Paller AS, Leffell DJ, Wolff K, eds. *Fitzpatrick's Dermatology in General Medicine*. 8th ed. New York, NY: McGraw-Hill Education; 2012.)

Candidiasis was ruled out by the absence of pseudohyphae and yeast on the PAS stain. The presence of gram-positive cocci favors **bullous impetigo** over **pemphigus foliaceus**. Occasionally, direct immunofluorescence is required for definitive diagnostic distinction. **Toxic epidermal necrolysis** can be distinguished from **bullous impetigo** by the presence of necrotic keratinocytes throughout the full thickness of the epidermis and not just limited to the granular layer or higher. An expanded differential diagnosis for subcorneal pustular conditions is present in Table 7-4C.

Table 7-4C. Differential Diagnosis of Subcorneal Pustules

Impetigo
Tinea and *Candida* spp
Scabies
Psoriasis and subcorneal pustular dermatosis
Drug eruption (drug-induced pemphigus, AGEP)
Neonatal pustular melanosis
Acropustulosis of infancy
Pemphigus (various types)
Gonococcemia
Mucha-Habermann disease
Late stages of intraepidermal blistering diseases

ANSWER 7-5: A.

This patient has **catscratch disease**, which is a condition caused by the same microorganism that causes **bacillary angiomatosis** (choice E). *Bartonella henselae* is a gram-negative pleomorphic bacillus, which is most frequently contracted from either bites or scratches from an inoculated cat. The initial small erythematous papulopustules of **catscratch disease** typically present 2 to 5 days after inoculation and resolve with scarring after 2 weeks. Around this time, massive regional lymphadenopathy may develop. Unlike **bacillary angiomatosis**, these lesions do not respond to antibiotic therapy and the lymphadenopathy will gradually resolve over a period of weeks or months. The organisms are extremely difficult to culture; however, a **Hanger-Rose test** will usually be positive if conducted within the first week of infection. Microscopically, early cutaneous lesions are characterized by dermal abscesses filled with necrotic debris and neutrophils surrounded by a palisade of histiocytes. The overlying epidermis exhibits reactive epidermal hyperplasia. A granulomatous inflammatory process predominates in older lesions, at which point identification of bacilli becomes more difficult. Similar lesions are seen in the affected lymph nodes, where the histiocytes may even form occasional giant cells. A GMS or Warthin-Starry stain may highlight the organisms in the skin biopsy or within the thickened hyalinized walls of lymph node vessels.

The cutaneous differential diagnosis includes any suppurative process for early lesions (ie, **folliculitis, cellulitis**) and any granulomatous process for older lesions (ie, **mycobacterial infections, fungal infections**). Clinical correlation and confirmation for the presence of the microorganism (ie, PCR if not visualized in the biopsy) is essential.

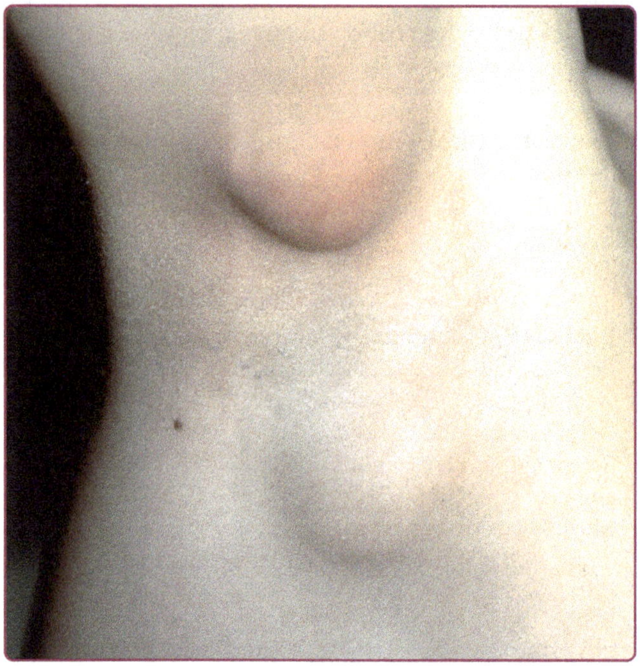

Bartonellosis: catscratch disease with axillary lymphadenopathy. Acute, very tender, axillary lymphadenopathy in a child; cat scratches were present on the dorsum of the ipsilateral hand. (Reproduced, with permission, from Goldsmith LA, Katz SI, Gilchrest BA, Paller AS, Leffell DJ, Wolff K, eds. *Fitzpatrick's Dermatology in General Medicine*. 8th ed. New York, NY: McGraw-Hill Education; 2012.)

ANSWER 7-6: B.

Cellulitis is an acute spreading of inflammation in the skin involving the deeper dermis and subcutaneous tissue (Table 7-6A). It typically arises in sites where skin integrity is compromised from other causes (ie, tinea, traumatic wound, stasis dermatitis, etc). Fever, chills, lymphangitis, leukocytosis, and regional lymphadenopathy may develop. The most common presentation is an ill-defined warm and tender, bright red, painful macule or indurated plaque. Epidermal changes such as scaling, pustules, and ulcers are not present in most patients but may occur in the later stages. Group A streptococci and *Staphylococcus aureus* are the most common etiologic agents. Other organisms implicated include *Haemophilus influenzae* Type B in facial cellulitis in children and HIV-infected patients, Group B streptococci in newborns, and *Streptococcus pneumoniae* in patients with diabetes mellitus or other immunocompromised states. *Staphylococcus epidermidis* is being recognized as a pathogenic agent in the setting of various immunocompromised states, including HIV and organ transplant patients. Biopsies are often not necessary unless an unusual (such as nonbacterial) pathogen or clinical mimic of cellulitis (such as malignancy) is suspected.

Table 7-6A. Infectious Cellulitis

Clinical Features
Bright red erythematous patches or plaques without epidermal change
Low yield of positive cultures after biopsy
Sharply demarcated raised edge on the facial "erysipelas" variant
Histopathologic Features
Diffuse dermal interstitial neutrophils
Dermal edema
Gram stain uncommonly demonstrates bacteria in dermis
Possible epidermal necrosis in later stages if severe

Histopathologic features are often not specific, and demonstration of bacteria is rare. Biopsies usually show diffuse infiltration of the dermis or underlying soft tissue by lymphocytes or neutrophils. Edema and extravasation of erythrocytes may be present. The epidermis is unremarkable except in the later stages, when intraepidermal pustules or necrotic foci may be present. Necrosis in the dermis and **secondary vasculitis** may also be found in late lesions. Special stains for Gram, AFB, or PAS may be needed.

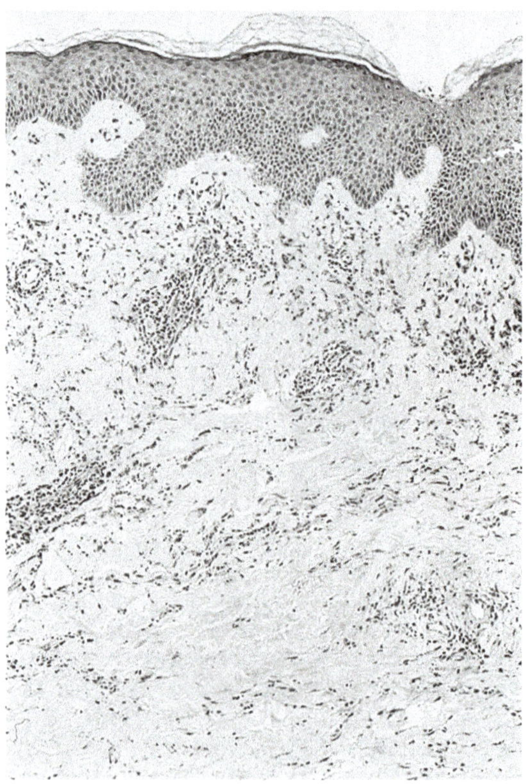

Infectious cellulitis. Perivascular and interstitial infiltrate of neutrophils and lymphocytes.

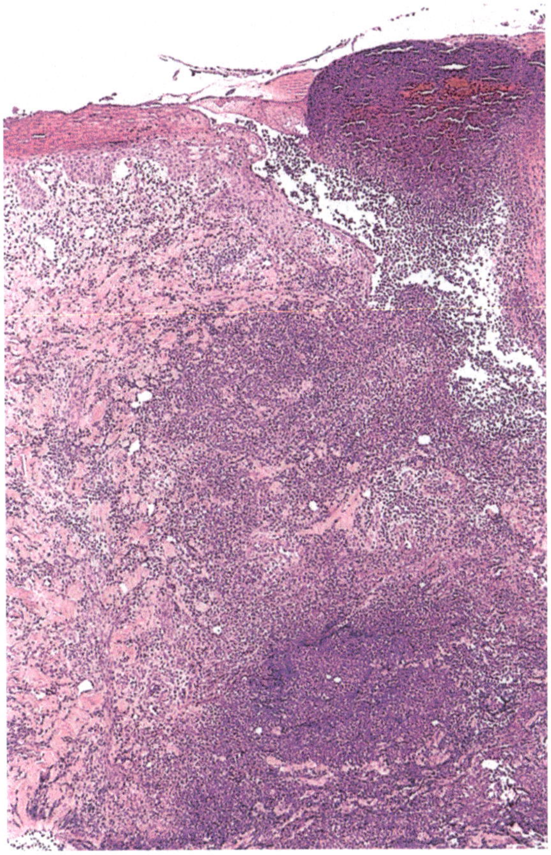

Staphylococcal furuncle. As in cellulitis, neutrophils are predominant in the dermis, but here they are dense and form a dermal abscess. Most are centered on follicles, which largely have been destroyed here.

The borders of **cellulitis** are not elevated or sharply demarcated, unlike **erysipelas**, which is a special type of superficial infectious cellulitis that occurs most commonly on the face. These lesions are well demarcated, rapidly advancing, red, and have an elevated margin. Vesicles and bullae may develop because of prominent dermal edema. The lesions tend to recur periodically in the same area. *S pyogenes* and rarely other streptococci or *S aureus* are responsible for **erysipelas**. As with other forms of **cellulitis**, the organisms may be difficult to demonstrate or culture. Skin biopsy cultures have a low yield (about 13%). Elevated serologic titers to **antistreptolysin O (ASO)** and **antideoxyribonuclease B (anti-DNase B)** are often helpful diagnostically. Constitutional symptoms, such as fever, malaise, headache, and vomiting, may occur. Bacteremia is noted in 5% of patients. Diabetes mellitus can be a predisposing factor. The histopathology of **erysipelas** is similar to other examples of **cellulitis**, but superficial dermal edema and lymphatic dilatation are often exceptionally prominent, even to the point of subepidermal blister formation. Fibrosis may occur in recurrent cases. The gram-positive cocci are very difficult to demonstrate with routine Gram stain. By definition, the inflammation does not extend into the subcutis.

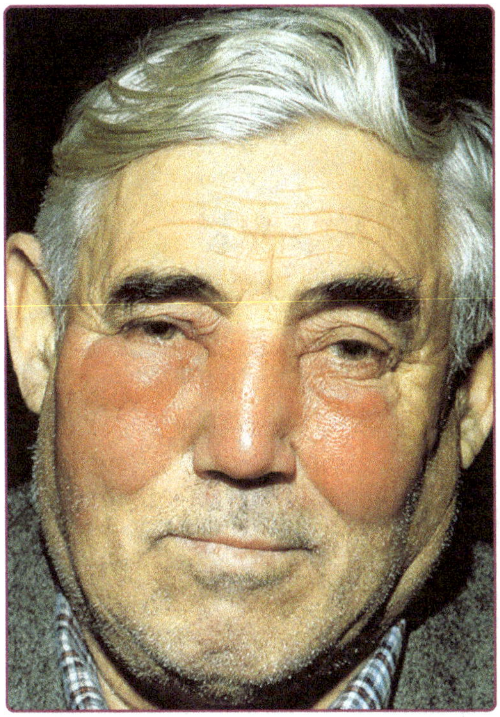

Erysipelas. Painful, edematous erythema with sharp margination on both cheeks and the nose. There is tenderness, and the patient has fever and chills. (Reproduced, with permission, from Goldsmith LA, Katz SI, Gilchrest BA, Paller AS, Leffell DJ, Wolff K, eds. *Fitzpatrick's Dermatology in General Medicine*. 8th ed. New York, NY: McGraw-Hill Education; 2012.)

Erysipeloid is derived from the clinical resemblance to **erysipelas** (hence the suffix *-oid*). This is a relatively rare **cellulitis** owing to the gram-positive bacillus *Erysipelothrix rhusiopathiae*, which is found in decaying animal matter. Although it grows in routine culture media, definitive identification depends on the clinician alerting the laboratory about the detection of this organism, which otherwise may resemble streptococci and diphtheroids. Cultures are best accomplished by skin biopsy taken from the advancing edge of the **cellulitis**. Clinically, **erysipeloid** usually develops on the hands and fingers of those who are injured after handling fish or other animal products. A purplish macule may arise at the site of injury. The lesions are otherwise erythematous macules or slightly elevated plaques, as with other forms of **cellulitis**, but there tends to be a central pallor or clearing and a slowly advancing edge. Constitutional symptoms are less common than with **cellulitis** secondary to streptococci and staphylococci. Lymphangitis and lymphadenitis are rare. In unusual cases, endocarditis may ensue. If untreated, **erysipeloid** tends to resolve spontaneously within 3 weeks, although relapses may occur. Biopsies of **erysipeloid** are similar to other forms of infectious **cellulitis**. Edema of the dermis may be prominent, and the diffuse inflammatory cells tend to be polymorphous, with superficial and deep perivascular lymphocytes and plasma cells as well as neutrophils. Organisms generally cannot be demonstrated with the Gram stain.

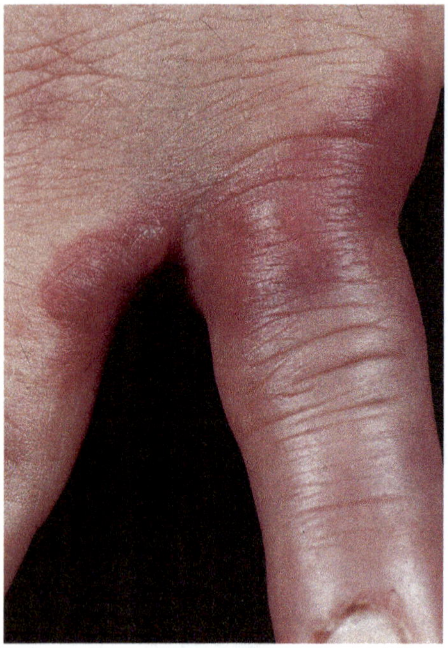

Erysipeloid of hand. A well-demarcated, violaceous, cellulitic plaque (without epidermal changes of scale or vesiculation) on the dorsa of the hand and fingers, occurred following cleaning fish; the site was somewhat painful, tender, and warm. (Reproduced, with permission, from Wolff K, Johnson RA, Saavedra AP. *Fitzpatrick's Color Atlas and Synopsis of Clinical Dermatology*. 7th ed. New York, NY: McGraw-Hill Education; 2013.)

Clinically, the wheals of **urticaria** are strikingly different than the lesions of **cellulitis**. Although microscopically both lesions exhibit interstitial infiltrates of neutrophils and edema, the extent of dermal edema is much greater than that seen in **urticaria**. Additionally, the neutrophilic infiltrates of urticaria are less robust than **cellulitis**. **Sweet syndrome** may clinically appear very similar to **cellulitis**; however, bacterial colonies, vasculitis (characterized by fibrin thrombi within vessels), and tissue necrosis are absent. By definition, **Sweet syndrome** and **pyoderma gangrenosum** must be negative for microorganisms.

ANSWER 7-7: C.

The biopsy reveals a denuded epidermal surface and pale superficial dermis consistent with necrosis and infarction. The blood vessels contain bright pink fibrin thrombi. This is a classic example of **ecthyma gangrenosum**. The adjective "gangrenosum" appended to "ecthyma" generally refers to severe, disseminated, ulcerative lesions in very ill patients owing to sepsis with *Pseudomonas aeruginosa*. This type of sepsis often occurs in those who are immunosuppressed from a wide variety of causes, and the condition often is fatal. Clinically, the ulcers may start as red macules, bullae, or pustules, but eventually they become covered with black eschars. Patients are very ill owing to sepsis and frequent **disseminated intravascular coagulation (DIC).** Microscopically, in most cases, the most striking change is extensive necrosis or ulceration of the epidermis and infarction of the dermis. The inflammatory infiltrate is usually composed of sparse lymphocytes or neutrophils, sometimes with vessel wall changes compatible with **vasculitis.** Gram-negative bacilli may sometimes be seen in the dermis in huge numbers as subtle light blue rods with routine H&E staining (even though staining with Gram stain shows a red color [gram negative]).

In regard to the differential diagnosis, cultures or special stains allow a definitive diagnosis. Extensive necrosis of the epidermis may occur in **toxic epidermal necrolysis (TEN), herpes simplex,** and **ecthyma;** however, these conditions lack the characteristic **thrombogenic vasculopathy** seen in **ecthyma gangrenosum.** Extensive dermal infarction is common with **pyoderma gangrenosum** and certain deep fungal infections, such as from ***Mucor, Rhizopus, Aspergillus,*** and ***Fusarium* infection. Pyoderma gangrenosum** is negative for microorganisms and fungal infections will reveal hyphae on PAS or GMS stains.

ANSWER 7-8: E.

The biopsy reveals epidermal necrosis and perivascular dermal mixed inflammatory infiltrates. The most striking changes are the fibrosis and diffuse inflammation in the adipose septa and the fascia. **Necrotizing fasciitis (NF)** is an acute, rapidly progressive deep infection of the fascia and soft tissue. Initially, it tends to largely spare the skin and underlying muscle. It usually occurs as a result of an injury, diabetes, alcoholism, peripheral vascular disease, malignancy, drug abuse, or immunosuppression. The origin of some cases is idiopathic because it can appear suddenly in young, healthy individuals. **Necrotizing fasciitis (NF)** is more common in children than in adults. Predisposing factors include varicella, intramuscular injections, penetrant gluteal trauma, dental abscess, and streptococcal toxic shock syndrome. The administration of nonsteroidal anti-inflammatory drugs may also contribute to the progression **NF** in children, especially when associated with varicella. Clinically, **necrotizing fasciitis** presents as a rapidly advancing, painful, indurated erythema that progresses to necrosis, blistering, and ulceration. The abdominal wall, perineum, and extremities are involved most commonly. Anaerobic infections may be foul smelling.

Early recognition based on signs and symptoms is potentially lifesaving. Although lab tests and imaging studies can confirm one's clinical impression, rapid treatment with antibiotics and surgery are crucial to improving survival (Table 7-8A).

A number of different organisms have been implicated, often growing synergistically. Streptococci, enterococci, *S aureus*, *Proteus* spp, and anaerobes such as *Peptostreptococcus*, *Bacteroides*, and *Clostridium* spp are common. When a mixed

Table 7-8A. Clinical Features Highly Suspicious for Necrotizing Fasciitis

- Rapid progression of erythema to bullae, ecchymosis, and necrosis or gangrene.
- The erythematous skin may develop a dusky blue discoloration. Vesicular and bullous lesions form over the erythematous skin, with some serosanguineous drainage. The bullae may become violaceous. The skin can become gangrenous and develop a black eschar.
- Edematous, wooden feel of subcutaneous tissues extending beyond the margin of erythema.
- High fevers and severe systemic toxicity.
- Unrelenting intense pain out of proportion to cutaneous findings.
- Pain progresses to cutaneous anesthesia as disease evolves. Anesthesia of the skin develops as a result of infarction of cutaneous nerves.
- Crepitus occurs when there is gas in the soft tissues.
- Unresponsive to empiric antimicrobial therapy.

infection is present, the term **"type I necrotizing fasciitis"** has been used. **"Meleney synergistic gangrene"** and **"Meleney ulcer"** are terms used for a similar type of mixed infection when it occurs in surgical wounds. **"Fournier gangrene"** is a related condition involving the genital area idiopathically or after trauma, surgery, urinary infection, appendicitis, or pancreatitis.

"Type II necrotizing fasciitis" infections are caused by group A streptococci or sometimes *S aureus*. Some authors have more strictly defined **necrotizing fasciitis** as this type only. The lay press has recently coined the term "flesh-eating bacteria" (usually referring to *Streptococcus*) for some of these rapidly progressive infections.

"Type III necrotizing fasciitis" is the fulminant form caused by marine organisms, such as *Vibrio vulnificus*, *Vibrio parahaemolyticus*, and *Vibrio alginolyticus*, either spontaneously or after a puncture wound.

Early antibiotic therapy, aggressive surgical debridement of necrotic tissue, and fasciotomy are important for successful treatment of necrotizing fasciitis. Magnetic resonance imaging and computed tomography scanning may help determine the depth of tissue necrosis for surgical management. The mortality rate is as high as 50%.

Microscopically, there is diffuse infiltration of the soft tissue and fascia with neutrophils and lymphocytes, with areas of necrosis, hemorrhage, and thrombosis. **Secondary vasculitis** may occur. In the late stages, only a few inflammatory cells may be present. Special stains may reveal organisms. Tissue culture is essential for identifying the causative organism and initiating the appropriate antibiotic therapy.

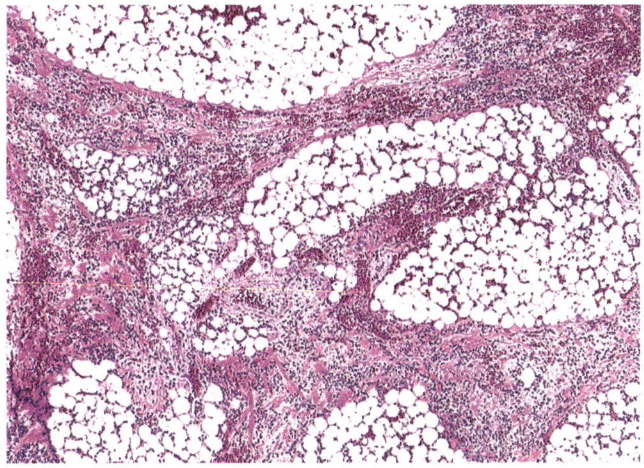

Necrotizing fasciitis. Higher power view showing diffuse hemorrhage and mixed inflammatory infiltrate in the fibrosing adipose septa and fascia.

In regard to the differential diagnosis, **necrotizing fasciitis** may be confused initially with any type of **panniculitis** or deep inflammatory condition, but the rapidly aggressive course makes the diagnosis more obvious. **Lupus panniculitis** and **eosinophilic fasciitis** are seldom mistaken for very long. Special stains and cultures are key to the latter distinction.

ANSWER 7-9: A.

This patient has **erythrasma**, which is caused by colonization of the skin by gram-positive rods called *Corynebacterium minutissimum* (Table 7-9A). This lipophilic bacterium frequently colonizes intertriginous skin of obese diabetic patients. The organism produces **porphyrins**, which result in the characteristic coral-red color under Wood lamp examination. Microscopically, the

Table 7-9A. Erythrasma

Clinical Features
- Red or brownish-red patches in moist intertriginous areas
- Characteristic coral-red fluorescence with Wood lamp

Histopathologic Features
- Filamentous gram-positive rods in stratum corneum seen with H&E, PAS, or Giemsa stains
- Minimal inflammation

Differential Diagnosis
- Nonspecific intertrigo
- Tinea, *Candida* spp
- Contact dermatitis

involved skin is acanthotic with hyperkeratosis and frequent cleft-like separations within the stratum corneum. Under close examination (or with a Gram stain), rod-shaped bacilli can be identified within the cornified layer. A minimal inflammatory response is elicited by the colonization of the bacteria. The coccobacilli and thin bacterial filaments may be barely visible with H&E stain but are seen more easily with the Gram, periodic acid-Schiff (PAS), Gomori methenamine silver (GMS), and Giemsa stains or with electron microscopy. Other species of *Corynebacteria* can colonize the skin, hair, and nails. *Corynebacteria* are difficult to speciate; many species are normal flora, and collectively, they have been known as **diphtheroids** or **coryneforms**. Besides this condition, they are implicated in **pitted keratolysis** and **trichomycosis**.

Pitted keratolysis is a superficial skin infection caused by various *Corynebacterium* spp, *Micrococcus sedentarius*, *Dermatophilus congolensis*, or *Actinomyces*. It is due to excessive heat and moisture and prolonged occlusion of the feet. The organisms apparently elaborate a proteinase that produces hundreds of tiny pits in the skin. Clinically, numerous 1- to 2-mm or larger asymptomatic pits occur in the whitish macerated stratum corneum of the soles, especially over pressure points. The feet may have a strong odor. Microscopically, coccobacilli and filaments are seen within the stratum corneum of the pits. They may be seen with H&E stain but are seen more clearly with Gram stain, as well as PAS, GMS, and Giemsa stains. There is no significant inflammatory reaction.

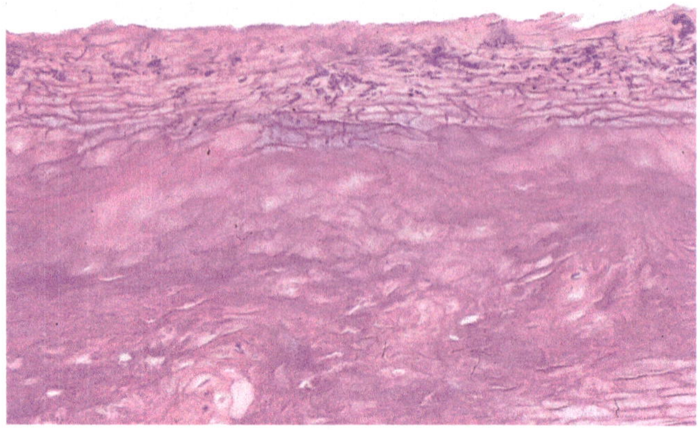

Pitted keratolysis, PAS stain. Coccobacilli and bacterial filaments are infiltrating the superficial stratum corneum.

Trichomycosis axillaris is a superficial bacterial colonization of the hair shafts in sweat gland–bearing areas, such as the armpits and the pubic area. It is a trivial disease of worldwide occurrence that is caused by *Corynebacterium tenuis*. The identification of specific species of this genus is not well delineated and is not done routinely; thus, the diagnosis generally is made clinically without culture or biopsy. *Corynebacteria* (coccobacilli and filaments) are seen within the concretion stuck to the hair. They stain weakly with H&E and are better seen with Giemsa stain or electron microscopy.

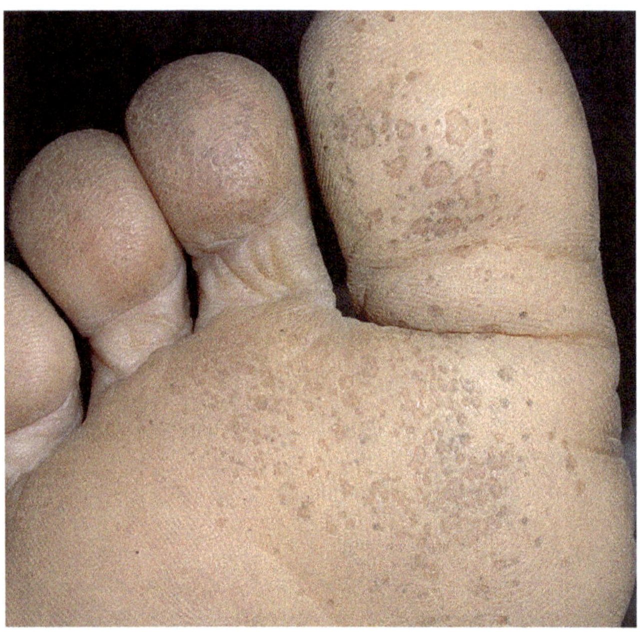

Pitted keratolysis on the pressure-bearing areas of the toes and the ball of the foot. (Reproduced, with permission, from Usatine RP, Smith MA, Mayeaux EJ Jr, Chumley HS, eds. *Color Atlas of Family Medicine*. 2nd ed. New York, NY: McGraw-Hill Education; 2012. Used with permission of Richard P. Usatine, MD.)

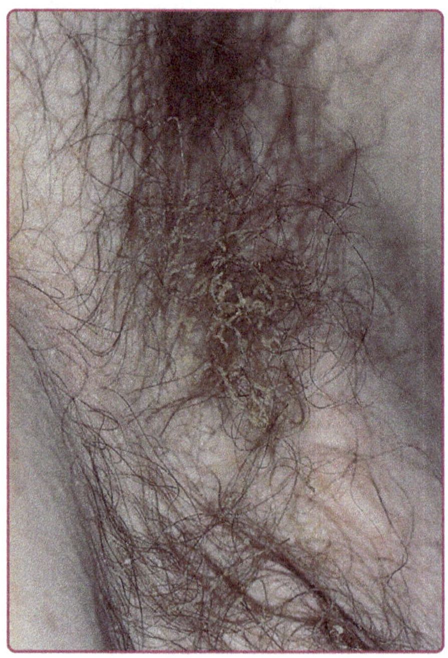

Trichomycosis axillaris. Tan-yellow concretions on the hair shafts of the axilla. (Reproduced, with permission, from Goldsmith LA, Katz SI, Gilchrest BA, Paller AS, Leffell DJ, Wolff K, eds. *Fitzpatrick's Dermatology in General Medicine*. 8th ed. New York, NY: McGraw-Hill Education; 2012.)

Patients with **erythrasma** may also have concomitant **trichomycosis axillaris.** The main differential diagnosis is **dermatophyte infection**, which will reveal much larger hyphae infiltrating the stratum corneum on PAS stain. Erythrasma may resemble **contact dermatitis** or **nonspecific intertrigo**. Some of these diseases may occur concomitantly with **erythrasma**. Concretions on the hairs are also seen with **white piedra (*Trichosporon cutaneum*)** on the scalp, mustache, or groin hairs. In **black piedra (*Piedraia hortae*),** concretions form on the scalp. Both of these fungi are larger than *Corynebacteria* and can be distinguished microscopically or by culture. Both white and black piedra mainly occur in South America. **Tinea** also most commonly involves scalp hair rather than axillary or groin hair. The diagnosis of **pitted keratolysis** is usually clinically straightforward and should not be confused with other causes of pits on the palms and soles, such as **Darier disease** and **basal cell nevus syndrome**. The hyphae of **tinea pedis** are larger. Cultures for fungus may be done if necessary. Most laboratories are not prepared to routinely identify the various causative agents of pitted keratolysis and will report "normal skin flora" or "diphtheroids."

ANSWER 7-10: B.

There are many different *Mycobacterium* species that may infect humans besides ***Mycobacterium tuberculosis*** and ***M leprae***. The Runyon classification into four groups of atypical mycobacteria is not as useful as it once was (Table 7-10A). Common organisms include ***Mycobacterium marinum*** (common "**swimming pool granuloma**"), ***Mycobacterium ulcerans*** (**Buruli ulcer** in Central Africa), ***Mycobacterium avium-intracellulare*** (**MAI**, especially with AIDS), and ***Mycobacterium fortuitum*** and ***Mycobacterium chelonae*** (rapid growers). Clinical lesions include solitary or multiple erythematous nodules, abscesses, ulcers, verrucous plaques, or sinus tracts. The **Buruli ulcer** is caused by infection with ***Mycobacterium ulcerans***. An early nodule at the site of trauma and subsequent painless ulceration characterizes this infection. The incubation period is approximately 3 months. Fever and constitutional findings are usually absent. The ulcer extends into the subcutaneous fat, and its margin is deeply undermined. Ulcerations may enlarge to involve an entire extremity. Legs more commonly involve sites of trauma; however, any site may be involved. As ulcerations heal, scarring and disabling deformities may occur. **Osteomyelitis** may develop in long-standing lesions. Histopathologically, the **Buruli ulcer** is characterized by coagulative necrosis, compared to the caseous necrosis seen in other forms of mycobacterial infection. Also contrasted with other forms of mycobacteria infection, these "atypical" acid-fast–positive bacilli are most frequently found in microabscesses or within vacuoles rather than within multinucleated giant cells. Fluorescent antibodies or PCR may be used for detection of the organism.

Table 7-10A. Atypical Mycobacteria

Clinical Features
- Ulcers, cysts, sinus tracts, or purulent nodules
- Multiple or solitary, systemic or cutaneous only
- May be sporotrichoid

Histopathologic Features
- Epidermis hyperplastic or ulcerated
- Suppurative and granulomatous inflammation with or without necrosis
- Acid-fast bacilli may be present
- Sometimes prominent fibrosis or granulation tissue

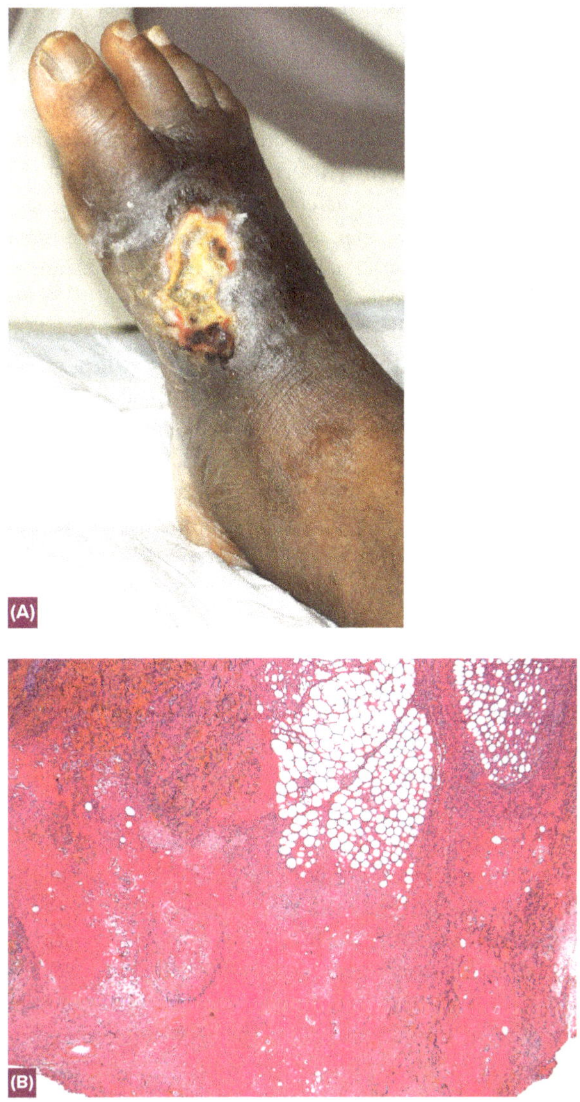

***Mycobacterium ulcerans*. (A)** Buruli ulcer on the foot. **(B)** Extensive coagulative necrosis throughout the dermis and subcutaneous fat.

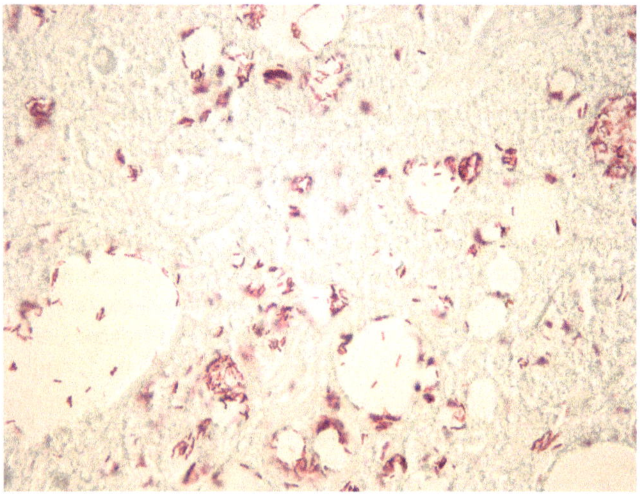

Mycobacterium ulcerans. Numerous vacuoles contain acid-fast bacilli (Ziehl-Neelsen stain).

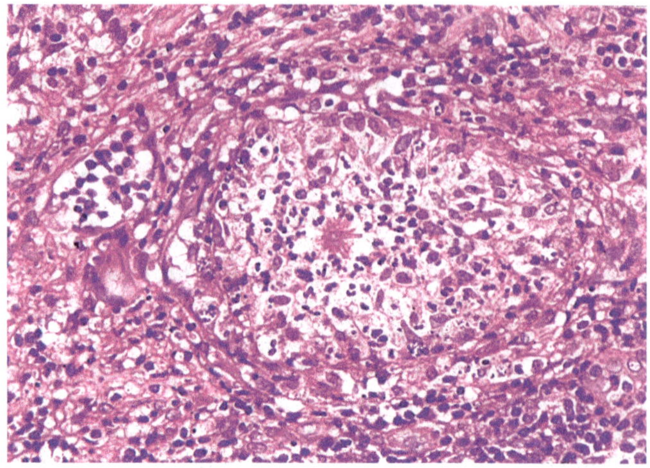

Sporotrichosis. Suppurative granuloma containing an asteroid body. (Used with permission of Dr S. Seopela.)

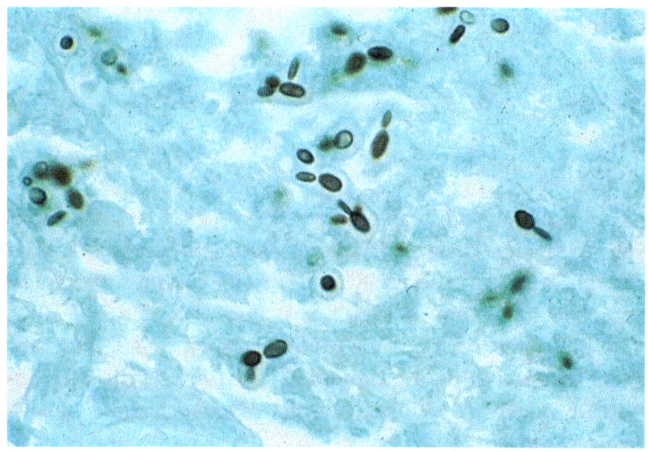

Sporotrichosis. Round to oval spore forms with budding demonstrated with Gomori methenamine silver stain. (Used with permission of Dr F. Von Lichtenberg.)

Sometimes mycobacterial infections spread in a **lymphocutaneous "sporotrichoid" pattern**, as demonstrated by the patient in question. ***Mycobacterium marinum*** is the most common mycobacterium to present in this fashion and is most commonly associated with the handling of fish or the cleaning of fish tanks. Once inoculated, a hard nodule typically develops at the site of inoculation weeks to months after infection. This nodule may drain seropurulent fluid and become ulcerated. Satellite lesions may follow along the lymphatic drainage system (**sporotrichoid spread**) with associated lymphadenopathy. The initial lesion may remain for several weeks and ultimately heals with scarring. This form of infection may become chronic if not treated. The clinical presentation of **lymphocutaneous spread** is also commonly seen in infections by ***Sporothrix schenckii, Leishmania braziliensis,*** and ***Nocardia brasiliensis***. Microscopically, the typical lesions of ***mycobacterium marinum*** show suppurative and granulomatous inflammation with or without caseation. The epidermis may be hyperplastic or ulcerated. Fibrosis and granulation tissue may be prominent. Various modifications of the Ziehl-Neelsen acid-fast stain or Fite stain may reveal the mycobacteria. ***Sporothrix*** is a dimorphic fungus that exists as a saprophytic mold in soil, wood, and decaying vegetative matter worldwide. There is often a history of traumatic inoculation of the organism into the skin (ie, prick from a thorn of a rose). The most important diagnostic use of a biopsy is for microbiologic cultures because the organism is rarely identified histopathologically. It is a fast-growing fungus; characteristic colonies become apparent within 3 to 5 days. The histopathologic findings are by and large nonspecific but typically also include a suppurative or granulomatous tissue reaction. If organisms are present, a fungal stain (PAS, GMS) may reveal them within asteroid bodies or in the tissue as round to oval spores. Cigar-shaped bodies are observed much less commonly. There may be single or multiple buds. No capsule is present.

Leishmania braziliensis is transmitted by the bite from a sandfly and typically presents with an ulcerated hard nodule that spreads in a **lymphocutaneous fashion ("sporotrichoid")**, several months after inoculation. The most common sites include the face and extremities. After the lesions heal, subclinical infection persists and after many years (3 to 20 years) the parasites gradually cause oral and nasal lesions that eventuate in severe damage to the mucous membranes. The histopathologic findings are nonspecific and typically include a suppurative or granulomatous tissue reaction. **Amastigotes** are identified within the macrophages of the infiltrate.

Nocardia brasiliensis is a gram-positive and acid-fast–positive filamentous rod-shaped bacteria. Although ***Mycobacteria*** and ***Nocardia*** are both acid-fast positive, ***Nocardia*** organisms are very long and filamentous. Cutaneous manifestations included cellulitis, pustules, ulcerations, pyoderma, subcutaneous abscesses, lymphocutaneous syndrome, and **mycetoma**. Disseminated disease may occur.

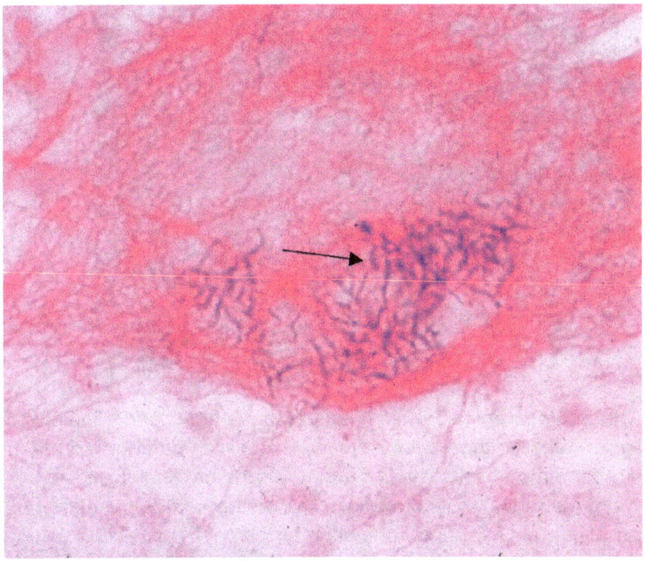

Nocardia braziliensis—H&E stain. Arrow points to area of filaments of gram-positive rods. An acid fast or Fite stain would stain the filamentous rods red. (Used with permission of Dr. Thomas Sellers, Emory University, Centers for Disease Control and Prevention.)

DDX for Lymphocutaneous "Sporotrichoid" Spread and Nodular Lymphangitis

Steve **M**artin **L**ikes **N**o**B**ody

Sporothrix schenckii
Mycobacterium marinum
Leishmania brasiliensis
Nocardia brasiliensis
Blastomyces dermatitidis

ANSWER 7-11: D.

This patient's biopsy reveals elongated granulomas infiltrating the dermis in a serpentine-like distribution. The granulomas have sparse lymphocytic mantles and are seen surrounding vessels and nerves. **Hansen disease (Leprosy)** affects millions of people worldwide (Table 7-11A). It is caused by ***Mycobacterium leprae***, which is a noncultivable, gram-positive, obligate intracellular, acid-fast bacillus. In the United States, it occurs mainly in immigrants from endemic areas, but some cases originate in Texas and Louisiana, perhaps from armadillo exposure. **Leprosy** affects multiple organs of the body, but clinical disease is most apparent in the skin, eyes, and peripheral nerves. Neuropathies may result in deformities of the distal extremities. **Leprosy** is divided into several types in the Ridley-Jopling classification based on the immune status of the patient. Ridley's construct is a six-member spectrum, ranging from high to low resistance, **TT (polar tuberculoid), BT (borderline tuberculoid), BB (borderline), BL (borderline**

Table 7-11A. Leprosy (Hansen Disease)

Clinical Features
- *Lepromatous*:
  - Multiple erythematous or hypopigmented smooth patches, plaques, or nodules, sometimes leonine facies
- *Tuberculoid*:
  - Hypopigmented scaly or annular patches or plaques, smaller in number than lepromatous, more hypoesthesia in the lesions
- *Borderline*:
  - Features intermediate between lepromatous and tuberculoid
- *Indeterminant*:
  - Early hypopigmented or erythematous macules
- *Lepra reaction (type I reaction)*:
  - Acute redness or pain in previously existing lesions
  - Erythema nodosum leprosum (type II reaction):
  - Acute onset of erythematous nodules in new sites not previously involved
- *Lucio phenomenon (type III or variant of II)*:
  - Acute onset of hemorrhagic plaques or ulcers

Histopathologic Features
- *Lepromatous*
  - Diffuse dermal infiltrate of foamy macrophages
  - Grenz zone separating the macrophages from the epidermis
  - Numerous AFB, often in clumps called globi
- *Tuberculoid*
  - Tuberculoid (epithelioid) granulomas without grenz zone
  - Granulomas often linear, following nerves
  - AFB rare or absent
- *Borderline*
  - Histology in between lepromatous and tuberculoid
- *Indeterminant*
  - Perivascular and/or perineural lymphohistiocytic inflammation
  - Few or no AFB
- *Type I reaction*
  - Histology as in borderline leprosy
- *Type II reaction*
  - Lepromatous leprosy plus leukocytoclastic vasculitis
- *Type III reaction*
  - Similar to type II, with greater tendency to thrombosis, necrosis, and ulceration

Differential Diagnosis
- *Lepromatous*
  - Leishmaniasis
  - Atypical mycobacteria
  - Histiocytic infiltrates
  - Xanthomas

Table 7-11A. Leprosy (Hansen Disease) *(continued)*

Granular cell tumors	
Clear-cell neoplasms	
Tuberculoid	
Tuberculosis	
Atypical mycobacteria	
Secondary and tertiary syphilis	
Noninfectious sarcoidal granulomas	
Sarcoidosis	Beryllium
Reaction to foreign agents	Zirconium
Silica	Keratin
Cutaneous Crohn disease	
Granulomatous cheilitis	
Rosacea	

lepromatous), LLs (subpolar lepromatous), and finally **LLp (polar lepromatous):** TT⇐BT⇔BB⇔BL⇔LLs,LLp.

Conceptually, **TT** and **LLp** are clinically stable, but, between the poles, the host response may change, as indicated by the arrows, upgrading (or reversing) to a state of higher resistance, often with devastating inflammation, or downgrading to a posture of lower resistance, usually silent but occasionally inflammatory. **BT** patients may upgrade to **TT**, thus, becoming stable, but **LLs** patients do not downgrade to **LLp** nor do **LLp** patients upgrade. ("**LL**" includes both **LLs** and **LLp** patients.) The host's granulomatous response is the result of the degree of cell-mediated immunity directed against ***M leprae***. The classification is determined primarily by clinical and histologic changes, bacillary numbers being a secondary consideration. Patients along the clinical spectrum of **leprosy** are presumed to be manifestations of evolving immune responses, which, based on environmental and genetic factors, will eventually gravitate toward one of the two poles.

The **tuberculoid (TT)** form occurs in those with intact cellular immunity, and patients tend to develop only one or a few lesions with prominent hypoesthesia and palpable peripheral nerves. The lesions may be annular or scaly or macular and hypopigmented.

Microscopically, **TT** is characterized by small, well-developed epithelioid granulomas that are surrounded by large lymphocytic mantles. Abundant **Langhans-type giant cells** and brisk lymphocyte exocytosis into the epidermis are usually found. The histopathology of **TT** may closely resemble **lupus vulgaris** (cutaneous *Mycobacterium tuberculosis*). Rarely caseation necrosis is seen. Acid-fast–positive bacilli are not found.

On the other end of the spectrum is **lepromatous leprosy (LL)**, in which patients are anergic and tend to develop widespread cutaneous lesions. These patients have impaired cellular immunity against ***M leprae*** and have high circulating antibodies. Although they are less likely to have hypoesthesia in the lesions, the peripheral nerves may still be enlarged with consequent neuropathies. Lesions of **lepromatous leprosy** include hypopigmented or erythematous macules, infiltrated erythematous nodules or plaques, leonine (lion-like) facies with

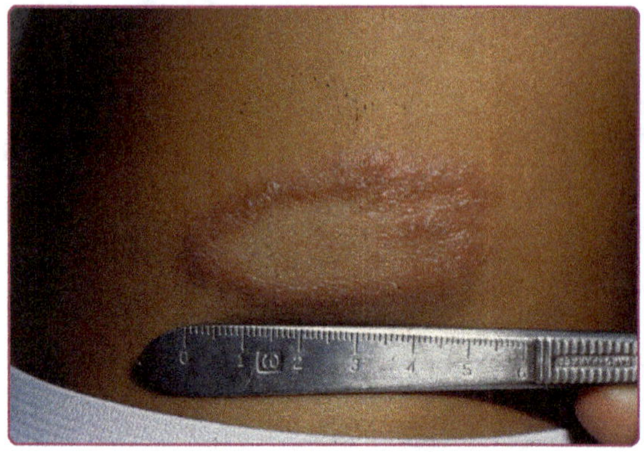

Tuberculoid leprosy (TT). A solitary, anesthetic, and annular lesion of polar tuberculoid leprosy (TT), which had been present for 3 months. Its sharp margins, erythema, and scale are more evident than its elevation. The central red dots are the sequelae or "footprints" of testing for pinprick perception when it is absent. (If present, the patient withdraws, preventing overly purpuric consequences.) The central portion of the lesion was slightly hypopigmented as compared to the surrounding normal skin. (Reproduced, with permission, from Goldsmith LA, Katz SI, Gilchrest BA, Paller AS, Leffell DJ, Wolff K, eds. *Fitzpatrick's Dermatology in General Medicine*. 8th ed. New York, NY: McGraw-Hill Education; 2012.)

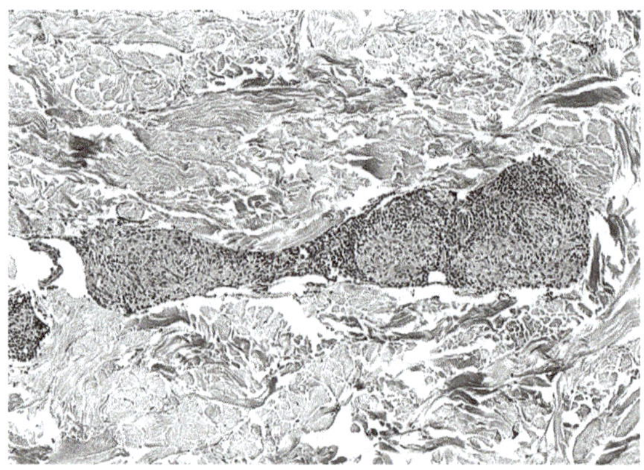

Tuberculoid leprosy. Linear granuloma with a robust lymphocytic mantel following the course of a nerve.

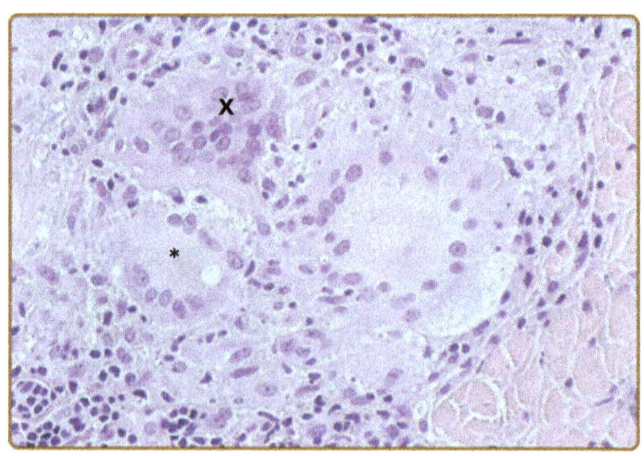

Tuberculoid leprosy. Mixture of Langhans-type (*) and foreign body giant cells (x). (Reproduced, with permission, from Goldsmith LA, Katz SI, Gilchrest BA, Paller AS, Leffell DJ, Wolff K, eds. *Fitzpatrick's Dermatology in General Medicine*. 8th ed. New York, NY: McGraw-Hill Education; 2012.)

a loss of eyebrows and eyelashes, and diffuse macular involvement of the skin resulting in a smooth surface. Microscopically, **LL** is characterized by diffuse or serpentine granulomas with minimal lymphocytic mantles. There is typically a Grenz zone separating the macrophages from the epidermis. The granulomatous infiltrates follow a perivascular and perineural distribution. The granulomas of older lesions exhibit a foamy appearance. Numerous bacilli are present within the granulomas. The Fite stain or modifications of it are recommended because the Ziehl-Neelsen method used for other acid-fast bacteria does not work as well. Immunostaining for acid-fast bacteria can enhance the ability to diagnose lesions containing few bacilli. In situ hybridization and PCR analysis of specimens are more sensitive and are available through the Hansen's Disease Center in Baton Rouge, Louisiana.

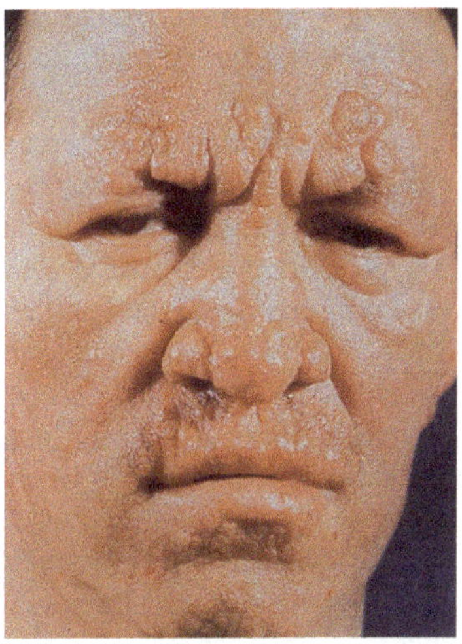

The leonine face of lepromatous leprosy. Multiple nodular skin lesions, particularly of the forehead, and loss of eyebrows. (Reproduced, with permission, from Levinson W, ed. *Review of Medical Microbiology and Immunology*. 13th ed. New York, NY: McGraw-Hill Education; 2012. Courtesy of Robert Gelber, MD.)

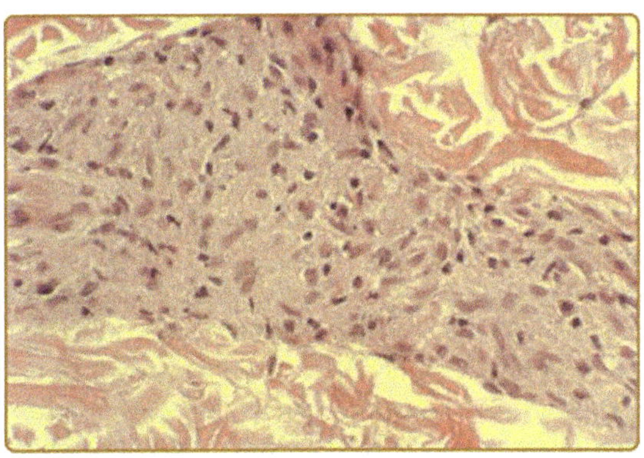

The histology of a young, active LL lesion. The undifferentiated macrophages have not been active for long enough to develop a characteristic "foamy" appearance. (H&E, 40× objective.) (Reproduced, with permission, from Goldsmith LA, Katz SI, Gilchrest BA, Paller AS, Leffell DJ, Wolff K, eds. *Fitzpatrick's Dermatology in General Medicine*. 8th ed. New York, NY: McGraw-Hill Education; 2012.)

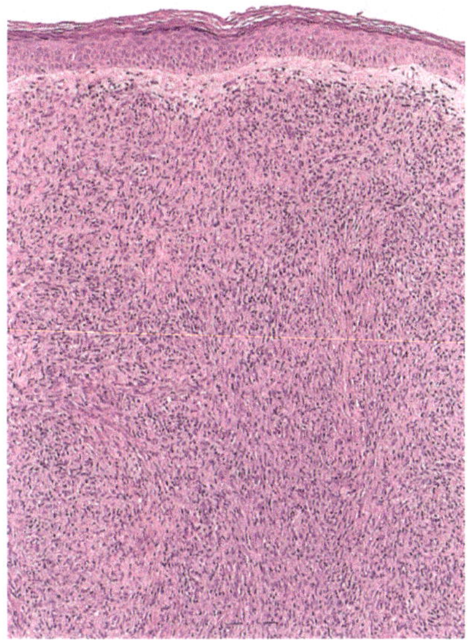

Lepromatous leprosy. Diffuse infiltration of the dermis by foamy macrophages separated from the dermis by a Grenz zone.

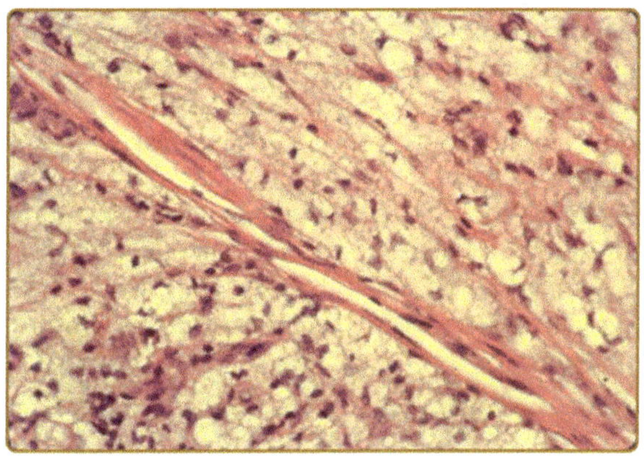

The histology of a very old and inactive LL lesion. The "foamy" change has become ubiquitous. (H&E, 40× objective.) (Reproduced, with permission, from Goldsmith LA, Katz SI, Gilchrest BA, Paller AS, Leffell DJ, Wolff K, eds. *Fitzpatrick's Dermatology in General Medicine*. 8th ed. New York, NY: McGraw-Hill Education; 2012.)

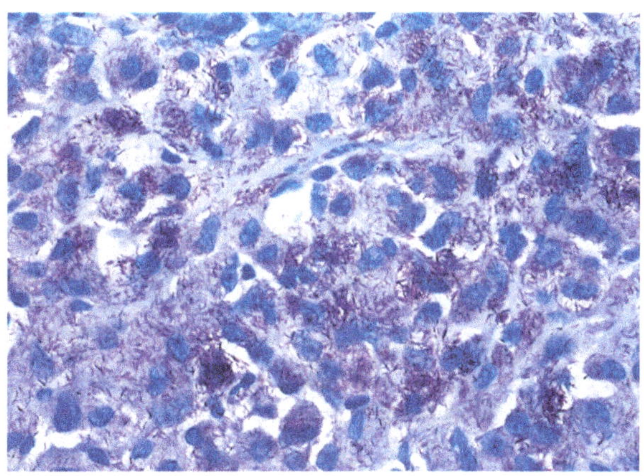

Lepromatous leprosy. Fite stain of numerous acid-fast bacilli, often clumped into globi.

In **borderline leprosy (BB)**, combined features of tuberculoid and lepromatous disease are seen.

Indeterminant leprosy represents early disease in patients living in populations where leprosy is prevalent; it is difficult to establish a definite diagnosis in some of these patients. They tend to have only a single or few hypopigmented or erythematous macules with or without hypoesthesia. The disease may heal spontaneously or may evolve into one of the other forms. **Histoid leprosy** refers to dermatofibroma-like nodules of **lepromatous leprosy.**

There are three types of **reactional leprosy**, and they occur with or without treatment, usually as a result of a change in the patient's immune status. The type I reaction (**Lepra reaction**) is called a "reversal reaction" when the patient is under treatment and has shifted toward the **tuberculoid spectrum** with greater immunity. It is called a "downgrading reaction" when untreated patients shift toward the **lepromatous pole.** Type I reactions involve swelling of previously existing cutaneous and neural lesions with associated constitutional symptoms.

Type II reactions (**erythema nodosum leprosum**) occur in **lepromatous** and **borderline lepromatous leprosy** patients. Tender new red plaques and nodules develop on normal skin, accompanied by constitutional symptoms. This type of reaction involves immune complexes with frequent **leukocytoclastic vasculitis.**

Type III reactions (**Lucio phenomenon**) occur only in patients with the diffuse form of **lepromatous leprosy.** Hemorrhagic plaques occur on the legs, arms, or buttocks. These may ulcerate eventually. There are usually no constitutional symptoms.

ANSWER 7-12: C.

Ringworm of the glabrous skin is called **tinea corporis;** it results from proliferation of fungi in the stratum corneum and may be caused by infection by any **dermatophyte**, with regional differences dictating the prevailing dermatophytic flora. Infection of the skin at the site of inoculation spreads centrifugally, followed by a secondary tissue response. The central area may clear as fungus is eliminated, with active proliferation continuing at the periphery, resulting in characteristic annular, scaly patches with raised erythematous or vesicular margins. The natural history varies depending on the attributes of the fungal species and the host. Most cases are caused by *T rubrum*, *T mentagrophytes*, and *M canis*. Special expressions of **tinea corporis** have been recognized. For example, *T rubrum* commonly causes extensive eruptions, sometimes with psoriasiform lichenified plaques and nodular granulomatous perifolliculitis (**Majocchi granuloma**).

Microscopically, dermatophytic infections display a spectrum of patterns depending on the causative agent and the host response. For example, dry, scaly patches and plaques, often caused by **anthropophilic dermatophytes**, show hyperkeratosis. Compact orthokeratosis, the presence of neutrophils within the stratum corneum, and the "**sandwich sign**" may also be clues to a dermatophyte infection. The sandwich sign denotes hyphae "sandwiched" in between a superficial normal-appearing basket-weave pattern of orthokeratosis in the stratum corneum and a deeper layer of abnormal stratum corneum showing either parakeratosis or compact hyperkeratosis. Variable spongiosis and occasional subcorneal or intraepidermal pustule formation may be seen. The dermis contains a mild perivascular inflammatory infiltrate consisting of lymphocytes, histiocytes, eosinophils, and neutrophils. **Zoophilic dermatophyte** infections tend to be more inflammatory with vesicle formation. Hyphae within the stratum corneum may be visible even with H&E stain if they are numerous, but they are seen more easily with periodic acid-Schiff (PAS) or methenamine silver staining (GMS). In **Majocchi granuloma** owing to *T rubrum*, **arthroconidia** and **mycelia** are seen in follicles, and there is a dermal infiltrate of lymphocytes, histiocytes, epithelioid cells, and often foreign-body giant cells. Rupture of the follicular wall releases conidia and mycelia, stimulating granuloma formation.

In regard to the differential diagnosis, cases in which the inflammation is minimal and hyphae are not visualized with routine staining, biopsy of **tinea corporis** may resemble that of normal skin. Lesions with hyperkeratosis, spongiosis, and mild inflammation may mimic **subacute spongiotic dermatitides** such as **nummular eczema, seborrheic dermatitis, contact dermatitis**, and the **herald patch** of **pityriasis rosea.** Zoophilic dermatophytic infections may be confused with **impetigo, cellulitis, folliculitis decalvans**, or other pustular infections. Potassium hydroxide preparations usually reveal fungal elements in skin scrapings from tinea corporis. Cultures should be obtained routinely and are positive in 5% to 15% of KOH-negative cases.

ANSWER 7-13: B.

Dermatophytic infection of the scalp, eyebrows, and eyelashes is called **tinea capitis** (Table 7-13A). The patient in question has "**black-dot ringworm,**" a form of large-spore **endothrix** infection. The most common etiologic agents for **tinea capitis** are *Trichophyton* and *Microsporum* species. *T tonsurans* has superseded *M audouinii* and *M canis* as the primary cause of this condition in the United States, as well as in most of North, Central, and South America. *M canis*, a zoophilic organism, is the pathogen for most cases in Europe, especially in Mediterranean and eastern countries. However, a shift in etiology toward anthropophilic dermatophyte species has been observed, especially in urban regions, where the incidence of tinea capitis due to *T tonsurans*, mostly in the United Kingdom, and *T soudanense* and *M audouinii*, in France, has increased significantly. Infection occurs via direct or indirect person-to-person contact. Unlike *Microsporum* infections, childhood *T tonsurans* infections do not always

Table 7-13A. Dermatophytoses

DISEASE	ORGANISM
Tinea capitis	
Small-spore ectothrix	*Microsporum audouinii,*[a] *M canis,*[z] *M gypseum,*[g] *M fulvum,*[g] *M ferrugineum*[a]
Large-spore endothrix	*Trichophyton tonsurans,*[a] *T violaceum,*[a] *T soudanense,*[a] *T gourvilii,*[a] *T yaoundei*[a]
Large-spore ectothrix	*T mentagrophytes* var *interdigitale,*[a] *T mentagrophytes* var *mentagrophytes,*[z] *T verrucosum,*[z] *T megninii*[a]
Tinea favosa	*T schoenleiniia (T violaceum, M gypseum rare)*
Tinea corporis	*T rubrum,*[a] *T mentagrophytes,*[z] *M canis, others*
Tinea faciei	*T mentagrophytes, T rubrum*[a]
Tinea barbae	*T mentagrophytes,*[z] *T verrucosum,*[z] *T rubrum,*[a] *T violaceum,*[a] *T megninii,*[a] *M canis*[z]
Tinea cruris	*T rubrum,*[a] *E floccosum,*[a] *T mentagrophytesa*
Tinea pedis	*T rubrum,*[a] *T mentagrophytes,*[a] *E floccosum*[a]
Tinea manuum	*T rubrum,*[a] *E floccosum,*[a] *T mentagrophytesa*[a]
Tinea unguium	*T rubrum,*[a] *T mentagrophytes,*[a.z] *(E floccosum,*[a] *T violaceum,*[a] *T schoenleinii,*[a] *T tonsuransa rare)*

Key: [a] = anthropophilic; [g] = geophilic; [z] = zoophilic.

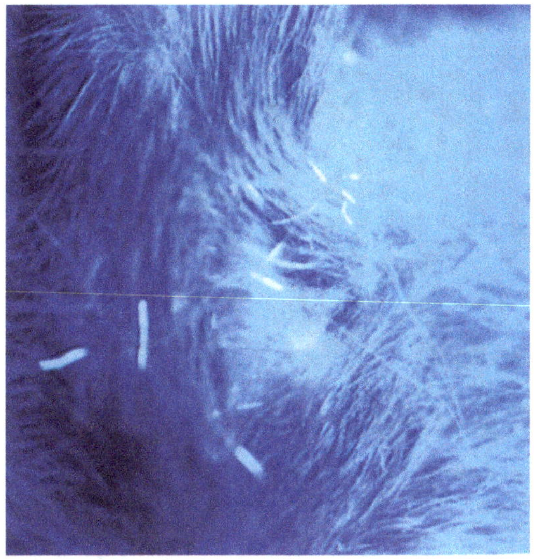

Tinea capitis. Close-up using an ultraviolet lamp (Wood light) reveals fluorescing hair fragments. The culture grew *Microsporum audouinii.* (Reproduced with permission from Willey J, Sherwood L, Woolverton C (eds). *Prescott's Principles of Microbiology.* 8th ed. New York: McGraw-Hill; 2011.)

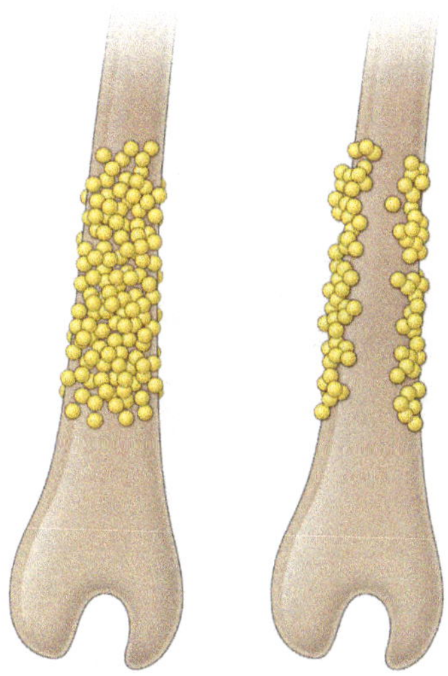

Dermatophytic folliculitis. Endothrix type (left): hyphae and arthroconidia occur within the hair shaft (intrapilary). Ectothrix type (right): mycelia and arthroconidia are seen on the surface of the hair follicle (extrapilary). (Reproduced, with permission, from Wolff K, Johnson RA, Saavedra AP. *Fitzpatrick's Color Atlas and Synopsis of Clinical Dermatology.* 7th ed. New York, NY: McGraw-Hill Education; 2013.)

resolve at puberty. Also, unlike *M canis*, *M audouinii*, and *M ferrugineum*, which show green fluorescence with Wood lamp, *T tonsurans* does not fluoresce. *T schoenleinii*, the etiologic agent of **tinea favosa**, shows a green-gray fluorescence with the Wood lamp.

Tinea capitis infections can be further divided based on how they invade the hair shaft (**ectothrix** vs **endothrix**). Whereas **ectothrix** infections are typically associated with inflammation and clinical erythema, **endothrix** infections may have little inflammation and no clinically appreciable erythema. In general, **tinea capitis** may be divided into **small-spore ectothrix, large-spore ectothrix, large-spore endothrix**, or **tinea favosa**.

Small-spore ectothrix is caused by *Microsporum* species. Infection begins with hyphal invasion of the hair follicles. Hyphae grow within the hair shaft toward the hair bulb. As the hair emerges from the follicle, it is covered with a mass of small arthrospores 2 to 5 μm in diameter. Clinical manifestations vary from mild inflammation, as seen in anthropophilic *Microsporum* species, to severe inflammatory reactions caused by the zoophilic and geophilic *Microsporum* species.

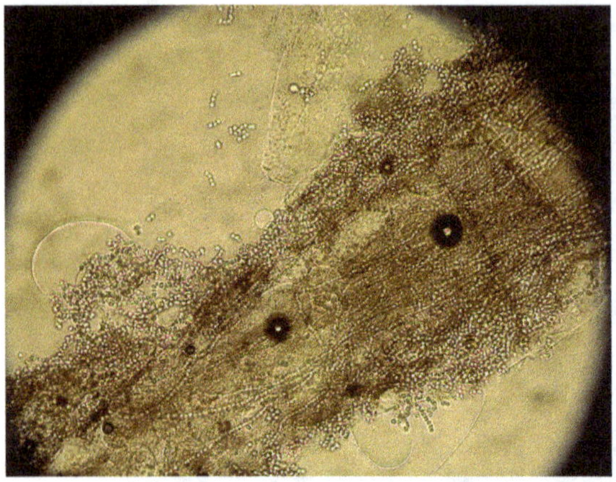

Small-spore ectothrix. *M canis* showing hyphae on the exterior of the hair at 40 power after adding Swartz-Lamkins fungal stain. (Reproduced, with permission, from Usatine RP, Smith MA, Mayeaux EJ Jr, Chumley HS, eds. *Color Atlas of Family Medicine*. 2nd ed. New York, NY: McGraw-Hill Education; 2012; Used with permission of Eric Kraus, MD.)

Gray-patch ringworm, typical of *M audouinii* infection, is characterized by patches of dull bristles of hair with slight erythema and mild scaling. All hairs in a given area are affected, and lesions spread in a characteristic ring formation. *M canis*, *M gypseum*, and *M fulvum*, the zoophilic and geophilic species, cause more host response, often leading to suppurative folliculitis or kerion formation, characterized by intense inflammation, pus, crusting, and matting of hairs.

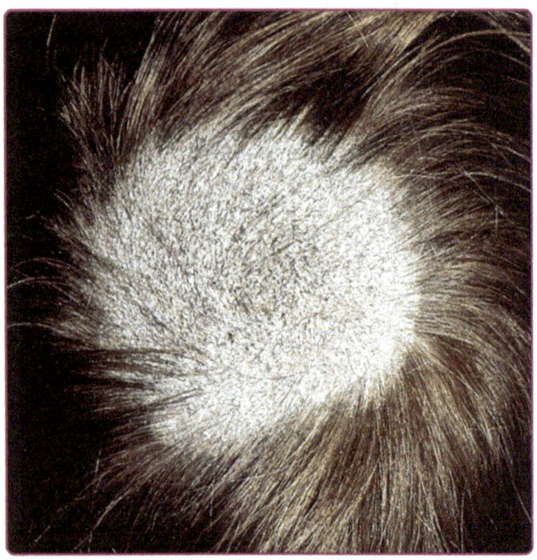

Tinea capitis "gray patch" type. A large, round hyperkeratotic plaque of alopecia due to breaking off of hair shafts close to the surface, giving the appearance of a mowed wheat field on the scalp of a child. Remaining hair shafts and scales exhibit a green fluorescence when examined with a Wood lamp. *Microsporum canis* was isolated on culture. (Reproduced, with permission, from Goldsmith LA, Katz SI, Gilchrest BA, Paller AS, Leffell DJ, Wolff K, eds. *Fitzpatrick's Dermatology in General Medicine*. 8th ed. New York, NY: McGraw-Hill Education; 2012.)

Large-spore ectothrix infections are caused by *T verrucosum* and *T mentagrophytes*. Whereas *T verrucosum* infections are characterized by arthroconidia 8 to 12 μm in diameter arranged in large, dense chains along hair, *T mentagrophytes* infections demonstrate arthroconidia 3 to 4 μm in diameter in chains along the external surface of the hair. It is most commonly associated with **tinea barbae** (ringworm of the beard and mustache). These organisms often cause suppurative folliculitis or **kerion** formation with subsequent atrophy of hair follicles, scarring, and patchy permanent **scarring alopecia**. Histologic examination of a **kerion** reveals a dense perifollicular and perivascular infiltrate of lymphocytes, neutrophils, plasma cells, and eosinophils in the dermis.

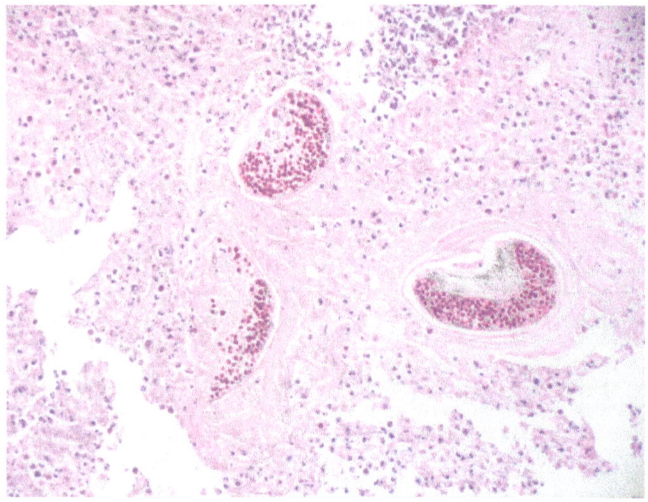

Kerion, caused by endothrix infection, PAS stain. Endothrix infection associated with robust necrotizing inflammatory infiltrates. The hair shafts contain numerous spores and hyphae.

Large-spore endothrix is caused by *T tonsurans* and *T violaceum* in the United States. In Africa, *T gourvilii*, *T soudanense*, and *T yaoundei* are common etiologic agents. These anthropophilic species produce **black-dot ringworm**, caused by intrafollicular hyphae that fragment into 5- to 8-μm-wide arthrospores within the shaft, often resulting in breakage at the level of the follicular ostium. The alopecic patches are smaller than in gray-patch ringworm, and not all hairs in the area are affected. Infections caused by *Trichophyton* species tend to be more inflammatory than those caused by *Microsporum* species, and **kerion** formation is often seen in association with *T violaceum*.

Tinea favosa (also called **"favus"**) is an uncommon clinical presentation that occurs mostly in Eurasia and Africa usually associated with *T schoenleinii*. *T violaceum*, *M gypseum*, and *M canis* have also been identified as causative agents of **favus**. Broad hyphae and air spaces develop within the hair shaft without arthrospores. Areas of scales, crusty debris, and masses of mycelium form cup-shaped **scutula** over the scalp. In **tinea favosa**, hyphae are present within the stratum

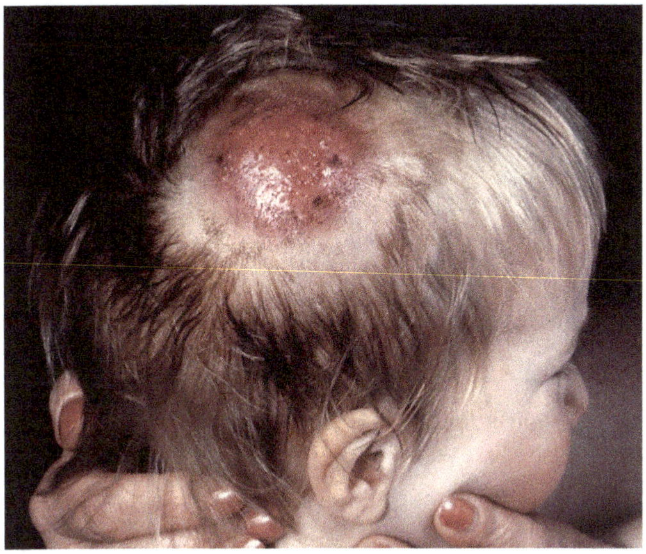

Tinea capitis with central kerion formation. (Reproduced with permission from Wolff K, Johnson R, Suurmond R: *Fitzpatrick's Color Atlas & Synopsis of Clinical Dermatology, 5th ed.* New York, McGraw-Hill, 2005.)

corneum, in hair shafts, and in **scutula,** which consist of tangled mycelial elements, sebum, debris, and scales forming a characteristic cup-shaped lesion. Follicular atrophy and a chronic dermal inflammatory infiltrate are present.

ANSWER 7-14: C.

The biopsy reveals numerous yeasts and branching **pseudohyphae** within the stratum corneum. The pseudohyphae are composed of elongated ellipsoids that remain attached to one other at constricted septations as they grow. **Candidiasis** is caused by dimorphic yeast-like fungi of the genus *Candida*, indisputably the single most important cause of **opportunistic mycoses** worldwide. More than 90% of invasive *Candida* infections can be attributed to five pathogenic species: *C albicans*, *C glabrata*, *C parapsilosis*, *C tropicalis*, and *C krusei*, although the list of reported species, now including *C guilliermondi*, *C lusitaniae*, *C kefyr*, *C rugosa*, *C famata*, *C inconspicua*, *C norvegensis*, and others, continues to expand. As opportunistic organisms, they depend on a change in host physiology, defenses, or normal flora to colonize, invade, and cause disease. The degree of virulence among species varies greatly, with *C albicans*, *C glabrata*, and *C tropicalis* being the most virulent. Less virulent species require greater host debilitation to cause disease.

Candida albicans is part of the normal flora of the gastrointestinal (GI) tract, oral cavity, and vagina. *C albicans* grows as a budding yeast; whereas hyphal forms are hallmarks of tissue invasion, blastoconidia are thought to be involved in hematogenous dissemination. In oral lesions, the finding of mycelia is useful in differentiating a pathogenic infection. Clinically, the expression of candidal infection may be divided into acute mucocutaneous forms, chronic mucocutaneous forms, and disseminated disease. In addition, cutaneous infection may result in **intertriginous candidiasis**, **paronychia, onychomycosis**, **diaper candidiasis**, and **candidal granuloma**. Cutaneous candidal infections generally produce erythema with moist exudates having irregular edges and satellite papules. Subcorneal pustules lead to superficial erosions and peeling.

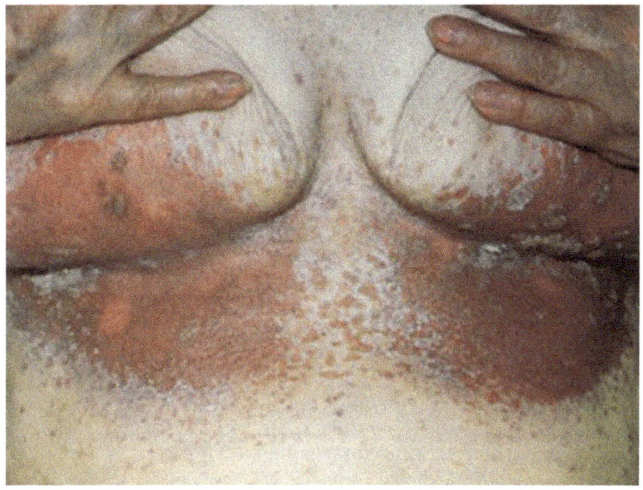

Candida intertrigo, with prominent satellite lesions at the margins. (Reproduced, with permission, from Wolff K, Goldsmith LA, Katz SI, et al. *Fitzpatrick's Dermatology in General Medicine*. 7th ed. New York: McGraw-Hill; 2008.)

Acute mucocutaneous candidiasis may present as **oral thrush**, which occurs most often in infants, elderly individuals, and patients with terminal or chronic illnesses (Table 7-14A). It is characterized by friable white plaques on the oral mucosa; unlike the plaques of **leukoplakia**, they can be scraped off easily, revealing an erythematous base. **Acute atrophic candidiasis** presents as a painful erythematous stomatitis. **Chronic atrophic candidiasis**, which is common among denture wearers, is characterized by asymptomatic erythema of the mucosa that bears the denture. Inhaled corticosteroids and HIV infection are also associated with chronic oral candidiasis. Other conditions involving the oral mucosa, such as **perlèche** (**angular cheilitis**), **leukoplakia,** HIV-associated **oral hairy leukoplakia**, and **median rhomboid glossitis**, may predispose the affected individual to mucosal invasion by *Candida* species.

Vulvovaginitis is characterized by pruritus; pain; and a thick, white exudate. **Balanitis**, more commonly seen in uncircumcised patients, produces white pustules or vesicles on the glans penis. Other acute mucocutaneous forms include infections of the GI tract, including esophagitis, gastritis, and peritonitis.

Chronic mucocutaneous candidiasis is a disorder of chronic, recurrent *Candida* infections of the skin, mucous membranes, and nails in patients with underlying defects in

Table 7-14A. Mucocutaneous Candidiasis

Clinical Features
Various acute forms are more common in infants, elderly, pregnant, and diabetic patients
Chronic mucocutaneous candidiasis
Often associated with cell-mediated immune deficiency
May involve genetic transmission
Candidal granuloma (rare)
Chronic atrophic candidiasis in denture wearers
Erythema with irregular margins, moist exudates, and satellite papules
Oral friable white plaques that can be scraped off easily
Histopathologic Features
Spores (3-6 μm), pseudohyphae, and hyphae seen in stratum corneum
Subcorneal pustules and vesicles
Candidal granuloma
Prominent hyperkeratosis and papillomatosis
Dense dermal infiltrate with giant cells
Differential Diagnosis
Dermatophyte infection
Impetigo
Subcorneal pustular dermatitis
Pustular psoriasis

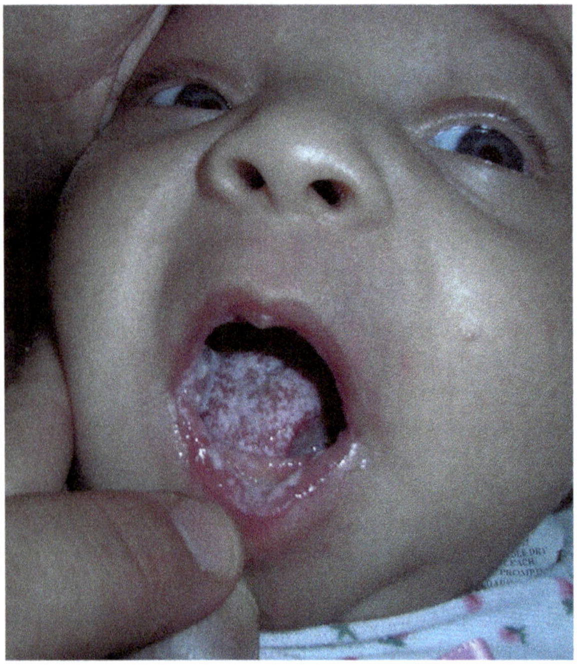

Thrush in an otherwise healthy infant. (Reproduced, with permission, from Usatine RP, Smith MA, Mayeaux EJ Jr, Chumley HS, eds. *Color Atlas of Family Medicine*. 2nd ed. New York, NY: McGraw-Hill Education; 2012. Used with permission of Richard P. Usatine, MD.)

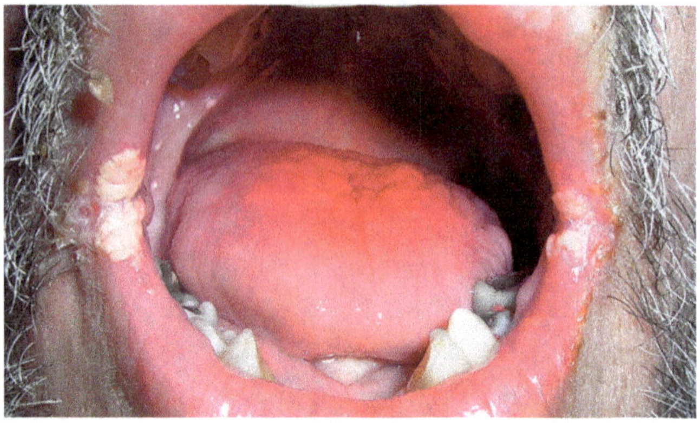

Severe angular cheilitis in HIV-positive man complicated by oral thrush. (Reproduced, with permission, from Usatine RP, Smith MA, Mayeaux EJ Jr, Chumley HS, eds. Color Atlas of Family Medicine. New York, NY: McGraw-Hill Education; 2009. Used with permission of Richard P. Usatine, MD.)

cell-mediated immunity. Lethal immune deficiencies involving dysgenesis of the thymus (**Nezelof syndrome, DiGeorge syndrome**, and the **Swiss type of agammaglobulinemia**) may present in childhood with mild candidiasis often limited to the oral cavity; death usually occurs before age 2 years from other infections. Nonlethal immune deficiencies also present early in life and include endocrinopathy, which is associated with candidiasis of the oral cavity, skin, and nails and appears to be genetically transmitted, and a rare variant called **candidal granuloma**, which presents with multiple hyperkeratotic, crusted plaques. Late-onset chronic mucocutaneous candidiasis is associated with thymoma and may accompany myasthenia gravis. AIDS is often associated with chronic mucocutaneous candidiasis and frequently involves the oral cavity and esophagus.

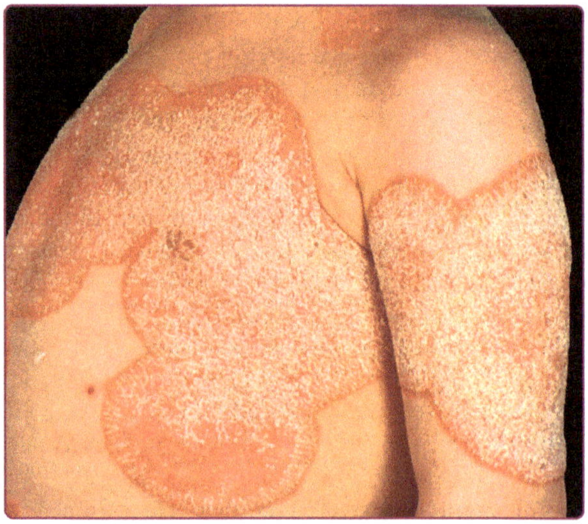

Chronic mucocutaneous candidiasis. Well-demarcated serpiginous lesions with massive scaling. Lesions look like psoriasis. (Reproduced, with permission, from Goldsmith LA, Katz SI, Gilchrest BA, Paller AS, Leffell DJ, Wolff K, eds. *Fitzpatrick's Dermatology in General Medicine*. 8th ed. New York, NY: McGraw-Hill Education; 2012.)

Disseminated candidiasis is associated with cutaneous manifestations in 10% to 13% of patients (Table 7-14B). These manifestations are highly variable, ranging from very few to numerous erythematous macules, papules, and nodules that may be associated with purpura, necrotic eschars, subcutaneous abscesses, ecthyma gangrenosum–like ulcers, and nodular folliculitis in heroin users. **Systemic candidiasis** with skin manifestations was caused by *C tropicalis* in 64% of patients. The triad of high fever, papular erythematous rash, and diffuse severe myalgias in neutropenic patients suggests disseminated disease.

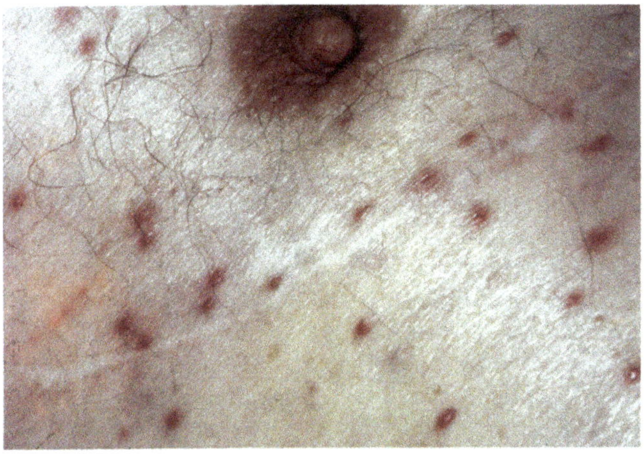

Widespread nodular skin lesions in a patient with disseminated candidiasis. (Reproduced, with permission, from Kantarjian HM, Wolff RA, Koller CA. *The MD Anderson Manual of Medical Oncology*. 2nd ed. New York, NY: McGraw-Hill Education; 2011.)

Table 7-14B. Disseminated Candidiasis

Clinical Features
Cutaneous findings in 10% to 13% of patients
Variable skin manifestations
C tropicalis in 64% of cases with skin manifestations
Triad of fever, papular erythematous rash, and diffuse severe myalgias in neutropenic patients is highly suggestive
Histopathologic Features
Pseudohyphae, hyphae, and spores (3-6 μm) in dermis often near blood vessels
Spores may show budding
Perivascular inflammatory infiltrate
Leukocytoclastic vasculitis
Differential Diagnosis
Aspergillus fumigatus
Histoplasma capsulatum
May be confused with *C glabrata*, which forms spores only

Systemic candidiasis is the most common invasive fungal infection in patients with cancer, burns, and AIDS or those undergoing organ transplantation. **Candidemia**, the most common clinical manifestation, occurs in 50% to 70% of patients with invasive **candidiasis**, and carries a mortality rate of about 40%, down from 80% in the 1970s; this decrease is attributed to early empirical antifungal and improved prophylactic treatment. Approximately 9% of hospital-acquired nosocomial bloodstream infections (BSIs) in the United States have been attributed to *Candida* species, making the genus the fourth leading cause of nosocomial bloodstream infections (BSI). *C glabrata* is a rising cause of **candidiasis** in neutropenic patients, especially with underlying hematologic malignancies, despite receiving fluconazole prophylaxis. Although a less common cause of *Candida* bloodstream infection in the rest of the world, *C glabrata* now ranks second to *C albicans* in the United States, with 20% to 24% of *Candida* BSIs due to this recently emerged opportunistic pathogen. Compared with isolates of *C glabrata* from Europe, Latin America, and the Asia-Pacific area, those from North America demonstrated lower susceptibility to azole antifungal agents.

Microscopically, the vesicles and pustules of **mucocutaneous candidiasis** are characterized by a subcorneal collection of lymphocytes and necrotic debris, with hyphae, pseudohyphae, and yeast cells confined to the stratum corneum. **Pseudohyphae** are chains of cells formed by the repeated budding of blastoconidia; although they are separated by septa, mother and daughter cells remain physically attached. Although *C glabrata* occurs as yeasts only, other species show numerous hyphae measuring 2 to 4 μm in diameter and a few spores that may show budding and measure 3 to 6 μm in diameter. The organisms stain well with PAS, methenamine silver, Gridley, and Gram stains.

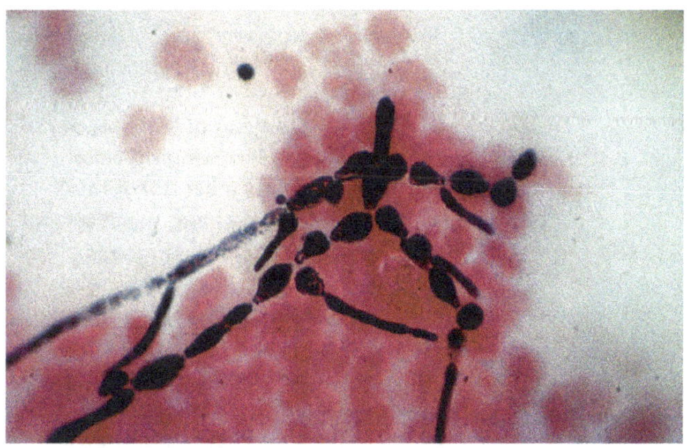

Gram stain of *Candida albicans*. Note the yeast cells and pseudohyphae. (Reproduced with permission from Nester EW, Anderson DG, Roberts CE Jr, Nester MT. *Microbiology: A Human Perspective*, 6th ed. New York: McGraw-Hill, 2008.)

In **candidal granuloma**, hyperkeratosis and papillomatosis are prominent, and parakeratosis and acanthosis may also be noted. A dense chronic inflammatory infiltrate with multinucleated giant cells may be found in the dermis and may extend into the subcutis. The histologic examination of

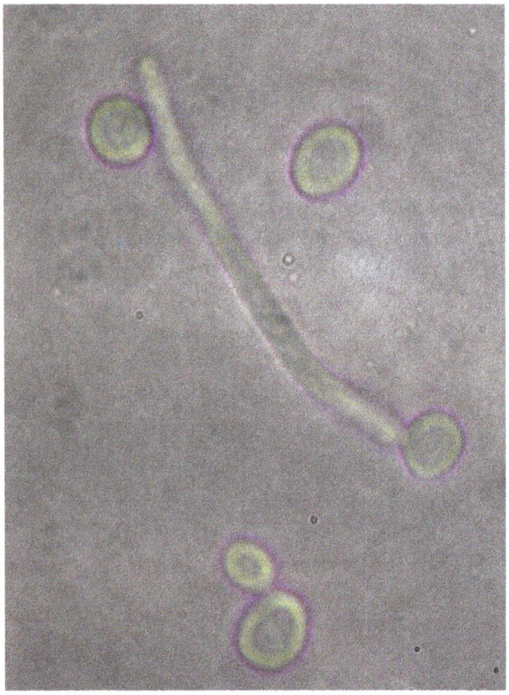

Candida germ tube, culture. Unlike other species of *Candida, Candida albicans* produces true hyphae as well as budding yeast cells and pseudohyphae in culture. After incubation in serum at 37°C for 60 to 90 minutes in the laboratory, clinical isolates of *Candida albicans* are stimulated to form hyphae, and this process is initiated by the production of germ tubes, which are thinner and more uniform than pseudohyphae (1000×). (Reproduced, with permission, from Carroll KC et al, eds. *Jawetz, Melnick & Adelberg's Medical Microbiology*. 26th ed. New York, NY: McGraw-Hill Education; 2013.)

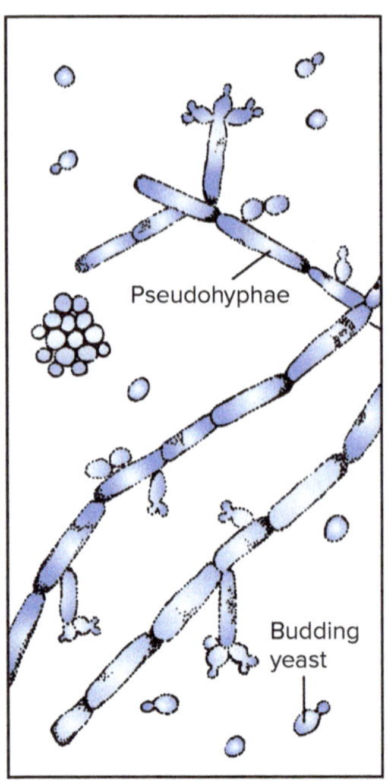

Drawing of KOH preparation showing mycelial forms (pseudohyphae) and budding yeast typical of *Candida albicans*. The pseudohyphae are elongated ellipsoids. The ellipsoid-shaped cells remain attached to one other at the constricted septations as they grow. Numerous foci of branching are a result. (Reproduced, with permission, from Nicoll D, Lu CM, Pignone M, McPhee SJ, eds. *Pocket Guide to Diagnostic Tests*. 6th ed. New York, NY: McGraw-Hill Education; 2012.)

disseminated candidiasis reveals *Candida* pseudohyphae and yeast cells within the dermis, often near or within blood vessels. Perivascular tissues and blood vessel walls may show edema. The epidermis is intact, and small foci of hemorrhage and fibrin exudate may be seen in the middle and lower dermis. The tissue response varies from a perivascular chronic inflammatory infiltrate to a **leukocytoclastic vasculitis** characterized by groups of neutrophils, nuclear debris, and necrosis in and around blood vessels.

In regard to the clinical differential diagnosis, **oral candidiasis** resembles or may coexist with **leukoplakia, squamous cell carcinoma**, or **herpes simplex**. Esophageal infection may mimic **cytomegalovirus, herpes simplex**, or **peptic ulcer esophagitis**. The histopathological differential diagnosis for a subcorneal pustule secondary to *Candida* infection includes **dermatophytic infection, impetigo, subcorneal pustular dermatitis,** and **pustular psoriasis**. **Candidiasis** may be differentiated from **dermatophyte** infection by the presence of spores and pseudohyphae. The best diagnostic test is the demonstration of pseudohyphal invasion on microscopic examination of mucocutaneous lesions. A positive culture may lend support but is not by itself diagnostic, since *Candida* is a part of normal mucocutaneous flora. The necrotic pustules and ulcerative plaques of **ecthyma gangrenosum,** characteristic of *Pseudomonas* septicemia, resemble the cutaneous findings of **disseminated candidiasis**. Although skin manifestations are relatively uncommon in **disseminated candidiasis**, biopsy of skin lesions is important because blood cultures are positive in only 25% of cases. When blastospores are not seen, *Candida* pseudohyphae may be confused with *Aspergillus* hyphae; however, the latter are gram negative. *C glabrata*, which does not form pseudohyphae, may resemble *Histoplasma capsulatum*, although the latter usually elicits a granulomatous rather than a pyogenic response. **Erythrasma** is caused by *Corynebacterium minutissimum*, which is a small gram-positive coccobacillus.

ANSWER 7-15: D.

The scraping illustrates the "spaghetti and meatballs" hyphae and spores characteristic of the genus ***Malassezia***. ***Malassezia*** are dimorphic, lipophilic yeasts that for reasons that remain unclear, transform from the saprophytic state in healthy skin to a pathogenic mycelial state. This genus, of the phylum *Basidiomycota*, was previously known in the literature as ***Pityrosporum***, with *P ovale* and *P orbiculare* identified on the basis of microscopic morphology as the pathogenic species. When the genus was initially divided on the basis of lipophilicity (requires lipid such as olive oil to grow), *M furfur* emerged as the predominant pathogenic species. A taxonomic revision with classification of the genus into seven species was carried out in 1996, when *M globosa*, *M obtusa*, *M slooffiae*, and *M restricta* were added to the genus, which had contained only three species: *M furfur*, *M pachydermatis* (the only nonlipid-dependent species), and *M sympodialis*.

Of the identified species, *M globosa*, *M sympodialis*, and *M furfur* probably cause most cases of **tinea versicolor**; *M globosa* is the predominant species associated with the condition in temperate climates. *M slooffiae*, *M restricta*, and *M obtusa* have also been implicated.

The patients illustrated in answer choices A and B have **tinea versicolor**, which is one of the most common pigmentary disorders in the world (Table 7-15A). It has an increased prevalence (up to 40%) in tropical areas owing to high temperature and humidity. In temperate zones, the incidence is higher during the warmer months of the year. The infection does not appear to be contagious and occurs under conditions permitting overgrowth of the fungus such as warm weather and continual perspiration. The typical presentation of **tinea versicolor** is scaly oval to round macules scattered over characteristic areas of the body, including the upper trunk, neck, and upper arms. The macules enlarge and may become either hypo- or hyperpigmented depending on natural skin color and sun exposure. The color of patches varies from almost white to pink to reddish brown or fawn colored. **Depigmentation** has been attributed to the production by the yeasts of dicarboxylic acids, such as azelaic acid, that competitively inhibits tyrosinase and may have a directly toxic effect on melanocytes. **Hyperpigmentation** appears to be related to an increase in melanosome size. Although most cases are asymptomatic, the major complaint is cosmetic because the fungus causes uneven tanning by filtering out ultraviolet radiation. The scale is characteristically described as dust-like or furfuraceous. Extensive scaling can be produced by lightly scraping a #15 scalpel blade over the involved skin. Patches may have a wrinkled surface appearance and this feature serves as a useful clinical pearl for the diagnosis.

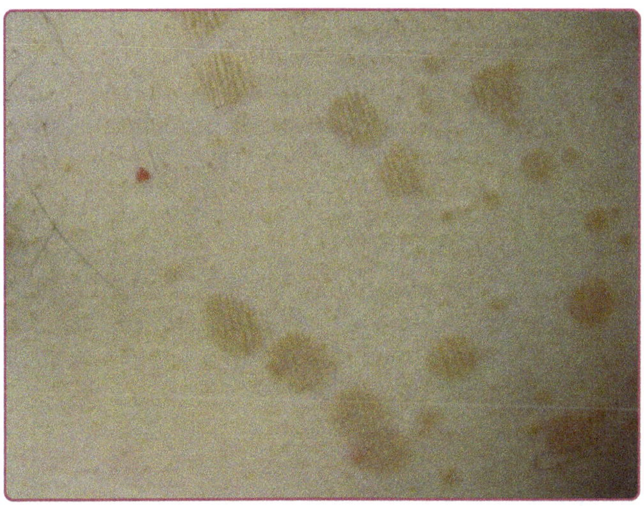

Pityriasis (tinea) versicolor. Macules and patches may have a wrinkled surface appearance. (Reproduced with permission from Goldsmith LA, Katz SI, Gilchrest BA, Paller AS, Leffell DJ, Wolff K, eds. *Fitzpatrick's Dermatology in General Medicine*. 8th ed. New York, NY: McGraw-Hill Education; 2012.)

Table 7-15A. Tinea Versicolor

Clinical Features
Caused by *Malassezia furfur* or *M ovalis*
Occurs in tropics and warm months of temperate zones
Age of onset usually in early twenties in temperate zones
Pale to brown, slightly scaling macules over the upper trunk
Histopathologic Features
Hyperkeratosis and slight acanthosis
Superficial dermal lymphohistiocytic infiltrate
Hyphae and spores seen in stratum corneum
Differential Diagnosis
Tinea corporis
Candidiasis
Spongiotic dermatitis

The presenting concern often relates to the cosmetic appearance of the eruption rather than any symptoms, since pruritus is usually mild or absent. The diagnosis made on clinical grounds is supported by Wood light (365 nm) examination which may show yellow-orange fluorescence thought to be due to the presence of **pteridine** and is confirmed by microscopic KOH examination of the scale. Tinea versicolor tends to recur in warmer months of the year.

Microscopically, the H&E findings of **tinea versicolor** are nonspecific and most commonly demonstrate hyperkeratosis, slight acanthosis, spotty pigmentation of the epidermal basal layer, and a superficial perivascular lymphohistiocytic infiltrate. PAS stain reveals numerous short, multibranching hyphae and spores (so-called "spaghetti and meatballs") within the stratum corneum. *Malassezia* species exhibit monopolar budding.

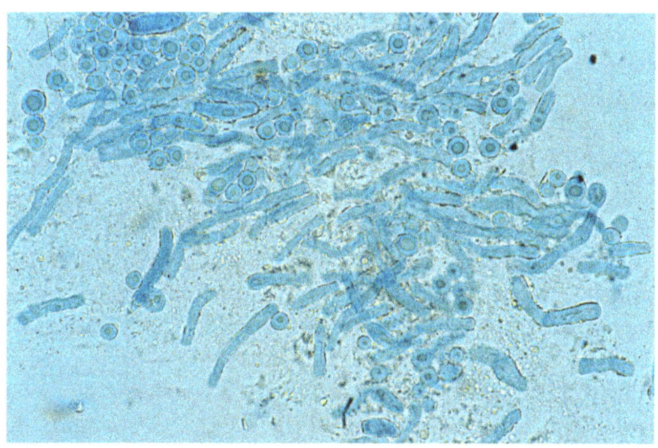

Malassezia. Potassium hydroxide preparation with pseudohyphae, showing "spaghetti and meatballs" pattern. (Reproduced with permission from Goldsmith LA, Katz SI, Gilchrest BA, Paller AS, Leffell DJ, Wolff K, eds. *Fitzpatrick's Dermatology in General Medicine*. 8th ed. New York, NY: McGraw-Hill Education; 2012.)

Table 7-15B. Malassezia (Pityrosporum) Folliculitis

Clinical Features
Caused by *Malassezia furfur* or *M ovalis*
Occurs in young to middle-aged adults
Pruritic papules on the trunk, shoulders, and occasionally the face
Occlusion and greasy skin may predispose to infection
Histopathologic Features
Numerous spores within dilated, plugged hair follicles
Neutrophils, lymphocytes, and histiocytes within follicles and in perifollicular regions
Foreign body reaction near ruptured follicles
Pools of mucin may be seen within follicles
Differential Diagnosis
Acneiform drug eruption
Dermatophytic or bacterial folliculitis
Follicular mucinosis
Acne vulgaris

The patient in answer choice C has ***Malassezia* folliculitis**, previously referred to as ***Pityrosporum* folliculitis** (Table 7-15B). The exact pathogenesis of this disease remains controversial. The initiating event may be follicular occlusion followed by overgrowth of the organism rather than direct invasion of the follicle. Predisposing factors appear to include occlusion and greasy skin. The condition has been associated with tetracycline antibiotics, corticosteroids, and immunosuppression in organ transplant patients. ***Malassezia* folliculitis** is a benign condition characterized by follicular papules and pustules occurring predominantly on the back and chest; it is more common in tropical climates and summer in temperate climates. The typical patient is a young to middle-aged adult with pruritic papules on the trunk, shoulders, and occasionally the face. Pustules, cysts, and "molluscoid" papules, which have a central depression similar to the papules of molluscum contagiosum, may also be seen.

Microscopically, most cases of ***Malassezia* folliculitis** show numerous spores inside the hair follicles that appear widely dilated and are plugged with keratinous material. Features of **secondary perforating folliculitis** may be present. Occasional hyphae have been noted within distended follicles. A perifollicular inflammatory cell infiltrate consisting of neutrophils, lymphocytes, and histiocytes is present in the intrafollicular and perifollicular regions, and pools of mucin, which may be confirmed by a colloidal iron stain, may be seen both within and around the follicles. A foreign body type of granulomatous reaction near a ruptured follicular wall has been reported. The **Splendore-Hoeppli phenomenon**, which is characterized by a homogeneous, partially laminated core containing *Malassezia* spores surrounded by a thin layer of darkly stained filaments, may occasionally be seen within the follicle.

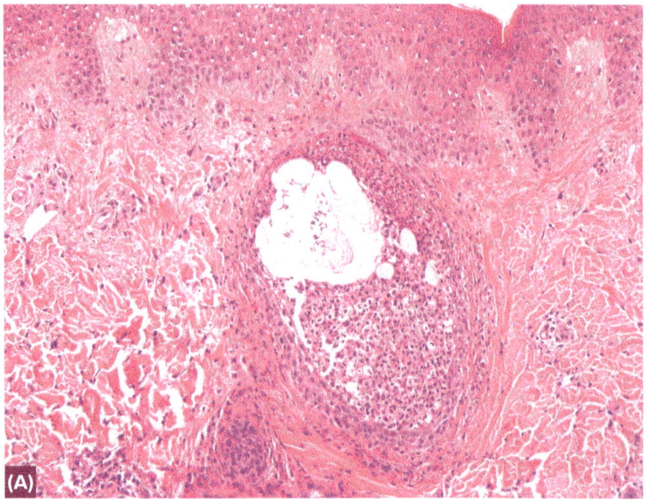

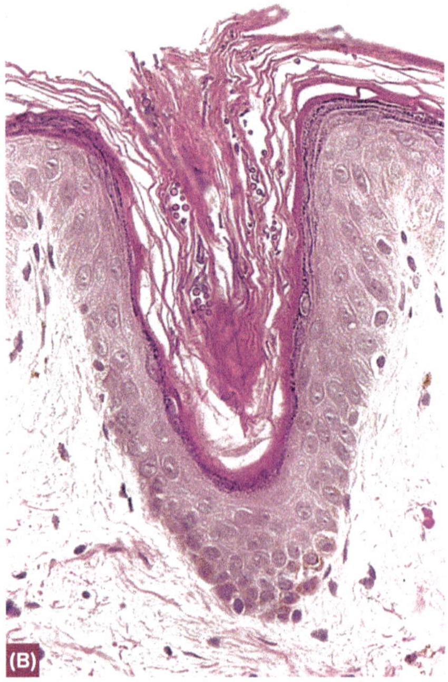

Malassezia (Pityrosporum) folliculitis. (A) The follicle is dilated and infiltrated by neutrophils, resulting in follicular pustule formation. There are Pityrosporum yeast forms present within the hair follicle. **(B)** Hyphae and spores in follicular orifice.

The patient illustrated in answer choice D has ***Candida* intertrigo**. The border is not well demarcated and there are satellite lesions. The hyperpigmentation is most likely attributed to post-inflammatory pigmentary alteration.

ANSWER 7-16: D.

The genus *Cryptococcus* includes two species of yeasts, which are known to be pathogenic in humans: *C neoformans* and *C gattii*. *C neoformans* is an important opportunistic infection worldwide in persons infected with HIV, and a recent outbreak of **cryptococcosis** in apparently immunocompetent persons on Vancouver Island, Canada, was attributed to *C gattii.* Attributed to widespread use of highly active antiretroviral therapy (HAART), the incidence of **cryptococcosis** declined in the United States during the 1990s, both in the general population in persons living with AIDS. Almost 90% of cases occurred in HIV-infected persons. **Cryptococcosis** is caused by *Cryptococcus* species, a saprophyte found worldwide in soil enriched by bird droppings (Table 7-16A). Humans are infected via environmental exposures. *Cryptococcus* is unencapsulated in nature; its smallest forms measure less than 2 μm, and thus it lodges in alveolar spaces after inhalation. Encapsulation occurs in the lung and is associated with increased virulence because phagocytosis is impaired by concealment by opsonizing antibodies. Adults with lymphoma, carcinoma, sarcoidosis, collagen vascular disease, AIDS or those who are on immunosuppressive therapy may show increased susceptibility to *Cryptococcus* infection.

Primary cutaneous cryptococcosis is a rare event that occurs after direct inoculation. Pulmonary infection often is transient or asymptomatic, and in most instances, **cryptococcosis** presents as **disseminated cryptococcosis** or **central nervous system cryptococcosis** (eg, as a chronic meningitis or a focal brain lesion resembling a tumor). The phenotypic switching in vivo that results in an altered capsular polysaccharide may inhibit phagocytosis by alveolar macrophages and is associated with an enhanced inflammatory response and greater lethality. Cutaneous lesions may appear as erythematous nodular firm, cystic-appearing excrescences; acneiform papules or pustules; crusted or infiltrating plaques; or cellulitis. Any of these lesions may ulcerate. In individuals with AIDS, numerous nodules resembling giant **molluscum contagiosum** are common. Serum latex agglutination is valuable in the diagnosis of active disease.

Microscopically, in the past, two distinct histopathologic patterns were described; a granulomatous pattern consisting of a dense mixed infiltrate with few organisms and a gelatinous pattern consisting of little inflammation and large numbers of spores. However, they may both be present and are not of recognizable clinical significance. The characteristic feature includes aggregates of encapsulated yeasts, often but not always with a granulomatous response and sometimes with necrosis. The yeast cells range from 2 to 15 μm in diameter and show narrow-based, unequal budding. The yeast cytoplasm stains with PAS or methenamine silver and the capsule with Alcian blue or mucicarmine. A combination of PAS and Alcian blue stains highlights the yeast cytoplasm in red and the capsule in blue. *C neoformans* stains black with the Fontana-Masson stain, a valuable feature in patients with AIDS who are infected with strains

Table 7-16A. Cryptococcosis

Clinical Features
- Caused by *Cryptococcus neoformans* var *neoformans in* >80% of cases
- *C neoformans* is found in soil contaminated with bird and bat excreta
- Usually inhaled, can disseminate to brain, meninges, and cerebrospinal fluid
- Skin involvement variable—papules, pustules, nodules, plaques, cellulitis
- Most common systemic fungal infection in AIDS patients
- Serum latex agglutination valuable in diagnosis of active disease

Histopathologic Features
- Large aggregates of encapsulated, budding, refractile yeast, 5-15 μm in diameter
- Variable granulomatous infiltrate of lymphocytes, histiocytes, multinucleated giant cells and neutrophils
- If infiltrate is dense, few organisms are seen; those present are smaller and may lie within macrophages
- Yeast stains with PAS, methenamine silver and Fontana-Masson
- Capsule stains with Alcian blue and mucicarmine

Differential Diagnosis
- Blastomycosis
- Histoplasmosis
- Lobomycosis

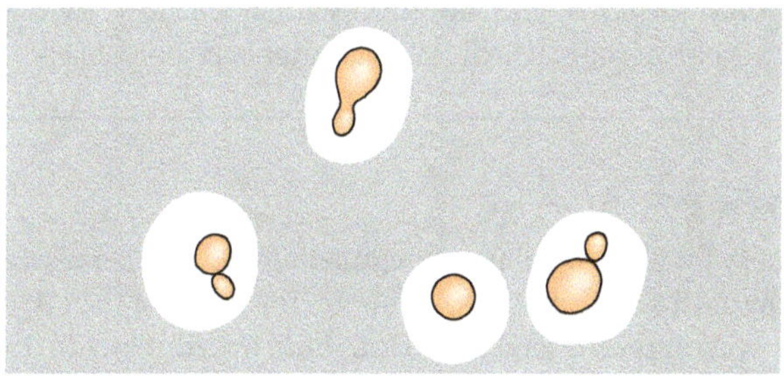

Drawing of *Cryptococcus neoformans*. India ink preparation shows budding yeasts with a wide capsule. India ink forms a dark background; it does not stain the yeast itself. (Reproduced with permission from Brooks GF et al: *Jawetz, Melnick & Adelberg's Medical Microbiology*. 19th ed. New York, NY: Appleton & Lange; 1991.)

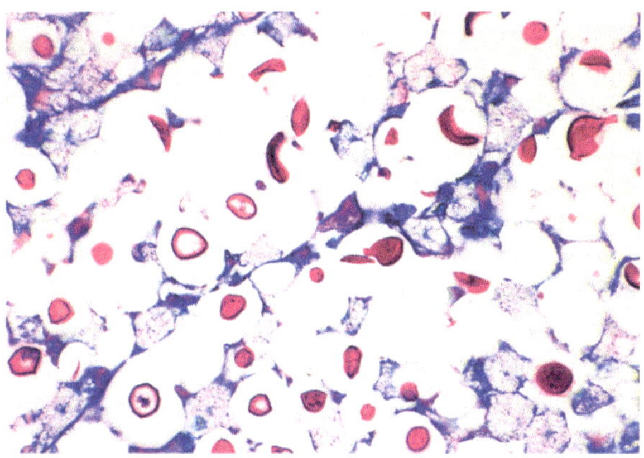

Cryptococcal meningitis. The *C neoformans* cells are stained red by this PAS (periodic acid-Schiff) stain. The capsule is not stained but is creating the halo around the organisms. Note the lack of inflammatory cells. (Reproduced, with permission, from Connor DH, Chandler FW, Schwartz DQA, Manz HJ, Lack EE (eds). *Pathology of Infectious Diseases*. Vol 1. Stamford, CT: Appleton & Lange; 1997.)

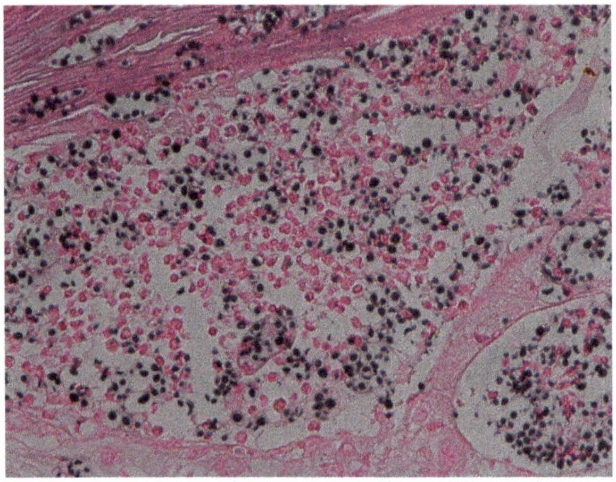

Crytococcus with Fontana-Masson stain. Note the black staining, consistent with melanin pigment.

of low virulence and relatively little capsular material. Variable acanthosis or ulceration of the overlying skin may be present.

The differential diagnosis among *C neoformans*, **histoplasmosis**, **blastomycosis**, and **lobomycosis** may be aided by the Fontana-Masson stain, which stains **cryptococci** alone black.

ANSWER 7-17: E.

The biopsy findings reveal **pseudoepitheliomatous hyperplasia** overlying a dense inflammatory infiltrate. The image of the PAS-stained section reveals large, spherical thick-walled yeasts (8-15 μm in diameter) admixed with neutrophilic and granulomatous infiltrates. The yeasts exhibit uniform "broad-based" budding. In contrast to fungal infections that preferentially develop in immunosuppressed individuals, **blastomycosis** (as well as **coccidioidomycosis, paracoccidioidomycosis,** and **histoplasmosis**) is endemic and can infect healthy individuals. First described in 1894 by Gilchrist, **blastomycosis** is caused by *Blastomyces dermatitidis*, a dimorphic fungus. Although called **North American blastomycosis** because the original cases clustered around states crossed by the Mississippi and Ohio Rivers, it has also been reported in South America, Europe, and Africa (Table 7-17A). *B dermatitidis* is found in the acidic soil of wooded areas. The typical patient is a man between 25 and 50 years of age with occupational or recreational exposure to the outdoors. **Blastomycosis** also occurs in dogs.

Primary cutaneous blastomycosis is a rare disorder that has been described after accidental inoculation in the laboratory or during an autopsy. An ulcerated verrucous plaque arises at the inoculation site followed by lymphangitis and nodules spreading in a **"sporotrichoid" lymphocutaneous distribution.** Spontaneous healing occurs in the ensuing months. The more common clinical forms of **blastomycosis** are the primary pulmonary, chronic cutaneous, and disseminated forms. Infection with *B dermatitidis* begins with inhalation of conidia. If not cleared by bronchopulmonary macrophages,

Table 7-17A. North American Blastomycosis

Clinical Features
Caused by *Blastomyces dermatitidis*
Dimorphic fungus, found in acid soil of wooded areas
Endemic in South Central and Southeastern United States
More common in men with a history of outdoor exposure
Age 25-50 years
Cutaneous involvement in 70% of patients with disseminated disease
Verrucous plaques with peripheral pustules—face, mucosa
Occasional ulcers
Erythema nodosum associated with pulmonary blastomycosis
Usually inhaled, may disseminate to bones and CNS
Histopathologic Features
Pseudoepitheliomatous hyperplasia
Intraepidermal and dermal neutrophilic microabscesses
Suppurative granulomatous infiltrate with giant cells
Spores are thick walled and 5-15 μm in diameter
Present extracellularly, within giant cells, epidermal and dermal abscesses, and granulomas
Buds are single and broad based
Differential Diagnosis
Coccidioidomycosis
Tuberculosis
Paracoccidioidomycosis
Chromoblastomycosis
Pyoderma gangrenosum
Halogenoderma

these conidia transform into yeast forms and multiply in the lung parenchyma, although **pulmonary blastomycosis** may heal spontaneously. Subsequent hematogenous dissemination may occur (**disseminated blastomycosis**). The clinical spectrum of **pulmonary blastomycosis** thus ranges from no symptoms whatsoever in up to 50% of those who have inhaled *Blastomyces* conidia or spores to an acute or chronic pneumonia. **Erythema nodosum** may occur during the resolving phase of the acute pneumonia. Patients with acute pneumonia may appear to recover but then return months later with disseminated infection. **Chronic pulmonary blastomycosis** is often associated with weight loss, fever, night sweats, chest pain, and hemoptysis. Chest radiographs are nondiagnostic and may reveal masses in 32% and alveolar infiltrates in 48% of patients as well as cavitation, pleural fibrosis, and hilar lymphadenopathy simulating **tuberculosis**. **Cutaneous blastomycosis** occurs from hematogenous spread in 70% of patients with **disseminated blastomycosis.** These patients develop verrucous plaques with peripheral pustules and occasional ulcerations on the face, mucous membranes, and arms. If **cutaneous blastomycosis** is present and there is no pulmonary disease, the latter is thought to have resolved spontaneously. Osteomyelitis occurs in 25% of patients with disseminated disease, most commonly affecting the spine, pelvis, skull, ribs, and long bones. Granulomas, suppuration, or necrosis can be contiguous between bone and adjacent soft tissues, leading to subcutaneous abscesses. CNS infections occur in fewer than 10% of patients and may be associated with meningitis and brain abscess formation. Infection may also involve the genitourinary tract.

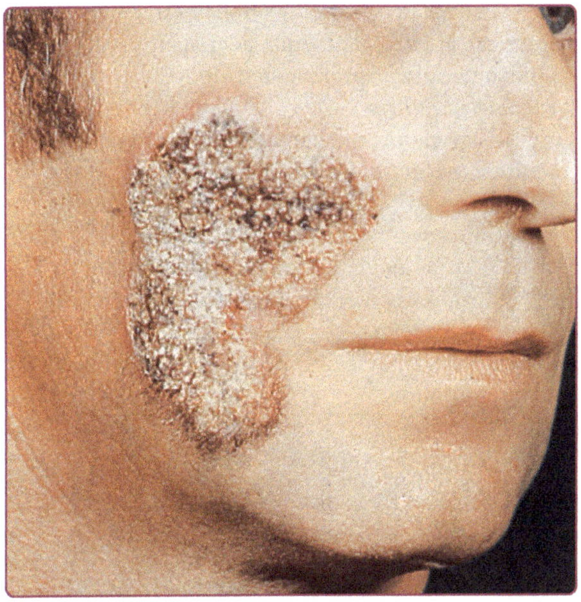

Blastomycosis. Chronic verrucous plaque on the cheek. (Reproduced, with permission, from Goldsmith LA, Katz SI, Gilchrest BA, Paller AS, Leffell DJ, Wolff K, eds. *Fitzpatrick's Dermatology in General Medicine*. 8th ed. New York, NY: McGraw-Hill Education; 2012.)

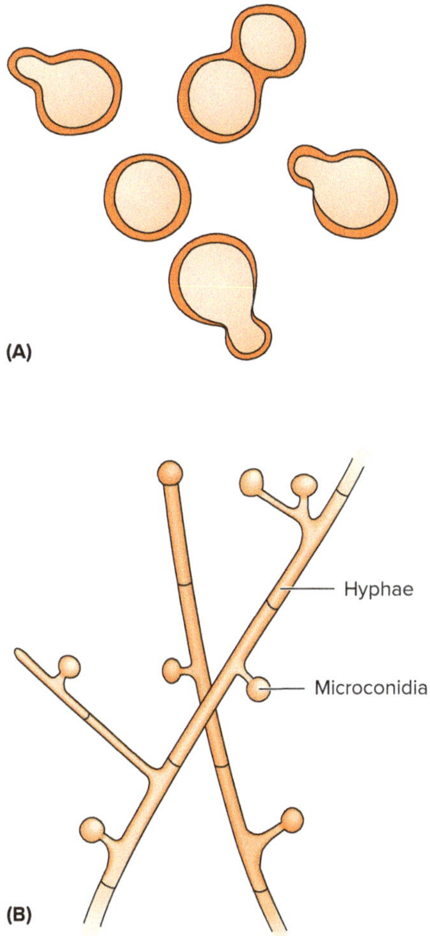

***Blastomyces dermatitidis*. (A)** Yeast with a broad-based bud at 37°C. **(B)** Mold with microconidia at 20°C. (Reproduced with permission from Brooks GF et al: *Jawetz, Melnick & Adelberg's Medical Microbiology*. 19th ed. New York, NY: Appleton & Lange; 1991.)

Serologic tests are of limited value at present because of a high rate of false-positive and false-negative results. Although a positive immunodiffusion test result is diagnostic, this test has false-negative results in 10% of patients with disseminated infection and 60% of patients with localized infection. A urinary antigen enzyme immunoassay with 92.9% sensitivity and 79.3% specificity has been developed, but there is significant cross-reactivity with histoplasmosis antigen. Diagnosis is made by histologic examination and fungal culture.

Biopsy of the active border of a plaque or of an ulcer reveals **pseudoepitheliomatous hyperplasia**. Intraepidermal and dermal neutrophilic abscesses also are seen. The dermis contains a granulomatous infiltrate consisting of lymphocytes, histiocytes, plasma cells, neutrophils, and multinucleated giant cells. *B dermatitidis* spores are seen free in the tissue or within giant cells within the foci of suppurative granulomatous inflammation and **pseudoepitheliomatous hyperplasia**. *B dermatitidis* spores measure 5 to 15 μm and have a thick wall consisting of the exterior and interior cell surfaces. An occasional single, broad-based,

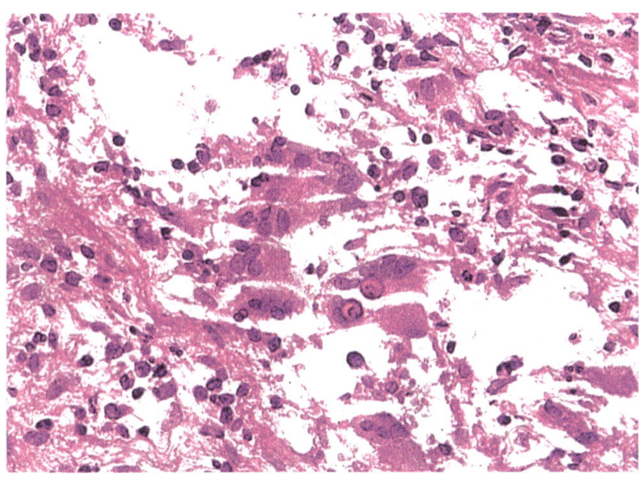

***Blastomyces dermatitidis*, PAS stain.** There are numerous large spherical yeasts present within multinucleated giant cells.

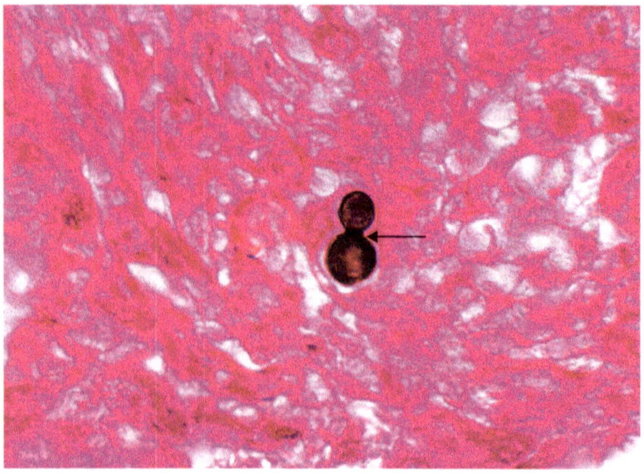

Blastomyces dermatitidis (PAS stain) broad-based budding yeast. Arrow points to the broad base of the budding yeast. (Used with permission of Dr L. Ajello, Public Health Image Library, Centers for Disease Control and Prevention.)

equal-sized bud is characteristic. Spores can be identified as an empty round space within the cytoplasm of giant cells using H&E stain; however, their visualization is enhanced with PAS or methenamine silver stains.

In regard to the differential diagnosis, **blastomycosis** may be distinguished from **coccidioidomycosis** by the greater number of intraepidermal microabscesses and the much smaller size of the spores (5-15 µm) compared with the large sporangia of *Coccidioides* species. Both conditions are associated with **pseudoepitheliomatous hyperplasia**. The etiologic agent of **paracoccidioidomycosis** has multiple buds with a narrow base as opposed to the broad-based buds of *B dermatitidis*. Whereas the **dematiaceous fungi** of **chromoblastomycosis** appear dark brown on H&E-stained sections, *B dermatitidis* lacks melanin pigment. This negative staining for melanin on Fontana-Masson is helpful in distinguishing blastomycosis from cryptococcus, which is positive. **Pyoderma gangrenosum** by definition lacks an infectious etiology.

ANSWER 7-18: D.

Paracoccidioidomycosis is endemic in the humid mountain forests of South and Central America, and it has also been reported in individuals who have previously spent time in these regions (Table 7-18A). It is the most common **systemic mycosis** in Latin America, with 10 million individuals, or about 10% of the endemic area's population, presently infected. Brazil accounts for 80% of reported cases, with the highest incidence in the tropical and subtropical forested areas of the southeast; Columbia and Venezuela have the next highest incidence. Infection occurs after inhalation of the mycelia or conidia of the dimorphic fungus, *Paracoccidioides brasiliensis*, the causative agent. The precise ecologic niche remains unknown. The organism has been isolated rarely from soil, which has generated debate about soil as the permanent habitat.

Table 7-18A. Paracoccidioidomycosis

Clinical Features
- Caused by *Paracoccidioides brasiliensis*
- Dimorphic soil fungus of subtropical South and Central America
- Infection occurs predominantly in men
- Pulmonary infection characterized by fever and weight loss
- Mucocutaneous involvement in 60% of cases
    - Ulcers of lip, tongue, palate
    - Verrucous plaques, usually on the head and neck
    - Cervical and submandibular adenopathy
    - Difficulty eating, speaking, breathing

Histopathologic Features
- Ulceration, pseudoepitheliomatous hyperplasia
- Granulomatous infiltrate
    - Lymphocytes, histiocytes, neutrophils, giant cells
    - Occasional necrosis, abscess formation
- Yeast seen intra- and extracellularly, and in giant cells
- Thick-walled, refractile, variably sized yeast measure 4-40 µm in diameter
- Yeast occur singly, in chains, or as a "captain's wheel" with multiple buds

Differential Diagnosis
- North American blastomycosis
- Lobomycosis
- Histoplasmosis
- Leishmaniasis

Clinically, **paracoccidioidomycosis** typically begins with primary pulmonary infection followed by dissemination to other organs with the development of ulcerative granulomas of the oral and nasal mucous membranes and sometimes other tissues, including the skin, lymph nodes, and adrenal glands. The infection may remain subclinical, with only a positive skin test reaction, or may progress to overt disease, usually with a long latency period. More than 90% of **paracoccidioidomycosis** cases occur in adults, with clinical disease rates highest in the 30- to 60-year-old age group. Although there are no gender differences in the rates of subclinical infections, as determined by positive paracoccidioidin skin test result, or in childhood disease, there is a striking male predominance of 13:1 in endemic areas and up to 150:1 in Columbia, Ecuador, and Argentina. The observed male predominance is thought to be most likely owing to inhibition by estrogens of conidium- and mycelium-to-yeast transformation. **Pulmonary**

paracoccidioidomycosis is characterized by cough, fever, night sweats, and anorexia. In some cases, it resolves without dissemination; however, it may become latent, with possible reactivation years later. Bilateral infiltrates, fibrosis, and cavitation may be seen on chest radiographs. Mucosal and skin involvement is common in progressive disease, occurring in 60% of patients. Progressive painful ulcers develop on the gingivae, tongue, lips, and palate and may lead to perforation of the palate or nasal septum. Cutaneous manifestations of **paracoccidioidomycosis** usually involve the face but may be disseminated. Acneiform papules or nodules slowly develop into crusted plaques with well-defined, raised borders. Complications including difficulty speaking, swallowing, and breathing; scarring fibrosis; and draining sinus tracts may be seen in the late stages of the disease. Lymphadenopathy, most often in the cervical and submandibular nodes, may occur in patients with disseminated disease. Hematogenous spread may lead to multiple organ involvement, including adrenal gland destruction, osteomyelitis, and CNS involvement.

High titers (1:1024) of complement-fixing antibodies to paracoccidioidin imply active disease. However, cross-reactivity to *H capsulatum*, *B dermatitidis*, and other fungal pathogens may make interpretation difficult. Some patients experience impaired delayed hypersensitivity. Immunodiffusion test results are positive in approximately 80% of patients with disease, although cross-reactivity remains a problem with some. Other immunologic assays in addition to a nested PCR assay may serve as useful diagnostic adjuncts.

Microscopically, ulceration is observed commonly, both in mucosal lesions and at the center of the verrucous and crusted plaques. **Pseudoepitheliomatous hyperplasia**, as well as a variable dermal granulomatous infiltrate consisting of lymphocytes, histiocytes, neutrophils, and multinucleated giant cells, characterizes long-standing plaques. Necrosis and abscess formation may be seen. T-cell subsets may play a role in immunoregulation because most cells in the granulomas are CD4+. *P brasiliensis* yeasts are seen readily in H&E-, methenamine silver–, or PAS-stained sections and may be seen intra- or extracellularly or within giant cells. *P brasiliensis* are thick-walled, refractile yeasts of variable size, 4 to 30 μm in diameter. They may be observed singly, in chains, or budding in the distinctive "captain's wheel" pattern with multiple, small, narrow-based buds surrounding a central large yeast.

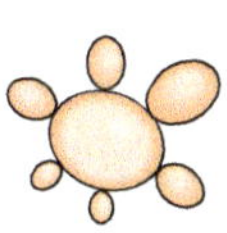

Paracoccidioides brasiliensis. Note the multiple buds of the yeast form of *Paracoccidioides*, in contrast to the single bud of *Blastomyces*. (Reproduced, with permission, from Levinson W, ed. *Review of Medical Microbiology and Immunology*. 13th ed. New York, NY: McGraw-Hill Education; 2012.)

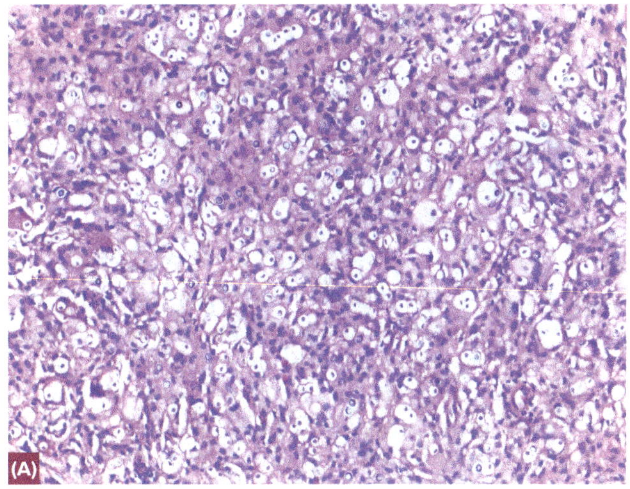

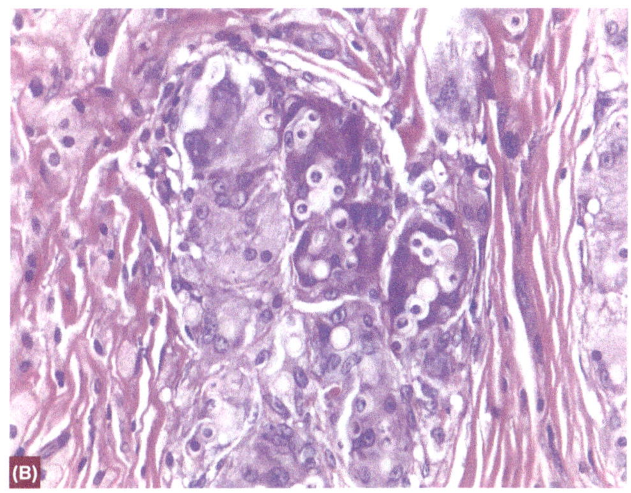

Lobomycosis. (A) Numerous intracellular yeasts arranged singly or in chains within macrophage vacuoles. Note the brown color of the yeasts, consistent with melanin. **(B)** Robust granulomatous response with numerous yeasts within giant cells. The yeasts divide with narrow-based budding." Courtesy of Robledo Fonseca, MD, Universidade Federal de Roraima.

The differential diagnosis includes other forms of systemic mycoses such as **North American blastomycosis, lobomycosis, histoplasmosis,** and **coccidioidomycosis.** If the yeasts occur singly or in chains, it may be difficult to distinguish the etiologic agent of **paracoccidioidomycosis** from those of **North American blastomycosis, lobomycosis,** and **histoplasmosis**. A diligent search for the characteristic "captain's wheel" is helpful. The agent of **North American blastomycosis** has a single broad-based bud as opposed to the narrow budding pattern of *P brasiliensis* and *Lacazia loboi.* The yeasts of *H capsulatum* are smaller (2-4 μm) than those of

P brasiliensis. **Coccidioidomycosis** is caused by *Coccidioides* species in which large spherical spores contain numerous small spherical endospores.

ANSWER 7-19: D.

The biopsy reveals numerous large spherical sporangia containing small round endospores. The sporangia are larger than the adjacent small vessels. A mixed inflammatory infiltrate is present. **Coccidioidomycosis** is endemic in the arid and semiarid regions of the southwestern United States and northern Mexico, and it also occurs in parts of Central and South America (Table 7-19A). The disease is a significant opportunistic mycosis in patients with HIV and organ transplant recipients. *Coccidioides* species are found in the soil, and pulmonary disease is caused by inhalation of contaminated dust. On the basis of genomic analyses, the genus has been divided into two species: *C immitis* (strains from California) and *C posadasii* (strains from outside California); there is no apparent difference in clinical expression caused by the two species. Three types of **coccidioidomycosis** have been described: pulmonary, cutaneous inoculation, and systemic. **Primary pulmonary coccidioidomycosis**, which is by far the most common form, occurs in about 40% of individuals exposed to *C immitis* and manifests 10 to 14 days after exposure with fever, chest pain, headache, and cough. Chest radiographs may show cavitary pulmonary lesions that usually resolve spontaneously in 3 to 4 months. Simultaneously or in the weeks after pulmonary infection, **erythema nodosum** and **erythema multiforme** may occur.

Table 7-19A. Coccidioidomycosis

Clinical Features
Caused by *Coccidioides immitis*
Endemic in arid regions of southwestern United States, Mexico, and South America
Dimorphic soil fungus, inhaled with dust
Frequency of systemic disease: <0.5% of patients with pulmonary disease develop systemic disease
Incidence
Filipinos > African Americans > Mexicans > Whites
20% Cutaneous involvement with disseminated disease
Granulomatous plaques, pustules, and nodules
Erythema nodosum, erythema multiforme
Coccidioidin skin test converts weeks following exposure, remains positive for years
Histopathologic Features
Acanthosis, intraepidermal microabscesses
Granulomatous infiltrate
Lymphocytes, histiocytes, neutrophils, giant cells
Eosinophils
Variable abscess formation and necrosis
Sporangia are rare but large, ≤ 80 μm in diameter
Numerous 1-4 μm endospores in sporangia
Present in giant cells or extracellularly
Differential Diagnosis
North American blastomycosis
Tuberculosis verrucosa cutis
Halogenoderma
Pemphigus vegetans

Only 0.1% to 0.5% of patients with pulmonary disease go on to develop **systemic coccidioidomycosis**, which may involve the skin, CNS, and musculoskeletal system. Systemic disease is more common in Filipinos, African Americans, and Mexicans and affects men more often than women, with the exception of pregnant women. **Systemic coccidioidomycosis** is associated with skin changes in about 20% of patients. These include granulomatous plaques, pustules, and nodules. **Erythema nodosum** is the most characteristic reactive cutaneous manifestation of disseminated infection, and it tends to occur 1 to 3 weeks after onset of illness. **Erythema nodosum** may have a protective effect against dissemination of coccidioidomycosis in pregnant women. An immunosuppressed state or immunosuppressive therapy may activate a latent pulmonary infection and result in systemic disease. **Primary cutaneous coccidioidomycosis** is quite rare; lesions clinically resemble the verrucous plaques of **primary cutaneous tuberculosis** and are often associated with lymphangitis and lymphadenitis 2 to 3 weeks after accidental inoculation.

If a patient has traveled to an endemic area and **coccidioidomycosis** is suspected, chest radiography and a coccidioidin skin test should be performed. The coccidioidin skin test becomes reactive 2 to 6 weeks after infection and remains positive for years; however, a negative test result does not rule out disease in immunosuppressed patients. Peripheral eosinophilia and eosinophilia of cerebrospinal fluid, the lungs, and other tissues may be seen in disseminated infection, most likely owing to increased interleukin-5 production. The presence of complement-fixing antibodies correlates strongly with systemic disease.

Microscopically, examination of the verrucous plaques of rare primary inoculation **coccidioidomycosis** reveals acanthosis and a diffuse, dense dermal infiltrate of neutrophils, lymphocytes, histiocytes, plasma cells, eosinophils, and giant cells. Spores are found within the giant cells and free in the tissue. In the verrucous plaques and papulonodules of **systemic coccidioidomycosis**, there is acanthosis and formation of intraepidermal microabscesses, although to a lesser degree than in **blastomycosis**. Endothelial cell proliferation and a perivascular acute and chronic inflammatory infiltrate are seen. In addition to perivascular inflammation, the dermis may contain a granulomatous infiltrate consisting of neutrophils, lymphocytes, histiocytes, plasma cells, eosinophils, and multinucleated giant cells. Within the granulomas, abscess formation and necrosis are seen, both in the verrucous plaques and in the subcutaneous abscesses noted clinically. Leukocytoclasia and focally altered collagen associated with increased dermal mucin may be seen in association with the granulomatous infiltrate. The sporangia of *Coccidioides* species are usually few in tissue sections, but when they are present, they are quite large and thick walled, measuring up to 80 μm. They contain numerous endospores measuring 1 to 4 μm and are present within the giant cells or free in the tissue. Although they may be seen with H&E-stained sections, PAS and methenamine silver highlight the endospores.

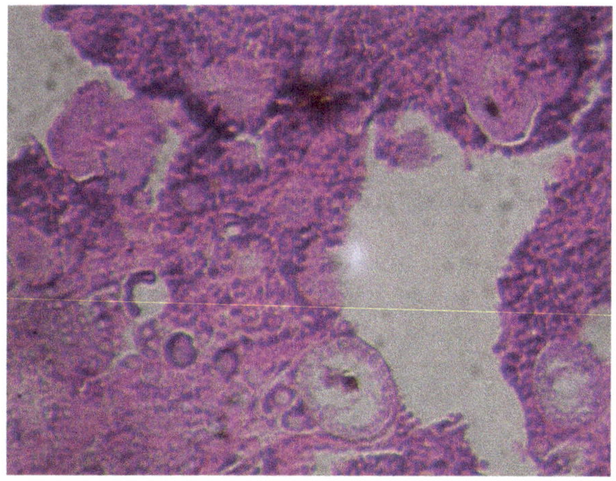

Coccidioides species. Large spherules containing endospores can be seen in this section of lung tissue. (H&E 200×.) (Reproduced, with permission, from Carroll KC et al, eds. *Jawetz, Melnick & Adelberg's Medical Microbiology*. 26th ed. New York, NY: McGraw-Hill Education; 2013.)

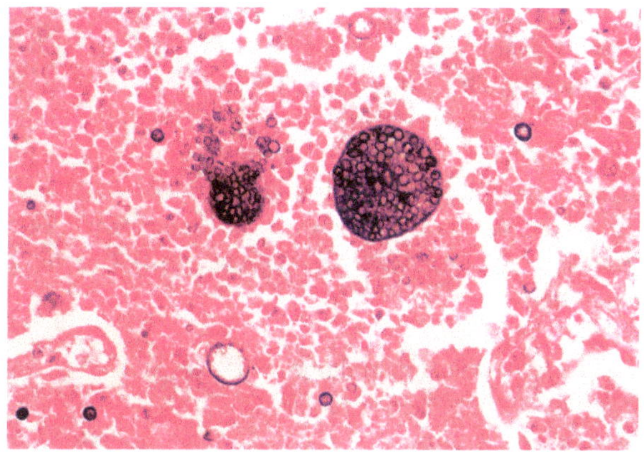

***Coccidioides immitis*, PAS stain.** Lung tissue with a large thick-walled spherule containing multiple endospores. The smaller spherule to its left has ruptured releasing endospores. (Reproduced, with permission, from Connor DH, Chandler FW, Schwartz DQA, Manz HJ, Lack EE, eds. *Pathology of Infectious Diseases*. Vol 1. Stamford, CT: Appleton & Lange; 1997.)

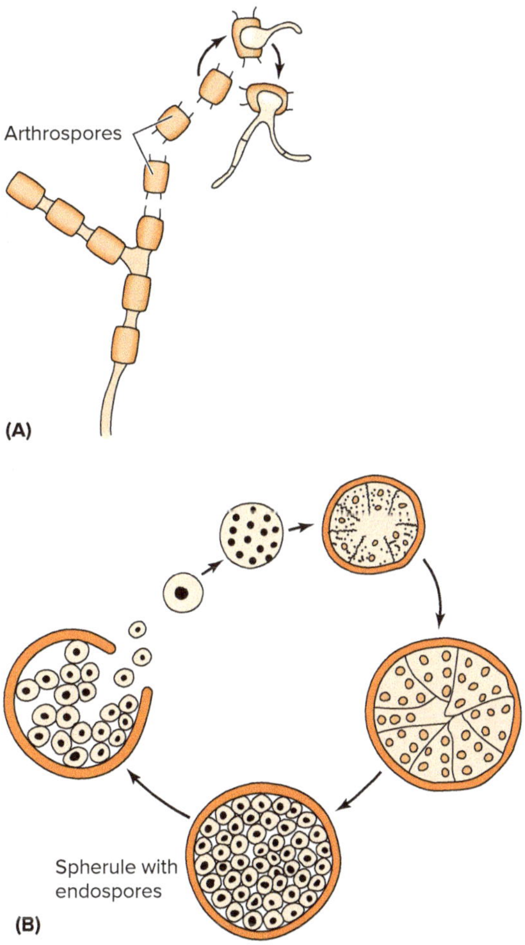

Stages of *Coccidioides immitis*. (A) Arthrospores form at the ends of hyphae in the soil. They germinate in the soil to form new hyphae. If inhaled, the arthrospores differentiate into spherules. **(B)** Endospores form within spherules in tissue. When spherules rupture, endospores disseminate and form new spherules. (Modified with permission from Brooks GF et al: *Jawetz, Melnick & Adelberg's Medical Microbiology*. 19th ed. New York, NY: Appleton & Lange; 1991.)

The differential diagnosis includes both infectious and noninfectious processes that exhibit **pseudoepitheliomatous hyperplasia**, intraepidermal microabscesses, and suppurative granulomas in the dermis and subcutis. The verrucous plaques may resemble those seen in **North American blastomycosis** but have fewer microabscesses. Methenamine silver (GMS) and PAS stains performed on multiple tissue sections should enable recognition of large sporangia containing endospores, which are not seen in **North American blastomycosis, histoplasmosis, lobomycosis**, or **paracoccidioidomycosis**. **Rhinosporidiosis** is a chronic granulomatous infection of the mucocutaneous tissues that affects humans and animals (Table 7-19B). The etiologic agent is *Rhinosporidium seeberi*, an organism that has never been cultured successfully in a cell-free medium, isolated from nature or transmitted to

Table 7-19B. Rhinosporidiosis

Clinical Features
Caused by *Rhinosporidium seeberi*
Highest prevalence in India and Sri Lanka
Nasal area involved in 70% of cases Large polypoid, globoid, pedunculated, mottled nodules
Conjunctiva involved in 15% of cases, more in drier climates
Sessile or stalked growth involving palpebral conjunctiva
Cutaneous infection rare
Autoinoculation more common than primary cutaneous origin
Papules evolve into verrucous nodules that may ulcerate
Hematogenous dissemination very rare
Numerous small (0.5-2.0 cm) nodules that may ulcerate
Other mucocutaneous sites in 8% of cases
Histopathologic Features
Mild hyperkeratosis, hyperplasia, and areas of thinning near sporangia
Sporangia (30-350 μm) in submucosa
Endospores (7-9 μm) within sporangia, free in tissue, and inside giant cells
Submucosal infiltrate of neutrophils, lymphocytes, histiocytes, plasma cells, and multinucleated giant cells
Prominent vascularity, hemorrhage, and hemosiderin disposition
Differential Diagnosis
Midline lethal facial granuloma
Cryptococcus neoformans
Coccidioides immitis
Spherules 30-60 μm, colorless, and flattened

experimental animals. Like *Coccidioides* species, *R seeberi* occurs in tissues as very large spherules, called *sporangia*, which typically measure 250 to 350 μm in diameter and contain endospores. However, phylogenetic analysis of *R seeberi*'s 18S SSU rDNA and that of 23 other microorganisms has led to the conclusion that the organism is not actually a fungus but rather belongs in a recently described group of fish parasites referred to as the DRIP clade (*Dermocystidium*, rosette agent, *Ichthyophonus*, and *Psorospermium*), located near the animal-fungal divergence nearly 1 billion years ago. Clinically, **rhinosporidiosis** is characterized by large polypoid growths that usually involve the nasal, ocular, or nasopharyngeal mucosa (not the skin). The disease affects both humans and animals and occurs most commonly in India, Sri Lanka, and other parts of South Asia, but it has also been reported elsewhere, including the Americas, Africa, and Europe. The modes of infection and transmission are unknown, although stagnant water and dust have been suspected as possible sources. The most commonly affected site is the nose, accounting for approximately 70% of cases. The presentation often involves unilateral obstruction or epistaxis, although bilateral involvement is common in the later stages. A blood-tinged mucoid discharge, often containing spores and sporangia, may be noted, and local pruritus is sometimes reported. Infection usually begins as a sessile tumor that may develop into a globoid pedunculated polyp weighing 20 g or more. The color, ranging from pink to red, is caused by vascularization and free blood. Macroscopically visible whitish spherules or round bodies representing bulging sporangia impart a mottled appearance to the polyp and give it a characteristic strawberry appearance. Septal perforation is common.

Microscopically, the surface of the polypoid mass is stratified squamous or columnar epithelium with slight hyperkeratosis and hyperplasia, although areas of thinning and erosion, particularly near mature sporangia, may be present. Numerous spores and sporangia in various developmental stages are noted in the submucosa, along with histiocytes, neutrophils, lymphocytes, and plasma cells; multinucleated giant cells, usually of the foreign body type, are seen occasionally. Whereas spores usually range from 7 to 9 μm in diameter, sporangia vary greatly in size from 60 to 450 μm or more in diameter; refractile spores may be noted free in tissue, often close to the surface, and within giant cells. Release of spores from a spherule appears to incite a neutrophilic response, and prominent vascularity, hemorrhage, and hemosiderin deposition are often seen. In addition to the neovascularization, necrosis and neutrophilic microabscesses may be seen. The walls of the spherules and spores stain with Gomori methenamine silver, Gridley, and PAS stains. *R seeberi* and *C immitis* both produce spherules in the yeast tissue phase; however, on direct examination, *R seeberi* spherules are globose, brown, and much larger than *C immitis* spherules, which are colorless, not perfectly spherical, and measure 30 to 60 μm in diameter.

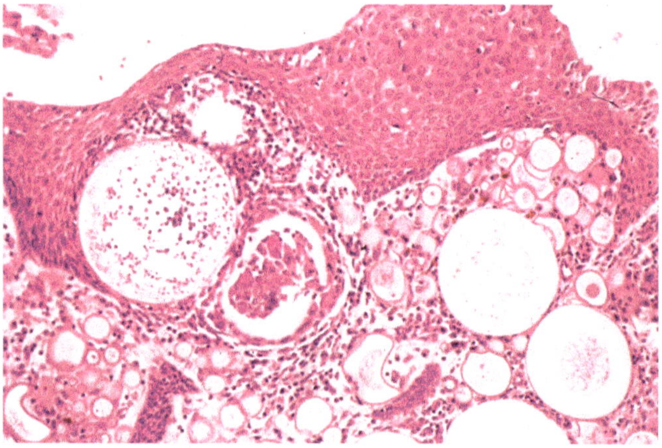

Rhinosporidiosis. Large sporangia are present in the nasal submucosa. (Used with permission of Dr F. Von Lichtenberg.)

ANSWER 7-20: A.

The biopsy reveals numerous small spherical organisms within macrophages. The GMS stain reveals scattered intracellular and extracellular spores in clusters and chains with narrow-based budding. The Giemsa-stained peripheral blood smear demonstrates intracellular yeast forms in a macrophage. **Histoplasmosis** is caused by two strains of the dimorphic fungus *H capsulatum* var *capsulatum* and var *duboisii* (associated with **African histoplasmosis**). The organism occurs worldwide, particularly in soil contaminated by bird and bat excreta. Despite the distinct clinical and histologic appearance of **African histoplasmosis**, *H capsulatum* var *capsulatum* and var *duboisii* are considered variants of the same species because their yeast forms appear identical after prolonged growth at 37°C.

Classic histoplasmosis is endemic in the Mississippi and Ohio River valleys, Central America, and parts of Southeast Asia and the Mediterranean basin, with a positive histoplasmin skin test result in up to 80% of the population in highly endemic areas (Table 7-20A). It occurs in four forms: primary cutaneous inoculation, acute pulmonary infection, chronic pulmonary infection, and disseminated disease. Before the advent of AIDS, **disseminated histoplasmosis** was a rare event, occurring in 1 in 100,000 to 1 in 500,000 persons per year. In endemic areas, **disseminated histoplasmosis** may affect 10% of AIDS patients, and for 75% of these, this will be their first manifestation of HIV infection. Since the introduction of HAART, **disseminated histoplasmosis** is less frequent in persons infected with HIV in the United States, but it continues to be a significant opportunistic infection in Central America.

Table 7-20A. Classic Histoplasmosis

Clinical Features
Occurs worldwide in soil containing bird excreta
Common in southeastern and midwestern United States, where 80% of population may have a positive historesultplasmin test
Pulmonary infection is portal of entry, asymptomatic in vast majority of cases
Disseminated disease characterized by
Mucosal ulcers
Cutaneous nodules, plaques, ulcers, pustules, panniculitis
Hepatosplenomegaly
Anemia, meningitis
Adrenal destruction
Histopathologic Features
H capsulatum var *capsulatum*, 2-4 μm in diameter, argyrophilic, with pseudocapsule
Leukocytoclastic vasculitis, granulomatous infiltrate, panniculitis, ulceration
Yeast present in histiocytes, giant cells, and yeast and extracellularly
Differential Features
Rhinoscleroma
Granuloma inguinale
Leishmaniasis
Cryptococcosis

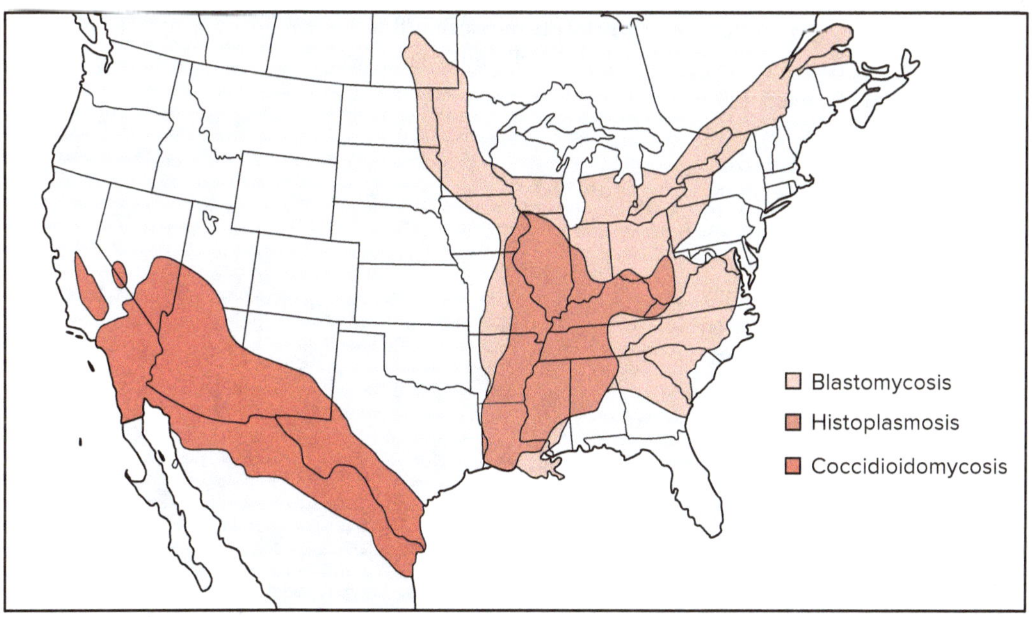

Geographic distribution of systemic fungal infections in the United States. (Reproduced, with permission, from Ryan KJ, Ray CG, et al, eds. Sherris Medical Microbiology, 6th ed. New York; NY: McGraw-Hill Education; 2014)

Primary cutaneous histoplasmosis is extremely rare and results from direct inoculation. It presents as a chancriform ulcer with associated regional lymphadenopathy. Its course may be self-limited, or it may progress to disseminated disease in immunocompromised individuals.

The vast majority of people who inhale *H capsulatum* spores remain asymptomatic. A minority of patients, after an incubation period of 3 weeks, develops flu-like symptoms. **Erythema nodosum** or **erythema multiforme** may occur during the recovery phase. Chest radiographs reveal hilar lymphadenopathy and small, scattered nodules that may heal with calcification.

Chronic pulmonary histoplasmosis occurs in older men who have a history of chronic obstructive pulmonary disease and is associated with fever, hemoptysis, and weight loss. Segmental interstitial infiltrates may progress to extensive fibrosis, cavitation, and destruction of lung tissue.

Disseminated histoplasmosis may develop in infants and immunocompromised individuals and may manifest as an indolent chronic illness or as a rapidly fatal one if left untreated. Hepatosplenomegaly, anemia, and fever may be the presenting signs of **acute disseminated histoplasmosis**. In later stages, endocarditis, meningitis, and adrenal gland destruction may be seen. Mucosal ulcerations occur in 60% of patients with disseminated disease and may involve the oral, nasal, GI, or genital mucosae. In contrast, cutaneous manifestations of **disseminated histoplasmosis** are present in fewer than 25% of patients. These manifestations range from **exfoliative erythroderma** to nodules, papules, ulcers, acneiform pustules, **erythema multiforme**, **erythema nodosum** panniculitis, and diffuse hyperpigmentation from **Addison disease**.

Microscopically, *H capsulatum* is a small yeast that is 2 to 4 μm in diameter that divides with narrow-based, unequal buds. Although it is called *capsulatum*, it lacks a true capsule, but its cell walls stain strongly with methenamine silver (GMS). It usually is seen within the cytoplasm of histiocytes, although it may be seen extracellularly or within giant cells. A halo-like clear space is sometimes seen separating the yeast wall from the macrophage cytoplasm. Biopsies of lesions from patients having **primary cutaneous histoplasmosis** and of the ulcers from patients with **disseminated histoplasmosis** reveal an underlying lymphohistiocytic infiltrate with *H capsulatum* within histiocytes faintly visible with H&E stain but strongly visible with the methenamine silver stain (GMS). The pattern of inflammation in patients with disseminated disease is variable and depends on the clinical presentation. Histopathologic examination of cutaneous papules and plaques reveals **leukocytoclastic vasculitis** consisting of a granulomatous infiltrate with multinucleated giant cells and variable foci of necrosis. In *Histoplasma* panniculitis, the dermal infiltrate extends into the subcutaneous fat, where the organisms may be seen. The diagnostic benchmark of all biopsies from histoplasmosis patients is the presence of numerous spores.

African histoplasmosis, which is endemic in Central and West Africa and on the island of Madagascar, is caused by *H capsulatum* var *duboisii* and occurs in two forms: localized and disseminated. The localized form is a chronic illness involving the skin, bone, and lymph nodes. Variable numbers of cutaneous papules and plaques may ulcerate, and purulent bone lesions may extend into the adjacent soft tissue, causing a subcutaneous abscess or a draining sinus tract. The disseminated form involves the liver, spleen, and other organs in addition to the features of the localized form and often is fatal.

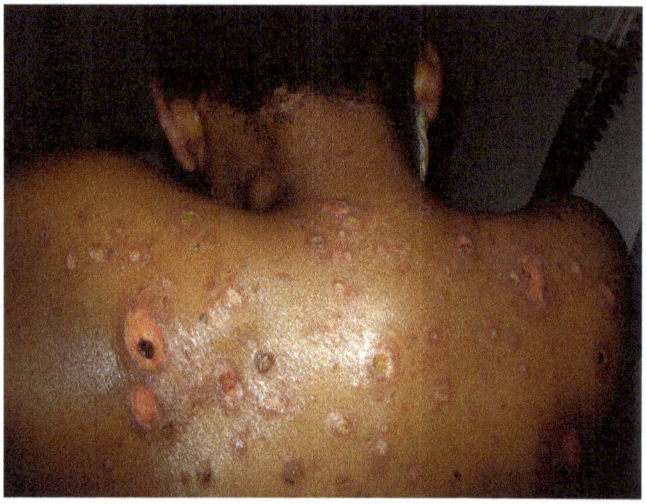

Disseminated histoplasmosis in HIV disease. Widespread cutaneous necrotic ulcers, infiltrated plaques, and cervical adenopathy. (Used with permission of Adam Lipworth, MD.)

Biopsies of cutaneous plaques of **African histoplasmosis** reveal a granulomatous infiltrate consisting of lymphocytes, histiocytes, neutrophils, and giant cells. Numerous larger organisms measuring 8 to 15 μm are present, mostly within the giant cells and histiocytes.

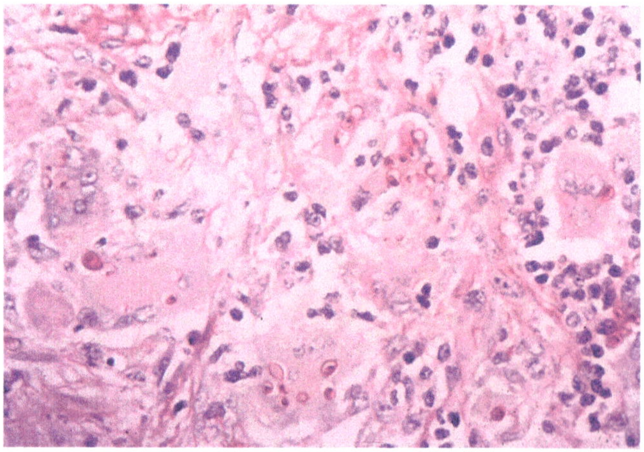

African histoplasmosis. Larger yeast forms within cells are demonstrated by Periodic acid-Schiff (PAS) staining with diastase, mostly within giant cells. (Used with permission of Dr J.R. Nethercott.)

The differential diagnosis for parasitized histiocytes includes **rhinoscleroma, granuloma inguinale,** and **leishmaniasis.** The histopathological distinction between **classical histoplasmosis** and **African histoplasmosis** is the larger sized yeasts in the African type. **Rhinoscleroma** is associated with a plasma cell–rich infiltrate, and the Donovan bodies (*Klebsiella granulomatis;* gram-negative rods) of **granuloma inguinale** do not stain with silver (GMS) or PAS stains. Also, *H capsulatum* lacks the kinetoplast of *Leishmania* **(leishmaniasis)**. Extracellular *H capsulatum* can be distinguished from extracellular **cryptococcosis** by the Fontana-Masson stain, which stains *Cryptococcus* species but not *H capsulatum.* Unlike the yeast forms of *Candida glabrata*, which are of similar size, the yeast forms of *H capsulatum* stain only weakly or not at all with the Gram stain. A commercially available DNA probe for *H capsulatum* grown in culture is highly specific and can confirm the presence of the fungus in culture.

ANSWER 7-21: B.

The biopsy reveals **pseudoepitheliomatous hyperplasia** and underlying suppurative and granulomatous dermatitis with round-pigmented spores (**Medlar bodies**). **Chromoblastomycosis** is primarily a disease of tropical and subtropical regions, but it may also occur in temperate climates (Table 7-21A). Its inoculation is typically related to penetrating wounds, splinters, and thorns and is associated with outdoor activity or agricultural work. Various saprophytic hypomycetatous fungi of the **Dematiaceae** (darkly pigmented fungi) family, including *Fonsecaea pedrosoi* (most common), *Phialophora verrucosa, Cladophialophora carrionii* (synonym *Cladosporium carrionii*), and less commonly, *Fonsecaea compacta* and *Rhinocladiella aquaspersa,* may cause chromoblastomycosis. The brown pigment is melanin and can be highlighted with a Fontana-Masson stain. Cultures of each of these organisms yield slow-growing green to black colonies that are distinguished from each other by the microscopic appearance of the fungi. These organisms have been isolated from decaying wood or soil.

Table 7-21A. Chromoblastomycosis

Clinical Features
- Caused by *Fonsecaea pedrosoi, Fonsecaea compactum, Cladosporium carrionii, Phialophora verrucosa, Rhinocladiella aquaspersa* most common
- Primary inoculation into skin; however, extremities are the most frequent site, often distal
- Verrucous plaques, nodules, tumors
- Scarring, central clearing

Histopathologic Features
- Pseudoepitheliomatous hyperplasia
- Suppurative granulomas
- Organisms do not require a special stain
  - Pigmented ("chestnut brown")
  - Sclerotic (septate) bodies
  - Medlar bodies ("copper pennies")

Differential Diagnosis
- Other infectious processes
  - Phaeohyphomycosis
  - Other deep fungi
  - Mycobacteria and atypical mycobacteria
- Halogenoderma
- Pyoderma gangrenosum

Dematiaceous Fungi That Cause Chromoblastomycosis

Pedro's Very Wet Compact Car

Fonsecaea ***pedro****soi*
Phialophora ***ver****rucosa*
Rhinocladiella ***aqua****spersa*
Fonsecaea ***comp****acta*
Cladophialophora ***car****rionii*

Clinically, the initial lesion is an erythematous papule that subsequently develops into one or multiple coalescing warty papules or plaques. Carrión described five clinical presentations: nodules, tumors, plaques, warty lesions, and scarring lesions. They typically occur on an extremity. The patients are usually otherwise well. Pruritus is frequently associated with the condition, and scratching may lead to satellite lesions. The disease rarely spreads to noncutaneous sites. A potential cutaneous complication is the development of **squamous cell carcinoma** in a long-standing lesion. KOH preparations may be diagnostic by revealing pigmented sclerotic **"Medlar" bodies**, since these structures are frequently transepidermally eliminated. The clinical differential diagnosis includes other fungal or mycobacterial infections, particularly **tuberculosis, leprosy,** and **blastomycosis**, as well as **leishmaniasis, botryomycosis,** and **tertiary syphilis**.

Microscopically, biopsy of a papule or plaque usually shows hyperkeratosis and epidermal hyperplasia, often with a pseudoepitheliomatous pattern, overlying a suppurative and granulomatous dermatitis. The organisms may vary in number but can be recognized easily on routine H&E-stained sections. The spores may be present free in tissue or located within giant cells. They are round to oval and bronze colored, measuring 6 to 12 μm in diameter, usually with a central septation. They have been called **Medlar bodies; sclerotic bodies;** or descriptively, "copper pennies."

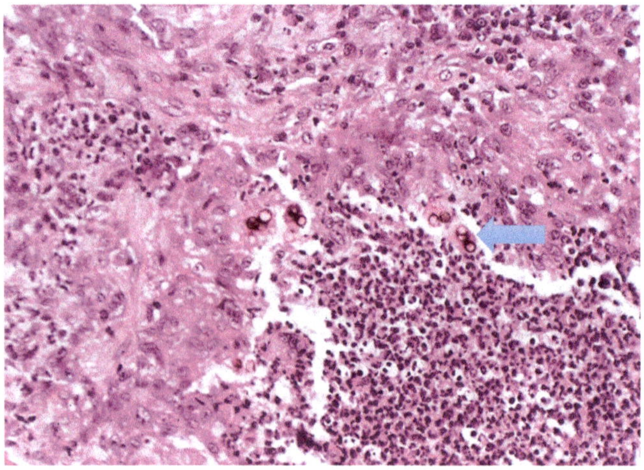

Chromoblastomycosis. Suppurative granuloma with pigmented sclerotic (Medlar) bodies. Note the spore with central septation (arrow).

In regard to the differential diagnosis, when septation is present within a dividing **Medlar body**, the findings are diagnostic and distinguish **chromoblastomycosis** from **phaeohyphomycosis**, in which budding occurs and the characteristic septations are not found. Ajello coined the term **phaeohyphomycosis** in 1974 to encompass infections caused by **dematiaceous** fungi that have hyphal elements and grow by budding (Table 7-21B). The most common fungi in this group are *Exophiala jeanselmei* and *Wangiella dermatitidis.* This form of **subcutaneous mycosis** results in a spectrum of clinical presentations; subcutaneous pseudocysts and ulcerated and verrucous lesions. In immunocompromised patients, dissemination may occur. Whereas *E jeanselmei* is typically present in phaeomycotic cysts, *W dermatitidis* is more often associated with ulcerating and verrucous lesions. This histopathologic reaction pattern is that of a suppurative or mixed inflammatory cell infiltrate with a granulomatous tissue reaction. There may be fibrous encapsulation of cyst-like lesions (**phaeomycotic cyst**). Foreign material, such as vegetable matter or a splinter, may occasionally be observed. **Pseudoepitheliomatous hyperplasia** and intradermal neutrophilic microabscesses may be seen at the surface of nodules or verrucous plaques. Fungi are typically abundant and often are located in or near suppurative foci. They are brown colored and measure 2 to 6 μm but may be larger. The fungi in **phaeohyphomycosis** are budding spores often producing chains and have abundant hyphal elements that may be septate (not septate spores) or branching or may exhibit pseudohyphae. Pigmentation may not always be obvious, and a Fontana-Masson stain may be needed to demonstrate melanin.

Table 7-21B. Subcutaneous Phaeohyphomycosis

Clinical Features
Caused by *Exophiala* and *Phialophora* species most commonly
Inoculation into skin
Extremities, particularly fingers, wrists, knees, ankles
Usually solitary nodule
Histopathologic Features
Usually circumscribed, encapsulated "phaeomycotic cyst"
Suppurative granuloma within "cyst"
Epidermis and dermis may be unaffected
Organisms: usually pigmented but not always
Morphologic spectrum
Budding yeast forms
Pseudohyphae
Candida-like hyphae with branching, septa, and in chains
Differential Diagnosis
Chromoblastomycosis
Mycetoma and related conditions
Candida species

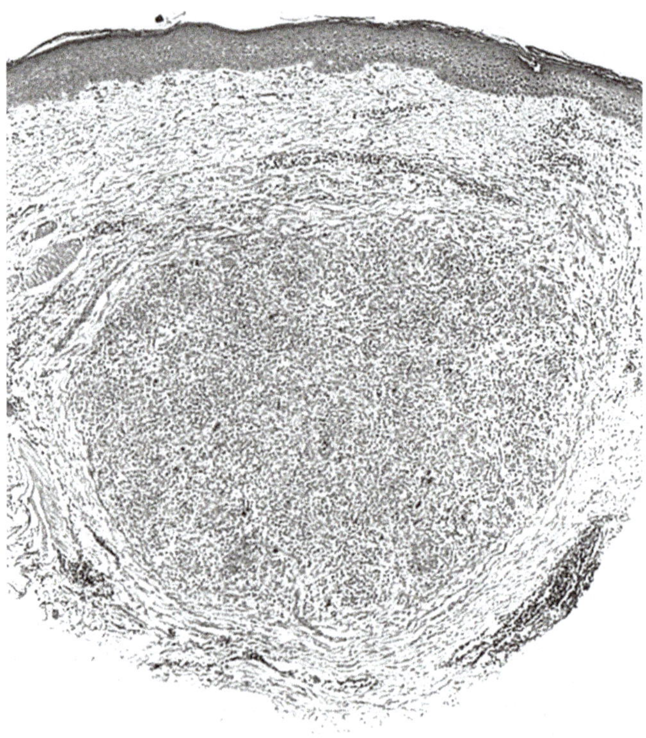

Phaeohyphomycosis. Well-circumscribed, cyst-like lesion in the deep dermis.

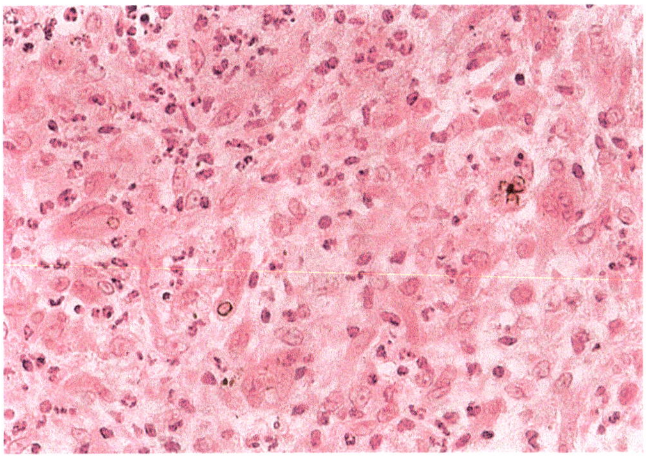

Phaeohyphomycosis. Neutrophilic and granulomatous infiltrates with pigmented budding yeast forms.

ANSWER 7-22: B.

The biopsy reveals a chronic inflammatory reaction with neutrophil abscesses, scattered giant cells, and fibrosis. Pigmented granules (grains) composed of hyphae are found in the center of the inflammation. **Mycetoma** is a chronic infectious disease localized to the skin or subcutaneous tissue. This disease is characterized by tumefaction, draining sinuses, and the presence and extrusion of aggregates (grains) of microorganisms (Table 7-22A). Whereas a fungus causes **eumycetoma**, **actinomycetoma** may be caused either by endogenous anaerobic bacteria (*Actinomyces* species), which is called **actinomycosis**, or by aerobic bacteria, including *Actinomadura* species, *Nocardia brasiliensis*, and *Streptomyces* species. **Mycetoma** is typically initiated by percutaneous trauma. **Mycetomas** have been classified into three different groups based on the micromorphology of their grains: **botryomycosis** (cocci or short rods), **actinomycetoma** (thin, branching, intertwined bacterial filaments), and **eumycetoma** (thick, branching, intertwined fungal filaments).

Eumycetoma is caused by a fungus and is endemic in equatorial Africa, the Middle East, India, and Mexico. The grains of fungi may be nonpigmented or pigmented (**dematiaceous fungus**). The most prevalent dematiaceous fungal agent of **eumycetoma** is *Madurella mycetomatis*, the predominant etiologic agent in India and Africa. A common nonpigmented etiologic agent of **eumycetoma** in North America is *Pseudallescheria boydii*. The asexual form of this organism is named *Scedosporium apiospermum*. Although not an endemic disease in the Amazon rainforest, where **actinomycetoma** is the more common type, true fungal **eumycetoma** in Brazil is most commonly caused by *Acremonium* species and *Madurella grisea*. Most affected patients live in tropical or subtropical regions. The etiologic agents of **eumycetoma** are usually associated with woody plants and soil. After the initial trauma, a small nodule develops that subsequently expands and frequently drains into a sinus tract. Sinuses rarely occur before 3 months' duration. Sinuses may

Table 7-22A. Clinical and Histopathologic Features of Mycetoma Grains[a]

ORGANISMS	HEMATOXYLIN AND EOSIN SECTION APPEARANCES
Eumycetoma	
Dark grains	Cement present, vesicles sometimes prominent
Madurella mycetomatis	Cement absent, compact outer layer
M grisea	Cement in outer zone, dark periphery with vesicular center
Leptosphaeria senegalensis	Cement absent, often hollow
Exophiala jeanselmei	Cement lacking, compact outer layer
Pyrenochaeta romeroi	
Pale grains	
Pseudallescheria boydii,	Compact, pigment lacking, interwoven fungal filaments (*Scedosporium*
Fusarium sp, Acremonium, Aspergillus nidulans, Neotestudina rosati	*apiospermum* may have prominent vesicles)
Actinomycetoma	
Pale (white to yellow) grains	Basophilic-stained fringe in layers
Actinomadura madura	Small, pale blue, eosinophilic fringe
Nocardia brasiliensis	
Yellow to brown grains	
Streptomyces somaliensis	Grains fractured, basophilic, or pink
Red to pink grains	
A pelletieri	Small, basophilic layers

Quick Fack

Helpful rules of thumb:
Black or dark grains are always produced by fungi.
Red grains are always produced actinomycetes.
But pale (white/yellow) grains may be produced by fungi, actinomycetes, or other bacteria.

close, and organisms may be discharged with subsequent healing. Many times new nodules form after the initial one has healed. With time, the lesions may extend deeply and involve bone (as in the patient in the question), forming cavities. Fungus may ultimately even spread via the lymphatics (sporotrichoid pattern) to visceral sites. Seventy percent of all **eumycetoma** involve the foot.

Microscopically, the typical finding includes an aggregate of microorganisms (grain) in a microabscess surrounded by granulation tissue and fibrosis. Neutrophils are often numerous, and a granulomatous tissue reaction is common. Eumycotic grains or granules (also known as "**sclerotia**") are poorly organized collections of about 5-μm-thick septate hyphal elements, which in the case of **dematiaceous** fungi are brown or black. **North America eumycetoma** caused by *Pseudallescheria boydii* characteristically produces pale or white grains. The micromorphology of the grains helps to distinguish **eumycetoma** from **actinomycetoma** and **botryomycosis**.

Actinomycetomas with draining sinus tracts are typically caused by *Actinomyces, Nocardia,* or *Streptomyces* species. **Actinomycosis** (infection with *Actinomyces* species) is a chronic suppurative infection noted for the production of "**sulfur granules**."

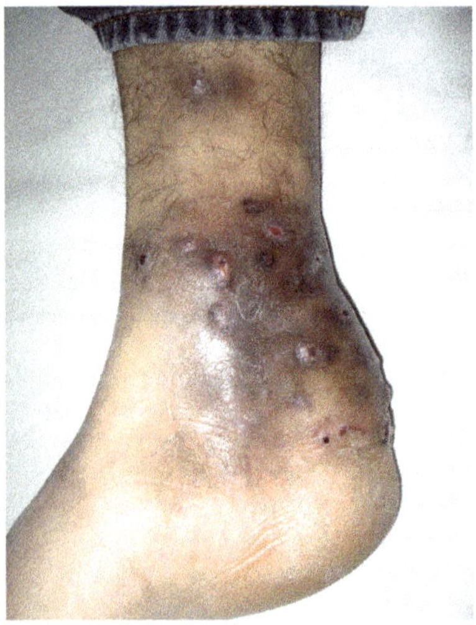

Mycetoma. A eumycetoma with typical chronic sinus drainages in the foot and ankle of a 33-year-old agricultural worker in Peru. Treatment was with itraconazole. (Reproduced, with permission, from Knoop KJ, Stack LB, Storrow AB, Thurman RJ. *The Atlas of Emergency Medicine*. 3rd ed. New York, NY: McGraw-Hill; 2010. Courtesy of Rob Griedanus, MD and Universidad Peruana Cayetano Heredia, Lima, Peru.)

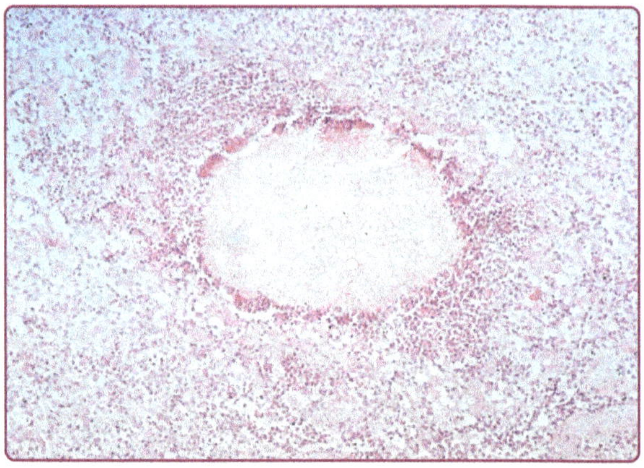

Pale eumycetoma grains of *Pseudallescheria boydii* (hematoxylin and eosin stain). (Reproduced, with permission, from Goldsmith LA, Katz SI, Gilchrest BA, Paller AS, Leffell DJ, Wolff K, eds. *Fitzpatrick's Dermatology in General Medicine*. 8th ed. New York, NY: McGraw-Hill Education; 2012.)

Several members of the order of Actinomycetales cause the disease, most commonly by *Actinomyces israelii*. They are anaerobic saprophytic gram-positive, acid–fast–negative bacteria present in the normal flora of the mouth and GI and urogenital tracts. Infection is often associated with mucosal trauma, such as from dental procedures or surgery. Three major clinical presentations have been described: cervicofacial, thoracic, and abdominal. The disease may also disseminate in immunocompromised patients. Cervicofacial **actinomycosis** accounts for more than 50% of cases. It typically occurs in the premandibular region as a discrete, slowly growing swelling. Subsequent abscess formation and drainage via sinus tracts are common. Potential complications include osteomyelitis. If infected oral material is aspirated, pulmonary infection may develop (thoracic form, 15% of **actinomycoses**). Abdominal infection usually occurs after traumatic rupture of the intestine. Appendicitis with perforation is the most common precipitating event. In recent years, an increase in the abdominal-pelvic form has been observed, possibly related to an increased and prolonged use of intrauterine devices. The lesion typically begins as a **cellulitis** with subsequent abscess formation and fibrotic induration. Discharge of the "**sulfur granules**" from sinus tracts is common. Unlike *Actinomyces,* which is part of the normal human microbial flora, *Nocardia* and *Streptomyces* species are free-living soil organisms. The majority of human infections in the United States are associated with members of the *Nocardia asteroids* complex. Other medically significant species include *N brasiliensis, N otitidiscaviarum,* and *N pseudobrasiliensis*. **Nocardiosis** is seen worldwide, infects predominantly immunocompromised individuals, and has a wide variety of clinical manifestations. **Nocardiosis** usually presents as pulmonary disease acquired through inhalation, with dissemination from the lungs manifested as bacteremia, empyema, brain abscess, pericarditis, synovitis, or soft tissue infection (which may present as **actinomycetoma** or **cellulitis**). Less frequently, primary cutaneous **nocardiosis** results from percutaneous trauma with soft tissue inoculation that induces

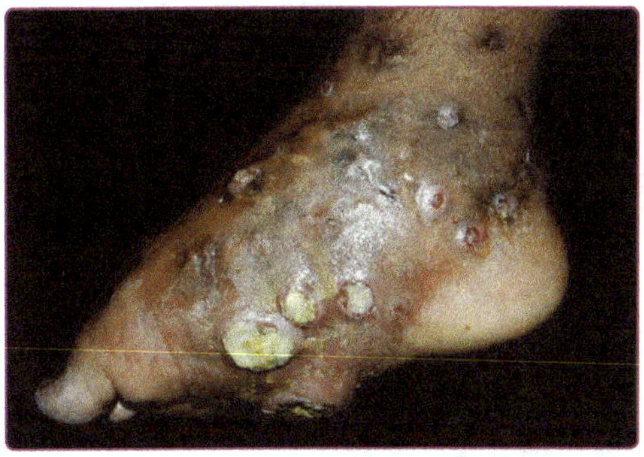

Actinomycetoma of the foot with multiple draining sites and pale yellow granules. (Reproduced, with permission, from Goldsmith LA, Katz SI, Gilchrest BA, Paller AS, Leffell DJ, Wolff K, eds. *Fitzpatrick's Dermatology in General Medicine*. 8th ed. New York, NY: McGraw-Hill Education; 2012.)

local abscess formation, even in healthy hosts. Skin involvement may occur via dissemination from another site, typically in an immunocompromised host. In immunocompromised hosts and those with multiple brain abscesses, the mortality rate of **disseminated nocardiosis** has been reported to be greater than 85%. *N brasiliensis* may be associated with a lymphocutaneous presentation (**sporotrichoid**). Thus cultures are important in defining the disease.

Histopathologically, aggregates of *Actinomyces* organisms appear as round to oval bodies up to 10 mm in diameter. The organisms may appear yellow on routine H&E stains

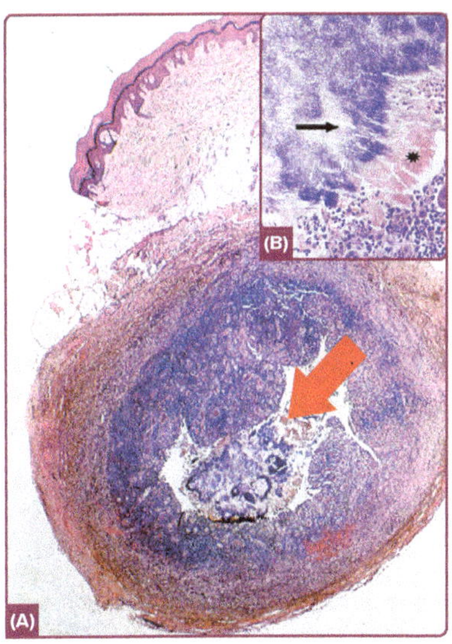

Actinomycetoma. (A) Skin biopsy shows the granule (*red arrow*) inside the inflammatory reaction (hematoxylin and eosin, 20×). **(B)** The contrast between the blue fibrillary material (*black arrow*), representing *Actinomyces* bacteria, and the eosinophilic proteinaceous material of the Splendore-Hoeppli phenomenon (*star*) (hematoxylin and eosin, 100×). (Reproduced, with permission, from Goldsmith LA, Katz SI, Gilchrest BA, Paller AS, Leffell DJ, Wolff K, eds. *Fitzpatrick's Dermatology in General Medicine*. 8th ed. New York, NY: McGraw-Hill Education; 2012.)

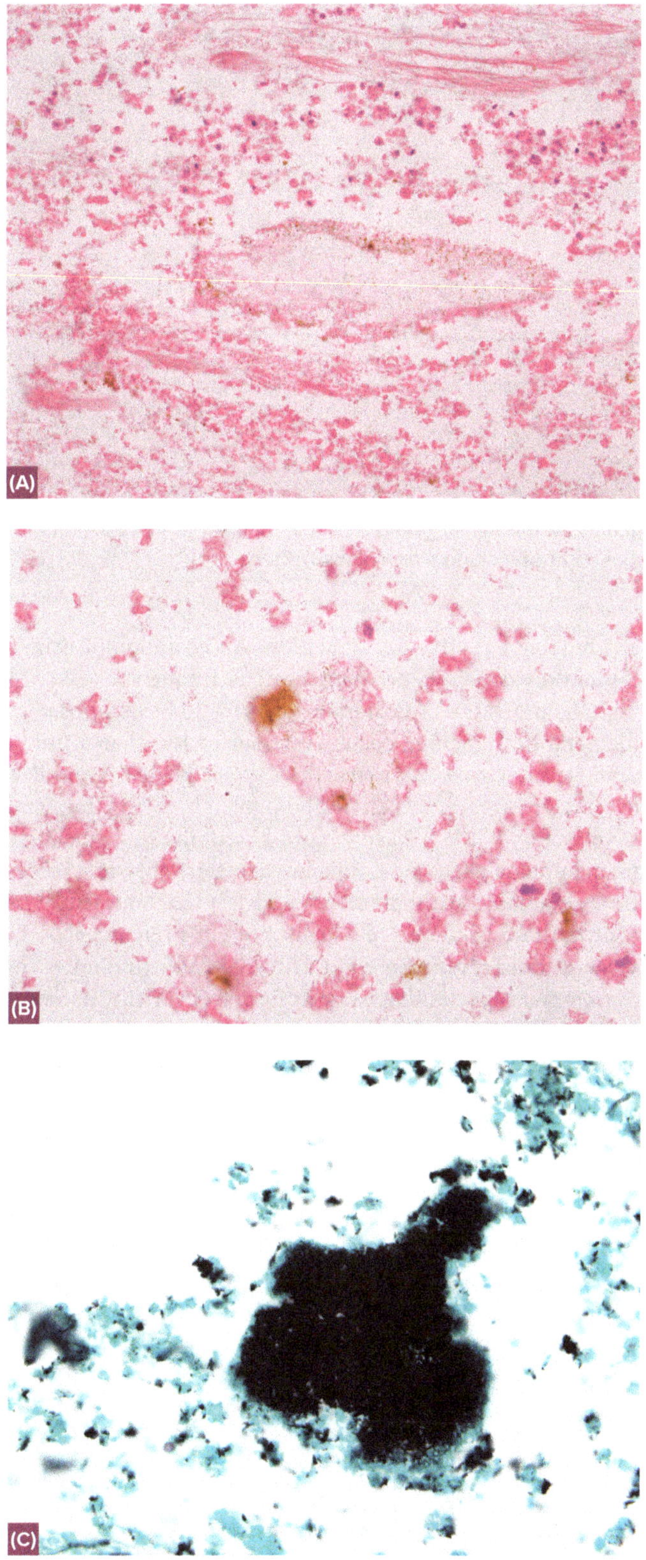

Actinomycosis. (A) The organisms may appear yellow on routine hematoxylin and eosin sections attributable to sulfur accumulation. **(B)** There is a focus of granular eosinophilia whereby higher power magnification discloses filamentous structures, some of which appear yellow. **(C)** The organisms are highlighted by a Gomori methenamine silver stain.

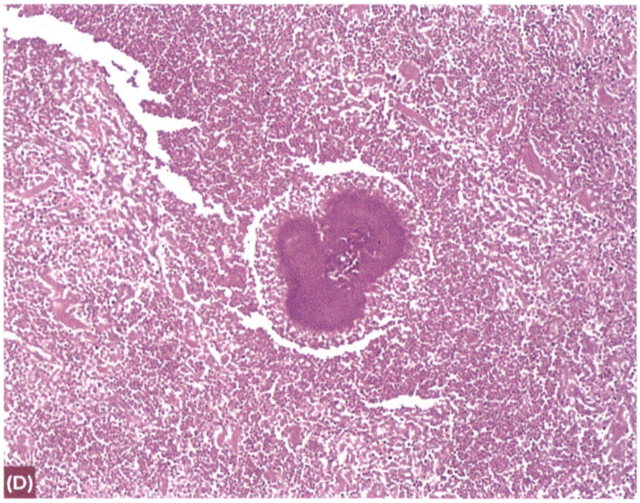

(D) Note the "sulfur granule" within the abscess that is composed of branching filamentous bacteria.

attributable to sulfur accumulation. An eosinophilic fringe (**Splendore-Hoeppli phenomenon**) is frequently seen. At high magnification, the granules are seen to be composed of filamentous branching bacteria measuring less than 1 μm in diameter. In tissue, these structures typically are surrounded by macrophages. They can be highlighted by both Gram and silver stains (GMS). *Nocardia* are basophilic gram-positive filamentous structures (1 μm in diameter) that are sometimes stainable with modified acid-fast methods (ie, Fite stain). These bacteria are usually present in aggregates. In **visceral nocardiosis**, in contrast to the "sulfur granules" of *Actinomyces* species that cause **actinomycosis**, the filaments in *Nocardia* tend to break up into short bacillary segments similar to *Mycobacterium tuberculosis*. However, in **mycetomas**, grains similar to the sulfur granules of *Actinomyces* may be formed. Tissue culture is recommended for definitive speciation.

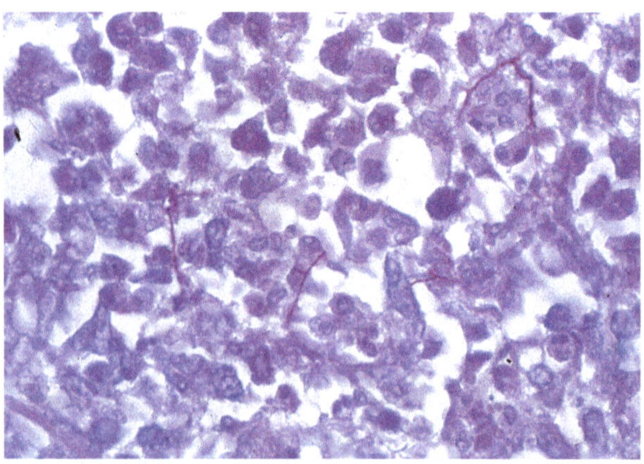

Visceral nocardiosis. Loose aggregates of filamentous bacteria stained with Fite-Faraco reaction (acid–fast positive). (Used with permission of Drs S. Lucas and F. Von Lichtenberg.)

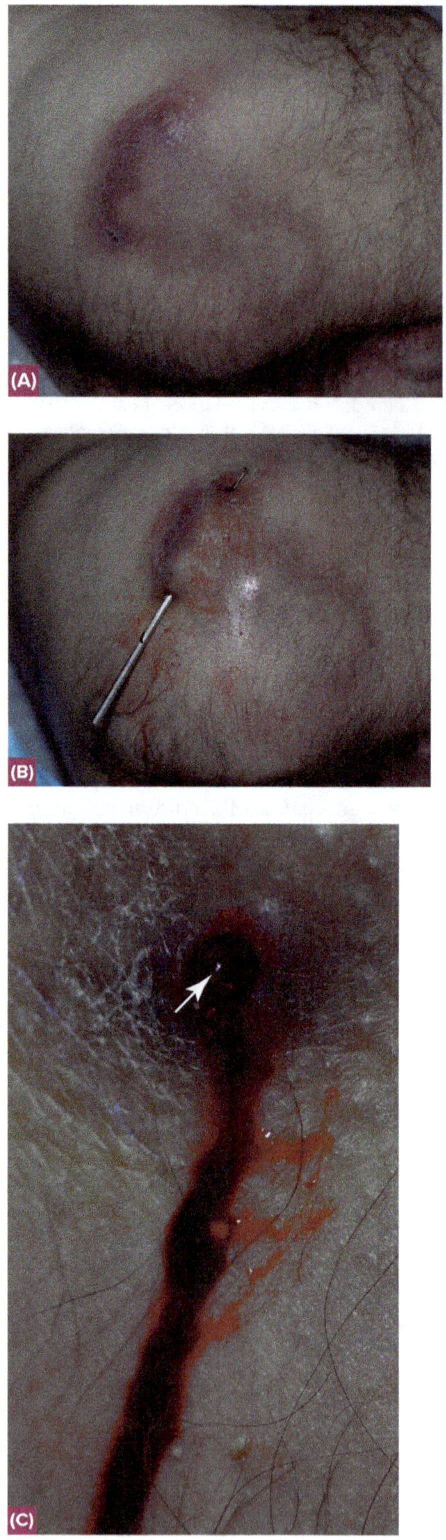

Chronic abscess, botryomycosis: MRSA 41-year old with HIV disease had an extensive abscess for months. **(A)** R-buttock abscess. **(B)** The abscess was drained and treated with linezolid. **(C)** The white grains noted in the drainage represent colonies of *S aureus*. (Reproduced, with permission, from Wolff K, Johnson RA, Saavedra AP. *Fitzpatrick's Color Atlas and Synopsis of Clinical Dermatology*. 7th ed. New York, NY: McGraw-Hill Education; 2013.)

Botryomycosis is an uncommon chronic bacterial infection usually caused by staphylococci and less commonly by other organisms such as *Pseudomonas*, *Proteus*, or *Escherichia coli*. Although the pathogenesis is poorly understood, reduced host resistance may perpetuate growth of lower-virulence organisms in a symbiotic fashion. There are two forms: visceral and integumental. The latter is the more common form and is often associated with trauma or foreign body or chronic wound contamination. Clinically, lesions may affect not only the skin but also the internal organs and bone. The skin lesions typically consist of small, tender nodules with seropurulent discharge from draining sinuses. Tonsillar **botryomycosis** may cause tonsillar hypertrophy.

Microscopically, common epidermal changes include hyperkeratosis, hyperplasia, and spongiosis. In the dermis, there is a mixed inflammatory cell infiltrate composed of neutrophils, lymphocytes, and histiocytes, often with granulation tissue. Within the inflammatory infiltrate, there are usually granules of tightly clustered gram-positive cocci. Sometimes the granules are surrounded by amorphous eosinophilic material, creating the so-called "**Splendore-Hoeppli phenomenon**". This effect of seemingly radiating lateral projections gives the granules a striking similarity to actinomycotic granules. The eosinophilic material has been found to contain immunoglobulins and is likely produced by the host's response to bacterial antigens. In some instances, *Pseudomonas* or *Proteus* species may cause the same phenomenon, giving rise to granules mimicking *Actinomyces* species. However, in those instances, the granules are composed of tight clusters of gram-negative rods (Table 7-22B).

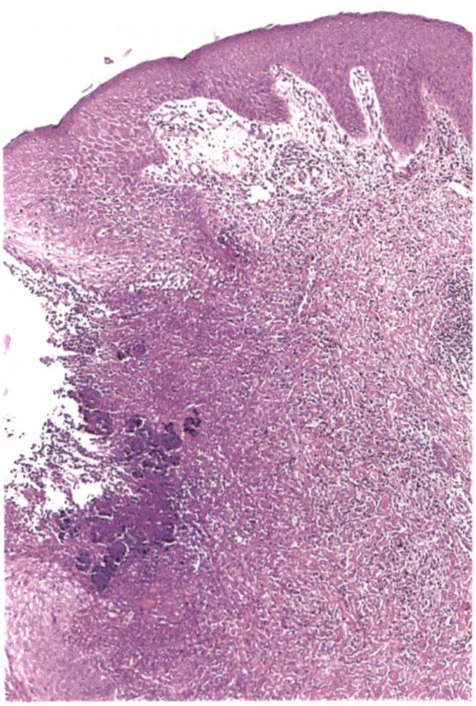

Botryomycosis. A group of basophilic granules lining an ulcer contains gram-positive staphylococci surrounded by acute inflammation.

Table 7-22B. Mycetoma (Eumycetoma and Actinomycetoma) and Botryomycosis

Clinical Features
- Caused by
  - True fungus (eumycetoma)
  - *Actinomyces, Nocardia, Streptomyces* (actinomycetoma)
  - *Staph, Pseudomonas, Proteus, E coli* (botryomycosis)
- Inoculation into skin after trauma; rare dissemination
- Localized infection of skin, subcutis, fascia, bone
- Tumefactive nodules
- Ulceration
- Draining sinuses with extrusion of sclerotia (grains, granules) in exudates
- Bone involvement is often extensive

Histopathologic Features
- Neutrophilic abscesses contain sclerotia (grains, granules)
- Surrounding granulation tissue
- Granulomatous inflammation
- Sinus tracts
- Organisms in sclerotia:
  - Eumycetoma; circumscribed mass of hyphae with or without pigment and associated host tissue or soil; distinction of organisms based on color, texture, shape, internal architecture
  - Actinomycetoma; often filaments in granules from *Actinomyces or Nocardia*, usually without pigment
  - Botryomycosis; gram-positive cocci or gram-negative rods, usually without pigment

Differential Diagnosis
- Other infections characterized by ulceration, tumefaction, draining sinuses
  - Chromoblastomycosis
  - Phaeohyphomycosis
  - Dermatophyte infection

Quick Fact

Special Stains for DDX in Mycetoma and Botryomycosis

Eumycetoma (*Pseudallescheria boydii*): branching filamentous hyphal structures >1 μm; PAS+, GMS+, Fontana-Masson−, Gram−, ABF(Fite)−

Eumycetoma (other, dematiaceous): branching filamentous hyphal structures >1 μm; PAS+, GMS+, Fontana-Masson+, Gram−, ABF(Fite)−

Actinomycetoma (*Actinomyces*): beaded and branching thin filamentous bacteria; Gram+, AFB(Fite)−, GMS+, PAS+/−, Fontana-Masson−

Actinomycetoma (*Nocardia*); beaded and branching thin filamentous bacteria; Gram+, AFB(Fite)+, GMS+, PAS+/−, Fontana-Masson−

Botryomycosis (*Staph*); cocci in clusters; Gram+, AFB(Fite)−, GMS−, PAS−, Fontana-Masson−

Botryomycosis (*Pseudomonas, Proteus, E coli*); bacilli; Gram−, AFB(Fite)−, GMS−, PAS−, Fontana-Masson−

ANSWER 7-23: D.

The patient's biopsy reveals an intravascular fungal infection in which large nonseptate hyphae invade through the blood vessels into the surrounding tissues. There is extensive vascular thrombosis with little inflammation. The hyphae branch at 90° angles. The findings are consistent with **Mucormycosis** (aka **Zygomycosis**) (Table 7-23A). This patient has the unusual combined presentation of both **rhinocerebral mucormycosis** and **subacute cutaneous mucormycosis**. The *Mucorales* are ubiquitous saprophytic organisms found in soil and on decomposing organic material such as fruit and bread. They can be cultured as normal flora from the feces and oral and nasal cavities of healthy individuals, but infection with tissue invasion occurs mainly in immunosuppressed patients. Large numbers of sporangiospores are released into the air and then inhaled, causing pulmonary and nasal sinus infection. Less commonly, ingestion or cutaneous inoculation may cause disease. Risk factors include diabetes mellitus, diabetic ketoacidosis, neutropenia, leukemia, burns, prior skin trauma, iron chelation therapy (deferoxamine or desferrioxamine), iron overload states, broad-spectrum antibiotic therapy, intravenous drug use, and the use of elasticized adhesive tape. Sporangiospores that have escaped host defense mechanisms may germinate into the hyphal form capable of invading blood vessels, which may lead to hematogenous dissemination or infarction and necrosis. Defects in macrophages or neutrophils increase an individual's susceptibility to systemic infection. Macrophages prevent the transformation of *Rhizopus* species, the most common etiologic agent of **mucormycosis**, from its yeast to its hyphal form. Neutrophils are able to damage the hyphal form.

The clinical forms of **mucormycosis** are rhinocerebral, pulmonary, GI, cutaneous, and disseminated. **Rhinocerebral mucormycosis** occurs most commonly in uncontrolled diabetics who rapidly develop fever, unilateral headache, periorbital or perinasal swelling, and drainage of discolored pus. If not treated with aggressive debridement and antifungal therapy, *Mucorales* species can invade brain tissue and bone and cause death within days. Pulmonary and gastrointestinal **mucormycosis** are the most common types that can progress to the disseminated form, which is 100% fatal if untreated and is associated with widespread abscess formation and necrosis of multiple organs, including the brain, heart, and spleen. Two variants of **cutaneous mucormycosis** have been described: subacute and rapidly progressive. The subacute form occurs in an otherwise healthy host exposed to contaminated adhesive tape and begins as vesicles and pustules that progress to eschars. The rapidly progressive form occurs in compromised patients and is characterized by an ecthyma-like necrotic black crust surrounded by **cellulitis**. If untreated, it may progress to disseminated disease. Unfortunately, serologic diagnostic tests are not clinically useful. Molecular techniques based on PCR restriction fragment length polymorphism have recently identified some of the major *Mucorales* species in histopathologic samples and are a continuing focus of laboratory research.

Table 7-23A. Mucormycosis

Clinical Features
- Most common pathogens: *Rhizopus, Absidia, Mucor*
- Mucorales are found in soil and in decomposing organic matter
- Risk factors: diabetes, leukemia, neutropenia, skin ulceration, burns, use of adhesive tape
- Ecthyma-like necrotic crust surrounded by cellulitis

Histopathologic Features
- Necrosis, thrombosis, infarction
- Large, broad ≤ 30 μm in diameter hyphae
- Hyphae branch at 90° angles and lack septa
- Hyphae often present in vessel walls

Differential Diagnosis
- *Conidiobolus*
- *Basidiobolus*
- Aspergillosis

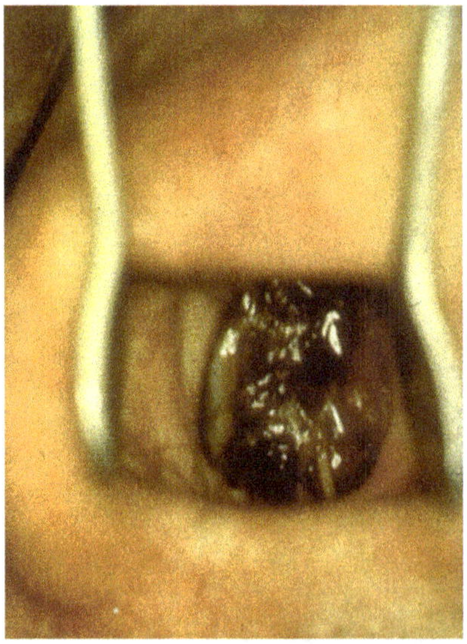

Mucormycosis sinusitis in a patient with diabetes showing the classic black nasal discharge. (Reproduced, with permission, from Usatine RP, Smith MA, Mayeaux EJ Jr, Chumley HS, eds. *Color Atlas of Family Medicine*. 2nd ed. New York, NY: McGraw-Hill Education; 2012. Used with permission of Randal A. Otto, MD.)

Microscopically, extensive necrosis and vascular damage characterize the eschar. Only the hyphal form of *Mucorales* species are seen in tissue. The hyphae are broad (≤30 μm in diameter) with bulbous lateral protrusions. They often appear hollow; lack microscopically visible septa; branch at variable up to 90° angles; and are visible with H&E, PAS, and methenamine silver stains. The organisms typically exhibit intravascular localization. At times, the infection may localize in the subcutis and be associated with a striking pattern of paucicellular necrotizing panniculitis.

The differential diagnosis includes **aspergillosis** and **fusariosis**. The hyphae of *Aspergillus* and *Fusarium* species are thinner, branch at an acute angle, show dichotomous branching, and often exhibit septa. Tissue culture is extremely helpful when hyphae are scarce or distorted in tissue.

Aspergillus species are ubiquitous saprophytes found in soil, air, and decaying organic matter. Hospital renovations or construction sites producing contaminated dust have been implicated in outbreaks of **aspergillosis**. **Aspergillosis** is a leading cause of opportunistic infection among immunocompromised patients, especially those with leukemia and solid organ or bone marrow transplant recipients (Table 7-23B). The incidence is increasing, and it is the second most common nosocomial fungal infection, exceeded only by **candidiasis**, in neutropenic hosts. Other risk factors for **aspergillosis** include AIDS and high-dose corticosteroid therapy. The true incidence is probably higher because many cases remain undiagnosed. *A fumigatus* is the most common human pathogen of the genus, followed by *A flavus*, *A niger*, and *A terreus*. Infections due to *A terreus* appear to be increasing in frequency and are of concern because of its apparently reduced susceptibility to amphotericin B compared with *A fumigatus*.

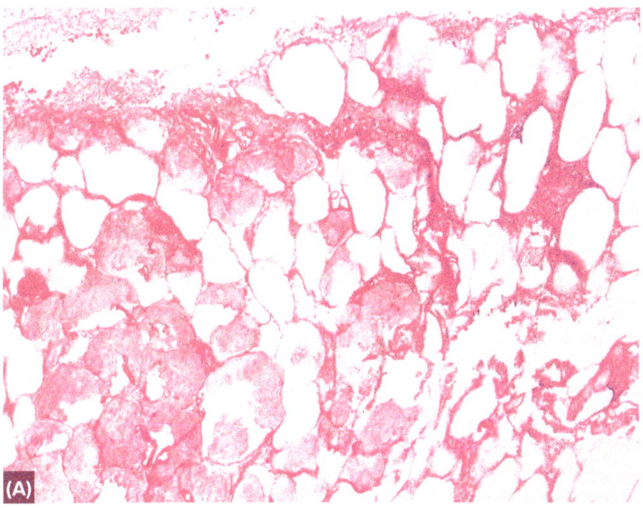

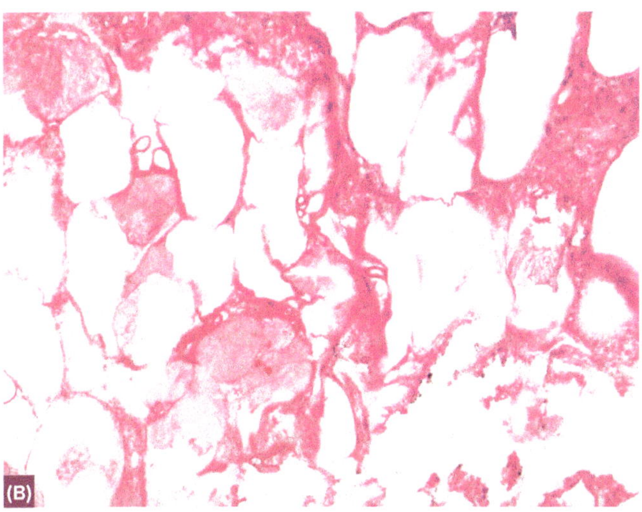

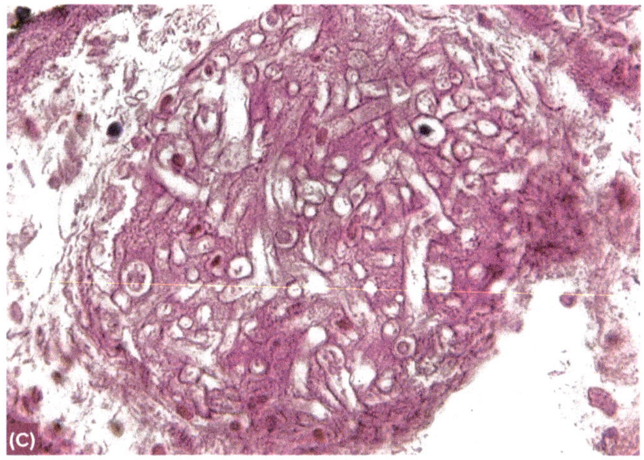

Mucormycosis. (A) There is striking paucicellular fat necrosis. Even at this power, numerous pleomorphic broad-based fungal elements are seen that appear as negative shadows, although with an eosinophilic membranous borders. **(B)** Higher power magnification reveals the extent of tissue infiltration by the organism, although with the prominent tissue necrosis attributable to angioinvasion. **(C)** Large, empty-appearing hyphae without septa show 90° branching.

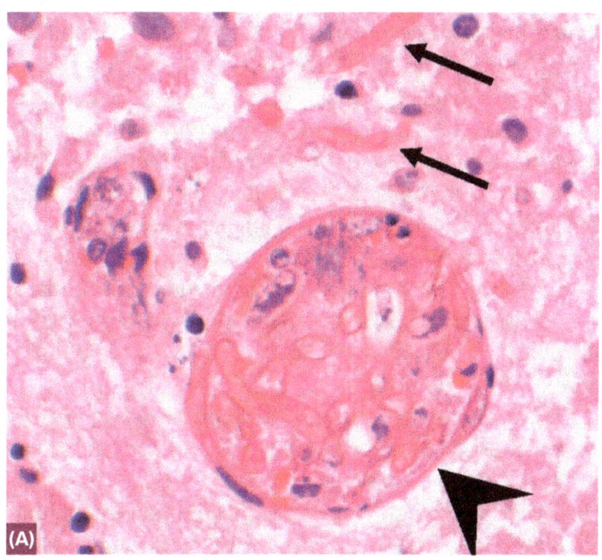

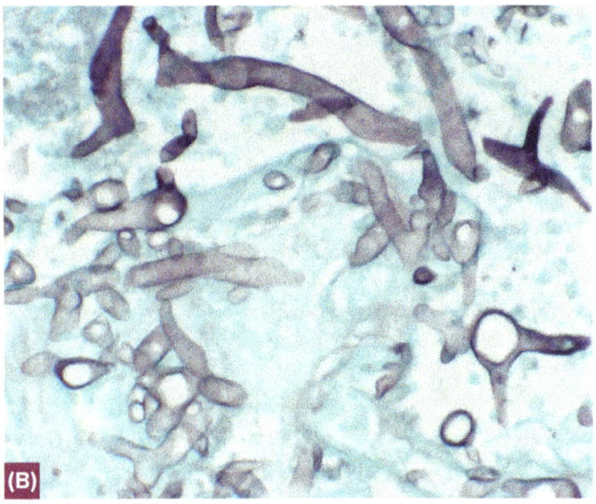

Histopathology sections of *Rhizopus oryzae* in infected brain. (A) Broad, ribbon-like, nonseptate hyphae in the parenchyma (*arrows*) and a thrombosed blood vessel with extensive intravascular hyphae (*arrowhead*) (hematoxylin and eosin). **(B)** Extensive, broad, ribbon-like hyphae invading the parenchyma (Gomori methenamine silver). (Reproduced, with permission, from Longo DL, Fauci AS, Kasper DL, Hauser SL, Jameson JL, Loscalzo J, eds. *Harrison's Principles of Internal Medicine*. 18th ed. New York, NY: McGraw-Hill Education; 2011.)

The respiratory tract is the usual portal of entry. Localized lung disease may occur as **allergic aspergillosis** in atopic individuals and as fungus balls (**aspergillosis**) or necrotizing pneumonia in patients with a history of lung disease such as **sarcoidosis, tuberculosis,** or **pneumoconioses**. In **acute invasive aspergillosis**, widespread growth of *Aspergillus* species in lung tissue leads to infarction. Hematogenous dissemination may affect multiple sites, including the CNS, eyes, heart, bone, kidneys, liver, spleen, and skin. **Cutaneous aspergillosis** may arise as a primary infection or secondary to disseminated disease. **Primary cutaneous aspergillosis** generally occurs in immunocompromised hosts at sites where the skin is disrupted by catheters, burns, or trauma or occluded by contaminated adhesive tape. It begins as an erythematous macule, papule, or nodule that may develop a hemorrhagic bulla with subsequent ulceration, resulting in a centrally necrotic eschar. KOH preparations from the intermediate-stage blister roof may reveal hyphae. **Cutaneous aspergillosis** may also disseminate in immunocompromised patients. In **disseminated aspergillosis**, cutaneous disease occurs in 5% to 11% of patients and presents as five main types: solitary necrotizing dermal plaque, subcutaneous granuloma or abscess, persistent maculopapular eruption with suppuration or necrobiosis, transient erythema or erythroderma, and progressive confluent granulomas.

In both primary and disseminated **cutaneous aspergillosis**, histopathologic examination of the dermis and subcutaneous fat reveals numerous septate hyphae (2-4 μm in diameter) that branch at a 45° angle and exhibit dichotomous branching. The hyphae are optimally visualized with methenamine silver

Table 7-23B. Aspergillosis

Clinical Features

- Ubiquitous in decaying organic matter, soil, and dust
- Caused by *Aspergillus flavus, A niger,* and *A fumigatus*
- Predisposing conditions: neutropenia, hematologic malignancy, organ transplantation–associated immunosuppression, chronic granulomatous disease
- Primary cutaneous aspergillosis associated with burns, catheter sites, hospital construction dust, and adhesive tape
- Primary cutaneous aspergillosis: ecthyma-like papule with central necrosis
- Lungs are usually portal of entry heading to disseminated disease, metastases in 5-11% of patients—necrotizing plaques, subcutaneous granulomas or abscesses, maculopapular eruption, erythema
- Hematogenous dissemination may involve CNS, liver, spleen, heart, kidneys, and eyes

Histopathologic Features

- Septate hyphae (2-4 μm diameter) that branch at a 45° angle, dichotomous
- Variable granulomatous infiltrate: neutrophils, lymphocytes, histiocytes, and giant cells
- In disseminated disease, hyphae may be intravascular and invade vessel walls

Differential Diagnosis

	Aspergillus	*Mucor*
Septa	Present	Absent
Diameter	2-4 μm	≤ 30 μm
	45°	90°
	Dichotomous	Bulbous lateral protrusions

or PAS stains. Ulceration; **pseudoepitheliomatous hyperplasia**; necrosis; and a granulomatous infiltrate of neutrophils, lymphocytes, histiocytes, and giant cells may be seen. In disseminated disease, hyphae may be seen within dermal vessels as well as invading vascular walls.

Fusariosis is caused by *Fusarium* species, a common soil fungus, and is responsible for a broad spectrum of human infections, including superficial, locally invasive, and disseminated infections, depending on host factors. Three species are implicated in human infections: *F solani, F oxysporum,* and *F moniliforme*. *Fusarium* species are frequent causes of corneal and nail infections and deep localized infections such as **mycetomas** (pale granules) and have emerged as a cause of **disseminated mycoses** among cancer patients undergoing chemotherapy and hematopoietic stem cell transplantation. Cutaneous infection may develop as a complication of ulcers, surgical trauma, and burns, especially in neutropenic patients. **Disseminated**

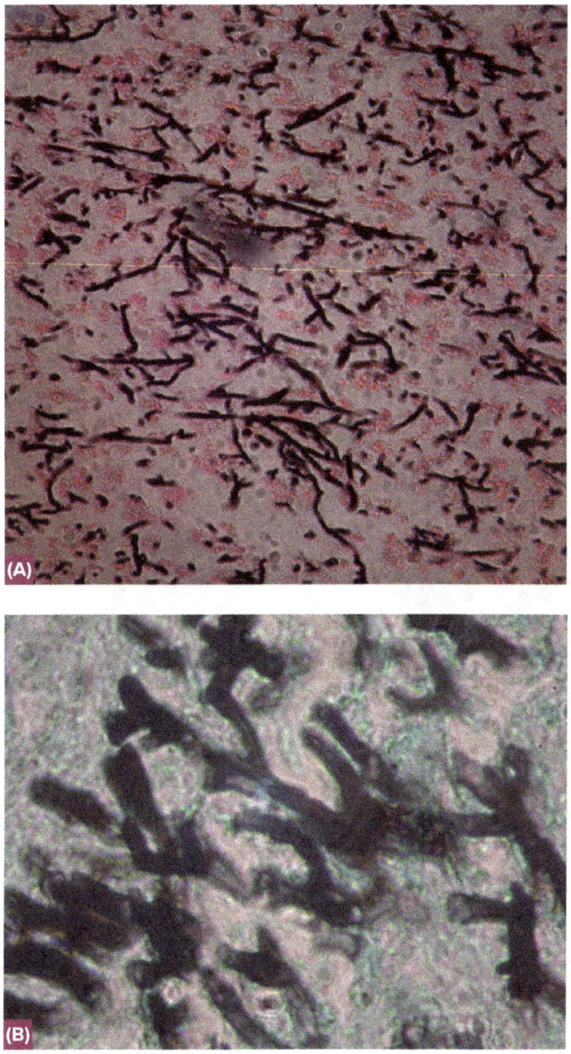

Invasive aspergillosis. (A) Uniform, branching (45°) septate hyphae (ca 4 μm in width) of *Aspergillus fumigatus* in lung tissue stained with Gomori methenamine silver (400×). **(B)** Similar preparation with Grocott stain. The hyphae are smaller than those observed in mucormycosis and exhibit 45° dichotomous branching (1000×). (Reproduced, with permission, from Carroll KC et al, eds. *Jawetz, Melnick & Adelberg's Medical Microbiology.* 26th ed. New York, NY: McGraw-Hill Education; 2013.)

fusariosis, similar to **aspergillosis**, may arise after pulmonary inhalation or as a result of spread of cutaneous disease. Risk factors for **fusariosis** include prolonged neutropenia and T-cell immunodeficiency. Similar to *Rhizopus* and *Aspergillus* species, *Fusarium* species are angioinvasive and lead to tissue infarction in neutropenic patients. However, unlike *Rhizopus* and *Aspergillus* species, *Fusarium* species continuously release spores, consisting of phialides and phialoconidia, into the blood; this intravascular adventitious sporulation is associated with a higher rate of positive blood cultures and dissemination of infection. The clinical presentation is usually fever in the setting of neutropenia; positive blood cultures, with or without lung or sinus involvement; and characteristic cutaneous lesions that range from subcutaneous painful lesions to an ecthyma gangrenosum-like necrotic lesion, which may be surrounded by a rim of erythema. The prognosis of **disseminated fusariosis** in neutropenic patients is poor.

The microscopic findings are similar to those of **aspergillosis**, both in culture and tissue sections. There is a striking tendency for the organism to exhibit angioinvasion with resultant ischemic necrosis of the skin and subcutis. *Fusarium* species have characteristic thick-walled swellings along the filaments. In culture *Fusarium* exhibits sickle-shaped, multiseptate macroconidia.

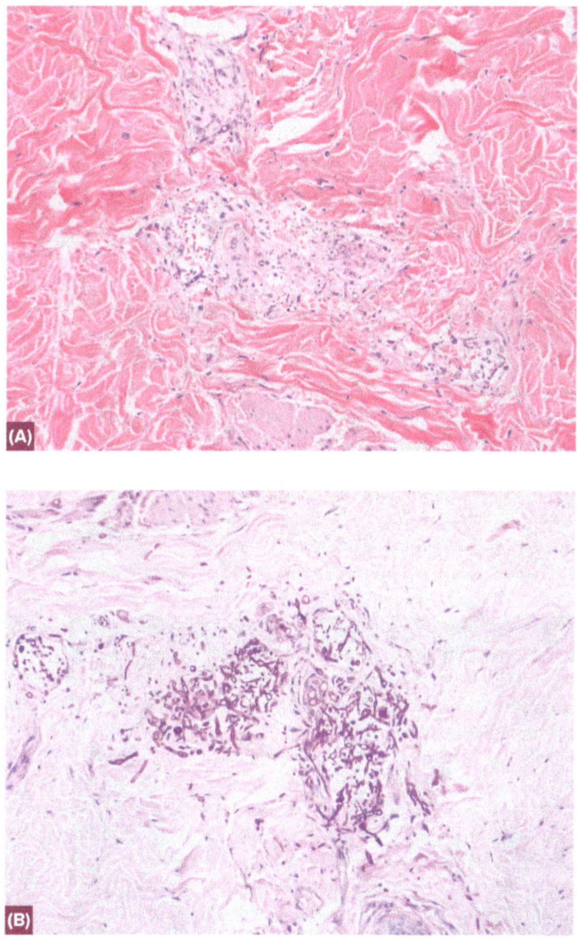

Fusariosis. (A) H&E revealing numerous angioinvasive hyphae. **(B)** The hyphae are septate and exhibit branching at 45° angles. Note the characteristic thick-walled swellings along the filaments.

ANSWER 7-24: C.

The biopsied lesion reveals superficial multilocular intraepidermal vesicles with reticular degeneration. The involved keratinocytes are enlarged with a decreased nucleus to cytoplasmic ratio and eosinophilic cytoplasm. Scattered lymphocytic infiltrates are seen in the superficial dermis. No viral inclusions are identified. **Hand-foot-and-mouth disease** is a mucocutaneous disorder that characteristically involves only a few localized sites and is most frequently caused by **coxsackie A viruses** and less commonly by **coxsackie B viruses** and **enteroviruses**. The disease is most common in children and is highly contagious. Most outbreaks occur between June and October. The illness begins with fever up to 101°F (38.6°C) with associated malaise, soreness of the throat and mouth, and refusal to eat. Cough, headache, diarrhea, and arthralgias may be present. Initially, small reddish macules appear on the oropharynx with evolution to small papulovesicles that are 1 to 3 mm in size. The latter lesions ulcerate with development of a yellow-gray base and a red peripheral rim. Ulcerations are most prevalent on the palate, buccal mucosa, tongue, and gingiva. The hands and feet are involved commonly, especially the sides and dorsa of the fingers and toes. As with mucosal lesions, initially there are reddish macules that evolve into oval or football-shaped vesicles with a surrounding red halo. Rarely, lesions may be disseminated, especially in patients with altered cutaneous barrier function, such as in atopics. The process usually resolves without incident after several days.

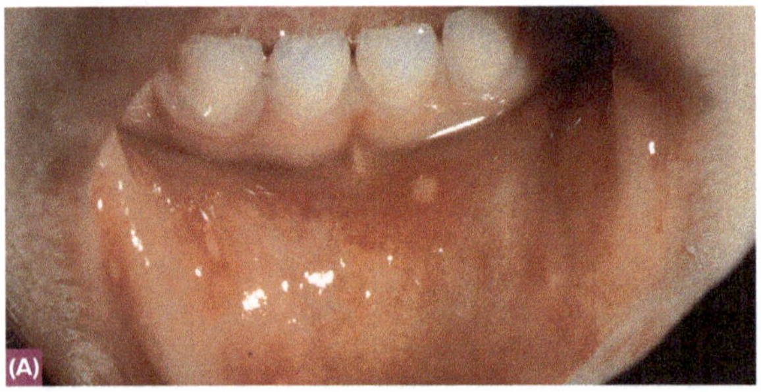

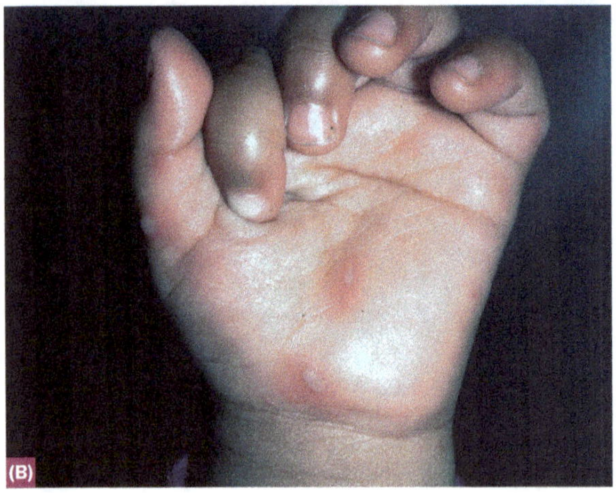

Hand-foot-and-mouth disease. (A) Multiple, superficial erosions with an erythematous halo on the lower labial mucosa; gingiva is normal. In primary herpetic gingivostomatitis, which presents with similar oral vesicular lesions, painful erosive gingivitis usually occurs as well. **(B)** Erythematous vesicular rash scattered on the palms consistent with coxsackievirus. (Part **(A)** reproduced, with permission, from Wolff K, Johnson RA, Saavedra AP. *Fitzpatrick's Color Atlas and Synopsis of Clinical Dermatology*. 7th ed. New York, NY: McGraw-Hill Education; 2013; part **(B)** reproduced, with permission, from Knoop KJ, Stack LB, Storrow AB, Thurman RJ. *The Atlas of Emergency Medicine*. 3rd ed. New York, NY: McGraw-Hill; 2010.)

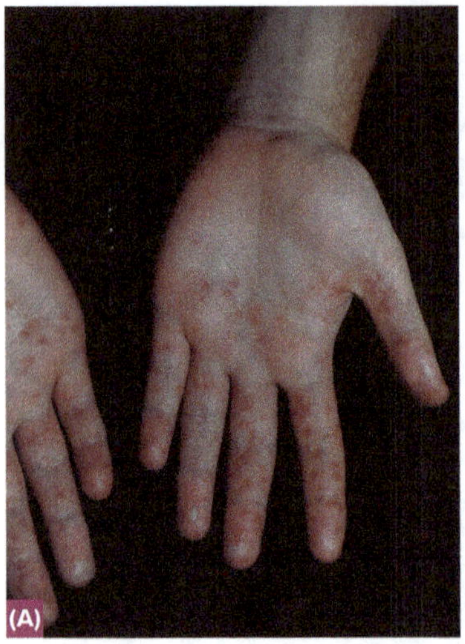

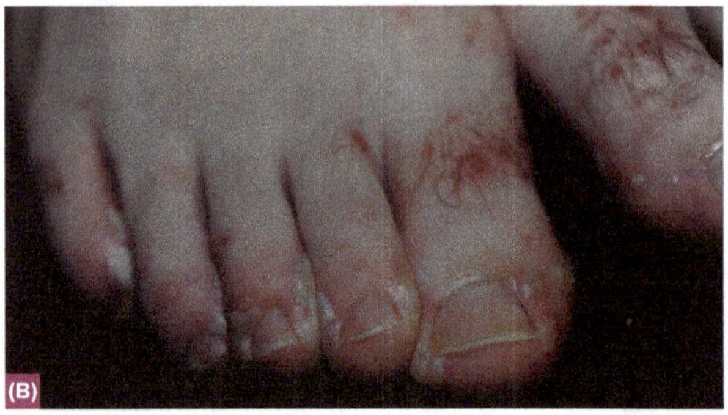

Hand-foot-and-mouth disease. A 21-year-old male with extensive blister formation on **(A)** palms and fingers, and **(B)** soles and toes. (Reproduced, with permission, from Wolff K, Johnson RA, Saavedra AP. *Fitzpatrick's Color Atlas and Synopsis of Clinical Dermatology*. 7th ed. New York, NY: McGraw-Hill Education; 2013.)

Microscopically, **hand-foot-and-mouth disease** is characterized by a variably intense inflammatory infiltrate in the superficial dermis consisting primarily of lymphocytes, but there may be variable numbers of neutrophils. The most prominent changes are in the epidermis in fully developed lesions, where there is intracellular edema (ballooning), spongiosis, and localized epidermal necrosis where cytolysis results in a reticular pattern of degeneration. Usually there is minimal epidermal hyperplasia. In time, there is confluent epidermal necrosis, crusting, and sloughing of degenerated epithelium with reepithelialization. Mucosal ulcers may appear quite similar to aphthous ulcers. There is a localized ulceration, beneath which there is an infiltrate of lymphocytes, plasma cells, and neutrophils.

In regard to the clinical differential diagnosis, other viral vesicular disorders that may be confused with **hand-foot-and-mouth disease** and include **varicella** and **herpes simplex virus (HSV) infection. Erythema multiforme** may also appear similar; especially when there is involvement of the palms and soles, however, exhibits true target lesions and is histopathologically characterized by cytotoxic interface dermatitis. Distinction of **hand-foot-and-mouth disease** from **herpes** is based on clinical features, balloon degeneration of keratinocytes, and absence of characteristic herpes viral cytopathic changes. Although **hand-foot-and-mouth disease** is has a viral etiology, no virus-specific cytopathic changes are present. Although **hand-foot-and-mouth disease** has a viral etiology, no virus-specific cytopathic changes are present. The histopathological differential diagnosis includes **acrodermatitis enteropathica** and **pellagra**, in which the microscopic findings are essentially identical. **Acrodermatitis enteropathica** is an autosomal recessive disorder of zinc absorption. It occurs in infants, bottle-fed with bovine milk, days to few weeks or in breast-fed infants, soon after weaning. Patches and plaques of dry, scaly, sharply marginated and brightly red, eczematous dermatitis evolving into vesiculobullous, pustular, erosive, and crusted lesions are seen. Initially the lesions occur in the perioral and anogenital areas. Later, lesions may extend to the scalp, hands, feet, flexural regions, and trunk. **Pellagra** is attributed to niacin deficiency and is characterized clinically by skin abnormalities, gastroenteritis, and encephalopathy (dermatitis, diarrhea, and dementia). The cutaneous features are often sunlight induced, appearing in the spring and summer and improving in winter. Pruritus and erythema occur initially on exposed areas, followed by vesicles, bullae, and largely symmetric, chronic, scaly, hyperpigmented, thickened sclerotic papules and plaques. Dusky erythema and powdery scaling of the nose, a scaling collarette around the neck with sternal extension (**Casal necklace**), glossitis, and mucous membrane ulcerations are also typical.

ANSWER 7-25: D.

Eight **herpes viruses** have now been defined. **Herpes simplex virus (HSV) 1 and 2** infections are characterized by an acute eruption of tense, umbilicated, grouped vesicles on an erythematous base, usually at or near a mucocutaneous junction (Table 7-25A). The onset is usually preceded by a prodrome of burning and itching a few hours before onset of the eruption. The vesicles appear in groups, are of pinhead size, and often later become seropurulent. Answer choice B illustrates **orolabial herpes simplex virus** in an adult woman showing a deroofed blisters (cold sore). **Primary genital HSV infection** occurs most commonly in young adults. It is transmitted through sexual contact and presents as a painful, erosive balanitis, vulvitis, or vaginitis. Individuals who have a primary attack are prone to recurrent attacks, which may have their onset shortly after the primary infection or may be delayed for months to years. There may be a "latency" period of variable duration between recurrences. A complication of **recurrent HSV** is the secondary development of **erythema multiforme**.

Table 7-25A. Herpes Simplex

Clinical Features
Localized clusters of vesicles usually on the lip (type 1) or genital mucosa (type 2)
Prodrome of burning a few hours before eruption
Primary and recurrent lesions
HSV type 1 usually above the waistline; HSV type 2 usually below the waist
Herpetic folliculitis
Herpetic whitlow (involvement of fingers)
Generalized and chronic localized herpes, often in immunocompromised hosts
Histopathologic Features
"Steel gray" nuclei of keratinocytes
Margination of chromatin and multinucleated epithelial giant cells
Eosinophilic intranuclear inclusions with clear halo
Intracellular edema and ballooning degeneration
Reticular degeneration and rupture of cell walls of epithelial cells
Acantholysis
Multiloculated intraepidermal vesicle formation
Lymphoid infiltrates, often rather dense in dermis
Infiltration of nerve twigs by infiltrate
Occasional lymphocytic and leukocytoclastic vasculitis

Other presentations of **HSV infection**, particularly in immunosuppressed patients, include **herpes folliculitis, herpetic whitlow** (HSV of the digits), **herpes cervicitis, herpes keratoconjunctivitis,** and **recurrent lumbosacral herpes** (low back and buttocks).

Kaposi varicelliform eruption or **eczema herpeticum** refers to secondary, usually widespread involvement of a primary dermatosis such as **atopic dermatitis, Darier disease, pemphigus foliaceus**, or other dermatitides complicated by HSV. Lesional skin or skin previously involved by the dermatitis is preferentially affected by typical vesicles of **HSV**. Vesicles are first confined to eczematous skin. In contrast to primary or recurrent **HSV eruptions**, in **eczema herpeticum**, lesions are not grouped but disseminated within the dermatosis and later spread to normal-appearing skin. "Punched-out" erosions may become confluent, producing large denuded areas. Successive crops of new vesiculation may occur. Common sites include the face, neck, and trunk.

Varicella is one of the most common childhood infections. The disease is caused by the **varicella-zoster virus (VZV),** which is a double-stranded DNA virus and is also a member of the family Herpesviridae (Table 7-25B). Airborne droplet infection is the usual route of transmission, although direct contact is another mode of spread. It is one of the most contagious of all infections. **Herpes zoster** represents

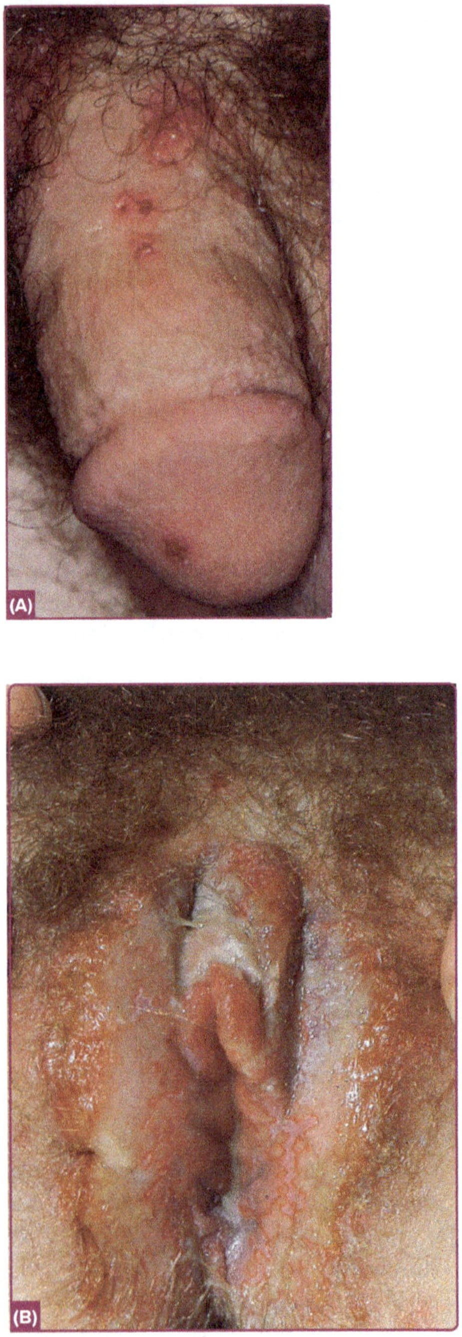

Genital herpes simplex infection. (A) Primary genital herpes with vesicles. **(B)** Primary herpetic vulvitis. (Reproduced, with permission, from Goldsmith LA, Katz SI, Gilchrest BA, Paller AS, Leffell DJ, Wolff K, eds. *Fitzpatrick's Dermatology in General Medicine*. 8th ed. New York, NY: McGraw-Hill Education; 2012. Part A Courtesy of Clyde S. Crumpacker, MD.)

reactivation of latent **varicella** infection that resides in sensory ganglia. The incubation period of **primary VZV infection ("chicken pox")** (answer choice A) ranges from 11 to 20 days and is followed by a prodrome of mild fever and malaise, often accompanied by photophobia. The eruption is characterized by crops of erythematous macules and papules

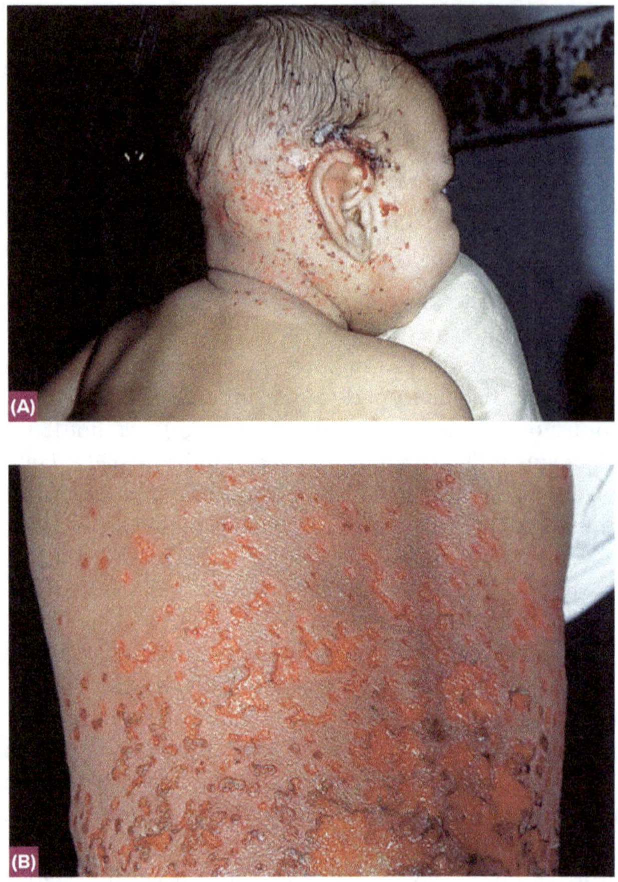

Eczema herpeticum. (A) Vesicles evolving into "punched-out" erosions. **(B)** Erosions may become confluent, producing large denuded areas. (Used with permission of Binita R. Shah, MD.)

Table 7-25B. Varicella (Chickenpox)

Clinical Features
Incubation period of 11-20 days
Mild fever, photophobia
"Dew drops on rose petal" vesicular eruption on face and trunk
Histopathologic Features
Same as HSV

on the trunk and face that evolve rapidly into vesicles of 1 to 3 mm in size with clear serous fluid surrounded by narrow red halos. The patient in answer choice A exhibits vesicles in different stages of maturation. Note the clear vesicle on an erythematous base ("dewdrop on a rose petal") in the center of the chest. The number of vesicles varies, ranging from only a few to several hundred. Older lesions crust and begin to heal usually within 1 week to 10 days.

Herpes zoster is manifest as a painful eruption of vesicles and occasionally papules on erythematous bases that develops within a sensory dermatome, usually on the trunk, but in some cases, the face, neck, or scalp may be involved (Table 7-25C). The patient in answer choice C exhibits vesicles in a classic thoracic dermatomal distribution. Usually, older individuals are affected, although patients with immunosuppression such as those with HIV infection also commonly develop the condition. **Herpes zoster** in HIV-infected patients may assume a number of unusual manifestations, especially persistent crusted, verrucous lesions.

Table 7-25C. Herpes Zoster

Clinical Features
Unilateral painful eruption of vesicles within a sensory dermatome
Ophthalmic branch of trigeminal nerve commonly involved
May be disseminated in immunocompromised patients
Histopathologic Features
Same as herpes simplex

Microscopically, there are essentially no significant differences between **HSV1, HSV2,** and **VZV infection**. The earliest change occurs in the epidermis, in which there is pallor and swelling of the cytoplasm of keratinocytes, imparting a "steel gray" appearance of nuclei. The nuclei also show margination of chromatin. Infected keratinocytes may fuse, forming characteristic multinucleated epithelial giant cells. Eosinophilic inclusion bodies usually surrounded by a clear halo may be observed in the nuclei of infected cells. Spongiosis and intracellular edema are also present in the epidermis and the epithelium of hair follicles. Infected keratinocytes characteristically develop intracellular edema, leading to ballooning degeneration, which is a feature of viral vesicles. Epithelial cells showing ballooning degeneration lose intercellular adhesions and thus become acantholytic. Intracellular edema also results in reticular degeneration and the rupture of cell walls. The latter phenomenon and acantholysis eventuate in multiloculated intraepidermal vesicles. In time, keratinocytes become necrotic and develop pyknotic nuclei and dense eosinophilic cytoplasm. There is a variably dense inflammatory infiltrate in the dermis consisting of lymphocytes, neutrophils, and occasionally eosinophils. Associated lymphocytic or **leukocytoclastic vasculitis** and inflammation are often within and around nerve twigs. Biopsy specimens from immunocompromised patients often demonstrate extensive infection of the epidermis with marked necrosis and involvement of cutaneous adnexal structures such as the hair follicles, sebaceous glands, and eccrine sweat units.

Quick Fact

HSV1, HSV2, and VZV share identical viral cytopathic changes and cannot be distinguished based on histopathology.

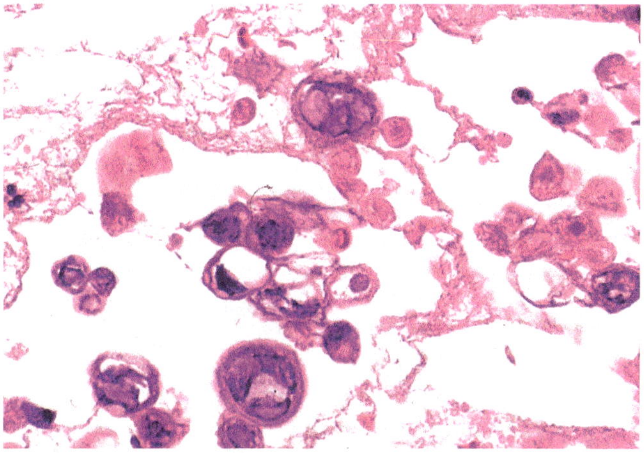

Herpes virus infection. The intraepidermal vesicle shows striking multinucleate giant cells. The nuclei within these giant cells exhibit molding and prominent ground-glass alteration of chromatin. There is also prominent reticular degeneration, resulting in the intraepidermal vesicle.

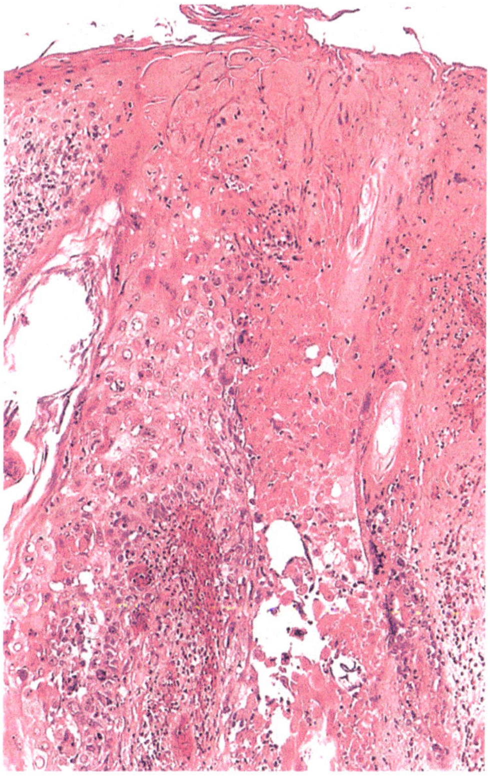

Herpes folliculitis. Edema and ballooning degeneration of follicular epithelial cells with vesicle formation are seen.

Table 7-25D. Viral Exanthems

DISEASES	ETIOLOGY	CLINICAL FEATURES	HISTOPATHOLOGIC FEATURES	DIFFERENTIAL DIAGNOSIS
Measles	Measles virus/RNA virus	Incubation period of 9-10 days Erythematous macules and papules first on the face then spread to neck, trunk, and extremities Koplik spots	Superficial psoriasiform spongiotic dermatitis with dyskeratotic keratinocytes Warthin-Finkeldey giant cells	Drug eruption, rubella, fifth disease, Kawasaki disease, scarlet fever
Rubella (German measles)	Rubella virus/RNA virus	"Butterfly" facial rash, Forschheimer spots, centrifugal spread, cervical and occipital lymphadenopathy (Winterbottom sign)	Sparse superficial perivascular dermatitis with slight spongiosis, Turk cells (atypical lymphocytes) in peripheral blood and in skin infiltrate	Scarlet fever, infectious mononucleosis, fifth disease, typhus, RMSF, secondary syphilis, and toxoplasmosis
Fifth disease (erythema infectiosum)	Parvovirus B19/DNA virus	Incubation period of 2 weeks "Slapped cheeks" sparing circumoral areas, reticulated erythematous eruption on extensor extremities	Sparse superficial perivascular dermatitis and focal spongiosis	Juvenile rheumatoid arthritis, erythema multiforme, rubella, bilateral facial erysipelas
Roseola (exanthem subitum)	HHV-6 DNA virus	Incubation period of 4-7 days Rose-pink macules and papules on trunk sparing face	Sparse superficial perivascular dermatitis	Rubella, measles, fifth disease, scarlet fever, and morbilliform drug eruptions
Hand-foot-and-mouth disease	Coxsackie virus A16, A5, A10, A7, A9, B1, B3, B5	Incubation period of 3-6 days; Papulovesicles and ulceration of palate buccal mucosa; "Football"-shaped vesicles on dorsa of fingers and toes	Spongiosis, ballooning, and epidermal necrosis with superficial perivascular dermatitis	Varicella, herpes simplex, erythema multiforme
Acute exanthem of HIV infection	HIV-1/RNA virus	Incubation period of 3-6 weeks; Morbilliform eruption involves trunk, chest, and upper arms	Superficial perivascular, dermatitis spongiosis, and necrotic keratinocytes	Drug eruption, CMV, infectious mononucleosis
Infectious mononucleosis	EBV/DNA virus	Pharyngitis, fever and cervical lymphadenopathy, splenomegaly, lymphocytosis, pinkish macules and papules on trunk and upper arms	Superficial perivascular, dermatitis spongiosis and parakeratosis, atypical lymphocytes in infiltrate	Drug eruption, CMV, toxoplasmosis
Acute exanthem of CMV	CMV/DNA virus	Similar to EBV "mononucleosis syndrome"	Similar to other viral exanthemata with characteristic "owl's eye" inclusions in cytoplasm and nuclei of endothelial cells	Infectious mononucleosis, toxoplasmosis

The patient in answer choice D exhibits a **morbilliform viral exanthem** attributed to **infectious mononucleosis** and concomitant amoxicillin therapy (Table 7-25D). **Infectious mononucleosis** is caused by the **Epstein-Barr virus (EBV)**, which is a member of the human herpesvirus family. It is an enveloped icosahedral DNA virus that grows well in B lymphocytes, leading to their immortalization. Infections typically develop in teens and young adults between ages 17 and 25 years. Infections occur less commonly in young children and are seen rarely before age 1 year or after age 40 years. There is a long incubation period of between 30 and 50 days. Administration of ampicillin and, less commonly, penicillin, cephalosporins, or tetracycline leads to the development of an **exanthematous eruption** (70%-100% of cases) that is usually more widespread and erythematous than the primary eruption. It usually develops 7 to 10 days after institution of the antibiotic. Periorbital edema is present in 25% to 30% of patients. Occasionally, jaundice, arthritis, and pneumonitis may be seen. **Viral exanthems** are generally nonspecific and may be associated with many viral infections such as **HIV, Human herpes virus 6 (HHV6),** and **Measles, Rubella, Parvovirus B19,** and **enteroviruses. Disseminated HSV** may rarely present with a diffuse eruption, but the eruption is more papulopustular with areas of ulceration (similar to eczema herpeticum). **Viral exanthems** are microscopically characterized by superficial perivascular lymphohistiocytic infiltrates with minimal epidermal involvement. Mild spongiosis or vacuolar interface dermatitis may be present. Although the lymphocytes of the infiltrate may exhibit atypical features (enlarged irregular nuclei), viral cytopathic changes are not characteristic for **EBV-associated viral exanthems.**

ANSWER 7-26: E.

The biopsy reveals a slightly acanthotic epidermis with swollen superficial keratinocytes containing bluish-gray cytoplasm and chunky keratohyaline granules. The keratinocyte nuclei are not pleomorphic and suprabasilar mitoses are not present. **Epidermodysplasia verruciformis** refers to a cutaneous eruption caused by specific subtypes of **HPV**, especially types 3, 5, and 10, in which patients have an abnormal propensity to develop cutaneous **squamous cell carcinoma** after ultraviolet irradiation. **Epidermodysplasia verruciformis** may be familial or sporadic. Familial cases usually demonstrate autosomal recessive inheritance, although an x-linked inheritance has also been reported. Affected individuals develop numerous red, flat to skin-colored, wart-like papules on sun-exposed surfaces. The condition is linked to defective cell-mediated immunity, with elucidation of mutations in *EVER1* and *EVER2* genes (band 17q25). Malignant transformation is common.

Microscopically, the hydropic superficial keratinocytes filled with gray-blue ("robin's egg blue") cytoplasm are pathognomonic. Other features of **HPV** infection such as chunky keratohyaline granules, peripherally marginated nuclear chromatin, and occasional multinucleation may be present. Evaluation for full-thickness keratinocytic atypia and suprabasilar mitoses is important to exclude evolution to **squamous cell carcinoma in situ.**

Answer choice E describes **Heck disease** (aka **focal epithelial hyperplasia**), in which patients develop pink-white, verrucous papules of the mucous membranes of the lip, tongue, or less commonly the buccal mucosa, floor of the mouth, and palate. It is associated with infection by HPV types 13 and 32. The lesions are painless and very contagious. Children and adolescents are most commonly affected. Microscopically, the oral squamous epithelium exhibits focal parakeratosis, hyperkeratosis, acanthosis, and marked papillomatosis. Basal cell hyperplasia with increased mitoses is common. The superficial keratinocytes exhibit isolated perinuclear cellular vacuolization (**koilocytosis**), cellular binucleation, and nuclear irregularities. Epithelial dysplasia is not present.

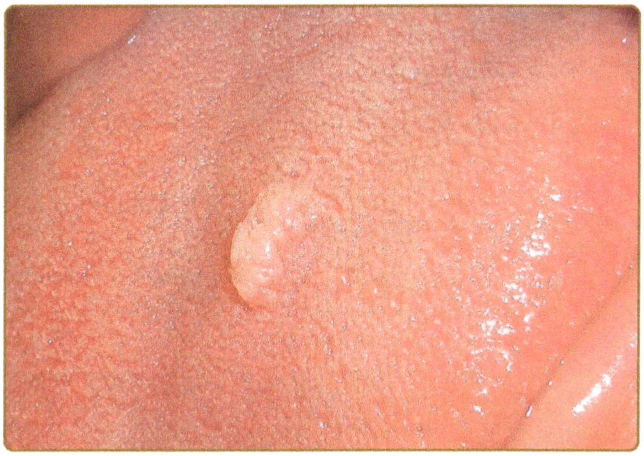

Focal epithelial hyperplasia (Heck disease). There is a pink verrucous papule on the tongue. (Courtesy of Shelly Abramowicz, Children's Hospital Boston, Boston, MA.)

ANSWER 7-27: F.

This patient's biopsy reveals full thickness keratinocytic atypia and numerous suprabasilar mitoses and dyskeratotic cells, consistent with **Bowenoid papulosis** (high grade squamous intraepithelial lesion [HGSIL], PeIN III). **Human papillomavirus infection (HPV)** is an extremely prevalent disorder and is one of the most common viral infections of human beings (Table 7-27A). The causative agents are small double-stranded DNA viruses that are 50 to 55 nm in diameter. More than 100 different strains have now been described. **HPV** is transmitted by close, repeated contact that is often sexual in nature, although patients may inoculate themselves and thus spread lesions from one body site to another. These viruses all have a tropism for epithelial cells and result in distinctive clinical presentations (Table 7-27B). After internalization, the virus

Table 7-27B. Human Papillomavirus Infection

CLINICAL FEATURES	HISTOPATHOLOGIC FEATURES	DIFFERENTIAL DIAGNOSIS
Condyloma acuminata Anogenital areas Soft sessile lesions smooth or digitated surface 3-5 mm Often multiple	*Condyloma acuminata* Polypoid configuration Epidermal hyperplasia Focal parakeratosis in invaginations of epidermis Koilocytes Dyskeratosis	*Condyloma acuminata* Bowenoid papulosis Squamous papilloma Verrucous carcinoma
Verruca vulgaris Exposed skin Fingers, hands, dorsal aspects; face Hyperkeratotic papules, plaques Solitary or grouped lesions Filiform variants on face Mosaic variants on palms and soles	*Verruca vulgaris* Hyperkeratosis Focal parakeratosis overlying epidermal papillomatosis Digitated epidermal hyperplasia Hypergranulosis Vacuolization of upper Malpighian layer with prominent keratohyaline granules Dilated vessels in dermal papillae	*Verruca vulgaris* Epidermal nevus Seborrheic keratosis
Verruca plana Face, extremities Skin-colored or brown, slightly elevated papules Barely palpable 1-3 mm Usually multiple or numerous	*Verruca plana* Basket-weave hyperkeratosis Often absence of parakeratosis Slight or no papillomatosis Hypergranulosis Vacuolated keratinocytes (Bird's-eye cells) in upper Malpighian layer	*Verruca plana* Seborrheic keratosis Stucco keratosis
Verruca plantaris Soles, particularly ball of foot Solitary often Firm papules or plaques Often marked hyperkeratosis	*Verruca plantaris* Hyperkeratosis Prominent papillomatosis Vacuolization of keratinocytes Prominent eosinophilic cytoplasmic inclusions at periphery of cell Rounded deeply basophilic nuclei	*Verruca plantaris* Punctate keratosis Verrucous carcinoma

Table 7-27A. Human Papillomavirus

Condyloma acuminatum HPV-6, -8, -11, -16, and -18
Verruca vulgaris HPV-1, -2, -3, and -4
Verruca plana HPV-3
Verruca plantaris and palmaris HPV-1, -2
Epidermodysplasia verruciformis HPV-3, -5, -12, -17, -19, and -29
Bowenoid papulosis HPV-16, -18
Verrucous carcinoma HPV-61, -11

enters the nucleus, eventuating in either productive infection or a period of latency. Once infected, the host almost always remains infected for life, irrespective of whether clinical lesions develop or not. In active infections, transcription of **HPV** takes place primarily in basal cells, and virion production occurs in the more differentiated layers of the epithelium. Thus, only the surface epithelium contains infectious viral particles.

In addition to causing verrucae and papillomata, HPV infection may lead to **squamous cell carcinoma**. Proteins produced by the oncogenic HPVs bind p53, a tumor suppressor gene product, resulting in unregulated cell growth and neoplasia. Particular **HPV** types tend to cause predictable lesions, but there is considerable overlap. Whereas types 6 and 11 generally induce benign lesions, types 16, 18, 31, and 33 are associated with potential for malignancy, especially types 16 and 18. Use of a quadrivalent **HPV** vaccine for types 6, 11, 16, and 18 has been shown to reduce the incidence of **HPV-associated anogenital disease** in young women.

Condyloma acuminata, also known as **genital warts**, is the most common venereal disease in the United States and poses a public health problem of major magnitude. The annual incidence of this disorder has been reported to be as high as 0.1% of the entire population. The incubation period varies from 3 weeks to 8 months, averaging 2.8 months. Men and women are affected similarly, and the median age of infection with **anogenital HPV** is 22 to 25 years. In men, the most common sites of involvement are the penis; urethra; scrotum; and perianal, anal, and rectal areas. Types 6, 8, and 11 **HPV** are the most common viral isolates from **anogenital condylomata**, followed by types 16 and 18. Clinically, lesions are usually manifest as soft, sessile tumors with surfaces that may be either smooth or markedly digitated with numerous finger-like projections. **Penile condylomata** are usually 3 to 5 mm in diameter and often occur in groups of three to four.

In women, the spectrum of clinical disease induced by **HPV** may be quite broad. Classic exophytic lesions of the external genitalia generally are readily recognized, although detection of other forms of **HPV** infection requires colposcopic and sigmoidoscopic examination. **Vulvar condylomata acuminata** appear as soft, whitish, sessile tumors with papillae or fine, finger-like projections seen most commonly in moist areas such as the introitus and labia. **Cervical condylomata** occur in 20% of women with **HPV** infection involving other areas of the genital tract. Papillary epithelial projections are usually present at the cervical transformation zone and involve the squamous epithelium on colposcopic examination. While **HPV** types 6, 8, and 11 are associated with benign epithelial proliferations, types 16 and 18 are associated with malignant transformation (as in the patient in question).

Microscopically, the **condyloma acuminatum** is a papular or nodular lesion with prominent acanthosis and often **koilocytosis**. Lesions are usually gently papillated and rounded, although they may be digitated ("church spires"). Lesions frequently have a striking resemblance to **seborrheic keratosis**. The epithelial retia are bulbous and branching and may simulate **pseudoepitheliomatous hyperplasia** in some cases. The cells of the upper portion of the epithelium have perinuclear vacuolization and round or "raisinoid" (crinkled) hyperchromatic nuclei. The latter cytopathic alteration is characteristic of **HPV** and constitutes **koilocytosis**. Often anisokaryosis of keratinocytes and dyskeratotic cells are present as well. In many cases, increased mitoses are also observed. The dermis or lamina propria appears edematous with dilated blood vessels and a variably intense lymphocytic infiltrate.

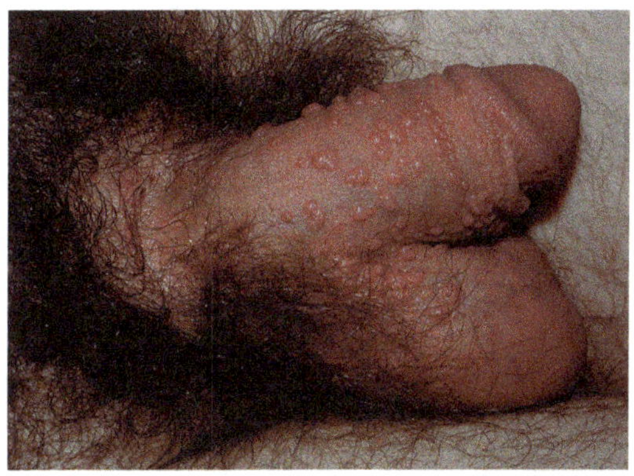

Condyloma acuminata. Numerous well-defined papules on the penis and scrotum. (Reproduced, with permission, from Wolff K, Johnson RA, Saavedra AP. *Fitzpatrick's Color Atlas and Synopsis of Clinical Dermatology*. 7th ed. New York, NY: McGraw-Hill Education; 2013.)

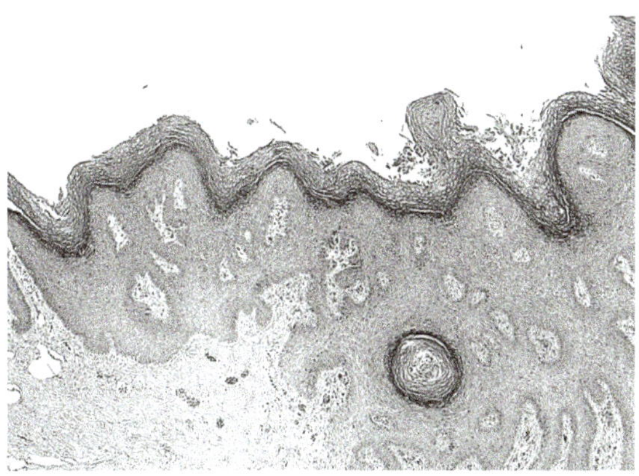

Condyloma acuminatum. The lesion shows hyperkeratosis, a polypoid configuration, and slight papillomatosis. Note the horn-cyst and resemblance to seborrheic keratosis.

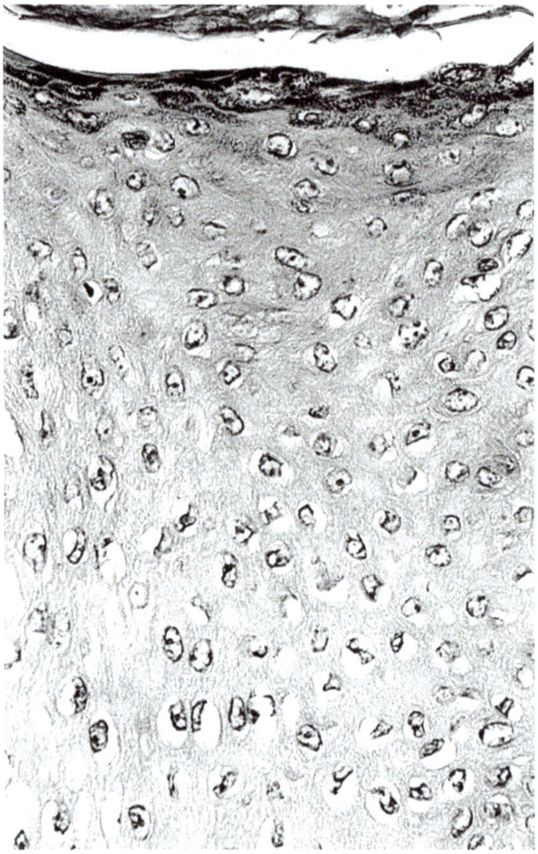

Condyloma acuminatum. This field shows koilocytes with the characteristic distortion of nuclear outlines. The nuclei are wrinkled (raisin-like) with clear perinuclear halos. Focal binucleation is present. The superficial granular layer keratinocytes contain large chunky keratohyaline granules.

Verrucae vulgares, or **common warts**, are the most common manifestation of **HPV** infection, occurring most frequently on the dorsal aspects of the fingers and hands. Clinically, they present as circumscribed, firm papules or plaques with a rough surface. They may occur singly or in groups and are caused most commonly by **HPV** types 1, 2, 3, and 4. **Filiform warts** are more slender and elongated, commonly localized to the eyelids and beard region.

Microscopically, **verruca vulgares** generally show epidermal hyperplasia with acanthosis, papillomatosis, and dilated blood vessels in the papillary dermis, intraepidermal hemorrhage, and parakeratosis. The **koilocytes** of **verrucae** contain enlarged, clumped keratohyaline granules that appear intensely basophilic. Vertical columns of parakeratosis are also present at the tips of individual digitations. There is often hemorrhage within the cornified layer at the tips of individual digitations. These changes are more pronounced in relatively early, well-developed lesions; however, involuted or older lesions often lack these characteristic features and rather demonstrate compact ortho- and parakeratosis with wedge-shaped hypergranulosis, slight papillomatosis, and acanthosis.

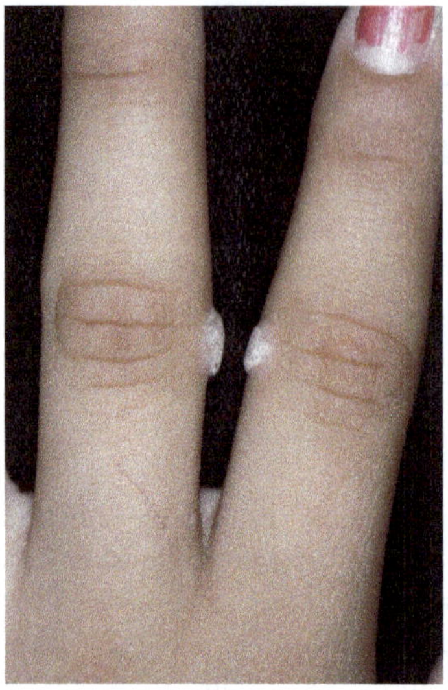

Verruca vulgaris. Warts may infect the skin on opposing digits causing "kissing warts." (Reproduced, with permission, from Usatine RP, Smith MA, Mayeaux EJ Jr, Chumley HS, eds. Color Atlas of Family Medicine. 2nd ed. New York, NY: McGraw-Hill Education; 2012. Used with permission of Richard P. Usatine, MD.)

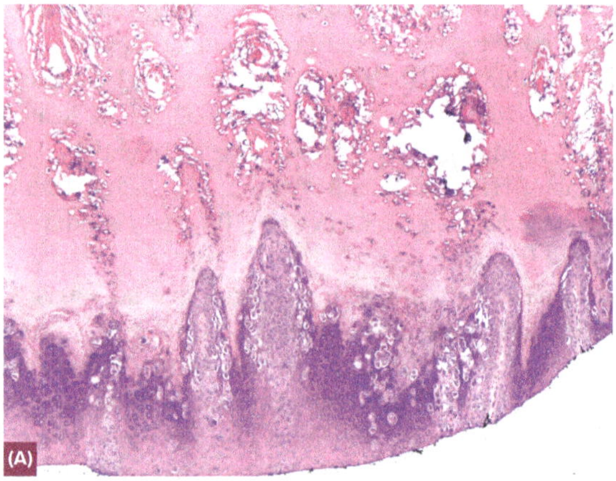

(A)

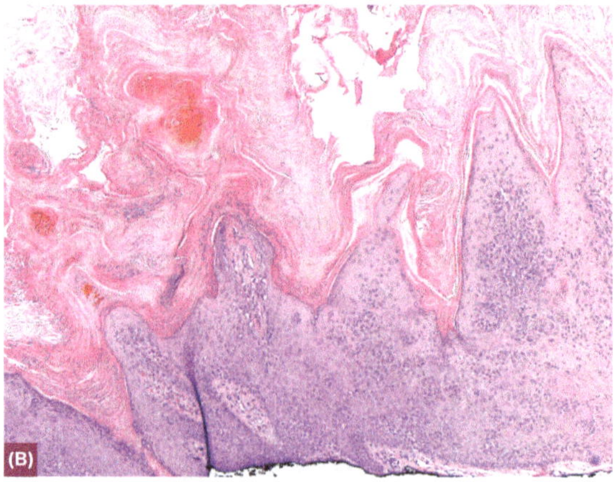

(B)

Verruca vulgaris. (A) There is acanthosis and "church spire–like" papillomatosis. The keratinocytes within the granular layer are enlarged with perinuclear halos and chunky keratohyaline granules. There is thick parakeratosis overlying the "church spires" containing foci of hemorrhage. **(B)**: Note the hemorrhagic infarcted tips, indicative of trauma.

Verruca plana, or **flat warts**, are a 1- to 3-mm, slightly elevated, skin-colored or slightly brownish papules. They are usually well demarcated and exhibit a minimally hyperkeratotic surface. They are often multiple and commonly involve the face or extremities.

Microscopically, **verruca plana** are only slightly elevated and show less pronounced or no papillomatosis compared with common verruca. In general, the stratum corneum has a basket-weave pattern of hyperkeratosis with little or no parakeratosis. Perhaps the most striking finding is the presence of vacuolated koilocytes (so-called "bird's-eye" cells) in the superficial malpighian layer of the epidermis.

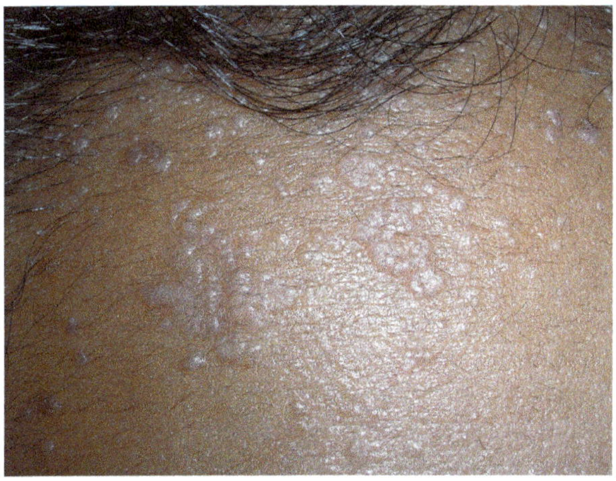

Flat warts on a patient's forehead. (Reproduced, with permission, from Usatine RP, Smith MA, Mayeaux EJ Jr, Chumley HS, eds. Color Atlas of Family Medicine. 2nd ed. New York, NY: McGraw-Hill Education; 2012. Used with permission of Richard P. Usatine, MD.)

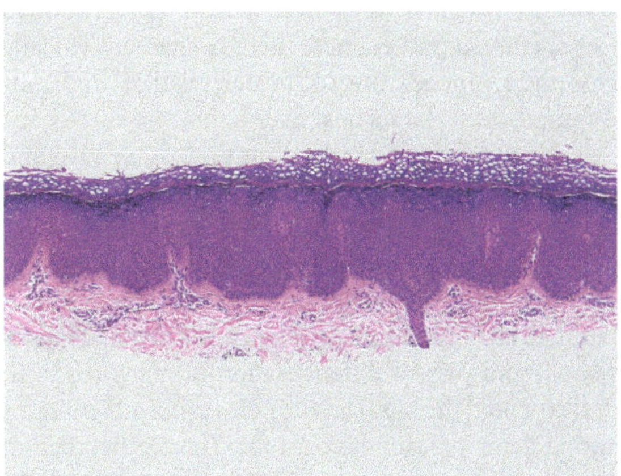

Verruca plana. The lesion demonstrates hyperkeratosis, hypergranulosis, slight acanthosis, and the characteristic vacuolated or "bird's-eye" cells in the uppaer spinous layer.

Warts on the soles (**verruca plantaris; aka myrmecia**) are variants of **verrucae vulgares**, most commonly occurring as solitary lesions on the ball of the foot, and they typically exhibit a markedly thickened cornified layer. **Mosaic warts** are coalesced clusters of warts on the sole; they are not generally as elevated as other **plantar verrucae**, possibly because of constant weight bearing. They tend to recur after removal, and because of the massive number of viral particles being shed, they tend to be more infectious than other verrucae. **Plantar warts** may lead to severe pain with walking and often pose a difficult therapeutic problem.

Microscopically, **plantar verrucae** show features similar to **verruca vulgaris**, although there may be less papillomatosis because the lesions tend to be endophytic. Parakeratosis containing large chunky keratohyaline granules are present with subjacent markedly thickened granular layer. **Koilocytes**, are located in the upper portion of the epidermis, especially the granular layer.

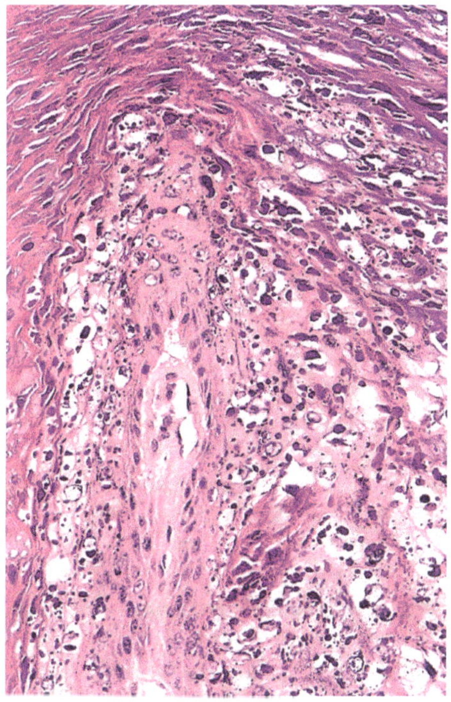

Verruca plantaris (myrmecia). The lesion exhibits hypergranulosis with prominent vacuolization of keratinocytes, many of which contain large keratohyalin granules.

Bowenoid papulosis refers to a localized form of **squamous cell carcinoma in situ** that develops as a consequence of infection by oncogenic **HPVs**, especially types 16 and 18. Lesions may clinically appear identical to **condylomata acuminata** but usually consist of small, brown, flat-topped papules involving the genital and perigenital areas. The condition is seen in both sexes but is more common in men. Lesions may become confluent and hyperplastic, and in some cases they may progress to fully developed **invasive squamous cell carcinoma**. The shaft of the penis is involved more commonly than the glans.

Microscopically, **bowenoid papulosis** demonstrates architectural features similar to condyloma acuminatum, but cytologically, the changes of a full thickness atypical keratinocytic proliferation and features of **squamous cell carcinoma in situ** are seen. Individual keratinocytes are large, hyperchromatic, and pleomorphic and are closely crowded together, and they fail to demonstrate normal maturation from the basal cell layer to the granular cell layer. Recently, a unified histopathological nomenclature for all HPV-associated preinvasive squamous lesions of the lower anogenital tract have been recommended (LAST). The nomenclature is similar to that used for the female cervix (grades I, II, and III). Lesions with full thickness keratinocyte atypia should be referred to as "high grade squamous intraepithelial lesion (HGSIL)" with secondary reference to anatomic site and grade (i.e. penis = PeIN III, vulva=VIN III, vagina = VaIN III, anus=AIN III). **Epidermodysplasia verruciformis** demonstrates papillomatosis, large vacuolated cells in the epidermis, and variable keratinocytic atypia. In some cases, there is an unusual form of dyskeratosis with corps rond-like bodies in the basket-weave stratum corneum.

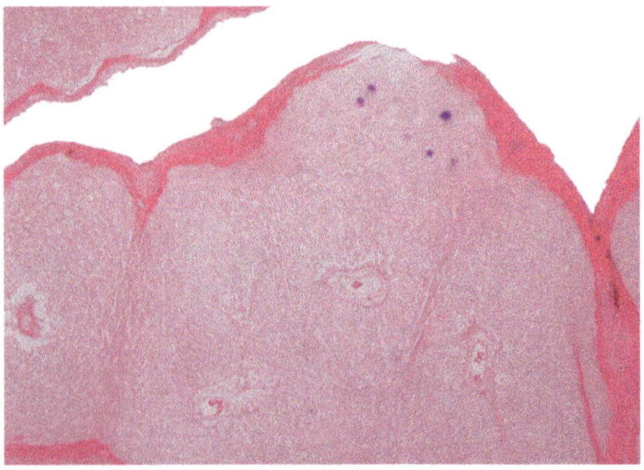

Condyloma acuminatum. In situ hybridization study for HPV detection demonstrates very focal staining of keratinocytes (blue nuclei) for the high-risk HPV strains 16 and 18.

Giant HPV-induced verrucous carcinomas are large, vegetating tumors developing most commonly in the genital and perigenital areas. Other sites include the oral mucosa and soles. These tumors appear as warts, which bluntly invade the underlying dermis. The lesions appear to "sink" down into the dermis and are frequently misdiagnosed on superficial biopsies.

ANSWER 7-28: C.

The patient's biopsy reveals marked inter- and intracellular edema, vacuolization, and ballooning degeneration, consistent with **Orf. Poxviruses** are the largest animal viruses and are the only viruses that are visible by light microscopy. Three groups affect humans: **orthopoxviruses** such as **variola** and **vaccinia**, which are ovoid and 300 by 250 nm in diameter; **parapoxviruses** such as those which cause **orf** and **milker's nodule**, which are cylindrical and 260 by 160 nm in diameter; and the **molluscum contagiosum** virus, which has an oval bullet shape and is 275 by 200 nm in diameter (Table 7-28A). Humans may also be affected by **tanapox**, which is somewhat similar to the **parapoxviruses**. These are complex DNA viruses that replicate in the cytoplasm and are adapted to proliferation in keratinocytes. Spread is primarily by direct contact with infectious

Table 7-28A. Poxvirus Infections

Poxvirus Infections
Orthopoxviruses
Variola
Vaccinia
Cowpox
Parapoxviruses
Orf
Milker's nodule
Tanapox
Virus of molluscum contagiosum

material from an infected individual or animal or via fomites, although **variola** is spread via aerosolized droplets.

Clinically, all of the **poxvirus** infections have prominent cutaneous manifestations. Although **smallpox** vaccination is no longer routine except in military settings, occasional infections with **vaccinia** are encountered. The most important manifestation is **eczema vaccinatum**, which represents a widespread eruption of edematous, inflamed lesions in individuals with altered cutaneous barrier function, such as those with atopic dermatitis. These patients usually have a high fever and lymphadenopathy. The condition may be fatal, and there is a 5% mortality rate.

Animal poxviruses may affect humans. Human **monkeypox** is indistinguishable clinically from **smallpox**, although there is more pronounced lymphadenopathy. **Cowpox** is primarily a disease of cattle, although humans may be infected on occasion. After an incubation period of 5 to 7 days, a papule develops that vesiculates, becomes pustular, and then ulcerates. The pustule, which is often umbilicated, is surrounded by a zone of erythema and edema. There is characteristically lymphangitis and lymphadenitis with fever, myalgia, and constitutional symptoms. Lesions heal over 3 to 4 weeks. Lesions are most commonly present on the hands, arms, or face and may be multiple.

Microscopically, the acute inflammatory **poxvirus** infections all have similar features and usually exhibit prominent spongiosis, ballooning degeneration, dermal edema, and acute inflammation. Individual lesions demonstrate changes that are distinct and permit differentiation in many cases. In **vaccinia** and **cowpox**, the basal layer of the epidermis contains large, eosinophilic cytoplasmic inclusions. There is necrosis of the epithelium with spongiosis; pallor of keratinocytes; and a dense infiltrate consisting mostly of neutrophils, lymphocytes, and some eosinophils. There are also extravasated erythrocytes in the dermis with prominent papillary dermal edema.

Orf is caused by a **parapoxvirus** that is widespread in sheep and goats, affecting mainly lambs and kids. Human lesions are caused by direct inoculation of infected material and are common among shepherds, veterinary surgeons, and other individuals with exposure to these animals. There is an incubation period of 5 to 6 days, after which a small, firm, red

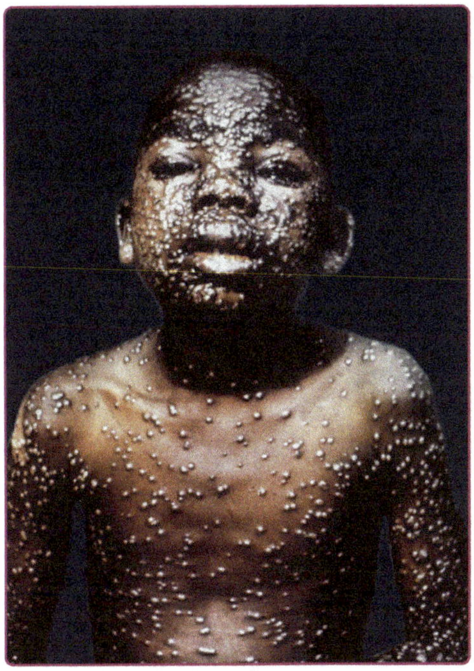

Small pox. Pustular smallpox lesions with characteristic highest density on the face and extremities. [Reproduced with permission from The Centers for Disease Control and Prevention (CDC) Public Health Image Library, Atlanta, GA, USA.]

or reddish-blue papule enlarges to form an umbilicated hemorrhagic pustule or bulla. The lesion enlarges to up to 3 to 5 cm in diameter and becomes crusted. A grayish to violaceous ring is surrounded by a zone of redness and warmth. The lesions are usually solitary or few in number and are located most commonly on the fingers, hands, or forearms. There may be tenderness and associated lymphangitis and regional adenitis with mild fever. Spontaneous recovery usually occurs within 3 to 6 weeks.

Microscopically, **Orf** demonstrates marked inter- and intracellular edema, vacuolization, and ballooning degeneration. A dense infiltrate is seen in the dermis that has a characteristic architecture, consisting mainly of histiocytes and macrophages centrally with lymphocytes and plasma cells at the periphery. Characteristically, there are very few neutrophils. There is also prominent vascularity with an increased number of small blood vessels, many of which show swelling and proliferation of endothelial cells. Ultrastructural studies show viral particles within the cytoplasm of degenerating epidermal cells.

Milker's nodule is also caused by a **parapoxvirus** that most commonly leads to infection of the teats and mouths of cattle so that milkers, farmers, and veterinarians are accidental hosts. The infection may be transmitted by contaminated fomites in some cases. There is an incubation period of 5 days to 2 weeks, after which a small, red papule develops that enlarges and becomes violaceous, firm, and slightly tender over the course of 1 week. The epidermis becomes opaque and grayish, and soon after, a crust develops centrally. As

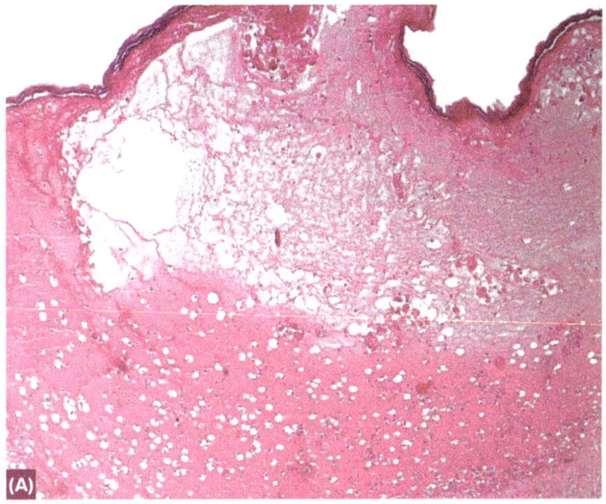

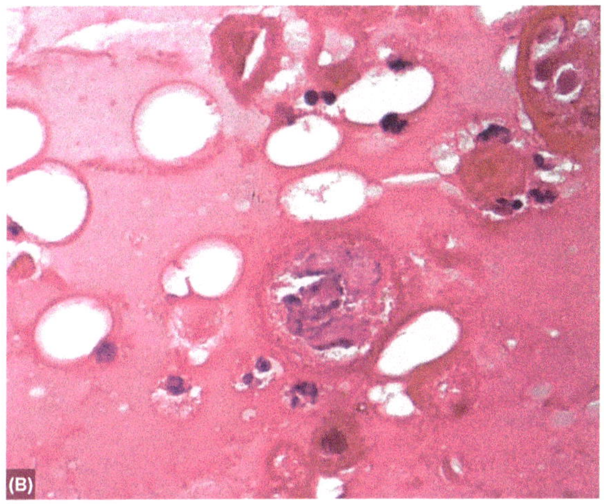

Smallpox. (A) This biopsy of smallpox shows a hemorrhagic necrolytic blister associated with striking acantholysis and marked epithelial degeneration. Although clinically the lesions may have a pustular appearance, the vesicles are actually composed of serum and necrotic cellular debris. **(B)** Higher power magnification reveals prominent intracytoplasmic and intranuclear inclusions with multinucleation.

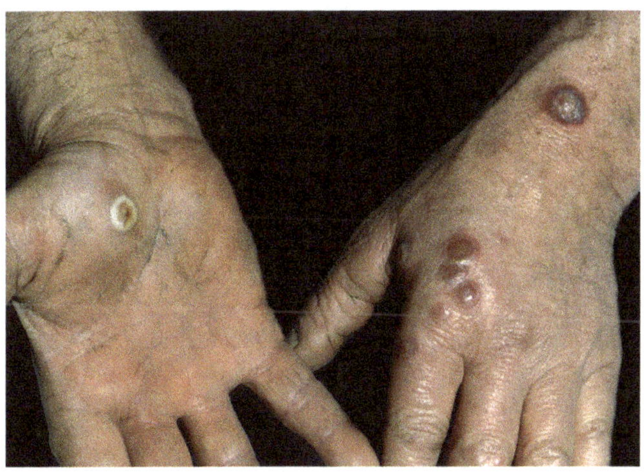

Orf. Multiple lesions on hands. Multiple blisters with target patterns in lesions on the hands of a sheep herder.

with other **poxvirus** infections, central umbilication is usually present. There is a surrounding zone of erythema, and there may be lymphangitis. Lesions resolve over 4 to 6 weeks without scarring. In contrast to **orf**, lesions are usually multiple and number between two and five but may be more numerous. The most common sites of involvement are the hands and fingers. Rarely, a more widespread papulovesicular eruption of the hands, arms, legs, and neck may develop.

Microscopically, **milker's nodule** is characterized by multilocular vesicle formation in the epidermis that is strikingly acanthotic. There is characteristically less ballooning degeneration than in **orf**. There is often marked parakeratosis, and eosinophilic cytoplasmic and intranuclear inclusions are seen commonly. The dermis is edematous, and there is an infiltrate of mononuclear cells that may be granulomatous.

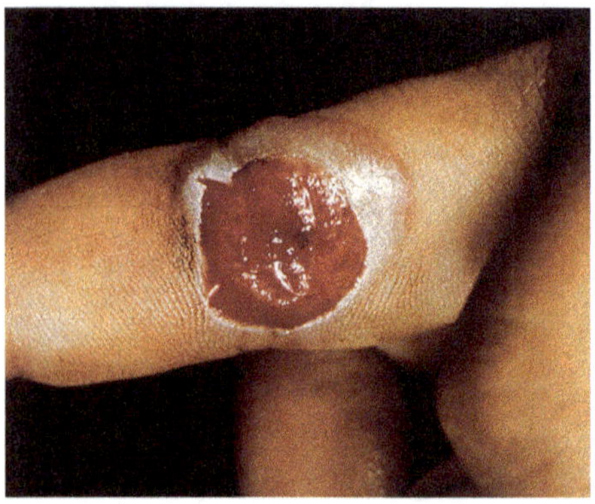

Milker's nodule on the finger. A single beefy eroded nodule on the finger of a dairy farmer at the site of inoculation. (Reproduced, with permission, from Wolff K, Johnson RA, Saavedra AP. *Fitzpatrick's Color Atlas and Synopsis of Clinical Dermatology.* 7th ed. New York, NY: McGraw-Hill Education; 2013.)

Molluscum contagiosum is the most common human disease induced by **poxviruses**. Infection occurs after contact with infected individuals and fomites. It is common in childhood, although it is rare under the age of 1 year. In children, the face, limbs, and trunk are involved commonly. A second peak occurs in young adults due to sexual transmission, with involvement of the genital and perineal skin. The face is involved commonly in HIV-infected patients. Any body site may be involved, including the mucous membranes. The incubation period ranges from 14 days to 6 months. The individual lesion is a translucent, skin-colored to whitish dome-shaped papule that is characteristically umbilicated with a central pore. Lesions range from 1 to 10 mm and may be significantly larger, sometimes resembling **keratoacanthoma**, especially in immunocompromised hosts. Small lesions may coalesce to form plaques. In time, the lesions may become inflamed, suppurative, and crusted before eventual resolution. Most cases are self-limited and resolve within 6 to 9 months, although some may persist for as long as 3 or 4 years.

Microscopically, the **molluscum contagiosum** virus initially enters basal keratinocytes and is accompanied by

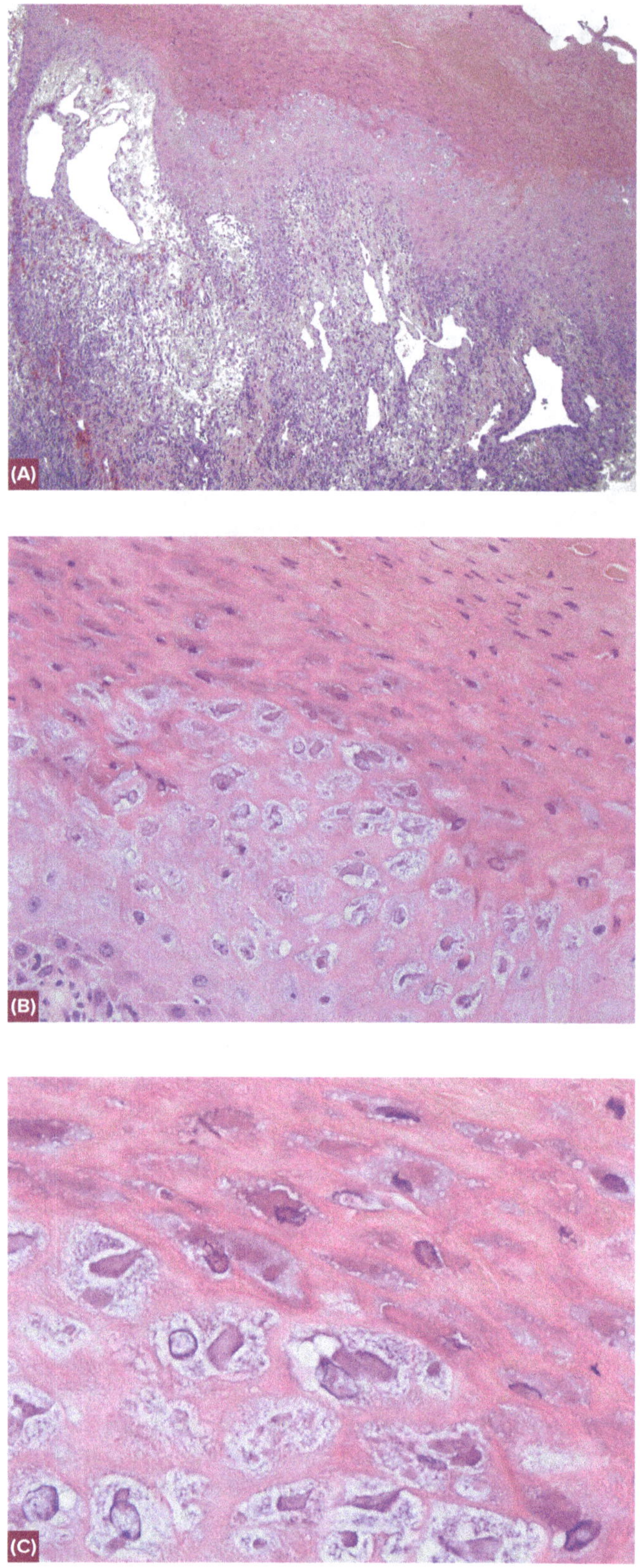

Milker's nodule. (A) Low-power view of a lesion of a milker's nodule shows a striking mononuclear cell dominant infiltrate with prominent vascularity and vascular ectasia. **(B), (C)** Prominent intracytoplasmic and nuclear eosinophilic inclusions are seen within the epidermal keratinocytes.

an increase in cell turnover, leading to epidermal proliferation. The basal layer remains intact, and cells at the core of the lesion become enlarged as a consequence of the accumulation of masses of viral material and appear as large, purplish red bodies (**molluscum bodies**) that are up to 25 μm in diameter. The proliferation has a distinct lobulated character with formation of a central crater that corresponds to the central umbilication observed clinically. Lesions typically have an exo- or endophytic appearance. Inflammatory changes in the dermis are usually minimal but may be pronounced when lesions rupture and discharge their contents.

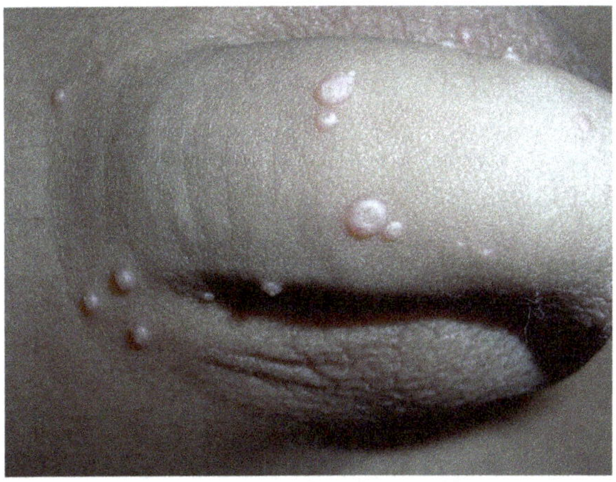

Molluscum contagiosum. There are numerous umbilicated papules on and around the penis of a young boy. There was no evidence for sexual abuse. (Reproduced, with permission, from Usatine RP, Smith MA, Mayeaux EJ Jr, Chumley HS, eds. *Color Atlas of Family Medicine*. 2nd ed. New York, NY: McGraw-Hill Education; 2012. Used with permission of Richard P. Usatine, MD.)

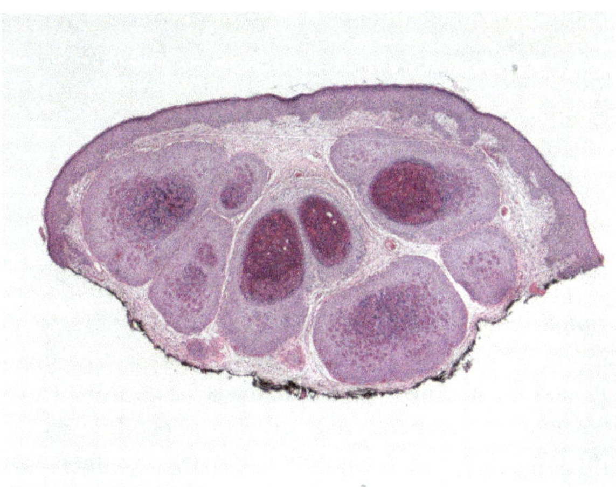

Molluscum contagiosum. Scanning magnification shows the characteristic lobular architecture of epithelium infected by molluscum contagiosum.

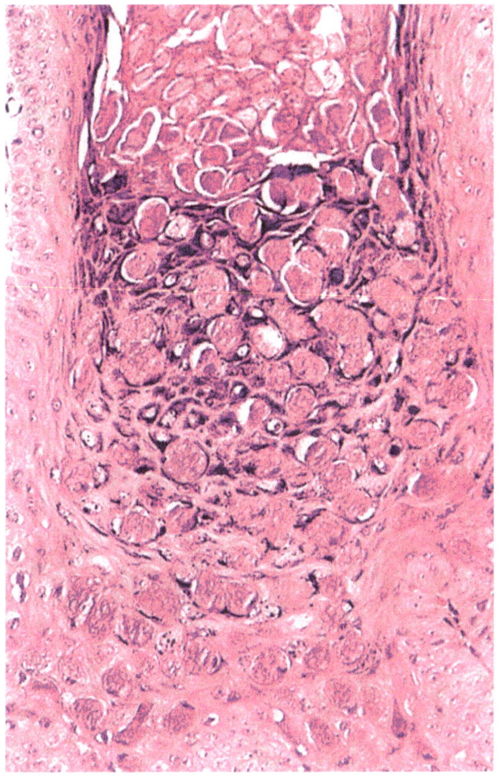

Molluscum contagiosum. The epithelial cells contain the characteristic eosinophilic cytoplasmic inclusion bodies. The nuclei are pushed to the periphery of the cell by the inclusion body.

Cytomegalovirus (CMV) is an enveloped DNA virus measuring 110 nm in diameter that is a member of the herpesvirus group. The virus is widespread, and subclinical infections are prevalent because most of the population at large demonstrates **CMV** antisera. Transmission is via body fluids, including saliva, blood, urine, semen, breast milk, and cervical secretions. Viral secretion may persist for years. Individuals at risk for clinical infections are those immunocompromised for one reason or another, such as those with HIV infection, transplant recipients, those undergoing chemotherapy, and pregnant women.

Clinically, although most cases are subclinical, a **mononucleosis syndrome** that is similar to that caused by **EBV** may develop. Affected patients develop fever, malaise, myalgias, lymphadenopathy, hepatosplenomegaly, and a sore throat without exudate. An exanthem manifest by an eruption of erythematous macules and papules that may be either urticarial or petechial may develop. The eruption may be precipitated by administration of ampicillin, as with **infectious mononucleosis**. A vasculitis with palpable purpura also has been reported. In patients with AIDS, **CMV** may cause chronic perineal and lower extremity ulcerations, chorioretinitis, gastroenteritis, pneumonia, and other visceral involvement. Fetal infection with **CMV** results in significant, often fatal developmental abnormalities. As with congenital rubella, extramedullary hematopoiesis may be seen in the skin as purplish papules and nodules.

Microscopically, the **acute viral exanthem** of **CMV** infection generally appears histopathologically similar to other **viral exanthemata**, with the possible exception of scattered enlarged fibroblasts or endothelial cells in the dermis. There is characteristically a sparse infiltrate of lymphocytes around blood vessels in the upper dermis with slight spongiosis. **CMV** does not infect keratinocytes, so epidermal changes are usually minimal. Virally infected cells in the dermis are characteristically enlarged one- to threefold and contain purplish crystalline inclusions in the cytoplasm and nuclei. These latter inclusions result in the characteristic "owl's eye" appearance of the cells. **CMV** vasculitis is a manifestation of endothelial cell infection with swelling, inflammation, and secondary vascular compromise. Ulcerations in immunocompromised hosts are usually not caused by **CMV** itself but by another agent such as herpesvirus with secondary colonization.

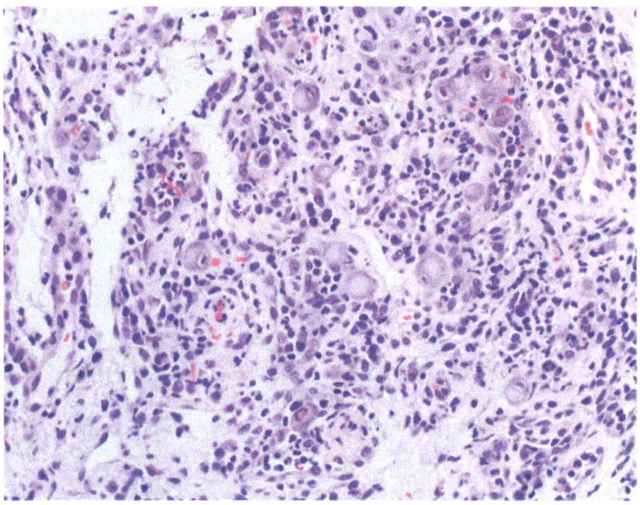

Cytomegalovirus (CMV) infection. These endothelial cells show classic cytopathic changes of CMV infection. The cells appear large, and there is a prominent "owl's eye" nucleoli and brightly eosinophilic intranuclear inclusions.

ANSWER 7-29: B.

Leishmaniasis is a spectrum of diseases caused by various species of the dimorphic protozoa *Leishmania* and is prevalent in tropical and neotropical areas of more than 70 countries throughout Asia, Africa, the Americas, and the Mediterranean, with up to 1.5 to 2.0 million new cases each year (Table 7-29A). The incidence and spread of the disease has increased due to global climate changes, migration and tourism, urbanization, and deforestation, as well as increased drug resistance. Approximately one-third of the world's HIV-infected population lives in zones endemic for **leishmaniasis**. Dogs, cats, and rodents typically serve as reservoirs. Humans acquire the infection from the bite of infected female sandflies carrying the flagellated **promastigote** forms in their gastrointestinal (GI) tract. The infective **promastigotes** enter at the inoculation (bite) site and invade reticuloendothelial cells. There they transform into aflagellate **amastigotes** and proliferate intracellularly until the cell ruptures. Although macrophages are the primary cells that

Table 7-29A. Leishmaniasis

Clinical Features
Spectrum of disease caused by multiple species of *Leishmania*
Old World cutaneous (*L tropica, L major, L aethiopica*)
Middle East, Africa, Asia, Mediterranean
Rural (moist), multiple, progress from papules to ulcer with spontaneous healing in 6 months
Urban (dry), single, on face, protracted course of up to 2 years or more
New World cutaneous and mucocutaneous (*L braziliensis, L tropica*)
Bay sore usually visceral (*L donovani*)
Histopathologic Features
Ulceration often
Histiocytic infiltrates with varying admixtures of lymphocytes, neutrophils, and plasma cells
Epithelioid granulomas on occasion (with greater immunity)
Intracellular organisms (amastigote forms—Leishman-Donovan bodies) varied in number depending on age of lesion and immunologic status of host
Amastigotes with round basophilic nucleus and small basophilic rodlike kinetoplast
Giemsa stain—nucleus purple and kinetoplast intense red or reddish-purple
Laboratory Evaluation
Giemsa, PAS, silver stains
Culture on NNN or Schneider *Drosophila medium*
Differential Diagnosis
American trypanosomiasis
Histoplasmosis
Rhinoscleroma
Granuloma inguinale
Leprosy
Atypical mycobacteriosis

harbor the parasites, phagocytosis by fibroblasts in the dermis and regional lymph nodes also occurs and may provide an important reservoir of organisms in latent disease. The incubation period for **cutaneous leishmaniasis** varies from 2 to 8 weeks but may be several months or years depending on the size of the inoculum and the immunologic status of the host.

Leishmania subgenera include *Leishmania* (which develop in the midgut and foregut of the sandfly) and *Viannia* (which develop in the hindgut and migrate to the mid and foregut). Three serologically and biochemically distinct species of *Leishmania*—*L tropica*, *L aethiopica*, and *L major*—are responsible for **Old World leishmaniasis**. They are transmitted by sandflies of the genus *Phlebotomus*. **New World leishmaniasis** with predominately cutaneous involvement is caused by multiple species of *L* (*Viannia*)—*L* (*V*) *braziliensis*, *L* (*V*) *guyanensis*,

L (V) peruviana, *L (V) panamensis*, and *L (V) columbiensis* and by *L* (L) *mexicana*, *L (L) amazonensis*, and other minor species. All of which are transmitted by sandflies of the genus *Lutzomyia*. *Leishmania (V) braziliensis* is the etiologic agent of **mucocutaneous leishmaniasis** and is also transmitted by the genus *Lutzomyia*. **Visceral leishmaniasis** is caused by *L donovani*, *L infantum*/*L chagasi* and *L (L) amazonensis*. Because of new genetic techniques and field testing, the taxonomy of *Leishmania* genera, subgenera, species, and subspecies is in flux.

Clinically, **Old World leishmaniasis** (ie, Baghdad boil, Biskra button, *Leishmania* tropica, Lahore sore, bouton d'orient or Oriental sore) is characterized by two types of lesions, moist (rural) and dry (urban). Moist lesions present as a slowly growing indurated red papule that may be intensely pruritic; multiple lesions are common. The papules enlarge in a few months to form nodules with an indurated border and dusky discoloration. These nodules tend to ulcerate within a few weeks, forming ulcers up to 5 cm in diameter with depressed granulating centers and raised indurated margins. Secondary bacterial infection is common after ulceration. Spontaneous healing usually occurs within 6 months, leaving a characteristic depressed, flattened white or pink cribriform scar. Dry lesions have a similar presentation but follow a more protracted course. Lesions are often single and occur primarily on the face. Progression to the nodular form does occur; however, the lesions do not ulcerate for several months. Healing may be delayed up to 2 years.

New World leishmaniasis encompasses several clinical entities. The "bay" sore typically occurs on the face as one or occasionally multiple erythematous plaques that typically do not ulcerate. "Apple jelly" nodules resembling **lupus vulgaris** are sometimes seen. The "Chiclero" ulcer is similar but is more often a single erythematous plaque that ulcerates; it affects the ear in 40% of patients and may cause extensive destruction of the cartilage. "Uta" presents as one or several papules on exposed sites; lesions usually ulcerate and are self-healing. In "pian bois," the patient has a single skin ulcer. Lymphatic spread may occur and result in widespread ulceration, but mucocutaneous involvement is extremely uncommon.

Leishmaniasis recidivans (lupoid leishmaniasis) is a relapsing form of the disease that may occur with any of the forms of **cutaneous leishmaniasis** but is usually secondary to *L tropica* infection. Most cases are in Iran and Iraq. Typically arising months to years after the primary lesion has healed, the disease presents as erythematous, sometimes circinate papules with a whitish scale. Lesions begin on the face, often at the edge of healed scars, and spread on an erythematous base. Patients are hypersensitive with good humoral and cellular immune (skin test) responses but are unable to completely eliminate the parasites. As the central lesion heals, active peripheral ones continue to form. The course is chronic and often relentless, lasting 20 to 40 years in some patients.

Disseminated cutaneous leishmaniasis presents as a single ulcer, nodule, or plaque on the face and other exposed areas. Nodular or plaque-like satellite lesions develop from the primary lesion and may disseminate over the entire body. Patients are anergic to leishmanial antigens and do not mount a specific cellular immune response to the infection. The organisms proliferate indefinitely, forming many lesions teeming with parasites.

Effective host response depends on both innate and adaptive immunity. Th1 (interferon-γ)-induced macrophage activation is required to kill the intracellular parasites. The Th2 (IL-4) response blunts tissue damage but promotes intracellular infection and increases the susceptibility to diffuse cutaneous (anergic) disease. In mucocutaneous disease, there is a mixed Th1/Th2 response with increased delayed-type hypersensitivity.

Microscopically, the diagnosis of **leishmaniasis** ultimately depends on isolation or identification of the organism from tissue. Common to all leishmanial lesions are dermal infiltrates of large histiocytes and varying numbers of organisms. The histiocytes range from 20 to 30 μm in diameter and have abundant cytoplasm. Organisms vary in number depending on the age of the lesion and the immunologic status of the host. They are more numerous in early lesions and those arising in immunocompromised hosts. **Amastigote** forms (**Leishman-Donovan bodies**) are generally found intracellularly, singularly, or in great numbers. In routine hematoxylin and eosin (H&E)–stained sections, **amastigotes** are 1 to 3 μm in diameter, round to oval, and nonencapsulated with a distinct cytoplasmic membrane. **Amastigotes** have a round basophilic nucleus approximately 1 μm in diameter and a small basophilic rod-like **kinetoplast**. In Giemsa-stained sections, the nucleus is purple, and the **kinetoplast** is an intense red or reddish purple. Various admixtures of lymphocytes, neutrophils, and plasma cells are also present. Areas of ulceration may have **pseudoepitheliomatous hyperplasia** (PEH) at the edge of the ulcer and show predominantly nonspecific inflammatory infiltrates. As the lesions age, there tends to be a gradual reduction in the number of both organisms and histiocytes. A granulomatous infiltrate containing epithelioid cells and multinucleated giant cells develops; caseous necrosis is notably absent.

Lesions in which organisms cannot be identified in histologic sections require additional studies. Species-specific PCR assays for the detection of *Leishmania* species have been developed and can be used with a number of specimens. The specificity and sensitivity of the current PCR technology generally exceed those of culture methods and histologic detection of parasites.

The histopathologic differential diagnosis includes **American trypanosomiasis, histoplasmosis, penicilliosis, rhinoscleroma, granuloma inguinale, leprosy,** and **atypical mycobacteriosis**. Each of these entities is characterized by an infiltrate of parasitized histiocytes admixed with chronic inflammatory cells. However, *Leishmania* **amastigotes** generally can be differentiated histopathologically from other organisms. Differentiation of *Leishmania* **amastigotes** from those of *Trypanosoma cruzi* may be quite difficult. *T cruzi* **amastigotes** are larger (3-5 μm) and round to oval with

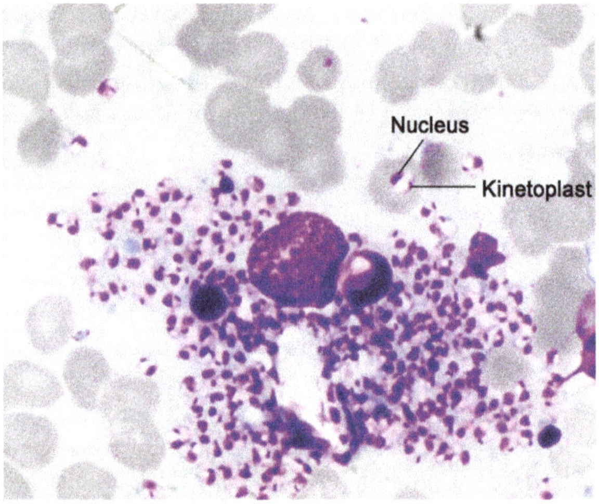

Leishmaniasis. A macrophage with numerous intracellular amastigotes (2-4 μm) in a Giemsa-stained splenic smear from a patient with visceral leishmaniasis. Each amastigote contains a nucleus and a characteristic kinetoplast consisting of multiple copies of mitochondrial DNA. A few extracellular parasites are also visible. (Reproduced, with permission, from Longo DL, Fauci AS, Kasper DL, Hauser SL, Jameson JL, Loscalzo J, eds. *Harrison's Principles of Internal Medicine*. 18th ed. New York, NY: McGraw-Hill Education; 2011.)

a distinct cytoplasmic membrane, a round nucleus, and a basophilic kinetoplast. Unlike *Leishmania* and *Histoplasma* species, *Trypanosoma* species are able to invade mesenchymal cells and are often seen in myocytes. **American trypanosomiasis (Chagas disease)** is transmitted by various species of the triatomid bugs (**reduviid bug**, "kissing bug," or "assassin bug") (Table 7-29B). The parasite multiplies and matures in the gastrointestinal tract of the insect. The infective **trypomastigotes** are located in the hindgut and are passed in the feces that are stimulated as the insect feeds. The infective feces contaminate the insect's bite site, conjunctivae, mucous membranes, or breaks in skin. **Trypomastigotes** are engulfed by histiocytes or actively invade histiocytes, adipose cells, and muscle cells immediately below the inoculation site. Intracellularly, they transform into **aflagellate amastigotes** and proliferate until the host cells rupture. Parasites are released to invade other cells and to enter the lymphatics or bloodstream and travel to distant sites. A primary lesion, the **trypanosomal chancre**, may appear at the bite site within 5 to 15 days. The painful chancre appears as a red-purple nodule 2 to 5 cm in diameter. It is well circumscribed and indurated and may have a surrounding white halo; ulceration may occur. The lesion persists for 2 to 3 weeks and subsides spontaneously.

Table 7-29B. Trypanosomiasis

Clinical Features
- Caused by *Trypanosoma gambiense* and *Trypanosoma rhodesiense:*
- African forms of the disease (Gambian and Rhodesian forms)
    - Trypanosomal chancre—painful red-purple nodule 2-5 cm at site of bites of tsetse flies
    - Evanescent circinate eruption resembling erythema multiforme
    - Urticaria, erythema nodosum, painful edemas
    - Lymphadenopathy
- Caused by *Trypanosoma cruzi:* American forms of the disease (Chagas disease)
    - Chagoma—erythematous indurated nodule at site of bite of reduviid bug
    - Acute, subacute, or chronic course
    - Fever, malaise, edema of face and extremities

Table 7-29B. Trypanosomiasis (*continued*)

Histopathologic Features
- Trypanosomal chancre and chagoma
    - Epidermal ulceration and hyperplasia
    - Infiltrate of histiocytes, plasma cells, and lymphocytes
    - Vasculitis
- Trypomastigotes with nucleus and kinetoplast that stain with
- Giemsa
    - Multiply in interstitium in cancer and intracellularly in chagoma

Laboratory Evaluation
- Giemsa, Wright, Romanowsky stains
- Culture *T brucei gambiense* and *T brucei rhodesiense* on Tobie and Weinman media or *T cruzi* on NNN medium

Differential Diagnosis
- Trypanosomal chancre
    - Syphilis
- Chagas disease
    - Leishmaniasis
    - Histoplasmosis
    - Rhinoscleroma
    - Granuloma inguinale

The diagnostic feature of **histoplasmosis** is the presence of yeast cells of *Histoplasma capsulatum* within histiocytes and occasionally within giant cells. In sections stained with H&E, yeast cells appear as 2- to 4-μm round to oval bodies surrounded by clear spaces. The yeasts of **penicilliosis** (*Penicillium marneffei*) are elongated ovals 2 to 4 μm that divide by transverse septae. Spores of both fungi are better visualized with methenamine silver stain. They are positive to periodic acid-Schiff (PAS).

In **rhinoscleroma**, the histiocytes (**Mikulicz cells**) range from 10 to 100 μm in diameter and have pale vacuolated cytoplasm containing the gram-negative bacilli *Klebsiella pneumoniae* **rhinoscleromatis**. The bacilli are 2 to 3 μm in length, appear round to oval in cross section, and stain poorly

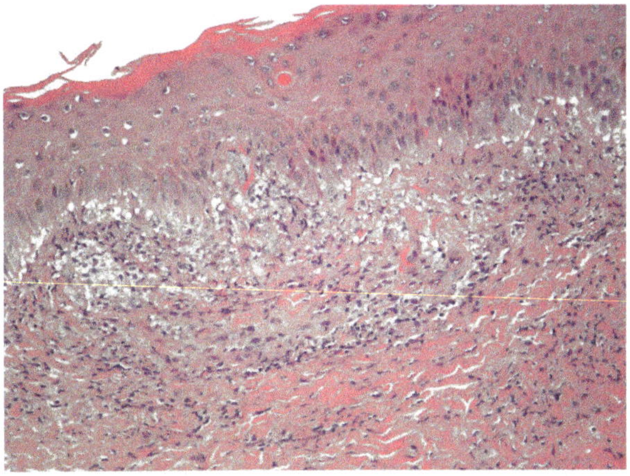

Chagas disease. In this case of Chagas disease, a predominance of mononuclear cells with epidermal hyperplasia and a suggestion of an ensuing interface dermatitis are observed. (Used with permission of Claudia I. Vidal, MD, PhD, Fellow, *Dermatopathology*, Mount Sinai School of Medicine.)

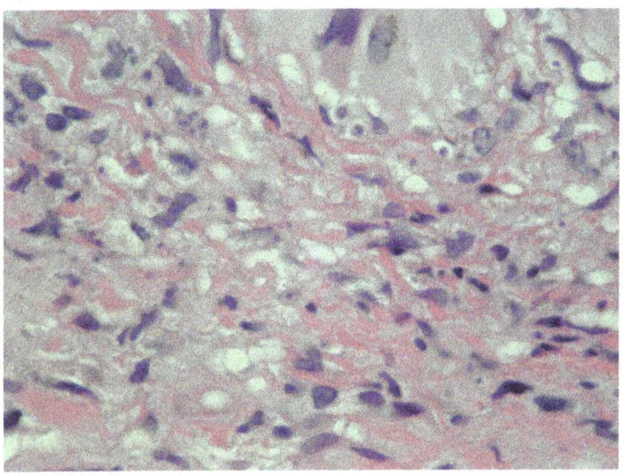

Chagas disease. Higher power magnification reveals structures highly reminiscent of those encountered in leishmaniasis. Note the small, rounded morphology with discrete centrally positioned nuclei and vertically oriented kinetoplasts. (Used with permission of Claudia I. Vidal, MD, PhD, Fellow, *Dermatopathology*, Mount Sinai School of Medicine.)

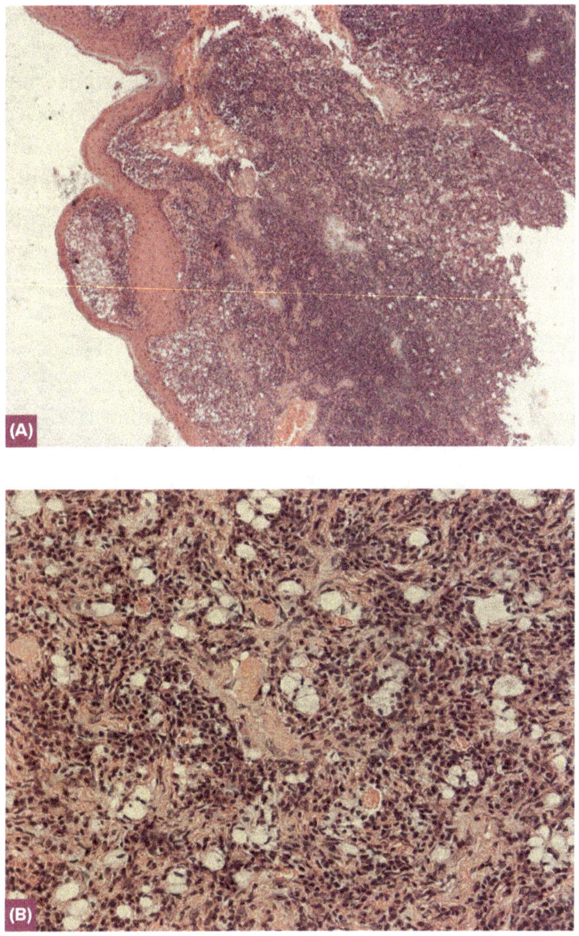

Rhinoscleroma (A) There is pseudoepitheliomatous hyperplasia with an underlying lymphoplasmacytic infiltrate admixed with numerous macrophages containing clear foamy cytoplasm (Mikulicz cells). **(B)** High power reveals the numerous plasma cells with Russell bodies and pale Mikulicz cells. A Warthin-Starry stain or Gram stain will reveal numerous rod-shaped bacteria within the pale cells." (Courtesy of David Molnar MD, Ist Dept. of Pathology and Experimental Cancer Research, Semmelweis Univ, Budapest.)

with routine H&E staining. The organisms are much better visualized with Warthin-Starry (WS) silver impregnation. The inflammatory infiltrate is rich in plasma cells with prominent Russell bodies.

The intracytoplasmic inclusions (**Donovan bodies**) in histiocytes of **granuloma inguinale** are small coccobacilli (1 to 2 μm in length). The multivacuolated histiocytes may be 20 μm or more in diameter. Vacuoles contain organisms (best seen with WS). The accompanying inflammatory infiltrate is rich in plasma cells with fewer lymphocytes and scattered neutrophils.

The histologic spectrum seen in **leprosy** varies with the type of disease. Histiocytes have abundant foamy or vacuolated cytoplasm, may be epithelioid, and are often separated from the epidermis by a narrow grenz zone. The histiocytes may be scattered among other inflammatory cells in the dermis or form granulomas. The granulomas tend to be elongated and course along nerves. Organisms stain poorly with Ziehl-Neelsen stain and are best seen with a Fite-Faraco acid-fast stain. They appear as red-staining bacilli measuring approximately 0.5 by 5.0 μm, primarily within histiocytes. **Atypical mycobacteriosis** also has a varied histologic appearance. Earlier lesions show dermal infiltrates of histiocytes, lymphocytes, and neutrophils with occasional microabscess formation. As the lesions age, epithelioid and tuberculoid type granulomas as well as **Langhans giant cells** are noted. Epithelial hyperplasia and hyperkeratosis may also be present. Variable numbers of organisms primarily within histiocytes are seen in acid-fast–stained sections.

Anti-leishmaniasis immunohistochemistry can differentiate *Leishmania* species from *T cruzi*, *H capsulatum*,

P marneffei, and *Toxoplasma gondii*. Although *H capsulatum*, *P marneffei*, and *T gondii* lack the characteristic kinetoplast found in *Leishmania* species, the **kinetoplasts** are sometimes difficult to identify on paraffin sections and are not observed in every parasite because of the plane of section. In the absence of immunohistochemical analysis using specific antibodies, it may be difficult to distinguish the **trophozoites** of *T gondii* from the **amastigotes** of *Leishmania* species.

ANSWER 7-30: D.

High-power examination of the patient's biopsy reveals multiple **trophozoites** with small, round, uniform nuclei rimmed by blue rings of chromatin along the nuclear membranes. Additionally, there is phagocytosis of red blood cells. The findings are consistent with **Amebiasis** (Table 7-30A). *E histolytica* is a pathogenic intestinal **amoeba** that is usually acquired via the fecal-oral route through ingestion of cysts. Prevalence rates are highest in areas where sanitation is poor, such as developing countries. Most infected individuals are asymptomatic cyst passers; the parasite resides in the colon but does not invade the mucosal tissues. Risk factors for disease include very young age (neonates); pregnancy and postpartum states; corticosteroids; and immunosuppression due to malnutrition, malignancy, chemotherapy, and HIV/AIDS. In most symptomatic patients, *E histolytica* causes colitis or proctitis, but severe cases may spread to the liver, lung, skin, or subcutaneous tissue. Cutaneous involvement results from several mechanisms, including direct extension of a bowel infection to the anogenital region; at sites of perforation or fistulization of hepatic, pleural, or enteric abscesses; and as a consequence of surgical interventions. Genital (cervical, vulvovaginal, or penile) ulcers may also occur, especially in patients who practice anal-receptive intercourse or have poor hygiene. Rare cases of primary inoculation of the skin of the orbit, face, and legs are reported from contact with contaminated material. Anogenital lesions present as serpiginous or spreading ulcers with well-demarcated, raised borders that are frequently undermined. The ulcer crater contains necrotic slough, a sanguinopurulent exudate, and granulation tissue. Ulcers are often painful and have a variable course (weeks to years). Rapid, fatal spread has been reported in young patients and those with compromised immune status. Some patients develop granulomas (**amebomas**), polypoid lesions, or marked **pseudoepitheliomatous hyperplasia** resembling a **condyloma** (which may be clinically mistaken for carcinoma). Infection and malignancy may coexist, and secondary bacterial infection occurs. Superficial lesions usually have concomitant visceral lesions with contiguous spread or perforation.

Table 7-30A. Entamebiasis

Clinical Features
Caused by *Entamoeba histolytica*
Increased frequency in patients with poor hygiene, severe dysentery, or immunosuppression
Due to direct extension of invasive intestinal disease (most common), rupture or fistulization of hepatic or pleural abscesses, direct contamination (rare)
Painful, necrotic ulcers
Epithelial hyperplasia common
Histopathologic Features
Ulcerative dermatitis with acute and chronic inflammation
Granulomata, marked pseudoepitheliomatous hyperplasia may be present
Trophozoites easily identified in tissues, ≥15-25 μm
Typical nuclear structure with smooth rim of chromatin on nuclear membrane
Laboratory Evaluation
Laboratory Evaluation
Direct smears stained with iron-hematoxylin or trichrome
Serologic tests are often nondiagnostic
Differential Diagnosis
Genital ulcer diseases

Microscopically, the lesions themselves are nonspecific. *E histolytica*, as the name implies, causes tissue lysis with ulceration. The ulcer has a necrotic base with acute and chronic inflammation, granulation tissue, and edema. In chronic lesions, granulomas and fibrosis may be prominent. Superficial lesions show spongiosis, **pseudoepitheliomatous hyperplasia**, liquefaction necrosis, ulceration, and fissures with invasive **trophozoites**. Varying degrees of acanthosis and papillomatosis are present at the epithelial margin. Deep lesions have deep dermal and subcutaneous liquefaction necrosis with suppuration and vasculitis. **Trophozoites** are seen in the areas of inflammation or at the interface between necrotic and viable tissue. They measure 15 to 25 μm, have fine granular cytoplasm and phagocytosed erythrocytes, and are usually isolated from the surrounding tissue by a small space (shrinkage artifact). The nucleus is small and round with a uniform blue ring of chromatin along the nuclear membrane; it may not be visible in all sections. The nucleus contains a single tiny karyosome that frequently is not observed. For the experienced observer, the organisms are seen easily with H&E staining but may be easier to locate using PAS stain. Material from the ulcer edge can also be examined directly using iron hematoxylin or trichrome stain.

In regard to the differential diagnosis, the ulcers of **amebiasis** must be differentiated from other anogenital or cutaneous ulcers (eg, **syphilis, chancroid,** or **herpes**) by biopsy or direct smear. Pseudoepitheliomatous lesions can mimic **squamous cell carcinomas** or **condylomata. Trophozoites** of *E histolytica* can be differentiated from macrophages by their nuclear configuration; the nuclei of macrophages are convoluted and have an irregular distribution of chromatin.

ANSWER 7-31: E.

The Gomori methenamine silver (GMS) impregnation of the olecranon bursa biopsy reveals numerous pleomorphic organisms with classic **morula** or "daisy" forms. **Protothecosis** is a rare exogenous, nontransmissible infection caused by the achlorophyllic algae *Prototheca wickerhamii* and *P zopfii* (Table 7-31A). Both species are ubiquitous in soil, contaminated water, and vegetation. The index case of human **protothecosis** was reported in a rice farmer from Sierra Leone in 1964. There are now more than 100 cases recorded in the world literature; they have come from almost all continents in both tropical and temperate climates. Cases have been reported in HIV-infected individuals. *Chlorella* species are chlorophyllic or green algae. Although **chlorellosis** has been described in several animal species, there is only one published report involving a human.

Three clinical syndromes are associated with *Prototheca* infection: a localized infection of the olecranon bursa in patients with normal immunity and an eczematoid dermatitis or disseminated disease in immunocompromised individuals. Disseminated infections have involved subcutaneous tissue, lymph nodes, deep organs, and meninges (in an HIV-infected individual). Use of topical steroids may predispose some individuals to a localized skin lesion. Many infections have been associated with trauma or contact with contaminated water, but the source of the infection is often unknown. **Protothecosis** of the olecranon bursa develops several weeks after injury to the elbow. There is local swelling or thickening of the bursa, development of draining sinuses, and epithelial hyperplasia. Systemic symptoms are not reported. In the cutaneous and subcutaneous forms, single or multiple lesions are seen, usually over an exposed surface of the body such as the face or limbs. The lesions develop slowly, spread centrifugally, and do not resolve. Typical lesions are indurated and maculopapular with an overlying crust and may have focal ulceration. Other reported presentations included verrucous, herpetiform, pyoderma-like, and chromomycosis-like eruptions.

Microscopically, in olecranon bursitis, the changes include areas of caseation necrosis surrounded by granulation tissue, Langhans giant cells, and fibrosis. *Prototheca* organisms are scattered throughout the areas of caseation. In cutaneous lesions, the inflammatory response varies from minimal to necrotizing granulomas and appears related to the depth of the invasion. The organisms may be in any or all layers of the skin and may be single or in clusters, extracellular, or within giant cells. Although the organisms are usually apparent on routine staining with H&E stain, they are much better seen with fungal stains such as GMS, PAS, and Gridley fungus. These spherical, unicellular organisms with hyaline **sporangia** reproduce asexually by internal septation and cytoplasmic cleavage. *P wickerhamii* is smaller and measures from 2 to 12 μm in diameter; *P zopfii* measures from 10 to 25 μm. *P wickerhamii* divides to form characteristic **morulas**, a form usually not produced by *P zopfii*. Fluorescence immunoassay aids in determining the species; specific antisera for each of the *Prototheca* species are available and can be used on either fresh or formalin-fixed tissue. *Chlorella* species are similar to *Prototheca* species but can usually be differentiated in tissue sections by immunohistochemical staining or the presence of chloroplasts (seen with the GMS and PAS methods or on electron microscopy). Material from skin scrapings, biopsies, and aspirates can be cultured on Sabouraud medium and require 1 to 2 days for growth. Differentiation is done by sugar assimilation tests.

In regard to the differential diagnosis, **Protothecosis** of the olecranon bursa is quite specific clinically and can be confirmed by biopsy, wet mount, or culture. Cutaneous **protothecosis** must be differentiated from other granulomatous diseases such as **cryptococcosis**, **coccidioidomycosis**, and **blastomycosis**. A biopsy or culture is required for definitive diagnostic distinction. *Prototheca* species are distinguished from *Cryptococcus neoformans*, *Coccidioides immitis*, *B dermatitidis*, and other fungi by the type of division. In rare cases mimicking **chromoblastomycosis** or if typical morula or septate forms are not seen, immunofluorescence studies can be performed.

Table 7-31A. Protothecosis and Chlorellosis

Clinical Features
Caused by *Prototheca wickerhamii* or *Prototheca zopfii*
Rare, ≈ 100 reported cases worldwide
Majority of cases in adults, men slightly > women
Associated with contaminated water or soil
Two syndromes:
Olecranon bursitis in immunocompromised host
Chronic eczematoid dermatitis
Histopathologic Features
Granulomatous inflammation, may have caseous necrosis in bursa
Severity of skin lesions related to depth of invasion
Organisms in areas of necrosis
Diagnostic features include
Size (*P wickerhamii*, 2-12 μm; *P zopfii* 10-25 μm)
Septation and morula formation
Stain well with fungal stains
Species identification by immunofluorescence
Confirmation by electron microscopy
Laboratory Evaluation
Culture on Sabouraud medium
Sugar assimilation
Differential Diagnosis
Olecranon bursitis is clinically unique
Granulomatous dermatitides (eg, fungal, mycobacterial)
Chromoblastomycosis

ANSWER 7-32: A.

Venereal syphilis, caused by *Treponema pallidum*, was a significant cause of morbidity and mortality in the early 20th century, although its incidence in the developed world has so diminished that many physicians are now unfamiliar with its manifestations. The incidence of acquired syphilis increased in the 1980s to 20 per 100,000 in North America. New diagnoses of syphilis increased eightfold in the United Kingdom between 1997 and 2002. By 2003, more than 60% of all reported cases of syphilis were believed to occur in men who have had sex with men. Spread of *T pallidum* usually occurs by contact between an infectious lesion and disrupted epithelium, either at sites of trauma incurred during sexual intercourse or at sites of concurrent chancroid and other genital sores. Coinfection with human immunodeficiency virus (HIV) is common, particularly in parts of Africa, where the incidence is up to 360 per 100,000, and the transmission rate is up to 60%.

The initial lesion of **primary syphilis,** the **chancre**, presents approximately 21 days after exposure at the inoculation site, as a painless, brown-red, indurated papule, nodule, or plaque up to 2 cm in diameter, in which organisms are identifiable (Table 7-32A). Multiple lesions or regional lymph node enlargement may be seen. After hematogenous dissemination of organisms, **secondary syphilis** occurs, resulting in widespread disease, with constitutional symptoms such as fever and malaise; generalized lymphadenopathy; and a disseminated eruption of red-brown macules, papules, papulosquamous lesions resembling guttate psoriasis, and rarely, pustules (Table 7-32B). Follicular-based annular or serpiginous lesions may be seen, particularly in recurrent attacks. Alopecia, **condyloma lata** (comprising confluent gray papules in anogenital areas), pitted hyperkeratotic palmoplantar papules (**syphilis cornee**), or, in severe cases, ulcerative lesions of **lues maligna** may develop. Shallow, painless ulcers sometimes are seen in mucosal surfaces.

Table 7-32A. Primary Syphilis

Clinical Features
- Painless papulonodular lesion
- Develops 21 days after exposure
- Lymphadenopathy in some cases

Histopathologic Features
- Frequent central ulceration
- Lateral psoriasiform hyperplasia
- Dense lymphoplasmacellular infiltrate
- Obliterative endovasculopathy

Differential Diagnosis
- Chancroid
- Zoon balanitis
- Insect-bite reaction
- Granuloma inguinale

Table 7-32B. Secondary and Tertiary Syphilis

Clinical Features
- Secondary
  - Fever
  - Generalized lymphadenopathy
  - Disseminated macular or papulosquamous eruption
  - Occasionally alopecia, pustules, hyperkeratotic palmoplantar pits, ulcers
- Tertiary
- Gummatous skin and mucosal lesions
  - Solitary or multiple nodules
  - Ulcerative subcutaneous lesions
- Cardiovascular disease
  - Syphilitic large-vessel aneurysms
- Neurologic disease
  - Tabes dorsalis
  - Meningoencephalitis

Histopathologic Features
- Psoriasiform hyperplasia
- Rare spongiform pustulation
- Vacuolar or lichenoid interface injury pattern
- Mixed lymphohistiocytic and plasmacellular infiltrate
- Granulomata
- Obliterative endovasculopathy

Differential Diagnosis
- Lichenoid dermatitides
- Psoriasiform dermatitides
- Tuberculoid leprosy
- Sarcoidal granulomatous dermatitides

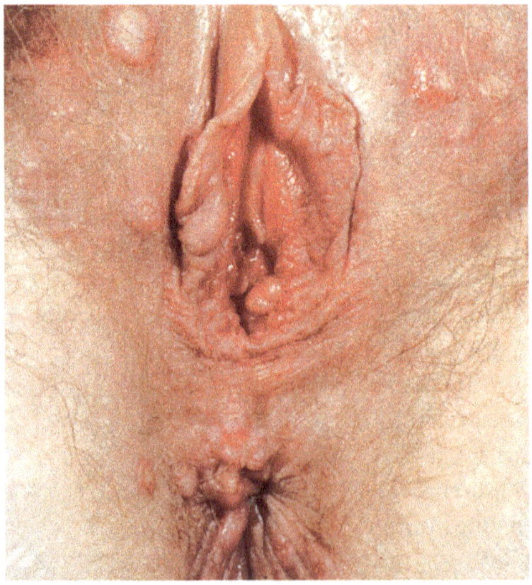

Condyloma Lata. Typical appearance of the verrucous, heaped up lesions of condyloma lata, a manifestation of secondary syphilis. (Reproduced, with permission, from Knoop KJ, Stack LB, Storrow AB, Thurman RJ. *The Atlas of Emergency Medicine*. 3rd ed. New York, NY: McGraw-Hill; 2010. Photo contributor: H. Hunter Handsfield. *Atlas of Sexually Transmitted Diseases*. New York: McGraw-Hill; 1992.)

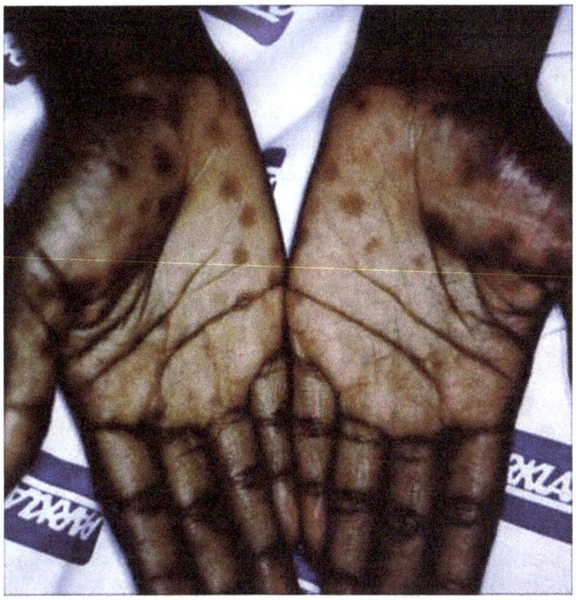

Secondary syphilis. Target lesions on the palms of a pregnant woman with secondary syphilis. (Reproduced, with permission, from Cunningham et al, eds. *Williams Obstetrics*. 24th ed. New York, NY: McGraw-Hill Education; 2014.)

Primary- and secondary-stage lesions that resolve without therapy may herald evolution into a latent phase, consisting of an early and late stage, and defined by an infection of less than or more than 1 year's duration. After a variable latent period, the patient enters the tertiary stage. **Tertiary syphilis** encompasses **gummatous** skin and mucosal lesions, termed **benign tertiary syphilis** as well as cardiovascular and neurologic manifestations. Skin lesions are solitary or multiple and consist of superficial nodular and deep gummatous subtypes, the former having smooth, atrophic centers with raised, serpiginous borders, and the latter manifesting as ulcerative subcutaneous swellings.

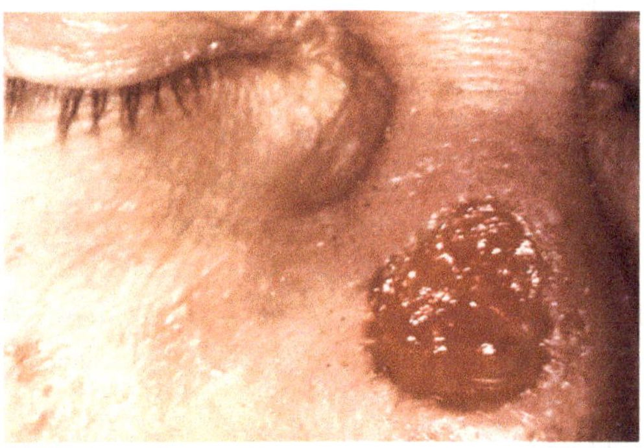

Tertiary syphilis. Gumma of the nose due to long-standing tertiary syphilis. (Used with permission of J. Pledger, Public Health Image Library, CDC.)

Congenital syphilis arises through transplacental infection and affects more than 50% of infants born to mothers with primary or secondary syphilis. The diagnosis is made when organisms are seen by dark-field, fluorescent antibody, or conventional histochemical methods. A presumptive case includes any infant born to a mother whose syphilis was inadequately treated or untreated at the time of birth or when an infant or child with a reactive treponemal test has any evidence of congenital syphilis, including physical signs, long-bone involvement radiologically, a reactive cerebrospinal fluid (CSF) **Venereal Disease Research Laboratories (VDRL) test**, an elevated CSF protein or white blood cell count, or quantitative treponemal titers four times higher than the mother's. Clinical signs include rhinitis, chancres, or a desquamative maculopapular rash.

Microscopically, **cutaneous syphilis** manifests as a perivascular infiltrate composed of lymphoid cells and often plasma cells. The late secondary and tertiary stages also show infiltrates of epithelioid histiocytes and giant cells. In all stages, endothelial swelling and proliferation are apparent. Autopsy studies on newborns with congenital syphilis show multiorgan involvement by an angioinvasive CD68-positive mononuclear cell infiltrate that imparts an "onion skin" morphology to involved vessels. Numerous spirochetes are usually detectable. Most HIV-infected patients exhibit a normal serologic response to *T pallidum* infection; however, in some HIV-positive patients with biopsy-proven secondary syphilis, both treponemal (FTA-ABS, MHA-TP, HATTS) and non-treponemal (VDRL, RPR) test results for syphilis have been reported as negative. The diagnosis of syphilis in seronegative HIV-infected patients depends on dark-field microscopy and histopathology of lesional biopsy tissue, with demonstration of spirochetes by silver stains (Warthin-Starry, Steiner), direct fluorescent antibody for *T pallidum* (DFA-TP), or spirochete immunohistochemical stain.

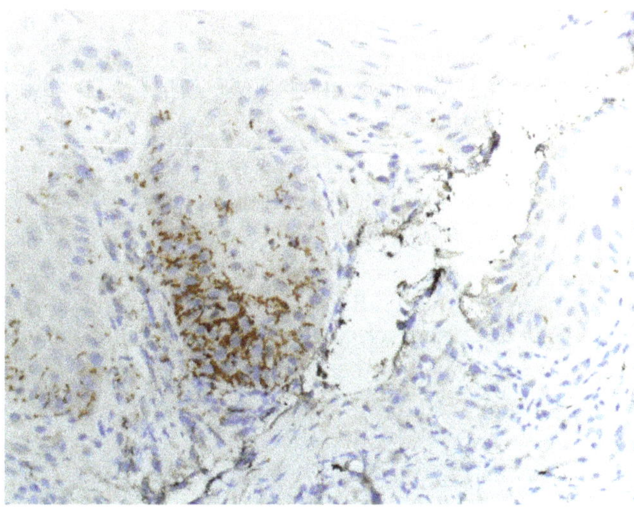

Immunohistochemical stain for spirochetes. There are numerous spirochetes in the superficial dermis and in between keratinocytes in the lower epidermis.

The **primary syphilitic chancre** manifests a variable histopathology, depending on whether the center or edge is biopsied; the center is often ulcerated, and the edges show acanthosis, spongiosis, and exocytosis of lymphocytes and neutrophils. The papillary dermis is edematous, and a dense dermal perivascular and interstitial lymphohistiocytic and plasmacellular infiltrate is present, often accompanied by neutrophils. An obliterative endarteritis, characterized by endothelial swelling and mural edema, completes the picture. With silver stains, immunofluorescent techniques, or immunohistochemical stains, spirochetes are usually seen within and around blood vessels and along the dermal-epidermal junction. In their full length, the spirochetes show 8 to 12 spiral convolutions, each roughly 1 μm in length. In evaluating biopsy specimens, histochemical stains, Warthin-Starry silver stains, and Steiner silver stains must be interpreted with caution because in addition to spirochetes, other structures and artifacts may be mistaken as *T pallidum*. Silver stains also decorate melanin and reticulin fibers, which must be differentiated based on recognition that melanin in the dendritic processes of melanocytes has a granular appearance and that reticulin fibers, although wavy, do not have a spiral architecture. Correlation with serology is prudent.

In regard to the differential diagnosis, the clinical differential diagnosis includes **chancroid, granuloma inguinale,** and **Zoon balanitis. Chancroid**, due to infection with *Haemophilus ducreyi,* is difficult to distinguish clinically from the syphilitic chancre. Chancroid lesions show dense lymphohistiocytic infiltrates with a paucity of plasma cells, granulomatous vasculitis, and an epidermal reaction pattern similar to the syphilitic chancre, consisting of psoriasiform epidermal hyperplasia and spongiform pustulation. A Giemsa, Alcian blue, or periodic acid-Schiff stain reveals coccobacillary forms between keratinocytes and along the dermal-epidermal junction. Spirochetes may coinfect chancroid lesions. Whereas **Zoon balanitis** may mimic those chancres, manifesting a lichenoid pattern of plasma cell-rich inflammation, the dermis is typically markedly sclerotic. Zoon balanitis will fail to show spirochetes. **Granuloma inguinale** is distinctive by virtue of manifesting **Donovan bodies. Yaws,** which is caused by *T pallidum pertenue*, is spread by casual contact between primary or secondary lesions and abraded skin. It classically affects the buttocks, legs, and feet of children and is most prevalent in warm, moist tropical climates. Seropositivity rates of up to 95% are seen in areas of Ecuador. *T pallidum pertenue* is indistinguishable microscopically from *T pallidum* but is distinctive by Southern blot analysis and by other molecular methods. Despite only minor sequence variation between the organisms, there are distinct differences between disease expressions of **yaws** and **syphilis**. For example, infants born to mothers with **yaws** do not produce IgM antibodies, and their organs, when examined by PCR methods and by animal inoculation studies, do not contain the spirochete. These findings emphasize the dermotropic, as opposed to organotropic, character of *T pallidum pertenue.*

BIBLIOGRAPHY

1. Agterof MJ, van der Bruggen T, Tersmette M, et al. Nocardiosis: a case series and a mini review of clinical and microbiological features. *Neth J Med.* 2007;65(6):199–202.
2. Amagai M, Yamaguchi T, Hanakawa Y, et al. Staphylococcal exfoliative toxin B specifically cleaves desmoglein 1. *J Invest Dermatol.* 2002;118: 845–850.
3. Amato VA, Tuon FF, Bacha HA, et al. Mucosal leishmaniasis. Current scenario and prospects for treatment. *Acta Trop.* 2008;105:1.
4. Amsbaugh S, Huiras E, Wang N, et al. Bacillary angiomatosis associated with pseudoepitheliomatous hyperplasia. *Am J Dermatopathol.* 2006;28:32–35.
5. Anstead GM, Graybill JR. Coccidioidomycosis. *Infect Dis Clin N Am.* 2006;20:621–643.
6. Antal GM, Lukehart SA, Meheus AZ. The endemic treponematoses. *Microb Infect.* 2002;4:83–94.
7. Antal GM, Lukehart SA, Meheus AZ. The endemic treponematoses. *Microbes Infect.* 2002;4:83–94.
8. Arend SM, Lavrijsen APM, Kuijken I, et al. Prospective controlled study of the diagnostic value of skin biopsy in patients with presumed meningococcal disease. *Eur J Clin Microbiol Infect Dis.* 2006;25:643–649.
9. Auluck A. Maxillary necrosis by mucormycosis. A case report and literature review. *Med Oral Patol Oral Cir Bucal.* 2007;12:E360–E364.
10. Bakleh M, Wold LE, Mandrekar JN, et al. Correlation of histopathologic findings with clinical outcome in necrotizing fasciitis. *Clin Infect Dis.* 2005;40:410–414.
11. Bingol-Kologlu M, Yildiza R, Alper B, et al. Necrotizing fasciitis in children: diagnostic and therapeutic aspects. *J Pediatr Surg.* 2007;42(11):1892–1897.
12. Bodey GP, Mardani M, Hanna HA, et al. The epidemiology of *Candida glabrata* and *Candida albicans* fungemia in immunocompromised patients with cancer. *Am J Med.* 2002;112(5):380–385.
13. Bonifaz A, Carrasco-Gerard E, Saul A. Chromoblastomycosis: clinical and mycologic experience of 51 cases. *Mycoses.* 2001;44:1–7.
14. Booton GC, Visvesvara GS, Byers TJ, et al. Identification and distribution of *Acanthamoeba* species genotypes associated with non-keratitis infections. *J Clin Microbiol.* 2005;43:1689.

15. Brown C, Kowalczyk A, Taylor E, et al. p53 represses human papillomavirus type 16 DNA replication via the viral E2 protein. *Virol J.* 2008;5:5

16. Bruns T. A kingdom revised. *Nature.* 2006;443: 758–761.

17. Chao S-C, Hsu MM-L, Lee JY-Y. Cutaneous protothecosis: report of five cases. *Br J Dermatol.* 2002;146:688.

18. Chayakulkeeree M, Perfect JR. Cryptococcosis. *Infect Dis Clin N Am.* 2006;20:507–544.

19. Chedid MBF, Chedid MF, Porto NS, et al. Nocardial infections: report of 22 cases. *Rev Inst Med Trop S Paulo.* 2007;49(4):239–246.

20. Chen CY, Chi KH, Alexander S, et al. The molecular diagnosis of lymphogranuloma venereum: evaluation of a real-time multiplex polymerase chain reaction test using rectal and urethral specimens. *Sex Transm Dis.* 2007;34:451–455.

21. 1. Chiller K, Selkin BA, Murakawa GJ. Skin microflora and bacterial infections of the skin. *J Invest Dermatol.* 2001;6:170–174.

22. Chuh A, Chan H, Zawar V. Pityriasis rosea—evidence for and against an infectious aetiology. *Epidemiol Infect.* 2004;132:381–390.

23. Conti Díaz IA. On the unknown ecological niche of *Paracoccidioides brasiliensis.* Our hypothesis of 1989: present status and perspectives. *Rev Inst Med Trop S Paulo.* 2007;49(2):131–134.

24. Crespo-Erchiga V, Florencio VD. Malassezia species in skin diseases. *Curr Opin Infect Dis.* 2002;15:133–142.

25. Dayal R, Agarwal M, Natrajan M, et al. PCR and in-situ hybridization for diagnosis of leprosy. *Indian J Pediatr.* 2007;74:645–648.

26. Durkin M, Witt H, LeMonte A, et al. Antigen assay with the potential to aid in the diagnosis of blastomycosis. *J Clin Microbiol.* 2004;42:4873–4875.

27. Enoch DA, Ludlam HA, Brown NM. Invasive fungal infections. a review of epidemiology and management options. *J Med Microbiol.* 2006;55:809–818.

28. Epps RE. Impetigo in pediatrics. *Cutis.* 2004;73:25–26.

29. Farina MC, Gegundez MI, Pique E, et al. Cutaneous tuberculosis: a clinical, histopathologic, and bacteriologic study. *J Am Acad Dermatol.* 1995;33:433–440.

30. Feng H, Shuda M, Chang Y. Clonal integration of a polyomavirus in human Merkel cell carcinoma. *Science.* 2008;319:1096–1100.

31. Fleming RV, Walsh TJ, Anaissie EJ. Emerging and less common fungal pathogens. *Infect Dis Clin N Am.* 2002;16:915–933.

32. Frantzeskaki F, Betrosian AP. Ecthyma gangrenosum: a rare manifestation of *Pseudomonas aeruginosa* sepsis in a critically ill adult patient. *Eur J Dermatol.* 2008;18:345–346.

33. Fredricks DN. Microbial ecology of human skin in health and disease. *J Invest Dermatol.* 2001;6: 167–169.

34. Frydenberg A, Starr M. Hand, foot, and mouth disease. *Aust Fam Physician.* 2003;32:594–595.

35. Fuchs J, Milbradt R, Pecher SA. Lobomycosis (keloidal blastomycosis): case reports and overview. *Cutis.* 1990;46:227–234.

36. Fustes-Morales A, Gutierrez-Castrellon P, Duran-Mckinster C, et al. Necrotizing fasciitis: report of 39 pediatric cases. *Arch Dermatol.* 2002;138:893–899.

37. Gaffin J, Gallagher J. Picture of the month. Blueberry muffin baby (extramedullary hematopoiesis) due to congenital cytomegalovirus infection. *Arch Pediatr Adolesc Med.* 2007;161:1102–1103.

38. Ghorpade A. Primary perianal perineo-crural postpederasty donovanosis. *Int J Dermatol.* 2007;46:855–857.

39. Gill MJ, Arlette J, Buchan KA, et al. Human orf. *Arch Dermatol.* 1990;126:356–358.

40. Ginter-Hanselmayer G, Weger W, Ilkit M, Smolle J. Epidemiology of tinea capitis in Europe: current state and changing patterns. *Mycoses.* 2007;50(Suppl 2): 6–13.

41. Gottlieb GJ, Ackerman AB. The "sandwich sign" of dermatophytosis. *Am J Dermatopathol.* 1986;8:347–350.

42. Guarner J, Zaki SR. Histopathology and immunohistochemistry in the diagnosis of bioterrorism agents. *J Histochem Cytochem.* 2006;54:3–11.

43. Gupta AK, Batra R, Bluhm R, et al. Skin diseases associated with *Malassezia* species. *Am Acad Dermatol.* 2004;51(5):785–798.

44. Gupta AK, Chaudhry M, Elewski B. Tinea corporis, tinea cruris, tinea nigra, and piedra. *Dermatol Clin.* 2003;21:395–400.

45. Gupta AK, Ryder JE, Summerbell RC. Onychomycosis: classification and diagnosis. ***J Drugs Derm.* 2004;3(1):51–56.

46. Gupta AK, Tu LQ. Dermatophytes: diagnosis and treatment. *J Am Acad Dermatol.* 2006;54:1050–1055.

47. Gutierrez ME, Canton A, Sosa N, et al. Disseminated histoplasmosis in patients with AIDS in Panama: a review of 104 cases. *Clin Infect Dis.* 2005;40:1199–1202.

48. Hackett BC, O'Connell K, Cafferkey M, et al. Tinea capitis in a paediatric population. *Ir Med J.* 2006;99(10):294–295.

49. Hadfield TL, McEvoy P, Polotsky Y, et al. The pathology of diphtheria [review]. *J Infect Dis.* 2000;181(Suppl):S116–S120.

50. Hajjeh RA, Sofair AN, Harrison LH, et al. Incidence of bloodstream infections due to *Candida* species and in vitro susceptibilities of isolates collected from 1998 to 2000 in a population-based active surveillance program. *J Clin Microbiol.* 2004;42(4): 1519–1527.
51. Harman RRM, English MP, Halford M, et al. Botryomycosis. *Br J Dermatol.* 1990;102:215–222.
52. Hart CA, Rao SK. Rhinoscleroma. *J Med Microbiol.* 2000;49:395–396.
53. Heffelfinger JD, Swint EB, Berman SM, et al. Trends in primary and secondary syphilis among men who have sex with men in the United States. *Am J Pub Health.* 2007;97:1076–1083.
54. Hibbett DS, Binder M, Bischoff JF et al. A higher-level phylogenetic classification of the Fungi. *Mycol Res.* 2007;111(5):509–547.
55. Hill HR, Kirkpatrick CH. Chronic mucocutaneous candidiasis. *Pediatr Infect Dis J.* 2001;20(2):197–206.
56. Hofman V, Brousset P, Mougneau E, et al. Immunostaining of visceral leishmaniasis caused by *Leishmania infantum* using monoclonal antibody (19-11) to the *Leishmania* homologue of receptors for activated C-kinase. *Am J Clin Pathol.* 2003;120:567.
57. Hu W, Nuovo G, Willen M, Somach S. Epidermodysplasia verruciformis in two half brothers with HIV infection. *J Cutan Med Surg.* 2004;8:357–360.
58. Jarman A, Duggal A, Korus L, Tredget EE. Toxic shock syndrome in an adult burn patient. *Burns.* 2007;33:1051–1053.
59. Joseph AK, Rosen T. Laboratory techniques used in the diagnosis of chancroid, granuloma inguinale, and lymphogranuloma venereum. *Dermatol Clin.* 1994; 12:1–8.
60. Kahawita IP, Lockwood DNJ. Towards understanding the pathology of erythema nodosum leprosum. *Transactions Royal Soc Trop Med Hygiene.* 2008;102:329–337.
61. Kapoor V, Travadi J, Braye S. Staphylococcal scalded skin syndrome in an extremely premature neonate: a case report with a brief review of the literature. *J Paediatr Child Health.* 2008;44:374–376.
62. Kauffman CA. Endemic mycoses: blastomycosis, histoplasmosis, and sporotrichosis. *Infect Dis Clin N Am.* 2006;20:645–662.
63. Kauffman CA. Histoplasmosis: a clinical and laboratory update. *Clin Microbiol Rev.* 2007;20(1):115–132.
64. Keeling PJ, Luker MA, Palmer JD. Evidence from beta-tubulin phylogeny that *Microsporidia* evolved from within the Fungi. *Mol Biol Evol.* 2000;17(1):23–31.
65. Kempf W, Burg G. Pityriasis rosea: a virus-induced skin disease? An update. *Arch Virol.* 2000;145: 1509–1520.
66. Kempf W, Kadin M, Kutzner H, et al. Lymphomatoid papulosis and human herpesviruses: a PCR-based evaluation for the presence of human herpesvirus 6, 7 and 8 and related herpesviruses. *J Cutan Pathol.* 2001;28:29–33.
67. Kidd SE, Hagen F, Tscharke RL, et al. A rare genotype of *Cryptococcus gattii* caused the cryptococcosis outbreak on Vancouver Island (British Columbia, Canada). *Proc Natl Acad Sci USA.* 2004;101(49):17258–17263.
68. Kroshinsky D, Grossman ME, Fox LP. Approach to the patient with presumed cellulitis. *Semin Cutan Med Surg.* 2007;26:168–178.
69. Leavell UW, Phillips IA. Milker's nodules. *Arch Dermatol.* 1975;111:1307–1311.
70. Leclerc S, Teixeira A, Mahe E, et al. Recurrent erysepelas: 47 cases. *Dermatology.* 2007;214:52–57.
71. Lee PL, Lemos B, O'Brien SH, et al. Cutaneous diphtheroid infection and review of other cutaneous Gram-positive Bacillus infections. *Cutis.* 2007;79:371–377.
72. Lupi O, Tyring SK, McGinnis MR. Tropical dermatology: fungal tropical diseases. *J Am Acad Dermatol.* 2005;53:931–951.
73. Magaña M, Magaña ML, Alcantara A, Perez-Martin MA. Histopathology of cutaneous amebiasis. *Am J Dermatopathol.* 2004;26:280.
74. Malani A, Hmoud J, Chiu L, et al. *Candida glabrata* fungemia: experience in a tertiary care center. *Clin Infect Dis.* 2005;41:975–981.
75. Mancini AJ. Bacterial skin infections in children. The common and the not so common [review]. *Pediatr Ann.* 2000;29:26–35.
76. Marques SA, Conterno LO, Sgarbi LP, et al. Paracoccidioidomycosis associated with acquired immunodeficiency syndrome: report of seven cases. *Rev Inst Med Trop São Paulo.* 1995;37:261–265.
77. Mohammed TT, Olumide YM. Chancroid and human immunodeficiency virus infection: a review. *Int J Dermatol.* 2008;47:1–8.
78. Nelson J, Stone M. Update on selected viral exanthems. *Curr Opin Pediatr.* 2000;12:359–364.
79. Neonate with staphylococcal scaled skin syndrome. *Arch Dis Childhood Fetal Neonatal Ed.* 2006;91:F25.
80. Nucci M, Anaissie E. Fusarium infections in immunocompromised patients. *Clin Microbiol Rev.* 2007;20(4):695–704.
81. Paniz-Mondolfi AE, Jaimes OR, Jones LD. Lobomycosis in Venezuela. *Int J Dermatol.* 2007;46:180–185.

82. Pardillo FEF, Fajardo TT, Abalos RM, et al. Methods for the classification of leprosy for treatment purposes. *Clin Infect Dis.* 2007;44:1096–1099.

83. Pereyra SB, Danielo CA, Ponssa GJ. Wade's histoid leprosy: three clinical presentations. *Int J Dermatol.* 2007;46:944–946.

84. Pfaller MA, Diekema DJ. Epidemiology of invasive candidiasis: a persistent public health problem. *Clin Microbiol Rev.* 2007;20(1):133–163.

85. Posnett DN, Yarilina AA. Sleeping with the enemy: endogenous superantigens in humans (letter, comment). *Immunity.* 2001;15:503–506.

86. Qian X, Jin L, Hayden R, et al. Diagnosis of cat scratch disease with *Bartonella henselae* infection in formalin-fixed paraffin-embedded tissues by two different PCR assays. *Diagn Mol Pathol.* 2005;14:146–151.

87. Quimby SR, Connolly SM, Winkelmann RK, Smilack JD. Clinicopathologic spectrum of specific cutaneous lesions of disseminated coccidiomycosis. *J Am Acad Dermatol.* 1992;26:79–85.

88. Rampf J, Essig A, Hinrichs R, et al. Lymphogranuloma venereum: a rare cause of genital ulcers in central Europe. *Dermatology.* 2004;209:230–232.

89. Reithinger R, Dujardin J-C, Louzir H, et al. Cutaneous leishmaniasis. *Lancet Infect Dis.* 2007;7:581.

90. Rhajaoui M, Nesereddin H, Azmi K, et al. New clinico-epidemiologic profile of cutaneous leishmaniasis, Morocco. *Emerg Infect Dis.* 2007;13:1358.

91. Rho N-K, Kim B-J. A corynebacterial triad: prevalence of erythrasma and trichomycosis axillaris in soldiers with pitted keratolysis. *J Am Acad Dermatol.* 2008;58(Suppl):S57–S58.

92. Rinaldi MG. Dermatophytosis: epidemiological and microbiological update. *J Am Acad Dermatol.* 2002;43(5):20–24.

93. Rogstad KE, Simms I, Fenton KA, et al. Screening diagnosis and management of early syphilis in genito-urinary medicine clinics in the UK. *Int J STD AIDS.* 2005;16:348–352.

94. Rosenberg AS, Morgan MB. Disseminated acanthamoebiasis presenting as lobular panniculitis with necrotizing vasculitis in a patient with AIDS. *J Cutan Pathol.* 2001;28:307.

95. Saubolle MA, Sussland D. Nocardiosis: review of clinical and laboratory experience. *J Clin Microbiol.* 2003;41(10):4497–4501.

96. Scheinfeld NS. Is blistering distal dactylitis a variant of bullous impetigo? *Clin Exp Dermatol.* 2007;32: 314–316.

97. Schwartz RA. Superficial fungal infections. *Lancet.* 2004;364:1173–1182.

98. Silva V, Pereira CN, Ajello L, Mendoza L. Molecular evidence for multiple host-specific strains in the genus *Rhinosporidium. J Clin Microbiol.* 2005;43(4):1865–1868.

99. Stone M, McGuire L, Moore M, et al. Bilateral nasal obstruction in a 50-year-old woman. *Pathology.* 2007;39:516–518.

100. Tajiri T, Tate G, Akita H, et al. Autopsy cases of fulminant-type bacterial infection with necrotizing fasciitis: group A (beta) hemolytic *Streptococcus pyogenes* versus *Vibrio vulnificus* infection. *Pathol Int.* 2008;58:196–202.

101. Tolat SN, Gokhale NR, Belgaumkar VA, et al. Disseminated cutaneous rhinosporidiomas in an immunocompetent male. *Indian J Dermatol Venereol Leprol.* 2007;73:343.

102. Torno MS, Babapour R, Gurevitch A, et al. Cutaneous acanthamoebiasis in AIDS. *J Am Acad Dermatol.* 2000;42:351.

103. Tuon FF. A systematic literature review on the diagnosis of invasive aspergillosis using polymerase chain reaction (PCR) from bronchoalveolar lavage clinical samples. *Rev Iberoam Micol.* 2007;24:89–94.

104. Vanittanakom N, Cooper CR, Fisher MC, Sirisanthana T. *Penicillium marneffei* infection and recent advances in the epidemiology and molecular biology aspects. *Clin Microbiol Rev.* 2006;19(1):95–110.

105. Varella TCN, Nico MMS. Erysipeloid. *Int J Dermatol.* 2005;44:497–498.

106. Vetrichevvel TP, Pise GA, Agrawal KK, Thappa DM. Cutaneous diphtheria masquerading as a sexually transmitted disease. *Indian J Dermatol Venereol Leprol.* 2008;74:187.

107. Ware AJ, Cockerel CJ, Skkiest DJ, et al. Disseminated sporotrichosis with extensive cutaneous involvement in a patient with AIDS. *J Am Acad Dermatol.* 1999;40(2):350–355.

108. Warnock DW. Trends in the epidemiology of invasive fungal infections. *Jpn J Med Mycol.* 2007;48:1–12.

109. Wicher K, Wicher V, Abbruscato F, Baughn RE. *Treponema pallidum* subsp. *pertenue* displays pathogenetic properties different from those of *T. pallidum* subsp. *pallidum. Infect Immun.* 2000;68:3219–3225.

110. Wohlrab J, Rohrbach D, Marsch WC. Keratolysis sulcata (pitted keratolysis): clinical symptoms with different histological correlates. *Br J Dermatol.* 2000;143: 1348–1349.

CHAPTER 8

Tumors of the Epidermis and Cysts

QUESTION 8-1.

A 4-year-old child presents with an enlarging subcutaneous swelling overlying the midline of the neck. The lesion is excised and the findings are illustrated below. Which of the following diagnoses is CORRECT?

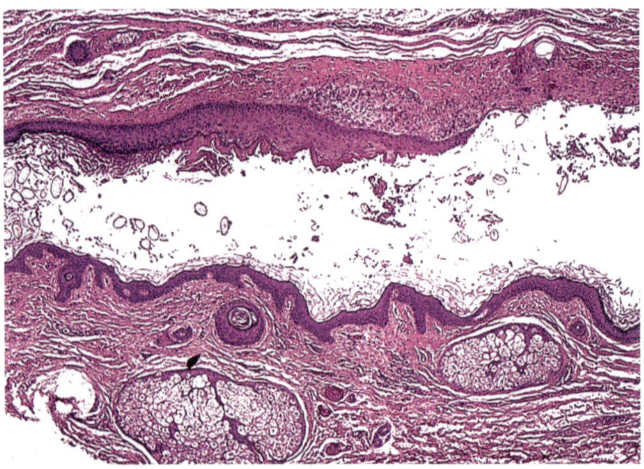

A) Epidermal inclusion cyst
B) Dermoid cyst
C) Branchial cleft cyst
D) Bronchogenic cyst
E) Thyroglossal duct cyst

QUESTION 8-2.

A 16-year-old patient who recently had dental work presents with a subcutaneous swelling in the right anterior neck. The lesion is excised revealing a squamous lined cyst with ulceration, and marked acute and chronic inflammation. Which of the following diagnoses is CORRECT?

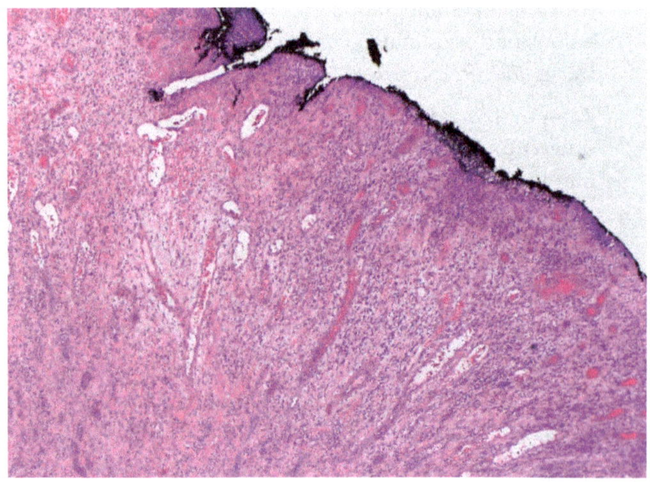

A) Bronchogenic cyst
B) Epidermal inclusion cyst
C) Cutaneous ciliated cyst
D) Submental draining sinus tract
E) Branchial cleft cyst

QUESTION 8-3.

A 13-year-old child presents with a rapidly enlarging subcutaneous swelling in the right lateral neck adjacent to the thyroid gland. The lesion is excised. The illustrated findings below include the cyst and the adjacent soft tissue. Which of the following diagnoses is CORRECT?

A) Thymic cyst
B) Branchial cleft cyst
C) Thyroglossal duct cyst
D) Bronchogenic cyst
E) Epidermal inclusion cyst

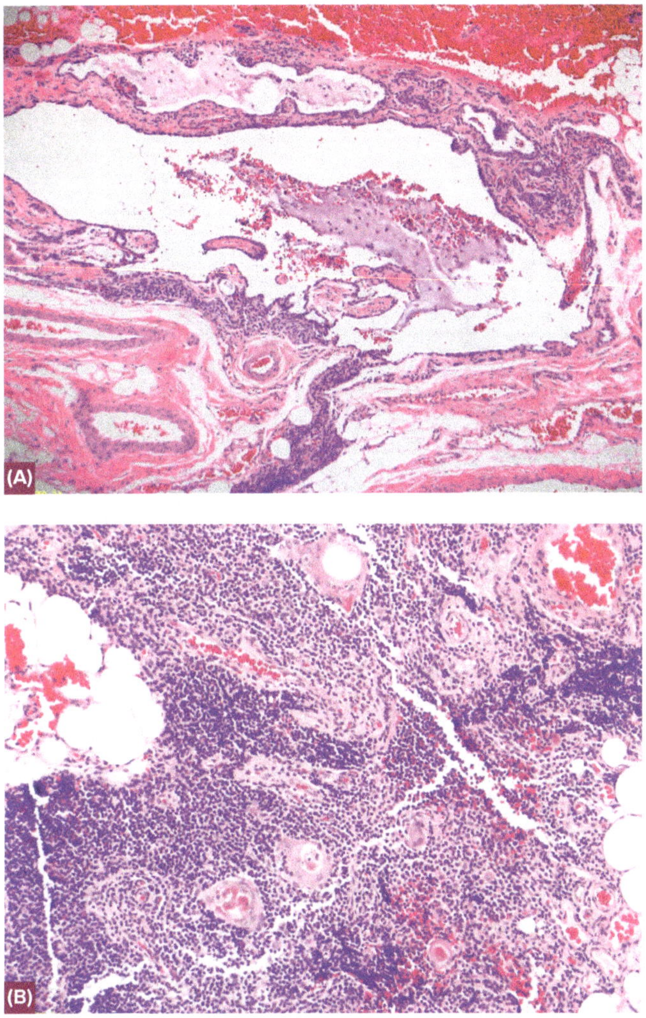

QUESTION 8-4.

The biopsy illustrated below is from a cyst on the leg of a young female. Which of the following additional features is MOST commonly associated with this lesion?

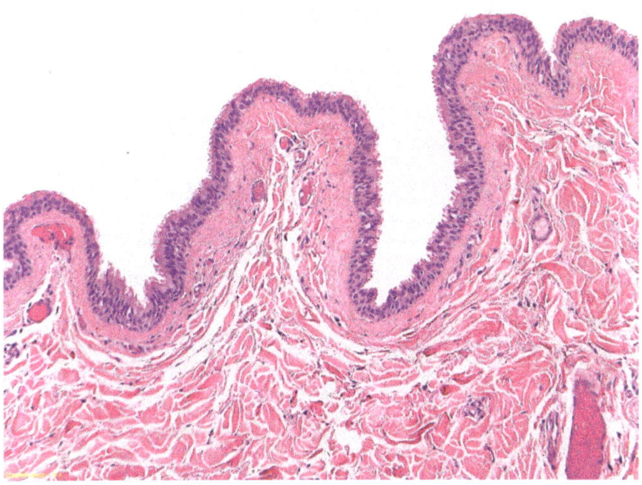

A) Decapitation secretions by the epithelial
B) Lymphoid aggregates
C) Cholesterol granulomas
D) Foci of squamous metaplasia
E) Muscle fibers surrounding the cyst

QUESTION 8-5.

An 18-year-old female develops a brown painful nodule within an umbilical scar. The lesion is biopsied and the findings are illustrated below. Which of the following statements regarding this condition is INCORRECT?

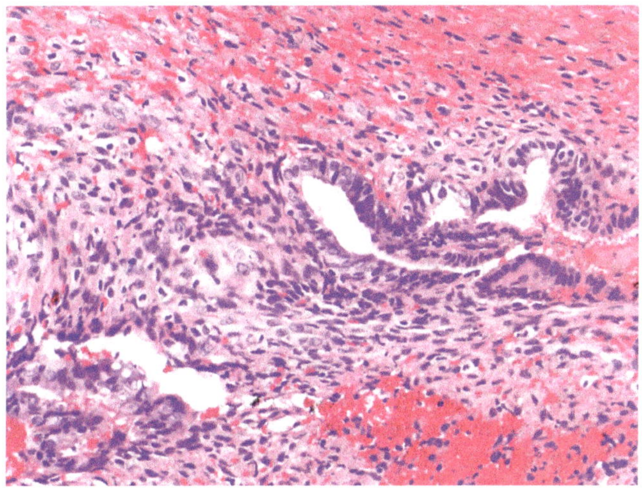

A) These cutaneous lesions, although rare, usually arise within cesarean section and periumbilical scars.
B) These patients experience monthly fluctuations in symptoms with occasional bleeding from the cyst.
C) The lesion is a form of foreign body reaction to a prior procedure.
D) These lesions may be found essentially anywhere.
E) Perl stain will reveal numerous blue granules throughout the lesion.

QUESTION 8-6.

An 11-year-old boy presents with a 3-mm solitary bluish cyst on the ventral shaft of the penis. The lesion is biopsied and the findings are illustrated below. Which of the following statements regarding this entity is INCORRECT?

A) These lesions are seen exclusively in males.
B) These cysts do not connect with the urethra.
C) These cysts are believed to arise from a small urothelial rest of the urethra.
D) Microscopically, the cysts appear empty due to the fluid leaking out after biopsy.
E) The epithelial lining exhibits apocrine decapitation-type secretion.

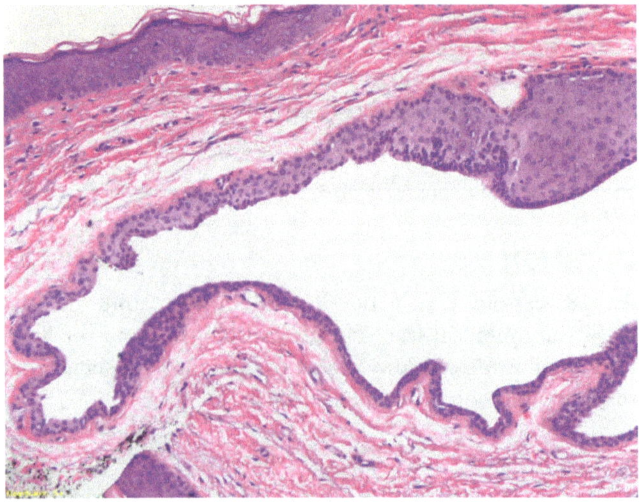

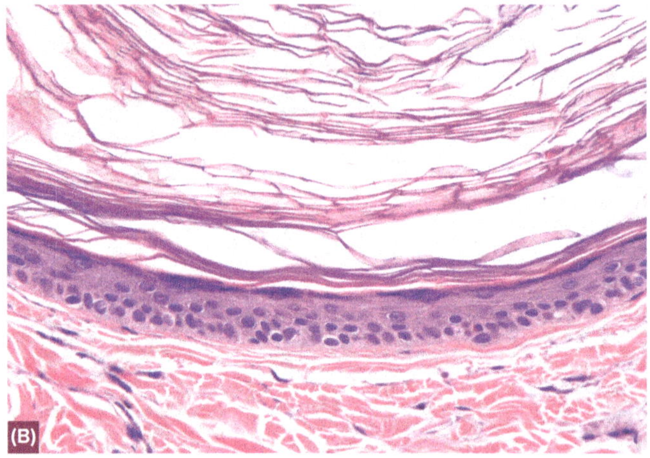

QUESTION 8-7.

A 16-year-old male develops an erythematous dome-shaped nodule on the back. The lesion has been present for several months. An excisional biopsy is performed. Which of the following statements regarding this entity is INCORRECT?

A) Cysts of acral sites with an identical histopathology are believed to arise from implantation of epidermis into the dermis through trauma.
B) The cyst in this patient is most likely due to cystic dilatation of the infundibular portion of a hair follicle.
C) Multiple cysts with identical histology frequently arise within scrotal skin, become calcified, and are referred to as "scrotal calcinosis."
D) Rupture of these cysts results in an intense foreign body giant cell reaction with fragments of keratin identified within giant cells.
E) The cyst lining is usually acanthotic with platelike extensions and accentuated rete ridges.

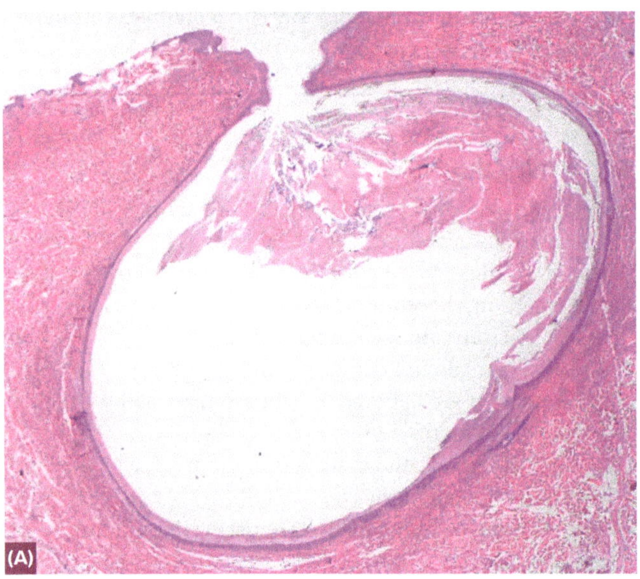

QUESTION 8-8.

A 38-year-old male presents with a two dome-shaped nodules on the scalp with alopecia. The lesion is excised and the findings are illustrated below. Which of the following statements regarding this lesion is INCORRECT?

A) These cysts are difficult to remove surgically and frequently require wide excision.
B) These cysts arise from portions of the hair follicle that lack an inner root sheath, such as the isthmus of anagen hairs or the sac surrounding catagen and telogen hairs.
C) Ruptured cysts produce a foreign body giant cell reaction accompanied by frequent calcification and occasionally ossification.
D) These cysts are frequently referred to as "sebaceous cysts."
E) Nuclear palisading of the basal layer is a characteristic feature.

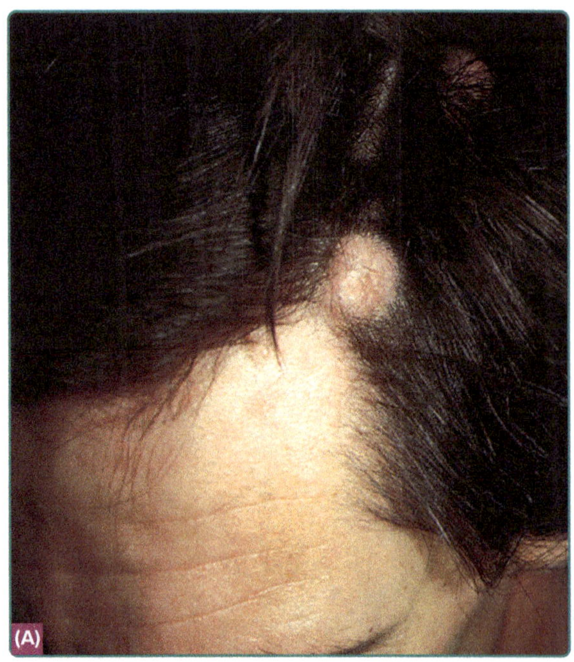

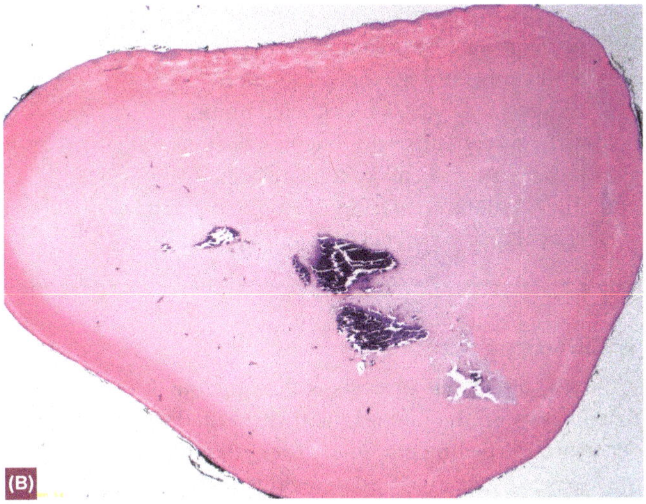

Reproduced, with permission, from Goldsmith LA, Katz SI, Gilchrest BA, Paller AS, Leffell DJ, Wolff K, eds. *Fitzpatrick's Dermatology in General Medicine*. 8th ed. New York, NY: McGraw-Hill Education; 2012.

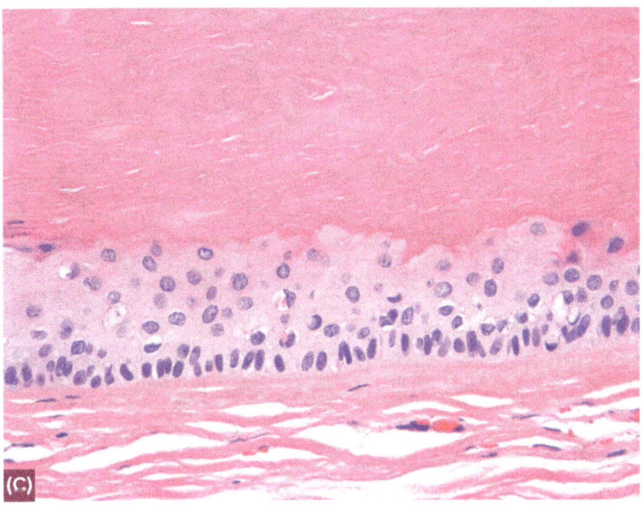

QUESTION 8-9.

An 11-year-old male presents with numerous diffuse small (1-3 mm) slightly pigmented dome-shaped papules on the anterior chest, abdomen, and extremities. He has an older sibling with a similar condition. One of the lesions is biopsied and the findings are illustrated below. Which of the following statements regarding this condition is INCORRECT?

A) This patient most likely has an autosomal dominant condition responsible for the numerous lesions.
B) Multiple lesions are associated with steatocystoma multiplex.
C) These lesions are thought to arise from the lower infundibular portion of the hair.
D) Fascicles of smooth muscle may be seen attaching to the outer cyst wall.
E) In the vast majority of cases, the cyst wall contains adnexal components such as sebaceous glands.

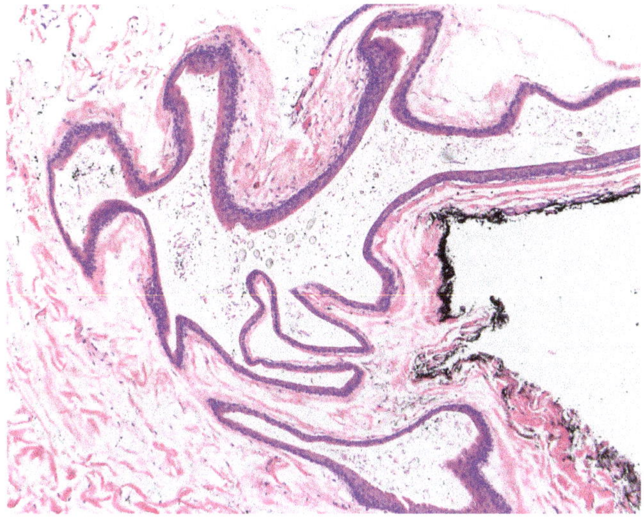

QUESTION 8-10.

A 13-year-old male patient presents with a white/yellowish nodule on the chest. The lesion is biopsied and the findings are illustrated below. Which of the following diagnoses is CORRECT?

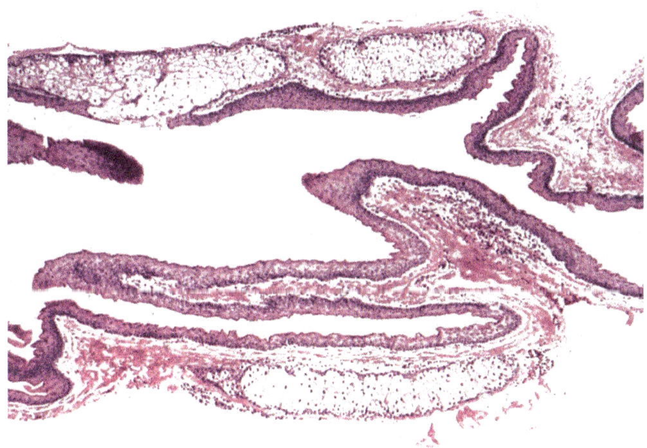

A) Epidermoid cyst
B) Milium cyst
C) Vellus hair cyst
D) Steatocystoma
E) None of the above

QUESTION 8-11.

A 33-year-old male in the US army presents with an erythematous and painful raised nodule in the sacrococcygeal region. The lesion is excised. Which of the following statements regarding this entity is INCORRECT?

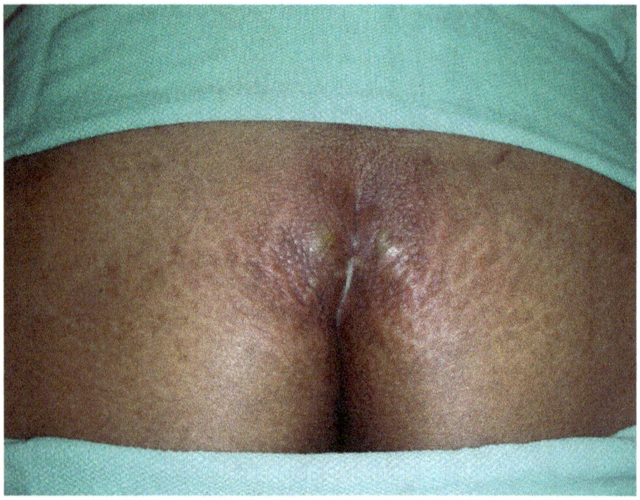

Reproduced with permission from Fitch MT, Manthey DE, McGinnis HD, et al: Videos in clinical medicine. *Abscess incision and drainage, N Engl J Med.* 2007 Nov 8;357(19):e20.

A) The most diagnostic feature is the presence of naked hair shafts embedded within the dermis admixed with inflammatory infiltrates.
B) These lesions are felt to represent draining sinus tracts as a result from penetration of the hair shafts into the skin.
C) Most frequently, numerous noncaseating granulomas surround a cyst wall that is commonly lined by squamous epithelium.
D) In the absence of a cyst lining or hair shafts, appropriate stains for microorganisms should be performed.

QUESTION 8-12.

A 36-year-old patient presents with a firm nodule on the dorsum of the right index finger next to the distal interphalangeal joint. Incision releases a clear gelatinous material. Which of the following statements regarding this entity is INCORRECT?

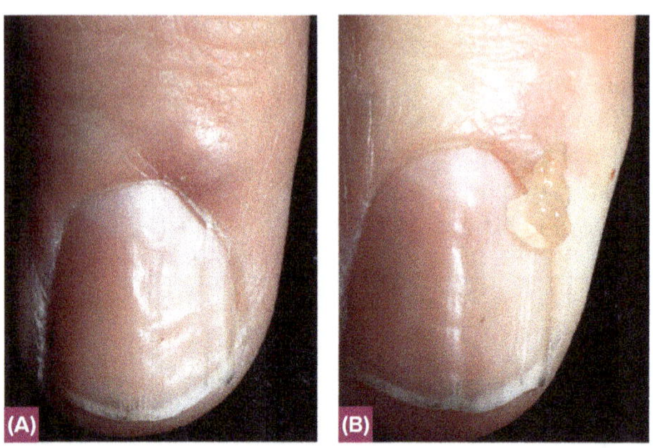

Reproduced with permission from Wolff K, Johnson RA, Saavedra AP. *Fitzpatrick's Color Atlas and Synopsis of Clinical Dermatology.* 7th ed. New York, NY: McGraw-Hill Education; 2013.

A) The cyst cavity frequently contains broad villous projections lined by inflammatory cells, reactive cuboidal epithelium, and fibrinous exudates.
B) The cyst wall lacks an epithelial lining.
C) The cyst contains acid mucin, which is highlighted by alcian blue and colloidal iron stains.
D) These lesions arise from the joint space and are freely attached via a pedicle.

QUESTION 8-13.

A 35-year-old female presents with numerous 1-2 mm dome-shaped cysts on the forehead and cheeks following a series of dermabrasion treatments. One of the cysts is biopsied. Which of the following statements regarding this entity is INCORRECT?

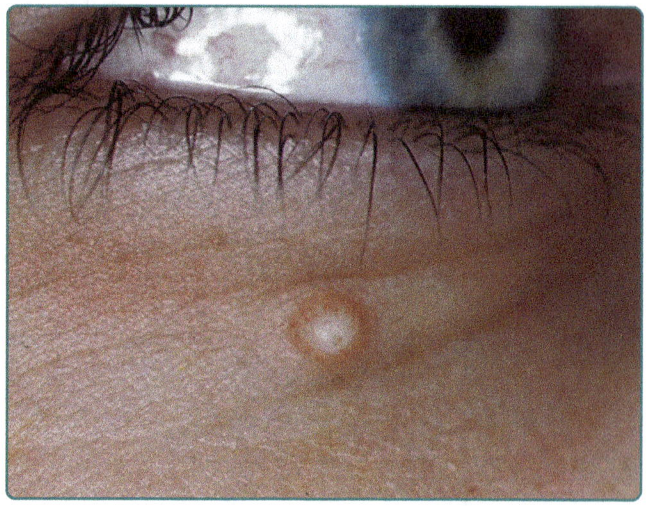

Reproduced, with permission, from Goldsmith LA, Katz SI, Gilchrest BA, Paller AS, Leffell DJ, Wolff K, eds. *Fitzpatrick's Dermatology in General Medicine.* 8th ed. New York, NY: McGraw-Hill Education; 2012.

A) Histopathologically, the cyst lining is identical to that of epidermoid cysts.
B) These lesions most commonly arise from the infundibular portion of terminal hairs.
C) Numerous cysts may develop in patients with bullous disorders such as porphyria cutanea tarda, epidermolysis bullosa, and cicatricial bullous pemphigoid.
D) Fragments of hair shaft are usually not identified within the cyst contents.
E) Adnexal structures such as sebaceous glands do not connect with the cyst wall.

QUESTION 8-14.

A 50-year-old male presents with a slow growing flesh-colored to brown papule on the face with a rolled smooth edge and a central hyperkeratotic plug. Foul-smelling cheesy material is expressed from the central crater with lateral compression.

The lesion is biopsied and the findings are illustrated below. Which of the following statements regarding this entity is INCORRECT?

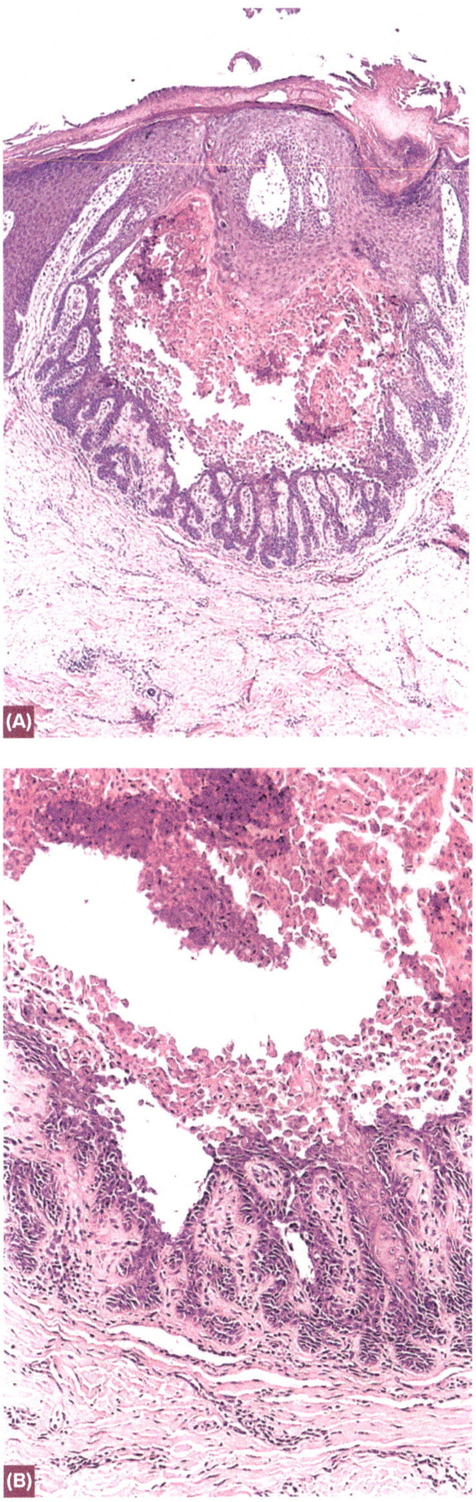

A) Oral lesions with this histopathology may arise secondary to irritation and trauma.
B) Glabrous lesions have a propensity to arise on sun-exposed areas correlating with prolonged UV light exposure.
C) An abnormality in the genes responsible for the production of keratins K1 and K10 has been reported in these lesions.
D) Glabrous lesions are usually associated with pilosebaceous structures and early changes are usually limited to the upper portions of the follicular infundibulum.
E) These lesions are usually accompanied by a moderate perivascular inflammatory infiltrate composed of lymphocytes, histiocytes, rare eosinophils, and occasional plasma cells.

QUESTION 8-15.

A 55-year-old patient presents with several “stuck on” flesh-colored and dark brown scaly lesions on the head and neck, trunk, and extremities. The palms or soles are spared. One of the lesions is biopsied and the findings are illustrated below. Which of the following statements regarding this entity is INCORRECT?

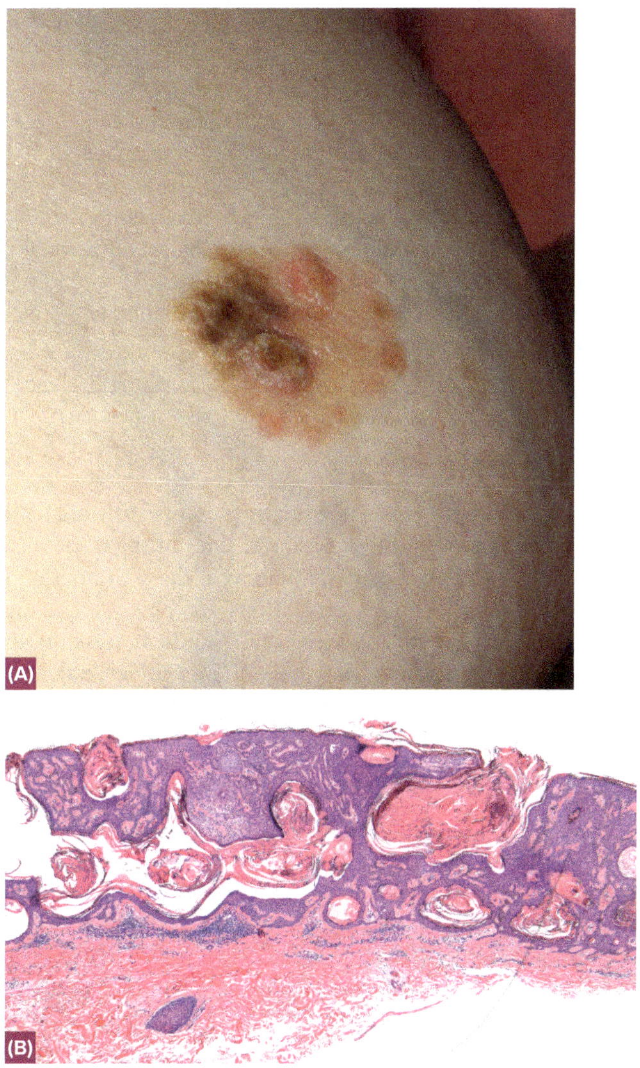

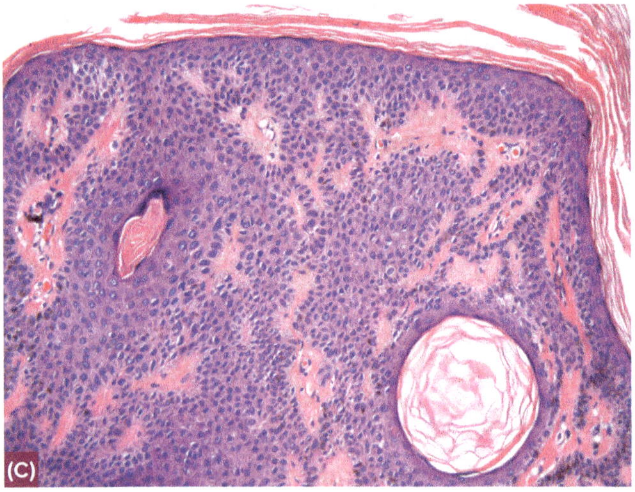

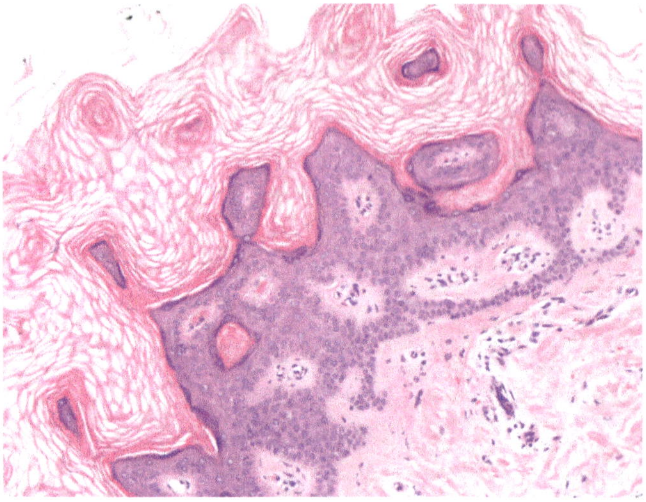

A) This represents the most common human neoplasm, and may be seen in approximately 20% of elderly patients.
B) The eruption of multiple lesions has been described in association with internal visceral malignancy, most commonly adenocarcinomas of the gastrointestinal tract.
C) Patients that have these lesions have an increased incidence of basal cell carcinoma, squamous cell carcinoma, eccrine porocarcinoma, melanoma, and keratoacanthoma.
D) Multiple histopathologic variants of this lesion exist, each with its own unique histopathological differential diagnosis.
E) This lesion represents a hamartoma and not true neoplasm.

QUESTION 8-16.

A 3-year-old obese Hispanic patient presents with bilateral hyperpigmentation of the axillae and sides of the neck with a velvety texture. There is accentuation of the skin lines and focal small papillomatous projections are present. During the physical exam you notice that the child is missing an iris of one eye (aniridia) and has mild swelling restricted to one side of the body. The mother reports that the child's urine has an abnormal color. Palpation of the abdomen and flank reveals a large firm mass. Examination of the mouth reveals mucosal surface hyperpigmentation. A skin biopsy of the neck is performed. Which of the following diagnoses is CORRECT?

A) Epidermal nevus
B) Dowling-Degos disease
C) Acanthosis nigricans
D) Confluent and reticulated papillomatosis of Gougerot and Carteaud
E) Dermatosis papulosa nigra

QUESTION 8-17.

A 50-year-old patient presents with a solitary, erythematous, moist, and smooth papule on the sole of the foot with well-circumscribed borders. There is blanching of the lesion with compression. A fine scale is also appreciated. The lesion is biopsied and the findings are illustrated below. Which of the following statements regarding this entity is INCORRECT?

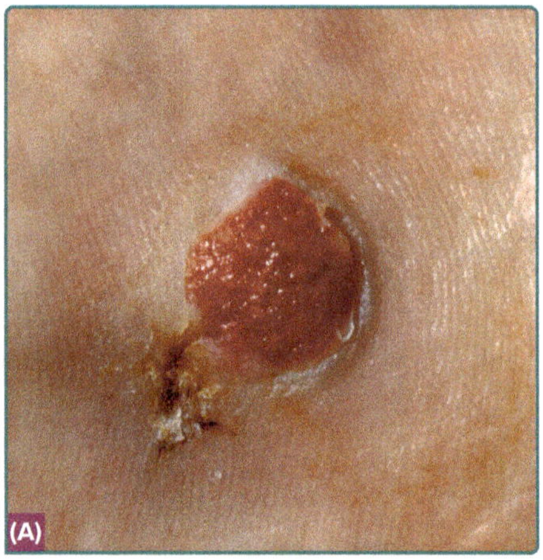

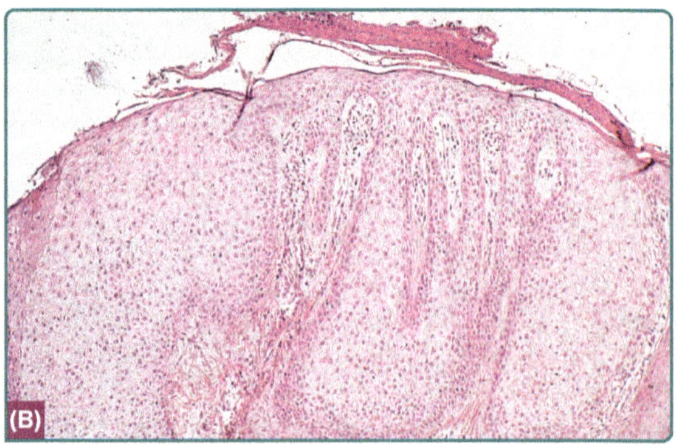

Reproduced, with permission, from Goldsmith LA, Katz SI, Gilchrest BA, Paller AS, Leffell DJ, Wolff K, eds. *Fitzpatrick's Dermatology in General Medicine*. 8th ed. New York, NY: McGraw-Hill Education; 2012.

A) This lesion is most likely inflammatory rather than neoplastic in nature.
B) A PAS stain will reveal bright eosinophilic cytoplasm in the pale cells, representing an increased glycogen concentration.
C) The pigmented variant of this lesion is colonized by melanocytes containing increased concentrations of melanin granules within elongated dendritic processes.
D) There is upregulation of keratinocyte growth factors present within these lesions.
E) These tumors are believed to be a variant of eccrine poroma.

QUESTION 8-18.

A 16-year-old patient presents with a linear arrangement of flesh colored to red papules on the left flank. The eruption has been present since the patient was a young child. Some of the papules have become dark-red to brown with scaling and crusting. You notice that the lesions follow Blaschko lines. A biopsy is performed and the findings are illustrated below. High-power examination reveals striking hypogranulosis with abrupt transition to thick eosinophilic parakeratosis. Which of the following diagnoses is CORRECT?

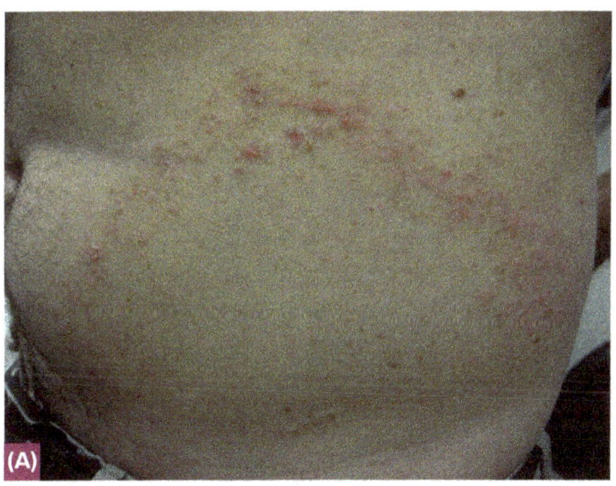

Reproduced, with permission, from Usatine RP, Smith MA, Mayeaux EJ Jr, Chumley HS, eds. *Color Atlas of Family Medicine*. 2nd ed. New York, NY: McGraw-Hill Education; 2012.

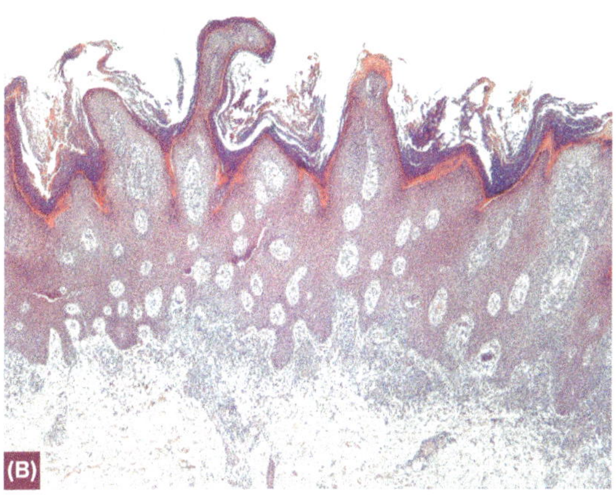

A) Prurigo nodularis
B) Verruciform xanthoma
C) Verruca vulgaris
D) Inflammatory linear verrucous epidermal nevus
E) Psoriasis vulgaris

QUESTION 8-19.

Which of the following biopsies illustrated below are diagnostic of actinic keratosis?

A)

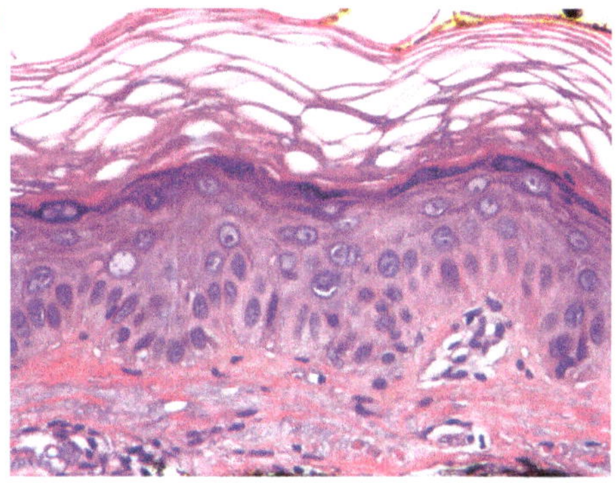

B)

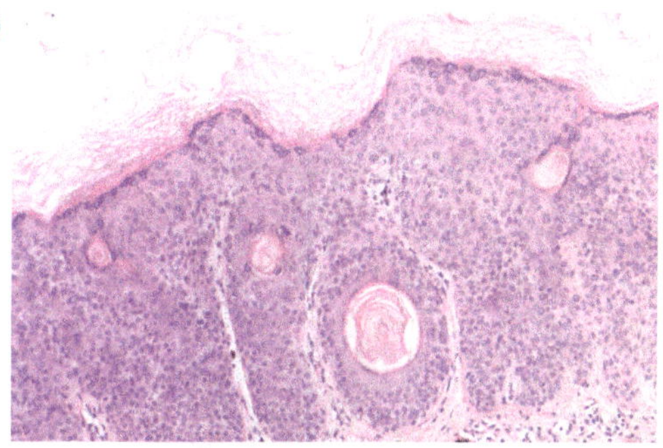

C)

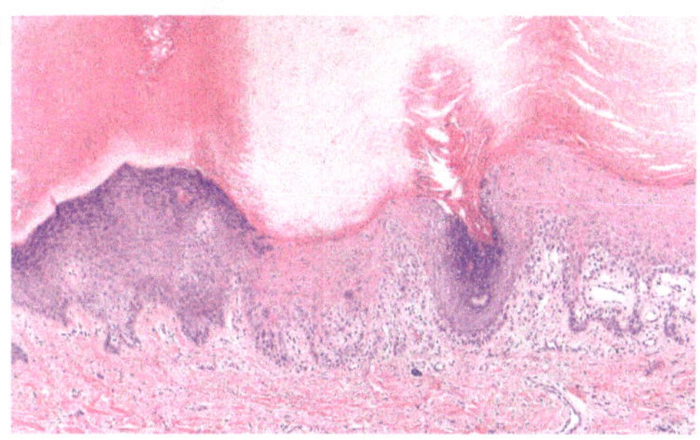

D)

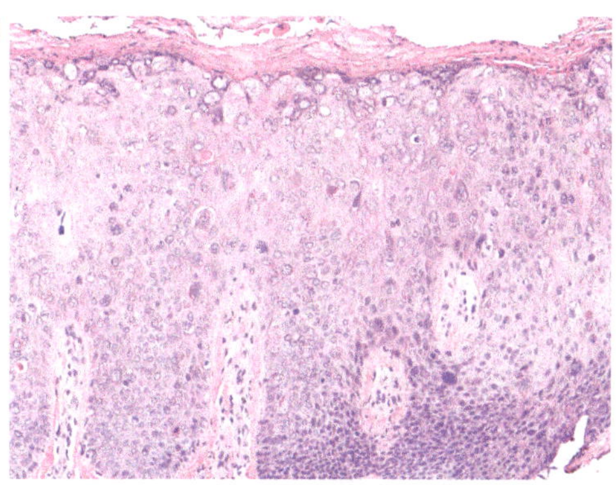

QUESTION 8-20.

An elderly man presents with multiple indurated and ulcerated nodules on the scalp. A biopsy is performed and the findings are illustrated below. Which of the following statements about this tumor is INCORRECT?

A) Tumors that arise on the ear, genitalia, and oral mucosa exhibit a significantly increased risk for aggressive clinical course.

B) Tumors that arise in association with radiation exposure, immunosuppression, and within chronic ulcers exhibit a dramatically increased risk for aggressive clinical course.

B) The tumor cells are positive for high molecular weight cytokeratin and negative for BerEP4 via immunohistochemistry.

C) These invasive tumors always arise within preexisting in situ tumors.

D) Risk factors for developing these tumors include chronic UV-light exposure, HPV infection, certain forms of chronic dermatitis, increased age, light skin pigmentation, immunosuppression, and genetic disorders such as xeroderma pigmentosum.

E) These tumors may uncommonly arise within cyst walls deep in the dermis or subcutis.

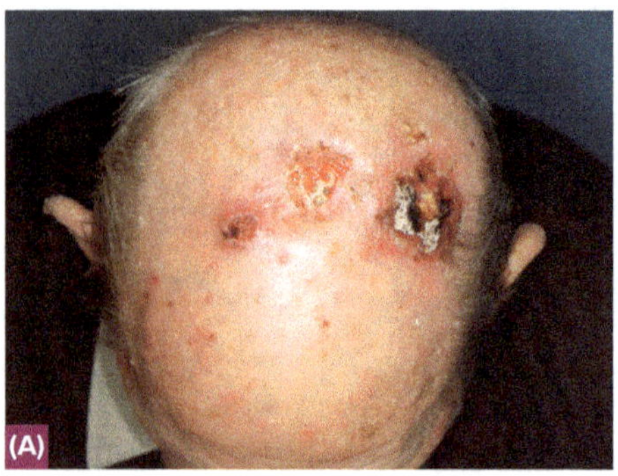
(A)

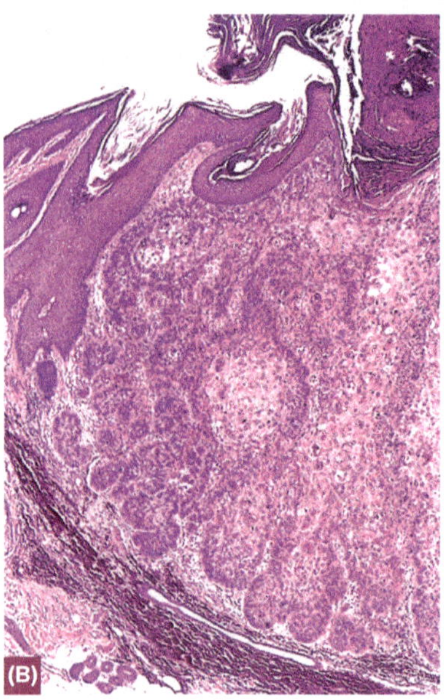
(B)

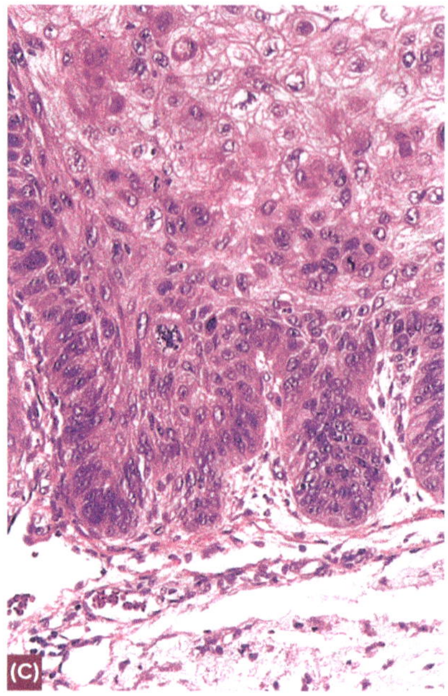
(C)

QUESTION 8-21.

A 60-year-old male presents with a rapidly enlarging smooth, hemispheric nodule with a central crater containing keratinous material. The lesion is biopsied and the findings are illustrated below. Which of the following statements regarding this tumor is INCORRECT?

A) A subset of these lesions will regress spontaneously or after injection with medications such as kenalog, methotrexate, or 5FU.

B) A subset of these tumors is persistent, exhibits malignant behavior, and therefore must be completely excised.

C) There is a nonfamilial syndrome characterized by a generalized eruption of smaller tumors (2-3 mm in diameter).

D) An eruptive form of these tumors may be seen following treatment for BRAF-positive melanoma.

E) These tumors classically arise on the soles, genitalia, and oral cavity, are usually slow growing, locally aggressive, and frequently misdiagnosed as warts on superficial biopsies.

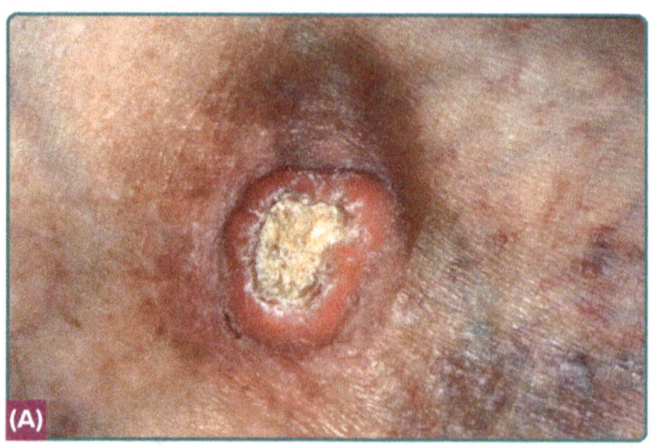
(A)

Reproduced, with permission, from Goldsmith LA, Katz SI, Gilchrest BA, Paller AS, Leffell DJ, Wolff K, eds. *Fitzpatrick's Dermatology in General Medicine*. 8th ed. New York, NY: McGraw-Hill Education; 2012.

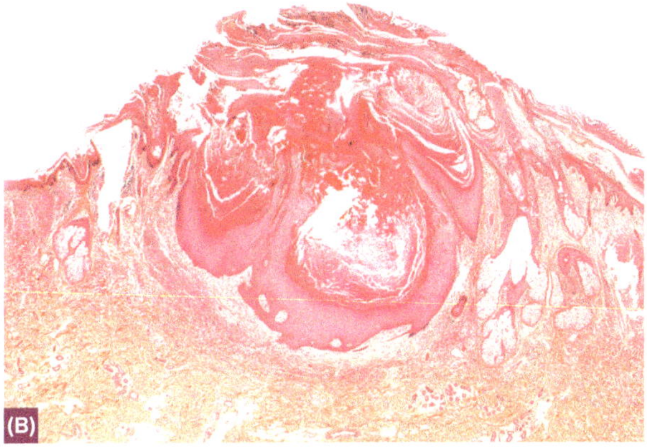

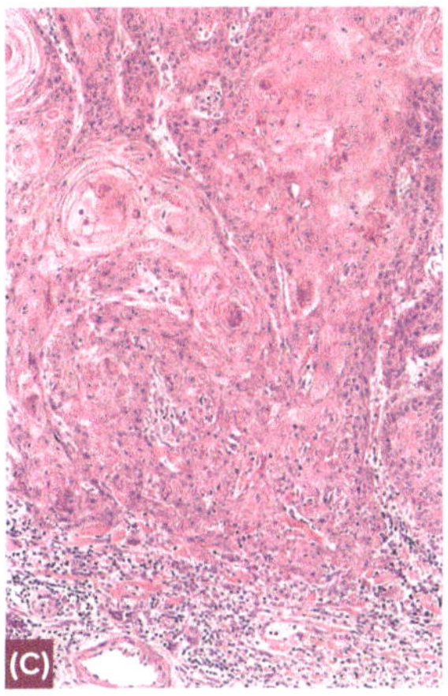

QUESTION 8-22.

A 35-year-old female presents with a painful, yellow nodule on the plantar surface with a hard central core. The lesion is biopsied and the findings are illustrated below. The central crater is surfaced by compact parakeratosis. Which of the following diagnoses is CORRECT?

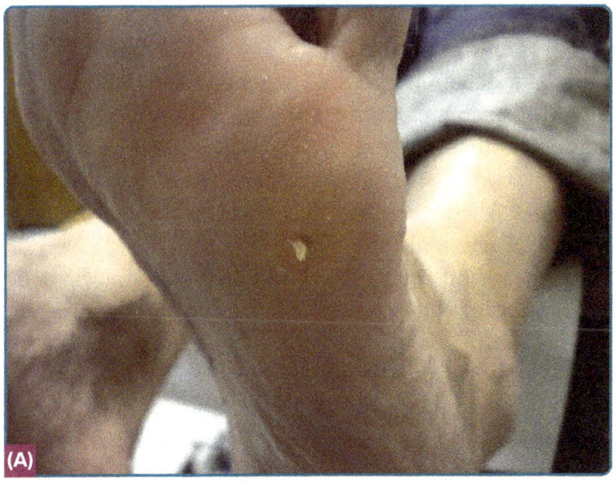

Reproduced, with permission, from Goldsmith LA, Katz SI, Gilchrest BA, Paller AS, Leffell DJ, Wolff K, eds. *Fitzpatrick's Dermatology in General Medicine.* 8th ed. New York, NY: McGraw-Hill Education; 2012.

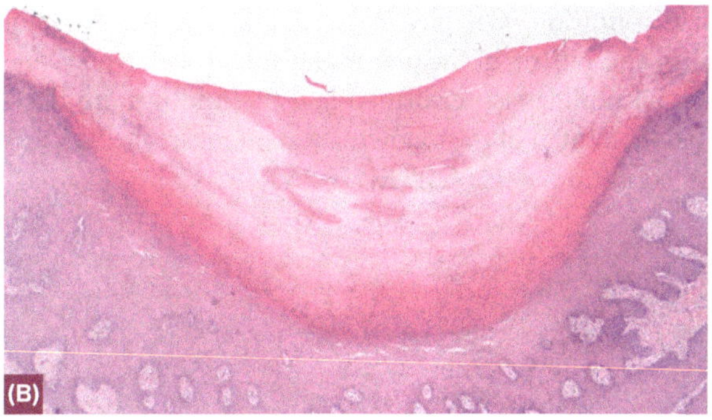

A) Verruca vulgaris
B) Callous
C) Squamous cell carcinoma in situ
D) Clavus
E) Porokeratosis

QUESTION 8-23.

An elderly women presents with a pink translucent macule with telangiectasias on the temple. A biopsy is performed and the findings are illustrated below. Which of the following regarding this tumor is INCORRECT?

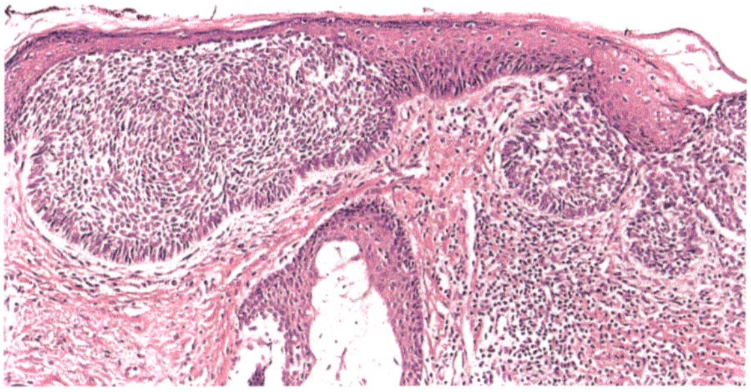

A) This tumor expresses BerEP4 and BCL2 via immunohistochemistry.
B) This particular tumor may be treated with topic imiquimod or 5-fluorouracil.
C) This particular tumor type has a propensity for multifocality.
D) This tumor is the most common malignant neoplasm in humans and is strongly associated with chronic UV exposure.
E) The epidermal changes are non-neoplastic and a reactive response to an underlying dermatofibroma.

QUESTION 8-24.

A 25-year-old female patient presents with numerous dome-shaped papules to soft nodular or flat plaques on the face and trunk. Additionally, the patient began to develop numerous nodular masses in the jaw around the age of 7, which have resulted in tooth loss. The patient reports that the father had a similar condition. On physical exam you notice skeletal anomalies and pitting of the palms and soles. A biopsy of one of the facial nodules is performed and the findings are illustrated below. Which of the following statements regarding this patient's condition is INCORRECT?

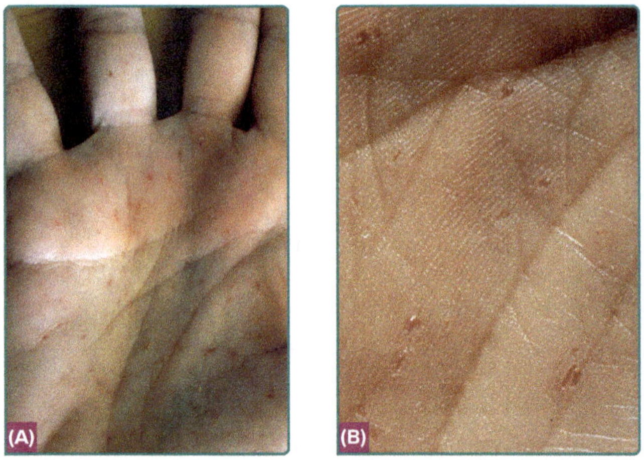

Reproduced, with permission, from Goldsmith LA, Katz SI, Gilchrest BA, Paller AS, Leffell DJ, Wolff K, eds. *Fitzpatrick's Dermatology in General Medicine*. 8th ed. New York, NY: McGraw-Hill Education; 2012.

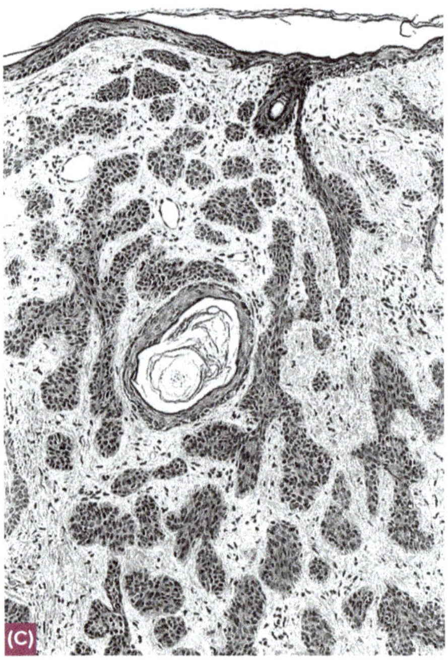

A) This is an autosomal dominant condition in which patients are born with a malfunctioning tumor-suppressor gene known as *PATCHED* on chromosome 9q22-q31.
B) The tumor imaged above is referred to as fibroepithelioma of Pinkus, and is the most common type of tumor associated with this condition.
C) Patients with this condition are associated with a markedly increased risk of metastasis of this tumor compared to the general population.
D) This patient is at an increased risk of developing rhabdomyosarcoma, ovarian fibrosarcoma, and leiomyosarcoma.
E) The nodular jaw masses are most likely keratinous cysts lined by epithelium containing an eosinophilic cuticle and lacking a granular cell layer.

ANSWERS

ANSWER 8-1: B.

Dermoid cysts are rare and result from aberrant sequestration of ectoderm into the dermis during embryogenesis. They present in children as enlarging subcutaneous swellings along an embryonic fusion plane. Commonly located around the eyes, they may erode into bone. Microscopically, they are lined by a thin stratified squamous epithelium, including a granular layer. They contain abundant loose lamellar orthokeratosis, as well as other normal cutaneous structures such as hair follicles, sebaceous lobules, eccrine glands, apocrine glands, or smooth muscle. The cyst lumen contains fragments of hair shaft.

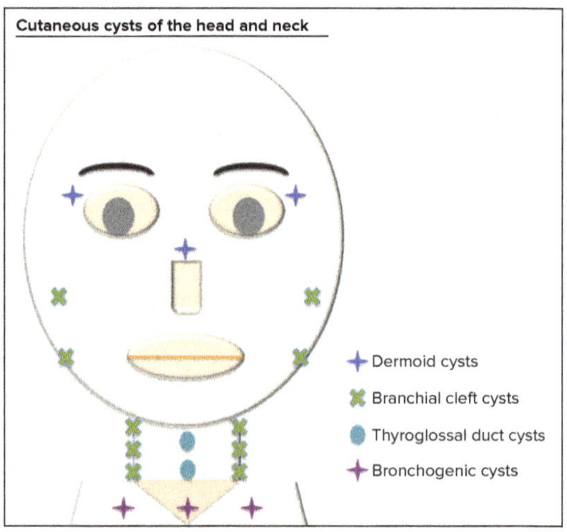

Epidermoid cysts may occur anywhere on the body at any age. Like **dermoid** cysts, microscopically they consist of a stratified, squamous epithelium with a granular layer and abundant laminated orthokeratin within the cavity. Unlike **dermoid cysts**, however, epidermoid cysts lack skin appendages and hair shaft material. They may occasionally rupture inducing a foreign body giant cell reaction.

Branchial cleft cysts are found in the lateral neck along the lymph node chain, on the mandible, or preauricular region. Failure of a portion of the second branchial cleft to involute completely during development results in formation of an epithelium-lined cyst with or without a sinus tract to the overlying skin. This type of cyst may be lined by various types of epithelium (squamous, respiratory, stratified cuboidal). Lymphoid follicles are found within the wall, but true encapsulated lymph node architecture is not identified. They can become tender, inflamed, or develop abscesses, especially during periods of upper respiratory tract infection, due to the lymphoid tissue located beneath the epithelium.

Bronchogenic cysts arise from abnormal ventral budding of the tracheobronchial tree. They are most commonly located on the suprasternal notch, and rarely on the anterior neck and chin. A fistulous tract may attach to the epidermis. They are lined by pseudostratified ciliated columnar epithelium with interspersed goblet cells, and the cyst wall often contains smooth muscle and mucous glands, and, rarely, cartilage.

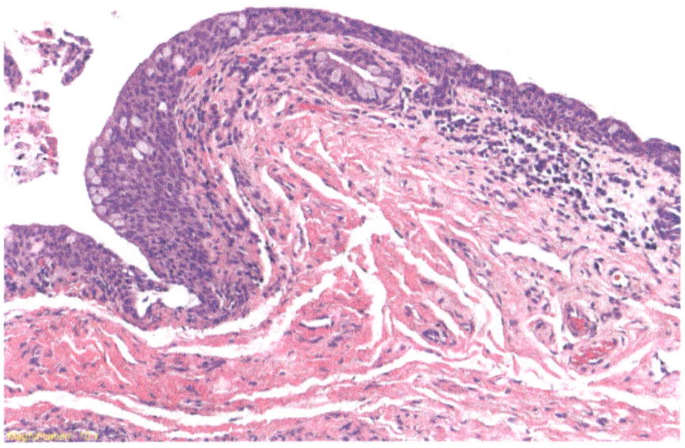

Bronchogenic cyst. High-power magnification shows cyst lining composed of ciliated pseudostratified epithelium with goblet cells. Focal areas of squamous metaplasia are present.

CLUES IN THE CYST WALL

Dermoid cyst
Normal cutaneous structures

Vellus hair cyst
Telogen-like hair follicles
Small arrector pili muscles
Melanocytes, Langerhans cells

Steatocystoma
Sebaceous glands

Thymic cyst
Lymphoid cells
Hassle corpuscles
Cholesterol granulomas

Bronchogenic cyst
Smooth muscle
Cartilage

Branchial cleft cyst
Abundant lymphoid tissue

Thyroglossal duct cysts
Thyroid follicles

Thyroglossal duct cysts are found on the anterior midline neck in young children. They represent remnants of the **thyroglossal duct** that have failed to migrate. Frequently there is a tract connecting these cysts to the hyoid bone, and therefore the cysts will characteristically move with swallowing. They are lined by simple cuboidal or columnar epithelium or stratified squamous epithelium that may contain some ciliated columnar cells. A pseudostratified columnar ciliated lining might also be observed. Thyroid follicles are characteristically present within the wall of the cyst and are the most characteristic feature. The thyroid follicles are composed of lobules of low cuboidal cells surrounding homogenous pink material (colloid).

ANSWER 8-2: D.

Submental draining sinus tract due to a dental abscess is usually lined by squamous epithelium and exhibits marked acute and chronic inflammation, characterized by neutrophilic and lymphohistiocytic infiltrates, respectively. The underlying stroma exhibits varying stages of granulation, characterized by loose collagen, numerous fibroblasts, and dilated vessels oriented perpendicular to the surface. Ulceration and acute and chronic inflammation are generally not features of the other entities, with the possible exception of ruptured epidermoid cysts and **branchial cleft cysts**. Furthermore, the keratinous contents of a ruptured cyst usually generate a striking foreign body giant cell reaction, a feature lacking in fistulas or sinus tracts. Clinical correlation may be required to distinguish from lymphoid follicle-containing **branchial cleft cysts.**

Branchial cleft cysts are found in the lateral neck along the lymph node chain, on the mandible, or preauricular regions. The cyst wall contains lymphoid follicles and is lined by various types of epithelium (squamous, respiratory, or stratified cuboidal). Acute inflammation (neutrophils) and erosion are not typical features.

Cutaneous ciliated cysts are rare and occur on the legs of females, although a few cases have been reported in men. Upon rupture they drain clear to amber fluid. They may be unilocular or multiloculated, and the epithelial lining is composed entirely of ciliated columnar epithelium that may have projections into the cyst lumen.

Bronchogenic cysts occur on the suprasternal notch and, rarely, on the anterior neck or chin. They have a respiratory lining, consisting of goblet cells filled with mucin, as well as ciliated pseudostratified columnar epithelium. Squamous metaplasia of the cyst wall may occur, resulting in both stratified squamous as well as ciliated columnar cells and goblet cells. Cartilage and smooth muscle are usually present.

ANSWER 8-3: A.

Thymic cysts are rapidly enlarging subcutaneous swellings that arise in children in the neck lateral to the thyroid glands. These cysts are lined by simple cuboidal epithelium with prominent lymphoid follicles in the wall. **Hassall corpuscles**, which are composed of concentric squamous epithelial cells with focal central apoptosis, are abundant. An additional finding is an occasional granulomatous inflammatory component with multinucleated giant-cell aggregates and cholesterol crystals. These cysts are considered a variant of **branchial cleft cyst**, since the thymus arises from the third branchial pouch. **Thymic cysts** are separated from this entity because **branchial cleft** cysts lack **Hassall corpuscles** and cholesterol granulomas.

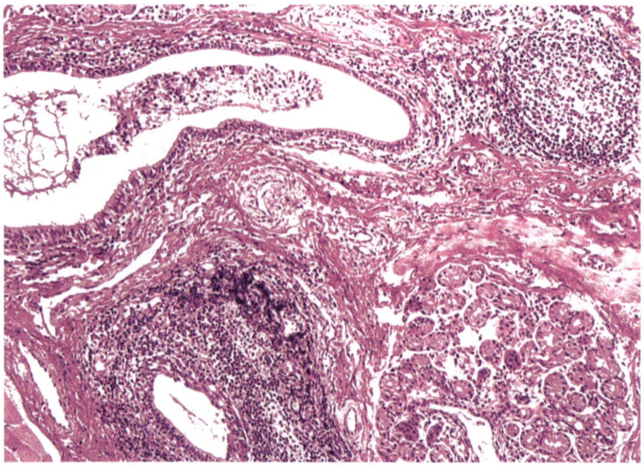

Branchial cleft cyst. The cyst is lined by respiratory-type epithelium. Note the lymphoid tissue surrounding the cyst wall. Hassall corpuscles are absent.

Thyroglossal duct cysts occur in the anterior midline of the neck and are lined by metaplastic stratified squamous epithelium and/or respiratory epithelium (ciliated pseudostratified columnar epithelium with goblet cells) and contain thyroid follicles within their walls.

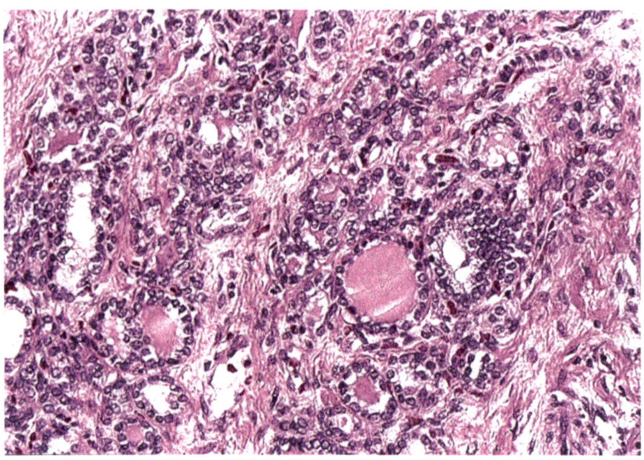

Thyroglossal duct cyst. Thyroid follicles are present near the wall of the cyst. The follicles are composed of lobules composed of circular glands containing eosinophilic colloid.

Bronchogenic cysts may contain cartilage and smooth muscle within their walls and do not have Hassall corpuscles, cholesterol granulomas, or associated lymphoid tissue.

Epidermoid cysts may occur anywhere on the body at any age. Microscopically, there is a squamous lining and the cyst is filled with thick acellular keratinous debris. However, they may occasionally rupture inducing a foreign body giant cell reaction with acute and chronic inflammation. They obviously lack Hassall corpuscles.

ANSWER 8-4: D.

Cutaneous ciliated cysts are uncommon lesions, and usually occur on the buttocks and lower extremities in young women. Occasionally they may arise within the vulva. Some authors have suggested that these cysts should be renamed **cutaneous Müllerian cysts** to reflect their presumed Müllerian duct origin. Others, however, citing the extremely rare occurrence of these lesions in men, too, suggest that these lesions arise from eccrine glands that have undergone ciliated metaplasia. They may be located in either the subcutis or deep dermis and may be either unilocular or multilocular. Papillary projections in the cyst lumen are characteristic, and the tissues surrounding the cyst are free of skin appendages, glandular elements, and muscle fibers. The lining of the cyst is a simple cuboidal to columnar ciliated epithelium, with some areas of pseudostratified ciliated epithelium. Occasionally areas with squamous metaplasia may be present.

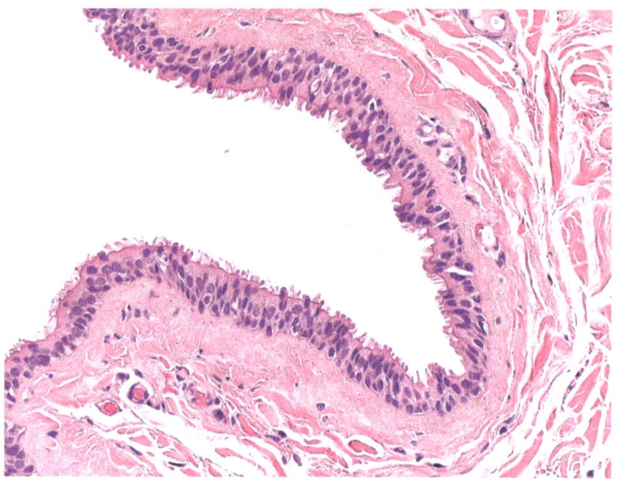

Cutaneous ciliated cyst. The cyst lining is composed of columnar epithelium with cilia. The adjacent stroma lacks adnexal structures, inflammation, and smooth muscle.

Like **bronchogenic cysts**, foci of squamous metaplasia can occur; however, lymphoid tissue is absent in **cutaneous ciliated cysts**. Cholesterol granulomas and Hassall corpuscles are observed in **thymic cysts**. The differential diagnosis also includes **hidrocystoma**; however, the absence of decapitation secretions in cutaneous ciliated cysts distinguishes these two entities. A summary of the clinical and histopathological features of cysts lined by mixed squamous and nonsquamous ciliated epithelium is provided in Table 8-4A.

Table 8-4A. Clinical and Histologic Features of Cysts Lined by Mixed Squamous and Nonsquamous Ciliated Epithelium

CYST	CLINICAL FEATURES	HISTOPATHOLOGIC FEATURES	OTHER FEATURES
Bronchogenic	Neck, but may occur on face, back, shoulder, abdomen	Ciliated lining with goblet cells, stratified squamous lining in some areas because of metaplasia	Wall may contain smooth muscle or cartilage
Branchial cleft	Jaw and preauricular area in areas of lymph nodes	Pseudostratified columnar epithelium with cilia and areas of stratified squamous epithelium	Lymphoid follicles are abundant and may be the predominant component
Ciliated (mucinous) cyst of vulva	Labia minoris	Mucin-containing cells with some cilia	Müllerian origin
Cutaneous ciliated	Buttocks, LE, women	Cuboidal or columnar single layer of ciliated cells	Same origin as ciliated cyst of vulva
Thyroglossal duct	Midline of neck	Cuboidal ciliated epithelium admixed with stratified squamous epithelium	Characteristic presence of thyroid follicles in cyst wall

Abbreviation: LE = lower extremities.

ANSWER 8-5: C.

This is an example of **cutaneous endometriosis**. These painful brown nodular lesions in the skin most frequently arise from ectopic implantation in cesarean and periumbilical scars; however, hematogenous dissemination may occur. Symptoms generally worsen during menstruation. The clinical differential diagnosis for umbilical cutaneous endometriosis includes **hemangioma, umbilical hernia, pyogenic granuloma, foreign body granuloma, keloids, omphalomesenteric duct cyst, urachal duct cyst, endosalpingiosis, irritated nevus, melanoma, primary carcinoma, sarcoma,** or a **Sister Mary Joseph nodule (umbilical metastasis of a visceral carcinoma).**

Umbilical Nodule DDX

Cutaneous endometriosis
Endosalpingiosis
Hemangioma
Umbilical hernia
Pyogenic granuloma
Foreign body granuloma
Keloid
Omphalomesenteric duct cyst
Urachal cyst
Irritated nevus
Melanoma
Primary carcinoma
Primary sarcoma
Sister Mary Joseph nodule (most commonly gastric, colon, ovarian, or pancreatic cancers)

Microscopically, **cutaneous endometriosis** is characterized by the presence of endometrial glands, short spindle cell stroma, and hemorrhage/hemosiderin in the mid- or deep dermis. In general two out of the three elements are needed to confidently establish a diagnosis. The glandular component is comprised of tall columnar epithelium with basophilic cytoplasm and basally located nuclei. Sometimes there can be marked mitotic activity, depending on the phase of the menstrual cycle. Menstrual bleeding into the dermis leads to hemosiderin deposition (which is seen with the Perl stain), scarring, and chronic inflammation.

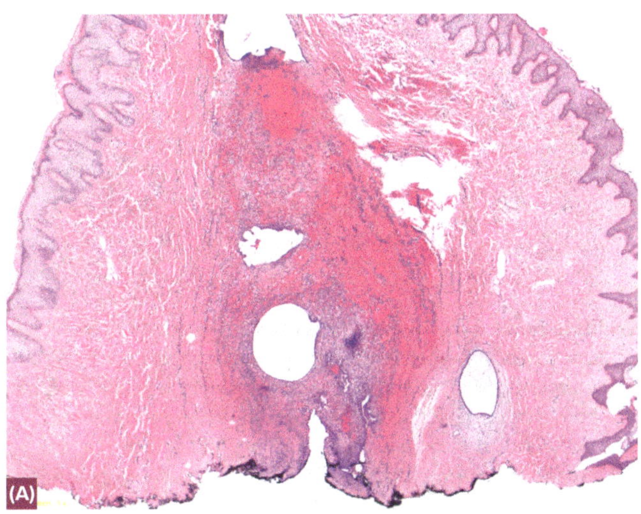

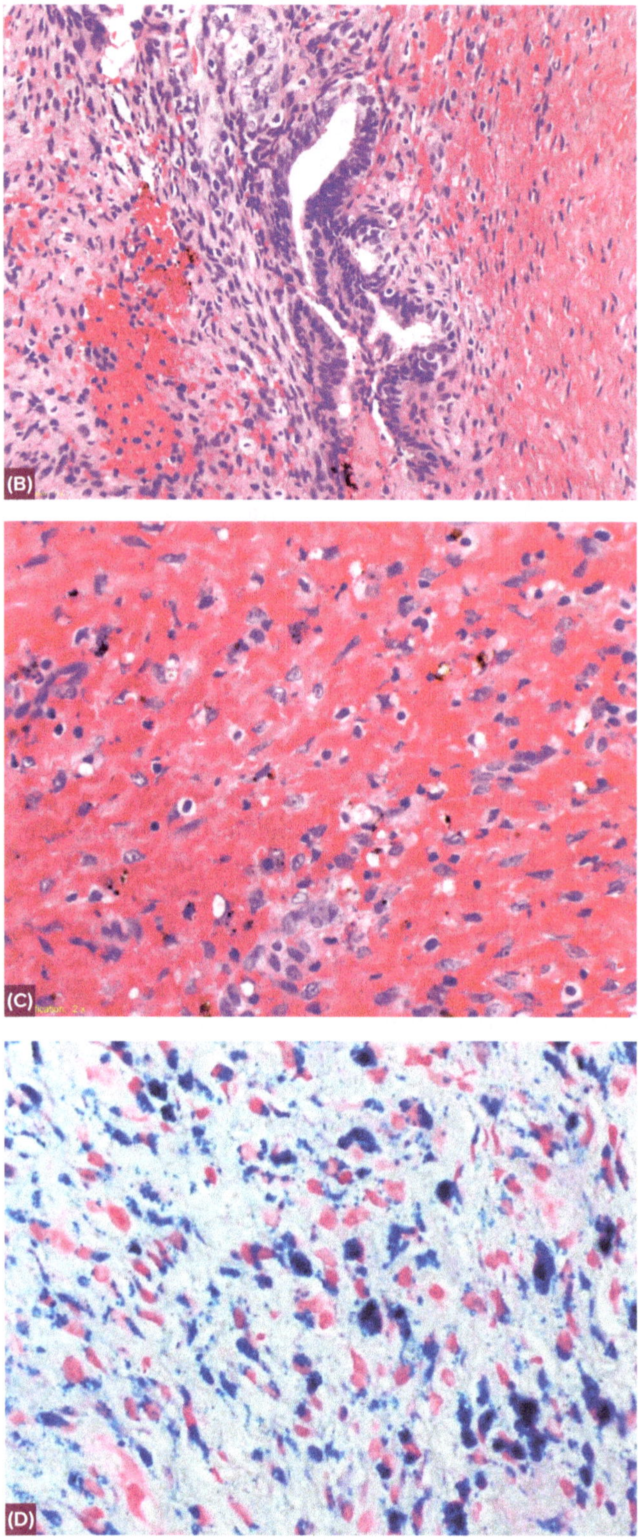

Endometriosis, proliferative phase. (A) Low power revealing a nodular focus of hemorrhage admixed with glandular and stromal elements. **(B)** The glands are composed of basaloid columnar epithelial cells, consistent with proliferative endometrium. The surrounding stroma is composed of short spindle cells. **(C)** Extravasated red blood cells and hemosiderin are present. **(D)** Perl stain highlights the hemosiderin granules in light blue.

Cutaneous endosalpingiosis is clinically indistinguishable from endometriosis. It may arise after salpingectomy for ectopic tubal pregnancy. It differs by the cyst epithelium being of fallopian tube differentiation with ciliated and nonciliated columnar cells and intercalary or peg cells.

Urachal cyst results from an incomplete urachal duct remnant. The urachus is the tube that connects the fetal bladder to the umbilicus. Persistent urachus presents during infancy with leakage of urine from the umbilicus. These cysts are characterized by urothelial lining of stratified transitional epithelium.

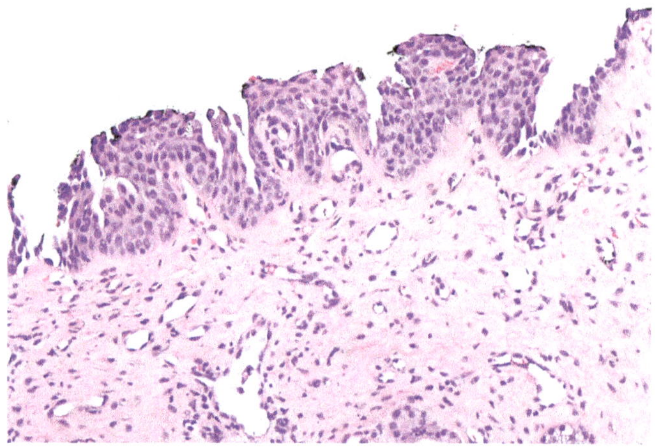

Urachal cyst. The cyst lining is composed of transitional-type urothelium.

Omphalomesenteric duct cyst results from faulty closure of the omphalomesenteric duct, which is the embryologic connection between the midgut and the yolk sac. They are characterized by ectopic gastrointestinal mucosa and must be distinguished from umbilical metastases of gastrointestinal adenocarcinoma.

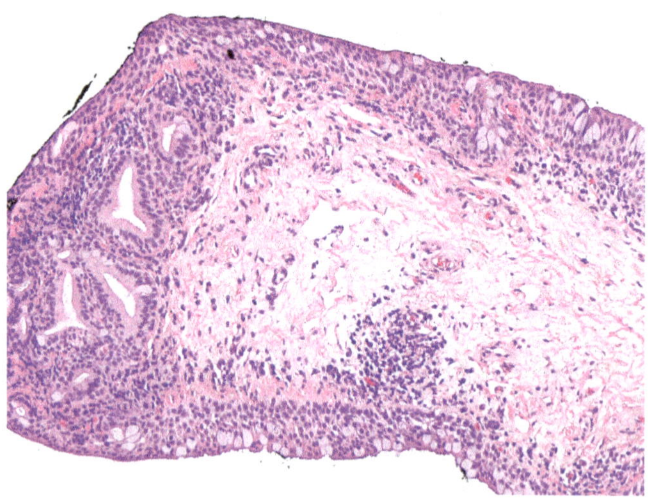

Omphalomesenteric duct cyst. The cyst wall lining is composed of intestinal-type glandular mucosa containing numerous goblet cells.

ANSWER 8-6: E.

Median raphe cysts occur exclusively in young males as a single bluish/translucent cyst on the ventral shaft of the penis. They are believed to arise from a small urothelial rest of the urethra. The clinical differential diagnosis for cysts of the penis included **glomus tumor, dermoid cyst, pilonidal cyst, epidermal cyst, urethral diverticulum**, and **steatocystoma**. Occasionally several cysts may be present in a linear configuration. Microscopically, the cysts are lined by transitional epithelium (urothelium) with occasional mucinous glands and a highly vascularized dermis. The epithelium varies in thickness, but typically does not exceed five cell layers, and in some areas a single layer may be observed consisting of fusiform cells. **Urethral diverticula** communicate with the urethra, not **median raphe cysts**. Distinguishing **median raphe cysts** from **apocrine hidrocystoma** can be difficult, and several reports of **apocrine hidrocystoma** of the penis may actually represent **median raphe cyst**. **Apocrine hidrocystomas** have an apical border of luminal cells, show “snouting” or apical decapitation secretion, and are GCDFP-15 positive.

Penile Cyst Clinical DDX

Median raphe cyst
Glomus tumor
Dermoid cyst
Pilonidal cyst
Epidermal cyst
Urethral diverticulum
Steatocystoma

ANSWER 8-7: E.

Epidermoid cysts are lined by an attenuated stratified squamous epithelium with a granular layer containing abundant laminated orthokeratotic contents. They are the most common type of cysts to be evaluated in the pathology laboratory. They most frequently present on the face, neck, back, and torso, and many authors prefer the term **infundibular cyst** or **follicular inclusion cyst**, since it is believed that they arise from the infundibular portion of the hair follicle. However, rarely these cysts may arise at acral sites or within scars, which are devoid of hair follicles. Therefore, cysts at these sites with identical lining are believed to arise from implantation of epidermis into the dermis through trauma. Some authors propose the term **epidermal inclusion cyst** for these cases. Therefore, the designation **epidermoid cyst** represents an “umbrella” term encompassing both entities. When multiple **epidermoid cysts** arise in scrotal skin and calcify, it is referred to as “**scrotal calcinosis**.” Rupture of **epidermoid cysts** results in an exuberant granulomatous foreign body giant cell reaction where flakes of keratin may be identified within giant cells. Fragments of hair shaft may also be seen in **infundibular cysts**. These lesions may occasionally communicate with the overlying epidermis, but the keratinous material results in attenuation (or stretching) of the epithelial lining. Occasionally, only cyst contents are present in the biopsy sample, which are characterized by loose flakes of orthokeratosis.

Dilated pore of Winer consists of a large cystic cavity filled with basket weave stratum corneum and a stenotic ostium communicating with the epidermal surface. The lesion extends into the dermis, with hyperplastic epithelium forming platelike extensions of elongated rete ridges. This is in contrast to the attenuated epithelial lining of an **epidermoid cyst**. **Pilar sheath acanthoma** is similar, but exhibits numerous eosinophilic staining lobular aggregates of cells that radiate outward from the cystic cavity into the surrounding dermis.

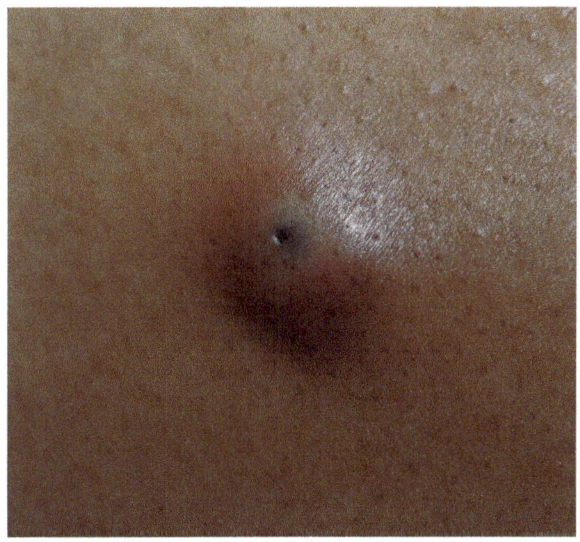

Epidermoid cyst. There is a dome-shaped nodule with a small opening communicating with the epidermal surface. (Reproduced, with permission, from Wolff K, Johnson RA, Saavedra AP. *Fitzpatrick's Color Atlas and Synopsis of Clinical Dermatology.* 7th ed. New York, NY: McGraw-Hill Education; 2013.)

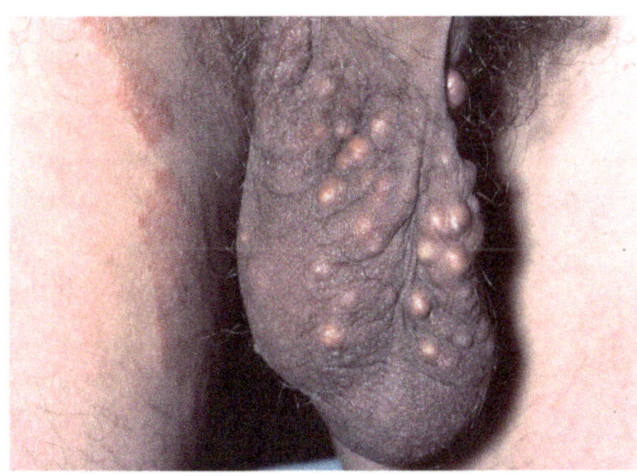

Scrotal calcinosis.

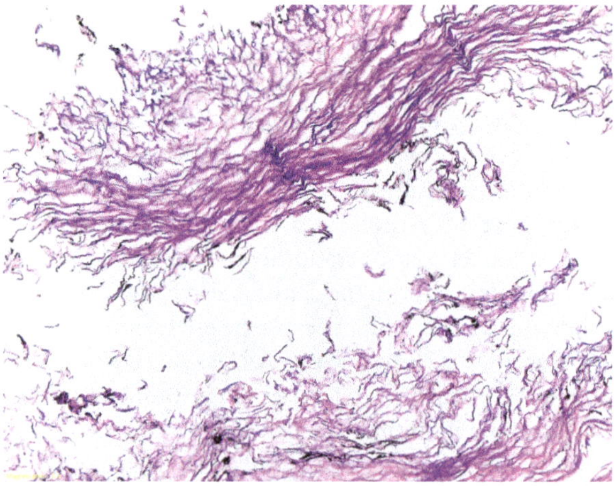

Contents of an epidermoid cyst.

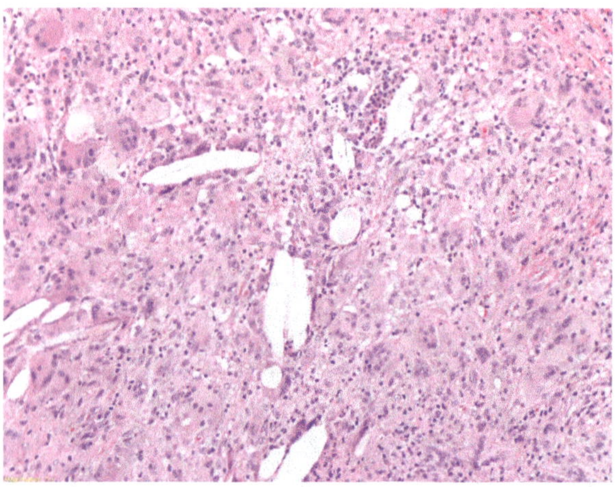

Ruptured infundibular cyst. Note the robust foreign body giant cell reaction to the flakes of keratin and naked hair shaft.

ANSWER 8-8: A.

Trichilemmal cysts (aka **pilar cysts**) are common lesions that arise predominantly on the scalp, but otherwise share clinical features similar to **epidermoid cysts**. There is a strong female preponderance. Lesions tend to be solitary; however, multiple cysts can occur. Unlike **epidermoid cysts**, where it may be difficult to completely remove the cyst lining with incision, **pilar cysts** frequently "pop out" with simple incision. **Pilar cysts** are lined by outer root sheath epithelium, hence arise within portions of the hair follicle that do not contain an inner root sheath, such as the isthmus of anagen hairs or from the sac surrounding catagen and telogen hairs. These cysts may be situated in the middle to deep reticular dermis or subcutis. There is abrupt keratinization of the inner surface of the cyst lining resulting in compact homogeneous keratin. A characteristic feature of **pilar cysts** is the apparent absence of intercellular bridges between the keratinocytes. Unlike **epidermoid cysts**, no granular cell layer is present and there is palisading of nuclei in the basal layer. When ruptured, a robust foreign body giant cell reaction with calcification occurs (Table 8-8A).

Follicular Origin of Cysts

FOLLICULAR INFUNDIBULUM
- Epidermoid cyst
- Milium
- Pigmented follicular cyst
- Vellus hair cyst

SEBACEOUS DUCT
- Steatocystoma

OUTER ROOT SHEATH
- Trichilemmal cyst

Table 8-8A. Clinical and Histologic Features of Cysts Lined by Stratified Squamous Epithelium

CYST	CLINICAL FEATURES	HISTOPATHOLOGIC FEATURES	OTHER FEATURES
Epidermoid inclusion (infundibular cyst)	Solitary or multiple, face, neck, torso; occasionally palms and soles	Stratified squamous lining with variably thick granular layer; loose, abundant laminated orthokeratin	Rupture associated with foreign body giant cell reaction, inflammation, and scarring
Pilar (trichilemmal)	Usually solitary, may be multiple, head and scalp	Stratified squamous lining of keratinocytes with poorly defined intercellular bridges Abrupt keratinization to compact keratin No or attenuated granular layer	Proliferating pilar tumor arises from the benign cystic counterpart
Vellus hair	Multiple, autosomal dominant or sporadic; trunk, chest, and extremities, small and may be pigmented	Small, dermally located, thin stratified squamous lining, characteristic presence of multiple vellus hairs in cyst lumen	Connection to a vellus hair may be identified

Table 8-8A. Clinical and Histologic Features of Cysts Lined by Stratified Squamous Epithelium *(continued)*

CYST	CLINICAL FEATURES	HISTOPATHOLOGIC FEATURES	OTHER FEATURES
Milium	Small, 1- to 2-mm papules, primary or associated with blistering disorders	Small cysts arising from infundibulum of vellus hairs, lined by thin stratified squamous lining	Milia secondary to scarring or bullous disease probably arise from eccrine ducts
Pigmented follicular	Solitary lesions on the face, M> > >F, deeply pigmented	Stratified squamous epithelium with numerous pigmented hair shafts in lumen	Connection to the surface of the epidermis usually observed
Hybrid	Rare, scalp or face, wide age range	Superior portion of cyst lined by stratified squamous epithelium, like an EC; sharp transition to lower portion showing trichilemmal keratinization	Hybrid cyst consisting of other combinations of hair follicle derivation may be seen
Proliferating epithelial cyst	Rare; 1:1.8 F:M ratio; pelvic, anogenital area, scalp, upper extremities, trunk	Acanthotic papillomatous or verrucous stratified squamous lining, atypia, mitotic figures may be present	Carcinomatous change may be seen, local recurrence relatively common, frequent connection with epidermis

ANSWER 8-9: E.

Vellus hair cysts most commonly present as multiple lesions as part of an autosomal dominant disease termed **eruptive vellus hair cysts (EVHCs)**. A sporadic form with solitary lesions also exists. Small pigmented cysts of red, brown, gray, or black coloration usually occur on the anterior chest, abdomen, extremities of patients within the first or second decade of life. The familial form has an association with **steatocystoma multiplex, trichostasis spinulosa**, and other heritable disorders, such as **pachyonychia congenital type 2 (PC-2)**. **PC-2** can result from mutations in genes encoding either keratin 17 (*KRT17*) or keratin 6B (*KRT6B*). Keratin 17 is expressed in the nail bed, hair follicles, and sebaceous glands, but not in stratified squamous epithelium.

Vellus hair cysts arise within the lower infundibular portion of the vellus hair follicle. The cyst wall lining is that of attenuated epithelium with a diminished granular layer, filled with keratinized debris and multiple vellus hair shafts. Frequently, the inner lining may contain an eosinophilic cuticle, identical to that seen in **steatocystomas** and normal sebaceous ducts. The cyst wall may contain telogen hair follicles as well as elongated fascicles of smooth muscle (erector pili), but lacks other adnexal components such as sebaceous glands or apocrine glands. Cysts with a similar lining that lack vellus hairs but do contain sebaceous glands are consistent with **steatocystomas. Steatocystomas**, in contrast, often have readily identifiable sebaceous glands in the cyst wall, as well as a pink cuticle on the luminal aspect of the epithelial lining. **Steatocystomas** lack vellus hair shafts.

ANSWER 8-10: D.

Steatocystomas may occur as solitary non-inherited cysts in adults referred to as **steatocystoma simplex**, or as numerous autosomal dominantly inherited cysts referred to as **steatocystoma multiplex**. These lesions appear clinically as small white/yellowish cysts in the axilla, groin, or chest. They usually occur during puberty suggesting some androgenic control. These lesions are thought to represent a hamartomatous condition of the pilar sebaceous junction, hence the frequent presence of erector pili smooth muscle in close proximity to the cyst wall. The cysts are lined by a thin stratified squamous epithelium, which lacks a granular cell layer and contains a crenulated eosinophilic cuticle on its surface, analogous to normal sebaceous duct lining. Lobules of sebaceous glands

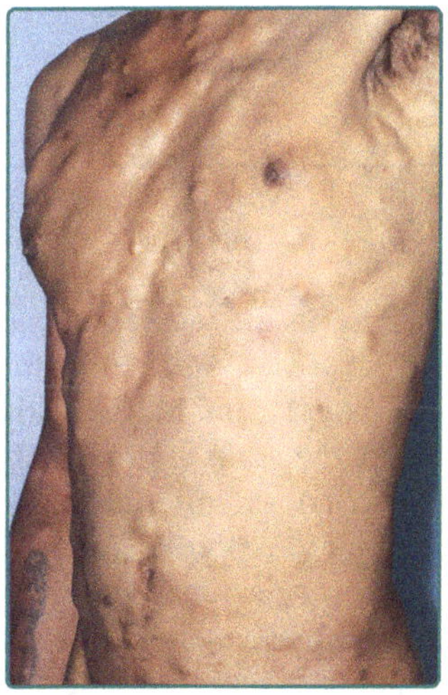

Steatocystoma multiplex. Multiple skin-colored cystic lesions on the trunk. (Reproduced, with permission, from Goldsmith LA, Katz SI, Gilchrest BA, Paller AS, Leffell DJ, Wolff K, eds. *Fitzpatrick's Dermatology in General Medicine*. 8th ed. New York, NY: McGraw-Hill Education; 2012.)

are frequently seen attached to the cyst wall; however, their presence is not required for diagnosis.

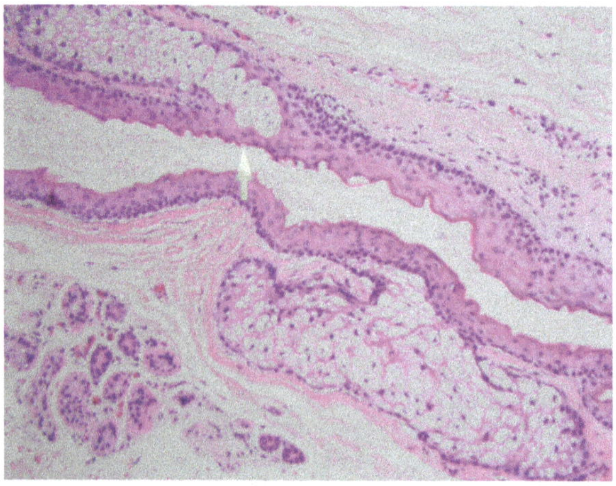

Steatocystoma. The cyst is lined by squamous epithelium without a granular cell layer. The inner lining is composed of an eosinophilic cuticle. Numerous sebaceous glands are present in the cyst wall (arrow).

Steatocystomas may be distinguished from **epidermoid cysts** by the thinner cyst wall lining, the presence of sebaceous glands within the wall, and the pink cuticle. Similarly, **milia** and **vellus hair cysts**, which are similar in size to **steatocystoma**, lack the sebaceous glands in the wall.

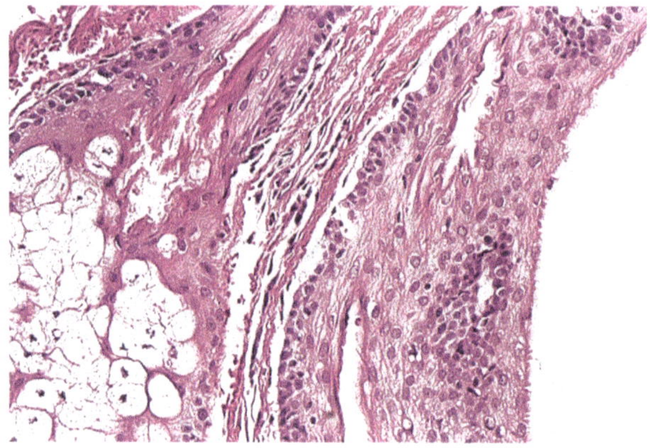

Steatocystoma. The cyst is lined by a wrinkled eosinophilic cuticle.

Table 8-10A. Clinical and Histologic Features of Cysts Lined by Stratified Squamous Epithelium and Containing Elements within the Cyst Wall

CYST	CLINICAL FEATURES	HISTOPATHOLOGIC FEATURES	OTHER FEATURES
Steatocystoma	Simplex (solitary) or multiplex (hereditary), axilla, groin, chest	Ruggated wall lined by very thin stratified squamous lining with glassy pink cuticle overlying the internal surface	Sebaceous glands arranged within the outer wall of the cyst
Dermoid	Infants and children; periocular, congenital, firm nodules, 1-4 cm	Unilocular cyst with stratified squamous lining; wall contains various appendageal elements such as hair follicles, sebaceous glands, eccrine glands	
Thymic cyst	Neck or anterior mediastinum	Unilocular or multilocular, cuboidal epithelium or stratified squamous, occasional ciliated cells	Thymic tissue may be identified in wall Pseudoepitheliomatous hyperplasia or even malignant transformation may occur, although rare

ANSWER 8-11: C.

Pilonidal cysts most commonly arise in the sacrococcygeal region of men, and can be seen as part of the "**follicular inclusion tetrad**" which consists of **acne conglobata, hidradenitis suppurativa, dissecting cellulitis of the scalp (aka perifolliculitis capitis abscedens et suffodiens)**, and **pilonidal cyst**. **Pilonidal cysts** are believed by many to represent acquired sinus tracts created by the reinsertion of penetrating hairs into the dermis inducing dense neutrophilic and lymphohistiocytic inflammatory infiltrates. Although these lesions may arise in a variety of clinical situations, constant friction or minor trauma at the site may induce reinsertion of hair shafts. Military personnel who frequently travel in jeeps through rocky terrain are notorious for developing these lesions. The cyst wall is lined by stratified squamous epithelium that in many cases may be obliterated or obscured by the inflammatory infiltrates resulting in a fibrous wall. The most diagnostic feature of a pilonidal cyst is the presence of naked hair shafts within the cyst surrounded by an inflammatory infiltrate. The differential diagnosis includes **cutaneous Crohn disease** and a deep dermal abscess. Fistula tracts from **Crohn disease** may arise in this location but will lack an epithelial cyst lining and will contain noncaseating granulomas, which should not be present in a **pilonidal cyst**. **Pilonidal cysts** contain multinucleated giant cell granulomas of the foreign body reaction. Special stains for microorganisms should be performed in lesions in which no cyst lining is identified to exclude a deep-seated infection.

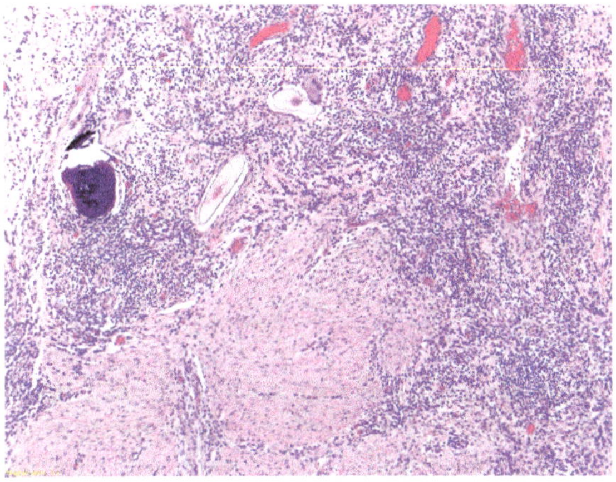

Pilonidal cyst. In this case the epithelial lining has been destroyed by the chronic inflammatory infiltrate. Notice the naked hair shafts surrounded by multinucleated giant cells and scar formation.

ANSWER 8-12: A.

Digital mucous cysts usually arise on the dorsal surface of the finger next to the distal interphalangeal joint. They arise from the adjacent joint space and frequently attach to the joint by a pedicle. An epithelial cyst lining is usually absent with the cyst walls being composed of compressed fibrous tissue. These well-circumscribed nodular lesions contain large amounts of acid mucopolysaccharides, which are highlighted by alcian blue and colloidal iron stains. The clinical location, as well as the sharply localized distribution of the mucin, distinguishes these lesions from focal papular mucinosis and myxedema, which may have a similar histopathology.

Metaplastic synovial cysts contain broad villi lined by inflammatory cells, reactive cuboidal epithelium, and fibrinous exudates. These cysts may arise at any site that has undergone trauma, such as sites with injection of air into tissue,

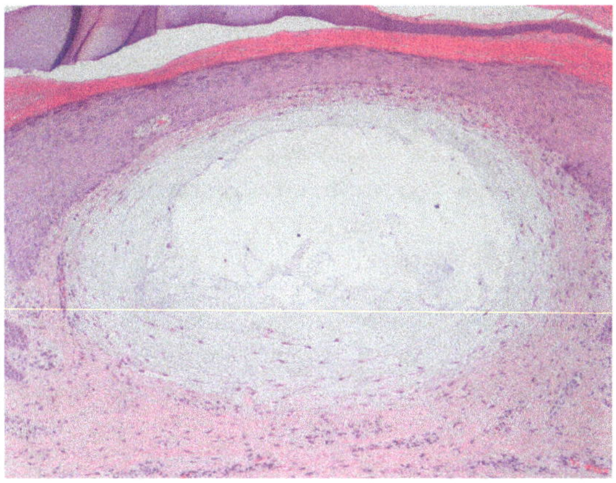

Digital mucous cyst. There is a circumscribed collection of dermal mucin without an epithelial lining.

surgical scars, and puncture wounds. They are located in the dermis and often communicate with the overlying epidermis through fistula tracts. Clinically they are easily mistaken for **suture granulomas, leiomyomas**, and **basal cell carcinomas**. The lining of the **metaplastic synovial cyst** is strikingly reminiscent of inflamed synovium (ie, **villous synovitis**). The central fibrous cores within the villi are composed of dense collagen and fibroblasts. Both the center fibroblasts and the cuboidal epithelial lining cells are positive for vimentin and negative for cytokeratins. **Digital mucous cysts** do not contain villous-like structures within the cyst contents.

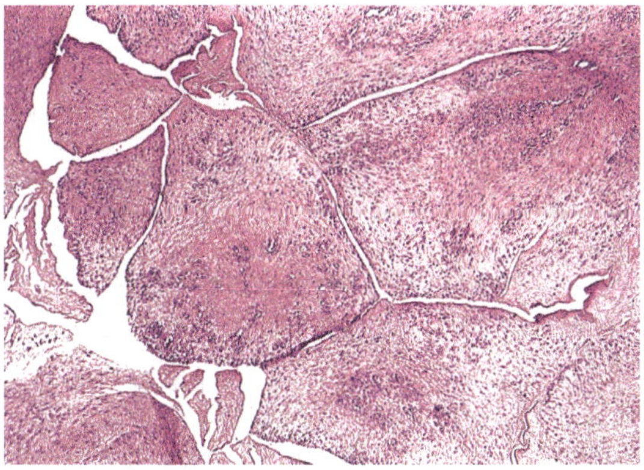

Metaplastic synovial cyst. Bulbous projections are lined by cuboidal cells reminiscent of inflamed synovium.

Table 8-12A. Clinical and Histologic Features of Cysts Not Lined by an Epithelium

CYST	CLINICAL FEATURES	HISTOPATHOLOGIC FEATURES	OTHER FEATURES
Digital mucous cyst	Dorsum of finger	Collagenous wall, lumen that contains acid mucopolysaccharides	Connected to the interphalangeal joint
Pseudocyst of auricle	Asymptomatic swelling of upper pinna of the ear	Cystic space within the cartilage associated with some degenerative changes	Most likely represents developmental defect in ear formation exacerbated by trauma

Table 8-12A. Clinical and Histologic Features of Cysts Not Lined by an Epithelium (*continued*)

CYST	CLINICAL FEATURES	HISTOPATHOLOGIC FEATURES	OTHER FEATURES
Metaplastic synovial cyst	Occur in areas of trauma or surgical sites	Villous projections into cystic cavity, lined by fibrinous exudate, epithelioid cells, inflammation	Immunocytochemically and histologically similar or identical to synovium
Pilonidal cyst	Sacrococcygeal area, but any area may be affected	Acute and chronic inflammation surrounding sinus tract or cystic cavity, hair shafts often identified	May rarely progress to squamous cell carcinoma

ANSWER 8-13: B.

Milia present as small, superficial, 1-2 mm cysts usually on the face. They may arise secondarily due to bullous disorders or trauma such as dermabrasion. The cysts are lined by a stratified squamous epithelium containing a granular cell layer and filled with keratinous debris. Primary **milium cysts** arise from the infundibular portion of vellus hairs, hence sharing the identical cyst lining of epidermoid cysts, which arise from terminal hairs. **Secondary milia** that occur after resolution of bullous lesions or trauma (such as dermabrasion) may occasionally arise from eccrine ducts. **Milium cyst** walls do not contain adnexal structures and the cavities lack fragments of hair shaft distinguishing these lesions from **dermoid cysts** and **vellus hair cysts**.

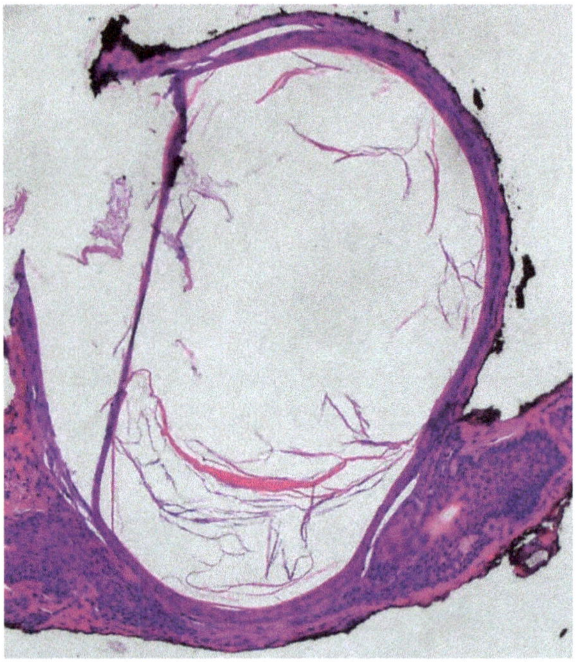

Milium cyst. A small cyst arising from the infundibular portion of a vellus hair that is lined by epithelium containing a granular layer.

ANSWER 8-14: C.

The biopsy reveals a single hair follicle enlarged into a "flask" shape. The lining epidermis shows dyskeratosis and acantholysis. The findings are consistent with a **warty dyskeratoma**, which falls under the general category of **specialized acanthomas**, which include **epidermolytic acanthoma, warty dyskeratoma, acantholytic acanthoma**, and **acantholytic dyskeratoma**. These lesions represent isolated solitary lesions with a histopathology analogous to several widespread counterparts. The glabrous lesions of **warty dyskeratoma** are usually associated with pilosebaceous structures and early changes are limited to the upper portion of the follicular infundibulum (Table 8-14A). However, oral lesions are rare but have been reported and present as small papules or nodules with a central crater. They may assume a papillomatous appearance and are flesh-colored to white. They are frequently

Table 8-14A. Warty Dyskeratoma

Clinical Features
Isolated lesions on the sun-damaged skin of middle-aged persons
Also seen on the oral mucosa
Papulonodule with central pore or umbilication
May discharge foul-smelling material
Histopathologic Features
Flask-shaped cystic invagination involving a pilosebaceous structure
Parakeratotic and hyperkeratotic material in infundibulum
Suprabasal acantholysis with villi and acantholysis
Dyskeratosis, corps ronds, and grains are present
Differential Diagnosis
Darier disease
Benign familial pemphigus
Pemphigus vegetans
Syringocystadenoma papilliferum

associated with irritation and trauma. There is an increased incidence of **warty dyskeratomas** arising in areas with chronic UV light exposure. **Warty dyskeratomas** are endophytic cystic invaginations usually based around follicular ostia in which the epidermis exhibits acantholysis and dyskeratosis analogous to that seen in **Darier disease**. **Corps ronds** and **corps grains** and overlying parakeratosis are observed. Non-endophytic variants with this histopathology are referred to as **acantholytic dyskeratomas**. If these lesions are widespread, the differential diagnosis includes either **Grover disease** or **Darier disease**. Both the **warty dyskeratoma** and **acantholytic dyskeratoma** frequently contain a mixed perivascular inflammatory infiltrate, which is uncommonly present in **Darier disease**. **Acantholytic acanthomas** are solitary lesions with the histopathology similar to that seen in **pemphigus vulgaris** or even **Hailey–Hailey disease,** in which there is marked hyperkeratosis, parakeratosis, and acantholysis present throughout most of the epidermis and accentuated in the granular and suprabasilar layers (Table 8-14B). If multiple lesions are present, the differential diagnosis includes **Grover disease, Hailey–Hailey disease,** and **pemphigus vulgaris**. **Epidermolytic acanthomas** are solitary lesions with the histopathologic features of **epidermolytic hyperkeratosis** analogous to that seen in **bullous congenital ichthyosiform erythroderma**, in which patients are born with critical rod domain mutations for both suprabasal keratins 1 and 10 (Table 8-14C). Clinical correlation is required for definitive diagnosis with all of these specialized acanthomas.

Table 8-14B. Acantholytic Acanthoma

Clinical Features
- Solitary, asymptomatic papule or nodule on the trunk
- 5-15 mm in diameter and hyperkeratotic
- Most common in middle-aged men

Histopathologic Features
- Acantholysis throughout most of the epidermis
- Hyperkeratosis, parakeratosis, and acanthosis
- Symmetric and circumscribed

Differential Diagnosis
- Pemphigus vulgaris, pemphigus vegetans, benign familial pemphigus, and Grover disease
- Acantholytic changes of seborrheic keratoses or actinic keratoses
- Warty dyskeratoma

Table 8-14C. Epidermolytic Acanthoma

Clinical Features
- Small, flat, or verrucous papules
- Most common on the extremities
- Occurs in middle-aged persons and more often in men than in women

Histopathologic Features
- Hyperkeratosis with dense, loosely packed keratinocytes
- Large, coarse basophilic granules in the granular layer with vacuolated keratinocytes
- Fine eosinophilic granules and strands in the spinous and granular layers
- Normal basal layer

Differential Diagnosis
- Epidermolytic hyperkeratosis seen in different cutaneous tumors and diseases
- Warts, particularly the palmoplantar type

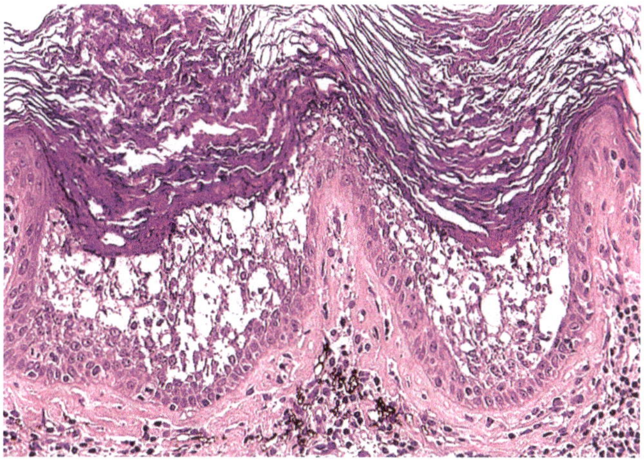

Epidermolytic acanthoma. The spinous and granular layers are vacuolated with enlarged keratohyaline granules. Hyperkeratosis is also present.

ANSWER 8-15: E.

This is an example of a **seborrheic keratosis**, which is a benign neoplasm in which clonality has been documented within keratinocytes (Table 8-15A). The **sign of Leser-Trélat** is a sudden eruption of numerous **seborrheic keratoses** in persons with concomitant cancers, most commonly **gastrointestinal adenocarcinomas**. Tumors arising in patients younger than 35 years of age are highly unusual. In these cases, clinical correlation to exclude **epidermal nevi, nevus sebaceus, acanthosis nigricans, confluent and reticulated papillomatosis of Gougerot and Carteaud**, and **Dowling-Degos disease** is required. There are numerous histologic variants of **seborrheic keratosis** including the **acanthotic, hyperkeratotic (papillomatous), adenoid (reticulated), clonal**, and **macular**. All of these variants share in common the characteristic pattern of acanthosis with hyperkeratosis, papillomatosis, and frequent horn cyst formation.

Table 8-15A. Seborrheic Keratosis

Clinical Features
Present on middle-aged and older patients on the head, neck, and trunk
Flesh-colored to black papules with a "stuck-on" appearance
From 1 mm to several centimeters in diameter and sharply demarcated
Smooth to warty with a crumbly texture
Histopathologic Features
Benign squamoid and basaloid proliferation with acanthosis, hyperkeratosis, papillomatosis, reticulation, and horn pseudocysts
Basal layer hyperpigmentation
Infiltrating lymphocytes in the dermis and epidermis
Differential Diagnosis
Hidroacanthoma simplex or eccrine poroma
Basal cell carcinoma
Fibroepithelioma of Pinkus
Epidermal nevus (particularly the inflammatory linear verrucous variant)
Acantholytic changes of isolated lesions

Seborrheic keratoses are frequently irritated and inflamed as well as pigmented, which are reasons for which these lesions are biopsied. Clinically they can be mistaken for **squamous cell carcinoma** and **basal cell carcinoma** as well as **melanocytic proliferations**. Irritated and inflamed lesions frequently exhibit various degrees of keratinocytic atypia characterized by apoptosis, acantholysis, scale crust, spongiosis, and squamous eddy formation. The degree of atypia may be marked and the threshold in which these lesions are designated as **squamous cell carcinoma in situ** is relatively an area of subjectivity. The cytologic atypia in **irritated and inflamed seborrheic keratosis** is generally uniform in contradistinction to the marked pleomorphism of **bowenoid squamous cell carcinoma**.

Histopathologic Variants of Seborrheic Keratosis

Acanthotic: This is the variant illustrated in the associated question and is one of the most common variants of **seborrheic keratosis**. On low power the lesion appears to have a smooth dome shape. The epidermis is broad and composed of basaloid cells. Horn cysts are present and may be very large. Hyperkeratosis and papillomatosis are minimal. The base of the lesion demonstrates a "flat bottom." Hyperpigmentation is usually visible along the basal layer but may involve the upper cell layers as well. Xanthoma cells have been reported in the papillary dermis underlying an **acanthotic seborrheic keratosis**.

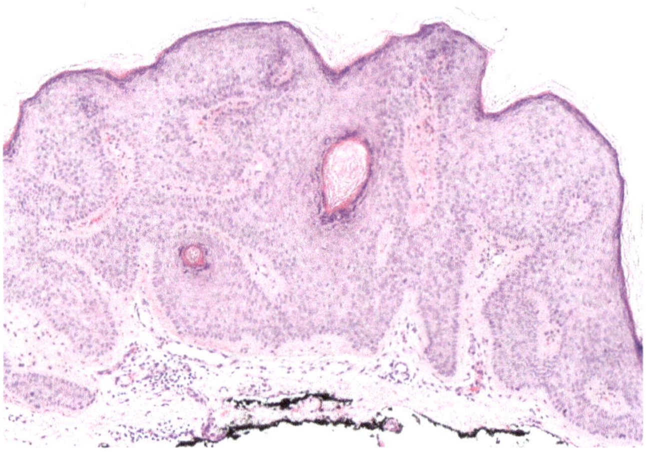

Acanthotic seborrheic keratosis.

Hyperkeratotic (Papillomatous): The epidermis shows a papillomatous, "church spire" proliferation, frequently with a "squared off" top. There is orthokeratotic and parakeratotic hyperkeratosis. The rest of the stratum malpighii is acanthotic with a basaloid and squamous cell proliferation. The stratum corneum is loosely laminated and interdigitated. The base of the lesion is flat. There is usually some hyperpigmentation along the basal layer. **Stucco keratoses** are probably variants of hyperkeratotic seborrheic keratoses. These lesions demonstrate regular, sharp, pointed papillomatosis. Pigment deposition is minimal. They may be indistinguishable from **acrokeratosis verruciformis of Hopf**.

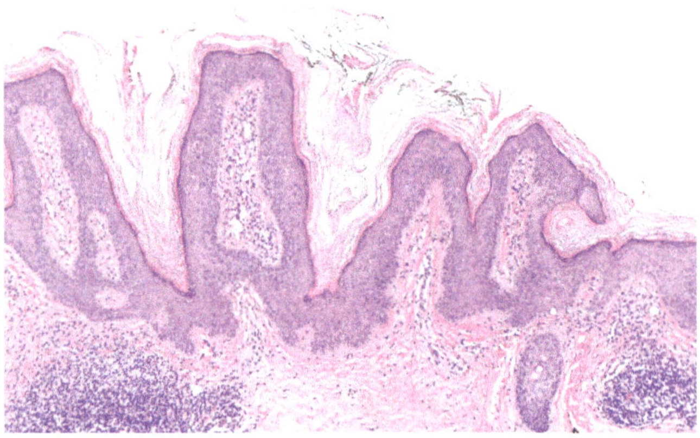

Papillomatous/hyperkeratotic seborrheic keratosis.

Adenoidal (Reticulated): In this variant, the epithelium is elongated and reticulated with moderate to prominent pigment deposition. Small horn pseudocysts are present. Epithelial anastomosis is common and surrounds some horn cysts. The pattern is reminiscent of a proliferative solar lentigo, and some investigators believe that these tumors are identical. This variant most closely resembles the epidermal lesions of **Dowling-Degos disease** or **fibroepithelioma of Pinkus**.

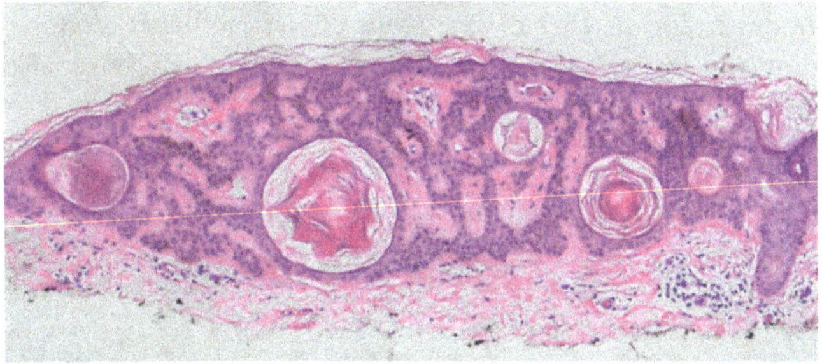

Adenoid/reticulated seborrheic keratosis.

Clonal: These **seborrheic keratoses** demonstrate a nesting pattern. The epidermis is mildly hyperkeratotic and acanthotic. Within the acanthotic epidermis are "clones" of basaloid epidermal cells surrounded by otherwise unremarkable keratinocytes. This pattern is termed the **Borst-Jadassohn phenomenon** and may be seen in other cutaneous tumors.

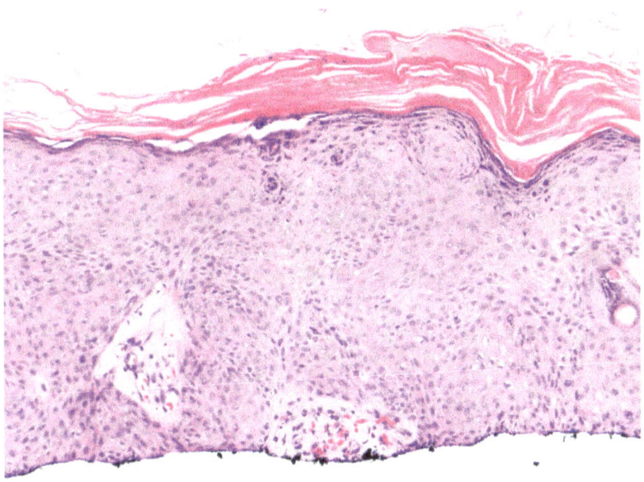

Clonal seborrheic keratosis with irritation (compact orthokeratosis and hypergranulosis).

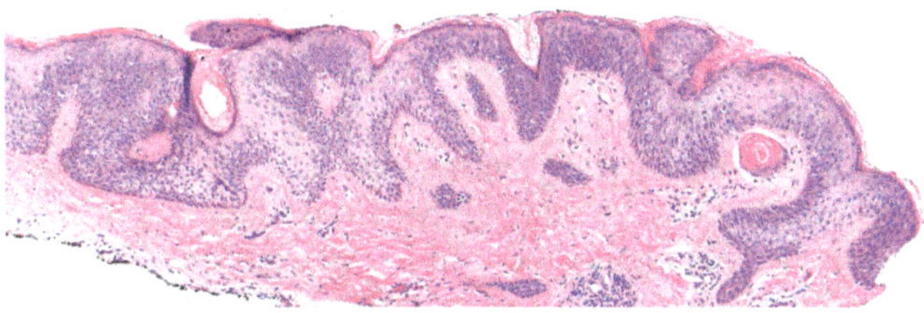

Macular seborrheic keratosis.

Macular: Also known as an "incipient" **seborrheic keratosis**, the macular variant demonstrates subtle changes. The epidermis is minimally acanthotic and hyperkeratotic. Epidermal proliferation is flat and even across the bottom. There may be increased basal layer pigmentation, but it is generally minimal and difficult to discern.

ANSWER 8-16: C.

This patient has **acanthosis nigricans**, which was initially reported by Pollitzer in 1890 (Table 8-16A). The condition is divided into four clinical categories: benign, malignant, syndromic, and obesity associated. The cutaneous changes of **acanthosis nigricans** are believed to result from prolonged growth factor stimulation of keratinocytes and dermal fibroblasts. There is an association with fibroblast growth factor receptor 3 gene mutations in children with familial disease. **Malignant acanthosis nigricans** in adults is typically associated with abdominal adenocarcinomas, such as **colorectal adenocarcinoma**. In pediatric cases, **gastric adenocarcinomas** as well as **osteogenic sarcoma**, and **Wilm tumors** are well represented. This patient most likely has **acanthosis nigricans** arising secondarily to a **Wilm tumor**. Certain medications associated with **acanthosis nigricans** include nicotinic acid, estrogens, systemic corticosteroids, heroin, insulin, pituitary extract, oral contraceptives, hydantoin-like derivatives, somatotropin, fusidic acid, and highly active antiretroviral therapy. The histopathologic features of **acanthosis nigricans** include regular papillomatosis, mild acanthosis, and hyperkeratosis. Although there are subtle histologic features indicative of **acanthosis nigricans**, the histomorphology is overall nonspecific and falls under the category of **"seborrheic keratosis-like" epidermal proliferations**. From

Table 8-16A. Acanthosis Nigricans

Clinical Features
Velvety plaques involving the axillae and neck
Mucosal lesions are seen
Associated with obesity, underlying malignancy, various syndromes, and drug intake
All ages are affected
Histopathologic Features
Papillomatosis, moderate hyperkeratosis, and a mildly thinned epidermis
Minimal basal layer hyperpigmentation and rare horn pseudocyst formation
Mild perivascular inflammation
Differential Diagnosis
Seborrheic keratoses (including stucco keratoses)
Epidermal nevi
Confluent and reticulate papillomatosis

a histopathologic perspective this category includes **epidermal nevus, acanthosis nigricans, confluent and reticulated papillomatosis of Gougerot and Carteaud, Dowling-Degos disease**, and **dermatosis papulosa nigra**. Since the histopathology of these conditions is essentially identical, clinical correlation is required for accurate diagnosis.

Epidermal nevi are hamartomatous proliferations of the epithelium that may be associated with different syndromes (Table 8-16B). Most tumors are isolated lesions that are present at birth or arise within the first few years of life. Others are associated with what is termed the **epidermal nevus syndrome**. These patients demonstrate defects of the central nervous system (CNS) (epilepsy, mental retardation), skeletal system (bone anomalies, cysts, and deformities), eyes (colobomas, cataracts, choristomas), and oral cavity (absent or malformed teeth). **Epidermal nevi** present as papules, nodules, and patches of verrucous epidermal hyperkeratosis. Comedo-like plugs and filliform hyperkeratosis have also been described.

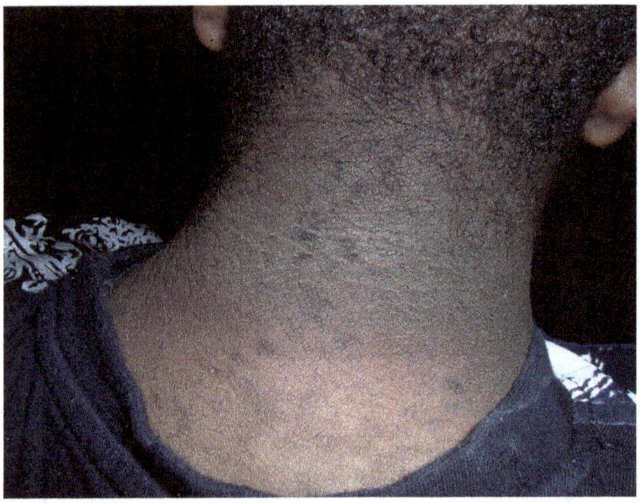

Acanthosis nigricans on the neck of a 15-year-old boy with no obesity or diabetes. His mother has very prominent acanthosis nigricans. (Reproduced, with permission, from Usatine RP, Smith MA, Mayeaux EJ Jr, Chumley HS, eds. *Color Atlas of Family Medicine*. 2nd ed. New York, NY: McGraw-Hill Education; 2012.)

Table 8-16B. Epidermal Nevus

Clinical Features
Verrucous brown papules and patches in an isolated or linear array
Some mild scaling and hyperkeratosis
Few symptoms
Histopathologic Features
Irregular epidermal hyperkeratosis, papillomatosis, hypergranulosis
Occasional parakeratosis and epidermolytic hyperkeratosis
Basal layer hyperpigmentation
Scant perivascular lymphohistiocytic inflammatory infiltrate
Differential Diagnosis
Seborrheic keratosis
Wart
Epidermolytic hyperkeratosis
Acrokeratosis verruciformis

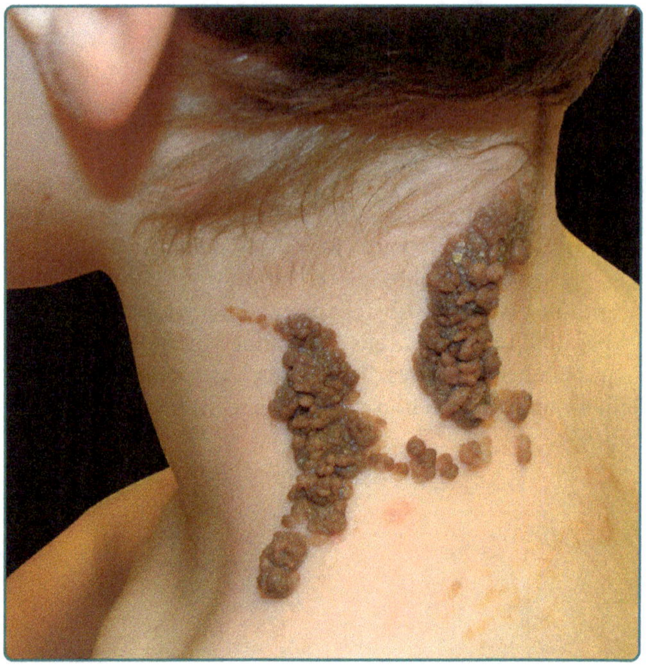

Epidermal nevus. Localized, closely set, skin-colored to brown verrucous papules, which coalesce to form well-demarcated papillomatous plaques. Linear configurations are common on the limbs as is distribution in Blaschko lines or in relaxed skin tension lines. (Reproduced, with permission, from Goldsmith LA, Katz SI, Gilchrest BA, Paller AS, Leffell DJ, Wolff K, eds. *Fitzpatrick's Dermatology in General Medicine*. 8th ed. New York, NY: McGraw-Hill Education; 2012.)

Gougerot and Carteaud initially described **confluent and reticulate papillomatosis (CARP)** in 1927 (Table 8-16C). This idiopathic disorder may represent an imbalance of the endocrine system, a variant of amyloidosis, an abnormal host response to colonization by *Pityosporum* organisms, or an inherited condition. It is currently believed to be a disorder of keratinization. The eruption occurs around adolescence, affects women more often than men, and blacks more often than whites. Although it is considered nonhereditary, familial cases have been reported. Summertime aggravation has been reported. The chest, upper arms, back, and neck are most commonly affected. Papules 1-2 mm in size emerge and enlarge to 4-5 mm. The eruption becomes confluent around the midline and more reticulated as it expands peripherally. Axillary

Table 8-16C. Confluent and Reticulate Papillomatosis

Clinical Features
Begins around adolescence
Women > men; blacks > whites
Small 45-mm patches of hyperpigmentation arising on the chest and back
Confluence of the lesions toward the midline
Histopathologic Features
Papillomatosis, hyperkeratosis, parakeratosis, and acanthosis
Increased basal layer pigmentation
Epidermal down-growths from between the rete ridges
Differential Diagnosis
Acanthosis nigricans
Dowling-Degos disease
Seborrheic keratoses

Table 8-16D. Dowling-Degos Disease

Clinical Features
Reticulate pigmentation of the flexures
Pitted perioral scars
Comedo-like lesions
Histopathologic Features
Mild hyperkeratosis
Slightly thinned epidermis
Downward projection of the epidermal rete ridges
Basal layer hyperpigmentation
Occasional small horn pseudocysts
Differential Diagnosis
Adenoid seborrheic keratosis
Solar lentigo
Acanthosis nigricans

lesions are slightly verrucous. Lesions are initially red to brown and become darker and grayer as they age. A true scale is not present, but scraping the lesions may yield a small amount of keratinous debris. Patients experience no symptoms, and mucosal involvement does not occur. After the eruption has reached its full expansion, it tends to remain unchanged.

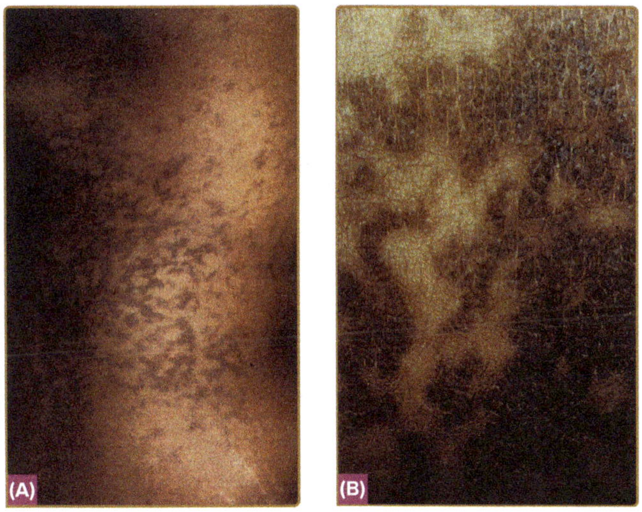

Confluent and reticulated papillomatosis of Gougerot and Carteaud. (A) Dark, scaly papules and plaques on the trunk, which become reticulated toward the periphery. **(B)** Close-up view of the distinctive, scaly, reticulated papules and plaques. (Reproduced, with permission, from Goldsmith LA, Katz SI, Gilchrest BA, Paller AS, Leffell DJ, Wolff K, eds. *Fitzpatrick's Dermatology in General Medicine*. 8th ed. New York, NY: McGraw-Hill Education; 2012.)

Dowling-Degos disease (**DDD**) is also known as **reticulate pigmented anomaly of the flexures** *or* **dark dot disease** (Table 8-16D). It is believed to be in a disease spectrum that includes **Haber syndrome, reticulate acropigmentation of Kitamura (RAPK), pigmentation reticularis faciei et colli with epithelial cystomatosis**, and **familial multiple follicular hamartoma.** It is inherited in an autosomal dominant fashion with variable penetrance and is more common in women. Mild mental retardation, non-scarring alopecia, and an association with human leukocyte antigen (HLA) B6 have been described. Two loci on chromosomes 12q and 17p13.3 are believed to be linked to this condition. The onset is typically in early adulthood. Clinically, affected patients have reticulate flexural pigmentation, infundibular cysts, breaks in dermatoglyphics, and pitted scars around the mouth. This scarring may extend onto the face. Comedo-like lesions have been described, and this condition has been confused with **chloracne.** Hypopigmented macules and papules have also been reported. **RAPK** shows symmetrical atrophic freckle-like lesions and pitting on the dorsal hands, feet, and sides of the neck. Slow, progressive hyperpigmentation of atrophic macules begins in adolescence and may be accentuated by sunlight. These lesions may eventually become gray-blue to black. Pigmented scars are found at the angles.

Dermatosis papulosa nigra was first described in 1925 by Castellani (Table 8-16E). It occurs almost exclusively in blacks, Filipinos, Mexicans, Vietnamese, and American Indians. Whites have been described with **dermatosis papulosa nigra**, but it is uncommon. Women are more commonly affected than men, and there seems to be a genetic component to this disease. An eruption of lesions associated with an **adenocarcinoma of the colon**, similar to the sign of **Leser-Trelat,** has been reported. Clinically, these lesions are found almost exclusively on the face. They are well demarcated, are 1-5 mm in diameter, and have a pedunculated appearance. Most are hyperpigmented, but some are flesh colored. They are rarely pruritic.

Table 8-16E. Dermatosis Papulosa Nigra

Clinical Features
- Small, dark, pedunculated papules on the face
- Restricted to blacks, Hispanics, Vietnamese, American Indians, and Filipinos

Histopathologic Features
- Epidermal acanthosis or reticulation with basal layer hyperpigmentation
- Polypoid appearance
- Inflamed lesions with spongiosis, exocytosis, and perivascular lymphocytes

Differential Diagnosis
- Fibroepithelial polyp
- Seborrheic keratosis, particularly the pedunculated variant

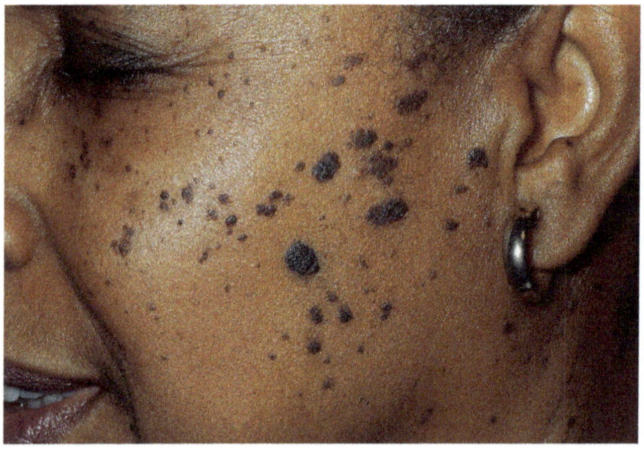

Dermatosis papulosa nigra. This consists of a myriad of tiny black lesions, some enlarging to more than a centimeter. This is seen in Black Africans, African Americans, and deeply pigmented South East Asians. (Reproduced, with permission, from Wolff K, Johnson RA, Saavedra AP. *Fitzpatrick's Color Atlas and Synopsis of Clinical Dermatology*. 7th ed. New York, NY: McGraw-Hill Education; 2013.)

ANSWER 8-17: E.

This is an example of a **clear cell acanthoma**, which was originally thought to represent a variant of **seborrheic keratosis**; however, recent studies suggest that these lesions may be inflammatory rather than neoplastic in nature (Table 8-17A). Upregulation of keratinocyte growth factor, a growth factor prominent in **psoriasis**, has been described in **clear cell acanthomas**. **Clear cell acanthomas** have been described in psoriatic plaques suggesting that they represent modified solitary lesions of **psoriasis**. Histopathologically, the epidermis is acanthotic with clear cell change that is sharply demarcated from the adjacent normal epidermis. These pale or clear cells have a polyhedral shape with PAS positive and diastase sensitive cytoplasm, indicating the presence of glycogen. Mitoses and cytologic atypia are uncommon. The lesions are frequently spongiotic and may have varying degrees of intraepidermal pustulation with neutrophilic parakeratotic scale crust. The pigmented variant of clear cell acanthoma shows increased melanosomes within dendritic melanocytes and not within keratinocytes.

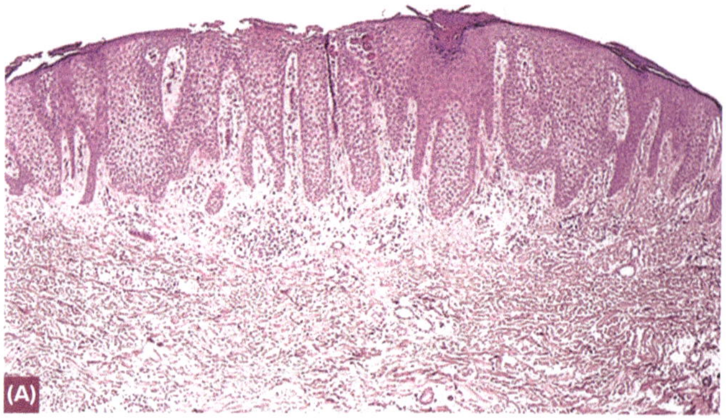

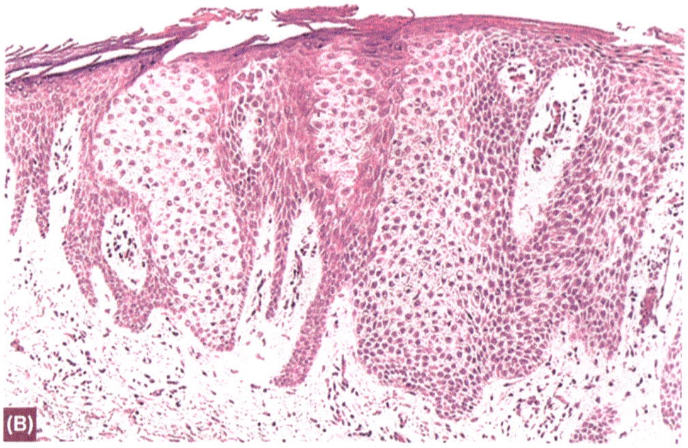

Clear cell acanthoma. (A) There is psoriasiform epidermal hyperplasia with overlying parakeratosis containing neutrophils. **(B)** Clear cell changes are well demarcated from the adjacent epidermis.

Table 8-17A. Clear Cell Acanthoma

Clinical Features
- Found on the lower extremity or foot in middle-aged or older patients
- Lesions are well demarcated and erythematous and have a moist surface
- A peripheral collarette of scale may be appreciated

Table 8-17A. Clear Cell Acanthoma *(continued)*

Histopathologic Features
Acanthosis with clear cell changes is present and is well demarcated from normal epithelium
Psoriasiform-like hyperplasia with some fusion of rete ridges
Infiltrating neutrophils in the epidermis
Clear cells are PAS positive and diastase resistant
Epidermal melanin absent
Differential Diagnosis
Seborrheic keratosis with clear cell changes
Eccrine poroma
Psoriasis vulgaris

The differential diagnosis includes **seborrheic keratosis, eccrine poroma**, and **psoriasis. Seborrheic keratosis** may have an increased intracellular glycogen but lack the sharply demarcated pale cells in the adjacent epidermis. Additionally, horn cysts and the flat bottom appearance of seborrheic keratosis are usually lacking. **Eccrine poromas** also exhibit a sharply demarcated cellular proliferation within the epidermis with elongation of the rete ridges; however, intraepithelial duct-like structures are present in eccrine poroma and absent in clear cell acanthoma. Additionally, **eccrine** poromas do not typically have clear cell changes. **Psoriasis vulgaris** demonstrates regular psoriasiform hyperplasia, prominent parakeratosis, and neutrophil microabscesses; clear cells are absent. **Clonal seborrheic keratosis** may appear similar with a sharp demarcation of the clonal keratinocyte proliferation. However, horn cysts are not present in **clear cell acanthomas**.

ANSWER 8-18: D.

The **inflammatory linear verrucous epidermal nevus (ILVEN)** is believed to be a variant of an **epidermal nevus** and was first reported by Unna in 1896 (Table 8-18A). These lesions arise early in life (half by 6 months of age), although onset during adulthood has also been reported. The legs and thighs are most commonly involved, but the lesions may also be seen on the arms, buttocks, groin, and genitalia. Some authors have postulated that the left side of the body is involved more frequently than the right, but others have disagreed. Females are more often affected than males. Intense pruritus is common. Associated arthritis, similar to that of **juvenile psoriatic arthritis**, has been reported. **ILVEN** begins as flesh colored to red papules that arise in a linear fashion. The papules become dark-red to brown with scaling and crusting. A tendency to follow Blaschko lines may be present. They may clinically resemble **eczematous dermatitis** or **psoriasis** and may develop a lichenoid appearance.

Table 8-18A. Inflammatory Linear Verrucous Epidermal Nevus

Clinical Features
Begins at an early age, often in the first year of life
Red to brown hyperkeratotic papules that coalesce into a linear lesion
Usually on the extremities, buttocks, and genitalia
Pruritus is common and may be intense
Histopathologic Features
Alternating hyperkeratosis and parakeratosis overlying an increased and decreased granular layer
Papillomatosis and psoriasiform hyperplasia
Exocytosis with microabscess formation
Perivascular and interface lymphocytic infiltrate
Differential Diagnosis
Psoriasis vulgaris
Chronic eczematous or contact dermatitis
Senescent wart

Controversy exists as to whether **ILVEN** represents a mosaic form of **psoriasis vulgaris.**

Microscopically, the epidermis shows exaggerated rete ridges with hyperkeratosis and parakeratosis. There is typically a sharp demarcation between the areas of parakeratosis with a decreased to absent granular layer and orthohyperkeratosis with an intact or accentuated granular layer. This alternating pattern of hypogranulosis–hypergranulosis and parakeratosis–orthokeratosis is characteristic of **ILVEN**. There is acanthosis with psoriasiform changes, mild-to-moderate papillomatosis, and an even elongation of the rete ridges. Mitotic activity may be brisk, but atypical mitotic figures are not seen. The dermis contains a perivascular and interface inflammatory infiltrate that may be quite brisk at times. An evaluation of the immunohistochemical properties of **ILVEN** compared with **psoriasis vulgaris** demonstrated increased keratin-10–positive keratinocytes and greater HLA-DR expression in the former but a markedly reduced number of Th17 lymphocytes relevant to the pathogenesis of the latter.

In regards to the differential diagnosis, it is important to be able to differentiate an **ILVEN** from **psoriasis, contact dermatitis, eczematous dermatitis, prurigo nodularis**, and **resolving warts. Psoriasis vulgaris** does not show the typical alternating parakeratosis and orthohyperkeratosis seen in ILVEN. Additionally, the dilated papillary dermal vessels, infiltrating neutrophils, neutrophil-rich Munro microabscesses, and thinned suprapapillary plates favor a diagnosis of psoriasis. **Chronic eczematous dermatitis** and **prurigo nodularis** are psoriasiform with mild spongiosis and exocytosis but typically do not show papillomatosis or the pattern of parakeratosis–orthokeratosis seen with ILVEN and have infiltrating eosinophils. **Senescent warts** often demonstrate papillomatosis but usually do not have psoriasiform changes and show parakeratosis emanating from the tips of the papillomatous projections. **Verruciform xanthoma** demonstrates similar areas of striking hypogranulosis/parakeratosis alternating with hypergranulosis/orthokeratosis; however, is polypoid with numerous foamy macrophages within the papillary dermis. These tumors most commonly arise in the oral mucosa and genitalia.

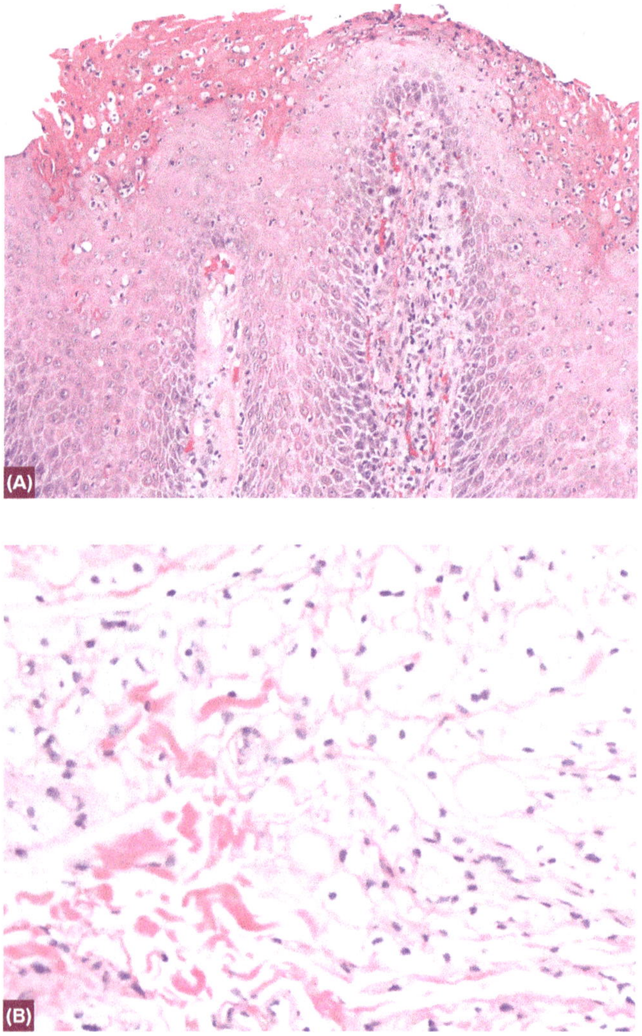

Verruciform xanthoma. (A) The epidermis exhibits papillomatosis with focal hypogranulosis and thick parakeratosis, identical to that of ILVEN. **(B)** Verruciform xanthoma contains pale foamy macrophages in the papillary dermis, which are absent in ILVEN.

ANSWER 8-19: C.

Actinic keratoses (AK) are UV-associated precancerous changes of the skin that are found in 11%-25% of the population and are most common in elderly patients (Table 8-19A).

Table 8-19A. Actinic Keratosis

Clinical Features
Small, erythematous keratotic lesions on the sun-damaged skin of elderly patients
Scale may be white to yellow-brown
Borders are sharply demarcated
Typically asymptomatic, but itching or tenderness may occur
Histopathologic Features
Hyperkeratosis with intermittent large parakeratotic nuclei
Keratinocyte atypia is prominent along the basal layer
Spongiosis in the immediate suprabasalar layer
Budding of basal layer keratinocytes into the dermis
Perivascular inflammation and solar elastosis
Differential Diagnosis
Squamous cell carcinoma in situ
Superficial basal cell carcinoma
Bowenoid papulosis
Spongiotic dermatoses

Some clinicians consider them to be equivalent to **squamous cell carcinoma in situ**. The surrounding clinically "normal" skin shows keratinocytic atypia, suggesting a UV-damage "field-effect" and a stepwise progression from subclinical to overt **squamous cell carcinoma in situ**. There is concern that these lesions will eventually convert to a frankly **invasive squamous cell carcinoma**. Among untreated lesions, this risk is approximately 1 per 1000 per year. Thick, hyperkeratotic, and ulcerative lesions are most at risk. About 20%-25% of patients with **actinic keratoses** eventually develop a **squamous cell carcinoma**. The estimated time of progression to **squamous cell carcinoma** is approximately 2 years.

Clinically, typical **actinic keratoses** are small, hyperkeratotic growths on sun-exposed surfaces in middle-aged and older patients. They are well demarcated from the surrounding skin and are slightly red. The overlying scale is white to gray or yellow. Most lesions are stable and less than 1 cm in size. Affected patients usually have a history of prolonged sun exposure or are those who tan poorly and freckle easily. Lesions are usually asymptomatic, but mild pruritus or tenderness may be present. Organ transplant recipients and other immunosuppressed patients may have many more and thicker lesions. In addition, a significant percentage of actinic keratoses from this patient population have demonstrated evidence of HPV DNA, a proposed cofactor in cutaneous carcinogenesis. The surrounding areas typically demonstrate overt evidence of long-standing actinic damage. Differentiation from a squamous cell carcinoma, particularly in thick lesions, may be impossible.

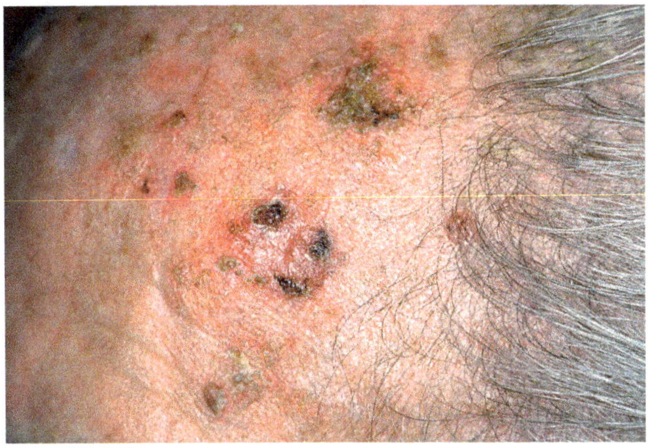

Actinic keratoses, close up. Grayish dirty-looking, tightly adherent scales on the forehead of an 80-year-old man. Abrading these hyperkeratoses is painful and leaves erosions. There is a small basal cell carcinoma at the border of the hairy scalp. (Reproduced with permission from Wolff K, Johnson RA, Saavedra AP. *Fitzpatrick's Color Atlas and Synopsis of Clinical Dermatology*. 7th ed. New York, NY: McGraw-Hill Education; 2013.)

Microscopically, the requisite criteria for **AKs** include partial thickness keratinocytic atypia and a background of solar elastosis. Lesions with full thickness keratinocytic atypia represent **squamous cell carcinoma in situ**. Proposals have been made for classifying the spectrum of these lesions similar to that of evolving carcinoma of the uterine cervix. These lesions are hyperproliferative with defective maturation and therefore are surfaced by varying degrees of dry parakeratosis and frequent loss of the granular layer. The parakeratotic nuclei may be large with oval or circular features. The basal layer becomes proliferative with slight budding into the dermis. Mild spongiosis above the atypical basal cells is common. The keratinocytes demonstrate increased mitotic activity with enhanced cytoplasmic eosinophilia compared to the surrounding cells. Enlarged nuclei with prominent nucleoli are also present. Acantholysis is seen as a focal occurrence or as a dominant process. Adnexal structures are usually spared with acrotrichia or acrosyringia showing a preserved granular layer and a normal orthokeratotic stratum corneum above it. Since the hair follicle outer root sheath and eccrine ductular stem cells reside deeper in the dermis they are less vulnerable to UV damage. When keratinocyte atypia involves the acrotrichia or acrosyringia and extends down the corresponding adnexal structures, one must be suspicious for evolution to squamous cell carcinoma in situ. The dermis demonstrates a mild superficial perivascular inflammatory infiltrate with some evidence of neoangiogenesis.

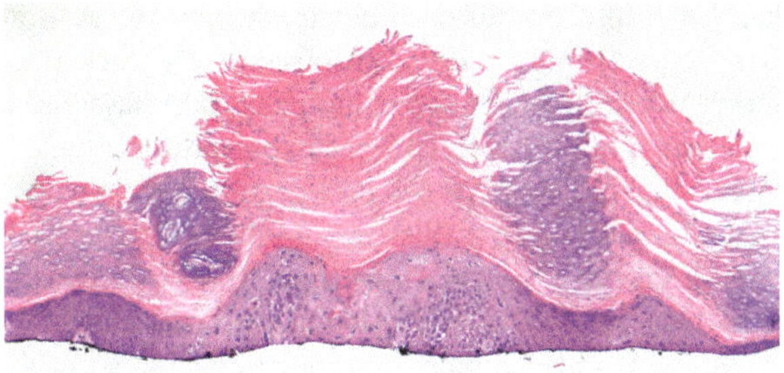

Actinic keratosis. The epidermis exhibits focal areas of partial thickness keratinocytic atypia with overlying hypogranulosis and dry parakeratosis. Note the focal sparing of the acrosyringia.

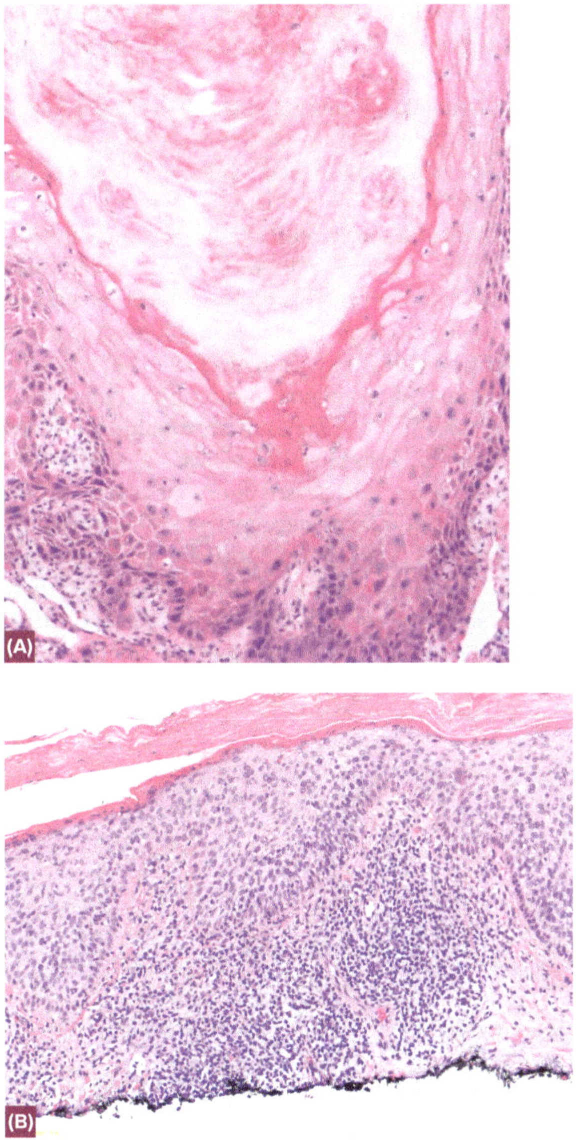

UV-associated squamous cell carcinoma in situ. (A) Note the full thickness keratinocytic atypia characterized by pleomorphic eosinophilic keratinocytes with absent granular layer and thick parakeratosis. **(B)** This example reveals full thickness keratinocytic atypia and numerous mitoses at all levels of the epidermis.

There are different histopathologic variants of **actinic keratoses. Hypertrophic actinic keratoses** have a thickened, acanthotic epidermis. Atypia is common along the basal layer but may be minimal. An overall irregular, psoriasiform hyperplasia may be seen. Papillomatous proliferation is more common in acral lesions, such as that seen in the correct answer choice C. The papillary dermis may show mild fibrosis with elongation of dermal capillaries. **Atrophic actinic keratoses** show a thinned and atrophic stratum malpighii, typically with substantive overlying hyperkeratosis. Atypical cells are found predominantly along the basal layer. **Acantholytic actinic keratoses** demonstrate widespread keratinocyte acantholysis. Dyskeratotic cells may be seen. **Actinic keratoses** with prominent epidermolysis are known as **epidermolytic actinic keratoses. Pigmented actinic keratoses** display moderate pigment incontinence and hyperpigmentation along the basal layer. Distinct nests of melanocytes are not present. The use of immunohistochemical stains for melanocytes has shown a varying ability to differentiate these lesions from more ominous melanocytic neoplasms such as lentigo maligna. **Actinic keratoses** with an interface inflammatory infiltrate are known as **lichenoid actinic keratoses.** Recognizing the atypical keratinocytes may be difficult. **Proliferative actinic keratoses** demonstrate elongated rete ridges with keratinocyte atypia and occasional adnexal involvement. The extension into the papillary dermis may be difficult to distinguish from **superficially invasive squamous cell carcinoma.** Although they may occur at any location, these lesions commonly arise within thickened acral skin such as that of fingers, toes, palms, and soles, where the cellular turnover rate is decreased due to increased concentrations of cytokeratins and desmosomal adhesion molecules. These lesions must be closely examined for areas of frank invasion at the base, even though full thickness atypia may not be present. More recent evaluations of proliferative actinic keratoses have concluded that they likely represent low-grade squamous cell carcinomas despite an absent in situ component.

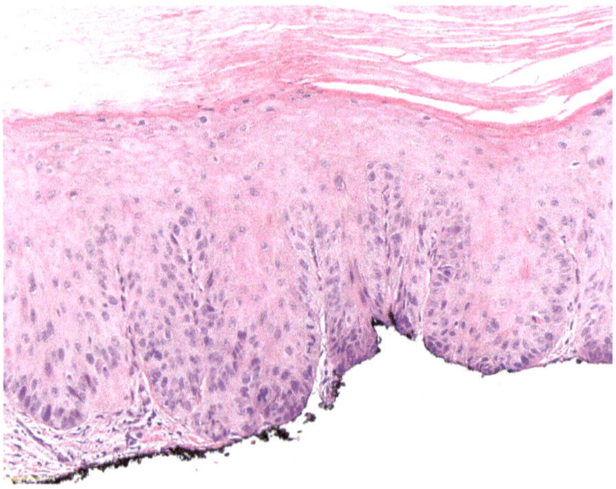

Hypertrophic actinic keratosis. There is partial thickness keratinocytic atypia involving a markedly acanthotic epidermis. Overlying thick hyperkeratosis is also present.

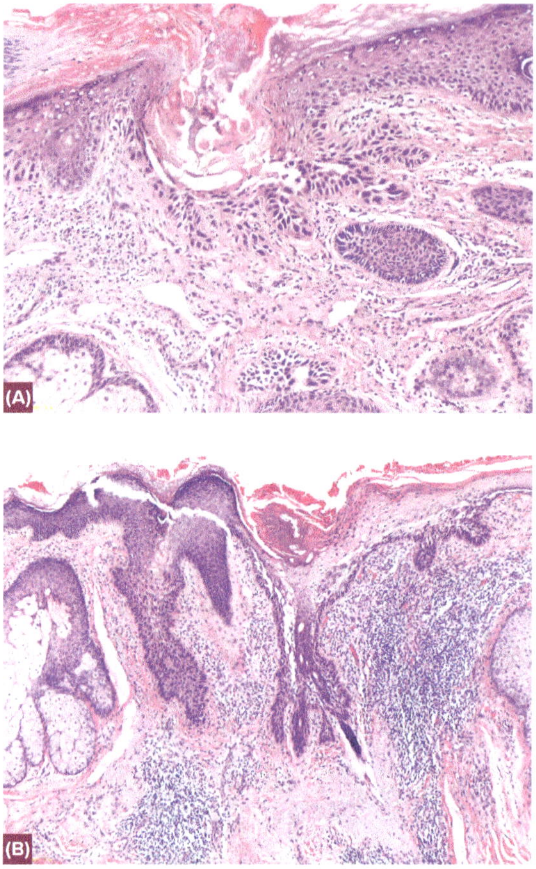

Proliferative actinic keratosis. (A) There is partial thickness keratinocytic atypia concentrated at elongated rete ridges extending into the papillary dermis. **(B)** Actinic keratosis with adnexal extension.

Answer choices A, B, and D are examples of **large cell acanthoma, clonal seborrheic keratosis**, and **bowenoid squamous cell carcinoma**, respectively. **Large cell acanthomas** are likely induced by prolonged sun exposure because it arises in areas of solar damage on elderly patients (Table 8-19B). These tumors may be a variant of **actinic keratosis** or **solar lentigo.** DNA analysis has shown that the cells are aneuploid or tetraploid and that abnormal clones are present. Most cases are single, but patients with multiple lesions have also been described. **Large cell acanthomas** have a benign and indolent clinical course. They are usually less than 1 cm in diameter and may be slightly hyperpigmented and occasionally hyperkeratotic. The histopathologic features are believed to be pathognomonic, being well-circumscribed with a clear demarcation between affected and uninvolved epidermis. Keratinocytes are enlarged with proportionally larger nuclei (normal nuclear to cytoplasmic ratio). These nuclei are pleomorphic but not hyperchromatic. Mitotic activity is not prominent, and the acrosyringia are spared. Rete ridges may be bulbous. The most distinguishing characteristic from **AK** is the presence of orthohyperkeratosis and a preserved granular layer. **Clonal seborrheic keratoses** demonstrate a nesting pattern. The epidermis is mildly hyperkeratotic with acanthosis. Within the acanthotic

Table 8-19B. Large Cell Acanthoma

Clinical Features
Arise on the sun-damaged skin of elderly patients
Lesions are slightly hyperpigmented, flat, and mildly hyperkeratotic
<1 cm in diameter
Histopathologic Features
Well-demarcated, enlarged keratinocytes and nuclei
Rare mitotic figures
Slight hyperkeratosis without parakeratosis
Bulbous rete ridges with mild hyperpigmentation along the basal layer
Solar elastosis and telangiectasias
Differential Diagnosis
Actinic keratosis
Seborrheic keratosis
Solar lentigo

epidermis are "clones" of basaloid monomorphous keratinocytes surrounded by otherwise unremarkable keratinocytes. This pattern is termed the **Borst-Jadassohn phenomenon** and may be seen in other cutaneous tumors. When irritated and inflamed, these lesions may exhibit eosinophilic cytoplasm and reactive cytologic atypia mimicking **squamous cell carcinoma.**

Bowen disease is believed by most investigators to be a unique form of **squamous cell carcinoma in situ** associated with HPV infection (Table 8-19C). This disease may also be more common in uncircumcised males. HPV 2, 16, 18, 33, 34, 57b, and 82 have been reported in **anogenital Bowen disease.** HPV types 23, 5, 16, 18, 20, 21, 31, 33, 34, 54, 56, 58, 61, 62, 73, and 82 have been described in extragenital disease, usually on the extremities. HPV-associated extragenital disease is linked to black race, an acral location, young age, and a hyperkeratotic or verrucous appearance.

There are two clinical variants of Bowen disease—that involving the anogenital area and that of glabrous skin. Anogenital disease involves the mucous membranes, but mucosal sites such as the oral cavity and conjunctiva are also involved. Glabrous lesions appear as slowly enlarging, well-demarcated patches or plaques. Some are large and poorly defined. Tumors display mild scaling or crusting. Verrucous and hyperkeratotic variants are seen. Most are flesh colored to erythematous and clinically mistaken for **basal cell carcinomas.** A pigmented variant has also been reported and may simulate melanocytic neoplasms. Most patches of **Bowen disease** are a few millimeters to a few centimeters in diameter. Patients are usually in the sixth to eighth decades of life. **Bowen disease** pursues a relatively benign course. Microscopically, these tumors are acanthotic with a striking loss of epidermal polarity in that normal and progressive keratinocyte maturation has ceased resulting in full thickness keratinocyte atypia. The tumor cells are basophilic and pleomorphic with frequent dyskeratotic keratinocytes and mitoses above the basal layer. Multinucleated

Table 8-19C. Bowen Disease

Clinical Features
Glabrous and anogenital patches a few centimeters in diameter
Well-demarcated and scaling with mild erythema
Patients are usually older, and lesions arise in sun-damaged areas
Women more often affected than men
Histopathologic Features
Epidermis demonstrates acanthosis and hyperkeratosis
Mild-to-moderate psoriasiform hyperplasia
Full-thickness epidermal atypia with dyskeratotic cells and atypical mitoses
Loss of epidermal polarity
Frequent involvement of adnexal structures
Differential Diagnosis
Bowenoid actinic keratoses and bowenoid papulosis
Extramammary Paget disease
Epidermotropic carcinoma metastatic to the skin
Erythroplasia of Queyrat
Podophyllin-treated condylomata acuminata

cells are common. Occasionally, scattered clusters of atypical cells may be seen throughout a normal epidermis, imparting a "windblown" appearance. This process is referred to as **Borst-Jadassohn phenomenon** and introduces **melanoma in situ, Paget disease**, and **clonal seborrheic keratosis** into the differential diagnosis. The stratum corneum is hyperkeratotic and usually parakeratotic. The parakeratosis may be extensive and platelike. Importantly, involvement of the adnexae, particularly pilosebaceous structures, may be present. The infundibulum, sebaceous glands, and external root sheath may be replaced by tumor cells. Dermal invasion occurs in 3%-5% of cases, most often in head and neck lesions in middle-aged to older men.

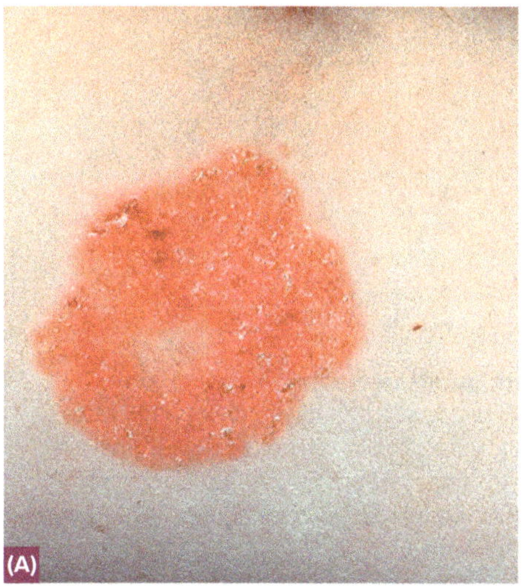
(A)

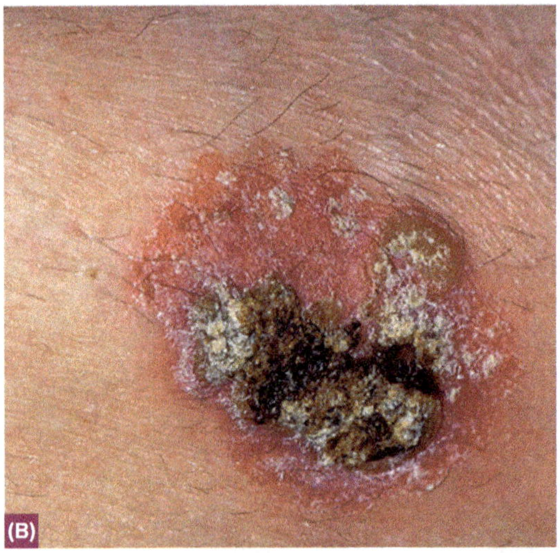

Squamous cell carcinoma in situ: Bowen disease. (A) A large, sharply demarcated, scaly, and erythematous plaque simulating a psoriatic lesion. **(B)** A similar psoriasiform plaque with a mix of scales, hyperkeratosis, and hemorrhagic crusts on the surface. (Reproduced, with permission, from Goldsmith LA, Katz SI, Gilchrest BA, Paller AS, Leffell DJ, Wolff K, eds. *Fitzpatrick's Dermatology in General Medicine*. 8th ed. New York, NY: McGraw-Hill Education; 2012.)

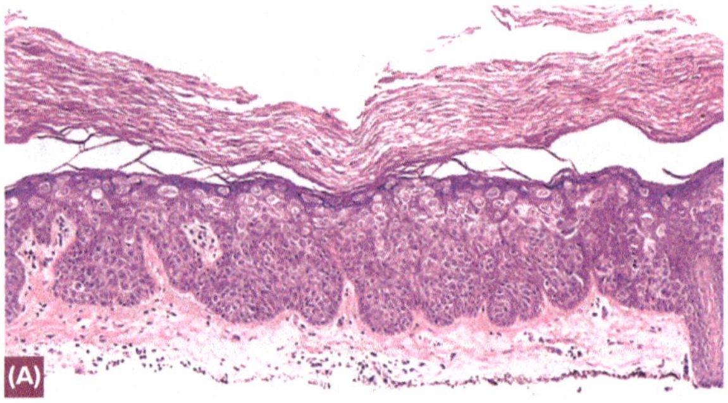

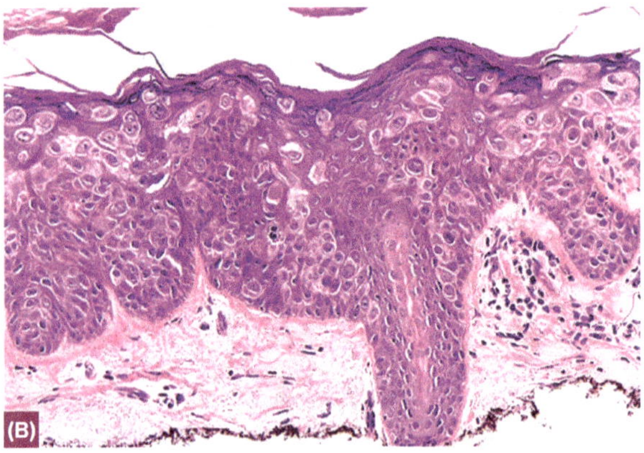

Bowen disease with Borst-Jadassohn phenomenon.
(A) The epidermis is psoriasiform and slightly hyperkeratotic. **(B)** Clusters of atypical keratinocytes are present scattered throughout the full thickness of the epidermis. Frequently scattered dyskeratotic keratinocytes and mitoses are present at all levels of the epidermis.

ANSWER 8-20: C.

Invasive squamous cell carcinomas are the second most common cutaneous malignancy (Table 8-20A). They account for about 20% of all skin cancers and are the most prevalent skin cancer in blacks. Risk factors for developing a **squamous cell carcinoma** include increased age, light skin pigmentation, immunosuppression, and genetic disorders such as **xeroderma pigmentosum**. The most common inciting cause of **cutaneous squamous cell carcinomas** is cumulative UV radiation (UVR) exposure. Sunlight is the greatest source of UVR, with UVB being the most damaging factor. Other etiologic factors include cigarette smoking, HPV infection (types 16, 31, and 34), and chronic dermatoses such as **porokeratosis, lupus erythematosus, lichen planus, lichen sclerosus, epidermolysis bullosa, erythema ab igne, dissecting cellulitis of the scalp, chromoblastomycosis, port wine stain, arteriovenous malformation, necrobiosis lipoidica**, and **nevus sebaceus**. Tumors that arise within the setting of immunosuppression, prior sites of ionizing radiation exposure, and within chronic ulcers and sinus tracts exhibit a markedly increased risk for recurrence and metastasis (regional lymph nodes in 36%-54% of cases). Deeper skin invasion and perineural invasion are associated with increased metastatic disease and recurrence rates. Tumors greater than 2 cm in diameter are twice as likely to recur and three times as likely to metastasize. Tumor thickness may be measured in millimeters similar to that for melanomas. **Squamous cell carcinoma**, occasionally arising from lesions of **bowenoid papulosis**, may arise on or near the mucosal surfaces of the anogenital region. These tumors demonstrate evidence of infection with HPV, particularly HPV-16. Other HPVs have also been identified, including types 18, 31, 33, 39, 52, and 67. Overall, metastatic disease is uncommon. The overall rate approximates 2% but is between 10% and 15% for lesions on the ears, genitalia, and oral mucosa. Metastases are more prevalent in tumors that are poorly differentiated, of long standing, and inadequately treated.

Clinically, most tumors are nodules with an overlying scale or scale crust. Scaly lesions that evolve into painful nodules represent transformation of **actinic keratosis** into **invasive squamous cell carcinoma**. Lesions are flesh colored, but some may be red to brown, and telangiectasias are present. Exophytic cauliflower-shaped lesions, indurated crusted plaques, ulceration, and subcutaneous nodules, may also be seen. Different histologic types may have more specific clinical features.

Microscopically, **squamous cell carcinoma** has been divided into five histologic categories: **conventional, spindle cell, acantholytic, keratoacanthomatous**, and **verrucous**. This is a useful paradigm for purposes of classification, but other histopathologic subtypes also exist. In **conventional squamous cell carcinoma** (the tumor in question), atypical, slightly epithelioid cells emanate from the epidermis and spread into the dermis. Nuclei are enlarged and pleomorphic. Atypical mitotic figures and keratin pearls are present.

Table 8-20A. Squamous Cell Carcinoma

Clinical Features
- Quickly growing, flesh-colored to red nodules on sun-exposed skin
- Overlying scale or crusting
- Lip lesions with atrophy, crusting, and ulceration
- Most commonly affect the head and neck of elderly patients
- Usually asymptomatic unless perineural invasion is present
- Ulcerating, papillomatous, and subcutaneous variants

Histopathologic Features
- Conventional
  - Aggregates of atypical epithelial cells invading the dermis
  - May derive from an actinic keratosis or Bowen disease
  - Variable mitotic activity, keratin pearl formation, premature cornification
  - Focal acantholysis or spindle cell proliferation
  - Nonspecific inflammatory infiltrate with lymphocytes and plasma cells
- Spindle cell
  - Spindle cells emanating from the basal layer and invading the dermis
  - Mitotic activity and atypia are present
  - Pleomorphic giant cells are occasionally seen
  - Cells are cytokeratin positive and occasionally vimentin positive
- Acantholytic
  - Lobules and nests of atypical, acantholytic keratinocytes
  - Premature cornification with free-floating neoplastic keratinocytes
- Signet ring
  - Atypical nuclei are displaced yielding a signet ring appearance
  - Paranuclear clear zone or nuclear displacement by eosinophilic globule
  - Strong staining for glycogen
- Pseudovascular
  - Proliferation of pleomorphic, atypical cells with "hobnail" appearance
  - Cellular aggregates with vascular appearance
  - Erythrocytes contained in pseudovascular spaces
  - Moderate to marked mitotic activity
- Subcutaneous
  - Intradermal aggregates of atypical, epithelioid cells
  - Mitotic activity and premature cornification variable
  - Atypical mitoses occasionally seen
  - Connection to epidermis or adnexal structures present on deeper sectioning

Differential Diagnosis
- Conventional
  - Pseudocarcinomatous hyperplasia
  - Inflamed seborrheic keratosis
  - Metatypical basal cell carcinoma
  - Inflamed wart
- Spindle cell
  - Spindle cell malignant melanoma
  - Atypical fibroxanthoma
- Acantholytic
  - Acantholytic dermatoses (Hailey–Hailey disease, pemphigus vulgaris, transient acantholytic dermatosis)
  - Angiosarcoma
- Signet ring
  - Metastatic gastric or colon carcinoma
  - Paget disease
  - Signet ring cell basal cell carcinoma
  - Myxoid liposarcoma
- Pseudovascular
  - Angiosarcoma
  - Atypical fibroxanthoma
- Subcutaneous nodular
  - Metastatic squamous cell carcinoma

Dyskeratotic and prematurely cornifying cells are seen. The depth of dermal invasion is variable. If deep enough, the tumor may show lateral spread upon reaching the fascial or capsular plane, muscle, periosteum, or perichondrium. The surface of the tumor is often hyperkeratotic with varying amounts of parakeratosis. Immunohistochemical staining for cytokeratin is positive for both high- and low-molecular-weight cytokeratins, but negative for BerEP4, unlike basal cell carcinomas, which are normally positive for BerEP4. Vimentin may also be positive in poorly differentiated spindle cell lesions. The marker p63 is very useful in distinguishing spindle cell variants from histologic mimics, including **atypical fibroxanthomas (AFXs)** and **desmoplastic melanomas**. Tumors that arise within the thickened skin of acral sites and within a background of **lichen simplex chronicus** or **lichen sclerosus** may exhibit invasion without establishing full thickness atypia (in situ component). Therefore, biopsies from these sites may require deeper levels and close inspection to identify **invasive squamous carcinoma** from mere **actinic keratosis**.

Special Variants of Squamous Cell Carcinoma

Spindle Cell: **Spindle cell squamous cell carcinomas (SCSCCs)** may be associated with previous trauma or radiotherapy. They are commonly ulcerated and are associated with high local recurrence rates but rare distant metastasis. Histopathologically, atypical spindle cells are seen emanating from the epidermis and intermingle with strands of collagen in a whorled fashion. They are arranged into intertwining fascicles and bundles. The surrounding stroma may be myxoid, and pleomorphic giant cells may be appreciated. Individual tumor cells are eosinophilic with hyperchromatic, elongated nuclei and multiple nucleoli. Mitotic activity with occasional atypical figures is present. Many **SCSCCs** stain for both cytokeratin and vimentin. This gradient between the two tumors may be explained by a metaplastic change with more mesenchymal differentiation in the **SCSCC**. Previously, spindle cell tumors taking up the vimentin stain were thought to be **atypical fibroxanthomas (AFX)**, and it is likely that many such tumors have been misdiagnosed. The use of high-molecular-weight cytokeratins such as 34βE12 and CK5/6 has been suggested for lesions failing to take up low-molecular-weight cytokeratin stains. Tumor cells are consistently negative for melanocytic markers (Melan-A, HMB45, S100).

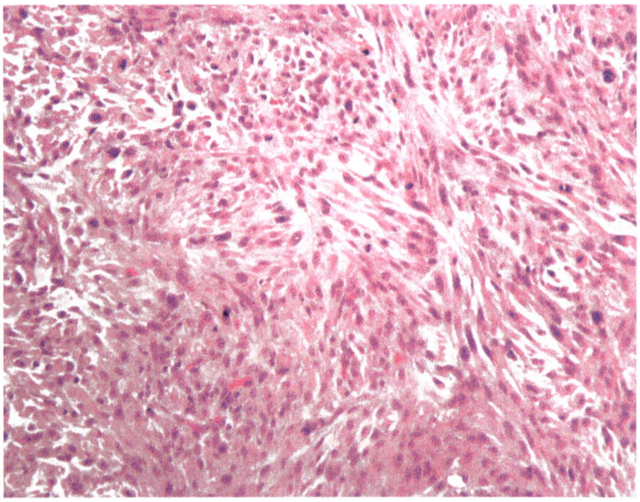

Spindle cell squamous cell carcinoma. Tumor cells are atypical and spindled in a slightly whorled fashion. Mitotic activity is brisk.

Acantholytic: The lesions typically arise on the head and neck as a nodule or ulcer in elderly men. They have been associated with recurrent tumors after radiation therapy and portend a better prognosis. Similar lesions have been described in the oropharynx, lung, larynx, vulva, and breast. The acantholysis is likely an accentuation of the same process seen in **actinic keratoses**. The tumor is arranged in cords and nests in a glandular (pseudoglandular) or adenoid pattern. Polygonal cells surround lumen-like spaces (pseudolumens) containing free-floating, neoplastic keratinocytes. Dyskeratotic cells may be few or abundant and are single or grouped.

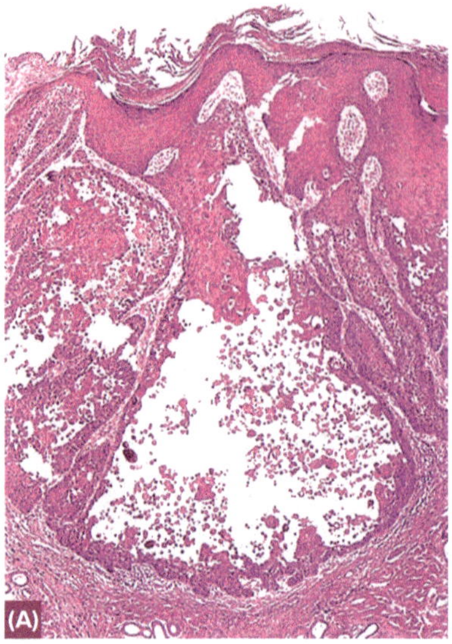

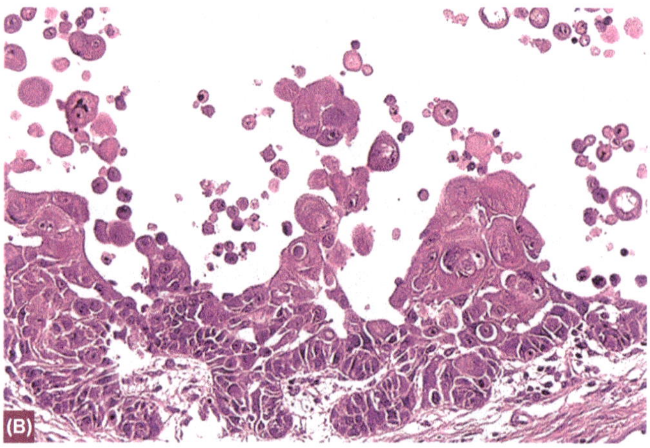

Acantholytic squamous cell carcinoma. (A) Aggregates of invading keratinocytes demonstrate acantholysis. **(B)** Enlarged, free-floating keratinocytes are present.

Subcutaneous: These tumors present as asymptomatic subcutaneous nodules on the head and neck. The overlying skin is unremarkable. This lack of epidermal connection introduces a **metastatic squamous cell carcinoma** into the differential diagnosis. **Subcutaneous squamous cell carcinomas** show an intradermal collection of atypical epithelioid cells with mitoses, premature cornification, and squamous eddies. These tumors most commonly arise within the epithelial lining of **epidermoid cysts** and have a high incidence of perineural invasion. **Malignant proliferating pilar tumors** are low-grade variants of **squamous cell carcinoma** with trichilemmal differentiation and may arise within **trichilemmal (pilar) cysts**.

Follicular squamous cell carcinomas: These tumors develop from the upper infundibular portion of hair follicles, showing full-thickness atypia and invasion of the adjacent dermis. In situ carcinoma of the epidermis may be absent. Immunohistochemical studies show positive staining with cytokeratin stains but not for epithelial membrane antigen, CEA, and vimentin.

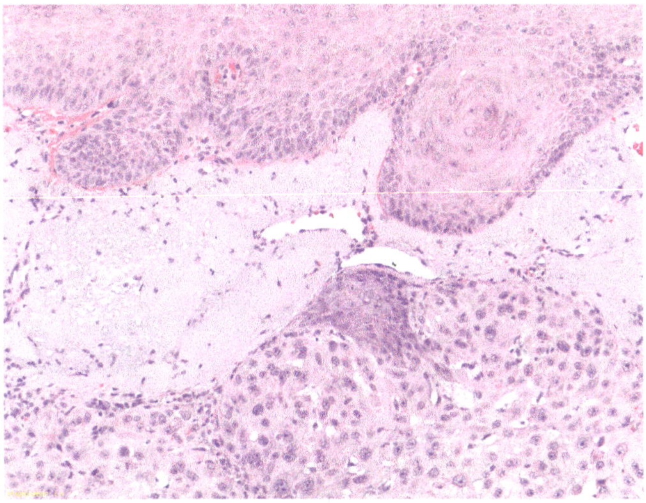

Follicular squamous cell carcinoma. There is an infiltrative mass of malignant squamous cells in the dermis arising from the follicular infundibulum. Note the absence of in situ carcinoma within the overlying epidermis. These tumors may be mistaken for metastatic squamous cell carcinomas; therefore, multiple deeper sections are needed to thoroughly evaluate for connection to hair follicles.

ANSWER 8-21: E.

Keratoacanthomas (KA) are rapidly growing cutaneous tumors with atypical histologic features that resolve leaving an atrophic scar (Table 8-21A). They are believed to represent a **low-grade squamous cell carcinoma** and typically arise as solitary lesions in sun-exposed sites; however, different clinical syndromes are associated with these tumors. **Multiple keratoacanthomas of Ferguson Smith** is an autosomal dominant disorder that begins in childhood to early adulthood. Numerous lesions arise and disperse over the years. This disorder must be differentiated from the **generalized eruptive keratoacanthomas of Grzybowski**. In this latter disease, the erupting **keratoacanthomas** are smaller (2-3 mm in diameter) and may number in the hundreds or thousands. Familial inheritance is not present, and pruritus is common. Facial involvement may be severe, resulting in ectropion and masked facies. Two additional syndromes, the **Muir–Torre syndrome** and **xeroderma pigmentosum**, demonstrate an increased incidence of tumor formation. **Eruptive KAs** have been reported in patients with melanoma treated with BRAF inhibitors. Clinically, **keratoacanthomas** typically arise on the sun-exposed skin of older persons although they have also been reported in children. The peak incidence begins in the sixth decade of life, and lesions are commonly found on the face, hands, and forearms in men and on the face and legs in women. Men are more commonly affected than women. Classical lesions pass through several stages of development. The initial or proliferative phase consists of a smooth, hemispheric nodule that enlarges rapidly over a 2- to 4-week period. These are flesh colored to slightly erythematous and asymptomatic. The next stage, the mature form, demonstrates a dome- or berry-shaped nodule with a central crater containing a plug of compact keratin. This stage lasts several weeks or months. The final phase is that of a resolving lesion. These keratoacanthomas resorb and expel the keratinous core. Over weeks to months, they become progressively more depressed and eventuate into a scar with variable atrophy. Regression may be augmented by injections with kenalog, methotrexate, or 5-fluorouracil (5-FU). Although **classic KAs** spontaneously regress, a subset of tumors persists and behaves like **conventional squamous cell carcinomas**, and therefore must be completely excised. No defined histopathologic criteria have been established to distinguish between regressing and persistent tumors.

Table 8-21A. Keratoacanthoma

Clinical Features
Flesh-colored to erythematous nodules with a central keratin plug
Typically present on middle-aged or older patients in sun-exposed sites
Resolving lesions are scarred and atrophic
Lesions may exist at previous sites of trauma or with various dermatoses
Histopathologic Features
Overlying epithelium forms "lips" with adjacent hypergranulosis and hyperkeratosis
Cutaneous plug is eosinophilic and parakeratotic
Infiltrating epithelium is eosinophilic and may be atypical with increased mitotic activity
Entrapped collagen and elastic fibers are seen
Horn pearls and neutrophilic or eosinophilic microabscesses are present
Differential Diagnosis
Conventional squamous cell carcinoma
Dilated pore or infundibular cyst
Resolving inflamed wart

Microscopically, early lesions demonstrate an invaginating epidermis with a keratin-filled crater. Adjacent epithelium shows acanthosis, hypergranulosis, and premature cornification. Parakeratosis may be present, but orthohyperkeratosis is the rule. Invaginating strands of epithelium may be carcinoma-like (pseudoepitheliomatous) and typically possess an eosinophilic or "glassy" appearance. Some acantholysis may be present. Fully developed keratoacanthomas have similar features that are more exaggerated. The overlying epidermis develops "lips" or buttresses surrounding the crateriform plug, which has expanded and consists of parakeratotic material. Epidermal proliferations become more exaggerated as they invade the dermis. Mitotic activity and atypical mitotic figures are more common, particularly at the edges of the epithelial proliferation. Intraepidermal neutrophilic and eosinophilic microabscesses are present. Horn pearls are seen. Within the epidermis, occasional fragments of entrapped collagen and elastin fibers are present. An inflammatory infiltrate is composed largely of lymphocytes, but eosinophils are also prominent. Neutrophils and plasma cells are present. The stroma may be granulomatous if epithelium has ruptured into the dermis and is being resorbed.

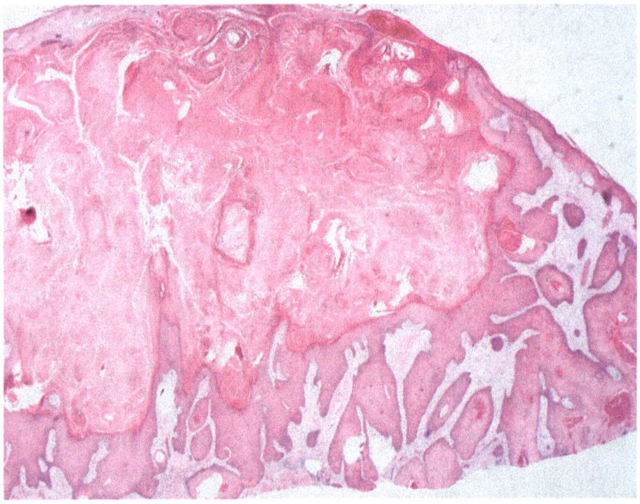

Keratoacanthoma. There is a squamous proliferation with a crateriform configuration, characterized by a central hyperkeratotic plug, and surrounding buttresses of squamous epithelium. Within the dermis the infiltrating keratinocytes are eosinophilic and variably atypical.

Table 8-21B. Verrucous Carcinoma

Clinical Features
Oral verrucous carcinoma
Gray or white warty growth on buccal or gingival mucosa
More common in older men
Plantar verrucous carcinoma
Painful, exophytic, verrucous mass on the heel, toe, or ball of foot
Extrude foul-smelling keratogenous material
Buschke–Loewenstein tumor
Polypoid mass on the glans penis in uncircumcised males
May ulcerate or form sinus tracts
May occlude structures such as the urethra
Histopathologic Features
Oral verrucous carcinoma
Hyperkeratosis with orthokeratosis
Rete pegs with pushing well-polarized base
Large cells with scattered mitoses
Plantar verrucous carcinoma
Exophytic and endophytic epithelial proliferation forming crypts and sinuses
Hyperkeratosis and parakeratosis
Infrequent mitoses
Buschke–Loewenstein tumor
Hyperplastic, exophytic epithelial proliferation with infrequent mitoses
Well-differentiated epidermal proliferation forming crypts and sinuses
Hypergranulosis with koilocyte-like changes
Differential Diagnosis
Low-grade squamous cell carcinoma
Warts or condyloma acuminata
Pseudoepitheliomatous hyperplasia

Choice E describes **verrucous carcinoma**, which is composed of three entities—**oral verrucous carcinoma, plantar verrucous carcinoma**, and the **Buschke–Loewenstein tumor** (Table 8-21B). Tobacco use (especially chewing), betel nut or leaf use, poor oral hygiene, **oral lichen planus, chronic candidiasis**, and malfitting dentures may induce oral forms of this tumor. HPV types 2, 6, 11, 16, and 18 have been associated with these lesions. The expression of c-*erb*B-3 oncogene has been described in **oral verrucous carcinoma. Plantar verrucous carcinoma** is a distinct type of **squamous cell carcinoma** of the sole. Abundant crypts and sinuses are present. This tumor is slow growing and rarely metastasizes but may display locally aggressive features. HPV-11 and -16 infection and increased oncogene activity have been reported in **plantar verrucous carcinoma. Buschke–Loewenstein tumors** appear as exophytic masses involving the anogenital mucosa. Most cases are due to infection with HPV type 6 or 11, although types 16 and 18 have been reported in lesions from HIV-positive patients. These tumors comprise 5%-25% of all penile malignancies. Some clinicians consider **Buschke–Loewenstein tumors** to be nothing more than very large **condyloma accuminata**. Most of these lesions pursue a banal course, but metastases to the lymph nodes, skin, and distant sites have been reported. Destruction and local compression of adjacent structures is more common.

Clinically, **verrucous carcinomas** are slow growing, locally destructive tumors that are frequently misdiagnosed and treated as **verruca**, unlike the rapidly evolving and regressing **keratoacanthoma. Oral verrucous carcinoma** presents as a slowly enlarging white to gray growth on the buccal or gingival mucosa of older men. The average age of affected patients is 65 years. Invasion into the cheek or mandible may be seen. **Plantar verrucous carcinoma** is a slow-growing, exophytic or polypoid tumor. It is most common on the heel or ball of the foot but has also been described on the toes, toe web spaces, leg, knee, wrist, finger, hand, axilla, abdominal wall, buttocks, nose, and scalp. Lesions are typically tender, pink to flesh colored, and well circumscribed at their borders. Most tumors have been treated as recalcitrant warts or corns for an extended period. **Plantar verrucous carcinoma** is more common in middle-aged to older men. Foul-smelling keratinous material is excreted through multiple sinus openings. Penetration of the tumor to the dorsum of the foot and involvement of the metatarsal bones has been described. Metastases are rare. The **Buschke–Loewenstein tumor** is a cauliflower-like polypoid excrescence that arises on the glans penis in uncircumcised men between the ages of 18 and 86 years. The prepuce, coronal sulcus, and perianal mucosa may also be involved. Lesions may ulcerate and form fistulous tracts. A foul smell is common. Compression of the urethra and other structures may occur. These tumors may involve the genitalia, perineum, and urethra. Perianal tumors have a higher degree of malignant degeneration but no increased mortality. Activities such as walking and defecation may become difficult. Persons predisposed to these lesions may have a particularly fulminant course. **Buschke-Loewenstein tumors** have a similar appearance in women.

Microscopically, the epithelium of the **verrucous carcinoma** shows acanthosis and papillomatosis with hyperkeratosis and parakeratosis overlying bulbous rete pegs, which invade the dermis in a "pushing" rather than an infiltrating manner. These rete pegs are blunt and well polarized. Nuclei and nucleoli are enlarged. Mitotic activity is present but is scattered. Parabasal mitoses are common. Formation of keratin pearls is infrequent. Acral and genital tumors typically exhibit hypergranulosis, imparting a histomorphology similar to that of verruca. In fact, superficially sampled lesions in which the base is not visualized are frequently misdiagnosed as verruca. An inflammatory infiltrate is seen and may be abundant if the keratin has been extruded into the dermis. Infiltration between bones and muscles may be appreciated.

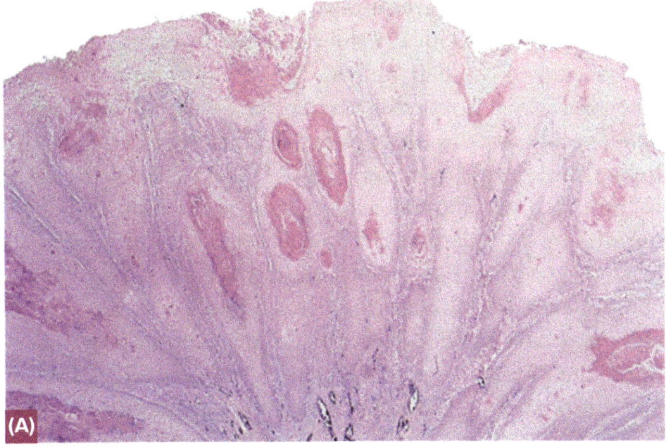

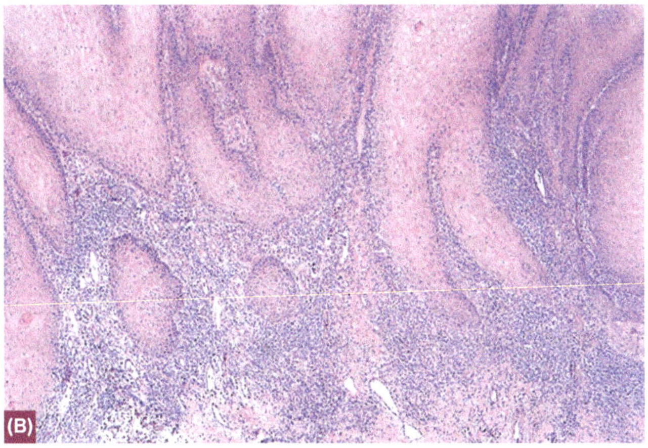

Oral verrucous carcinoma. (A) The epidermis is verrucous and hyperkeratotic. **(B)** Rete pegs with atypia and pushing, bluntly invasive borders.

ANSWER 8-22: D.

Clavi (corns) are hyperkeratotic lesions of the feet and are seen only in people who wear ill-fitting shoes (Table 8-22A). They are a consequence of persistent frictional injury and are typically painful. Women are affected more often than men. Underlying bony prominences and other orthopedic abnormalities exert pressure through the skin. Clinically, lesions are yellow to brown with a central core. Hard corns are burnished with a smooth surface. Soft corns are macerated and sodden. Microscopically, tumors are endophytic with a cup-shaped depression. A thick parakeratotic plug is seen. The spinous and granular layers are decreased.

In regards to the differential diagnosis, these tumors should be differentiated from **warts, calluses, porokeratosis,**

Table 8-22A. Clavus (Corn)

Clinical Features
Yellow to brown hyperkeratotic lesion on the feet
May be hard with a smooth surface (hard corn) or macerated and sodden (soft corn)
Women more commonly affected than men
Histopathologic Features
Concave, cup-shaped depression with hyperkeratosis and parakeratosis
Spinous and granular layer decreased
Differential Diagnosis
Wart
Callus
Porokeratosis

and **squamous cell carcinomas** with cutaneous horn formation. **Verruca** may show a concave depression, but the granular layer is usually accentuated rather than diminished. **Calluses** also demonstrate concave depression and typically show hypergranulosis and less parakeratosis (Table 8-22B). **Porokeratoses** are hyperkeratotic with coronoid lamellae. However, these lesions are not endophytic and demonstrate focal areas of dyskeratotic keratinocytes. Frequently, **squamous cell carcinomas** and **actinic keratoses** may be surfaced by a markedly thickened parakeratotic stratum corneum (**cutaneous horn**) (Table 8-22C). These lesions exhibit full thickness and partial thickness keratinocytic atypia, respectively.

Table 8-22B. Callus

Clinical Features
Flesh-colored to yellow or brown hyperkeratotic lesions on the palms and soles
Elevated, hard, dry, and usually asymptomatic
Histopathologic Features
Hyperkeratotic stratum corneum with variable parakeratosis
Cup-shaped depression with hypergranulosis and accentuated spinous layer
Differential Diagnosis
Clavus
Wart

Table 8-22C. Cutaneous Horn

Clinical Features
Hyperkeratotic gray to yellow masses on the face, scalp, hands, and ears
The lesion's height is at least half the diameter of the base
Histopathologic Features
Compact stratum corneum in a conical formation
Lamellated with occasional parakeratosis
Underlying lesions are typically actinic keratoses, warts, squamous cell carcinomas, or seborrheic keratoses
Differential Diagnosis
Wart
Inflamed seborrheic keratosis

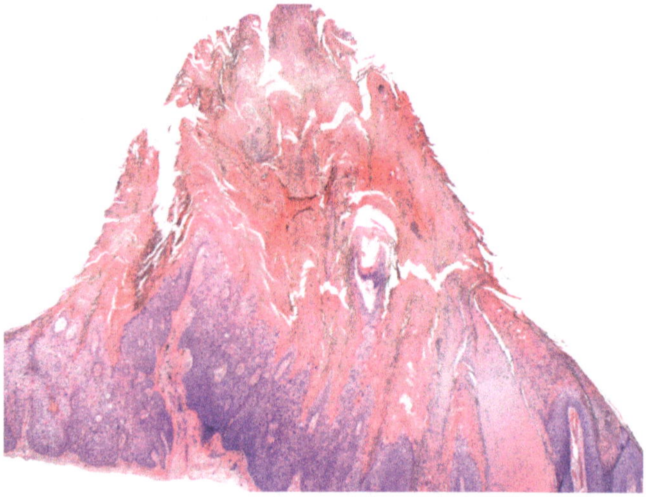

Squamous cell carcinoma in situ with cutaneous horn. The cutaneous horn demonstrates compact hyperkeratosis and parakeratosis with underlying squamous cell carcinoma in situ.

ANSWER 8-23: E.

Basal cell carcinoma is the most common malignant disease in humans and accounts for 50% of all cancers in the United States (Table 8-23A). **Basal cell carcinomas** typically begin after age 30 years and peak at age 70 years. Intense intermittent sun exposure has been correlated with a greater risk of tumor development compared with continuous sun exposure. Anatomic areas with increased sebaceous gland concentration are more likely to be involved, such as the head and neck. Risk factors for **basal cell carcinoma** include exposure to arsenic, psoralens, irradiation, coal tar derivatives, and UV light. Immunocompromised patients are at increased risk for **basal cell carcinoma** perhaps due to impaired cell-mediated immunity and an increased susceptibility to oncogenic viruses. There is some evidence that **nodular basal cell carcinomas** are more strongly associated with occupational sunlight than the superficial variant. **Basal cell carcinomas** are believed to derive from the epidermis, specifically the basal cell layer and the outer root sheath of the hair follicle. The cells of origin are likely pluripotential and may be progenitor epithelial cells in the case of adults or primary epithelial germ cells in the case of **linear unilateral basal cell nevi**. The expression of CD10 in **basal cell carcinomas** supports the contention that these tumors are of follicular derivation. Anti-keratin antibodies have shown that **basal cell carcinomas** possess a keratin component that is not normally found in the basal layer and stain similarly to the lower part of the hair follicle epithelium. The presence of cytokeratin 15 in **trichoepitheliomas** and its relative absence in **basal cell carcinomas** suggest

Table 8-23A. Basal Cell Carcinoma

Clinical Features
- Flesh-colored to pearly, raised papules and nodules on sun-exposed sites
- May bleed or ulcerate and occasionally destroy contiguous structures
- Indurated plaques are seen
- Superficial variant with erythema, scaling, and some epidermal breakdown
- Pigmented variant with hyperpigmentation, at times very black

Histopathologic Features
- Nodular
  - Small to large aggregates of basaloid cells emanating from the epidermis or follicular structures
- Peripheral palisading, stromal retraction, and mitoses are present
  - Necrosis, apoptosis, calcification, and mucin production are variable
  - Focal accumulation of melanin in the pigmented variant
  - Discrete areas of clear cell changes in clear cell variant
- Superficial
  - Small, discrete islands of basaloid cells present intermittently along the basal layer
  - Prominent peripheral palisading and stromal retraction
  - Peritumoral mucin production
- Keratotic infundibulocystic (pilar)
  - Keratin-filled cysts with features suggesting follicle derivation
  - Reticulated basaloid cells with some mitotic activity and mucin production
  - Stromal retraction is unusual
- Infiltrative, morpheaform
  - Small islands of basaloid cells with an angulated and "spiky" configuration
  - Poor peripheral palisading and minimal stromal retraction
  - Fibrotic and variably mucinous stroma
  - Deep infiltration and poor circumscription
- Fibroepithelioma of Pinkus
  - Aggregates of basaloid cells in the uppermost dermis
  - Extension into the dermis of elongated strands of palisading basaloid cells
  - Mucin in the dermis and stromal fibromucinous changes
  - "Glandular" appearance to the tumor at low power
- Metatypical
  - Tumor nests with more eosinophilic characteristics
  - Poor peripheral palisading and stromal retraction
  - Keratin pearls, increased mitotic activity, and premature cornification

Differential Diagnosis
- Nodular, micronodular
  - Eccrine spiradenoma
  - Nodular hidradenoma
  - Trichoepithelioma or trichoblastoma
- Superficial
  - Actinic keratosis
  - Seborrheic keratosis
- Keratotic, infundibulocystic
  - Trichoepithelioma or trichoblastoma
  - Basaloid follicular hamartoma
  - Reticulated seborrheic keratosis
- Infiltrative, morpheaform
  - Microcystic adnexal carcinoma
  - Desmoplastic trichoepithelioma
- Adenoid, fibroepithelioma of Pinkus
  - Primary cutaneous adenoid cystic carcinoma
  - Malignant mixed tumor of the skin (malignant chondroid syringoma)
  - Aggressive digital papillary adenocarcinoma
- Clear cell
  - Sebaceous adenoma
  - Tricholemmoma
  - Clear cell hidradenoma
  - Clear cell acanthoma
  - Balloon cell nevus and balloon cell melanoma
- Metatypical
  - Squamous cell carcinoma

that these malignancies arise infrequently from the so-called "bulge region" of the hair follicle. More recent evidence suggests that **basal cell carcinomas** differentiate toward follicular matrix cells. The oncogene BMI-1 is upregulated by the sonic hedgehog pathway and is strongly expressed in **basal cell carcinomas**, implying an association in pathogenesis between the former and latter.

Clinically, typical lesions are flesh colored or translucent to slightly erythematous papules and nodules with raised, rolled borders. Bleeding and crusting are occasionally seen. Telangiectasias may be present, particularly at the borders. Some lesions ulcerate, but significant scaling is unusual.

If untreated, large tumors destroy structures such as the ears, eyes, and nasal passages. Different variants may

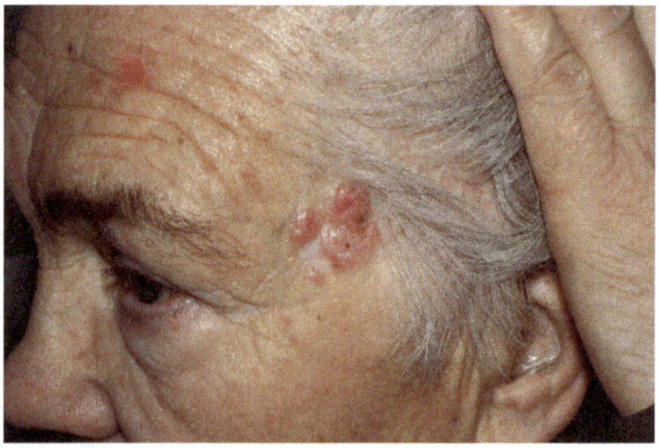

Nodular basal cell carcinoma. Nodular pinkish translucent tumor with telangiectasias.

have different clinical presentations. **Pigmented basal cell carcinomas** are more common in blacks and Hispanics. They present as variably pigmented nodular lesions and may simulate melanocytic tumors. The hyperpigmentation may be light brown to dark black and involve all or only parts of the lesion. The **desmoplastic basal cell carcinoma** has an actively spreading, indurated border with an atrophic or scar-like border. **Multicentric (multifocal, "field-fire") basal cell carcinoma** shows grouped tumors arising close to each other. Finally, the **linear variant of BCC** demonstrates a longitudinal arrangement of tumoral deposits with a predilection for the periocular region, perhaps propagated by the Koebner phenomenon. Overall, **metastatic basal cell carcinoma** is an extremely rare occurrence, with fewer than 300 cases reported in the literature. Different growth patterns of **basal cell carcinoma** have been documented to exhibit unique biological behavior. Indolent "low-risk" patterns include **superficial-multifocal BCC** and **nodular BCC.** Locally aggressive "high-risk" variants include **infiltrative, micronodular**, and **desmoplastic/morpheaform basal cell carcinomas.** These "high-risk" patterns have an increased incidence of perineural invasion and local recurrence, and therefore are typically removed via Mohs micrographic surgery. **Metatypical (basosquamous) basal cell carcinoma** exhibits squamous differentiation and behaves similar to **squamous cell carcinomas** with possible (but low) risk for distant metastasis. **Nodular basal cell carcinoma** is the most common histologic subtype. The vertical depth of invasion has been positively correlated with male gender, increased horizontal diameter, and more aggressive tumor subtypes such as **micronodular** or **infiltrative basal cell carcinoma.**

Basal cell proliferations with peripheral cell palisading but absent stromal retraction are occasionally seen in the epidermis overlying a **dermatofibroma.** These changes may represent proliferating epidermal basal cells or follicle induction by underlying stroma. Stromal retraction artifact and necrotic tumor cells support a diagnosis of **basal cell carcinoma.**

Quick Fact

- **Low-risk BCC**
  - Superficial (may be treated with topical therapy)
  - Nodular (surgical destruction)
- **High-risk BCC** (Mohs micrographic surgery)
  - Infiltrative
  - Micronodular
  - Desmoplastic
- **Metastatic potential**
  - Metatypical

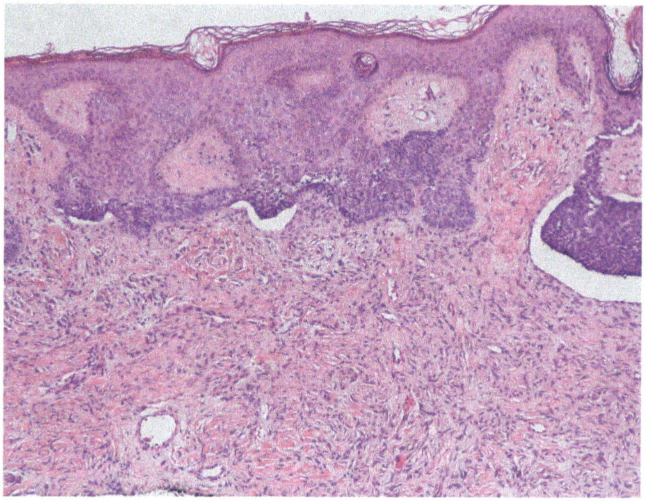

Dermatofibroma with epidermal induction. There is a spindle cell proliferation admixed with dermal fibrosis, consistent with a dermatofibroma. The overlying epidermis is acanthotic with expanded bulbous rete ridges lined by palisading basal cells. Note the absent tumor cell necrosis and tumoral mucin. This case exhibited tumor retraction artifact, which is absent in most cases of dermatofibroma-associated basal cell induction.

Basal Cell Carcinoma Growth Patterns (Variants)

Superficial: (The tumor in question). This variant is sometimes referred to as **superficial multicentric** since the tumor serpiginously winds through the epidermis revealing separate scattered foci of tumor along the undersurface of the epidermis, making margin assessment on bisected biopsy specimens inaccurate. Nests of basaloid cells extend from the epidermis and hair follicle epithelium. Tumor islands are relatively small and tend to have a broad base of attachment to the epidermis. Neoplastic cells resemble primordial germ cells. Peripheral palisading is usually prominent, and the surrounding stroma is somewhat blanched due to the presence of mucin. Tumor lobules have a well-rounded and well-defined peripheral contour. Retraction spaces are usually prominent. Mitotic activity and scattered necrotic tumor cells are usually present. Clinically, this pattern appears as erythematous patches or plaques with mild-to-moderate scaling, superficial ulcerations, and well-defined borders. If the growth pattern is restricted to superficial pattern only, topical therapy with imiquimod or 5-fluorouracil may be appropriate. Tumors with nodular or more aggressive patterns must be treated with destructive therapy (ie, curettage) or excision.

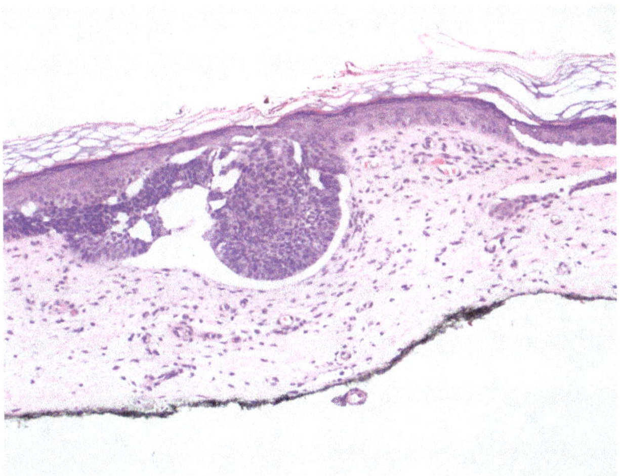

Basal cell carcinoma, superficial multifocal pattern. There are basaloid nests underlying the epidermal surface with prominent tumor-stromal retraction artifact.

<u>**Nodular:**</u> Tumors demonstrate dermal aggregates of basophilic staining neoplastic cells with well-defined contours. Palisading of the peripheral row of cells is usually obvious, and retraction from surrounding stroma is seen. Aggregates of cells that have become particularly large may demonstrate central necrosis with eosinophilic, granular features presumably due to an outstripping of the growing nodule's blood supply. Mucin may be present within the aggregates of neoplastic cells, and when exaggerated, form large pools, giving the tumor a "cystic" structure. The surrounding stroma tends to be myxoid in nature and slightly fibrotic. Calcification may be present, particularly in long-standing lesions, although this phenomenon reportedly has a proclivity for more aggressive histologic subtypes. Mitotic activity and keratinocyte necrosis are usually mild but may be marked in more aggressive lesions. Occasionally, tumors may demonstrate a reticulated configuration of basaloid cells extending into the dermis where the strands are several cells wide and may show significant peripheral palisading and stromal retraction. Tumors may on occasion exhibit variable cytomorphology including clear cell (PAS+/glycogen+), sebaceous, pigmented, and pleomorphic types. Unlike growth pattern, these cytologic variants have no bearing on behavior, management, or prognosis with the exception of squamous differentiation (**Metatypical BCC**), which is discussed later. **Nodular patterns of basal cell carcinoma** require destruction through curettage or excision.

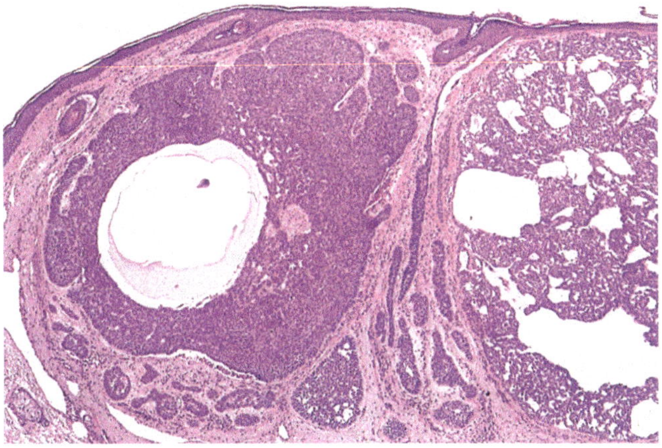

Nodular basal cell carcinoma. The tumors are composed of dermal nodular aggregates of atypical basaloid cells with peripheral palisading, stromal retraction artifact, and mucin production.

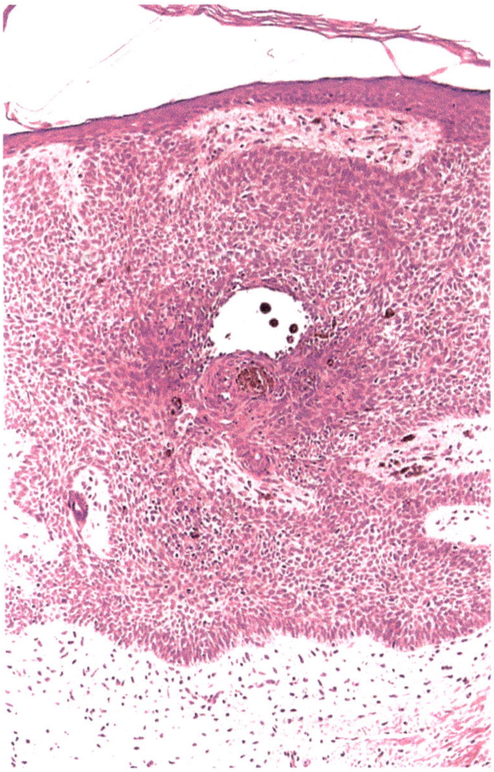

Pigmented nodular basal cell carcinoma. The features are similar to those of nodular basal cell carcinoma. Melanin pigment is present within basaloid cells and dermal macrophages.

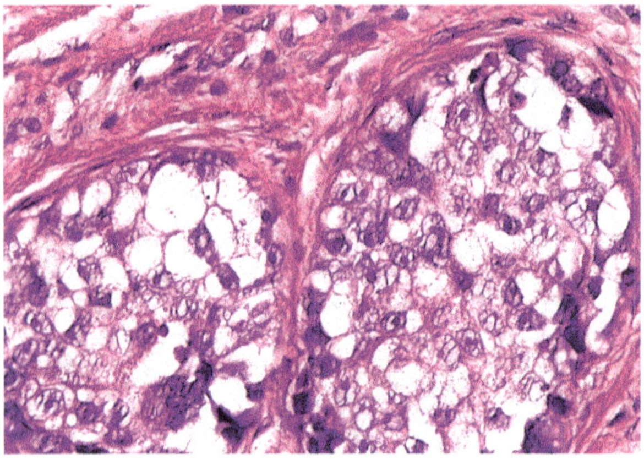

Basal cell carcinoma with sebaceous differentiation. Aggregates of nodular basal cell carcinoma show sebaceous differentiation. The clear cytoplasm is lipid and not glycogen.

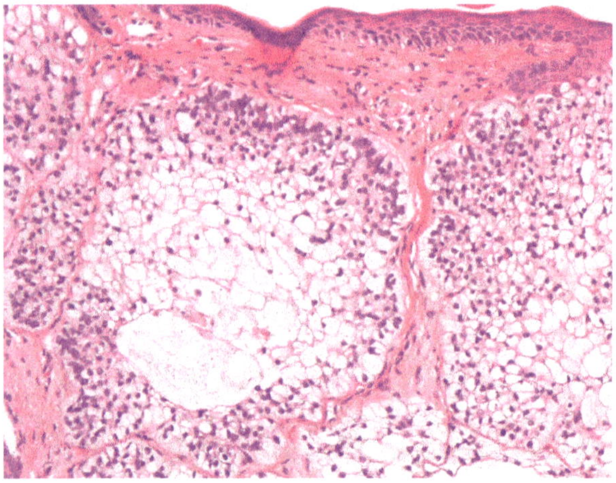

Clear cell basal cell carcinoma. Aggregates of clear tumor cells are seen in association with lobules of nodular basal cell carcinoma. PAS stain will reveal increased amounts of pink glycogen.

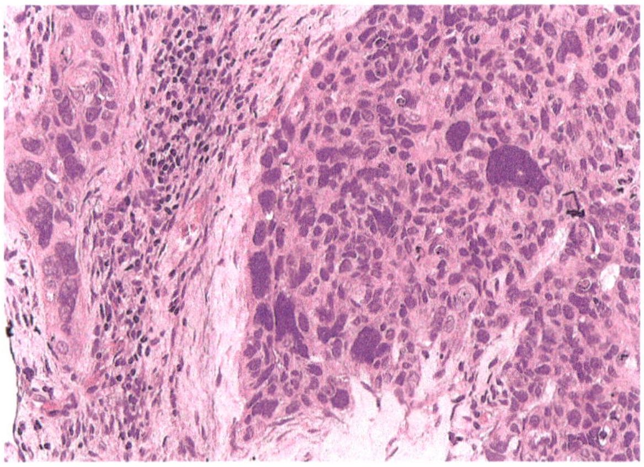

Pleomorphic basal cell carcinoma. Enlarged nuclei and giant cells are present within lobules of nodular basal cell carcinoma.

Micronodular: These tumors are plaque-like, indurated, firm, and poorly defined. Typically, they are difficult to remove and have an increased incidence of recurrence. Histopathologically, **micronodular basal cell carcinomas** demonstrate rounded nodules of tumor similar to the nodular variant but are smaller. They are approximately the size of hair bulbs and display minimal palisading. Tumor nodules are widely dispersed in an asymmetric pattern. Retraction spaces are uncommon as the tumor nodules are characteristically wrapped in their own stroma. The surrounding stroma is collagenous and slightly myxoid, particularly adjacent to the tumor nodules. The presence of smooth muscle actin within the malignant cells is thought to facilitate invasion and has been correlated with a more aggressive clinical picture.

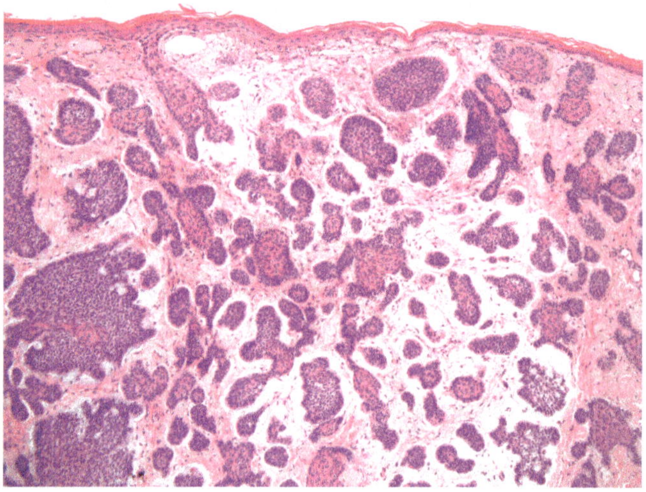

Micronodular basal cell carcinoma. Small nests of atypical basaloid cells proliferate in a myxoid stroma. This pattern is considered "high risk" for perineural invasion and local recurrence.

Infiltrative: **Infiltrative basal cell carcinomas** exist on the continuum between the **nodular** (nodulo-infiltative variants) and **morpheaform variants** both histopathologically and clinically. These tumors are composed of atypical basaloid cells in varying sized nodules and islands with irregular, jagged peripheral contours. Elongated strands four to eight cells wide invade the deeper dermis. The surrounding stroma is fibrous but minimally mucinous. Peripheral palisading and stromal retraction are less prominent. The tumor is poorly circumscribed. Invasion of the subcutis and muscle is occasionally appreciated. Inflammation is minimal. This tumor is more aggressive, more difficult to eradicate, and capable of greater destruction than **nodular variants of BCC**. Clinically, **infiltrative basal cell carcinomas** are yellow-white in color without a sharply defined or rolled border. Tumors blend imperceptibly with the surrounding skin.

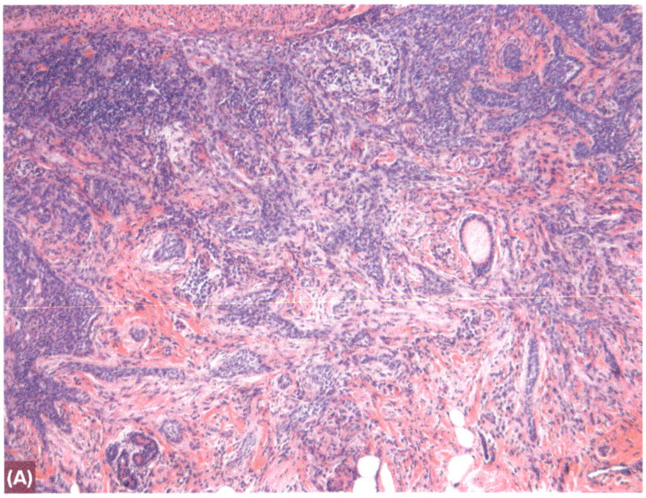

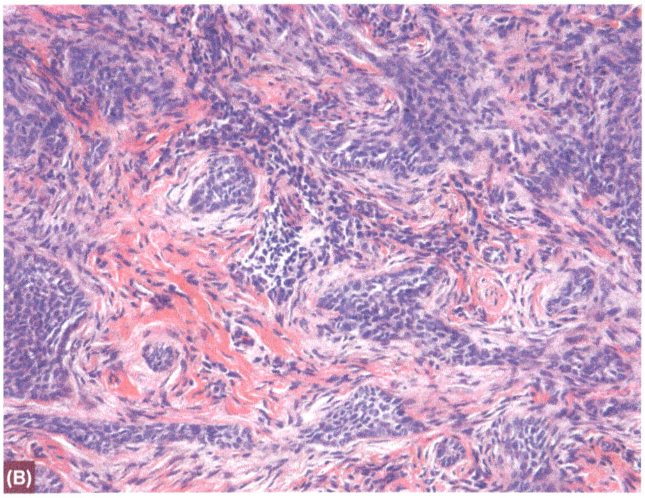

Infiltrating basal cell carcinoma. (A) Linear strands and islands of atypical basaloid epithelium are present. **(B)** The atypical basaloid epithelium exhibits some peripheral palisading of nuclei. The tumor stroma is slightly sclerotic.

Desmoplastic (Morpheaform/Sclerosing): Sclerosing basal cell carcinomas are also known as **morpheaform (morpheic), fibrosing, scirrhous**, or **desmoplastic BCC** and comprise up to 5% of all lesions. Tumors are white or yellow and are fibrotic. They are usually macular and rarely ulcerate or bleed. No particular anatomic site is preferred. Tumor islands are small, thin, and elongated. They tend to be less than five cells in width and possess sharp, angulated ends. Peripheral palisading is absent, and stromal retraction is rare. Mitotic activity is usually present but is not marked. The surrounding dermis is fibrous and dense to the point of sclerosis. Tumors are usually poorly circumscribed and may invade deeply into the muscle and fat. Typically, they are difficult to remove and have an increased incidence of perineural invasion and recurrence. The histopathological differential diagnosis includes **microcystic adnexal carcinoma** (MAC) and **desmoplastic trichoepithelioma** (DTE). Unlike **MAC** and **DTE**, these tumors do not contain CEA+ lumens and scattered CK20+ Merkel cells, respectively. The extent of tumor involvement is typically much greater than what can be appreciated clinically, and therefore the preferred management is via Mohs micrographic surgery.

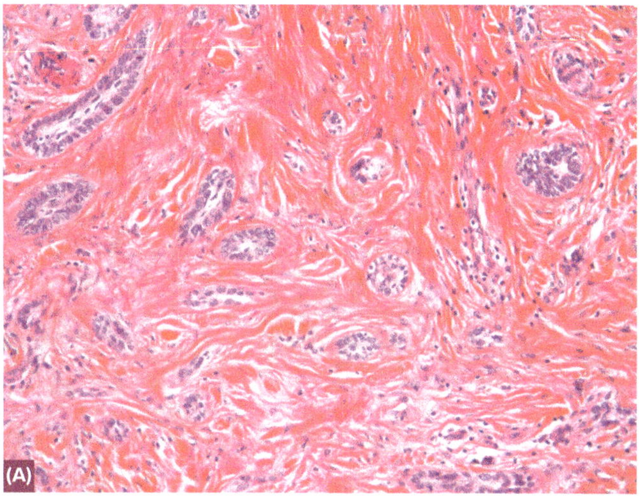

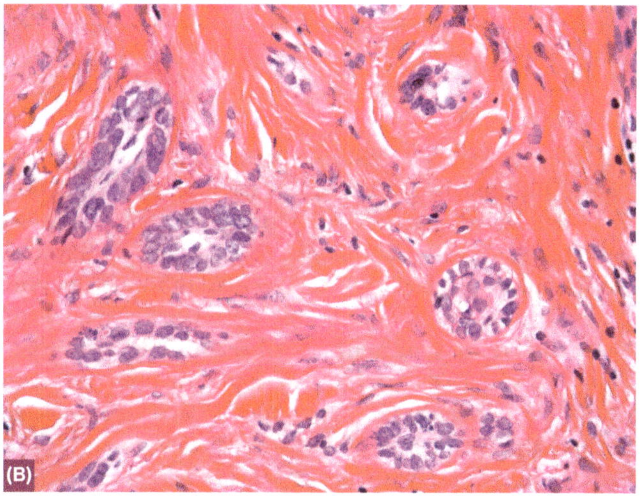

Desmoplastic basal cell carcinoma. (A) and **(B)** Aggregates of atypical basaloid tumor cells are rounded or elongated and isolated in a sclerotic background.

Metatypical (Basal Cell Carcinoma with Squamous Differentiation): This subtype of **basal cell carcinoma** has been the source of some confusion regarding its histologic features. It is probably best to use this designation when evaluating a **basal cell carcinoma** with features intermittent between **nodular basal cell carcinoma** and **squamous cell carcinoma**. These tumors have basaloid cells with variable eosinophilic features, prominent mitotic activity, and numerous apoptotic cells. Peripheral palisading and stromal retraction are rare to absent. Nuclei are enlarged, and some spindling of cells may be seen. Premature cornification is common, and keratin pearls are occasionally seen. These tumors tend to be more aggressive, with a greater incidence of perineural and lymphatic spread. They may grow with the speed of **squamous cell carcinomas** and have clinical features of both tumor types.

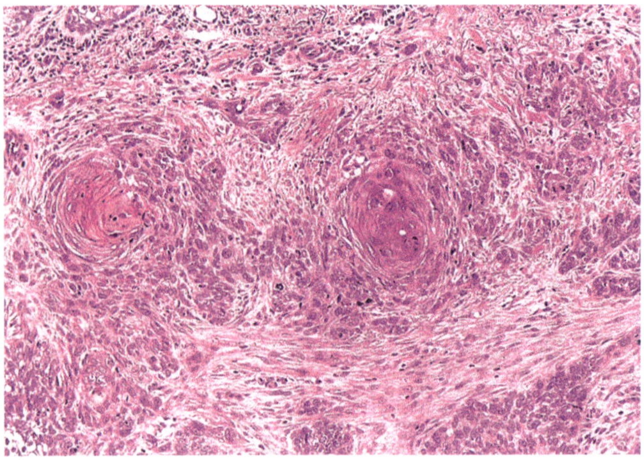

Metatypical basal cell carcinoma. Tumor islands are slightly basaloid with absent palisading and stromal retraction. Dyskeratosis and keratin pearl formation are seen.

ANSWER 8-24: B.

The biopsy reveals a basaloid proliferation with connection to the epidermal surface. The basaloid cells proliferate in a reticulated manner and form small cysts. Adjacent perifollicular-type stroma is not present. The findings are consistent with **basal cell carcinoma, infundibulocystic type**. This condition is referred to as **Gorlin syndrome, basal cell nevus syndrome**, or **Gherkin-Goltz syndrome** (Table 8-24A). This complex of symptoms is inherited as an autosomal dominant trait, but about 35%-50% of affected patients represent new mutations. The disease usually begins between 17 and 35 years of age but has been described in children as young as 2 years. Disease activity is increased at puberty. The prevalence is approximately 1 in 56,000. Because of the relatively young age of affected patients, there is not a strong association between cumulative sun exposure and tumor development. However, in susceptible persons, sun exposure does exacerbate the development of **basal cell carcinomas**. A malfunctioning tumor-suppressor gene known as *PATCHED* on chromosome 9q22-q31 is believed to cause this condition. Unlike **conventional basal cell carcinomas**, which have an extremely low rate of distant metastasis, patients with this syndrome have an increased incidence of **metastatic basal cell carcinoma**. Neoplasms also reported in patients with **nevoid basal cell carcinoma syndrome** include

Table 8-24A. Nevoid Basal Cell Carcinoma

Clinical Features
Numerous flesh-colored to brown papules 1-10 mm in diameter
Develops on the face and trunk beginning around puberty
Autosomal dominant inheritance
Jaw and cutaneous cysts, skeletal anomalies (particularly bifid ribs), ectopic central nervous system calcification, and palmar or plantar pitting
Histopathologic Features
Basal cell carcinomas
Essentially identical to those found idiopathically
Most commonly nodular and superficial variants
Calcification and pigment deposition are more common
Jaw and cutaneous cysts
Epithelial lining with granular layer similar to infundibular cysts
Epithelial lining with corrugated, compact lining similar to steatocystomas
Cutaneous pits
Sharply defined absence of keratin and thinned epidermis at base of pit
Diminished or absent granular layer
Differential Diagnosis
Basal cell carcinomas
Eccrine spiradenoma
Nodular hidradenoma
Trichoepithelioma or trichoblastoma
Jaw and cutaneous cysts
Dilated pore
Dermoid cyst
Cutaneous pits
Pitted keratolysis

rhabdomyosarcoma, ovarian fibrosarcoma, and **leiomyosarcoma**. Clinically, the features of **nevoid basal cell carcinoma syndrome** are divided into five major categories. The first is the presence of numerous **basal cell carcinomas**. These may range from a few to 1000 and are similar to routine **basal cell carcinomas**. They may be very small and flesh colored to brown. Tumors appear as dome-shaped papules to soft nodular or flat plaques on the face and trunk. Lesions vary from 1 to 10 mm and may be clinically mistaken for **skin tags, nevi, molluscum contagiosum**, or **hemangiomas**. These tumors may be aggressive, particularly when they involve the embryonic clefts of the face. The second feature is the development of numerous cysts, particularly **epithelium-lined**

jaw cysts. These lesions begin to develop after age 7 years and may cause pain, tooth shifting, drainage, and jaw swelling. **Cutaneous cysts** may also be present and arise on the trunk and limbs in about 50% of affected patients. These cysts contain thick, discolored liquid with features similar to **steatocystomas**. Intermittent **milium cysts** are present in 35%-50% of patients. Skeletal anomalies are prevalent in this syndrome and include bifid ribs, frontal bossing of the skull, bridging of the sella turcica, and spinal deformities. Intracranial calcification, particularly of the falx cerebri, is seen. **Medulloblastomas, meningiomas**, and **craniopharyngiomas** have been reported in patients with this condition. Finally, pitting of the palms and soles is seen. These pits are 1-3 mm in depth and 2-3 mm in diameter. They develop during the second decade of life.

The cutaneous cysts are similar to infundibular cysts (**epidermoid cysts**). These tumors have an epithelial lining with a distinct granular layer and produce keratin. Some cysts, however, resemble **keratinous jaw cysts**. These lesions show a festooned or corrugated epithelium two to five cells thick that lacks a granular layer. These features are similar to those of **steatocystomas**, but sebaceous glands are absent. **Cutaneous pits** demonstrate a sharply defined absence of keratin. The epidermis is thinned at the base, and the rete ridges proliferate irregularly. The granular layer is diminished. These pits are believed to result from premature desquamation of the keratinocytes.

Histopathologically, the **basal cell carcinomas** of **Gorlin syndrome** are identical to those found in patients without this syndrome. The tumors are most commonly of the nodular and superficial subtype with the morpheaform, infiltrative, and fibroepithelial variants less likely. A rare manifestation of **nodular basal cell carcinoma**, referred to as **infundibulocystic basal cell carcinoma**, is commonly seen in these patients, in which reticulated strands of atypical basaloid epithelium connect with the overlying epidermis. Scattered small cysts lined by tumor cells are also present. Calcification and pigment deposition may be increased. Neuroendocrine tumor differentiation (uptake by chromogranin and neuron-specific enolase stains) has been reported in a patient with metastatic disease. A **carcinosarcoma** with features of a basal cell carcinoma and fibrosarcoma has been reported in a patient with this syndrome.

Although **fibroepithelioma of Pinkus** may be seen in **Gorlin syndrome**, it is not the most characteristic pattern of basal cell carcinoma. Pinkus initially described **fibroepithelioma of Pinkus** in 1953. They typically arise on the lumbosacral regions as pink to flesh-colored nodules with a constricted base. Elongated, branched, and trabecular strands of basaloid cells extend deep into the dermis and proliferate symmetrically. Horn cysts may be present, and palisading is seen. Stromal retraction is uncommon. The surrounding stroma is fibromucinous, and stromal–stromal separation may be present. Some controversy exists as to whether this tumor represents a **basal cell carcinoma** or a benign adnexal neoplasm with follicular differentiation such as a **trichoepithelioma** or **trichoblastoma**. Androgen receptors, occasionally found on **basal cell carcinomas**, have been noted with increased frequency in **fibroepitheliomas of Pinkus** compared with **trichoepitheliomas** or **trichoblastomas** but have also demonstrated retention of Merkel cells, a feature of benign follicular tumors. Low levels of staining with Ki-67 and p53 and significant numbers of cells expressing cytokeratin 20 have been reported in these tumors, supporting the contention that they more closely resemble **trichoblastomas** than **basal cell carcinomas**.

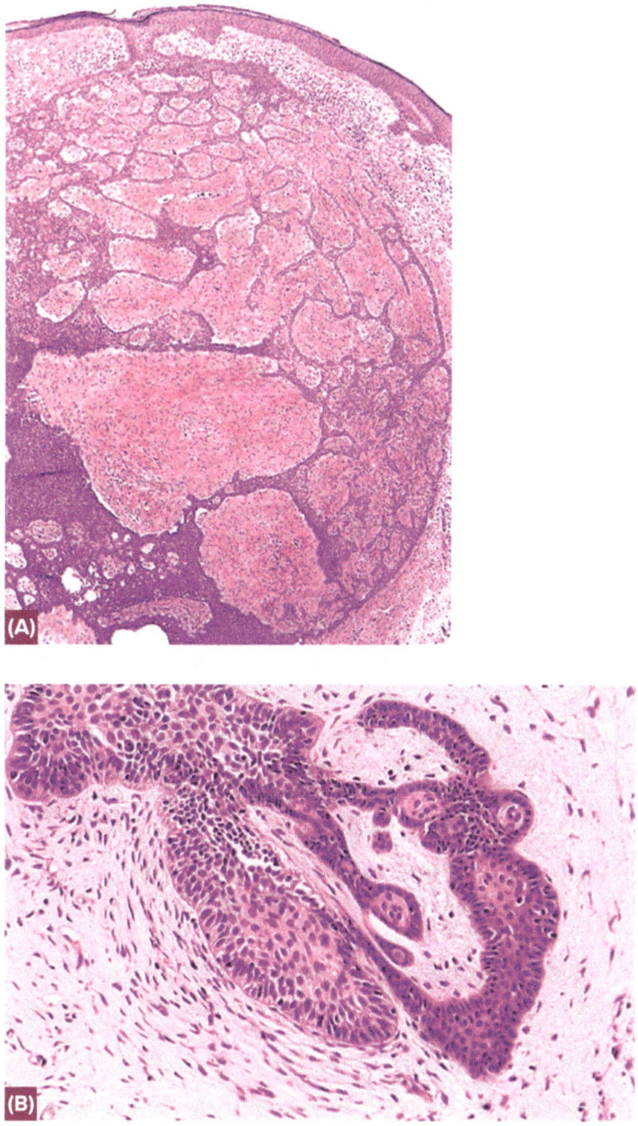

Fibroepithelioma of Pinkus. (A) The tumor proliferates symmetrically as reticulated strands of basaloid cells surrounding fibromucinous stroma. **(B)** The tumor is a biphasic epithelial-stromal neoplasm similar to trichoepithelioma and trichoblastoma, but exhibits malignant cytomorphology with occasionally scattered necrotic tumor cells.

BIBLIOGRAPHY

1. Al-Enezi A, Huber AM, Krafchik BR, et al. Inflammatory linear verrucous epidermal nevus and arthritis: a new association. *J Pediatr.* 2001;138:602–604.
2. Anadolu R, Boyvat A, Calikoglu E, et al. Buschke-Loewenstein tumour is not a low-grade carcinoma but a giant verruca. *Acta Dermato Venereol (Stockh).* 1999;79:253–254.
3. Ansai S, Kimura T, Hayashi M. Fatal genital verrucous carcinoma. *Am J Dermatopathol.* 2007;29:68–71.
4. Ansarin H, Daliri M, Soltani-Arabshahi R. Expression of p53 in aggressive and non-aggressive histologic variants of basal cell carcinoma. *Eur J Dermatol.* 2006;16:543–547.
5. Ashton MA. Cutaneous ciliated cyst of the lower limb in a male. *Histopathology.* 1995;26:467–469.
6. Aslan F, Demirkesen C, Baatay P, et al. Expression of cytokeratin subtypes in intraepidermal malignancies: a guide for differentiation. *J Cutan Pathol.* 2006;33:531–538.
7. Aydogan K, Ozbek S, Balaban AS, et al. Irritated seborrhoeic keratosis presenting as a cutaneous horn. *J Eur Acad Dermatol Venereol.* 2006;20:626–628.
8. Azuma Y, Matsukawa A. Warty dyskeratoma with multiple lesions. *J Dermatol.* 1993;20:374–377.
9. Bahcekapili D, Buyukbabani N, Saglik E, et al. Seborrhoeic dermatosis arising on a nevus sebaceous. *J Eur Acad Dermatol Venereol.* 2006;20:875–877.
10. Bale AE, Gailani MR, Leffell DJ. Nevoid basal cell carcinoma syndrome. *J Invest Dermatol.* 1994;103:126S–130S.
11. Bhattacharjee P, Leffell D, McNiff JM. Primary cutaneous carcinosarcoma arising in a patient with nevoid basal cell carcinoma syndrome. *J Cutan Pathol.* 2005;32:638–641.
12. Bhawan J, Dayal Y, Gonzalez-Serva A, Eisen R. Cutaneous metaplastic synovial cyst. *J Cutan Pathol.* 1990;17:22–26.
13. Bigby SM, Charlton A, Miller MV, et al. Biphasic sarcomatoid basal cell carcinoma (carcinosarcoma): four cases with immunohistochemistry and review of the literature. *J Cutan Pathol.* 2005;32:141–147.
14. Bowen AR, LeBoit PE. Fibroepithelioma of Pinkus is a fenestrated trichoblastoma. *Am J Dermatopathol.* 2005;27:149–154.
15. Braun-Falco M, Ring J. Enhanced cytoplasmic expression of desmocollin 3 in epidermal rete ridges of Dowling-Degos disease. *Br J Dermatol.* 2003;149:1293–1295.
16. Cambiaghi S, Brusasco A, Grimalt R, et al. Acantholytic dyskeratotic epidermal nevus as a mosaic form of Darier's disease. *J Am Acad Dermatol.* 1995;32:284–286.
17. Cassarino DS, DeRienzo DP, Barr RJ. Cutaneous squamous cell carcinoma: a comprehensive clinicopathologic classification. Part 1. *J Cutan Pathol.* 2006;33:191–206.
18. Cassarino DS, DeRienzo DP, Barr RJ. Cutaneous squamous cell carcinoma: a comprehensive clinicopathologic classification. Part 2. *J Cutan Pathol.* 2006;33:261–279.
19. Clausen OP, Aass HC, Beigi M, et al. Are keratoacanthomas variants of squamous cell carcinoma? A comparison of chromosomal aberrations by comparative genomic hybridization. *J Invest Dermatol.* 2006;126:2308–2315.
20. Cohen PR, Schulze KE, Nelson BR. Basal cell carcinoma with mixed histology: a possible pathogenesis for recurrent skin cancer. *Dermatol Surg.* 2006;32:542–551.
21. Consigli JE, Gonzalez ME, Morsino R, et al. Generalized eruptive keratoacanthoma (Grzybowski variant). *Br J Dermatol.* 2000;142:800–803.
22. Coskey RJ, Mehregan AH. The association of basal cell carcinomas with other tumors. *J Dermatol Surg Oncol.* 1987;13:553–555.
23. Cox NH, Long E. Dowling-Degos disease and Kitamura's reticulate acropigmentation: support for the concept of a single disease. *Br J Dermatol.* 1991;125:169–171.
24. Cuesta KH, Palazzo JP, Mittal KR. Detection of human papillomavirus in verrucous carcinoma from HIV-seropositive patients. *J Cutan Pathol.* 1998;25:165–170.
25. Davis KA, Mock CN, Versaci A, Lentrichia P. Malignant degeneration of pilonidal cysts. *Am Surg.* 1994;60:200–204.
26. Diaz-Cascajo C, Borghi S, Weyers W, et al. Follicular squamous cell carcinoma of the skin: a poorly recognized neoplasms arising from the wall of hair follicles. *J Cutan Pathol.* 2004;31:19–23.
27. Eiberg H, Hansen L, Hansen C, et al. Mapping of hereditary trichilemmal cyst (*TRICY1*) to chromosome 3p24-p21.2 and exclusion of beta-*CATENIN* and *MLH1*. *Am J Med Genet A.* 2005;133(Suppl A):44–47.
28. Ersoy-Evans S, Sahin S, Mancini AJ, et al. The acanthosis nigricans form of epidermal nevus. *J Am Acad Dermatol.* 2006;55:696–698.
29. Fuchs A, Marmur E. The kinetics of skin cancer: progression of actinic keratosis to squamous cell carcinoma. *Dermatol Surg.* 2007;33:1099–1101.
30. Grimalt R, Gelmetti C. Eruptive vellus hair cysts: case report and review of the literature. *Pediatr Dermatol.* 1992;9:98–102.
31. Hafner C, Hartmann A, van Oers JM, et al. FGFR3 mutations in seborrheic keratoses are already present in flat lesions and associated with age and localization. *Mod Pathol.* 2007;20:895–903.
32. Hafner C, van Oers JM, Hartmann A, et al. High frequency of FGFR3 mutations in adenoid seborrheic keratoses. *J Invest Dermatol.* 2006;126:2404–2407.

33. Hallerman C, Gunawan B, Bertsch HP. No chromosomal imbalances in seborrheic keratoses detectable by comparative genomic hybridization. *J Invest Dermatol.* 2004;123:1204–1205.
34. Happle R. Epidermal nevus syndromes. *Sem Dermatol.* 1995;14:111–121.
35. Heaphy MR, Ackerman AB. The nature of solar keratosis: a critical review in historical perspective. *J Am Acad Dermatol.* 2000;43:138–150.
36. Heaphy MR, Millns JL, Schroeter AL. The sign of Leser-Trelat in a case of adenocarcinoma of the lung. *J Am Acad Dermatol.* 2000;43:386–390.
37. Ihm CW. Squamous eddies in irritated seborrheic keratosis. *Am J Dermatopathol.* 2007;29:28–31.
38. Kamiya M, Takeuchi Y, Katho M, et al. Expression of p73 in normal skin and proliferative lesions. *Pathol Int.* 2004;54:890–895.
39. Kato N, Ueno H. Infundibulocystic basal cell carcinoma. *Am J Dermatopathol.* 1993;15:265–267.
40. Katona TM, Ravis SM, Perkins SM, et al. Expression of androgen receptor by fibroepithelioma of Pinkus: evidence supporting classification as a basal cell carcinoma variant? *Am J Dermatopathol.* 2007;29:7–12.
41. Ko CJ, Iftner T, Barr RJ, et al. Changes of epidermodysplasia verrucifomis in benign skin lesions: the EV acanthoma. *J Cutan Pathol.* 2007;34:44–48.
42. Koreda S, Horiguchi Y, Ueda M, et al. Basal cell carcinoma cells resemble follicular matrix cells rather than follicular bulge cells: immunohistochemical and ultrastructural comparative studies. *Am J Dermatopathol.* 1998;20:362–369.
43. Kovacs D, Cota C, Cardinali G, et al. Expression of keratinocyte growth factor and its receptor in clear cell acanthoma. *Exp Dermatol.* 2006;15:762–768.
44. Kurban RS, Bhawan J. Cutaneous cysts lined by nonsquamous epithelium. *Am J Dermatopathol.* 1991;13:509–517.
45. Kurokawa I, Nakai Y, Nishimura K, et al. Cytokeratin and filaggrin expression in nevus comedonicus. *J Cutan Pathol.* 2007;34:338–341.
46. Kurokawa I, Yokoyama T, Nishimura K, et al. Pinkus tumor may originate from intraepidermal eccrine ducts and proliferate in the dermis. *Oncol Rep.* 2007;17:49–54.
47. Lee SH, Choi EH, Lee WS, et al. Confluent and reticulated papillomatosis: a clinical, histopathological, and electron microscopic study. *J Dermatol.* 1991;18:725–730.
48. Lober BA, Lober CW. Actinic keratosis is squamous cell carcinoma. *S Med J.* 2000;93:650–655.
49. Lubbe J, Kormann A, Adams V, et al. HPV-11 and HPV-16–associated oral verrucous carcinoma. *Dermatology.* 1996;192:217–221.
50. Miller SJ. Biology of basal cell carcinoma (part I). *J Am Acad Dermatol.* 1991;24:1–13.
51. Miller SJ. Biology of basal cell carcinoma (part II). *J Am Acad Dermatol.* 1991;24:161–175.
52. Mishalani SH, Lones MA, Said JW. Multilocular thymic cyst. *Arch Pathol Lab Med.* 1995;119:467–470.
53. Morgan MB, Stevens GL, Somach S, et al. Carcinoma arising in epidermoid cysts: a case series and aetiological investigation of human papillomavirus. *Br J Dermatol.* 2001;145:505–506.
54. Morillo V, Manrique P, De Miguel E, et al. Nevus comedonicus with epidermolytic hyperkeratosis. *Eur J Derm.* 2007;17:176–177.
55. Moy RL. Clinical presentation of actinic keratoses and squamous cell carcinoma. *J Am Acad Dermatol.* 2000;42(Suppl):S8–S10.
56. Nakamura S, Nisioka K. Enhanced expression of p16 in seborrhoeic keratosis: a lesion of accumulated senescent epidermal cells in G1 arrest. *Br J Dermatol.* 2003;149:560–565.
57. Neuhaus IM, LeBoit PE, McCalmont TM. Seborrheic keratosis with basal clear cells: a distinctive microscopic mimic of melanoma in situ. *J Am Acad Dermatol.* 2006;54:132–135.
58. Nyquist GG, Mumm C, Grau R, et al. Malignant proliferating pilar tumors arising in KID syndrome: a report of two patients. *Am J Med Genet A.* 2007; 143(Suppl A):734–741.
59. Ohtake N, Kubota Y, Takayama O, et al. Relationship between steatocystoma multiplex and eruptive vellus hair cysts. *J Am Acad Dermatol.* 1992;26:876–878.
60. Papadavid E, Pignatelli M, Zakynthinos S, et al. The potential role of abnormal E-cadherin and α-, β- and Γ-catenin immunoreactivity in the determination of the biological behaviour of keratoacanthoma. *Br J Dermatol.* 2001;145:582–589.
61. Pelucchi C, Di Landro A, Naldi L, et al. Risk factors for histological types and anatomic sites of cutaneous basal-cell carcinoma: an Italian case-control study. *J Invest Dermatol.* 2007;127:935–944.
62. Perez GL, Peters MS, Reda AM, et al. Mast cells, neutrophils and eosinophils in prurigo nodularis. *Arch Dermatol.* 1993;129:861–865.
63. Pulitzer M, Desman G, Busam KJ. CK7 expression in primary cutaneous squamous cell carcinoma. *J Cutan Pathol.* 2010 Sep;37(9):966–972.
64. Queille S, Luron L, Spatz A, et al. Analysis of skin cancer risk factors in immunosuppressed renal transplant patients shows high levels of UV-specific tandem CC to TT mutations of the p53 gene. *Carcinogenesis.* 2007;28:724–731.

65. Reguiai Z, Cribier B, Derancourt C, et al. Multiple spreading epidermolytic acanthomas of the genital and perigenital skin. *Dermatology*. 2005;211:152–154.
66. Rubin AI, Chen EH, Ratner D. Basal-cell carcinoma. *N Engl J Med*. 2005;353:2262–2269.
67. Satyaprakash A, Sheehan, DJ, Sangueza O. Proliferating trichilemmal tumors: a review of the literature. *Dermatol Surg*. 2007;33(9):1102–1108.
68. Sau P, Graham JH, Helwig EB. Proliferating epithelial cysts: clinicopathological analysis of 96 cases. *J Cutan Pathol*. 1995;22:394–406.
69. Schell BJ, Rosen T, Rady P, et al. Verrucous carcinoma of the foot associated with human papillomavirus type 16. *J Am Acad Dermatol*. 2001;45:49–55.
70. Schlauder SM, Calder KB, Moody P, et al. HER2 and EGFR expression in cutaneous spindle cell carcinoma. *Am J Dermatopathol*. 2007;29:559–563.
71. Schwartzberg JB, Ricotti CA, Ballard CJ, et al. Eruptive dermatosis papulosa nigra as a possible sign of internal malignancy. *Int J Dermatol*. 2007;46:186–187.
72. Sexton M, Jones DB, Maloney ME. Histologic pattern analysis of basal cell carcinoma. *J Am Acad Dermatol*. 1990;23:1118–1126.
73. Shah V, Shet T. Scrotal calcinosis results from calcification of cysts derived from hair follicles: a series of 20 cases evaluating the spectrum of changes resulting in scrotal calcinosis. *Am J Dermatopathol*. 2007;29(2):172–175.
74. Sinha S, Schwartz RA. Juvenile acanthosis nigricans. *J Am Acad Dermatol*. 2007;57:502–508.
75. Sonkoly E, Muller A, Lauerma AI, et al. IL-31: a new link between T cells and pruritus in atopic skin inflammation. *J Aller Clin Immunol*. 2006;117:411–417.
76. Stern JB, Haupt HM, Smith RRL. Fibroepithelioma of Pinkus: eccrine duct spread of basal cell carcinoma. *Am J Dermatopathol*. 1994;16:585–587.
77. Stosiek N, Ulmer R, von den Driesch P, et al. Chromosomal mosaicism in two patients with epidermal verrucous nevus. *J Am Acad Dermatol*. 1994;30:622–625.
78. Takenouchi T, Nomoto S, Ito M. Factors influencing the linear depth of invasion of primary basal cell carcinoma. *Dermatol Surg*. 2001;27:393–396.
79. Tilli CMLJ, Van Steensel MAM, Krekels GAM, et al. Molecular aetiology and pathogenesis of basal cell carcinoma. *Br J Dermatol*. 2005;152:1108–1124.
80. Ting PT, Kasper R, Arlette JP. Metastatic basal cell carcinoma: report of two cases and literature review. *J Cutan Med Surg*. 2005;9:10–15.
81. Tsao H. Update on familial cancer syndromes and the skin. *J Am Acad Dermatol*. 2000;42:939–969.
82. Tschen JP, Cohen PR, Schultze KE, et al. Pleomorphic basal cell carcinoma: case reports and review. *South Med J*. 2006; 296–302.
83. Tsubota A, Akiyama M, Sakai K, et al. Keratin 1 gene mutation detected in epidermal nevus with epidermolytic hyperkeratosis. *J Invest Dermatol*. 2007;127:1371–1374.
84. Van der Putte SCJ, Toonstra J. Cutaneous "bronchogenic" cyst. *J Cutan Pathol*. 1985;12:404–409.
85. Vissers WH, Muys L, Erp PE, et al. Immunohistochemical differentiation between inflammatory linear verrucous epidermal nevus (ILVEN) and psoriasis. *Eur J Dermatol*. 2004;14:216–220.
86. Walsh SN, Hurt MA, Santa Cruz DJ. Psoriasiform keratosis. *Am J Dermatopathol*. 2007;29:137–140.
87. Williams K, Anderson ND, Babar K, et al. The hybrid epidermoid and apocrine cyst. The combination of apocrine hydrocystoma and epidermoid inclusion cyst. *Am J Dermatopathol*. 1996;518(4):364–366.
88. Wong T-Y, Suster S. Tricholemmal carcinoma: a clinicopathologic study of 13 cases. *Am J Dermatopathol*. 1994;16:463–473.
89. Wy YH, Hsiao PF, Lin YC. Verruciform xanthoma-like phenomenon in seborrheic keratosis. *J Cutan Pathol*. 2006;33:373–377.
90. Yabe T, Furukawa M. The origin of pilonidal sinus: a case report. *J Dermatol*. 1995;22:696–699.
91. Yada K, Kashima K, Daa T, et al. Expression of CD10 in basal cell carcinomas. *Am J Dermatopathol*. 2004;26:463–471.
92. Youn M, Hann SK, Moon TK, Lee MG. Acantholytic dyskeratotic epidermal nevus induced by ultraviolet B radiation. *J Am Acad Dermatol*. 1998;39:301–304.
93. Zedek DC, Langel DJ, White WL. Clear-cell acanthoma versus acanthosis: a psoriasiform reaction pattern lacking tricholemmal differentiation. *Am J Dermatopathol*. 2007;29:378–384.
94. Zheng S, Adachi A, Shimizu M, et al. Human papillomaviruses of the mucosal type are present in some cases of extragenital Bowen's disease. *Br J Dermatol*. 2005 Jun;152(6):1243–7.
95. Zvulunov A, Anichai D, Grunwald NH, et al. Cutaneous bronchogenic cysts: delineation of a poorly recognized lesion. *Pediatr Dermatol*. 1998;16(4):277–281.

CHAPTER 9

Adnexal Tumors

QUESTION 9-1.

A 16-year-old female presents with multiple flesh-colored to yellow papules under the lower eyelids that range from 1 to 2 mm. One of these lesions is biopsied and is illustrated below. Immunohistochemistry reveals the basolateral cell layer of the tubules to stain positive for EMA and the inner ductal lining staining positive for CEA. Which of the following diagnoses is CORRECT?

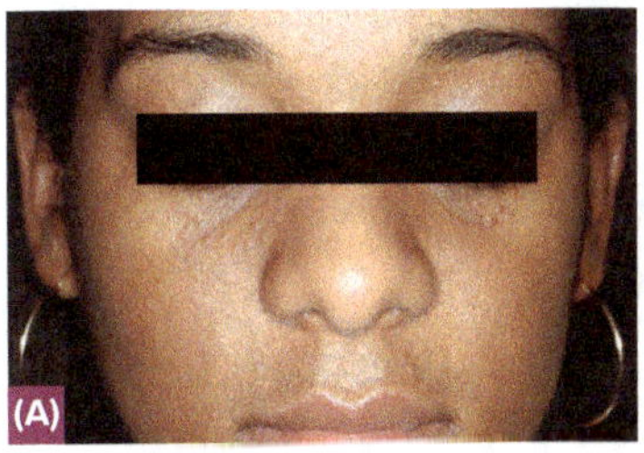

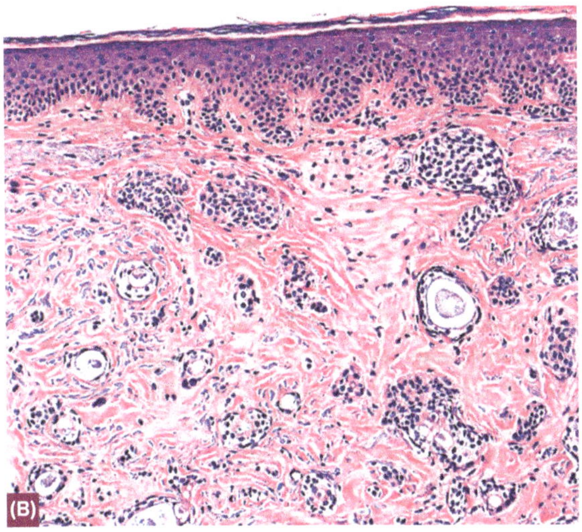

A) Trichoepithelioma
B) Syringoma
C) Microcystic adnexal carcinoma
D) Desmoplastic basal cell carcinoma
E) Milium cyst

QUESTION 9-2.

A 76-year-old patient presents with a painless, firm, slightly pedunculated flesh-colored to slightly pigmented nodule on the sole of the foot measuring 1 cm. The lesion is well demarcated with a peripheral "moat-like" change. A biopsy is performed and the findings are illustrated below. Which of the following diagnoses is CORRECT?

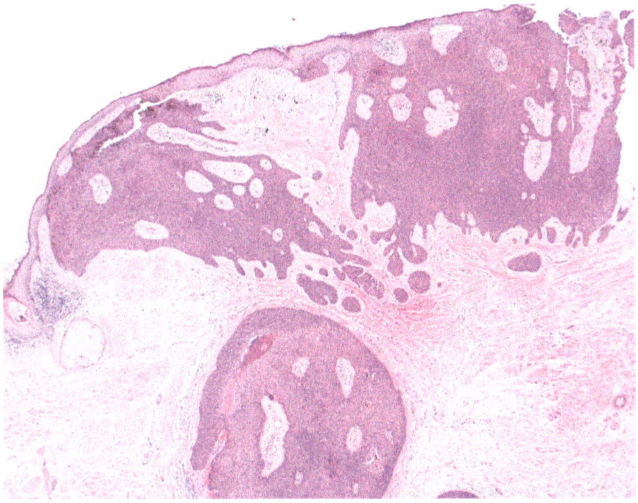

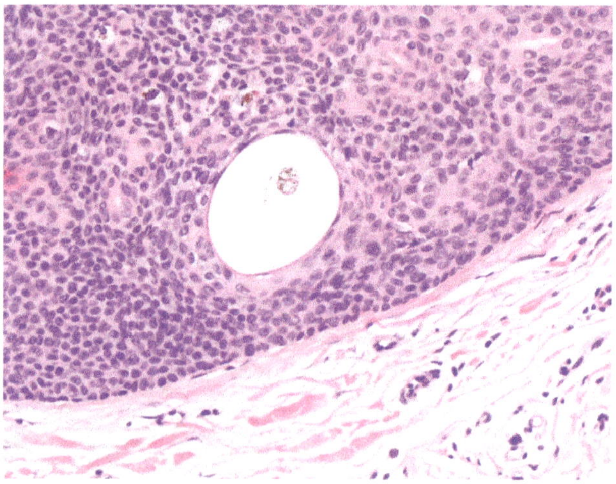

A) Eccrine poroma
B) Invasive squamous cell carcinoma
C) Basal cell carcinoma
D) Tumor of the follicular infundibulum
E) Trichilemmoma

QUESTION 9-3.

A patient presents with two eroded hyperkeratotic nodular plaques on the left upper extremity measuring approximately 3 cm in diameter. The patient has thickened palms and soles, sparse hair, multiple eyelid cysts and is missing some teeth. A biopsy is performed and the findings are illustrated below. The thin anastomosing strands of epithelium contain lumina lined by eosinophilic cuticles. Which of the following diagnoses is CORRECT?

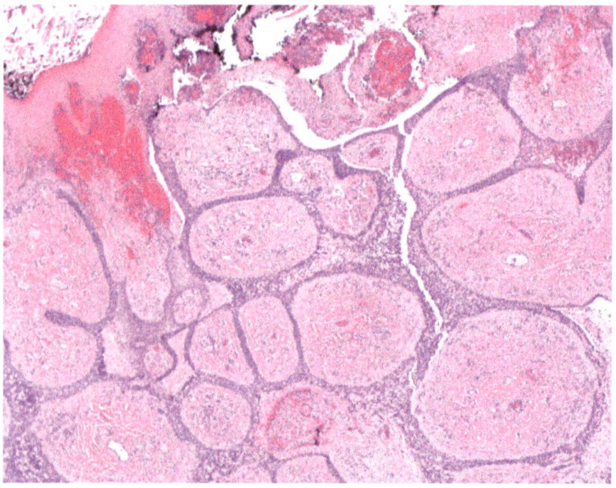

A) Fibroepithelioma of Pinkus
B) Eccrine syringofibroadenoma
C) Reticulated seborrheic keratosis
D) Pseudoepitheliomatous hyperplasia
E) None of the above

QUESTION 9-4.

A 55-year-old male patient presents with numerous dome-shaped smooth nodules on the scalp of varying sizes. There are also tumors on the face and upper body. His mother as well as two of his children also have similar lesions. Which of the following statements regarding this patient's tumor is INCORRECT?

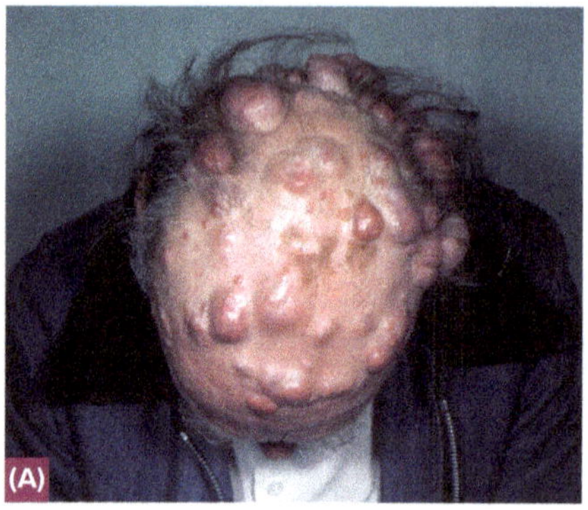

(A)

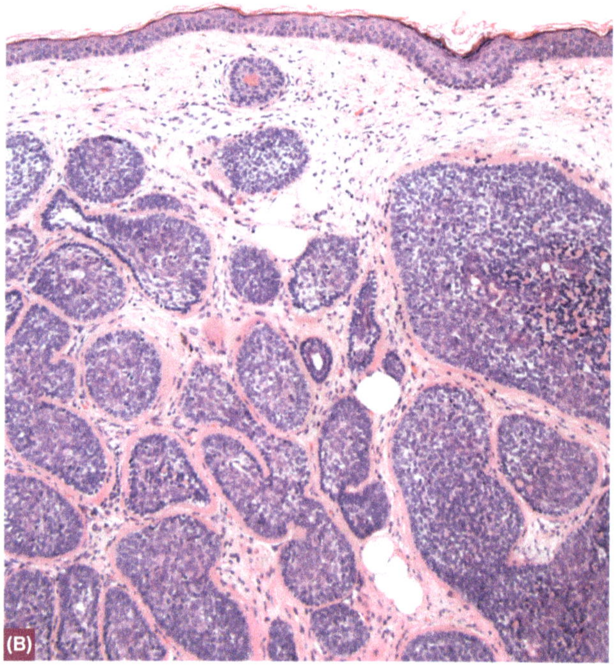

(B)

A) This is an autosomal dominant syndrome in which patients may also develop multiple trichoepitheliomas and eccrine spiradenomas.
B) The presence of small, detached tumor islands in the subcutis represents malignant transformation.
C) A PAS stain with diastase digestion will highlight an eosinophilic hyaline sheath encasing the tumor lobules as well as globules dispersed within the tumor.
D) This familial tumor syndrome is associated with *CYLD1* mutations.
E) The tumors always lack a connection with the overlying epidermis.

QUESTION 9-5.

A 16-year-old patient presents with a 1-cm painful solitary intradermal nodule on the arm. The lesion is excised and the findings are illustrated below. Immunohistochemical stains reveal CK7+ and CD45+ cells within the tumor mass. Which of the following diagnoses is CORRECT?

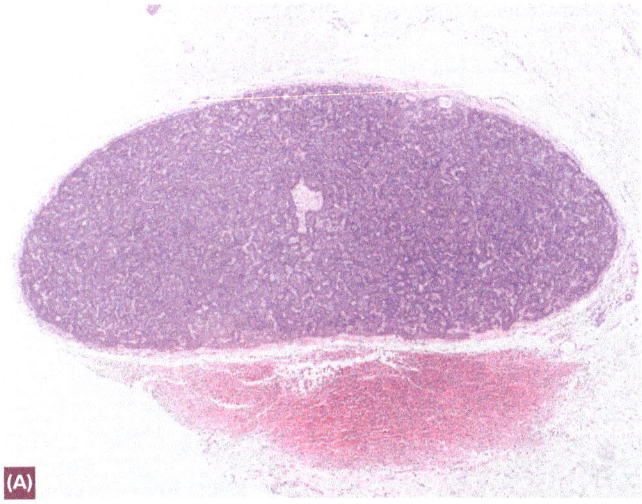

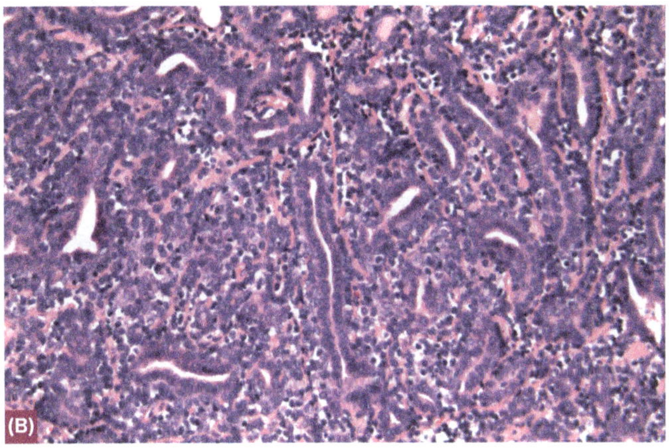

A) Cylindroma
B) Glomus cell tumor
C) Spiradenoma
D) Basal cell carcinoma
E) Merkel cell carcinoma

QUESTION 9-6.

A patient presents with a 1-cm cutaneous nodule. A biopsy is performed and the findings are illustrated below. Which of the following diagnoses is CORRECT?

A) Chondroid syringoma
B) Squamous cell carcinoma
C) Basal cell carcinoma
D) Nodular hidradenoma
E) Trichilemmoma

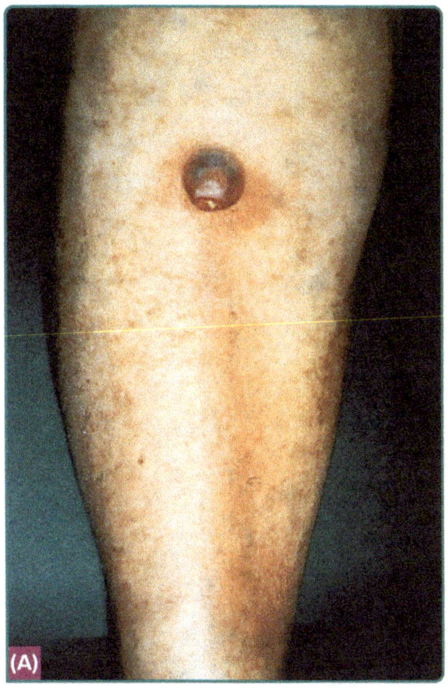

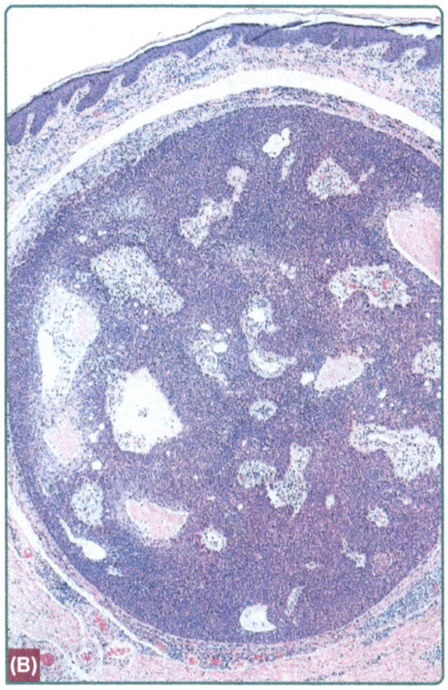

Reproduced, with permission, from Goldsmith LA, Katz SI, Gilchrest BA, Paller AS, Leffell DJ, Wolff K, eds. *Fitzpatrick's Dermatology in General Medicine*. 8th ed. New York, NY: McGraw-Hill Education; 2012.

QUESTION 9-7.

A 16-year-old male presents with an enlarging linear crusted plaque on the forehead that contains several small opening that drain clear malodorous fluid. He reports that the lesion has been present for many years and has recently begun to slowly enlarge. There is no pain or pruritus. A biopsy is performed and the findings are illustrated below. Which of the following statements regarding this entity is INCORRECT?

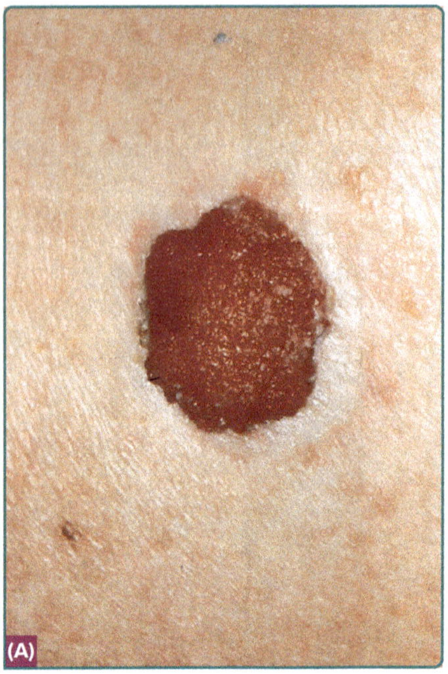

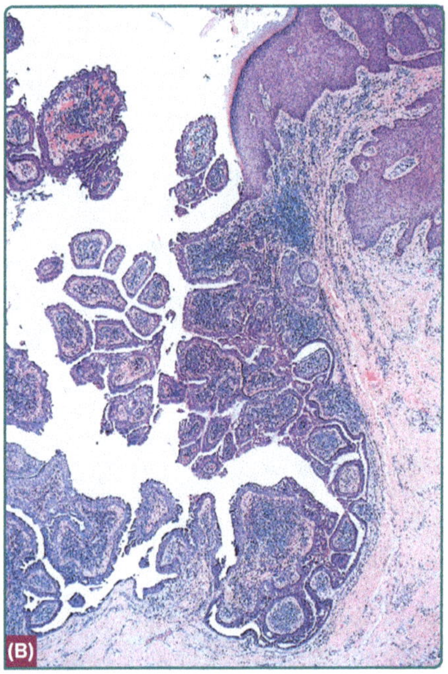

Reproduced, with permission, from Goldsmith LA, Katz SI, Gilchrest BA, Paller AS, Leffell DJ, Wolff K, eds. *Fitzpatrick's Dermatology in General Medicine*. 8th ed. New York, NY: McGraw-Hill Education; 2012.

A) These tumors may arise in conjunction with a wide variety of other adnexal tumors including nevus sebaceous, apocrine nevus, tubular apocrine adenoma, apocrine hidrocystoma, clear cell syringoma, eccrine nevus, verrucous carcinoma, and apocrine or eccrine adenocarcinoma.
B) Plasma cell infiltrates within the stroma of the papillary structures are a highly diagnostic feature of this lesion.
C) Some studies have shown that mutations in tumor suppressors PTCH and p16 may play a role in the evolution of these tumors.
D) These lesions may demonstrate both apocrine and eccrine differentiation.
E) The fact that the lesion has been increasing in size suggests malignant degeneration, which is a common occurrence in these tumors.

QUESTION 9-8.

A female patient presents with a 1-cm pedunculated nodule on the scalp that has been present for many years. The lesion is biopsied and the high magnification findings are illustrated below. At low magnification the tubules are closely arranged into a well-circumscribed nodule within the dermis. Which of the following diagnoses is CORRECT?

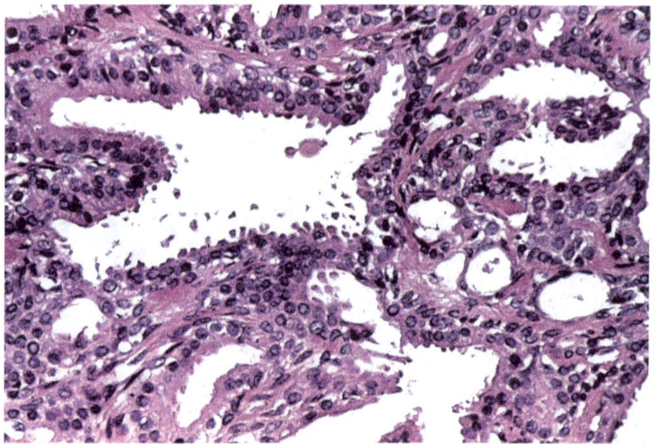

A) Ductopapillary apocrine adenocarcinoma
B) Tubular apocrine adenoma
C) Syringocystadenoma papilliferum
D) Hidradenoma papilliferum
E) Papillary eccrine adenoma

QUESTION 9-9.

A 35-year-old female presents with a small, unilateral, asymptomatic, flesh-colored nodule on the labia majora. The lesion is biopsied and the findings are illustrated below. Which of the following diagnoses is CORRECT?

A) Syringocystadenoma papilliferum
B) Hidradenoma papilliferum
C) Tubular apocrine adenoma
D) Metastatic colorectal adenocarcinoma
E) None of the above

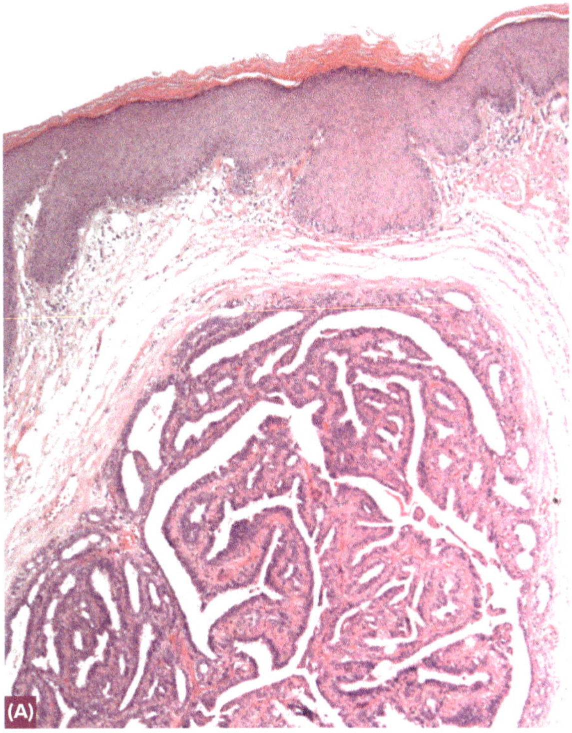

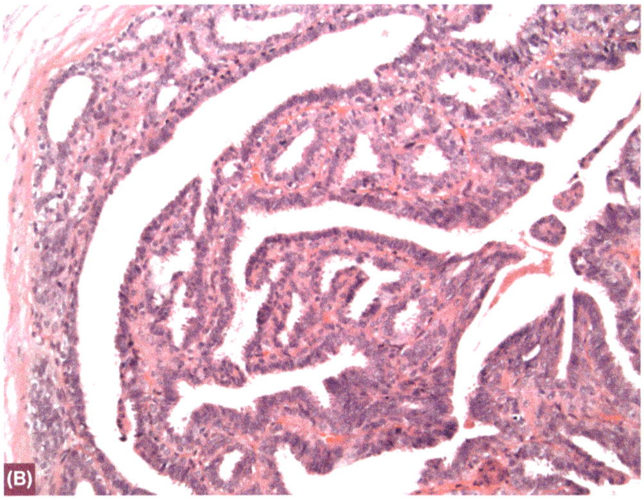

QUESTION 9-10.

A 45-year-old patient presents with a 1-cm firm nodule on the nose. The lesion is biopsied and the findings are illustrated below. Which of the following statements regarding this tumor is INCORRECT?

A) This is an example of carcinosarcoma, in which the tumor stem cells undergo divergent differentiation at a morphological level into dissimilar malignant tissue types.

B) Immunohistochemical staining characteristically reveals the epithelial cells to express androgen receptor (AR), EMA, GCFP-15, CK7, and CD117.

C) Partial sampling of these tumors may be misdiagnosed as osteoma cutis or lipoma.

D) Reassuring features of benignity include well-circumscribed tumor growth combined with the absence of nuclear pleomorphism, mitoses, and necrosis.

E) Although of apocrine differentiation, the basolateral tumor cells express p63 via immunohistochemistry, distinguishing it from metastatic mammary adenocarcinoma.

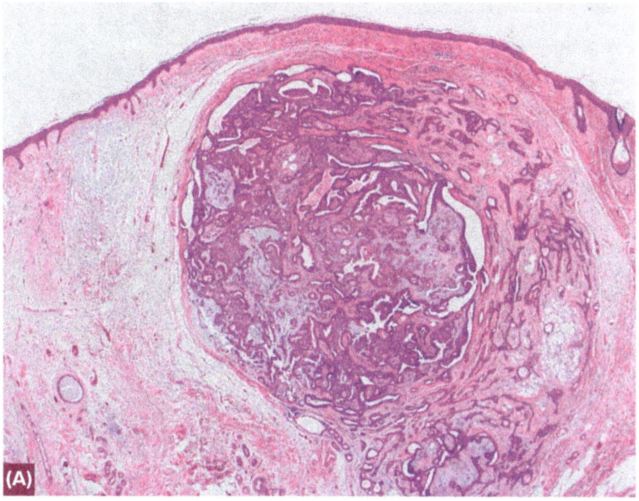

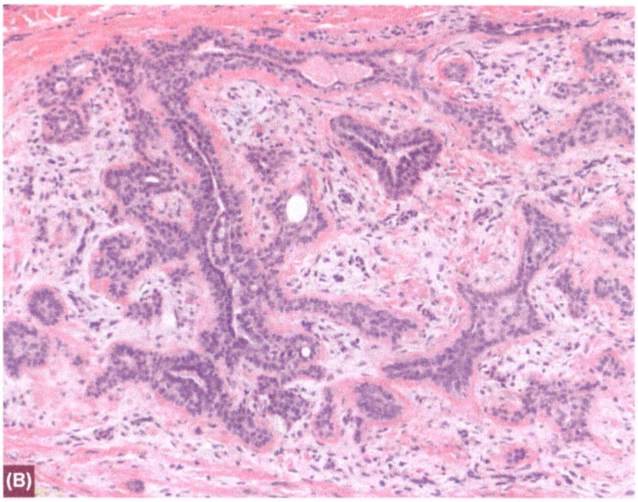

QUESTION 9-11.

A patient presents with a 7-mm papule on the face with a blue hue. The lesion is biopsied and the findings are illustrated below. Which of the following statements regarding this lesion is INCORRECT?

A) When similar lesions occur on the penis they are referred to as median raphe cysts.

B) Immunohistochemistry will reveal the epithelial cells to express GCFP-15.

C) These lesions are considered to be cystic adenomas and not retention cysts.
D) These lesions most frequently present as multiloculated cysts lined by one or two cell layers without papillary structures.
E) Eyelid lesions may arise within the Moll glands.

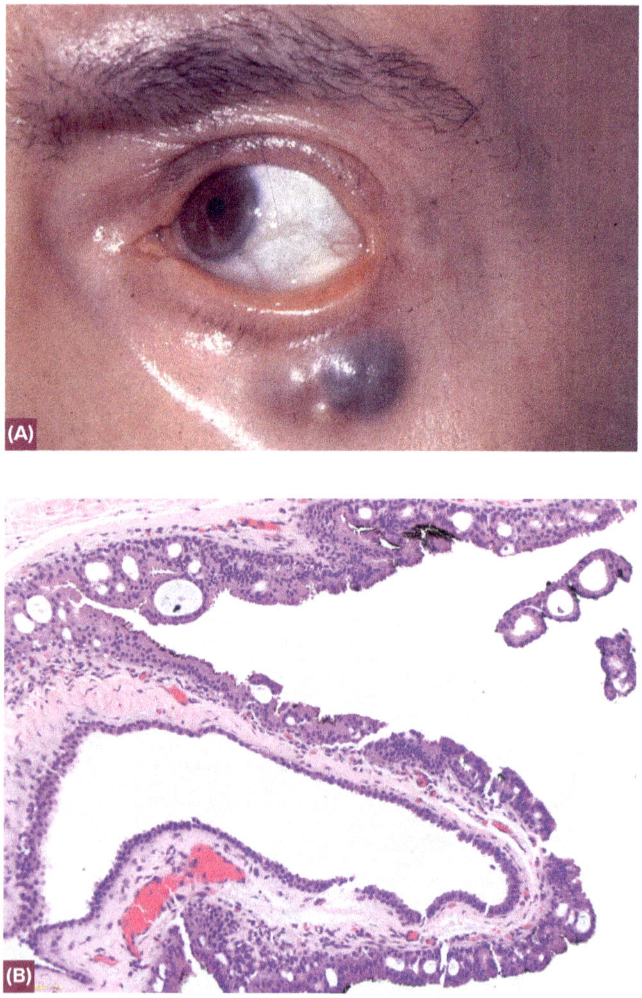

Reproduced with permission from Desman GT, Ozerdem U, Shin SJ: Neighboring look-a-likes: distinguishing between breast and dermatologic lesions, Adv Anat Pathol 2014 Jul;21(4):228-247

QUESTION 9-12.

A 39-year-old female presents with a nodular thickening of the nipple with serous discharge. She reports that the lesion was initially red and swollen and eventually eroded. A biopsy is performed and the findings are illustrated below. Which of the following diagnoses is CORRECT?

A) Tubular carcinoma of the breast
B) Paget disease
C) Erosive adenomatosis of the nipple
D) Hidradenoma papilliferum
E) Microcystic adnexal carcinoma

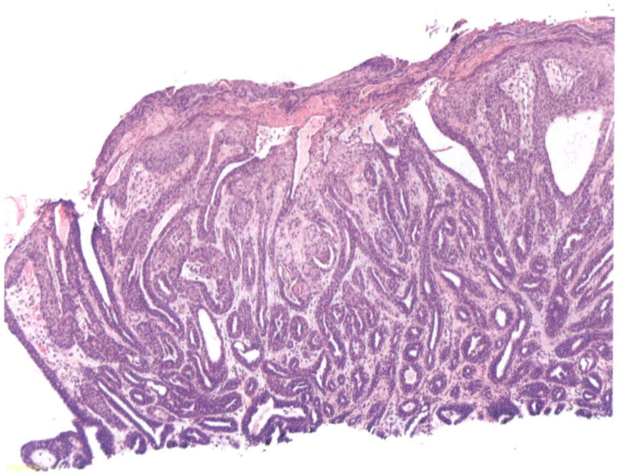

QUESTION 9-13.

Malignant eccrine and apocrine neoplasms may arise de novo or through transformation from benign tumor counterparts. Which of the following tumors arises de novo without an associated benign precursor?

A) Clear cell hidradenocarcinoma
B) Porocarcinoma
C) Carcinoma ex eccrine spiradenoma
D) Malignant mixed tumor
E) Microcystic adnexal carcinoma

QUESTION 9-14.

A 58-year-old female presents with a long-standing, slow-growing, crusted nodule on the scalp. A biopsy is performed and the findings are illustrated below. Which of the following statements regarding this tumor is INCORRECT?

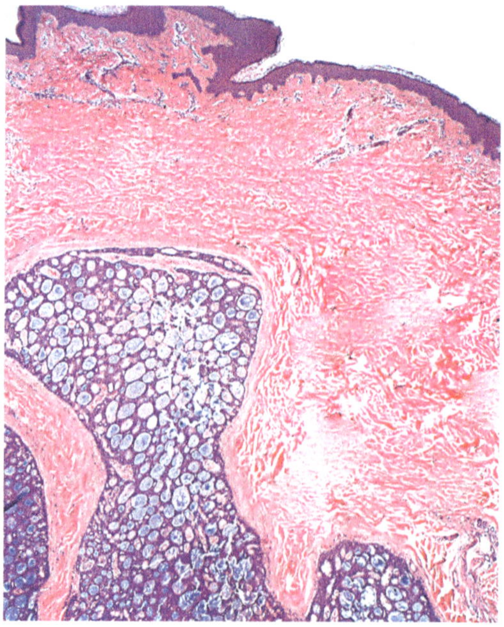

A) These tumors are strongly associated with mutations in the PTCH tumor suppressor gene.
B) Tumors with identical histomorphology most commonly arise in the salivary glands, respiratory tract, or breast.
C) Immunohistochemistry reveals the tumor cells to express cytokeratin and CD117 with variable luminal staining for EMA, CEA, SMA, and S100.
D) These tumors have a high rate of local recurrence, but a low rate of distant metastasis.
E) Perineural invasion is a very common finding in these tumors.

QUESTION 9-15.

A 55-year-old Caucasian male presents with a solitary, 2-cm nodule localized to the volar skin between the nail bed and distal interphalangeal joint of the index finger. The lesion is biopsied and the findings are illustrated below. Which of the following statements regarding this tumor is INCORRECT?

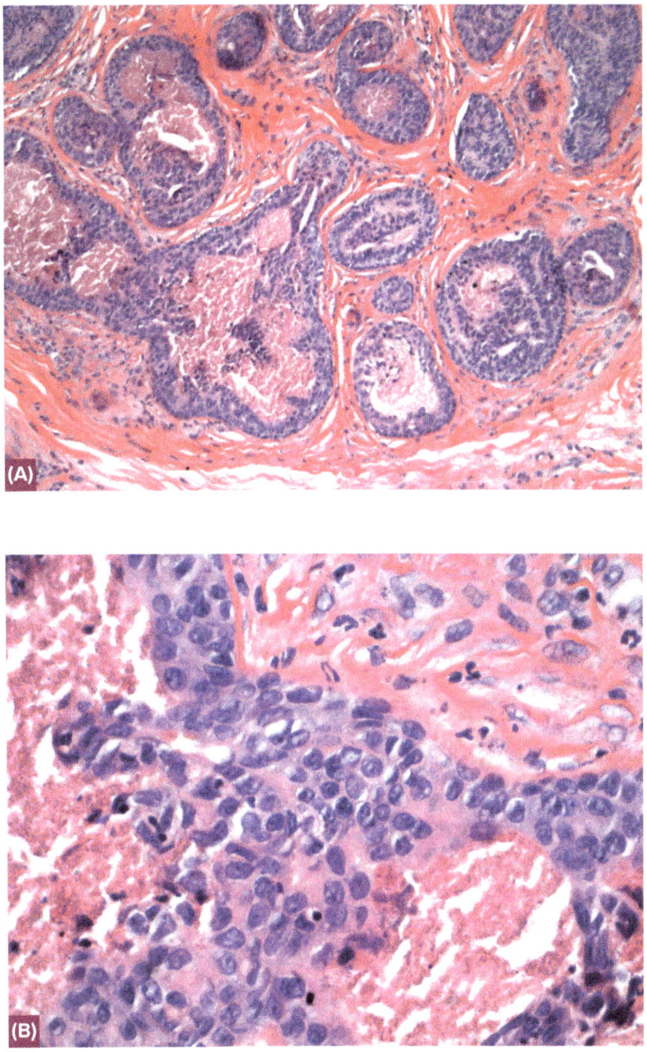

A) This is an aggressive neoplasm with a local recurrence rate of 50% and a distant metastasis rate of 15%.
B) Digital amputation may be necessary for the management of this neoplasm.
C) These tumors occasionally communicate with the overlying epidermis and may be predominantly solid.
D) Immunohistochemistry will reveal the tumor cells to express keratin, S-100, and CEA.
E) These tumors frequently arise in association with preexisting benign adenomas.

QUESTION 9-16.

A middle-aged female presents with a solitary, slowly growing mass measuring 5 cm in diameter on the scalp that has been present for many months. The lesion is biopsied and the findings are illustrated below. By immunohistochemistry, the tumor cells are positive for cytokeratin, EMA, CEA, ER, PR, c-erbB-2, p63, and S-100. Which of the following diagnoses is CORRECT?

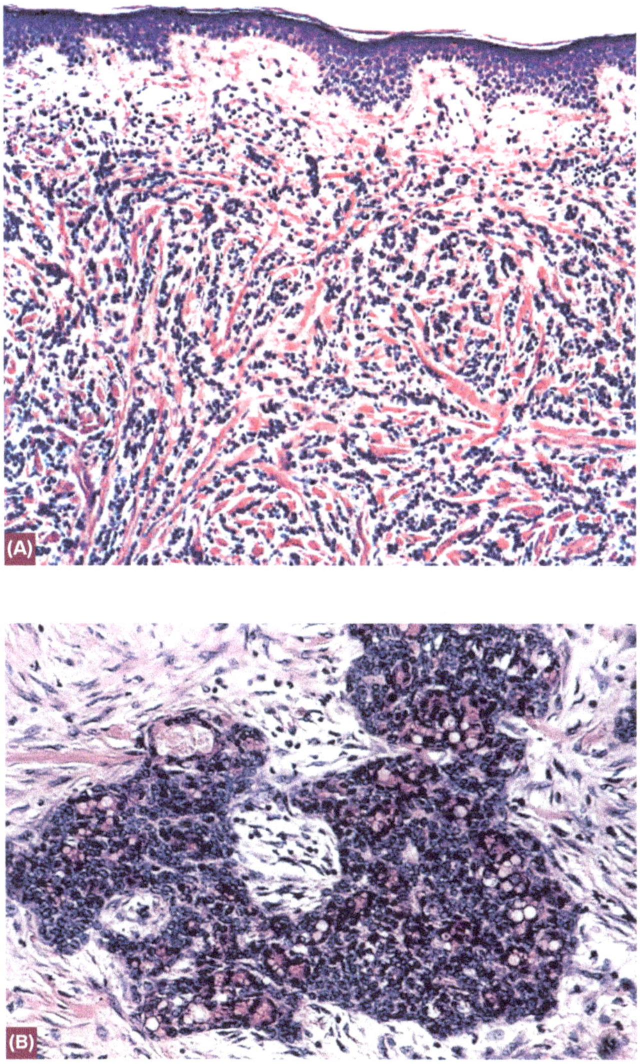

A) Desmoplastic basal cell carcinoma
B) Poorly differentiated squamous cell carcinoma
C) Ductal eccrine adenocarcinoma
D) Metastatic mammary carcinoma
E) Carcinoma ex spiradenoma

QUESTION 9-17.

A 73-year-old patient presents with an ulcerated verrucous plaque on the lower extremity. The lesion has been present for many years but has recently enlarged and become painful. A biopsy is performed and the findings are illustrated below. Which of the following diagnoses is CORRECT?

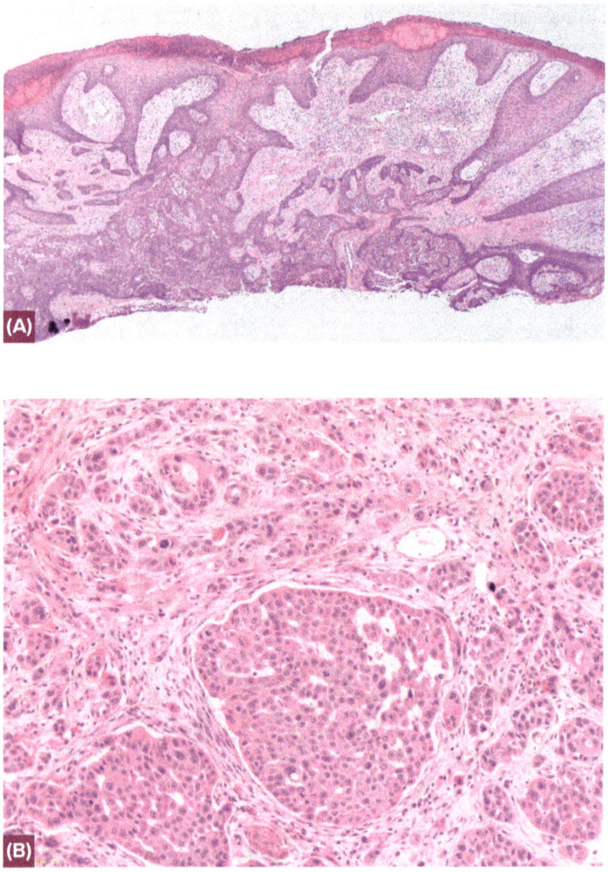

A) Invasive squamous cell carcinoma
B) Hidroacanthoma simplex
C) Hidradenocarcinoma
D) Eccrine porocarcinoma
E) Metastatic adenocarcinoma

QUESTION 9-18.

A 32-year-old female presents with a slow-growing, firm, indurated plaque with indistinct borders on the upper lip. A deep punch biopsy is performed and the findings are illustrated below. Immunohistochemical stains reveal the epithelial structures to stain for high-molecular-weight cytokeratin (K903) and the cystic structures stain for CEA. There is p63 expression of basolateral cells but not the luminal cells. There is no staining with BerEP4 or CK20. Which of the following diagnoses is CORRECT?

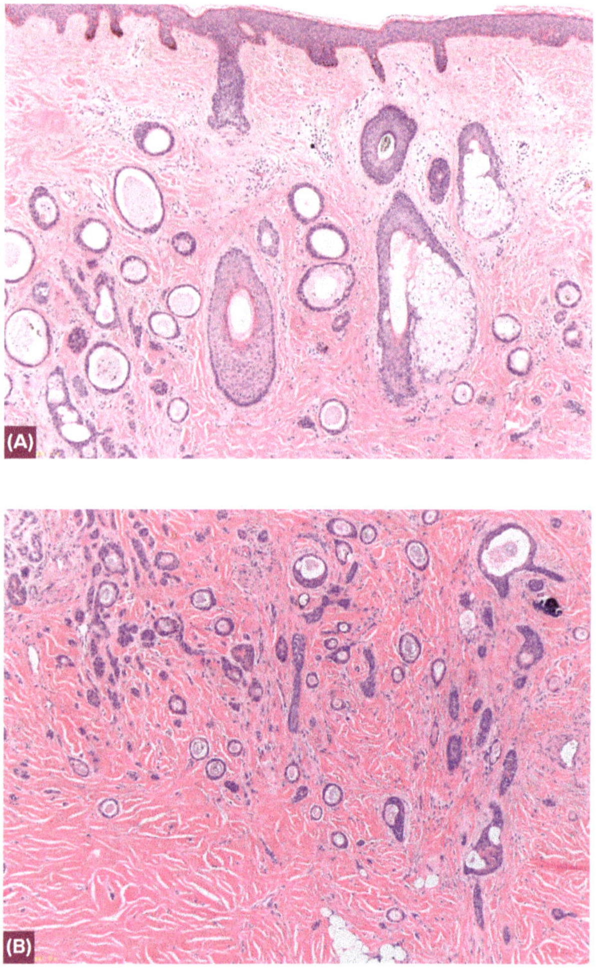

A) Microcystic adnexal carcinoma
B) Syringoma
C) Desmoplastic trichoepithelioma
D) Desmoplastic basal cell carcinoma
E) Primary cutaneous adenosquamous carcinoma

QUESTION 9-19.

Which of the following locations are apocrine adenocarcinomas LEAST likely to occur?

A) External meatus of the ear
B) Axilla
C) Anogenital region
D) Lower extremity
E) Face

QUESTION 9-20.

A 66-year-old African American patient presents with a 2-cm, slightly discolored, sponge-like nodule on the eyelid. The lesion is excised and the findings are illustrated below. Immunohistochemistry reveals the epithelial tumor cells to express CK7, p63, GCFP-15, ER, and PR. Which of the following statements regarding this tumor is INCORRECT?

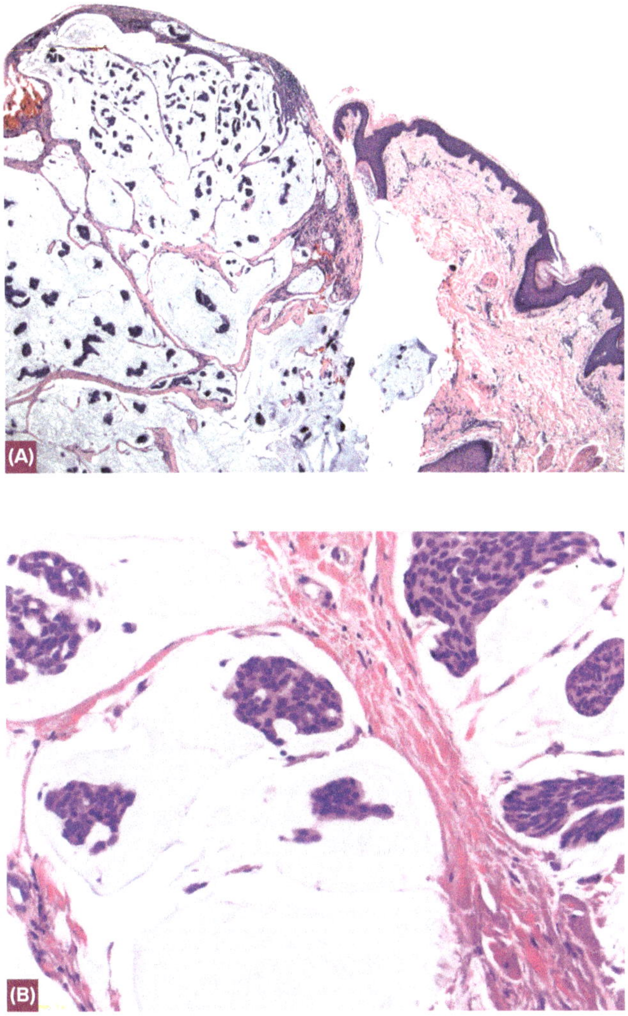

A) These tumors have a high rate of local recurrence, but low rate of lymph node and distant metastasis.
B) These primary cutaneous tumors arise de novo without an associated benign counterpart.
C) Mucicarmine, PAS with diastase (dPAS), colloidal iron, and Alcian blue stains will highlight the pools of positively staining material in this tumor.
D) This tumor most likely represents a cutaneous metastasis from gastrointestinal, breast, or ovarian origin.
E) Occasionally the epithelial cells of this tumor may exhibit neuroendocrine differentiation with synaptophysin and chromogranin expression.

QUESTION 9-21.

A 70-year-old male presents with a moist, well-demarcated, eroded, oozing plaque on the scrotum. A biopsy is performed and the findings are illustrated below. Immunohistochemical stains reveal the tumor cells to be positive for GCDFP-15 and CK7, and negative for CK20 and S100. Which of the following statements regarding this condition is CORRECT?

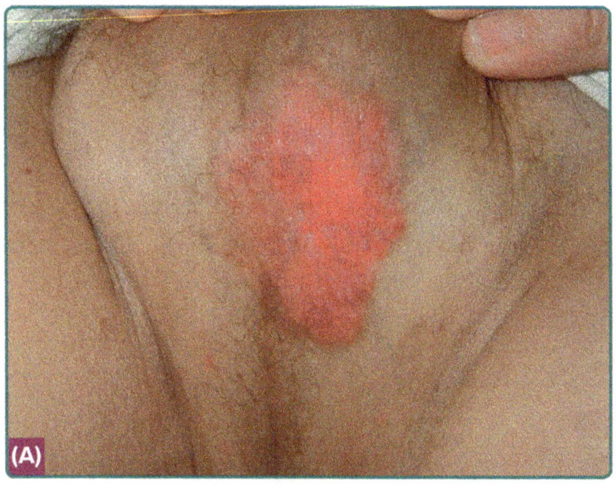

Reproduced, with permission, from Goldsmith LA, Katz SI, Gilchrest BA, Paller AS, Leffell DJ, Wolff K, eds. *Fitzpatrick's Dermatology in General Medicine*. 8th ed. New York, NY: McGraw-Hill Education; 2012.

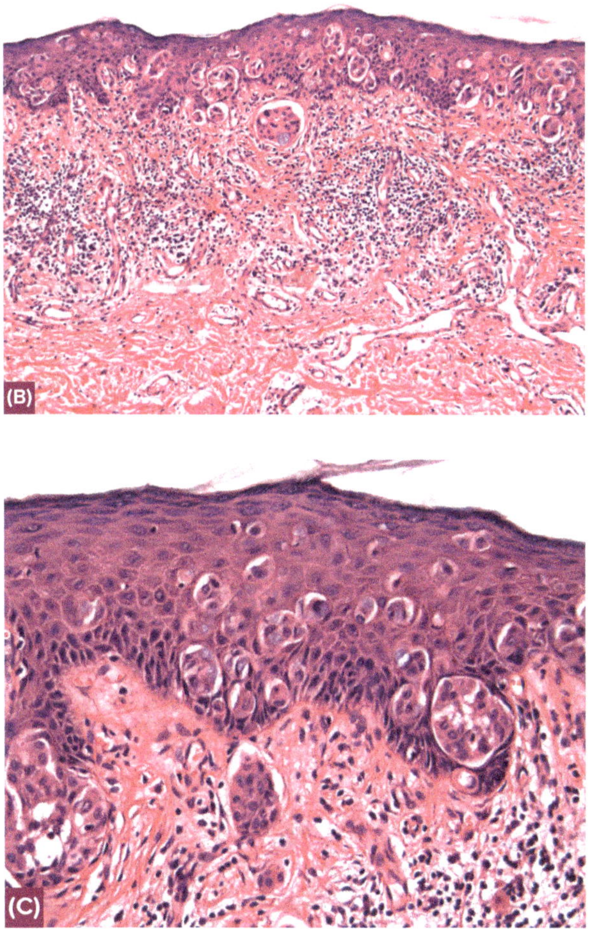

A) A mucicarmine stain will be positive for mucin within the tumor cells.
B) This lesion is always associated with an underlying visceral malignancy.
C) This is an example of an epidermotropic metastasis of urothelial carcinoma.
D) The scattered tumor cells throughout the epidermis are malignant melanocytes.
E) The tumor cells scattered throughout the epidermis are consistently positive for CEA.

QUESTION 9-22.

A 76-year-old patient presents with a localized eruption of yellowish-tan umbilicated papules on the forehead. One of the lesions is biopsied and the findings are illustrated below. Which of the following diagnoses is CORRECT?

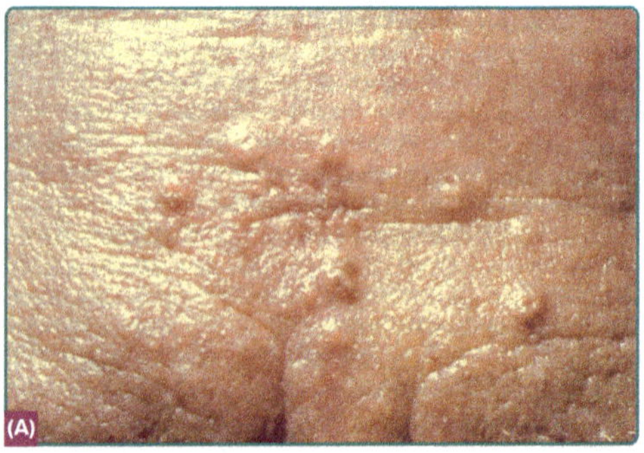

(A)

Reproduced, with permission, from Goldsmith LA, Katz SI, Gilchrest BA, Paller AS, Leffell DJ, Wolff K, eds. *Fitzpatrick's Dermatology in General Medicine*. 8th ed. New York, NY: McGraw-Hill Education; 2012.

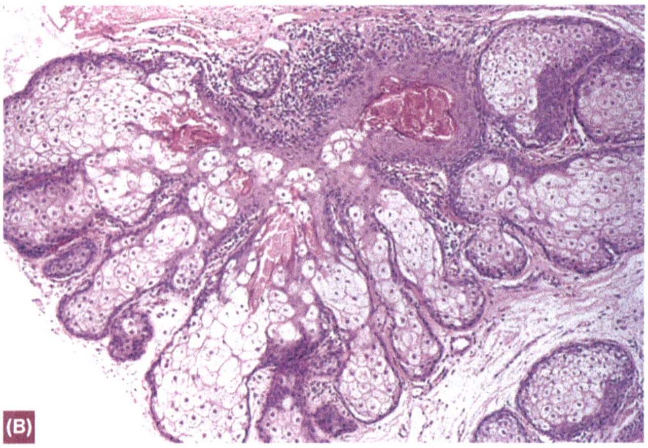

(B)

A) Sebaceous adenoma
B) Sebaceous hyperplasia
C) Basal cell carcinoma with sebaceous differentiation
D) Nevus sebaceus of Jadassohn
E) Montgomery tubercle

QUESTION 9-23.

An elderly female patient presents with a solitary, pale-yellow, nodular facial papule that is slowly enlarging. The lesion is biopsied and the findings are illustrated below. Immunohistochemical stains for MLH1, MSH2, MLH6, and PMS2 reveal absent nuclear staining for MSH2. Which of the following diagnoses is CORRECT?

A) Sebaceous adenoma
B) Sebaceous hyperplasia
C) Sebaceoma
D) Sebaceous carcinoma
E) Basal cell carcinoma with sebaceous differentiation

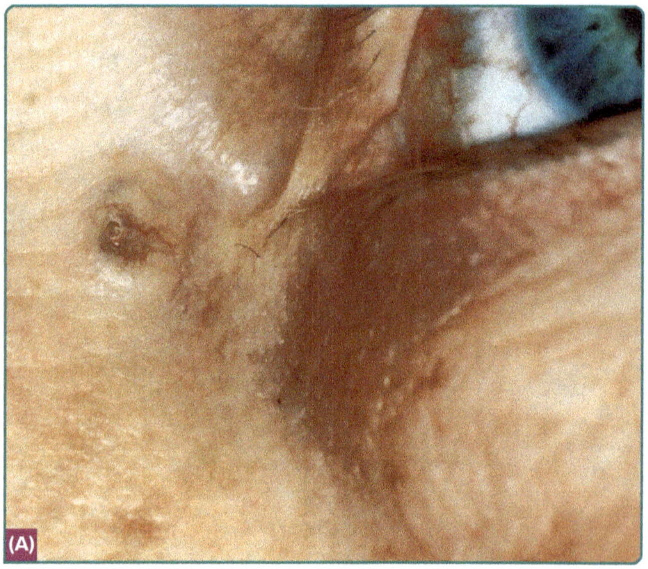

(A)

Reproduced, with permission, from Goldsmith LA, Katz SI, Gilchrest BA, Paller AS, Leffell DJ, Wolff K, eds. *Fitzpatrick's Dermatology in General Medicine*. 8th ed. New York, NY: McGraw-Hill Education; 2012.

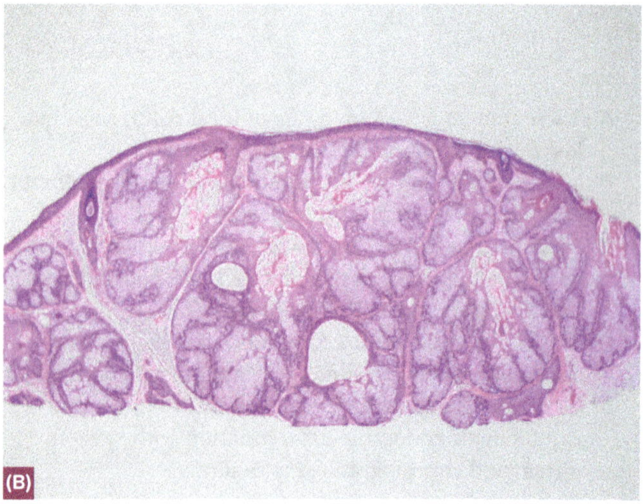

(B)

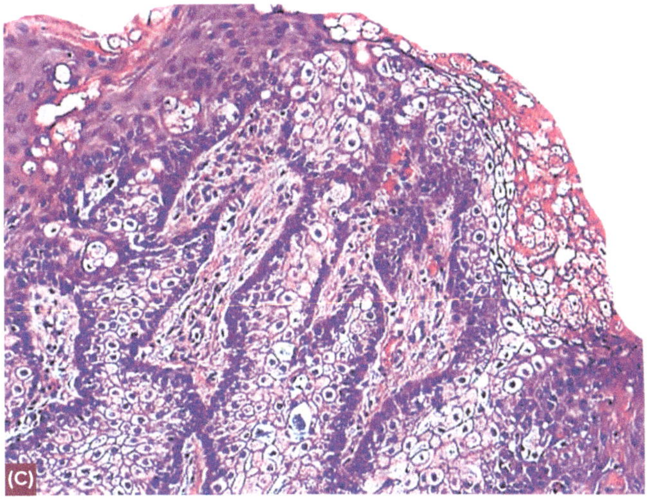

(C)

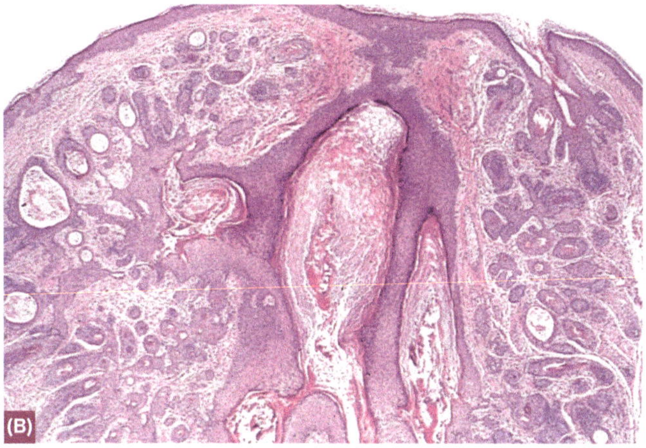

(B)

QUESTION 9-24.

A 45-year-old patient presents with a solitary, small, skin-colored, dome-shaped papule on the face. There is a central pore with an emerging tuft of small white hairs. The lesion is biopsied and the findings are illustrated below. Which of the following diagnoses is CORRECT?

A) Trichofolliculoma
B) Dilated Pore of Winer
C) Pilar sheath acanthoma
D) Keratoacanthoma
E) Trichoadenoma

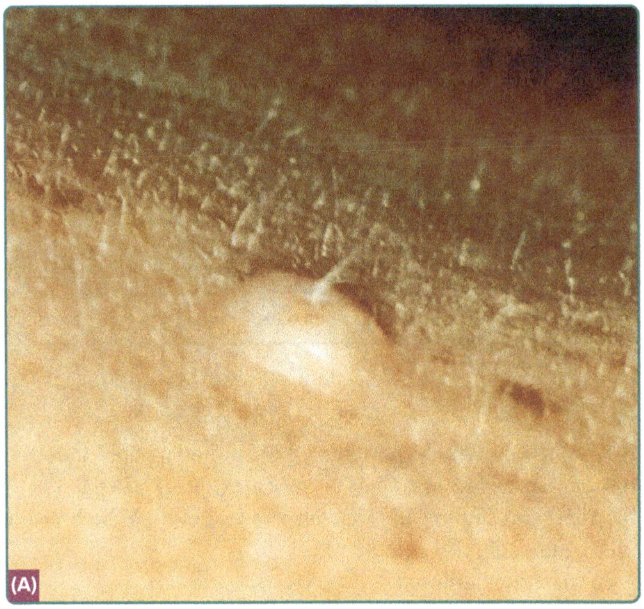

(A)

Reproduced, with permission, from Goldsmith LA, Katz SI, Gilchrest BA, Paller AS, Leffell DJ, Wolff K, eds. *Fitzpatrick's Dermatology in General Medicine*. 8th ed. New York, NY: McGraw-Hill Education; 2012.

QUESTION 9-25.

A 35-year-old male presents with multiple rounded, skin-colored, firm, 4-mm papules on the nasolabial folds. One of the papules is biopsied and is illustrated below. Which of the following statements regarding these tumors is INCORRECT?

A) Multiple lesions are frequently associated with an autosomal dominant inheritance pattern, in which these tumors may arise in association with numerous syringomas.
B) Solitary lesions are much more frequent than multiple lesions.
C) A giant solitary variant of this lesion occurs later in life and arises most commonly on the thigh and perianal regions.
D) These lesions rarely exhibit aggressive biological behavior.
E) Occasionally, rupture may result in giant-cell reaction and dystrophic calcification.

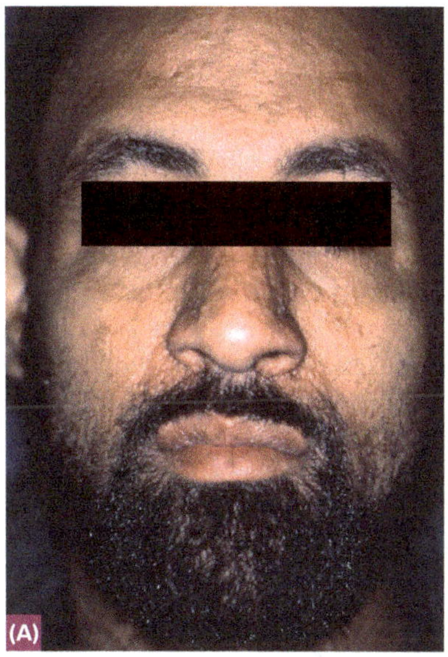

(A)

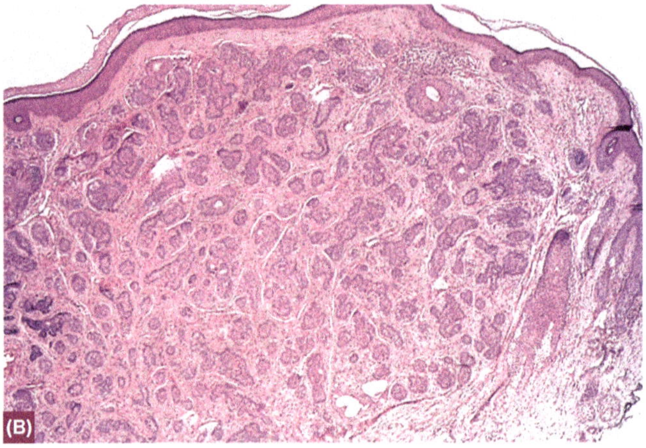

(B)

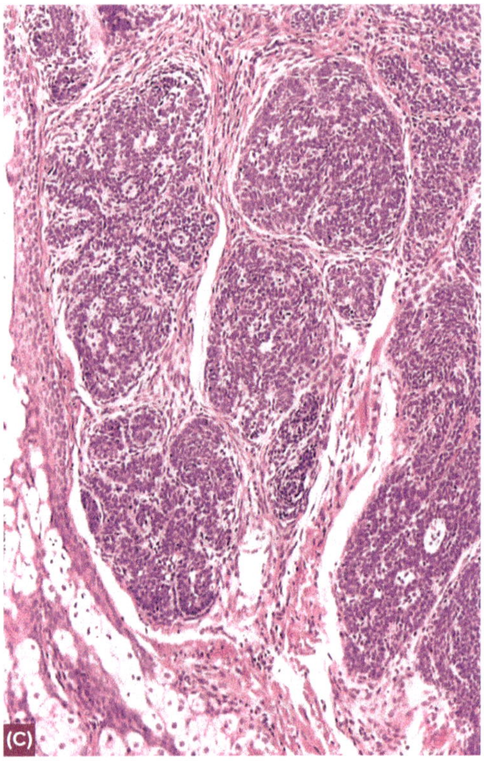

(C)

QUESTION 9-26.

A 62-year-old Asian patient presents with a nontender mass on the eyelid. Several prior biopsies produced diagnoses of chalazion; however, the mass is persistent and enlarging. An excisional biopsy is performed and the findings are illustrated below. Which of the following statements regarding this tumor is INCORRECT?

- **A)** This malignant tumor is always associated with microsatellite instability and Muir-Torre syndrome.
- **B)** These tumors are associated with an approximate risk of 30% to 40% for local tumor recurrence, 25% to 35% for distant metastases, and 10% to 20% for tumor-related death.
- **C)** These tumors are positive for both EMA and BerEP4 via immunohistochemistry in the majority of cases.
- **D)** These tumors commonly exhibit intraepidermal colonization, mimicking extramammary Paget disease or superficial spreading melanoma.
- **E)** These tumors are frequently immunoreactive for c-*erb*B-2 oncoprotein.

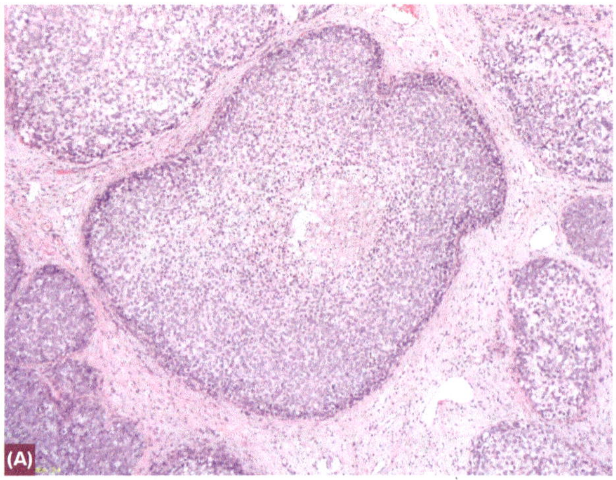

(A)

Reproduced with permission from Desman GT, Ozerdem U, Shin SJ: Neighboring look-a-likes: distinguishing between breast and dermatologic lesions, Adv Anat Pathol 2014 Jul;21(4):228-247

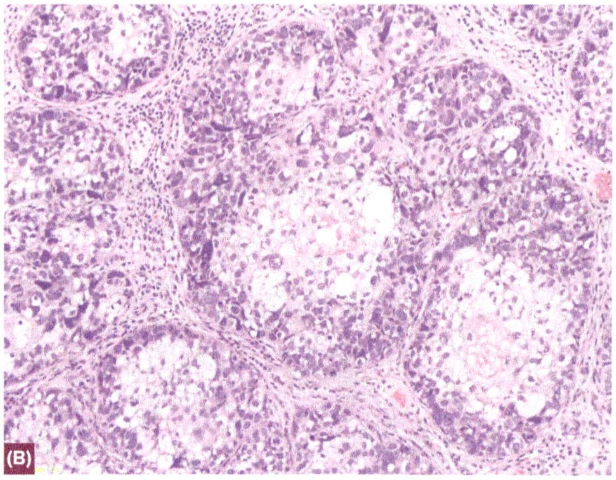

(B)

QUESTION 9-27.

A 45-year-old female presents with a solitary papulonodular tumor measuring less than 1 cm on the neck. The lesion is biopsied and the findings are illustrated below. Which of the following diagnoses is CORRECT?

- **A)** Trichofolliculoma
- **B)** Tumor of the follicular infundibulum
- **C)** Basal cell carcinoma, superficial growth pattern
- **D)** Trichilemmoma
- **E)** Reticulated seborrheic keratosis

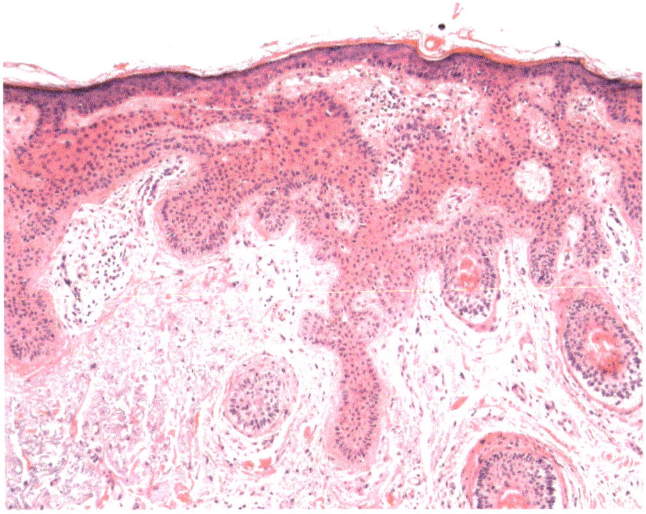

QUESTION 9-28.

A patient presents with multiple 3-mm nodules on the face. Additionally, there are numerous translucent punctate keratoses of the palms and soles, and hyperkeratotic, flat-topped papules on the dorsa of the hands and forearms. The oral mucous membranes are covered by numerous coalescent papules, resulting in a "cobblestone" appearance. There is a strong family history of breast cancer and visceral hamartomas. One of the lesions is biopsied and the findings are illustrated below. Which of the following diagnoses is CORRECT?

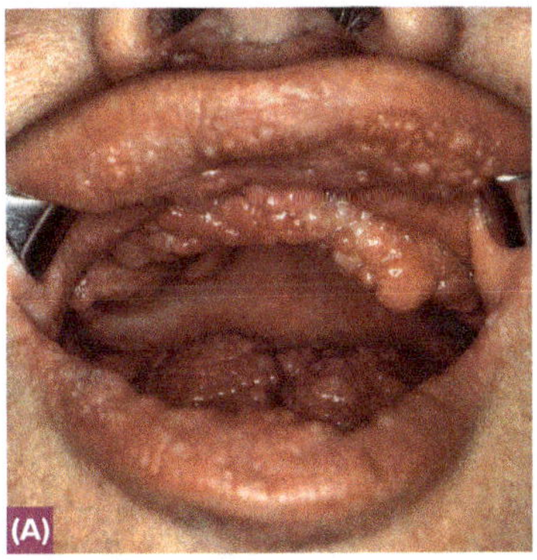

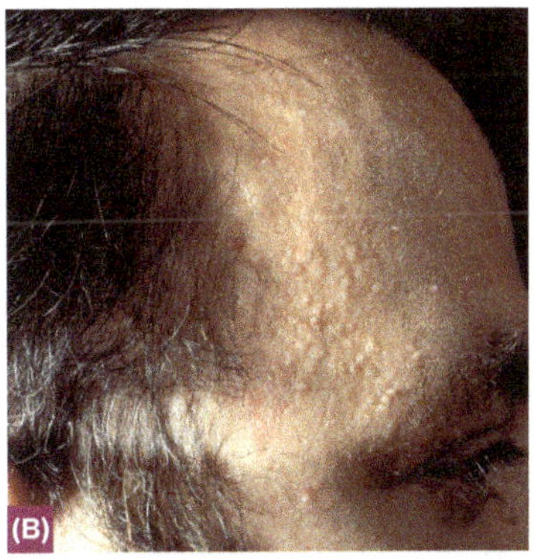

Reproduced with permission from Wolff K, Johnson RA, Saavedra AP. *Fitzpatrick's Color Atlas and Synopsis of Clinical Dermatology*. 7th ed. New York, NY: McGraw-Hill Education; 2013.

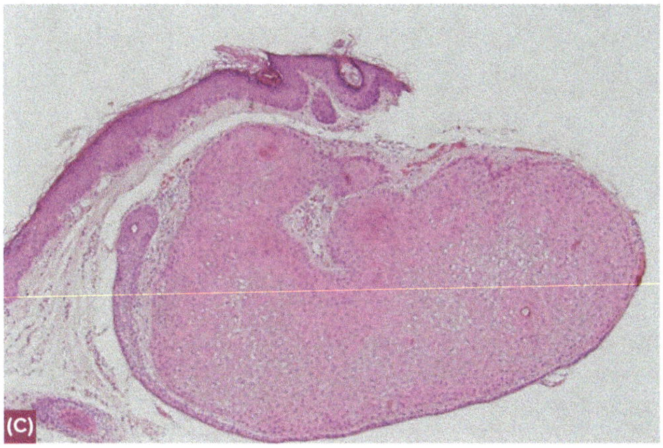

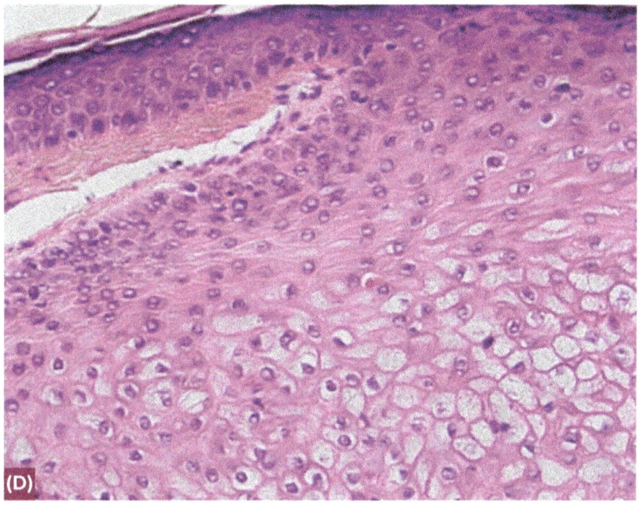

A) Verruca vulgaris
B) Basal cell carcinoma
C) Well-differentiated sebaceous carcinoma
D) Trichilemmoma
E) Squamous cell carcinoma

QUESTION 9-29.

A 34-year-old female presents with a 5-mm firm nodule with central induration in the malar region. The lesion is biopsied and the findings are illustrated below. Immunohistochemical staining for CK20 reveals rare scattered positive cells throughout the tumor. Which of the following diagnoses is CORRECT?

A) Microcystic adnexal carcinoma
B) Trichoepithelioma
C) Desmoplastic basal cell carcinoma
D) Desmoplastic trichoepithelioma
E) Syringoma

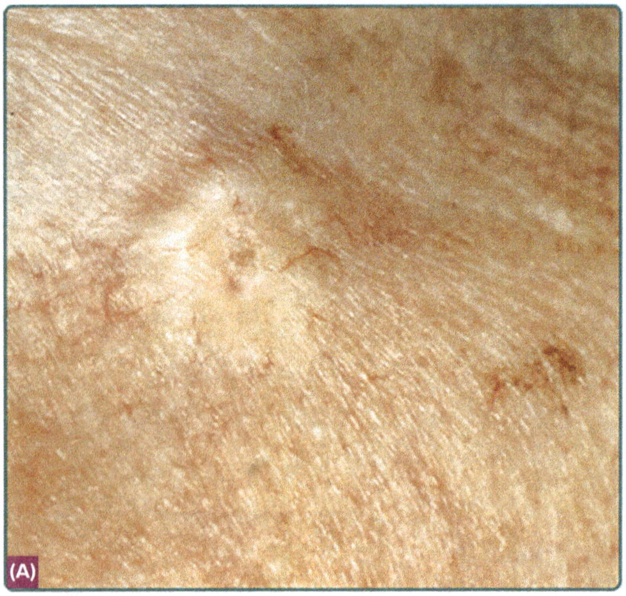

Reproduced, with permission, from Goldsmith LA, Katz SI, Gilchrest BA, Paller AS, Leffell DJ, Wolff K, eds. *Fitzpatrick's Dermatology in General Medicine*. 8th ed. New York, NY: McGraw-Hill Education; 2012.

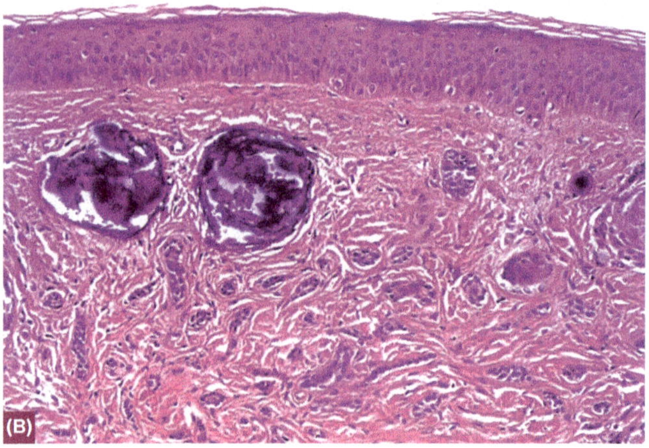

QUESTION 9-30.

A 17-year-old boy presents with a 5.5-cm firm deep-seated nodule on the right arm with slight reddish discoloration. He reports that the lesion had been present for over a year and measured approximately 2 cm, but began to rapidly grow over the past 6 weeks. The lesion is biopsied and the findings are illustrated below. Scattered mitoses are identified within the basophilic epithelium. Which of the following statements about this patient's tumor is INCORRECT?

A) This tumor is associated with frequent calcification, occasional stromal ossification, and foreign body giant cell reaction.

B) The recent increase in size, mitotic activity, and eosinophilic necrosis (illustrated in image C) indicates that this tumor is malignant.

C) The fact that this tumor is composed predominantly of eosinophilic keratinized cells over basaloid cells signifies that this tumor is long standing.

D) These tumors are associated with mutations in beta-catenin.

E) On rare occasion, these tumors may perforate through the dermis and epidermis.

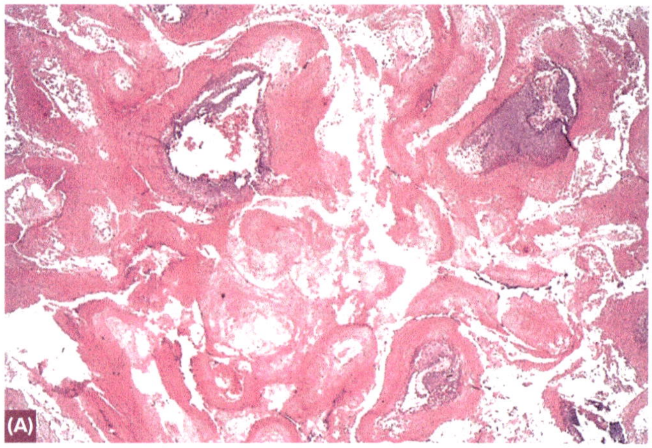

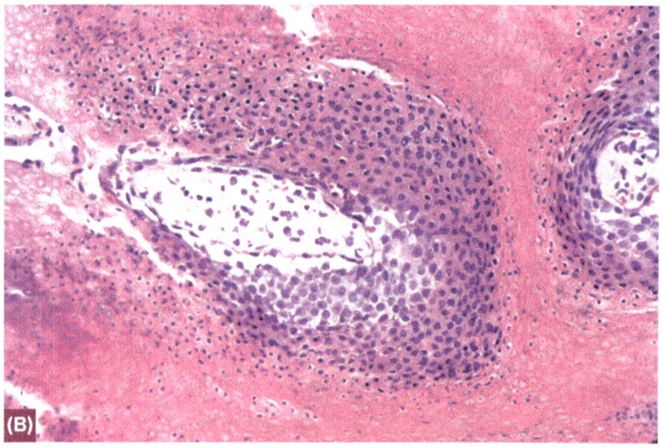

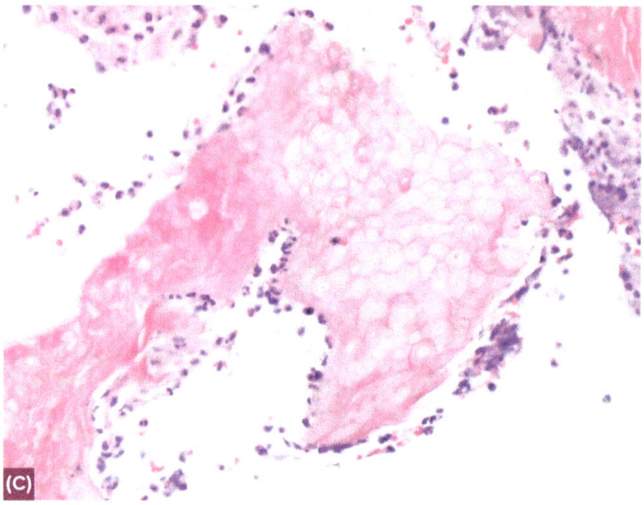

QUESTION 9-31.

An 80-year-old female presents with an enlarging lobulated mass on the scalp with focal ulceration. The lesion is biopsied to reveal a well-circumscribed cystic tumor. The findings are illustrated below. Which of the following statements regarding this lesion is CORRECT?

A) Nuclear atypia and focal keratinization of individual cells resulting in "squamous eddy" formation defines the lesion as an invasive squamous cell carcinoma.
B) These tumors most commonly arise on the scalp of elderly males.
C) This tumor is frequently associated with adjacent benign cysts of similar differentiation.
D) Multiple lesions on the face are associated with Cowden disease.
E) The pattern of growth, not the cytomorphology, defines the benignancy versus malignancy in these neoplasms.

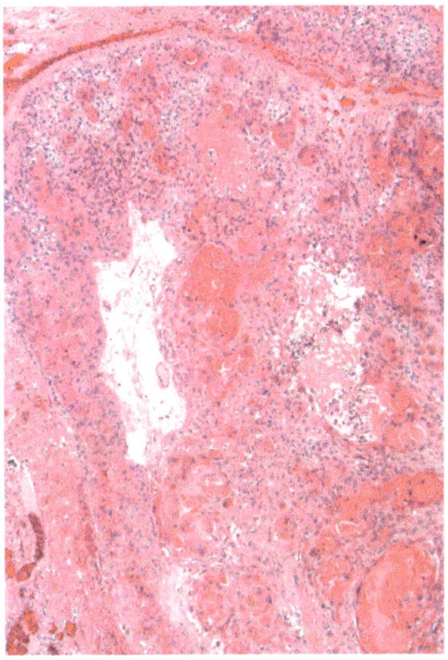

QUESTION 9-32.

An elderly patient presents with a pigmented nodule on the scalp with alopecia. The tumor has been slowly growing over a period of years and is not associated with pain. A biopsy is performed and the findings are illustrated below. Which of the following diagnoses is CORRECT?

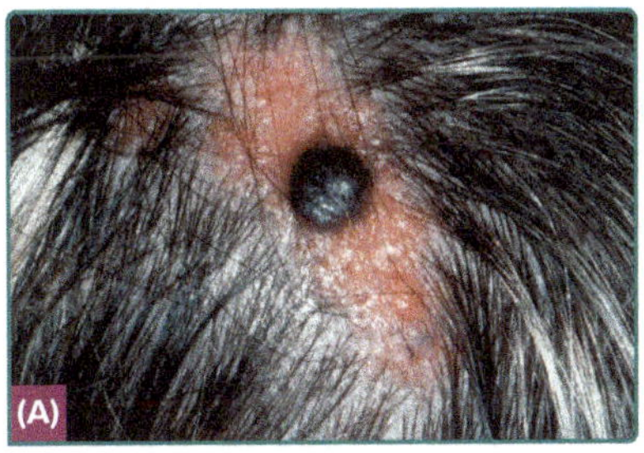

(A)

Reproduced, with permission, from Goldsmith LA, Katz SI, Gilchrest BA, Paller AS, Leffell DJ, Wolff K, eds. *Fitzpatrick's Dermatology in General Medicine.* 8th ed. New York, NY: McGraw-Hill Education; 2012.

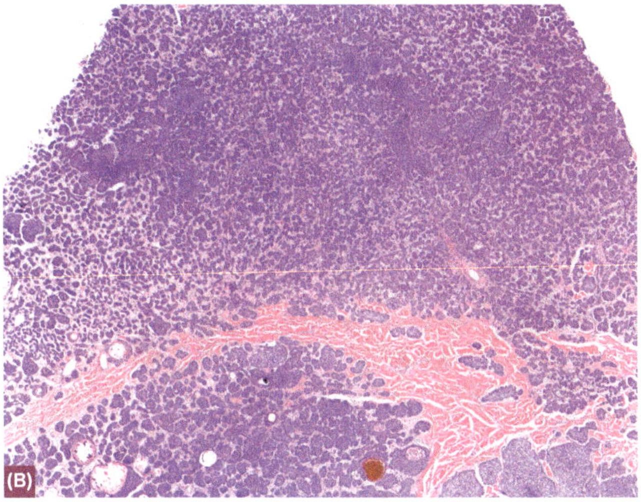

(B)

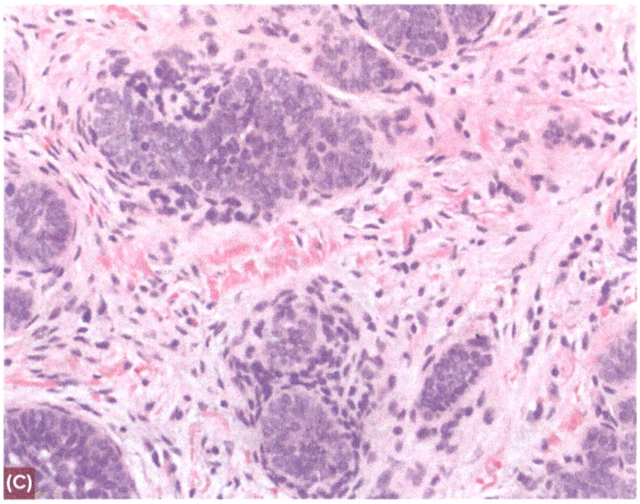

(C)

A) Basaloid follicular hamartoma
B) Basal cell carcinoma, micronodular pattern
C) Cutaneous lymphadenoma
D) Trichoblastoma
E) Malignant proliferating pilar tumor

QUESTION 9-33.

A 27-year-old patient presents with numerous small grouped papules on the head and neck. The papules appear to be folliculocentric. Additionally, there are numerous skin tags at flexural sites. There is a family history of similar cutaneous lesions as well as pneumothorax and "kidney tumors" in both the father and an older sibling. A biopsy of one of the papules is performed and the findings are illustrated below. Which of the following statements regarding this patient's condition is INCORRECT?

A) This patient has an autosomal dominant condition attributed to mutations in the *FLCN* gene.
B) The biopsied lesion is a fibrofolliculoma.

C) Patients with this condition frequently present with hypomelanotic macules that appear brighter than the normal skin when examined under a Wood lamp.
D) The "kidney tumors" described in the patient's family members most likely represent renal cell carcinomas.

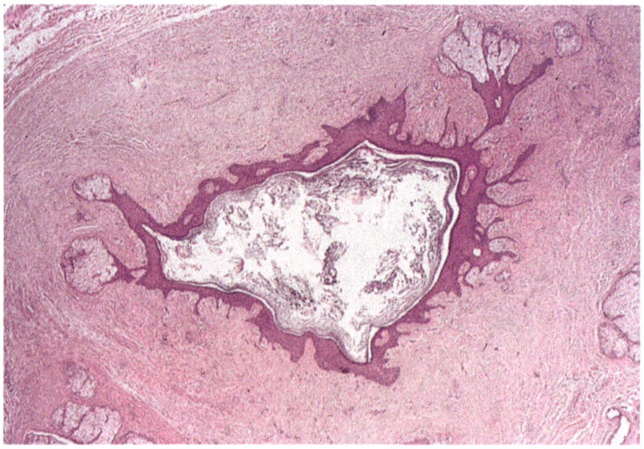

ANSWERS

ANSWER 9-1: B.

These lesions are **syringomas**, which most commonly present as multiple clustered white-yellow papules predominantly on the lower eyelids of young women (Table 9-1A). There is debate as to whether they are hamartomas versus neoplasms since solitary lesions also commonly present in the head and neck region. Generalized and eruptive forms exist that most commonly present on the chest, neck, and forearms. Microscopically, the tumor is composed of superficial dermal cords and tubules with a "tadpole" or "comma-shaped" appearance. The tubules are composed of two rows of cells with the apical layer frequently containing vacuolated or even clear cytoplasm due to secondary glycogen accumulation. **Clear cell syringoma** with abundant accumulations of glycogen is associated with glucose intolerance and **diabetes mellitus**. An eosinophilic cuticle usually lines the inner ductules, identical to that of normal eccrine sweat ducts, and the lumens contain eosinophilic to amphophilic secretions. **Syringomas** are believed to be of eccrine derivation. Immunohistochemistry will reveal the basolateral cells to express p63 and EMA, and the inner cuticular lining is highlighted by CEA.

Table 9-1A. Syringoma

Clinical Features
Usually multiple
Plaque-like, milia-like, linear, and eruptive variants
Upper cheeks, below eyelids, genitalia, thighs
Small, discrete, whitish or yellowish papules, 1-4 mm in diameter
Histopathologic Features
Superficial dermal well-defined tumor
Small tubule or epithelial aggregates, often comma shaped
Central lumina with luminal cuticle
Polygonal or flattened tumor cells with eosinophilic or clear cytoplasm
Absence of cytologic atypia, mitoses, and infiltrative growth
Differential Diagnosis
Basal cell carcinoma
Desmoplastic trichoepithelioma
Microcystic adnexal carcinoma

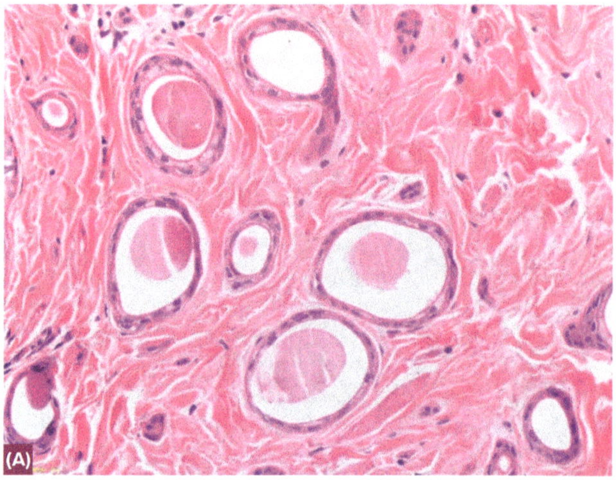

Reproduced with permission from Desman GT, Ozerdem U, Shin SJ: Neighboring look-a-likes: distinguishing between breast and dermatologic lesions, Adv Anat Pathol 2014 Jul;21(4):228-247

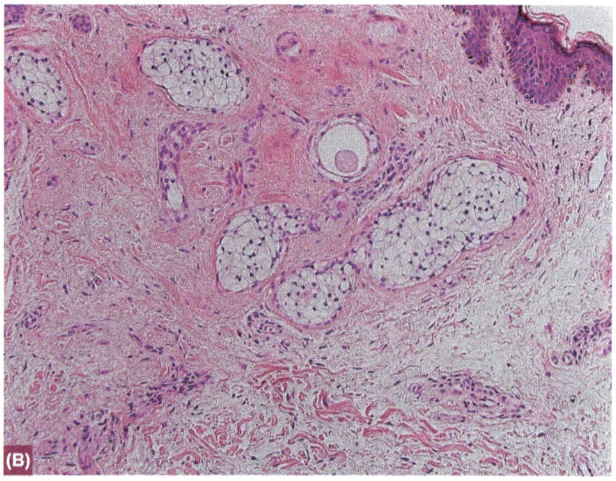

Syringoma. (A) There are numerous tubules, some of which contain tapered ends imparting a "tadpole" appearance. Note the eosinophilic secretion present within the lumen. **(B)** Clear cell syringoma composed of tubules and lobules containing two or more cell layers with abundant clear cytoplasm.

The histopathological differential diagnosis includes **desmoplastic trichoepithelioma (DTE), desmoplastic basal cell carcinoma,** and **microcystic adnexal carcinoma** (MAC). The most immediate finding supporting **syringoma** is that the other tumors in the differential diagnosis most commonly present as solitary lesions. When **syringoma** arises as a solitary lesion, the index of suspicion should be raised for the other tumors in differential diagnosis. Occasionally, the tubules of syringomas reside close to an irritated or traumatized epidermis and may exhibit keratinization, which may be confused with the horn cysts of **trichoepithelioma**. Additionally, the cords of **syringoma** may be embedded in a dense stroma, and therefore confused with both the **desmoplastic basal cell carcinoma** and **desmoplastic trichoepithelioma. Desmoplastic basal cell carcinomas** and **desmoplastic trichoepitheliomas** do not contain central lumens lined by an eosinophilic cuticle staining immunohistochemically for CEA. Although **MAC** also contains CEA positive lumens, **syringomas** are much smaller and more symmetric and do not extend into the deep dermis and/or subcutis. However, any solitary syringomatous lesion that has extension to the base must be reexcised for further evaluation to rule out **microcystic adnexal carcinoma. Syringoma** may be distinguished from **MAC** by its superficial and well-demarcated configuration versus the deep infiltration of reticular dermis, subcutaneous fat, skeletal muscle, and cutaneous nerves seen in **MAC**. Lastly **MAC** and **desmoplastic BCC** may reveal cytologic atypia with occasional necrotic tumor cells. **Syringoma** is a benign tumor and hence lacks the perineural invasion frequently seen in **MAC** and **desmoplastic BCC. Milium cysts** are follicular inclusion cysts of vellus hairs and contain keratinous material and are lined by an epithelium that contains a granular cell layer. They do not exhibit a "comma-shaped" pattern of growth.

ANSWER 9-2: A.

This is a classic example of **eccrine poroma**, which is a benign tumor with eccrine sweat duct differentiation involving both the epidermis and dermis (Table 9-2A). Tumors that arise within acrosyringia, where the sweat duct enters the epidermis, are referred to as **hidroacanthoma simplex**, and typically present as a solitary hyperkeratotic plaque on the extremities of middle-aged and elderly females. The histopathologic features of **hidroacanthoma simplex** include intraepidermal "lakes" of compact, monotonous polyhedral cells with bland nuclei and moderate amounts of amphophilic cytoplasm, resembling "mosaic tiles." The tumor cells are sharply demarcated from the adjacent epidermal keratinocytes. Peripheral palisading of the nuclei is not a feature. Small punched-out duct-like structures are randomly dispersed throughout the tumor. Mitoses are rare.

Tumors that arise solely within the dermis are referred to as **dermal duct tumor** and clinically present as a nondescript nodule. Frequently both intraepidermal and dermal tumor

Table 9-2A. Eccrine Poroma

Clinical Features
- Hidroacanthoma simplex
  - Lower extremities common
  - Slightly raised verrucous plaques
  - Skin-colored or brownish
- Poroma and dermal duct tumor
  - Palms, soles, other sites
  - Papules or nodules
  - May have verrucous or moist, eroded surface

Histopathologic Features
- Hidroacanthoma simplex
  - Discrete intraepidermal nests of basaloid cuboidal cells
  - Association with sweat ducts
- Poroma
  - Anastomosing ribbons of cuboidal epithelium, sharply demarcated from epidermis
  - Ductal structures
  - Vascular stroma
  - Uniformity of cuboidal epithelial cells
  - Occasional focal atypia and mitoses
- Dermal duct tumor
  - Rounded lobules of epithelium in dermis with little or no epidermal connection

Differential Diagnosis
- Hidroacanthoma simplex
  - Clonal seborrheic keratosis
  - Squamous cell carcinoma in situ
  - Basal cell carcinoma
  - Paget disease
  - Melanoma
- Poroma
  - Acrospiroma
  - Basal cell carcinoma
  - Porocarcinoma

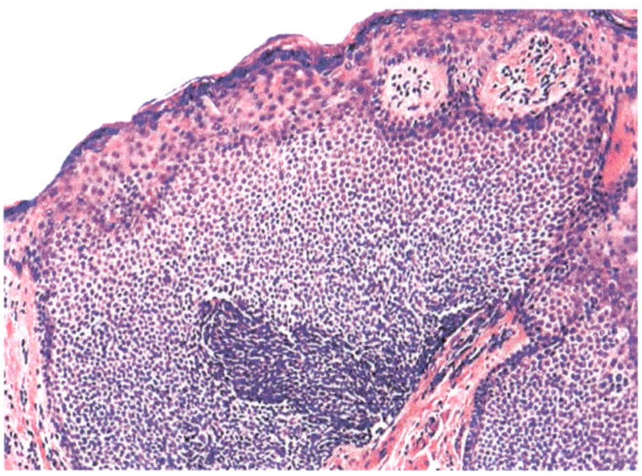

Intraepidermal poroma (hidroacanthoma simplex). The epidermis is expanded by a monotonous population of small basaloid cells.

nodules are present, in which case they are referred to simply as **poroma**. Clinically, these tumors typically present as a brownish raised friable papule or plaque with sharp demarcation or peripheral moat-like change. In general all forms of **poroma** may arise in any location where the skin contains high concentrations of eccrine sweat glands. The soles of the feet are most commonly affected in **poroma** and **dermal duct tumor**. **Dermal duct tumors** and **eccrine poromas** have similar cytomorphology to **hidroacanthoma simplex** and their tumor lobules contain duct-like structures. The deeper tumor cells may contain larger amounts of eosinophilic cytoplasm and "squamatization." The characteristic surrounding stroma is fibrovascular. Immunohistochemical stains reveal the tumor cells to express CK7 and p63 with EMA and CEA highlighting the duct-like foci.

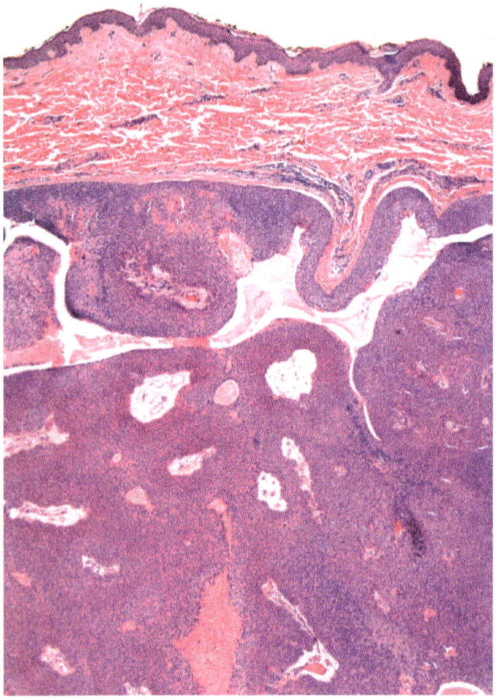

Intradermal poroma (dermal duct tumor). Nests of cytologically uniform cells do not communicate with the overlying epidermis. Small, irregular, duct-like spaces are evident.

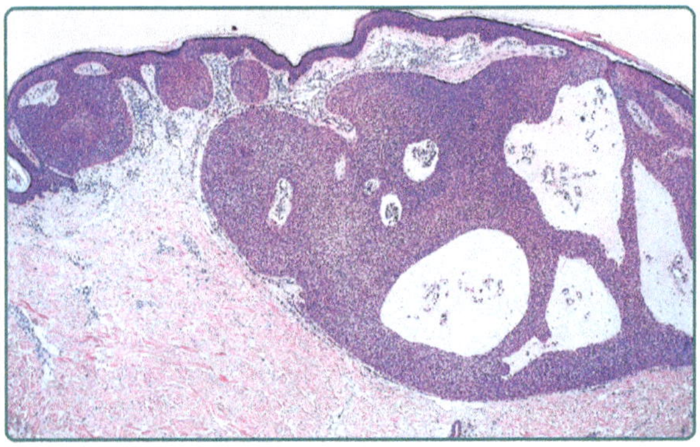

Eccrine poroma. Nodular aggregations of basaloid cells extend from the epidermis into the superficial dermis. Note the intratumoral stroma composed of loose fibromyxoid material and clusters of dilated vessels. (Reproduced, with permission, from Goldsmith LA, Katz SI, Gilchrest BA, Paller AS, Leffell DJ, Wolff K, eds. *Fitzpatrick's Dermatology in General Medicine*. 8th ed. New York, NY: McGraw-Hill Education; 2012.)

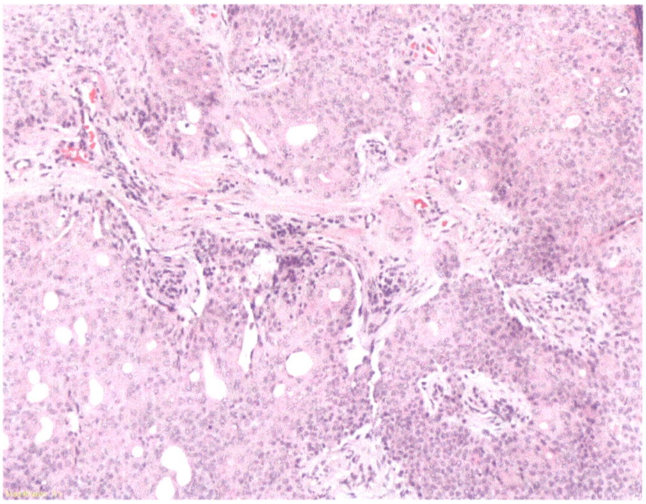

Eccrine poroma, high power. The tumor cells may occasionally contain abundant eosinophilic cytoplasm imparting a "squamoid" appearance. Note the numerous duct-like structures throughout the tumor. (Reproduced with permission from Desman GT, Ozerdem U, Shin SJ: Neighboring look-a-likes: distinguishing between breast and dermatologic lesions, Adv Anat Pathol 2014 Jul;21(4):228-247)

The most important histopathologic feature that distinguishes **poroma** from the other answer choices is the fact that those tumors lack ductular structures. Additionally, **poroma** differs from **basal cell carcinoma** by displaying fairly uniform anastomosing cords of epithelium, a lack of peripheral palisading of nuclei and separation artifact, and a uniformity of cuboidal cells without mitotic activity or tumor cell necrosis. **Poroma** differs from **trichilemmoma** and **tumor of the follicular infundibulum** by the lack of a hyalinized basement membrane at the periphery of the tumor, the degree of dyskeratosis noted in **trichilemmoma**, and often a greater depth of involvement than typically observed in **trichilemmoma** and **tumor of the follicular infundibulum**. **Squamous cell carcinomas** exhibit cytologic atypia with mitotic activity.

ANSWER 9-3: B.

This is an example of **eccrine syringofibroadenoma**, which is a very rare tumor usually presenting as a solitary hyperkeratotic nodular plaque on one extremity measuring several centimeters. Microscopically, these lesions are composed of slender anastomosing epithelial acrosyringeal cords extending downward from the epidermal surface.

The cords contain lumina lined by an eosinophilic cuticle. The thin net-like cords are embedded in a dense fibrous stroma with prominent lymphoplasmacytic infiltrates. The lesion is similar to the **fibroadenoma** of the breast. These lesions are typically sharply circumscribed and lack nuclear atypia and mitotic activity in either component. It is likely that the stroma is "induced" by the epithelial proliferation in **syringofibroadenoma**, as is thought to be true of its counterpart in the breast. The major lesions to be considered in the histopathological differential diagnosis include **fibroepithelioma of Pinkus**, **pseudoepitheliomatous hyperplasia**, and a reticulated form of **seborrheic keratosis**. The **syringofibroadenoma** differs from these entities by demonstrating a uniform population of cuboidal basaloid cells and the presence of ducts in the anastomosing bands of epithelium. **Eccrine syringofibroadenomatosis** (multiple lesions) have been associated with **inherited palmar-plantar keratodermas** and **Schopf-Schulz-Passarge syndrome (SSP). SSP syndrome** is a very rare syndrome characterized by thickened skin on palms and soles, missing teeth, sparse hair, and eyelid cysts.

ANSWER 9-4: B.

The tumor is an **eccrine cylindroma** (Table 9-4A) and this patient has **Brooke-Spiegler syndrome,** which is an autosomal dominant syndrome characterized by multiple **cylindromas**, **trichoepitheliomas**, and **eccrine spiradenomas** on the scalp, face, and upper body associated with mutations in the *CYLD1* gene. When numerous on the scalp, they may be referred to clinically as **turban tumors**. Sporadic solitary tumors are much more common and are not inherited. They are most common on the face, head, and neck of young adults. There is a strong predilection for females. The histopathologic features consist of angular nests that are molded to one another in a "jigsaw puzzle" configuration. The nests are located in the dermis and occasionally the subcutis without attachment to the epidermal surface. The nests are surrounded by dense eosinophilic basement membrane material composed of type IV collagen and laminin that stains with PAS with diastase. This basement membrane material may be present as small globules within the tumor islands (similar to **adenoid cystic carcinoma** or **eccrine spiradenoma**). The tumor is composed of two cell populations: compact basaloid cells and polygonal cells with amphophilic cytoplasm. Nucleoli are inconspicuous and mitotic activity is rare. Small buds of tumor trailing off from the tumor mass are common and should not be interpreted as malignant transformation. The histopathological differential diagnosis includes **eccrine spiradenoma** and **basal cell carcinoma (BCC).** There may be considerable overlap between **cylindroma** and **spiradenoma**, and some tumors may be hybrid lesions. The essential discriminating feature is the mosaic pattern of many small epithelial aggregates in **cylindroma** versus the isolated rounded tumor lobules that are often few in number in **spiradenoma. BCC** differs from **cylindroma** by showing frequent origin from the epidermis, peripheral palisading of nuclei, separation artifact (from the surrounding stroma), a mucinous stroma, and necrosis and mitoses.

Table 9-4A. Eccrine Cylindroma

Clinical Features
- Head, neck especially scalp
- Multiple tumors (turban tumors)
  - Autosomal dominant
- Association with eccrine spiradenomas and trichoepitheliomas (Brook syndrome)

Histopathologic Features
- Mosaic or jigsaw puzzle pattern of tumor islands
- Tumor aggregates delimited by basement membrane material that also results in "hyaline" droplets within aggregates
- Basaloid tumor aggregates with two cellular populations
  - Outer layer composed of small, round cells with scant cytoplasm
  - Inner layer comprised of larger polygonal cells with more abundant cytoplasm
- Irregular pattern at periphery of tumor (budding)
- Occasional mitotic figures

Differential Diagnosis
- Basal cell carcinoma
- Eccrine spiradenoma

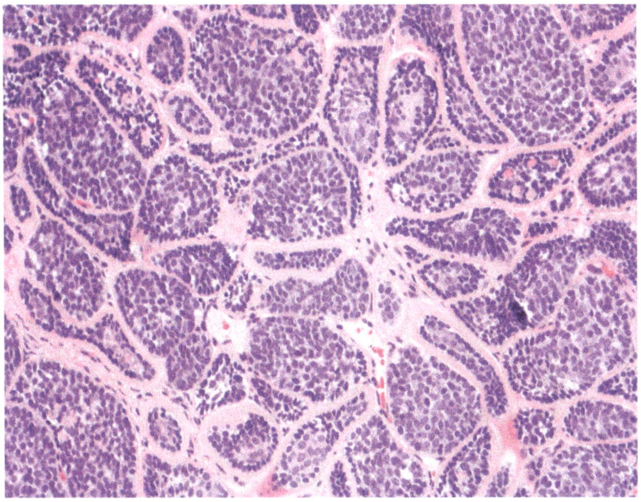

Cylindroma. There are numerous basaloid lobules closely arranged in a "jigsaw puzzle" configuration. A band of bright pink hyalinized basement membrane surrounds the individual tumor lobules. (Reproduced with permission from Desman GT, Ozerdem U, Shin SJ: Neighboring look-a-likes: distinguishing between breast and dermatologic lesions, Adv Anat Pathol 2014 Jul;21(4):228-247)

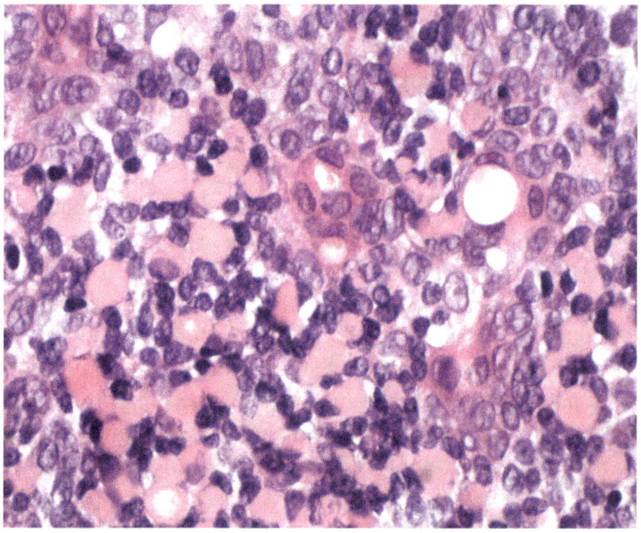

Cylindroma. Hyaline basement membrane material is regularly dispersed in a basaloid cell population.

ANSWER 9-5: C.

This is a classic presentation of **eccrine spiradenoma** (Table 9-5A). These painful solitary nodular lesions usually arise in young adults and may rarely occur in clusters in a zosteriform distribution. The other tumors that commonly present as painful nodules include **glomus cell tumors, angiolipomas,** and **angioleiomyomas.** Microscopically, **spiradenomas** are composed of well-circumscribed, frequently encapsulated, dark, hypercellular, intradermal nodules without connection to the overlying epidermis ("blue balls"). Similar to **cylindroma**, the individual rounded lobules may trail off at the periphery and should not be misinterpreted as invasion. They are composed of a two cell type population: (1) peripheral, small, dark basophilic cells with depleted cytoplasm and occasional nuclear palisading adjacent to a vascularized stroma, and (2) central cords, lobules, or occasionally tubules of slightly larger cells with more cytoplasm and somewhat vesiculated nuclei. In cases without lumina, a rosette arrangement may be seen. By electron microscopy, these cells are immature but may exhibit varying degrees of eccrine duct and eccrine secretory differentiation. Intratumoral vascular spaces are often dilated and are most numerous at the periphery of tumor cell clusters. These channels may become cystic and contain lymphatic fluid, erythrocytes, or both. Hyalinized stromal globules similar to **cylindroma** may be present within the lobules. A diffuse T-cell infiltrate is also commonly seen, which will be positive for CD45 and CD3 by immunohistochemistry. The glandular tumor cells are positive for CK7 and p63. These lesions may arise in large numbers in patients with **familial cylindromas**. **Spiradenoma** and **cylindroma** may have considerable overlapping histopathologic features. In general, **spiradenomas** are distinguished from **cylindromas**

Table 9-5A. Eccrine Spiradenoma

Eccrine Spiradenoma
Clinical Features
Trunk
Ventral surfaces
Skin-colored or bluish with cystic or sponge-like consistency
Painful or tender
Histopathologic Features
Rounded tumor lobules, often large and few in number
No epidermal connection or jigsaw puzzle pattern
Tumor lobules delimited by basement membrane material and contain hyaline droplets
Smaller outer cell
Larger inner polygonal cells
Often highly vascular and infiltrated by lymphocytes
Overlap with eccrine cylindroma
Differential Diagnosis
Basal cell carcinoma
Eccrine cylindroma
Vascular and glomus tumors

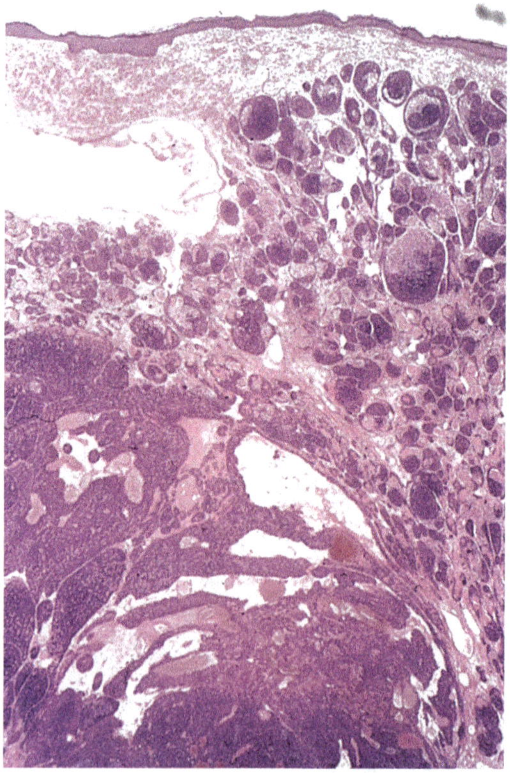

Spiradenoma. An organoid pattern of epithelial cells is interrupted by dilated/cystic intratumoral vascular channels. Note how small well-circumscribed lobules trail off at the periphery of the tumor.

by their lack of a "jigsaw" configuration at low power. Additionally, **cylindromas** are not painful and lack dilated/cystic intratumoral vascular channels. Both **spiradenoma** and **glomus tumors** may be vascular. **Spiradenomas**, in general, are distinguished from **glomus tumors** by the presence of a capsule of hyalinized basement membrane, hyaline globules within the tumor, the two cell populations, and the presence of occasional tubular structures. Superficial biopsies may resemble **BCC** due to the palisading of the dark cells, but **spiradenomas** lack dermal retraction and mucin. **Merkel cell carcinomas** also fall into the "blue balls in the dermis" histopathological category, but are invasive and not encapsulated, lack tubules, and are composed of overtly malignant cells with nuclear molding, crush artifact, and numerous mitoses and necrotic cells. Malignant transformation of spiradenomas may occur in long-standing lesions, in which case the cytomorphology is obviously anaplastic.

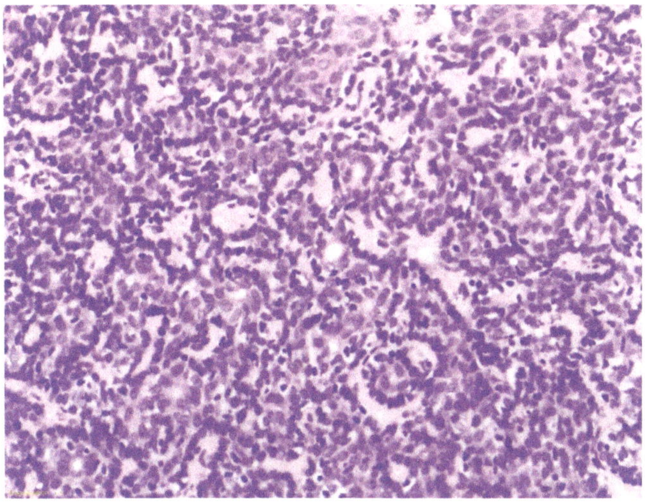

Spiradenoma. High-power image revealing numerous basophilic cells arranged in lobules with scattered duct-like structures. Note the permeation of the tumor by smaller hyperchromatic lymphocytes.

Table 9-6A. Eccrine Hidradenoma (Acrospiroma)

Clinical Features
Wide age range
Women > men
Almost any location
Papule or nodule, 1-2 cm
Often skin colored
Histopathologic Features
Frequent origin from epidermis
Large lobular epithelial aggregates, well demarcated
Often solid nodules of cuboidal cells with varying degrees of squamous differentiation and clear cell change
Occasional focal spindled epithelial cells
Ductal structures
Cystic spaces
Focal decapitation secretion
Variable focal cytologic atypia and occasional mitoses
Variable hyalinized stroma
Differential Diagnosis
Eccrine poroma
Mixed tumor
Squamous cell carcinoma

ANSWER 9-6: D.

This is a **nodular hidradenoma (acrospiroma)**, which most often presents a solitary nodule or cystic lesion measuring 1 to 2 cm in diameter (Table 9-6A). They may occur in any location. The pathogenesis is uncertain; however, most cases exhibit evidence of eccrine differentiation. Occasional cases with apocrine, squamous, and mucinous differentiation have been reported. The histopathologic features include well-circumscribed epithelial lobules surrounded by a fibrovascular or hyalinized stroma in the dermis or occasionally the subcutis. Connection with the overlying epidermis may be seen and may result in ulceration. The well-circumscribed tumor lobules are frequently solid; however, occasionally large cystic areas, squamous metaplasia with squamous eddies, and/or eccrine ductal differentiation with eosinophilic cuticles may be seen. The tumor has a biphasic cellular population: (1) round or polygonal cells with amphophilic cytoplasm and vesicular elongated grooved nuclei and conspicuous nucleoli, and (2) clear cells containing eccentric small hyperchromatic nuclei. The dominant cell type determines the adjectival modifier of **"nodular"** versus **"clear cell" hidradenoma**. A pigmented variant contains sparse melanocytes and melanin pigment within epithelial cells. Occasionally, the dense hyalinized stroma in the central portions of the tumor may result in angular arrangements of the tumor lobules, imparting a "pseudoinvasive" growth pattern. Mitoses are rare. Although local recurrence is rare, tumor nodules that exhibit budding or irregular peripheral cords, focal nuclear pleomorphism, and increased mitoses (1-2 per 10 high-power fields) should be reexcised to exclude **well-differentiated hidradenocarcinoma**. Immunohistochemical stains reveal the tumor cells to express p63 and AE1/AE3 with luminal staining for EMA and CEA. A PAS stain will highlight the clear cells, consistent with glycogen accumulation. Approximately half of cases harbor the t(11:19) chromosomal translocation, particularly in the clear cell variant.

The histopathological differential diagnosis includes **chondroid syringoma (mixed tumor), squamous cell carcinoma, basal cell carcinoma**, and **trichilemmoma**. On occasion, there may be overlap between **hidradenoma** and

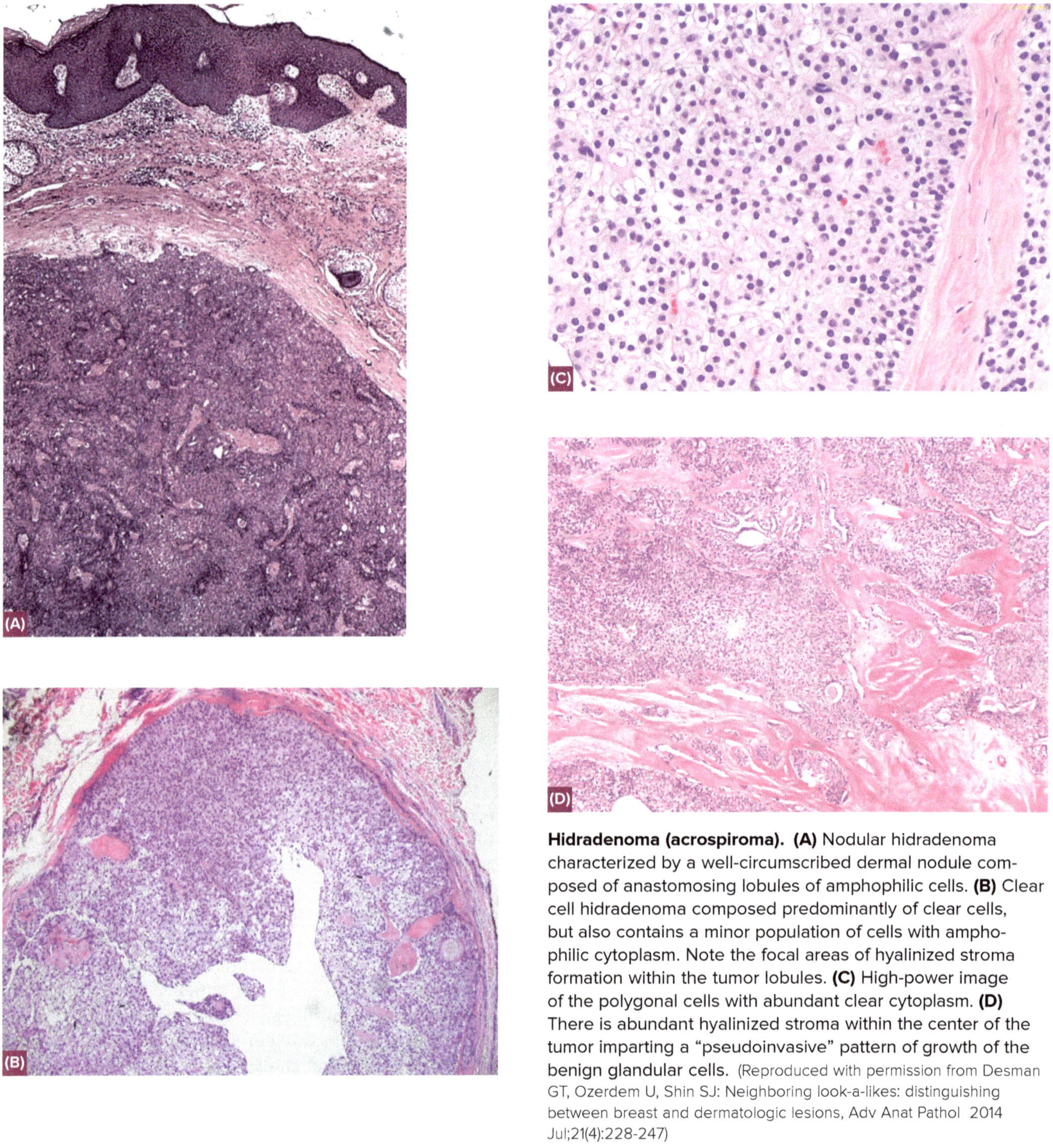

Hidradenoma (acrospiroma). (A) Nodular hidradenoma characterized by a well-circumscribed dermal nodule composed of anastomosing lobules of amphophilic cells. **(B)** Clear cell hidradenoma composed predominantly of clear cells, but also contains a minor population of cells with amphophilic cytoplasm. Note the focal areas of hyalinized stroma formation within the tumor lobules. **(C)** High-power image of the polygonal cells with abundant clear cytoplasm. **(D)** There is abundant hyalinized stroma within the center of the tumor imparting a "pseudoinvasive" pattern of growth of the benign glandular cells. (Reproduced with permission from Desman GT, Ozerdem U, Shin SJ: Neighboring look-a-likes: distinguishing between breast and dermatologic lesions, Adv Anat Pathol 2014 Jul;21(4):228-247)

mixed tumor, with both lesions frequently showing prominent cystic spaces, hyalinized stroma, and anastomosing cords of epithelium. The final categorization must be based on the prominence of the stromal component in relationship to the other features present. Thus, for a diagnosis of **mixed tumor**, a lesion should exhibit a rounded configuration with a significant component of stroma, whether it is chondroid, myxoid, or hyalinized. In contrast, **hidradenomas** primarily exhibits nodular aggregates of epithelium. A proportion of **hidradenomas** may show prominence of squamous differentiation, raising the possibility of **squamous cell carcinoma**. However, careful examination should disclose the lack of significant cytologic atypia and the presence of other features typical of **hidradenoma**, including ductal structures, cystic spaces, variable degrees of clear cell change, and a hyalinized stroma. **Hidradenoma** differs from **basal cell carcinoma** by the lack of peripheral palisading of nuclei, separation artifact, a mucinous stroma, and the overall basaloid appearance of the tumor that typifies **basal cell carcinoma**. **Trichilemmoma** also frequently exhibits clear cell change due to accumulations of cytoplasmic glycogen; however, **hidradenomas** only rarely connect with the overlying epidermis, contain lumina, and lack peripheral nuclear palisading along a thickened eosinophilic basement membrane. **Metastatic clear cell renal cell carcinoma** and **seminoma** may be distinguished from **clear cell hidradenoma** by immunohistochemical carbonic anhydrase IX and PLAP expression, respectively. There is considerable overlap between **eccrine hidradenoma (acrospiroma)** and the **eccrine poroma** group. In some instances, a tumor may present with an intraepidermal portion resembling **poroma (hidroacanthoma simplex)** and with a deeper dermal component typical of **hidradenoma (acrospiroma)**. The final diagnosis may be based on the predominant features present.

ANSWER 9-7: E.

Syringocystadenoma papilliferum (SPAP) is a distinctive lesion that is largely, but not exclusively, restricted to the skin of the head and neck and particularly affects the scalp (Table 9-7A). It is one of several neoplasms that may be associated with **nevus sebaceus of Jadassohn**, but it most often

Table 9-7A. Syringocystadenoma Papilliferum

Clinical Features
- Head and neck, especially scalp
- Solitary verrucous-like plaque or nodule
- Often moist or oozing surface
- Often 2-3 cm
- Frequently congenital and associated with nevus sebaceus

Histopathologic Features
- Epidermal cystic invagination lined by squamous epithelium with transition to epithelial lining with two cell layers
- Often verrucous epidermal surface
- Cystic invagination contains papillary projections lined by luminal columnar cells and inner cuboidal cells
- Decapitation secretion
- The stroma of the papillary epithelial structures contains numerous plasma cells
- Background nevus sebaceus common

Differential Diagnosis
- Nevus sebaceus
- Hidradenoma papilliferum

Quick Fact:

SPAP ("SS")

Syringocystadenoma papilliferum

Slides into the dermis from the epidermis

occurs as a sporadic tumor. Rarely, a linear or agminated extracranial configuration is encountered. These tumors present as linear papules or plaques, and approximately half of cases are present at birth or early childhood. During puberty, these tumors may gradually enlarge and become hyperkeratotic. Malignant degeneration into **syringocystadenocarcinoma papilliferum** is extremely rare with signs of malignant behavior including rapid growth, ulceration, pain, and pruritus. There is a low risk of regional lymph node metastases, while distant metastases have not been reported. **SPAP** may be seen in conjunction with a wide variety of other adnexal tumors including **nevus sebaceous, apocrine nevus, tubular apocrine adenoma, apocrine hidrocystoma, clear cell syringoma, eccrine nevus, verrucous carcinoma,** and **eccrine** or **apocrine adenocarcinoma**. Molecular studies have demonstrated loss of heterozygosity for tumor suppressor genes PTCH and p16.

Microscopically, **SPAP** is characterized by one or more duct or tubular structures extending downward from the epidermis ending in a cystic dilatation containing papillary structures whose fibrovascular cores contain numerous plasma cells. The tubules, cysts, and papillary structures are lined by a double layer epithelium composed of basilar cuboidal cells and an inner columnar layer of secretory cells. The glandular epithelium may have both apocrine and/or eccrine differentiation. The tumor epithelial cells express AE1/AE3, EMA, and CEA. There is variable GCFP-15 expression.

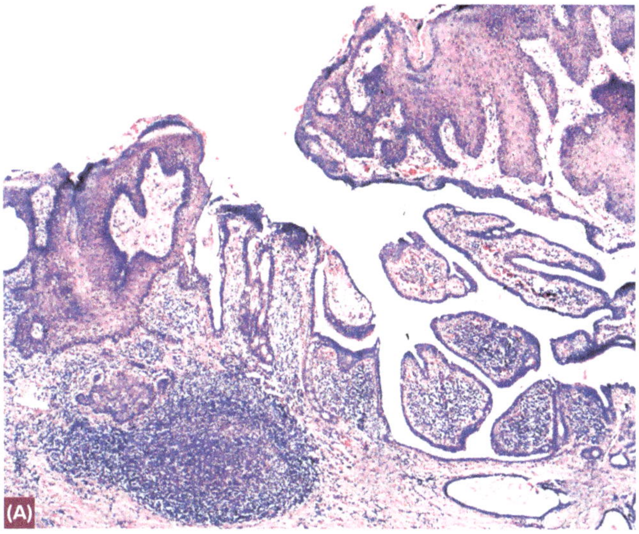

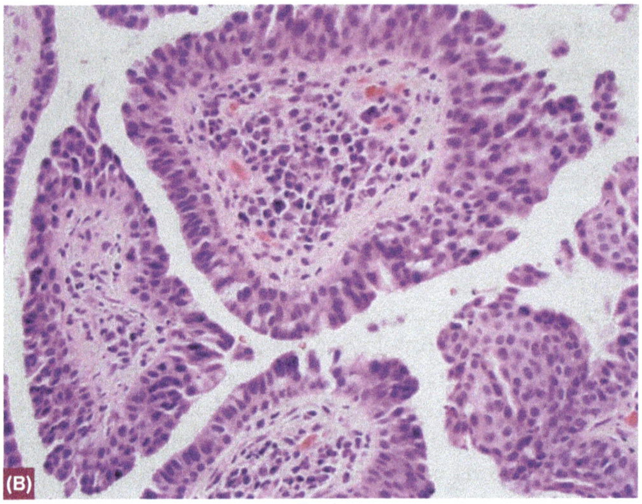

Syringocystadenoma papilliferum. (A) A papillary proliferation lines a semicystic depression in the dermis that is in continuity with the epidermis. **(B)** Low columnar cells with apocrine-type secretion line inflamed fibrovascular cores. The cores are populated by a plasma cell–rich mononuclear infiltrate.

The histopathological differential diagnosis includes **hidradenoma papilliferum** (HP). **SPAP** can be distinguished from **HP** in almost all cases by its epidermal invagination, verrucous surface alteration, and a location on the head or neck.

ANSWER 9-8: B.

Tubular apocrine adenoma (aka apocrine adenoma, tubulopapillary adenoma) is a rare benign tumor, which shows a female predominance, a wide age distribution, and most commonly arises on the scalp. Lesions have been described at a number of sites including the face, eyelid, axilla, leg, and genitalia. These tumors frequently arise in a background of **nevus sebaceus** and sometimes **syringocystadenoma papilliferum (SPAP).** These tumors are benign with a low rate of local recurrence after excision. Microscopically, low-power examination reveals a well-circumscribed intradermal nodule composed of closely arranged lobules and tubules. Epidermal connection is absent except for tumors that arise in continuity with a **syringocystadenoma papilliferum** or **nevus sebaceus**, in which case communication with the epidermis may occur through duct-like structures or dilated follicular infundibula. The nodule is composed of variably sized, well-formed tubules lined by a multi- or double epithelial cell layer of cuboidal to low columnar cells with eosinophilic cytoplasm and uniform round to oval nuclei. Solid, cribriform, and micropapillary configurations of hyperplastic epithelium may fill the tubules. True papillary structures with fibrovascular cores are not present, but may be seen in cases arising in association with **syringocystadenoma papilliferum**. The apical cells show apocrine decapitation secretion while the basolateral cells are flattened myoepithelial cells. There is no nuclear pleomorphism and mitoses are rare. Immunohistochemical studies have documented the epithelial cells to express EMA and CEA, and GCFP-15. The myoepithelial cells express S-100 protein and SMA.

The differential diagnosis includes **syringocystadenoma papilliferum (SPAP), papillary eccrine adenoma, hidradenoma papilliferum,** and **ductopapillary apocrine adenocarcinoma**. Although **tubular apocrine adenoma** frequently arises in association with **SPAP**, distinguishing features of **tubular apocrine adenoma** include an intradermal tumor that lacks connection with the epidermal surface, lacks true papillae with fibrovascular cores, and the absence of a plasma cell–rich inflammatory cell infiltrate. **Papillary eccrine adenomas** occur almost exclusively on the extremities and lack apocrine-type decapitation secretion. Occasional tumors may show features of both eccrine and apocrine differentiation. **Hidradenoma papilliferum** also lacks a connection with the epidermal surface, but most commonly arises in the perineal and perianal areas and contains true papillary structures with fibrovascular cores.

ANSWER 9-9: B.

Hidradenoma papilliferum (HP) typically presents as a small, unilateral, asymptomatic, flesh-colored nodule in middle-aged women on the labia majora, perineal or perianal regions (Table 9-9A). Rare cases of perineal and arm tumors have been reported in men. This benign neoplasm develops from the anogenital apocrine glands. Microscopically, a well-circumscribed tumor nodule is confined to the dermis and is surrounded by a fibrous capsule. If an overlying epidermal connection is present, one must consider **syringocystadenoma papilliferum (SPAP).** The central portion of the nodule consists of an anastomosing pattern of numerous glandular structures and papillary folds. The papillary structures contain fibrovascular cores that are usually devoid of an inflammatory cell infiltrate. The lumina are made of a double layer of cells: an inner layer of secretory cells demonstrating decapitation secretion, and an outer layer of cuboidal myoepithelial cells. Most cases exhibit high cellularity and

> **Quick Fact:**
>
> **HP ("HH")**
>
> Hidradenoma papilliferum
>
> Hidden in the dermis

Table 9-9A. Hidradenoma Papilliferum

Clinical Features
Women, almost exclusively
Vulva, rarely other sites such as breast, eyelid, ear canal
Dome-shaped nodule with occasional bleeding pain, usually solitary
Histopathologic Features
Well-circumscribed dermal nodule, solid or cystic
Usually no epidermal connection
Complex pattern of anastomosing papillary structures, tubules
Epithelial lining with myoepithelial cells and luminal columnar or cuboidal cells
Decapitation secretion
Occasional slight nuclear pleomorphism, mitoses
Differential Diagnosis
Syringocystadenoma papilliferum
Tubular apocrine adenoma

asymmetry, which should not be confused with malignancy. Focal keratinization may be seen in the peripheral epithelium. Malignant transformation to **adenosquamous carcinoma** or **squamous cell carcinoma** has been reported in the literature. Immunohistochemical studies have documented the epithelial cells to express low-molecular-weight keratin, EMA, CEA, and GCFP-15. Estrogen and to a lesser extent progesterone receptors are positive. Androgen receptor is expressed in a minority of tumors. The myoepithelial cells express S-100 protein and SMA.

In regard to the histopathological differential diagnosis, the major entities to be considered include **SPAP** and other **apocrine adenomas**, such as **tubular adenoma**. In general, **HP** is distinguished from **SPAP** by its well-demarcated nodular appearance in the dermis without epidermal connection, localization to the vulvar and perineal area, and almost exclusive occurrence in women. Unlike **HP**, **SPAP** connects with the overlying epidermis and its fibrovascular cores contain plasma cells. **Tubular apocrine adenoma** also presents as a dermal nodule composed of glandular structures, but unlike HP, the tubules and glands contain micropapillary structures without fibrovascular cores. The occasional appearance of **HP** in males, particularly in the anal skin, may cause confusion with **well-differentiated colorectal neoplasms**. Careful attention to the cytologic, architectural, and immunohistochemical features of the tumor in question should be sufficient to make this diagnostic separation. In particular, hormonal receptor proteins and p63 are present in **HP** but not in intestinal tumors.

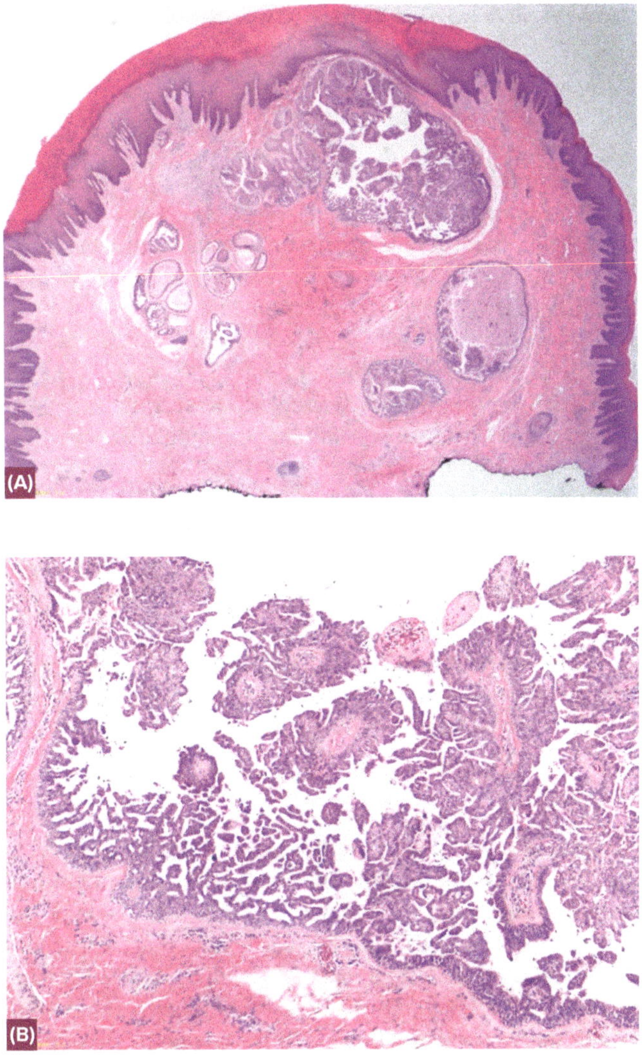

Hidradenoma papilliferum. (A) This intradermal lesion is composed of variably sized cystic spaces into which papillary cellular proliferations project. The tumor does not connect with the overlying epidermal surface. **(B)** Frond-like growth with micropapillary and true papillary structures with fibrovascular cores are present. The fibrovascular cores are devoid of inflammatory cells. The epithelial cells exhibit decapitation.

ANSWER 9-10: A.

Mixed tumor of the skin (MTS), also referred to as **chondroid syringoma**, is a benign adnexal neoplasm that most commonly arises on the head and neck as a nondescript 0.5 to 2 cm firm dermal or subcutaneous nodule (Table 9-10A). Tumors less commonly arise on the trunk and extremities. Patients are typically in the fourth and fifth decades of life. This tumor is the prototype for the frequent biphasic nature of benign cutaneous adnexal neoplasms, in which the tumor stem cells undergo divergent differentiation at a morphological level into dissimilar tissue types. Microscopically the

Table 9-10A. Mixed Tumor (Chondroid Syringoma)

Clinical Features
Head and neck, especially face
Men > women
Firm dermal or subcutaneous nodule
Histopathologic Features
Well-circumscribed dermal or subcutaneous lobular tumor
Only rare epidermal connection
Stromal component: variable chondroid, mucinous, hyalinized, or osteoid matrix
Epithelial component heterogeneous: eccrine, apocrine, sebaceous, pilar, simple glandular, or squamous differentiation
Often small tubular lumina lined by cuboidal epithelium or complex pattern of anastomosing tubular lumina lined by one or two cell layers that are cuboidal or columnar
Occasional prominent cystic spaces
Differential Diagnosis
Cutaneous chondroma
Eccrine acrospiroma

tumor is composed of an intradermal or subcutaneous well-circumscribed, multilobulated nodule with two common cellular components: (1) epithelial tubules lined by cuboidal apocrine ductal cells and (2) basophilic mucoid/pseudocartilaginous spindled stromal cells with retraction spacing (resembling lacunae). The epithelial tubules are composed of two or more cuboidal cell layers with oval nuclei, inconspicuous nucleoli, and a moderate amount of eosinophilic or clear cytoplasm with an outer row of flattened myoepithelial cells. The epithelium may form small ductules, tubules with partial branching, solid nests, or even as single cells. Other metaplastic epithelial components include eccrine, sebaceous, pilar, mucinous, clear cell, spindle cell, or simple glandular differentiation. Metaplastic stromal components include matrix of fibroblastoid, chondroid, myoid, myoepithelioid, lipoid, or even osteogenic appearance. Variable mixtures of these elements may be present within a single tumor. Occasionally, large stromal components are predominant, and with partial sampling may result in a misdiagnosis of **chondroma, osteoma cutis**, or **lipoma.** The overall features reassuring of benignity are the well-circumscribed tumor growth combined with the absence of nuclear pleomorphism, mitoses, and necrosis. Tumors with extensive trailing elements beyond the tumor capsule or foci with enhanced cytologic atypia (usually of the myoepithelial cells) are referred to as **atypical mixed tumors**; however, they display a benign clinical course. By immunohistochemistry the apical tumor cells are typically positive for keratin, EMA, CEA, CD117, CK7, GCFP-15, and androgen receptor (AR), whereas the basolateral myoepithelial cells are positive for p63, S100, vimentin, and occasionally smooth muscle actin (SMA). Stromal cells are vimentin and S-100 protein positive. Occasionally, distinction of apocrine tumors from **metastatic breast adenocarcinoma** can be difficult. While most apocrine tumors (including breast carcinoma) are negative for p63, the mixed tumor of skin expresses p63 in the myoepithelial layer. This double layer of distinct cell types is an additional feature supporting benignancy versus the single cell type seen in malignant tumors. Lastly, mixed tumors typically lack immunoreactivity for Brst-2, ER, and PR.

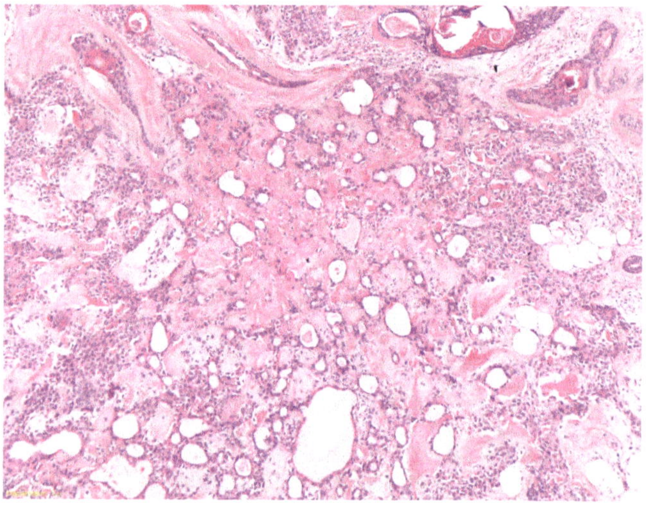

Mixed tumor of the skin (chondroid syringoma). There is a relatively heterogenous tumor in regard to epithelial and stromal elements. Similar to hidradenoma, the central portion of the tumor occasionally contains hyalinized stroma which may impart a "pseudoinvasive" pattern of the glandular growth. The surrounding architecture is still that of a relatively well-circumscribed nodule.

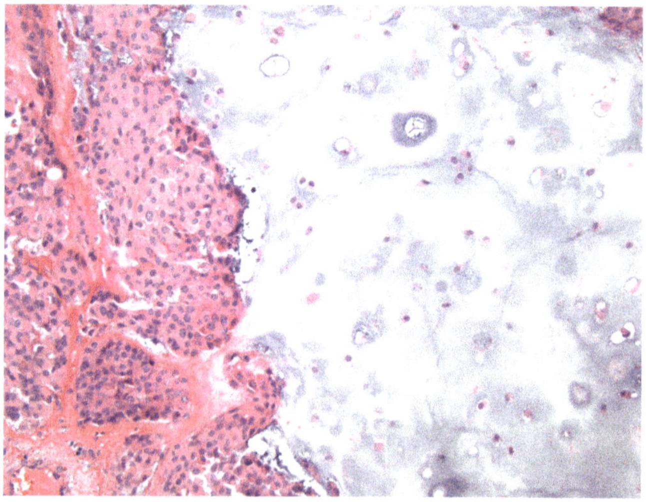

Mixed tumor of the skin (chondroid syringoma). High-power focus revealing a chondromyxoid stroma containing scattered solitary plasmacytoid-appearing myoepithelial cells.

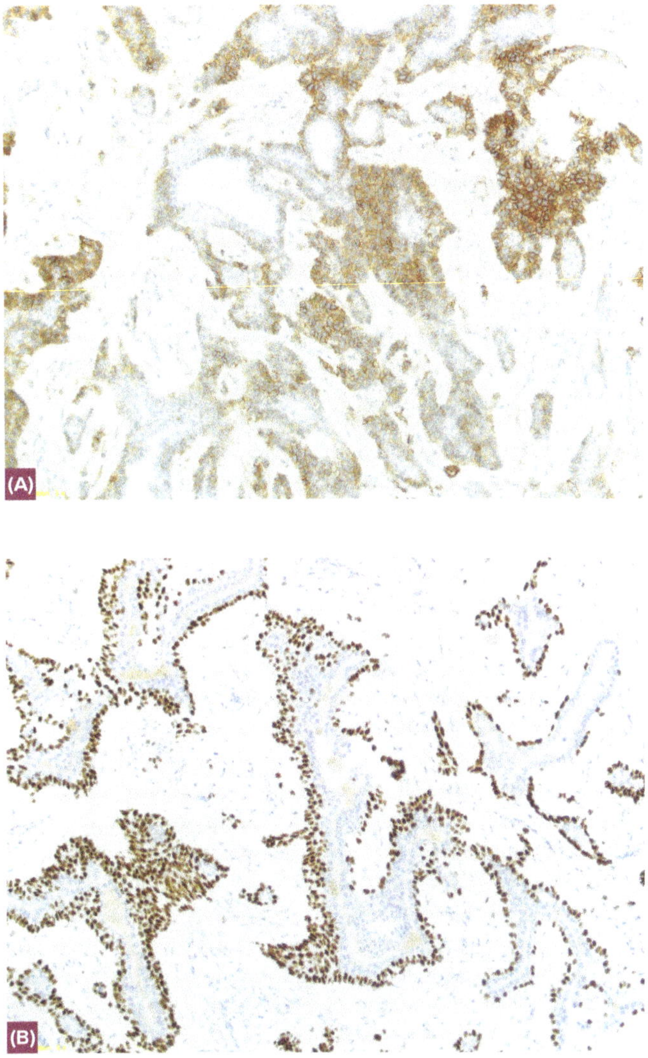

Mixed tumor of the skin (chondroid syringoma), immunohistochemistry. (A) The apical cells express CK7. **(B)** The basolateral myoepithelial cells are positive for p63.

Answer choice A describes the features of **carcinosarcoma (metaplastic carcinomas)**, which are rare tumors with both malignant epithelial and mesenchymal elements. They arise de novo without a preexisting benign component, unlike **malignant mixed tumors of the skin,** which arise in association with **benign mixed tumors.** Carcinosarcomas are seen in other organ systems such as the bladder, breast, kidney, cervix, uterus, and gallbladder. **Cutaneous carcinosarcomas** present as eroding and ulcerating nodules on the skin of older patients. Some patients have reported rapid growth. Death from metastatic spread has been described, although cutaneous lesions seem to pursue a less aggressive course than their visceral counterparts. Lesions larger than 40 mm reportedly demonstrate a worse clinical outcome. **Carcinosarcomas** have been reported in patients with the **nevoid basal cell carcinoma syndrome** and **Brooke-Spiegler syndrome** (Table 9-10B). Microscopically, basaloid and squamoid cells with stromal retraction, peripheral palisading, and mucin deposition form the superficial aspects of these tumors. In the deeper dermis, sarcomatous changes appear and consist of spindled cells with nuclear atypia and mitotic activity. These two cell populations are usually easily distinguished. The basaloid and squamoid cells are cytokeratin positive, but the sarcomatous cells are not. Similarly, sarcomatous cells are vimentin positive, but epithelial cells are negative. These mesenchymal components are believed to represent sarcomatous metaplasia of malignant epithelial cells. Poorly differentiated epithelial components can be found in some tumors and may reportedly be highlighted using a p63 stain. **Basal cell carcinoma, squamous cell carcinoma, malignant eccrine spiradenoma, cylindrocarcinoma,** and **eccrine porocarcinoma** have been described in carcinosarcomas. The mesenchymal portion of these neoplasms most often demonstrates **osteosarcomatous** (80%) and **chondrosarcomatous** (40%) differentiation; however, **rhabdomyosarcomatous**, **angiosarcomatous**, **fibrosarcomatous**, and **atypical fibrous histiocytoma-like** features have been described as well. Tumors derived from the epidermis (**basal cell carcinoma** and **squamous cell carcinoma**) reportedly arise more commonly in older patients and have a better 5-year disease-free survival than those with adnexal components. **Malignant mixed tumors** exhibit a malignant epithelial component and a benign mesenchymal component. The malignant cells can have glandular **(malignant mixed tumor)** or myoepithelial derivation **(myoepithelial carcinoma).**

Quick Fact

- **Mixed tumor of skin**
  - Benign epithelial and stromal elements
- **Malignant mixed tumor of skin**
  - Malignant epithelial but benign stromal elements
- **Carcinosarcoma**
  - Malignant epithelial and stromal elements

Table 9-10B. Carcinosarcoma

Clinical Features
Solitary nodules with epidermal ulceration and breakdown on the skin of elderly patients
Histopathologic Features
Two types of cellular proliferation: basaloid or squamoid cells with palisading, retraction, and surrounding fibromucinous stroma (cytokeratin positive and vimentin negative)
Second cell type composed of atypical spindle-shaped cells (cytokeratin negative and vimentin positive)
Differential Diagnosis
Malignant mixed tumor of the skin
Malignant fibrous histiocytoma

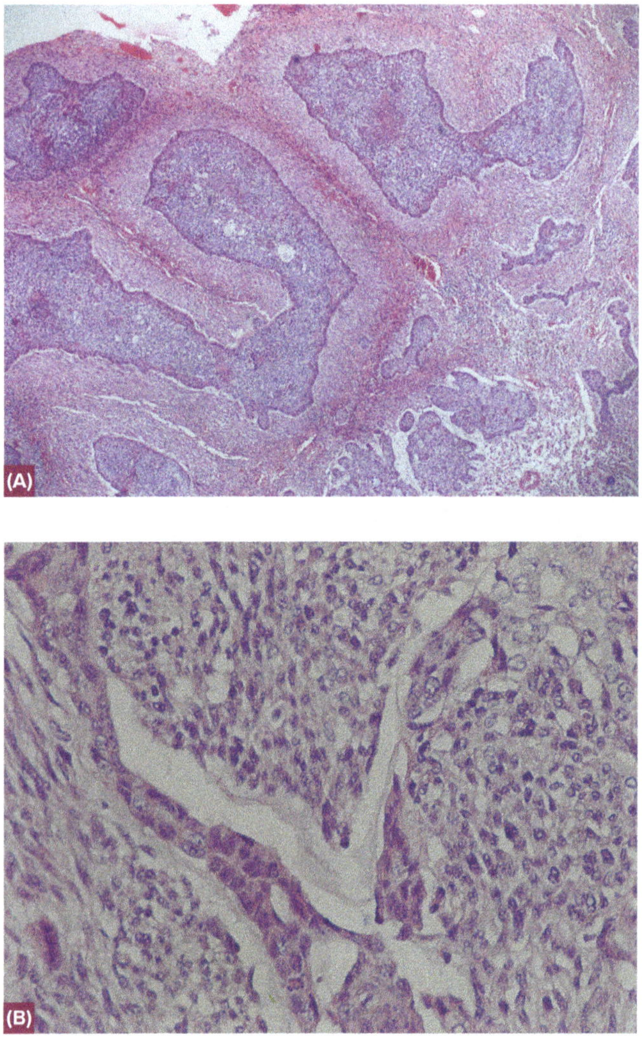

Basal cell carcinosarcoma. (A) There is a tumor composed of distinct basaloid and spindle cell components. **(B)** High power reveals the highly cellular malignant mesenchymal component with mitoses. There are strands of malignant basaloid epithelium with focal necrotic keratinocytes.

ANSWER 9-11: A.

This lesion is an **apocrine cystadenoma**, which is a cystic dilatation of apocrine sweat ducts with papillary, micropapillary, and adenoid epithelial hyperplasia most commonly arising on the face; however, involvement at other sites such as the head, neck, upper trunk, genitalia, and perineum has been documented (Table 9-11A). Cystic lesions without papillary or adenoid architecture are simply referred to as **hidrocystomas**, which are more common. The cyst lining is composed of one or two layers of cuboidal cells with eosinophilic cytoplasm and apocrine decapitation secretion (snouts). Immunohistochemistry will reveal the epithelial cells to stain for GCFP-15. Additionally, similar to other primary apocrine tumors of the skin, the tumor cells may contain focal hemosiderin pigment, a finding not seen in cutaneous metastases of mammary carcinoma. Clinically, these lesions present as skin-colored-to-bluish, translucent papules or nodules with frequent multiloculation. Most authors support a neoplastic derivation for these lesions. Eyelid lesions arising in association with Moll glands are well described in the literature. **Median raphe** cysts arise on the ventral penis and are derived from urothelial rests that may only mimic apocrine differentiation.

Table 9-11A. Eccrine and Apocrine Hidrocystoma or Cystadenoma

ECCRINE	APOCRINE
Clinical Features Usually adults Men = Women Periorbital sites but also head and neck, upper trunk Solitary > multiple Solitary almost exclusively Skin-color or bluish papules, nodules Commonly translucent Often <1 cm but rarely ≤ 7 cm Precipitated or exacerbated by heat	*Clinical Features* Usually adults Men = Women Periorbital sites but also head and neck, upper trunk Solitary > multiple Solitary almost exclusively Skin-color or bluish papules, nodules Commonly translucent Often <1 cm but rarely ≤ 7 cm Precipitated or exacerbated by heat
Histopathologic Features Often dilated cystic structure in dermis Epithelial lining: One or two cell layers Cuboidal or flattened Squamous metaplasia Hyperplasia of lining	*Histopathologic Features* Often dilated cystic structure in dermis Epithelial lining: Two cell layers Luminal cell is columnar or cuboidal with decapitation secretion Outer layer composed of myoepithelial cells (cuboidal or flattened) Hyperplasia of lining with papillary projections, folding Occasional mitoses, slight pleomorphism
Differential Diagnosis Other cysts, epidermoid cyst	*Differential Diagnosis* Other cysts Papillary adenoma Ductopapillary carcinoma

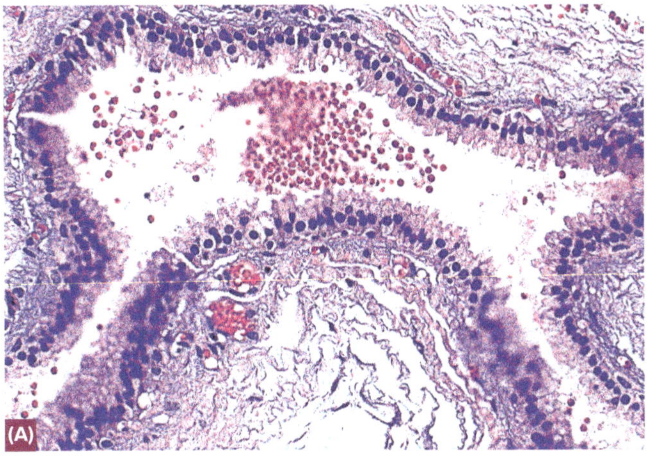

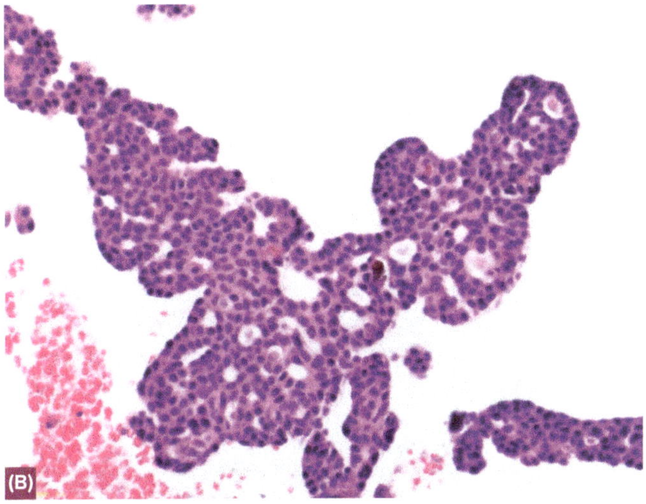

Apocrine hidrocystoma. (A) Hidrocystomas are simple cysts of the sweat gland apparatus formed by dilatation of sweat ducts with secondary epithelial proliferation. The presence of cuboidal eccrine or low columnar apocrine epithelium with decapitation secretion (snouts) further defines these cystic lesions. **(B)** Papillary fronds of apocrine cystadenoma with central hemosiderin deposition.

ANSWER 9-12: C.

Erosive adenomatosis of the nipple (EAN), also referred to simply as **nipple adenoma,** typically presents as an ill-defined mass centered under the areolar complex in middle-aged to elderly females. The lesion frequently distorts the nipple and may be associated with eczematous dermatitis of the surrounding nipple skin, clinically resembling **mammary Paget disease**. The histopathologic features include a vaguely nodular proliferation of small glands and tubules centered on large lactiferous ducts that connect with the overlying nipple skin. The glandular structures may dissect in between smooth muscle bundles in the nipple skin, mimicking invasion. Two cell layers line the glands: basal cells with pale cytoplasm and apical cells with eosinophilic cytoplasm and frequent apocrine snouts.

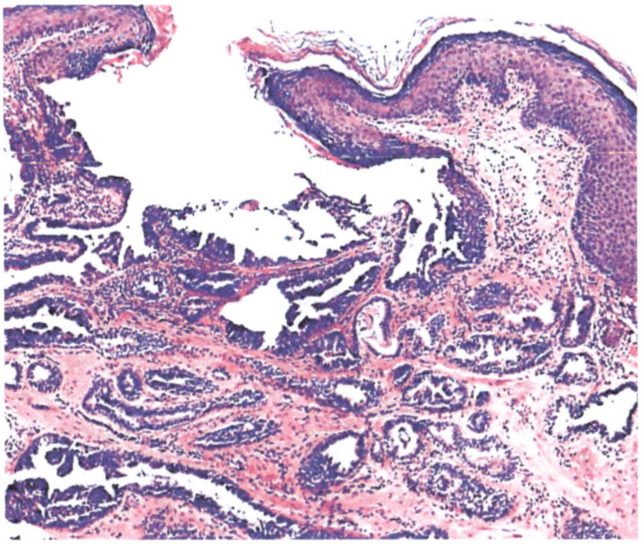

Erosive adenomatosis of the nipple (nipple adenoma). Ductular and papillary proliferations are centered on large ducts and lactiferous sinuses beneath the skin of the nipple.

In regard to the differential diagnosis, these lesions may be distinguished from **hidradenoma papilliferum** by their location and overlying connection to the epidermis. **Microcystic adnexal carcinoma**, as well as **tubular carcinoma of the breast**, must be considered in the differential diagnosis. The demonstration of muscle-specific actin-positive basal cells in each of the proliferating glands in **EAN** distinguishes it from those pathologic alternatives. **Paget disease of the nipple** is characterized by small clusters and solitary units of large epithelioid cells randomly scattered throughout the epidermis. It is considered in the clinical differential diagnosis, but not the histopathological differential diagnosis.

ANSWER 9-13: E.

Malignant eccrine poroma (porocarcinoma), malignant eccrine spiradenoma and cylindroma (carcinoma ex eccrine spiradenoma and cylindroma), malignant mixed tumor (malignant chondroid syringoma), and **malignant clear cell hidradenoma (clear cell hidradenocarcinoma)** may arise within long-standing benign counterparts. **Ductal apocrine adenocarcinoma, ductopapillary adenocarcinoma, eccrine ductal adenocarcinoma, syringoid eccrine carcinoma, microcystic adnexal carcinoma, primary cutaneous mucinous carcinoma, adenoid cystic carcinoma**, and **aggressive digital papillary adenocarcinoma** are known to only arise de novo without a benign precursor.

ANSWER 9-14: A.

Primary cutaneous adenoid cystic carcinoma (ACC) is an extremely rare neoplasm most commonly arising on the scalp or chest with a slow-growing yet locally aggressive behavior. Perineural invasion is very common. The tumor has counterparts in other organ systems such as the salivary gland, breast, and respiratory tract, and genitourinary tract; however, unlike the salivary gland tumors, primary cutaneous tumors have a local recurrence rate of 50%, but rarely metastasize.

This neoplasm is believed to demonstrate eccrine differentiation since it is composed of a "pure" population of monomorphic basaloid cells that are arranged in tubules, elongated nests, and cords. Ductal lumina may be formed by the neoplastic elements, or they may enclose "cylinders" or "pseudolumina" of mucoid matrix with a lightly basophilic hue that stains with Alcian blue. Another common feature is the deposition of linear profiles or globules of PAS-positive brightly eosinophilic basement membrane material in the intercellular spaces. Nuclei are compact, with dispersed chromatin and indistinct nucleoli; mitoses are sparse. Cytoplasm is scant and amphophilic. There is an absence of peripheral nuclear palisading and stromal retraction artifact. The cribriform nests described above are the most common growth pattern encountered and are the most diagnostically distinctive; however, tubular and solid forms exist. Immunohistochemistry reveals the tumor cells to express cytokeratin 7 and CD117 with "true luminal" staining for EMA and CEA, and "pseudoluminal" staining for SMA, p63, and S100.

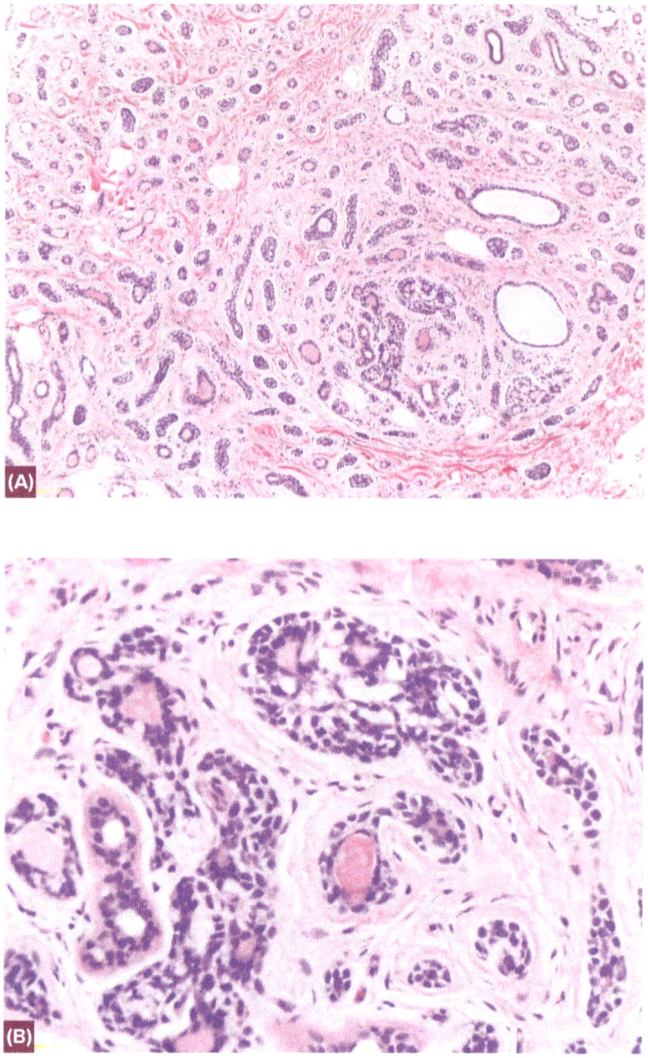

Adenoid cystic carcinoma, tubular pattern. (A) There are numerous tubules and cords with two cell layers infiltrating the dermis. **(B)** Focal cribriform formation and complex glandular structures are present.

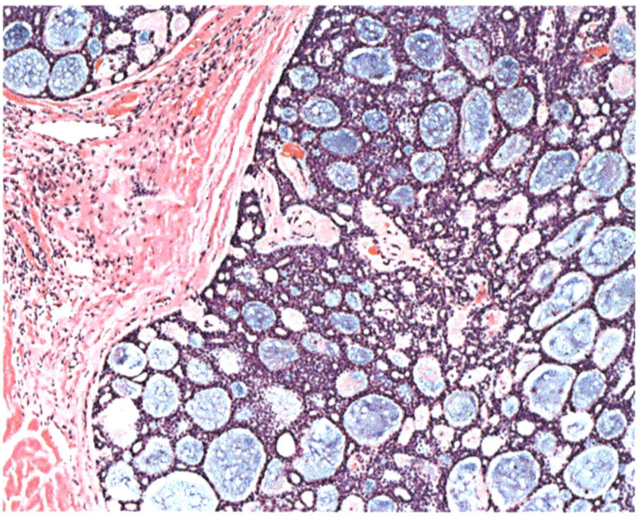

Adenoid cystic carcinoma, cribriform pattern. Large angular clusters of basaloid cells are dispersed in the dermis. Uniform, rounded cylinders (pseudolumens) containing dermal mucin and other stromal elements interrupt the monomorphic basaloid nests. Smaller true lumens are also present.

The differential diagnosis mainly includes **adenoid basal cell carcinoma,** which is associated with mutations in the tumor suppressor gene PTCH. Importantly, the dermal stroma adjacent to clusters of tumor cells in **ACC** does not show retraction artifact or fibromyxoid alteration, as seen in **basal cell carcinomas**. This is a crucial distinction because most tumors thought to be cutaneous **ACCs** are actually **adenoid BCCs**. The overall growth pattern of both of those tumor types is infiltrative, and permeation of vascular adventitia and perineural spaces is potentially common to both of them as well. Additional minor points of difference between **ACCs** and **adenoid BCCs** is that the latter neoplasm manifests the regular presence of apoptotic cells in the center of tumor cell nests and may even show cohesive foci of geographic necrosis, but those observations are rare in **ACCs**. Moreover, **BCCs** of all types commonly display evidence of multilinear differentiation (eg, a mixture of adenoid and pilar-keratotic foci) and may contain true melanin pigment. Such attributes are again not part of the morphologic spectrum of **ACC**. Whenever it is needed, immunostaining is again capable of distinguishing between these tumors; whereas **adenoid BCC** is epithelial membrane antigen (EMA) negative, **ACC** regularly expresses that marker. Moreover, immunoreactivity for keratin-7 or CD117 favors a diagnosis of **ACC**.

ANSWER 9-15: E.

The biopsy reveals solid nests and tubules containing papillary structures. At higher magnification, areas of mitotic activity are associated with atypical cells with vesicular nuclei and prominent nucleoli. The lumens contain eosinophilic gritty necrosis. The findings are consistent with high-grade **papillary digital eccrine adenocarcinoma** (Table 9-15A). In 1987, Kao and coworkers published the seminal description of a distinctive group of eccrine neoplasms that are unique to the distal extremities, particularly the digits. Although these tumors were originally segregated into two groups by those authors—as **"aggressive digital papillary adenomas"** and "**aggressive** digital **papillary adenocarcinomas**"—it is now considered that they represent points in the same continuum of what is basically a family of universally malignant neoplasms. Thus, the more unifying term of **papillary digital eccrine adenocarcinoma (PDEA)** in reference to such lesions is preferable. No benign precursor lesion exists for this malignant tumor as they always arise de novo. These tumors present as a solitary, firm, tan or pink, rubbery nodule on the acral extremities. Specifically, the most common location is the volar surface of the skin between the nail bed and distal interphalangeal joint, clinically mimicking a **digital mucous cyst**. While the lesions are generally asymptomatic, patients may experience pain, bleeding, ulceration, and rarely, limited range of motion. **PDEAs** are highly aggressive tumors with frequent local recurrence and metastases. The local recurrence rate is nearly 50% after surgical excision, with recurrence occurring as early as 2 months to 9 years. Metastases occur in approximately 15% of cases, with the most common site being the lung. Other sites of metastases include lymph nodes, brain, kidney, bone, or retroperitoneum. These tumors should be treated aggressively with excision or digital amputation. Annual monitoring for metastatic disease, including physical examination and chest x-ray, is recommended for 10 years after diagnosis.

On scanning microscopy, **PDEAs** feature the formation of macropapillae that project into large cystic spaces and, in addition, contain solid nests and tubules composed of polygonal cells that irregularly infiltrate the surrounding dermis and subcutis. Involvement of the underlying bone may sometimes be present as well. Nuclear characteristics are bimorphic; one subgroup of **PDEAs** (so-called **aggressive papillary digital adenomas/low-grade PDEA**) shows dispersed chromatin, small or indistinct nucleoli, and limited mitotic activity and may accordingly be considered as the low-grade member of the spectrum under consideration here. However, the second variant (**so-called aggressive digital papillary adenocarcinomas/high-grade PDEA**) manifests vesicular nuclei, prominent nucleoli, numerous atypical mitotic figures, and foci of spontaneous geographic necrosis. The latter tumor is a more poorly differentiated form of **PDEA**. Perineural and lymphatic invasion may be observed regardless of tumor grade, but only poorly differentiated tumors in this category will produce distant metastases. Squamous metaplasia, and clear, ovoid, possibly myoepithelial cells are seen more often in low-grade than in high-grade **PDEA**.

Table 9-15A. Papillary Digital Eccrine Adenocarcinoma

Clinical Features
- Elderly individuals
- Digits, palms, soles
- Firm nodules

Histopathologic Features
- Micropapillae projecting into cystic spaces
- Solid nests and tubules composed of polygonal cells
- Infiltration of surrounding tissue
- Nuclear features varying from dispersed chromatin and small nucleoli to vesicular nuclei with prominent nucleoli

Differential Diagnosis
- Hidradenoma papilliferum

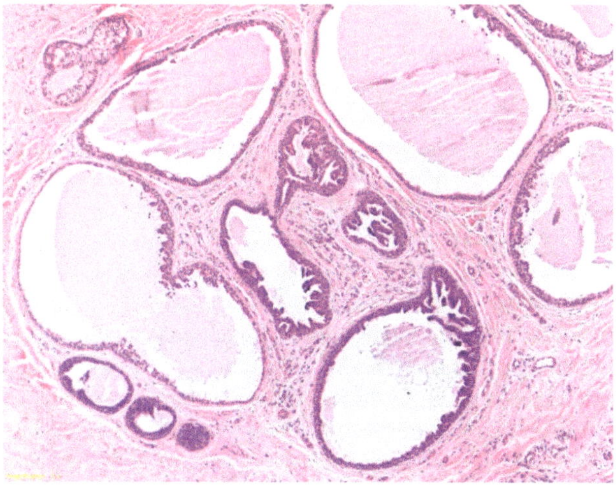

Papillary digital eccrine adenocarcinoma, low grade. The dilated tubules are lined by papillary and micropapillary structures. There is mild cytologic atypia and the lumens contain eosinophilic secretions and not gritty tumor necrosis. (Reproduced with permission from Desman GT, Ozerdem U, Shin SJ: Neighboring look-a-likes: distinguishing between breast and dermatologic lesions, Adv Anat Pathol 2014 Jul;21(4):228-247)

ANSWER 9-16: C.

The biopsy reveals a proliferation of solid cords and ductules composed of pleomorphic cellular elements. Infiltrative angular nests with numerous cribriform ducts are also present. Stromal desmoplasia is prominent. The combined clinical, histopathological, and immunohistochemical findings are consistent with **ductal eccrine carcinoma (DEA)** (Table 9-16A). **Ductal eccrine carcinoma** is perhaps the most common of the **de novo eccrine carcinomas.** Its histopathologic features are virtually identical to those seen in "conventional" **invasive ductal carcinoma of the breast**, metastases of which, for obvious reasons, represent the principal differential diagnostic consideration. Obtaining a detailed clinical history of the skin lesion in question is therefore most important. **DEA** is virtually always a solitary, slowly growing mass on the scalp, head, neck, or extremities that measures up to 5 cm in diameter and has been present for many months or even years before the patient seeks medical attention. In contrast, **metastases of mammary carcinoma** are typically multiple and occur in "crops" that manifest a rapid clinical evolution. The reason for emphasis on historical data is that, as one might expect, the detailed pathologic (ultrastructural and immunohistochemical) features of ductal breast and eccrine carcinomas are identical; this synonymity even extends to the expression of estrogen and progesterone receptors by both tumors. One distinguishing feature is that **DEAs** often express p63, and when present, is a helpful marker since mammary carcinomas are negative for p63. **DEA** is notable for a relatively high rate of metastasis, that is, approximately half of the cases metastasize.

The salient microscopic characteristics of **DEA** include the proliferation of solid cords or tubules of obviously atypical polygonal cells that randomly infiltrate the dermal connective tissue. Focal formation of ductal lumina is often apparent, and entrapped eccrine ducts may sometimes demonstrate the changes of carcinoma in situ. The intratumoral stroma is variably desmoplastic and may contain chronic inflammatory cells. When such features are prominent (as they are in only a minority of cases), one can be somewhat confident of the primary nature of the neoplasm; however, their absence does not conversely equate with a diagnosis of metastatic disease. Nuclear chromatin is either dense or vesicular, and prominent nucleoli are commonly present; mitotic activity is almost always appreciable but may be limited in scope. Cytoplasm is usually amphophilic, and small intracytoplasmic vacuoles may be evident; well-defined areas of overtly squamoid differentiation are sometimes seen in **DEA** as well, such that differential diagnosis with a form of **squamous cell carcinoma** may be considered.

One variant of **DEA** that is site related has been termed **ductal eccrine adenocarcinoma with fibromyxoid stroma (DEAFS).** In the past, this lesion was probably included under the rubrics of **malignant chondroid syringoma** or **syringoid carcinoma**, and occurs more commonly on the distal extremities (particularly the sole of the foot). As its name implies, **DEAFS** differs from "usual" **DEA** by its possession of a uniformly fibromyxoid stroma that recalls one of the attributes of **cutaneous mixed tumor**. Other peculiarities of this tumoral subtype are its ability to communicate with the surface epithelium in a similar manner to that of **poroma** and to be composed of compact, almost basaloid cells. Because of the concatenation of these features (ie, a fibromyxoid matrix and an epidermal connection to cords of relatively small polyhedral cells), a mistaken diagnosis of **BCC** may also be rendered in such cases. When selected circumstances (such as limited,

Table 9-16A. Ductal Eccrine Adenocarcinoma

Clinical Features
Solitary, slow-growing tumor
≤5 cm in diameter
Approximately 50% metastatic
Histopathologic Features
Solid cords and tubules of polygonal cells
Ductal structures
Variable squamous differentiation
Infiltrating features
Variably desmoplastic stroma
Cytologic atypia
Mitotic figures usually readily apparent
Differential Diagnosis
Metastatic adenocarcinoma, particularly breast carcinoma
Basal cell carcinoma
Squamous cell carcinoma

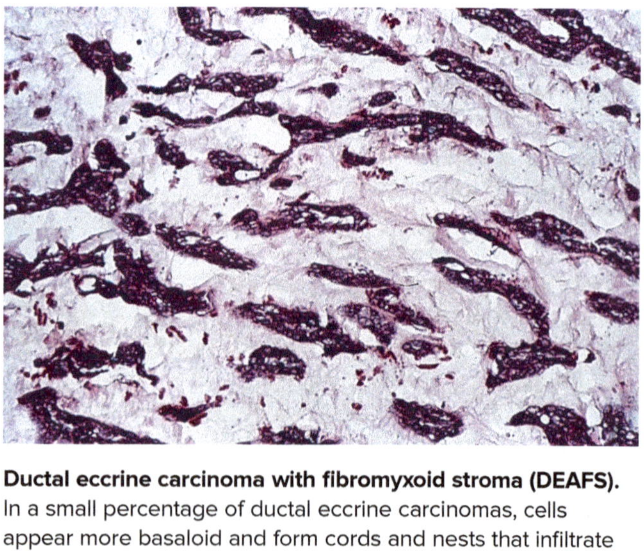

Ductal eccrine carcinoma with fibromyxoid stroma (DEAFS). In a small percentage of ductal eccrine carcinomas, cells appear more basaloid and form cords and nests that infiltrate a fibromyxoid matrix.

artifactually distorted biopsy material) make it necessary, the latter problem can be addressed by performing immunostains for EMA. Virtually all forms of sweat gland carcinoma are EMA positive, but BCCs are consistently nonreactive for that determinant.

Malignant degeneration within preexisting **eccrine cylindromas** and **spiradenomas** has been well documented. These lesions clinically present as a rapid expansion within a previously indolent cutaneous nodule of long standing, with or without ulceration or pain. For this diagnosis to be accepted pathologically, there must be remnants of the "parent" lesion along with a carcinomatous component in the excised tissue, or one must be able to confirm that a banal cylindroma or spiradenoma was removed previously from the exact site at which a sweat gland carcinoma is now present. The malignant elements most often assume the character of an undifferentiated carcinoma, showing sheets or clusters of nondescript but highly anaplastic epithelioid, stellate, or fusiform tumor cells with marked anisonucleosis, nucleolar prominence, cellular pleomorphism, and brisk mitotic activity. As such, the image of a "sarcomatoid" carcinoma may be encountered. Less commonly, more definable carcinoma morphotypes are reflected in the malignant components of **carcinoma ex cylindroma** or **spiradenoma (CECS)**; these may include **squamous carcinoma** or **pure adenocarcinoma** (Table 9-16B). One behavioral peculiarity of **CECS** merits some attention; that is, there may be an inexplicable disparity between the grade of the carcinomatous elements and the biologic evolution of the neoplasm. Several examples have been reported in which highly undifferentiated forms of CECS were attended by a lack of metastasis and long-term disease-free survival.

Table 9-16B. Carcinoma Ex Dermal Cylindroma and Eccrine Spiradenoma

Clinical Features
Long-standing lesion with recent enlargement, ulceration, pain
Common disparity between high-grade appearance of tumor and lack of aggressive behavior
Histopathologic Features
Remnant of benign cylindroma or spiradenoma
Anaplastic epithelium in sheets or nests
Epithelioid, stellate, or fusiform tumor cells with pronounced cytologic atypia
Resemblance to squamous cell carcinoma, adenosquamous carcinoma, adenocarcinoma, clear cell adenocarcinoma, sarcomatoid carcinoma
Prominent mitotic rate
Differential Diagnosis
Any anaplastic tumor

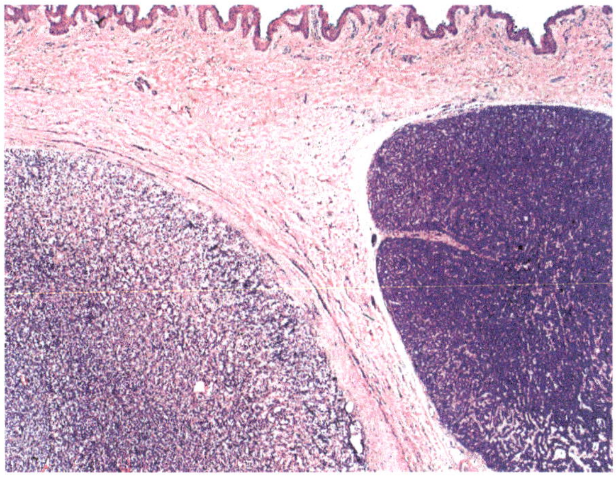

Carcinoma ex eccrine spiradenoma. Invasive carcinoma is juxtaposed with residual benign spiradenoma.

ANSWER 9-17: D.

The biopsy reveals an infiltrative epithelial proliferation extending downward from the epidermal surface. The invasive component at the base of the specimen is composed of pleomorphic nests and cords of epithelial cells with eosinophilic cytoplasm. Numerous mitoses and necrotic tumor cells are present. The tumor contains numerous duct-like structures. The findings are consistent with **eccrine porocarcinoma** (Table 9-17A). **Eccrine porocarcinoma** presents

Table 9-17A. Eccrine Porocarcinoma

Clinical Features
Older individuals, often >60 years
Lower extremities, head and neck, upper extremities, trunk
Verrucous papule or nodule ≤5 cm in diameter
High rate of local recurrence
Regional lymph node metastases
Tendency to multiple epidermotropic metastases
Histopathologic Features
Many features in common with poroma
Infiltrative features
Desmoplastic stroma often
Tumor necrosis
Cytologic atypia
Mitoses
Extensive clear cell change frequent
Differential Diagnosis
Eccrine poroma
Squamous cell carcinoma
Malignant acrospiroma
Malignant trichilemmoma
Amelanotic melanoma

as a verrucous plaque or nodule with frequent ulceration, commonly measuring up to 5 cm in diameter and localized to the lower extremities, head and neck, upper extremities, and trunk. In general, these tumors tend to present in older individuals, most frequently in the seventh decade of life. In many cases, there is a history of a relatively long-standing lesion. The onset of rapid growth and pain should raise suspicion for malignancy. **Eccrine porocarcinomas** are notable for the high frequency of local recurrence, regional lymph node metastases, and a peculiar tendency for multiple epidermotropic metastases. **Eccrine porocarcinoma** is closely related clinically and histopathologically to ordinary **eccrine poroma**. The points of histologic dissimilarity between the benign and malignant lesions in this category include the presence in **porocarcinomas** of infiltrative growth (with desmoplastic stromal response); spontaneous tumor necrosis; obvious global cytologic anaplasia with high nucleus-to-cytoplasmic ratios and nucleolation; extensive clear cell change; or perineural or vascular invasion. Not all those features need to be present to assign a diagnosis of malignancy; in fact, infiltrative growth is sufficient unto itself in this regard. Akalin and colleagues have shown that both **poroma** and **porocarcinoma** may demonstrate mutant p53 protein immunohistochemically; thus, that determinant is not useful in a distinction between the two tumor types. As expected, **invasive porocarcinoma** may have both intraepidermal (hidroacanthoma simplex like) and dermal components (dermal duct tumor like). However, unlike the case in question, a solely intraepidermal form of the tumor has been recognized (termed **malignant hidroacanthoma simplex**) that falls into the category of Borst-Jadassohn lesions. As such, it shows the clonal, micronodular growth of atypical polygonal cells within the surface epithelium, yielding nests of tumor cells that are sharply marginated from adjacent keratinocytes. In these cases where luminal structures are not apparent, it may be necessary to perform immunohistochemical stains, in which case **porocarcinoma** is positive for CEA and S100 and other histologic look-alikes such as clonal **Bowen disease (squamous cell carcinoma in situ)** or **seborrheic keratosis** are negative for CEA and S100. **Melanoma in situ** may resemble these intraepithelial tumors but are CEA negative and S-100 protein positive. In addition, the scattering of single malignant cells throughout the epidermis—as typically seen in **Paget disease** of the skin or **amelanotic superficial spreading malignant melanoma**—is not a feature of **porocarcinoma**. The last of these considerations is particularly important in cases of **porocarcinoma** in which the neoplastic cells acquire melanin pigment (often causing clinicians to make a diagnosis of melanoma), a well-recognized but rare potentiality of that tumor. **Metastatic carcinomas** involving the epidermis have only reported in a few cases and are considered exceptionally rare. In any event, recent publications have suggested that immunohistochemical staining for keratins 5/6, p63 protein, and podoplanin (D2-40) might be useful in the differential diagnosis of adnexal carcinoma versus metastatic carcinoma in the skin. All three of those markers are more often observed in primary cutaneous adnexal tumors.

In regard to the differential diagnosis, mainly intraepidermal forms of **porocarcinoma** must be distinguished from **hidroacanthoma simplex, squamous cell carcinoma in situ, mammary and extramammary Paget disease**, and **melanoma**. Deeper forms of the tumor must be distinguished from **invasive squamous cell carcinoma, malignant acrospiroma (hidradenocarcinoma),** and **cutaneous metastasis**. In general, **eccrine porocarcinoma** is characterized by a small cuboidal cell population as opposed to somewhat larger cells in conventional **squamous cell carcinoma**. **Porocarcinoma** also shows prominent ductal or tubular structures. Squamous cell carcinomas may have acantholytic foci, but lack true luminal structures. Immunohistochemical staining with CEA may be helpful in these cases, which will highlight the luminal foci. While CK7 is positive in eccrine epithelium and negative in squamous epithelium, poorly differentiated squamous cell carcinomas may positively express CK7 in approximately 25% of cases; therefore this marker should be used with caution in differentiating between invasive porocarcinoma and poorly differentiated squamous cell carcinomas. **Porocarcinomas** also have more frequent epidermal involvement as opposed to a more prevalent dermal location of **malignant acrospiroma (hidradenocarcinoma)**. Finally, in rare instances, **cutaneous metastases** must be differentiated from **porocarcinoma**. Careful clinicopathologic correlation may be needed to arrive at a final diagnosis.

ANSWER 9-18: A.

The biopsy reveals small, rounded, or syringoid profiles consisting of basaloid and squamoid cells, some with keratinization. The tubules loosely infiltrate a markedly sclerotic dermis. As the tumor cells infiltrate into the deeper dermis they become markedly smaller and widely scattered. The findings are consistent with **microcystic adnexal carcinoma** (Table 9-18A). **Microcystic adnexal carcinoma (MAC),** also referred to as **sclerosing sweat duct carcinoma, malignant syringoma,** or **syringoid carcinoma**, is a malignant tumor with mixed eccrine and pilar differentiation. They usually present as a solitary indurated plaque or nodule involving the face, particularly the upper lip, but also in other locations such as the axilla. These tumors are generally perceived as slow-growing indolent tumors and may develop in individuals of any age, but especially in young women. The rate of local recurrence approaches 50%, but true metastasis is vanishingly rare, if it truly exists at all. A causal association with prior therapeutic irradiation has been noted in the past several years.

Microscopically, **MAC** is composed of syringoma-like profiles of bland cuboidal epithelial cells, generally lacking nucleoli and mitotic activity, which infiltrate the dermis and subcutis in a random and permeative fashion. These cellular aggregates are occasionally punctuated by microcystic arrays containing pilar-type (trichilemmal) keratin. Infiltration of perineural sheaths, vascular adventitia, and even subjacent muscle is a common finding. The neoplastic cells may focally aggregate themselves into whorled, concentric profiles in

Table 9-18A. Microcystic Adnexal Carcinoma

Clinical Features
- Adults, age 20-76 years
- Women = men
- Face, especially upper lip, axilla
- Slowly developing indurated plaque or nodule
- Skin-colored, yellowish
- Local recurrence common
- Metastasis rare

Histopathologic Features
- Small epithelial aggregates with keratinous cysts, especially superficially
- Solid epithelial islands and cords, some with lumina
- Fibrotic to densely sclerotic stroma
- Deeply invasive with frequent infiltration of subcutis, skeletal muscle, and nerves
- Minimal or low-grade atypia
- Mitotic figures generally uncommon

Differential Diagnosis
- Syringoma
- Desmoplastic trichoepithelioma
- Morpheaform basal cell carcinoma
- Papillary eccrine adenoma

the dermis. Secretory material can also be observed in the lumina of the syringoma-like foci. Interestingly, despite the obviously aggressive nature of this tumor, it lacks the immunohistochemical expression of markers (such as p53 protein, Ki-67, bcl-2, and c-erbB-2 protein) that usually correlate with adverse biologic behavior. In accord with the general capacity for divergent differentiation in **MAC**, it should come as no surprise that occasional examples demonstrate sebaceous foci as well as eccrine and pilar elements.

The differential diagnosis of **MAC** does not include **metastatic carcinomas of visceral origin**, since metastases would be expected to show a more confined growth pattern and a higher degree of cytologic anaplasia. Instead, other lesions that must be considered include **conventional syringoma, desmoplastic trichoepithelioma** (DTE), **morpheaform/desmoplastic basal cell carcinoma** (BCC), and **primary adenosquamous carcinoma** (ASC) of the skin. Both conventional **syringoma** and **DTE** are distinguishable from **MAC** simply by attention to adequate clinical information. All are predominantly facial lesions, but whereas the first two tumors are small, exquisitely circumscribed papulonodular lesions, **MAC** is an ill-defined fixed plaque. **Syringomas** commonly present as multiple clustered papules, in contrast to a solitary lesion. Analogous to the clinical presentation, microscopically **syringoma** and **DTE** show a profile in which the dermal tumor is broader than it

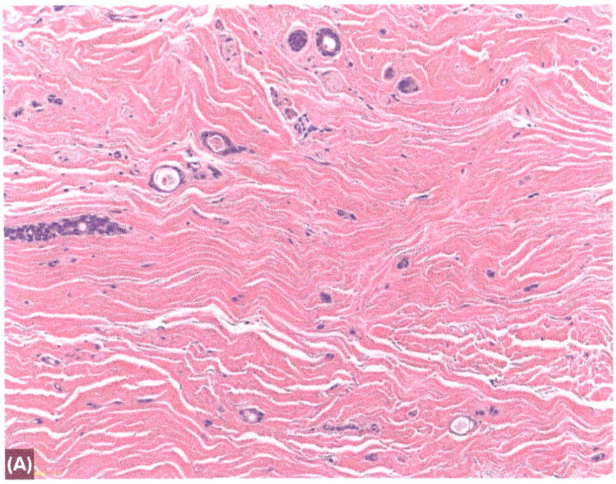

Reproduced with permission from Desman GT, Ozerdem U, Shin SJ: Neighboring look-a-likes: distinguishing between breast and dermatologic lesions, Adv Anat Pathol 2014 Jul;21(4):228-247

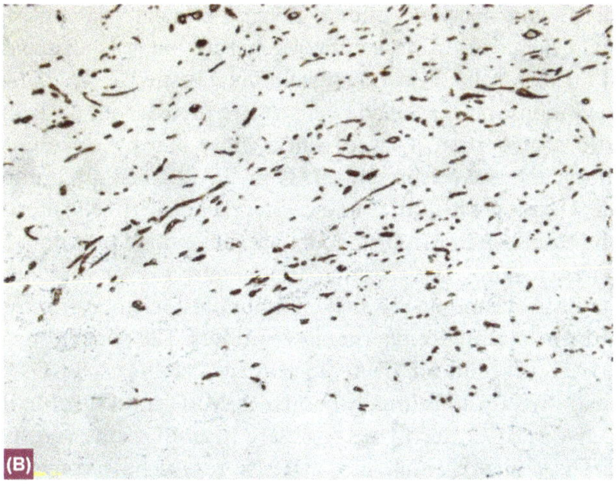

Microcystic adnexal carcinoma. (A) At the deep portion of the tumor small cords and nests are identified scattered throughout a sclerotic dermis. **(B)** Immunohistochemical stain for pan-cytokeratin highlights the extent of tumor invasion throughout the dermis.

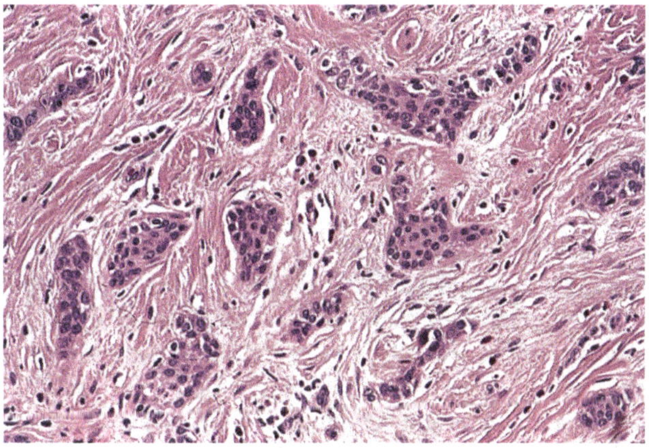

Microcystic adnexal carcinoma. The absence of microcysts typifies a subset of microcystic adnexal carcinomas. Small angular clusters in these lesions are associated with a desmoplastic stromal response. The term ***sclerosing sweat duct carcinoma*** has been applied to such tumors.

is deep, with sharply defined peripheral borders. In contrast, **MAC** extends to the base of even generous biopsy specimens and "trickles off" into the surrounding tissue. Given these observations, one can readily appreciate the wisdom of diagnostic equivocation if faced with a shave biopsy containing a tumor that may represent **MAC** in the absence of clinical data. **Desmoplastic BCC** shows more branched solid nests than those seen in **MAC**, and luminal differentiation is not an apparent feature. Rarely, tumor-stromal retraction artifact may be seen in **desmoplastic BCC**. Immunohistochemical stains may be helpful in deciphering these tumors. The ductular foci of **MAC** will stain for CEA, whereas the keratocysts of **DTE** are negative. CK15 is usually positive in **MAC** and **DTE**, but is negative in **BCC**. Ber-EP4 is expressed in all **BCCs**, a majority of **DTEs**, and rarely in **MACs**. CD23 expression has a converse utility. P63 expression should be seen in all tumor cells of **DTE** and **BCC**, whereas only the basolateral cells are positive in **MAC**. **DTE** contains CK20-positive Merkel cells scattered throughout the tumor, which are absent in **MAC** and **BCC**.

ANSWER 9-19: D.

Apocrine adenocarcinomas are most frequent in the breast and are rare in the skin. In skin, they are typically found in regions endowed with apocrine glands such as the axilla and anogenital region. The ceruminous glands of the external auditory meatus and Moll glands of the eyelids are modified apocrine glands. They may be seen arising on the scalp in association with nevus sebaceus. **Apocrine adenocarcinomas** have been reported to occur at other various sites, but only in isolated cases. Cases of **bilateral axillary apocrine adenocarcinoma** associated with **apocrine hyperplasia** have been reported, as well as carcinomas arising within **tubular apocrine adenomas** and **syringocystadenoma papilliferum**. Intralymphatic cutaneous metastatic disease similar to that of **inflammatory breast carcinoma** has also been described. These tumors occur in the elderly with a very high frequency of metastasis. The main differential diagnosis is **metastatic apocrine breast carcinoma**. **Apocrine adenocarcinomas** characteristically exhibit morphologic plasticity often revealing foci with variable differentiation, making the distinction of **primary cutaneous carcinoma** versus **cutaneous metastasis** extremely difficult. In general there are four types of apocrine carcinoma with reproducible histomorphology. Two forms may be reliably diagnosed as primary cutaneous malignancies: **ductopapillary apocrine carcinoma (DPAC)** (Table 9-19A) and the **apocrine type of extramammary Paget disease**. The other two forms closely mimic metastatic adenocarcinoma: **ductal apocrine adenocarcinoma (DAA)** and **primary signet ring cell carcinoma** of the skin. Unfortunately both **primary cutaneous apocrine adenocarcinomas** and **metastatic mammary adenocarcinomas** are typically negative for p63, unlike most cutaneous sweat gland neoplasms, and both tumors typically express GCFP-15. **Ductal apocrine adenocarcinoma (DAA)** is composed of infiltrative tubules (with occasional cribriform architecture), cords, and single cells with distinct cell borders, abundant pink dPAS+ cytoplasm with decapitation secretion, atypical central to eccentric vesicular nuclei, and prominent nucleoli. The myoepithelial layer is generally absent in the regions of infiltration and may be highlighted by a negative actin-smooth muscle stain. Some lesions may show continuity with the overlying epidermis with intraepidermal spread manifesting as **Paget disease**. Micropapillary structures within **ductopapillary apocrine adenocarcinomas (DPAC)** are a feature favoring primary cutaneous origin since **metastatic mammary adenocarcinoma** typically lacks this feature. Additionally, **breast adenocarcinomas** tend to be positive for

Quick Fact

- **Histopathological Dx of Primary Apocrine Adenocarcinoma**
  - Ductopapillary apocrine adenocarcinoma
  - Extramammary Paget disease, apocrine type
- **Histopathological Dx Indistinguishable from Metastatic Mammary Adenocarcinoma**
  - Ductal apocrine adenocarcinoma
  - Primary signet ring cell adenocarcinoma

Table 9-19A. Ductopapillary Apocrine Carcinoma

Clinical Features
Older individuals
Eyelids, axillae, genitoperineal skin
Solitary multinodular lesion, usually a few cm in diameter
Association with nevus sebaceus and extramammary Paget disease
Frequent lymph node metastases and visceral metastases in 40% of cases
Histopathologic Features
Similar to digital papillary eccrine carcinoma
Polygonal cells with finely granular eosinophilic cytoplasm
Often decapitation secretion
Infiltration of surrounding tissue
Cytologic atypia and mitoses
Prussian blue iron stain positive in 40%-50%
Gross cystic disease fluid protein-15 positive
Differential Diagnosis
Digital papillary eccrine carcinoma
Hidradenoma papilliferum

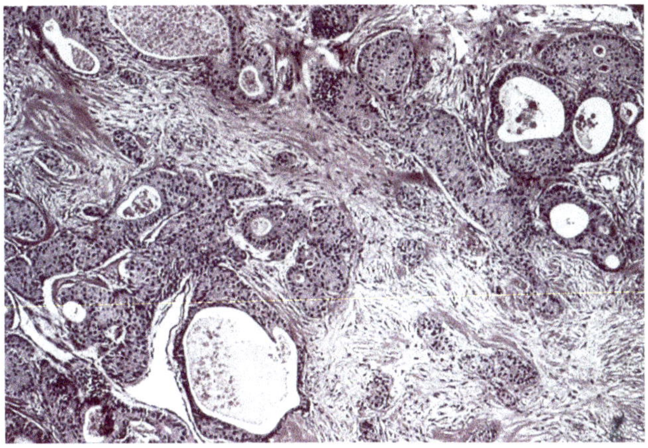

Ductopapillary apocrine adenocarcinoma. Note the infiltrative glands composed of atypical cells with abundant eosinophilic cytoplasm.

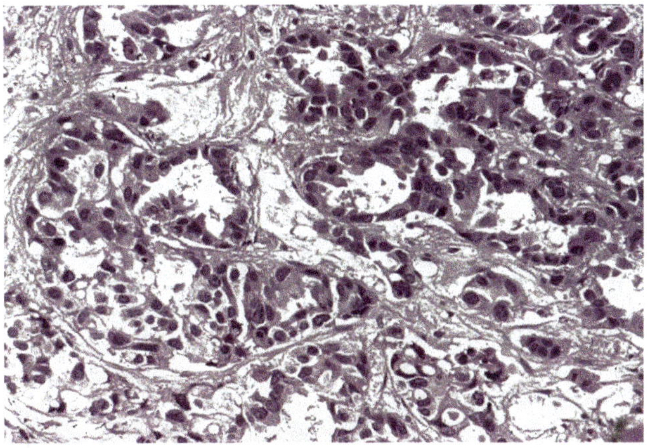

Ductopapillary apocrine adenocarcinoma. Note the micropapillary structures within the glandular lumens.

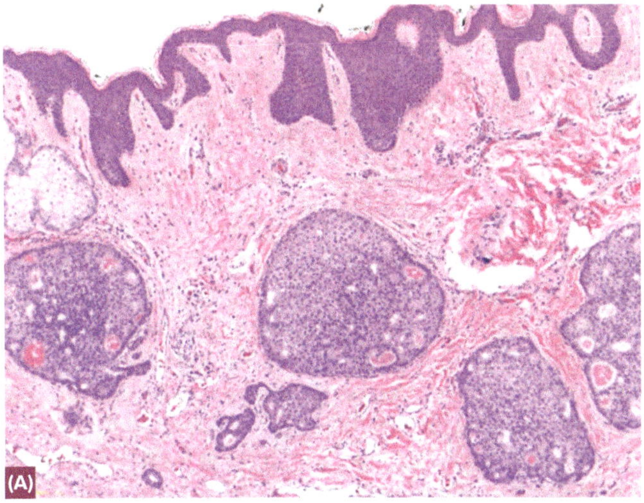

Reproduced with permission from Desman GT, Ozerdem U, Shin SJ: Neighboring look-a-likes: distinguishing between breast and dermatologic lesions, Adv Anat Pathol 2014 Jul;21(4):228-247

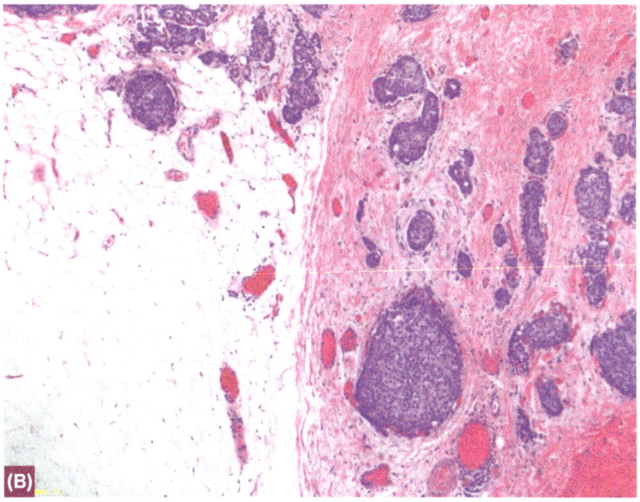

Ductal apocrine adenocarcinoma. (A) Solid and cribriform nests are present in the dermis with focal areas of infiltrative growth. **(B)** The tumor is seen invading into the underlying subcutaneous fat, identical to the growth pattern seen in mammary carcinoma.

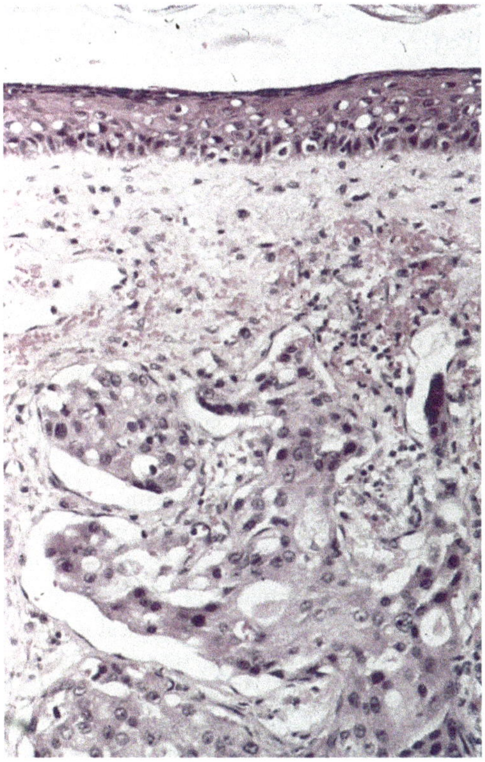

Ductal apocrine carcinoma. Vascular infiltration is a common feature in apocrine carcinomas.

ER and PR, whereas **primary cutaneous adenocarcinomas** tend to be positive for AR. Lastly, **primary cutaneous apocrine adenocarcinomas** frequently contain iron granules, which are absent in **metastatic mammary adenocarcinomas**. Clinical correlation is required for definitive distinction.

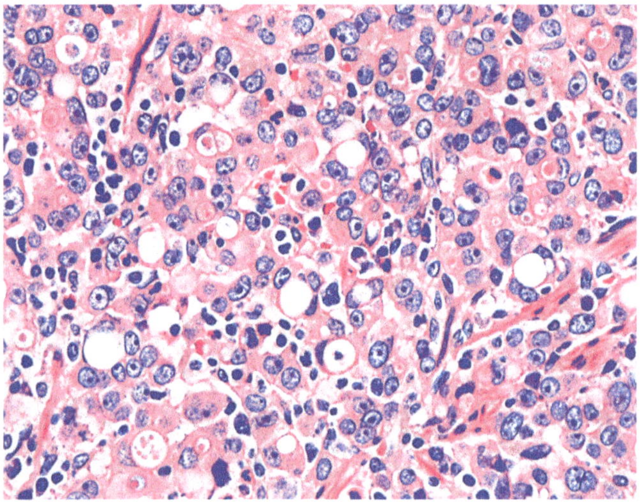

Primary signet ring-cell carcinoma of the skin. Intracytoplasmic mucin droplets displace the nucleus, yielding the characteristic signet ring cell appearance.

Table 9-20A. Mucinous Carcinoma of the Skin

Clinical Features
Older individuals (50-70 years)
Head and neck, especially eyelids, scalp
Skin-colored or discolored nodule ≤3 cm in diameter
Recurrences common
Low rate of metastasis
Histopathologic Features
Aggregates of epithelial cells in lakes of mucin
Epithelial nests may be solid, contain lumina, or show cribriform patterns
Minimal cytologic atypia
Mitoses uncommon
Differential Diagnosis
Metastases from the breast, gastrointestinal tract, and ovary (unlikely)
Myxoid melanoma

ANSWER 9-20: D.

Primary cutaneous mucinous carcinoma is a distinctive tumor often presenting on the face and especially the eyelids as a skin-colored or occasionally slightly discolored nodule, measuring up to 3 cm in diameter (Table 9-20A). In many cases, the tumor has a soft or sponge-like consistency. The vast majority of tumors develop in older individuals in the sixth and seventh decades of life. It is possible that these tumors may be more common in men and African Americans. In general, **mucinous carcinoma** is prone to local recurrence but has a relatively low rate of regional lymph node metastasis. These tumors arise de novo without an associated benign counterpart, making histopathological distinction from **colloid carcinoma of the breast** extremely difficult when they arise in the axilla. Occasionally connection with the overlying epidermis provides the evidence for primary cutaneous derivation. The typical histopathologic features include large extracellular pools of epithelial mucin in the dermis and occasionally the subcutis. The mucin pools typically dissect through the tissue and contain irregular nests and small clusters of amphophilic polygonal cells with oval nuclei and small nucleoli. Mitoses and perineural and lymphovascular invasion are rare. The mucin stains with mucicarmine, colloidal iron, Alcian blue, and PAS with diastase. Immunohistochemistry reveals the tumor cells to express CK7, p63, GCFP-15, ER, and PR. Cutaneous metastases of **mucinous carcinoma of gastrointestinal, breast,** and **ovarian origin** are almost nonexistent. Additionally, **colloid carcinomas of the breast** and **mucinous gastrointestinal carcinomas** are typically negative for p63. Similar to **colloid carcinomas of the breast, cutaneous mucinous carcinoma** may show neuroendocrine differentiation immunohistochemically, with reactivity for such markers as synaptophysin and chromogranin in the tumor cells.

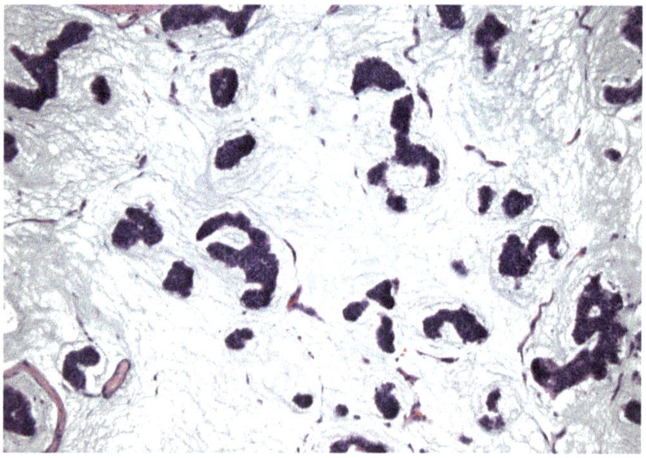

Mucinous carcinoma of the skin. Mucin pools dissect through the dermis. As in mucinous carcinomas in other sites, cords of malignant epithelial cells may only sparsely populate areas of the lesion.

ANSWER 9-21: A.

The biopsy reveals large epithelioid cells with clear cytoplasm scattered singly and in clusters throughout the epidermis. The nuclei are large and pleomorphic. The cytoplasm contains basophilic vacuoles, consistent with epithelial mucin. The combined clinical, histopathological, and immunohistochemical findings are consistent with **primary extramammary Paget disease**. Today's conventional dogma still teaches that **mammary Paget disease** and **extramammary Paget disease** of the skin represents two separate diseases (Table 9-21A). Whereas **mammary Paget disease (MPD)** is said to emanate from the "migration" of neoplastic cells into the epidermis

Table 9-21A. Mammary and Extramammary Paget Disease

MAMMARY	PRIMARY EXTRAMAMMARY
Clinical Features	
Age 40-60 years	Often age 50 years
Women >> men	Women ≥ men
Nipple and areolae	Vulva, penis and scrotum, perineum, umbilicus, axillae, eyelid, ear canal
Erythematous oozing or scaling plaque	Erythematous oozing or scaling plaque
Histopathologic Features	
Hyperkeratosis, parakeratosis	
Epidermal hyperplasia	
Epidermis permeated by aggregates of polygonal cells and single cells with abundant pale-staining or eosinophilic cytoplasm	
Lumen formation may occur	
Vesicular nuclei with prominent nucleoli	
Intracellular mucin stained by PAS-D, mucicarmine, Alcian blue in 50%-60% of cases	
Immunoreactivity for CEA, GCDFP-15, and keratin-7	
Differential Diagnosis	
Squamous cell carcinoma in situ	
Pagetoid melanoma	

from an underlying carcinoma of the breast, **extramammary Paget disease (EPD)** is thought to originate within the epidermis by the proliferation of primitive native stem (basal) cells with the potential for glandular differentiation. It must be acknowledged that other cellular lineages are occasionally manifested in **Paget disease,** including sebaceous, eccrine, and visceral-enteric pathways. However, these account for a small minority of cases.

Mammary Paget disease is a rare neoplastic phenomenon where solitary and occasionally small clusters of malignant glandular cells colonize the skin of the nipple. It is almost always associated with an underlying **breast adenocarcinoma,** and therefore generally believed to represent epidermotropic metastasis to the skin. **Extramammary Paget disease** typically involves the vulva, perianal region, scrotum, and occasionally the penis. The pathogenesis of **extramammary Paget disease** remains controversial and some authors have tried to further divide this condition into either primary or secondary forms. Lesions of **primary extramammary Paget disease** are not associated with an underlying adenocarcinoma and hence some propose that the malignant cells originate within the epidermis by the proliferation of primitive native stem cells with the potential for glandular differentiation. The malignant cells exhibit features of apocrine differentiation, and therefore other authors argue in favor of a unifying concept for primary cutaneous origin. **Secondary extramammary Paget disease** is most commonly attributed to **epidermotropic metastasis of colorectal** or **urothelial carcinomas.** Rarely mentioned in the literature is the fact that many **primary cutaneous malignant adnexal neoplasms** may seed epidermotropic metastases to the skin. The most common of these tumors are **apocrine carcinomas;** however, **sebaceous carcinomas** and **eccrine carcinomas** have been reported to manifest **Paget disease.** The most common location for **sweat carcinoma-associated Paget disease** is the axilla. Clinically, both mammary **Paget disease** and **extramammary Paget disease** present as red and eczematous scaling lesions on the involved areas of skin. The histopathologic features for all types include scattered large epithelioid cells arranged in the epidermis in a "buckshot" distribution. The cells are dispersed singly or in small clusters, have pale amphophilic and vacuolated cytoplasm, and contain eccentrically placed nuclei with vesicular chromatin. The overlying epidermis is frequently acanthotic with overlying hyperkeratosis. The histochemical stains PAS, mucicarmine, and Alcian blue will usually highlight intracytoplasmic mucin. Immunohistochemical stains reveal the tumor cells of **mammary Paget disease** and **primary extramammary Paget disease** to express AE1/AE3, CK7, CAM 5.2, and EMA. Staining for CEA is variable. GCFP-15 is usually positive in mammary and primary extramammary Paget disease but negative in secondary disease. The forms of Paget disease with apocrine differentiation (**mammary, primary extramammary, and apocrine carcinoma associated**) are typically negative for p63 expression. Additionally, the majority of these cases are also negative for PR and ER, but are positive for AR and Her-2/neu. **Secondary extramammary Paget disease** attributed to epidermotropic metastasis of **colorectal adenocarcinoma** and **urothelial carcinoma** will be CK7 negative/CK20 positive and CK7 positive/CK20 positive, respectively. While **colorectal adenocarcinomas** are also p63 negative, the majority of **urothelial carcinomas** are p63 positive.

Quick Fact

- **Mammary Paget disease**
  - CK7+, CK20−, p63−
- **Primary extramammary Paget disease (apocrine differentiation)**
  - CK7+, CK20−, p63−

<u>Secondary Paget disease:</u>

- **Epidermotropic colorectal adenocarcinoma**
  - CK7−, CK20+, p63−
- **Epidermotropic urothelial carcinoma**
  - CK7+, CK20+, p63+
- **Epidermotropic cutaneous apocrine carcinoma**
  - CK7+, CK20−, p63−

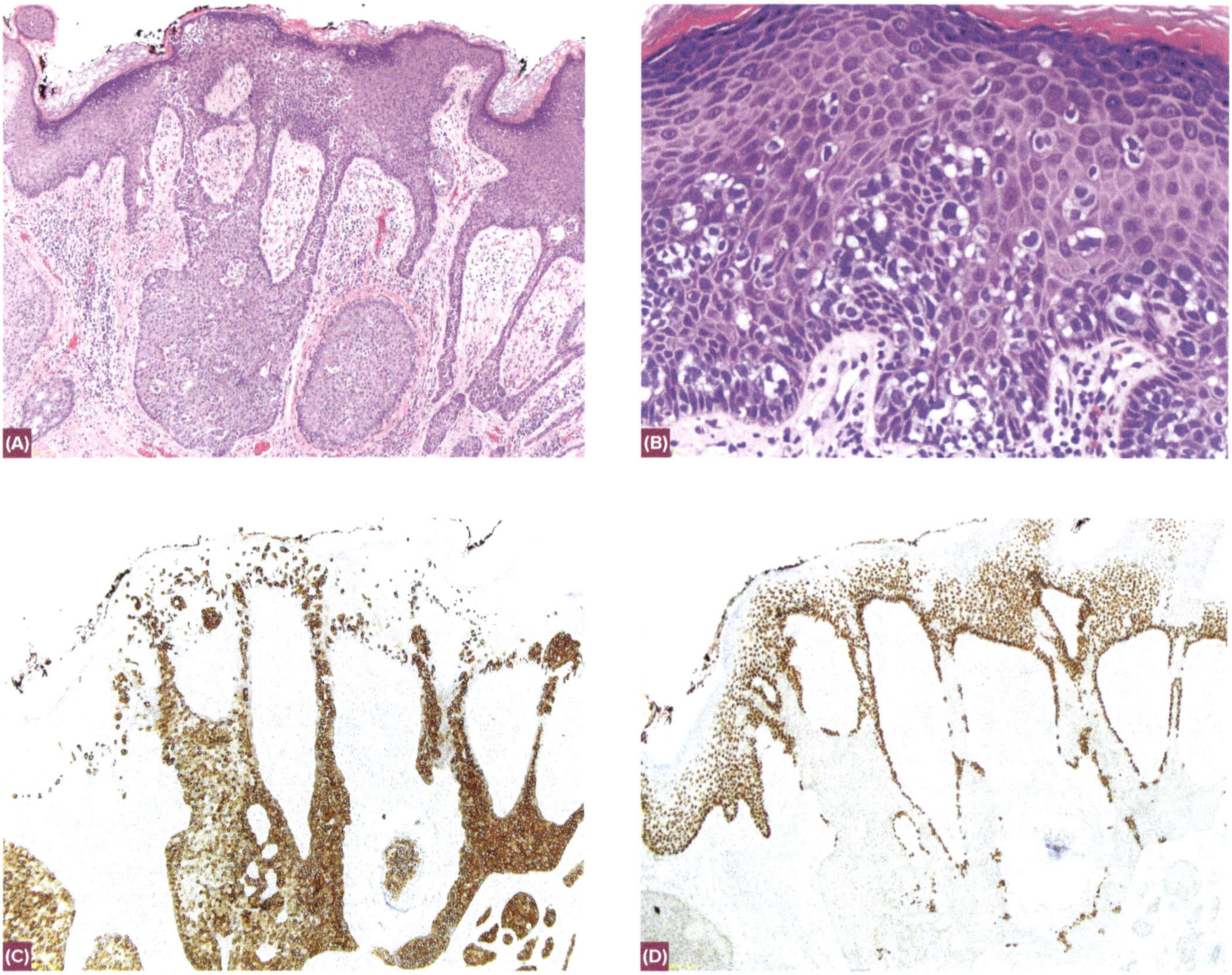

Ductal apocrine carcinoma with overlying Paget disease of the axilla. **(A)** The dermis contains a ductal apocrine adenocarcinoma where the malignant cells are seen colonizing the sweat ducts and infiltrating the epidermis in a scattered "buckshot" distribution. **(B)** Malignant epithelioid cells are scattered throughout the epidermis with a distinct cytomorphology from the adjacent keratinocytes. **(C)** The tumor cells are strongly and diffusely positive for CK7. **(D)** The epidermal keratinocytes and peripheral lining cells of the sweat ducts express p63, but the tumor cells are negative.

ANSWER 9-22: B.

Sebaceous hyperplasia (SH) usually presents on the face or eyelids, but occasionally affects the mammary areola or genital skin with the potential for confluence (Table 9-22A). The lesion may also clinically resemble the papulonodular profile of **basal cell carcinoma (BCC),** and rare forms have been termed **linear (zosteriform) or giant solitary sebaceous hyperplasia (SH).** Because **SH** does not involute clinically, most pathologists believe that it is probably a benign neoplasm rather than a form of hyperplasia.

Microscopically, one may define SH by the presence of four or more sebaceous lobules attached to the infundibulum of each hair follicle-sebaceous unit seen in the biopsy specimen. The cells comprising the lobules are predominantly fully mature sebocytes, showing compact nuclei and abundant multivacuolated clear cytoplasms. However, a thin rim of solitary basaloid cells is often present at the periphery of the sebocytic aggregates. The overlying epidermis may be atrophic in unusually expansive examples of **SH**. By definition the sebaceous lobules do not connect directly with the epidermal surface.

In regard to the differential diagnosis, the primary entities to be considered are **sebaceous adenoma (SA)** and **nevus sebaceus (NS).** The lobules of both **SA** and **NS** connect directly

Table 9-22A. Sebaceous Hyperplasia

Clinical Features
Older individuals
Face, mammary areola, genital skin
Yellowish to tan papules, often umbilicated
Rare linear or giant forms
Histopathologic Features
Single follicular canal opens to umbilicated epidermal surface
Four or more sebaceous lobules attached to central infundibulum of sebaceous follicle
Fully mature sebaceous lobules composed of sebocytes with compact nuclei and abundant multivacuolated clear cytoplasm
Differential Diagnosis
Sebaceus adenoma
Nevus sebaceus

with the overlying epidermal surface, rather than with the hair follicle as seen in SH. **Sebaceous adenoma** is distinguished from **SH** by showing a larger basaloid germinative component (from two layers up to half of the sebaceous lobules) than is observed in SH. **Nevus sebaceus** differs from **SH** by its general breadth, the presence of hamartomatous (rudimentary) folliculosebaceous units, papillomatous epidermal hyperplasia, and frequent apocrine elements (Table 9-22B). **NS** is typically present at birth and gradually enlarges thereafter. It produces a localized area of alopecia or is a tan-brown, roughly surfaced plaque in the skin of the face or neck that becomes overtly verrucoid during puberty. A minor proportion of these lesions are also associated with multisystem abnormalities, including structural oculocerebrocranial defects that may cause seizures, mental retardation, and visual field defects. A variety of cutaneous tumors have been reported to arise potentially in **NS**, including **BCC, trichilemmoma (TL), proliferating pilar tumor, syringocystadenoma papilliferum, apocrine adenoma, SA, sebaceous carcinoma,** and **pilar leiomyoma.** It has been suggested that these contextual proliferations are not truly neoplastic in nature, but rather are hamartomatous in keeping with the general character of **NS**. This is an attractive hypothesis, but it is one that the author believes to be oversimplified. Several examples have been documented wherein **NS** gave rise to undisputed neoplasms that demonstrated aggressive behavior, including **squamous cell carcinoma, basal cell carcinoma**, and **ductal apocrine adenocarcinoma.**

Table 9-22B. Nevus Sebaceus of Jadassohn

Clinical Features
Congenital onset
Head and neck, usually scalp; upper trunk
Oval or elongated yellowish or tan-brown alopecic plaque
Rough to verrucous surface
An association with other developmental abnormalities, including oculocerebrocranial defects that may result in seizures, mental retardation, visual field lost
Histopathologic Features
All ages
Rudimentary hair follicle structures with basaloid epithelium resulting in clinical alopecia
Variable papillomatosis of epidermis and sebaceous gland underdevelopment or prominence
After puberty
Prominent papillomatosis of epidermis
Prominence of sebaceous glands
Prominent apocrine glands in a subset
Development of various hamartomas and tumors
Basaloid (basal cell) hamartomas
Trichilemmoma
Proliferating pilar tumor
Syringocystadenoma papilliferum
Apocrine hamartomas or adenomas
Sebaceous hamartomas or adenomas
Basal cell carcinoma
Ductal apocrine adenocarcinoma
Differential Diagnosis
Epidermal nevus
Verruca
Sebaceous hyperplasia
Sebaceous adenoma

Quick Fact

- **Sebaceous proliferations that connect through the hair follicle**
  - Normal sebaceous glands
  - Sebaceous hyperplasia
  - Sebaceous carcinoma
- **Sebaceous proliferations that connect with the epidermal surface**
  - Montgomery tubercle
  - Nevus sebaceus of Jadassohn
  - Sebaceous adenoma
  - Sebaceoma
  - Sebaceous carcinoma

Montgomery tubercles are specialized sebaceous glands of the areola surrounding the nipple. These glands clinically correlate with the numerous papules typically seen in the areola, and on the nipple itself. They may become exposed and raised when the nipple is stimulated, especially during pregnancy. Microscopically, the glands are small and lined

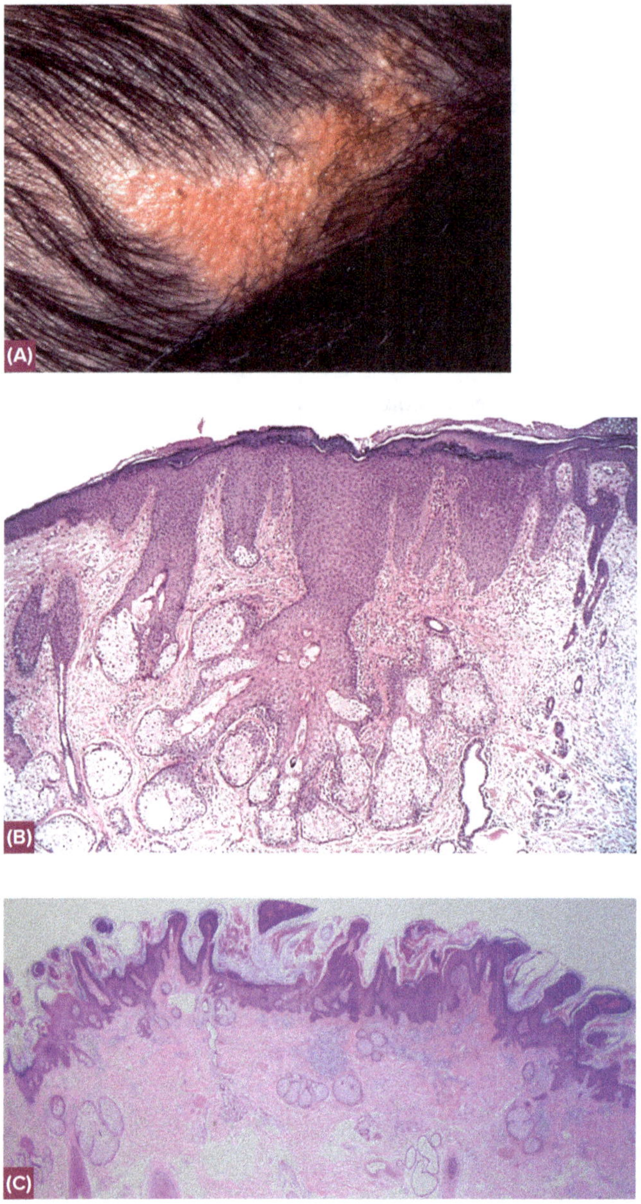

Nevus sebaceus of Jadassohn. (A) A linear, slightly yellowish, well-defined alopecic plaque involving the scalp. **(B)** The epidermis is acanthotic with an accompanying proliferation of sebaceous and apocrine glands that connect directly with the overlying epidermal surface and lack an association with hair follicular structures. **(C)** In this example the epidermis is papillomatous and the dermis contains numerous sebaceous and apocrine glands without association with hair follicles. Both types of these glands are seen directly emptying onto the epidermal surface.

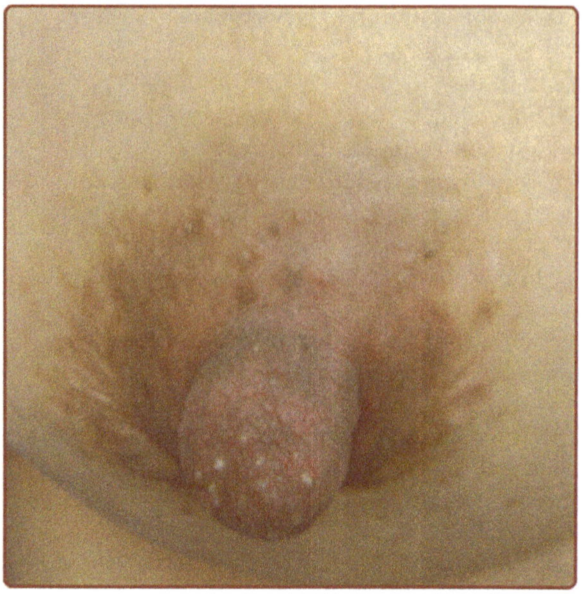

Montgomery tubercles. The sebaceous glands of the nipple and areola, which are responsible for lubricating the breast during breast-feeding, enlarge during pregnancy. (Reproduced, with permission, from Goldsmith LA, Katz SI, Gilchrest BA, Paller AS, Leffell DJ, Wolff K, eds. *Fitzpatrick's Dermatology in General Medicine.* 8th ed. New York, NY: McGraw-Hill Education; 2012.)

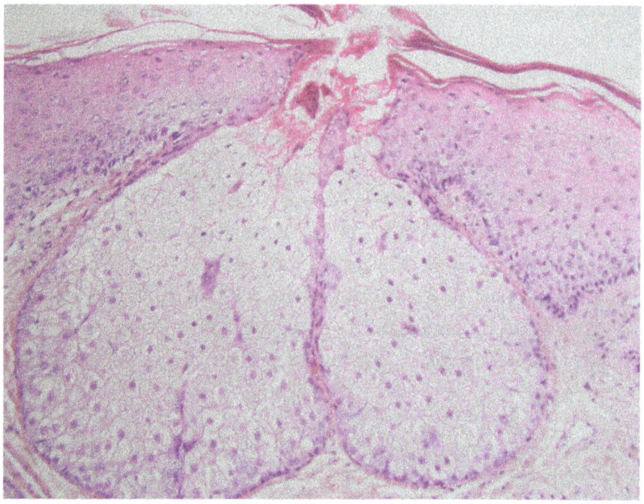

Montgomery tubercle. There are two sebaceous lobules lined by a single layer of basaloid germinative epithelium. The glands empty directly onto the epidermal surface.

by one or two basaloid (germinative) cell layers and numerous central clear sebocytes, identical to normal sebaceous glands. A feature distinctive from **normal sebaceous glands** and **sebaceous hyperplasia** is that the glands connect directly with the epidermal surface, similar to **nevus sebaceus** and **sebaceous adenoma**.

ANSWER 9-23: A.

Sebaceous adenoma (SA) typically presents as a solitary yellow-tan papule that slowly enlarges with time (Table 9-23A). The face is most commonly affected, but other locations have been described. The lesion typically makes its appearance after the age of 50 years. This tumor ranges in size from less than

Table 9-23A. Sebaceous Adenoma

Clinical Features
- Patient often older than 50 years of age
- Head and neck, especially face
- Yellowish nodule
- Usually <1 cm but can be ≥5 cm
- Association with Muir-Torre syndrome (sebaceous neoplasms, squamous cell carcinomas, and visceral carcinomas [laryngeal and gastrointestinal])

Histopathologic Features
- Classical type
  - Well-defined enlarged sebaceous lobules
  - Frequent attachment to epidermis with epidermal thinning
  - Fully mature sebocytes
  - Lobules may contain duct-like structures
- Variant type (Muir-Torre)
  - Sharp demarcation of lobules may be lacking
  - Lobules show admixture of peripherally located basaloid epithelium (≤50%) centrally mature sebocytes
  - Basaloid epithelium may show slight nuclear pleomorphism, distinct nucleoli, and occasional mitoses

Differential Diagnosis
- Sebaceous hyperplasia
- Basal cell carcinoma with sebaceous differentiation

1 cm (the usual size) to greater than 5 cm in maximum dimension. Clinical misdiagnosis of SA as **basal cell carcinoma (BCC)** is a common problem. There may be an association with **Muir-Torre syndrome (MTS),** wherein the patient has metachronous or synchronous visceral malignancies and cutaneous SAs, **sebaceous carcinomas (SCs), BCCs with sebaceous differentiation**, or **squamous carcinomas** of the **"keratoacanthoma"** type. Malignant tumors of internal organs in **MTS** are most often carcinomas of the larynx and gastrointestinal tract, but virtually any visceral site may be affected; rarely, nodal or extranodal malignant **lymphomas** may be encountered as well. **Muir-Torre syndrome** is a microsatellite instability syndrome in which nucleotide mismatch repair is disrupted. Immunohistochemical staining for MLH1, MSH2, MSH6, and PMS2 will reveal preserved nuclear staining in normal tissue, but in Muir-Torre syndrome nuclear staining is lost. The SAs seen in this context may either be "classical" microscopic lesions or may demonstrate histologic peculiarities and thus be labeled as **sebaceous adenomas, MTS variant.**

The microscopic characteristics of "classical" **sebaceous adenoma** are probably the most clear-cut of any sebaceous proliferation, except for **sebaceous hyperplasia**. They are represented by the sharply circumscribed proliferation of enlarged sebaceous lobules, comprised by fully mature sebocytes, frequently attenuating the overlying epidermis, and attaching to its basal aspect. A fibrous pseudocapsule commonly surrounds the lesion and attests to its slow growth, as do appendageal "collarettes" that may form at the periphery of the tumors. The cellular lobules are lined by two or more layers of basaloid (germinative) epithelium comprising less than 50% of the tumor. SA may contain duct-like structures into which holocrine secretion occurs; this phenomenon may result in the formation of intralesional cysts. Modest nucleolar prominence may be appreciated in the constituent cells of SA, but nuclear hyperchromasia or pleomorphism

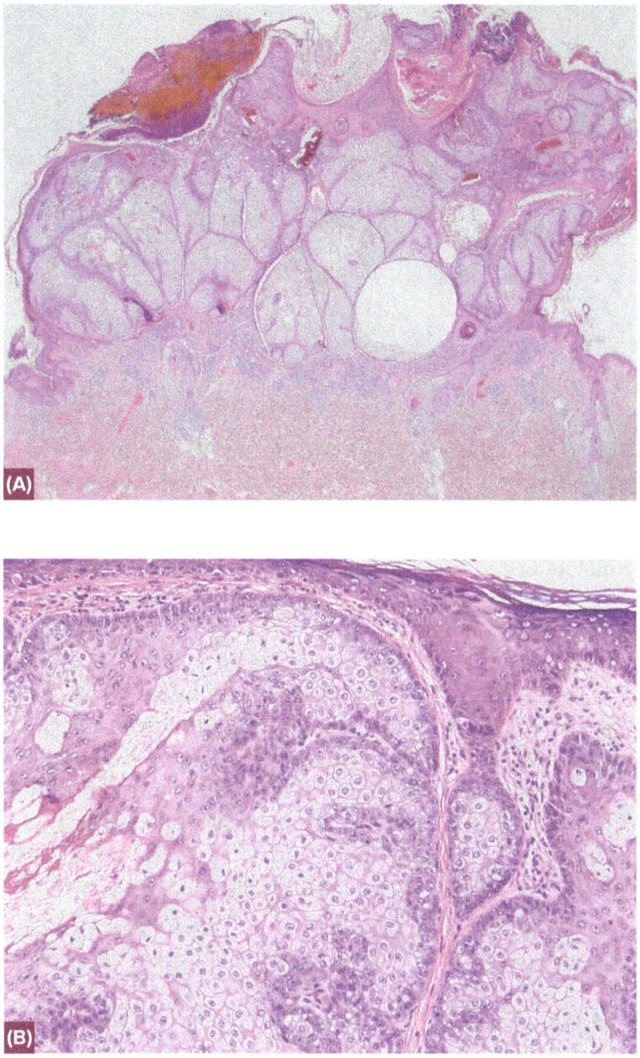

Classic sebaceous adenoma. (A) There is a nodular proliferation composed of several sebaceous lobules pushing up the epidermis, resulting in a polypoid configuration. **(B)** The lobules are centrally filled with numerous clear sebocytes and lined by more than two layers of germinative epithelium. However, the germinative component accounts for less than 50% of the tumor. The lobules connect directly with the overlying epidermal surface.

and mitotic activity are only rarely observed. On the other hand, the **"MTS variant" of SAs** differs from the preceding descriptions in several regards. First, the tumor lobules may lack the exquisite demarcation from the adjacent dermis that is shown by classical SA. Instead small nests of sebocytes and germinative cells may be present descending into the dermis. Second, the component cellular lobules are composed of an admixture of peripherally disposed basaloid, germinative-type epithelial cells—often with mild nuclear pleomorphism, distinct nucleoli, and modest mitotic activity—and centrally mature sebocytes.

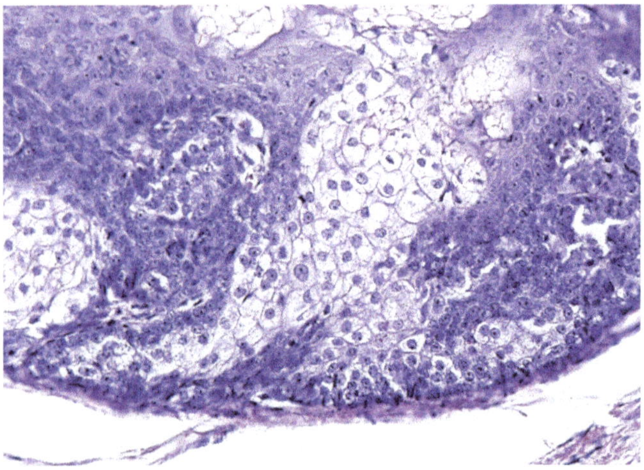

Sebaceous adenoma, Muir-Torre variant. At high magnification, an admixture of basaloid cells and sebocytes replace the more orderly transition seen in classic sebaceous adenoma. Nonetheless, the cells are benign, and most sebocytes assume a mature phenotype.

In regard to the differential diagnosis, **Muir-Torre–type SAs** may be difficult to distinguish diagnostically from **basal cell carcinoma with sebaceous differentiation** (BCCSD) (also known as **sebaceous epithelioma**). The salient points of difference between these tumors are subtle but reproducible; whereas **BCCSD** manifests an at least focally fibromyxoid stroma and epithelial-stromal "clefts," in similarity to ordinary **basal cell carcinoma**, **Muir-Torre sebaceous adenoma**

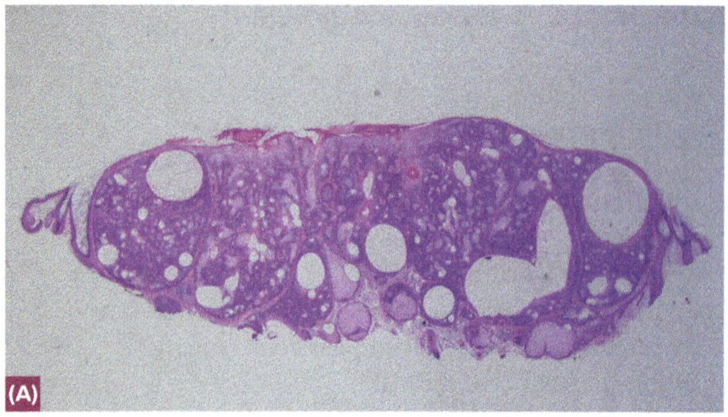

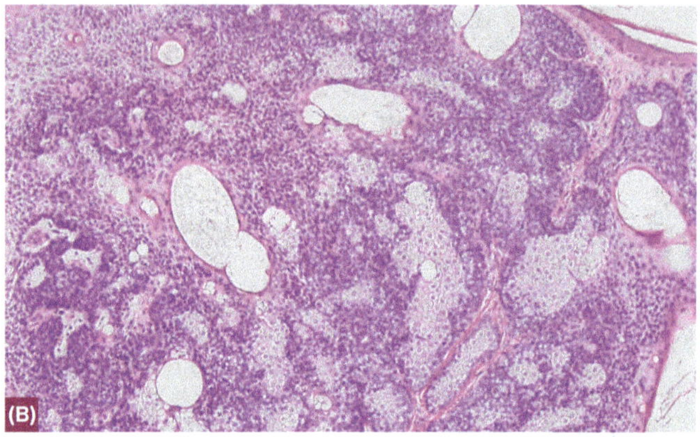

Sebaceoma. **(A)** Numerous lobules are present in the dermis with direct connection to the overlying epidermis. Even at low power, the tumor is composed predominantly of basaloid cells. Note the numerous sebaceous ducts scattered throughout the tumor, some of which are markedly dilated. **(B)** The tumor is composed of a disorganized mixture of germinative basaloid cells and mature sebocytes. The basaloid component comprises greater than 50% of the tumor cell populace.

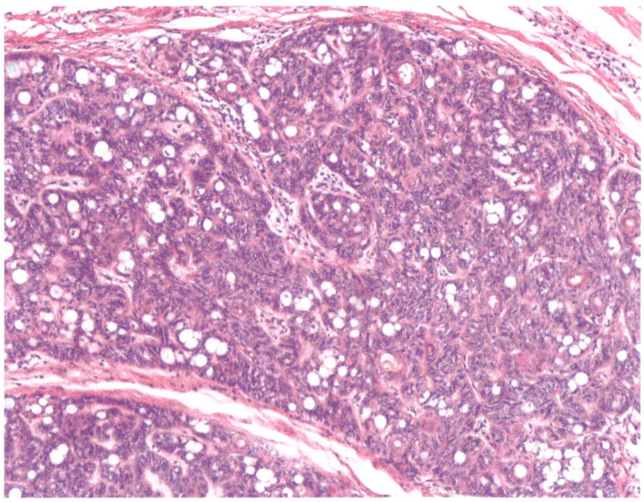

Sebaceoma, rippled pattern. A reticulated growth pattern of basaloid cells with focal sebocyte differentiation embedded in a dense hyalinized stroma.

Quick Fact

- **Sebaceous Adenoma**
  - Basaloid cells comprise >2 layers but less than 50% of total tumor mass.
- **Sebaceoma**
  - Basaloid cells comprise >50% of total tumor mass
  - Scattered pale sebocytes may be scattered throughout the tumor

does not. Moreover, **BCCSD** is dominated by its basaloid cell constituents, with only a minor proportion of sebocytic elements. **Sebaceous adenomas**, whether classic or Muir-Torre type, contain no more than 50% germinative-type cells. The tumor called **sebaceoma** was first described by Troy and Ackerman and is also associated with microsatellite instability. Microscopically, they are characterized by lobules composed of a disorganized mixture of sebocytes and germinative basaloid cells in excess of 50% of the total tumor cell populace. Kiyohara and colleagues have described an unusual variant in which a "rippled" microscopic image is observed, with aligned tumor cell nuclei simulating the Verocay bodies of **schwannomas**. Similar lesions have been documented by Kazakov et al, who also noted a resemblance to the organoid growth patterns of neuroendocrine tumors in some cases.

ANSWER 9-24: A.

The biopsy reveals a dilated infundibulum supporting a complex proliferation of small germinative hair elements and small follicles. **Trichofolliculoma** occurs on the face of adults and histopathologically consists of a large intradermal squamous-lined cyst filled with keratinous material and fragments of hair shaft (Table 9-24A). If a central pore is present, the cyst communicates with the epidermal surface. Radiating from the wall of the cyst, connected by strands of epithelium, are well-developed secondary hair follicles with papillae, an inner and outer root sheath, and embedded sebaceous glandular cells.

Table 9-24A. Trichofolliculoma

Clinical Features
Usually adults
Head and neck, especially the nose
Small skin-colored papule or nodule, usually solitary
Central keratinous plug with vellus hairs
Histopathologic Features
Dilated hair follicle structure opening to surface
Infundibulum or isthmic-type epithelium
Secondary follicular structures radiate (or "bud") from the central structure
The secondary follicles show varying degrees of differentiation from germinative to formation of mature hair
An organoid fibrous stroma surrounding the follicle structure, well-demarcated from adjacent dermis
Considerable heterogeneity of epithelial cells
Isthmic, clear cells with peripheral nuclear palisading, basaloid matrical cells
Differential Diagnosis
Trichoepithelioma
Basal cell carcinoma
Fibrofolliculoma

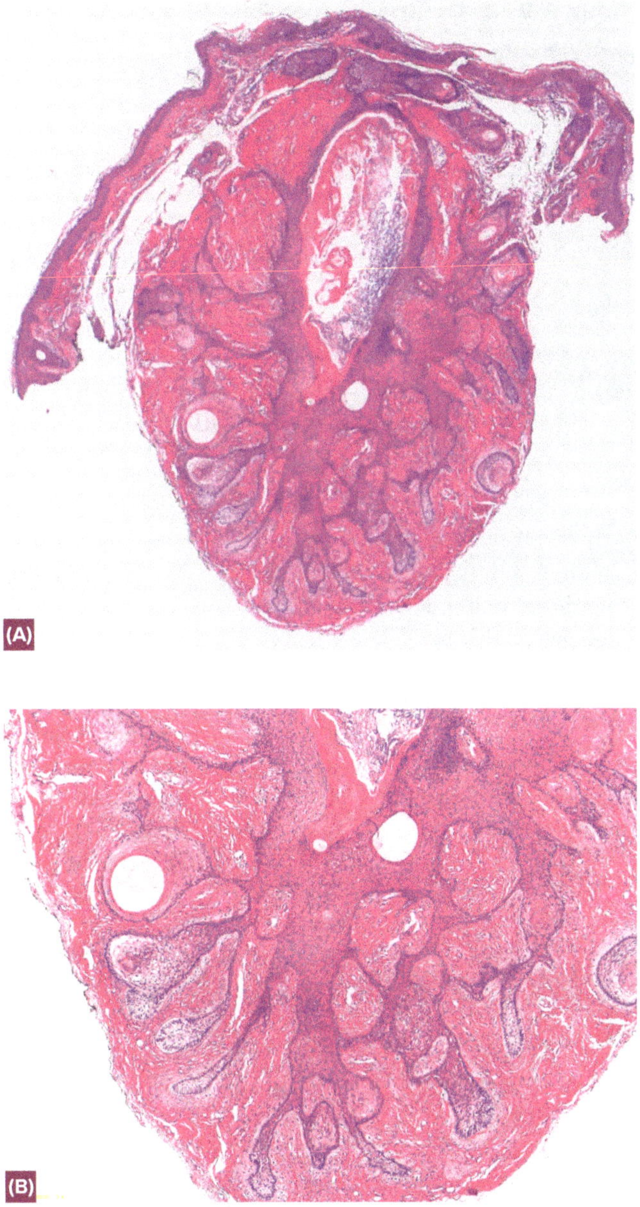

Trichofolliculoma. (A) There is a cystic follicular infundibulum with radial strands of outer root sheath epithelium terminating in vellus hairs and occasional horn cysts. **(B)** Both basaloid clusters and small immature vellus hair follicles are surrounded by follicular stroma.

Dilated pore of Winer (DPW) and **pilar sheath acanthoma** (PSA) appear clinically similar and both are also composed of a large squamous-lined cyst filled with keratinous debris (Table 9-24B). The **dilated pore of Winer** shows a markedly dilated follicular infundibulum with hyperplasia at the base and atrophy at the ostium. Although **DPW** characteristically opens at the epidermal surface through a cystic infundibulum, cross sections of the intradermal component may be difficult to distinguish from **pilar sheath acanthoma**.

Table 9-24B. Comparison of Pilar Sheath Acanthoma and Dilated Pore of Winer

PILAR SHEATH ACANTHOMA				DILATED PORE OF WINER
		Clinical Features		
	⇐	Middle-aged or elderly patients	⇒	
	⇐	Women equal to men	⇒	
	⇐	Face, especially upper lip	⇒	
	⇐	Solitary tan-ink papule or plaque	⇒	
	⇐	Central keratotic plug or comedone	⇒	
	⇐	*Histopathologic Features*		
	⇐	Central infundibular microcyst	⇒	
	⇐	Cystic opening to epidermal surface	⇒	
	⇐	Keratinous material in cyst	⇒	
	⇐	Polygonal cells in epithelial lining with variably pale or clear cytoplasm (containing glycogen) or basaloid appearance	⇒	
	⇐	Bland cytologic characteristics	⇒	
	⇐	**No hair formation**	⇒	
Epithelial wall proliferative with lobular cellular buds Proliferative buds may contain keratinous accumulations				Greater cystic opening to surface Cystic wall less proliferative than PSA
		Differential Diagnosis		
		Epidermoid cyst Trichofolliculoma Perifollicular fibroma Fibrofolliculoma		

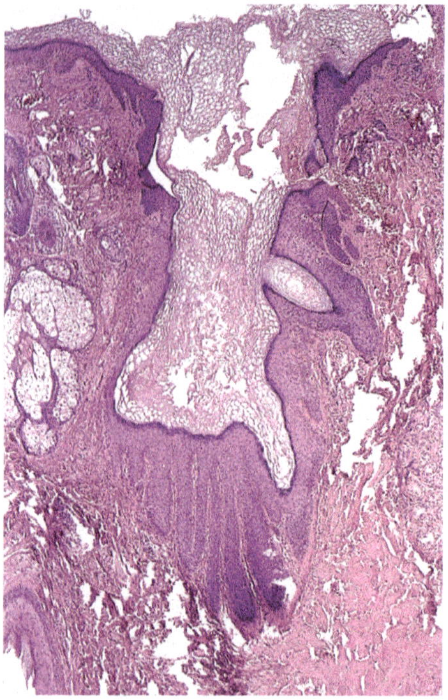

Dilated pore of Winer (DPW). There is a dilated pore that opens onto the epidermal surface via a stenotic infundibulum. The epithelial lining is hyperplastic with acanthosis of the outer root sheath epithelium and elongated rete ridges.

The **pilar sheath acanthoma** contains a larger irregular branching cystic cavity. In contrast to the thin epithelial strands seen in the **trichofolliculoma**, the **pilar sheath acanthoma** contains numerous lobulated masses of outer root sheath epithelium with peripheral palisading. Unlike **trichofolliculoma**, **pilar sheath acanthoma** lacks hair bulb formation. It is worth mentioning that in cases of **pilar sheath acanthoma** that are sectioned tangentially or do not reveal the cystic cavity may be mistaken for **squamous cell carcinoma**.

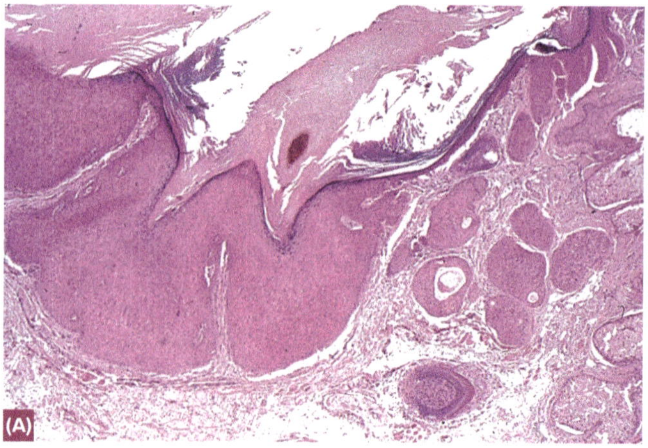

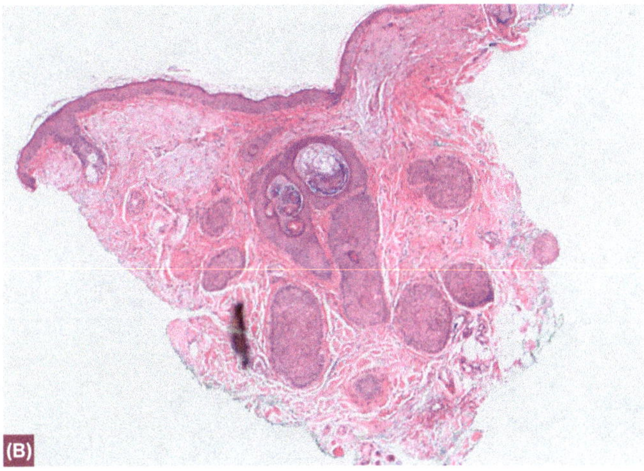

Pilar sheath acanthoma. (A) A central microcyst derived from the infundibulum (complete with epidermal-type keratinization) has areas of acanthosis (left) with small radiating lobules of keratinocytes budding into the dermis (right). **(B)** The dilated follicular infundibulum contains numerous radiating lobules of outer root sheath epithelium without hair bulb formation.

Trichoadenoma (TA) is an infrequently encountered neoplasm that is represented clinically by a nondescript solitary nodule in the skin of the head, neck, or trunk (Table 9-24C). It generally measures less than 1 cm in greatest dimension. Microscopically, there is a dermal proliferation of microcystic arrays composed of trichilemmal keratinizing epithelium, separated from one another by fibroblastic stroma. The keratin-filled cysts are comprised by polyhedral cells typically devoid of keratohyaline granules. However, occasionally keratohyaline granules may be present as these tumors typically arise at the junction of the follicular infundibulum and isthmus. Nuclei are bland, without nucleoli or mitotic figures. There are no basaloid elements, and only a minor component of non–cyst-forming epithelial cells, in the form of solid "buds" from microcysts, is apparent.

Table 9-24C. Trichoadenoma

Clinical Features
Usually adults
Head, neck, and trunk
Nondescript papule <1 cm
Histopathologic Features
Dome shaped
Symmetric
Keratinous cysts lined by uniform cuboidal cells
Eosinophilic or clear cytoplasm
Granular layer
No basaloid epithelium
Differential Diagnosis
Syringoma
Trichoepithelioma, especially desmoplastic type
Microcystic adnexal carcinoma
Tumor of the follicular infundibulum
Basal cell carcinoma

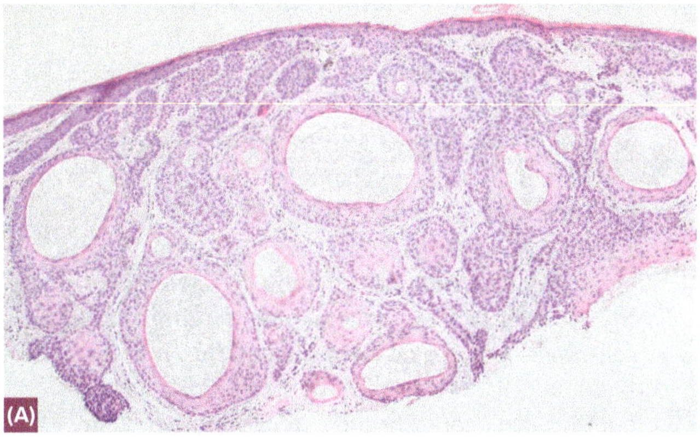

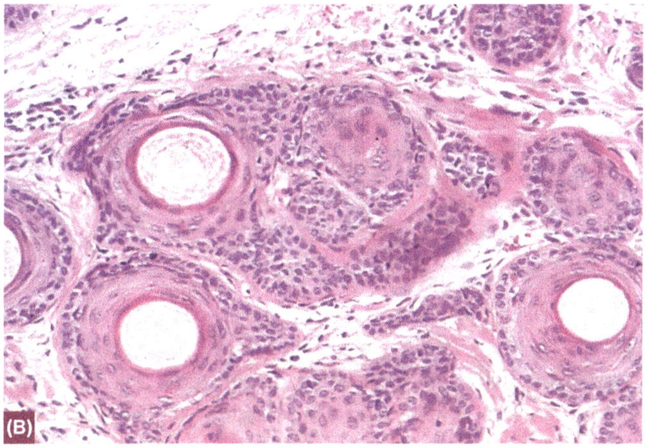

Trichoadenoma (of Nikolowski). (A) A nodular growth of keratinizing epithelium surrounded by perifollicular stroma. Trichoadenoma is distinguished from dilated pore and pilar sheath acanthoma by the presence of trichilemmal type keratin lining the small horn cysts within the radial arrays. **(B)** Note the horn cysts lined by pink trichilemmal keratinization.

ANSWER 9-25: A.

The biopsy reveals a lobular proliferation of basaloid cells inducing its own tumoral stroma that sharply demarcates the lesion from dermal collagen. The epidermis is not involved. Several lobules contain dilated horn cysts containing keratinous material without hair shafts. This is a classic example of multiple **trichoepitheliomas (TE)** (Table 9-25A). These lesions rarely, if ever, transform into **basal cell carcinoma**. TE of the "classical" type is usually seen as a solitary, slowly growing, flesh-colored nodule in the skin of the face, which typically arises during childhood. The clinical distinction between solitary TE and BCC is nearly impossible in some cases. Multiple TEs are seen in the **Brooke-Fordyce ("epithelioma adenoides cysticum")**

Table 9-25A. Trichoepithelioma

Clinical Features
- Children and adults
- Solitary or multiple ("epithelioma adenoides cysticum"—Brooke-Fordyce syndrome)
- Head and neck, especially face
- Skin-colored papule or nodule, pearly appearance
- Usually <1 cm
- Multiple TE associated with multiple cylindromas, spiradenomas, salivary glandular tumors, trichilemmomas, or basal cell carcinomas

Histopathologic Features
- Organoid arrangement of mature collagenous hypocellular stroma about lobules of uniform basaloid cells, well-demarcated from surrounding dermis
- Basaloid cells tend to show peripheral palisading of nuclei, lacelike or cribriform in patterns, and hair matrix–like differentiation
- Keratinous microcysts frequent
- Often hair papilla–like structures ("mesenchymal papillary bodies") in stroma adjacent to hair matrical–like epithelium
- Minimal or no mitotic figures and necrotic cells

Differential Diagnosis
- Trichofolliculoma
- Basal cell carcinoma

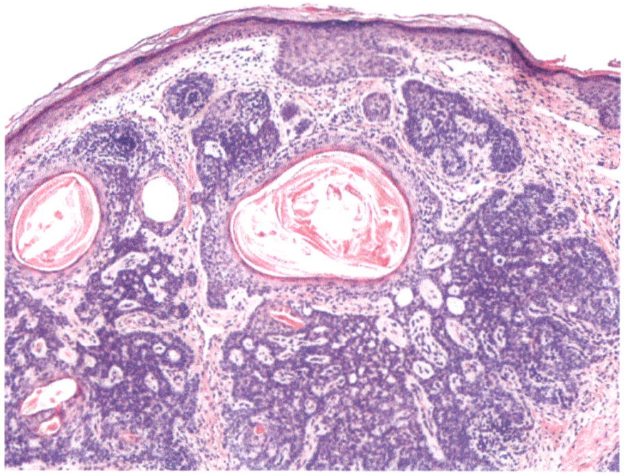

Trichoepithelioma. There are several basaloid nests in the dermis with focal horn cyst formation. The basaloid nests are wrapped tightly by a cellular fibrous stroma. Dermal mucin is absent. Additionally, the tumor cells exhibit low-grade atypia and lack necrotic cells and significant mitotic activity. (image courtesy of Rajendra Singh, MD, Icahn School of Medicine at Mount Sinai)

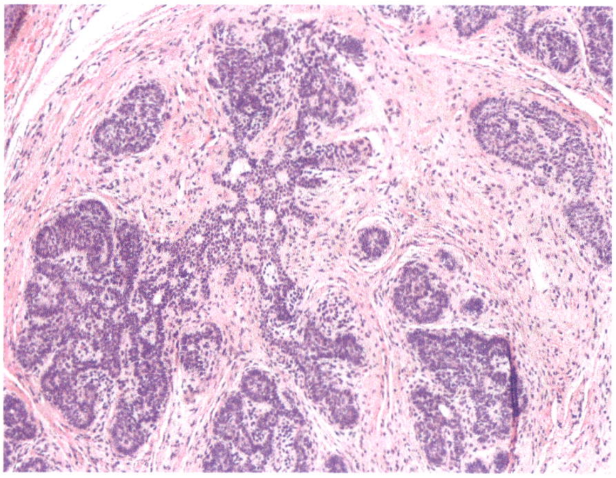

Immature trichoepithelioma. Solid and reticulated basaloid proliferations devoid of keratocyst formation comprise the dominant growth pattern.

syndrome, which is transmitted in an autosomal dominant fashion. In that disease complex, TEs may literally cover the face, with each lesion being smaller than 1 cm, and extracranial skin fields may be involved as well. It is interesting that multiple TEs may coexist with multifocal **cylindromas, spiradenomas, salivary glandular "dermal analogue tumors"** (which resemble cylindromas), **trichilemmomas,** or **basal cell carcinomas**, in the context of the **Brooke-Fordyce** or **Cowden syndromes** or in related, "derivative" genodermatoses. Systemic conditions that may potentially coexist with multifocal trichoepitheliomatosis include the **Rombo syndrome** (milia, hypotrichosis, atrophoderma, TEs, BCCs, and vasodilatation with cyanosis), systemic lupus erythematosus, and myasthenia gravis.

Regardless of whether they are sporadic or syndromic tumors, TEs have the same histopathologic characteristics. They are composed of lobular arrays of relatively uniform basaloid cells in the dermis, separated from one another by mature, collagenous, hypocellular stroma. The lobular constituents often connect to one another focally and contain variably sized keratinous microcysts mantled by cells showing infundibular or isthmic differentiation. These keratocysts frequently rupture and produce dystrophic calcifications. The cited distinction is also particularly difficult in TEs that lack obvious keratinous microcyst formation and are composed of solidly cellular basaloid clusters; such variants have been termed **immature TEs**.

A key distinction between TE and BCC is the biphasic nature (epithelial-stromal elements), absence of stromal retraction and dermal mucin, and absent mitoses and tumor cell necrosis in TE. Genetic analysis has affirmed a synonymity between classical sporadic TE and BCC, both of which demonstrate the same chromosomal deletion at 9q22.3. In contrast, syndromic (Brooke-Fordyce) TE appears to have a different genetic constitution, featuring mutations in the *CYLD* gene at 16q12-13. Investigators have attempted to use immunostains for bcl-2 protein and CD34 to separate TE from BCC; reported observations in those studies have included a lack of bcl-2 protein in TE and the regular presence of that marker in BCC and the presence of CD34 in the stroma immediately adjacent to cellular clusters in TE but not in BCC. Regardless, dermatologists aim to conservatively but completely excise both tumor types and should do so.

ANSWER 9-26: A.

The biopsy reveals discrete tumor lobules separated by a nondesmoplastic fibrous stroma.

The lobules are composed of markedly pleomorphic tumor cells with both basophilic and clear cytomorphology. Numerous mitoses and necrotic tumor cells are present. There is central gritty comedo-type tumor necrosis. **Sebaceous carcinomas (SC)** are typically seen in middle-aged or elderly patients, with a mean age of 62 years (Table 9-26A). For unexplained reasons, ocular neoplasms show a marked predilection for Asian individuals. These patients present with nontender masses at the eyelid margin or in the conjunctiva, and, as such, they are commonly misdiagnosed as having **chalazions, blepharitis**, or **conjunctivitis**. Multicentricity is observed in 5% to 10% of cases, and other ophthalmologic conditions confused with **sebaceous carcinoma** include **cicatricial ocular pemphigoid, basal cell carcinoma** (BCC) or **squamous cell carcinoma (SCC),** and **cutaneous horn**. Traditionally, **sebaceous carcinomas** have been considered in two categories: ocular and extraocular. The proposed justification for this paradigm was based on a putative difference in the behavior of these two groups of tumors; it was contended that ocular sebaceous carcinomas had a more aggressive nature than that of extraocular lesions. However, a redactive examination of the pertinent literature fails to support that premise. Both ocular and extraocular sebaceous malignancies are attended by an approximate risk of 30% to 40% for local tumor recurrence, 25% to 35% for distant metastases, and 10% to 20% for tumor-related death. Hence, there is in fact no inherent biologic difference between them, with the exception that an ocular location is, by far, more common than an origin in the skin outside of the eyelids and whereas **extraocular sebaceous carcinomas** are strongly associated with **Muir-Torre syndrome**, **ocular sebaceous carcinomas** less frequently demonstrate microsatellite instability. In reference to extraocular tumors, most **SCs** are seen on the head and neck followed, in relative order, by the trunk, genitalia, and extremities. They present as relatively nondescript nodular masses that are occasionally painful or rapidly growing. A proportion of tumors are ulcerated at presentation. Ho and colleagues have suggested that the sentinel lymph node biopsy technique should be used in cases of sebaceous carcinoma. However, there is no evidence that lymphadenectomy improves the survival of patients with this tumor type.

Table 9-26A. Sebaceous Carcinoma

Clinical Features
Middle-aged and elderly patients (mean age, 62 years)
Predilection for Asians
Ocular (eyelids) more often than extraocular sites (head and neck more often than trunk, genitalia, extremities)
Nontender mass
Histopathologic Features
Pagetoid spread of atypical epithelial cells within epidermis or conjunctival epithelium
Lobular dermal aggregates of variably atypical polyhedral cells
Central necrosis ("comedo" pattern) common
Well-differentiated tumors: cells with abundant multivacuolated cytoplasm, vesicular nuclei, and discernible nucleoli
Poorly differentiated tumors: nondescript cells with high nucleus-to-cytoplasmic ratios, prominent nuclear pleomorphism, prominent nucleoli, prominent mitotic activity
Basaloid SC: small cells with scanty cytoplasm, peripheral palisading, nuclear anaplasia
Squamoid SC: prominent squamous metaplasia with keratin pearls
Sarcomatoid SC: spindle cell features
Differential Diagnosis
Balloon cell melanoma
Clear cell squamous cell carcinoma
Clear cell basal cell carcinoma
Clear cell eccrine carcinoma
Trichilemmal carcinoma
Metastatic clear cell carcinomas of visceral origin

The microscopic characteristics of **sebaceous carcinoma** include the presence of lobular dermal aggregates of variably atypical polyhedral cells separated from each other by fibrovascular stroma that lacks obvious desmoplasia. The resulting image is that of an organoid neoplasm. Central portions of the tumor cell nests may become necrotic, yielding a "comedo" pattern on scanning microscopy.

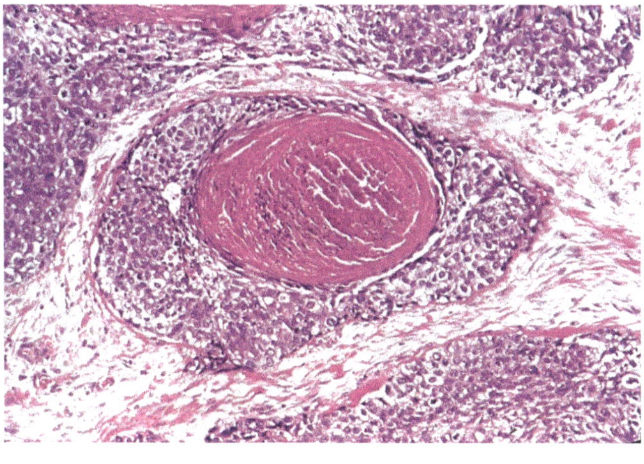

Sebaceous carcinoma with central comedo-like necrosis. Comedo-like necrosis may be conspicuous in high-grade lesions.

Cytologically, the constituent elements of **well-differentiated sebaceous carcinomas** show abundant multivacuolated lucent cytoplasms and oval vesicular nuclei with discernible nucleoli but sparse mitoses.

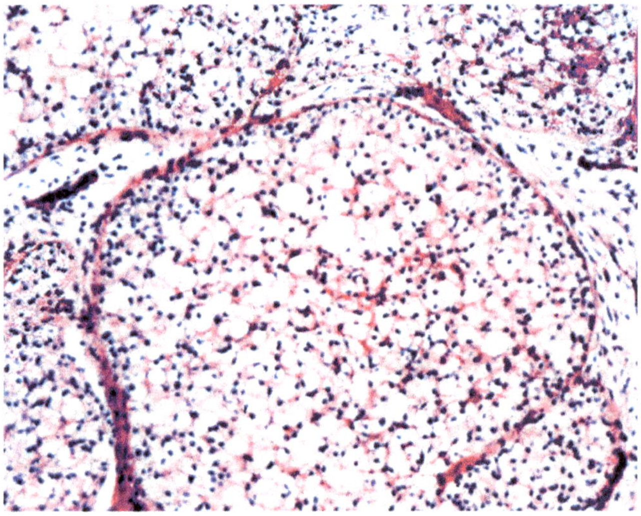

Well-differentiated sebaceous carcinoma. The tumor consists of discrete lobules of clear cells separated by nondesmoplastic stroma.

At the other end of this spectrum, **poorly differentiated sebaceous carcinomas** are composed of more nondescript cells with high nucleus-to-cytoplasmic ratios, more prominent nuclear pleomorphism, prominent nucleoli, brisk mitotic activity with possibly atypical division figures, and amphophilic to basophilic cytoplasm. Intracellular compartmentalized vacuoles are not nearly as prominent in the latter lesions and may require the use of special techniques—such as oil red O or Sudan IV stains on fresh tissue or EMA immunostains in paraffin sections—to highlight their presence. In further reference to immunohistology, no single marker is currently available that is specific for sebaceous differentiation.

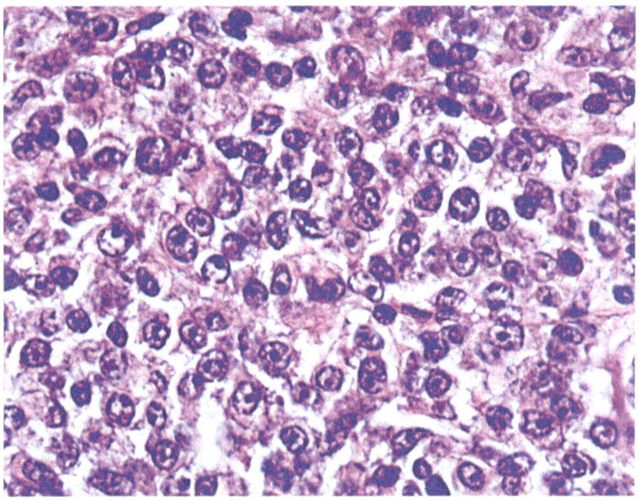

Poorly differentiated sebaceous carcinoma. The tumor consists predominantly of cells with less well-defined intracytoplasmic compartments, although at lower power elements may be admixed. Nuclei are pleomorphic with striking atypia.

Grading of **sebaceous carcinomas** is accomplished most reproducibly using tumor growth patterns rather than nuclear features. Neoplasms that are composed of generally rounded, demarcated, roughly equally sized lobules of cells are graded as I/III, and those that show an admixture of rounded and distinct infiltrative and confluent cell nests are graded as II/III. Grade III/III sebaceous carcinomas feature the presence of highly permeative cellular aggregates with jagged profiles or demonstrate medullary sheet-like growth. The tumor in the associated question is a Grade II/III. Regardless of grade, all examples of **sebaceous carcinoma** share a possible association with epidermotropism or **secondary extramammary Paget disease** (EPD) of the sebaceous type where the surface

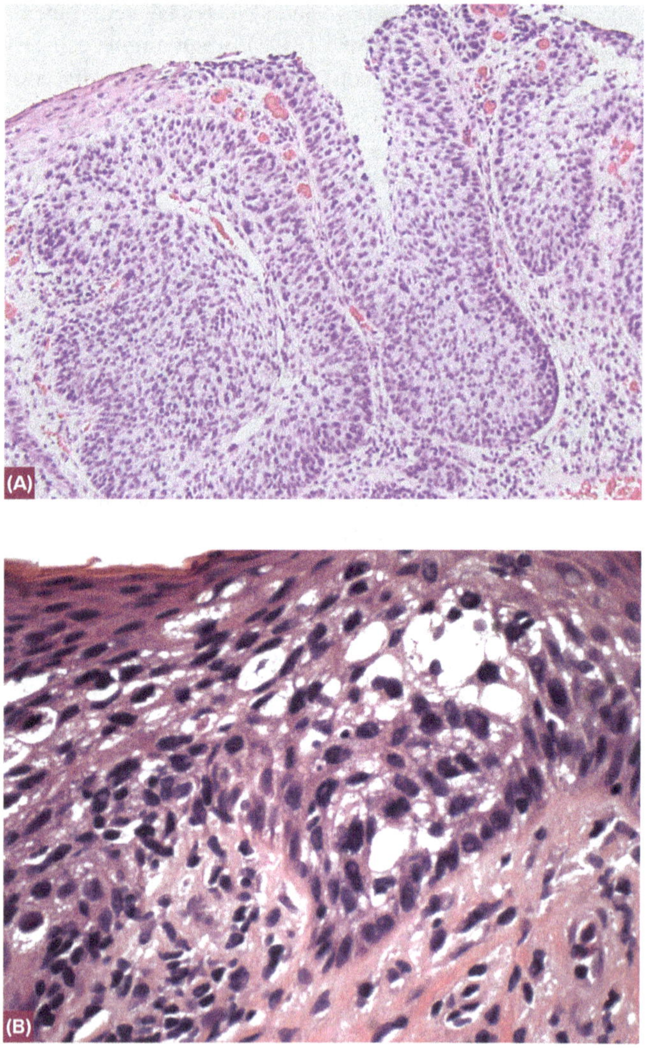

Sebaceous carcinoma with intraepidermal colonization (so-called extramammary Paget disease, sebaceous type). **(A)** There is a dermal-based tumor with focal connection to the overlying epidermal surface. **(B)** Tumor cells containing abundant multivacuolated cytoplasm colonize the epidermis. The nuclei are large with variably prominent nucleoli and few mitoses.

Table 9-26B. Special Stains in the Differential Diagnosis of Clear Cell Cutaneous Tumors

TUMOR	PAS-d	PAS-s	AE13/14	S-100	EMA[a]	CEA	CA-125	CA19-9
TLC	0	+	+	0	+	0	0	0
HBCC	0	+/−	0	0	0	0	0	0
HSCC	0	+/−	0	0	+/−	0	0	0
CCEC	0	+	0	+/−	+	+/−	0	0
SC	0	+/−	0	0	+	0	0	0
BCM	0	+/−	0	+	0	0	0	0
MCCA	+/−	+/−	0	+/−	+	+/−	+/−	+/−

Key:
PAS-d = Periodic acid-Schiff (PAS) stain with diastase digestion
PAS-s = PAS stain without diastase digestion
AE13/14 = Pilar-selective keratin immunostains
S-100 = S-100 protein
EMA = Epithelial membrane antigen
CEA = Carcinoembryonic antigen
TLC = Trichilemmal carcinoma
HBCC = Hydropic basal cell carcinoma
HSCC = Hydropic squamous cell carcinoma
CCEC = Clear cell eccrine carcinoma
SC = Sebaceous carcinoma
BCM = Balloon cell melanoma
MCCA = Metastatic visceral clear cell adenocarcinomas
[a]EMA reactivity in sebaceous carcinomas is uniquely multivacuolated within the cytoplasm of the tumor cells.

epidermis contains scattered malignant tumor cells overlying the main dermal tumor mass. From a practical perspective, the pathologist should especially consider an underlying **invasive oculocutaneous sebaceous carcinoma** whenever a conjunctival or eyelid biopsy demonstrates such pathologic changes because its relationship with intraepithelial neoplasia is strongest in those sites. Outside of the ocular region, however, **extramammary Paget disease (EPD)** that does not label for epithelial mucin content or apocrine-selective immunohistologic markers may also have this association.

In regard to the differential diagnosis, as one might expect, the pathologic differential diagnosis of **sebaceous carcinoma** is broad, encompassing virtually all of the malignant clear cell tumors of the skin (Table 9-26B). These include entities such as **balloon cell melanoma, clear cell squamous carcinoma, clear cell basal cell carcinoma, clear cell eccrine carcinoma, trichilemmal carcinoma** (TLC), and **metastatic clear cell carcinomas of visceral origin (ie, clear cell renal cell carcinoma)**. With the possible exception of selected **balloon cell melanomas**, however, none of these neoplasms exhibit the particular vacuolization pattern that is seen in sebocytes, which is a multivesicular "bubbly" compartmentalization of the cytoplasm of each cell, rather than a unilocular vacuole. As discussed, immunostains for EMA or histochemical analyses for neutral lipid may be necessary to confirm the presence of the former of these two patterns. Furthermore, **sebaceous carcinoma** lacks several specialized protein products that may be seen in sweat gland tumors or metastatic visceral carcinomas; included among these are CEA, S-100 protein, gross cystic disease fluid protein-15, CA-125, and CA19-9. Recently, Sramek et al have examined the utility of two particular markers—EMA and BER-EP4—in the differential diagnosis of **sebaceous carcinoma, basal cell carcinoma,** and **squamous carcinoma**. Those authors found that EMA+/BER-EP4+ tumors were **sebaceous carcinomas**, EMA+/BER-EP4- tumors were **squamous cell carcinomas**, and EMA-/BER-EP4+ neoplasms were **basal cell carcinomas**. Additionally, **sebaceous carcinomas** are positive for androgen receptor (AR), which is negative in **SCC** and **BCC**. Cho and colleagues have also observed frequent immunoreactivity for c-*erb*B-2 oncoprotein in **sebaceous carcinomas.**

ANSWER 9-27: B.

Tumor of the follicular infundibulum (**TFI**) is also known as **infundibuloma** (Table 9-27A). It is a relatively uncommon lesion that shows a marked predilection for middle-aged or elderly women and presents as a solitary papulonodular tumor measuring less than 1 cm in greatest dimension. Multiplicity is rarely seen but has indeed been reported, and there may be an association with concomitant **nevus sebaceous** or **Cowden syndrome**.

Microscopically, **TFI** is typified by a subepidermal plate of compact eosinophilic polyhedral cells that forms a latticework structure connecting to the stratum basalis multifocally. The lesion is sharply demarcated laterally. Peripherally disposed tumor cells in the constituent cellular

Table 9-27A. Tumor of the Follicular Infundibulum

Clinical Features
Middle-aged or elderly patients
Women more often than men
Head and neck
Solitary papule or nodule
Usually <1 cm
Histopathologic Features
Well demarcated
Subepidermal plate of compact polyhedral cells
Multifocal connection to overlying epidermis by strands of epithelium
Peripheral palisading of nuclei
Variable clear cell change (glycogen)
Cytologic atypia usually absent
Differential Diagnosis
Trichilemmoma
Basal cell carcinoma

cords may demonstrate nuclear palisading and contain glycogen, in likeness to the trichilemmal sheath. A prominent layer of eosinophilic basement membrane material is often seen surrounding the cords as well. Nuclei are bland, and mitotic activity and necrosis are consistently absent. Hair is not formed in **TFI**, but "bystander" follicles may be entrapped in the tumor, and intralesional acrosyringia are seen in some examples. Cribier and Grosshans found that there is an accentuated deposition of dermal elastic tissue immediately beneath **TFIs**. An infundibular nature for the lesion is more inferential than proven, and it is predicated largely on the microanatomic relationship of **TFI** to the acrotrichium.

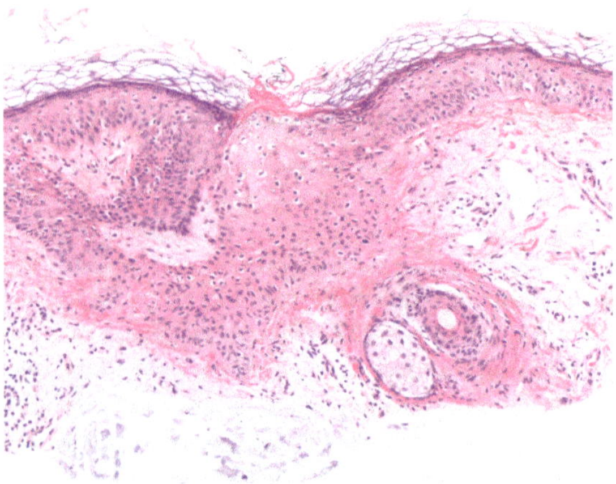

Tumor of the follicular infundibulum. There are anastomotic strands of epithelium extending downward from the epidermal surface. The epithelial strands are composed of bright eosinophilic keratinocytes lined by a layer of keratinocytes with peripheral palisading. Stromal retraction artifact and dermal mucin are absent.

In regard to the differential diagnosis, distinguishing **TFI** from **superficial basal cell carcinoma** (**BCC**) may be challenging in selected cases. Both tumors exhibit peripheral palisading of tumor nuclei; however, **TFI** is more highly differentiated with regular formation of basement membrane and more voluminous eosinophilic cytoplasm. Stromal retraction artifact, dermal mucin, and necrotic tumor cells are absent in **TFI**. Lastly it differs from **BCC** in being negative with the BER-EP4 antibody immunohistochemically. **Trichofolliculoma** is a cystic lesion with radiating strands of outer root sheath epithelium terminating in vellus hair bulbs. **TFI** is not cystic and although it may occasionally entrap hair structures, it does not produce hair bulbs. **Reticulated seborrheic keratosis** may impart a very similar appearance; however, they lack peripheral palisading of tumor nuclei and frequently contain horn cysts. **TFI** is actually considered by many to be a variant of **trichilemmoma**; however, **trichilemmomas** demonstrate large plate-like lobules of outer root sheath epithelium instead of thin strands.

ANSWER 9-28: D.

The biopsy reveals a plate-like epithelial proliferation extending downward from the epidermal surface. The epithelial cells are polygonal in shape and contain abundant amounts of eosinophilic and clear cytoplasm. Rare dyskeratotic keratinocytes are present. **Trichilemmomas** are common lesions that usually occur on the face singularly (Table 9-28A). When they are multiple, they are usually associated with **Cowden disease**, which is an autosomal dominant syndrome of multiorgan hamartomas. This condition is important to recognize clinically, since these patients have a high incidence of **breast carcinoma**. Multiple oral lesions may be seen in these patients. Additionally, these patients frequently develop multiple **storiform collagenomas**.

Microscopically, one to two lobules of epithelium are seen descending from the epidermis and pushing into the dermis in regions surrounding hair follicles. Abundant glycogenization may be present, giving the cytoplasm a clear appearance. PAS and PAS-diastase stains will reveal bright pink and clear cytoplasm, respectively, compatible with glycogen. The periphery of the tumor lobules is lined by palisading basaloid cells with a "glassy pink" basement membrane. Interestingly, although derived of outer root sheath epithelium, these lesions do not exhibit trichilemmal or pilar keratinization, but epidermoid keratinization with keratohyaline granules and may produce a cutaneous horn. Occasionally, rare dyskeratotic keratinocytes may be present in these tumors, reflective of the normal involuting catagen phase of the hair cycle.

In **desmoplastic trichilemmomas**, irregular bundles of dense stroma may form within the center of the tumor lobules and disrupt the epithelium, imparting a "pseudoinvasive"

Table 9-28A. Trichilemmoma

Clinical Features
Adults
Head and neck, especially upper lip and nose
Keratotic pink papules
Solitary or multiple
Association with Cowden syndrome
Multifocal hamartomatous polyposis of the intestines
Increased risk of breast carcinoma and other internal malignancies
Autosomal dominant
Histopathologic Features
Verrucous surface configuration often
Lobular proliferation of polygonal cells with variably clear cytoplasm (containing glycogen)
Peripheral palisading of nuclei
Occasional apoptotic bodies
Lobules bounded by eosinophilic basement membranes
Differential Diagnosis
Tumor of the follicular infundibulum
Inverted follicular keratosis
Verruca
Eccrine acrospiroma
Basal cell carcinoma

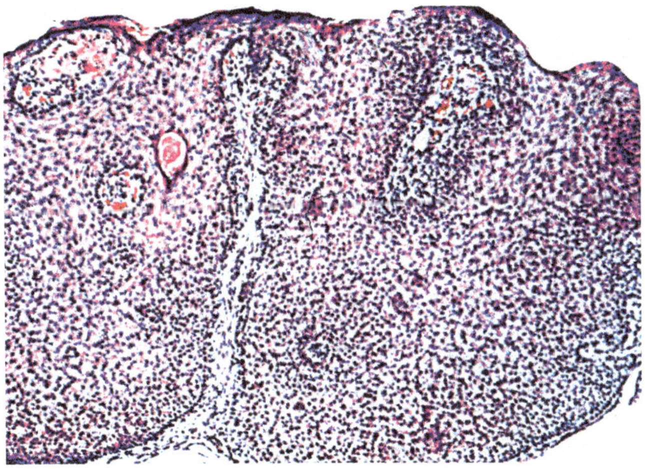

Trichilemmoma with extensive clear cell change. A lobular proliferation of bland cells with clear cytoplasm is surrounded by a peripheral row of basaloid cell with peripheral palisading and a thick eosinophilic basement membrane. Note the absence of tumor retraction artifact, dermal mucin, or necrotic tumor cells.

Quick Fact

- Desmoplastic trichilemmoma is CD34+
- Trichilemmal carcinoma is CD34–

pattern of growth. Therefore, these lesions may mimic **invasive squamous cell carcinoma (SCC);** however, the peripheral aspects of the tumor are well circumscribed. In cases where these pseudoinvasive foci are located at the peripheral tumor-dermal interface, immunohistochemical staining with CD34 may be helpful. **Trichilemmomas** will stain positive for CD34, while **squamous cell carcinomas** are negative for CD34. **Malignant trichilemmal carcinomas** are rare, usually slow growing, and are essentially **squamous cell carcinomas.** These lesions are invasive with glycogenization and marked cytologic atypia with occasional pagetoid spread into the adjacent epidermis resembling **melanoma** or other tumors in the intraepidermal epithelioma category (ie, **extramammary Paget disease**).

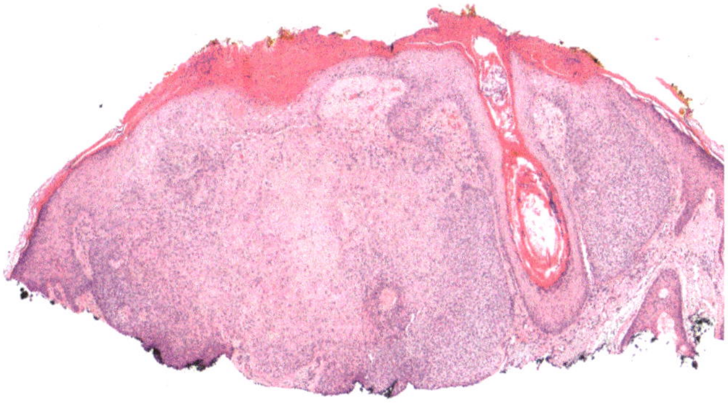

(A)

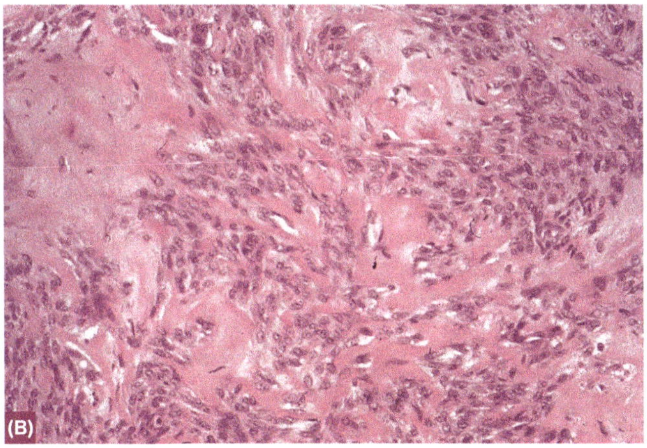

(B)

Desmoplastic trichilemmoma. (A) There is a well-circumscribed tumor extending downward from the epidermal surface composed of pale, glycogen-rich epithelium. In the central portions of the tumor, hyalinized stroma distorts the epithelium and separates it into strands. **(B)** High-power image of the center of the tumor lobule containing nests and cords of epithelial cells that infiltrate a dense fibromyxoid of collagenous stroma, mimicking invasion. The peripheral aspects of the tumor are well circumscribed.

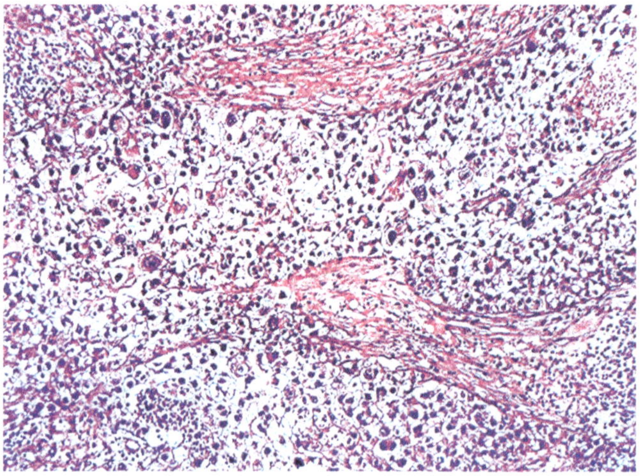

Trichilemmal carcinoma. Infiltrating lobules of malignant tumor cells containing glycogenated clear cytoplasms are associated with a focally prominent inflammatory infiltrate and a desmoplastic stroma.

In regard to the differential diagnosis, **trichilemmoma** shows significant overlap with **tumor of the follicular infundibulum (TFI).** Whereas **trichilemmoma** is notable for a lobular configuration, **TFI** has a reticular pattern with interconnecting epithelial cords. **Basal cell carcinomas (BCC)**, especially the clear cell variant, may resemble **trichilemmoma**; however, **BCC** exhibits stromal retraction artifact with dermal mucin, necrotic and mitotic tumor cells, and lacks a thickened eosinophilic basement membrane. Whereas **BCC** expresses bcl2 via immunohistochemistry, **trichilemmoma** is negative. Lesions with extensive clear cell change may also resemble **well-differentiated sebaceous carcinoma (SC)**; however, **SC** does not contain glycogen and lacks a thickened eosinophilic basement membrane. Two histologically similar pilar proliferations, namely, **follicular verruca vulgaris** and **inverted follicular keratosis** (which may, in fact, be one and the same lesion), must be considered. In general, **trichilemmoma** differs from the latter entities by the lack of squamous eddies and overt keratinization.

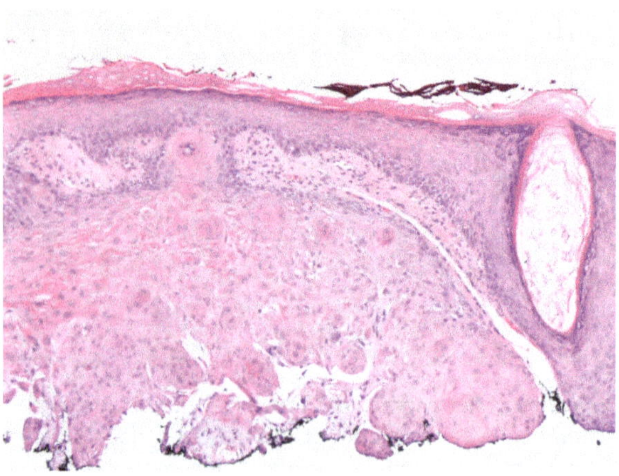

Inverted follicular keratosis. There is a well-circumscribed dermal nodule extending downward from the epidermal surface. The central epithelial cells contain bright eosinophilic cytoplasm. Numerous whorled squamous clusters ("squamous eddies") are present, but the tumor is well circumscribed without peripheral invasive growth, and lacks significant cytologic atypia and mitotic activity.

ANSWER 9-29: D.

The biopsy reveals numerous cords of basaloid epithelium embedded within a sclerotic stroma. Two large keratocysts contain calcified material. Stromal retraction artifact and dermal mucin are absent. The combined clinical, histopathological, and immunohistochemical findings are consistent with a **desmoplastic trichoepithelioma** (Table 9-29A). **Desmoplastic trichoepithelioma (DTE)** is considered by some to be a nonfamilial solitary variant of **trichoepithelioma (TE)**; however, others question its nosological relatedness to **TE**. This tumor is almost always located on the central face, occurs in early adulthood, and is much more common in females. More histopathological than clinical dissimilarities can be seen between **TE** and **DTE**. Microscopically, **DTE** is characterized by a discoid lesion in the dermis that is wider than it is deep and whose lateral margins are sharply circumscribed. The dermal nodule is composed of basaloid cords of two to three layers thick with horn cysts embedded in a dense sclerotic stroma.

Table 9-29A. Desmoplastic Trichoepithelioma

Clinical Features
Young to middle-aged adults
Women more often than men
Central face, especially the cheeks
Solitary, often skin-colored or slightly yellowish plaque
Raised borders and slightly depressed central area
Firm or scar like
Histopathologic Features
Discoid lesion in upper dermis with well-defined margins
Narrow linear or slightly branching cords of compact polygonal cells
Keratinous microcysts often filled with calcified material
Densely collagenized stroma surrounds epithelial elements
Dystrophic calcification
Foreign body giant cell reaction to keratin
No appreciable cytologic atypia or mitotic activity
Differential Diagnosis
Morphea form basal cell carcinoma
Syringoma

Occasionally, cyst rupture may result in giant-cell reaction and dystrophic calcification. **TE** usually presents as multiple papules involving the nasolabial folds of the central face and is microscopically characterized by a lobular/organoid proliferation of basaloid cells that induce their own cellular tumoral stroma, sharply demarcating the lesion from the surrounding dermis. In small specimens, the immunophenotype of **DTE** is helpful in making its distinction from the principal histopathologic differential diagnostic alternatives: **desmoplastic/morpheaform basal cell carcinoma** (BCC) and **microcystic adnexal carcinoma** (MAC). **Desmoplastic** BCC simulates **DTE** in exhibiting narrow, slightly branching cords of epithelial cells embedded in a dense collagenous stroma—often with epithelial cords connecting to the overlying epidermis. However, **BCC** is poorly circumscribed and lacks horn cysts. Additionally, **BCC** exhibits individual cell necrosis, mitoses, tumor-stromal retraction artifact, and dermal mucin. It must be noted that **desmoplastic BCC** may occasionally lack tumor-stromal retraction artifact and dermal mucin due to the encroachment of the dense collagenous stroma. Frequently the stroma in **desmoplastic BCC** has a fibromyxoid quality. Immunohistochemistry with CK20 will reveal rare scattered Merkel cells within **DTE**, whereas Merkel cells will be absent in **BCC**. **MAC** deeply infiltrates the dermis and occasionally the subcutis, usually exhibits true lumen formation with eosinophilic secretions, and often exhibits marked squamous metaplasia. None of these features are seen in **desmoplastic trichoepithelioma.** The lumen-like structures of **MAC** will express CEA and EMA via immunohistochemistry. All three of the tumors under discussion may be labeled with BER-EP4, albeit in differing proportions **(BCC > DTE > MAC).** However, epithelial reactivity for EMA and neuroendocrine markers is unique to **DTE** in this narrow setting.

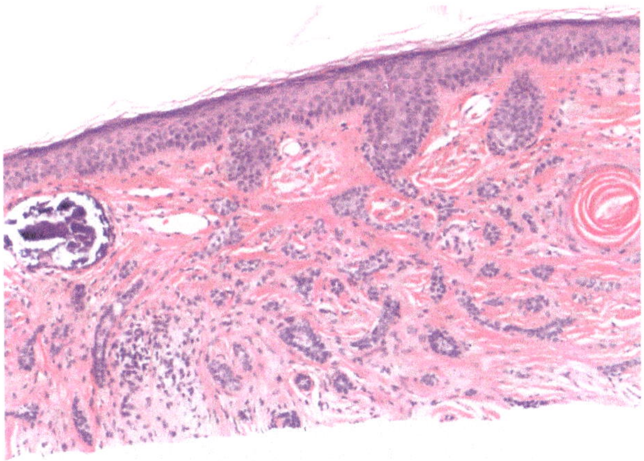

Desmoplastic trichoepithelioma. There are numerous curved basaloid strands embedded within a dense collagenous stroma. The cords focally connect with the overlying epidermal surface. Additionally, horn cysts are present, one of which is calcified (upper left). Lastly, the tumor cells lack mitoses and individual cell necrosis.

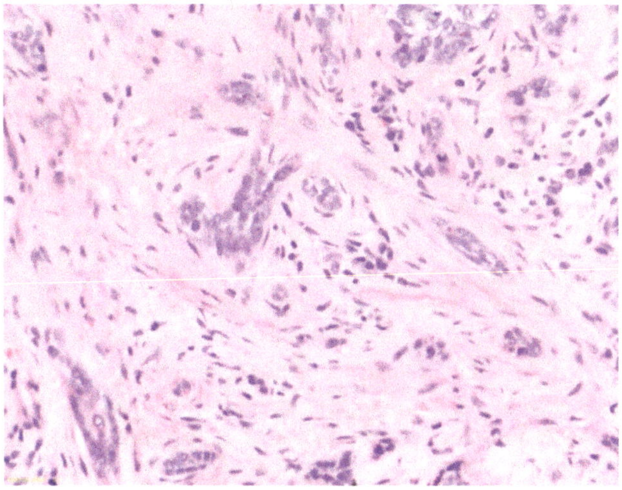

Desmoplastic basal cell carcinoma. There are numerous infiltrative strands of basaloid epithelium embedded within a dense collagenous stroma. Horn cysts are absent. There is significant cytologic atypia characterized by mitoses and numerous necrotic tumor cells. (Reproduced with permission from Desman GT, Ozerdem U, Shin SJ: Neighboring look-a-likes: distinguishing between breast and dermatologic lesions, Adv Anat Pathol 2014 Jul;21(4):228-247)

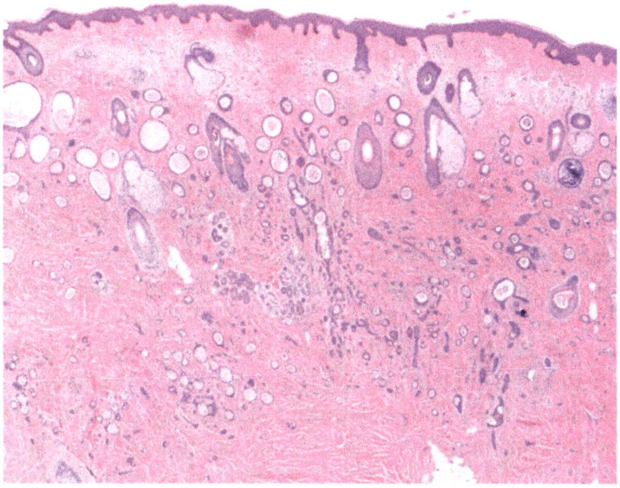

Microcystic adnexal carcinoma. There are numerous ductules and cords of basaloid epithelial cells embedded within a dense collagenous stroma. The tumor does not connect with the overlying epidermal surface and the tubules contain eosinophilic secretions. A few of the ductules contain keratinous debris due to squamous metaplasia, equivalent to horn cysts. The tumor extends into the deep dermis where the tubules and cords become smaller and exhibit a more infiltrative pattern of growth.

ANSWER 9-30: B.

The biopsy reveals occasional islands of basaloid cells resembling hair matrix that abruptly transition into abundant eosinophilic keratinous debris. The eosinophilic

Table 9-30A. Pilomatricoma

Clinical Features
- Children and adolescents, but any age may be affected
- Head and neck most common
- Solitary slowly developing hard nodule, usually deeply seated

Histopathologic Features
- Well-defined lobular tumor in dermis or subcutis
- Initially the tumor may be cystic with infundibular and germinative-matrical cellular components
- Germinative-matrical cells are uniform basaloid cells with monotonous round nuclei, dark chromatin, and small nucleoli
- Prominent mitotic activity
- Transition of matrical epithelium to "ghost" or "shallow" cells that exhibit an imprint of a nucleus that has been lost
- Formation of hard nail-like keratin
- Progressive loss of basaloid epithelium
- Foreign body giant cell reaction to keratin
- Calcification, ossification

Differential Diagnosis
- Basal cell carcinoma
- Pilomatrix carcinoma

material contains pale spaces with retained cellular outlines and absent nuclear chromatin ("ghost cells"). The overall tumor is composed predominantly of matrical keratin. The findings are consistent with an "ancient" **pilomatricoma (PM)** (Table 9-30A). **Pilomatricoma (aka pilomatrixoma** and **calcifying epithelioma of Malherbe)** is a benign hair matrix neoplasm. These lesions occur in the first two decades of life in 60% of cases and typically presents as a slowly growing, deeply seated, cystic nodule in the skin of the head, neck, and extremities. Other locations have been reported. Occasionally, the tumor may undergo a rapid increase in size due to rupture and hematoma formation. These tumors are strongly associated with mutations in the beta-catenin gene.

Microscopically, several stages of development have been observed for **pilomatricoma (PM),** and distinctive clinicopathologic variants of the tumor also exist. Ackerman had suggested that **PM** begins as a subepidermal cyst that is lined in part by infundibular-type epithelium and, in its inferior-peripheral aspects, by germinative-matrical cells of the hair bulb. The latter elements are the most distinctive component of this neoplasm; they are represented by compact basaloid polygonal cells with monotonous round nuclei, dark chromatin, small nucleoli, often-brisk mitotic activity, and amphophilic cytoplasm. The peripherally disposed germinative cells blend into an intermediate zone nearer the cyst lumen, where nuclei variably assume a washed-out, ghost-like appearance and the cytoplasm becomes more uniformly cornified and eosinophilic. This is not tumor necrosis, but matrical keratinization. In the center of the lesion, **"ghost cells"** are seen exclusively, which often undergo regional dystrophic calcification. Immunohistochemistry will reveal nuclear and cytoplasmic beta-catenin expression within the germinative (basaloid) epithelial cells.

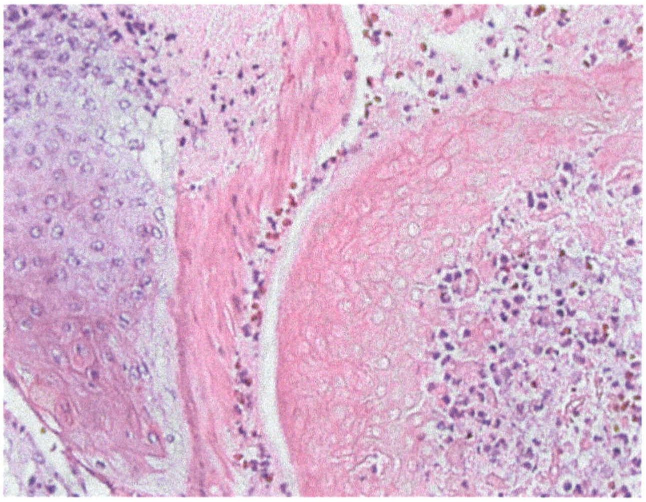

Matrical keratinization. There are islands of basophilic epithelium with adjacent portions of eosinophilic keratinous material maintaining observable cellular outlines. The pale empty spaces correlate with the location where once viable nuclei resided ("ghost cells").

With the passage of time, the number of basaloid cells in **PM** decreases progressively, eventually to be replaced entirely by aggregates of ghost cells, calcium deposits, and even foci of metaplastic bone. Extravasated keratin often elicits a foreign body–type giant cell reaction in the surrounding dermis; in fact, these changes may dominate old or **"ancient" PMs.** Moreover, extensive secondary heterotopic ossification may simulate the appearance of a cutaneous osteoma if attention is not paid to residual basaloid or ghost cell elements. Histologic variants of **PM** include a "perforating" form of the tumor in which it is seemingly eliminated through the overlying epidermis. Transepidermal extrusion therefore would appear to be one way in which **PMs** resolve or mature; conversely, transformation of the lesion into an osteocalcific mass is the apparent outcome for those neoplasms that are retained in the dermis.

Invasive PM differs from ordinary type **PM** only in demonstrating irregular "budding" cellular growth into the surrounding stroma at the periphery of the lesion, much in the same way that **low-grade malignant proliferating**

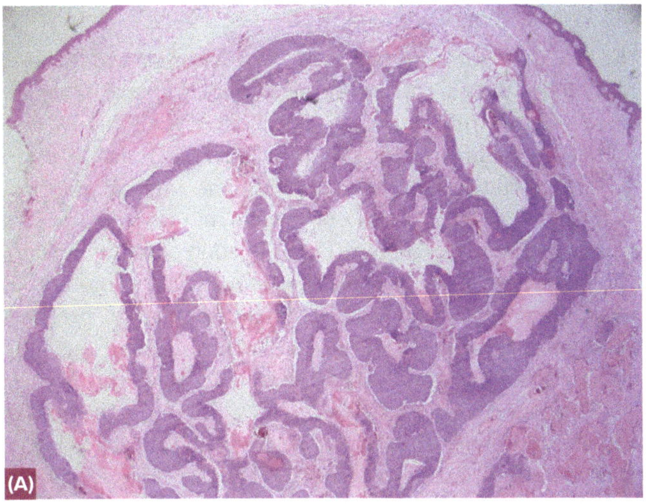

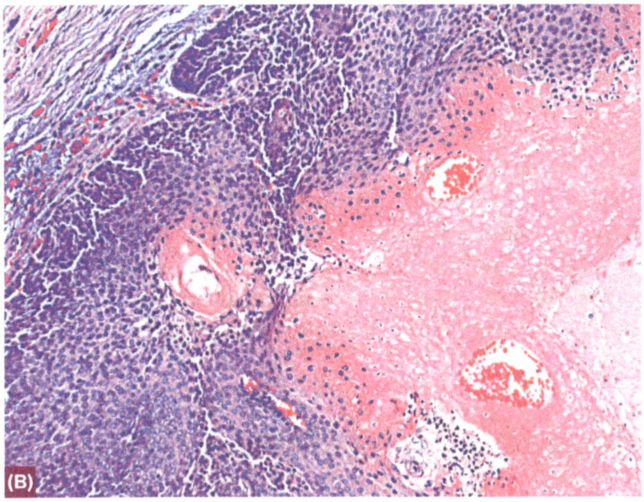

Pilomatricoma, early. (A) There are irregular nests of basophilic epithelium containing eosinophilic keratinous material. **(B)** High power reveals a tumor composed peripherally of basaloid germinative cells, which undergo matrical keratinization into eosinophilic material with clear spaces (where nuclei once resided). These areas of eosinophilic material are referred to as "ghost cells" since they maintain their cellular outlines without nuclei.

pilar tumor infiltrates the dermis or subcutis. On the other hand, **overt pilomatrix carcinoma (PMC)** is typified by broad zones of geographic necrosis; infiltrative growth; and, most important, an alteration in the cytologic features of the tumor cells. They acquire high nucleocytoplasmic ratios, obviously vesicular nuclear chromatin, and large nucleoli, and as such resemble the neoplastic elements of **lymphoepithelioma-like carcinomas** of the skin. However, the retention of focal ghost or shadow cell keratinization betrays the matrical differentiation of **PMC**. Behaviorally, **invasive PM** has the potential for local recurrence but not for distant metastasis. In contrast, **PMC** may spread secondarily to the regional lymph nodes or the viscera, and tumor-related fatality obviously is a possibility under those circumstances (Table 9-30B).

Table 9-30B. Invasive Pilomatricoma and Pilomatrix (Matrical) Carcinoma

INVASIVE PILOMATRICOMA	PILOMATRIX CARCINOMA
Clinical Features	
Features similar to pilomatricoma	Adults Face, trunk, and extremities Nodules, possibly ulcerated
Histopathologic Features Features similar to pilomatricoma except invasion of surrounding tissue at periphery of tumor by irregular cords of cells	Large tumors with atypical matrical epithelium and shadow cells Zones of geographic necrosis Infiltrative growth Sheets of atypical epithelium High nucleus-to-cytoplasmic ratios Vesicular nuclear chromatin Large nucleoli Prominent mitoses
Differential Diagnosis Pilomatricoma	Lymphoepithelioma-like carcinoma of the skin Metastatic undifferentiated carcinoma

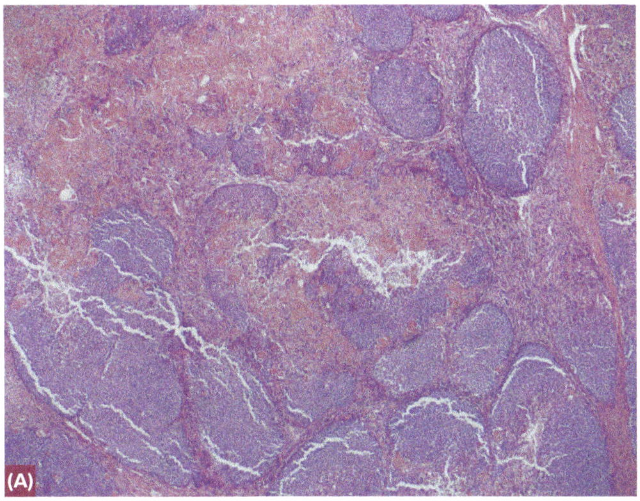

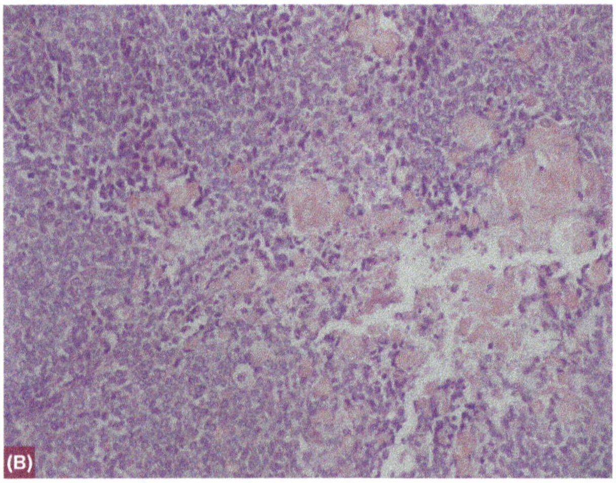

Invasive pilomatricoma. (A) There are numerous basaloid nests with an invasive pattern of growth throughout the dermis. **(B)** Focal areas of matrical keratinization are present.

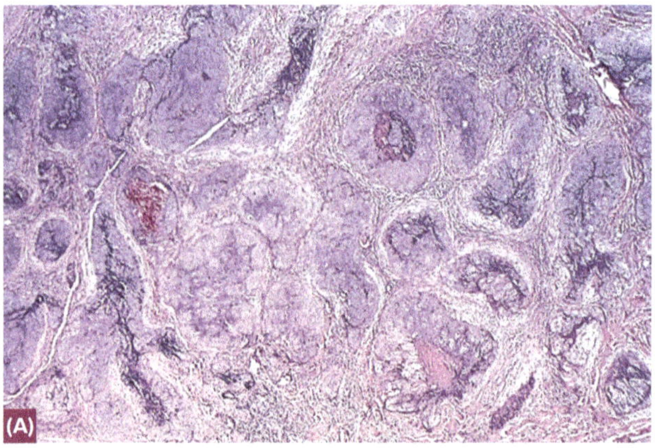

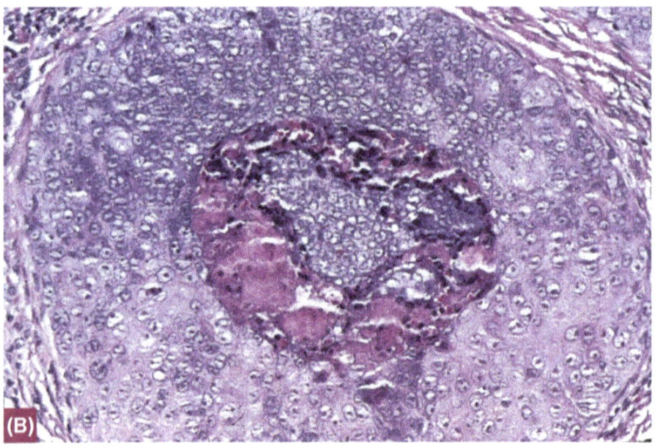

Pilomatrix carcinoma. (A) Irregular nests and lobules of large polygonal cells infiltrate dermis. The cytoplasm is pale amphophilic, and central zones of necrosis are evident. **(B)** Large polygonal cells with high nucleus-to-cytoplasmic ratios, indistinct cell membranes (syncytial), large vesicular nuclei, prominent nucleoli, and amphophilic cytoplasm are present. Central zones of eosinophilic necrosis are present. Matrical keratin containing "ghost cells" is absent.

ANSWER 9-31: E.

The biopsy reveals a central cystic area encompassed by nests and cords of keratinizing epithelial cells. There is abrupt keratinization without a granular cell layer resulting in compact eosinophilic keratin without pale spaces (pilar keratin). Squamous eddies are present within the internal portions of the cystic cavity. The tumor is well circumscribed with a rounded peripheral contour (upper portion of biopsy image). This lesion is not an **invasive squamous cell carcinoma** but a **benign proliferating trichilemmal cyst (benign proliferating pilar tumor; BPPT)** (Table 9-31A). These frequently ulcerated lesions occur in the scalp of the elderly with a female predominance in 80% of cases. These lesions, unlike **trichilemmomas**, are not associated with Cowden disease. They are almost exclusively solitary, but rare cases have been reported to contain adjacent **benign trichilemmal cysts**. They occur as a subcutaneous nodule composed of variably sized lobules of squamous epithelium. It is characterized by peripheral basal cells abruptly differentiating into squamous cells with marked glycogenization, which abruptly mature into eosinophilic amorphous keratin without keratohyalin granules. A distinct "glassy" layer of stroma sharply demarcates the lesion, separating it from **invasive squamous cell carcinoma.** The lesions may exhibit mild nuclear atypia with squamous eddie formation. These lesions recapitulate outer root sheath epithelium, hence the abrupt keratinization and glycogenization. Dystrophic calcification of the amorphous keratin component is common. The cytologic features of

Table 9-31A. Benign Proliferating Pilar Tumor

Clinical Features
Usually older individuals
Women more often than men
Scalp most common site
Often large exophytic tumors, measuring ≤10 cm in diameter
Recurrence after removal is infrequent
Metastases to regional lymph nodes occur rarely
Histopathologic Features
Lobular proliferation of squamous epithelium with trichilemmal differentiation
Usually well demarcated at periphery
A trichilemmal cyst remnant usually present
The epithelium often shows
Variable clear cell change
Disordered proliferation
Nuclear pleomorphism
Prominent nucleoli
Mitoses
Differential Diagnosis
Squamous cell carcinoma

BPPT differ substantially from those of other **benign pilar cysts** in that they often include nuclear pleomorphism, vesicular nuclear chromatin, prominent nucleoli, and brisk mitotic activity (up to 10 per 10 high-power [×400] fields). Because of this constellation of findings, it is easy to understand why a number of such tumors have been confused with **SCCs** in the past. Nevertheless, it must be reiterated that the architecture of **BPPT**, rather than its cytomorphology, is of paramount behavioral importance. If the lesion shows a well-demarcated, generally rounded interface with the surrounding connective tissue, it will behave in a benign fashion. Alternatively, infiltrative margins should be viewed with concern. Foci of dystropic calcification are common in the stroma and within the cell nests of **BPPT**, and areas of "abrupt" trichilemmal keratinization are regularly interspersed throughout the lesion.

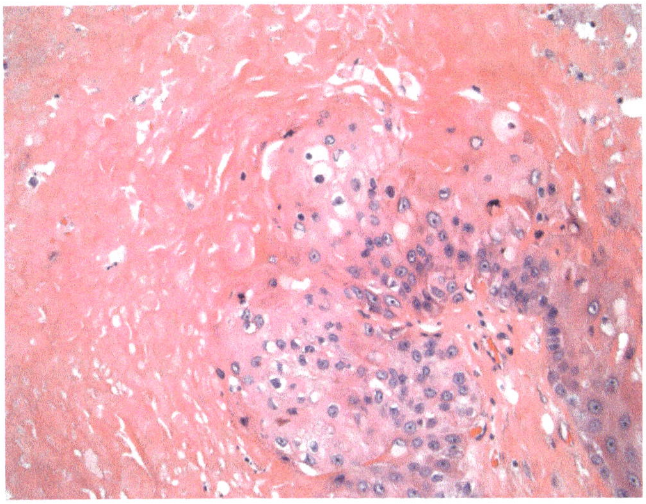

Benign proliferating pilar tumor. Abrupt (trichilemmal) keratinization typifies this lesion. Cells are relatively uniform in size, the cytoplasm is clear or weakly eosinophilic, and mild cytologic atypia and mitotic activity may be seen.

In regard to the differential diagnosis, the principal distinction is between **malignant proliferating pilar tumor (MPPT)** and **squamous cell carcinoma** (**SCC**). The basic clinicopathologic profile attending **malignant proliferating pilar tumor**, also known as malignant trichilemmal cyst, and malignant pilar tumor is basically identical to that which was delineated previously in reference to **BPPT** (Table 9-31B). That is true, at least in part, because it appears that some **MPPTs** arise in transition from **BPPT**, in a manner similar to that attending sweat gland carcinoma ex dermal cylindroma or eccrine spiradenoma. The first pathologic issue that must be addressed in connection with MPPT is the caution with which it should be diagnosed. Brownstein and Arluk properly drew attention to the fact that **BPPTs** have cytologic features that, at first glance, suggest an interpretation of carcinoma. However, as stated previously, the pattern of growth is of greater importance in determining the biologic potential of pilar neoplasms

Table 9-31B. Malignant Proliferating Pilar Tumor (MPPT)

Clinical Features
Similar to benign proliferating pilar tumor (BPPT)
Middle-aged to elderly females
Scalp
Nodules, often ulcerated
Histopathologic Features
Low-grade MPPT: features similar to BPPT except
Irregular invasion of surrounding connective tissue by irregularly shaped and sized cords of epithelium
High-grade MPPT
Lack of lobular growth pattern of BPPT
Foci of geographic necrosis
Cellular anaplasia
Abnormal mitotic figures
Spindle cell transformation
Differential Diagnosis
Low-grade MPPT
Squamous cell carcinoma
High-grade MPPT
Poorly differentiated eccrine ductal carcinoma
Metastatic carcinoma with squamous metaplasia

of this type. With that caveat in mind, there are two forms of **MPPT** with dissimilar behavioral attributes. The first is a close mimic of **BPPT**, except for the fact that **low-grade MPPT** demonstrates irregular invasion of the surrounding and intervening connective tissue by irregularly shaped and sized cords and nests of neoplastic cells. The cytologic attributes and the remaining architectural features of **low-grade MPPT** are synonymous with those of **BPPT**. In contrast, **high-grade MPPT** lacks the lobular growth pattern of **BPPT** and demonstrates foci of obvious geographic necrosis. Moreover, it shows a much more anaplastic cytologic image with striking nuclear pleomorphism, abnormally shaped mitotic figures, and potential spindle cell transformation. Separation of **MPPT** into the mentioned subtypes facilitates the prognostication of these lesions. Low-grade tumors are expected to show the potential for local recurrence only (which may, nevertheless, be mutilating and difficult to control), whereas high-grade neoplasms also possess the capability for distant metastasis.

The overall growth pattern of **squamous cell carcinomas** (SCC) is typically infiltrative, unlike that of **BPPT**, and **SCC** does not feature the presence of pilar-type keratinization. **Primary cutaneous SCCs** typically contain an overlying component of **squamous cell carcinoma in situ**. Distinction of **metastatic** SCC and **MPPT** may be impossible without clinical correlation. Last, the clinical history has an important role in this contextual diagnosis because **BPPT** typically evolves over a much longer period of time than **SCC** does.

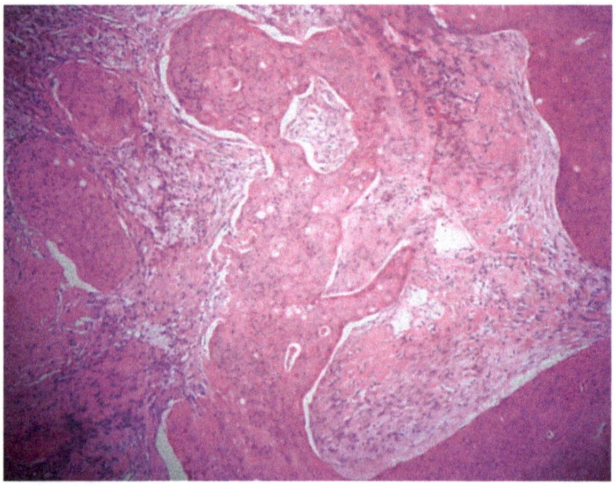

Malignant proliferating pilar tumor, low grade. At the peripheral aspect of dermal cystic proliferation are invasive tongues of bright pink squamous epithelium.

ANSWER 9-32: D.

The biopsy reveals a dermal-based tumor that extends into the deep dermal-subcutaneous interface. There are solid basaloid nests lined by a peripheral layer of cells containing palisading nuclei. No stromal retraction artifact or dermal mucin is present. The tumor nests are surrounded by a condensed spindle cell stroma reminiscent of dermal papillae. The findings are consistent with **trichoblastoma (TBL)**, which was first described by Headington who brought two salient elements of this lesion into focus. These are (1) its relatively primitive histologic appearance, resembling that of the embryonic hair, and (2) other morphologic attributes that suggest an epithelial-stromal interaction as the underlying mechanism for the peculiar image of this tumor (Table 9-32A). Depending on whether the epithelium or stroma is predominant in neoplasms in this category, additional diagnostic modifications, such as **TBL** or **trichoblastic fibroma,** may be used as desired. However, it should be stressed that regardless of such nuances, the basic designation of TBL is associated with a distinctive, well-recognized, visual, and clinicopathologic profile. TBL may arise in almost any skin field, except possibly in the distal extremities. It is generally a solitary, nondescript, nodular lesion that is situated at any level of the dermis; the size is usually less than 2 cm, but "giant" tumors of this type have been documented. No syndromic associations pertain.

Microscopically, TBL is a basaloid proliferation in which the neoplastic cells are arranged in cords, sheets, or discrete clusters. The most common of these patterns is the first, in which strands of two to three cells in thickness anastomose with one another and are separated by cellular stroma. A hyaline membrane may invest the cellular cords as well, and globular deposits of eosinophilic matrix may be seen between them or in the adjacent stroma. Hair differentiation is evident, either as immature cellular clusters that bud from the mass and are indented by stroma in the manner of a primitive hair papilla and hair bulb or as more mature proliferative foci that resemble hair root structures. Occasional examples of TBL may exhibit the formation of melanin pigment, as described by Aloi and coworkers. A multinodular variant of TBL showing desmoplastic stroma has been reported by Chan and colleagues; this lesion also differed from classical forms of the tumor in showing small foci of keratinization, mucomyxoid stromal alteration, and focal spindle-cell differentiation with infiltration of perineural spaces and arrector muscles. Despite these worrisome findings, the clinical evolution was innocuous.

Table 9-32A. Trichoblastoma and Related Tumors

Clinical Features
Adults
Women = men
Almost any location, especially the face and scalp
Usually does not involve distal extremities
Solitary nondescript papule or nodule
Usually <2 cm, but may be giant
Histopathologic Features
Well-demarcated from surrounding tissue
Symmetric
Basaloid epithelial proliferation in cords, sheets, or discrete clusters
Fibrotic investment of epithelium
Follicular germinative epithelium
Peripheral palisading of nuclei
Follicular differentiation resembling hair bulbs and papillae
Keratinous cysts on occasion
Fibrotic stroma
Occasional necrosis
Limited numbers of mitoses
Differential Diagnosis
Basal cell carcinoma

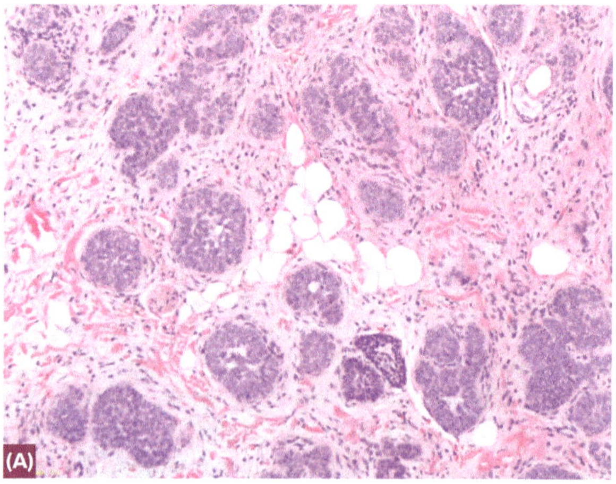

Reproduced with permission from Desman GT, Ozerdem U, Shin SJ: Neighboring look-a-likes: distinguishing between breast and dermatologic lesions, Adv Anat Pathol 2014 Jul;21(4):228-247

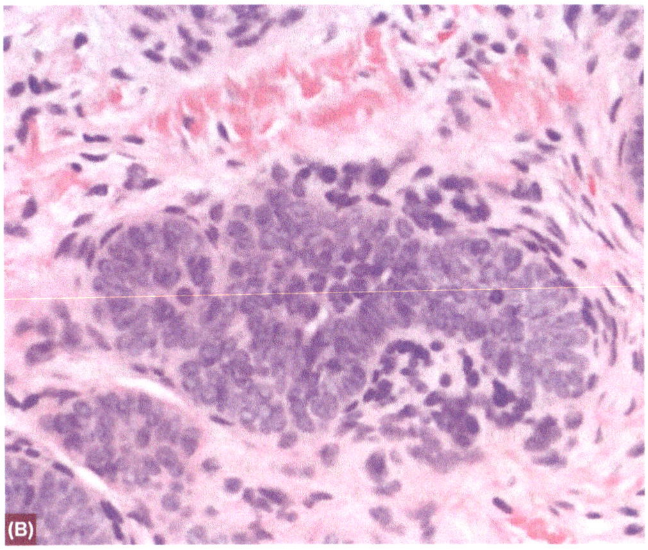

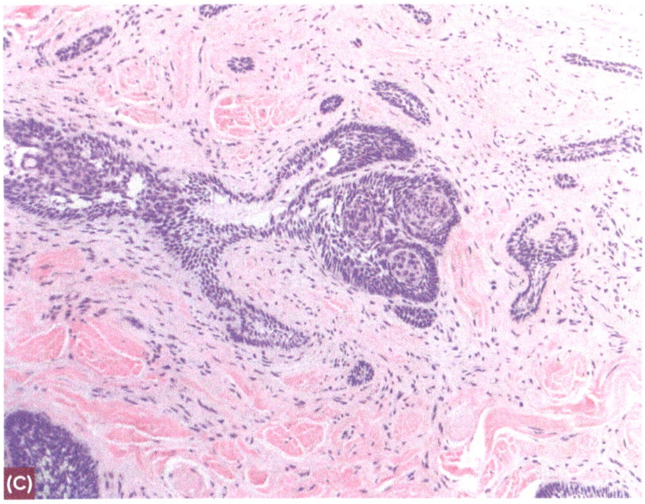

Trichoblastoma. (A) There are clusters and nests of basaloid epithelium with peripheral palisading; however, stromal retraction artifact and dermal mucin are absent. **(B)** Condensed fibrous stroma surrounds the basaloid cells and indents the epithelium reminiscent of the dermal papilla of the normal hair follicle. **(C)** There are basaloid cords surrounded by fibrous stroma. Foci reminiscent of hair bulbs containing dermal papillae are present.

In regard to the differential diagnosis, depending on its particular histologic constituency, the differential diagnosis of TBL encompasses **basal cell carcinoma** (BCC) of the nodular, micronodular, and morpheaform types, **basaloid follicular hamartoma** (BFH) (Table 9-32B), and **cutaneous lymphadenoma**. Of these, the most difficult distinction is between TBL and BFH because of their shared potential for cellular growth in single-file strands and an "interactive" interface between epithelial and stromal cells in those lesions. **Basaloid follicular hamartoma (BFH)** is generally regarded today as a malformative developmental lesion rather than a true neoplasm.

Table 9-32B. Basaloid Follicular Hamartoma

Clinical Features
Children or adults
Any location
Solitary or multiple forms: localized, linear, or generalized
Papules, plaques
Comedones, keratotic plugs
Alopecia may occur
Histopathologic Features
Folliculocentric
Proliferation of bland uniform basaloid cells in cords and aggregates
Organized fibrous stroma
Adenoid or reticulated patterns
Small keratinous cysts
Calcification may occur
Differential Diagnosis
Fibroepithelioma of Pinkus
Superficial basal cell carcinoma
Trichoepithelioma
Reticulated seborrheic keratosis

However, it should be noted in that regard that this condition may develop for the first time during adulthood. It likewise may be linear or regionalized, pale or erythematous, plaque-like or papular, and solitary or generalized. Some examples of BFH have caused alopecia or arisen in patients with myasthenia gravis. The microscopic features of **BFH** include a folliculocentric proliferation of bland, uniform basaloid cells that are arranged in cords and clusters and separated from each other by an organized fibrous stroma. Adenoid or reticulated

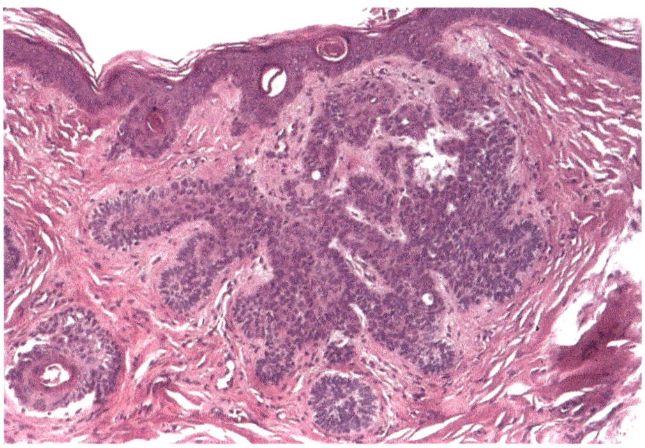

Basaloid follicular hamartoma. A small folliculocentric proliferation of basaloid cells is present separated by fibrous stroma.

patterns can often be appreciated in the epithelial component, and small keratinous cysts may be evident as well. These may become calcified; vellus hairs or sebaceous glands may also be included in **BFH**. **TBL** contains structures resembling embryonic hair follicles which are not present in **BFH**. A key distinction of **TBL** and **BFH** from **basal cell carcinoma** is the absence of necrotic tumor cells. Additionally, **BCC** exhibits tumor-stroma retraction artifact and dermal mucin.

Cutaneous lymphadenoma (CL) was first described by Santa Cruz and colleagues in 1991 as a dermal neoplasm with a distinctive histologic appearance. Many believe it to be a benign lesion related to **TBL**. **CL** typically presents as a slow-growing, nondescript, nonulcerated, flesh-colored nodule in the skin of the head and neck in young or middle-aged adults (average age, 40 years). The maximum tumor diameter is usually no larger than 2 cm. No syndromic associations have been

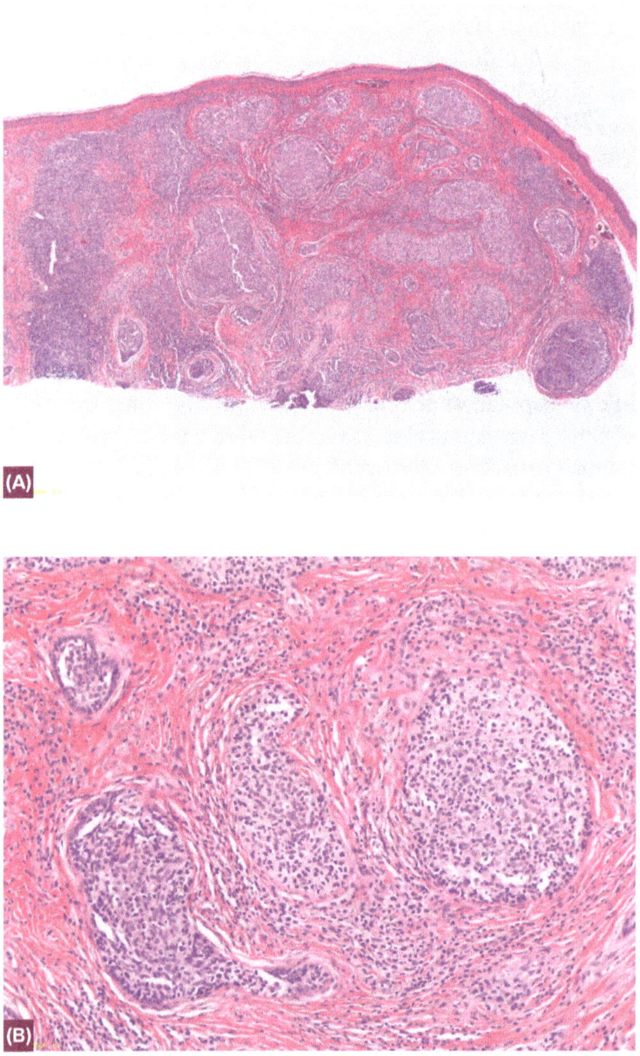

Cutaneous lymphadenoma. (A) A lobular growth pattern is visible on low-power microscopy. **(B)** Some of the tumor cell nests demonstrate slight dyscohesion. Numerous mature lymphocytes are interspersed among bland epithelioid tumor cells.

reported in connection with lymphadenoma of the skin, and it is cured by simple excision. The typical microscopic image of **CL** closely simulates that of intradermal thymic tissue. It is characterized by rounded lobules of uniform, cytologically bland basaloid cells, with numerous interspersed mature lymphocytes. Lymphoid cells may also be seen in the intervening stroma. The neoplastic cell groups tend to conform to one another, and peripherally located cells within them have a tendency to palisade. Foci of keratinization and apparent ductal differentiation have been reported as well, and occasional lesions in this group may demonstrate a subepidermal network of cells similar to that seen in **tumor of the follicular infundibulum (TFI).** The tumor cells in **CL** have open nuclei with discernible nucleoli, but mitotic activity and apoptosis are sparse. Immunophenotyping of the lesion shows diffuse keratin reactivity, with specific antibodies to CK20, demonstrating the presence of scattered positivity (putatively representing Merkel cell differentiation). Intratumoral lymphoid cells are predominantly T cells, with the majority labeling for CD3, CD5, CD43, and CD45R0. A generous number of apparent Langerhans cells, which stain for CD1a and S-100 protein, are also usually observed. Intralesional histiocytes that label for CD68, with or without CD30, have also been reported. **Trichoepitheliomas** and classical **TBL** do not exhibit an investment by lymphocytes, as seen in **CL**. Additionally, **CL** lacks a specialized peritumoral stroma component. **CL** may resemble **lymphoepithelioma-like carcinoma of the skin (LELCS);** however, the latter is characterized by frankly malignant cytology and pattern of growth.

ANSWER 9-33: C.

The biopsy reveals a perifollicular fibrous proliferation with a central dilated follicle. Thin septa of proliferating epithelium containing sebaceous lobules divide the fibrous mantle. The findings are consistent with a **fibrofolliculoma.** This patient most likely has **Birt-Hogg-Dubé syndrome,** which is an autosomal dominant condition attributed to mutations in the *FLCN* gene which codes for the protein **folliculin** (possibly a tumor suppressor protein). These patients are prone to developing **renal cell carcinomas** and pulmonary cysts which frequently result in spontaneous pneumothorax. Cutaneous perifollicular stromal tumors are most common manifestation of the disease. Outside of Birt-Hogg-Dubé syndrome, tumors demonstrating differentiation toward the stromal elements that are associated with developing hair follicles are extremely rare. Moreover, their clinical presentations and histologic images are quite similar. The lesions grouped in this category include **trichodiscoma, perifollicular fibroma**, and **fibrofolliculoma** (Table 9-33A). Many believe these tumors to represent a spectrum of the same tumor.

Trichodiscoma was so named because this tumor was presumed to show differentiation toward the hair discs, or Haarscheibe. In normal skin, the latter structures are receptor

Table 9-33A. Comparison of Trichodiscoma, Perifollicular Fibroma, and Fibrofolliculoma

TRICHODISCOMA		PERIFOLLICULAR FIBROMA		FIBROFOLLICULOMA
		Clinical Features		
	⇐	Usually adults Head and neck, trunk, extremities Often multiple May be generalized Small skin-colored papules, flat or dome shaped	⇒	
		Histopathologic Features		
Stromal component expands dermis, forming nodule		Stromal component: stroma composed of delicate collagen bundles, scattered fibroblasts, mucin deposition, and numerous microvessels Stromal component oriented about central hair follicle		Well-demarcated stromal component oriented about central hair follicular infundibular structure Thin epithelial cords extend from infundibular structure into surrounding stroma The cords have an anastomosing pattern

complexes composed of nerve ends and supporting fibrovascular stroma, which are associated with intraepidermal Merkel cells. In reality, no objective evidence supports the presence of morphologic or functional attributes of the hair disc in trichodiscoma. Clinically, this neoplasm becomes manifest as a grouping of otherwise banal small nodules in the skin, most often in the head and neck region but also possibly in other locations, in patients of virtually any age. These nodules may be grouped in a regional fashion, or the patient may have a generalized trichodiscomatosis. Contrary to what may be expected intuitively because of its putative relationship with the Haarscheibe, trichodiscoma is not a painful lesion. There may be an association between this lesion and other follicular malformations or neoplasms in the same individual. The histologic diagnosis of trichodiscoma is predicated on the presence of a superficial dermal "plate" of paucicellular fibrovascular tissue containing nerve twigs (seen only by silver impregnation stains), stromal mucin, and elastin. The overlying epidermis is attenuated, and hair follicles are usually present at the periphery

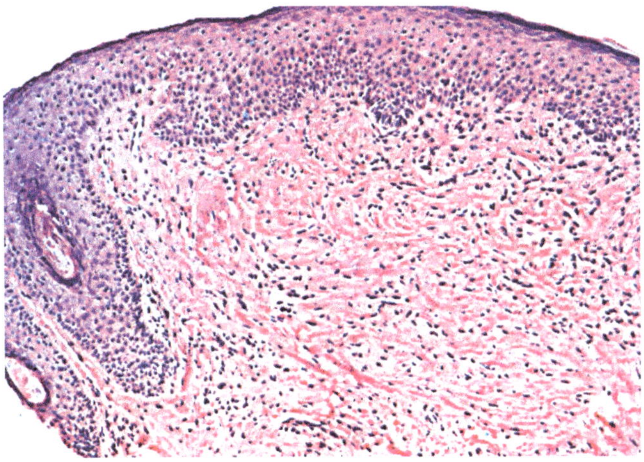

Trichodiscoma. A superficial plate of paucicellular fibrous stroma expands the corium. The lesion is bordered by a hair follicle.

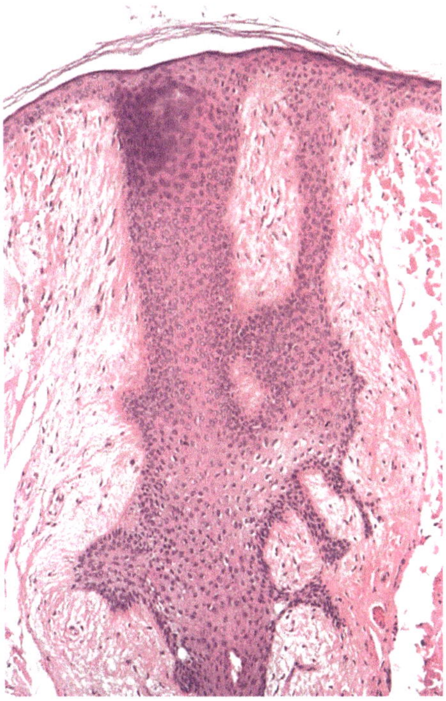

Perifollicular fibroma. The perifollicular mesenchyme is expanded by a paucicellular fibrous stroma similar to that seen in trichodiscoma.

of the dermal abnormality. Interestingly, immunostains show an absence of Merkel cells in the overlying epithelium, contrary to theoretical predictions.

Perifollicular Fibroma (PF) is also primarily a fibroblastic proliferation, with clinical features that are similar, if not identical, to those of trichodiscoma. In the past, much literature was devoted to a consideration of whether PF was kin to **fibrous papule** of the face and **adenoma sebaceum (fibrous papule of the face associated with tuberous sclerosus)**. Answer choice C describes the so-called ash leaf spots of tuberous sclerosus. Inasmuch as those proliferations are basically angiofibromatous, we do not recognize any relatedness between them and PF. The latter lesion differs from them histologically in showing a vaguely nodular proliferation of bland, paucicellular fibrous stroma—with or without mucin deposition—around hair follicles. This process assumes a lamellar image and may or may not be associated with fibrosis of the adjacent interfollicular dermis as well. Junkins-Hopkins and Cooper have considered the significance of a multiplicity of PFs, revisiting traditional teaching that this finding was sometimes associated with **familial colonic polyposis** and an increased risk of colorectal carcinoma. Those authors concluded that the latter paradigm was erroneous and that multiple **fibrofolliculomas** (vide infra), as seen with multiple **trichodiscomas** and **acrochordons** in the autosomal dominant **Birt-Hogg-Dubé syndrome,** were the real culprits in regard to related colonic pathology.

Fibrofolliculoma is similar to **PF** clinicopathologically but differs from that tumor in being associated with central follicular dilatation or distortion and showing interanastomosing septa of follicular epithelium that traverse the lamellated fibrous mantle around the affected pilosebaceous unit or units. Weintraub and Pinkus have referred to this as an "epithelial net." Besides the previously mentioned role played in the **Birt-Hogg-Dubé syndrome**, **fibrofolliculoma** may also be linked in selected patients to the concurrent presence of **connective tissue nevi.**

BIBLIOGRAPHY

1. Abesamis-Cubillan E, El-Shabrawi-Caelen L, LeBoit PE. Merkel cells and sclerosing epithelial neoplasms. *Am J Dermatopathol.* 2000;22:311–315.
2. Akalin T, Sen S, Yuceturk A, Kandiloglu G. p53 protein expression in eccrine poroma and porocarcinoma. *Am J Dermatopathol.* 2001;23:402–406.
3. Aloi F, Tomasini C, Pippione M. Pigmented trichoblastoma. *Am J Dermatopathol.* 1992;14:345–349.
4. Ambrojo P, Caballero-Martinez AA, Sanchez-Yus E, Furio V. Clear cell syringoma. *Dermatologica.* 1989;178:164–166.
5. Ansai S, Hashimoto H, Aoki T, et al. A histochemical and immunohistochemical study of extraocular sebaceous carcinoma. *Histopathology.* 1993;22:127–133.
6. Ansai S, Watanabe S, Aso K. A case of tubular apocrine adenoma with syringocystadenoma papilliferum. *J Cutan Pathol.* 1989;16:230–236.
7. Argenyi AZ, Nguyen AV, Balogh K, et al. Malignant eccrine spiradenoma: a clinicopathologic study. *Am J Dermatopathol.* 1990;12:335–343.
8. Baptista AP, Silva LGE, Born MC. Proliferating trichilemmal cyst. *J Cutan Pathol.* 1983;10:178–187.
9. Brook JD, Fitzpatrick JE, Golitz LE. Papillary mesenchymal bodies: a histological finding useful in differentiating trichoepitheliomas from basal cell carcinomas. *J Am Acad Dermatol.* 1989;21:523–528.
10. Brownstein MH. Basaloid follicular hamartoma: solitary and multiple types. *J Am Acad Dermatol.* 1992;27:237–240.
11. Carlsten JR, Lewis MD, Saddler K, et al. Spiradenocylindrocarcinoma: a malignant hybrid tumor. *J Cutan Pathol.* 2005;32:166–171.
12. Chan JK, Ng CS, Tsang WY. Nodular desmoplastic variant of trichoblastoma. *Am J Surg Pathol.* 1994;18:495–500.
13. Chibber V, Lyle S, Mahalingam M. Ductal eccrine carcinoma with squamous differentiation: apropos a case. *J Cutan Pathol.* 2007;34:503–507.
14. Chiller K, Passaro D, Scheuller M, et al. Microcystic adnexal carcinoma: forty-eight cases, their treatment, and their outcome. *Arch Dermatol.* 2000;136:1355–1359.
15. Cho KJ, Khang SK, Koh JS, et al. Sebaceous carcinoma of the eyelids: frequent expression of c-*erb*B-2 oncoprotein. *J Korean Med Sci.* 2000;15:545–550.
16. Cribier B, Grosshans E. Tumor of the follicular infundibulum: a clinicopathologic study. *J Am Acad Dermatol.* 1995;33:979–984.
17. DeFrancesco V, Frattasio A, Pillon B, et al. Carcinosarcoma arising in a patient with multiple cylindromas. *Am J Dermatopathol.* 2005;27:21–26.
18. Diaz-Cascajo C, Borghi S, Rey-Lopez A, Carretero-Hernandez G. Cutaneous lymphadenoma: a peculiar variant of nodular trichoblastoma. *Am J Dermatopathol.* 1996;18:186–191.
19. Diaz-de-Leon E, Carcangiu ML, Prieto VG, et al. Extramammary Paget disease is characterized by the consistent lack of estrogen and progesterone receptors but frequently expresses androgen receptor. *Am J Clin Pathol.* 2000;113:572–575.
20. Duke WH, Sherrod TT, Lupton GP. Aggressive digital papillary adenocarcinoma (aggressive digital papillary

adenoma and adenocarcinoma) revisited. *Am J Surg Pathol.* 2000;24:775–784.

21. Farina MC, Pique E, Olivares M, et al. Multiple hidrocystoma of the face: three cases. *Clin Exp Dermatol.* 1995;20:323–327.
22. Gerber PA, Schulte KW, Ruzicka T, Bruch-Gerharz D. Eccrine porocarcinoma of the head: an important differential diagnosis in the elderly patient. *Dermatology.* 2008;216:229–233.
23. Gould E, Kurzon R, Kowalczyk AP, Saldana M. Pilomatrix carcinoma with pulmonary metastases: a report of a case. *Cancer.* 1984;54:370–372.
24. Grouls V. Tricholemmale Keratose und tricholemmales Karzinom. *Hautarzt.* 1987;38:335–341.
25. Hara K. Mixed tumors of the skin: a histopathological, enzyme-histochemical, and immunohistochemical study. *Histopathology.* 1995;26:145–152.
26. Hartschuh W, Schulz T. Merkel cells are integral constituents of desmoplastic trichoepithelioma: an immunohistochemical and electron microscopic study. *J Cutan Pathol.* 1995;22:413–421.
27. Harvell JD, Kerschmann RL, LeBoit PE. Eccrine or apocrine poroma? Six poromas with divergent adnexal differentiation. *Am J Dermatopathol.* 1996;18:1–9.
28. Henner MS, Shapiro PE, Ritter JH, et al. Solitary syringoma: a report of five cases and comparison with microcystic adnexal carcinoma. *Am J Dermatopathol.* 1995;17:465–470.
29. Ho VH, Ross MI, Prieto VG, et al. Sentinel lymph node biopsy for sebaceous cell carcinoma and melanoma of the ocular adnexa. *Arch Otolaryngol Head Neck Surg.* 2007;133:820–826.
30. Hoang MP, Dresser KA, Kapur P, et al. Microcystic adnexal carcinoma: an immunohistochemical reappraisal. *Mod Pathol.* 2008;21:178–185.
31. Hoang MP, Dresser KA, Kapur P, et al. Microcystic adnexal carcinoma: an immunohistochemical approach. *Mod Pathol.* 2008;21:178–185.
32. Horn TD, Vennos EM, Bernstein BD, Cooper PH. Multiple tumors of follicular infundibulum with sweat duct differentiation. *J Cutan Pathol.* 1995;22: 281–287.
33. Housholder MS, Zeligman I. Sebaceous neoplasms associated with visceral carcinomas. *Arch Dermatol.* 1980;116:61–64.
34. Hunt SJ, Kilzer PB, Santa Cruz DJ. Desmoplastic trichilemmoma: histologic variant resembling invasive carcinoma. *J Cutan Pathol.* 1990;17:45–52.
35. Hurt MA. Pilar sheath acanthoma (lobular infundibuloisthmicoma). *Am J Dermatopathol.* 1996;18:435.
36. Inaloz HS, Chowdhury MM, Knight AG. Cutaneous lymphadenoma. *J Eur Acad Dermatol Venereol.* 2001;15:481–483.
37. Inglefield CJ, Muir IF, Gray ES. Aggressive pilomatricoma in childhood. *Ann Plast Surg.* 1994;33:656–658.
38. Isaacson D, Turner ML. Localized vulvar syringomas. *J Am Acad Dermatol.* 1979;1:352–356.
39. Ivan D, Nash JW, Prieto VG, et al. Use of p63 in distinguishing primary and metastatic cutaneous adnexal neoplasms from metastatic adenocarcinoma to skin. *J Cutan Pathol.* 2007;35:474–480.
40. Junkins-Hopkins JM, Cooper PH. Multiple perifollicular fibromas: review of a case and analysis of the literature. *J Cutan Pathol.* 1994;21:467–471.
41. Kaddu S, Soyer HP, Cerroni L, et al. Clinical and histopathological spectrum of pilomatricoma in adults. *Int J Dermatol.* 1994;33:705–708.
42. Kaddu S, Soyer HP, Hodl S, Kerl H. Morphological stages of pilomatricoma. *Am J Dermatopathol.* 1996;18:333–338.
43. Kanitakis J, Zambruno G, Euvrard S, et al. Eccrine syringofibroadenoma. *Am J Dermatopathol.* 1987;9:37–40.
44. Kao GF, Laskin WB, Weiss SW. Eccrine spiradenoma occurring in infancy, mimicking a mesenchymal tumor. *J Cutan Pathol.* 1990;17:214–219.
45. Katoh N, Hirano S, Hosokawa Y, et al. Mucinous carcinoma of the skin: report of a case with DNA cytofluorimetric study. *J Dermatol.* 1994;21:117–121.
46. Kazakov DV, Bisceglia M, Spagnolo DV, et al. Apocrine mixed tumors of the skin with architectural and/or cytologic atypia: a retrospective clinicopathologic study of 18 cases. *Am J Surg Pathol.* 2007;31:1094–1102.
47. Kazakov DV, Calonje E, Zelger B, et al. Sebaceous carcinoma arising in nevus sebaceus of Jadassohn: a clinicopathologic study of five cases. *Am J Dermatopathol.* 2007;29:242–248.
48. Kazakov DV, DV, Belousova IE, Bisceglia M, et al. Apocrine mixed tumor of the skin ("mixed tumor of the folliculosebaceous-apocrine complex"). Spectrum of differentiation and metaplastic changes in the epithelial, myoepithelial, and stromal components based on a histopathologic study of 244 cases. *J Am Acad Dermatol.* 2007;57:467–483.
49. Kazakov DV, Kutzner H, Rutten A, et al. Carcinoid-like pattern in sebaceous neoplasms: another distinctive, previously unrecognized pattern in extraocular sebaceous carcinoma and sebaceoma. *Am J Dermatopathol.* 2005;27:195–203.
50. Kazakov DV, Kutzner H, Spagnolo DV, et al. Sebaceous differentiation in poroid neoplasms: report of 11 cases,

including a case of metaplastic carcinoma associated with apocrine poroma (sarcomatoid apocrine porocarcinoma). *Am J Dermatopathol.* 2008;30:21–26.

51. Kazakov DV, Mikyskova J, Kutzner H, et al. Hidradenoma papilliferum with oxyphilic metaplasia: a clinicopathologic study of 18 cases, including detection of human papillomavirus. *Am J Dermatopathol.* 2005;2:102–110.
52. Kazakov DV, Mukensnabl P, Michal M. Tubular adenoma of the skin with follicular and sebaceous differentiation: a report of two cases. *Am J Dermatopathol.* 2006;28:142–146.
53. Kazakov DV, Soukup R, Mukensnabl P, et al. Brooke-Spiegler syndrome: report of a case with combined lesions containing cylindromatous, spiradenomatous, trichoblastomatous, and sebaceous differentiation. *Am J Dermatopathol.* 2005;27:27–33.
54. Kazakov DV, Suster S, LeBoit PE, et al. Mucinous carcinoma of the skin, primary and secondary: a clinicopathologic study of 63 cases with emphasis on the morphologic spectrum of primary cutaneous forms—homologies with mucinous lesions in the breast. *Am J Surg Pathol.* 2005;29:764–782.
55. Kiyohara T, Kumakiri H, Kuwahara H, et al. Rippled-pattern sebaceoma: a report of a lesions on the back with a review of the literature. *Am J Dermatopathol.* 2006;28:446–448.
56. Koh BK, Choi JM, Yi JY, et al. Recurrent primary cutaneous adenoid cystic carcinoma of the scrotum. *Int J Dermatol.* 2001;40:724–725.
57. Krahl D, Sellheyer K. Monoclonal antibody Ber-EP4 reliably discriminates between microcystic adnexal carcinoma and basal cell carcinoma. *J Cutan Pathol.* 2007;34:782–787.
58. Kuan SF, Montag AG, Hart J, et al. Differential expression of mucin genes in mammary and extramammary Paget's disease. *Am J Surg Pathol.* 2001;25:1469–1477.
59. Kwon TJ, Ro JY, Mackay B. Clear-cell carcinoma: an ultrastructural study of 57 tumors from various sites. *Ultrastruct Pathol.* 1996;20:519–527.
60. Laing V, Knipe RC, Flowers FP, et al. Proliferating trichilemmal tumor: report of a case and review of the literature. *J Dermatol Surg Oncol.* 1991;17:295–298.
61. Letizia C, Marcheggiano A, DeToma G, et al. Mixed type sweat gland adenoma: a case report. *Ann Ital Med Intern.* 1993;8:248–249.
62. Liang H, Wu H, Giorgadze TA, et al. Podoplanin is a highly sensitive and specific marker to distinguish primary skin adnexal carcinomas from adenocarcinomas metastatic to skin. *Am J Surg Pathol.* 2007;31:304–310.
63. Liang H, Wu H, Giorgadze TA, et al. Podoplanin is a highly sensitive and specific marker to distinguish primary skin adnexal carcinomas from adenocarcinomas metastatic to skin. *Am J Surg Pathol.* 2007;31: 304–310.
64. Liu HN, Chang YT, Chen CC, Huang CH. Histopathological and immunohistochemical studies of poroid hidradenoma. *Arch Dermatol Res.* 2006;297:319–323.
65. Long SA, Hurt MA, Santa Cruz DJ. Immature trichoepithelioma: report of six cases. *J Cutan Pathol.* 1988;15:353–358.
66. Mambo NC. The significance of atypical nuclear changes in benign eccrine acrospiromas: a clinical and pathological study of 18 cases. *J Cutan Pathol.* 1984;11:35–44.
67. Manivel JC, Wick MR, Mukai K. Pilomatrix carcinoma: an immunohistochemical comparison with benign pilomatrixoma and other benign lesions of pilar origin. *J Cutan Pathol.* 1986;13:22–29.
68. Matsumoto M, Ishiguro M, Ikeno F, et al. Combined Bowen disease and extramammary Paget disease. *J Cutan Pathol.* 2007;34(Suppl 1):47–51.
69. Matt D, Xin H, Vortmeyer AO, et al. Sporadic trichoepithelioma demonstrates deletions at 9q22.3. *Arch Dermatol.* 2000;136:657–660.
70. McCalmont TH. A call for logic in the classification of adnexal neoplasms. *Am J Dermatopathol.* 1996;18(2):103–109.
71. McKee PH, Fletcher CDM, Stavrinos P, Pambakian H. Carcinosarcoma arising in eccrine spiradenoma: a clinicopathologic and immunohistochemical study of two cases. *Am J Dermatopathol.* 1990;12:335–343.
72. McNiff JM, Eisen RN, Glusac EJ. Immunohistochemical comparison of cutaneous lymphadenoma, trichoblastoma, and basal cell carcinoma: support for classification of lymphadenoma as a variant of trichoblastoma. *J Cutan Pathol.* 1999;26:119–124.
73. Michaelsson G, Olsson E, Westermark P. The Rombo syndrome: a familial disorder with vermiculate atrophoderma, milia, hypotrichosis, trichoepitheliomas, basal cell carcinoma, and peripheral vasodilatation with cyanosis. *Acta Dermatol Venereol.* 1981;61:497–503.
74. Michal M, Lamovec J, Mukensnabl P, Pizinger K. Spiradenocylindromas of the skin: tumors with morphological features of spiradenoma and cylindroma in the same lesion: report of 12 cases. *Pathol Int.* 1999;49:419–425.
75. Miettinen M, Lasota J. KIT (CD117): a review on expression in normal and neoplastic disease and mutations and their clinicopathologic correlation. *Appl Immunohistochem Molec Morphol.* 2005;13:205–220.

76. Nakhleh RE, Swanson PE, Wick MR. Cutaneous adnexal carcinomas with mixed differentiation. *Am J Dermatopathol.* 1990;12:325–334.

77. Ogunrinade K, Blobstein SH, Desman GT. Agminated syringocystadenoma papilliferum: a new clinical presentation of a rare benign adnexal neoplasm. *Dermatol Online J.* 2013 August 15;19(8):19270.

78. Ohtsuka H, Nagamatsu S. Microcystic adnexal carcinoma: review of 51 Japanese Patients. *Dermatology.* 2002; 204(3):190–3.

79. Pariser RJ. Multiple hereditary trichoepitheliomas and basal cell carcinomas. *J Cutan Pathol.* 1986;13:111–117.

80. Patrizi A, Neri I, Marzaduri S, et al. Syringoma: a review of twenty-nine cases. *Acta Derm Venereol.* 1998;78:460–462.

81. Patterson JW, Straka BF, Wick MR. Linear syringocystadenoma papilliferum of the thigh. *J Am Acad Dermatol.* 2001;45:139–141.

82. Pizinger K, Michal M. Malignant cylindroma in Brooke-Spiegler syndrome. *Dermatology.* 2000;201:255–257.

83. Pruzam DL, Esterly NB, Prose NS. Eruptive syringoma. *Arch Dermatol.* 1989;125:1119–1120.

84. Pylyser K, DeWolf-Peeters C, Marien K. The histology of eccrine poroma: a study of 14 cases. *Dermatologica.* 1983;167:243–249.

85. Regauer S. Extramammary Paget's disease—a proliferation of adnexal origin? *Histopathology.* 2006;48:723–729.

86. Reis-Filho JS, Silva P, Milanezi F, Lopes JM. Hyaline cell-rich chondroid syringoma: case report and review of the literature. *Pathol Res Pract.* 2002;198:755–764.

87. Robson A, Greene J, Ansari N, et al. Eccrine porocarcinoma (malignant eccrine poroma): a clinicopathologic study of 69 cases. *Am J Surg Pathol.* 2001;25:710–720.

88. Robson A, Lazar AJF, Ben-Nagi J, et al. Primary cutaneous apocrine carcinoma: a clinicopathologic analysis of 24 cases. *Am J Surg Pathol.* 2008;32:682–690.

89. Rockerbie N, Solomon AR, Woo TY, et al. Malignant dermal cylindroma in a patient with multiple dermal cylindromas, trichoepitheliomas, and bilateral dermal analogue tumors of the parotid gland. *Am J Dermatopathol.* 1989;11:353–359.

90. Rosen LB. A review and proposed new classification of benign acquired neoplasms with hair follicle differentiation. *Am J Dermatopathol.* 1990;12:496–516.

91. Rutten A, Burgdorf W, Hugel H, et al. Cystic sebaceous tumors as marker lesions for the Muir-Torre syndrome: a histopathologic and molecular genetic study. *Am J Dermatopathol.* 1999;21:405–413.

92. Rutten A, Hantschke M, Angulo J, Requena L. Clear-cell dermal duct tumor: another distinctive, previously underrecognized cutaneous adnexal neoplasm. *Histopathology.* 2007;51:805–813.

93. Rutten A, Requena L. Sweat gland carcinomas of the skin. *Hautarzt.* 2008;59:151–160.

94. Sakai H, Satoh K, Manabe A, et al. Eccrine squamous syringometaplasia and syringomatous hyperplasia in association with linear scleroderma. *Dermatology.* 2002;204:136–138.

95. Salhi A, Bornholdt D, Oeffner F, et al. Multiple familial trichoepithelioma caused by mutations in the cylindromatosis tumor suppressor gene. *Cancer Res.* 2004;64:5113–5117.

96. Sanchez-Yus E, Requena L, Simon P, Sanchez M. Complex adnexal tumor of the primary epithelial germ with distinct patterns of superficial epithelioma with sebaceous differentiation, immature trichoepithelioma, and apocrine adenocarcinoma. *Am J Dermatopathol.* 1992;14:245–252.

97. Sarivya D, Ruth K, Adams-McDonnell R, et al. Clinicopathologic correlation of cutaneous metastases: experience from a cancer center. *Arch Dermatol.* 2007;143:613–620.

98. Sau P, Lupton GP, Graham JH. Pilomatrix carcinoma. *Cancer.* 1993;71:2491–2498.

99. Schell H, Haneke E. Tricholemmal carcinoma: report of 11 cases. *Hautarzt.* 1986;37:384–387.

100. Schulz T, Hartschuh W. Folliculosebaceous cystic hamartoma is a trichofolliculoma at its very late stage. *J Cutan Pathol.* 1998;25:354–364.

101. Sieron J, Thein T, Pirsig W, Hemmer J. The Nikolowski trichoadenoma: a rare tumor of the ENT area. *Laryngorhinootologie.* 1993;72:140–142.

102. Sington J, Chandrapala R, Manek S, Hollowood K. Mitotic count is not predictive of clinical behavior in hidradenoma papilliferum of the vulva: a clinicopathologic study of 19 cases. *Am J Dermatopathol.* 2006;28:322–326.

103. Smith KJ, Williams J, Corbett D, Skelton H. Microcystic adnexal carcinoma: an immunohistochemical study including markers of proliferation and apoptosis. *Am J Surg Pathol.* 2001;25:464–471.

104. Southey MC, Young MA, Whitty J, et al. Molecular pathologic analysis enhances the diagnosis and management of Muir-Torre syndrome and gives insight into its underlying molecular pathogenesis. *Am J Surg Pathol.* 2001;25:936–941.

105. Souvatzidis P, Sbano P, Mandato F, et al. Malignant nodular hidradenoma of the skin: report of seven cases. *J Eur Acad Dermatol Venereol.* 2008;22:549–554.

106. Spielvogel RL, Austin C, Ackerman AB. Inverted follicular keratosis is not a specific keratosis but a verruca vulgaris (or seborrheic keratosis) with squamous eddies. *Am J Dermatopathol.* 1983;5:427–442.

107. Sramek B, Lisle A, Loy T. Immunohistochemistry in ocular carcinomas. *J Cutan Pathol.* 2008;35:641–646.

108. Starink TM, Kisch LS, Meijer CJLM. Familial multiple trichodiscomas: a clinicopathologic study. *Arch Dermatol.* 1985;121:888–891.

109. Starink TM, Lane EB, Meijer CJ. Generalized trichoepitheliomas with alopecia and myasthenia gravis: clinicopathologic and immunohistochemical study and comparison with classic and desmoplastic trichoepithelioma. J Am Acad Dermatol. 1986;15:1104–1112.

110. Starink TM, Meijer CJLM, Brownstein MH. The cutaneous pathology of Cowden's disease: new findings. J Cutan Pathol. 1985;12:83–93.

111. Stefanato CM, Finn R, Bhawan J. Extramammary Paget disease with underlying hidradenoma papilliferum: guilt by association? Am J Dermatopathol. 2000;22:439–442.

112. Takei Y, Fukushiro S, Ackerman AB. Criteria for histologic differentiation of desmoplastic trichoepithelioma (sclerosing epithelial hamartoma) from morphea-like basal cell carcinoma. *Am J Dermatopathol.* 1985;7:207–211.

113. Tellechea O, Reis JP, Marques C, Baptista AP. Tubular apocrine adenoma with eccrine and apocrine immunophenotypes or papillary tubular adenoma? *Am J Dermatopathol.* 1995;17:499–505.

114. Troy JL, Ackerman AB. Sebaceoma: a distinctive benign neoplasm of adnexal epithelium differentiating toward sebaceous cells. Am J Dermatopathol. 1984;6:7–13.

115. Urso C, Bondi R, Paglierani M, et al. Carcinomas of sweat glands: report of 60 cases. Arch Pathol Lab Med. 2001;125:498–505.

116. Van der Walt JD, Rohlova B. Carcinomatous transformation in a pilomatrixoma. *Am J Dermatopathol.* 1984;6:63–69.

117. Weedon D, Bell J, Maize J. Matrical carcinoma of the skin. J Cutan Pathol. 1980;7:39–42.

118. Weiss J, Heine M, Grimmel M, Jung EG. Malignant proliferating trichilemmal cyst. J Am Acad Dermatol. 1995;32:870–873.

119. Wick MR, Cooper PH, Swanson PE, et al. Microcystic adnexal carcinoma: an immunohistochemical comparison with other cutaneous appendage tumors. Arch Dermatol. 1990;126:189–194.

120. Wick MR, Ockner DM, Mills SE, et al. Homologous carcinomas of the breasts, skin, and salivary glands: a histologic and immunohistochemical comparison of ductal mammary carcinoma, ductal sweat gland carcinoma, and salivary duct carcinoma. *Am J Clin Pathol.* 1998;109:75–84.

121. Wick MR, Swanson PE, LeBoit PE, Cooper PH. Lymphoepithelioma-like carcinomas of the skin with adnexal differentiation. J Cutan Pathol. 1991;18:93–102.

122. Wick MR, Swanson PE: "Carcinosarcomas"—current perspectives and a historical review of nosological concepts. Semin Diagn Pathol. 1993;10:118–127.

123. Wollina U, Rulke D, Schaarschmidt H. Dermal cylindroma: expression of intermediate filaments, epithelial and neuroectodermal antigens. Histol Histopathol. 1992;7:575–582.

124. Wong TY, Reed JA, Suster S, et al. Benign trichogenic tumors: a report of two cases supporting a simplified nomenclature. *Histopathology.* 1993;22:575–580.

125. Ye J, Nappi O, Swanson PE, Patterson JW, Wick MR. Proliferating pilar tumors: a clinicopathologic study of 76 cases with a proposal for definition of benign and malignant variants. *Am J Clin Pathol.* 2004;122:566–574.

CHAPTER 10

Melanocytic Proliferations

QUESTION 10-1.

A 30-year-old Caucasian male presents with multiple stellate brown macules on the shoulder after a severe sunburn from last summer. The lesions are all of about the same size and are sharply marginated. A biopsy is performed and the findings are illustrated below. Melan-A stain reveals a normal concentration of intraepidermal melanocytes. Which of the following diagnoses is CORRECT?

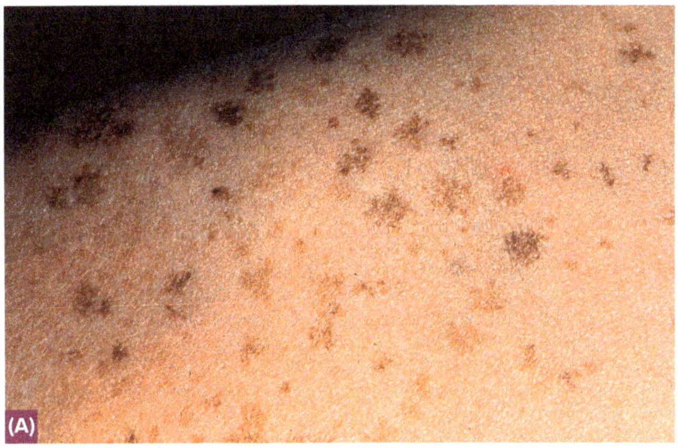

(A)

Reproduced with permission from Wolff K, Johnson RA, Saavedra AP. *Fitzpatrick's Color Atlas and Synopsis of Clinical Dermatology.* 7th ed. New York, NY: McGraw-Hill Education; 2013.

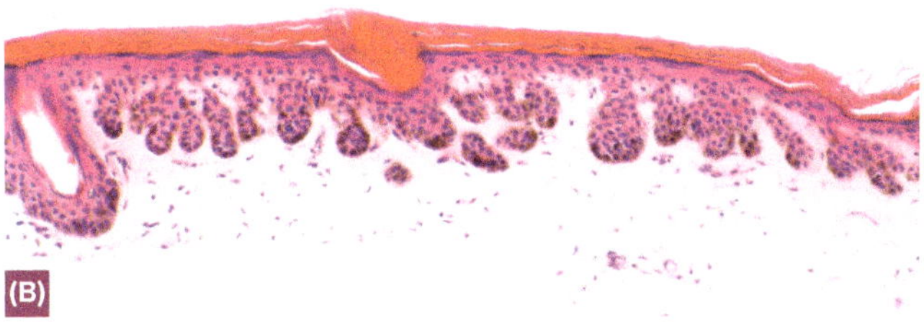

(B)

A) Pigmented actinic keratosis
B) Lentigo maligna melanoma
C) Solar lentigo
D) Junctional melanocytic nevus
E) Freckle

QUESTION 10-2.

A young adult patient presents with a well-circumscribed, dark, uniformly pigmented macule on the shoulder. The lesion has been present for several years. A biopsy is performed and the findings are illustrated below. Melan-A stain reveals a slight increase in dendritic melanocytes along the basal layer. Which of the following diagnoses is CORRECT?

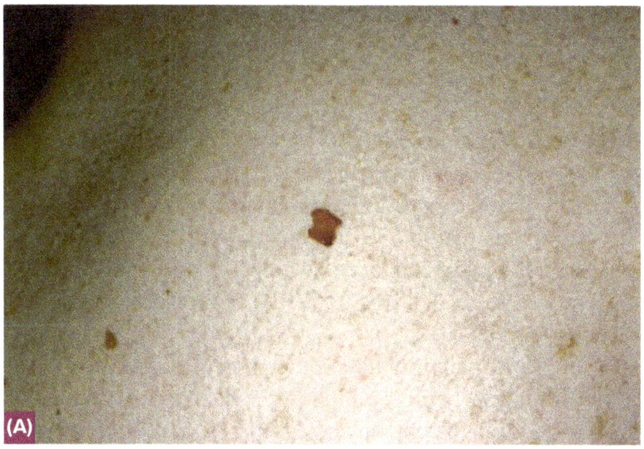

(A)

Courtesy of S Goldstein.

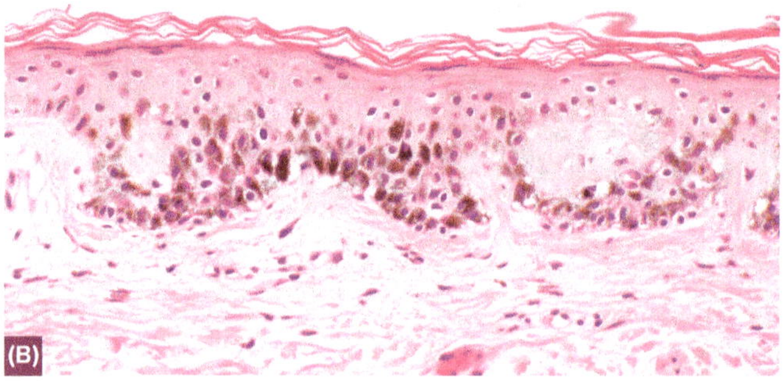

A) Lentigo simplex
B) Junctional nevus
C) Freckle
D) Primary acquired melanosis
E) Melanotic macule

QUESTION 10-3.

Which of the following statements regarding benign acquired neoplastic melanocytic proliferations is INCORRECT?

A) Pigmented macules are typically histopathologically characterized by either lentiginous or nested melanocytes along the basal layer of the epidermis.
B) Pigmented papules are typically histopathologically characterized by nested melanocytes along the basal layer of the epidermis and within the dermis.
C) Lightly pigmented or flesh-colored papules are typically histopathologically characterized by nests of melanocytes within the dermis only.
D) The presence of mitoses in basal layer melanocytes indicates malignant transformation.
E) As melanocytes descend into the deeper aspects of the dermis, there is a shift in cellular morphology and gene expression toward neural differentiation.

QUESTION 10-4.

A 35-year-old patient presents with a uniformly dark brown papule with well-circumscribed borders on the arm (Fig. 10-4 (A)). The lesion measures approximately 5 mm in diameter. The patient claims that the lesion appeared several years ago and has remained unchanged. A biopsy is performed and the findings are illustrated (Fig. 10-4 (B)). Which of the following diagnoses is CORRECT?

A) Common acquired junctional melanocytic nevus
B) Common acquired compound melanocytic nevus
C) Intradermal melanocytic nevus
D) Compound dysplastic nevus
E) Malignant melanoma, superficial spreading type

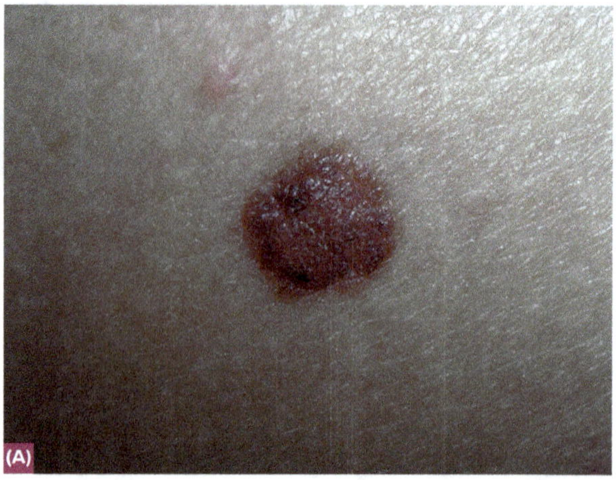

Reproduced, with permission, from Usatine RP, Smith MA, Mayeaux EJ Jr, Chumley HS, eds. *Color Atlas of Family Medicine*. 2nd ed. New York, NY: McGraw-Hill Education; 2012.

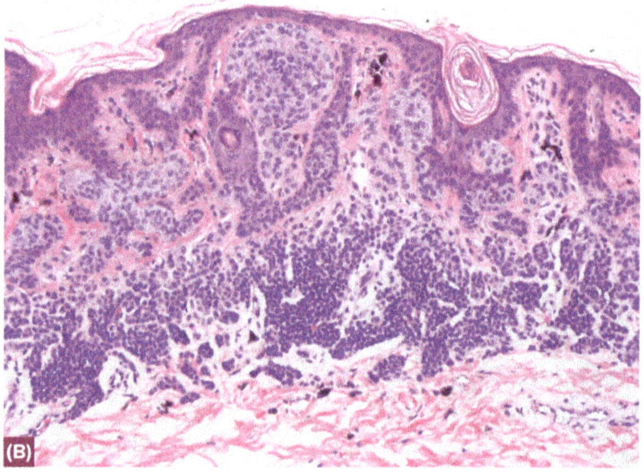

QUESTION 10-5.

A patient presents with a dome-shaped nodule on the forehead. Some focal areas with scattered pigmentation are noted. A biopsy is performed and the dermatopathologist reports a diagnosis of intradermal melanocytic nevus. Features that support this benign diagnosis include absent dermal melanocytic mitoses and so-called "maturation" with dermal descent. Various portions of the lesion are illustrated below. Going from superficial to deep, which of the following sequences accurately reflects normal "maturation" with descent?

A) B, C, D
B) D, C, B
C) D, B, C
D) C, D, B
E) B, D, C

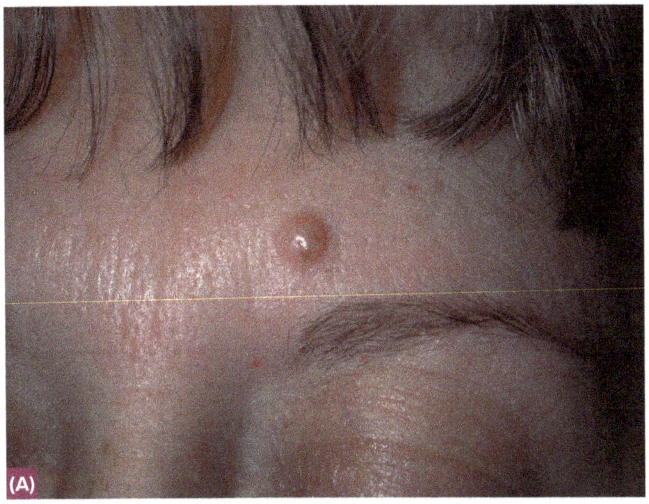

Reproduced, with permission, from Usatine RP, Smith MA, Mayeaux EJ Jr, Chumley HS, eds. *Color Atlas of Family Medicine*. 2nd ed. New York, NY: McGraw-Hill Education; 2012.

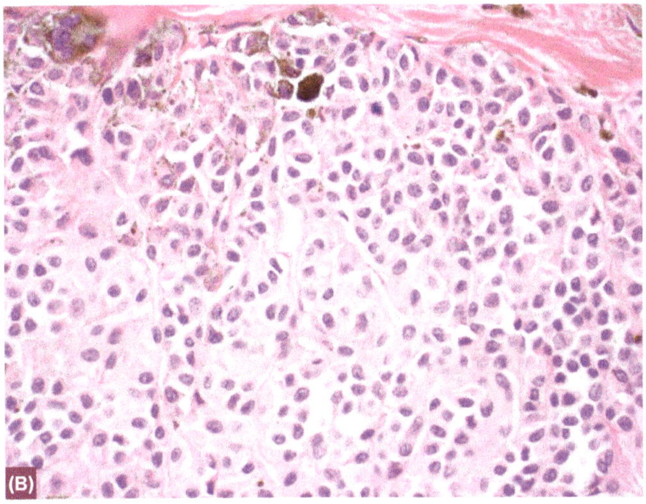

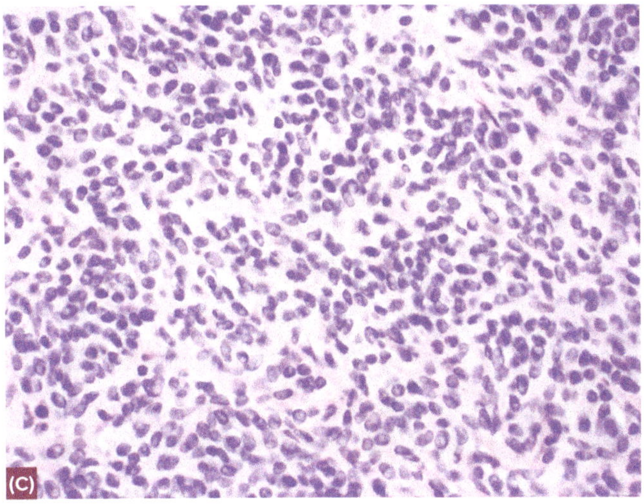

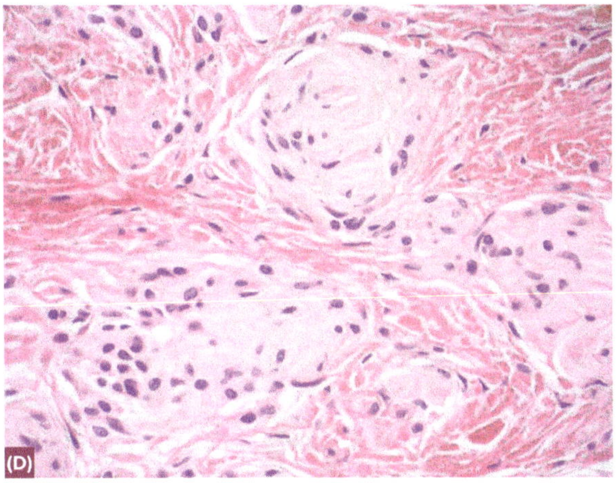

QUESTION 10-6.

Malignant melanoma has been historically categorized into the subtypes listed below. Please match the following descriptions that best coincide with the features of these melanoma subtypes.

I. Superficial spreading melanoma
II. Lentigo maligna
III. Acral (and mucosal) lentiginous melanoma
IV. Nodular melanoma

A) This form of melanoma is associated with chronic UV-light exposure, develops in elderly patients, and typically has a prolonged radial growth phase. These tumors are uncommonly associated with melanocytic nevi and tend to lack *BRAF* mutations.
B) This form of melanoma is associated with intermittent UV-light exposure, develops in relative young individuals, has a frequent association with atypical melanocytic nevi, and is associated with a high frequency of *BRAF* mutations.
C) This form of melanoma develops in relatively sun-protected sites, has a high frequency of chromosomal aberrations, generally lacks BRAF mutations, and occasionally has c-KIT mutations.
D) This form of melanoma is considered aggressive with no adjacent intraepithelial component. It is thought by many to be a final common pathway of rapid tumor progression irrespective of the intraepithelial pattern or location.

QUESTION 10-7.

An adult patient with a family history of malignant melanoma in a sibling presents with over 100 pigmented lesions on the chest, abdomen, and back. The clinically abnormal lesions are circled with black marker. The cluster of lesions in circle #2 is illustrated at high magnification below. The largest lesion is biopsied and the findings are also illustrated below. Which of the following statements regarding the biopsied lesion is INCORRECT?

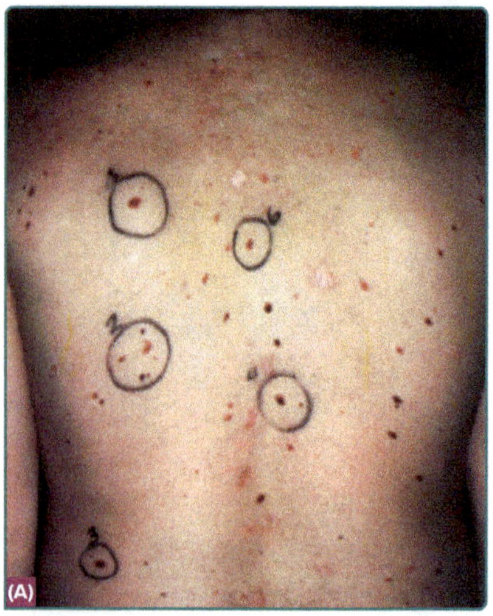

(A)

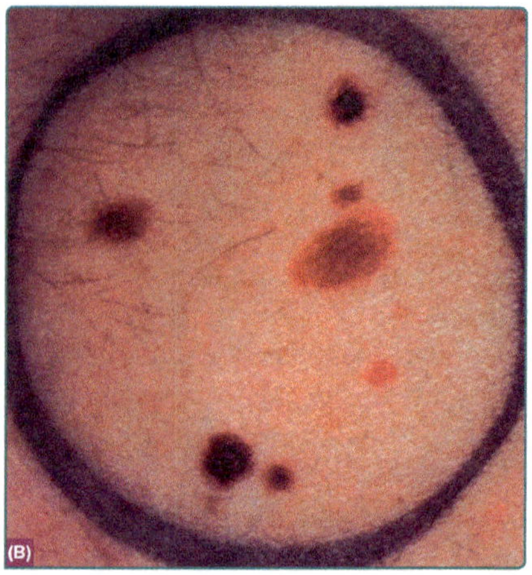

(B)

Reproduced, with permission, from Goldsmith LA, Katz SI, Gilchrest BA, Paller AS, Leffell DJ, Wolff K, eds. *Fitzpatrick's Dermatology in General Medicine*. 8th ed. New York, NY: McGraw-Hill Education; 2012.

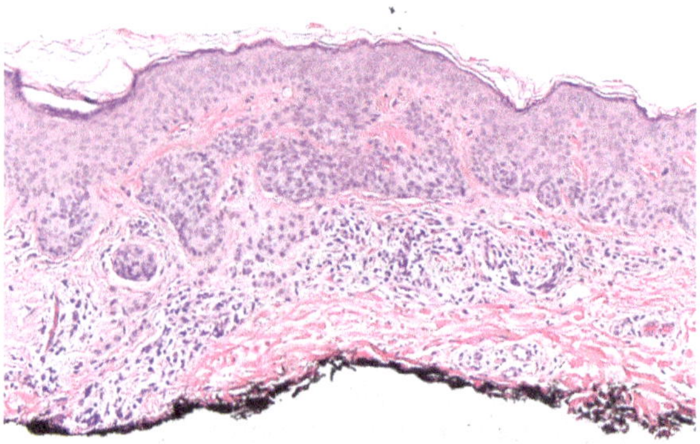

(C)

A) This lesion represents a type of melanocytic tumor that was first recognized during the clinical assessment of melanoma-prone families.

B) Several lines of evidence suggest that intense intermittent ultraviolet light (UV) exposure is important in the etiology of these lesions.

C) The usual clinical criteria for the diagnosis of these lesions are two obligate features: diameter in one dimension of at least 5 mm and a prominent flat component, and two of three other features: asymmetric outline, indistinct borders, and variable pigmentation.

D) Cytologic atypia of melanocytes is frequently encountered at the junctional component of these lesions.

E) This histopathologic diagnosis is based exclusively on cytologic atypia of melanocytes.

QUESTION 10-8.

A 30-year-old male presents with a pigmented lesion of the chest. He reports that the lesion has recently changed in size and shape. A biopsy is performed and the findings of the central and peripheral portions of the lesion are illustrated below, respectively. A Melan-A stain reveals focal areas of confluent melanocytic growth within the epidermis, but no pagetoid melanocytes. The melanocytic proliferation extends to the peripheral biopsy edges. Which of the following statements regarding this lesion is CORRECT?

A) This is a compound nevus with architectural disorder and severe cytologic atypia and should be re-excised with a 5-mm margin.

B) This is a common acquired compound melanocytic nevus that requires no further surgical management.

C) This is malignant melanoma, superficial spreading type, and should be conservatively re-excised.

D) This is a compound nevus with architectural disorder and mild cytologic atypia and should be re-excised with a 5-mm margin.

E) This is a compound nevus with architectural disorder and severe cytologic atypia that requires no further surgical management.

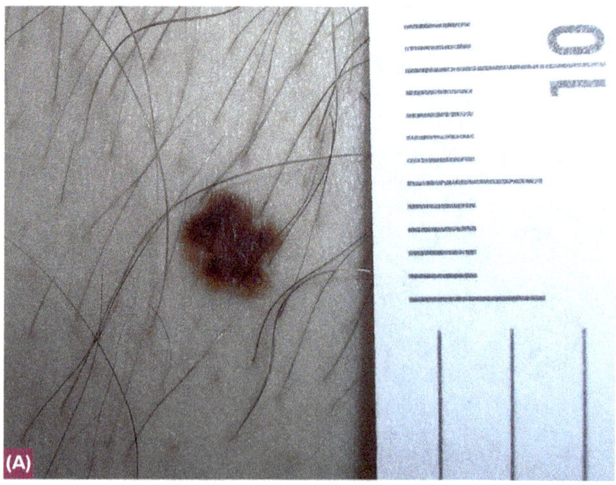

(A)

Reproduced, with permission, from Usatine RP, Smith MA, Mayeaux EJ Jr, Chumley HS, eds. *Color Atlas of Family Medicine*. 2nd ed. New York, NY: McGraw-Hill Education; 2012.

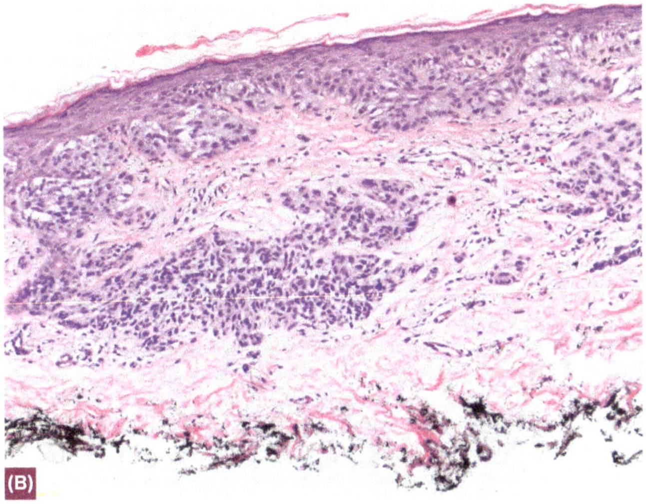

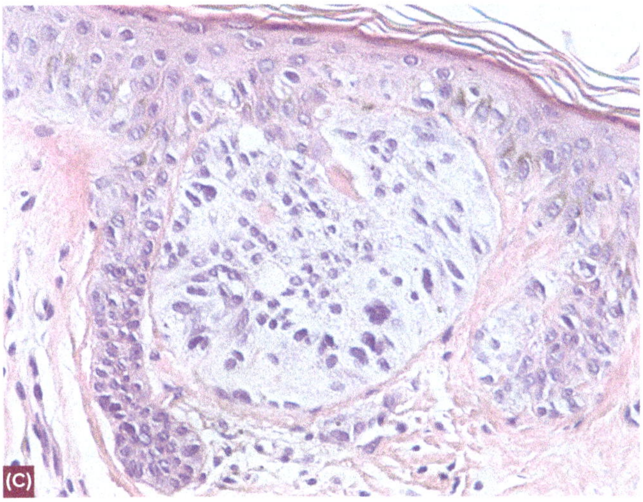

QUESTION 10-9.

In recent years, extensive investigation into the molecular basis of melanoma has unearthed novel findings regarding the natural history of these lesions. While many questions remain unanswered, this information has created a revolution in melanoma diagnostics and biologically targeted treatment. Which of the following statements regarding the molecular aspects of benign and malignant melanocytic proliferations is INCORRECT?

A) Melanocytic nevi are true neoplasms driven by oncogenic mutations.

B) While approximately 95% of malignant melanomas harbor chromosomal aberrations, benign nevi lack chromosomal aberrations or have a very restricted set that usually do not overlap with malignant melanoma.

C) There is an association with certain melanoma mutations and types of exposure to UV-light.

D) The so-called "maturation with dermal descent" of melanocytic nevi is a reflection of cellular senescence and the inability to divide.

E) Tumors with gains in isochromosome 11p (*HRAS* oncogene) are associated with malignant biological behavior.

QUESTION 10-10.

A 22-year-old female presents with several pigmented papules surrounded by a hypo- or amelanotic peripheral border. A few completely depigmented areas are present. A biopsy of one of the pigmented lesions is biopsied and the findings are illustrated below. Combined Melan-A/Ki67 immunostain reveals absent mitotic activity within dermal melanocytes. Which of the following statements regarding these lesions is INCORRECT?

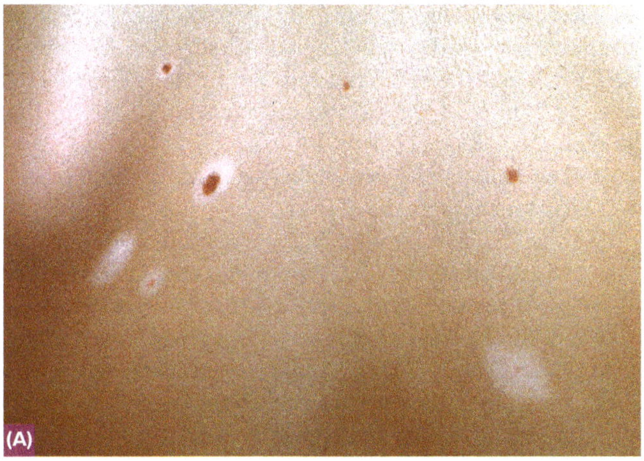

Reproduced, with permission, from Usatine RP, Smith MA, Mayeaux EJ Jr, Chumley HS, eds. *Color Atlas of Family Medicine*. 2nd ed. New York, NY: McGraw-Hill Education; 2012.

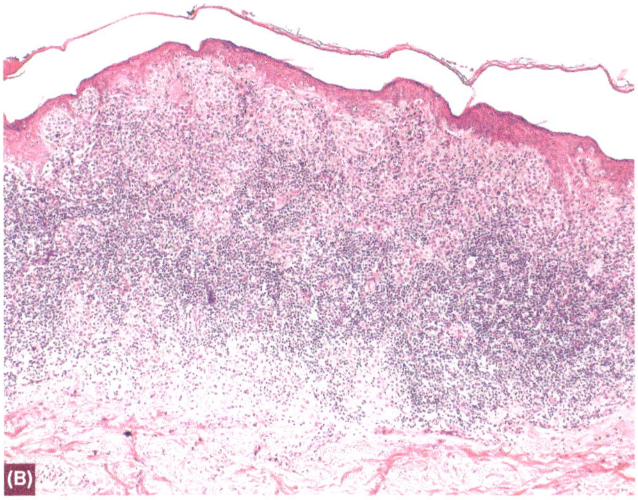

A) This rare phenomenon occurs most commonly in adults younger than 20 years of age.
B) There is an association with this condition and vitiligo.
C) This phenomenon typically occurs in acquired nevi, is of sudden onset, and frequently results in partial or complete involution of the pigmented lesions.
D) Most of the infiltrating cells in the biopsy are T lymphocytes and macrophages possibly directed against melanocyte antigens.
E) This phenomenon most likely represents malignant transformation and the onset of melanoma with regression.

QUESTION 10-11.

A patient presents with a pigmented lesion on the sole of the foot. Dermoscopy reveals a parallel network of pigment in the furrows (valleys) rather than the ridges. The findings are illustrated below. Note the white eccrine gland openings on the ridges, which are wider than the furrows. A biopsy is performed and the findings are also illustrated (Fig. 10-11 B and C). Which of the following statements regarding this lesion is INCORRECT?

A) These tumors may occasionally contain scattered melanocytes above the basal layer.
B) These lesions typically contain organized columns of melanin pigment within the stratum corneum.
C) This is an example of acral lentiginous melanoma.
D) The clinical features of these lesions are extremely valuable in determining benignancy versus malignancy.
E) This type of melanocytic proliferation may also arise on the palms, elbows, and knees.

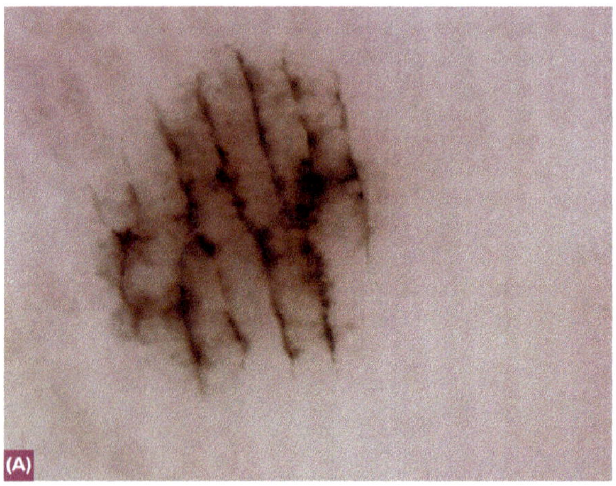
(A)

Reproduced, with permission, from Usatine RP, Smith MA, Mayeaux EJ Jr, Chumley HS, eds. *Color Atlas of Family Medicine*. 2nd ed. New York, NY: McGraw-Hill Education; 2012.

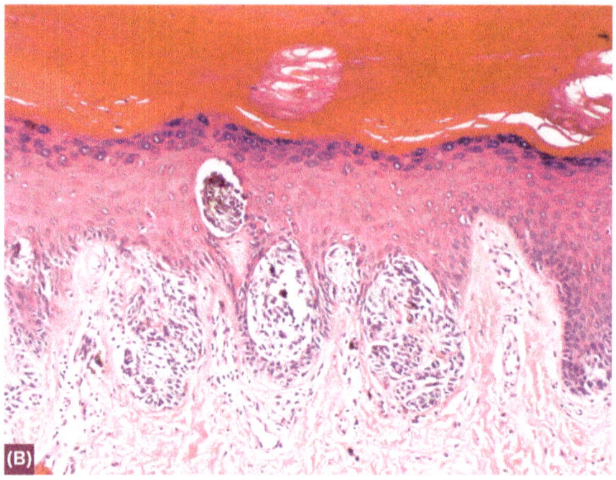
(B)

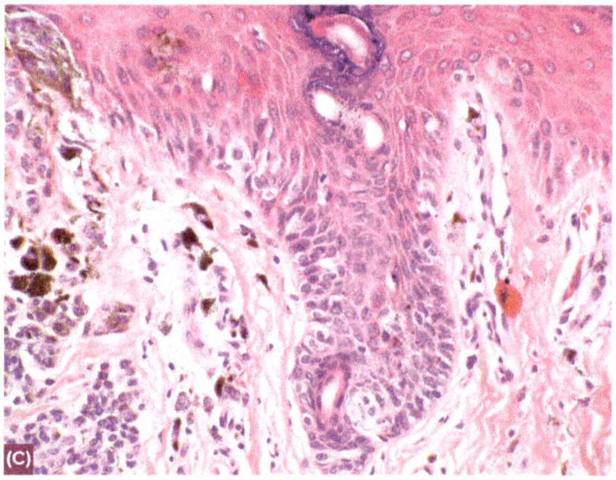
(C)

QUESTION 10-12.

A 30-year-old female presents with a 7 mm pigmented macule on the labia majora with fairly regular borders. There is significant pigment heterogeneity with tan, brown, and red areas. A biopsy is performed and the findings are illustrated below. Combined Melan-A/Ki67 stain (red/brown, respectively) is also illustrated below. Which of the following diagnoses is CORRECT?

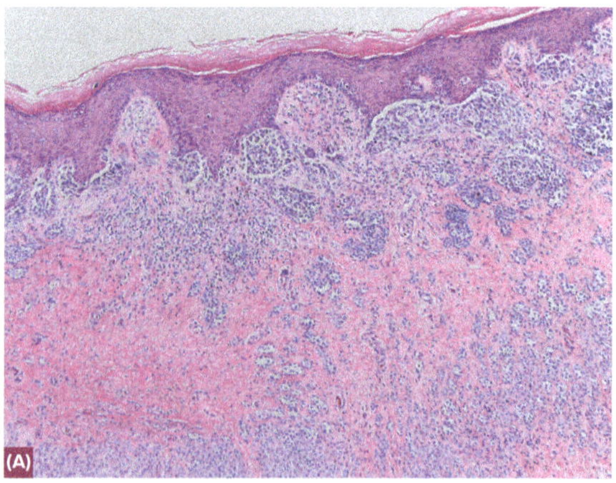
(A)

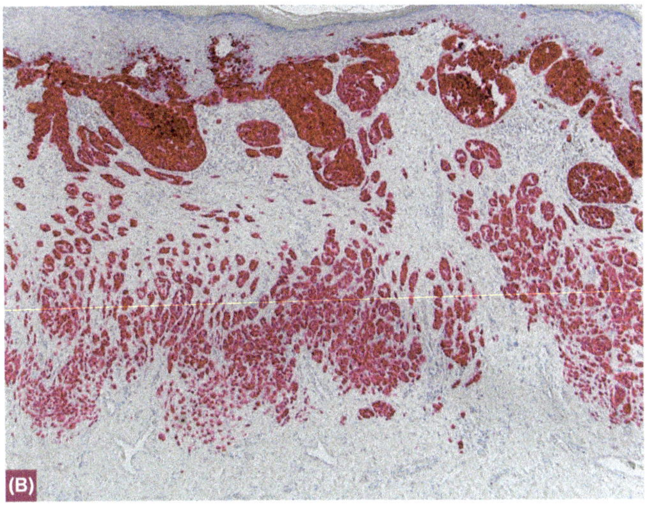
(B)

A) Compound genital melanocytic nevus
B) Benign vulvar melanosis
C) Mucosal lentigo
D) Malignant genital melanoma
E) Spitz nevus

QUESTION 10-13.

A 7-year-old boy presents with a 1.7 cm pigmented hairy plaque on the buttock. A biopsy is performed and the findings are illustrated below. Which of the following statements regarding this lesion is INCORRECT?

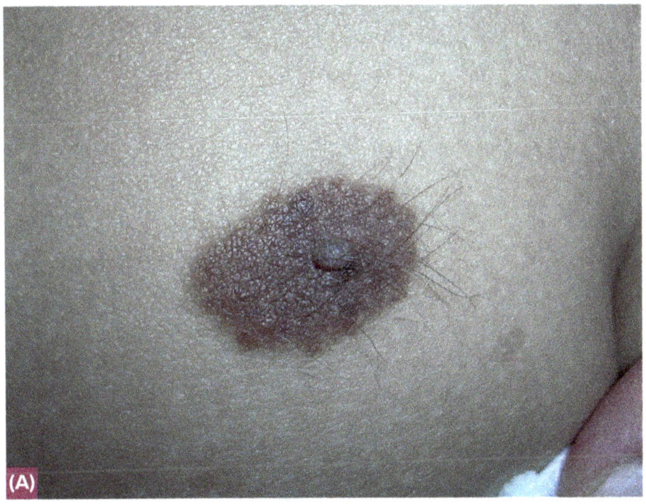
(A)

Reproduced, with permission, from Usatine RP, Smith MA, Mayeaux EJ Jr, Chumley HS, eds. *Color Atlas of Family Medicine*. 2nd ed. New York, NY: McGraw-Hill Education; 2012.

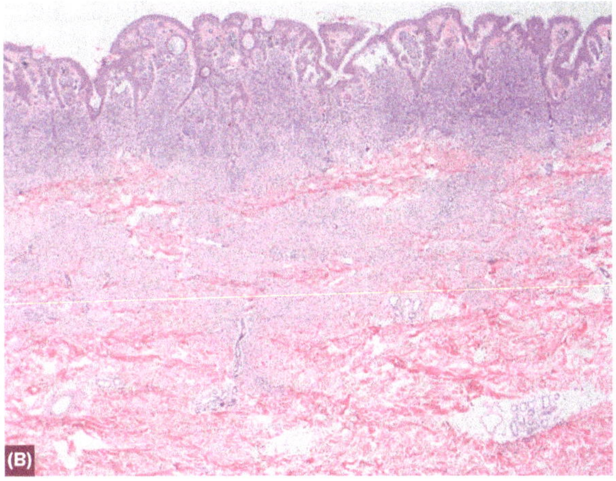
(B)

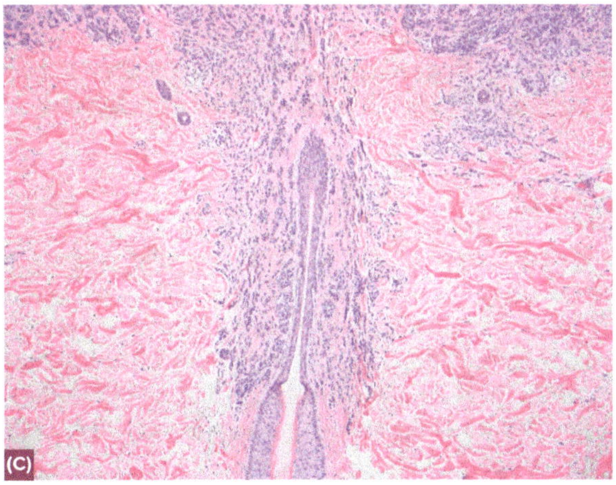
(C)

A) It is likely that this lesion has been present since birth.
B) Lesions on the face with this histomorphology are commonly acquired later in life.
C) This is an example of vertical growth phase melanoma arising within a common acquired compound melanocytic nevus.
D) These lesions commonly exhibit infiltration of perineurium and vascular walls by nevus cells.
E) When these lesions measure less than 20 cm in diameter, they are believed to carry a low risk for aggressive biological behavior.

QUESTION 10-14.

Which of the following statements regarding the pathological staging (pTNM) of malignant melanoma is INCORRECT?

A) The most important criteria for pathological tumor (pT) staging are anatomic compartment involved (Clark level), the presence or absence of ulceration, and the number of dermal mitoses.

B) Tumor thickness is measured microscopically in millimeters from the granular layer of the epidermis to the deepest focus of tumor cells.

C) Microsatellitosis is defined as the presence of tumor nests in the dermis or subcutis measuring greater than 0.05 mm in diameter, but separated from the main tumor by at least 0.3 mm of normal tissue on the section in which the Breslow measurement is taken.

D) Tumor regression carries adverse prognostic importance when it is complete or involves greater than 75% of the tumor.

E) The recommended approach for assessing dermal tumor mitotic activity is to search diligently throughout the dermis at 40× magnification for the focus of highest mitotic activity (so-called "hot-spot"), then measure additional separate fields (usually about 4 to 5) for an evaluation of 1 mm^2; the field diameter of a microscope be formally calibrated using a stage micrometer to determine the number of high-power fields that equates to a square millimetre.

QUESTION 10-15.

An elderly female presents with a large irregular pigmented patch on the cheek. The lesion has been present for several years and has slowly continued to grow in size. Dermoscopy reveals pigmented rhomboid structures. A biopsy is performed and the findings of the H&E and Melan-A stained sections are illustrated below. Which of the following diagnoses is CORRECT?

A) Solar lentigo
B) Melanoma in situ, lentigo maligna type
C) Superficial pigmented actinic keratosis
D) Lentiginous junctional melanocytic nevus
E) Chronic photoactivation of melanocytes

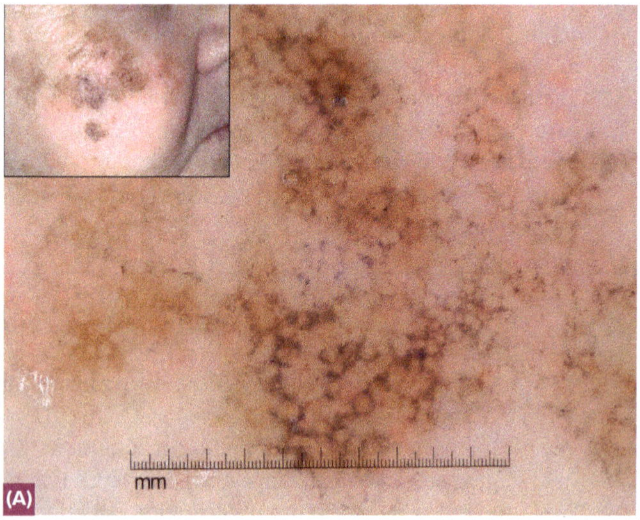

Reproduced, with permission, from Usatine RP, Smith MA, Mayeaux EJ Jr, Chumley HS, eds. *Color Atlas of Family Medicine*. 2nd ed. New York, NY: McGraw-Hill Education; 2012.

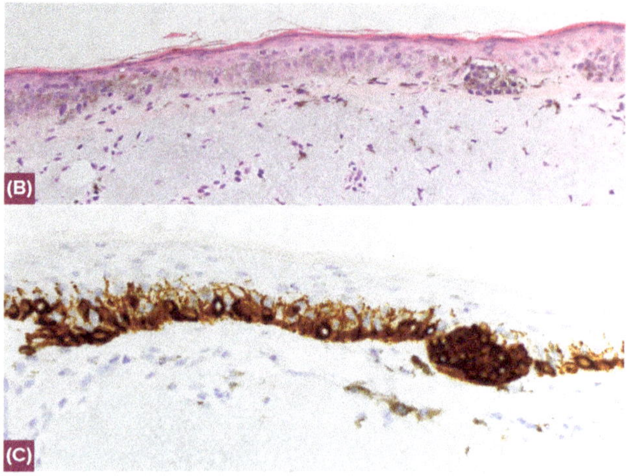

QUESTION 10-16.

An infant presents with a large area of pigmentation involving the majority of the skin of the chest, abdomen, and back. There is hypertrichosis in the portion involving the lower back. Numerous satellite lesions are present. Within the large pigmented region are a few nodular lesions. Biopsies of the flattened pigmented (image #1) and nodular pigmented areas (images #2 and 3) are performed and illustrated below. The nodular lesion contains two mitoses per mm^2. Which of the following statements regarding the biopsied nodular lesion is CORRECT?

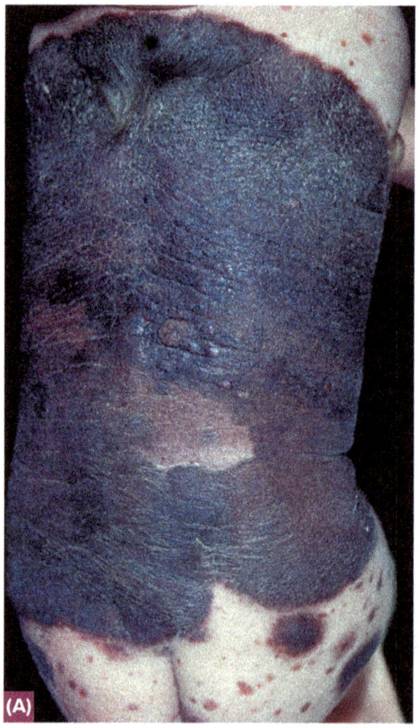

Reproduced, with permission, from Wolff K, Johnson RA, Saavedra AP. *Fitzpatrick's Color Atlas and Synopsis of Clinical Dermatology*. 7th ed. New York, NY: McGraw-Hill Education; 2013.

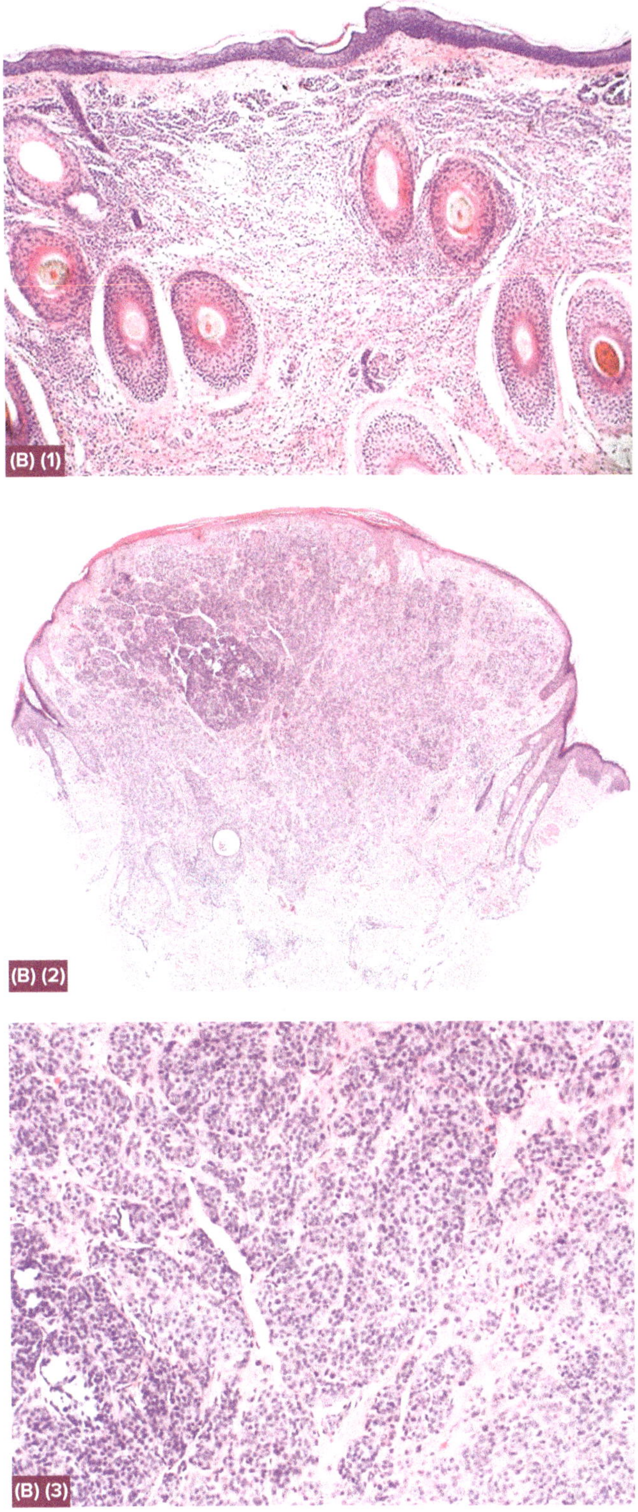

(B) (1) (B) (2) (B) (3)

A) This is an example of small cell malignant melanoma arising within a giant congenital nevus.
B) This is an example of an indolent proliferative dermal melanocytic nodule arising within a giant congenital nevus.
C) Both lesions are examples of conventional benign giant congenital nevus.
D) This is an example of cellular blue nevus arising within a giant congenital nevus.

QUESTION 10-17.

A 20-year-old woman presents with unilateral hyperpigmentation around the orbita that extends into the sclera. The lesion has been present since birth. A biopsy is performed and the findings are illustrated below. Immunohistochemical stain for HMB45 reveals positive expression within the pigmented spindle cells. Which of the following diagnoses is CORRECT?

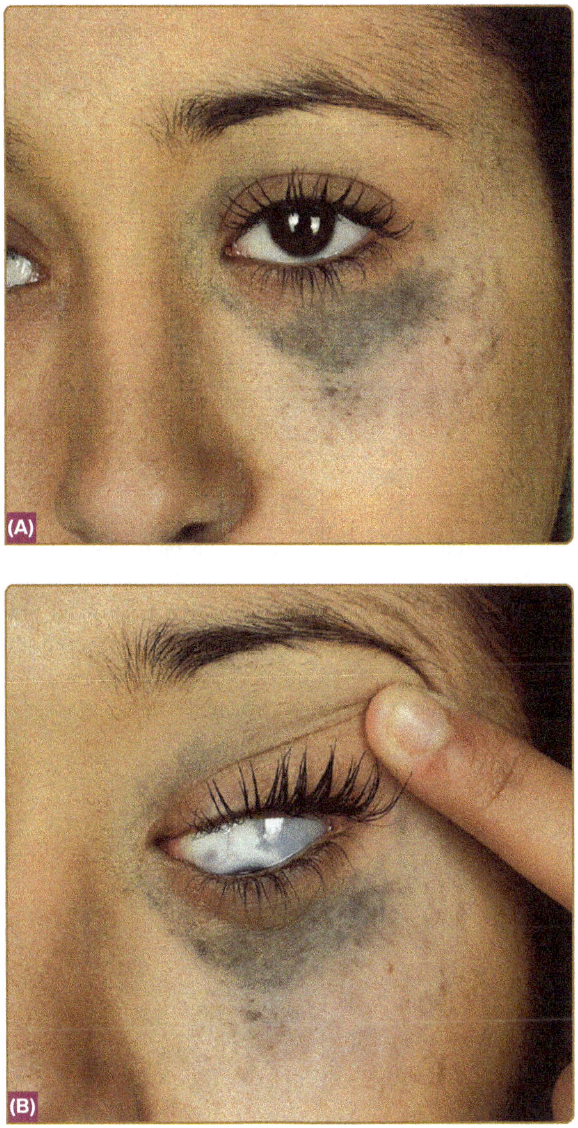

(A) (B)

Reproduced, with permission, from Goldsmith LA, Katz SI, Gilchrest BA, Paller AS, Leffell DJ, Wolff K, eds. *Fitzpatrick's Dermatology in General Medicine*. 8th ed. New York, NY: McGraw-Hill Education; 2012.

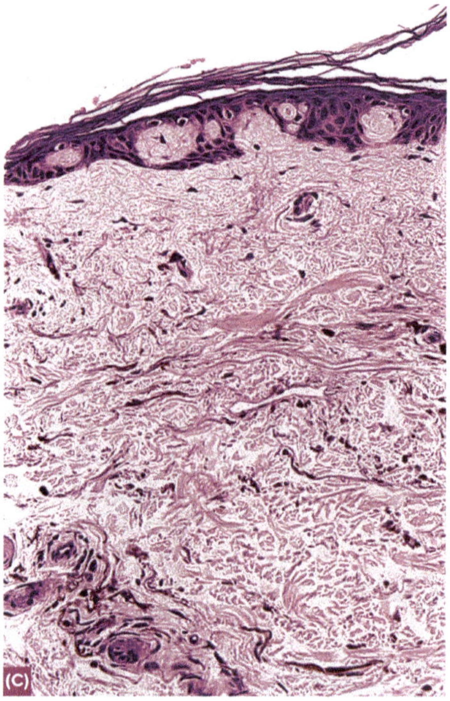

A) Nevus of Ito
B) Nevus of Ota
C) Mongolian spot
D) Common blue nevus
E) Primary acquired melanosis of the conjunctiva

QUESTION 10-18.

A 27-year-old female presents with a 1.5 cm pigmented plaque on the left buttock. A biopsy is performed and the findings of the H&E (Fig. 10-18 (B)-(D)) and combined Melan-A/Ki67 (brown/red) stained sections are illustrated (Fig. 10-18 (E)). Total body examination reveals no other pigmented lesions and there is no family history of melanoma. Which of the following diagnoses is CORRECT?

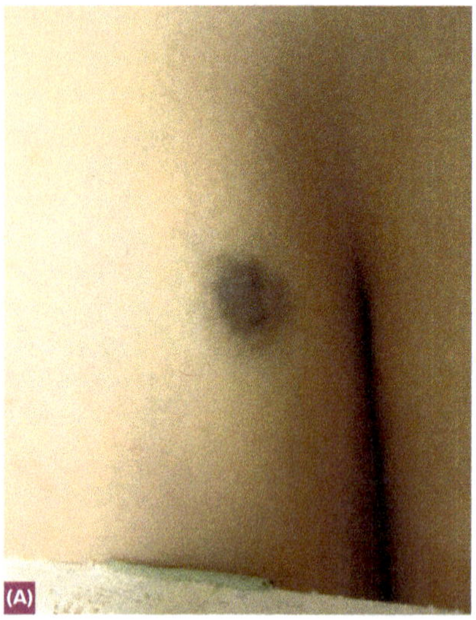

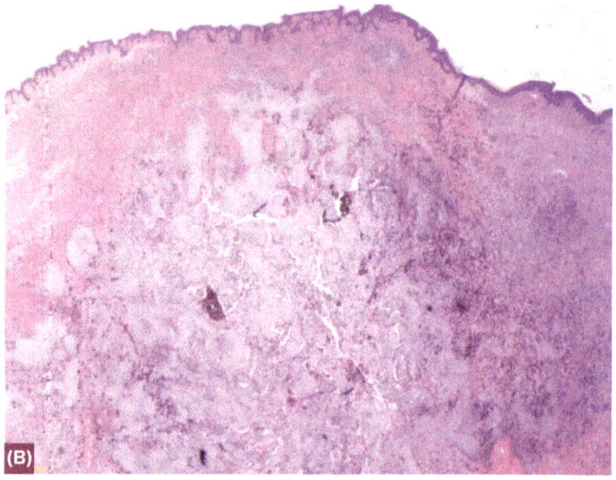

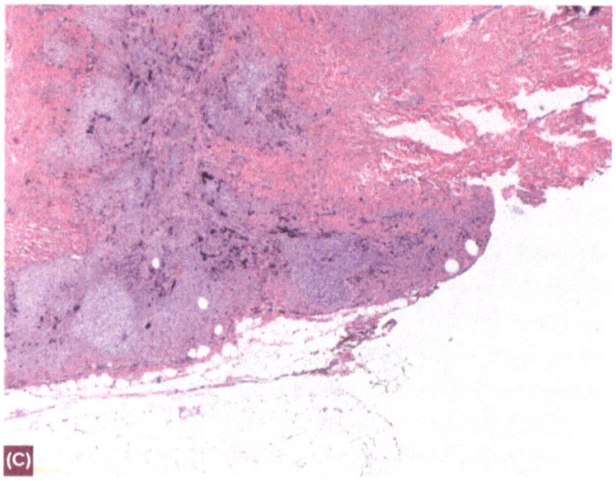

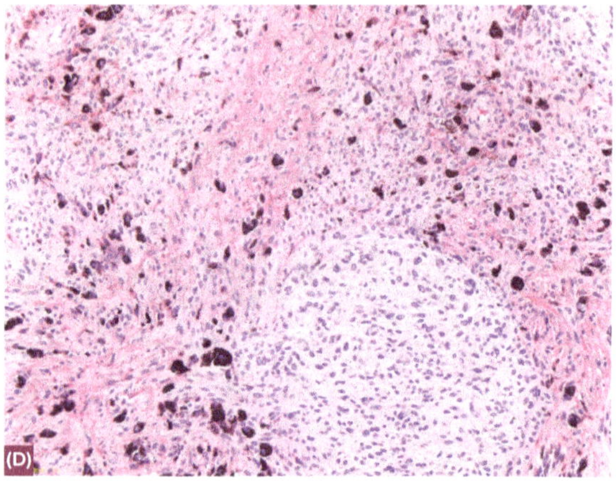

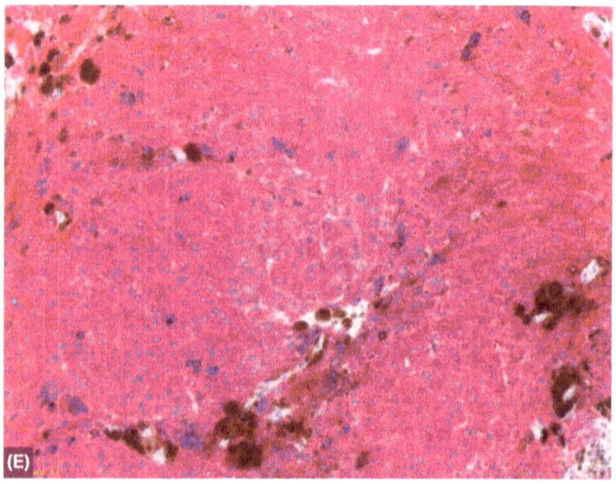

A) Metastatic melanoma
B) Cellular blue nevus
C) Melanocytic nevus with phenotypic heterogeneity
D) Blue nevus-like melanoma (malignant blue nevus)
E) Sclerosing blue nevus

QUESTION 10-19.

A 17-year-old obese female patient presents with multiple lentigines and a 1.2 cm symmetrical blue-black nodule on the upper extremity. She has a history of glucose intolerance and amenorrhea. Her mother has a similar body habitus, multiple lentigines, and history of atrial fibrillation and hirsutism. An excisional biopsy of the large nodule is performed and the findings are illustrated below. Combined Melan-A/Ki-67 immunostain reveals no mitotic activity. Which of the following statements regarding this tumor is INCORRECT?

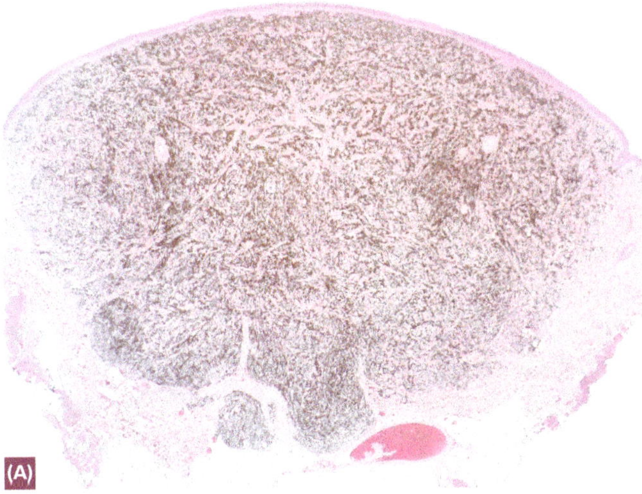
(A)

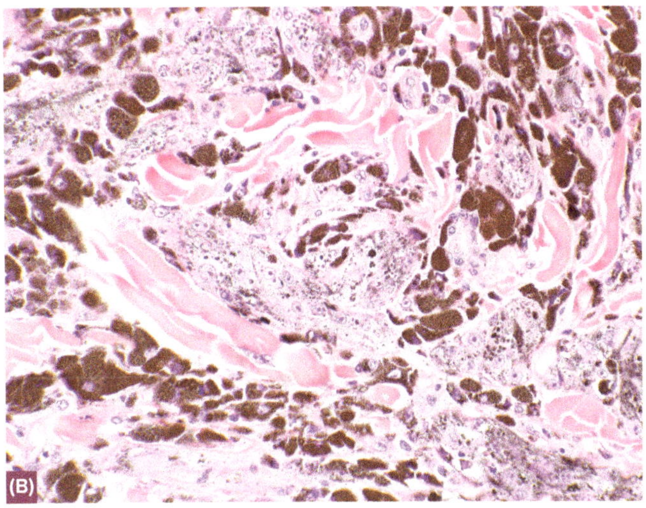
(B)

A) This tumor may arise in association with Carney complex.
B) These tumors are associated with mutations in the *PRKAR1A* (protein kinase A regulatory subunit 1α) gene.
C) This tumor is histopathologically similar to a melanocytic neoplasm that arises in gray horses and laboratory animals; however, it appears to have a different molecular origin.
D) These tumors may be sporadic and associated with a high incidence of lymph node metastasis, but overall indolent clinical course.
E) This tumor is an example of a pilar neurocristic hamartoma.

QUESTION 10-20.

An 18-year-old female presents with a 0.4 cm flesh-colored papule on the nose. She reports that the lesion rapidly developed over the course of a year, but has remained stable over the past 4 years. Dermoscopy reveals scattered dot-like blood vessels. A biopsy is performed and the findings are illustrated below. The tumor measures 1 mm in thickness but is confined to the dermis. A single dermal bipolar mitosis is present. Ulceration is absent. Which of the following statements regarding this lesion is INCORRECT?

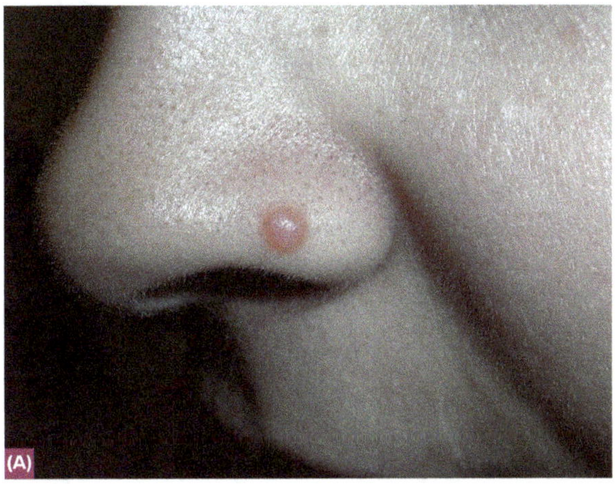
(A)

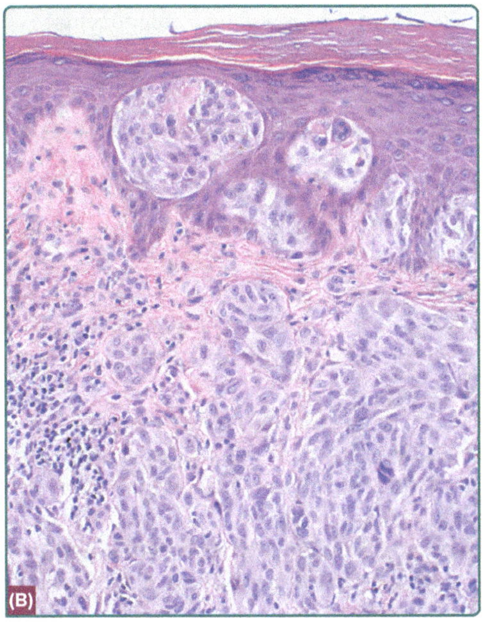
(B)

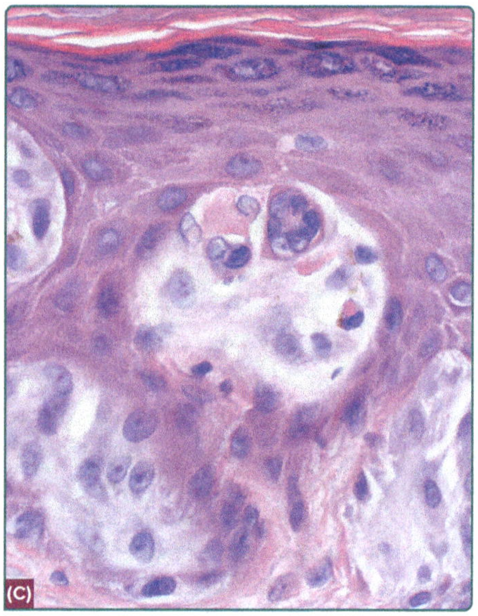

Part **(A)** reproduced, with permission, from Usatine RP, Smith MA, Mayeaux EJ Jr, Chumley HS, eds. *Color Atlas of Family Medicine*. 2nd ed. New York, NY: McGraw-Hill Education; 2012; parts **(B), (C)** reproduced, with permission, from Goldsmith LA, Katz SI, Gilchrest BA, Paller AS, Leffell DJ, Wolff K, eds. *Fitzpatrick's Dermatology in General Medicine*. 8th ed. New York, NY: McGraw-Hill Education; 2012.

A) This type of melanocytic proliferation is characterized by a unique form of cytologic atypia.
B) Features that correspond with a benign clinical course include: patient age less than 10 years, lesional symmetry, sharp lateral demarcation, size (<1 cm), maturation with dermal descent (zonation), lack of deep extension (subcutis), lack of ulceration, lack of significant pagetoid spread, and lack of mitoses in the deepest component.
C) These tumors may rarely occur in either grouped (agminate) or disseminated patterns.
D) These tumors frequently contain eosinophilic amorphous globules at the dermal–epidermal junction that are composed of basement membrane components.
E) This tumor should be re-excised with wide surgical margins.

QUESTION 10-21.

While examination of H&E stained sections remains the gold standard for deciphering the biological behavior of melanocytic proliferations, various immunohistochemical stains are an important adjunct in establishing a diagnosis. Which of the following statements regarding the role of various immunohistochemical stains is INCORRECT?

A) Melan-A (MART-1) is a specific marker for melanocytic differentiation that stains melanocyte cytoplasms and highlights the density and location of melanocytes within the epidermis and dermis.
B) S100 is a cytoplasmic and nuclear stain that is highly sensitive but nonspecific for melanocytic differentiation. It is most useful in identifying primary and metastatic melanomas that have lost expression for other melanocytic markers.
C) Sox-10 is a nuclear stain that is highly sensitive but nonspecific for melanocytic differentiation since it also stains cells with peripheral nerve sheath differentiation.
D) Microphthalmia-associated transcription factor (MITF) is a nuclear and weakly cytoplasmic stain that is specific for melanocytic differentiation and highlights the density and location of melanocytes within the epidermis and dermis.
E) gp100 (HMB45) is a cytoplasmic stain that is specific for malignant melanocytes within intraepidermal and dermal compartments.

QUESTION 10-22.

You receive a slide consultation from a colleague without any clinical history. The sample is limited and the findings of the H&E and Melan-A stained sections are illustrated below. Which of the following additional findings would increase your suspicion for malignant melanoma?

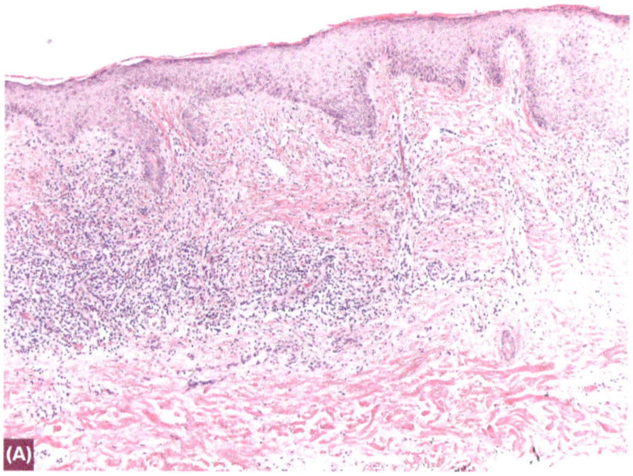

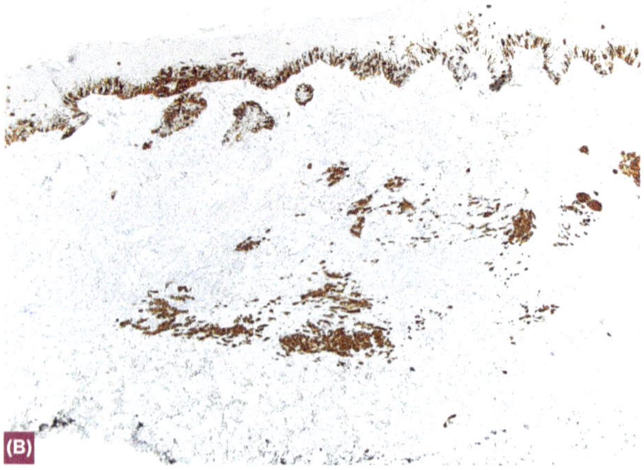

A) The development of new pigmentation was clinically present within the scar of a prior biopsy performed less than 6 months ago.

B) The pigment was clinically present beyond the scar of a biopsy performed several years ago.
C) The lesion was present for many years within the umbilicus and there is no history of prior biopsy at the site.
D) There are well-defined junctional and dermal nests of melanocytes without pagetoid ascent in the regions peripheral to the dermal fibrosis.
E) Clinically, the pigmented area measures 4 mm in greatest diameter.

QUESTION 10-23.

An 85-year-old female presents with a very hard, bluish-black nodule on the cheek. Palpation reveals the induration to extend beyond the clinical pigmentation. A biopsy is performed and the findings of the H&E, Melan-A (brown), and S100 (red) stained sections are illustrated (Fig. 10-23 (B)-(E)). Which of the following diagnoses is CORRECT?

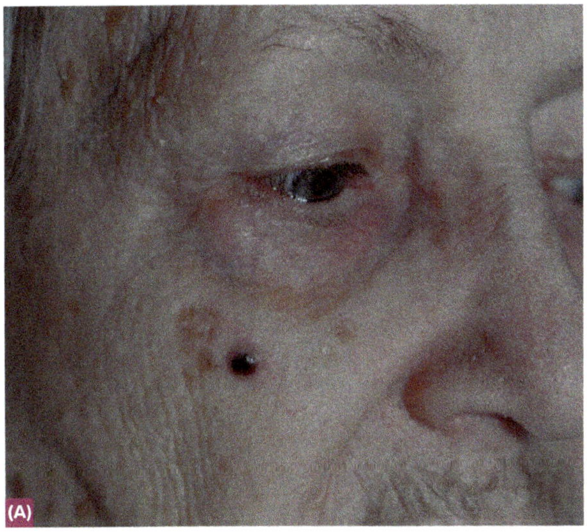

Reproduced with permission from Wolff K, Johnson RA, Saavedra AP. *Fitzpatrick's Color Atlas and Synopsis of Clinical Dermatology.* 7th ed. New York, NY: McGraw-Hill Education; 2013.

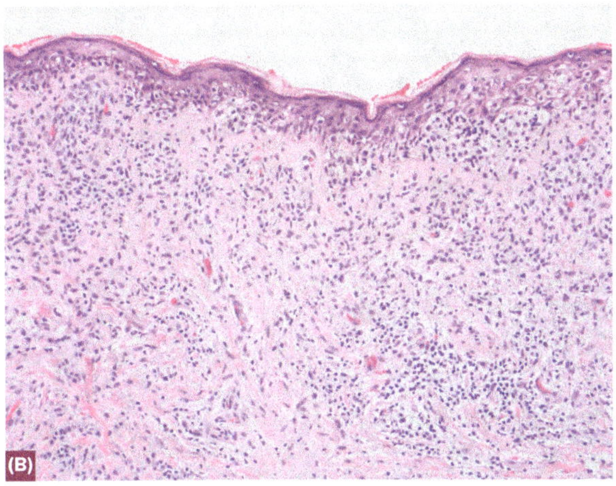

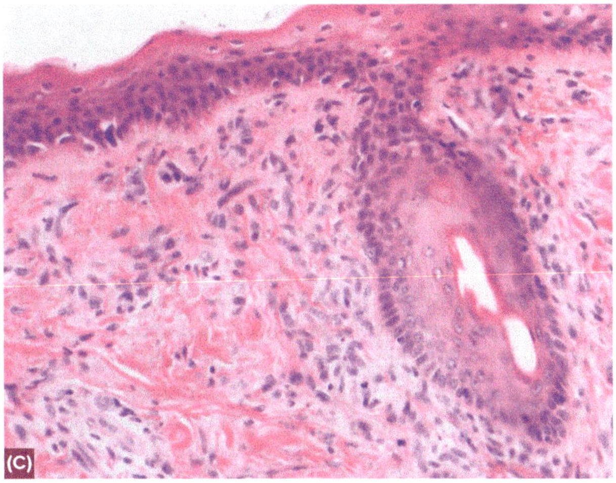

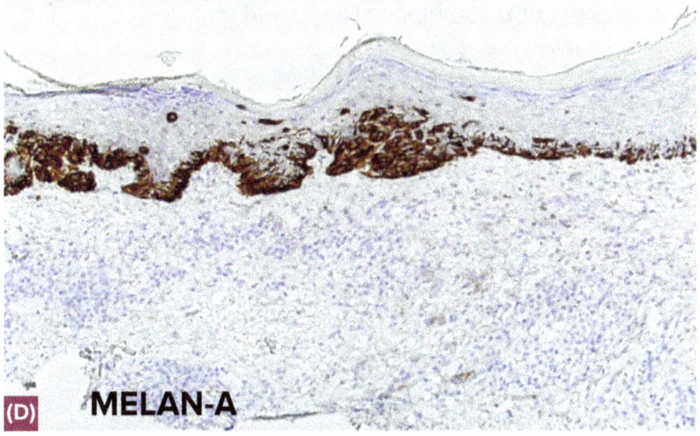

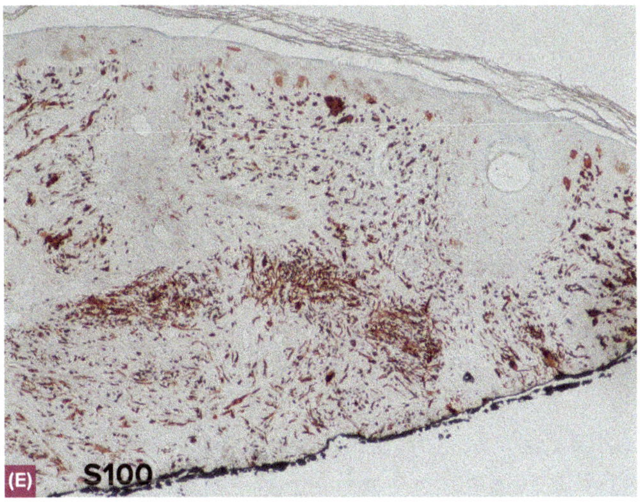

A) Desmoplastic Spitz nevus
B) Melanoma in situ, lentigo maligna type
C) Recurrent nevus phenomenon
D) Desmoplastic melanoma
E) Sclerosing blue nevus

QUESTION 10-24.

A 9 year-old patient presents with a 1.2-cm dome-shaped pink nodule on the upper back with slight pigmentation. The patient cannot recall how long the lesion has been present. The tumor is excised and the findings are illustrated below. Fig. 10-24 (D) is a high-power representation of the base of the tumor at the dermal–subcutis interface. Sentinel lymph node biopsy was performed and reveals a focus of tumor within the peripheral lymph node sinus. Immunohistochemistry reveals strong p16 expression within both the cutaneous tumor and lymph node deposit. Fluorescent in situ hybridization (FISH) is performed on the main tumor and lymph node deposit and reveals increased copy numbers of 11p and normal copy numbers of 9p21. Which of the following diagnoses is MOST appropriate?

A) Desmoplastic melanoma
B) Desmoplastic Spitz nevus
C) Atypical Spitz tumor
D) Malignant melanoma with spitzoid features

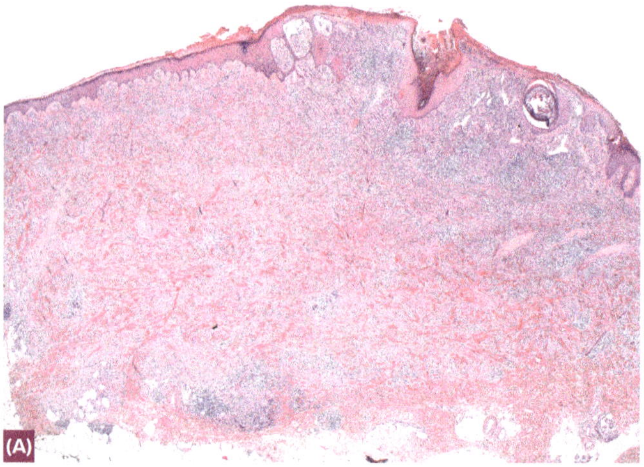

(A)

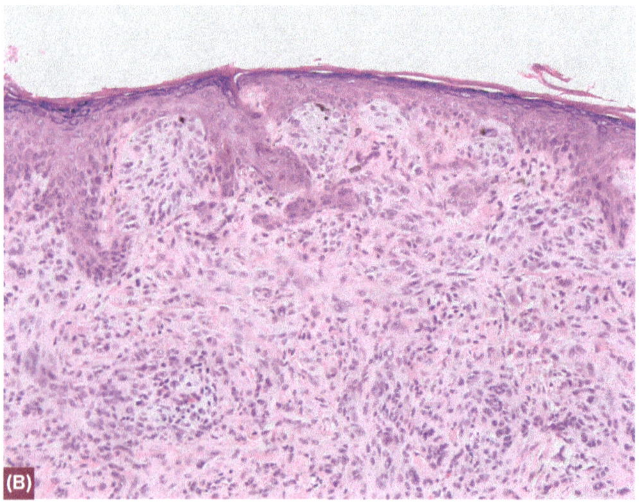

(B)

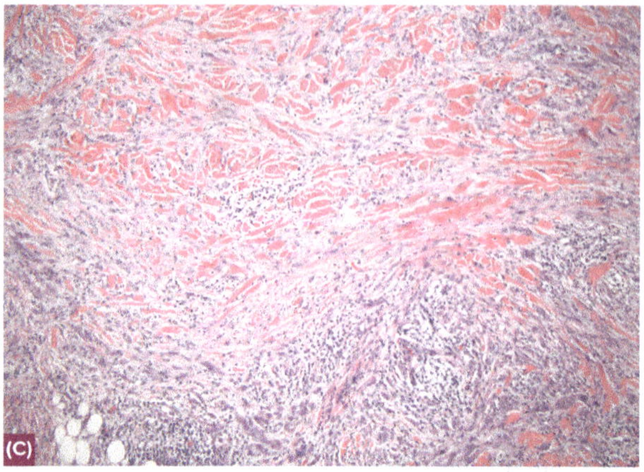

(C)

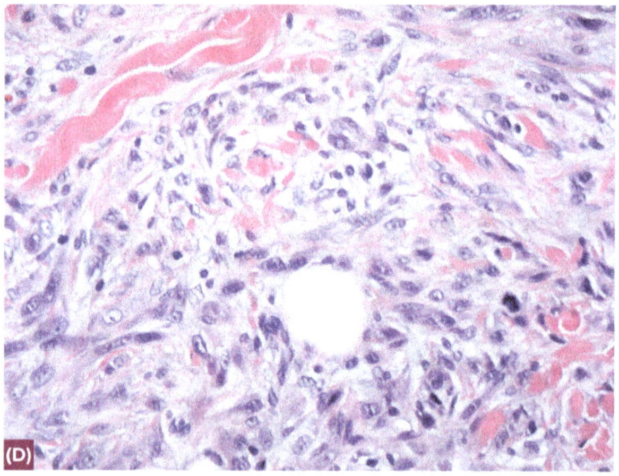

(D)

QUESTION 10-25.

A 22-year-old female presents with a rapidly growing darkly pigmented 0.6 cm plaque on the lower leg. Dermoscopy reveals a relatively symmetric lesion with peripheral streaks of the pseudopod type. A biopsy is performed and the findings are illustrated below. Which of the following diagnoses is CORRECT?

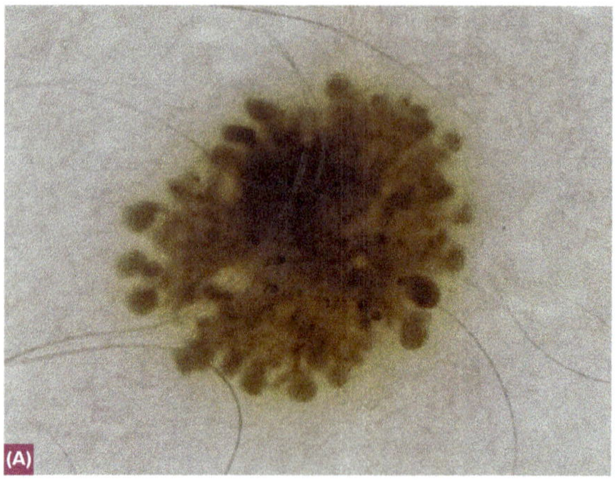

(A)

Reproduced, with permission, from Usatine RP, Smith MA, Mayeaux EJ Jr, Chumley HS, eds. *Color Atlas of Family Medicine*. 2nd ed. New York, NY: McGraw-Hill Education; 2012.

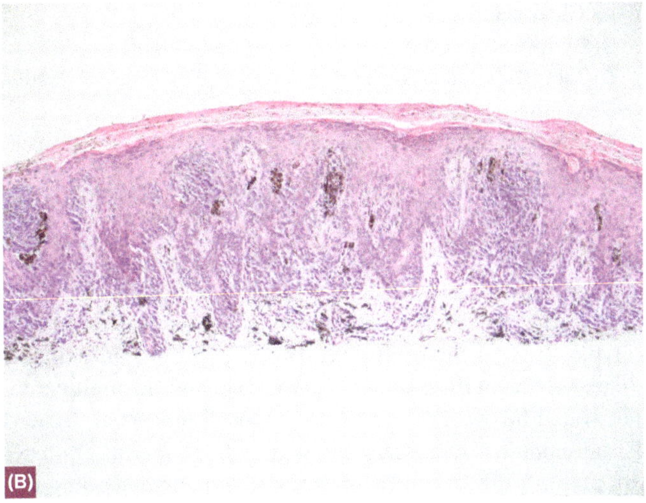

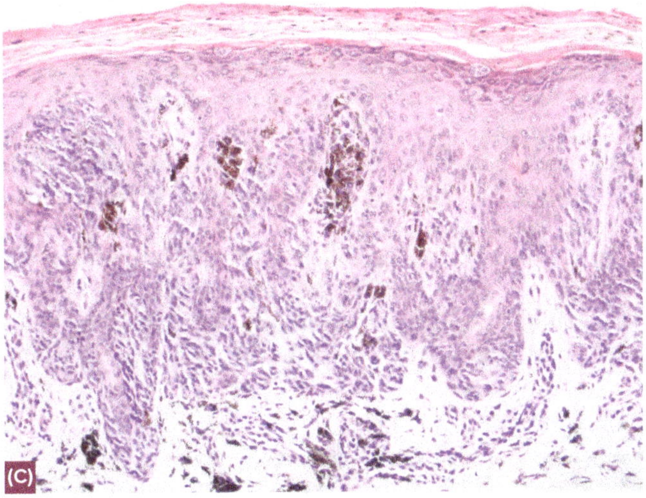

A) Malignant melanoma, superficial spreading type
B) Malignant melanoma, lentigo maligna type
C) Pigmented spindle cell nevus of Reed
D) Compound dysplastic nevus
E) Plexiform spindle cell nevus

QUESTION 10-26.

A 32-year-old patient presents with 1.2 cm slightly asymmetric pink nodule on the dorsal hand. Dermoscopy is performed (insert in upper corner) and reveals numerous vascular structures. There is palpable axillary lymphadenopathy. An excision is performed and the findings are illustrated below. The tumor cells are positive for Melan-A. The tumor measures 1.8 mm in thickness. Additionally, a fine needle aspiration (FNA) of the axillary lymph nodes reveals cells with similar cytomorphology to the cutaneous tumor. Which of the following statements regarding this tumor is INCORRECT?

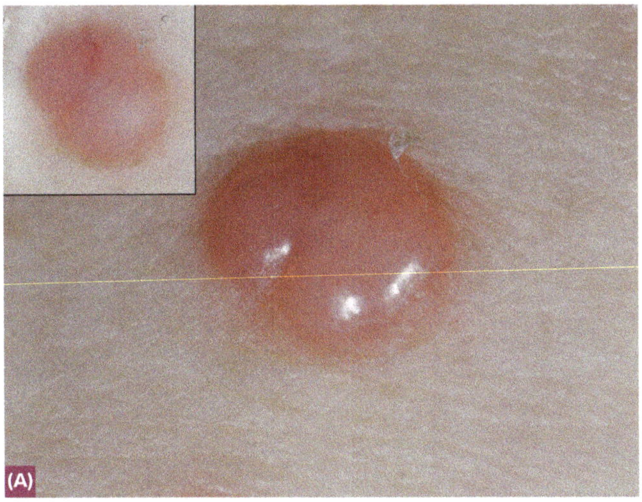

Reproduced, with permission, from Usatine RP, Smith MA, Mayeaux EJ Jr, Chumley HS, eds. *Color Atlas of Family Medicine.* 2nd ed. New York, NY: McGraw-Hill Education; 2012.

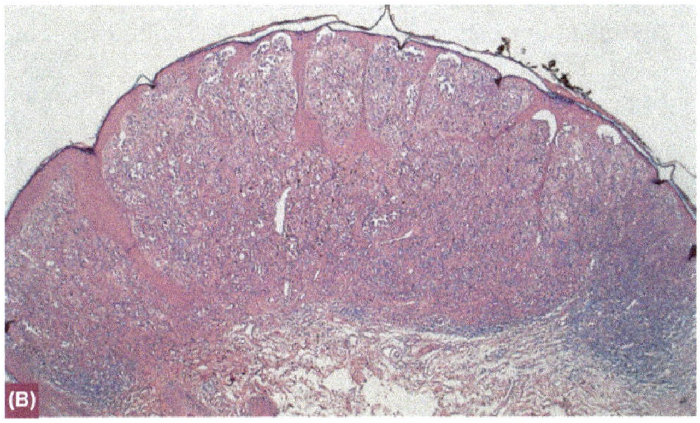

Reproduced, with permission, from Goldsmith LA, Katz SI, Gilchrest BA, Paller AS, Leffell DJ, Wolff K, eds. *Fitzpatrick's Dermatology in General Medicine.* 8th ed. New York, NY: McGraw-Hill Education; 2012.

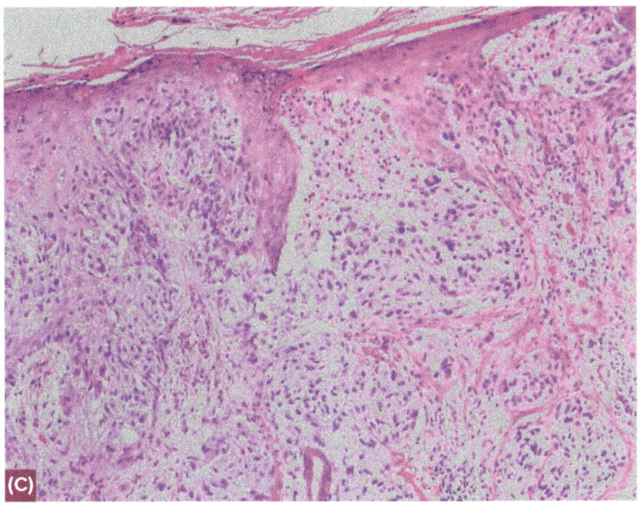

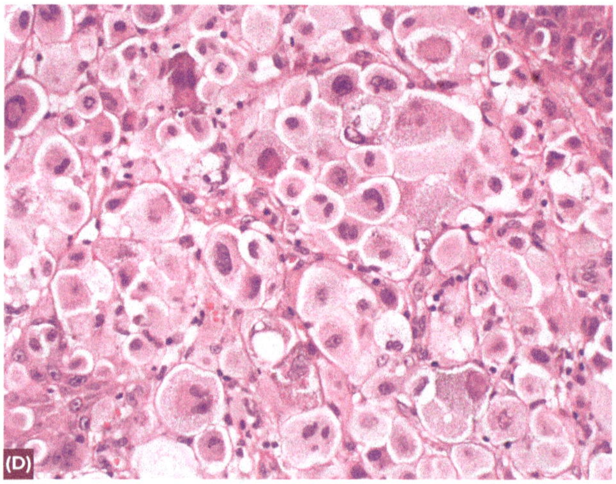

A) This is an atypical Spitz tumor and despite the lymph node involvement, this patient has a favorable prognosis.
B) This tumor should be widely re-excised with a 1-2 cm margin of full thickness normal skin.
C) This tumor may harbor gains in 8q24 via fluorescent in situ hybridization (FISH).
D) Serum lactate dehydrogenase levels will most likely be greater than 200-225 U/L.
E) Before any additional surgery is performed the patient should undergo imaging studies (ie, chest x-ray, CT, MRI, PET).

QUESTION 10-27.

A 35-year-old female patient presents with a slowly enlarging, deep-seated mass in close proximity to the Achilles tendon. The lesion is excised and the histopathological findings are illustrated below. The tumor cells positively express vimentin, S-100, HMB45, and Melan-A (MART-1). FISH analysis reveals a t(12;22) translocation resulting in an ATF-1-EWS gene fusion. Which of the following diagnoses is CORRECT?

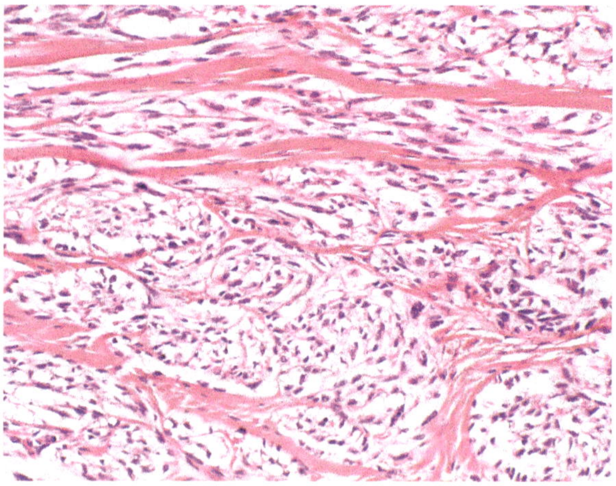

A) Clear cell sarcoma
B) Synovial sarcoma
C) Metastatic melanoma
D) Epithelioid sarcoma
E) Atypical cellular blue nevus

QUESTION 10-28.

A patient presents with several blue-black nodules scattered throughout the axilla, trunk, and neck. The patient had an "atypical" nevus removed several years ago from the axilla. A biopsy of one of the nodules is performed and the findings are illustrated below. The tumor is composed of several dermal-based nodules with scattered pigment. Numerous mitoses are present. Which of the following statements regarding this patient's condition is INCORRECT?

A) Fontana-Masson stain will label the pigment dark black, consistent with melanin.
B) These tumors represent satellite metastases of malignant melanoma and are associated with an overall poor prognosis.
C) Rarely, these tumors may exhibit epidermotropism with junctional nests and pagetoid cells scattered throughout the epidermis.
D) D2-40 and CD31 immunohistochemical stains may reveal intravascular deposits of tumor cells.
E) If tumor deposits are present within regional lymph nodes, they will most likely be present within the lymph node parenchyma or medullary sinus.

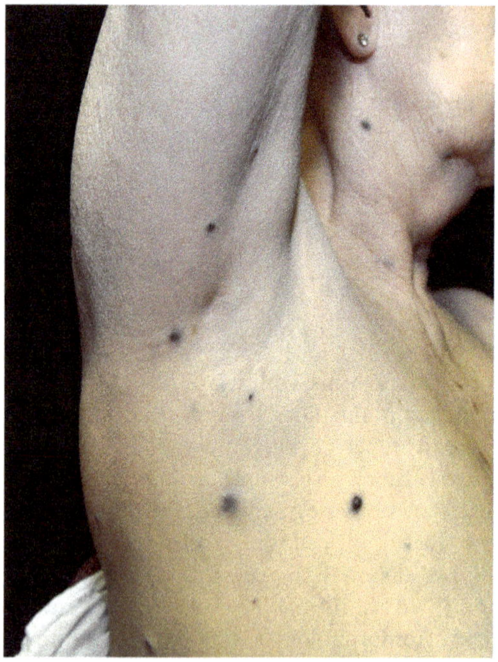

Reproduced, with permission, from Usatine RP, Smith MA, Mayeaux EJ Jr, Chumley HS, eds. *Color Atlas of Family Medicine*. 2nd ed. New York, NY: McGraw-Hill Education; 2012.

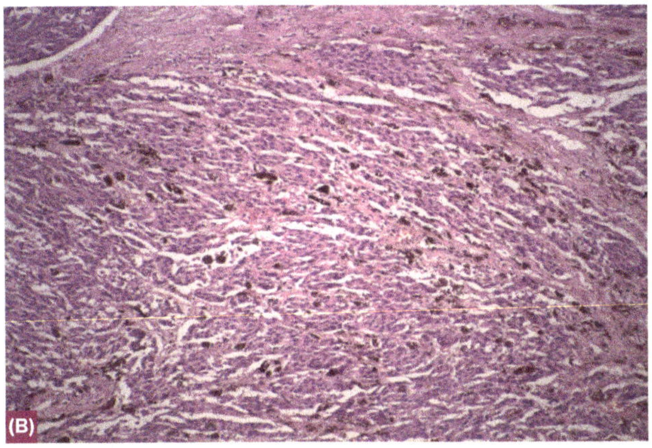

Reproduced, with permission, from Kemp WL, Burns DK, Travis Brown TG. *Pathology: The Big Picture*. 1st ed. New York, NY: McGraw-Hill Education; 2008.

QUESTION 10-29.

A 56-year-old patient presents with hyperpigmentation of the nail and nail bed. A biopsy of the nail plate (Fig. 10-29 (B)) and nail matrix (Fig. 10-29 (C)) is taken from the proximal nail fold and the findings are illustrated. Which of the following diagnoses is CORRECT?

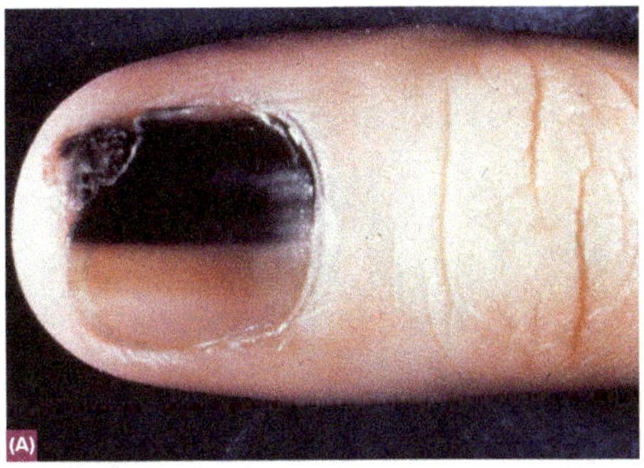

Reproduced, with permission, from Usatine RP, Smith MA, Mayeaux EJ Jr, Chumley HS, eds. *Color Atlas of Family Medicine*. 2nd ed. New York, NY: McGraw-Hill Education; 2012.

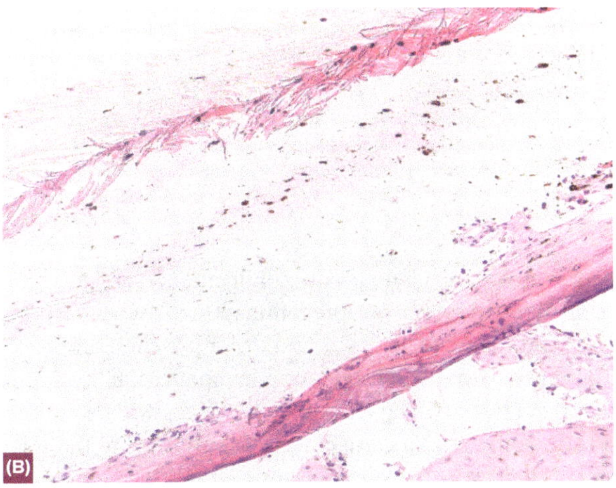

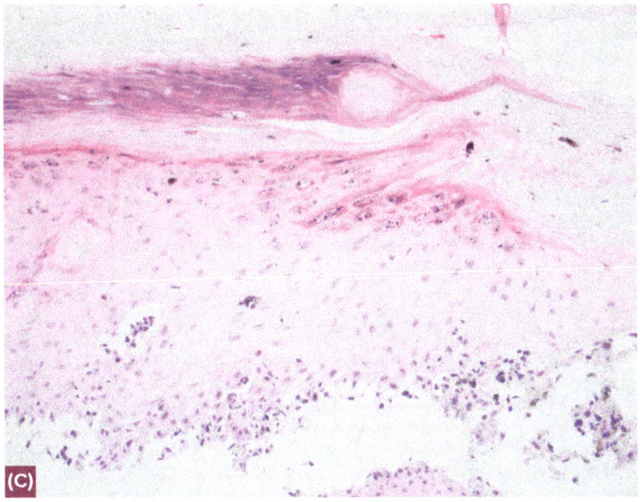

A) Subungual lentigo
B) Lentiginous subungual nevus (acral nevus)
C) Subungual melanotic macule
D) Subungual acral lentiginous melanoma
E) Melanonychia associated with drug therapy

QUESTION 10-30.

A 53-year-old patient presents with lightly pigmented nodule on the back measuring 1 cm in diameter. The patient cannot recall how long the lesion has been present. A full body examination reveals only a few small ordinary nevi. No other clinically atypical lesions are identified. A biopsy is performed and the findings are illustrated below. Which of the following diagnoses is MOST appropriate?

A) Minimal deviation melanoma
B) Nevoid melanoma
C) Common acquired intradermal melanocytic nevus
D) Nodular epithelioid Spitz tumor with loss of BAP1 expression
E) Metastatic melanoma

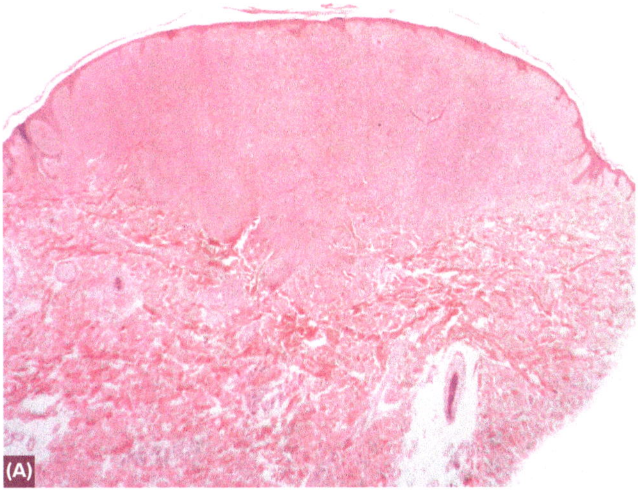

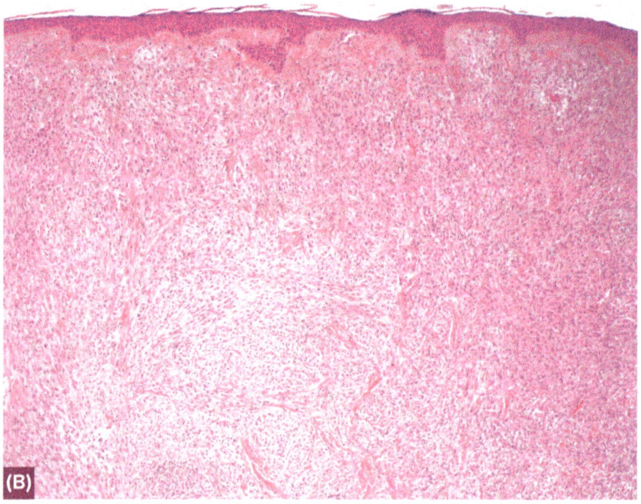

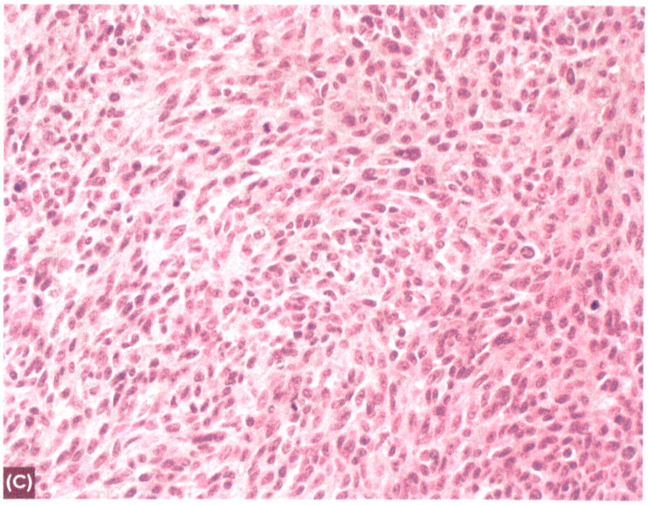

ANSWERS

ANSWER 10-1: C.

Solar lentigo occurs on sun-exposed skin in more than 90% of the white population older than age 60 years but may be observed in much younger individuals as well. **Solar lentigines** are distinguished from common **freckles** by their persistence despite absence of sun exposure. Solar lentigines are prominent in **xeroderma pigmentosum**. The **photochemotherapy-induced (PUVA) lentigo** has been observed in patients receiving long-term methoxypsoralen PUVA for psoriasis. Carriers of one or two of the melanocortin-1-receptor (MC1R) gene variants have a 1.5- to 2-fold increased risk for the development of numerous solar lentigines. Clinically, solar lentigines are well-circumscribed, round, oval, or irregularly bordered macules of yellow, tan, or brown color, varying in size from about 1 to 3 cm in diameter, with a tendency to confluency. Solar lentigines occur on sun-exposed areas, predominantly the dorsal aspects of hands and forearms, the face, and the upper chest and back. The "sunburn," hypermelanotic, or "ink spot" solar lentigo is characterized by a striking jet-black color and a stellate outline. The PUVA lentigo has a close clinical resemblance to the solar lentigo, particularly the hypermelanotic type.

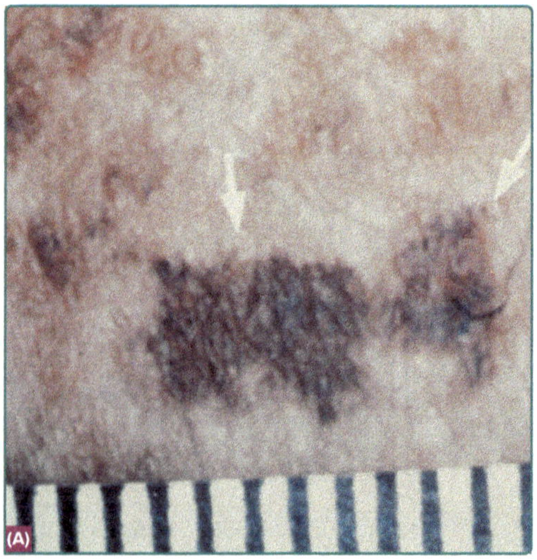

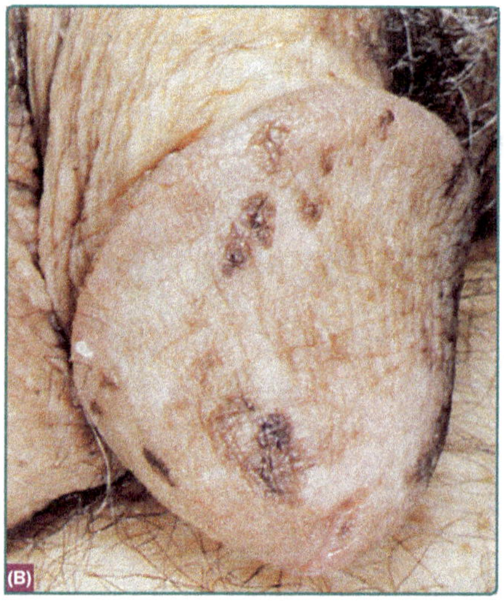

Photochemotherapy (psoralen and ultraviolet A light [PUVA])-induced lentigines. (A) on the buttock and **(B)** penis of a 57-year-old white man who had received PUVA for psoriasis several times per week for 5 years. The PUVA lentigines appeared between 1 and 2 years after PUVA therapy was begun. The current recommendation is to shield the male genitalia during PUVA therapy to prevent squamous cell carcinoma of the penis and scrotum. (Reproduced, with permission, from Goldsmith LA, Katz SI, Gilchrest BA, Paller AS, Leffell DJ, Wolff K, eds. *Fitzpatrick's Dermatology in General Medicine*. 8th ed. New York, NY: McGraw-Hill Education; 2012.)

Microscopically, in general, the solar lentigo is characterized by increased melanin pigment within keratinocytes. The lesions are most notable for elongated, club-shaped epidermal rete ridges, and basal layer hyperpigmentation most prominent at the tips of the rete. The epidermis between rete ridges is usually flattened. There may also be hyperkeratosis and slight basal keratinocyte atypia (orthokeratosis rather than the parakeratosis seen in actinic keratosis) and rather prominent elongation and anastomosis of rete. The basal layer melanocytes are typically not increased in number, unless the lesions are arising in chronically sun-damaged skin with underlying melanocyte hyperplasia. On occasion, there is slight cytologic atypia of basilar melanocytes, consistent with photoactivation. Solar elastosis is almost always present. The solar lentigo may show transitions to reticulated seborrheic keratosis, large cell acanthoma, and lichenoid keratosis. Some solar lentigines develop associated lichenoid dermatitis and hence are termed **lichenoid keratosis (lichen planus-like keratosis)**. The PUVA lentigo occasionally exhibits lentiginous melanocytic hyperplasia and low-grade cytologic atypia of melanocytes.

Quick Fact

Solar Lentigo

- Pigmented keratinocytic proliferation
- Precursor to pigmented seborrheic keratosis
- May become inflamed resulting in a lichenoid keratosis
- May occasionally contain increased numbers of atypical melanocytes when arising in a background of chronic sun damage, hence the differential diagnosis in those instances may include lentigo maligna

The differential diagnosis includes **solar intraepidermal melanocytic proliferations with atypia (SIMPs with atypia or which probably represents a precursor to or overlaps with lentigo maligna)** involving sun-exposed skin and pigmented actinic keratosis. **Pigmented actinic keratosis** is also a pigmented keratinocytic proliferation; however, by definition, significant keratinocytic atypia is not present in solar lentigo. **Junctional melanocytic nevi** are composed of nests of melanocytes typically situated at the tips of the rete ridges. Although the tips of the rete may be somewhat bulbous in solar lentigo, the bulbs are composed of pigmented keratinocytes and not melanocytes. If true nests of melanocytes were present, the appropriate designation would be **lentiginous junctional melanocytic nevus**. In general, **lentigo maligna**, particularly when present on the central face, in contrast to solar lentigo, is characterized by absence or diminution of the epidermal rete pattern (effacement of the epidermis). In addition, in **SIMP (precursor lentigo maligna)**, in contrast to solar lentigo, there is an increased concentration of basilar melanocytes, occasional junctional nests, and prominent involvement of adnexal epithelium by the lentiginous proliferation of melanocytes. The characteristic **"lentiginous growth pattern"** refers to a single file confluent growth of melanocytes along the basal layer. Melanocytes may or may not be present above the layer (**"pagetoid melanocytosis"**). Finally, lentigo maligna is characterized by greater cytologic atypia of basilar melanocytes than should be seen in solar lentigo. Nonetheless, on occasion, one may encounter lesions transitional between solar lentigo and lentigo maligna (especially solar lentigos arising in chronically sun-damaged skin). Sampling errors may pose a diagnostic pitfall, especially lesions sampled from the face and other areas of chronic exposure. The clinician may have biopsied a paucicellular focus of an otherwise more cellular melanocytic lesion. Additionally, the cellular density may vary within a biopsy. Correlation with the clinical features (size, outline, color, etc) greatly enhances interpretation of histopathologically subtle alterations. Occasionally, multiple "mapping" biopsies may be needed to definitively exclude lentigo maligna in clinically large atypical lesions.

ANSWER 10-2: A.

The biopsy reveals elongated epidermal rete and basal layer hyperpigmentation, most prominently involving the lowermost aspects of the rete. There are increased numbers of small cells along the basal layer surrounded by clear halos, consistent with melanocytes. Melanocytes, unlike keratinocytes, lack structural keratin filaments and frequently shrink during tissue processing resulting in the clear "halo" space. Note that the nuclei are much smaller than those of the adjacent keratinocytes. This is a reassuring feature that the melanocytes are not atypical. No nests of melanocytes are present. The findings are consistent with **lentigo simplex**, which is a regular, well-circumscribed macule measuring 1-5 mm in diameter and having a uniform light brown, brown, or dark brown color. The **simple lentigo** of **lentigo simplex** may occur in a localized or in a widespread pattern as in **lentiginosis profusa** or in association with certain syndromes, as for example, **LEOPARD** (lentigines, electrocardiographic conduction abnormalities, ocular hypertelorism, pulmonary stenosis, abnormal genitalia, retardation of growth, and deafness), **multiple lentigines, LAMB** (lentigines, atrial myxomas, cutaneous papular myxomas, blue nevi), or **Peutz–Jeghers**. Certain pigmented macules may involve mucosal sites such as the conjunctiva, oral mucosa, the vermillion border of the lip, and genitalia. Multiple lentigines may involve the oral mucosa and vermillion border as part of the **Peutz–Jeghers syndrome**. **Mucosal lentigines** are clinically similar to their cutaneous counterparts. The borders are generally regular and well defined. Occasional lesions on the genitalia in particular are notable for a mottled appearance and large size, measuring up to 5 cm in greatest diameter. The latter clinical appearance suggests melanoma; however, biopsies of such lesions generally do not show atypical changes histopathologically. These lesions rarely eventuate in melanoma (Table 10-2A).

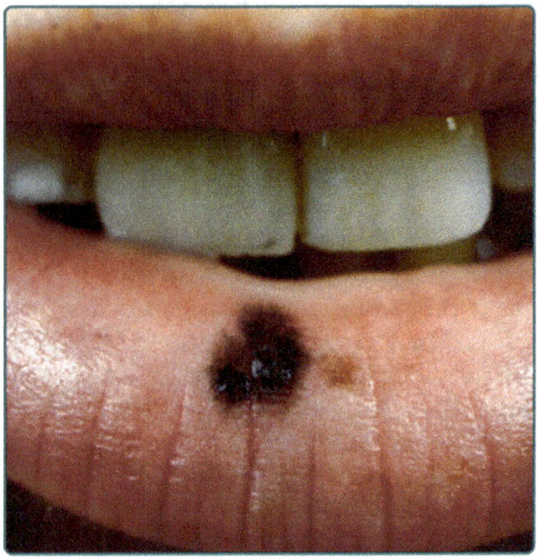

Labial melanotic macule. Pigmented macule appearing 5 years earlier, on the lower lip of a 26-year-old white woman. (Reproduced, with permission, from Goldsmith LA, Katz SI, Gilchrest BA, Paller AS, Leffell DJ, Wolff K, eds. *Fitzpatrick's Dermatology in General Medicine*. 8th ed. New York, NY: McGraw-Hill Education; 2012.)

The **simple lentigo** is defined histopathologically by three features: (1) increased frequency of basilar melanocytes compared with adjacent normal skin, (2) elongated, club-shaped epidermal rete, and (3) basilar hyperpigmentation of epidermal keratinocytes that may extend into the upper portion of the epidermis and stratum corneum. There is increased melanin and an increased frequency of melanocytes at the tips of the elongated epidermal rete with diminished frequency proceeding upward along the sides and between the rete. Nests of melanocytes are not present. The histologic spectrum of these lesions arising in mucosal epithelium may vary from slight acanthosis of epithelium, the presence or absence of club-shaped rete, and the presence or absence of basilar melanocytic hyperplasia. The lesions without melanocytic hyperplasia may be designated as a **melanotic macule** or **melanosis**. Lesions with melanocytic hyperplasia are best termed **lentigines**. Conjunctival lesions with melanocytic hyperplasia are referred to as **primary acquired melanosis (PAM)**. As with other simple lentigines, hyperpigmentation of the basilar epithelium is present.

In regards to the differential diagnosis, **simple lentigo** must be discriminated from a **freckle** and **solar lentigo**. Simple lentigo differs from freckles because of elongated epidermal rete ridges and an increased frequency of basilar melanocytes. Freckles are temporally associated with sun exposure. The simple lentigo does not usually have rete ridges as elongated and showing anastomosis or solar elastosis to the degree observed in solar lentigo. In addition, melanocytic hyperplasia may not be present in solar lentigo. The absolute

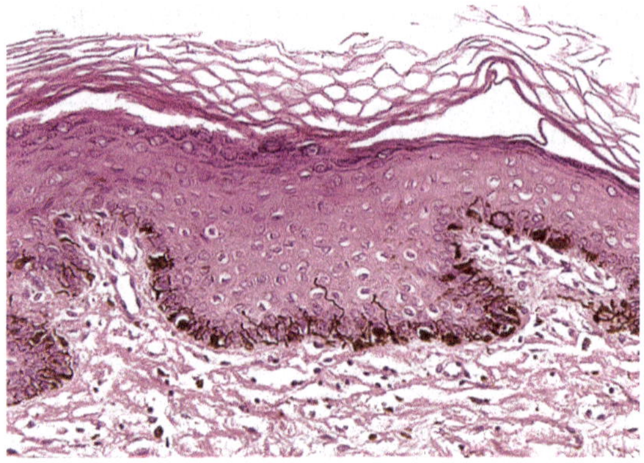

Penile lentigo. There are slightly increased numbers of basilar melanocytes with dendritic morphology.

Table 10-2A. Syndromes Associated with Lentigines

SYNDROME	CLINICAL FEATURES
Laugier–Hunziker syndrome	1. Sporadic 2. Melanonychia, mucosal and cutaneous lentigines 3. Not associated with hamartomas or malignant tumors
Peutz–Jeghers syndrome	1. Autosomal dominant; mutation in STK11/LKB1 gene 2. Mucosal and cutaneous lentigines 3. Hamartomatous gastrointestinal polyps
Carney complex	1. Autosomal dominant; mutation in PKAR1A gene 2. Cardiocutaneous type, also called LAMB syndrome (Lentigines, atrial myxomas, mucocutaneous myxomas, blue nevi) 3. Multiple endocrine neoplasia type, also called MEN type (Pigmented nodular adrenocortical disease, pituitary adenomas, gonadal and thyroid tumors, and schwannomas)
Leopard syndrome	1. Autosomal dominant; mutation in PTPN11 gene 2. Lentigines 3. ECG abnormality 4. Ocular hypertelorism 5. Pulmonic stenosis 6. Abnormality of genitalia 7. Retarded growth, skeletal abnormalities 8. Deafness

Quick Fact

Lentigo Simplex

- Pigmented keratinocytic and melanocytic lesion
- Precursor to junctional melanocytic nevus
- Mucosal lesions of large clinical size must be biopsied to exclude lentiginous melanoma.

distinction is sometimes difficult if not impossible. The theoretical importance lies with the concept that lentigo simplex is a pigmented lesion attributed to melanocyte hyperplasia and a precursor to **junctional melanocytic nevus**. Therefore, a common dilemma is differentiating a simple lentigo from a typical melanocytic nevus or dysplastic nevus. The **melanocytic nevus** is distinguished by the presence of junctional nests. The differential diagnosis for mucosal lesions includes melanocytic nevi of mucosal sites, atypical melanocytic proliferations, and melanoma. In general, as with melanocytic lesions located on other sites, progressively greater clinical atypicality raises concern about atypical histologic changes and melanoma. Histopathologically, **atypical melanocytic proliferations** and **melanoma** on mucosae are characterized by progressively greater frequency of basilar melanocytes and prominent cytologic atypia. In the case of melanoma, the basilar melanocytes often reach confluence along the basal layer in a lentiginous (single file) pattern. The melanocytes exhibit continuous marked cytologic atypia. Pagetoid spread is variable and may be absent, minimal, or prominent.

ANSWER 10-3: D.

Lentigines (lentigo simplex and **mucosal lentigo)** and **melanocytic nevi** are thought to represent progressive stages of melanocyte migration and proliferation in the skin (Table 10-3A). The precise location of the melanocyte stem cell reservoir has not been definitively established. In 1893, Paul Gerson Unna devised the theory that **melanoblasts** or related precursor cells migrate from the neural crest and take residence in the epidermis early in development (**Unna theory**). Proliferation of these cells in the basilar epidermis may give rise sequentially to lentigo and the three subsequent stages of the melanocytic nevus. The proliferation of melanocytes as clusters or nests within the epidermis defines the junctional nevus. Occasionally, a combination of increased single cell (lentiginous) and nested melanocytes is present. These lesions are often referred to as **lentiginous junctional nevi** or "**jentigos**." The term "**nevus cell**" describes the cells within these nests or clusters. These cells are closely related to melanocytes but are perhaps functionally altered by the aggregative pattern of growth. These cells tend to lose the dendritic processes that are characteristic of solitary basilar melanocytes and assume a more rounded (epithelioid) cytomorphology. In general, these

Table 10-3A. Histologic Criteria for the Classification of Melanocytic Nevi

I. Location of melanocytes in the skin (depth)
  A. Superficial
    - Intraepidermal
    - Papillary dermis
    - Upper half of reticular dermis
  B. Deep
    - Lower half of reticular dermis
    - Subcutaneous
    - Fascial

II. Disposition of melanocytes
  A. Intraepidermal
    1. Basilar melanocytes (single cell pattern)
      a. Normal numbers
      b. Increased frequency
        - With elongated rete (lentiginous)
        - Without elongated rete
    2. Pagetoid pattern
    3. Nested pattern
        - With lentiginous (single file) pattern
        - Without lentiginous (single file) pattern
  B. Dermal
    1. Diffuse, interstitial
    2. Patchy perivascular, periadnexal, perineurial
    3. Wedge pattern (deep apex of nests, fascicles of melanocytes extend into reticular dermis or subcutaneous fat)
    4. Plexiform pattern (discreet nests, fascicles associated with neurovascular or adnexal structures of reticular dermis with intervening normal dermis)
    5. Bulbous aggregates, nodules (cellular nests or fascicles with rounded contours, usually extending into reticular dermis, subcutis)
    6. Alveolar pattern
    7. Maturation or differentiation

III. Stroma
  - Desmoplasia, sclerosis

IV. Cell type
  - Small round or oval cells
  - Fusiform or spindle cell
  - Epithelioid cell (abundant cytoplasm, overall enlarged)
  - Dendritic cell (lengthy, delicate cellular processes)
  - Intermediate, difficult to classify cell types
  - All with varying degrees of melanization

cells have more abundant cytoplasm, somewhat larger nuclei, and somewhat more prominent nucleoli compared with the dendritic basilar melanocytes. Ultrastructurally, nevus cells contain single melanosomes in all stages of development similar to melanocytes. Thus, many authors consider nevus cells to be melanocytes and dismiss the need for alternative nomenclature.

Quick Fact

Lentigines and Acquired Melanocytic Nevi

- Lentigo → Junctional Nevus → Compound Nevus → Intradermal Nevus

Based on **Unna theory**, the presumptive natural history of melanocytic nevi includes proliferation within the epidermis as junctional nests (**junctional melanocytic nevus**) and subsequent migration or "dropping off" of nests of nevus cells into the papillary dermis, resulting in a **compound melanocytic nevus**. According to this hypothesis, eventually proliferation of all intraepidermal melanocytes ceases and the nevi become entirely intradermal (**intradermal melanocytic nevus**). Low levels of mitotic activity within intraepidermal melanocytes are normal in benign nevi. Nevus cells entering the dermis have a reduction in both proliferation and metabolic activity except for the formation of melanosomes. Mitotic activity within dermal melanocytes should not be present, or exceptionally rare. Thus, the cellularity of a nevus tends to decrease with age; because of this cessation of replication, the nevus cells are gradually replaced by mesenchymal elements—fibrous matrix, mucin, and fat. Most dermal nevi are believed to undergo progressive involution, perhaps via acrochordons and eventual shedding. This developmental sequence may be arrested at any point such that a lentigo, junctional nevus, or compound nevus may persist indefinitely.

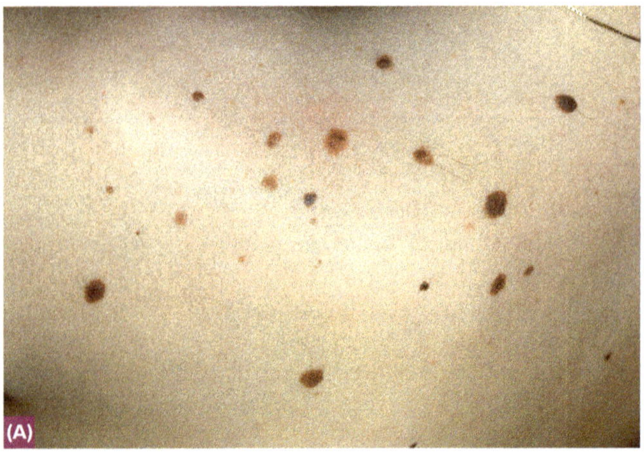
(A)

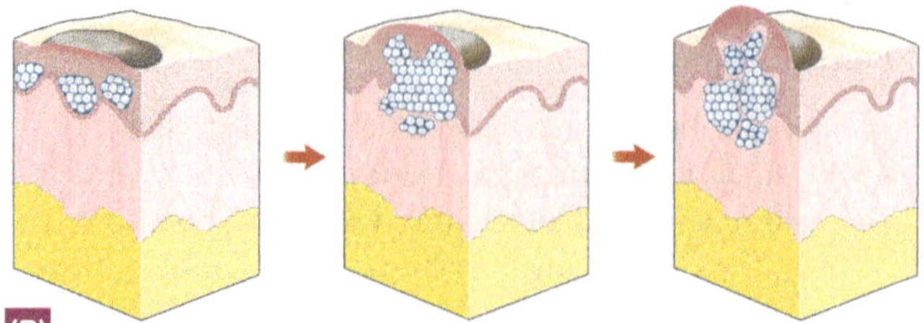

(B)

(A) Multiple melanocytic nevi on the shoulder of a 32-year-old female. Most of these nevi are junctional nevi; some are slightly elevated and thus compound nevi. Note relatively uniform shape and color of the lesions. Because of different developmental stages, they are of varying size ranging from 1 to 4 mm in diameter and they are regular and have a relatively uniform shape. **(B) Junctional nevi** arise at dermal–epidermal junction and are intraepidermal, pigmented, and flat. In **compound nevi**, nevus cells have descended into the dermis and are thus both intraepidermal and dermal. The dermal melanocytes result in increased dermal mass and produce the raised papule appreciated clinically. In **dermal nevi**, all nevus cells are now in the dermis and produce less amounts of melanin pigment. Additionally, the pigmented cells are further away from the epidermis. Dermal nevi are thus skin-colored, pink, or only slightly tan. As they still grow and expand into the dermis, they lift the lesion upward and are thus usually dome-shaped or papillomatous. (Reproduced, with permission, from Wolff K, Johnson RA, Saavedra AP. *Fitzpatrick's Color Atlas and Synopsis of Clinical Dermatology*. 7th ed. New York, NY: McGraw-Hill Education; 2013.)

ANSWER 10-4: B.

The biopsy reveals individual nests of melanocytes within the tips of the rete ridges and within the superficial dermis. The dermal component extends laterally beyond the overlying junctional component, consistent with a **common acquired compound melanocytic nevus** (Table 10-4A). The developmental biology and natural history of **acquired melanocytic nevi** remains poorly understood. The overriding importance and significance of studying benign melanocytic nevi (among all benign melanocytic lesions in general) is their relationship to melanoma. Benign melanocytic nevi are closely linked to melanoma in three important ways; they may be (1) clinical and histologic mimics of melanoma, (2) precursors to melanoma, or (3) clinical and histologic markers of increased risk for melanoma.

The prevalence of nevi is related to age, race, and genetic and environmental factors. Very few nevi are present in early childhood, but they increase in number, reaching a peak in the third decade of life, and tend thereafter to disappear with increasing age. There is a period of particularly rapid development of nevi at puberty. In general, the greatest numbers of melanocytic nevi are noted among individuals aged 20-29 years, and there are no substantial differences between men and women. Whites, in general, have greater numbers of nevi

Table 10-4A. Common Acquired Melanocytic Nevi

Clinical Features
Onset childhood, adolescence, third decade, or later
3-6-mm macule, papule (slight to clear elevation), often dome shaped, globoid, polypoid, or papillomatous
Round, oval
Symmetric
Well-defined regular borders
Homogenous tan, brown, dark brown
Slight accentuation of skin cleavage lines with oblique lighting
Histopathologic Features
Symmetry
Well-circumscribed
Regular arrangement of junctional nests of nevus cells, if present
Fairly uniform size, shape, position of nests
Nests usually at tips of epidermal rete
Usually cohesive nests
Generally no pagetoid spread
Nevus cells usually confined to papillary dermis or superficial reticular dermis
Usual transition or maturation from epithelioid to lymphocytoid to spindled nevus cells
Mitotic figures uncommon or rare in dermis
Usually only minimal nuclear pleomorphism
Differential Diagnosis
Lentigo
Atypical (dysplastic) nevus
Melanoma

than do darker-skinned groups such as blacks and Asians. Furthermore, a greater prevalence of nevi is associated with lighter skin color in whites. The frequency of melanocytic nevi on the palms and soles, nail beds, and conjunctivae is also related to race; nevi on these surfaces are more prevalent in blacks than in whites. Common acquired nevi range from small (2-6 mm in diameter), well-circumscribed pigmented macules to raised, flesh-colored lesions, defined by the location of aggregations of "nevus cells" in the skin. Although many nevi display slight asymmetry, the borders are usually regular and well defined.

The factors determining the baseline histopathological phenotype of common acquired nevi include age and programmed natural history; regional microanatomy; genetic factors; physiologic, hormonal, and immunologic factors; environmental factors such as sun exposure, trauma, and other insults; and other poorly understood factors. Microscopically, melanocytic nevi are usually symmetric and well circumscribed. The junctional component as a general rule does not extend peripherally beyond a dermal component, if present. The surface profile may vary from being almost flat to dome shaped, polypoid, or papillomatous and tends to correlate with type of nevus; for example, **junctional nevi** are relatively flat, **compound nevi** are slightly raised, and **dermal nevi** are often dome shaped, polypoid, or papillomatous. This surface configuration also correlates with anatomic location. Most **acral nevi** are relatively flat or slightly raised junctional or compound nevi. In contrast, many nevi on the head and neck, and to a lesser extent on the trunk, are dome shaped or polypoid. The junctional nevus has nesting of nevus cells within the epidermis. A junctional nest or **thèque** contains three to five or more nevus cells in close apposition that are cohesive and usually above the basement membrane. The size, shape, location, and spacing of these nests tend to be regular. The junctional nests are usually located on the tips of elongated rete rather than on the sides or between rete. Whereas the compound nevus has nevus cells within the dermis as well as junctional nesting, the dermal (or intradermal) nevus has no intraepidermal component. Most nevi are compound; on serial sectioning, 80% of apparent dermal nevi have junctional nests. Common acquired nevi are generally confined to the adventitial dermis (the finely textured collagenous stroma comprising the papillary dermis and surrounding adnexal structures and blood vessels). Dermal nevi mainly proliferate in and expand the papillary dermis, resulting in progressive elevation of nevus contours commensurate with the volume of nevus cells.

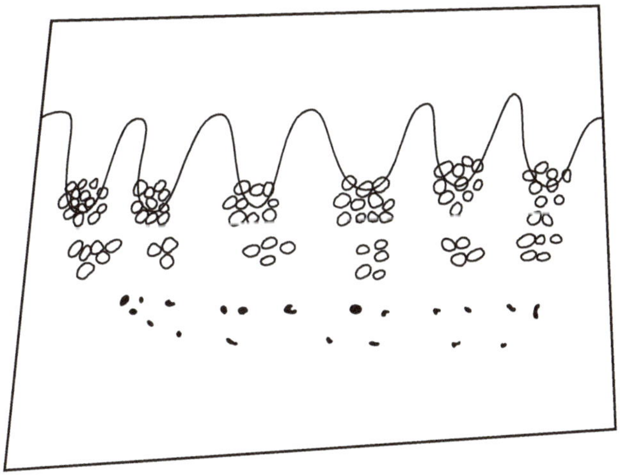

Common acquired compound melanocytic nevus. Note the evenly dispersed nests of nevomelanocytes at the tips of rete ridges. The peripheral aspects of the junctional component are vertically uniform with the underlying dermal component. The dermal melanocytes become progressively smaller with descent into the dermis.

In regards to the differential diagnosis, the main considerations are **dysplastic nevus** and **malignant melanoma** (superficial spreading type). The tumor illustrated in the biopsy lacks a junctional "shoulder" of nevomelanocytes, fusion of rete ridges by bridging nevomelanocytic nests, and papillary dermal fibroplasia. These are the main architectural

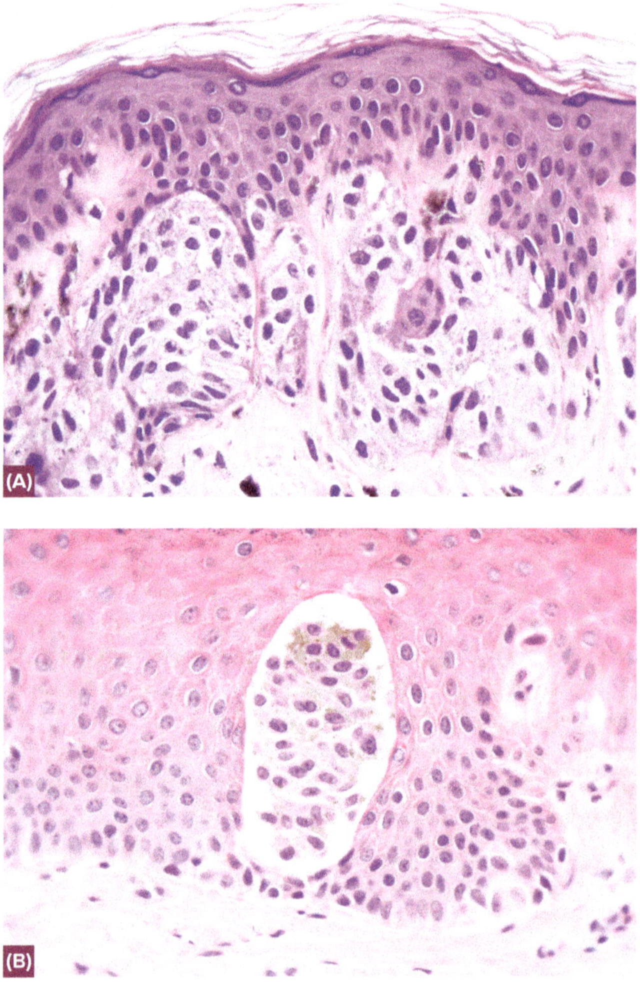

(A) Lentiginous compound nevus. The epidermis shows lentiginous and junctional nested patterns of melanocytes. A few nests are present in the papillary dermis. **(B) Junctional nevus.** Discohesive nest of epithelioid (type A) nevus cells.

features of a so-called "**dysplastic nevus.**" **Superficial spreading melanoma** reveals confluent growth of intraepidermal melanocytes with effacement of the epidermis (loss of rete ridges) and scattered melanocytes above the basal layer (pagetoid ascent). Additionally, the melanocytes in the dermis of melanoma lack maturation with dermal descent and may contain scattered mitoses.

ANSWER 10-5: A.

Nevus cells within junctional nests or the superficial dermis exhibit cohesive rounded nesting, a tendency to synthesis of melanin, and cytologic characteristics of epithelial cells and have been termed **epithelioid** or **type A cells** (image #1). The latter features refer to the abundant pinkish cytoplasm and the rounded or polygonal configuration of the cells. In general, the nuclei are slightly larger than those of basilar melanocytes. The nuclei have a uniform deposition of chromatin, generally with a ground glass basophilic appearance and delicate nuclear membranes. Small nucleoli may also be observed. **Type B nevus cells** in the papillary dermis, usually subjacent (deep) to the **type A cells**, resemble lymphocytes (image #2). This is caused by a smaller amount of cytoplasm and the tendency to form more compact cords and nests of cells. Generally, the latter nevus cells do not synthesize melanin or form rounded nests. On occasion, these cells may closely resemble lymphocytes. The final stage of maturation is that of **type C nevus cells** (image #3) with elongated or spindle-shaped morphology and separation by delicate fibrous tissue. These latter cells have considerable resemblance to fibroblasts or Schwann cells.

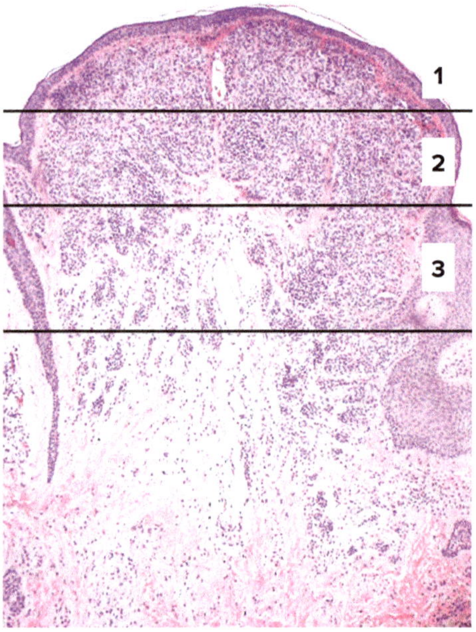

Intradermal nevus. Maturation with dermal descent. Zones 1, 2, and 3 typically contain the type A, B, and C melanocytes, respectively.

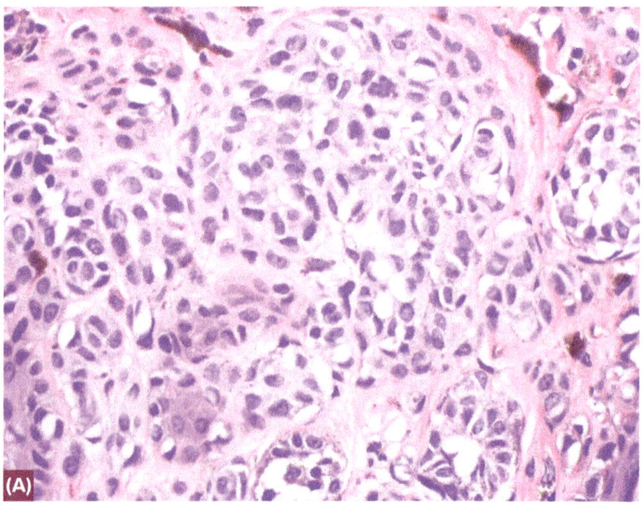

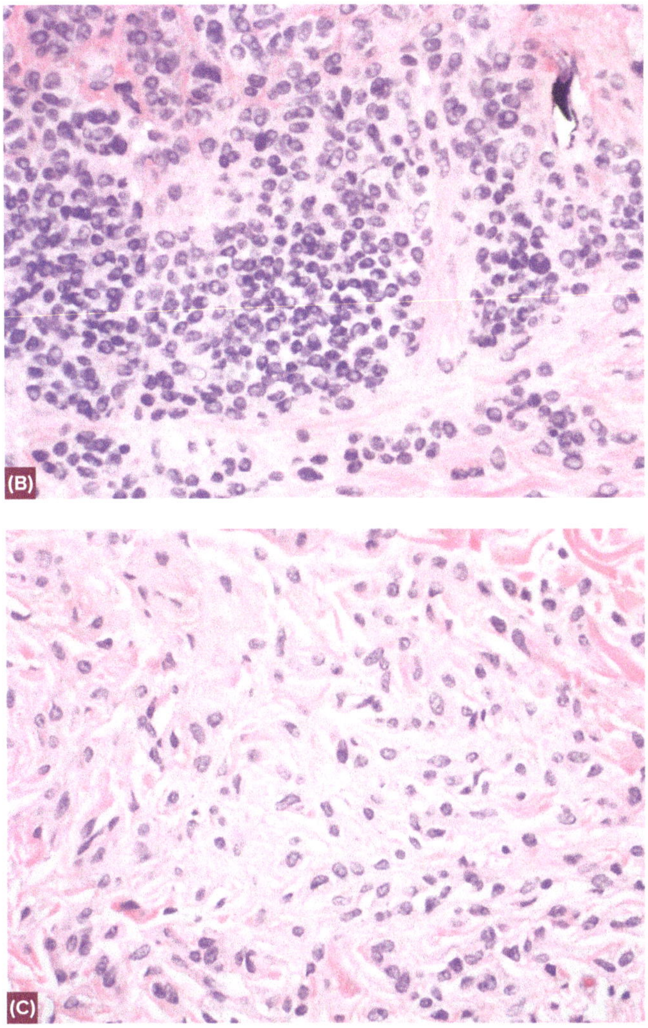

Melanocytic maturation with dermal descent. (A) Type A melanocytes. These round (epithelioid) cells have enlarged nuclei and abundant cytoplasm, often containing melanin pigment. **(B) Type B melanocytes.** These cells have somewhat smaller nuclei and scant amounts of cytoplasm, resembling lymphocytes. **(C) Type C melanocytes** have small nuclei and large amounts of pink cytoplasm, resembling Schwann cells.

Giant cells are observed in **melanocytic nevi** and **melanoma**. **Nevus giant cells** are principally of two types. One type contains tightly packed nuclei with scant cytoplasm and has been called a "mulberry" type giant cell. The molding of nuclei may lead to misinterpretation as a bizarre, **atypical nevus cell**. This cell type is often in the dermal component of a nevus. The nuclear chromatin typically has a smudgy appearance, correlating with cellular senescence. The second type has a peripheral, wreathlike arrangement of nuclei with central pink or slightly bluish cytoplasm. The latter cell type may closely simulate or on occasion be identical to a **Touton giant cell**. This particular giant cell is commonly observed in junctional nests.

Another common feature, the pseudonuclear inclusion, is an invagination of cytoplasm that on cross-section seems to lie within the nucleus and has the same staining properties as the nevus cell cytoplasm, often a pale or "dusty" ground glass appearance.

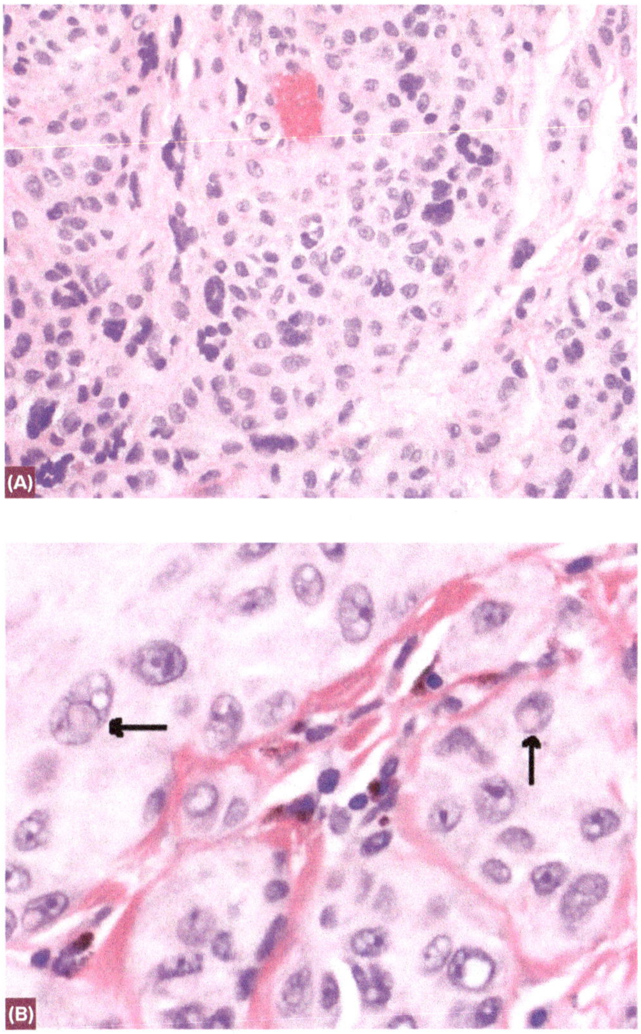

(A) Multinucleated giant type A melanocytes. Numerous multinucleated giant "mulberry" cells. **(B) Nuclear pseudoinclusions**. Melanocytes with amphophilic pseudonuclear inclusions (arrows).

ANSWER 10-6: I-B, II-A, III-C, IV-D.

The morphologic spectrum of **cutaneous melanoma** may be described according to the number of phenotypic characteristics: (1) the location of melanoma cells in the skin, whether intraepidermal, dermal, subcutaneous, or soft tissue; (2) the disposition and frequency or density of melanocytes in these domains, for example, **pagetoid** (dispersion of single and small groups of melanocytes throughout epidermis), **lentiginous** (a basilar epidermal single-cell proliferation of melanocytes), or **nested** arrangements of cells in the epidermis, single-cell infiltrating, or aggregative (nodular) patterns in the dermis and subcutis; (3) unusual histologic features or stromal alterations, such as verrucous, papillomatous, or polypoid epidermal surface configurations; desmoplasia, myxoid stroma, neurotropism, neurogenic or neural differentiation; and resemblance to melanomas developing in animals, experimentally or spontaneous; and (4) cytologic features such as epithelioid, spindled, dendritic, nevus-like, small, clear, balloon, Spitz nevus-like and other cell types (Table 10-6A).

Because nearly all melanomas are initiated in and localized to the epidermis (or epithelium) for some period of time, a classification of melanoma based on the presence or absence and patterns of intraepidermal involvement was developed and has been used for some time. One idea behind such a classification was that particular intraepidermal patterns (also termed **radial** or **horizontal growth phases**) might correlate with differences in etiology and possibly prognosis. **Radial growth phase** is a concept of expansile growth of melanocytes horizontal to and within the epidermal surface. The ability to develop metastatic potential in these lesions is considered low. When the proliferation is confined to the intraepidermal compartment, the phenomenon is equivalent to **melanoma in situ**. **Vertical growth phase** refers to the downward infiltration of malignant melanocytes into the dermis and metastatic potential. Four clinicopathologic subtypes of melanoma have been proposed.

Melanoma with an adjacent lentiginous intraepidermal component of sun-exposed skin (so-called **lentigo maligna melanoma**) may be distinct from other forms of melanomas with intraepithelial components (the pagetoid and acral forms of melanoma) because of its strong correlation with cumulative sunlight exposure, onset in older persons, and uncommon association with melanocytic nevi. These lesions most commonly occur on the head and neck and are associated with a prolonged radial growth phase. Furthermore, this group of melanomas seems to have significantly fewer chromosomal aberrations compared with **acral and mucosal melanomas**, an absence of *BRAF* mutations, frequent gains in CCND1 and regions of chromosome 22, and losses of chromosome 4q.

Table 10-6A. Historical Classification of Malignant Melanoma

Presence of radial growth phase
- Superficial spreading
- Lentigo maligna
- Acral lentiginous
- Unclassified

Absence of radial growth phase
- Nodular melanoma

Superficial spreading melanomas are characterized by adjacent pagetoid intraepidermal components. These tumors have been reported to correlate with intermittent sunlight exposure, develop in relative young individuals, have a frequent association with **atypical nevi**, and are associated with a high frequency of *BRAF* mutations.

Acral (and mucosal) melanomas develop in relatively sun-protected sites, have a high frequency of chromosomal aberrations, and generally lack *BRAF* mutations.

"Nodular" melanoma (NM) is described as having no adjacent intraepithelial component and is thought by many to be a final common pathway of rapid tumor progression irrespective of the intraepithelial pattern or location. By definition, **nodular melanomas** lack a radial growth phase and exhibit vertical growth only.

Although no correlation between intraepidermal pattern (so-called **radial growth phase**) and prognosis has been established, some evidence shows that etiologic factors might still explain some of the morphologic patterns of melanoma, as discussed above. Nevertheless, an objective assessment of the classification of melanoma according to intraepidermal pattern or growth phase has not been clearly validated. The reasons for this view are (1) the tremendous morphologic heterogeneity of melanoma; (2) morphologic patterns may correlate with anatomic site; (3) the intraepithelial components of many melanoma are not easily classified (because of overlapping features), and classification is not reproducible; (4) some intraepithelial components are difficult to recognize as either clearly benign, that is, a potential precursor such as atypical nevus, or malignant; and (5) the idea that nodular melanomas develop as de novo invasive tumors without any initial intraepithelial melanocytic proliferation is theoretically possible but has not been proved.

Despite the drawbacks in the current classification of melanoma outlined above, melanoma nonetheless still seems to have distinct developmental pathways that are related to genetic and other host factors interacting with the environment.

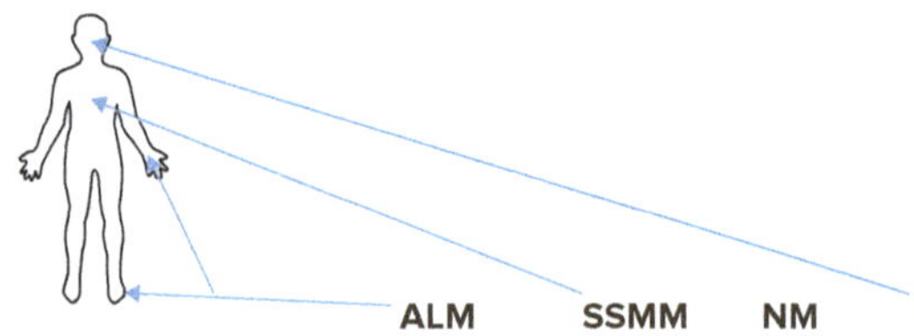

	ALM	SSMM	NM	LMM
Radial growth phase	Always	Always	Never	Always
Sun damage	None	Acute	+/–	Chronic
Relative frequencies	4%	67%	10%	9%

ALM = Acral lentiginous malignant melanoma

SSMM = Superficial spreading malignant melanoma

NM = Nodular melanoma

LMM = Lentigo maligna melanoma

ANSWER 10-7: E.

The patient has numerous pigmented lesions with lesion-to-lesion variability. A closer view of a cluster of lesions marked as #2 on the back reveals numerous lesions of different sizes, colors, and shapes, with differing amounts of asymmetry, and indistinct borders. Only the largest lesion meets all of the criteria for a clinical **dysplastic (atypical) nevus**. The biopsy reveals fusion of junctional nests of nevomelanocytes bridging two or more rete ridges. Additionally, the junctional melanocytic component extends laterally (on the right) beyond the dermal melanocytic component ("**junctional shoulder**"). Lastly, there is drape-like papillary dermal fibrosis and mild dermal inflammatory infiltrates. The combined clinical and histopathologic findings are consistent with a **compound dysplastic nevus** (aka **compound melanocytic nevus with architectural disorder and cytologic atypia**).

Throughout this discussion, the terms "**atypical nevus**" and "**dysplastic nevus**" will refer to clinical and histopathologic diagnoses, respectively. Since the description of **atypical or "dysplastic" melanocytic nevi (DMN)** in the setting of melanoma-prone families about 30 years ago and subsequently in individuals outside such kindreds, these lesions have remained highly controversial. This has largely resulted from the failure to reach consensus about the nature of these lesions, an inability to formulate precise criteria for recognition, and a lack of understanding about their biologic significance. Specifically, this relates to criteria for individual lesions and for the so-called "**dysplastic nevus syndrome**," that is, what minimal essential clinical morphologic criteria are needed for diagnosis of an individual lesion and how many clinically "**atypical nevi**" are needed to equate "**dysplastic nevus syndrome**." One particular problem dating back to the original studies on "**atypical nevi**" in hereditary kindreds has been the tendency to consider that histopathologic diagnosis of DMN as the gold standard; however, it has been shown that the histopathologic features ascribed to DMN lack specificity.

To appreciate the nature of the problem, one must emphasize the considerable clinical and histopathologic heterogeneity among benign melanocytic nevi in general. This is present to such a degree that there is substantial disagreement among many as to how to categorize a significant proportion of nevi with atypical, aberrant, or unusual features and their importance as risk markers for and precursors to melanoma. Furthermore, some authors consider "**dysplastic nevi**" to be distinctly different from other unusual nevi, such as small congenital-pattern nevi and nevi occurring on particular anatomic sites ("**special sites nevi**"), such as acral skin, the vulva, scalp, and so on, despite the frequent presence of histomorphologic features ascribed to "dysplastic" nevi in these other nevi. In principle, we contend that all melanocytic nevi, even normal-appearing ones, may demonstrate atypical histologic features intermediate between banal nevi and melanoma. Until recently the biologic significance of such abnormal histopathologic features had not been established. However, a recent case-control study involving the grading of histologic atypia ("dysplasia") in a series of melanocytic nevi by 13 pathologists has shown that nevi with moderate to severe atypia versus nevi with lesser degrees of atypia are an independent risk factor for melanoma.

It is difficult to estimate the prevalence or melanoma risk related to these lesions, except in the instance of specific clinical morphologic features and numbers of nevi. Thus, many studies have established that irrespective of histology, melanoma risk is directly related to numbers of ordinary nevi (>50 or 100 on the total skin surface), the presence and number of "atypical nevi" as defined by size (eg, >5, 6, or 8 mm), irregular or ill-defined borders, variation in color, macular component, and the like. Based on studies of hereditary melanoma kindreds, the presence of "atypical nevi" on individuals in these kindreds confers a significantly increased risk for the development of melanoma. In fact, the presence of "atypical nevi" in this setting confers a 48.9% cumulative risk for developing melanoma by age 50 years. In prospective follow-up, only family members with "atypical nevi" developed melanoma; those without "atypical nevi" (ie, common acquired nevi only) did not develop melanoma. Individuals in the general population also have "atypical nevi," which also serve as markers for increased melanoma risk, although not nearly so great as in "dysplastic nevus syndrome." Estimates of the relative risk for melanoma in persons with sporadic "atypical nevi" may be in the range of 7%-20%. "Atypical nevi" tend to have periods of relative stability and periods of increased activity, when several new nevi appear and existing nevi change in color, size, or appearance. The reasons for the increased rate of change are not understood. Anecdotally, the changes can occur after increased sun or UV exposure, or in times of hormonal/growth changes such as puberty and pregnancy. Although the majority of "atypical nevi" occur on the trunk, these nevi also show a peculiar propensity for the scalp, female breasts, buttocks, and dorsal surfaces of the feet. "Atypical nevi" tend to show considerable variation in size, shape, and coloration from nevus to nevus. Additionally, they are usually larger than common acquired nevi and smaller than melanoma (but not necessarily so) and generally measure 3-12 mm or larger. They often show asymmetry, often have irregular and ill-defined borders, and have a relatively flat surface (at least part of the lesion is entirely flat). The surface may also be "pebbled" or have a cobblestoned appearance. "Atypical nevi" generally have a more complex color than do ordinary nevi. There are often more than two colors present (ie, tan, brown, dark brown), and the colors have an irregular or haphazard pattern.

It seems logical that histopathologically, dysplastic nevi (DMN) should be associated with increased risk for evolution into melanoma. However, this has not been convincingly demonstrated until recently and requires more detailed study. Furthermore, studies examining the relationship between "atypical melanocytic nevi" and histopathologic DMN have shown a poor correlation. Therefore, the "dysplastic" nevus

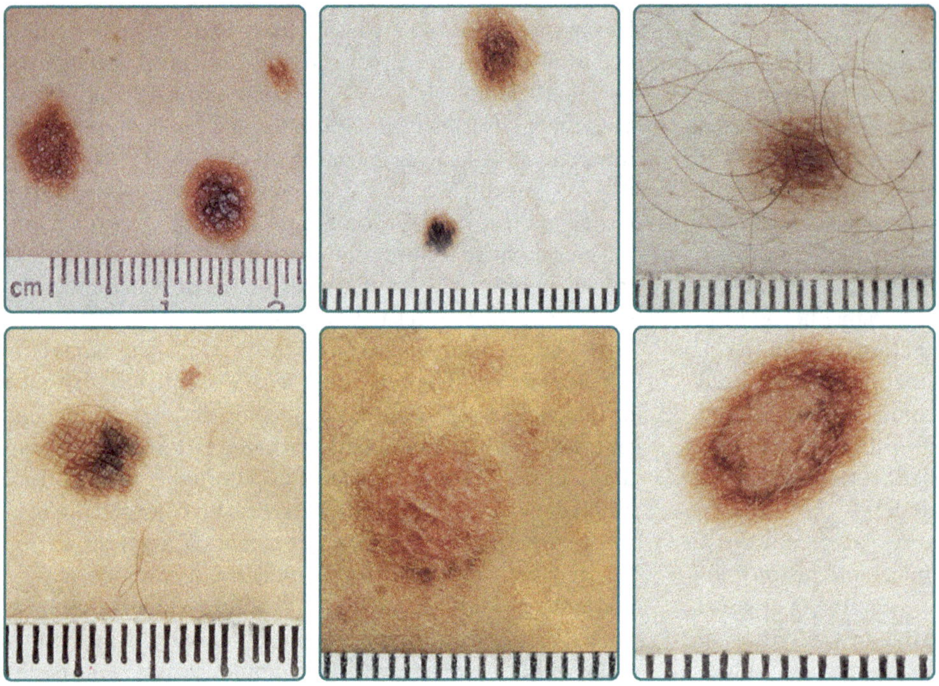

Atypical nevi have two obligate features: diameter in one dimension at least 5 mm and a prominent flat component, and two of three other features: irregular asymmetric outline, indistinct borders, and variable pigmentation. (Reproduced, with permission, from Goldsmith LA, Katz SI, Gilchrest BA, Paller AS, Leffell DJ, Wolff K, eds. *Fitzpatrick's Dermatology in General Medicine*. 8th ed. New York, NY: McGraw-Hill Education; 2012.)

cannot be considered a distinct clinicopathologic entity because the histopathologic features ascribed to histopathologic DMN lack specificity, as already mentioned. Currently, melanoma risk assessment of patients is based solely on clinical morphologic parameters of nevi—that is, total numbers of nevi on the skin surface and the presence and numbers of "atypical nevi"—along with other factors such as personal and family history of melanoma.

Therefore, at present, this category of dysplastic/atypical melanocytic nevi undoubtedly encompass a large and heterogeneous group of nevi, including (1) nevi with atypical clinical features that have been termed simply "atypical nevi," (2) nevi with abnormal histopathologic features ("dysplastic nevi"), (3) nevi with both abnormal clinical and histopathologic features, and (4) nevi with histopathologic features that are equivocal or of unknown significance. The immediate significance of such lesions is whether they are markers of increased melanoma risk; whether they are precursors of melanoma; and in practical terms, their histologic distinction from outright melanoma. These lesions occasionally progress to melanoma and thus may serve as precursors to melanoma. This progression has been observed through the use of serial photographs and the documentation histologically of focal melanoma developing in an otherwise stable DMN. Various authors have also reported remnants of DMN associated with melanoma with an average frequency of approximately 33%. A confounding problem in this situation is the inability in all instances to clearly distinguish the intraepidermal component of melanoma from DMN. Because of the controversy surrounding these nevi, a National Institutes of Health Consensus Conference recommended that the term **dysplastic nevus** be abandoned in favor of "**nevus with architectural disorder or cytologic atypia.**"

Microscopically, the determination of benignancy from malignancy of nevomelanocytic proliferations is based on the proper assessment of both architectural and cytologic atypia. Atypical architectural features include confluent growth, pagetoid ascent, and lack of maturation with dermal descent (when a dermal component is present), while atypical cytologic features include increased cellular size, pleomorphism, prominent nucleoli, and dermal mitoses (when a dermal component is present). The architectural disorder characteristically present in DMN is along the spectrum between that seen in benign common acquired nevi and malignant melanoma. The majority of DMN, perhaps 80%, are compound; the remainder are junctional. Most are relatively flat with only slight expansion of the papillary dermis by limited dermal components. Many (but not all) DMN are lentiginous, that is, the epidermal rete ridges are elongated, are often club shaped, and are accompanied by single cell melanocytic hyperplasia, and the epidermis has increased melanin content. Many heavily pigmented DMN also contain melanin macroglobules in the basilar epidermis, an entirely nonspecific finding. Typically, compound DMN have lateral extension and poor circumscription of the intraepidermal components. The latter features refer to the intraepidermal melanocytic component extending laterally or peripherally beyond the papillary dermal nevus elements (the "**shoulder**" **phenomenon**) and gradually diminishing in cellularity without clear-cut demarcation. Cytologic atypia is frequently present in this "shoulder" region, hence implying biological instability in these foci and the need

Quick Fact

Dysplastic Nevus

- Microscopic diagnosis rendered by assessment of architectural and cytologic features of melanocytes
- Architectural features:
  - Variation in the size, shape, and placement of junctional nests
  - Fusion of rete ridges by nests of nevomelanocytes
  - Papillary dermal fibroplasia
- Cytologic features:
  - Mild
  - Moderate
  - Severe

for re-excision when moderate or severe cytologic atypia extends to the peripheral biopsy edges. Junctional DMN by definition cannot display a lateral "shoulder" but tend to be poorly circumscribed. The nests of nevomelanocytes are disorganized and irregular with focal confluence. Compared with typical nevi, junctional nests in DMN tend to vary significantly in size, shape (ovoid, elongate, or confluent along the dermal–epidermal junction), and spacing (nests are not present at equidistant intervals). Instead of being located at the tips of rete, junctional nests are irregularly distributed on the sides and between rete, often with no regular pattern ("irregularly irregular"). The focal areas of confluence are typically in the form of fusion of rete ridges via confluent nests. This "**bridging of rete ridges**" by nevomelanocytes often appears as slight horizontal spindling of nested nevomelanocytes. The nuclei within these vacuolated cells are commonly pleomorphic with angulated contours. Lastly, DMN exhibit papillary dermal mononuclear cell infiltrates, fibroplasia, and prominent vascularity. The fibroplasia is concentric eosinophilic fibrosis, which is hyalinized collagen that is compactly disposed about the epidermal rete ridges. **Lamellar fibroplasia** is less prevalent and notable for delicate stacking of horizontally disposed collagen, subjacent to the epidermal rete ridges. Mesenchymal spindle cells typically line these filamentous strands of collagen. Both patterns of fibroplasia may be present in the same lesion or occur separately. Although upward migration of melanocytes (**pagetoid ascent**) throughout the epidermis is not a common feature of DMN, it is seen on occasion but is often limited, focal, or orderly in appearance.

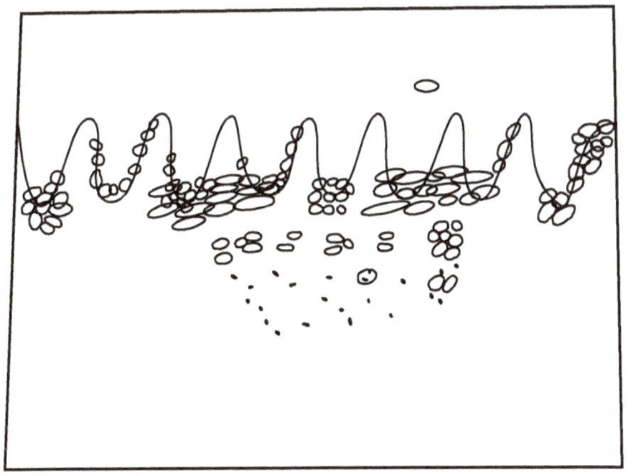

Compound dysplastic nevus. There is a lentiginous and nested intraepidermal melanocytic proliferation. Bridging nests of slightly spindled nevomelanocytes fuse the rete ridges. The junctional component extends peripherally beyond the underlying dermal component. Only rare (ie, one or two) pagetoid melanocytes are present.

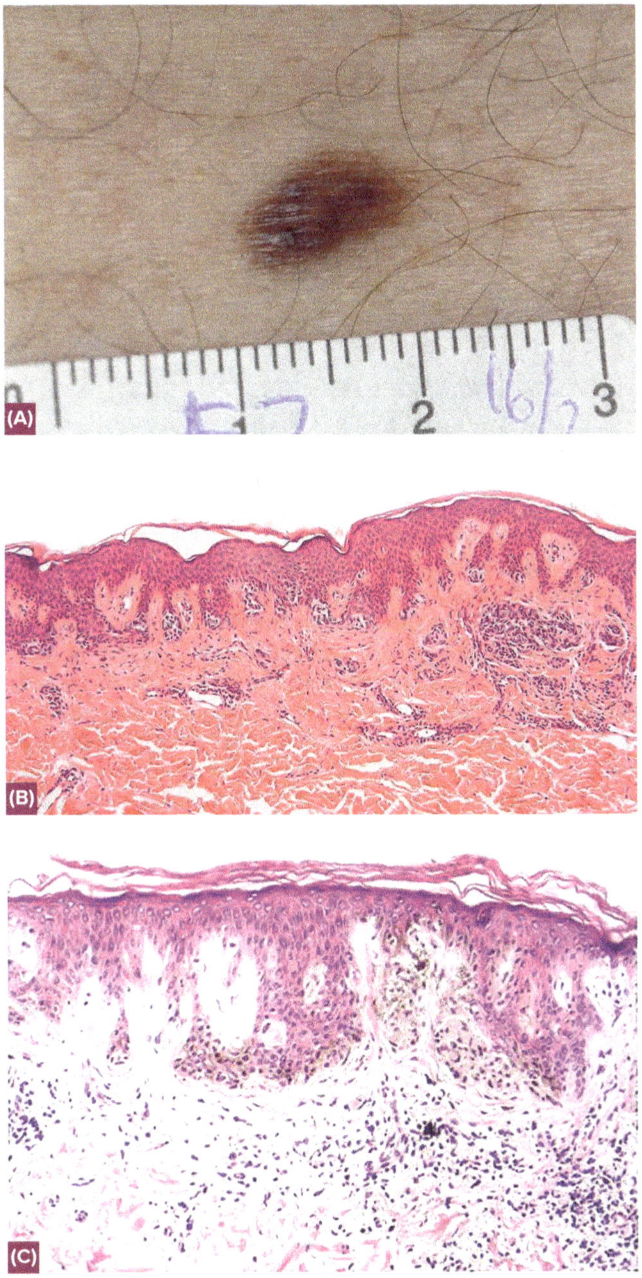

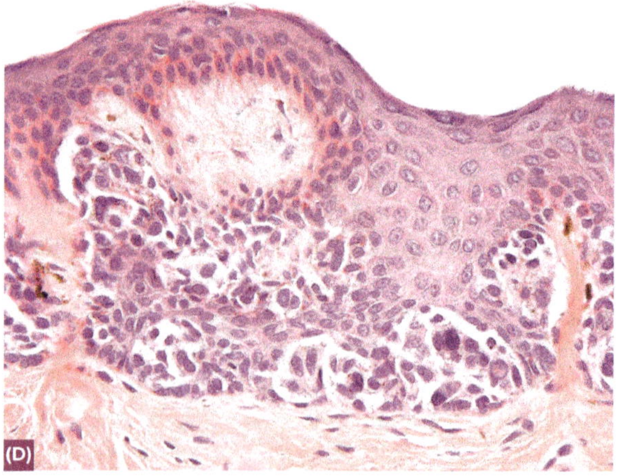

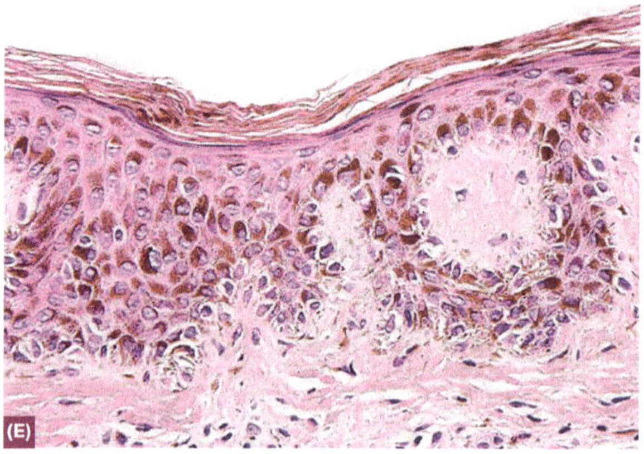

Compound nevus with architectural disorder and cytologic atypia (dysplastic nevus). (A) Clinically atypical compound melanocytic nevus. The lesion measures about 1 cm in greatest diameter, exhibits slight asymmetry, and has some variation in color. **(B)** This field demonstrates the lateral extension of the intraepidermal component (to the left) beyond the dermal nevus component (right side of the field). **(C)** Disordered junctional nested pattern. There is variation in the size, shape, and placement of junctional nests. A sparse lymphocytic infiltrate is present in the superficial dermis. **(D)** Higher magnification shows irregular junctional nesting and horizontal confluence of melanocytes at the dermal–epidermal junction. Cytologic atypia of melanocytes is evident at this magnification. Fibroplasia is present in the papillary dermis. **(E)** Disordered lentiginous pattern. The basilar melanocytes reach confluence along the rete ridges. (Part **(A)**: Used with permission of P Guitera and SW Menzies, Sydney Melanoma Diagnostic Centre and Dermatology Department, Royal Prince Alfred Hospital, NSW, Australia.)

ANSWER 10-8: A.

If the lesion meets the architectural criteria for **dysplastic nevus**, the cytologic atypia must be properly assessed. All three architectural features attributed to **dysplastic nevi (DMN)** are present in this case (ie, junctional shoulder of nevomelanocytes, fusion of rete ridges by nevomelanocytes, and superficial dermal fibrosis). A fundamental criterion for DMN is variable (or discontinuous) cytologic atypia of intraepidermal melanocytes. This refers to intraepidermal melanocytes that are not uniformly atypical but tend to vary from cell to cell as to the degree of nuclear atypia. In general, this nuclear atypia is a continuum and is characterized by gradual nuclear enlargement, pleomorphism, variation in nuclear chromatin pattern, and the eventual development of prominent nucleoli. The beginnings of nuclear atypia may be almost imperceptible and may not be reproducible. Commonly with slight or **mild cytologic atypia**, the cells show retraction of cytoplasm, and the size of the melanocytic nuclei is increased and approximates that of or is slightly larger than the nuclei of spinous layer keratinocytes. With **moderate cytologic atypia**, the nuclei are somewhat larger than the nuclei of spinous layer keratinocytes, and the nucleoli are more commonly visible. With **severe cytologic atypia**, the melanocytes may contain abundant cytoplasm, which often has a granular eosinophilic appearance or may contain finely divided ("dusty") melanin. The nuclei may be enlarged to twice the size of spinous layer keratinocyte nuclei or larger. Nucleoli are often enlarged and may be eosinophilic. The ultimate end point is a uniformly atypical population of cells, which marks the development of melanoma. The cell types that comprise DMN include basilar melanocytes with retracted cytoplasm; small, rounded nevus cells; spindle cells; sometimes pigmented cells; and epithelioid cells. Whereas the basilar melanocytes with retraction of cytoplasm are often observed in predominantly lentiginous forms of DMN, the epithelioid cell type is often present in a much less prevalent, predominantly nested form of DMN (so-called "**epithelioid cell dysplasia**").

Since the "shoulder" of junctional melanocytes in the **dysplastic nevus** may represent a region of biological instability, lesions in which moderate to severe cytologic atypia extend to the lateral biopsy edges should be re-excised. This is to ensure that the "most worrisome" portions of the lesion are completely removed. It is important to emphasize that numerous studies have demonstrated extremely low interobserver reproducibility in the grading and categorization of cytologic atypia in various types of atypical and dysplastic nevi, reinforcing the need for the developing future diagnostic adjuncts. The following guidelines are suggested: (1) severely atypical or high-grade **DMN** should be recognized because of their overlap with **melanoma in situ** (Table 10-8A). Such lesions should be completely excised with margins of at least 5 mm. (2) DMN with moderate atypia that extend to the biopsy edges should be completely removed with clear margins (conservative; ie, 3-mm margin). Because DNA aneuploidy has been documented in such lesions, they may have a greater potential for progression to melanoma than less atypical lesions. In addition, these nevi with moderate to severe atypia appear to be risk markers for melanoma, and one of the authors has observed such nevi with positive margins to recur as melanoma (RL Barnhill, unpublished observations, 2009). (3) DMN with slight or minimal atypia need not have re-excision if the bulk of the lesion has been removed, even if the biopsy edges are involved. Such lesions are common, and reproducible

Table 10-8A. Comparison of Severely Atypical Melanocytic Nevus and Melanoma

SEVERELY ATYPICAL MELANOCYTIC NEVUS	IN SITU OR MICROINVASIVE MELANOMA
Some asymmetry	Prominent asymmetry
Poorly circumscribed	Poorly circumscribed
Rete ridges preserved	Tendency to loss or effacement of rete ridges
Some maintenance of nevus nesting pattern and order	Loss of orderly nesting pattern
Some diminished cohesion of nests	Diminished cohesion of nests may be prominent
Lentiginous melanocytic proliferation concentrated on rete ridges	Loss of rete-oriented melanocytic proliferation
Pagetoid spread absent, minimal, or not prominent	Pagetoid spread prominent
Discontinuous cytologic atypia	Fairly uniform (continuous) cytologic atypia
Often some maturation of dermal component	Often no maturation of dermal component
Usually no mitoses in dermal component	Uncommon mitoses in dermal component (microinvasive melanoma)
Usually perivascular lymphocytic infiltrates	Tendency to band-like lymphocytic infiltrates

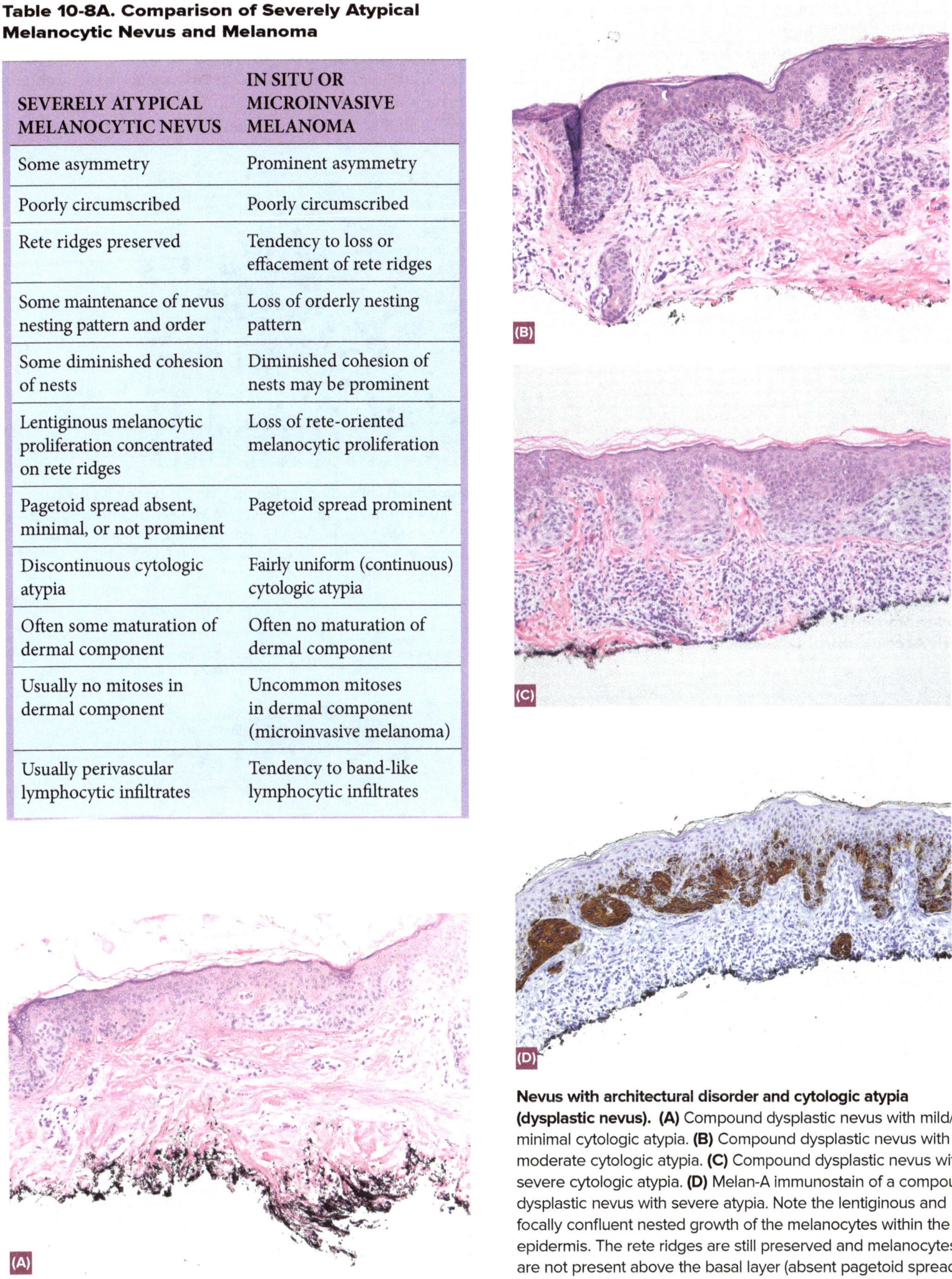

Nevus with architectural disorder and cytologic atypia (dysplastic nevus). (A) Compound dysplastic nevus with mild/minimal cytologic atypia. **(B)** Compound dysplastic nevus with moderate cytologic atypia. **(C)** Compound dysplastic nevus with severe cytologic atypia. **(D)** Melan-A immunostain of a compound dysplastic nevus with severe atypia. Note the lentiginous and focally confluent nested growth of the melanocytes within the epidermis. The rete ridges are still preserved and melanocytes are not present above the basal layer (absent pagetoid spread).

distinction from lentiginous nevi with architectural disorder and no cytologic atypia may not be possible. In general, slightly atypical DMN do not exhibit DNA aneuploidy (Table 10-8B).

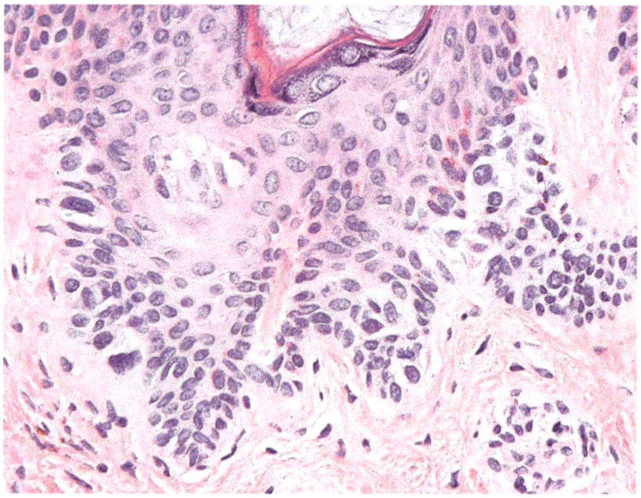

Junctional nevus with architectural disorder and severe cytologic atypia (dysplastic nevus). Note the severe cytologic atypia of lentiginous melanocytes. Some nuclei are more than twice the size of adjacent keratinocytic nuclei.

Table 10-8B. Histopathologic Reporting of Atypical Melanocytic (Dysplastic) Nevi (Melanocytic Nevi with Architectural Disorder and Cytologic Atypia)*

GRADE OF LESION	SUGGESTED RE-EXCISION IF MARGINS INVOLVED
Low-grade lesions	
Junctional or compound nevus with architectural disorder (no cytologic atypia)	No
Junctional or compound nevus with architectural disorder and mild/minimal cytologic atypia	No, if bulk of lesion removed
High-grade lesions	
Junctional or compound nevus with architectural disorder and moderate cytologic atypia	Yes, conservative*
Junctional or compound nevus with architectural disorder and severe cytologic atypia	Yes, with about 5-mm margins

*These suggested therapies are based on the presence of nuclear aneuploidy in such lesions. However, the grading of atypia in nevi has not been standardized and remains controversial; A reporting schema for melanocytic lesions: the MPATH-Dx schema has recently been developed by a National Institutes of Health-funded group. Implementation of this system would simplify classification and management of cutaneous melanocytic lesions.

The pathologist should communicate directly to the clinician in clear and unambiguous language the nature of the lesion and its significance, regardless of terminology used (ie, **Clark nevus, dysplastic nevus, nevus with architectural and cytologic atypia**). In one sense, the significance of the individual lesion is related to the degree of histologic

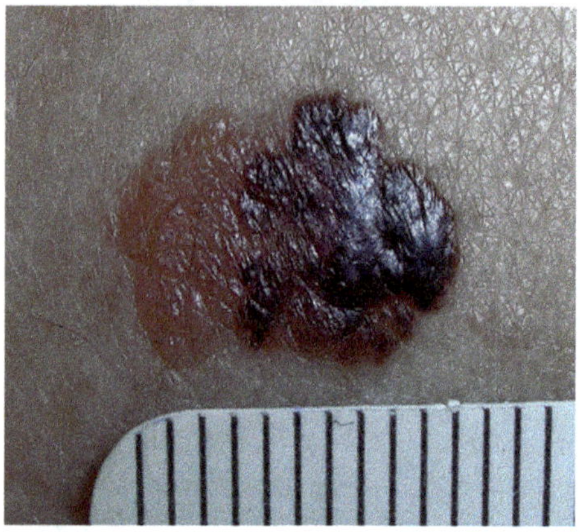

Superficial spreading melanoma on the back with ABCDE features of melanoma. (Reproduced, with permission, from Usatine RP, Smith MA, Mayeaux EJ Jr, Chumley HS, eds. *Color Atlas of Family Medicine*. 2nd ed. New York, NY: McGraw-Hill Education; 2012. Used with permission of Richard P. Usatine, MD.)

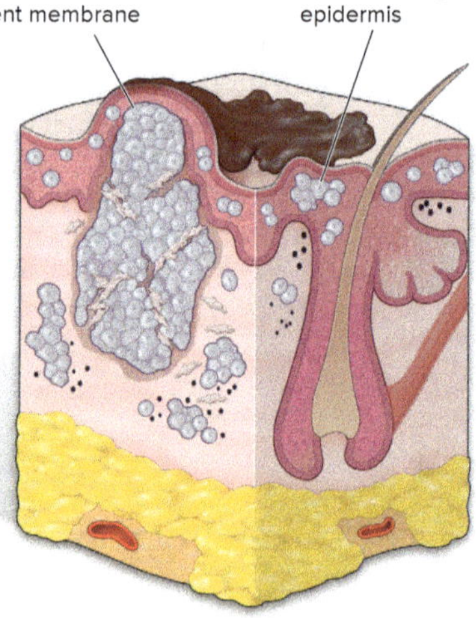

Superficial spreading melanoma. The border is irregular and elevated throughout its entirety; biopsy of this plaque surrounding the large nodule shows a pagetoid distribution of large melanocytes throughout the epidermis in multiple layers, occurring singly or in nests, and uniformly atypical (radial growth phase). On the left is a large nodule, and scattered throughout the surrounding portion of the plaque are smaller papular and nodular areas (vertical growth phase). The nodules may also show epithelioid, spindle cells, or small malignant melanocytes as in lentigo maligna melanoma and nodular melanoma. (Reproduced, with permission, from Wolff K, Johnson RA, Saavedra AP. *Fitzpatrick's Color Atlas and Synopsis of Clinical Dermatology*. 7th ed. New York, NY: McGraw-Hill Education; 2013.)

atypia (architectural and cytologic) in that lesion and its risk for progression to melanoma. The immediate concern is to ensure proper management of the individual lesion and the need for additional therapy (ie, surgery), if any, is communicated to the clinician. In another sense, the significance of a dysplastic melanocytic nevus must be viewed from the perspective of global melanoma risk in the patient. Thus, the significance of the individual dysplastic nevus can be viewed in quantitative terms and is directly related to the degree of histologic atypia (eg, moderate to severe vs slight or no atypia), family history of melanoma, family history of clinically "atypical nevi," personal history of melanoma, the patient's nevus phenotype (total number of typical and atypical nevi on the skin surface), the degree of atypia of previously removed nevi, and other risk factors for **superficial spreading melanoma** (Table 10-8C).

The histologic guidelines listed in the table represent the most common presentation. However, there is considerable variation among these features.

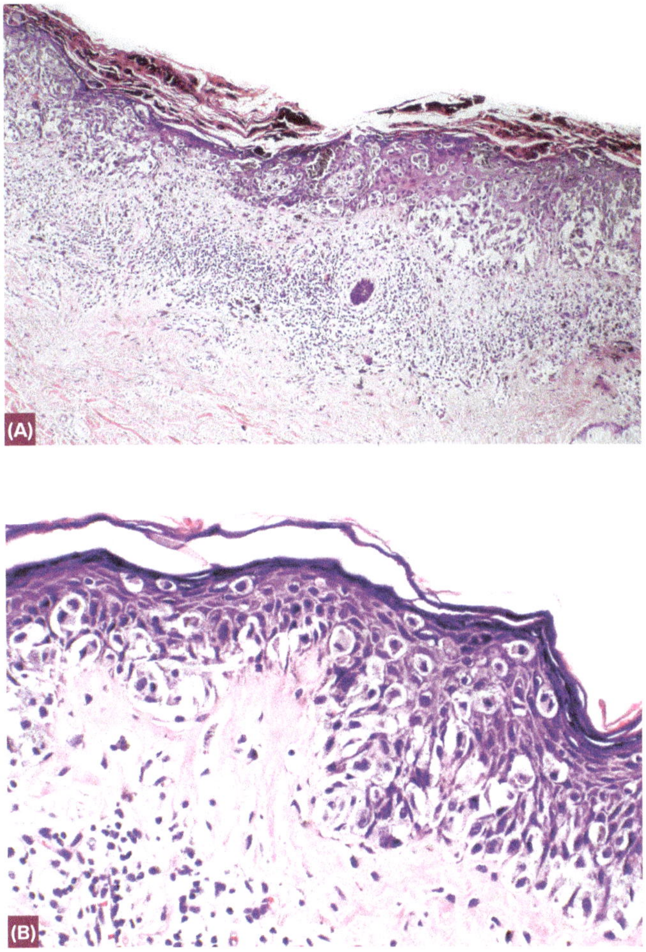

Superficial spreading melanoma (Pagetoid melanoma). **(A)** Pagetoid melanocytosis of epithelioid cells throughout epidermis. **(B)** Higher magnification shows the striking density of epithelioid melanoma cells within the epidermis and the degree of involvement of the superficial epidermis.

Table 10-8C. SUPERFICIAL SPREADING MELANOMA (PAGETOID MELANOMA)

Clinical Features
- In general, onset after puberty, but all ages affected
- Most frequent ages 30-70 years
- Whites >> Africans, Asians
- Women ≥ men
- Most common sites: lower extremities and trunk of women and trunk (back) of men
- Pain, pruritus
- Size often >1 cm (range: 2 mm->15 cm)
- Initially macular; later stages may be papular and nodular
- Asymmetry
- Irregular and often notched borders
- Complexity and variation in color often with admixtures of tan, brown, black, blue, gray, white, red
- May be entirely skin-colored (amelanotic) or black
- Ulceration and bleeding may be present

Histopathologic Features
- Architecture
  - Asymmetry
  - Heterogeneity of lesion
  - Large size (>6 mm) but many exceptions
  - Poor circumscription of proliferation
  - Melanin not uniformly distributed
- Organizational abnormalities of intraepidermal component
  - (1) Pagetoid spread
    - Upward migration of melanocytes in random pattern, single cells predominate over nests
    - Cells often reach granular and cornified layers
  - (2) Lentiginous melanocytic proliferation
    - Melanocytes reach confluence
    - Nesting of melanocytes (sun-damaged skin)
    - Melanocytes not equidistant
    - Proliferation of melanocytes along adnexal epithelium
  - (3) Nesting pattern
    - Variation in size, shape, placement of nests
    - Nests replace large portions of squamous epithelium
    - Diminished cohesiveness of cells in nests
    - Confluence of nests
- Loss of epidermal rete pattern (effacement)
- Mononuclear cell infiltrates, often band like
- Fibroplasia of papillary dermis
- Regression frequently present
- Cytology
  - (1) Nuclear changes
    - Majority of melanocytes uniformly atypical
    - Nuclear enlargement

Table 10-8C. SUPERFICIAL SPREADING MELANOMA (PAGETOID MELANOMA) *(continued)*

- Nuclear pleomorphism (variation in sizes and shapes)
- Nuclear hyperchromasia with coarse chromatin
- One or more prominent nucleoli

(2) Cytoplasmic changes
- Abundant granular eosinophilic cytoplasm in epithelioid cells
- Finely divided ("dusty") melanin
- Variation in size of melanin granules
- High nuclear to cytoplasmic ratios in spindle cells
- Retraction of cytoplasm

Mitoses (in dermal component)
Atypical mitoses
Necrotic cells

Invasive component usually in dermis

Architecture
- Tumefactive cellular aggregates
- Pushing, expanding pattern without regard for stroma
- Hypercellularity
- Less host response

Cytology
- As above
- Increased nuclear to cytoplasmic ratios
- Mitoses in dermal component
- Atypical mitoses
- Necrotic cells

Differential Diagnosis

Melanocytic tumors
- Atypical (dysplastic) melanocytic nevus
- Halo nevus with atypia
- Spitz nevus or tumor
- Pigmented spindle cell nevus
- Recurrent melanocytic nevus
- Other melanocytic nevi with prominent pagetoid spread

Nonmelanocytic tumors
- Squamous cell carcinoma
- Paget disease, mammary or extramammary
- Sebaceous carcinoma
- Cutaneous T-cell lymphoma
- Epidermotropic eccrine carcinoma
- Metastatic carcinoma, other
- Angiosarcoma
- Kaposi sarcoma
- Leiomyosarcoma
- Atypical fibroxanthoma
- Malignant fibrous histiocytoma

ANSWER 10-9: E.

Distinct sets of genetic alterations have been shown in **melanomas** with respect to their relationship with UV-light exposure. Interestingly, these UV-light associated groups of melanoma and genetic alterations roughly mirror (implied histopathologic correlation with location) the classical melanoma subtypes (ie, **lentigo maligna, superficial spreading**, and **acral** and **mucosal lentiginous melanomas [nodular excluded]**).

The autonomous (but limited) proliferation of benign nevus cells is typically driven by oncogenic mutations (usually point mutations) such as ***NRAS*** and ***BRAF***, both of which have been shown to be associated with a rounded (epithelioid) cytomorphology. Melanomas that arise in association with intermittent intense sun exposure (ie, several "bad" sunburns) also harbor *BRAF* and *NRAS* mutations. **Superficial spreading melanoma** is the classic subtype associated with **atypical nevi**. Supporting this theory of **melanomagenesis** are data derived from molecular studies and chromosomal rearrangement analysis. Comparative genomic hybridization (CGH) and DNA microarray technology have established that approximately 95% of malignant melanomas have chromosomal aberrations. Benign nevi lack chromosomal aberrations or have very restricted sets that don't overlap. As an example, approximately 20% of **Spitz nevi** have gains in isochromosome 11p (containing ***HRAS***), which is associated with an indolent clinical course.

As mentioned above, the initial melanocyte/nevus cell proliferation is driven by oncogenic point mutations. The reason frequent chromosomal aberrations are seen in **melanoma** and not **benign nevi** is due to increased cell cycle control in nevi. As cells continually divide, the **telomeres** flanking the chromosomes become progressively shorter. **Senescence** is the essential mechanism that prevents cellular division beyond a critically shortened telomere length. This is typically accomplished by upregulation of tumor suppressor genes such as *p53 & RB* pathway (including p16), which permanently arrests cell division. This phenomenon is reflective of "dropping off" of junctional melanocytes into the dermis with subsequent descending maturation and absent mitoses.

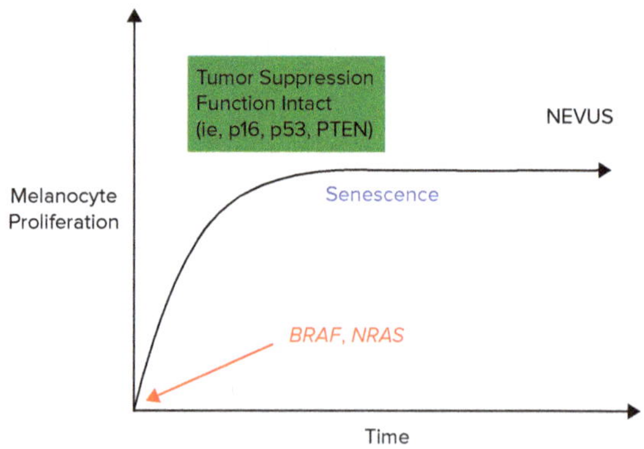

Benign melanocytic nevus. Oncogenic mutations (ie, point mutations in *BRAF* or *NRAS*) drive melanocytic proliferation. However, tumor suppressor function is upregulated as telomeres before shorter with each division, locking cells into senescence.

Loss of **tumor suppressor gene** function allows proliferation beyond the replication limit (complete loss of telomeres) and places cells in "**crisis**." Without intact telomeres, open DNA ends are prone to forming end-to-end chromatid fusions resulting in a cascade of gross chromosomal alterations. Crisis cells carry on division but show high rates of apoptosis (apoptosis > proliferation), due to large numbers of lethal cellular mutations. **Regression**, which we attribute to an immunologic response, may potentially be a reflection of this phenomenon. Eventually, stable clones are formed with rapid autonomous growth and aggressive biological behavior (**malignant melanoma**).

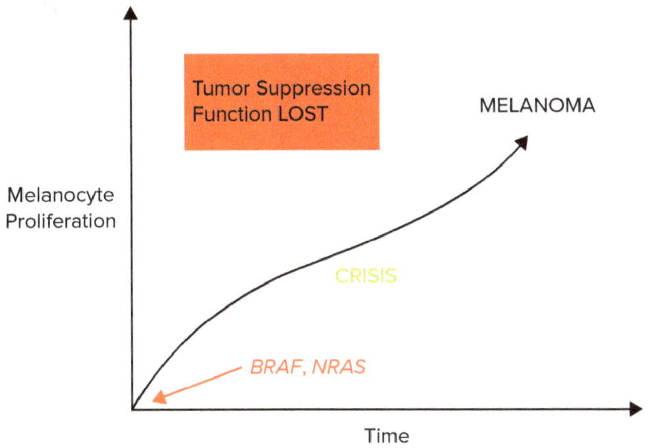

Malignant melanoma. Oncogenic mutations (ie, point mutations in *BRAF* or *NRAS*) drive melanocytic proliferation. Tumor suppressor function is compromised and cells continue dividing despite critically shortened telomeres. Once the telomeres are completely depleted, numerous structural chromosomal aberrations begin to form (crisis). Genomically stable clones eventually emerge as malignant melanoma.

Loss of **tumor suppressor** function may occur at a much later point in time within preexisting "stable" **melanocytic nevi**. One point of theoretical interest is the junctional "shoulder" of **dysplastic nevi** with frequent increased cytologic atypia. This expanded radial growth of intraepidermal melanocytes without an underlying dermal component may signify a genetic event in which the melanocytes have impaired ability to enter **senescence**. Melanomas that arise within "dysplastic nevi" frequently do so within these peripheral aspects.

In the study by Curtin et al melanomas ($n = 126$) were evaluated for genome-wide alterations in DNA copy number and *BRAF* and *NRAS* mutations. Their initial analysis divided these melanomas into four groups (**chronic sun exposure, intermittent sun exposure, acral sites**, and **mucosal sites**). On the basis of changes in the number of copies of DNA alone, samples could be correctly classified into the four groups with an overall 70% accuracy. The ***CCND1*** locus (cyclin-D1 protein) was frequently gained in the melanoma specimens from skin with chronic sun-induced damage. These tumors lacked ***BRAF*** mutations in 74% of cases. These tumors most frequently arose in the skin of the head and neck, the location

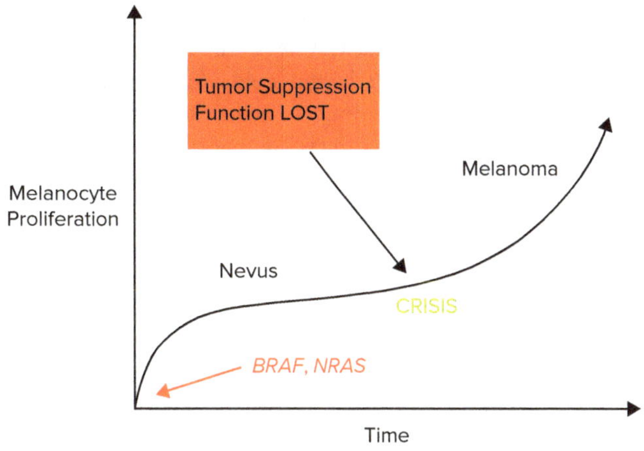

Melanoma arising within a preexisting nevus. Oncogenic mutations (ie, point mutations in *BRAF* or *NRAS*) drive melanocytic proliferation. Tumor suppressor function is initially intact and the cells enter senescence; however, at a later point in time tumor suppressor function is lost and cells continue dividing and eventually leading to crisis. Genomically stable clones eventually emerge as malignant melanoma.

most typical for **lentigo maligna melanoma**. Interestingly, **lentigo maligna melanomas** arise as single cell proliferations usually without associated preexisting melanocytic nevi. They also found that melanomas arising in chronically UV-damaged and intermittently UV-damaged skin harbored overall fewer chromosomal aberrations than those at relatively sun-protected sites (mucosal > acral).

Recently fluorescence in situ hybridization using a four probe test has been introduced for the evaluation of cutaneous melanocytic lesions. Initial studies have shown that gains in 11q13 and 6p25 and losses of 6q23 were 87% sensitive and 95% specific in distinguishing melanomas from melanocytic nevi. However, the utilization of FISH testing for melanocytic lesions in general requires more detailed investigation. In contrast, array comparative genomic hybridization allows for genome-wide analysis of chromosomal gains and losses, and a more robust test for many difficult melanocytic lesions.

ANSWER 10-10: E.

Scanning magnification of the biopsy shows dense mononuclear cell infiltrates that obscure junctional and papillary dermal nests of nevus cells. Junctional and dermal nests of melanocytes are present; however, confluent intraepidermal growth and pagetoid ascent are not present. Maturation of dermal nevus cells in the dense inflammatory infiltrate is preserved. The findings are consistent with a **halo nevus**. **Halo nevi** are almost always acquired, but any type of nevus or melanocytic lesion may develop a clinical **halo** or histologic **halo reaction**. Halo nevi generally affect individuals younger than age 20 years, and the overall incidence is probably less than 1%. There is no difference in incidence between males and females. Approximately 20% of individuals with halo nevi have **vitiligo**, and halo nevi have an association with **melanoma** and **atypical (dysplastic) nevi**. The natural history of halo nevi has not been well documented. However, in general, the hypopigmentation is thought to develop over weeks to months. The central nevus may persist, or more likely, undergoes involution over months to years. The depigmentation has been ascribed to (1) an immune response against antigenically altered (perhaps atypical) nevus cells or to (2) cell-mediated or humoral (antibody-mediated) reaction against nonspecifically altered melanocytes and possible cross-reactivity with melanocytes at a distant site or sites.

Clinically, the central melanocytic nevus may be relatively flat or raised and dark brown to pink, and exhibits surface scale or crusting. The central nevus is surrounded by a well-circumscribed annulus of hypo- or depigmented skin, commonly measures 3-6 mm in largest diameter, has regular and well-defined borders, and has a homogeneous coloration. These clinical findings are reassuring for a benign process. The subsequent course of a halo nevus is variable. Both the central nevus and the halo may persist or regress completely. The central nevus may not change or may become irregularly pigmented or pink or red. Probably more than half of all halo nevi undergo **complete regression**. The period of time associated with nevus regression varies from months to as long as several years. Halo nevi are most typically located on the upper back but may be found in any location. Approximately 25%-50% of affected individuals have two or more halo nevi.

Microscopically, the **halo nevus** may be junctional, compound, or dermal. In the fully evolved stages, the central nevus is associated with a well-circumscribed, dense, almost band-like infiltrate of mononuclear cells, almost exclusively lymphocytes and histiocytes, which occupies the papillary dermis and permeates nests of nevus cells. It is often difficult to distinguish nevus cells from surrounding mononuclear cells. Degenerating nevus cells can sometimes be identified in this zone. Homogeneous eosinophilic (apoptotic) bodies, representing degenerated cells, are often observed near the dermal–epidermal junction. Occasional nevus cells within the infiltrate show prominent eosinophilic cytoplasm and enlarged nuclei and may sometimes be pleomorphic. In some instances, the melanocytes closely resemble the cells in **Spitz nevi**, and thus such lesions may be confused with a **Spitz nevus**. Although most halo nevi demonstrate no obviously atypical nevus cells, some display varying degrees of cytologic atypia potentially ranging from slight to severe. The cytologic alteration is often reactive, but legitimate atypical halo nevi occur (equivocal for melanoma). Occasionally rare mitoses are observed in the dermal component of halo nevi and should prompt careful study to exclude **melanoma**. In general, more than two dermal mitoses render the lesion sufficiently atypical to warrant complete re-excision. Ki67 immunostain will label numerous dividing lymphocytes and macrophages; therefore, a combined Melan-A/Ki-67 (red and brown chromagen) is essential to properly assess dividing melanocytes. The peripheral zones of the nevus, corresponding to the clinical halo,

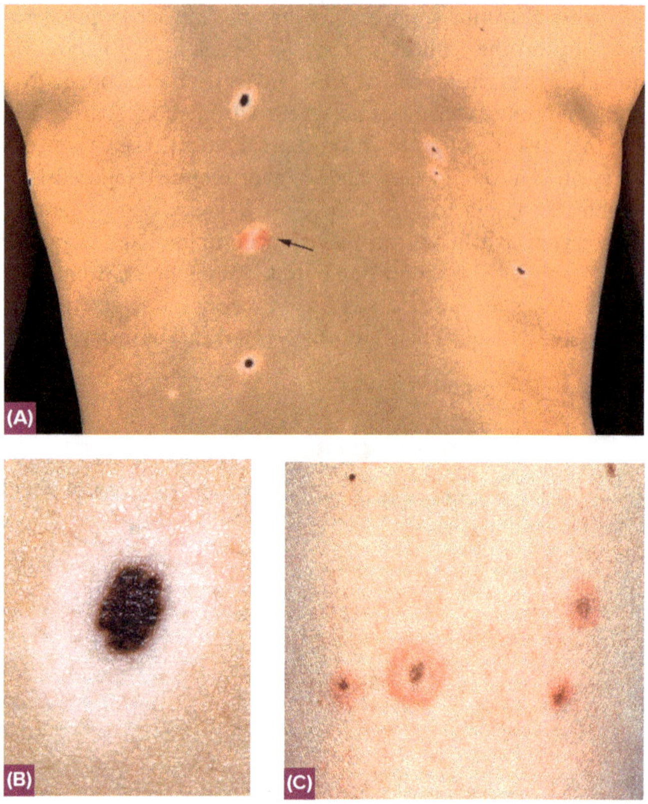

Halo nevi. (A) Halo melanocytic nevus on the back of a 22-year-old female. There are five halo nevi, all with a pigmented dot-like central junctional or compound nevi surrounded by a hypo- or amelanotic halo. The arrow indicates one lesion where the central nevus has completely regressed; the reddish color indicates telangiectasia. **(B)** Larger magnification of a halo nevus. The nevus is a junctional nevus that is surrounded by a hypomelanotic (almost white) halo. **(C)** Several tan junctional nevi are surrounded by an erythematous halo. This is the early stage of halo development. The erythematous rim will later turn white. (Reproduced, with permission, from Wolff K, Johnson RA, Saavedra AP. *Fitzpatrick's Color Atlas and Synopsis of Clinical Dermatology*. 7th ed. New York, NY: McGraw-Hill Education; 2013.)

show diminished or absent basilar melanocytes and melanin in the basal layer; the central part of the lesion may also show the latter features. The papillary dermis in this annulus may also demonstrate slight reparative alteration of the stroma, but usually no inflammatory cell infiltrates are found.

With **complete regression**, all nevus cells are destroyed, with resulting thickening of the papillary dermis, occasional delicate fibroplasia and frequent mucinous alteration, vascular ectasia, variable residual lymphocytic infiltrates, and melanophages. There may be complete depigmentation of the epidermis. Occasional nevi with typical hypopigmented halos do not exhibit cellular infiltrates. Most of the infiltrating cells in halo nevi are T lymphocytes and monocytes or macrophages. There are approximately equal numbers of helper or inducer (CD4+) and cytotoxic or suppressor (CD8+) T cells. The nevus cells also express class I human leukocyte antibody

Table 10-10A. Comparison of Halo Nevus and Malignant Melanoma

	HALO NEVUS	MELANOMA
Clinical Features	Central nevus 3-6 mm in size Symmetry of central nevus and halo Regular borders Uniform color of central nevus—tan, brown, or pink—and halo; hypo- or depigmentation	Usually >6 mm Asymmetry Irregular borders Haphazard or irregular color
Histopathologic Features	Symmetry Usually well circumscribed Mononuclear cell infiltrate orderly with well-defined inferior margin Maturation or differentiation of nevus elements Apoptosis of nevus cells common Rete ridges maintained Little or no cytologic atypia commonly Few mitoses in dermal component Atypical mitoses usually absent	Asymmetry Poorly circumscribed Often variation in pattern of infiltrate Usually little or no maturation Apoptosis may be observed Effaced rete ridges common Prominent cytologic atypia Mitoses in dermal component frequent Atypical mitoses may be observed

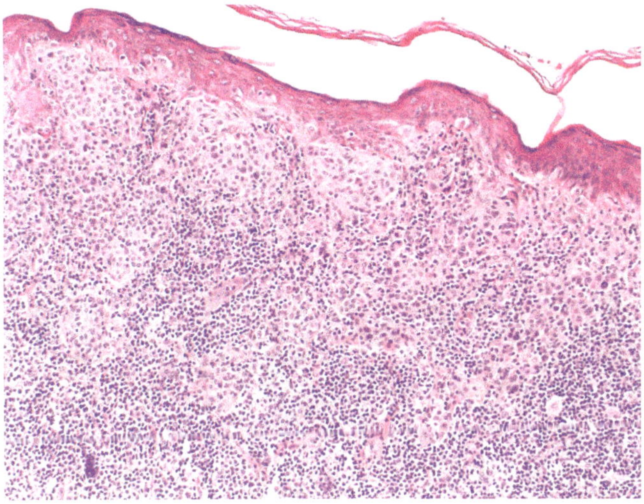

Halo nevus. There is a band-like lymphohistiocytic infiltrate with interface activity along the dermal–epidermal junction. The dermal melanocytes exhibit preserved maturation with dermal descent.

(HLA) antigens to a much greater extent than class II HLA antigens. These findings suggest a specific cell-mediated immune response in halo nevi.

In regards to the differential diagnosis, the **halo nevus** (benign nevus with regression) must primarily be distinguished from melanoma with regression (Table 10-10A). This distinction is not a significant problem for halo nevi showing little or no cytologic atypia. Such halo nevi generally are small (ie, <5-6 mm), symmetric, display maturation, and have an orderly appearance compared with melanoma. Halo nevi are notable for the symmetry and well-defined inferior margin of the mononuclear cell infiltrate contained in the papillary dermis. An important feature is the maturation of nevus cells. Although rare mitotic figures may be noted in the dermal component of any melanocytic lesion, including halo nevi, more than a few mitoses (typically >2), mitoses in the deepest dermal cells, and atypical mitoses are of particular concern.

ANSWER 10-11: C.

The biopsy reveals a lentiginous and nested compound melanocytic proliferation with a single melanocytic nest located above the basal layer. Confluent growth of melanocytes is absent and the epidermal architecture is preserved. The findings are consistent with an **acral melanocytic nevus (AMN)**. Melanocytic nevi of acral skin (sometimes referred to as atypical acral melanocytic nevi) may be defined as to their localization to glabrous (non-hair bearing) skin, the entire surface of the hands and feet (including hair-bearing dorsal aspects), or potentially inclusive of other sites such as the elbows and knees. Recently an additional subset of atypical lesions comprised predominately of atypical nevi from the distal lower extremities with features of acral nevi has been described. Without question, the histology of **acral nevi** involving glabrous skin is influenced by the **dermatoglyphics** (the ridges and furrows of skin lines), the thick stratum corneum, the concentration of eccrine glands, absence of hair follicles, and other factors such as repetitive mechanical trauma. The major clinical concern with AMN is their distinction from **acral melanoma**. Clinically, acral melanocytic nevi are usually acquired macular or only slightly elevated, uniform brown or dark brown lesions commonly indistinguishable from **simple lentigines**. They may exhibit striking striate appearances (linear pigment patterns) corresponding to the dermatoglyphics (ie, the skin lines of glabrous skin).

They are usually relatively small (<5-7 mm), well-circumscribed, and symmetrical lesions with regular borders. Nonetheless, congenital and atypical clinical variants occur and show a spectrum of abnormalities, including larger diameter, asymmetry, irregular borders, and variation in pigment patterns that require histologic distinction from melanoma.

Microscopically, at scanning magnification, the most typical **AMNs** usually measure 2-8 mm (mean, about 5 mm) in diameter, are symmetrical, well circumscribed, and have a relatively flat or slightly elevated topography. The vast majority are junctional or compound nevi, and a small proportion is entirely dermal. AMN usually demonstrates regular junctional nesting of melanocytes with absent to low-grade cytologic atypia. Junctional nests may be large, vertically oriented, and show transepidermal elimination (nests located high up within the epidermis). A characteristic property of AMN is the presence of occasional pagetoid melanocytes and vertically oriented melanin columns in the stratum corneum. For this reason, some refer to these lesions as **melanocytic acral nevus with intraepidermal ascent of cells** (**MANIAC**). The dermal components, if present, are usually limited to the papillary and superficial reticular dermis. Importantly, AMN may commonly exhibit features that raise suspicion for melanoma such as large diameter (>6-7 mm), asymmetry (≤44% cases), poor circumscription (≤63% cases), lentiginous melanocytic proliferation (≤54% cases), pagetoid melanocytosis (up to 86.5% cases), architectural disorder (5.4% in one study), and moderate to severe cytologic atypia. It is of interest that the abnormal features of asymmetry, poor circumscription, and absence of melanin columns correlate with plane of section of AMN parallel to skin lines (vs symmetry, sharp circumscription, and the presence of melanin columns correlating with plane of section perpendicular to skin lines).

In regards to the differential diagnosis, as with all melanocytic nevi, there is considerable heterogeneity of AMN, and a number of variants are observed on a regular basis, including **lentiginous AMN, AMN with architectural disorder and cytologic atypia, congenital pattern nevi at acral locations, pigmented spindle cell nevi**, and **Spitz nevi** or **Spitz tumors**. Suffice to say that AMN, as with all

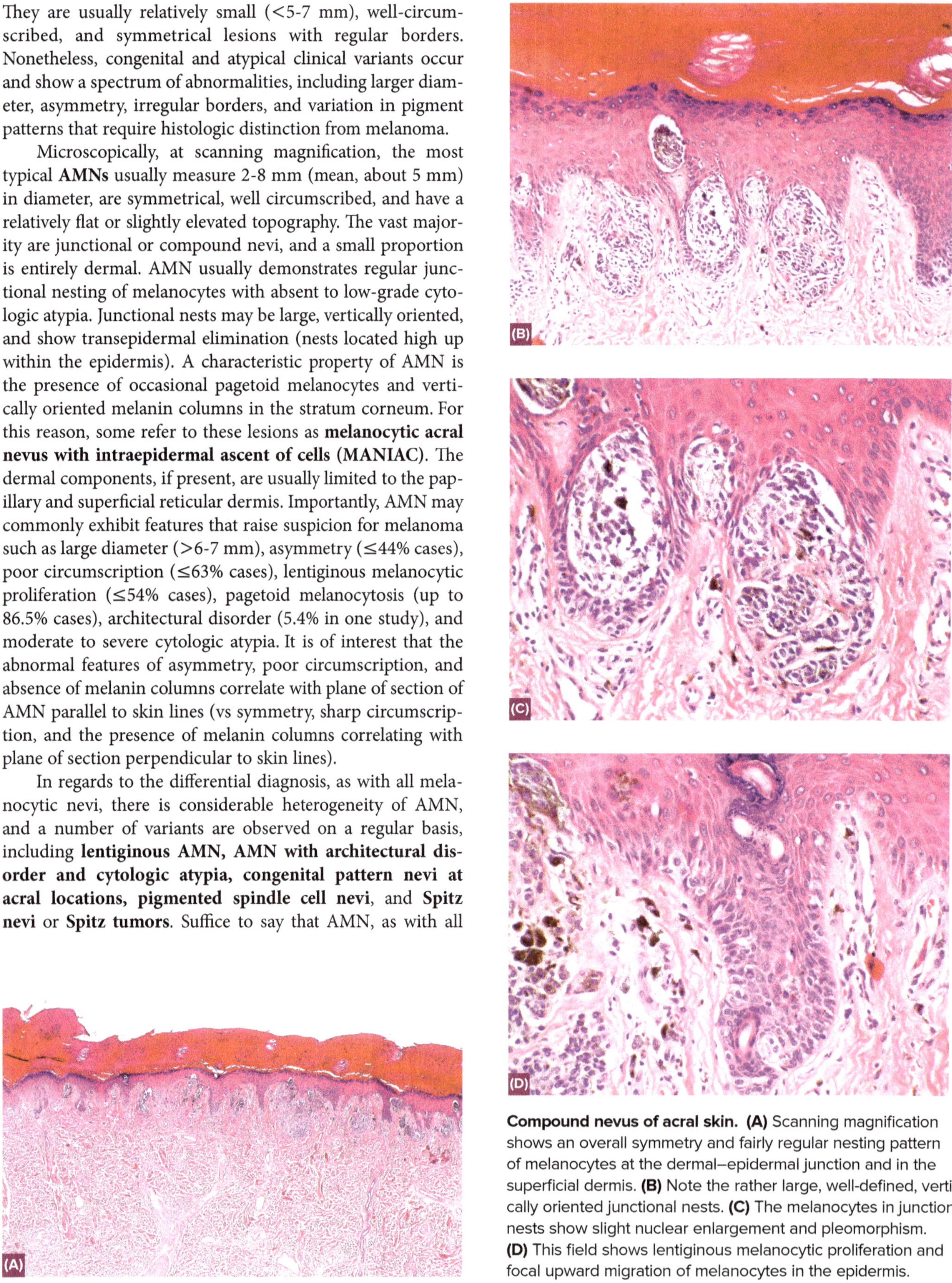

Compound nevus of acral skin. (A) Scanning magnification shows an overall symmetry and fairly regular nesting pattern of melanocytes at the dermal–epidermal junction and in the superficial dermis. **(B)** Note the rather large, well-defined, vertically oriented junctional nests. **(C)** The melanocytes in junctional nests show slight nuclear enlargement and pleomorphism. **(D)** This field shows lentiginous melanocytic proliferation and focal upward migration of melanocytes in the epidermis.

nevi, exhibit a broad spectrum of architectural and cytologic phenotypic variations that have not been sufficiently studied to establish their biologic significance. The fundamental problem is the distinction of AMN and their (many and atypical) variants from **acral melanoma**. Multiple standard criteria are needed because no single criterion is sufficient for this distinction, and there are exceptions to every criterion. Thus, the greatest diameter (eg, <5-6 mm vs >7 mm), symmetry versus asymmetry, sharp circumscription versus poor circumscription, degree of irregular and discohesive junctional nesting patterns, degree of lentiginous melanocytic proliferation, degree and proportion of lesion involved by pagetoid melanocytosis, nondisruption of epidermis versus effacement and obliteration of epidermis, degree of cytologic atypia of melanocytes, and degree of host response present are among the most important criteria. Particular features favoring an **acral melanocytic nevus** are small size (<5 mm), symmetry, sharp circumscription, large and vertically oriented junctional nests, transepidermal elimination of junctional nests, lentiginous melanocytic proliferation confined to (and not contiguous between) the epidermal retia, minimal pagetoid scatter, discrete organized melanin columns in the cornified layer, and absent or only slight to moderate cytologic atypia. On the other hand, **acral melanomas** usually exhibit size larger than 7 mm, asymmetry, poor circumscription, contiguous lentiginous melanocytic proliferation, more developed pagetoid spread, and high-grade cytologic atypia compared with acral nevi. Melanomas that arise within preexisting acral melanocytic nevi are most frequently of the superficial spreading type. **Acral lentiginous melanomas (ALM)** most frequently arise de novo and are characterized by a lentiginous (single file) proliferation of atypical melanocytes along the basal layer with occasional nesting and pagetoid ascent. In addition to epithelioid melanocytes, large numbers of atypical intraepidermal melanocytes have preserved dendritic processes that often extend throughout the epidermis and reach the granular layer. Melanin pigment is clumped and haphazardly arranged in the stratum corneum in acral lentiginous melanoma, in contrast to the organized columns in AMN. In invasive ALM, the dermal melanocytic component frequently exhibits a spindled cytomorphology. On occasion, **desmoplastic melanomas** may arise at these sites and may arise in association with acral lentiginous melanoma in situ. It is important to realize that a small proportion of acral melanocytic lesions prove to be so difficult that they cannot be confidently interpreted as benign or malignant (equivocal). Such lesions should be reported descriptively and excised with adequate margins, and the patients should be followed cautiously for lesional recurrence.

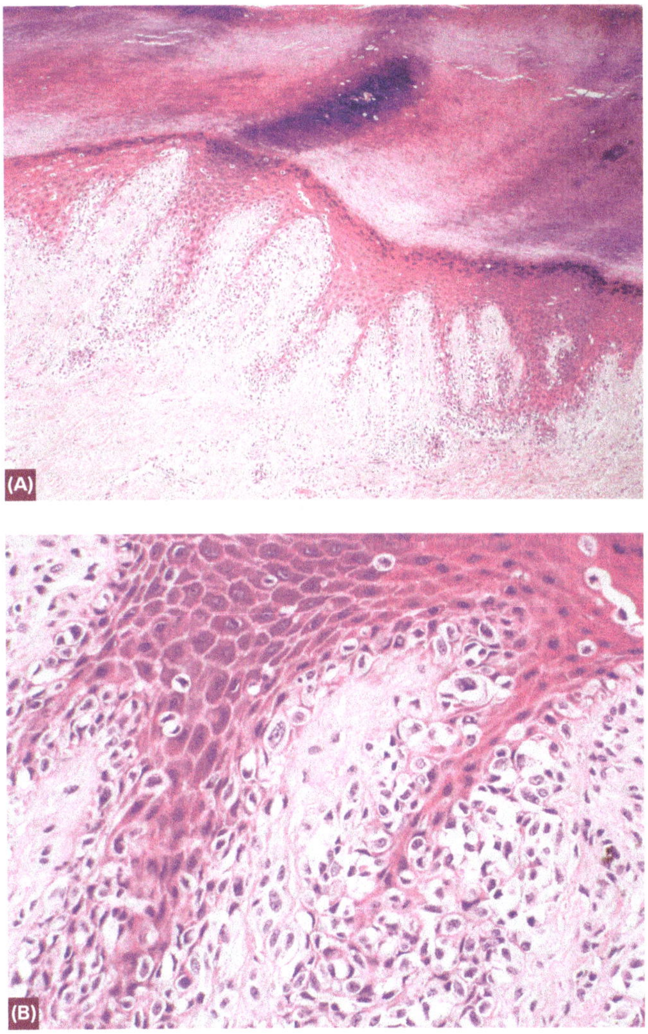

Acral lentiginous melanoma in situ. (A) The epidermal is hyperplastic and exhibits characteristic lentiginous proliferation of pleomorphic melanoma cells. **(B)** Note the confluence of severely atypical melanocytes along the dermal–epidermal junction.

ANSWER 10-12: A.

The biopsy reveals a lentiginous compound melanocytic proliferation with large junctional nests and focal areas of confluent growth. The dermal melanocytes exhibit maturation with descent into a markedly sclerotic dermis. The combined Melan-A/Ki67 stain reveals rare melanocytes above the basal layer; however, no dermal mitotic activity is present. The findings are consistent with a **compound genital melanocytic nevus**. The anatomic location of melanocytic nevi influences their histopathology and importantly may introduce particular histological properties that require distinction from melanoma. Over the past two decades, **acral nevi** and **vulvar nevi** have received the most detailed study in this regard. However, recent reports have suggested that melanocytic nevi from practically every anatomic region exhibit histologic properties that mark them as unique. Unfortunately, at present, there are no sufficiently large, comprehensive and rigorously controlled studies that provide any definitive conclusions about the differences in baseline histology among nevi from many different anatomic sites in relationship to age, gender, the considerable heterogeneity of nevi, and other factors. Because the latter data are lacking, one has the fundamental problem of defining how common acquired (or banal) nevi, clinically and histologically atypical nevi, and **"special sites" nevi** differ (Table 10-12A). Ultimately, the issue is clarifying and quantifying the biologic significance of the various phenotypic properties of melanocytic nevi. Locations most commonly associated with "special site" nevi include the acral surfaces, genital skin, flexural skin, breast, milkline, umbilicus, and scalp. Many of the studies reported thus far have not addressed inherent biases such as the origin of study subjects (ie, population-based vs various referral biases), how nevi have been selected for removal, and insufficient numbers of study subjects.

Melanocytic nevi, including common acquired, congenital, Spitz, blue nevi, and so on, involving the vulva have been detected in about 2.3% women undergoing routine examination. Particular melanocytic nevi occurring on the vulva estimated to comprise about 5.1% of vulvar nevi in one study, the

Table 10-12A. Unusual Genital or Flexural Melanocytic Nevus ("Special Sites Nevus")

Clinical Features
Occurrence in premenopausal women (range: 14-40 years of age)
Often enlarged, ≤10 mm in diameter
Other features not well studied
Histopathologic Features
Symmetry
Usually well circumscribed
Enlarged junctional nests with diminished cohesion
Lentiginous melanocytic proliferation
Confluence of cells, nests along dermal–epidermal junction
Variation in size, shape, position of junctional nests
Extension of intraepidermal component along adnexal epithelium
Generally no pagetoid spread
Generally no lateral extension
Fibroplasia common, often lamellar
Lymphocytic infiltrates
Cytologic atypia, often slight to moderate
Somewhat enlarged intraepidermal melanocytes, often abundant cytoplasm
Multinucleate nevus giant cells
Maturation of nevus cells common
Differential Diagnosis
Vulvar melanoma
Spitz nevus
Atypical nevus

male genitalia such as the scrotum (and in other flexural locations such as the umbilicus and axillae) are thought to have distinctive histopathologic features compared with most nevi from other sites. As with all melanocytic lesions, how such nevi are selected for removal may influence these observations. In fact, one may observe these features in nevi from any site, although probably much less commonly. The significance of the clinical and histologic features of such **genital nevi** in terms of melanoma risk and association with an atypical nevus phenotype has not been completely elucidated and requires further study. Some of the unusual genital nevi previously reported exhibit features intermediate between ordinary nevi and melanoma, and thus, share features with so-called **"dysplastic" nevi**. Irrespective of site or nomenclature, particular nevus phenotypic characteristics such as diameter larger than 8 mm, irregular borders, irregular coloration, and moderate to severe cytologic atypia of melanocytes are established risk factors for **genital melanoma**. However, of critical importance is the knowledge that such peculiar genital nevi may exhibit features that may result in misinterpretation as melanoma with potential catastrophic consequences (wide excision) for children, adolescents, and women of any age (ie, nevus located near clitoris or urethra). Although there are insufficient data at present to be certain as to the biologic potential of such nevi, there is no evidence of either documented progression to melanoma or metastases from such lesions. In only one instance has local recurrence occurred after removal of a vulvar nevus with positive surgical margins.

Clinically, such nevi are observed in women age 6-54 years (median, 26 years) in one study. Vulvar nevi range in size from 2 to 20 mm (mean, 6 mm; median, 5 mm) and commonly involve the labium majus, mons pubis, labium minus, clitoris, and perineum. They are often relatively flat, but not necessarily so; they generally have fairly regular borders; and often have a complex mahogany color, that is, an admixture of tan, brown, and red. Among 56 recently reported genital nevi, 45% were judged to be clinically atypical.

Microscopically, at scanning magnification, these **genital nevi** (also referred to as **"atypical" genital nevi** [AGN]) possess an overall symmetry and are well circumscribed. The most notable features include enlarged junctional nests; variation in the size, shape, position, and reduced cohesion of junctional nests; often-horizontal confluence and bridging of nests; and intraepidermal melanocytes that are slightly enlarged with abundant eosinophilic cytoplasms resembling the epithelioid cells in **Spitz nevus**. Cytologic atypia of melanocytes is usually present and generally of slight to moderate degree in about 80% of cases but may be severe on occasion. Focal pagetoid melanocytosis and lentiginous melanocytic proliferation are rare or absent. Scalp, breast, and milkline nevi are rather similar to genital nevi. **Umbilical nevi** are often distinctive because of dermal scarring. Because of their localization to skin folds (**flexural site nevi**), **axillary nevi** commonly have polypoid or papillomatous surface topographies.

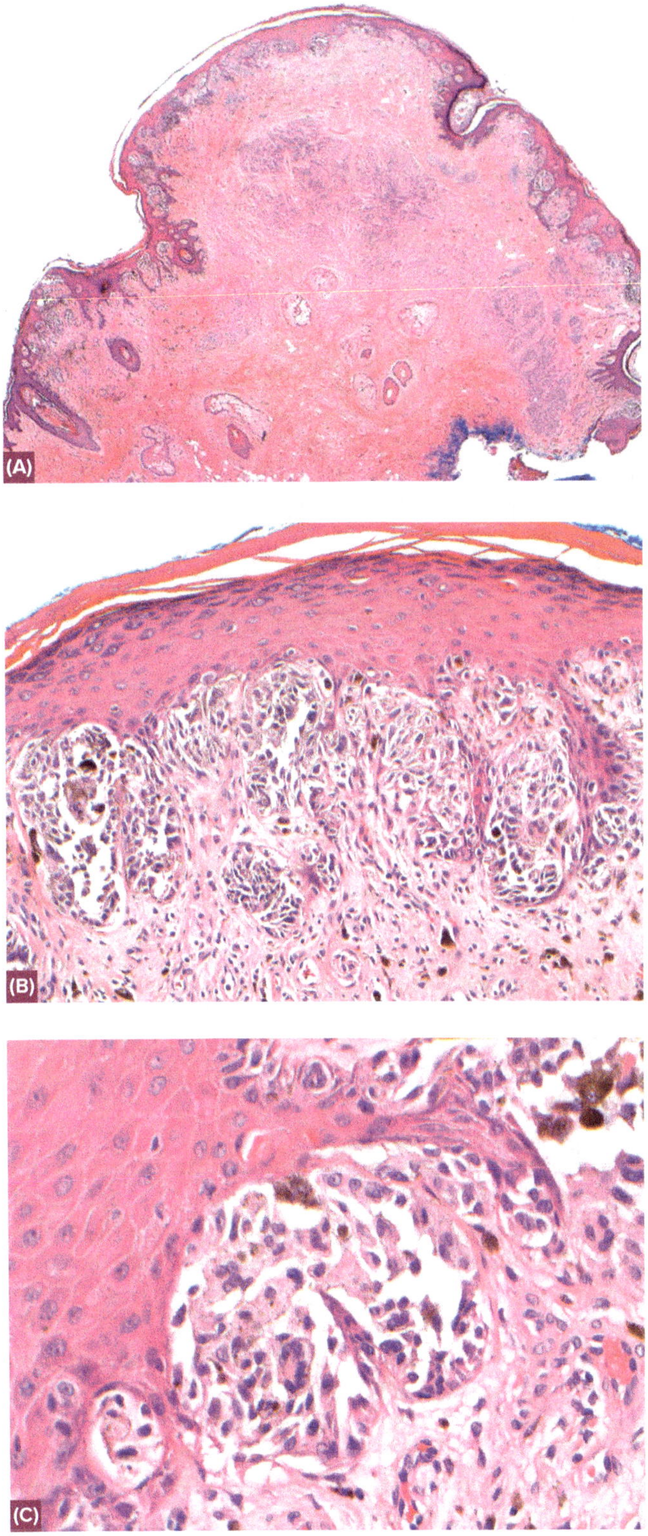

Compound nevus of the vulva (genital nevus). (A) The nevus is large and shows a protuberant ("mushroom-like") topography with bulky dermal component. **(B)** Note the large confluent nests of nevus cells along dermal–epidermal junction. **(C)** The melanocytes are enlarged epithelioid cells with abundant cytoplasms and display some nuclear enlargement and variation in nuclear contours. Multinucleate forms are present.

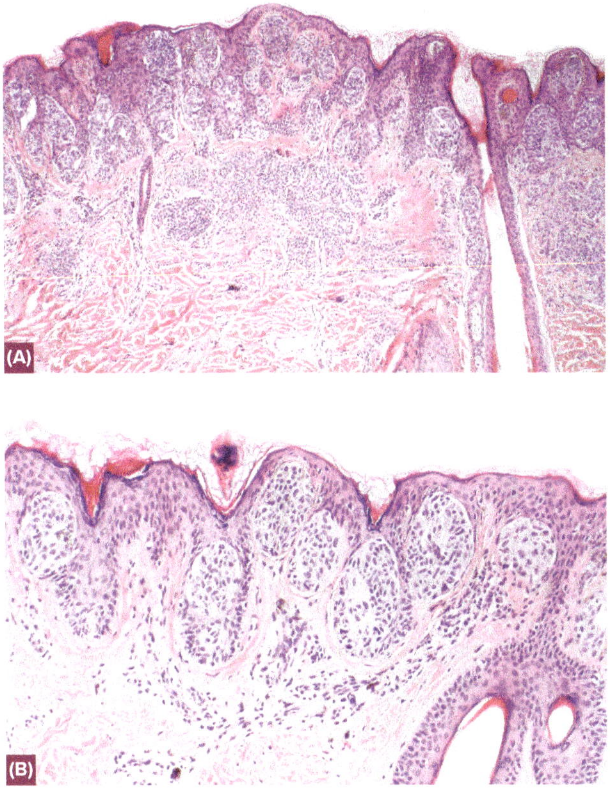

Compound nevus from the scalp. (A) The nevus demonstrates large confluent nests of nevus cells along dermal–epidermal junction with bridging and prominent cellularity. The lesion also characteristically shows involvement of the reticular dermis and follicular epithelium by nests of melanocytes suggesting a "congenital pattern." However, the nevus fails to show pagetoid melanocytosis, effacement of the epidermis, or dermal mitoses. **(B)** The melanocytes are enlarged, round to ovoid cells with some nuclear enlargement and pleomorphism.

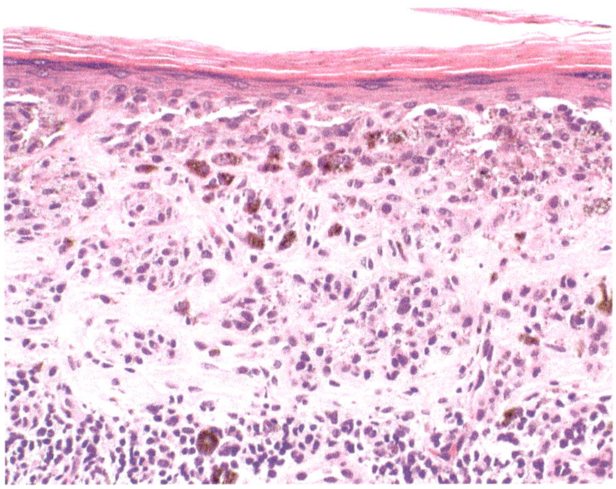

Compound nevus from the umbilicus. The lesion shows some effacement of the epidermis and strikingly confluent and hypercellular junctional nesting of melanocytes. The melanocytes exhibit nuclear enlargement and pleomorphism. The nevus otherwise shows maturation and no other characteristics suggesting melanoma.

The differential diagnosis for **genital nevus** includes **genital melanoma, common acquired nevus**, and **Spitz nevus/Spitz tumor**. Although abnormal architecture and cytologic atypia may be present in AGN, these features are not as developed as in melanoma. **Genital melanoma** usually demonstrates larger diameter, asymmetry, poor circumscription, confluent proliferation of basilar intraepidermal melanocytes, prominent pagetoid spread, greater cytologic atypia, and more developed host response. Moreover, vulvar melanoma is rare and occurs in older women (average age, about 65 years) compared with these AGN. Although AGN are not considered "dysplastic" by many, such a distinction may lack credibility for many lesions because of commonly shared features. Thus, in a general sense, both AGN and **"dysplastic" nevi** qualify as nevi exhibiting architectural disorder and cytologic atypia. **Spitz nevi** and tumors are recognized by typical architecture and enlarged monomorphous epithelioid or fusiform cells. **Benign vulvar melanosis** is a pigmented macule involving the vulvar skin with melanin pigment present in keratinocytes. When a slight increase in basilar melanocytes is present, the lesions are referred to as **mucosal lentigo**. Both **vulvar melanosis** and **mucosal lentigo** lack nests of melanocytes.

ANSWER 10-13: C.

The biopsy reveals a broad, yet symmetric, compound melanocytic proliferation without a peripheral junctional "shoulder" of melanocytic nests. The dermal melanocytes are arranged in sheets and small nests with preserved maturation with descent. These dermal melanocytes track along hair follicles and eccrine ducts into the deep dermis. The findings are consistent with a **compound congenital melanocytic nevus**. The term **congenital nevus** denotes presence at birth. However, **congenital melanocytic nevi (CMN)** also frequently differ from common acquired nevi because of overall size, depth of involvement by nevus cells, adnexal or vascular involvement, and diversity of neurocristic differentiation. Most melanocytic nevi greater than 1.5 cm in diameter are probably congenital. However, smaller CMN may be indistinguishable from acquired nevi. The significance of CMN, particularly the larger varieties, relates to their risk for progression to melanoma and cosmetic disfigurement. There is considerable controversy surrounding the melanoma risk and management of CMN. Accurate estimates of melanoma risk associated with CMN are difficult to obtain. The potential risk is probably related to the size of the CMN; that is, the larger the nevus, the greater the risk. The prevalence of relatively **small congenital melanocytic nevi** is approximately 1%; consequently, these nevi are fairly common. However, one particular problem associated with estimating melanoma risk in these nevi is the lack of specificity of histologic features for CMN of this size. At present, melanoma risk associated with small- and medium-sized CMN is thought to be low. The clinical characteristics of CMN are related to size and age. **Small congenital nevi** smaller than 1.5 cm in greatest diameter may be indistinguishable from **common acquired nevi**, and documentation at birth may be the only means of confirming a congenital origin (Table 10-13A). In general, CMN in the range of 1.5-10 or 20 cm in diameter have a well-circumscribed, elongated or oval clinical morphology, and an orderly distribution of pigment. Most of these nevi are brown but range in color from tan to dark brown or black. A speckled or mottled appearance is also common, and many have coarse, terminal hair follicles.

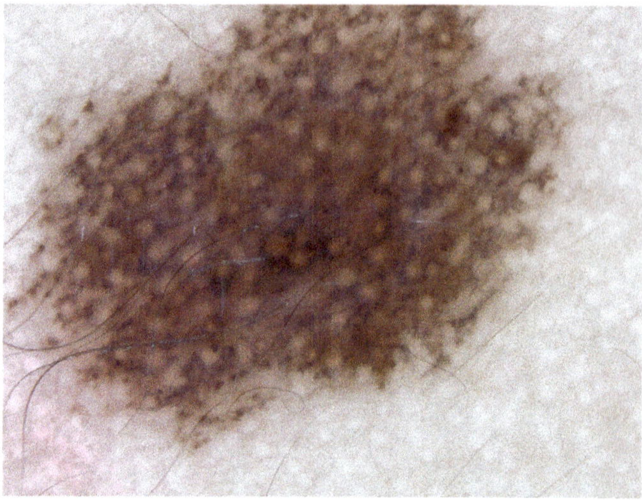

Dermoscopy of congenital melanocytic nevus. Note the pseudonetwork (netlike pattern) made by white adnexal openings within this congenital nevus. The central globules of pigment correspond to junctional melanocytic nests. (Reproduced, with permission, from Usatine RP, Smith MA, Mayeaux EJ Jr, Chumley HS, eds. *Color Atlas of Family Medicine*. 2nd ed. New York, NY: McGraw-Hill Education; 2012.)

The microscopic characteristics observed in **congenital melanocytic nevus** are related primarily to the size of the nevus and to a lesser degree to the age of the individual. Evidence now suggests that the depth of nevus cell involvement throughout the dermis and subcutis is established early and remains for the most part unchanged. However, the superficial (intraepidermal and superficial dermal) components of a CMN may mature in some instances. It is believed that immature, disordered patterns such as pagetoid spread, large irregular nests, and cytologic atypia do diminish (or mature) with time. However, the latter conclusion must be made with some circumspection because of the rather prominent morphologic heterogeneity throughout many CMN. Some **small CMN** may be entirely junctional and indistinguishable from **common acquired nevi**. Many small nevi, particularly those measuring less than 1.5 cm in diameter, also demonstrate what has been termed a superficial pattern (ie, junctional nests alone or a compound or entirely dermal pattern with aggregates of nevus cells extending to no greater depth than the upper half of the reticular dermis). Such a

Table 10-13A. Small- and Medium-Sized Congenital Nevi

Clinical Features
May occur anywhere, but head and neck common
Symmetry
<1.5-20 cm
Round, oval, elongated
Tan, brown, dark brown, often mahogany, or black
Slightly raised plaque
Pebbled or rugose surface
Often coarse hairs
Histopathologic Features
Often lentiginous melanocytic hyperplasia
Junctional, compound, or dermal
Small congenital nevi (<1.5 cm)
Involvement of upper half of reticular dermis common
- Interstitial pattern
- Perivascular, periadnexal pattern
Medium-sized congenital nevi (1.5-20 cm)
Involvement of reticular dermis, particularly lower half
- Diffuse dermal involvement by nevus cells
- Interstitial pattern
- "Inflammatory" pattern
Nevus cells within appendages, blood vessels, nerves
Differential Diagnosis
Becker nevus
Atypical (dysplastic) nevus
Epidermal nevus
Congenital lentigo
Melanoma

pattern may be seen in a significant percentage of common acquired nevi. Up to 28% of acquired nevi may also exhibit nevus cells extending into the lower two-thirds of the reticular dermis. Histopathologic features considered characteristic of CMN include involvement of the lower third of the reticular dermis by nevus cells, close association of nevus cells with or within appendageal structures, and neurovascular structures at the mid-reticular dermal level or deeper. In contradistinction to acquired nevi, CMN are notable for nevus cells being disposed, "fanning out," or splaying collagen bundles of the reticular dermis as single cells, files, sheets, and cords of cells (two cells in tandem). CMN also show a typical pattern of maturation of nevus cells from superficial to deep dermis. Near the epidermal surface, nevus cells tend to be aggregated in nests and may exhibit epithelioid cell features. With increasing depth, the nevus cells often demonstrate greater separation (ie, splaying) and slightly diminished cellular and nuclear sizes. Extension of nevus cells into the subcutaneous fat is also a common feature, particularly in larger varieties of congenital nevi. With increasing sizes of CMN, there is greater tendency for deep dermal, appendageal structures, and neurovascular involvement. However, even some congenital nevi less than 1.5 cm in diameter tend to involve eccrine and follicular units at the mid-reticular dermal level or deeper, much more commonly than acquired nevi. Because of histologic overlap between small CMN and acquired nevi, there are no features with 100% specificity and 100% sensitivity for recognition of small CMN. Nonetheless, the presence of nevus cells in the lower half of the reticular dermis, in an appendageal or neurovascular pattern, or both will enable one to detect a majority of small CMN. Absence of the latter features does not preclude a congenital origin. It is important to mention that **acquired melanocytic nevi of the face** also frequently exhibit tracking of melanocytic nests along adnexal structures, therefore, a diagnosis of congenital nevus should not be made in this location without clinical correlation. In general, it is recommended for the pathologist to report melanocytic lesions with these features as junctional/compound/intradermal melanocytic nevus with congenital features, defaulting to clinical correlation for definitive classification.

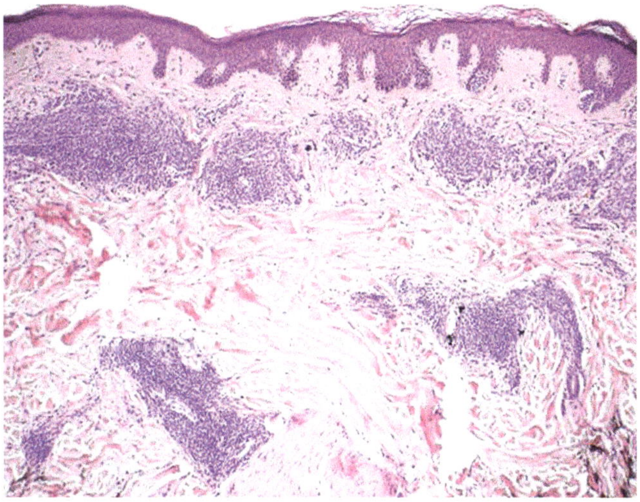

Small congenital nevus. Discrete nests of nevus cells are present in the dermis and track along adnexal structures.

ANSWER 10-14: A.

The pTNM Staging System of the American Joint Committee on Cancer (AJCC) and the International Union Against Cancer (UICC) for malignant melanoma was recently updated in 2009. The "p" stands for the pathological staging (vs clinical) and includes microstaging of the primary tumor (pT), regional lymph nodes (pN), and distant metastases (pM). In general, **malignant melanoma staging** is typically reported using a synoptic format (Table 10-14A). The criteria with (*) are essential and directly influence the pT stage of melanoma.

Table 10-14A. Malignant Melanoma; Sample Synoptic Report

SUBTYPE: (ie, Superficial spreading, lentigo maligna, acral-lentiginous, mucosal-lentiginous, nodular, desmoplastic, unclassified, other)
ANATOMIC LEVEL (CLARK LEVEL):
____ I (Melanoma in situ)
____ II (Melanoma present in but does not fill papillary dermis)
____ III (Melanoma fills and expands papillary dermis)
____ IV (Melanoma invades reticular dermis)
____ V (Melanoma invades subcutis)
*BRESLOW THICKNESS: ___mm
*ULCERATION: (Not identified, present)
*MITOTIC INDEX: (None identified, 1 per mm^2, >1 per mm^2)
*MICROSATELLITOSIS: (Not identified, present)
*LYMPHOVASCULAR INVASION: (Not identified, present)
ANGIOTROPISM: (Not identified, present)
TUMOR INFILTRATING LYMPHOCYTES: (Not identified, present-nonbrisk, present-brisk)
TUMOR REGRESSION: (Not identified, present-minor <75% of tumor, present-major >75% of tumor)
GROWTH PHASE: (Radial, vertical)
*MARGINS: (Completely excised, melanoma extends to the peripheral/deep margins)

Parameters without asterisks (*) are not required. Although these nonessential parameters may be clinically important, they have yet to be validated or are not regularly used in patient management.

The proper assessment of **malignant melanoma** requires a complete excision specimen since shave biopsies and punch biopsies may not sample the deep and peripheral aspects of the tumor, respectively. The World Health Organization (WHO) classification of variants of malignant melanoma include: **superficial spreading melanoma, nodular melanoma, lentigo maligna melanoma, acral-lentiginous melanoma, mucosal-lentiginous melanoma, desmoplastic/neurotropic melanoma, melanoma arising from blue nevus (malignant blue nevus), melanoma arising from a giant congenital nevus, melanoma in childhood, nevoid melanoma**, and **melanoma unclassified**. Despite ongoing research

Table 10-14B. Anatomic (Clark) Levels

Level I: Intraepidermal tumor only (in situ)
Level II: Tumor presents in but does not fill and expand papillary dermis
Level III: Tumor fills and expands papillary dermis
Level IV: Tumor invades into reticular dermis
Level V: Tumor invades subcutis

to correlate molecular abnormalities (ie, *BRAF* mutations) with histopathologic features, the melanoma subtype currently has no bearing on tumor stage.

Tumor thickness **(Breslow thickness)** has been consistently shown to be the most important prognostic factor, and therefore forms the basis for pT stratification. Although assessment of anatomic compartment involved by tumor **(Clark level)** has also been commonly used to indicate depth of invasion of the primary tumor, it has been found to be less predictive of clinical outcome than mitotic activity (Table 10-14B). Accordingly, Clark levels have been replaced in the new 7th edition TNM classification system by tumor mitotic rate for subclassifying pT1 lesions (pT1a or pT1b). In cases of pT1 melanoma (Breslow thickness 1 mm or less) without ulceration and where mitotic activity cannot be determined, Clark level IV or V may serve as tertiary criteria for upstaging lesions to pT1b, and therefore their inclusion into the pathology report is still recommended. The distinction of T1a versus T1b is clinically significant, since the AJCC recommends consideration of sentinel node examination for melanomas staged T1b and above.

Primary tumor thickness (Breslow thickness), ulceration, and dermal mitotic activity are the three criteria most directly affecting the pathological tumor stage. Maximum tumor thickness is measured by using an ocular micrometer positioned perpendicular to the overlying epidermis. The thickness should be measured from the granular layer of the epidermis to the deepest focus of malignant tumor cells. If the tumor is ulcerated, the tumor should be measured from the ulcer base to the deepest focus. If the tumor is transected at the base, the measured depth should be indicated as "__ mm, at least" with a comment explaining the limitation of thickness assessment due to partial sampling. Rarely, cases of melanoma tracking down adnexal structures may invade radially into the adventitial dermis (dermis surrounding adnexae). The most common subtypes to exhibit this phenomenon are **lentigo maligna** and **acral lentiginous melanomas**. In this situation, the ocular micrometer should be oriented parallel to the epidermal surface and the initial measurement should be made from the inner root/outer root sheath interface to the most radial distance of tumor. If the tumor extends beyond the adventitial dermis and into the reticular dermis, the conventional perpendicular measurement should be performed and both radial and vertical measurements reported.

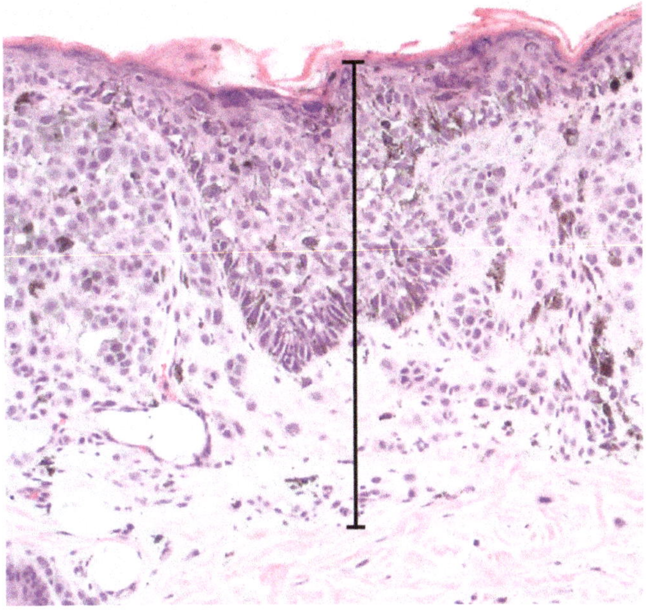

Breslow thickness of invasive melanoma. The measurement is taken in millimeters from the granular layer of the epidermis to the deepest invasive aspect.

Ulceration is an important prognostic factor in cutaneous melanoma without metastasis (changes pT stage from T1a to T1b if present). Tumor ulceration is defined as a full-thickness epidermal defect with fibrinous exudate and neutrophils, not attributed to trauma or prior procedure to the area. Overall, for patients without metastatic disease, the 10-year survival rate is 50% for ulcerated tumors and 78% for non-ulcerated tumors. A significantly worse prognosis and a higher risk of metastatic disease have been demonstrated for ulcerated versus non-ulcerated tumors of equivalent thickness via Cox regression analyses of prognostic factors in cutaneous melanoma. Additionally, there is a positive correlation between ulceration and thickness (median 3-mm thickness for ulcerated tumors vs median 1.3-mm thickness for non-ulcerated tumors). Nevertheless, the adverse prognostic significance of ulceration has been shown to be independent of tumor thickness. For melanomas measuring 1.0 mm or less in thickness (**thin melanomas**), the depth of invasion is more predictive of survival outcome than ulceration. In contrast, for melanomas measuring greater than 1.0 mm (**thick melanomas**), ulceration is more predictive for survival than thickness. Recent studies suggest that ulceration may lose its independent prognostic significance when dermal mitotic activity is present.

The identification of one or more dividing dermal melanocytes per square millimeter (mm^2) is an important adverse prognostic factor for cutaneous melanoma (changes pT1 lesions from pT1a to pT1b). The recommended approach for assessing dermal tumor mitotic activity is to search diligently throughout the dermis at 40× magnification for the focus of highest mitotic activity (so-called "hot-spot"), then measure four additional separate fields (five fields in total for an evaluation of 1 mm^2). The field diameter of the microscope objective should be formally calibrated using a stage micrometer in order to determine the number of high-power fields that equates to a square millimetre. If no mitotic activity can be identified, then five random 40× fields should be examined.

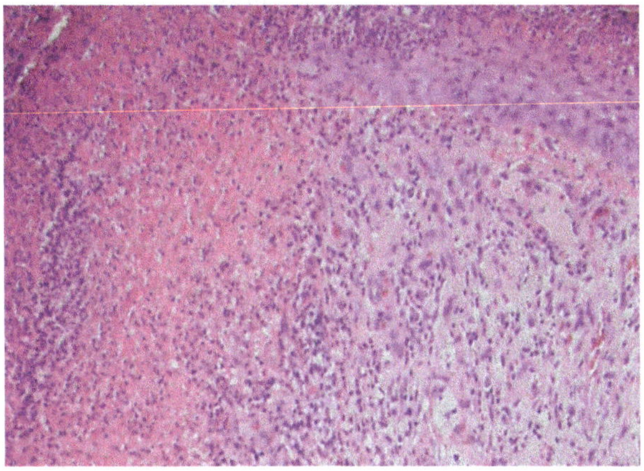

Ulcerated melanoma. Note the complete replacement of the epidermis by fibrinopurulent exudate with neutrophils.

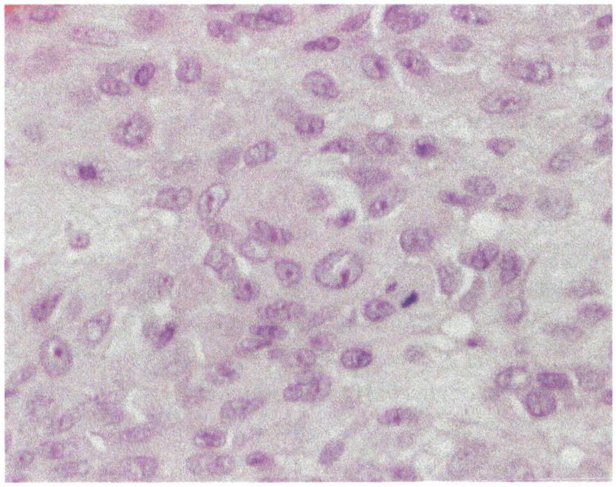

Mitotic activity. This melanoma contains at least one mitotic figure within one high-power field (40×). A total of about five high-power fields should be examined for an assessment of mitoses per mm^2, depending upon the calibration of the microscopic field.

Additional parameters found to negatively impact prognosis include **in-transit metastasis, satellitosis**, and **microsatellitosis**. The two former parameters are clinically evaluated, while microsatellitosis is histopathologically evaluated. All three parameters directly impact pN staging (pN2c). **Microsatellitosis** is defined as the presence of tumor nests in the dermis or subcutis measuring greater than 0.05 mm in diameter, but separated from the main tumor by at least 0.3 mm of normal tissue. **Satellitosis** is clinically defined as a separate tumor focus located within 2 cm of the primary tumor. **In-transit metastasis** is clinically defined as intralymphatic tumor spread 2 cm beyond the primary tumor site, but not beyond the nearest regional lymph node basin. The presence of any of these three parameters is associated with a poor prognosis and an analysis of the available data by the AJCC Melanoma Staging Committee revealed no significant difference in survival between these parameters. The presence of any of these features is associated with a prognosis equivalent to multiple lymph node metastases.

In regards to **lymphovascular invasion, perineural invasion,** and **angiotropism**, lymphovascular invasion has been found to correlate independently with worse overall survival, while **perineural invasion** is associated with an increased risk for local recurrence (especially **desmoplastic-neuroid melanomas**). Angiotropism is defined microscopically as the presence of melanoma cells disposed along the abluminal surfaces of vascular channels in a pericytic location in invasive melanomas. Angiotropism is the microscopic marker of extravascular migratory tumor spread. This type of tumor spread is predictive for the development of microscopic satellites, satellite metastases, in transit metastases, and both regional lymph node and distant metastases. Angiotropism is also predictive of diminished disease-free survival. **Tumor-infiltrating lymphocytes** and **regression** are separate histopathologic parameters. While regression of >75% of the total tumor mass is associated with a worse prognosis, it is the paucity of tumor infiltrating lymphocytes that has adverse prognostic significance. **Regression** is histopathologically characterized by the replacement of tumor cells by lymphocytic inflammation. The epidermis is typically attenuated and the dermis contains non-laminated fibrosis with lymphohistiocytic inflammatory infiltrates, melanophages, and telangiectasia. When total regression occurs and only clusters of melanophages are present, the condition is referred to as **tumoral melanosis**. In this situation, a measurement of thickness of melanophages should be taken in an attempt to assess the potential thickness of the melanocytic proliferation. **Tumor-infiltrating lymphocytes (TIL)** are semiquantitatively assessed as either not identified, present-nonbrisk, or present-brisk. Although the dermis may contain lymphocytes, the inflammatory cells must infiltrate the tumor to qualify as TIL. Nonbrisk TIL is defined as focal lymphocyte infiltration or lymphocytes incompletely surrounding the tumor mass. Brisk TIL is defined as either diffuse infiltration of the entire base of the vertical growth phase melanoma or throughout the entire tumor mass.

Again, the prognostic significance of melanoma subtype is less than the growth patterns (radial vs vertical) and depth of infiltration (Breslow thickness). **Radial growth phase** is defined as melanoma that is generally wider than it is deep. One commonly applied criterion for radial growth phase is the presence of melanoma in situ that extends three or more rete ridges beyond the invasive component. This phase is typically seen in thin melanomas (<1 mm) and therefore is associated with a better outcome. **Vertical growth phase** is considered an adverse prognostic factor and is defined as the presence of one or more dermal clusters larger than the largest intraepidermal cluster and/or the presence of any mitotic activity in the dermis.

A summary of the (pT) AJCC staging for primary malignant melanoma is provided in Table 10-14C.

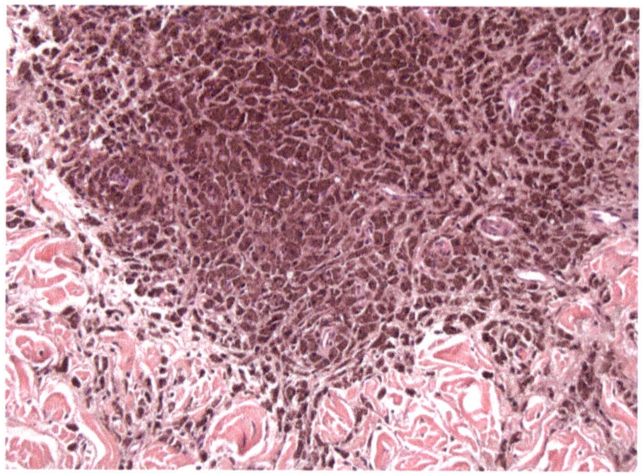

Total regression of melanoma (tumoral melanosis). The pigmented cells are actually melanin-containing macrophages. A Melan-A immunostain was performed using red chromogen and revealed the absence of dermal melanocytes.

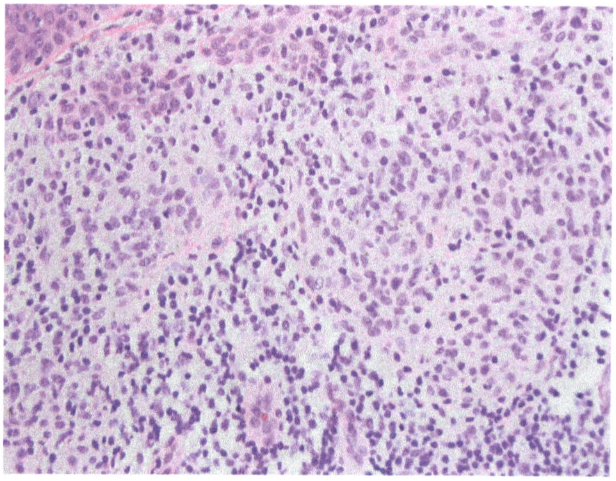

Tumor-infiltrating lymphocytes, brisk. Note the diffuse infiltration of the tumor by small lymphocytes.

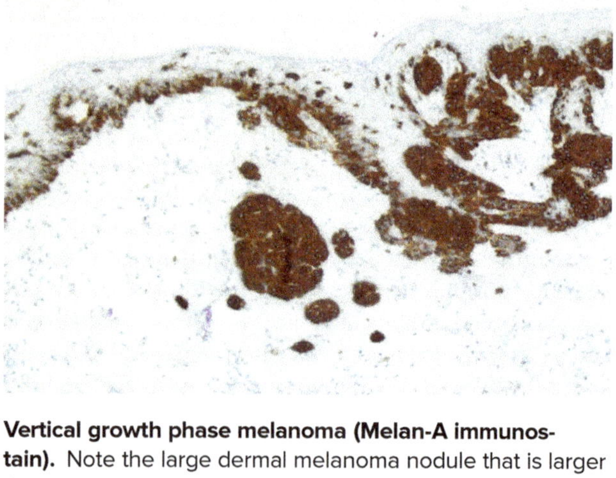

Vertical growth phase melanoma (Melan-A immunostain). Note the large dermal melanoma nodule that is larger than any of the overlying intraepidermal clusters. The epidermis contains numerous pagetoid melanocytes.

Table 10-14C. Primary Tumor (pT) Staging Criteria for Malignant Melanoma

pTX: Primary tumor cannot be assessed (eg, shave biopsy or regressed melanoma)
pT0: No evidence of primary tumor
pTis: Melanoma in situ (ie, not an invasive tumor: anatomic level I)
pT1: Melanoma 1.0 mm or less in thickness, with or without ulceration
- pT1a: Melanoma 1.0 mm or less in thickness, no ulceration, <1 mitoses/mm^2
- pT1b: Melanoma 1.0 mm or less in thickness with ulceration and/or 1 or more mitoses/mm^2

pT2: Melanoma 1.01-2 mm in thickness, with or without ulceration
- pT2a: Melanoma 1.01-2.0 mm in thickness, no ulceration
- pT2b: Melanoma 1.01-2.0 mm in thickness, with ulceration

pT3: Melanoma 2.01-4.0 mm in thickness, with or without ulceration
- pT3a: Melanoma 2.01-4.0 mm in thickness, no ulceration
- pT3b: Melanoma 2.01-4.0 mm in thickness, with ulceration

pT4: Melanoma greater than 4.0 mm in thickness, with or without ulceration
- pT4a: Melanoma greater than 4.0 mm in thickness, no ulceration
- pT4b: Melanoma greater than 4.0 mm in thickness, with ulceration

ANSWER 10-15: B.

The biopsy reveals a confluent melanocytic proliferation with lentiginous and focally nested architecture. The basal layer keratinocyte to melanocyte ratio is approximately 1:1. The epidermis is attenuated and there is marked solar elastosis. The nest of melanocytes is present along an attenuated epidermis and not at the tip of a rete ridge. A few scattered melanophages are present in the dermis. The findings are consistent with **melanoma in situ, lentigo maligna type. Lentigo maligna (LM)** is a subtype of melanoma with a prolonged radial growth phase (melanoma in situ) that may progress to **invasive lentigo maligna melanoma (LMM)** with time (Table 10-15A). Invasive lentigo maligna melanoma constitutes 10-15% of cutaneous melanomas. Both in situ (LM) and invasive lentigo maligna melanoma (LMM) are diagnosed most commonly in the seventh to eighth decades in an older population than other types of melanoma. It is uncommon before the age 40. The most common location is on the chronically sun-exposed skin of the face, such as the cheeks, nose, neck, scalp, and ears. Its pathogenesis

Table 10-15A. Lentigo Maligna Melanoma

Clinical Features
- Age 60-70 years
- Men = women
- Sun-exposed surfaces: cheek (most common), nose, forehead, ears, neck, dorsal surfaces of hands
- 0.2-20 cm
- Initial tan macule suggesting a varnish-like stain
- Tan, brown, black macule or patch (black flecks characteristic) (early lesions)
- Pink, gray, white with progression and areas of regression
- Papule or nodule, pigmented or amelanotic (advanced)
- Ulceration, bleeding
- Asymmetry
- Irregular, notched borders

Histopathologic Features
- Effacement and thinning of epidermis common
- Prominent solar elastosis
- Solar intraepidermal melanocytic neoplasia (lentigo maligna):
  - (1) Solar intraepidermal melanocytic proliferation (insufficient for melanoma in situ)
    - Lentiginous melanocytic proliferation
    - Pleomorphic melanocytes (variable cytological atypia)
    - Extension of melanocytic proliferation downward along appendages
    - Usual absence of nesting and pagetoid spread
  - (2) Melanoma in situ
    - Contiguous or near contiguous lentiginous melanocytic proliferation
    - Intraepidermal nesting of melanocytes
    - Pagetoid spread
    - Prominent extension of melanocytic proliferation downward along appendages, often with nesting
    - Significant cytologic atypia
    - Melanocytes somewhat spindled to increasingly epithelioid

Pigmented spindle cell variant (often on ears)
- Prominent intraepidermal discohesive nesting of atypical spindle cells
- Spindle cells often comprise invasive component but polygonal, small cells common
- Appendage-associated nesting of atypical melanocytes suggests invasion and may be florid (not true invasion)
- Partial regression relatively common
- Precursor nevus present about 3% of cases
- Desmoplasia, neurotropism, angiotropism common

Table 10-15A. Lentigo Maligna Melanoma *(continued)*

Differential Diagnosis
- Solar lentigo
- Solar melanocytic hyperplasia (photoactivation)
  - De novo
  - Occurrence with nevi, fibrous papule, basal cell carcinoma, actinic keratosis, etc
- Atypical intraepidermal melanocytic proliferation, not otherwise specified
- Solar lentiginous junctional or compound melanocytic nevi with or without atypia (may overlap atypical [dysplastic] nevi)
- Pigmented spindle cell nevus
- Pigmented actinic keratosis
- Squamous cell carcinoma, spindle cell type
- Atypical fibroxanthoma
- Cellular neurothekeoma
- Malignant peripheral nerve sheath tumor
- Angiosarcoma
- Kaposi sarcoma
- Leiomyosarcoma

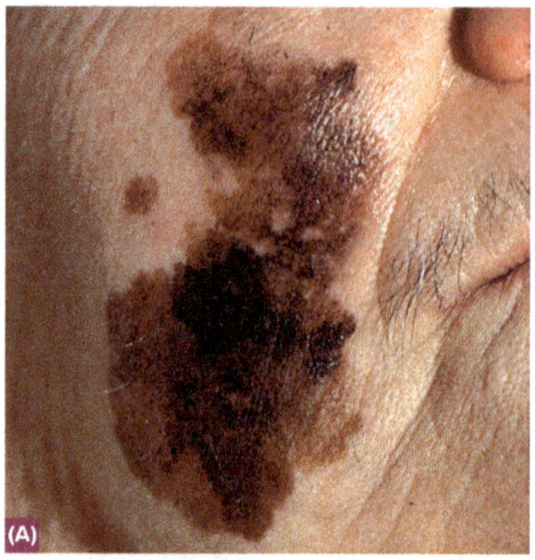

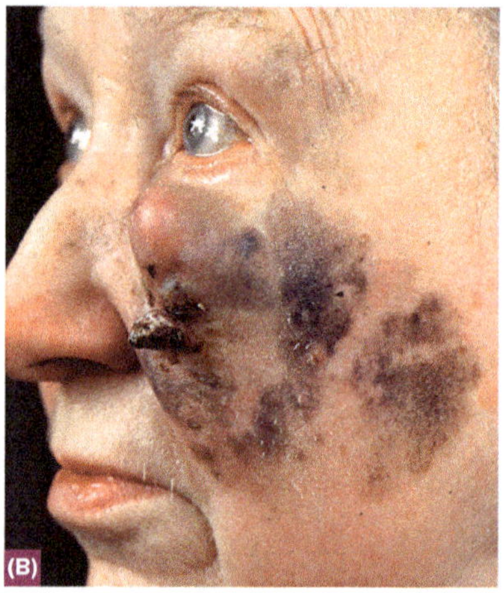

Lentigo maligna melanoma. (A) A very large lentigo maligna on the right cheek with the typical variegation in color (tan, brown, black) and highly irregular shape. The lesion is flat, macular, and thus represents an in situ melanoma. **(B)** The classically macular lentigo maligna is highly irregular in shape and variegated in color. However, there is a bluish component and a large pink nodule in the infraorbital region, indicating a switch from the radial to the vertical growth phase and thus invasiveness: the lesion is now called lentigo maligna melanoma. (Reproduced, with permission, from Wolff K, Johnson RA, Saavedra AP. *Fitzpatrick's Color Atlas and Synopsis of Clinical Dermatology*. 7th ed. New York, NY: McGraw-Hill Education; 2013.)

is thought to be related to cumulative sun exposure rather than intermittent exposure. LM is a flat, slowly enlarging, brown, freckle-like macule with irregular shape and differing shades of brown and tan, usually arising in a background of photodamage. In the past it was also referred to in the medical literature as **Hutchinson freckle**. The lifetime risk of invasive melanoma developing from LM is estimated to be low but the invasive component is potentially lethal. LMM is frequently larger than LM and may continue to be macular in early lesions, although a nodular portion is often seen within the macule later. Both LM and LMM often have clinically ill-defined borders, which may be obscured by background actinic damage consisting of lentigines, pigmented actinic keratoses, or ephelides. LM and LMM are associated with significantly higher rates of extensive subclinical lateral growth, resulting in higher recurrence rates with standard recommended margins and failure to completely excise the lesion. LM and LMM have the least common association with nevi, at 3% of cases, but the highest rate of association with **desmoplastic melanoma**.

In addition to a mainly basilar proliferation of melanocytes, involvement of appendageal structures, atrophy and effacement of the epidermis, and marked solar elastosis also characterize this form of melanoma. However, the presence of the latter changes may simply be related to the anatomic site; the skin of the cheeks in older individuals usually exhibits a flattened epidermis and prominent solar elastosis. There may be prominent involvement of appendageal epithelium with large cellular nests. Recognition of prominent appendageal involvement by melanoma is of critical importance so that the lesion is not misdiagnosed as invasive rather than simply as intraepithelial or in situ. The most typical cell type has retracted cytoplasm and often an elongate, stellate, or spindled configuration and a high nuclear-to-cytoplasmic ratio. The nuclei are commonly pleomorphic and hyperchromatic. With progression, the cells become more epithelioid in appearance and exhibit nuclear enlargement and prominent nucleoli. Another characteristic feature is the presence of prominent spindle cell differentiation with formation of confluent fascicles of spindle cells along the dermal–epidermal junction and appendages. Extension of melanoma into the dermis may be difficult to recognize because of prominent cellularity of the stroma and activation of mesenchymal cells. The invasive dermal component is frequently composed of spindle cells occurring either singly or in bundles with varying stromal desmoplasia and invasion of nerve twigs. However, the invasive component may contain any cell type. Invasion of the dermis may originate from appendageal-associated melanoma cells or nests. In the latter instances, the depth of invasion (Breslow thickness) should not be measured from the granular layer of the epidermis because this value would overestimate tumor depth. The measurement of tumor thickness instead should ideally be taken from the granular layer of the hair follicle or sweat gland.

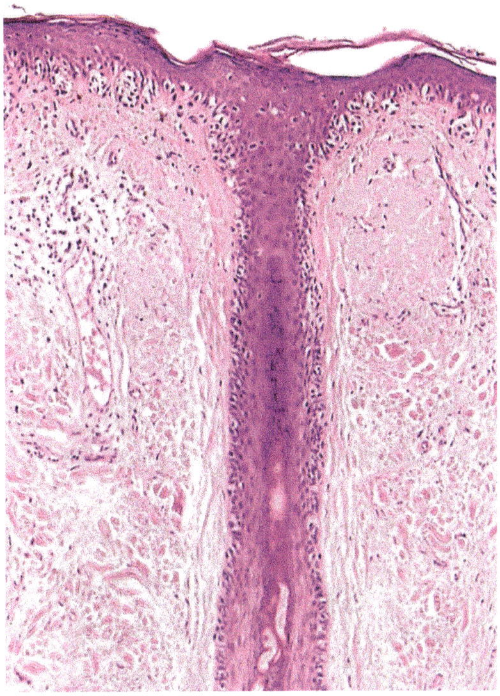

Lentigo maligna (melanoma in situ). There is a striking basilar proliferation of atypical melanocytes (stellate cells with retracted cytoplasm) in both the epidermis and the follicular epithelium.

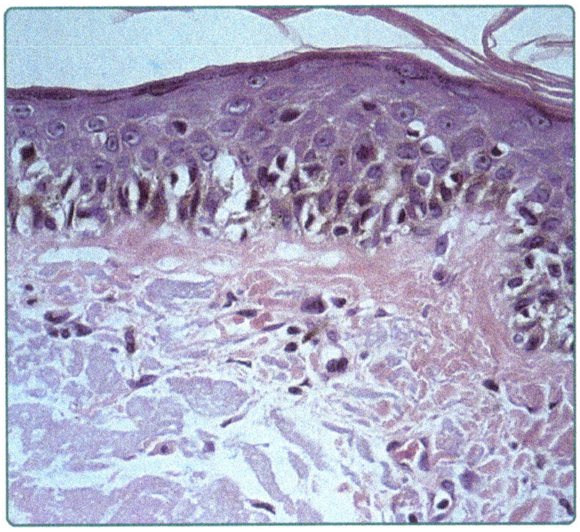

Lentigo maligna. This is a confluent lentiginous proliferation of pleomorphic melanocytes in the basal layer of an atrophic epidermis in sun-damaged skin. There are "back-to-back" melanocytes in a single file line along the basal layer. (Reproduced, with permission, from Goldsmith LA, Katz SI, Gilchrest BA, Paller AS, Leffell DJ, Wolff K, eds. *Fitzpatrick's Dermatology in General Medicine*. 8th ed. New York, NY: McGraw-Hill Education; 2012.)

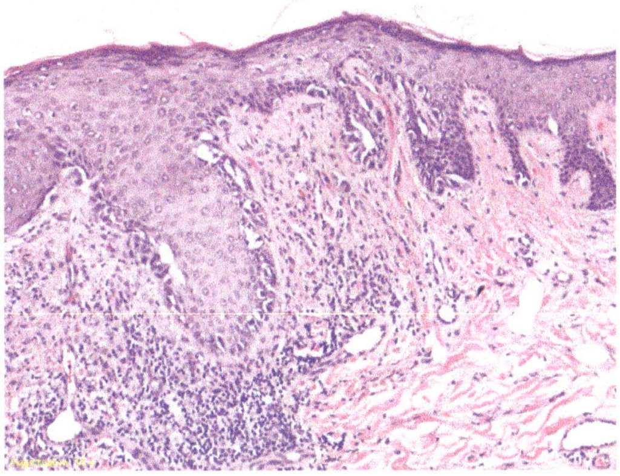

Lentigo maligna (melanoma in situ). Note the single file proliferation of severely atypical melanocytes along the basal layer.

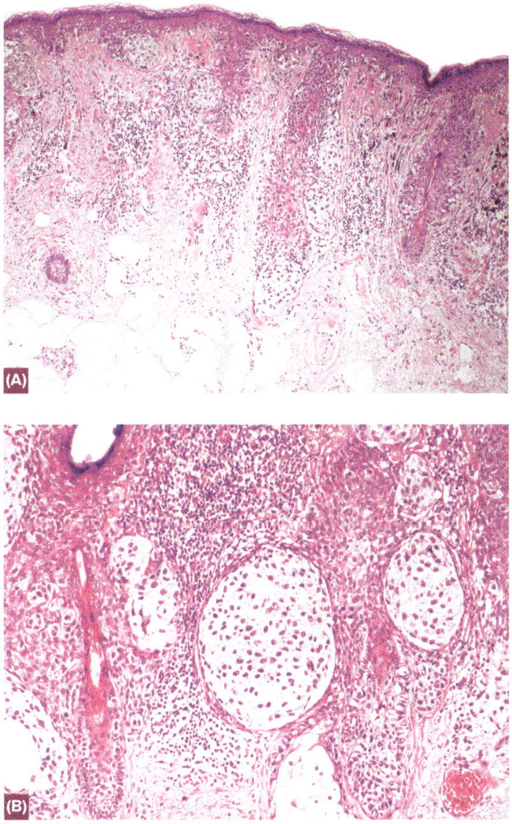

Lentigo maligna (melanoma in situ) and invasive lentigo maligna melanoma (LMM). (A) Lentigo maligna. This lesion shows not only lentiginous melanocytic proliferation but also significant nesting of melanoma cells involving the epidermis and particularly the follicular epithelium. **(B)** Invasive lentigo maligna melanoma (LMM). There is a confluent single-file proliferation of atypical melanocytes extending along the outer root sheath epithelium, consistent with melanoma in situ. The overlying epidermis (not visualized) contains an identical proliferation. Invasive nests and clusters of melanoma cells are present in the adjacent superficial dermis. These cells are outside of the adventitial dermis and therefore Breslow thickness should be measured from the granular layer of the overlying epidermis.

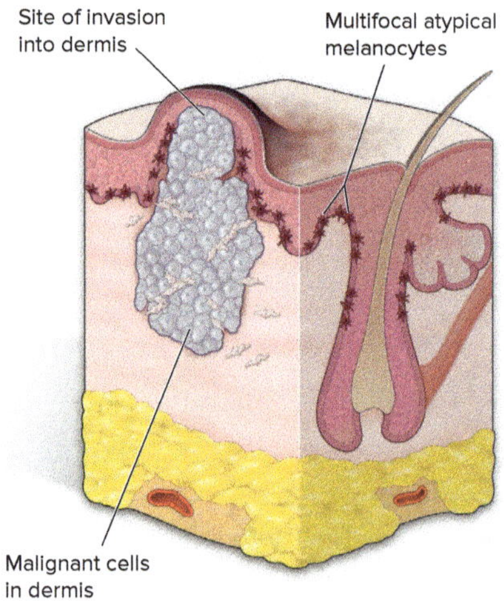

Invasive lentigo maligna melanoma (LMM). Illustrated on the right of the lesion is a large, variegated, freckle-like macule (not elevated above the plane of the skin) with irregular borders; the tan areas show increased numbers of melanocytes, usually atypical and bizarre, and are distributed single file along the basal layer; at certain places in the dermis, malignant melanocytes have invaded and formed nests (radial growth phase). At the left is a large nodule that is heavily pigmented and composed of epithelioid cells that have invaded the dermis (vertical growth phase). (Reproduced, with permission, from Wolff K, Johnson RA, Saavedra AP. *Fitzpatrick's Color Atlas and Synopsis of Clinical Dermatology*. 7th ed. New York, NY: McGraw-Hill Education; 2013.)

The assessment of surgical margins of LM poses a diagnostic challenge in many cases. Since these lesions arise in a background of chronic sun damage, the definitive distinction between the **"trailing edge" of melanoma in situ** and **chronic photoactivation of melanocytes (solar melanocytic hyperplasia, SMH)** may be extremely subtle if not impossible. Furthermore, the skin at these sites has typically been exposed to uniform amounts of UV-radiation, representing a "field effect" and possible multifocal disease. In many instances, all of the chronically sun-exposed skin in a patient may exhibit varying degrees of chronic photoactivation of melanocytes (SMH). If the peripheral surgical margins are "over called" as LM, the surgeon may end up chasing a never-ending surgical margin and removing excessive amounts of facial skin. If the peripheral surgical margins are "under called" as chronic photoactivation of melanocytes (SMH), the tumor will most likely recur. In general, the normal ratio of basal keratinocytes to melanocytes in facial and genital skin is approximately 4:1. In unequivocal LM (in situ), the ratio is 1:1. Chronic photoactivation of melanocytes (SMH) typically results in a ratio in between these two figures. Recently, several studies have evaluated the localized expression of **soluble adenylyl cyclase (sAC)** via immunohistochemistry in benign and malignant melanocytic proliferations and have identified a differential localization pattern of sAC within benign and malignant melanocytes. While benign melanocytes exhibit a perinuclear dot-like staining pattern, malignant melanocytes exhibit a pannuclear staining pattern. Although larger studies are needed for proper validation, the findings are promising as potential diagnostic adjunct in determining melanoma and margin assessment. For situations where lesions exhibit an increased density of basal layer melanocytes with cytologic atypia yet are equivocal for a diagnosis of melanoma in situ, some dermatopathologists recommend the term **solar intraepidermal melanocytic proliferation with atypia (SIMP with atypia)** followed by grading of cytologic atypia (slight, moderate, or severe) according to guidelines proposed for atypical nevi.

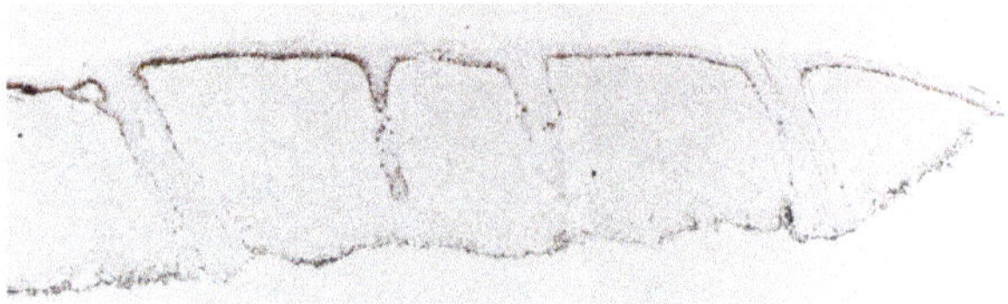

Melan-A stain of lentigo maligna (in situ) with trailing edge. Compared to the density of atypical melanocytes on the left (melanoma in situ), there is a gradually reduced concentration of melanocytes on the right. The absolute distinction between the "trailing off" of melanoma in situ and chronic photoactivation of melanocytes (hyperplasia) is extremely difficult.

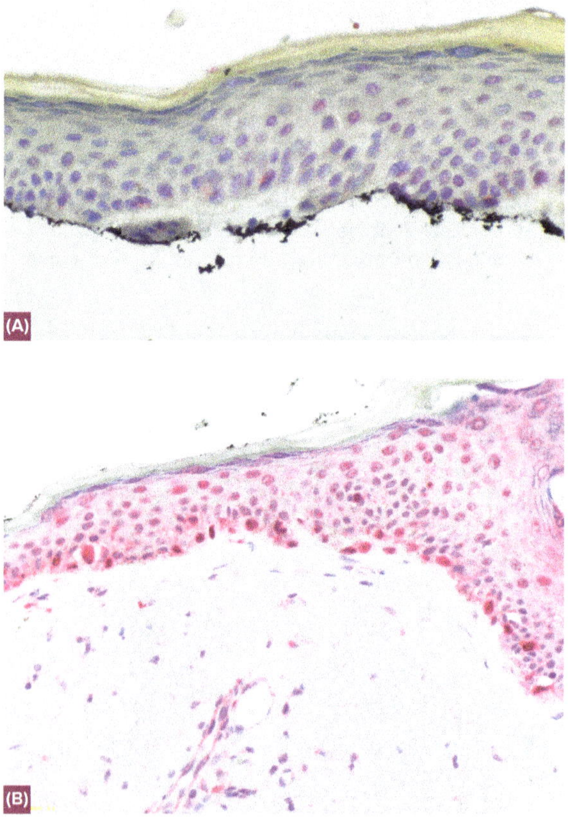

Immunohistochemical staining for soluble adenylyl cyclase (sAC). (A) Benign facial skin reveals occasional melanocytes along the basal layer with a perinuclear staining pattern. **(B)** Lentigo maligna cells exhibit a striking pannuclear staining pattern.

In regards to the other answer choices, **solar lentigo** is characterized by increased pigment within keratinocytes and varying degrees of melanocyte hyperplasia. There is typically minimal cytologic atypia of melanocytes and the concentration lacks confluence. **Spreading pigmented actinic keratosis** is similar to solar lentigo; however, there is additional partial thickness keratinocytic atypia. Although a nested focus of melanocytes is present along the basal layer, the dominant pattern is single-file lentiginous growth. Additionally, the epidermis is attenuated and the nest is not present at the tip of a rete ridge. Overall, the proliferation is confluent and therefore cannot be a **benign melanocytic nevus**.

ANSWER 10-16: B.

The biopsy from the diffuse more flattened pigmented area (image #1) reveals an intradermal population of nevus cells diffusely infiltrating the dermis with maturation. The nevus cells show small, fairly uniform nuclei. These findings are consistent with a **giant congenital intradermal nevus** (Table 10-16A). The nodular lesion reveals asymmetric and hypercellular aggregates of relatively small melanocytes (image #2). Although there is some maturation, the melanocytes have a monomorphous appearance and exhibit some nuclear enlargement and pleomorphism, and nucleoli are present (image #3). These findings are consistent with a **proliferative dermal melanocytic nodule arising within a giant congenital nevus.**

Giant congenital melanocytic nevi (CMN) are rare, with an incidence of approximately 1 in 20,000 births. Very high estimates of melanoma risk associated with large or giant CMN are partially explained by referral bias. On the other hand, a number of studies confirm substantial melanoma risk linked to large or giant (>20 cm) CMN. A lifetime risk of approximately 6.3% has been estimated from the Danish Birth Registry. A recent prospective study involving 92 patients with large or giant CMN demonstrated a cumulative 5-year life-table risk of 4.5% and a standardized morbidity ratio of 239 for the development of melanoma. Giant CMN often involve a large portion of the dorsal surface of the individual and are most commonly raised and exhibit a variably papular, lumpy, rugose, or even verrucous surface. The skin surface may be shiny or contain numerous terminal hairs. Soft tissue hypertrophy may mimic changes found in neurofibromatosis. The color is most often dark brown or black, but considerable variegation of pigment is often noted. Giant CMN are also remarkable for scattered, smaller satellite nevi on the skin surface beyond the **garment nevus**.

Microscopically, **giant CMN** (>20 cm) tend to exhibit distinctive features. Probably the most characteristic feature is the diffuse proliferation of nevus cells throughout the reticular dermis with frequent extension into the subcutaneous fat. There is usually a grenz zone separating the epidermis from the dermal infiltration of nevus cells; however, junctional nests may be noted. In fact, unlike small- and medium-sized CMN, giant CMN are most commonly intradermal. In contrast to the **superficial spreading type of melanoma** that commonly arises in **small and medium CMN**, melanomas arising in association with **giant CMN** tend to be dermal only (**nevoid melanoma**). The nevus cells of giant CMN tend to infiltrate collagen in an orderly and uniform pattern. The nevus cells also often extend along the fibrous trabeculae of the subcutaneous fat and occasionally infiltrate fat lobules. Aggregates of nevus cells also tend to cuff or infiltrate follicular epithelium, sebaceous glands,

Table 10-16A. Large or Giant Congenital Nevi

Clinical Features
Symmetry
>20 cm
Involvement of major anatomic area, segmental
Often dorsal involvement
Occasional congenital deformities
Well-defined borders
Brown, dark brown, black
"Animal pelt" feature, rugose, doughy
Soft tissue hypertrophy
Hypertrichosis
Scattered satellite nevi distant from giant nevus
Involvement of meninges common for head and neck nevi
Histopathologic Features
Lentiginous melanocytic hyperplasia common
Usually compound or dermal
Reticular dermal involvement, usually superficial and deep
- Diffuse
- Interstitial
- Perivascular, periadnexal
Subcutaneous involvement, septal >> lobular
Maturation
Neural differentiation, neuroid, or neurofibroma-like pattern on occasion
Wagner-Meissner–like corpuscles
Fascial or muscle involvement
Cellular nodules in reticular dermis on occasion
Blue nevus component on occasion
Spindle and epithelioid cell nevus component on occasion
Hamartomatous elements
- Cartilaginous differentiation
- Adipose differentiation
Differential Diagnosis
Becker nevus
Neurofibromatosis
Melanoma
Peripheral nerve sheath tumors

eccrine ducts and glands, the perineurium of nerve twigs, and the walls of vascular structures. The perivascular and periadnexal cuffing by nevus cells may closely resemble an inflammatory process such as a gyrate erythema. In contrast to **Unna theory** of an intraepidermal melanocytic stem cell and its role in the development of common acquired nevi, dysplastic nevi, and intraepidermal melanomas, substantial evidence supports an alternate theory that, in fact, a stem cell population may be located deep within the dermis, such that nevus formation involves a bottom-to-top migration of melanocytes. This is supported by the distinct embryologic origin of the melanocyte, the neural crest cell, which differs from the ectodermal origin of the dermis and epidermis. In 1984, Stewart F. Cramer developed the ***Hochsteigerung*** or "upward climbing" theory, which proposes that nevi inception and development reflects a recapitulation of embryogenesis such that melanocytes migrate upward alongside the nerve fibers that ascend through the dermis. Relative to other types of nevi, congenital nevi are particularly likely to be associated with **capsular nevi**, a phenomenon whereby melanocytes involve the capsules of local lymph nodes in a manner that may be mistaken for **metastatic melanoma** during sentinel lymph node biopsy due to the Melan-A and S-100 positivity of these cells. While the precise mechanism by which these nevus cells become deposited in lymph nodes is controversial, the two leading theories involve an aberration in the embryologic melanocyte migration from the neural crest to the skin, or embolic transfer of cells from cutaneous sites via lymphatic vessels. Again, congenital nevi commonly demonstrate focal dermal melanocyte clusters protruding into lymphatic vessels. A subset of large or giant CMN are also characterized by spindle cell or neuroidal differentiation resembling a neurofibroma (**neuroid CMN**). The constituent cells have a wavy configuration and are embedded in a delicate stroma. Neural differentiation resembling neural tubules or pseudo-Meissnerian structures may also occur. Such nevi may be associated with congenital anomalies such as club foot and spina bifida. Large CMN may also show a variety of other patterns, suggesting that they are indeed hamartomas of neural crest differentiation. Such nevi may contain heterologous elements such as cartilage, bone, adipose tissue, vascular malformation, hemangioma, lymphangioma, mastocytoma, and schwannoma. Foci suggesting **blue nevus, cellular blue nevus (CBN), Spitz nevus**, and other nevus variants are occasionally noted. Importantly, foci of hypercellularity are also sometimes noted within the dermal population of cells.

All varieties of **congenital nevi** may exhibit varying degrees of architectural and cytologic atypia of both the intraepidermal and dermal components. Perhaps one of the most common findings is lentiginous melanocytic proliferation, which may occur with or without variation in junctional nesting or cytologic atypia of the intraepidermal melanocytes. Another common finding, particularly in CMN in individuals younger than age 10 years, especially in the first year of life, is upward migration of intraepidermal melanocytes (pagetoid ascent). Although the latter changes may be alarming, the proliferation is usually orderly, often confined to the lower half of the epidermis, and with cytologic atypia absent or of low grade. One may encounter a spectrum of atypicality within the intraepidermal component, ranging from little or no atypia to frank melanoma in situ. Large or giant CMN may give rise to dermal or subcutaneous **proliferative melanocytic nodules**. Such proliferations may occur superficially or deeply and be composed of epithelioid, spindled, or small cells. Varying degrees of cytologic atypia; mitotic activity; and, occasionally, necrosis may be observed. Most of these cellular aggregates tend to blend with the surrounding nevus. The vast majority of such proliferations, particularly in the neonatal period, are biologically benign, despite their atypical histologic features. Small round cell tumors should be evaluated especially carefully for malignancy. Many of these nodular proliferations are composed of enlarged epithelioid or spindled cells containing granular cytoplasmic melanin. Usually, the melanin does not have the finely divided ("dusty") character observed in melanoma cells. The nuclei also tend to be uniform compared with the pleomorphism and clumped chromatin of melanoma cells.

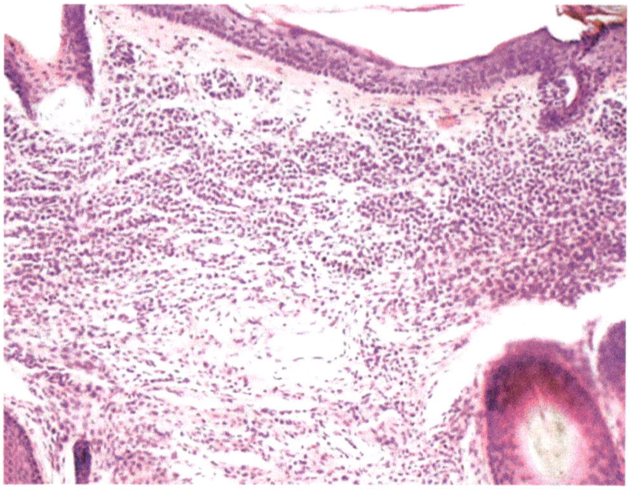

Giant congenital intradermal nevus. Note the sheets of bland melanocytes in the dermis with infiltration of collagen in an orderly and uniform pattern.

Conventional melanoma originating from an intraepidermal location occurs most commonly in relatively **small CMN**. Such melanomas are usually of the **superficial spreading (pagetoid) or nodular type**. However, such melanomas are uncommonly observed in large and giant CMN. The great majority of melanomas developing in the **giant CMN** are dermal and composed of epithelioid cells, spindle cells, or small round cells resembling malignant lymphoma. Some melanomas may have the characteristics of **malignant blue nevus (MBN)** or **malignant epithelioid schwannoma**. Such tumors usually manifest cohesive cellular nodules distinctly different from the surrounding nevus, substantial nuclear pleomorphism, necrotic cells, mitotic activity, and striking cellularity. Interpretation of such tumors may be exceedingly difficult,

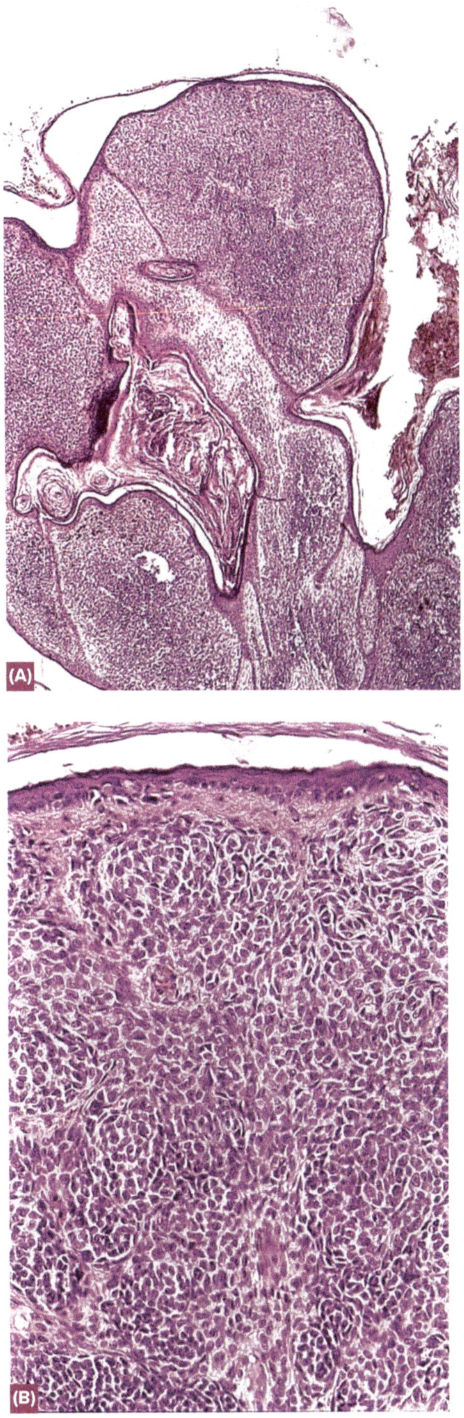

Small cell melanoma. (A) Diffuse sheet of small cells in the dermis. **(B)** Uniform population of cells resembling lymphoma. The patient died of metastases.

and a final diagnosis of benign or malignant tumor may not be possible. Melanomas developing in newborns and infants younger than 1 year of age are extremely rare, and such a diagnosis must always be seriously questioned. Furthermore, the vast majority of epithelioid and spindle cell nodular proliferations developing in CMN, particularly in young individuals, are benign or not aggressive. A prudent approach is to ensure complete surgical removal of such **proliferative melanocytic nodules** and to carefully monitor the patient for recurrence or metastasis. On the other hand, many of the true biologic melanomas arising in **giant CMN** are of the small cell type (**small cell melanoma**). The cells are disposed in sheets in a delicate myxoid stroma. The cells are closely crowded; have minimal cytoplasms; and contain small round or slightly oval nuclei with dense, uniformly dispersed chromatin. The cells take on the appearance of lymphoblastic lymphoma or comparable "blastic" tumors. Mitotic figures and nuclear debris are also commonly observed.

ANSWER 10-17: B.

The biopsy reveals a scattered dermal-confined population of heavily pigmented melanocytes with a spindled cytomorphology. Dermal sclerosis is absent. The histopathological findings are consistent with a **dermal melanocytosis**, and in this clinical setting is consistent with **nevus of Ota**. The classification of **dermal melanocytoses** and **blue nevi** is based on assessing a number of features, including clinical appearance; anatomic site of lesion; localization in the reticular dermis, subcutis, and the like; the extent to which the lesion is made up of dendritic, spindle-shaped, or epithelioid melanocytes; the degree of cellularity of the lesion; and the degree of fibrosis (sclerosis) (Table 10-17A). The bluish appearance of these various lesions is primarily related to the depth of melanin in the dermis and the **Tyndall phenomenon**. The longer wavelengths of visible light penetrate the reticular dermis and are absorbed by the melanin. However, the shorter wavelengths representing the bluish part of the color spectrum do not penetrate so deeply and are reflected back from the superficial dermis and epidermis. The **dermal melanocytoses** and **blue nevi** are thought to result from the dermal arrest of cells migrating from the neural crest. In contrast to ordinary nevi, it is believed that these migratory cells never reach the epidermis but instead give rise to melanocytic lesions with varying degrees of cellularity and melanization.

The **dermal melanocytoses** are composed of six clinical entities that are related because they are all essentially bluish macular lesions that histologically demonstrate scattered dendritic melanocytes in the reticular dermis with little or no stromal alteration.

Nevus of Ota (Nevus Fuscoceruleus Ophthalmomaxillaris) is a hamartomatous or nevoid condition that usually presents at birth or in childhood as a unilateral speckled bluish macule involving the periorbital region, forehead, temple, cheek, or nose, corresponding to the distribution of the first two branches of the trigeminal nerve. Examination may also disclose involvement of the sclera, conjunctiva, cornea, retina, or oral and nasal mucosa. Brownish lentigo-like lesions and bluish papules or nodules are occasionally associated with nevus of Ota.

Table 10-17A. Differential Features of Dermal Melanocytoses

FEATURE	MONGOLIAN SPOT	NEVUS OF OTA	NEVUS OF ITO
Onset	Birth or soon after	Birth or soon after	Birth or soon after
Size	5 cm	5 cm	5 cm
Color	Gray-tan, slate blue	Brown, slate blue	Brown, slate blue
Surface	Macular	Macular, rarely discrete papules	Macular, rarely discrete papules
Hair	Normal for site	Normal for site	Normal for site
Distribution	Midline	Unilateral	Unilateral
Number	Single, can be multiple	Single	Single
Site	Lumbosacral	First and second division trigeminal nerve	Shoulder and upper arm
Racial incidence	Asians and dark-skinned races	Asians and dark-skinned races	Asians and dark-skinned races
Familial incidence	Common	Rare	Rare
Gender	No difference	80% in females	80% in females
Age of appearance	At birth	60% at birth	60% at birth
Spontaneous fate	Usually disappears during first few years of life	Persist; rarely disappear	Persist; rarely disappear
Tendency to malignancy	Never reported	Rare	Rare
Histopathologic Features	Scattered dermal melanocytes in lower half of dermis in low concentrations	Moderate number of dermal melanocytes in upper dermis	Moderate number of dermal melanocytes in upper dermis
Ultrastructure	Fully developed melanocytes with only mature melanosomes; virtually no premelanosomes	Fully developed melanocytes with only mature melanosomes; virtually no premelanosomes	Fully developed melanocytes with only mature melanosomes; virtually no premelanosomes

Nevus Fuscoceruleus Zygomaticus (Acquired nevus of Ota-like macules, Sun nevus) is characterized by acquired bilateral bluish macules in the zygomatic areas of the face. It is considered a variant of **nevus of Ota**. The condition usually does not become apparent until the second decade of life, and is much more common in Chinese and Japanese women.

Acquired Dermal Melanocytosis of the Face and Extremities is a disorder associated with bilateral bluish or brownish discoloration of the face of adults, somewhat similar to **nevus of Ota**. Additionally, it is associated with involvement of the extensor surfaces of the upper extremities and possibly the palms.

Nevus of Ito (Nevus Fuscoceruleus Acromiodeltoideus) is closely related to **nevus of Ota**, but is distinguished by its unilateral distribution involving the supraclavicular, scapular, or deltoid regions.

Mongolian spots are oval or round, often poorly defined, macules (approximately 1-10 cm) varying in color from slight gray to blue-black or dark brown, most often affecting the lumbosacral region, but they may also be seen in other (ectopic or aberrant) locations. These lesions are present at birth but usually spontaneously regress by age 3-4 years. **Mongolian spots** are observed primarily in persons of color.

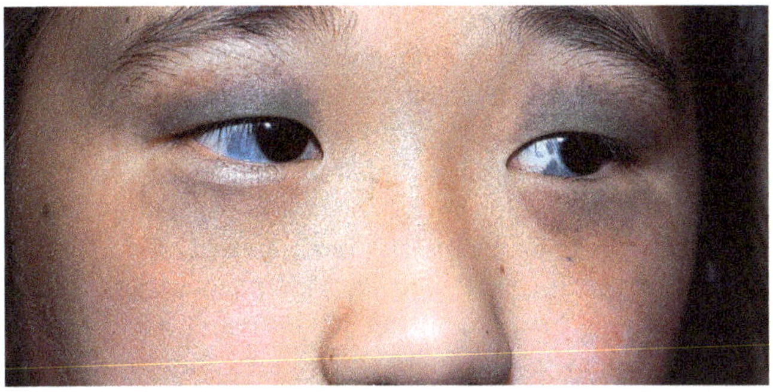

Acquired nevus of Ota-like macules (Sun nevus). Note the bilateral bluish macules in the zygomatic regions of this Asian female patient. The pigment first became clinically noticeable in her early teen years. (Reproduced with permission from Wolff K, Johnson RA, Saavedra AP. *Fitzpatrick's Color Atlas and Synopsis of Clinical Dermatology*. 7th ed. New York, NY: McGraw-Hill Education; 2013.)

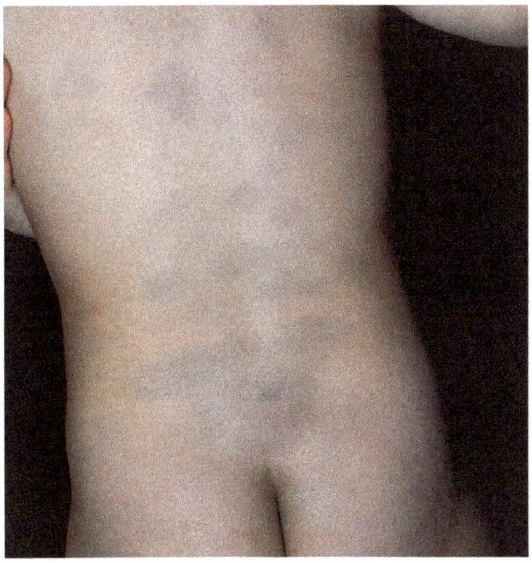

Mongolian spots. Multiple, ill-defined, bluish lesions are scattered on the back of this Japanese child. They were present at birth. Most of these lesions disappeared later in childhood. (Reproduced with permission from Wolff K, Johnson RA, Saavedra AP. *Fitzpatrick's Color Atlas and Synopsis of Clinical Dermatology.* 7th ed. New York, NY: McGraw-Hill Education; 2013.)

Dermal Melanocyte Hamartoma describes a small number of developmental abnormalities usually present at birth and exhibiting extensive involvement of the skin.

Common blue nevus usually presents as a well-demarcated, slightly raised, or dome-shaped bluish papule. The color is usually a uniform slate gray, blue-black, or black. The borders are generally regular, and these nevi usually measure less than 1 cm in diameter. They are primarily located on the dorsal aspects of the hands and feet or may involve the face and scalp. The onset is generally in childhood but may occur later in life. Melanoma has only rarely been reported to originate from this type of blue nevus.

Microscopically, this form of **blue nevus** shows an aggregation of dendritic melanocytes that alters the normal configuration of the dermis. The lesion may occur anywhere in the reticular dermis and even in the papillary dermis, but it most commonly involves the superficial dermis. In general,

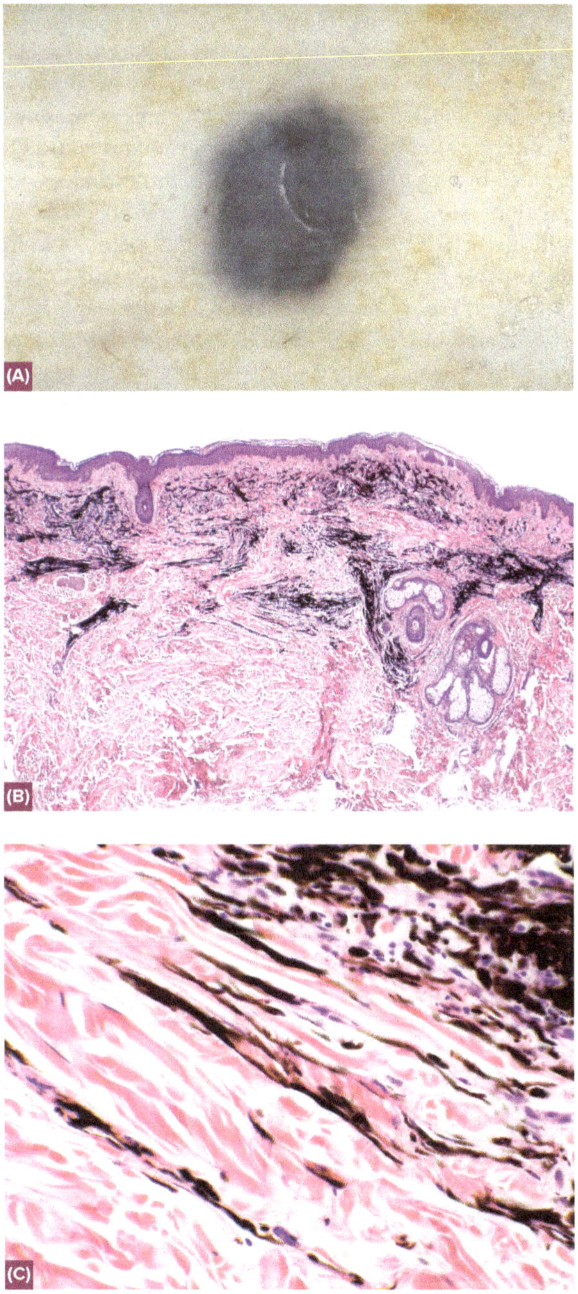

Blue nevus, common type. (A) The lesion shows a small diameter, symmetry, well-defined borders, and uniform blue color with dermoscopy. **(B)** The nevus is composed of pigmented dendritic melanocytes disposed in fascicles. **(C)** The dendritic melanocytes have long cellular processes that are heavily melaninized. The dermis is slightly collagenized. (Part **(A)**: Used with permission of P Guitera and SW Menzies, Sydney Melanoma Diagnostic Centre and Dermatology Department, Royal Prince Alfred Hospital, NSW, Australia.)

there are bundles of dendritic cells with frequent aggregation about appendages and neurovascular bundles. The cells are generally bipolar or stellate and characterized by lengthy dendritic processes. Most cells contain a dense accumulation of relatively fine melanin granules. The nuclei are ovoid with uniform chromatin patterns. **Melanophages** are usually present and may be the principal cell type in some cases. Variable degrees of fibrosis are also present.

In regards to the differential diagnosis, the **dermal melanocytoses** share the same dendritic cell type noted in **common blue nevi**. The **blue nevus** differs from the former entities by a greater concentration of dendritic melanocytes and is usually accompanied by varying degrees of fibrosis and melanophage accumulation. However, the papular and nodular lesions within nevus of Ota or nevus of Ito are histopathologically indistinguishable from this variant of blue nevus. An important feature of these pigmented dendritic melanocytes is their strong expression of HMB45, best highlighted with red chromogen. Lastly, the differential diagnosis might also include primary or metastatic **melanoma**, possibly with some degree of regression. In general, **blue nevi** can be distinguished from **melanoma** by their small size, overall symmetry, lack of cytologic atypia, and absence of mitotic activity and necrosis.

Quick Fact

- Dermal melanocytoses lack sclerosis
- Blue nevi, common type, contain increased numbers of pigmented spindled/dendritic melanocytes and usually have a sclerotic dermis.
- The dendritic melanocytes of both conditions express HMB45 as well as Melan-A and S100.

In regards to the differential diagnosis of pigmented lesions of the conjunctiva, the **dermal melanocytoses** and **blue nevi** exhibit a blue discoloration clinically. This is in contrast to the more brown discoloration of **conjunctival melanosis** and **conjunctival nevi**.

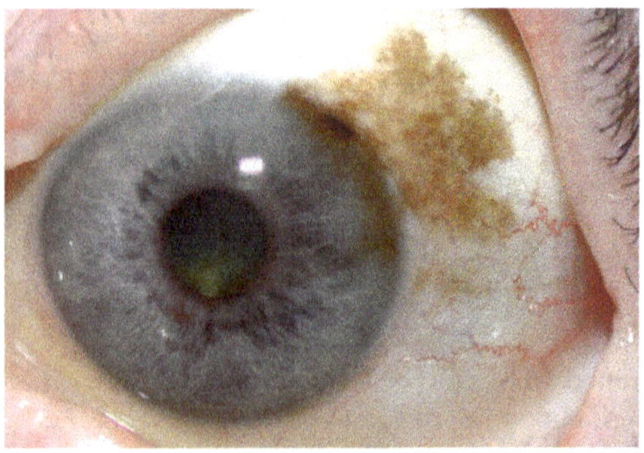

Conjunctival primary acquired melanosis (PAM). Note the discoloration is brown, in contrast to the blue discoloration of dermal melanocytoses. (Reproduced, with permission, from Riordan-Eva P, Cunningham ET Jr. *Vaughan & Asbury's General Ophthalmology*. 18th ed. New York, NY: McGraw-Hill; 2011.)

Melanosis (pigmentation) of the conjunctiva may be congenital or acquired. **Congenital melanosis of the conjunctiva** is typically bilateral and occurs more commonly in patients with pigmented skin. **Primary acquired melanosis of the conjunctiva (PAM)** is typically unilateral. Both lesions are histopathologically similar to **solar lentigo simplex** with melanin containing basal keratinocytes and slight lentiginous hyperplasia of melanocytes. Additionally, both lesions are considered benign and not premalignant. Occasionally, acquired lesions may exhibit varying degrees of melanocytic atypia (**primary acquired melanosis with atypia**), such as epithelioid cytomorphology and focal high-density lentiginous growth. These lesions should be closely followed clinically. Lesions with severe cytologic atypia, confluent growth, and pagetoid ascent should be classified as **conjunctival melanoma in situ. Conjunctival nevi** exhibit nested proliferations of nevomelanocytes similar to **common acquired nevi** of the skin. Approximately 75% and 25% of cases of **conjunctival melanoma** arise within preexisting **PAM** or **nevi**, respectively.

Post-inflammatory pigmentary alteration with scattered melanophages may histopathologically resemble **blue nevi** or **dermal melanocytoses**; however, the pigmented cells in this condition are macrophages and will be negative for Melan-A and HMB45.

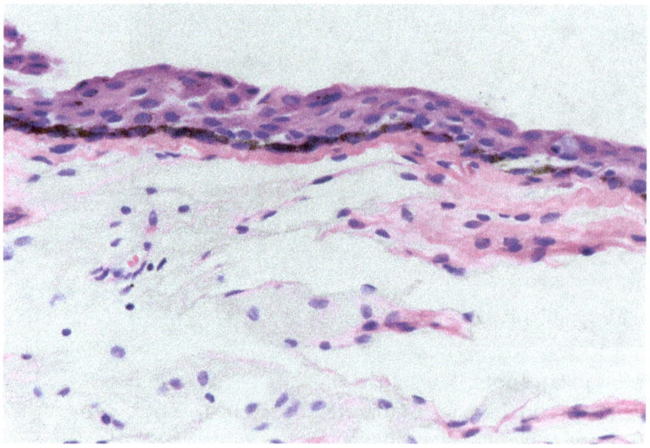

Primary acquired melanosis of the conjunctiva. Note the pigmentation within basal keratinocytes. Melan-A stain will reveal occasional dendritic melanocytes confined to the basal layer. (Used with permission of Adrienne Jordan, MD, New York Eye and Ear Infirmary of Mount Sinai, New York, NY.)

ANSWER 10-18: B.

The biopsy reveals a large lobular proliferation of hyperpigmented spindle cells and larger hypopigmented polygonal and rounded cells. The proliferation has both bulbous and fascicular patterns of growth and abuts the subcutis. The combined Melan-A/Ki67 stain (red/brown chromogen, respectively) reveals no brown nuclear staining within any of the cells with red cytoplasmic staining; therefore, the cells are melanocytes without mitotic activity. The brown cytoplasmic staining is melanin pigment and not chromogen deposition from the immunohistochemical stain. The findings are consistent with a **cellular blue nevus**. Historically, the classification of blue nevus has included two principal variants: the more prevalent **common blue nevus (BN)** and the relatively uncommon, larger variant, the **cellular blue nevus (CBN)**. However, examination of sufficient numbers of blue nevi reveals that there is indeed a morphologic spectrum rather than necessarily two well-defined subtypes. The morphologic features that account for the spectrum of blue nevi include the relative number and density of dendritic and spindled melanocytes, oval or fusiform melanocytes, melanophages, the degree of fibrosis, the disposition and relationship of the latter components, and the overall size of the lesion. The spindle cells may be individually disposed or arranged in fascicles or in compact nests. In **sclerosing blue nevi**, the fibrous component is conspicuous relative to the sparse number of spindle/dendritic melanocytes. These tumors are frequently mistaken for **dermatofibromas** with hemosiderin pigment (**hemosiderotic dermatofibroma**). Finally, some blue nevi contain cellular elements observed in other nevi such as **common acquired nevi** or **Spitz nevi** and have been designated as "**melanocytic nevi with phenotypic heterogeneity**" or **"combined" nevi** (Table 10-18A). The classification of blue nevi is based on the predominant histopathologic features.

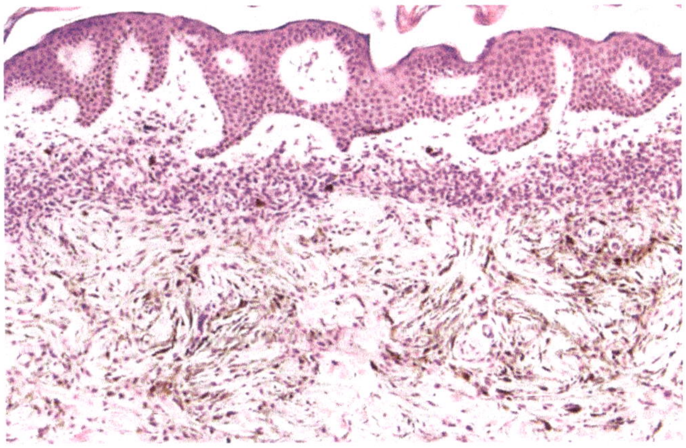

Melanocytic nevus with phenotypic heterogeneity ("combined melanocytic nevus"). This lesion has features of both an ordinary compound nevus with underlying blue nevus component. Note the well-defined zone of small nevus cells in superficial dermal overlying the blue nevus.

Cellular blue nevi are generally 1-3 cm in diameter with a blue, blue-black, or black coloration (Table 10-18B). Their surface is usually smooth but may be uneven. They most commonly involve the buttocks, sacral area, scalp and face, and dorsa of the feet and hands. They are generally diagnosed between the ages of 10 and 40 years and in rare instances may be congenital. They are usually asymptomatic. Rarely, these lesions may undergo transformation to melanoma (**blue nevus-like melanoma, malignant blue nevus; MBN**). Incomplete excision of **CBN** is rarely associated with recurrence. Microscopically, there is a continuum from ordinary blue nevi to "cellular" blue nevi, as discussed previously. However, no criteria have been established as to what proportion of a blue nevus should consist of fusiform cells to qualify as a CBN. The following criteria are proposed for diagnosis of CBN: the lesion should occupy the reticular dermis, at least one-third to one-half of the lesion should contain oval to fusiform cells, and the overall architecture should be multilobular or plexiform with deep involvement of the reticular dermis or subcutis.

Table 10-18A. Melanocytic Nevus with Phenotypic Heterogeneity (Combined Nevus)

Clinical Features
- Any age (birth to old age) but usually <40 years of age
- Women > men
- Head and neck (especially for blue nevus variants), upper trunk, proximal extremities
- Often component of blue, blue-black
- May have small (1-5 mm) blue, blue-black focus in ordinary nevus
- Size <6-7 mm in most instances

Histopathologic Features
- Symmetric
- Well circumscribed
- Orderly arrangements of cells
- Two or more of the following:
  - (1) Ordinary nevus component
  - (2) Pigmented dendritic melanocytes
  - (3) Pigmented spindle or epithelioid cells
  - (4) Amelanotic spindle cells
  - (5) Spitz nevus cells
- Ordinary nevus component often overlies or is adjacent to other component
- Deep involvement occurs often
- Plexiform configuration on occasion

Differential Diagnosis
- Cellular blue nevus
- Melanoma

CBN may show single or multiple lobular masses with a well-defined horizontal inferior margins that parallel or bulge into the subcutaneous fat. Extension into the subcutaneous fat may also occur.

CBN are heterogeneous, and their morphologic limits have not been clearly defined. For example, the distinction from ordinary blue nevi, some pigmented peripheral nerve sheath tumors, and other unusual melanocytic nevi may be problematic. Essential for the diagnosis are cellular foci of round, oval, elongate, or fusiform cells that constitute at least one-third to one-half, if not most, of the tumor. These cells are arranged in a number of patterns and vary considerably as to melanin content. As opposed to the frequent diffuse distribution of melanin-laden dendritic melanocytes in the ordinary

Table 10-18B. Cellular Blue Nevus

Clinical Features
- Onset: birth, childhood, adolescence
- Age: mean, 33 years (range: birth to 85 years)
- Site: buttocks, sacrococcygeal area, forearm or wrist, leg, ankle, foot, scalp, face
- Gray-blue to blue-black papule, nodule
- Usually well circumscribed
- Regular borders
- Size: ≥ 0.3-3 cm

Histopathologic Features
- Symmetry
- Localization to reticular dermis
- Often deep extension with bulging, nodular configuration, rounded, well-demarcated inferior margin
- Heterogeneity of patterns
    - Biphasic pattern most common:
        - (1) Melanin-laden dendritic melanocytes and fibrosis
        - (2) Bundles of amelanotic fusiform cells
    - Alveolar pattern:
        - Fascicles or nests of fusiform cells compartmentalized by fibrous trabeculae
    - Fascicular pattern
        - Fascicles of spindle cells often with clear cytoplasm and prominent schwannian differentiation
    - Cellular blue nevus with atypical features (atypical cellular blue nevus)
        - Large size (1-2 cm)
        - Marked cytologic atypia
        - Increased mitotic rate
        - Necrosis
        - Infiltration of surrounding tissue
    - Lacunae-containing melanophages
    - Cystic degeneration in central part of nevus with loose edematous stroma
    - Few or no mitotic figures
    - Necrosis absent or uncommon

Differential Diagnosis
- Blue nevus-like melanoma, (malignant blue nevus)
- Metastatic melanoma
- Clear cell sarcoma

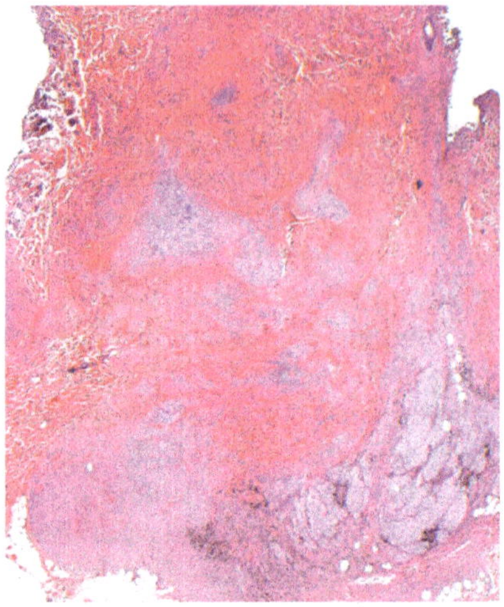

Blue nevus, cellular variant. This lesion occupies the entire dermis. The superficial eosinophilic portion of the lesion corresponds to that of a common blue nevus whereas the deeper pale-staining areas correspond to densely cellular nests and fascicles of spindled melanocytes.

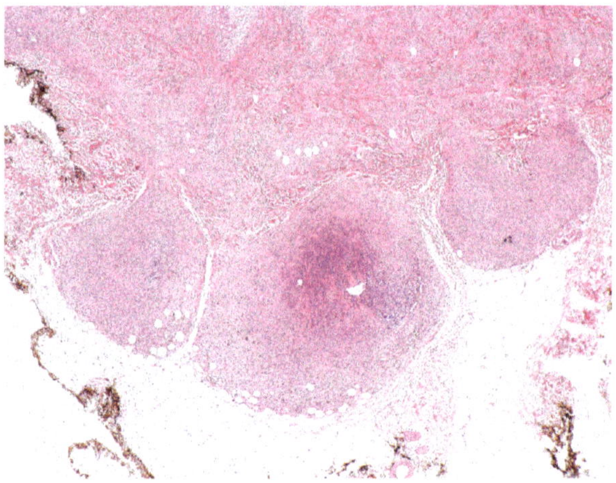

Blue nevus, cellular variant. Characteristic bulbous configuration of cellular blue nevus extending into subcutis.

type of blue nevus, the fusiform cells of CBN are usually disposed in variably organized nests or bundles. These bundles may or may not be encapsulated by fibrous tissue. There may be linear or concentric arrangements of cells within these nests. Pigmented dendritic melanocytes (identical to common BN) and melanophages are often present in the peripheral fibrous tissue surrounding the cellular fascicles. The sizes of fascicles or nests may vary considerably. Fascicles of spindle cells may have schwannian differentiation and may merge with and infiltrate cutaneous nerves. Perhaps two-thirds or so of CBN have a so-called "biphasic" pattern, that is, a separate component of common blue nevus (pigmented dendritic melanocytes, variable sclerosis, and melanophages), in addition to the cellular areas. These areas are often in the superficial dermis overlying or at the periphery of cellular lobules.

The cells comprising the "cellular" foci are most often spindle shaped but may also be round or oval. These cells are usually somewhat enlarged but may be relatively small. The cells' boundaries are often ill defined, and the cytoplasm is usually clear, vacuolated, slightly eosinophilic, or bluish. The fusiform cells do not contain readily apparent melanin by conventional microscopy. Because of the paucity or absence of melanin, these cellular foci appear pale or clear on scanning magnification, in contrast to the often heavily pigmented areas containing dendritic melanocytes, melanophages, and sclerosis. These pale areas are quite helpful in recognizing CBN. However, the degree of melanization may vary from barely visible fine granular melanin to heavy pigmentation obscuring cytologic detail. Usually, the small dendritic melanocytes and melanophages contain the heaviest deposition of melanin. However, the latter cells are usually located in peripheral fibrous trabeculae or in areas of sclerosis.

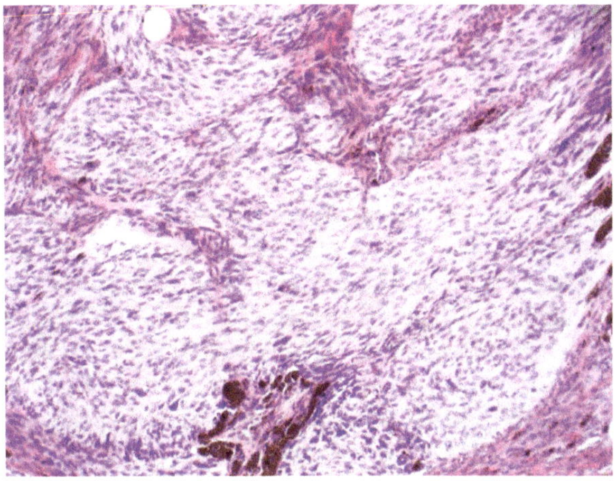

Blue nevus, cellular variant. Discrete fascicles of ovoid and fusiform melanocytes with clear cytoplasms partitioned by fibrous trabeculae. Note the heavily pigmented cells at the periphery of the lobules.

The nuclei of the cells within the "cellular" foci are commonly enlarged, and the chromatin tends to be evenly dispersed with one or more small nucleoli. Minimal or low-grade nuclear pleomorphism is noted in many CBN. However, this should not be pronounced. Similarly, occasional mitoses are noted in many CBN. As a general rule, if two or more mitoses are present per mm^2, the lesion should be carefully evaluated for other corroborating evidence of malignancy.

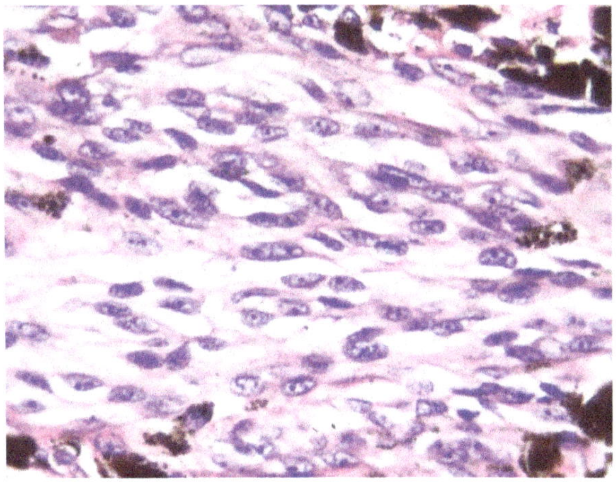

Blue nevus, cellular variant. The fusiform melanocytes display fairly uniform nuclei.

On occasion, foci of CBN may be detected in regional lymph nodes, such as the axillary or inguinal lymph nodes proximal to a CBN on an extremity. These nodal foci of CBN have most commonly involved the subcapsular peripheral sinuses and parenchyma of the lymph nodes, which are sites involved by metastatic cancer, but also the lymph node capsule. Explanations for such nodal involvement include benign metastases and aberrant histogenesis of CBN in lymph nodes. The latter phenomenon should be recognized, carefully assessed, and not misdiagnosed as **metastatic melanoma** or MBN. Similarly, a cutaneous lesion should not be misdiagnosed as MBN simply because of the lymph node involvement.

Atypical variants of CBN (**atypical cellular blue nevus**) may be extremely difficult or impossible to distinguish from melanoma (**malignant blue nevus; MBN**) (Table 10-18C). Morphologic criteria are not clearly established for such atypical variants, and their biologic potential often cannot be predicted. However, they are generally characterized by large size (>1-2 cm), deep extension, large expansile nests of spindle cells, prominent cellularity and cytologic atypia, necrosis, infiltration of adjacent tissue, and significant mitotic activity (usually $>2/mm^2$). It cannot be overemphasized that although MBN is exceedingly rare, **atypical CBN** should be completely excised and the patient monitored very carefully for recurrence. Metastases from such lesions have been observed after the passage of several years (as long as 15 years). Thus, because of the unusual nature of these lesions, their rarity, and the lack of long-term follow-up, the biologic potential of atypical forms of CBN is largely unknown and requires further study.

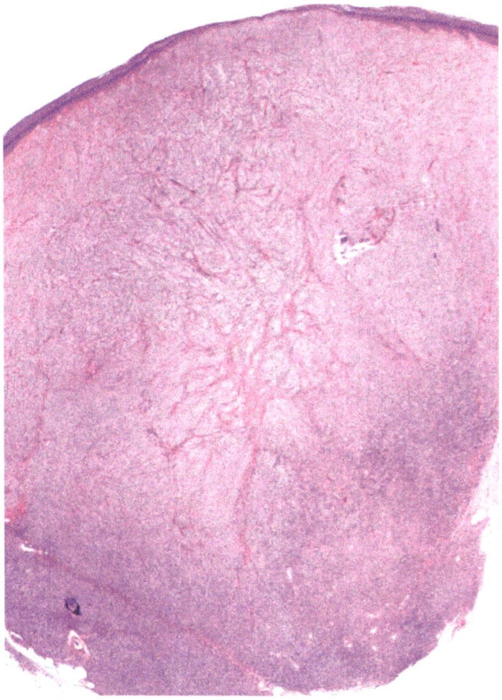

Atypical cellular blue nevus. Note the uniformly and highly cellular nodular nature of the lesion without typical zonation of superficial common and deep cellular blue nevus components.

Table 10-18C. Comparison of Cellular Blue Nevus and Blue nevus-like melanoma, (malignant blue nevus)

CELLULAR BLUE NEVUS	BLUE NEVUS-LIKE MELANOMA, (MALIGNANT BLUE NEVUS)
Clinical Features	
Mean age, 33 years (range: birth to 85)	Extremely rare: mean age, 46 years
Women > men	Men > women
Buttocks, sacrococcygeal area, extremities	Scalp most common site
Size: 1.8 cm (1-2 cm)	Size: 2.9 cm (1.3-4 cm)
Blue, blue-gray, blue-black plaque or nodule	Blue, blue-black nodule
Histopathologic Features	
Component of ordinary blue nevus in 60%	Blue nevus component, cellular in 92%
Symmetry	Asymmetry
Lobular or multilobular	Lobular or multilobular
Cytologic atypia, low grade or absent	Substantial cytologic atypia in some
Mitoses <1 or 2/mm^2	Mitoses usually > 2 and often 5 or more per mm^2.
Usually no atypical mitoses	Atypical mitoses may be present
Necrosis uncommon	Necrosis in 33%
	Pronounced heterogeneity in most tumors (1) Frankly malignant component in some—severely atypical epithelioid or spindle cells with prominent nucleoli (2) Confluent sheets of spindle cells suggesting sarcoma (3) Presentation of "atypical cellular blue nevus"

The differential diagnosis of CBN (and atypical CBN) includes malignant blue nevus (malignant melanoma arising in association with CBN), **epithelioid blue nevus, deep penetrating nevus**, and **metastatic melanoma**. The clinical history of a long-standing blue nevus with subsequent change or finding an associated benign blue nevus remnant (usually CBN) is extremely important for the diagnosis of MBN. Without such a clinical history or finding, MBN cannot be distinguished from conventional melanoma, whether primary or metastatic. An important feature ruling out a metastatic melanoma in this case is the biphasic nature ("cellular" and common "spindled/dendritic" areas) of the tumor. Metastatic melanomas are typically composed of one cell type. Additionally, this lesion lacks the cytologic atypia (pleomorphism, prominent nucleoli, and mitoses) one would expect to see in metastatic melanoma.

Malignant melanoma originating from or associated with a preexisting blue nevus (commonly a CBN) or closely resembling a blue nevus was first delineated by Allen and Spitz under the term "**malignant blue nevus.**" The term has been controversial, and many have called for its abandonment. Nonetheless, this appellation continues to be used in the literature because this variant of melanoma has a unique developmental basis (ie, origin from a BN, a rather distinctive clinicopathologic phenotype, and possibly prognostic differences from conventional melanoma, although this has not been definitively proven). So-called MBN are extremely rare, with fewer than 100 cases thus far being reported. Clinically, the average age at diagnosis is about 46 years, two-thirds of the patients are men, and the commonest site is the scalp. MBN most frequently presents as blue or blue-black plaques or nodules ranging from 1 to 4 cm (mean, 2.9 cm) that are often multinodular. There is usually a history of recent enlargement or change in a previously stable blue nevus. MBN usually are highly aggressive with metastasis to lymph nodes and a variety of visceral sites.

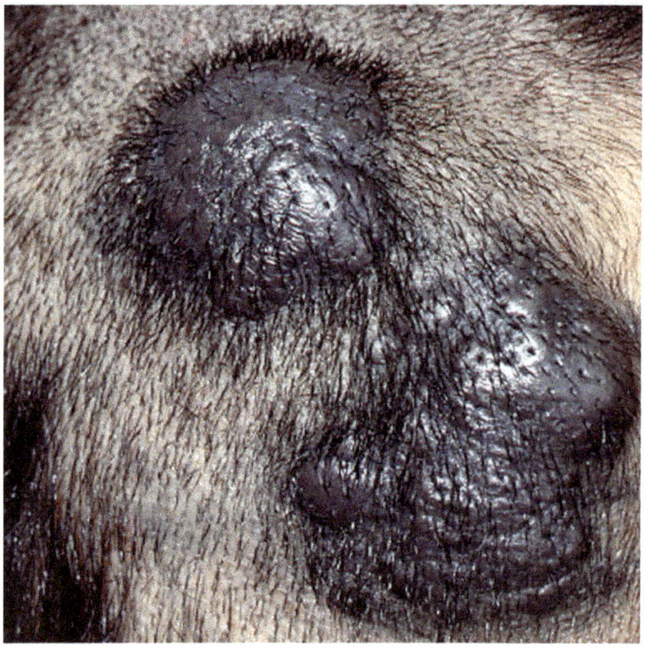

Blue nevus-like melanoma (malignant blue nevus). There is a recently enlarging multinodular blue-black lesion on the scalp. (Reproduced with permission from Wolff K, Johnson RA, Saavedra AP. *Fitzpatrick's Color Atlas and Synopsis of Clinical Dermatology*. 7th ed. New York, NY: McGraw-Hill Education; 2013.)

Microscopically, MBN usually presents in one of three patterns: (1) a lesion with an overtly malignant component juxtaposed to a benign blue nevus component, usually a

CBN; (2) a more subtle sarcoma-like presentation (without florid benign and malignant components) initially suggesting CBN but exhibiting large densely cellular fascicles or nodules of spindle cells that on closer inspection have mitoses and sufficient atypicality for malignancy and are distinctly more abnormal than the usual small fascicular or alveolar patterns in CBN; or (3) a lesion of "atypical blue nevus" that subsequently results in malignant behavior. In the most common presentation, MBN are characterized by nodular or multinodular aggregations of spindle cells in tightly packed fascicles in the dermis and often the subcutis. By definition, there is sparing of the epidermis. Occasional epithelioid cells and multinucleate giant cells are encountered. Melanin pigment and cytoplasmic vacuolization are noted in approximately two-thirds of cases. Necrosis, a feature previously thought characteristic of MBN, is observed in only about one-third of cases. In general, there is striking cytologic atypia, prominent nuclear pleomorphism, infrequent mitotic figures (about one to two mitoses/mm^2) and uncommonly atypical mitoses. Most MBN have a component of CBN, but elements of common blue nevus may also be observed.

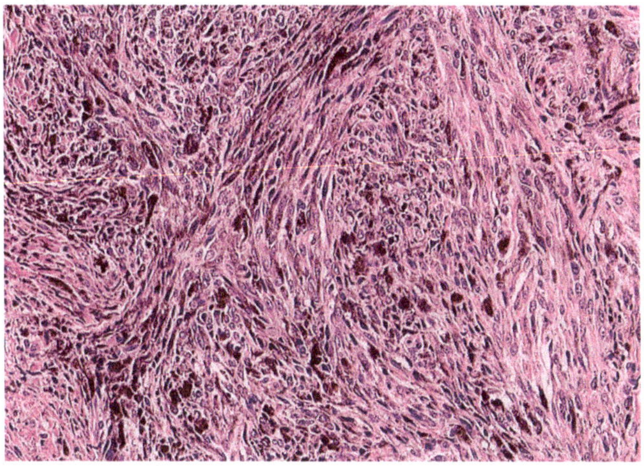

Malignant blue nevus, sarcoma-like presentation. Fascicular arrangements of atypical spindle cells, many of which contain melanin, can be observed in this field.

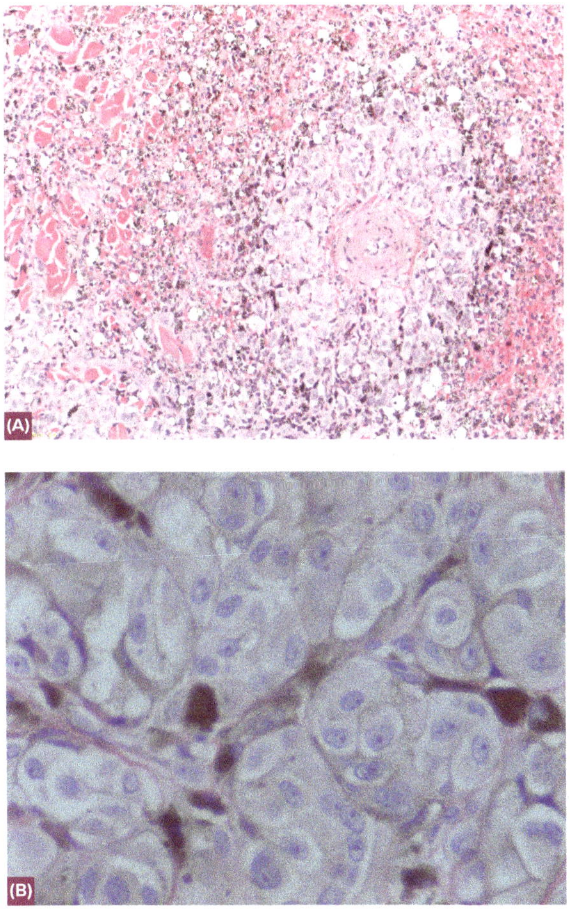

Malignant blue nevus, overt melanoma arising within CBN. (A) There are features of conventional cellular blue nevus juxtaposed to an overtly malignant component. **(B)** The malignant cells exhibit marked pleomorphism, enlarged nuclei, and prominent nucleoli. Up to three mitoses per mm^2 were identified in this lesion.

ANSWER 10-19: E.

The clinical features of the patient and the mother are highly suspicious for **Carney complex**. The biopsy reveals a large, poorly defined, yet symmetrical dermal-based proliferation of pigmented melanocytes. The melanocytes are large and epithelioid with large, round, pleomorphic nuclei containing large nucleoli. There is a mixture of heavily pigmented and slightly pigmented cells. The findings are consistent with an **epithelioid blue nevus**, which is a variant of blue nevus that has been described in association with the **Carney complex**. This syndrome is autosomal dominant and characterized by multiple **lentigines**, **psammomatous melanotic schwannomas, myxomas** involving the skin, heart, and breast, and endocrine tumors of the adrenal cortex, pituitary, testis, and thyroid. Carney complex is associated with point mutations in the *PRKAR1A* (protein kinase A regulatory subunit 1α) gene located on 17q22-24 (loss of tumor suppressor function). Nonetheless, such **blue nevi** occur outside the latter syndrome. Additional controversial neoplasms have been reported in the literature as "**pigmented epithelioid melanocytoma**" and "**animal-type melanoma**." These sporadic tumors will be discussed later. In addition to features of an ordinary blue nevus, epithelioid blue nevi often show epidermal thinning and effacement or sometimes hyperplasia. The epithelioid melanocytes of two types: (1) heavily pigmented polygonal cells with nuclei largely obscured by melanin granules and (2) lightly pigmented polygonal cells often with large vesicular nuclei and prominent nucleoli. Rare mitotic figures are observed in a significant proportion of cases. The presence of mitotic figures should prompt careful study for other atypical features and the possibility of melanoma.

The recently reported entity "pigmented epithelioid melanocytoma" shares features with if not being identical to epithelioid blue nevus. Previously, a subset of heavily pigmented sporadic tumors with similar histomorphology (yet with increased cytologic atypia) was reported in the literature as "animal-type melanoma." This designation was derived from a shared histomorphology with pigmented tumors arising in gray horses and laboratory animals; however, these animal tumors have a different molecular basis. The designation of "pigmented epithelioid melanocytoma" is meant to encompass the spectrum between epithelioid blue nevus and animal melanoma. These lesions have demonstrated a significant frequency of sentinel lymph node involvement (47% in one study) perhaps comparable to **Spitz tumors**. Even with lymph node disease, these tumors appear to be more indolent than conventional melanoma and may have a better prognosis, as most patients reported in the literature have done well. However, poor outcomes with distant metastatic disease and death have occurred. While there is loss of expression of protein kinase A regulatory subunit 1α (R1alpha) in lesions of pigmented epithelioid melanocytoma and epithelioid blue nevus of Carney complex, pigmented epithelioid melanocytoma shows loss of heterozygosity in 17q22-24 but no PRKAR1A point mutations. Although some proportion of both epithelioid blue nevi (and pigmented epithelioid melanocytomas) demonstrate atypical features, including cytologic atypia and increased mitotic rates, that raise concern as to their biologic potential, progression to overt malignancy has only rarely been documented and usually after one or more recurrences. Therefore, these tumors must be completely excised and the patients closely monitored for recurrence.

Pilar neurocristic hamartoma is a rare congenital lesion characterized by multiple perifollicular papules occupying an area of skin measuring several centimeters in diameter. Individual papules vary in color from tan to blue or black. There is some similarity to patch and plaque-like blue nevi in humans and pigmented epithelioid melanocytomas.

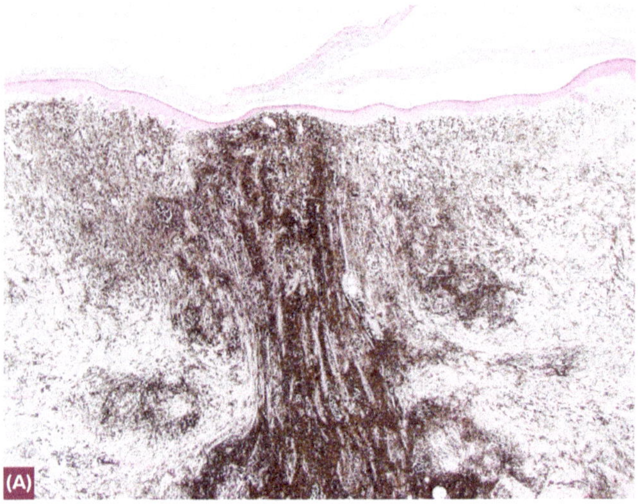

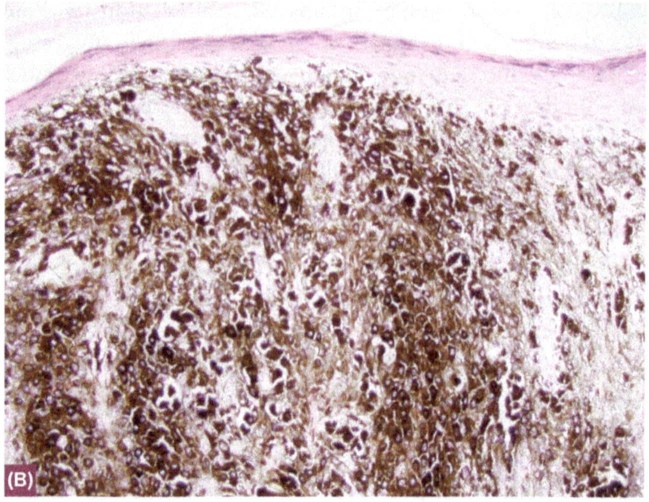

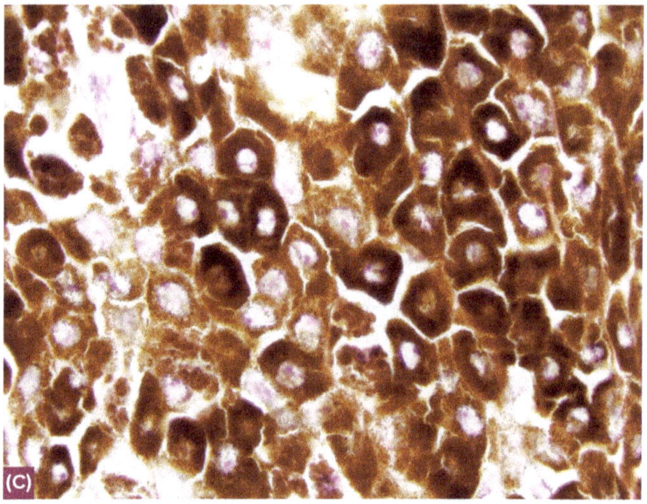

Pigmented epithelioid melanocytoma/animal type melanoma. (A) There is a poorly circumscribed dermal-based melanocytic proliferation that extends into the deep dermis. **(B)** The overlying epidermis is attenuated. **(C)** The melanocytes are all heavily pigmented and exhibit mild nuclear pleomorphism. No mitotic activity is present.

The most characteristic feature is prominent perifollicular accumulations of dendritic melanocytes showing extension to nearby eccrine ducts. The intervening reticular dermis contains scattered pigmented dendritic cells resembling a Mongolian spot.

ANSWER 10-20: E.

Spitzoid melanocytic proliferations have occupied a special niche in the melanocytic neoplastic system for many years, and increasing evidence suggests that they are a biologically unique melanocytic neoplasm (Table 10-20A). Yet there are still many unresolved questions with respect to the biologic nature, natural history, and biologic potential of spitzoid melanocytic lesions in general.

Table 10-20A. Spitz Nevus or Tumor

Clinical Features
Configuration: plaque, papule, or nodule, often dome shaped
Size: small (usually <1 cm)
Profile: smooth surface topography
Color: pink or red; darker forms occur
Age: majority in children and adolescents
Location: face and extremities most common
Number: usually solitary; rare multiple forms occur
Symptoms: commonly asymptomatic; rarely pruritic
History of growth: months; usually <1 year
Histopathologic Features
Cytologic features
Spindle or epithelioid cell type[a]
Overall monomorphous population of cells[a]
Occasional striking pleomorphism in a minority of cells
Architectural features
Symmetry[a]
Sharp lateral demarcation[a]
Zonation in depth (eg, "maturation")[a]
Orderly nondisruptive infiltration of collagen by Spitz nevus[a] cells
Other helpful diagnostic features
Absent or rare, but not atypical, mitoses in deep parts[a]
Giant nevus cells
Irregular contours of growth at deep margin[a]
Kamino bodies
Paucity or absence of single cell upward spread
Junctional clefts
Loss of cohesion between cells (retraction spaces)
Perivascular or diffuse inflammatory infiltrate
Superficial distribution of pigmentation
Telangiectasia and edema
Epidermal hyperplasia
Differential Diagnosis
Melanocytic lesions
Malignant melanoma
Atypical nevi with features of Spitz nevus
Variants of nevi with spindle or epithelioid cells
Pigmented spindle cell nevus
Desmoplastic Spitz nevus
Plexiform spindle cell nevus or deep-penetrating nevus
Cellular blue nevus
Various "combined" nevi
Nonmelanocytic lesions
Juvenile xanthogranuloma
Epithelioid cell histiocytoma
Reticulohistiocytoma
Cellular neurothekeoma

[a]Most helpful features.

The **Spitz nevus** (or **Spitz tumor**) has been recognized for well over a century but was first definitively characterized in 1948 by Sophie Spitz. Spitz believed that such lesions represented a juvenile counterpart of melanomas occurring in adults. **Spitz tumors** are usually acquired but may be congenital. The characteristics that set this nevus apart from other nevi are large epithelioid or spindle cells in varying proportions and frequent misdiagnosis as melanoma.

Clinically, **Spitz nevi** most often present as a solitary; asymptomatic; red, pink, or flesh colored; hairless; dome shaped; smooth nodule measuring less than 1 cm in diameter. Some lesions may be tan, brown, or even black in color. Pedunculated and polypoid forms occur. Spitz nevi may involve any site; however, there is a predilection for the face and the extremities. They may be slightly more common in females. Multiple Spitz nevi may occur in either a grouped (agminate) or disseminated pattern. The disseminated type is characterized by numerous, up to hundreds of Spitz tumors all over the body, typically sparing the palms, soles, and mucous membranes.

The vast majority of lesions with characteristics of Spitz nevi are benign. However, because of the histopathologic resemblance of Spitz nevi to some malignant melanomas, the presence of atypical variants, and rare metastases from such lesions, there is some justification for the belief that melanoma may uncommonly or rarely develop in association with Spitz nevi. The exact nature and classification of these lesions await definitive study.

Microscopically, spitzoid lesions, similar to other melanocytic lesions, occur along a histologic continuum of benign, atypical, and malignant and must be evaluated using all clinical, histopathologic, and other criteria available. After examination, one can usually assign a given lesion to one of three categories: (1) **Spitz nevus**; (2) Spitz tumors with one or more atypical features (**atypical Spitz tumor**), including those with indeterminate biologic or malignant potential; and (3) malignant melanoma with Spitzoid cytomorphology (**spitzoid melanoma**). Coming back to Question 10-20, this lesion is most consistent with a benign compound Spitz nevus.

The authors believe that it is overly simplistic to impose an (often arbitrary) interpretation of either "Spitz nevus" or malignant melanoma on every spitzoid lesion. This approach is not satisfactory for patient care and does not provide a realistic methodology for dealing prospectively with such a difficult problem. Such an exercise undoubtedly results in both the overdiagnosis of melanoma and under-recognition of atypical or ambiguous lesions requiring more medical attention. Patients may unfairly suffer the psychological burden of a grave diagnosis and be subjected to overly aggressive and potentially harmful therapies. Conversely, some proportion of patients will have the false and unjustified assurances of a benign diagnosis and may not receive appropriate treatment and follow-up.

The most distinctive histopathologic feature and an absolute prerequisite for diagnosis is the presence of large epithelioid or spindle-shaped melanocytes. The "**epithelioid Spitz nevus cells**" are large, round, oval, polygonal, rhomboidal, or polyangular cells with distinct cellular borders.

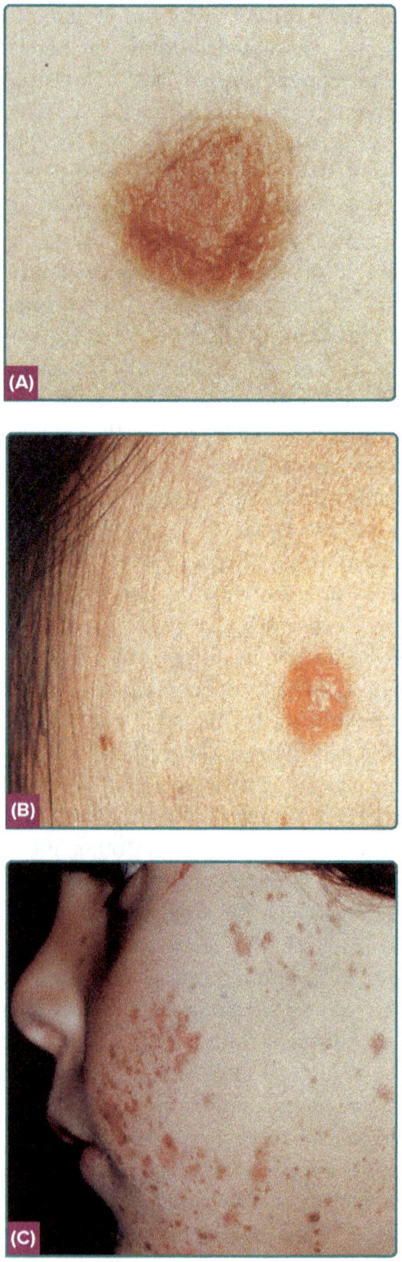

Spitz nevi. (A) Pink plaque, which appeared de novo over an 8-week period, becoming more elevated with time, in the preauricular area of a 4-year-old white boy. **(B)** Dome-shaped pink papule, which appeared de novo over a 2-week interval 4 months before, on the forehead of a 5-year-old white boy. **(C)** Agminated Spitz tumors. Numerous grouped pink papules and plaques, appearing at age 6 months, on the face of a 4-year-old white boy. (Reproduced, with permission, from Goldsmith LA, Katz SI, Gilchrest BA, Paller AS, Leffell DJ, Wolff K, eds. *Fitzpatrick's Dermatology in General Medicine*. 8th ed. New York, NY: McGraw-Hill Education; 2012.)

The "**spindled Spitz nevus cells**" are elongated, fusiform, and often plump and may exhibit dendrites. Both cell types possess centrally located nuclei, comparable in size to or even larger than the nuclei of keratinocytes. The nuclear contours are typically smooth and regular. The chromatin pattern is usually finely dispersed ("hollowed out") or slightly vesicular. Typically, a distinct, single, centrally located, round eosinophilic or amphophilic nucleolus is present. Multinucleated cells are often seen when epithelioid forms constitute the predominant cell type. The cytoplasms of both spindle and epithelioid cells are usually abundant with a homogeneous eosinophilic or bluish, sometimes "ground glass" appearance. Melanin is typically absent or scarce. The two cell types may be admixed in varying proportions, but either may occur alone. Regardless of the proportion of spindle or epithelioid cells, one of the most characteristic features of Spitz nevus is the uniformity of the cells and nuclei. From side-to-side, in horizontal zones, the cells tend to show a strikingly uniform appearance and size. In all age groups, Spitz nevi with predominant spindle cell morphology are the most common type and are especially prevalent in adults. Spitz nevi of the epithelioid cell type are observed mainly in children.

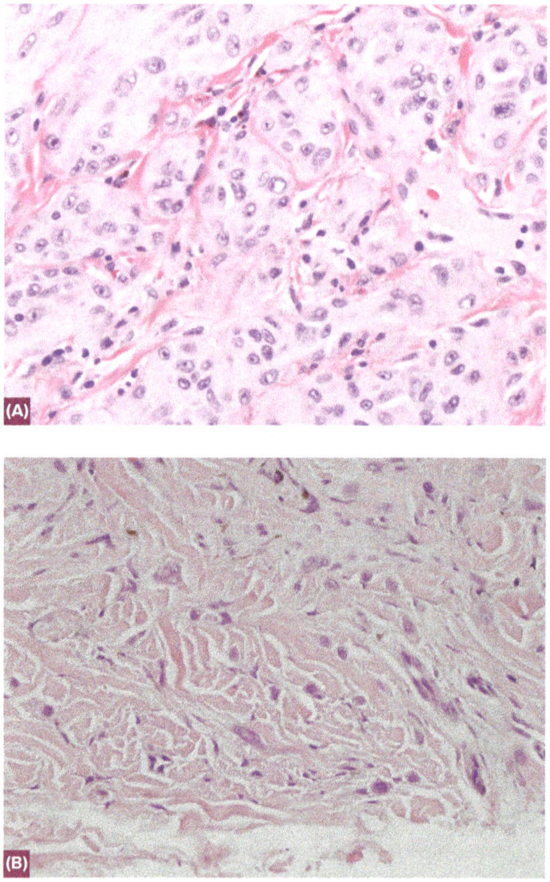

Spitzoid cytomorphology. (A) Epithelioid Spitz cytomorphology. There are oval-shaped cells containing abundant eosinophilic to amphophilic cytoplasm. The nuclei are enlarged and contain finely dispersed ("hollowed out") chromatin and a single prominent nucleolus. A few rare eosinophilic nuclear pseudo-inclusions are present, which represent cytoplasmic invagination over the nucleus. **(B)** Spindle Spitz cytomorphology. The cells exhibit similar cytoplasms and nuclei to the epithelioid form, but have a spindled shape. Note the uniformity of the cytomorphology ("typically atypical"). (Image B Used with permission of Claudia Vidal, MD, PhD, St. Louis University School of Medicine.)

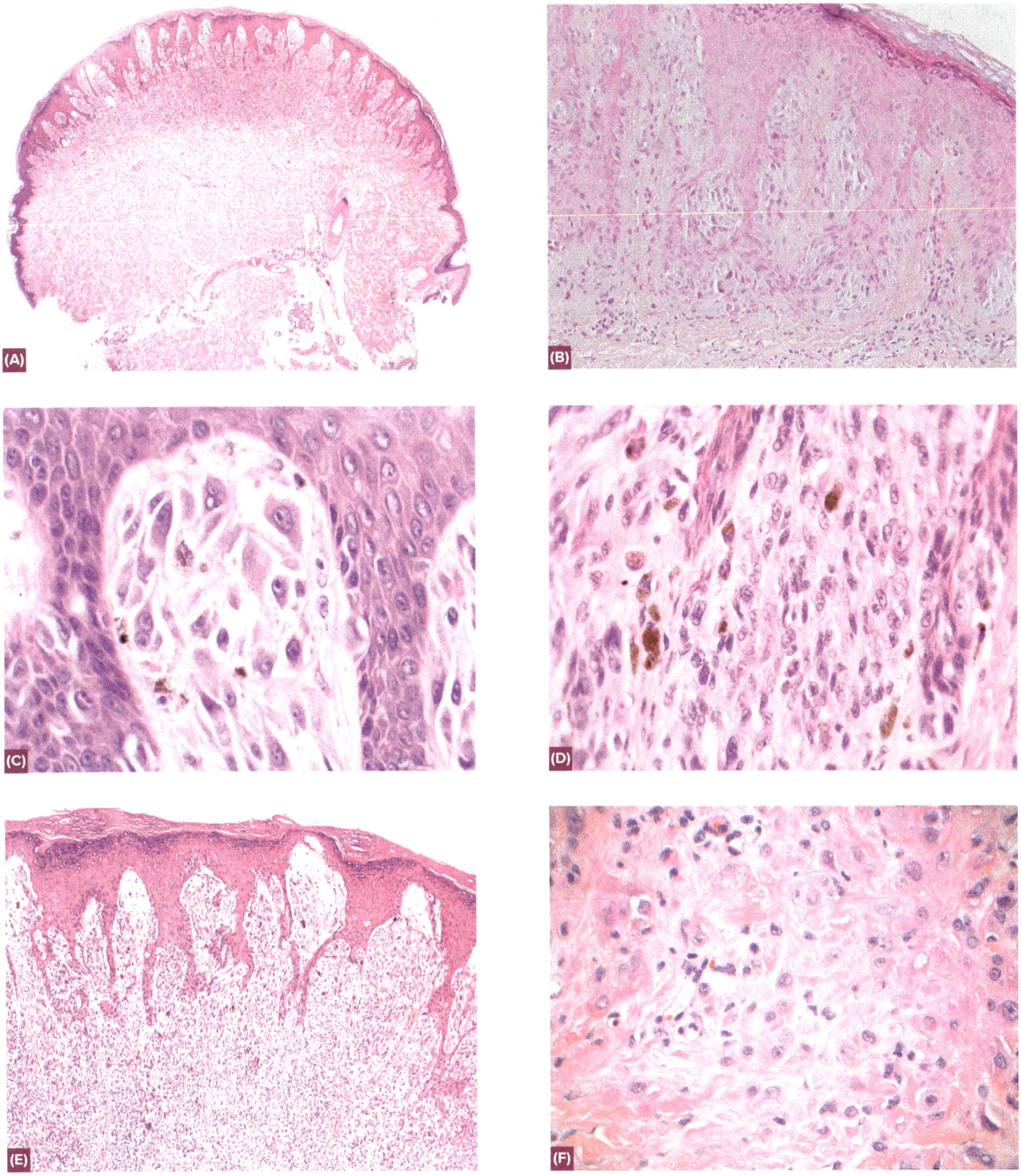

Spitz nevus. **(A)** Note the small diameter, dome-shaped morphology, striking symmetry from side to side, and sharp lateral demarcation. **(B)** The elongated junctional nests are oriented perpendicular (vertical) to the epidermal surface and exhibit large cleft-like retraction spaces. **(C)** Large epithelioid cells and spindle cells in the papillary dermis. Note the angular contours of the cells; some are triangular, some are rhomboidal, and some are polygonal in morphology. The cytoplasm is pink with a ground glass appearance. Many nuclei contain prominent nucleoli. **(D)** Fascicles of spindle cells with abundant cytoplasms. Note the striking uniformity of the spindle cells. The cells have abundant pink cytoplasms. Also note uniformity of nuclei with evenly dispersed chromatin. **(E)** Superficial portion of Spitz nevus demonstrating vertically oriented, predominately spindled melanocytes and progressive dispersion (maturation) of the melanocytic aggregates with depth. **(F)** Base of Spitz nevus shows orderly infiltration of collagen by individual cells (maturation).

Although spindle or epithelioid cells are a prerequisite for diagnosis, they must appear in an appropriate architectural arrangement to properly designate a lesion as a benign nevus. The majority of Spitz nevi (≥66% or more) are compound, 5%-10% are junctional, and 12%-20% are dermal. The major architectural criteria for benignity include: symmetry, sharp lateral demarcation, size (generally <1 cm in diameter), maturation (zonation), lack of deep extension, lack of ulceration, lack of significant pagetoid spread, and few or no deeply located mitoses. Additionally, lesions arising in individuals younger than 10 years of age are significantly more likely to have a benign clinical course. The characteristic architectural features that accompany Spitz nevi include elongated junctional and dermal nests arranged in a vertical orientation. This is different from the frequent parallel spindling of nests seen in **dysplastic nevi**. At the dermal–epidermal junction, the fascicles or nests of spindle cells are often separated by a cleft-like retraction space from the adjacent epidermis, a result of tissue shrinkage during processing. Unlike melanomas, which typically consume the overlying epidermis and efface the rete ridges, Spitz nevi are associated with epidermal hyperplasia. Eosinophilic amorphous globules (**Kamino bodies**), either singly or in aggregates, at the dermal–epidermal junction occur frequently in Spitz nevi and are useful because they are found less frequently in patients with melanoma. However, they are nonspecific. Ultrastructurally, these Kamino bodies are composed of amorphous masses and bundles of filaments. Immunohistochemically, they contain basement membrane components, including collagen types IV and VII, as well as laminin. Degenerate material derived from melanocytes and keratinocytes may also be present. Several Kamino bodies are present within the junctional nests of the lesion in the question. Like benign common acquired nevi, maturation with dermal descent should be present. Whether or not these lesions arise from an intraepidermal stem cell (top-to-bottom) or a dermal stem cell (bottom-to-top) remains to be answered; however, this zonation or layering of melanocytes with differing morphology is important in confirming benign biological behavior. The cytologic features of the spindle or epithelioid cells change from superficial to deep, leading to a gradient in cell size and shape, such as from large, plump cells at the top to smaller or more slender cells at the bottom. With this zonation, the cellular elements exhibit a nondisruptive insinuation among collagen bundles without induction of new stroma. If melanin is present in Spitz nevi, it is largely confined to cells immediately subjacent to the epidermis.

Mitoses in Spitz nevi are variable, but are typically rare or absent. Combined Melan-A/Ki-67 immunostain typically should not label greater than 10% of the dermal melanocyte nuclei. When mitoses are present, they most commonly occur in the upper portion of the lesion and are usually bipolar. Although an occasional mitosis in the deeper parts of the lesion or a rare atypical mitosis may be observed, they should nonetheless prompt careful evaluation for melanoma. Pagetoid spread of single melanocytes occurs less often in Spitz nevus than in melanoma. Upward migration of melanocytes in Spitz nevus usually takes the form of transepidermal elimination of nests of two or more cells. Additionally, the pagetoid melanocytes tend to be located within the central portions of the lesion. Similar to congenital nevi, Spitz nevi have a propensity to involve hair follicles and eccrine ducts. In most instances, intraepidermal fascicles of cells track along the adventitial sheaths of appendageal structures into the papillary dermis and often into the reticular dermis.

Although there are no standard recommendations in regards to surgical management of spitzoid neoplasms, a wide excision on the face for a benign Spitz nevus is excessive and inappropriate. It is generally recommended to completely remove all Spitz nevi/tumors, but this lesion could be easily managed with small conservative re-excision.

ANSWER 10-21: E.

Routine light microscopy remains the gold standard for deciphering between benign and malignant melanocytic proliferations, in which architectural and cytologic features are independently assessed to formulate a prediction of biological behavior. The adjunct of immunohistochemistry has been a major advancement in interpreting melanocytic lesions. Additionally, these immunohistochemical stains play an important role in identifying benign and malignant melanocyte deposits within lymph nodes. Melanocyte specific markers are most useful in highlighting the location and density of melanocytes within the epidermis and dermis. The most frequently used melanocyte specific stains are **Melan-A (MART-1)** and **microphthalmia-associated transcription factor (MITF)**, which stain melanocyte cytoplasm and nuclei, respectively. The overall sensitivity of Melan-A is high in primary melanoma (85%-95%), but is considerably reduced in metastatic melanomas (57%-92%), poorly differentiated melanomas, and melanomas with a spindle cell cytomorphology. It is worth mentioning that Melan-A reacts with PEComas, clear cell sarcomas, and some adrenal cortical and gonadal steroid tumors. MITF also has a reported high sensitivity (81%-100%) for primary melanomas with epithelioid cytomorphology; however, its expression is also substantially reduced in melanomas with spindle cell cytomorphology.

S100 and **Sox-10** are sensitive but nonspecific markers for melanocytic differentiation and are most useful in examining poorly differentiated and spindle cell primary melanomas and metastatic melanomas where the tumors have lost expression of melanocyte specific markers (ie, Melan-A, MITF). S100 is a cytoplasmic and nuclear stain and SOX-10 is a nuclear stain. S100 has a low specificity and stains Langerhans cells, lymph node dendritic cells, some histiocytoses, some myoepithelial

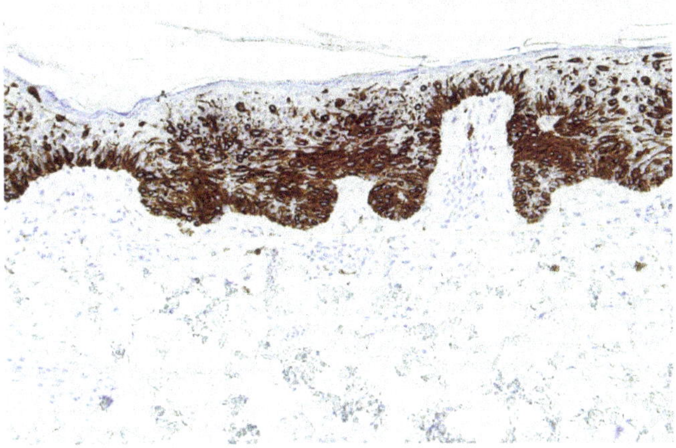

Melan-A immunohistochemical stain with brown chromogen. Note the cytoplasmic staining within melanocytes. In this case of melanoma in situ, superficial spreading type, the stain is extremely helpful in highlighting the increased density of melanocytes as well as extensive pagetoid ascent. There are a few pigmented melanophages in the dermis with a lighter shade of brown than the immunohistochemical chromogen.

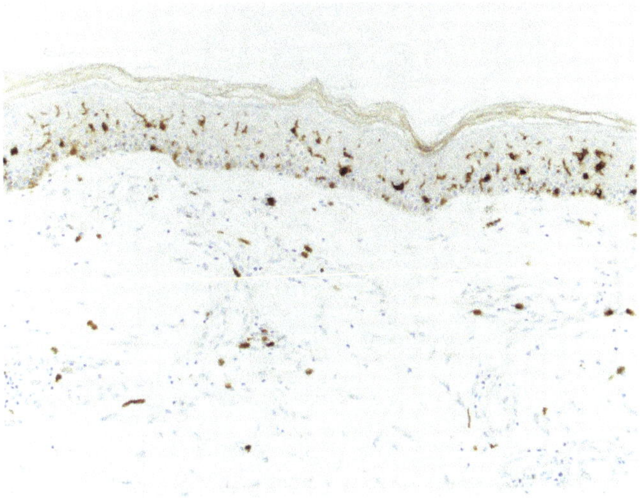

S100 immunohistochemical stain with brown chromogen. This is an example of normal skin. There is cytoplasmic staining and nuclear staining within both basal layer melanocytes and upper spinous Langerhans cells. Additionally, there are scattered dermal histiocytes that are staining. This lack of specificity makes S100 a rather unhelpful marker in the interpretation of primary melanocytic proliferations.

cells, and cells with peripheral nerve sheath differentiation. This high sensitivity is helpful in identifying benign and malignant melanocyte deposits within lymph nodes; however, the proper interpretation may be difficult since lymph nodes also contain numerous Langerhans cells and antigen presenting dendritic cells. SOX-10 has a similar sensitivity but a higher specificity when interpreting lymph nodes since it is not expressed in Langerhans cells, antigen presenting dendritic cells, or other histiocytoses. An overall advantage of markers with nuclear staining (MITF and SOX-10) versus cytoplasmic staining (Melan-A and S100) is in the setting of heavily pigmented cells where brown cytoplasmic melanin pigment may be difficult to distinguish from chromogen.

While the above markers are extremely helpful in identifying melanocytes and highlighting their densities and distributions (architectural features), they provide little information regarding their cytology or biological nature. In regards to a "cytologic" or biological melanocyte marker, **gp100 (HMB45)** is positively expressed in the cytoplasm of fetal melanocytes but not normal adult melanocytes. However, junctional (intraepidermal) and papillary dermal nevus cells are positive for HMB45, as they are benign melanocytic neoplasms. The expression is typically lost as the intradermal nevus cells descend into the dermis. Preserved expression within the descending deeper dermal melanocytes is a useful confirmation of invasive melanoma. The major drawback to the application of this stain is lack of differential staining in benign nevi and radial growth phase melanoma/melanoma in situ (both will be positive). Additionally, HMB45 is frequently expressed in normal melanocytes within or near recent surgical scar beds of tumor re-excisions or trauma. Thus, HMB45 is an antigen that appears in adult intraepidermal melanocytes during stimulation and benign and malignant transformation, and is therefore not a useful marker for diagnosing melanoma in situ or superficially invasive melanoma. Additionally, HMB45 is strongly expressed in the heavily pigmented spindled melanocytes of blue nevi, dermal melanocytoses, and plexiform spindle cell nevi/ tumors. Therefore, while the interpretation of HMB45 expression may be helpful in some situations, one must take into account other factors such as scar formation, patient age, and cytomorphology. Lastly, positive expression of HMB45 in deposits of melanocytes located within lymph nodes is helpful in establishing a diagnosis of metastatic melanoma. Again, the interpretation must be approached with caution since various forms of blue nevi frequently deposit in lymph nodes and will also express HMB45. Clinical pathological correlation is always recommended.

Proliferation markers such as **Ki-67** may provide additional information as, for example, labeling indices below 5% favoring benign lesions versus those above 15%-25% favoring melanomas. The use of other biomarkers such as loss of expression of **p16** and **cyclin-dependent kinase 4** and increased expression of **cyclin D1** favor melanoma versus benign or atypical melanocytic lesions. The antigen localization of **soluble adenylyl cyclase (sAC/R21)** has also been reported to differentiate benign (perinuclear dot staining) and malignant (pannuclear staining) melanocytes. Additional larger studies will be needed to better determine sensitivity and specificity of these markers and their eventual use in routine practice.

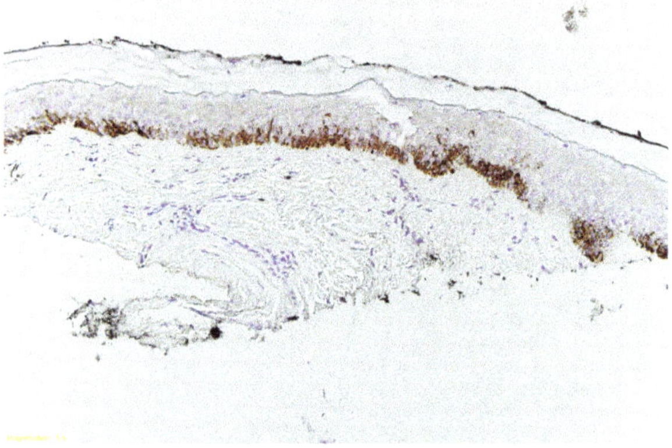

HMB45 immunohistochemical stain with brown chromogen. This is an example of benign "paracicatricial" melanocytic hyperplasia overlying a dermal scar. Note the positive cytoplasmic expression in these benign "activated" melanocytes. Without the proper context, this lesion could easily be misdiagnosed as lentigo maligna.

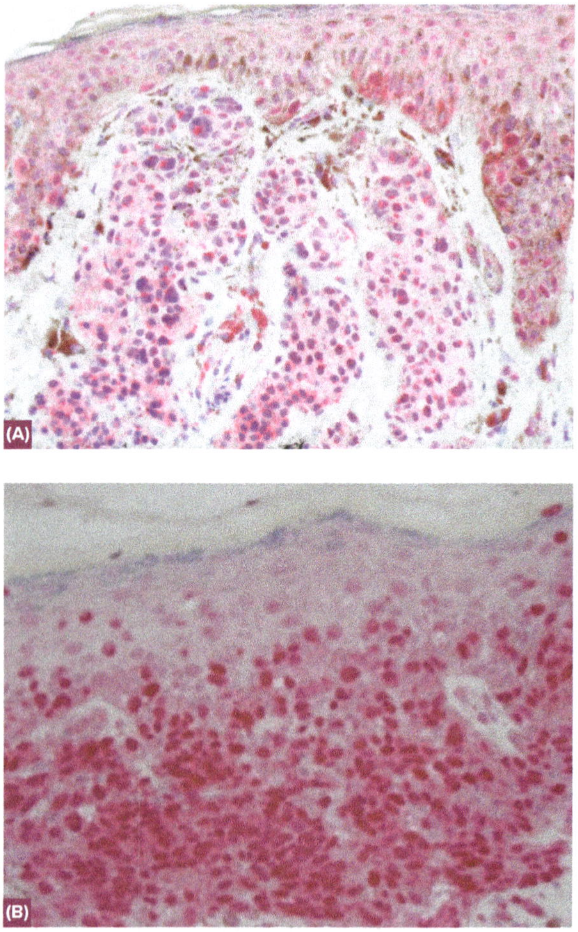

Soluble adenylyl cyclase (sAC/R21) with red chromogen. (A) Benign intradermal nevus with discrete perinuclear dot staining. **(B)** Malignant melanoma with strong pannuclear staining.

Finally, **comparative genomic hybridization (CGH)** has demonstrated that increased numbers and types of chromosomal aberrations (both losses and gains of DNA copy number) in melanocytic lesions may facilitate the diagnosis of melanoma and its distinction from other melanocytic neoplasms. CGH may help define the developmental pathways of melanoma.

ANSWER 10-22: B.

The biopsy reveals a slightly attenuated epidermis with a lentiginous melanocytic proliferation, occasional junctional nests, and rare pagetoid melanocytes. There is dermal fibrosis, vertical dilated vessels, and scattered inflammatory cells. At the base of the fibrosis are nests and solitary units of small melanocytes. This is an example of a **recurrent/residual compound congenital nevus**; however, clinical pathologic correlation, review of the prior biopsy material, and examination of areas present outside of the scar bed are needed to establish a definitive diagnosis (Table 10-22A). The recurrent melanocytic nevus (**recurrent nevus phenomenon**) shows pigmentation at the site of previous nevus removal or biopsy. Most of the recurrences have followed a shave excision. Approximately 50% of cases recur within 6 months. This phenomenon is thought to result from an intraepidermal proliferation of residual melanocytes, possibly from nearby sweat ducts, hair follicles, or intraepidermal melanocytes.

Clinically, these lesions are characterized by circumscribed hyperpigmentation within a scar from the previous surgical procedure for nevus removal or from other forms of trauma to the area. The lesion is usually macular and exhibits variable irregularity of borders and pigment pattern. Most recurrent nevi measure 4-6 mm in diameter and almost all are smaller than 1.5 cm.

Table 10-22A. Recurrent Melanocytic Nevus

Clinical Features
Onset about 6 weeks-6 months after previous surgery
Macular pigmentation
Limited to scar
4-6 mm (usually <1.5 cm)
Often some irregularity of borders
Histopathologic Features
Effacement of epidermis
Dermal scar
Intraepidermal melanocytic proliferation limited to area above scar
Lentiginous or nested pattern of intraepidermal melanocytes
Variable cytologic atypia, usually low grade
Differential Diagnosis
Atypical (dysplastic) nevus
Melanoma

Histopathologic examination usually reveals intraepidermal melanocytic proliferation confined to the area above a dermal scar. There is effacement of the epidermal rete ridge pattern and a variable lentiginous or nested intraepidermal proliferation of melanocytes. Occasional melanocytes may be present above the basal layer. This latter feature may also be focally present (ie, one to two cells) in **irritated nevi** exhibiting regular columns of pigment in the stratum corneum. Since the healing process distorts the architecture of the lesion, the distinction from malignant melanoma may be extremely difficult. The melanocytes often contain abundant melanin and relatively uniform nuclei but occasionally exhibit low-grade cytologic atypia. Dysplastic nevi tend to recur with fairly similar grades of cytologic atypia compared with the original lesion removed. Frequently, residual dermal nevus cells are seen beneath the superficial dermal scar.

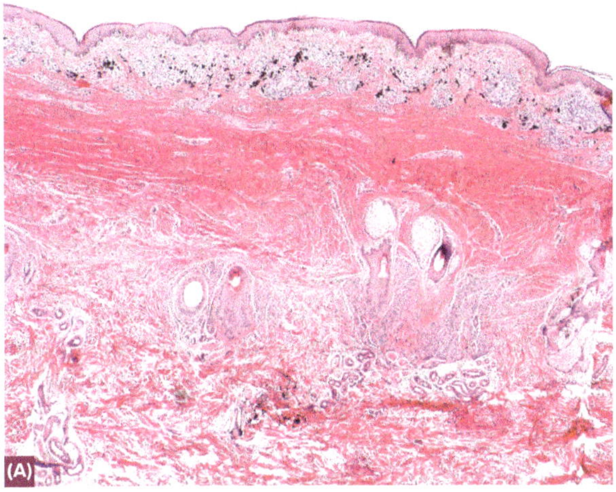

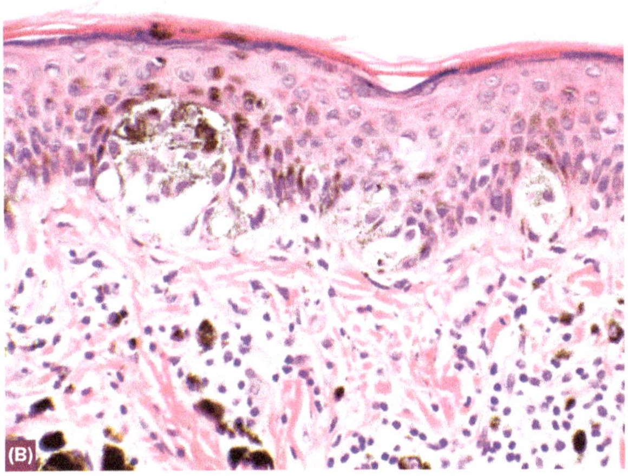

Recurrent melanocytic nevus. (A) Scanning magnification shows regenerative melanocytic proliferation along and subjacent to the effaced epidermis. A dermal scar lies between the epidermis, the regenerative superficial melanocytic dermal elements, and the original dermal nevus component previously biopsied (lower center of the field). **(B)** There is irregular single-cell and nested melanocytic proliferation at the dermal–epidermal junction. However, significant cytologic atypia of melanocytes is absent.

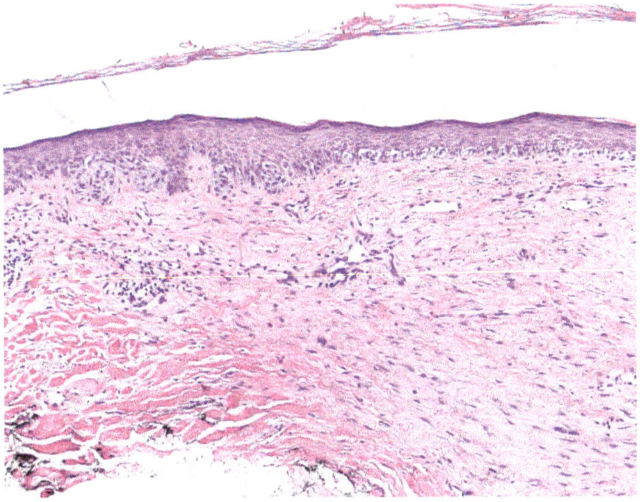

Residual melanocytic nevus with adjacent recurrent nevus phenomenon.

The differential diagnosis includes recurrent atypical (dysplastic) nevus, reactive lentiginous melanocytic proliferations developing in excision scars, and recurrent melanoma. In general, **recurrent melanocytic nevus** is usually but not always confined to the area of the surgical scar, appears within 6 months of surgery, and exhibits well-defined margins and a banal histologic picture. Recurrent atypical (dysplastic) nevi may have greater cytologic atypia than conventional recurrent nevi. Clinical features suggesting melanoma include irregular pigmentation, recurrence beyond the confines of the surgical scar, and a longer interval to recurrence (>6 months). Melanocytic lesions with similar forms of architectural distortion may be seen in other settings of fibrosis such as lichen sclerosus, fibrous papules, dermatofibromas, and the umbilicus. Review of the previous biopsy is mandatory to rule out an atypical proliferation, particularly melanoma. Re-excision of a recurrent nevus is not necessary unless abnormal features are present, for example, extension of distorted melanocytic architecture beyond the surgical scar or substantial cytologic atypia.

ANSWER 10-23: D.

The biopsy reveals a lentiginous and partially intraepidermal melanocytic proliferation involving an attenuated epidermis with scattered pagetoid melanocytes. This population of cells is nicely highlighted by the Melan-A stain. However, there is a subtle spindle cell population occupying the dermis accompanied by sclerosis and loose lymphocytic aggregates. These cells are negative for Melan-A but are strongly positive for S100. The findings are consistent with the **pure type of desmoplastic melanoma** arising in association with **lentigo maligna**.

Desmoplastic melanoma (DM) is a rare variant of cutaneous melanoma first reported by Conley et al in 1971 (Table 10-23A). In one population-based study, the general

Table 10-23A. Desmoplastic Neurotropic Melanoma

Clinical Features
- Age 60-65 years
- Men ≥ women
- Sun-exposed skin, head and neck, but also acral, mucosal sites
- Firm nodule
- Flesh-colored or with pigmented lesion (29%-43%)
- 1-3 cm
- Occasional dysesthesias, nerve palsies

Histopathologic Features
- Intraepidermal melanocytic proliferation in >75%
  - Solar melanoma in situ, most common
- Fibrous nodule in dermis and possibly subcutis
- Often absence of pigment
- Fascicles of atypical spindle cells
- Schwannian, perineurial differentiation
- Neurotropism common (perineurial and endoneurial invasion)
- Patchy lymphoid infiltrates common
- Variable myxoid stroma
- Occasional mitoses in dermis

Differential Diagnosis
- Sclerosing blue nevi including variants with hypercellularity
- Desmoplastic (sclerosing) Spitz nevus
- Neurothekeoma, particularly cellular variants
- Malignant peripheral nerve sheath tumors
- Myxoma
- Dermatofibroma
- Dermatofibrosarcoma protuberans
- Atypical fibroxanthoma
- Malignant fibrous histiocytoma
- Scar
- Fibromatosis
- Spindle cell squamous cell carcinoma
- Leiomyosarcoma

Immunohistochemistry
- S-100 protein +
- Vimentin +
- p75 neurotrophin receptor +
- Sox10 +
- HMB45, MART-1, MIFT, tyrosinase often –
- Leu 7 –
- Keratin –

prevalence of DM was estimated as 1% of all cutaneous melanomas. It has become increasing evident that DM is a distinctive clinicopathologic variant of melanoma with unique biological characteristics. Of course, one must bear in mind that DM exhibits a histopathologic continuum of features shared with other melanoma subtypes, and their properties are directly related to the criteria used to define DM and how rigidly they are applied. The phenotype of the tumor corresponds to the neuroectodermal origin of the melanocyte and thus may include any combination of conventional melanoma; desmoplasia; neurotropism (perineural and intraneural invasion); neural differentiation (both schwannian and perineural/neurofibroma-like); and less commonly, neuroendocrine, myofibroblastic, or other diverse forms of mesenchymal differentiation. Although DM most frequently arises in association with lentiginous melanomas, de novo variants of DM also occur. The pathogenesis of desmoplasia and the true nature of the spindle cells in DM remain a subject of controversy. Some authors maintain that the fibroplasia results from the induction of collagen synthesis by benign fibroblasts, but others believe that melanoma cells function as adaptive fibroblasts to promote collagenization in these tumors. The latter conclusion is based on ultrastructural and immunohistochemical studies and the fact that melanocytes are capable of collagen production, as well as melanin synthesis and schwannian differentiation.

In general, DM clinically presents in older white individuals (mean age, about 65 years) and is more common in men than in women. It involves predominately sun-exposed skin of the head and neck region, often presenting clinically as a nondescript raised, firm nodule or sometimes depressed indurated plaque that is amelanotic or associated with variable pigmentation. DM is usually not recognized until late compared with conventional melanomas. Palpation typically reveals a hard indurated surface extending beyond the clinical pigmentation. DMs may also involve acral and mucosal sites less frequently and ultimately any cutaneous site. The irregular and variegated features of an associated intraepithelial component, such as melanoma in situ of lentigo maligna or acral lentiginous types, and may be the most clinically visible feature of DM. Difficulty in recognizing DM, clinically and histopathologically, usually causes a delay in recognition and appropriate surgery.

The essential histopathologic criteria for DM are (1) individual spindle cells and variably sized fascicles of spindle cells interspersed among (2) dense collagenous ("desmoplastic") fibers involving a significant proportion of the melanoma. The mere presence of spindled melanoma cells alone is thus not sufficient for the diagnosis of DM. The proportion of such melanomas showing a sclerosing spindle cell component may range from less than 10% to more than 80% or 90% (ie, virtually all of the neoplasm). Thus, some proportions of DM are biphasic (ie, they show a desmoplastic component associated with another distinct melanoma component, often of the conventional type). How much of a melanoma must be "desmoplastic" to qualify as "DM," and does this differential composition of desmoplastic versus conventional components effect the potential biologic behavior and prognosis? Although most authors have not directly specified their threshold definitions for DM, one can infer that a large proportion (perhaps well over 50% of the lesion) should have the desmoplastic phenotype. To more precisely address this issue of composition of DM and its biologic and prognostic implications, Hawkins et al have recently proposed subclassifying DM as pure DM (>80%-90% of the lesion being DM) and mixed DM (10%-<50% desmoplasia). The preliminary results from this latter study suggest that this subclassification may have practical utility in terms of being reproducible and potentially delineating biologic and prognostic differences between these subgroups of DM. More detailed studies will be needed to verify the latter findings given the inherent heterogeneity of melanoma and DM and interobserver reproducibility. It is certain that it is desirable to arrive at a consensus as to how DMs are defined and perhaps subclassified based on tumor phenotypic properties.

DMs are usually diagnosed at an advanced stage because they are usually at least 4 or 5 mm in thickness and Clark level IV or V. Because of misdiagnosis, they are commonly first recognized as recurrent or metastatic tumors. DM frequently recurs locally. Based on a series of 45 cases, local recurrence was associated with the following factors: failure to correctly diagnose the tumor, inadequate surgery (resection margins <1 cm), location on the head and neck, anatomic level V, and thickness greater than 4 mm. Additional factors contributing to this high local recurrence rate include the difficulty of assessing the margins, nerve infiltration, and the fact that the tumor cells are usually amelanotic.

Despite the significantly high local recurrence rate, it is held that distant spread is less common despite a typically advanced tumor thickness. Therefore, the prognosis of DM is generally regarded as being more favorable than conventional melanomas for a given tumor thickness. A review of the literature, encompassing a total of 703 patients, documented a local recurrence rate of 26.2%, a nodal metastatic rate of 7.1%, and a rate of systemic metastasis of 19.8%. Another study of 129 DM patients with a mean tumor thickness of 4.2 mm reported 5- and 10-year rates of survival of 76% and 64%, respectively. It has further been reported that DM lesions greater than 4 mm in thickness demonstrate a 60% 5-year survival compared with 40% in non-DMs. Again, it is important to emphasize that the histopathological definition of DM is not clearly defined and therefore one must bear this in mind when interpreting these statistical findings. A recent study engaged in a nuanced examination of the histopathologic features of DM and their prognostic significance. They subdivided cases of DM into "pure" and "mixed" subtypes. They reported that patients classified as having pure DM showed a significantly lower incidence of lymph node metastasis and a lower 5-year melanoma-specific mortality compared with the patients with mixed DM. Furthermore, they discovered that the melanoma-specific mortality rate was equal between the pure DM and conventional melanoma patients, despite a threefold higher median tumor depth in the former. Interestingly, they also reported that the lymph node metastases in the patients with mixed DM were characterized by the non-desmoplastic component of the primary mixed DM lesions. Therefore, it may be reasonable to subclassify these lesions as Hawkins et al have suggested.

Microscopic examination of a typical DM at scanning magnification usually discloses a fibrous nodule suggesting a scar or fibroma that displaces the normal dermal collagen or lamina propria and often extends into subcutaneous fat. In many instances, relatively dense perivascular or nodular lymphocytic aggregates are present.

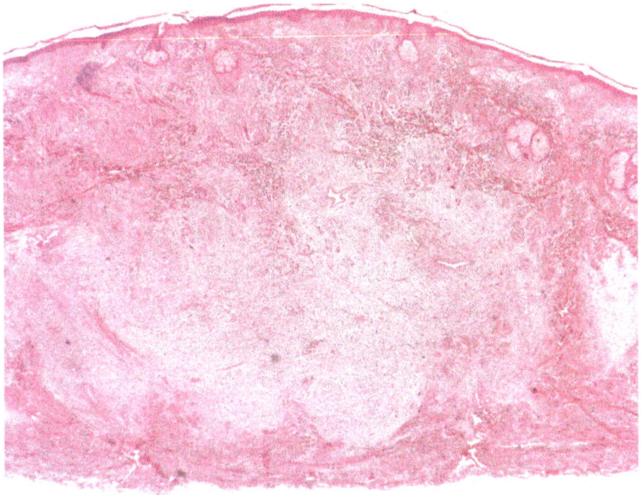

Desmoplastic melanoma, low power examination. Fibrotic nodule occupies dermis.

An intraepidermal melanocytic proliferation is observed in a range from less than 50% to about 75% of cases. The most common pattern is lentigo maligna, but the intraepidermal component may encompass any form on melanoma in situ. The histopathological appearance of the invasive or dermal/subcutaneous component of DM varies along a spectrum in regards to overall cellularity and degree of cytologic atypia. In the **pure form of DM**, solitary units of spindle cells are arranged haphazardly within a dense collagenous stroma throughout the dermis and possibly subcutis.

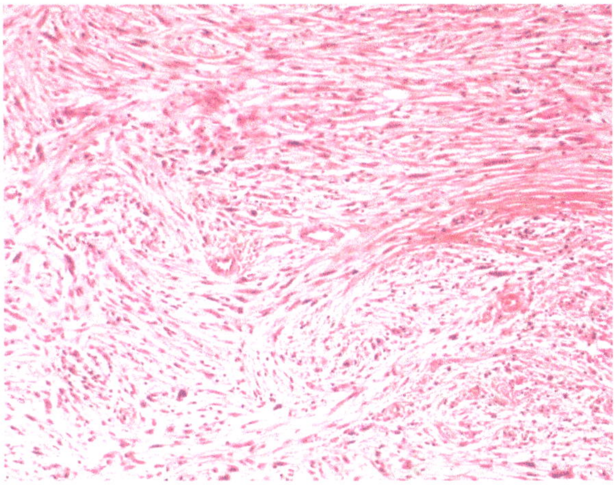

Desmoplastic melanoma, pure type. Storiform (haphazardly arranged) fascicles of atypical spindled melanocytes are embedded within a dense fibrous stroma.

The nuclei exhibit variable pleomorphism. Although most nuclei are enlarged and exhibit tapering contours, they may also exhibit wavy, plump, or multinucleate giant cell morphologies. Most DMs lack pigment, but occasional cells may contain fine melanin granules within cellular processes.

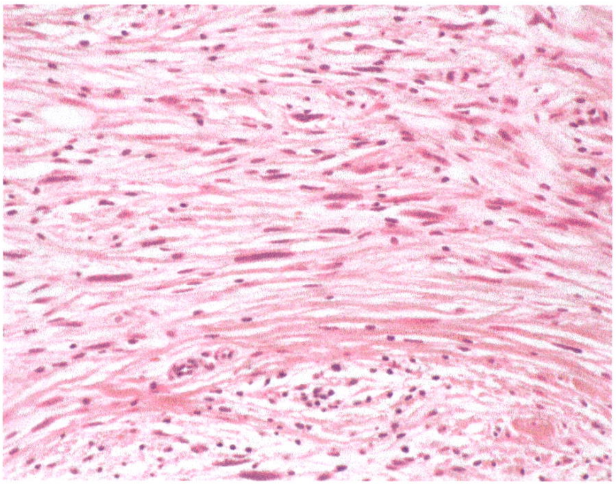

Desmoplastic melanoma, pure type. Note the spindle cells containing large pleomorphic nuclei with tapering contours.

The tumor stroma is usually fibrous, but myxoid alteration is occasionally encountered and uncommonly may be prominent. A finding typical of DM and useful in its recognition is the presence of variably dense perivascular lymphocytic infiltrates that are usually scattered throughout the tumor. The tumor cells in DM are also notable for angiotropism on occasion. Mitotic figures can usually be found even in the most paucicellular forms of this tumor.

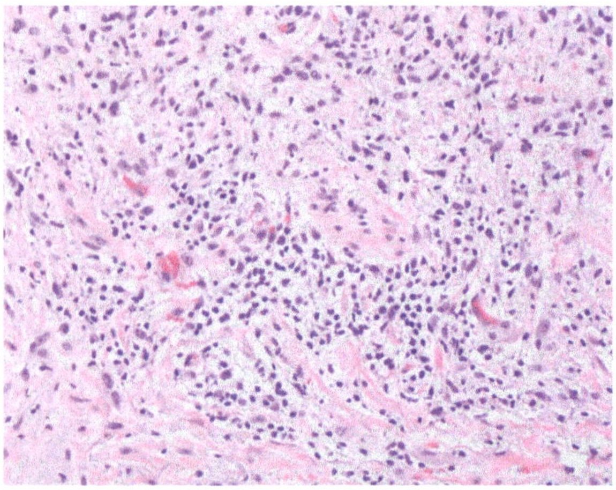

Desmoplastic melanoma. There are aggregates of lymphocytes admixed with the spindled melanocytic component.

The term "**neurotropism**" refers to the involvement of perineurium or endoneurium of cutaneous nerves by melanoma cells. There may be considerable thickening of the perineurium and expansion of the endoneurial space by the

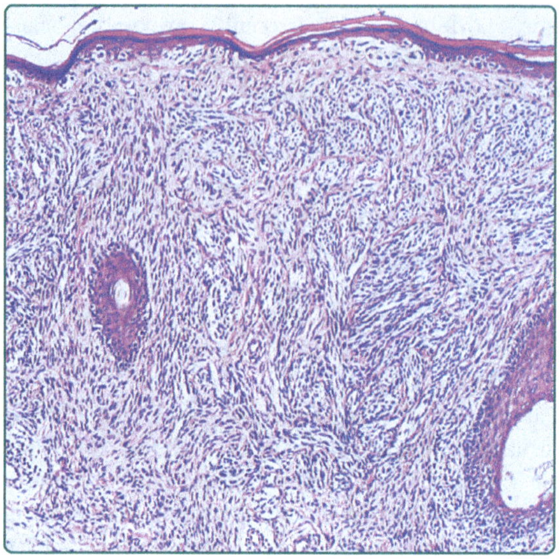

Desmoplastic melanoma, mixed type. There is an invasive spindled melanocytic infiltrate with minimal sclerotic collagen. The spindle cells are present in nests as well as solitary units and exhibit a plump cytomorphology. There is an overlying intraepidermal component of conventional lentigo maligna. (Reproduced, with permission, from Goldsmith LA, Katz SI, Gilchrest BA, Paller AS, Leffell DJ, Wolff K, eds. *Fitzpatrick's Dermatology in General Medicine*. 8th ed. New York, NY: McGraw-Hill Education; 2012.)

tumor involvement. Extension of tumor along the cutaneous nerves may, however, be extensive and subtle. Histologic clues to nerve involvement include the presence of hyperchromatic spindle cells in the perineurium or endoneurium and mucinous alteration of the nerve. Careful examination of cutaneous nerves at the surgical margins is mandatory to assess adequate excision. Neurotropism is strongly associated with local recurrence and overall worse outcome. Melanoma spindle cells involving cutaneous nerves usually show nuclear enlargement, hyperchromatism, and pleomorphism.

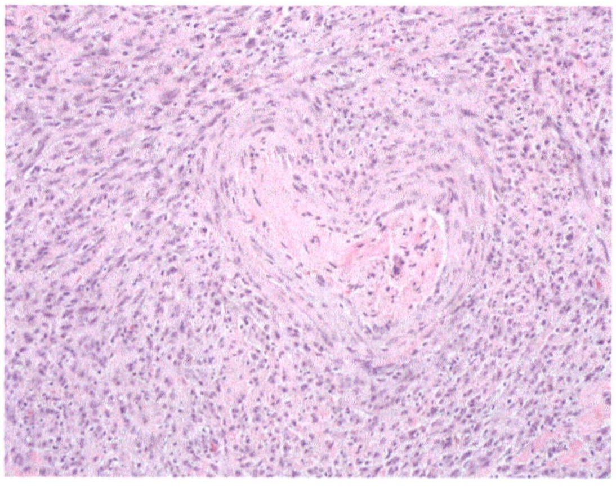

Desmoplastic melanoma with neurotropism. There are numerous spindled melanocytes encasing a nerve with infiltration of the perineurium.

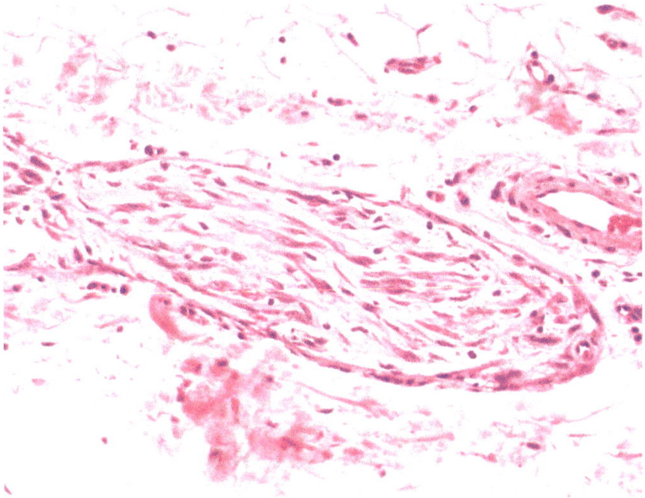

Desmoplastic melanoma with neurotropism. In this example there is subtle perineural and intraneural infiltration of the nerve by spindled melanocytes.

In regards to the differential diagnosis, the spectrum of tumors potentially confused with desmoplastic and neurotropic melanoma is varied and includes spindle cell proliferations and tumors with a fibrous appearance. The principal lesions to be considered include **sclerosing blue nevus, desmoplastic Spitz nevus, neurothekeoma, malignant peripheral nerve sheath tumor, dermatofibroma, atypical fibroxanthoma, malignant fibrous histiocytoma, scar, fibromatosis, myxoma, spindle cell squamous cell carcinoma**, and **leiomyosarcoma.** The intraepidermal lentiginous melanocytic proliferation commonly found in DM is characteristically absent in the other conditions. Because of the serious consequences of DM, immunohistochemistry is needed in most cases to confirm the diagnosis. Almost 100% of desmoplastic-neurotropic melanomas demonstrate immunoreactivity with antibodies against vimentin, S-100 protein, SOX-10, and p75 neurotrophin receptor, but uniquely, almost all are negative for HMB45, MART-1 (Melan-A), MITF (microphthalmia transcription factor), and tyrosinase. If there is positive immunostaining for HMB45 and the latter markers in DM, it involves non-desmoplastic foci only, such as an intraepidermal component or superficial dermal focus of conventional melanoma cells. A battery of markers must be used to evaluate such tumors. Other antibodies with variable reactivity with DM are neuron-specific enolase and NK1/C3. Antibodies against keratin, desmin, actin, and Leu-7 (specific for peripheral nerve sheath differentiation but negative in melanocytic tumors) are negative in DM.

Sclerosing blue nevus and **desmoplastic Spitz nevus** are both characterized by an orderly infiltration of the fibrotic stroma and an overall benign cytologic appearance. Mitotic figures, usually encountered in DM, are exceedingly rare or absent in sclerosing blue nevus, but early forms of DM may be exceedingly difficult to distinguish from sclerosing blue nevus, and it is vital to weigh all clinical and histologic features. For example, DM in a young individual on an anatomic site other than the head and neck or acral areas is highly unusual, and such circumstances argue against a diagnosis of DM. Sclerosing blue nevus will be positive for HMB45 and Melan-A, whereas DM will be negative.

Desmoplastic Spitz nevus typically presents as a firm, dome-shaped, flesh-colored papule or nodule, measuring up to 1 cm in greatest diameter; is most often located on the extremities; and suggests a dermatofibroma (Table 10-23B). This variant of Spitz nevus primarily affects adults, with a peak incidence in the third decade of life. The desmoplastic Spitz nevus is histopathologically characterized by symmetry, a wedge-shaped configuration, and infiltration of the dermis by relatively monotonous epithelioid or spindle cells, allowing its distinction from DM in most instances. DM may also show a fascicular arrangement of cells that is generally lacking in desmoplastic Spitz nevus. Desmoplastic Spitz nevus also shows maturation, that is, isolation of individually smaller cells with increasing depth versus little or no such transition in DM. The cell types in the two processes tend to be rather different. Whereas desmoplastic Spitz nevi contain typical large epithelioid or fusiform cells, DM is notable for pleomorphic spindle cells often with hyperchromatic nuclei. Desmoplastic Spitz nevus will be positive for Melan-A, in contrast to DM, which will be negative (Table 10-23C).

Table 10-23B. Desmoplastic Spitz Nevus

Clinical Features
Firm papule or nodule
Adults (peak incidence in third decade of life)
Most commonly located on extremities
Histopathologic Features
Spindle or epithelioid cells
Predominantly intradermal location of melanocytes
Sometimes junctional component
Dermal stroma with increased collagen
Usually circumscribed, but with ill-defined borders
Often vaguely wedge shaped
Usually diffuse distribution of cells with low cell density
Typically small nests and single melanocytes
Maturation often present
Mitoses absent or rare
Multinucleate giant cells not uncommon (usually superficial)
Melanin usually sparse or absent
Differential Diagnosis
Desmoplastic melanoma
Sclerosing blue nevus
Dermatofibroma
Epithelioid cell histiocytoma

Table 10-23C. Desmoplastic Spitz Nevus versus Desmoplastic Melanoma

	DESMOPLASTIC SPITZ NEVUS	DESMOPLASTIC MELANOMA
Preferred site	Extremities	Chronically sun-exposed skin such as the head and neck
Preferred age group	Early adulthood	Late adulthood
Melanocytic atypia		
Intraepidermal	Rare	Common
Dermal	Not uncommon, but usually slight	Common, often more than slight
Mitoses	Rare	Variable
Necrosis	Absent	Occasional
Maturation	Common	Uncommon

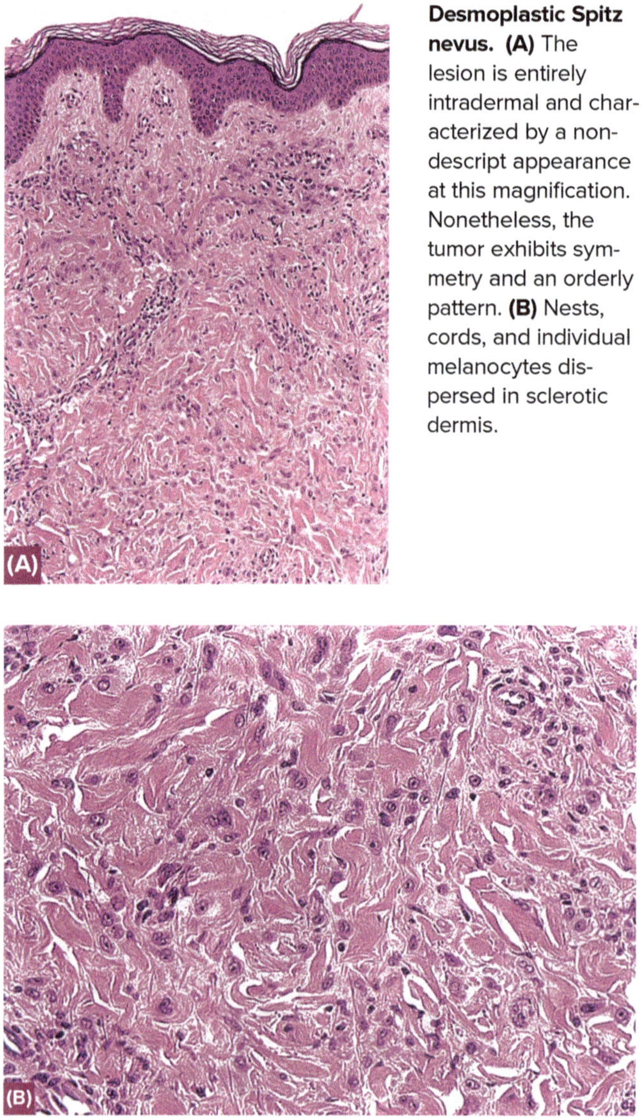

Desmoplastic Spitz nevus. (A) The lesion is entirely intradermal and characterized by a nondescript appearance at this magnification. Nonetheless, the tumor exhibits symmetry and an orderly pattern. **(B)** Nests, cords, and individual melanocytes dispersed in sclerotic dermis.

Relatively cellular variants of **neurothekeoma** may suggest DM. Neurothekeoma commonly arises in the head and neck region, as does DM. Neurothekeoma generally occurs in young individuals (average age, 20 years), does not demonstrate an intraepidermal melanocytic proliferation, and is typified by a lobular architecture in the dermis. Concentric and fascicular arrangements of cells are often noted in neurothekeoma, the constituent cells may be epithelioid or bipolar, and stellate and multinucleate forms are seen. Low-grade nuclear pleomorphism and occasional mitotic figures are occasionally encountered. Distinction from DM is based on a regular, organized appearance; orderly infiltration of the dermis; and a lesser degree of cytologic atypia. Immunohistochemistry is not as helpful in distinguishing cellular neurothekeoma from DM. **Cellular neurothekeoma** is typically positive for NKI/C3 and microphthalmia transcription factor (MITF) and usually negative for S100. While DM is typically negative for MITF, it may occasionally express NKI/C3, and almost always expresses S100. SOX-10 is an additional differential marker as it is negative in cellular neurothekeoma and almost always positive in DM.

Because of prominent schwannian differentiation, discrimination of **desmoplastic–neurotropic melanoma** from **peripheral nerve sheath tumors** may be difficult or impossible. All clinical and histologic characteristics must be considered. Tumors of the head and neck of elderly patients associated with lentiginous melanomas are usually not a diagnostic problem. Tumors in other anatomic sites without an intraepidermal component cause difficulty, and immunohistochemistry may be of particular value in them.

Lesions demonstrating fibrous or fibrohistiocytic differentiation figure prominently in the differential diagnosis of DM and include dermatofibroma (fibrous histiocytoma), juvenile xanthogranuloma, dermatofibrosarcoma protuberans, atypical fibroxanthoma, superficial forms of malignant fibrous histiocytoma, scar, and fibromatosis. These lesions

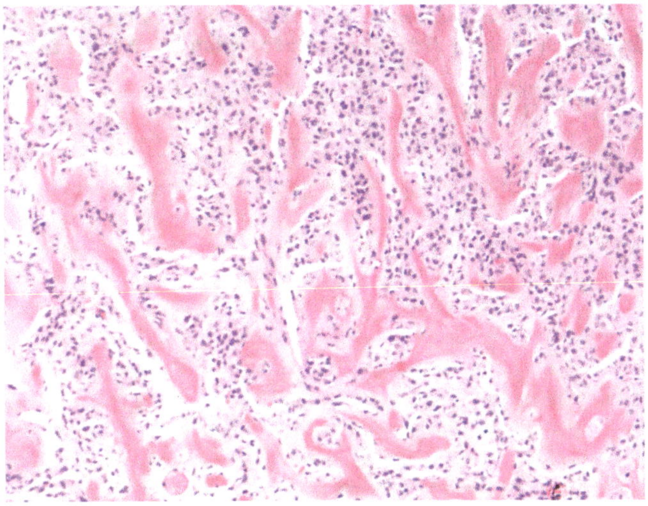

Cellular neurothekeoma. There are lobules and fascicles of epithelioid cells embedded in a thick collagenous stroma.

generally lack intraepidermal melanocytic proliferation, melanin pigment, and neurotropism. Atypical fibroxanthoma and malignant fibrous histiocytoma enter the differential diagnosis and often require immunohistochemical evaluation, although they may contain xanthoma cells, which are not usually seen in DM. While fibrohistiocytic tumors express markers such as Factor XIIIa, CD34, CD10 and CD68, these markers are typically negative in DM.

DMs with extensive mucin may raise problems of differential diagnosis, suggesting, for example, a **myxoma**. However, myxomas generally lack the cytologic atypia and neurotropism of desmoplastic–neurotropic melanoma, and the myxomatous variants of DM usually have zones of prominent cellularity. Myxomas are negative for S100 and may express CD34 in approximately 50% of cases.

Spindle cell squamous carcinoma and **cutaneous leiomyosarcoma** may be confused with DM, but each fails to demonstrate intraepidermal melanocytic proliferation and melanin synthesis. Squamous cell carcinoma may show keratinization, dyskeratosis, and intercellular bridges. Leiomyosarcoma may exhibit the cytologic characteristics of smooth muscle cells ("box car nuclei" with blunt tips), but immunohistochemistry may be essential to finalize the diagnosis. By definition, squamous cell carcinomas are cytokeratin+ and S100–, where DM is cytokeratin– and S100+.

ANSWER 10-24: C.

The biopsy reveals a large asymmetric compound melanocytic proliferation with spitzoid cytomorphology. The junctional component contains large nests of spindled melanocytes with vertical orientation to the epidermal surface. The epidermis is hyperplastic rather than attenuated and is not "consumed" by the tumor cells. Additionally, no lentiginous or pagetoid growth of these melanocytes is present. Ulceration is absent. The dermal component extends peripherally beyond the intraepidermal component and also extends into the deep dermis/subcutis interface. The cells become smaller at the base of the lesion; however, a single mitosis is present in the deep tumor aspect. Based on histopathology alone, the findings are best categorized as an **atypical Spitz tumor** (Table 10-24A). The relevance of the FISH findings, p16 immunohistochemical expression, and lymph node involvement will be discussed later.

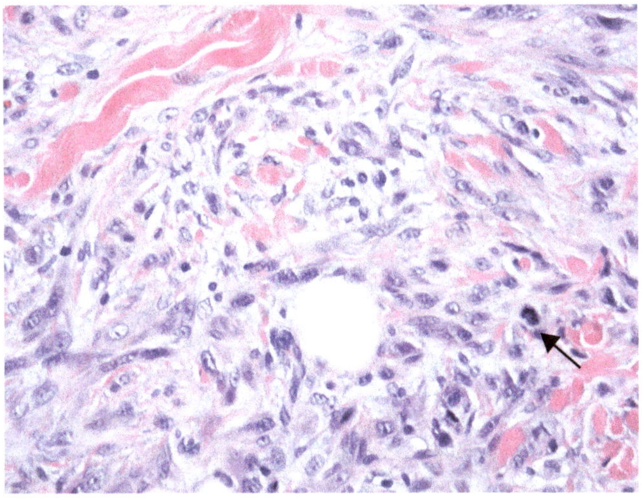

Atypical Spitz tumor. Note the single mitosis in this deep tumor component.

Similar to conventional "atypical" or "dysplastic" nevi, the "atypical" designation for Spitz tumors implies indeterminate biological behavior (borderline malignant potential). This "gray zone" of histomorphology may encompass a large number of worrisome features that overall fall short of a diagnosis of melanoma. **Spitz nevi** (totally benign) or **atypical Spitz tumors** (borderline malignant potential) are not uncommon yet remain controversial because there is no consensus concerning standardized criteria for recognizing or categorizing such lesions. In general, atypical features may be subdivided into those involving primarily the epidermis or the dermis or subcutis. The essential criteria for an "atypical" diagnosis are (1) large diameter (>1 cm), asymmetry, ulceration, epidermal effacement (or "consumption"), disordered architectural patterns of the intraepidermal component and (2) cytologic atypia of melanocytes beyond what is considered acceptable for a Spitz nevus (admittedly a subjective assessment).

A grading protocol for evaluating Spitz tumors with atypical features in children and adolescents was proposed by Spatz-Barnhill et al (Table 10-24B). The grading scheme attempts to estimate potential risk for metastases based on cumulative scores from quantifiable or objective parameters, including diameter (< or >1 cm), the presence or absence of ulceration, depth, mitotic rate per mm^2, and age (younger than or older than 10 years).

Table 10-24A. Spitz Nevus/Tumor with Atypical Features

I. Intraepidermal variant
- A. Architectural disorder
  1. Disordered intraepidermal melanocytic proliferation[a]
     - a. Lentiginous or single-cell pattern[a]
     - b. Disordered junctional nesting[a]
       - Variation in size, shape, orientation, spacing, cellular cohesion of nests
       - Horizontal confluence and bridging of nests
     - c. Pagetoid spread
  2. Asymmetry
  3. Poorly circumscribed
  4. Lateral extension of intraepidermal component ("shoulder phenomenon")
- B. Cytologic atypia[a]
  1. Nuclear pleomorphism
  2. Variation in nuclear chromatin patterns
  3. Nuclear enlargement
  4. Variation in nucleoli
- C. Host response
  1. Patchy to band-like mononuclear infiltrates in papillary dermis
  2. Fibroplasia

II. Dermal variant
- A. Architectural disorder[a]
  1. Expansile nodules
  2. Increased cellularity
  3. Loss of cellular cohesion
  4. Asymmetry
  5. Deep extension
  6. Lack of maturation or orderly infiltration of collagen
  7. Ulceration
  8. Necrosis
- B. Cytologic atypia (as above)
- C. Mitotic activity
  1. Numerous mitoses
  2. Mitoses at base of lesion
  3. Atypical mitoses
- D. Host response
  1. Prominent mononuclear cell infiltrates
  2. Formation of tumor stroma

[a]Essential criteria for diagnosis.

Table 10-24B. Assessment of Atypical Spitz Tumors in Children and Adolescents for Risk for Metastasis

PARAMETER	SCORE
Age (years)	
0-10	0
11-17	1
Diameter (mm)	
0-10	0
>10	1
Involvement of subcutaneous fat	
Absent	0
Present	2
Ulceration	
Absent	0
Present	2
Mitotic activity (mm^2)	
0-5	0
6-8	2
>9	5
Total score and risk for metastasis	
0-2: Low risk	
3-4: Intermediate risk	
5-11: High risk	

As already alluded to, abnormal properties of the dermal component include large diameter; asymmetry; cohesive cellular nodules; increased cellularity; deep extension into the lower most dermis or subcutis; lack of maturation or orderly infiltration of collagen; cytologic atypia; and mitotic activity (especially deep). Because of the rarity of such lesions and the lack of sufficient follow-up in many instances, the significance of these various features has not been elucidated. There is little question that the cumulative presence of these various features in any given lesion is highly worrisome for melanoma and that as these features increase in number and severity, the likelihood of malignancy increases.

In evaluating such lesions, a number of factors should be weighed in the final interpretation. Clinical factors such as the age of the patient, location of the tumor, clinical appearance, history of recent change in long-standing stable lesions, size larger than 1 cm, and family history of melanoma should be carefully considered. The older the patient, especially individuals older than age 30 to 40 years, the greater the likelihood of malignancy. As a general rule, one's threshold for diagnosing melanoma in such lesions should correlate inversely with the age of the patient, that is, a high threshold for very young individuals and a lower threshold for elderly individuals. The location of atypical tumors on sites less commonly involved by Spitz nevus, such as the back, is also another such factor suggesting careful scrutiny of the lesion for melanoma. If after weighing these factors, a clear-cut diagnosis of melanoma cannot be made, a practical approach is to communicate this situation to the clinician and patient.

Although the intraepidermal component in the case in question lacks significant architectural disorder, we will briefly discuss the features of "atypical intraepidermal Spitz tumors." The **atypical pagetoid Spitz nevus** is a distinctive variant of the intraepidermal subtype with a prominent pagetoid pattern. This variant may occur anywhere but is most commonly encountered on the lower extremities of young women. The most important reason for recognizing this lesion is its frequent misdiagnosis as in situ or microinvasive melanoma of the superficial spreading type. Most lesions measure less than 5 or 6 mm. Scanning magnification usually discloses a mainly intraepidermal proliferation of enlarged epithelioid and polygonal cells usually devoid of melanin with an overall symmetry from side to side and reasonably well-defined margins. However, some lesions have ill-defined margins. Many of these lesions show a combination of both a single cell and nested proliferation of epithelioid melanocytes. The single-cell proliferative pattern is often both basilar and pagetoid and commonly varies within the lesion. Typical junctional nests of epithelioid cells with associated clefting are also usually present and may be quite small in size. Nests of cells or single Spitz nevus cells may or may not be present in the papillary dermis. Often, the degree of pagetoid spread is focal or limited; however, it may be prominent in some lesions, raising the possibility of superficial spreading melanoma in situ.

Compound and dermal Spitz nevi and their atypical variants must also be discriminated from invasive melanoma. The absence or incomplete development of major diagnostic features, such as symmetry or sharply demarcated lateral borders, are of concern and should prompt a careful search for features of melanoma. Even if symmetry and sharp lateral demarcation are observed, the presence of extensive pagetoid spread, the lack of maturation in depth, prominent cellularity of the dermal component, nuclear pleomorphism of more than a small proportion of cells, cohesive cellular nodules in the dermis, or deeply located (albeit rare) mitoses are worrisome. Detailed knowledge of diagnostic criteria and their relative weight are critical in the histologic assessment of such atypical lesions. When an atypical lesion is present, it is appropriate to indicate whether the lesion is low grade (ie, only limited abnormal features are present) or high grade (ie, whether its features approach malignancy). Depending on the severity of the atypia, one should acknowledge that melanoma cannot be completely excluded. A diagnosis of malignancy should not be made unless there is sufficient histopathologic and other evidence so that overtreatment and undue psychological burden for the patient can be avoided.

Since there is so much variability in melanocyte cytomorphology (ordinary nevus vs Spitz vs melanoma, etc) additional diagnostic adjuncts have been sought out to better define these tumors. Molecular techniques have recently shed more light on the biological nature of Spitz tumors. In particular, *HRAS* activation by either point mutation or copy number increases in isochromosome 11p has been reported in a significant number of indolent Spitz tumors (estimated at 20%), and this finding has yet to be reported in **spitzoid melanomas**. It has been speculated that *HRAS* activation in the absence of cooperating additional genetic alterations may drive partially transformed melanocytes into senescence or a stable growth arrest and be partially responsible for the spitzoid cytomorphology. Although these molecular findings seem promising, future studies are required to definitively assess the biological behavior of Spitz tumors. While gains in isochromosome 11p have been shown to be associated with indolent biological

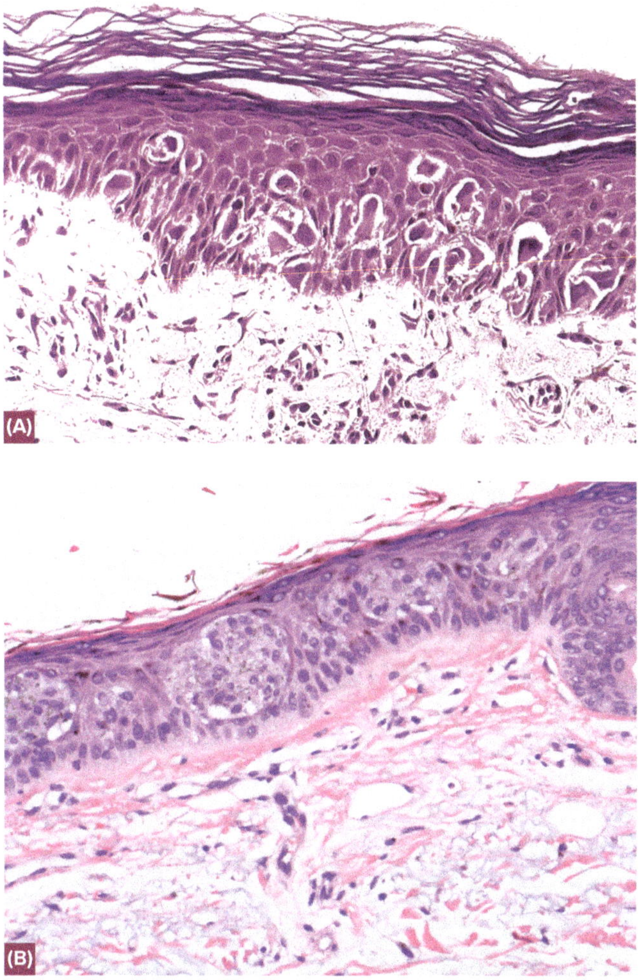

Pagetoid Spitz nevus (atypical) versus superficial spreading melanoma in situ. (A) Atypical pagetoid Spitz nevus. Pagetoid spread suggests melanoma in situ. However, note the characteristic cytologic details of Spitz nevus cells. The cells are polyangular and contain abundant ground glass cytoplasm, and the nuclei have dispersed chromatin. In general, pagetoid melanocytosis is limited to the lower half of the epidermis; whereas, in melanoma pagetoid cells extend to the granular layer. Little to no melanin pigment is present. Probably one of the most helpful findings is the rather small size of the lesion (<5-6 mm). **(B)** Melanoma in situ, superficial spreading type. There are nests and solitary melanocytes above the basal layer. The melanocytes have a rounded epithelioid morphology with melanized cytoplasm and hyperchromatic nuclei.

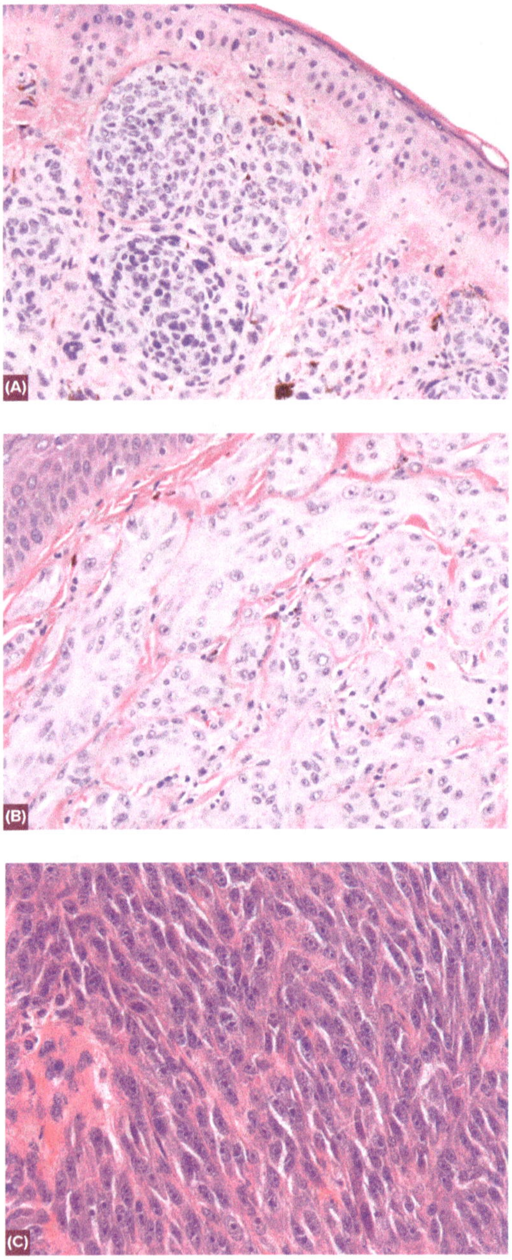

Spectrum of melanocyte cytomorphology. (A) Common acquired dermal nevus. These type A melanocytes are round (epithelioid) and contain melanized cytoplasm and nuclei without prominent nucleoli. **(B)** Dermal Spitz nevus. The cells are epithelioid and spindled with abundant eosinophilic "glassy" cytoplasm. Although the nuclei are enlarged, the nucleus to cytoplasmic ratio is not increased. The nuclei contain dispersed chromatin (vesicular or "hollowed out" appearance). Prominent nucleoli are present. **(C)** Malignant melanoma, nodular type. The melanocytes are round to elongated with amphophilic to basophilic granular cytoplasm and markedly enlarged nuclei with prominent nucleoli. The nucleus to cytoplasmic ratio is markedly increased. Although the nuclear pleomorphism is not dramatic in this example, the other cytologic features are overtly malignant. (Part **(C)** reproduced, with permission, from Kemp WL, Burns DK, Travis Brown TG. *Pathology: The Big Picture*. 8th ed. New York, NY: McGraw-Hill Education; 2008.)

behavior, they have only be found in approximately 20% of cases. The use of the standard FISH probe set (11q, 6p, 6q, and centromere 6) for identifying spitzoid melanomas only has a sensitivity of approximately 70%. Recently, several studies have evaluated the role of 9p21 (CDKN2A) in an expanded set of FISH probes. The 9p21 allele corresponds with the p16 tumor suppressor protein. When combined with the standard melanoma FISH probe set, the homozygous loss of 9p21 (CDKN2A) holds promise for the recognition of potentially aggressive or malignant spitzoid neoplasms. The recent report of TERT promoter mutations in atypical spitzoid lesions may have even greater predictive value for aggressive behavior. Several studies have applied p16 immunohistochemical staining to these tumors as a surrogate for FISH. While the positive expression of p16 implies retained function of 9p21, a recent study concluded that expression of p16 alone does not differentiate between Spitz nevi and Spitzoid melanoma. Loss of p16 expression has been reported in Spitz nevi with low-risk features as well as malignant melanoma; therefore, loss of p16 expression alone is not specific for malignancy. Although further studies are needed to determine the precise probe sets that will allow definitive assessment of benignity versus malignancy in spitzoid melanocytic lesions, the molecular findings present in this case are reassuring for indolent biological behavior.

Melanocytic lesions classified as Spitz nevi have been reported to spread to regional (including sentinel) lymph nodes. These metastasizing melanocytic lesions, albeit resembling in many ways Spitz nevi, often tend to be unusually large, deep, and ulcerated, and possibly also show other atypical features. Further studies are needed to clarify the nature of these tumors; however, until definitive information is available, such tumors must be considered potentially aggressive and managed on a case-by-case basis. The application of sentinel lymph node biopsy (SLNB) to atypical spitzoid melanocytic lesions as a means of obtaining more information about the biologic characteristics of such lesions may appear to have some rational basis. However, there are fundamental questions that must be addressed about this issue.

Since melanocytes normally exhibit migratory behavior, their presence in lymph nodes is not uncommon. Lymph node excisions for other various malignancies occasionally reveal deposits of benign melanocytes in the lymph node capsule or sinus (**capsular nevi**). Therefore, the presence of melanocyte deposits in lymph nodes does not equate to a diagnosis of **metastatic melanoma**. One must have a much better understanding of the metastatic process in general versus nonmalignant cellular migration and spread for the presence of ectopic cells in lymph nodes and other sites. The nature and significance of SLN deposits associated with all melanocytic lesions require much more rigorous study and analysis. Finally, only a study of sufficient numbers of patients with long-term follow-up will provide the data to definitively know the biologic nature of many SLN deposits associated with various spitzoid lesions, if they are inherently different from conventional melanomas, and if they potentially have

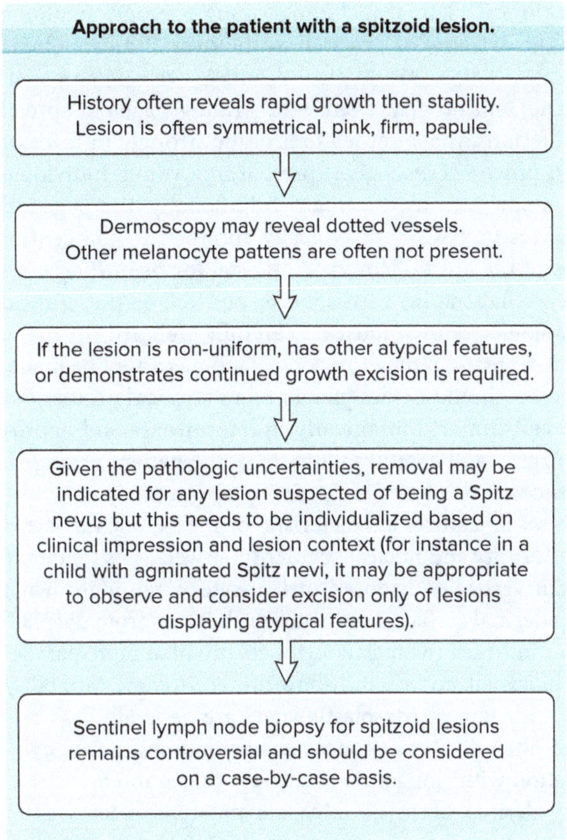

Approach to the patient with a spitzoid lesion. (Reproduced, with permission, from Goldsmith LA, Katz SI, Gilchrest BA, Paller AS, Leffell DJ, Wolff K, eds. *Fitzpatrick's Dermatology in General Medicine*. 8th ed. New York, NY: McGraw-Hill Education; 2012.)

better prognoses. Thus, without such data, it is impossible to know, in general, the true biologic significance of spitzoid deposits in SLN. However, data are available from the patients thus far reported in the literature. Among these patients, mostly children and adolescents, who have undergone sentinel lymph biopsy for spitzoid melanocytic tumors (probably a heterogeneous group of typical and atypical spitzoid lesions and possibly some true melanomas), approximately 50% of the patients have shown positive SLNB. In most instances, the tumor deposits have been microscopic and generally have involved the parenchyma or subcapsular sinuses of the SLN. With completion lymphadenectomy, very few patients have showed any further nodal involvement, usually only a single additional node being involved. At this point apparently none of the patients have shown any further disease progression with follow-up ranging from months to several years. Although these data are preliminary and not yet conclusive due to lack of consensus interpretation of the primary spitzoid neoplasms and sufficient long-term follow-up, the patients appear to show no progression of disease, and thus the positive SLN does not correlate with risk of further metastatic disease. As a result, the data suggest that many SLN deposits from spitzoid tumors are probably benign or at least biologically indeterminate. Consequently, atypical Spitz tumor deposits in SLNs may possibly have a different biology or significance than metastases from conventional melanoma.

ANSWER 10-25: C.

The biopsy reveals a compound melanocytic proliferation composed of large nests of spindled melanocytes containing abundant melanin pigment. These nests are situated predominantly at the sides of the rete ridges and exhibit a perpendicular orientation to the epidermal surface. Scattered pagetoid melanocytes are present in the granular layer and clumps of melanin pigment are present in the stratum corneum. Numerous melanophages are present in the dermis. The findings are consistent with a **pigmented spindle cell nevus of Reed.**

The **pigmented spindle cell nevus (PSCN)** is a distinctive clinicopathologic entity that is important to recognize because of its frequent confusion with melanoma (Table 10-25A). PSCN usually presents as a symmetric, sharply circumscribed, dark brown or black papule or nodule. It is typically a small lesion, often measuring less than 0.6 cm in diameter. PSCN is preferentially located on the extremities. It appears to affect women slightly more often than men.

Microscopically, these lesions are usually relatively small, strikingly well circumscribed, and remarkable for a slightly elevated, flat-topped plaque-like appearance of the epidermis. Although the PSCN may be compound, most cases are entirely junctional. If papillary dermal involvement occurs, the base of PSCN is typically broad with pushing borders. The PSCN contains uniform, delicate spindle cells present in tightly packed fascicles. These fascicles tend to have a fairly uniform and symmetric spacing and size within the epidermis and are often vertically oriented. The fusiform cells are often slightly more slender than the spindle cells of "classic" Spitz nevus. Their nuclei are equal in size or smaller than the nuclei of adjacent keratinocytes. The nucleoli are usually inconspicuous. Some PSCN, particularly in children, may show florid upward migration of single melanocytes closely simulating melanoma in situ. Also in contrast to ordinary Spitz nevus, melanocytes of PSCN contain variable amounts of granular melanin. Heavy pigmentation may also involve the adjacent keratinocytes, cornified layer, and papillary dermis.

There is a histopathologic continuum between **Spitz nevus** and PSCN. One will encounter many nevi showing varying degrees of transition between these two poles of the spectrum. For example, some nevi may exhibit slender spindle cells typical of PSCN yet at the same time contain somewhat larger fusiform cells and epithelioid cells that are less heavily melanized. Like conventional Spitz nevi, atypical features may be present in PSCN similar to the atypical forms of Spitz nevus. However, most atypical variants of PSCN are primarily intraepidermal. Some overlap may occur with conventional atypical (dysplastic) nevi.

In regards to the differential diagnosis, PSCN and its atypical variants must be distinguished from in situ

Table 10-25A. Pigmented Spindle Cell Nevus of Reed (Pigmented spindle cell tumor)

Clinical Features
Peak incidence in third decade of life
Most often located on extremities (especially thighs)
Women ≥ men
Small (usually <0.6 cm)
Symmetry
Pigmented (usually evenly, often heavily), often dark brown, black, or blue black
Sharply circumscribed
Papule or nodule
History of recent onset
Histopathologic Features
Junctional or compound nevus
Predominantly spindle cells, but occasionally epithelioid cells
Spindle cells more slender and delicate than in Spitz nevi
Uniform population of cells from side to side
Symmetric configuration
Predominance of junctional nests or fascicles
Typically ovoid nests with fusiform cells oriented vertically
Often confluence of nests leading to irregular shapes
Sharp lateral borders, occasional lentiginous lateral spread
Usually abundant coarse melanin
Uniform nuclear features
Decrease in cell size from top to bottom ("maturation")
Mitoses not uncommon in intraepidermal component
Absent or rare dermal mitoses
Differential Diagnosis
Lentiginous melanoma, particularly lentigo maligna
Pagetoid melanoma
Atypical (dysplastic) nevus

or microinvasive melanoma and from dysplastic nevus. PSCN (particularly atypical forms of PSCN) and lentiginous melanocytic proliferations of sun-exposed skin (ie, lentigo maligna) may occasionally show considerable similarity. Both are typically composed of pigmented spindle cells that may be arranged in junctional nests and may involve skin appendages. Discrimination of the two is based on clinical features, the usual small size, sharp circumscription, predominantly nested pattern, and uniformity of cell type in PSCN.

PSCN and atypical variants of PSCN are often confused with pagetoid variants of melanoma (superficial spreading type) because of prominent pagetoid spread. One must again rely on clinical factors, including young age and anatomic site (ie, the extremities), as well as the overall morphologic appearance. PSCN are typically small, well-demarcated, symmetric, and orderly. Even with striking pagetoid spread in some lesions, the latter features argue strongly in favor of a benign process, especially if present in a young individual and on a site such as the thigh. Additionally, the pagetoid melanocytes in PSCN are typically confined to the central portions of the lesion. However, atypical forms of PSCN are extremely challenging to diagnose, and all of the clinical and histologic features must be carefully weighed. In many instances, a clear-cut diagnosis of melanoma cannot be made. Such lesions should be designated as an **atypical pigmented spindle cell tumor, biologically indeterminate** and appropriate surgery and careful follow-up of the patient arranged. Recurrence of such lesions appears to be extremely rare.

The same features characteristic of PSCN, such as cytologic uniformity and nuclear regularity, as well as its tendency to contain vertically disposed melanocytes ("raining down") to the epidermal surface, help distinguish PSCN from dysplastic nevus, in which the melanocytes are oriented more parallel to the epidermal surface and show more cytologic variability and atypia. Atypical (dysplastic) nevi are generally less cellular and often display a pronounced lentiginous melanocytic proliferation with elongation of the rete ridges and associated papillary dermal fibrosis, which are not typical features of PSCN. However, some atypical forms of PSCN show substantial overlap with conventional atypical nevi. Discrimination of the two lesions thus may not be reproducible. Such lesions may be designated as PSCN with atypical features or as atypical (dysplastic) nevus with features of PSCN.

Plexiform spindle cell nevus (PLXSCN) is closely related to PSCN, Spitz tumors, blue nevus, and **deep penetrating nevus (DPN)** (Table 10-25B). However, it must be emphasized that plexiform spindle cell nevi/tumors are not variants of blue nevus. They differ from deep penetrating nevi based their distinctive plexiform architecture and often superficial location in the dermis. The lesions thus far reported have occurred in young adults (mean age, 22.5 years) and have involved the shoulders and back. Clinically, the lesions are raised and bluish or black, suggesting blue nevus, an atypical nevus, or melanoma. Microscopically, most lesions are slightly raised, symmetric, and exhibit a plexiform configuration in the reticular dermis. In a minority of cases, they may be both plexiform and wedge-shaped, as observed in so-called deep penetrating nevus. The most striking feature is the plexiform arrangement of fascicles of pigmented spindle cells that track along adnexal structures and neurovascular bundles. Other common features include junctional nests, diffuse involvement of the superficial dermis, and infiltration of cutaneous nerves and arrector pili muscles. The spindle cells contain abundant granular melanin and oval or elongate nuclei with delicate chromatin patterns and inconspicuous nuclei. As many as two-thirds of PLXSCN are biphasic (combined) and most frequently associated with an overlying or adjacent conventional acquired nevus. Occasional low-grade cytologic and rare mitotic figures (usually no more than $2/mm^2$) are observed. Rare atypical variants of plexiform spindle cell nevus occur and are designated atypical plexiform spindle cell tumor. These neoplasms exhibit atypical features such as greater mitotic activity, increased cellularity/nodular confluence, and more concerning cytological atypia. Rare high-grade PLXSCT suggesting melanoma may be seen. Potential risk markers for malignancy include patient older than 40 years, lesional diameter greater than 5 mm, asymmetry, biphasic or aberrant architecture, increased cellularity or odular configuration, mitotic rate greater than 2 to 5/mm2, and high-grade cytological atypia. Plexiform spindle cell nevus is distinctive strikingly but overlaps with DPN in about one third of cases. Deep penetrating nevus differs from PLXSCN because of its (1) architecture, which is wedge shaped and not inherently plexiform, and (2) conspicuous depth, that is, involvement of deep reticular dermis and subcutaneous fat.

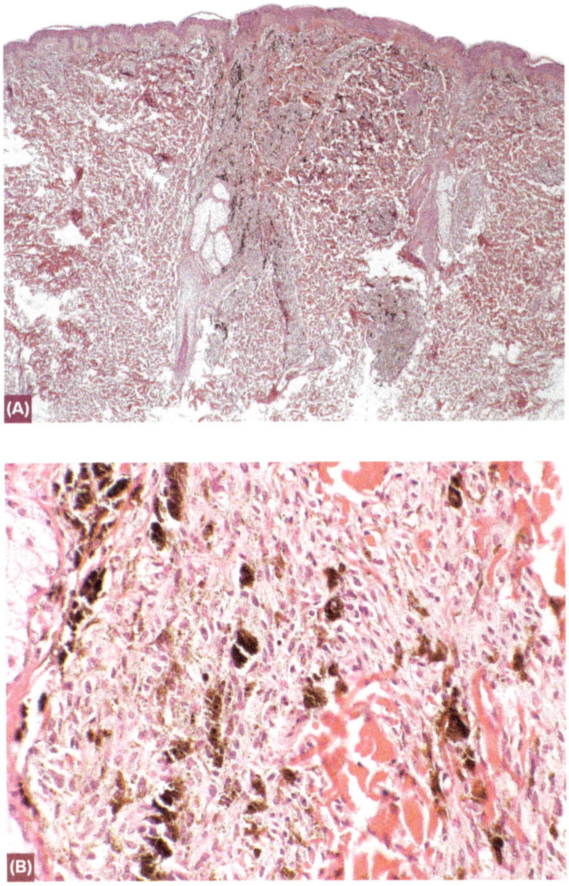

Plexiform spindle cell nevus. (A) Characteristic appearance on scanning magnification of fascicles of pigmented spindle cells in plexiform arrangement. The fascicles are associated with appendages, blood vessels, and nerves. There is normal collagen separating these cellular aggregates. **(B)** This field shows a bundle of uniform-appearing fusiform cells. The cells contain fine granular melanin and monotonous nuclei with dispersed chromatin.

Because of the unusual nature of these nevi, the immediate concern is melanoma, whether primary or metastatic. Particular features that aid in this differential diagnosis are the usual size being less than 6 or 7 mm (almost always <1 cm), overall symmetry, non-disruptive growth patterns, lack of high-grade atypia, and lack of significant mitotic activity. Nonetheless, some of these nevi are quite challenging because of large size, confluent masses of cells without evidence of maturation, and cytologic atypia. As a result, the biologic potential of a small minority of such lesions may be difficult to predict. Rare instances of lymph node metastases have been observed in both plexiform spindle cell nevus and DPN. Similar to atypical Spitz tumors, atypical plexiform spindle cell neoplasms with [these] lymph node [deposits] these deposits typically exhibit an indolent biological course. Regardless, the most appropriate management is to communicate to the clinician the uncertain potential for aggressive behavior.

Table 10-25B. Plexiform Spindle Cell Nevus[a]

Clinical Features
Age range, 10-30 years, but any age may be affected
Site: face, upper trunk, proximal extremities
Size: <1 cm
Raised lesions with bluish color
Histopathologic Features
Symmetric
Well circumscribed
Plexiform configuration in all cases
Wedge shaped in deep reticular dermis/fat in about one third of cases
Extension of cellular fascicles into deep dermis or subcutis
Pigmented spindle cells in fascicles associated with neurovascular bundles
Occasional junctional nests
Diffuse involvement of superficial dermis
Occasional cytologic atypia
Differential Diagnosis
Spitz nevus
Cellular blue nevus
Melanoma

[a]Plexiform spindle cell nevus overlaps with deep-penetrating nevus in about one third of cases. PLEXSCN shows a striking plexiform configuration that is not always present in deep penetrating nevus. Neither does the plexiform nevus always extend as deeply as deep-penetrating nevus.

ANSWER 10-26: A.

Scanning magnification discloses a raised, dome-shaped tumor exhibiting some asymmetry. The epidermis over the tumor is thin and partially effaced, but ulceration is absent. There is upward migration of melanocytes in the epidermis,

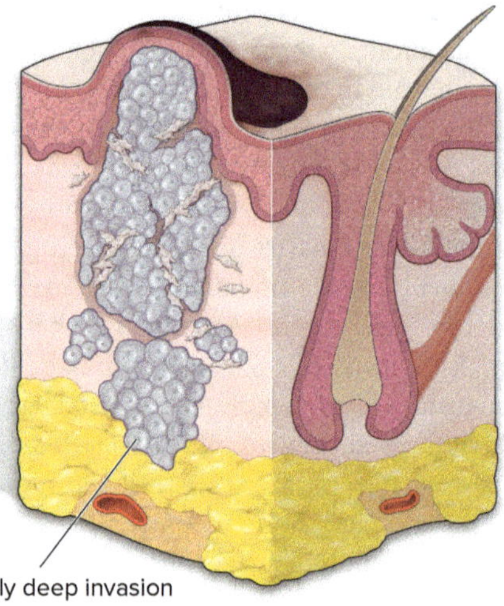

Nodular melanoma. This tumor arises at the dermal–epidermal junction and extends vertically in the dermis (vertical growth phase). The epidermis lateral to the areas of this invasion does not demonstrate atypical melanocytes. As in lentigo maligna melanoma and superficial spreading melanoma, the tumor may show large epithelioid cells, spindle cells, small malignant melanocytes, or mixtures of all three. (Reproduced, with permission, from Wolff K, Johnson RA, Saavedra AP. *Fitzpatrick's Color Atlas and Synopsis of Clinical Dermatology*. 7th ed. New York, NY: McGraw-Hill Education; 2013.)

but intraepidermal spread does not extend beyond the dermal margins of the tumor. The dermal component is composed of a cohesive nodule and smaller nests of tumor cells that have a pushing or expansile pattern of growth. The tumor cells are epithelioid without melanin pigment. The nuclei are markedly pleomorphic and hyperchromatic. Several cells contain prominent nucleoli and several mitoses are present (two mitoses are present in the high power [40×] image of the question). The findings are consistent with an amelanotic **nodular melanoma** with lymph node metastasis (Table 10-26A).

In regards to the differential diagnosis, NM may be confused with metastatic melanoma, Spitz nevus, atypical cellular blue nevi, squamous cell carcinoma, atypical fibroxanthoma, fibrous histiocytoma, leiomyosarcoma, myofibroma, cellular capillary hemangioma, and Kaposi sarcoma. **Amelanotic melanomas** (absent clinical pigment) are frequently clinically misdiagnosed as Spitz tumors, pyogenic granuloma, or other vascular tumor. While the tumor cells in this case exhibit abundant eosinophilic cytoplasm, there are numerous mitoses and the extent of nuclear pleomorphism and hyperchromatism are consistent with overt malignancy. Additionally, the tumor consumes the epidermis and there is extensive pagetoid ascent. Lastly, the melanocytes do not mature with descent into the dermis; therefore this tumor cannot be classified as anything but melanoma. **Metastatic melanoma** is typically a dermal-based lesion without an overlying intraepidermal component; however, exceptionally rare cases of **epidermotropic metastatic melanoma** involving the papillary dermis may prove impossible to distinguish from NM without proper

Table 10-26A. Conventional Melanoma with Little or No Adjacent Intraepidermal Component ("Nodular" Melanoma)

Clinical Features
- Age 30-70 years (often 40-50 but any age)
- Men = women
- Any site, especially trunk dorsal surfaces of hands
- 0.4-5 cm
- Often rapid evolution, eg, 4 months-2 years
- Papule or nodule, pigmented or amelanotic (advanced)
  - Often protuberant, polypoid
  - Black, blue-black, pink
- Ulceration, bleeding
- Asymmetry but symmetry may be present
- Often well-defined borders

Histopathologic Features
- Dome-shaped polypoid or sessile tumor often
- May be pedunculated
- Asymmetry with exceptions
- Epidermis commonly thinned, effaced, ulcerated
- Overlying intraepidermal component may or may not be present and usually does not extend peripherally beyond dermal invasive tumor
- Pagetoid spread, lentiginous melanocytic proliferation, intraepithelial nesting may be present
- Cohesive aggregate or aggregates of tumor cells fill subjacent dermis, subcutis
- Usually no maturation
- Host response at base or tumor-infiltrating lymphocytes common
- Epithelioid cells often comprise invasive component but spindle cells, small cuboidal cells common and often heterogeneity is present
- Partial regression relatively uncommon
- Precursor nevus present in about 6% of cases

Differential Diagnosis
- Spitz tumor
- Pigmented spindle cell nevus
- Atypical halo-like nevus
- Metastatic melanoma
- Cellular blue nevus with atypia
- Squamous cell carcinoma
- Adnexal carcinomas
- Atypical fibroxanthoma
- Fibrous histiocytoma
- Adult xanthogranuloma
- Lymphoma, particularly large cell anaplastic variants
- Cellular neurothekeoma
- Malignant peripheral nerve sheath tumor
- Capillary hemangioma
- Malignant glomus tumor or with atypia
- Angiosarcoma
- Kaposi sarcoma
- Leiomyosarcoma

clinical workup and clinical correlation. In general, melanoma metastases are often fairly monomorphous with little stromal response, whereas NMs are often polymorphous (pleomorphic) and exhibit greater stromal response. Distinction may be impossible in certain cases, and discrimination must rely on clinical information and the patient's clinical course. Recently, several studies have documented gains in 8q24 in **amelanotic nodular melanomas**. Additionally, copy number gains in 11q13 and 8q24 were predictive of metastatic disease.

Over the past 20-30 years, there has been extensive investigation of prognostic factors in melanoma using large databases and multivariate techniques. The most powerful predictors of survival from many such studies have been the thickness of the primary melanoma and the stage or extent of disease, that is, localized tumor, nodal metastases, and distant metastases (Table 10-26B).

Although a number of studies have described "breakpoints" for tumor thickness and prognosis—for example, patients with melanomas smaller than 0.76 mm have an almost 100% 5-year survival rate—good evidence now suggests that this inverse relationship between thickness and survival is essentially linear. Although thickness is the best prognostic factor available for localized melanoma, occasional melanomas defy this relationship (ie, thin melanomas that metastasize and thick ones that do not). A number of other factors have also been reported to influence outcome in patients with localized melanoma, particularly surface ulceration, mitotic rate, and microscopic satellites (localized metastases). However, these various factors largely derive their effect from a correlation with melanoma thickness and generally fail to remain significant after multivariate analysis. The presence or absence of melanoma involving regional lymph nodes has now been established as the most significant prognostic factor for survival in melanoma. **Sentinel lymph node biopsy** should be recommended to patients with localized cutaneous melanoma measuring 1 mm or greater in thickness. However, sentinel lymph node biopsy may be considered for melanomas measuring less than 1 mm in thickness if additional high-risk parameters are present (ulceration, one or more dermal mitoses). The incidence of sentinel lymph node metastasis is about 15% for thick melanomas (≥1-mm thick) and 4%-6% in so-called thin melanomas (<1-mm thick). The use of immunohistochemical stains (ie, HMB-45, Melan-A, S100, etc) dramatically increases the sensitivity of detection of microscopic melanoma metastases and are highly recommended in the examination of sentinel lymph nodes. It is important to mention that unlike sentinel lymph node biopsy and surgical removal of lymph node disease in breast carcinomas, which is both prognostic and therapeutic, sentinel lymph node biopsy in melanoma is for prognostication only. Therefore, one must be cognizant of the potential morbidity associated with the lymph node biopsy procedure (ie, lymphedema, etc) when consulting patients regarding the procedure. After regional lymph node metastases have developed, 5-year survival decreases to the range of approximately 10%-50% and is largely related to the number and extent of lymph nodes involved. If positive disease is present in the sentinel lymph node biopsy, a complete lymph node dissection is recommended for final staging. The median survival for patients with distant metastases is approximately 6 months. The only factors influencing the time to death include the number of metastatic sites, surgical resectability of the metastases, duration of remission, and location of metastases—that is, nonvisceral (skin, subcutaneous tissue, distant lymph nodes) versus visceral sites (lung, liver, brain, bone).

Table 10-26B. Histopathologic Reporting of Melanoma

Essential information
1. Diagnosis: Malignant melanoma, in situ or invasive
2. Measured depth (in mm)
3. Presence of histologic ulceration
4. Mitotic rate (per mm^2)
5. Presence of microscopic satellites
6. Adequacy of surgical margins
Other prognostic information reported to be significant in some databases
Clark level: I, II, III, IV, V
Tumor-infiltrating lymphocytes
Angiotropism
Vascular or lymphatic invasion
Desmoplasia-neurotropism
Degree of regression, particularly >50% of lesion
Radial or vertical growth phase
Histologic subtype

Elevated serum **lactate dehydrogenase levels (LDH)** which have been found through numerous studies have been found to be a stage-independent prognostic factor for decreased survival in melanoma. In these studies, pretreatment LDH elevation has been defined as serum levels greater than 200-225 U/L or as levels elevated above the laboratory reference range. It has been recommended to repeat the LDH testing after at least 24 hours when an initial result demonstrates any elevation above reference range. Another serum prognostic marker is albumin, which has been shown to be an independent adverse prognostic factor for stage IV melanomas when levels are decreased (≤3.5-4.0 g/dL).

Since the patient has clinical and cytopathological findings (FNA) consistent with lymph node metastasis, a systemic workup for distant metastases (ie, chest x-ray, CT scan, MRI, PET, etc) should be performed as soon as possible for proper staging. Patients with metastatic disease are candidates for chemotherapy and radiation. Tumor sections may now be tested for various oncogene mutations (ie, *BRAF, NRAS, c-kit*, etc) and treated with biological agents targeting cells harboring such mutations (ie, Vemurafenib). Lastly, another biologic agent known as Ipilimumab targets and blocks a protein receptor that downregulates the immune system (CTLA-4), allowing upregulated cytotoxic T-cell mediated destruction of the tumor cells.

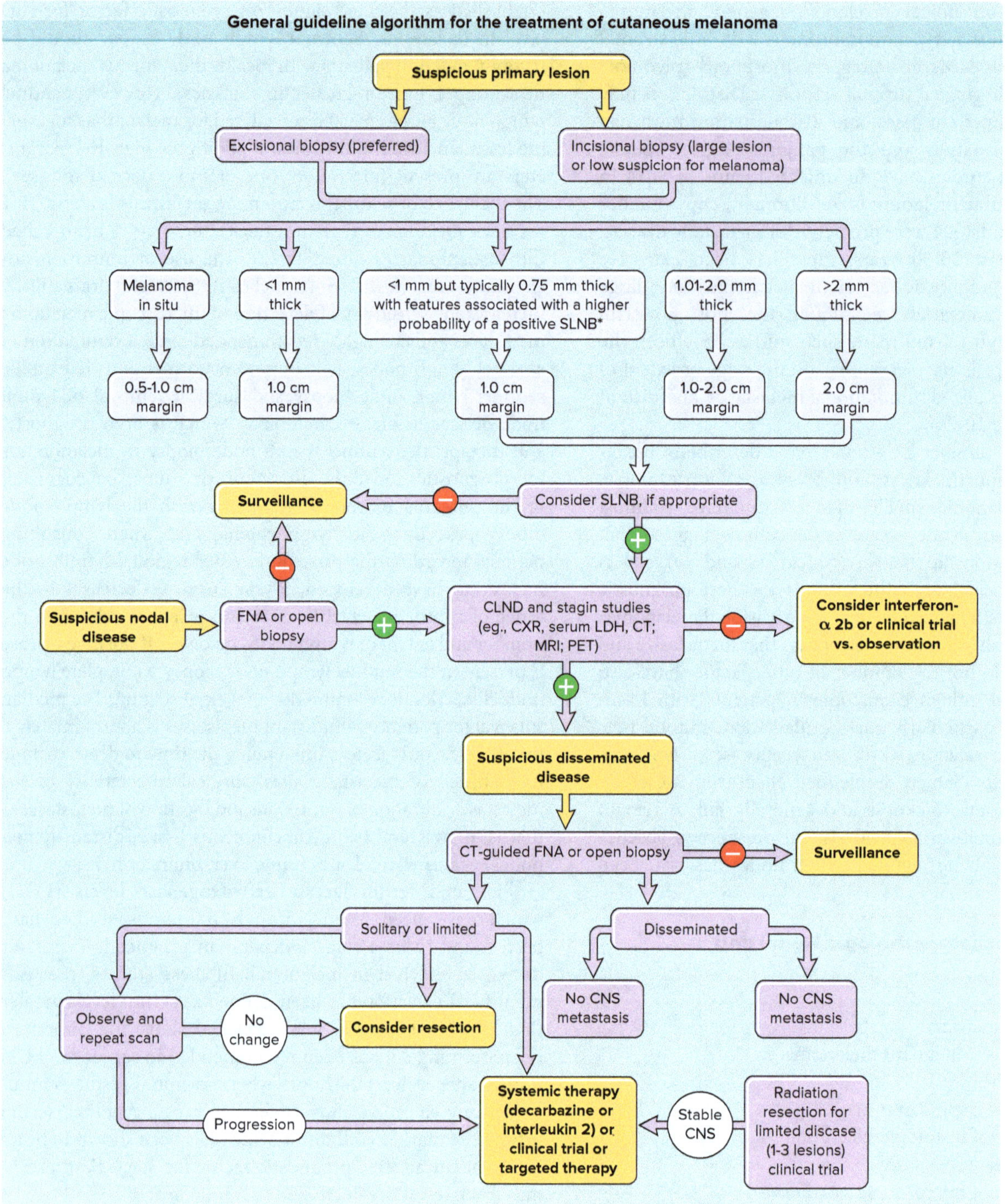

General guideline algorithm for the treatment of cutaneous melanoma. *Ulceration, extensive vertical regression to at least 1-mm thick, young patient age, high mitotic rate, especially in younger persons, shave biopsy with positive deep margin, presence of angio-lymphatic invasion, and Clark level IV. CLND = completion lymph-node dissection; CNS = central nervous system; CT = computed tomography; CXR = chest x-ray; FNA = fine-needle aspiration; LDH = serum lactate dehydrogenase; MRI = magnetic resonance imaging; PET = positron emission tomography; and SLNB = sentinel-lymph-node biopsy. A minus sign indicates no evidence of disease, and a plus sign evidence of metastasis. Patients who are candidates for SLNB should be referred to a surgeon experienced in performing the procedure so that the benefits and complications can be fully discussed. (Reproduced, with permission, from Tsao H, Atkins MB, Sober AJ. Management of cutaneous melanoma. *N Engl J Med.* 2004;351:998.)

ANSWER 10-27: A.

Clear cell sarcoma (melanoma of soft parts) has been a perplexing tumor because of its origin in soft tissue, classification in the past as synovial sarcoma or fibrosarcoma, and a pattern of biologic behavior that is consistent with a sarcoma (Table 10-27A). However, clear cell sarcoma (CSS) has also been considered an unusual variant of melanoma. At present, CCS is recognized as a distinct clinicopathologic entity, particularly because of an apparently tumor-specific translocation involving chromosomes 12 and 22 in 60%-75% of cases. The latter translocation is characterized by the fusion of a portion of the activating transcription factor gene (*ATF-1*) on the long arm of chromosome 12 (12q13.1-13.2) and the Ewing sarcoma oncogene (EWS) on chromosome 22 (22q13). This translocation has not been identified in conventional melanoma when studied by reverse transcriptase polymerase chain reaction and fluorescent in situ hybridization. CCS develops in young adults between the ages of 20 and 40 years and most commonly involves the distal extremities (the foot being the most common site). The tumor typically presents as a slowly enlarging, deep-seated mass because of its association with tendons and aponeuroses, and there may be occasional tenderness or pain. CCS is slightly more prevalent in women. Local recurrences are frequent, with 70% of patients in one series experiencing at least one recurrence during a mean period of 4.2 years. The recurrences are often multiple and followed by less-frequent regional node and lung metastases. In the series above, 43% of the individuals died of metastases.

Table 10-27A. Clear Cell Sarcoma

Clinical Features
Ages 20-40 years
Women ≥ men
Distal extremities, the foot most commonly involved
Deep location—tendons and aponeuroses
Slowly enlarging mass
Tenderness, pain
Histopathologic Features
Multilobulated tumor
Oval or fusiform cells in nests and fascicles
Fibrous trabeculae separate cellular aggregates
Clear or eosinophilic cytoplasm
Multinucleate giant cells
Melanin in over half of cases
Immunohistochemistry
S-100 protein+
HMB45+
MART-1+
Electron Microscopy
Premelanosomes
Melanosomes
Differential Diagnosis
Metastatic melanoma
Cellular blue nevus
Malignant blue nevus
Malignant peripheral nerve sheath tumor
Epithelioid sarcoma
Synovial sarcoma
Fibrosarcoma

Microscopically, the tumor is characterized by a well-circumscribed, multilobulated appearance. Oval or fusiform cells with clear or eosinophilic granular cytoplasm are arranged in well-defined nests and fascicles. Tumor aggregates are generally compartmentalized by fibrous tissue of variable thickness that merges with aponeurotic or tendinous structures. There is variation in nuclear size and shape, and the nuclei are notable for vesicular qualities and prominent nucleoli. Distinctive multinucleate giant cells occur in about two-thirds of cases. Melanin may be detected in approximately half of these tumors. Special stains yield more tumors containing melanin. Most tumors react with antibodies to vimentin, S-100 protein, HMB45, MART-1, tyrosinase, and neuron-specific enolase. Cytokeratin, epithelial membrane antigen, or leukocyte common antigen are not expressed. Melanosomes and premelanosomes are noted on electron microscopy.

In regards to the differential diagnosis, CCS may be confused with **cellular blue nevus, malignant blue nevus, metastatic melanoma, malignant peripheral nerve sheath tumor, epithelioid sarcoma, synovial sarcoma,** and **fibrosarcoma.** The tumor probably most closely resembles **atypical cellular blue nevus** and **malignant blue nevus**, but the latter do not usually occur in soft tissue. CCS is further distinguished by the typical clinical presentation in young adults, involvement of distal extremities, typical histology, immunohistochemistry, and (if necessary) the ATF-1-EWS fusion gene. **Epithelioid sarcoma** and **synovial sarcoma** immunostain with cytokeratin and epithelial membrane antigen but not with S-100 protein, with some exceptions for synovial sarcoma. Both tumors are negative for Melan-A and HMB45. Lastly synovial sarcoma is associated with a t(X;18) translocation.

Quick Fact

- **Cellular blue nevus**
  - Buttock
- **Malignant blue nevus**
  - Scalp
- **Clear cell sarcoma**
  - Distal extremity

ANSWER 10-28: B.

This is a classic example of **metastatic melanoma** (Table 10-28A). Melanoma may spread through lymphatic channels, by direct extravascular migratory spread, or hematogenously and thus may occur in any site of the body. Much remains to be learned about the mechanisms of melanoma metastasis. Metastases are more frequent to lymph nodes, skin, and subcutaneous tissue (nonvisceral sites) than to visceral organs. Lymph nodes are the most common site of metastases, and 60%-80% of patients with metastatic melanoma develop **lymph node metastases.** The lymph node groups most commonly involved are ilioinguinal, axillary, intraparotid, and cervical lymph nodes. The metastatic tumor may be clinically apparent (**macroscopic melanoma metastasis**) or detected only by histologic examination (**microscopic melanoma metastasis**). Although no obvious lymph node involvement is present in this patient, there is a high probability for microscopic metastases within the regional lymph nodes since multiple cutaneous metastases are present. Lymph node micrometastases are typically present within the lymph node parenchyma or sinus and exhibit overt malignant cytomorphology. Although not relevant to the staging of this patient in question, it is important to emphasize that collections of small benign melanocytes are occasionally seen within lymph nodes (sentinel or other) draining the skin. These aggregates, referred to as "**capsular nevi**" or "**nodal nevi**," are usually small and inconspicuous but may occupy as much as one-third of a lymph node. They are usually located in the fibrous capsule or trabeculae of the node rather than the medullary sinus or lymph node parenchyma. Their bland appearance, their frequent resemblance to nevus cells, and their location in the fibrous capsule of the lymph node help to distinguish them from micrometastases and suggest that many are nodal nevi. There has been considerable debate as to whether these nodal melanocytic lesions derive from aberrant migration of melanoblasts from the neural crest during embryogenesis or represent lymphatic spread from a benign cutaneous nevus.

Nearly 50% of patients with metastatic melanoma develop **cutaneous metastases**, which may occur in the area of locoregional lymphatic drainage or at a remote location. Two subtypes of regional cutaneous metastases are arbitrarily distinguished by their distance from the primary melanoma:

(1) **Cutaneous satellite metastases:** discontinuous tumor cell aggregates located in the dermis or subcutis within 2 cm of the primary tumor.

(2) **In-transit metastases:** tumor cell aggregates are located more than 2 cm away from the primary melanoma. This finding has poor prognostic implications because the majority of patients with such lesions develop disseminated metastatic disease.

The scattered tumor nodules in the patient in question are located farther apart than 2 cm and therefore represent in-transit metastases. Although virtually any organ may be involved, the most common first sites of visceral metastases reported in clinical studies are the lung (14%-20%), liver (14%-20%), brain (12%-20%), bone (11%-17%), and intestine (1%-7%); first metastases at other sites are very rare (<1%).

Microscopically, metastatic melanoma tends to grow in nests, sheets, or fascicles, often with an infiltrative border, pleomorphism, mitoses, and necrosis. Cytologically, epithelioid or spindle cells are commonly found in metastatic melanoma. Melanin, which greatly facilitates the recognition of metastatic melanoma, may be apparent, subtle, or absent (**amelanotic melanoma**). Primary tumors generally display more pleomorphism than metastatic lesions, which often appear as an atypical but rather monomorphous population of cells. Primary tumors tend to show more variation in the

Table 10-28A. Primary Cutaneous Melanoma versus Cutaneous Metastasis

	PRIMARY MELANOMA	CUTANEOUS METASTASIS
Location of tumor	Usually both dermis and epidermis	Dermis and/or subcutis
If epidermal involvement	Usually prominent; pagetoid horizontal and vertical spread commonly present; usually epidermal component extends laterally beyond dermal component	Usually dermal component extends laterally beyond epidermal component; pagetoid spread less common
Size	Nearly always >0.4 cm and usually >1.0 cm	Often small; may be <1.0 cm and occasionally <0.3 cm
Epidermal collarette	Usually less common	More likely present
Cytology	Usually pleomorphic	Usually monotonous
Reactive fibrosis	May be marked	Usually mild
Angiotropism	Perhaps less commonly seen	Usually present

overall composition of the lesion. There is often more fibrosis and more of an inflammatory host response. Although primary melanomas tend to have an intraepidermal component and melanoma metastases tend to be dermal-based or subcutaneous-based nodules, rare exceptions exist. Primary melanomas with little or no intraepidermal component are referred to as **nevoid melanoma** (or solitary dermal melanoma) and metastases with an intraepidermal component are referred to as **epidermotropic melanoma metastasis**. When deciding whether a melanocytic tumor is a metastasis or a primary lesion, one must weigh the histologic appearance against a detailed clinical history to arrive at the correct diagnosis. The importance of having precise clinical information is mandatory because there are exceptions to all of the guidelines for diagnosis mentioned above.

As mentioned above, a common problem is distinguishing a rare **epidermotropic metastasis** from a **primary melanoma** (or possibly a nevus in some instances). Cutaneous metastases usually lie within the reticular dermis or subcutis and only rarely involve the overlying epidermis, whereas primary cutaneous melanomas typically have an intraepidermal component. Metastases tend to be smaller (often <4 mm) than primary tumors (usually >4 or 5 mm). In cases of metastatic melanoma showing epidermotropism, the epidermal component is usually relatively limited compared with the dermal component. If the dermal metastasis is superficial, the overlying epidermis may be thinned, and the lateral borders may show hyperplastic, elongated rete ridges turned inward, forming a collarette. Angiotropic melanoma cells are more likely to be found in and around a metastatic lesion than near a primary tumor.

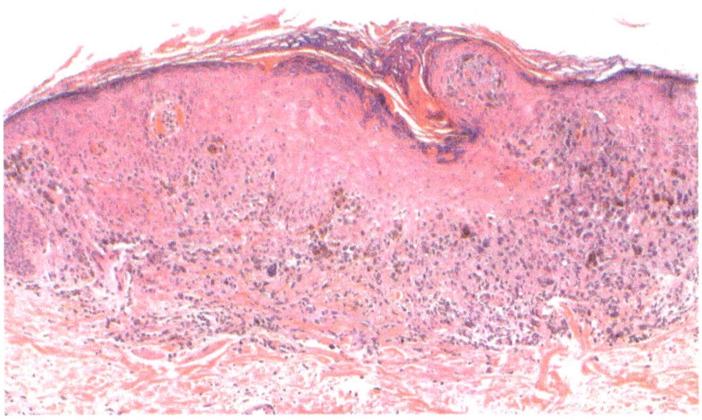

Epidermotropic metastatic melanoma. There is focal involvement of epidermis. The metastasis resembles a compound nevus; however, the lesion exhibits angiotropism, which is an important finding supporting a metastasis.

Approximately 4%-12% of patients with melanoma develop metastases without a clinically detectable primary tumor. Although it is possible that some melanomas may arise de novo within a lymph node, dermal, subcutaneous, or visceral site, it is generally believed that many of these cases are related to complete regression of a primary cutaneous melanoma. **Metastatic melanomas with an unknown primary site** are twice as common in men than in women, which is in agreement with the observation that tumor regression is more commonly observed in men than in women. The most common site of presentation is in lymph nodes (64%), and 21% of the cases present with visceral metastases.

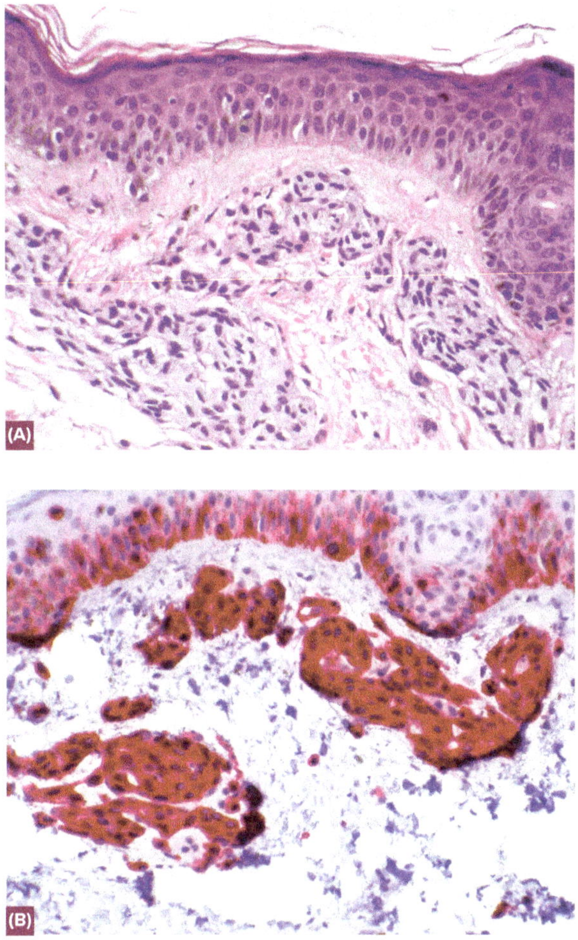

Angiotropic melanoma. (A) Melanoma cells cuff microvessels in a pericytic location in the superficial dermis. **(B)** Melan-A (red) immunostain reveals melanoma cells arrayed along external surfaces of [vascular] channels.

ANSWER 10-29: D.

Clinically, there is **longitudinal melanonychia** characterized by two broad bands of black and brown pigment. A portion of the nail plate has chipped away revealing underlying pigmentation of the nail bed epithelium, which extends onto the hyponychium. The biopsy reveals irregular scattered clusters of melanin pigment throughout the entire nail plate and a lentiginous proliferation of small dendritic melanocytes along the basal layer of the nail matrix epithelium. Scattered foci of pagetoid ascent are present. The findings are consistent with **acral lentiginous melanoma in situ**, at least (Table 10-29A).

Table 10-29A. Acral Melanoma

Clinical Features
- Age 60-70 years
- Men = women
- Equal incidence in all racial groups
- Most prevalent form of melanoma in Africans, Asians, Native Americans, other peoples of color
- Glabrous (volar) skin and nail unit
  - Palms, soles, digits, 85% of AM
  - Nail unit, 15%
- Feet, 90% of cases
  - Soles, 68%-71%
  - Toes, 11%
  - Nail units, 16%-20%
- Hands, 10% of cases
  - Palms, 4%-10%
  - Fingers, 2%
- Size 0.3-12 cm
  - Often ≥0.7 cm
  - <0.7 cm with irregular borders, color, or "parallel ridge" pattern on epiluminescence microscopy
- Often jet-black macule early, but also tan, brown, gray, blue, pink, white
- Pigmented or amelanotic papule or nodule (advanced) with ulceration, bleeding, eschar
- Irregular borders, notching

Histopathologic Features
- Prominent acanthosis with elongated epidermal rete common
- Thickened stratum corneum
- Contiguous or near contiguous lentiginous melanocytic proliferation in almost all lesions
- Intraepidermal melanocytes appear to lie in lacunae (clear spaces)
- Variable cytologic atypia with minimal atypia in early lesions
- Pagetoid spread (particularly in more advanced lesions)
- Intraepidermal nesting (particularly in more advanced lesions)
- Proliferation of melanocytes downward along eccrine ducts (even into deep dermis and subcutis)
- Pronounced pagetoid spread, large intraepidermal nests, significant numbers of melanocytes in stratum corneum in advanced lesions
- Polygonal to spindled melanocytes often with prominent dendrites
- Nuclear enlargement, hyperchromatism, pleomorphism prominent
- Invasive component
  - Cohesive nests, sheets of cells, or loosely aggregated files of cells
  - Spindle cells common but also polygonal, small, and highly pleomorphic cells are noted
  - Nevoid and sarcomatoid variants occur
- Desmoplasia, neurotropism, angiotropism common

Differential Diagnosis
- Melanotic macule
- Lentigo
- Atypical intraepidermal melanocytic proliferation, not otherwise specified
- Acral melanocytic nevus with or without atypia (may overlap atypical [dysplastic] nevus)
- Pigmented spindle cell nevus
- Squamous cell carcinoma, spindle cell type
- Atypical fibroxanthoma
- Cellular neurothekeoma
- Malignant peripheral nerve sheath tumor
- Angiosarcoma
- Kaposi sarcoma
- Leiomyosarcoma

Answer choices A, B, C, and D are conditions frequently associated with longitudinal melanonychia. The longitudinal pigmented streaks are the result of melanin granules in the growing plate derived from the segment of matrix involved by the melanocytic activation or proliferation. The current workup of melanonychia includes careful clinical assessment, dermoscopy, and one of three types of matrical biopsy (punch, shave, or lateral longitudinal). Longitudinal melanonychia is a brown-black band that indicates a melanin-producing lesion of the nail matrix located in the proximal nail fold. The same type of lesion in the distal nail bed, a non–plate-forming portion of the nail, results in a pigmented spot that is discrete and immobile. **Melanotic macule, subungual lentigo**, and **subungual nevi** may all produce a band that is narrow, sharply circumscribed, and homogeneous. The early phase of **acral lentiginous melanoma** may present as longitudinal melanonychia that is broader than 5 mm and associated with nail dystrophy, a bleeding mass, and **Hutchinson sign** (spread of pigmentation in the nail folds).

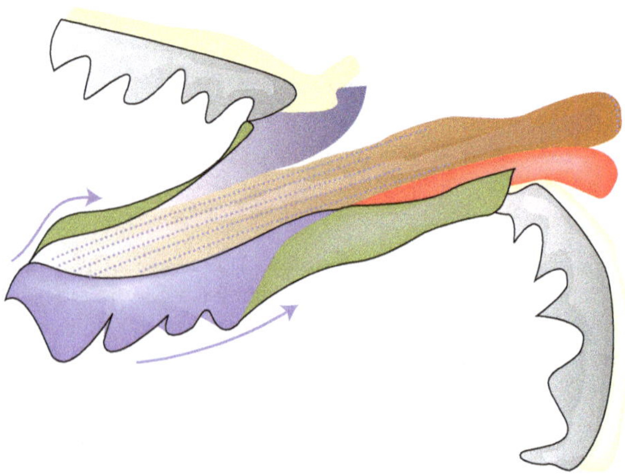

Nail plate biopsy for melanin. The understanding that the most superficial sheets originate in the proximal matrix and the deepest ones from the distal matrix allows for "histographic mapping" of melanin pigment to the matrical onychometameres containing the pigment-producing lesion.

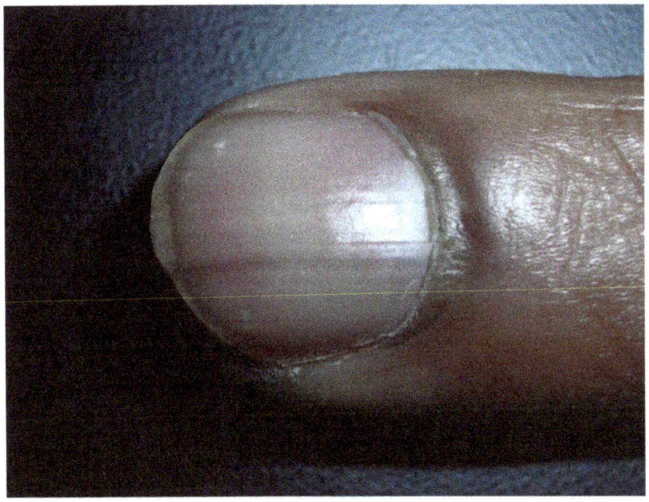

Benign longitudinal melanonychia. Note the color band is translucent. (Used with permission of Richard P. Usatine, MD.)

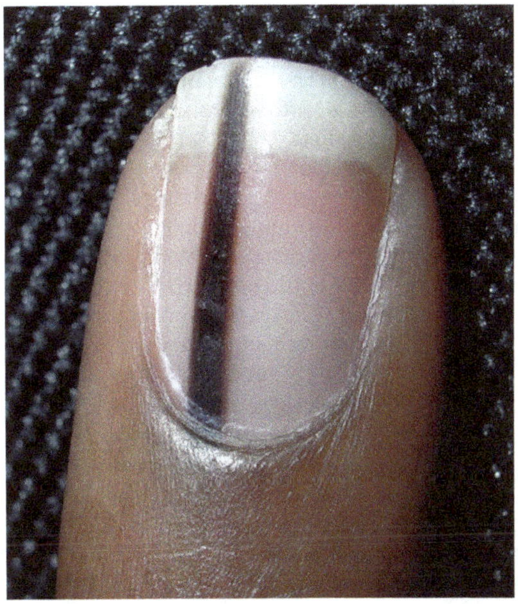

Longitudinal melanonychia. A single dark band of nail pigment appearing in the matrix region and extended to the tip of the nail. This is concerning for melanoma. The widening of the band in the proximal nail shows that the melanocytic lesion in the matrix is growing. This young woman had a biopsy that showed a benign nevus. (Reproduced, with permission, from Usatine RP, Smith MA, Mayeaux EJ Jr, Chumley HS, eds. *Color Atlas of Family Medicine*. 2nd ed. New York, NY: McGraw-Hill Education; 2012. Used with permission of Richard P. Usatine, MD)

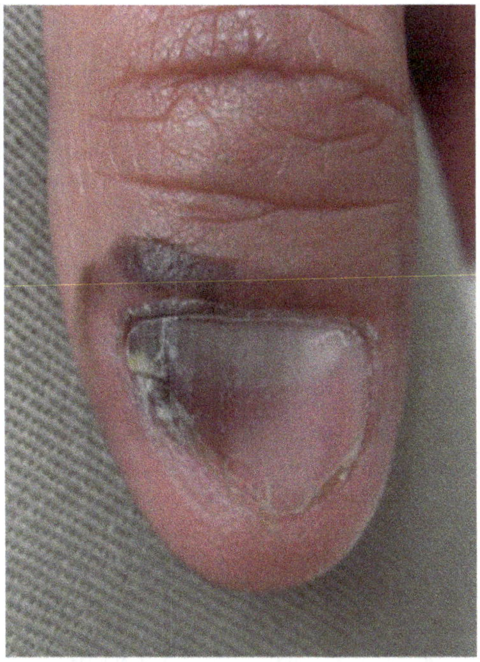

Acral lentiginous melanoma of the thumb with a very positive Hutchinson sign. Note how the pigmented band extends onto the proximal nail fold. The pigmented nail streak is greater than 3 mm in width. (Reproduced, with permission, from Usatine RP, Smith MA, Mayeaux EJ Jr, Chumley HS, eds. *Color Atlas of Family Medicine*. 2nd ed. New York, NY: McGraw-Hill Education; 2012. Used with permission of Robert T. Gilson, MD.)

Microscopically, melanocytic hyperplasia or **melanotic macule**, which may be the equivalent of an **ephelis (freckle)**, shows hyperpigmentation either with or without a (functional) slightly increased numbers of melanocytes. It is essentially a well-demarcated pigmented macule in the matrix. A simple **subungual lentigo** exhibits an increased number of melanocytes singly disposed in a variably hyperplastic epithelium. These two entities tend to appear early in life. The acquired or congenital melanocytic nevus, which is uncommon in the nail unit, contains nests of melanocytes in variably hyperpigmented rete ridges. Most of the **subungual nevi** are junctional and only rarely compound. Blue nevus shows up very rarely in subungual location. Biopsy of the nail plate in **acral lentiginous melanoma** will reveal melanin granules distributed broadly and, more important, irregularly throughout the whole thickness of the plate. This is a reflection of the usually wide and lengthy extension of the primary lesion. A problem in its recognition is the relatively uniform pattern of normal melanocytes near the junction of the nail matrix (practically always the source of melanoma in situ). Additionally, a suprabasal location of normal melanocytes throughout the lower half of the matrix has been described. However, in melanoma in situ, the process may be cellular, and nuclear pleomorphism and other signs of malignancy may be obvious (prominent nucleoli, increased or abnormal mitoses, longitudinally branching dendritic melanocytes). Unfortunately, in some instances a diagnosis of **"atypical" lentiginous melanocytic proliferation** (equivocal for melanoma) may be the most accurate interpretation of biopsy findings. Regardless of the terminology applied to such a lesion, complete removal of the lesion is mandatory. However, dermoscopy has been claimed as a means of follow-up in some instances. **Hutchinson sign** may be seen histopathologically as the continuation of the same matrical or bed-extended proliferation of melanocytes in the epidermoid epithelia of eponychium and hyponychium or the epidermis of the nail folds. The presence of microscopic

Hutchinson sign in proximal or lateral nail fold epithelia, but not so in the hyponychium (which is still part of the matrical stream of cells and keratins), is a valuable microscopic sign of melanoma. Extension of atypical melanocytes into subungual epidermoid inclusions (adnexal-like extension) may show greater relative thickness than actual malignant melanocytes in the subungual stroma. Limitations to the value of the Hutchinson sign is its presence in some nevi, so far only dermoscopically proven, or the existence of a **pseudo-Hutchinson sign** given by pigmented Bowen disease or by overly transparent nail folds that would appear falsely pigmented.

In regards to the differential diagnosis, the **longitudinal melanonychia** derived from neoplastic disorders (**lentigo** and **nevus**) must be distinguished from the same phenomenon secondary to the freckle-like lesions with hyperactive melanocytes (**melanotic macules**). The latter lesions may be related to ethnicity (Africans and Asians), may be spontaneous or congenital, may develop after trauma (such as friction or radiation), or may be associated with **Laugier–Hunziker syndrome**. These benign causes of longitudinal melanonychia have, in turn, to be distinguished from **acral lentiginous melanoma in situ**, also characterized by a pigmented band. However, this band usually is wider, darker or variegated, and less well circumscribed than a benign pigmented band. It reflects a larger, more irregular, and heterogeneous neoplasm of the matrix. High-density proliferations of atypical melanocytes with elongated dendritic extensions and pagetoid scatter should be considered melanoma in situ or at least "atypical." Drug-associated hyperpigmentation of the nail most frequently results in transverse pigmentation. Melanocytic hyperplasia is not associated with **drug-associated melanonychia**.

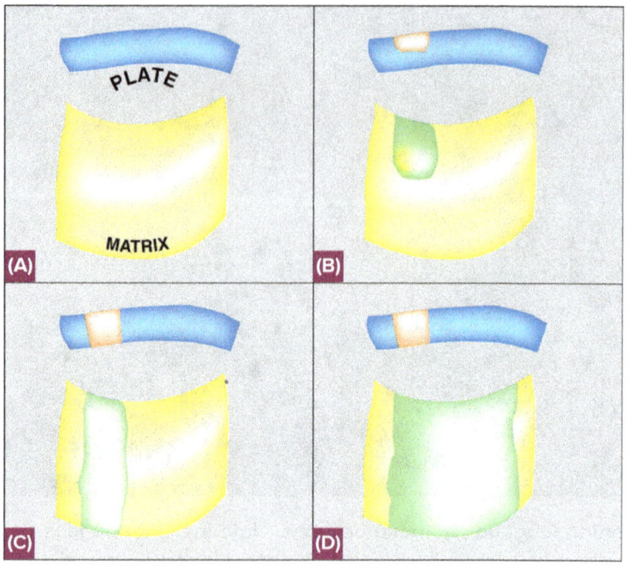

Dimensions of a matrical melanocytic lesion by means of analysis of a nail plate biopsy (NPB). The percentage of matrix involved by a pigment-producing lesion is manifested in an NPB. Correlation with clinical or histologic width of the pigmented band allows for a full picture of matrical involvement. **(A)** The plate is a mirror of the matrix, although 10-13 times thinner. **(B)** A small proximal matrical lesion produces a limited focus melanization of the upper plate sheets (eg, a lentigo). **(C)** A narrow but full-length matrical lesion will induce melanin throughout the entire vertical thickness of the plate (eg, a nevus). **(D)** A long and broad matrical lesion will give rise to a wide and full-thickness melanin trail in the plate (eg, melanoma). (The nail plate is depicted in the coronal view, matrix viewed en face [ie, from above].)

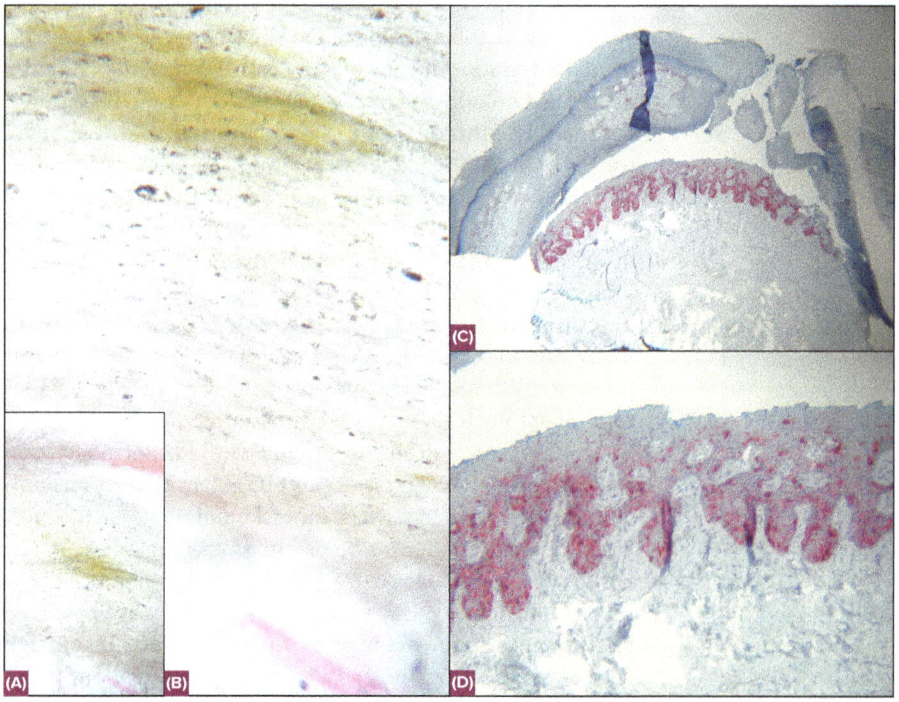

Nail plate biopsy for melanin in melanoma in situ. Low power **(A)** and higher power **(B)** Fontana-Masson stain shows full-thickness involvement by coarse melanin granules, most noticeable in the lower 87% of the plate. Low **(C)** and high **(D)** power longitudinal nail biopsy with immunoperoxidase stain for MART-1 reveals malignant melanoma in situ, extending as Hutchinson sign into the proximal nail fold.

ANSWER 10-30: B.

The biopsy reveals a diffuse, sheetlike, dermal-based melanocytic proliferation with little to no maturation with dermal descent. Six mitoses are identified within the high-power photograph. The findings are consistent with **nevoid melanoma** (Table 10-30A). It is well established that melanoma may show differentiation along the lines of almost every variant of benign melanocytic nevus or tumor. Thus a subset of melanomas closely resembles melanocytic nevi. Hence, the rubric "nevoid" melanoma has appeared in the literature as a direct result of this fundamental diagnostic problem of differentiating melanoma from nevus. In this chapter "nevoid" melanoma (NM) is defined as a group of melanomas that more or less recapitulate the architectural configuration and cytomorphology of melanocytic nevi yet concomitantly demonstrate histologic criteria for, and the biologic behavior of, melanoma. Because many such lesions are not diagnosed initially and are detected only in retrospect, the histologic diagnosis of NM remains controversial, and consensus criteria have not been well established. Suffice to say that nevoid melanoma remains a subject of ongoing research. In any case, this problem of the distinction of melanoma from nevus is among the most treacherous diagnostic problems in all of dermatopathology, and as such, carries significant medicolegal implications.

In very broad terms, the term "**nevoid melanoma**" could encompass any form of melanoma having some resemblance to or mimicking any type of melanocytic nevus. A variety of other terms have been used to describe this general group of melanomas, depending on how stringent are the criteria for inclusion, examples include **verrucous melanoma, spitzoid melanoma (SM)**, and **small cell melanoma**. Some nevoid melanomas might also be characterized as having a small diameter and also being comprised of small melanoma cells (ie, small cell melanoma). However, this chapter uses the term rather restrictively to describe melanomas that closely resemble ordinary dermal nevi or less commonly compound nevi. Nevoid melanomas generally fall into two groups: (1) those with a raised, dome-shaped, or polypoid (nodular non-verrucous) configuration that resemble a predominately dermal nevus and (2) those with a distinctly papillomatous or verrucous surface. Nevoid melanomas have no distinctive clinical features compared with conventional melanomas; however, verrucous or papillomatous variants may suggest a verruca, seborrheic keratosis, or warty nevus. Most tumors reported have been in adults.

The essential histopathologic criteria for diagnosis are as follows:

(1) At scanning magnification, the lesion has a striking resemblance to an ordinary compound or dermal nevus.
(2) An overall symmetry (some asymmetry may be present).
(3) A rather sharp circumscription at the peripheries of the lesion.
(4) The absence of or often only a limited intraepidermal component, commonly with little or no pagetoid spread.
(5) A monomorphous population of nevus-like cells in the dermis usually characterized by a confluent or sheet-like growth pattern in some portion of the lesion.
(6) Absent or minimal "maturation" with dermal descent.
(7) Dermal mitotic figures.

It is worth mentioning that some have applied the term "nevoid melanoma" to lentiginous junctional or compound melanocytic proliferations that are composed of melanocytes with overtly malignant melanocytes, but lack of confluent growth or pagetoid ascent. These lesions closely resemble atypical junctional nevi.

Table 10-30A. Nevoid Melanoma

Clinical Features
Women = men
All ages, but commonly fifth decade of life
Occurs anywhere, but trunk and lower extremities most common
No distinctive features, but may have verrucous appearance
Any size, often relatively small diameter but ≥2 cm
Histopathologic Features
Striking resemblance to banal compound or dermal nevus at scanning magnification
Symmetry common
Well-circumscribed lateral margins
Pagetoid spread not common
Often limited intraepidermal component
Relatively small nevus-like cells, monomorphous appearance
Some maturation may be present but often incomplete or absent
Single-cell infiltration at base
Cytologic atypia
Nuclear pleomorphism
Angulated nuclei
Hyperchromatism
Prominent nucleoli may be present
Mitoses in dermal component, particularly deep
Infiltration of adnexal structures
Little or no inflammation
Differential Diagnosis
Melanocytic nevus, especially papillomatous dermal nevus
Metastatic melanoma
Minimal deviation melanoma (MELTUMP)
Nodular epithelioid tumor with loss of BAP1 expression

There may be no intraepidermal melanocytic component in the majority of cases. The intraepidermal component, if present, may be subtle or limited in nature. One may observe melanocytes arranged as single cells, as junctional nests, or as both along the dermal–epidermal junction. The latter nesting may result in confluence of nested aggregates of melanocytes replacing the basilar portion of the epidermis. The epidermis is frequently effaced, thinned, and associated with dermal–epidermal separation. Pagetoid spread may be present in a small proportion of cases and is an important finding in confirming a diagnosis of melanoma; however, it is often not a conspicuous feature.

The principal architectural finding in the dermis includes a sheetlike or confluent arrangement of relatively small cuboidal or polygonal melanocytes closely mimicking nevus cells. Often the dermal melanocytic population fills the papillary dermis and is closely opposed to the epidermis, resulting in a strikingly crowded or hypercellular appearance. This is in contrast to the nested melanocytes seen in conventional dermal nevi. In some lesions, one may observe fairly discrete nesting of melanocytes in some areas; however, other parts of the lesion usually demonstrate the confluence and hypercellularity that favors melanoma. Although the lateral margins are commonly well demarcated, the base of the melanoma is often poorly defined and characterized by the presence of single cells infiltrating collagen. Although the absence of maturation with dermal descent raises suspicion for melanoma, in many cases the melanocytes extend into the reticular dermis with some diminished cellular density as well as some reduction in cellular and nuclear sizes (suggesting some degree of maturation). Furthermore, the heterogeneity of the lesion is another feature consonant with melanoma. In most instances, there is no host inflammatory response.

The melanocytes comprising NM, at least in the superficial part of the lesion and perhaps throughout, are generally polygonal or epithelioid cells (mimicking the so-called type A or epithelioid nevus cells), sufficiently small to suggest nevus cells. They nonetheless demonstrate definite, but sometimes subtle, nuclear enlargement, pleomorphism, and often hyperchromatism; rather prominent nucleoli may be present. Many NMs may exhibit some degree of maturation with dermal descent; nonetheless, major clues to diagnosis of NM are the presence of definite nuclear pleomorphism, particularly irregular nuclear contours, hyperchromatism, and nucleoli and continued pigment synthesis in the deepest parts of the dermal component. Commonly, one observes well-defined nests of relatively small cuboidal cells in the deepest portions of NM with the latter characteristics.

One of the most important, and sometimes the single most important, criterion for diagnosis is the presence of mitoses in the dermal component. This finding is often the first clue to considering melanoma in the differential diagnosis. The presence of one or a small number of dermal mitoses does not constitute sufficient evidence for diagnosis of melanoma, but it should prompt the histopathologist to search for additional criteria for melanoma and to either confirm or exclude the diagnosis (if possible). Mitoses are present in virtually all cases of NM, and their absence should provoke skepticism about melanoma. The mitotic rate is commonly relatively low, often less than 6/mm. Increasing mitotic rate, deeply situated mitoses, and atypical forms also provide progressively more support for NM. The presence or absence of mitotic figures in the deepest portion of a lesion can be a decisive factor in confirming or ruling out NM (Table 10-30B).

Many have proposed the term **"melanocytic tumor of undetermined malignant potential"** (MELTUMP) for

Table 10-30B. Comparison of Nevoid Melanoma and Melanocytic Nevus

NEVOID MELANOMA	MELANOCYTIC NEVUS
Clinical Features	
Older age	Younger age
Larger size (0.5 cm-2 cm)	Smaller size (<6 mm)
Some variation in color	More homogenous color
Greater asymmetry	Less asymmetry
Histopathologic Features	
Greater asymmetry	Symmetry
Less well circumscribed	Well circumscribed
Greater likelihood of pagetoid spread	Little or no pagetoid spread
Intraepidermal basilar melanocytic proliferation common	Basilar proliferation less common
Infiltration of adnexae	No infiltration of adnexae
Reduced or no maturation	Maturation
Mitoses in dermis	Usually no dermal mitoses
Atypical mitoses	No atypical mitoses
Deep infiltration of dermis	No deep infiltration

dermal-based melanocytic tumors with histopathologic features equivocal for melanoma. MELTUMP has been used to describe atypical Spitz tumors (both epithelioid and spindled), atypical cellular blue nevi, and atypical intradermal melanocytic proliferations. The systematic use of the term MELTUMP potentially risks creating an artificial category or "dumping ground" reserved for all borderline or ambiguous melanocytic lesions. Alternatively appropriate are less formalized simple descriptive terms such as "atypical dermal melanocytic neoplasm, biologically indeterminate" and an appended discussion of the differential diagnosis. Another term used to describe these lesions is **"minimal deviation melanoma" (MDM)**, which connotes a subset of melanocytic proliferations presumably characterized by lesser cytologic atypia and a better prognosis compared with conventional melanomas. Thus, central to the concept of MDM is the presence of a cohesive nodule of dermal tumor cells. The growth pattern of such a nodule potentially indicates aggressive properties, such as potential for recurrence or metastasis. Also implicit is the presence of a cell type lacking the characteristics of "fully evolved" melanoma cells. The cell types presumed to occur in MDM resemble ordinary nevus cells, spindled melanocytes, and epithelioid cells as from Spitz nevi. Dermal mitotic activity is typically rare (one or two mitoses) or absent. Because of the lack of specific histologic criteria and objective markers, data are not available that confirm or refute MDM as an entity.

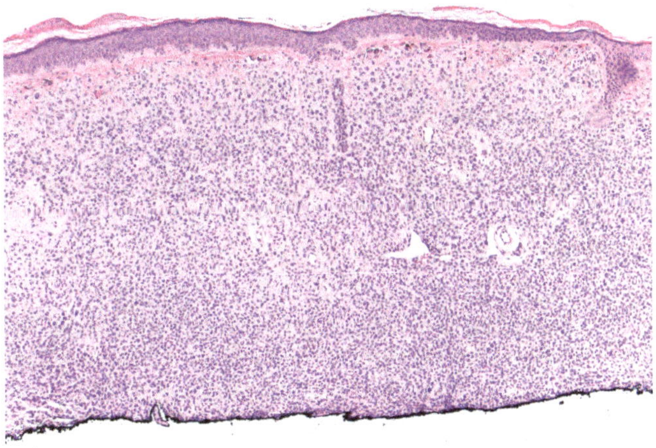

Dermal melanocytic neoplasm with indeterminate biological potential. There is a dermal-based, diffuse, sheetlike, population of melanocytes with limited maturation with dermal descent. Overt malignant cytologic atypia is not present. No dermal mitotic activity is identified. The lesion illustrates that not all atypical melanocytic lesions can be easily classified as "benign" or "malignant".

Recently a subset of atypical dermal epithelioid cell tumors with loss of BAP1 (BRCA1-Associated Protein 1) expression has been described. These tumors have been referred to as **"nodular epithelioid cell tumor with loss of BAP1 expression."** BAP1 is a known tumor suppressor that can be detected via nuclear staining with a BAP1 immunohistochemical stain. Loss of BAP1 will result in negative staining. These tumors have also been found to harbor $BRAF^{V600E}$ oncogene mutations. Although these tumors may occur sporadically, they also arise frequently as part of a familial cancer syndrome. Presence of multiple BAP1-loss melanocytic lesions should raise concern about a possible germline mutation. Germline mutations of BAP1 confer increased susceptibility for the development of several other tumors including uveal melanoma, mesothelioma, and clear cell renal cell carcinoma. However, the complete spectrum of tumors associated with these germline mutations is not yet known. Microscopically these atypical epithelioid Spitz tumors are characterized by a dermal nevus-like silhouette containing varying populations of hyperchromatic nevus cell-like and large atypical epithelioid spitzoid cells. The large spitzoid cells contain oval vesicular nuclei with "hollowed out" chromatin, distinct nucleoli, and abundant eosinophilic cytoplasm. The large epithelioid cells characteristically show loss of nuclear expression of BAP1. There is typically minimal to absent maturation with dermal descent.

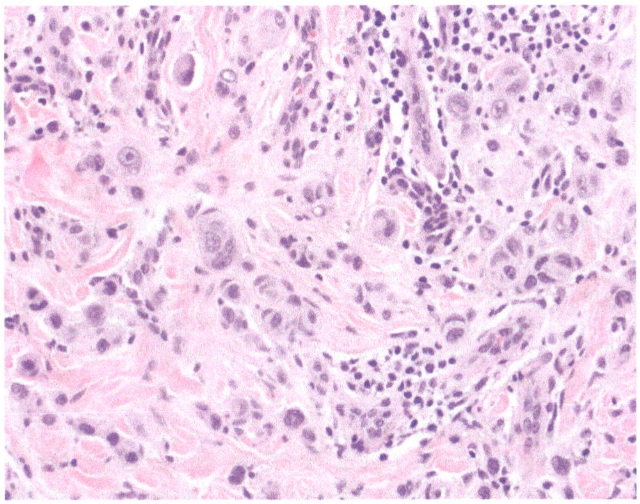

Nodular epithelioid cell tumor with loss of BAP1 expression. There is a mixed population of ordinary type A melanocytes admixed with enlarged epithelioid spitzoid melanocytes with "hollowed out" chromatin, prominent nucleoli, and abundant eosinophilic cytoplasm.

In regards to the differential diagnosis, the principal dilemma is discrimination of **nevoid melanomas** from **benign melanocytic nevi** (especially papillomatous dermal nevi) and **metastatic melanoma**. One's confidence in rendering a diagnosis of nevoid melanoma directly correlates with the number of abnormal features present. The following attributes are of critical importance in distinguishing NM from a nevus: (1) dermal mitoses, usually multiple and scattered throughout the lesion, are probably mandatory for the diagnosis. The higher the absolute mitotic rate and the more deeply located the mitoses, the more certain the diagnosis. However, the presence of rare mitoses, particularly in nevi in young or pregnant individuals and in nevi without atypia, must be interpreted with caution and are not proof of NM. (2) Dermal aggregates or fascicles of melanocytes showing high density and confluence, having a sheetlike appearance throughout, or showing both features. The dermal population often demonstrates a monotonous appearance with minimal to absent maturation with dermal descent. (3) Cytologic atypia of melanocytes is mandatory for the diagnosis. By definition, there are lesser degrees of atypia than in conventional melanomas. Careful scrutiny at higher magnifications is necessary to establish the presence of cytologic atypia. Differentiating **nevoid melanoma** from **metastatic melanoma** relies mostly on clinical correlation. While most metastatic melanomas exhibit overtly malignant large melanocytes, rare exceptions exist. In general, the melanocytes of NM may be relatively small compared with the usual enlarged epithelioid melanoma cells in metastatic melanoma.

BIBLIOGRAPHY

1. Bahrami A, Lee S, Wu G, et al. Congenital low-grade pigment-synthesizing melanocytic neoplasm with protein kinase C alpha (PRKCA) fusion: report of two cases. *JAMA Dermatol.* 2015. In press.
2. Bald T, Quast T, Landsberg J, et al. Ultraviolet-radiation-induced inflammation promotes angiotropism and metastasis in melanoma. *Nature.* 2014 Mar 6;507(7490):109–113.
3. Balin SJ, Barnhill RL. Chapter 113. Benign Melanocytic Neoplasms. In: Bolognia J et al, eds. *Dermatology.* 4th ed. London: Harcourt Press; 2015.
4. Balin SJ, Barnhill RL. The clinical presentation of the high-mitotic-rate melanoma. *JAMA Dermatol.* 2014 Oct 1;150(10):1047. doi:10.1001/jamadermatol.2014.924. PubMed PMID: 25142555.
5. Barnhill R, Lemaitre S, Levy-Gabriel C, et al. Satellite metastases in rapidly fatal conjunctival melanoma: implications for angiotropism and extravascular migratory metastasis. *Pathology.* Submitted. 2015.
6. Barnhill R, Lugassy C, Battistella A, et al. Angiotropism in uveal melanoma: frequency and effects of sampling in 90 cases. International Society of Ocular Oncology. June 2015.
7. Barnhill R, Lugassy C, Lemaitre S, Levy-Gabriel C, Desjardins L, Cassoux N. Satellite metastases in rapidly fatal conjunctival melanoma: implications for angiotropism and extravascular migratory metastasis. International Society of Ocular Oncology. June 2015.
8. Barnhill RL, Busam KJ, From L, Bagot M, Lugassy C, Berwick M. Inter-observer concordance for the recognition of angiotropism in human melanoma. *Pigment Cell Mel Res.* 2011;24:582–583.
9. Barnhill RL, Cerroni L, Cook M, et al. State of the art, nomenclature, and points of consensus and controversy concerning benign melanocytic lesions: outcome of an international workshop. *Adv Anat Pathol.* 2010;17(2):73–90.
10. Barnhill RL, Chastain MA, Jerdan MS, et al. Angiotropic neonatal congenital melanocytic nevus: how extravascular migration of melanocytes may explain the development of congenital nevi. *Am J Dermatopathol.* 2010;32(5):495–499.
11. Barnhill RL, Kutzner H, Schmidt B, et al. Atypical spitzoid melanocytic neoplasms with angiotropism: a potential mechanism of loco-regional involvement. *Am J Dermatopathol.* 2011;33:236–243.
12. Barnhill RL, Mihm MC. Chapter 1.4: Malignant Melanoma. In: Weinzweig J, ed. *Plastic Surgery Secrets.* 2nd ed. 2010.
13. Barnhill RL, Sarantopoulos P, Gupta K. Less common variants of cutaneous melanomas. In: Sharfman W, ed. *Emerging Cancer Therapeutics.* Springer; 2013.
14. Barnhill RL. Editor in Chief. *Dermatopathology.* 3rd ed. New York, NY: McGraw-Hill Inc.; 2010.
15. Barnhill RL. Editor in Chief. Piepkorn M, Busam KJ, Co-Editors. *Pathology of Melanocytic Nevi and Melanoma.* 3rd ed. New York, NY: Springer; 2014.
16. Broekaert SMC, Roy R, Okamoto I, et al. Genetic and morphologic features for melanoma classification. *Pigment Cell Melanoma Res.* 2010;23:763–770.
17. Cerroni L, Barnhill R, Elder D, et al. Melanocytic tumors of uncertain malignant potential (MELTUMPs): results of a tutorial held at the XXIX Symposium of the International Society of Dermatopathology in Graz, October 2008. *Am J Surg Pathol.* 2010;34(3):314–326.
18. Fan Y, Lee S, Wu G, et al. TERT promoter hypermethylation is the underlying mechanism for telomerase activation in subsets of malignant melanoma. *J Invest Dermatol.* 2015. In Press.
19. Frangos JE, Duncan LM, Piris A, et al. Increased diagnosis of thin superficial spreading melanomas: a 20-year study. *J Am Acad Dermatol.* 2011 Dec 7. [Epub ahead of print] PubMed PMID: 22153791.
20. Gerami P, Barnhill RL, LeBoit PE, Schneider P, Guitart J. Superficial melanocytic neoplasms with pagetoid melanocytosis: a study of inter-observer concordance and correlation with FISH. *Am J Surg Pathol.* 2010;34(6):816–821.

21. Gerami P, Busam K, Cochran A, et al. Histomorphologic assessment and interobserver diagnostic reproducibility of atypical spitzoid melanocytic neoplasms with long-term follow-up. *Am J Surg Pathol.* 2014 Mar 10. [Epub ahead of print]

22. Gerami P, Cooper C, Bajaj S, et al. Outcomes of atypical spitz tumors with chromosomal copy number aberrations and conventional melanomas in children. *Am J Surg Pathol.* 2013 Sep;37(9):1387–1394.

23. Gerami P, Scolyer RA, Xu X, et al. Risk assessment for atypical spitzoid melanocytic neoplasms using FISH to identify chromosomal copy number aberrations. *Am J Surg Pathol.* 2013 May;37(5):676–684.

24. Gould Rothberg BE, Bulloch KJ, Fine JA, Barnhill RL, Berwick M. Red meat and fruit intake is prognostic among patients with localized cutaneous melanomas more than 1 mm thick. *Cancer Epidemiol.* 2014 Oct;38(5):599–607. doi:10.1016/j.canep.2014.08.005. Epub 2014 Sep 5. PubMed PMID: 25194935.

25. Hung T, Argenyi Z, Berwick M, et al. Cellular blue nevomelanocytic lesions: analysis of clinical, histological, and outcomes data in 37 cases. *Am J Dermatopathol.* 2015. In press.

26. Hung T, Morin J, Munday WR, Mackenzie IR, Lugassy C, Barnhill RL. Angiotropism in primary cutaneous melanoma with brain metastasis: a study of 20 cases. *Am J Dermatopathol.* 2013 Aug;35(6):650–654.

27. Hung T, Yang A, Binder SW, Barnhill RL. Cutaneous ciliated cyst on the finger: a cutaneous mullerian cyst. *Am J Dermatopathol.* 2012 Jan 11. [Epub ahead of print] PubMed PMID: 22240776.

28. Hung T, Yang A, Mihm MC, Barnhill RL. Plexiform spindle cell nevus and atypical variants: report of 128 cases. *Hum Pathol.* 2014 Sep 2. pii: S0046-8177(14)00353-0. doi:10.1016/j.humpath.2014.08.009. [Epub ahead of print] PubMed PMID: 25300464.

29. Knezevich SR, Barnhill RL, Elder DE, et al. Variability in mitotic figures in serial sections of thin melanomas. *J Am Acad Dermatol.* 2014 Sep 16. pii: S0190-9622(14)01787-3. doi:10.1016/j.jaad.2014.07.056. [Epub ahead of print] PubMed PMID: 25239732.

30. Kokta, V, Hung T, Al Dhaybi R, Lugassy C, Barnhill R. High prevalence of angiotropism in congenital melanocytic nevi: an analysis of 54 cases. *Am J Dermatopathol.* 2012 Jul 5. [Epub ahead of print]

31. Landsberg J, Tuting T, Barnhill RL, Lugassy C. The role of neutrophilic inflammation, angiotropism and pericytic mimicry in melanoma progression and metastasis. *J Invest Dermatol.* 2015. In Press.

32. Lee S, Barnhill RL, Dummer R, et al. TERT promoter mutations are predictive of aggressive clinical behavior in patients with spitzoid melanocytic neoplasms. *Sci Rep.* 2015 Jun 10;5:11200. doi:10.1038/srep11200. PubMed PMID: 26061100; PubMed Central PMCID: PMC4462090.

33. Lugassy C, Lazar V, Dessen P, et al. Gene expression profiling of human angiotropic primary melanoma: selection of 15 differentially expressed genes potentially involved in extravascular migratory metastasis. *Eur J Cancer.* 2011;47:1267–1275.

34. Lugassy C, Péault B, Wadehra M, Kleinman HK, Barnhill RL. Could pericytic mimicry represent another type of melanoma cell plasticity with embryonic properties? *Pigment Cell Melanoma Res.* 2013 Sep;26(5):746–754.

35. Lugassy C, Wadehra M, Li X, et al. Pilot study on "pericytic mimicry" and potential embryonic/stem cell properties of angiotropic melanoma cells interacting with the abluminal vascular surface. *Cancer Microenviron.* 2013 Apr;6(1):19–29.

36. Lugassy C, Zadran S, Bentolila LA, et al. Angiotropism, pericytic mimicry and extravascular migratory metastasis in melanoma: an alternative to intravascular cancer dissemination. *Cancer Microenviron.* 2014 Oct 12. [Epub ahead of print] PubMed PMID: 25304454.

37. Michael Y. Xiong MY, Rabkin MS, et al. Diameter of dysplastic nevi is a more robust biomarker of increased melanoma risk than degree of histological dysplasia: a case-control study. *J Am Acad Dermatol.* 2014 Dec;71(6):1257–1258.e4. doi:10.1016/j.jaad.2014.07.030. Epub 2014 Nov 15.

38. Mravic M, Asatrian G, Soo C, et al. From pericytes to perivascular tumours: correlation between pathology, stem cell biology, and tissue engineering. *Int Orthop.* 2014 Feb 25. [Epub ahead of print]

39. Palmieri G, Sarantopoulos P, Barnhill R, Cochran A. Molecular pathology of melanocytic skin cancer. In: *Skin Cancer: A Practical Approach.* Springer; 2012.

40. Piepkorn MW, Barnhill RL, Elder DE, et al. The MPATH-Dx reporting schema for melanocytic proliferations and melanoma. *J Am Acad Dermatol.* 2014 Jan;70(1):131–141.

41. Piepkorn MW, Barnhill RL, Elder DE. Reply: surgical margins for possibly malignant melanocytic lesions and the overdiagnosis of melanoma. *J Am Acad Dermatol.* 2014 Sep;71(3):590. doi:10.1016/j.jaad.2014.05.031. PubMed PMID: 25128110.

42. Shen J, Shrestha S, Yen YH, et al. Pericyte antigens in angiomyolipoma and PEComa family tumors. *Med Oncol.* 2015 Aug;32(8):210. doi:10.1007/s12032-015-0659-y. Epub 2015 Jun 30. PubMed PMID: 26123600.

43. Su A, Low L, Li X, Zhou S, Mascarenhas L, Barnhill RL. De novo congenital melanoma: analysis of 2 cases

with array comparative genomic hybridization. *Am J Dermatopathol.* 2014 Jul 21. [Epub ahead of print] PubMed PMID: 25051103.

44. Wang YT, Geng B, Yoo KY, et al. Cutaneous granulomas and epidermodysplasia verruciformis in early onset combined immunodeficiency syndrome. *Am J Dermatopathol.* 2014 Feb;36(2):179–183.

45. Wilmott J, Haydu L, Bagot M, et al. Angiotropism is an independent predictor of microscopic satellites in primary cutaneous melanoma. *Histopathology.* 2012 Mar 30. doi:10.1111/j.1365-2559.

46. Zadran S, McMickle R, Shackelford D, Kleinman H, Barnhill R, Lugassy C. Monitoring extra-vascular migratory metastasis (EVMM) of migrating cancer cells using an in vitro co-culture system. *Protoc exch.* 2013 Nov 22;2013. pii: 2867.

CHAPTER 11

Tumors of Mesenchymal Origin

QUESTION 11-1.

Which of the following regarding normal vessels is INCORRECT?

A) Endothelial cells express CD31, CD34, von Willebrand factor, and *Ulex europaeus* lectin-1.
B) Pericytes and smooth muscle cells express smooth muscle actin and α-smooth muscle actin.
C) Lymphatic endothelial cells express LYVE-1 and podoplanin (D2-40).
D) Endothelial cells play an important role in antigen presentation and cytokine secretion.
E) Both large arteries and veins contain a prominent internal elastic lamina that can be highlighted with an elastic stain.

QUESTION 11-2.

Which of the following histopathologic features is NOT associated with vascular malignancy?

A) Small round vessels in a lobular distribution with flat endothelial cells containing inconspicuous nucleoli.
B) Prominent anastomosing angular vascular channels with plump endothelial cells containing conspicuous nucleoli.
C) Angular vessels lined by compact endothelial cells that exhibit multilayering or "piling up" on one another.
D) Solid areas composed of polygonal and/or spindled endothelial cells with intracytoplasmic lumina containing red blood cells
E) Irregular angulated vessels extending into the subcutis with intraluminal papillary growth and endothelial tufting.

QUESTION 11-3.

You are covering for a fellow physician's practice and as you are preparing to see a 3-year-old female patient for the first time, you notice in her chart that she presented at 12 months of age with a red to purplish rubbery nodule on the cheek that developed during her first weeks of life. The mother reported that the tumor evolved from a pink macule that gradually increased in size. The lesion was not ulcerated and did not interfere with any vital structures such as the eyes or airways. Your colleague reported in the chart that the lesion blanched with compression and no intervention was pursued. When you examine the child you notice that the lesion has now disappeared with only residual redundant skin. Although the lesion was not biopsied, the images below represent what the tumor would have looked like microscopically at 6 months (image A), 12 months (image B), and at its current state (image C). Which of the following statements regarding this tumor is INCORRECT?

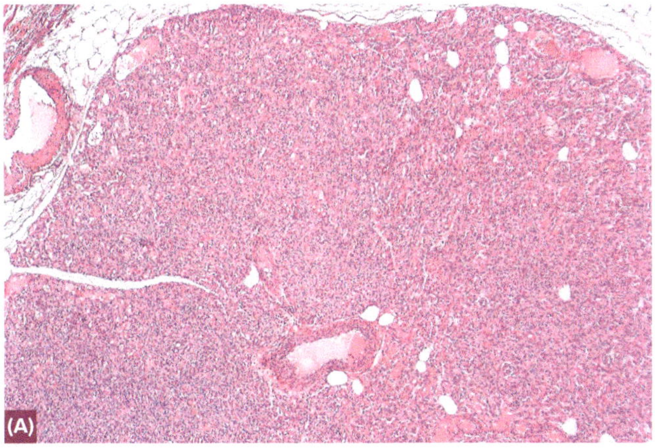
(A)

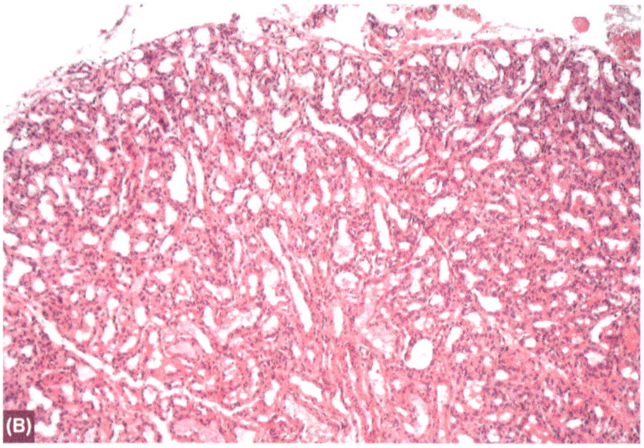

(B)

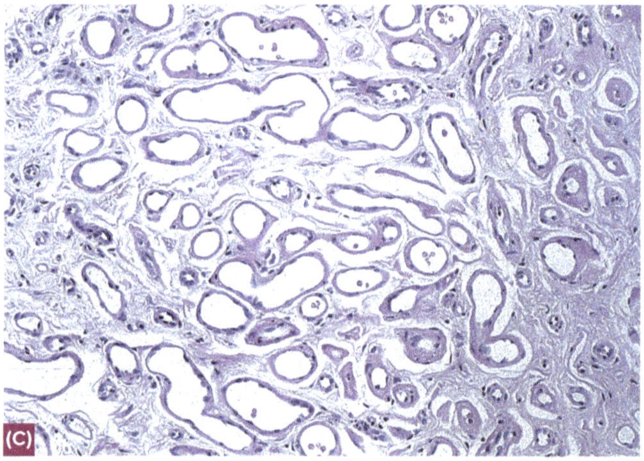

(C)

A) These tumors are typified by a fairly predictable natural history in the great majority of cases, which includes rapid proliferation and enlargement in the first 8 to 12 months of life (the proliferative phase) and regression over a period of 1 to 5 years (the involutional phase).

B) Approximately 10% of these tumors will require intervention, often because of ulceration, local destructive effects such as impingement on vital structures, or shunting of blood and high-output cardiac failure.

C) There is an association of these tumors with very low birth weight (<1 kg) and a history of chorionic villous sampling.

D) These tumors are associated with entrapment of platelets, thrombocytopenic coagulopathy, and potentially life-threatening hemorrhages.

E) These tumors have the unique immunophenotype of GLUT-1, merosin (α-laminin), and Lewis Y antigen expression.

QUESTION 11-4.

A 75-year-old golfer presents with a solitary, dark-blue, 0.7-mm papule on the cheek. The lesion blanches with compression. A biopsy is performed and the histopathology is illustrated below. Which of the following statements regarding this lesion is INCORRECT?

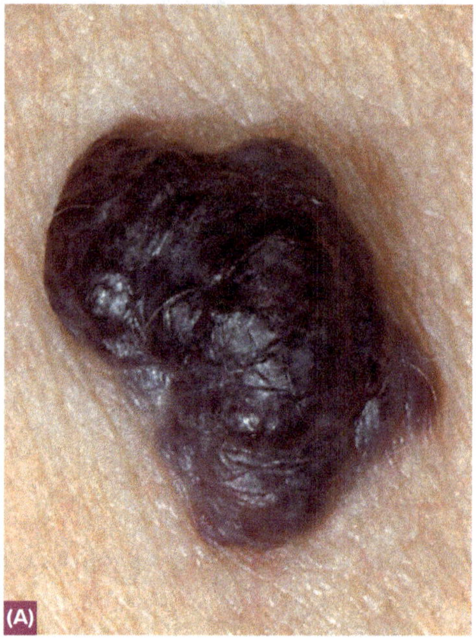

(A)

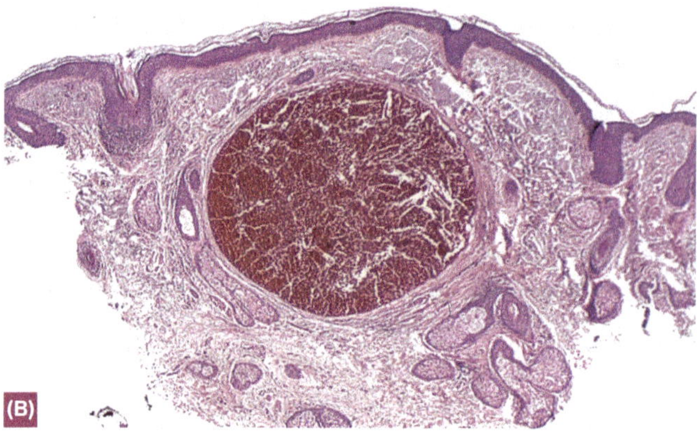

(B)

A) This is a benign neoplasm of postcapillary venule differentiation.

B) These lesions most commonly arise in chronically sun-damaged skin such as the ear, lip, face, and neck.

C) Occasionally these lesions may become thrombosed and clinically mistaken for a melanoma.

D) Pyogenic granulomas have been reported to arise within these lesions post cryosurgery.

E) Although a single layer of endothelium lines this lesion, smooth muscle elements may occasionally be associated with the vessel wall.

QUESTION 11-5.

A 23-year-old patient presents with a small (<1cm) blue-red nodule on the right index finger at the base of the nail. There is paroxysmal pain, tenderness, and temperature sensitivity. The lesion is biopsied and the histopathology is illustrated below. Which of the following statements regarding this lesion is INCORRECT?

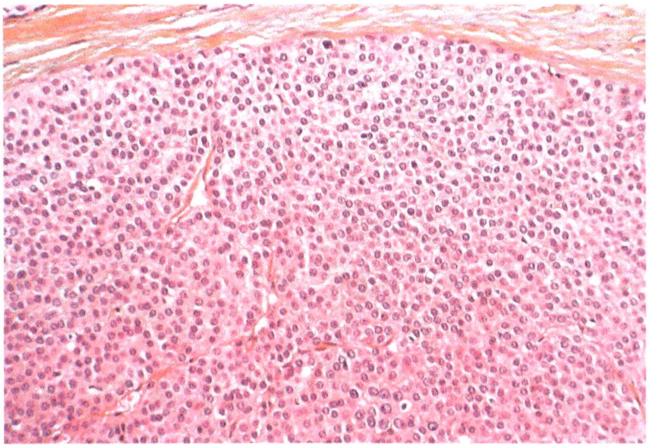

A) This is a benign neoplasm derived from capillary pericytes, which regulate arteriovenous shunting of blood and temperature regulation.
B) Subungual lesions that measure greater than 2 cm in diameter should be excised to exclude malignant transformation.
C) The lesional cells express vimentin, smooth muscle actins, and variably desmin, but are negative for von Willebrand factor, cytokeratin, and S-100 protein.
D) The presentation of multiple lesions suggests vascular malformation instead of neoplasia and is associated with an autosomal dominant inheritance pattern in 64% of cases.
E) Superficially situated lesions with malignant-appearing histologic features show less aggressive behavior than similar-appearing lesions at deep locations.

QUESTION 11-6.

A 3-year-old pale and lethargic patient presents with soft, blue to purple nodules and plaques on the neck, upper limbs, trunk, and perineum that have a compressible quality and increase in size with venous pressure or when dependent. The mother reports that the lesions have been present since birth and are occasionally painful with increased sweating around the site. She also reports that the child frequently has black tar-like stools with occasional bright red blood. One of the nodules is excised and the histopathological findings are illustrated below. Which of the following statements regarding this lesion is INCORRECT?

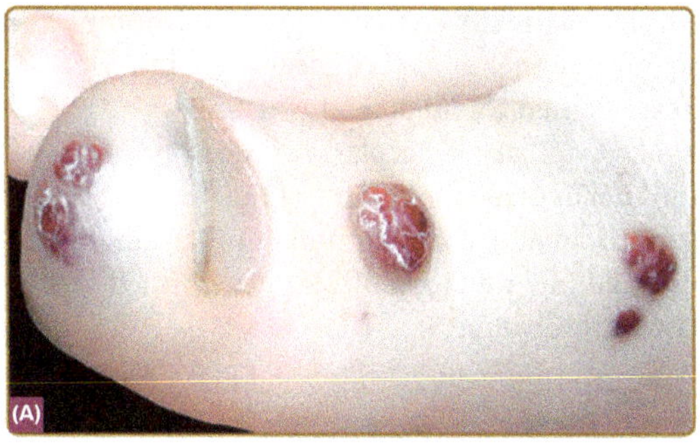

Reproduced, with permission, from Goldsmith LA, Katz SI, Gilchrest BA, Paller AS, Leffell DJ, Wolff K, eds. *Fitzpatrick's Dermatology in General Medicine*. 8th ed. New York, NY: McGraw-Hill Education; 2012.

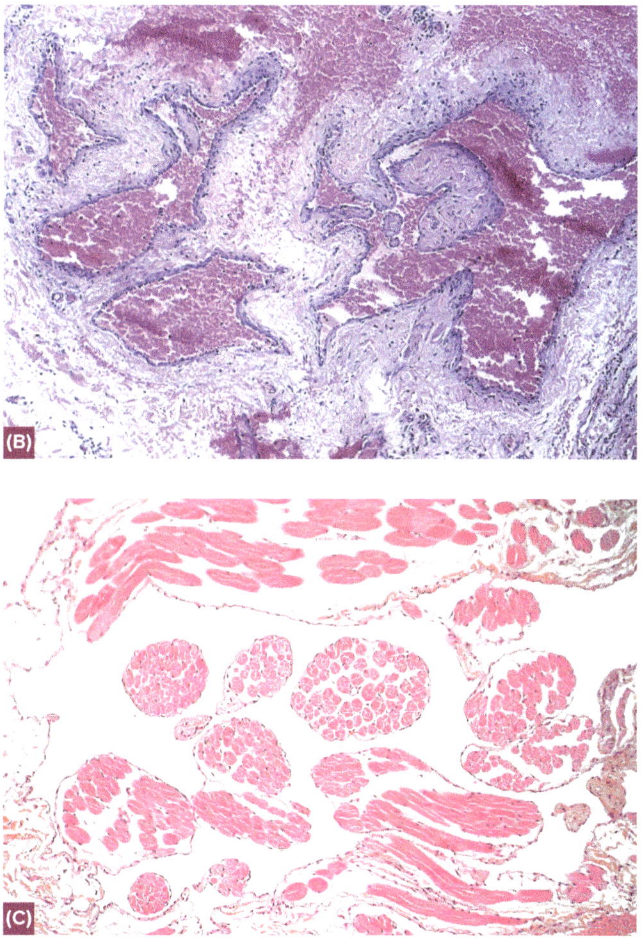

A) This patient has a syndrome in which multiple lesions are also present throughout the gastrointestinal tract, central nervous system, liver, and spleen with subsequent chronic blood loss and iron deficiency anemia.
B) Vascular lesions with similar histomorphology may be seen in Maffucci syndrome.
C) The lumina of the dilated vessels frequently contain numerous lymphocytes or lymphocytic aggregates within the vicinity of the malformed vessels. Additionally, EVG stain will reveal a thick internal elastic lamina within the vessel walls.

D) These lesions frequently contain organized thrombi, which manifest either as concentrically hyalinized structures, calcified round phleboliths, or as intravascular papillary hyperplasia of Masson.
E) A familial mucocutaneous variant of this patient's syndrome has an autosomal dominant inheritance pattern related to a mutation of *Tie2* gene, which is located on chromosome 9.

QUESTION 11-7.

Which of the following clinical presentations is NOT associated with the histopathological findings illustrated below?

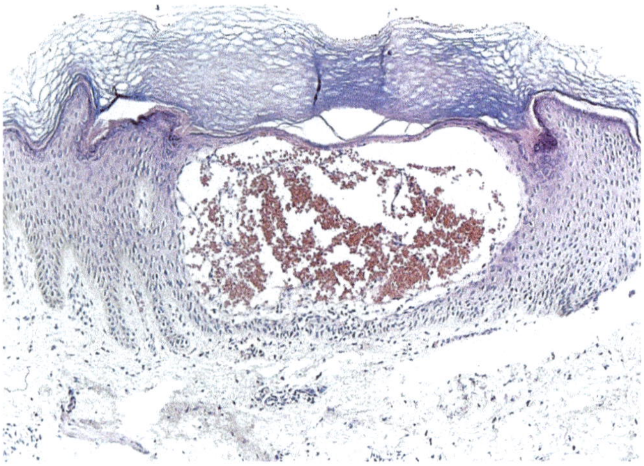

A) Hyperkeratotic lesions on the dorsal fingers and toes.
B) Dark red papules involving of the scrotum and vulva.
C) Multiple tumors arising in association with lysosomal storage disease (ie, Fabry disease, fucosidosis, and rarely β-galactosidase deficiency).
D) Multiple lesions arranged in groups or bands on an extremity.
E) Multiple tumors arising in association with a multisystem disorder consisting of polyneuropathy, organomegaly, endocrinopathy, and IgM paraproteinemia.

QUESTION 11-8.

A 22-year-old presents with unilateral pink to reddish keratotic papules and nodules on the face in the second and third trigeminal distribution. The patient reports that the lesions have been present since birth, but were originally flat faint red macules. The lesions have occupied the same proportion of the patient's face since birth. According to the patient, a biopsy was performed at birth and systemic workup was performed (image A). You perform another biopsy (image B). Which of the following statements regarding these lesions is INCORRECT?

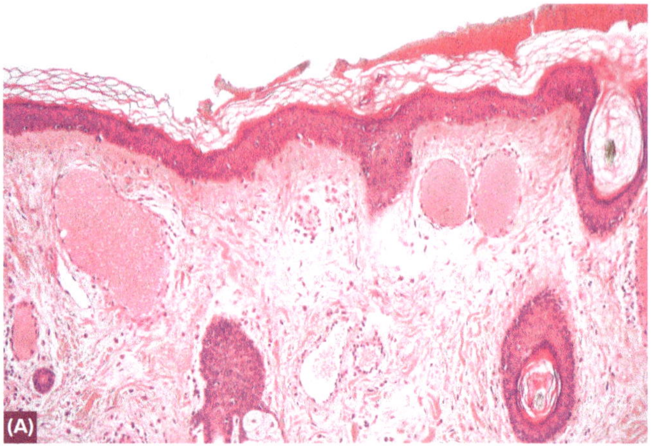
(A)

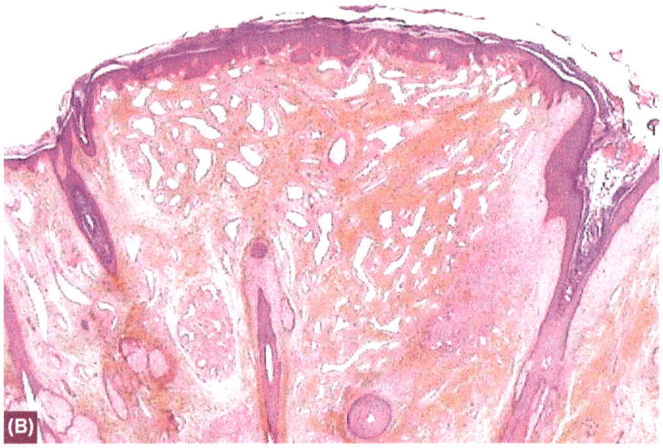
(B)

A) In the head region and especially the mandibular area, these lesions may be associated with underlying soft tissue and bone hypertrophy.
B) This condition represents a malformation of the Sucquet-Hoyer canal and is occasionally associated with angiolymphoid hyperplasia with eosinophilia, verruciform xanthoma, and basal cell carcinoma.
C) These lesions represent a form of capillary vascular malformation.
D) Pyogenic granulomas arise within these lesions more frequently than normal skin.
E) These lesions are associated with Sturge-Weber and Klippel-Trenaunay syndromes.

QUESTION 11-9.

Which of the following clinical presentations is MOST likely associated with the vascular lesion illustrated below?

A) A Japanese patient with multiple punctate to several-millimeter-sized, red and violaceous papules favoring the trunk and proximal limbs. The patient also has polyneuropathy, organomegaly, endocrinopathy, and an IgM-protein spike.

B) A child with slowly enlarging dull red-to-brown papules and plaques on the neck and upper truck. Peripheral blood analysis reveals a consumptive thrombocytopenia and coagulopathy.
C) A child with an enlarging intradermal and subcutaneous swelling of the head, neck, or extremities. There may be possible lymph node involvement; however, the long-term prognosis is excellent with complete excision.
D) A solitary, rapidly growing, dark red, polypoid lesion with ulceration on the finger following trauma.

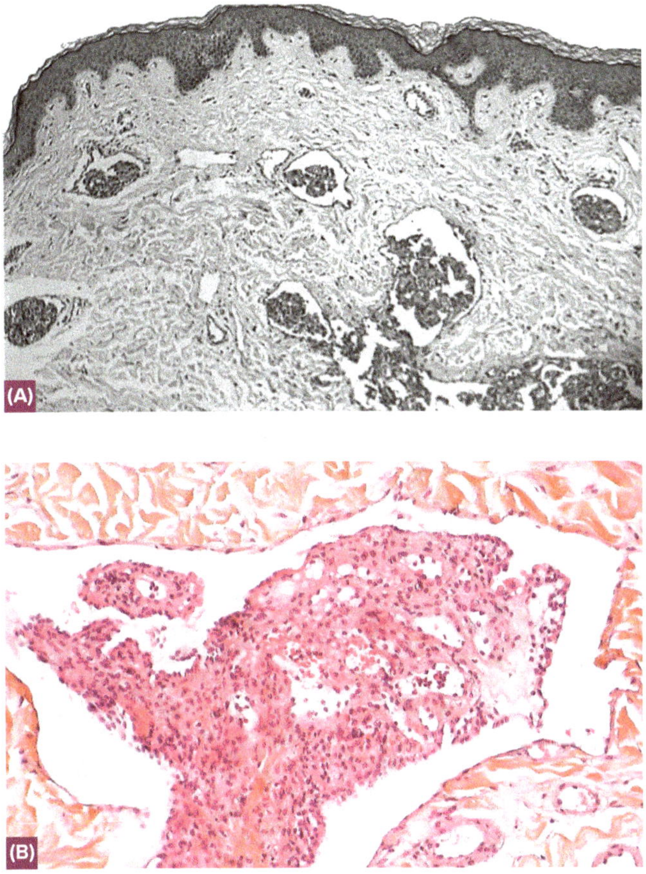

QUESTION 11-10.

An HIV positive patient presents with a solitary, rapidly growing, dark red, polypoid, vascular lesion with superficial ulceration on the tip of the finger following trauma. The lesion is biopsied. Which of the following regarding this lesion is INCORRECT?

A) Most lesions arise spontaneously without a known cause, but others are associated with trauma, cast immobilization, antiretroviral therapy, and various medications (ie, retinoids and minocycline).
B) The lesional endothelial cells are immunoreactive for ER and PR, suggesting hormonal influence in the formation of these lesions.
C) Oral mucosal lesions are strongly associated with pregnancy and female gender.
D) Satellite lesions on the upper back and trunk following surgical or laser excisions are well documented.
E) The rapid growth of these lesions may result from decreased apoptosis associated with increased expression of the Bcl-2 family of apoptotic-regulatory proteins.

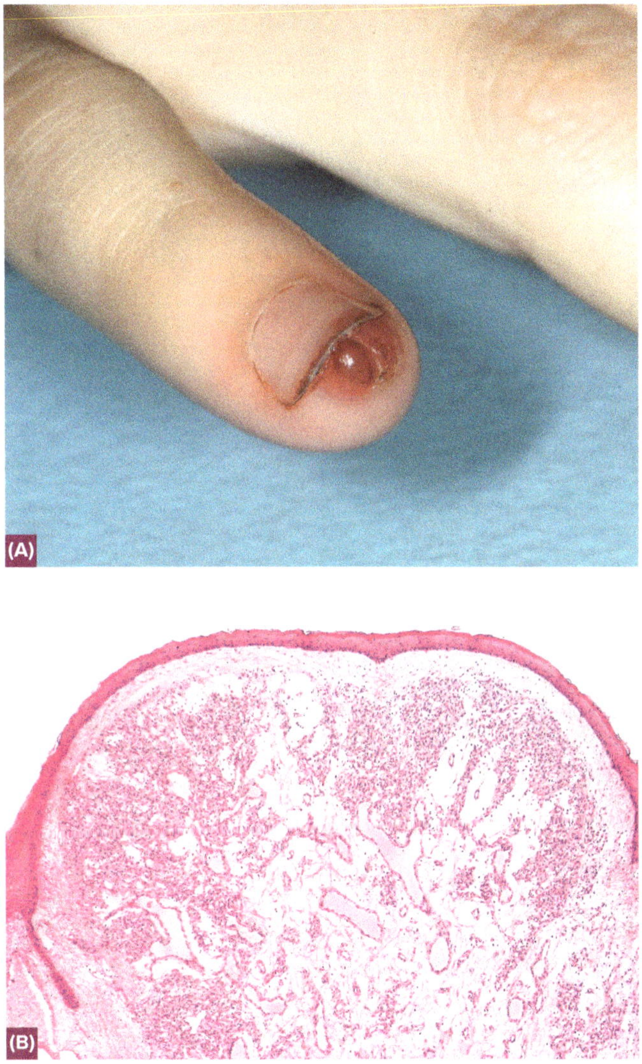

QUESTION 11-11.

A 32-year-old female presents with a pink to red-brown plaque on the ear. The lesion is mostly asymptomatic with only occasional mild pruritus. A biopsy is performed and illustrated below. Mitoses are present (5 per 10 high-power fields); however, atypical mitoses and "piling up" of endothelial cells are absent. Immunohistochemical stains reveal the endothelial cells to express common endothelial markers (CD31, CD34, von Willebrand factor) and focal epithelial keratins CK19 and CK7. Which of the following diagnoses is CORRECT?

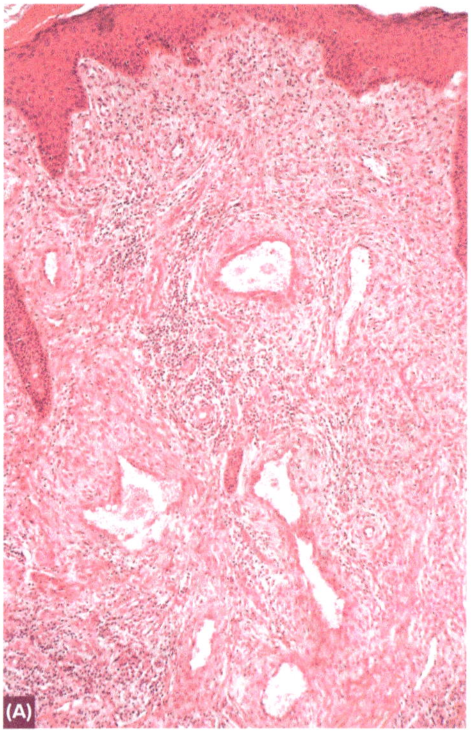

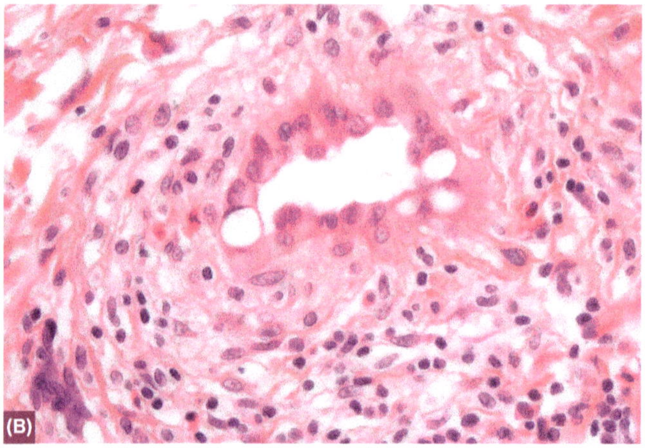

A) Epithelioid hemangioma
B) Epithelioid angiosarcoma
C) Kimura disease
D) Epithelioid hemangioendothelioma
E) Hobnail hemangioma

QUESTION 11-12.

A 55-year-old male with a history of mycosis fungoides treated with topical nitrogen mustard presents a new onset of diffuse uniform bright to dull red papules ranging in size from 2 to 10 mm. He reports that he originally developed a few of these lesions on the trunk 20 years ago and then noticed a few more several years later. The tumors are persistent and have remained stable in terms of size and shape. You tell the patient that this is an eruptive variant of the most common adult vascular tumor, and that this eruptive phenomenon is likely attributed to the use of topical nitrogen mustard. One of the lesions is biopsied. An incidental varicose vein is noted adjacent to one of the tumors. Which of the following images MOST accurately represents the biopsied lesion?

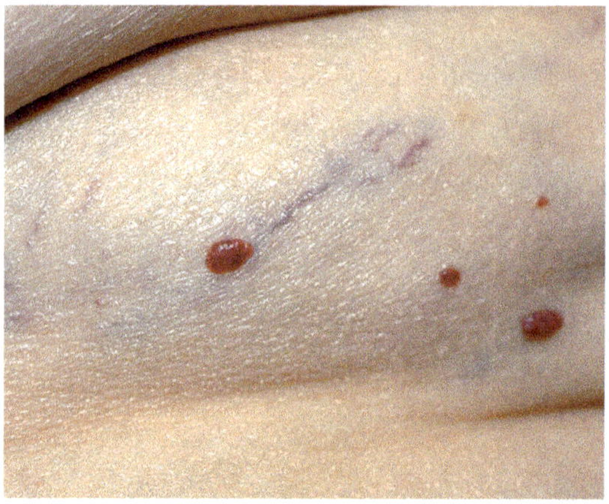

Reproduced, with permission, from Wolff K, Johnson RA, Saavedra AP. *Fitzpatrick's Color Atlas and Synopsis of Clinical Dermatology*. 7th ed. New York, NY: McGraw-Hill Education; 2013.

A)

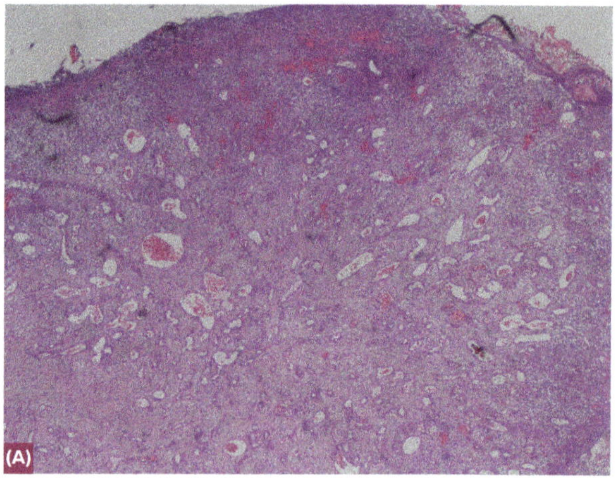

B)

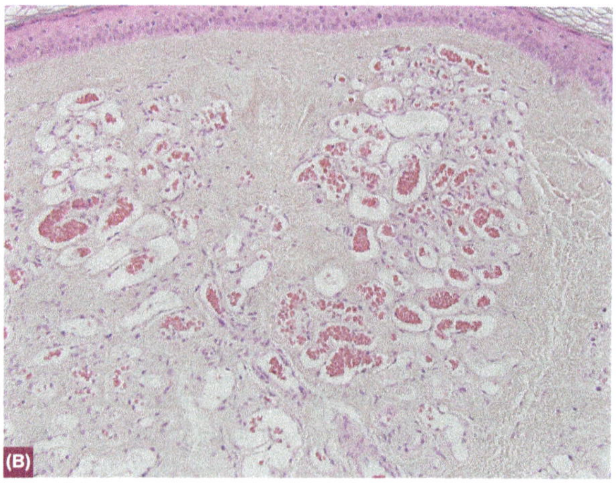

C) 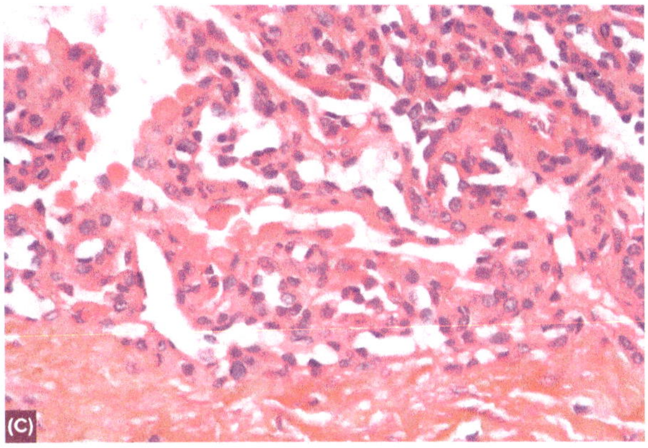

D) 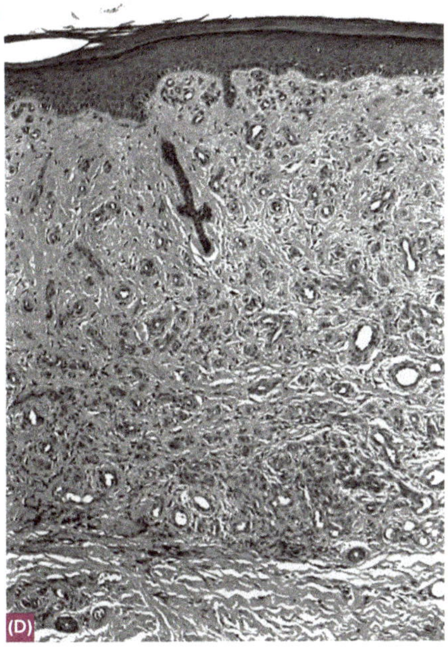

QUESTION 11-13.

A 32-year-old female patient presents with a solitary, annular, violaceous papule on the upper thigh measuring 2 to 3 mm in diameter. There is both a surrounding pale rim and a more peripheral ecchymotic ring resembling a "bull's eye." This ring expands peripherally and eventually disappears. She reports cyclic changes in the clinical appearance, sometimes during the menstrual cycle. The lesion is biopsied and the findings are illustrated below. Image B is a low-power view of the lesion. Image C is high-power view of the deep aspects of the lesion. Immunohistochemistry reveals the endothelial cells to express CD31 and D2-40 but no expression of HHV-8. Which of the following diagnoses is CORRECT?

A) Acquired progressive lymphangioma
B) Early Kaposi sarcoma
C) Retiform hemangioendothelioma
D) Targetoid hemosiderotic hemangioma
E) Microvenular hemangioma

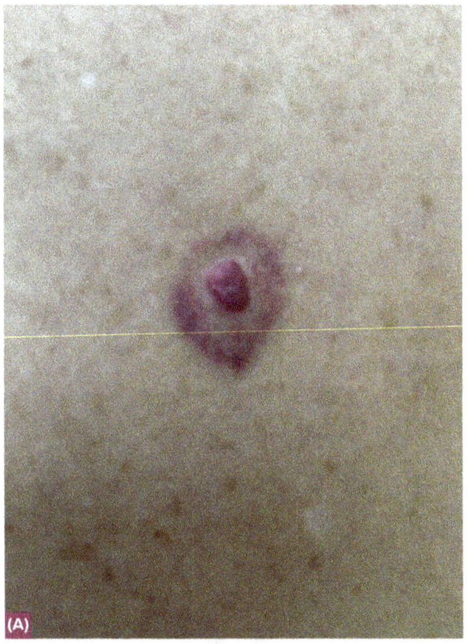

Courtesy of Robert Phelps, MD, Icahn School of Medicine at Mount Sinai, New York, NY.

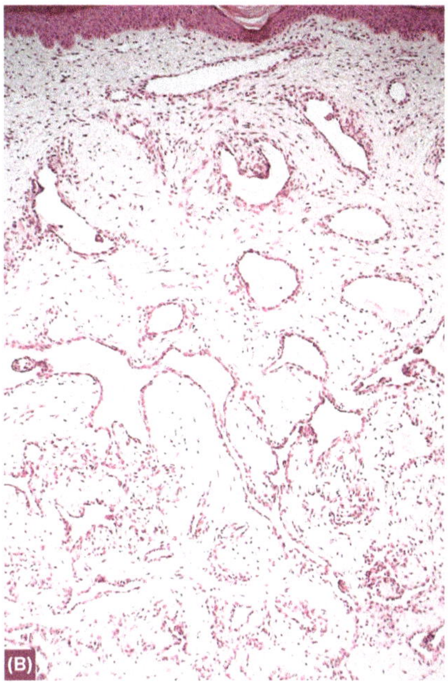

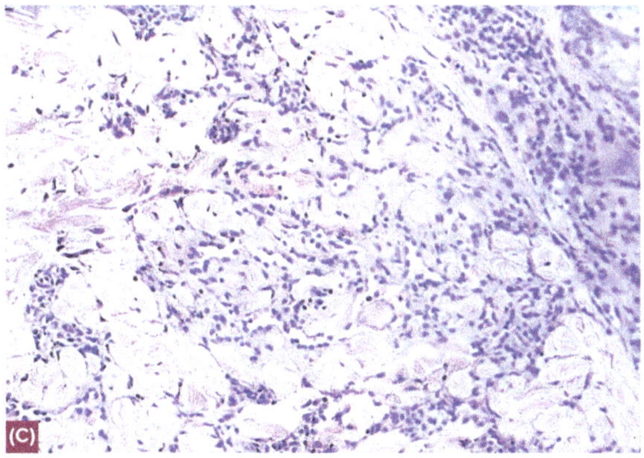

QUESTION 11-14.

A 28-year-old male patient with acute myelogenous leukemia presents with a solitary, asymptomatic, 0.5 cm, enlarging, purple to red plaque on the upper right extremity. The lesion is biopsied and the findings are illustrated below. Red blood cell extravasation and hemosiderin pigment are not identified. Which of the following diagnoses is CORRECT?

- A) Microvenular hemangioma
- B) Targetoid hemosiderotic hemangioma
- C) Kaposi sarcoma
- D) Stasis changes
- E) Reactive angiogenesis within a dermal scar

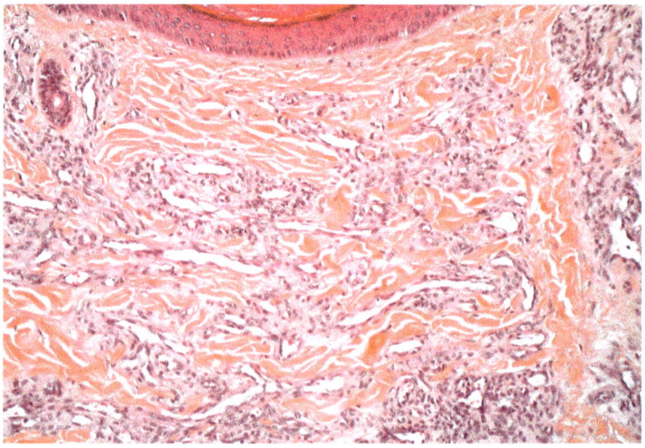

QUESTION 11-15.

A 1-year-old patient presents with a slowly enlarging cluster of dull red-to-brown plaques on the upper trunk that measure approximately 6 cm in total. The mother reports increased sweating from the area. Peripheral blood analysis reveals striking thrombocytopenia. The lesion is excised and upon microscopic examination the proliferation is found to extend into the deep dermis. There is no ulceration and no epidermal collarette. There are small circumscribed, cellular, capillary tufts dispersed as "cannonballs" throughout the dermis. Crescentic cleft–like vessels are found at the periphery of some of the capillary tufts. Scattered mitoses are identified but cytologic atypia is absent. Reticulin stain reveals a rich network of reticulin that ensheathes individual endothelial cells. The larger well-formed vascular channels are positive for *Ulex europaeus* lectin and von Willebrand factor. *Ulex europaeus* lectin also outlines the capillaries of the vascular tufts. D2-40 is expressed in a minor proportion of endothelial cells. Which of the following diagnoses is CORRECT?

- A) Glomeruloid hemangioma
- B) Pyogenic granuloma (lobular capillary hemangioma)
- C) Tufted angioma (angioblastoma)
- D) Low-grade angiosarcoma
- E) Infantile hemangioma

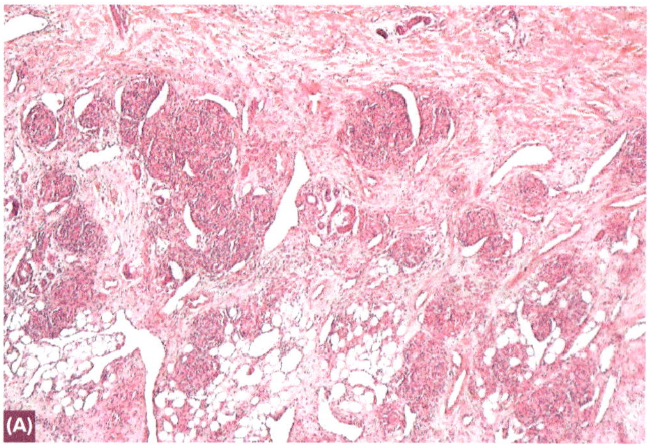

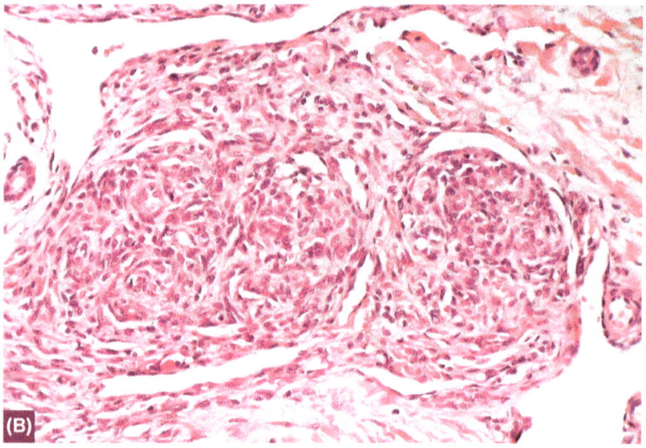

QUESTION 11-16.

A 2-month-old female patient presents with an unknown life-threatening coagulation disorder characterized by very low platelet count ($<5{,}000/mm^3$), low fibrinogen, high D-dimers, and anemia. Clinical examination reveals an indurated, ill-defined, violaceous mass occupying the perineum that is warm and tender. An emergent platelet transfusion is performed and the tumor diminishes rapidly in size but fails to show complete regression. A biopsy is then performed. The tumor cells are negative for HHV8 by immunohistochemistry. Which of the following diagnoses is CORRECT?

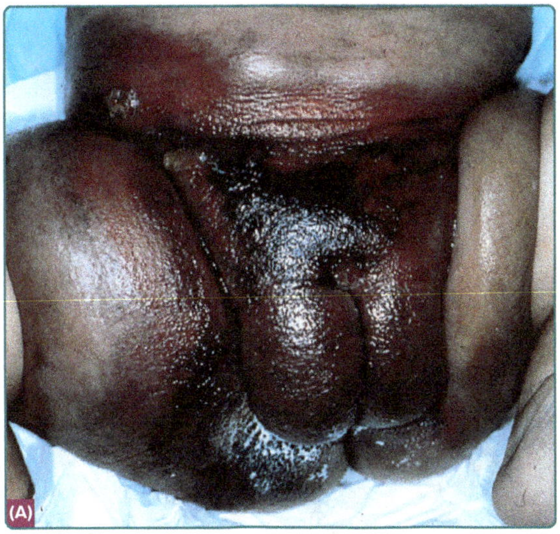

Reproduced, with permission, from Goldsmith LA, Katz SI, Gilchrest BA, Paller AS, Leffell DJ, Wolff K, eds. *Fitzpatrick's Dermatology in General Medicine*. 8th ed. New York, NY: McGraw-Hill Education; 2012.

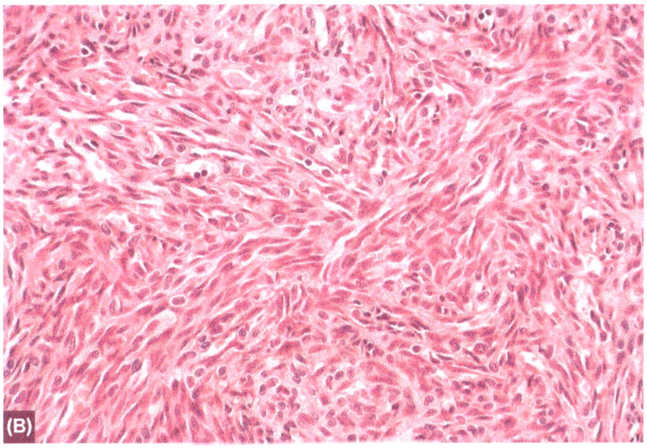

A) Targetoid hemosiderotic hemangioendothelioma
B) Infantile hemangioma
C) Kaposiform hemangioendothelioma
D) Spindle cell hemangioma
E) Kaposi sarcoma

QUESTION 11-17.

What is the MOST likely clinical presentation of the lesion imaged below?

A) A 56-year-old patient with cirrhosis presents with numerous slightly elevated erythematous puncta-containing arrays of peripherally radiating fine vessels. The lesions are pulsatile on diascopy, blanch with pressure, and upon release refill rapidly with blood flow originating from their centers.
B) A 6-month-old infant presented with a rapidly enlarging red plaque on the face. However, the patient is now 6 years of age and the lesion has resolved with only slight atrophy at the site.
C) A patient presents with a common, solitary, eroded, dusky red vascular nodule on the tip of a finger that bleeds spontaneously or after minor trauma. A collar of hyperplastic epidermis surrounds the lesion.
D) A 7-year-old presents with a large erythematous patch following the distribution of the trigeminal nerve. There is involvement of the eye and leptomeninges as well as superficial calcifications of the brain, contralateral hemiparesis, muscular hemiatrophy, epilepsy, and mental retardation.
E) A 40-year-old male patient presents with numerous red, violaceous, and black papules on the scrotum. They blanch upon diascopy.

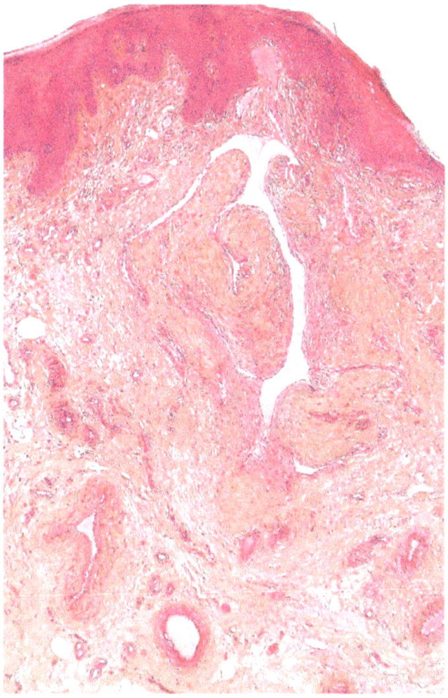

QUESTION 11-18.

A 6-year-old patient presents with diffuse swelling of the neck. Palpable lymphadenopathy is present in the adjacent region. The neck lesion is biopsied and the findings are illustrated below. Which of the following diagnoses is CORRECT?

A) Papillary intralymphatic angioendothelioma
B) Glomeruloid hemangioma
C) Lymphatic malformation
D) Intravascular papillary endothelial hyperplasia
E) Retiform hemangioendothelioma

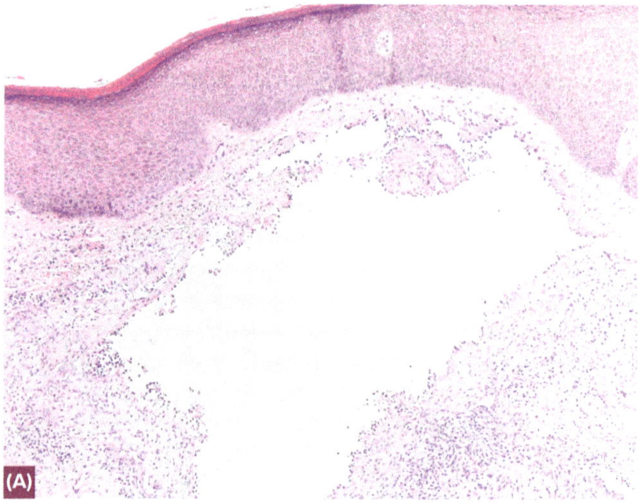

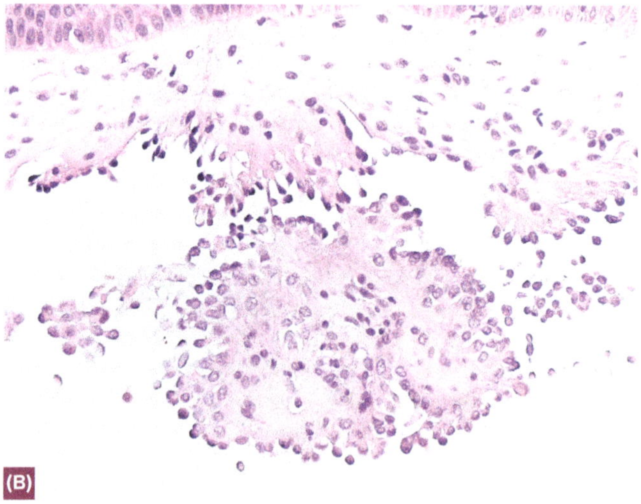

QUESTION 11-19.

A 60-year-old female patient with a history of mammary carcinoma of the right breast presents with extensive erythema studded with papules and violaceous nodules. A biopsy is performed and the findings are illustrated below. Which of the following statements regarding this tumor is INCORRECT?

A) This is an example of an atypical vascular lesion (AVL) associated with prior radiation exposure.

B) These tumors more commonly arise at cutaneous sites of prior ionizing radiation exposure and chronic lymphedema.

C) These tumors are strongly associated with *MYC* amplification.

D) Spontaneous tumors have a predilection for the head and neck region of males.

E) In addition to vascular markers, occasionally these tumors may express cytokeratin via immunohistochemistry.

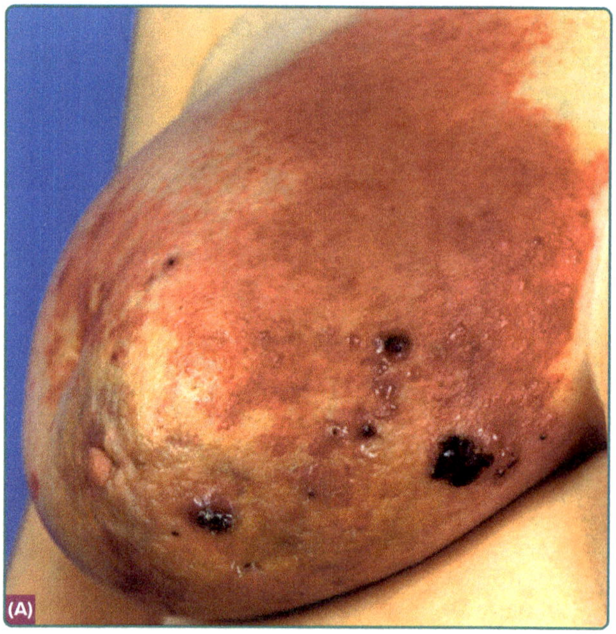

Reproduced, with permission, from Goldsmith LA, Katz SI, Gilchrest BA, Paller AS, Leffell DJ, Wolff K, eds. *Fitzpatrick's Dermatology in General Medicine*. 8th ed. New York, NY: McGraw-Hill Education; 2012.

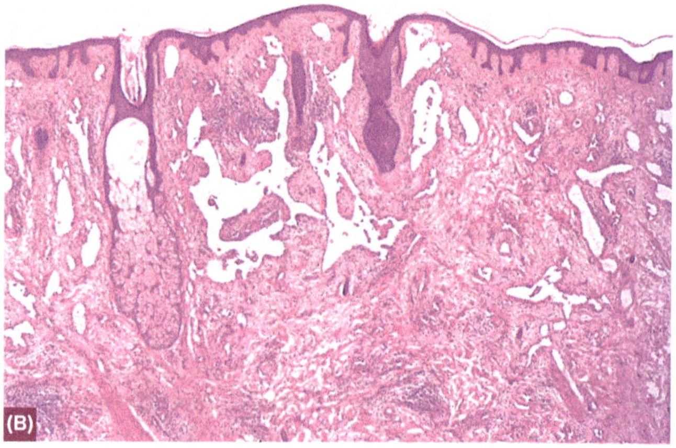

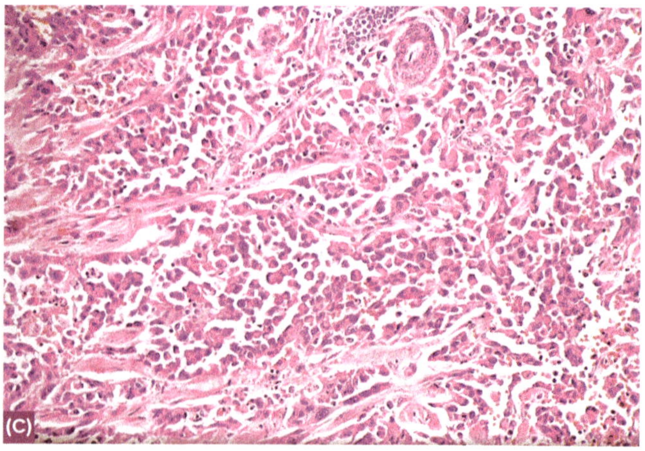

QUESTION 11-20.

An 11-month-old infant presents with an oval plaque-like tumor of pink to purple color with telangiectasias on the cheek. The tumor has been present since birth. It is warm on palpation. Magnetic resonance imaging (MRI) reveals the lesion to occupy the dermis and subcutis. Ultrasonography reveals irregular high-flow vessels with arterial aneurysms. A biopsy is performed and the findings are illustrated below. Which of the following statements regarding this tumor is INCORRECT?

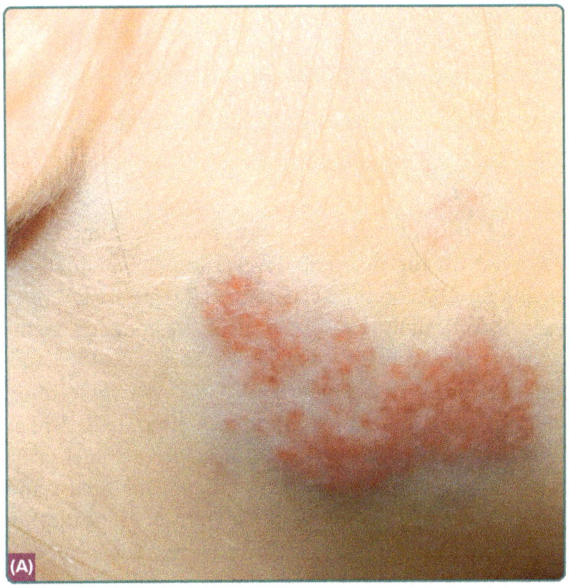
(A)

Reproduced, with permission, from Goldsmith LA, Katz SI, Gilchrest BA, Paller AS, Leffell DJ, Wolff K, eds. *Fitzpatrick's Dermatology in General Medicine*. 8th ed. New York, NY: McGraw-Hill Education; 2012.

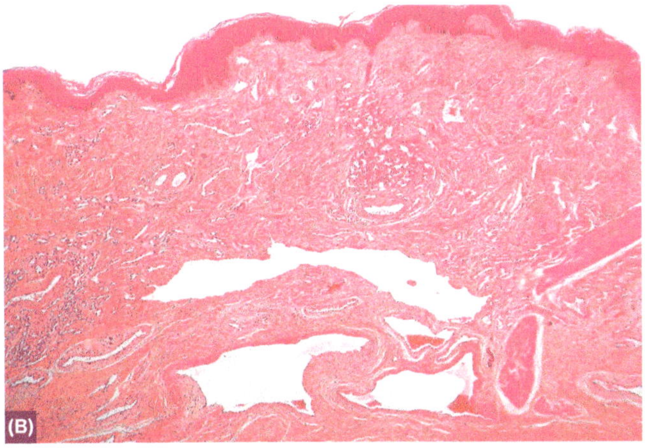
(B)

A) This is a vascular malformation that will most likely not regress over time.
B) High-power examination will most likely reveal the endothelial cells to have eosinophilic cytoplasmic inclusions, and dark, round nuclei protruding into the lumen with a hobnail pattern.
C) The endothelial cells will be negative for GLUT-1 expression via immunohistochemistry.
D) When these tumors contain central areas of depression, they are associated with rapid involution.
E) This tumor is associated with trauma at delivery and will contain numerous scattered neutrophils and a fibromyxoid stroma.

QUESTION 11-21.

Which of the following statements regarding malignant mesenchymal neoplasms is INCORRECT?

A) Malignant tumors tend to exhibit an infiltrative growth pattern into the surrounding tissues.
B) Malignant tumors tend to be highly cellular with numerous mitotic figures.
C) Cellular pleomorphism is the most sensitive and specific finding for diagnosing malignant mesenchymal tumors.
D) Malignant tumors confined to the dermis tend to have a significantly better prognosis than tumors arising or extending into the subcutis and/or fascia.
E) Malignant tumors frequently exhibit areas of tumor necrosis.

QUESTION 11-22.

A 5-year-old presents with a firm, nontender, erythematous nodule on the ear that gradually developed after ear piercing. The lesion has grown well beyond the site of initial piercing. The lesion is excised and the findings are illustrated below. Which of the following diagnoses is CORRECT?

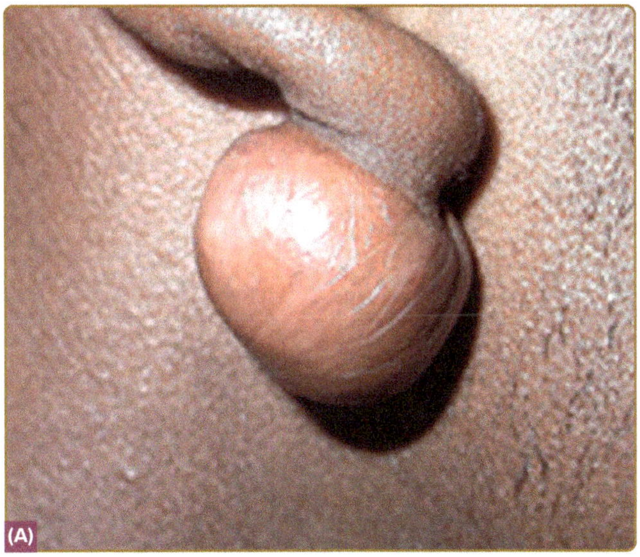
(A)

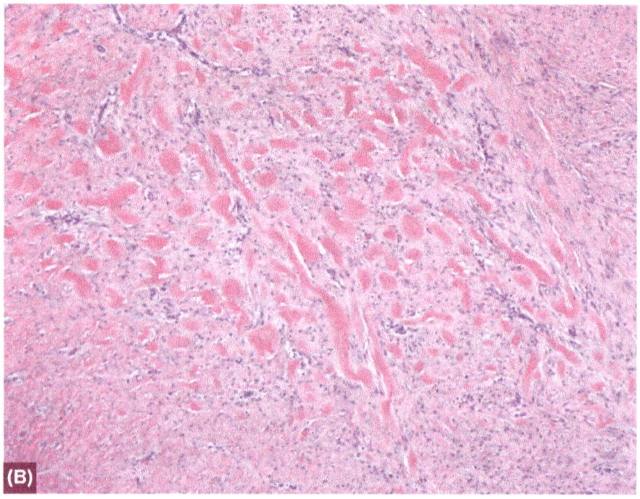

Part **(A)** reproduced, with permission, from Goldsmith LA, Katz SI, Gilchrest BA, Paller AS, Leffell DJ, Wolff K, eds. *Fitzpatrick's Dermatology in General Medicine*. 8th ed. New York, NY: McGraw-Hill Education; 2012.

A) Hypertrophic scar
B) Dermatofibroma
C) Fibroepithelial polyp
D) Keloid
E) Juvenile hyaline fibromatosis

QUESTION 11-23.

Which of the following statements regarding the lesion illustrated below is INCORRECT?

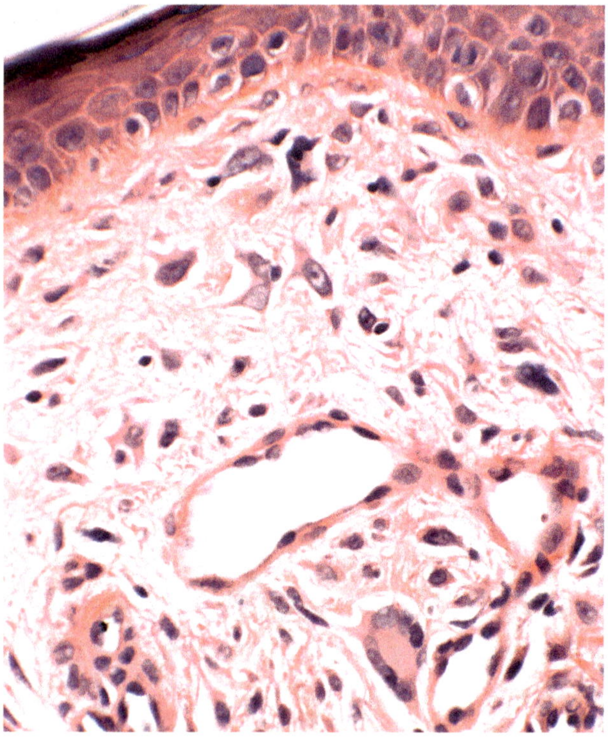

A) This tumor typically presents as a solitary firm papule on the nose or central face.
B) Multiple lesions are associated with an autosomal dominant neurocutaneous syndrome caused by mutations in the *TSC1* (hamartin) or *TSC2* (tuberin) gene.
C) These lesions may present as multiple tiny papules, usually no more than a few millimeters in diameter, circumferentially distributed on the glans penis.
D) These lesions may present as smooth, shiny, flesh-colored nodules that arise from the nail folds typically during the peripubertal period.
E) The stellate tumors cells are characteristically positive for S100 via immunohistochemistry.

QUESTION 11-24.

A 23-year-old patient presents with multiple tiny flesh-colored papules on the face and several larger 0.5- to 1-cm slow-growing nodules on the head and neck region and upper extremities. Additionally, examination of the mucous membranes reveals numerous tiny papules of the gingival, palatal, and lingual surfaces that coalesce, giving a "cobblestone" appearance. The patient reports that the father had similar lesions and expired at an early age from colorectal adenocarcinoma. The family history is also significant for breast and endometrial adenocarcinoma in the paternal grandmother and a sister with papillary thyroid carcinoma. You notice in the chart that a prior skin biopsy of a malar papule revealed a trichilemmoma. A biopsy of one of the larger arm nodules is performed and the findings are illustrated below. Which of the following diagnoses is CORRECT?

A) Tuberous xanthoma
B) Storiform collagenoma
C) Dermatomyofibroma
D) Keloid
E) Sclerosing perineurioma

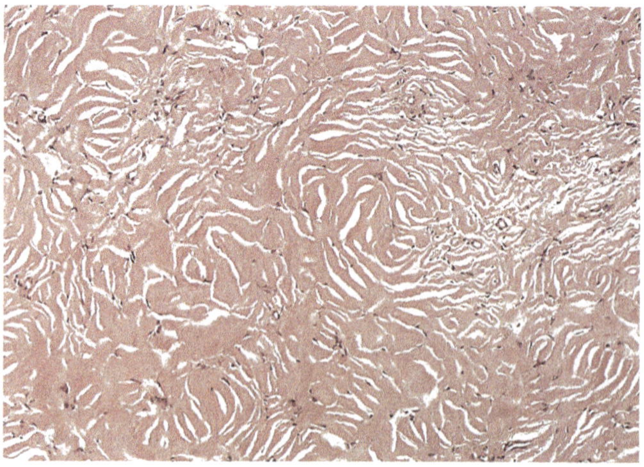

QUESTION 11-25.

A 24-year-old male patient presents with a small painless slow-growing nodule on the hand measuring 2 cm in diameter. An incisional biopsy is performed and the tumor appears to be a solitary nodule attached to the tendon. Low-power microscopic examination reveals a well-circumscribed nodule. Which of the following diagnoses is CORRECT?

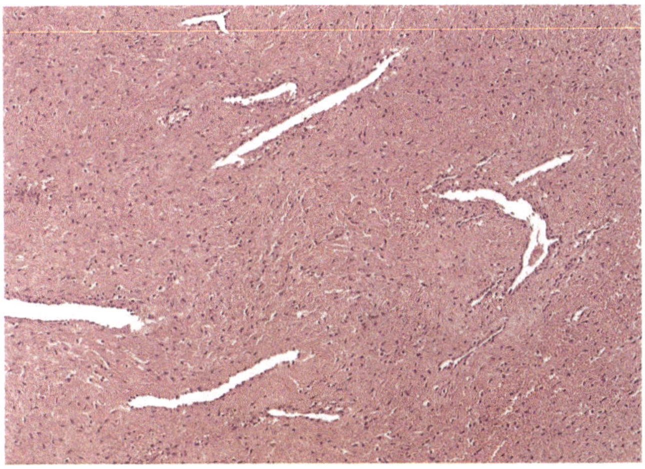

A) Giant cell tumor of tendon sheath
B) Superficial fibromatosis
C) Nodular fasciitis
D) Fibroma of tendon sheath
E) Angioleiomyoma

QUESTION 11-26.

A young female patient presents with a firm, 1-cm, flesh-colored nodule on the upper thigh. The lesion is biopsied and reveals a spindle cell proliferation arising in the mid-dermis that extends into the septum of the subcutaneous layer. Immunohistochemistry reveals the tumor cells to positively express factor XIIIa, stromelysin, and D2-40. The tumor cells are negative for CD34, CD31, and S100. Which of the following diagnoses is CORRECT?

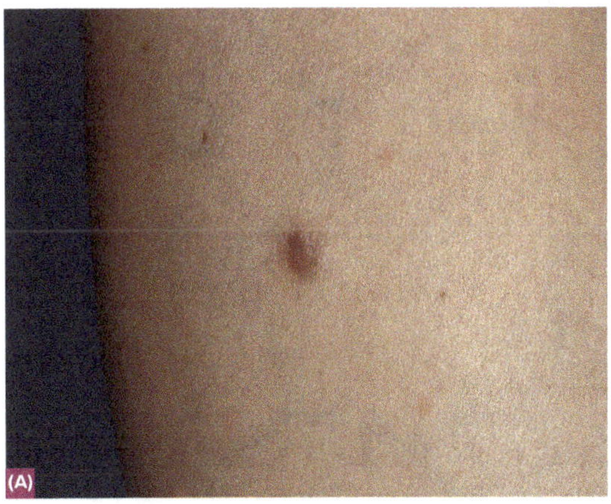

(A)

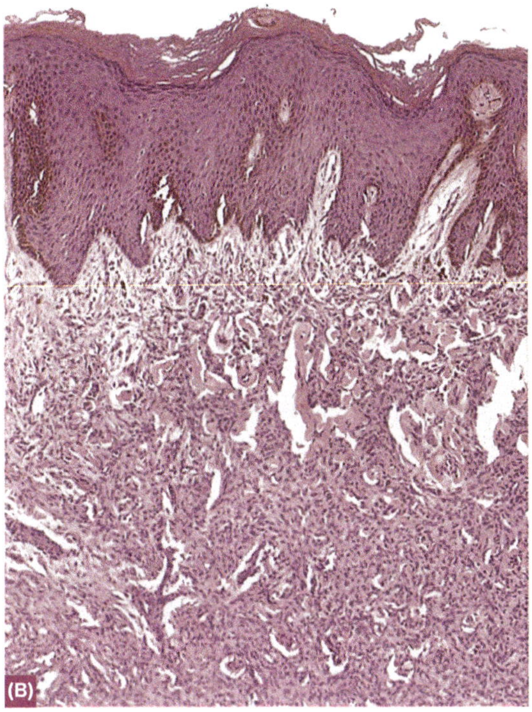

(B)

A) Dermatofibrosarcoma protuberans
B) Dermatofibroma
C) Spindle cell hemangioma
D) Desmoplastic Spitz tumor
E) Leiomyosarcoma

QUESTION 11-27.

A 57-year-old male with dermatoheliosis and a history of solar keratoses, invasive and in situ squamous carcinoma, and basal cell carcinoma presents with a rapidly enlarging eroded nodule on the vertex of the scalp. A biopsy is performed and the findings are illustrated below. Immunohistochemistry reveals the tumors to be negative for S100 and cytokeratin and positive for CD10. Which of the following statements regarding this entity is INCORRECT?

A) This tumor must be completely excised for definitive classification and to prevent local recurrence.
B) If the tumor is confined to the dermis, there is little risk for metastasis.
C) The presence of focal tumor necrosis is suggestive for high-grade malignancy and significant risk for metastasis.
D) Although vascular invasion is a common finding, there is little correlation with risk for metastasis.
E) The tumor cells are frequently positive for CD99, calponin, vimentin, α_1-antitrypsin, and α_1-antichymotrypsin.

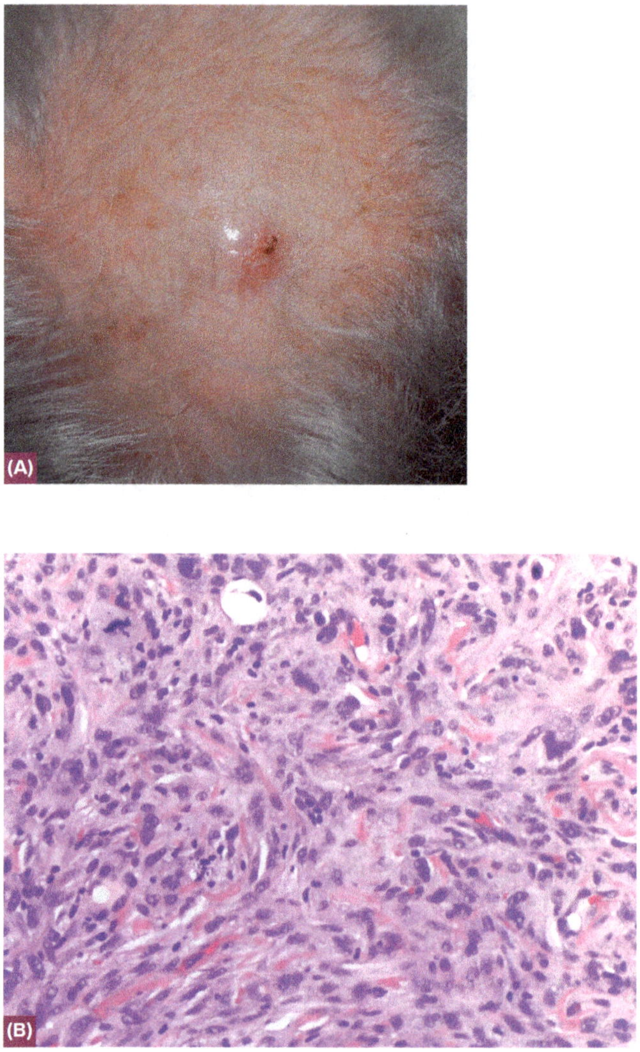

Part **(A)** reproduced, with permission, from Wolff K, Johnson RA, Saavedra AP. *Fitzpatrick's Color Atlas and Synopsis of Clinical Dermatology*. 7th ed. New York, NY: McGraw-Hill Education; 2013.

QUESTION 11-28.

A 30-year-old patient presents with an ill-defined firm indurated plaque on the upper back. The lesion is biopsied and the findings are illustrated below. The spindle cells extensively infiltrate the subcutaneous fat. Immunohistochemistry reveals the tumor cells to strongly and diffusely express CD34. Which of the following statements regarding this tumor is INCORRECT?

A) The tumor is generally locally aggressive only; however, if not completely excised, recurrence with increased cellularity and the ability to metastasize may occur.

B) A pigmented variant of this tumor contains entrapped HMB45+, Melan-A+, and S100+ spindled melanocytes.

C) This tumor is associated with a t(17;22) chromosomal translocation resulting in a monomorphic cell population.

D) This tumor typically occurs in much younger patients and may feature focal areas with pseudovascular spaces lined by floret-like giant cells embedded in a characteristic myxoid matrix.

E) Mohs micrographic surgery provides the best means for removal with clear margins.

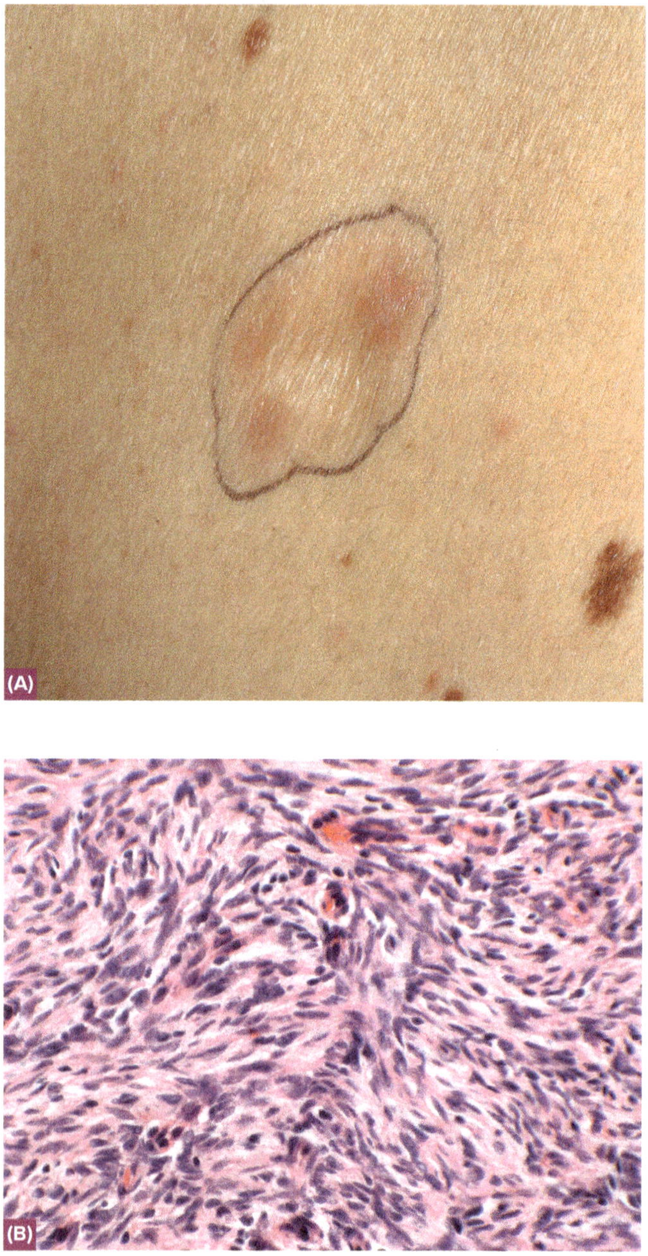

QUESTION 11-29.

A 1-year-old patient presents with 1 cm, asymptomatic nodule located on the lateral aspect of a finger. A biopsy is performed and the findings are illustrated below. Eosinophilic cytoplasmic inclusions are noted in some of the cells that stain with

Masson trichrome stain and smooth muscle actin. The tumor eventually regresses spontaneously. Which of the following diagnoses is CORRECT?

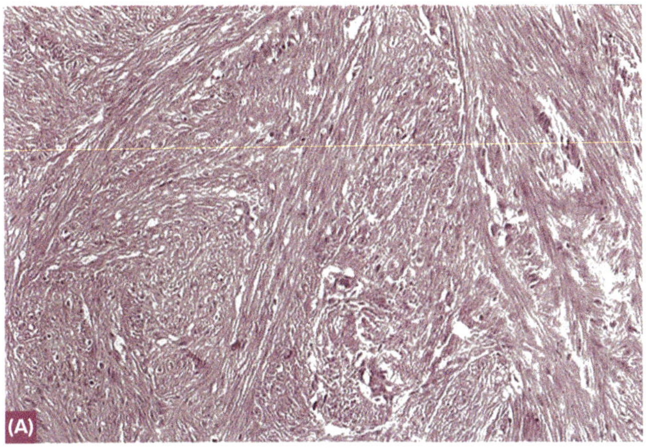

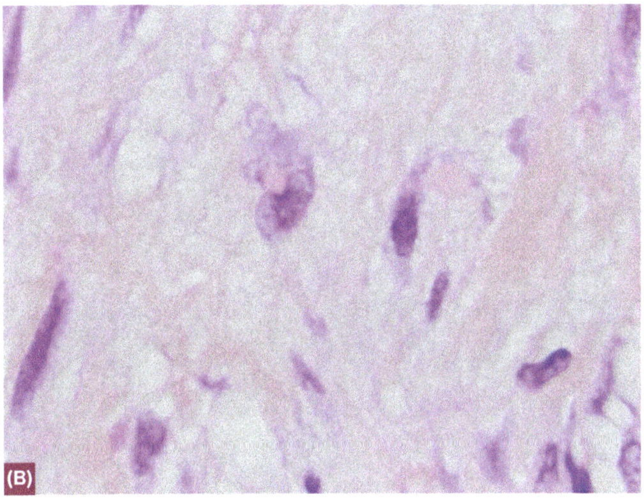

A) Infantile digital fibromatosis
B) Fibrous hamartoma of infancy
C) Plexiform fibrohistiocytic tumor
D) Angiomatoid fibrous histiocytoma
E) Solitary myofibroma

QUESTION 11-30.

A patient presents with a painful rapidly enlarging nodule on the forearm. An excision is performed and reveals an infiltrative proliferation involving the subcutis with separate areas of high and low cellularity. A high-power view of one of the paucicellular areas is illustrated below. Which of the following diagnoses is CORRECT?

A) Myxofibrosarcoma
B) Nodular fasciitis
C) Myxoma
D) Myxoid liposarcoma
E) Fibrosarcoma

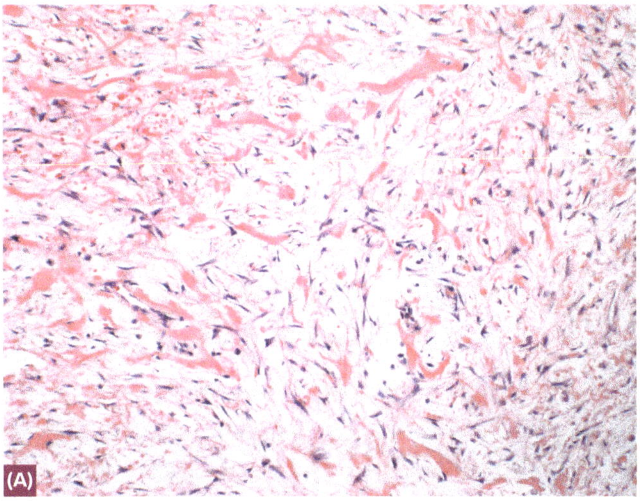

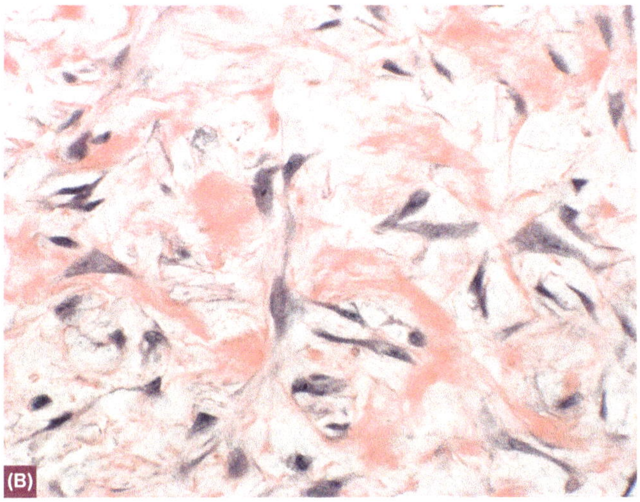

QUESTION 11-31.

A 27-year-old male presents with a 3-cm nodule on one of his toes. Focal ulceration is noted. A biopsy is performed; the findings are illustrated below. PAS, Gram, and Fite stains are negative for microorganisms. Immunohistochemistry reveals the tumor cells to positively express vimentin, CD34, pancytokeratin, and EMA. There is no expression for CD68, CD31, Fli-1, S100, HMB45, Melan-A, SMA, or desmin. Nuclear expression of INI-1 is lost. Which of the following diagnoses is CORRECT?

A) Metastatic squamous cell carcinoma
B) Metastatic melanoma
C) Epithelioid sarcoma
D) Rheumatoid nodule
E) Plexiform fibrohistiocytic tumor

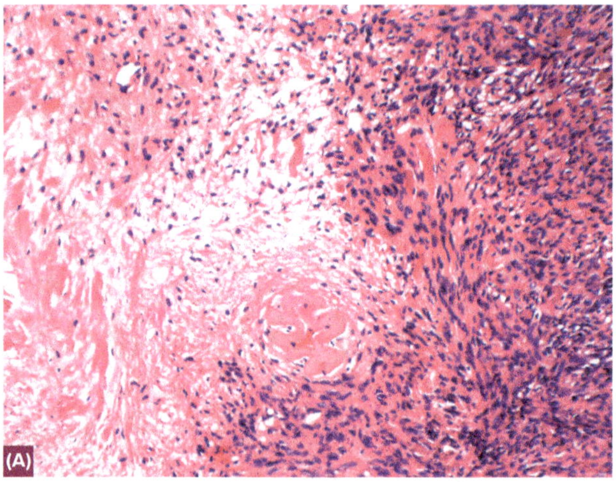

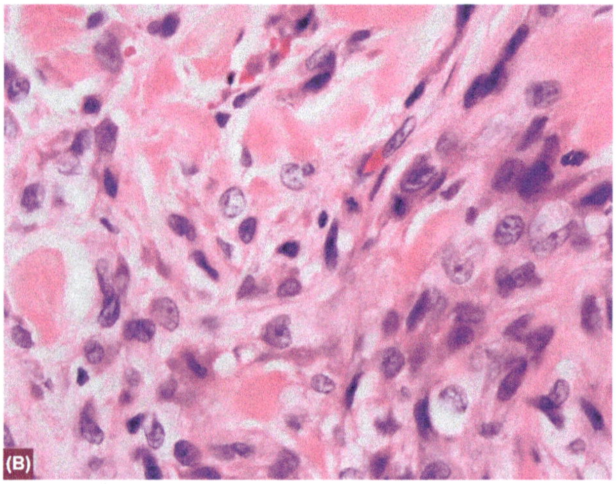

QUESTION 11-32.

A 55-year-old patient presents with a soft, 1-cm, compressible nodule on the upper thorax. The lesion is excised and reveals a well-circumscribed tumor nodule encased by a thin fibrous capsule. A high-power image of the tumor cells is illustrated below. Which of the following diagnoses is CORRECT?

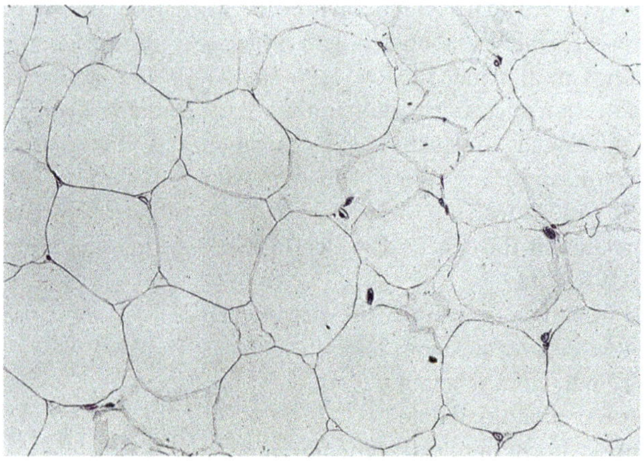

A) Nevus lipomatosus superficialis
B) Lipoma
C) Hibernoma
D) Nodular-cystic fat necrosis
E) Well-differentiated liposarcoma (WDL)/atypical lipomatous tumor (ALT)

QUESTION 11-33.

A 24-year-old patient presents with multiple painful soft nodules on the forearm. One of the tumors is excised and the histopathologic findings are illustrated below. The first image (A) is from the periphery of the lesion and the second image (B) represents the center of the lesion. Which of the following diagnoses is CORRECT?

A) Angiolipoma
B) Spindle cell lipoma
C) Capillary hemangioma
D) Kaposi sarcoma
E) Hibernoma

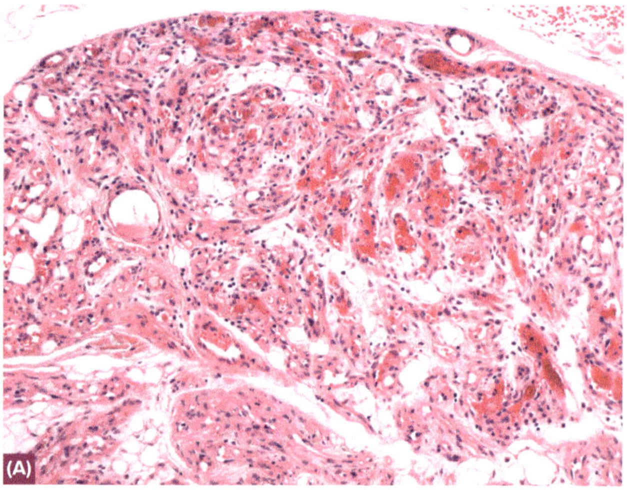

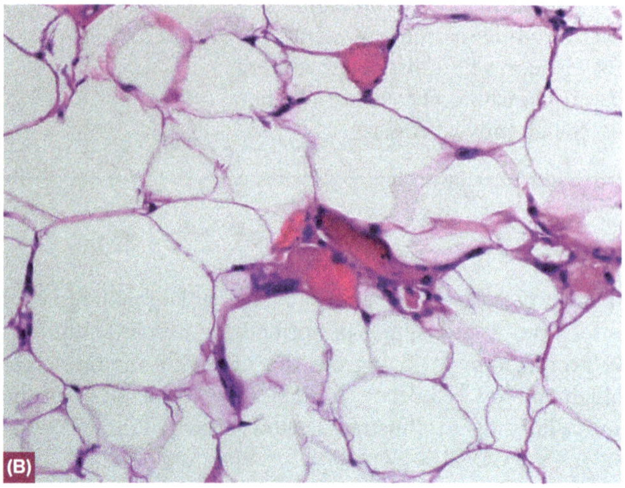

QUESTION 11-34.

A 50-year-old male patient presents with a solitary, 4 cm subcutaneous mass in the posterior neck. The tumor is excised and the histopathological findings are illustrated below. At low magnification, the tumor is circumscribed and lacks adnexal structures. Immunohistochemistry reveals the tumor spindle cells to positively express CD34. There is no expression of MDM2 or CDK4. Which of the following diagnoses is CORRECT?

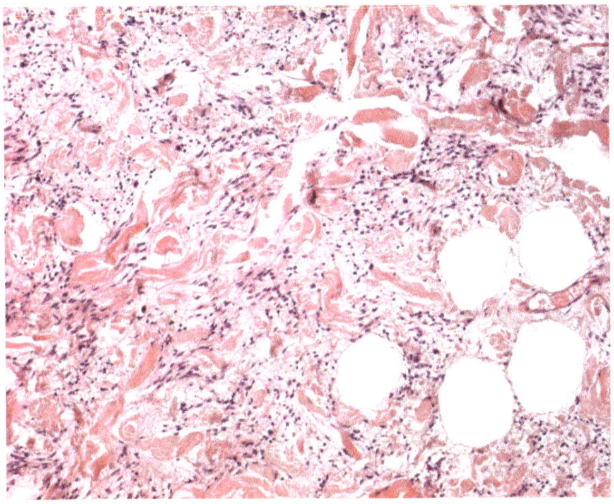

A) Dermatofibrosarcoma protuberans
B) Pleomorphic lipoma
C) Spindle cell lipoma
D) Myxoid liposarcoma
E) Solitary fibrous tumor

QUESTION 11-35.

A 50-year-old patient presents with a 10-cm soft nodule on the upper shoulder. The lesion is excised to reveal a well-circumscribed fatty mass in the subcutis. Immunohistochemistry reveals nuclear staining for MDM2 and CDK4 within tumor cells. Which of the following diagnoses is CORRECT?

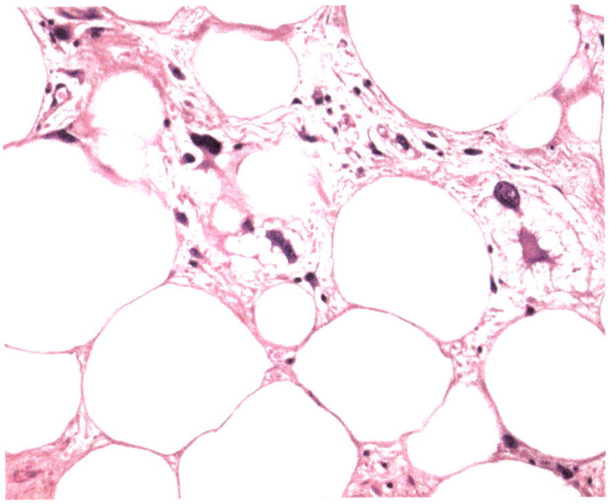

A) Lipoblastoma
B) Pleomorphic lipoma
C) Atypical lipomatous tumor
D) Dedifferentiated liposarcoma
E) Round cell liposarcoma

QUESTION 11-36.

A 17-year-old male presents with an ill-defined hyperpigmented plaque on the shoulder. The lesion was not present at birth but began to develop over the last few years. You notice that the patient has scoliosis and ipsilateral breast hypoplasia. A biopsy is performed and the findings are illustrated below. The loosely arranged fascicles are positive for smooth muscle actin and desmin via immunohistochemistry. Which of the following diagnoses is CORRECT?

A) Pilar leiomyoma
B) Congenital smooth muscle hamartoma
C) Accessory nipple
D) Dermatomyofibroma
E) Nevus lipomatosus superficialis

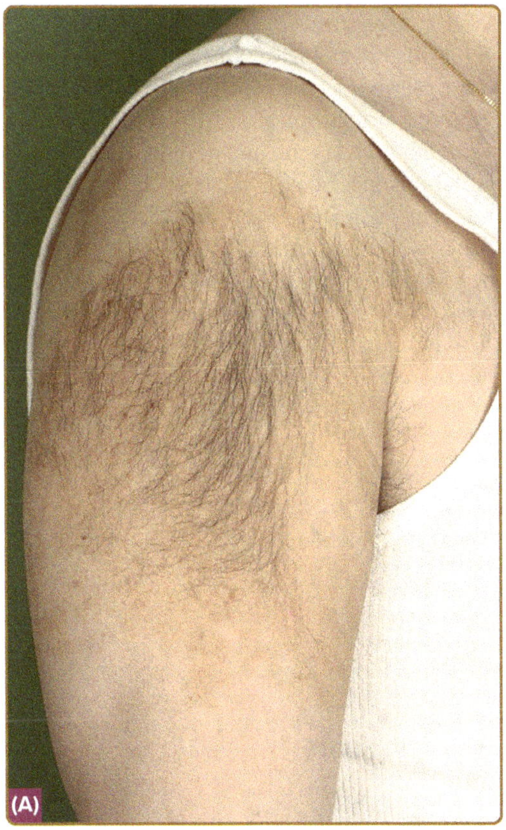

Reproduced, with permission, from Goldsmith LA, Katz SI, Gilchrest BA, Paller AS, Leffell DJ, Wolff K, eds. *Fitzpatrick's Dermatology in General Medicine*. 8th ed. New York, NY: McGraw-Hill Education; 2012.

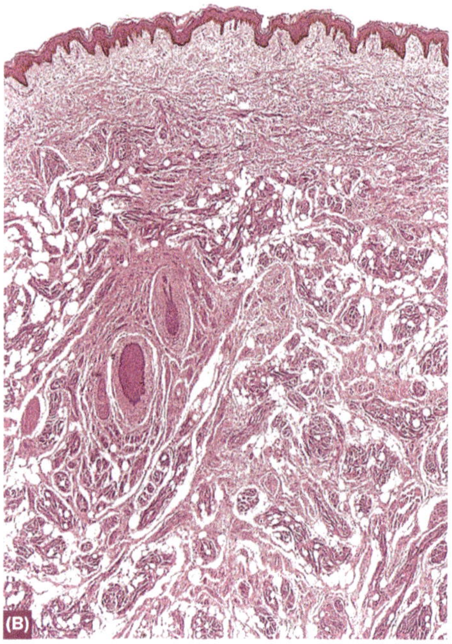

(B)

QUESTION 11-37.

A 47-year-old patient presents with a solitary painful nodule on the lower extremity measuring 6 cm in diameter. The lesion is excised and the histopathological findings are illustrated below. The spindle cell proliferation is confined to the superficial dermis. Immunohistochemical stains reveal the tumor cells to express smooth muscle actin and desmin. Ki-67 reveals positive nuclear staining in greater than 10% of the tumor cells. Which of the following diagnoses is CORRECT?

A) Atypical leiomyomatous tumor
B) Symplastic pilar leiomyoma
C) Angioleiomyoma
D) Vascular leiomyosarcoma
E) Dermatofibrosarcoma protuberans

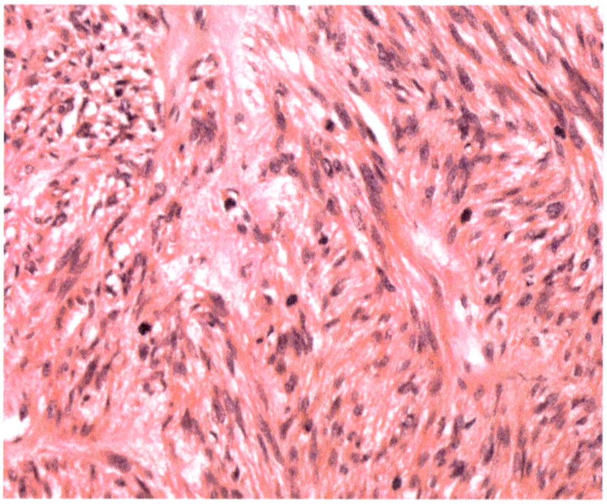

QUESTION 11-38.

Which of the following statements regarding peripheral nerves is INCORRECT?

A) The architectural arrangement of normal peripheral nerves, from smallest to largest component is as follows: unmyelinated axon, Schwann cell myelin sheath, endoneurium, epineurium, and perineurium.
B) Unmyelinated axons express PGP9.5 via immunohistochemistry.
C) Schwann cells express S100 via immunohistochemistry.
D) Endoneurium is composed of CD34+ fibroblasts, capillaries, and mast cells.
E) The perineurium is composed of a specialized cell type, the "perineurial cell," that is EMA+ and in continuity with the pia-arachnoidal lining of the CNS.

QUESTION 11-39.

A 45-year-old patient presents with a solitary, small (4-mm), skin-colored, rubbery, dome-shaped, asymptomatic papule on the face. The lesion is biopsied and the findings are illustrated below. The peripheral rim surrounding the tumor is EMA+ and the central tumor cells are S100+ and PGP9.5+. Which of the following diagnoses is CORRECT?

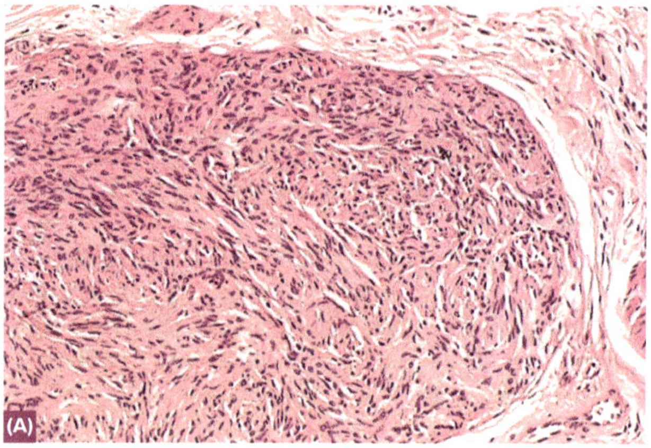

(A)

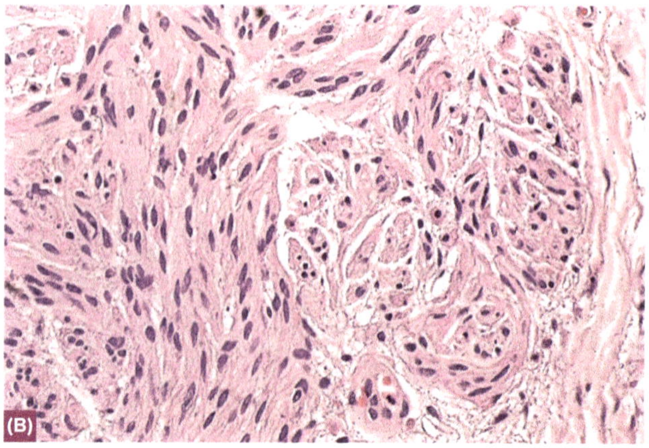

(B)

A) Leiomyoma
B) Palisaded and encapsulated neuroma
C) Schwannoma
D) Neurofibroma
E) Malignant peripheral nerve sheath tumor

QUESTION 11-40.

A patient presents with several rubbery, dome-shaped, skin-colored nodules on the back. There is invagination of the nodules when pressed with a finger. Additionally, numerous small, pigmented macules are noted diffusely on the trunk. A biopsy of one of the rubbery nodules is performed and the findings are illustrated below. Immunohistochemistry with S100, EMA, vimentin, CD117, and PGP9.5 reveals the tumor to be composed of a mixture of different cellular elements. Which of the following diagnoses is CORRECT?

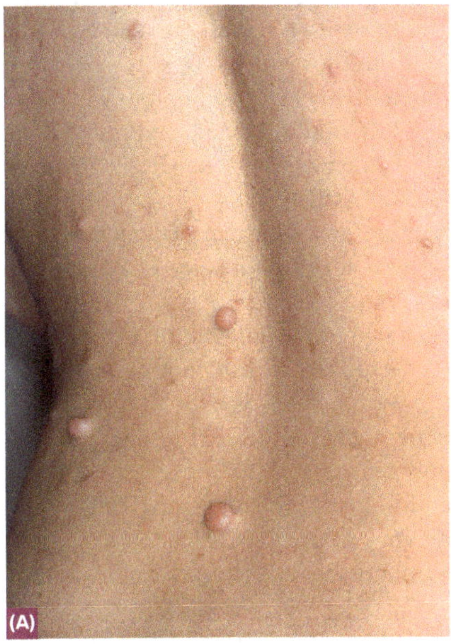
(A)

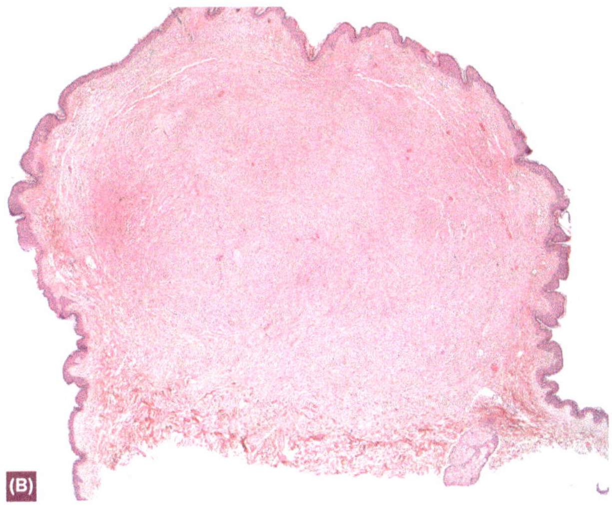
(B)

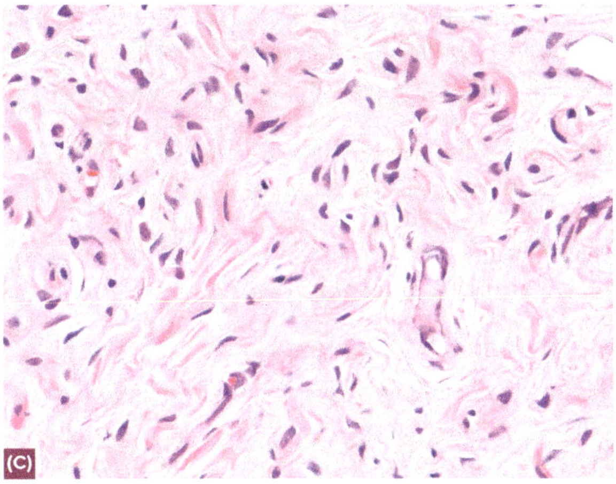
(C)

A) Dermatofibroma
B) Plexiform fibrohistiocytic tumor
C) Neurotized intradermal melanocytic nevus
D) Traumatic neuroma
E) Neurofibroma

QUESTION 11-41.

Which of the following statements regarding this tumor is INCORRECT?

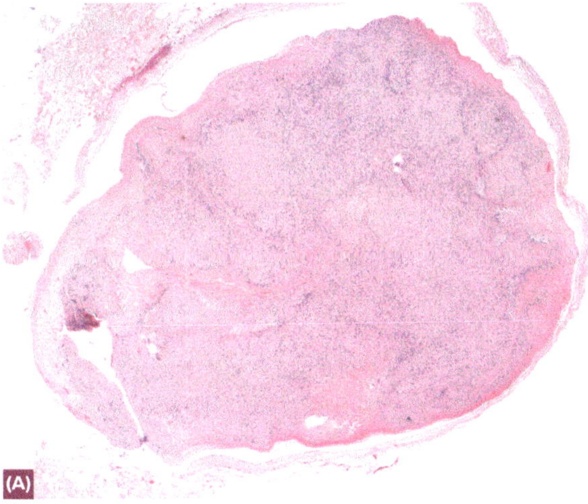
(A)

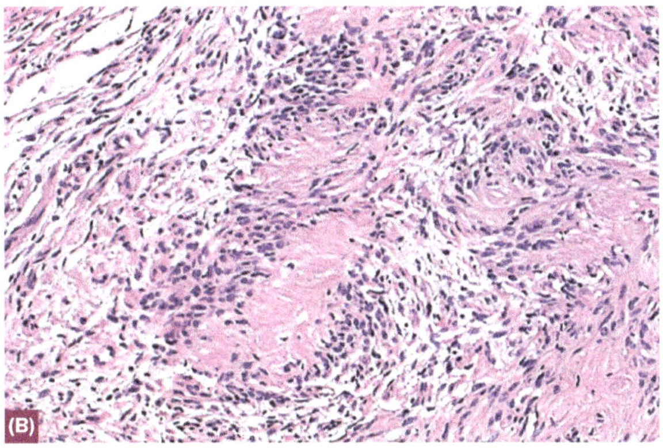
(B)

A) A rare pigmented (melanotic) variant of this tumor may occur sporadically or in association with multiple lentigines, cutaneous and visceral myxomas, blue nevi, and endocrine hyperactivity in patients with Carney complex.
B) There is an autosomal dominant condition where numerous tumors arise along cranial nerve VIII.
C) Immunohistochemistry will reveal the tumor cells to express S100 with a peripheral EMA-positive capsule.
D) Focal areas of cytologic atypia signify malignant transformation.
E) These tumors may exhibit a plexiform growth pattern without axonal nerve fibers.

QUESTION 11-42.

A 23-year-old female presents with a 1.5-cm, firm, pink nodule on the nose. The lesion is biopsied and the findings are illustrated below. Rare mitoses are identified. The tumor cells are positive for NKI/C3, smooth muscle actin, microphthalmia transcription factor (MITF), PGP 9.5, and neuron-specific enolase (NSE) via immunohistochemistry. There is no staining with S100 or HMB45. Which of the following diagnoses is CORRECT?

A) Cellular neurothekeoma
B) Nerve sheath myxoma
C) Granular cell tumor
D) Spitz nevus
E) Malignant peripheral nerve sheath tumor

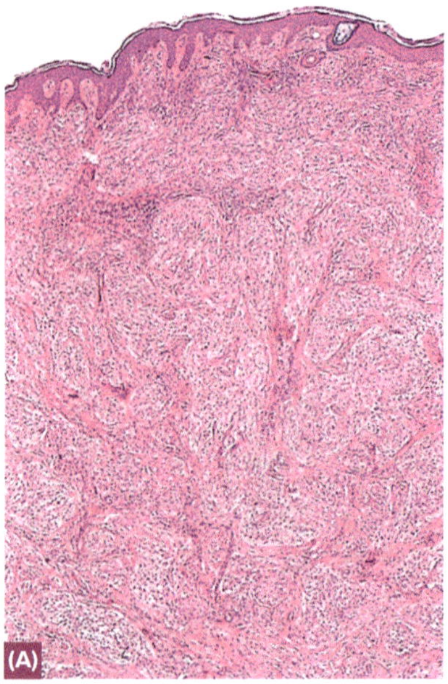

(A)

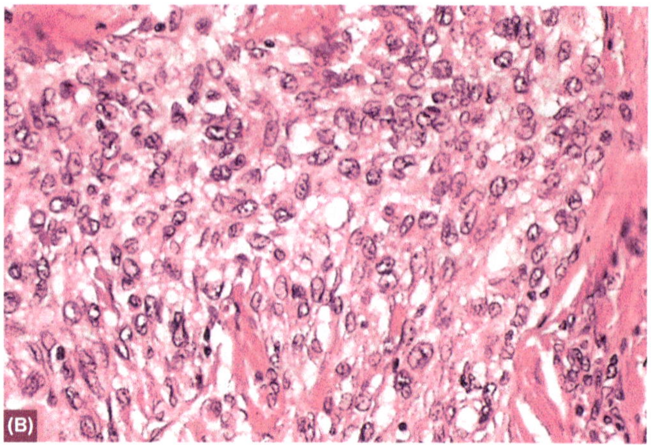

(B)

QUESTION 11-43.

A 66-year-old patient with a history of numerous nonmelanocytic skin tumors presents with a solitary, rapidly growing, pink to violaceous nodule on the arm. A biopsy is performed and the findings are illustrated below. The tumor cells reveal clumped paranuclear CK20 and CAM5.2 expression via immunohistochemistry. Which of the following statements regarding this tumor is INCORRECT?

A) This is an extremely aggressive primary cutaneous neoplasm with a 5-year survival for stage I disease estimated at only 81%.
B) Recent studies suggest genomic integration of a polyomavirus may be linked to the pathogenesis of these neoplasms.
C) These tumors frequently also express chromogranin, synaptophysin, and neuron-specific enolase.
D) Tumors with identical histomorphology that fail to express CK20, but are positive for CK7 and TTF1, most likely represent cutaneous metastases of Ewing sarcoma.
E) Sentinel lymph node biopsy is recommended due to the high incidence of lymph node metastasis.

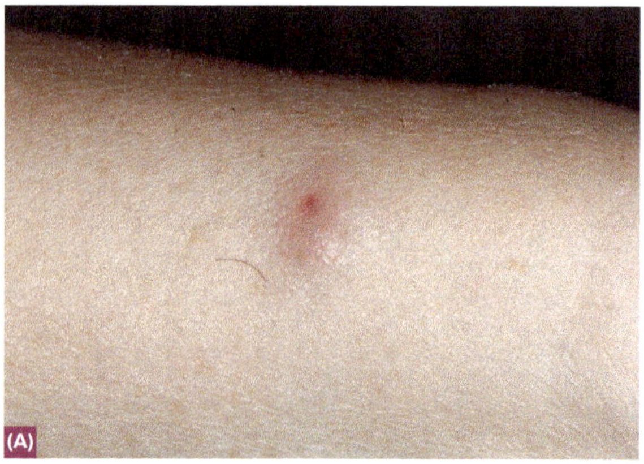

(A)

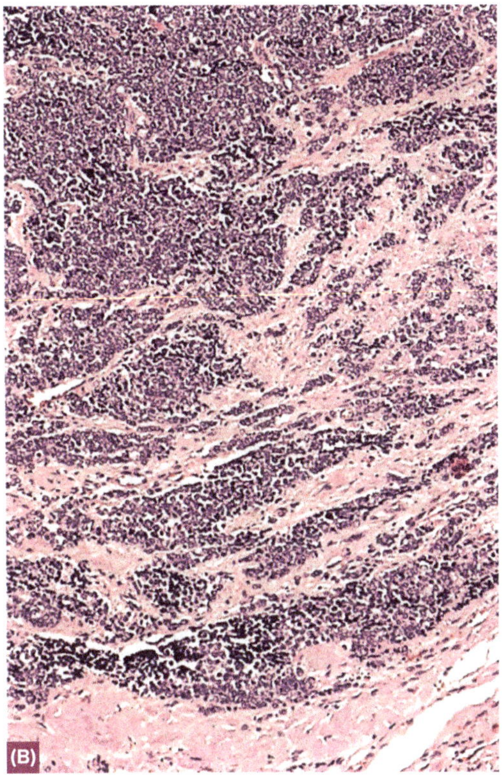

(B)

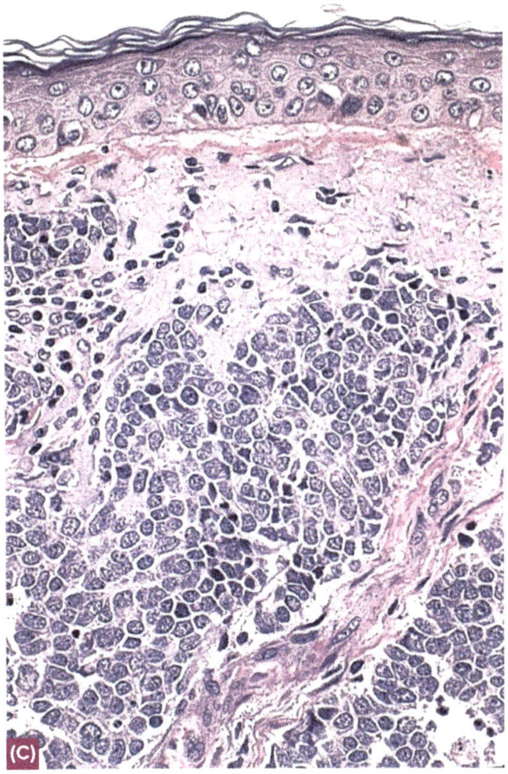

(C)

ANSWERS

ANSWER 11-1: E.

Endothelial cells line the vast majority of vascular channels, and with the exception of small lymphatics, sinuses, and sinusoids, also contain a peripheral layer of **pericytes** or smooth muscle cells. Endothelial cells express the so-called *vascular markers* CD31, CD34, von Willebrand factor, and *Ulex europaeus* lectin-1. Pericytes and smooth muscle cells contain contractile proteins (smooth muscle actin and α-smooth muscle actin). **Lymphatic endothelial cells** express lymphatic vascular endothelial hyaluronan receptor-1 (LYVE-1) and podoplanin (D2-40). Activated blood endothelial cells may, however, weakly express these two markers. Small lymphatics lack pericytes, and larger ones demonstrate irregular media made of smooth muscle cells.

There is undoubtedly considerable heterogeneity of endothelial and smooth muscle cell phenotypes and functions in normal vessels that remain poorly understood. It is certain that there are specialized functions of endothelial cells, including antigen presentation, secretion of cytokines, and so on, beyond the simple and obvious properties of maintenance of blood or lymph circulation. Veins lack an **internal elastic lamina.**

ANSWER 11-2: A.

Benign vascular lesions may be either true neoplasms that arise postnatally or vascular malformations that are present at birth. Although by definition vascular malformations are present at birth, they may not manifest clinically until later in life. In regard to histopathology, benign lesions have a relatively circumscribed architecture with rounded or rounded and linear vessels of arterial, capillary, venous, or mixed differentiation. The endothelial cells may be flat or plump with protrusion into the vascular lumens. An important feature of benign lesions is that the endothelial cells are spaced apart from one another. Malignant vascular tumors contain well-formed, anastomosing vascular channels that typically form angulated channels that dissect in between collagen bundles and frequently extend into the subcutis. Some tumors may exhibit areas of solid growth and may contain necrosis. In these solid tumor areas, regular vascular channels can be very difficult to identify. The endothelial cells of malignant vascular tumors are enlarged and have an increased nuclear-to-cytoplasmic ratio with hyperchromatic or vesicular nuclei. Prominent nucleoli may be found in high-grade lesions. Small intracytoplasmic lumens may sometimes be seen within individual tumor cells. Poorly differentiated tumors may have polygonal, spindle, or multinucleated endothelial cells with intracytoplasmic globules.

Table 11-2A. SSVA Classification Scheme for Vascular Anomalies

VASCULAR ANOMALIES	
VASCULAR TUMORS	VASCULAR MALFORMATIONS
Benign: Hemangioma Intermediate or borderline: Hemangioendothelioma Malignant: Angiosarcoma	Low flow: Capillary Venous Lymphatic High flow: Arteriovenous

These histopathological features correlate with biological behavior (Table 11-2A). The general classification of vascular neoplasms is as follows:

(1) **Hemangioma**: Benign
(2) **Hemangioendothelioma**: Intermediate malignant behavior (increased incidence of local recurrence, possible metastasis)
(3) **Angiosarcoma**: Malignant (high rate of local recurrence, metastasis, and death from disease)

ANSWER 11-3: D.

This patient has an **infantile hemangioma (IH)** (aka **hemangioma of infancy, juvenile hemangioma, strawberry hemangioma**), which is the most common tumor of infancy (Table 11-3A). Whites are most commonly affected relative to other racial groups, and girls outnumber boys by a ratio of 3:1. This patient's clinical course is typical; however, in some patients multiple large lesions can arise with complications. Blanching heralds involution, and the lesion may disappear without any residual scar. Large lesions may regress with distended redundant skin. More than 50% of patients have complete regression by age 5 years and up to 90% by age 10 years. Approximately 90% of **IH** are associated with no adverse effects in children and do not necessitate any treatment. The remaining 10% require intervention, often because of ulceration or local destructive effects such as impingement on vital structures (ie, airway or the eye). In addition, large or multiple **IH** may result in shunting of blood and **high-output cardiac failure**. Contrary to what was thought until recently, **IH** is not associated with entrapment of platelets, thrombocytopenic coagulopathy, and potentially life-threatening hemorrhages (ie, **Kasabach-Merritt syndrome**). These complications are associated with **tufted angiomas** and **kaposiform hemangioendotheliomas.** There is an association with very low birth weight (<1 kg) and chorionic villous sampling. There are many disparate hypotheses with regard to the pathogenesis of **IH**.

Table 11-3A. Infantile Hemangioma

Clinical Features
- Incidence at birth, 1%-2% and 12% by 1 year
- Most develop in the first month of life or in the first year
- Females outnumber males by a ratio of 3:1
- Whites are most commonly affected racial group
- Head and neck most common sites but may occur anywhere
- Present initially as pink or pale macular lesions that usually become red to purple nodules
- Involution occurs with the development of whitish streaks
- Natural history
  - Rapid proliferation and enlargement in the first 8-12 months of life
  - Regression of the lesion over 1-5 years or longer
- Occasional lesions may be life threatening
  - Impingement on vital structures such as an airway
  - Ulceration, infection, visceral location, hemorrhage, congestive heart failure

Histopathologic Features
- Proliferative phase
  - Highly cellular lobules separated by fibrous septa
  - Thick-walled afferent or efferent vessels
  - Lobules contain uniform endothelial cells with an admixture of pericytes and mast cells
  - Mitoses are common
  - Inconspicuous vascular lumina
  - With time, the lobules become less cellular and vascular lumina become more prominent
- Involuting phase
  - Vascular lobules composed almost entirely of microvessels
  - Gradual replacement of lobules by fibrous or fatty stroma
- All phases: expression of GLUT-1 in endothelial cells

Differential Diagnosis
- Congenital hemangioma
- Kaposiform hemangioendothelioma
- Tufted angioma
- Pyogenic granuloma
- Nonvascular tumors
- Vascular malformations

Because of their unique clinical presentation and course, these tumors are rarely biopsied. In the initial **proliferative phase**, there is a dense cellular proliferation of uniform capillaries grouped in lobules occupying the dermis and frequently the subcutaneous fat. Vascular lumina may be difficult to discern, but the highly organized architecture can be highlighted with reticulin stains. The mitotic rate of

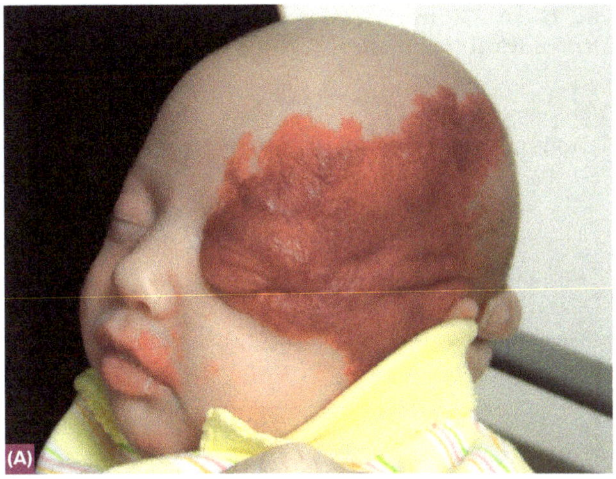

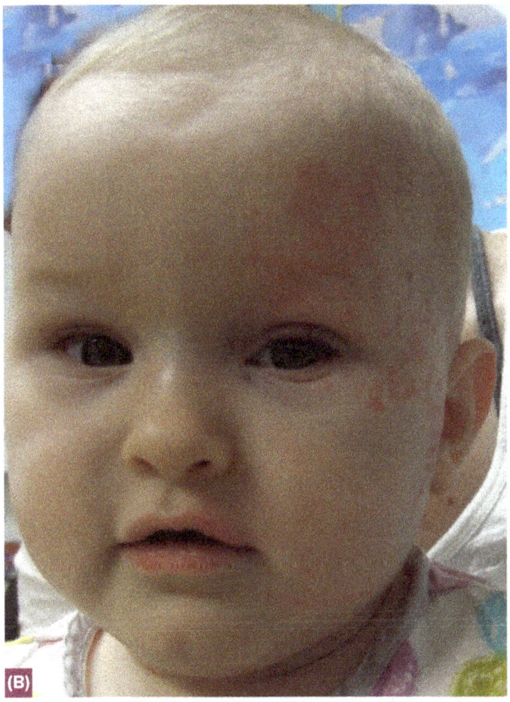

Large infantile hemangioma in which the child does not have the PHACE syndrome. However, urgent therapy was needed to shrink this hemangioma. **(A)** Before propranolol therapy. **(B)** After propranolol therapy. (Reproduced, with permission, from Usatine RP, Smith MA, Mayeaux EJ Jr, Chumley HS, eds. *Color Atlas of Family Medicine*. 2nd ed. New York, NY: McGraw-Hill Education; 2012.)

endothelial cells and pericytes is usually significant at this stage. The vessels may penetrate the perineurium or endoneurium of small nerves; in this setting, this feature is not indicative of malignancy. With time, the lobular character of the tumor becomes more evident, the degree of cellularity diminishes, and the vascular lumina are readily identified. In the **involution phase**, the vascular lobules are gradually replaced by fibrous tissue or fat, with hyalinization of the rare persisting capillaries. At all stages of evolution there is expression of common endothelial antigens; however, these tumors uniquely express erythrocyte-type glucose transporter molecule isoform 1 **(GLUT-1)**, merosin (α-laminin), Lewis Y antigen, and FcγRII (CD32). This phenotype is shared by the endothelial cells of the placenta and with respect to GLUT-1 and merosin by those of blood-tissue barriers.

The differential diagnosis includes **congenital hemangioma, kaposiform hemangioendothelioma, tufted angioma (TA), pyogenic granuloma (PG),** and **vascular malformations.** The clinical presentation and GLUT-1 immunohistochemical expression generally excludes these entities.

ANSWER 11-4: A.

This is an example of a **venous lake**, which is an acquired vascular malformation and not a neoplasm (Table 11-4A). These lesions are usually solitary and arise within chronically sun-damaged skin of the head and neck in elderly patients probably from lack of support from the surrounding tissue (solar elastosis). Clinically these lesions are easily distinguished from **melanomas** by their blanching with compression; however, this feature may be impaired if the vascular lumen contain a thrombus. Microscopically, the lesion is a solitary ectatic vascular space localized to the superficial to middle dermis and is usually lined by a single layer of endothelium; however, smooth muscle elements may occasionally be associated with the wall of the vessel. The surrounding dermis usually shows solar elastosis and diminished collagen. In regard to the differential diagnosis, this lesion is distinctive; however, other vascular ectasias might be considered. **Pyogenic granulomas** arising after cryosurgery has been reported.

Table 11-4A. Venous Lake

Clinical Features
Predilection for exposed ("weathered") skin of elderly individuals—face, ears, lips
Dark-blue papule, 3-10 mm, can appear suspicious for melanoma
Histopathologic Features
Dilated thin-walled vascular channel in dermis
Uncommon smooth muscle in wall
Occasional intraluminal thrombosis
Solar elastosis and lack of supporting dermal collagen
Differential Diagnosis
Telangiectases
Venous malformation

ANSWER 11-5: A.

This is a classic example of a **glomus tumor**, which typically produces a triad of symptoms, including pain that may be paroxysmal, tenderness, and temperature sensitivity (Table 11-5A). **Glomus cells** are modified smooth muscle cells concentrated at the arterial end of the **Sucquet-Hoyer canal**, and are responsible for shunting of blood and

Table 11-5A. Glomus Tumor and Glomuvenous Malformation

Clinical Features
- Glomus tumor
  - Adults
  - Nail beds, pads of fingers and toes, volar surfaces of hands and feet, ears, center of face
  - Blue-red nodule
  - <1 cm
  - Pain, often paroxysmal
  - Tenderness
  - Temperature sensitivity
- Glomuvenous malformation
  - Childhood common
  - Proximal >> distal sites
  - Regional or disseminated
  - Familial in 64% of cases
  - Bluish nodules
  - Often >1 cm
  - Often asymptomatic

Histopathologic Features
- Solitary type
  - Dermal or subcutaneous
  - Well circumscribed
  - Encapsulated usually
  - Nests and sheets of monotonous round or cuboidal cells
  - Glomus cells cuff small vascular channels
  - Round nucleus with amphophilic or eosinophilic cytoplasm
  - Smooth muscle may be present (glomangiomyoma)
  - Nerve fibers present
  - Occasional myxoid stroma
- Multiple type
  - Large, irregularly shaped vascular channels (glomangioma)
  - Usually fewer layers of glomus cells cuffing vessels
  - Glomus cells may blend with smooth muscle (glomangiomyoma)
- Immunohistochemistry
  - Positive for vimentin, smooth- or pan-muscle actin, myosin, desmin (variable)
  - Negative for von Willebrand factor–related S-100 protein

Table 11-5A. Glomus Tumor and Glomuvenous Malformation (*continued*)

Differential Diagnosis
- Adnexal tumor
  - Eccrine acrospiroma
  - Chondroid syringoma (mixed tumor)
- Mastocytoma
- Melanocytic nevi (pseudoangiomatous)
- Cavernous malformation
- Hemangiopericytoma
- Angioleiomyoma

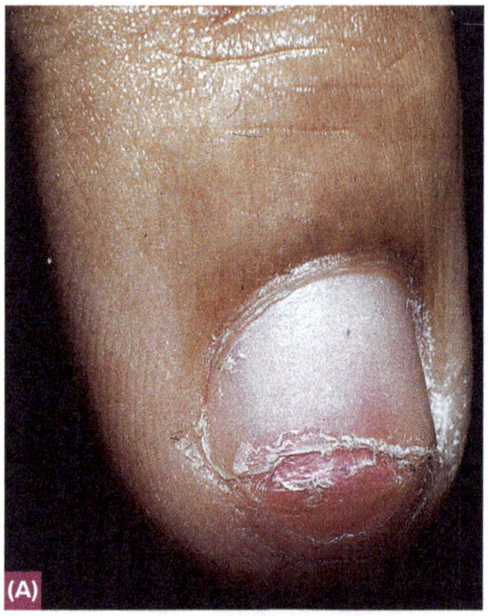

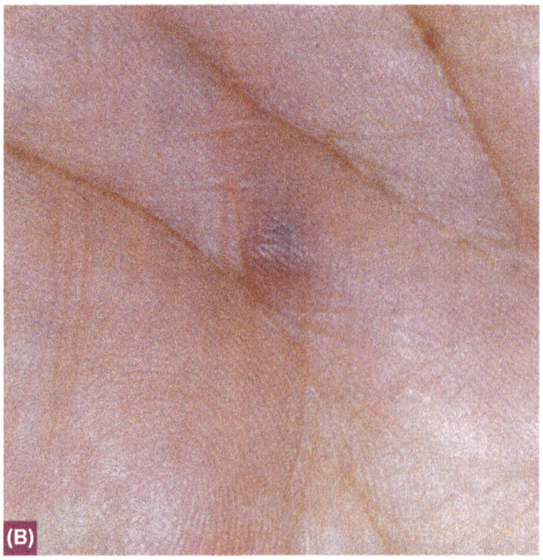

Glomus tumor. (A) There is an exquisitely painful subungual nodule of reddish color. Pain becomes paroxysmal when exposed to cold temperatures. **(B)** Hard bluish nodule on the palm. (Reproduced, with permission, from Wolff K, Johnson RA, Saavedra AP. *Fitzpatrick's Color Atlas and Synopsis of Clinical Dermatology.* 7th ed. New York, NY: McGraw-Hill Education; 2013.)

thermoregulation. Lesions may be classified into solitary and multiple types. **Solitary glomus tumors** are neoplasms that arise most commonly in the nail beds, pads of the fingers and toes, volar sides of the hands and feet, and center of the face in adults. The multiple types, referred to as **glomuvenous malformations (GVM),** are believed to represent vascular malformations with a frequent autosomal dominant inheritance pattern. GVM most often present in childhood, only rarely occur subungually, and may be subdivided anatomically into regional or disseminated variants. In general, GVM tend to be larger than solitary glomus tumors, may reach several centimeters in size, or more rarely present as large plaque-like lesions that may be congenital. Unlike venous malformations, they lack a cobblestone appearance. **Glomangiosarcoma**, or **malignant glomus tumor**, is rare and typically arises within a preexisting glomus tumor. These tumors have a high local recurrence rate with rare metastasis.

The typical glomus cell is round or cuboidal with a round nucleus in amphophilic to eosinophilic cytoplasm and occurs in monotonous nests and sheets that are interrupted by blood vessels, around which the glomus cells may form collars. Solitary glomus tumors are usually encapsulated, contain numerous small blood vessels, and are associated with ample nerve fibers. GVM are composed of large, irregularly shaped vascular spaces that may resemble those of a venous malformation. These spaces may be filled with blood or contain organized thrombi. Typically, only a few layers of glomus cells surround these large spaces, and some vessels may lack glomus cells.

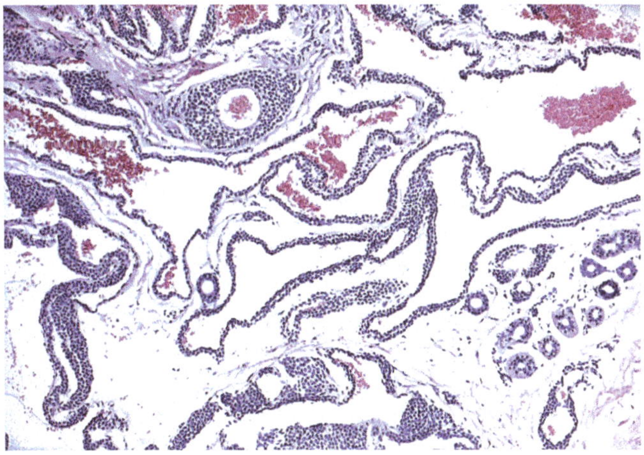

Glomuvenous malformations (glomangioma). Cavernous vascular channels that resemble a venous malformation are present and are lined by several layers of glomus cells, sometimes scant in number.

In contrast to the solitary tumors, nerve fibers about multiple glomus tumors are few. Glomangiosarcomas are characterized by short spindle cells, disordered arrangements of cells, moderate pleomorphism, single large nucleoli, and numerous mitoses. Recently, criteria for malignant glomus tumor (reserved for lesions with marked risk of metastasis) have been proposed: (1) greater than 2 cm size and a deep location or (2) atypical mitotic figures or (3) moderate to high nuclear grade and greater than or equal to 5 mitotic figures per 50 hpf. Unusual or atypical glomus tumors failing to meet these criteria did not metastasize and were classified as **glomus tumor of uncertain malignant potential**. At present, evidence suggests that superficially situated glomus tumors with malignant-appearing histologic features show less aggressive behavior than similar-appearing tumors in deep locations. Immunohistochemically, glomus tumors express vimentin, muscle actins, myosin, pericellular collagen type IV, and variably desmin but are negative for von Willebrand factor, cytokeratin, and S-100 protein. These features suggest that glomus tumors are not derived from capillary pericytes, as was once thought, but instead derive from smooth muscle cells of the vascular part of the **neuromyoarterial glomus** which regulates arteriovenous shunting of blood and temperature regulation.

ANSWER 11-6: C.

This patient has **blue rubber bleb nevus syndrome**, which is characterized by numerous **venous malformations (VM)** (aka **cavernous hemangiomas/malformations**) of the skin, gastrointestinal tract, central nervous system, liver, and spleen (Table 11-6A). Most cases occur sporadically. Patients may exhibit pain and **hyperhidrosis** from the cutaneous lesions and melena and anemia from those situated in the GI tract. Rupture of lesions at other sites can result in blindness, cognitive changes, and paralysis. Most commonly, gastrointestinal lesions exhibit slow chronic bleeds with **melena** and **iron deficiency anemia**.

Familial mucocutaneous venous malformations are related to a mutation of *Tie2* gene, which is located on chromosome 9. The principal findings typifying **Maffucci syndrome** include four varieties of vascular lesions: venous malformations, lymphatic malformations, phlebectasias, and **spindle cell hemangiomas**. Nonvascular lesions include multiple **enchondromas** and bony deformities resulting from nonossifying cartilage in the metaphyses of growing bones, frequent fractures of bone from the latter defects, and the frequent development of **chondrosarcoma** and **angiosarcoma** in up to 50% of affected individuals.

> **Quick Fact**
>
> **Syndromes Associated with Venous Malformations**
>
> Very Mild Bloody Mary
> V = Venous
> M = Malformation
> B = Blue Rubber Bleb Syndrome
> M = Maffucci Syndrome

Table 11-6A. Venous Malformation

Clinical Features
Onset commonly at birth or in childhood
Involve head and neck most commonly, but may occur anywhere
Soft, blue to purple nodules, masses, or plaques
Compressible and rubbery, inflate when dependent
Sometimes associated with lymphatic malformation (venolymphatic malformation)
Rarely familial (mucocutaneous venous malformation)
Associated with particular syndromes:
Blue rubber bleb nevus syndrome: autosomal dominant; venous malformations involving the skin, gastrointestinal tract, liver, spleen, and central nervous system; pain and hyperhidrosis; melena and anemia
Maffucci syndrome: venous malformations, rarely lymphatic malformations, and phlebectasias; spindle cell hemangioma; multiple enchondromas and bony deformities from nonossifying cartilage; high risk of chondrosarcoma and increased risk of angiosarcoma
Histopathologic Features
Location usually in deep dermis or subcutis
Generally diffuse; rarely circumscribed
Vascular channels are dilated and often encased in fibrous tissue
Vessels contain single layer of endothelium surrounded by fibrous tissue in vessel wall
Smooth muscle may be observed in the vessel wall but is often inconspicuous
Differential Diagnosis
Lymphatic malformation
Glomuvenous malformation (glomangioma)
Port wine stain
Arteriovenous and other malformations
Involuting juvenile capillary hemangioma

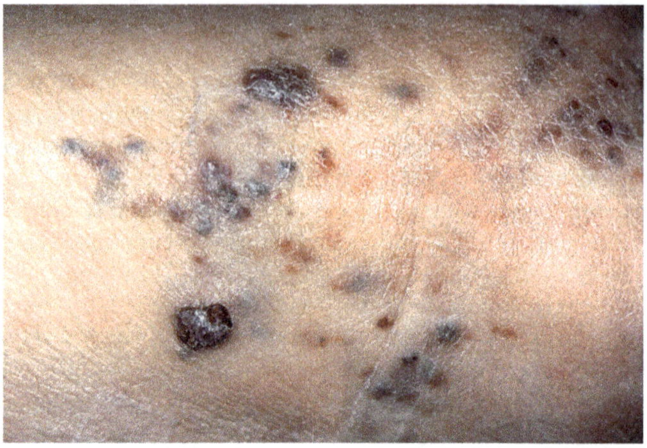

Blue rubber bleb nevus. A spontaneously painful and tender capillary-venous malformation. There are a number of compressible bluish-violaceous papules and nodules on the upper arm. (Reproduced, with permission, from Wolff K, Johnson RA, Saavedra AP. *Fitzpatrick's Color Atlas and Synopsis of Clinical Dermatology*. 7th ed. New York, NY: McGraw-Hill Education; 2013.)

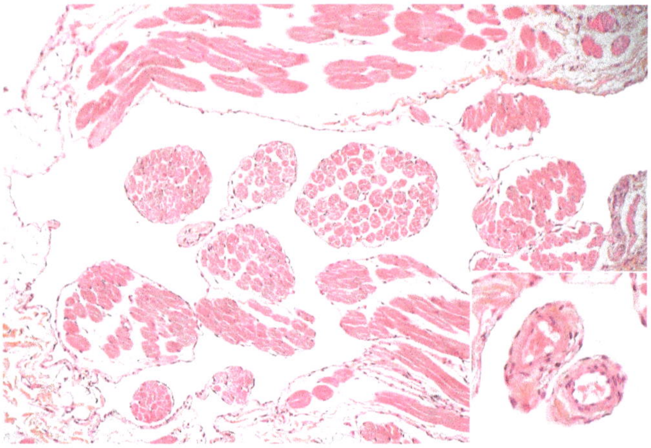

Venous malformation. The vascular channels form a complex network of open vessels dissecting the tissue and encasing normal structures such as hair follicles, arterioles, and cutaneous smooth muscle bundles. Microvessels are encases by the malformation (inset).

VMs are usually situated in the dermis and subcutis and are generally diffuse. The vascular channels form a complex network of slit-like, stellate, or open vessels dissecting the tissues and encasing normal structures such as hair follicles, nerves, arterioles, and cutaneous smooth muscle. The vessels exhibit a single layer of endothelium surrounded by a thin or relatively thickened layer of fibrous tissue. Various amounts of smooth muscle elements may be observed in the fibrous lining of the vessels; this smooth muscle component may be focal or extensive. VMs frequently contain organized thrombi, which manifest both as concentrically hyalinized structures and calcified round **phleboliths** or as **intravascular papillary hyperplasia of Masson.**

It must be emphasized that VMs may occur as a component of many complex or combined VMs or as part of many of the syndromes described above. Thus, for example, one may observe capillary-venous, lymphatico-venous malformations, or even more complex combinations of channels. In regard to the histopathological differential diagnosis, VMs must be distinguished from **lymphatic malformations (LM).** An LM may have a very similar and sometimes identical architecture as a VM, and histologic distinction of the two may not be possible without additional information. LMs may contain blood due to intralesional hemorrhage before or during surgery. Distinction is possible only if the lumina contain numerous lymphocytes or if lymphocytic aggregates are present in the

Table 11-6B. Angiomatosis of Soft Tissue

Clinical Features
- Usually presents in children and young adults
- Soft tissue mass, generally tender or painful
- High recurrence rate

Histopathologic Features
- Ill-defined infiltrating contours
- Made of veins with uneven walls, honeycomb cavernous spaces, thick onion-bulb vessels, lymphatics and lymphocytes aggregates
- Rarely capillary-sized vessels

Differential Diagnosis
- Intramuscular hemangioma
- Venous malformations
- Lymphatic malformations
- Soft tissue tumor
- Angiolipoma

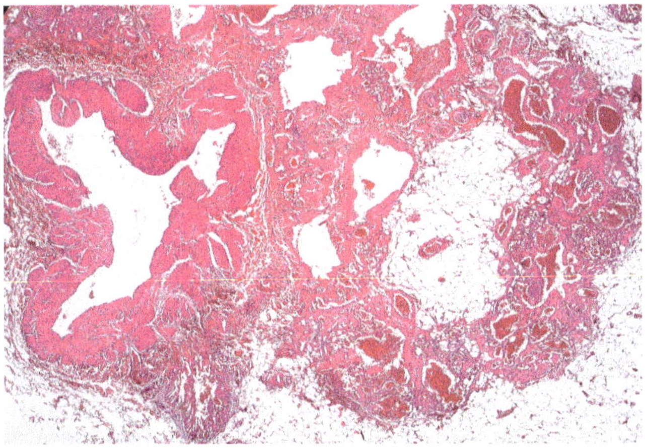

Angiomatosis of soft tissue. The dermis and subcutis contain multiple discrete nodules composed of an admixture of veins and cavernous vascular spaces.

vicinity of the malformed vessels. Encasing of normal elements within the vascular lumina is a feature more commonly noted in VM than in LM.

Other tumors that present as deep-seated vascular nodules include **angiomatosis of soft tissue,** and **arteriovenous malformation**. **Angiomatosis of soft tissue (AST)** is a relatively rare and probably underrecognized condition that usually presents in children or young adults with persistent swelling or pain in the soft tissue, muscle, and dermis (Table 11-6B). Nearly two-thirds of the cases involve the extremities, but all body areas may be affected. Occasional lesions extend into bone. Angiomatosis is associated with a very high rate of recurrence, with up to 90% in one series. Recurrence of AST is probably due to underestimation of the extent of the lesions and incomplete resection. AST often affects several adjacent tissue types but may be confined to one tissue. Microscopically, AST is characterized by infiltration of the dermis and soft tissue by multiple discrete nodules composed of an admixture of veins, cavernous vascular spaces, and thick-walled vessels with onion-skin concentric appearance. The veins demonstrate media of uneven thickness with fissures and muscular pads. Slit-like, tortuous, thin-walled vessels directly branch from their walls of these veins. In addition to such veins, aggregates of open vessels separated by thin fibrous septa in a honeycomb pattern are frequently seen. Distinction between AST and other subcutaneous or intramuscular vascular malformations (mainly **venous malformation**) essentially depends on the presence of the rather characteristic constellation of findings that defines AST.

Arteriovenous malformation (AVM) is a high-flow lesion and contains direct arteriovenous communications or fistulas (Table 11-6C). AVM is present at birth but is

Table 11-6C. Arteriovenous Malformation (Not Otherwise Specified)

Clinical Features
- Present at birth; generally undetected
- Equally affects both genders
- Becomes apparent during childhood or adulthood
- Pulsation, murmur, or both generally present
- May progress after trauma or hormonal change
- May be stages according to Schobinger:
  - Stage I: quiescent, asymptomatic
  - Stage II: progression and expansion
  - Stage III: destruction with necrosis and hemorrhage
  - Stage IV: high output cardiac failure

Histopathologic Features
- Ill-defined infiltrative lesion
- Composed of arteries, veins, arterialized veins, and unclassified vessels
- Variable capillary component
- Abnormal vessels evenly distributed, with round or oval contours and relatively thick wall
- Arteriovenous communications on elastic stains

Differential Diagnosis
- Capillary malformation in AVM quiescent stage
- Venous malformation

often undetected or masquerades as a capillary malformation (port wine stain). AVM becomes clinically apparent in childhood or adolescence, and only 20% are detected during adulthood. AVM may affect the skin, soft tissue, viscera, bone, and brain. **Capillary steal syndrome** may develop with skin atrophy, ulceration, pain, and sudden life-threatening hemorrhage. Microscopically, AVM are ill-defined lesions comprised of vessels of different calibers and thicknesses evenly distributed throughout the affected tissues and accompanied by variable amounts of fibrosis. The thickness of the vessel walls is generally proportionate to the diameter of the lumen but may vary from one segment to another of the same vessel section. Some dilated vessels with thin walls, resembling those of VM, may also occur. The type and structure of the vessels wall is best visualized with elastin stains, which show arteries, veins with thickened walls, and a majority of abnormal unclassified or intermediate vessels with defective elastic architecture. Direct communications between arteries and veins or unclassified vessels may be seen, especially on elastin stains. A capillary component is present in some cases, either as ill-defined capillary lobules, especially in the skeletal or cutaneous muscles, or as sheets of individual or anastomosing capillaries in the dermis. These capillaries may be found even without a history of ulceration. Mitoses, without abnormal figures, may be numerous in the capillary component. Hypervascularization of the subcutaneous fat lobules occurring adjacent to AVM is frequent and may mimic angiolipoma.

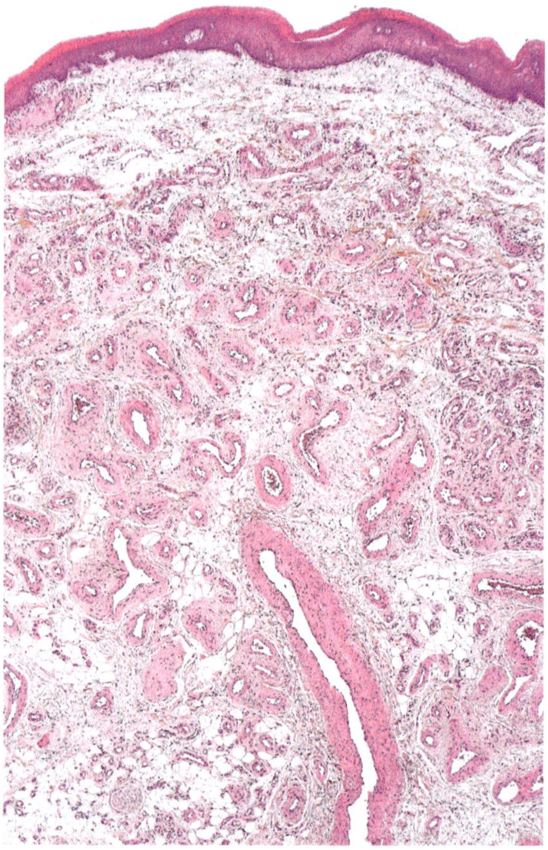

Arteriovenous malformation. Vessels of different calibers and thicknesses are evenly distributed throughout the affected tissues and are accompanied by variable amounts of fibrosis.

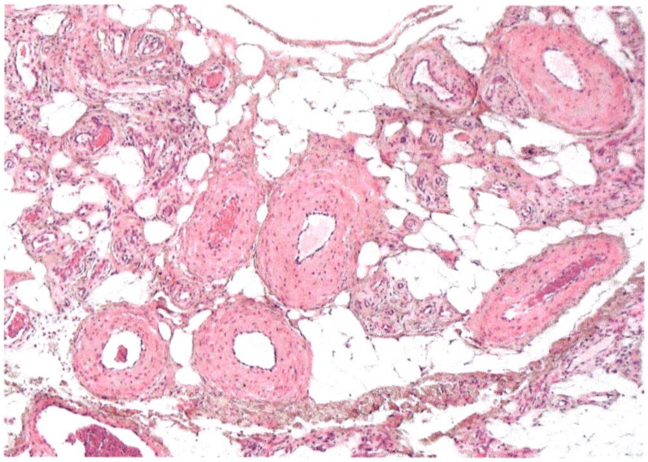

Arteriovenous malformation. The thickness of the vessel walls is generally proportionate to the diameter of the lumen but may vary from one segment to another of the same vessel section.

ANSWER 11-7: E.

The lesion in the image is an **angiokeratoma**, which is a form of telangiectasia characterized by ectatic, thin-walled vascular spaces in the papillary dermis and is intimately associated with and variably encased by a hyperplastic epidermis. Fibrin thrombi in various degrees of organization may be present. **Angiokeratomas** traditionally occur as five clinical variants.

(1) **Mibelli type**, characterized hyperkeratotic lesions on the dorsal fingers and toes.
(2) **Fordyce type,** characterized by involvement of the scrotum and vulva.
(3) **Angiokeratoma corporis diffusum (ACD),** a lysosomal storage disease inherited as an X-linked recessive disorder in Fabry disease (α-galactosidase A deficiency) but also seen with the autosomal recessive disorder, fucosidosis (α-L-fucosidase deficiency), and rarely with β-galactosidase deficiency, alone or in combination with neuraminidase deficiency.
(4) **The solitary or multiple type**, which may involve any site but favors the lower extremities.
(5) **Angiokeratoma circumscriptum**, characterized by lesions in groups or bands usually on an extremity. In contrast to the fundamental telangiectatic nature of the other variants of angiokeratoma, the fifth type of angiokeratoma—angiokeratoma circumscriptum—may demonstrate a deep component composed of a variable admixture of dilated capillaries, lymphatics, and veins. These lesions are best classified as hyperkeratotic capillary, lymphatic, venous, or combined vascular malformations.

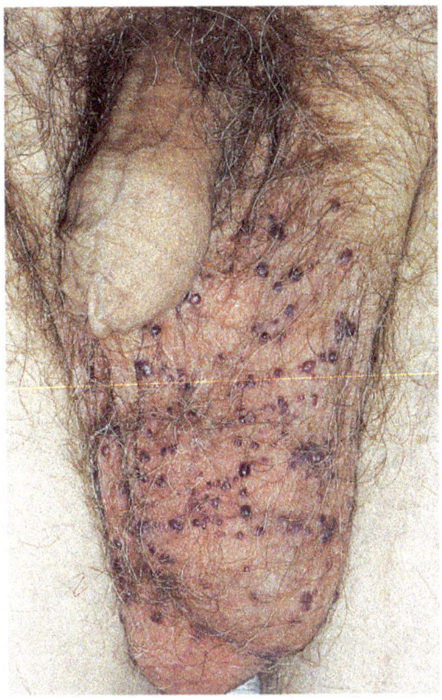

Angiokeratoma of Fordyce. Numerous red to violaceous papules on the scrotum. The lesions blanch under diascopy. (Reproduced, with permission, from Wolff K, Johnson RA, Saavedra AP. *Fitzpatrick's Color Atlas and Synopsis of Clinical Dermatology*. 7th ed. New York, NY: McGraw-Hill Education; 2013.)

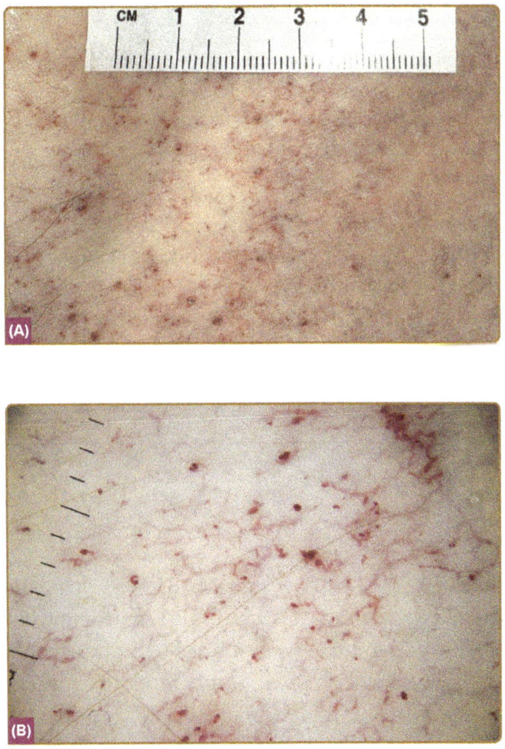

Angiokeratoma corporis diffusum. (A) Angiokeratomas and telangiectatic vessels on the flank in a patient with angiokeratoma corporis diffusum. **(B)** Dermatoscopic view showing angiokeratomas and upper dermal vessel tortuosity. (Reproduced, with permission, from Goldsmith LA, Katz SI, Gilchrest BA, Paller AS, Leffell DJ, Wolff K, eds. *Fitzpatrick's Dermatology in General Medicine*. 8th ed. New York, NY: McGraw-Hill Education; 2012.)

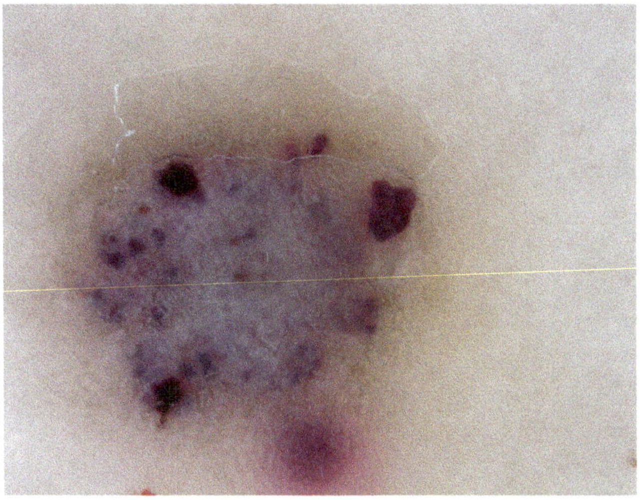

Solitary angiokeratoma. Angiokeratoma showing purple and black lacunae. (Used with permission of Richard P. Usatine, MD.)

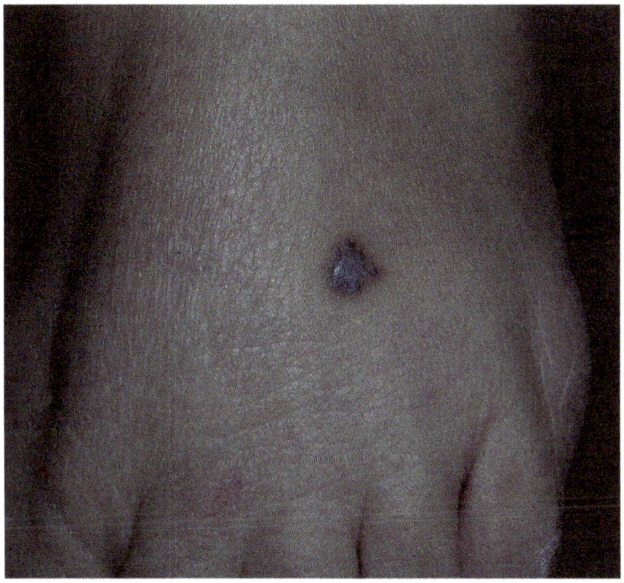

Angiokeratoma circumscriptum. Hyperkeratotic, blue-black papules and plaques. (Used with permission of Richard P. Usatine, MD.)

Angiokeratomas usually manifest no symptoms; however, with local trauma, they may become irritated and can bleed, given their highly vascular nature. The diagnosis of angiokeratoma is seldom difficult, and the clinical setting allows for appropriate subclassification. It is important to recognize angiokeratomas with enzyme deficiencies because of the obvious systemic implications.

The histopathological differential diagnosis for angiokeratoma includes **verrucous hemangioma (VH),** which is an uncommon vascular lesion that tends to arise at or near birth or in childhood (Table 11-7A). The most common site is the lower extremity, particularly distally. VH typically occurs

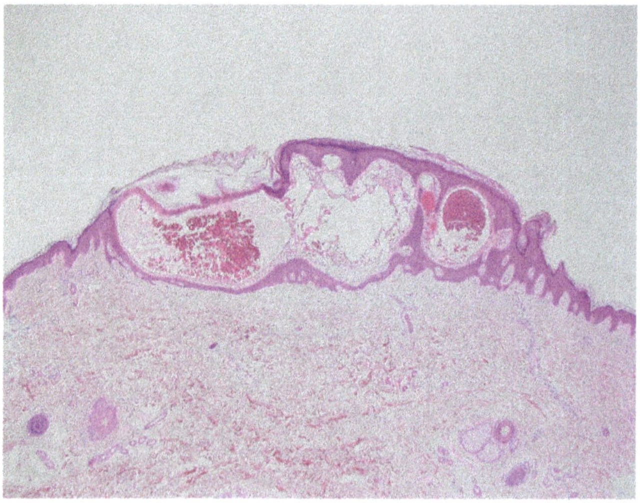

Angiokeratoma. There are capillaries and postcapillary venules packed into the papillary dermis just beneath and bulging into the epidermis, leading to hyperkeratosis.

Table 11-7A. Verrucous Hemangioma

Clinical Features
- Origin in infancy and childhood
- Distal lower extremity
- Hyperkeratotic angiomatous papules
- Grouped, discrete to confluent, sometimes linear or serpiginous
- Verrucous appearance developing over time

Histopathologic Features
- Capillary to venous vascular proliferation
- Pandermal involvement with extension into the subcutis
- Lateral extension into clinically normal-appearing skin
- Reactive acanthosis, papillomatosis, and hyperkeratosis
- Occasional inflammatory crusting or ulceration

Differential Diagnosis
- Angiokeratomas
- Angiokeratoma circumscriptum
- Angioma serpiginosa
- Cutaneous keratotic hemangioma

as unilateral, grouped, sometimes linear or serpiginous, discrete to confluent, hyperkeratotic angiomatous papules. Early lesions are bluish-red, well demarcated, soft, and compressible. Over time, VHs gradually enlarge, satellite nodules may arise, and ultimately a verrucous hyperkeratotic appearance develops. The linearity of VH has been theorized to reflect genetic mosaicism. VH enlarge proportionately with body growth and tend to recur after surgical excision. Accordingly, they are best removed early in life when they are still small. In contrast to **angiokeratomas,** which respond to various superficial means of therapy, removal of VH requires a deep and relatively wide surgical excision. Otherwise, the lesions are apt to recur. Microscopically, the epidermis shows papillomatous hyperplasia and is intimately associated with ectatic vascular channels containing erythrocytes. The features are indistinguishable from angiokeratoma. However, a deep vascular component is present.

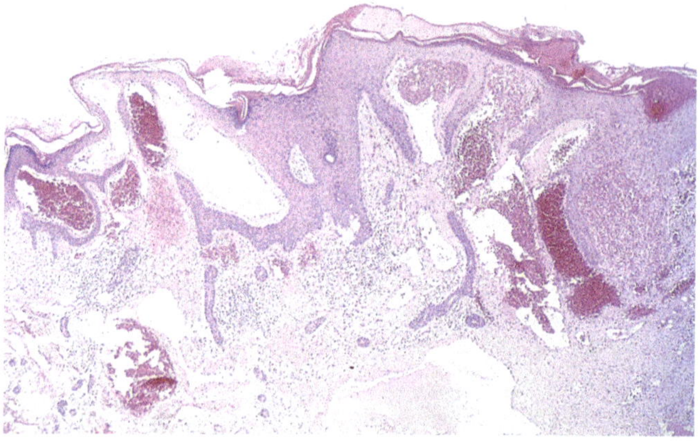

Verrucous hemangioma. The epidermis shows papillomatous hyperplasia and is intimately associated with ectatic vascular channels containing erythrocytes. The features are indistinguishable from angiokeratoma. However, a deep vascular component is present.

Choice E describes the **glomeruloid hemangiomas** associated with **POEMS syndrome**. These lesions are characterized by miniature glomeruloid vascular tufts located within ectatic vessels and may contain PAS-positive eosinophilic globules.

ANSWER 11-8: B.

This is a classic example of **port-wine stain (PWS)** or **nevus flammeus**, which is a **congenital capillary malformation** (Table 11-8A). These lesions are present at birth and mainly involve the head and neck with often a unilateral distribution but may occur anywhere. PWS, at birth, present as pink to reddish macules that are often irregular in configuration. The lesions grow proportionately with the child, and their color tends to darken with progressive nodularity and hyperkeratosis in adulthood. Papulonodular lesions of the head and neck tend to arise within the area of the second and third branches of the trigeminal nerve. In the mandibular region, PWS may be associated with underlying soft tissue and bone hypertrophy (**hypertrophic PWS**).

Table 11-8A. Capillary Malformations

Clinical Features
- Onset at birth
- Often involves head and neck but may occur anywhere
- Pink macular lesions but may become papular and keratotic
- Persistent lesions, such as the port wine stain, are associated with particular syndromes
  - Cobb syndrome: arteriovenous malformation in spinal cord and port wine stain in corresponding dermatome
  - Sturge-Weber syndrome: unilateral port wine stain involving the ophthalmic branch of trigeminal cranial nerve; seizures, hemiparesis, hemiplegia from vascular malformation of contralateral leptomeninges; occasional vascular malformations in other sites such as the choroid; mental retardation; glaucoma
  - Klippel-Trenaunay-Weber syndrome: unilateral hypertrophy of a limb (bone and soft tissue overgrowth); varicosities; venous malformation, lymphatic malformation on occasion; arteriovenous malformation often present; other vascular malformations on occasion
  - Parkes-Weber syndrome: unilateral limb hypertrophy; multiple arteriovenous fistula or arteriovenous malformation; lymphatic malformation on occasion
  - Capillary malformation arteriovenous malformation syndrome: small patchy port wine stains associated with arteriovenous fistulas or arteriovenous malformations, hereditary, caused by mutations in the *RASA1* gene

Histopathologic Features
- Widely dilated thin-walled venules in upper dermis or throughout reticular dermis

Differential Diagnosis
- Arteriovenous malformation, when in quiescent stage
- Telangiectases
- Spider angioma

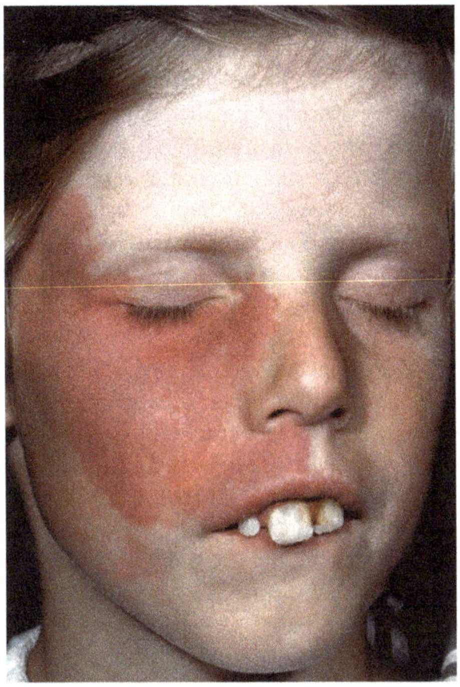

Port-wine stain in a child. Sharply marginated, port-wine red macule occurring in a distribution of the second branch of the trigeminal nerve in a child. (Reproduced, with permission, from Wolff K, Johnson RA, Saavedra AP. *Fitzpatrick's Color Atlas and Synopsis of Clinical Dermatology*. 7th ed. New York, NY: McGraw-Hill Education; 2013.)

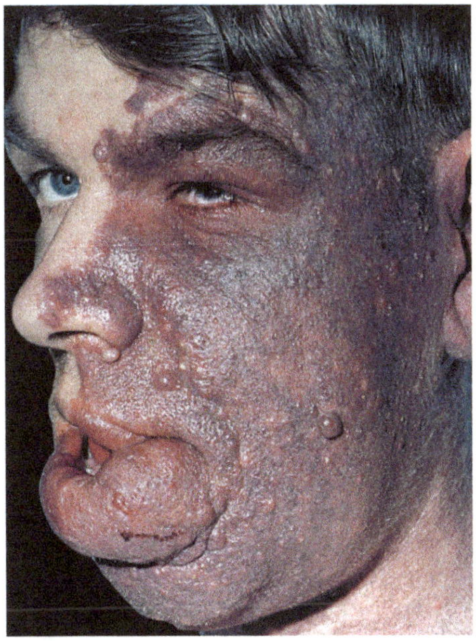

Hypertrophic port-wine stain in an adult. With increasing age, the color deepens and papular and nodular vascular lesions develop within the previously macular lesion, causing progressively increasing disfigurement. (Reproduced, with permission, from Wolff K, Johnson RA, Saavedra AP. *Fitzpatrick's Color Atlas and Synopsis of Clinical Dermatology*. 7th ed. New York, NY: McGraw-Hill Education; 2013.)

The literature sometimes refers to resolving lesions affecting the midline of the head, such as the forehead, eyelids, and glabella (the so-called "**salmon patch**"), or nape ("**stork bite**") as port-wines stains. These lesions, however, are not true vascular malformations and represent a form of temporary vasodilatation which gradually lightens and disappears in the postnatal period or generally before 5 years of age. There is a higher incidence of **pyogenic granulomas** arising within lesional skin compared with normal skin.

The essential findings of early lesions are widely dilated, thin-walled capillaries or venules scattered throughout the upper dermis or the entire reticular dermis. A decrease in the number of capillary-associated small nerves has been suggested to explain the vascular dilation. Papular or nodular lesions developing in PWS are composed of a proliferation of thin-walled vascular channels with lumina that vary in size or sometimes exhibit thicker walls (image B in question), histopathologically simulating **acral arteriovenous malformation (aAVM)**. Unlike aAVM, the walls of PWS are thin and lack the thick smooth muscle characteristic arteries. In **hypertrophic PWS**, nodular aggregates of venous-like channels may be found in the deep dermis and subcutis. Other vascular ectasias, such as **generalized essential telangiectasia, hereditary benign telangiectasia, hereditary hemorrhagic telangiectasia** (HHT), **unilateral nevoid telangiectasia,** and **spider angioma**, enter into the differential diagnosis. PWS differs from the other conditions based on congenital onset, rather distinctive macular to papular clinical lesions, and fairly discrete dilated capillaries or postcapillary venules in the upper reticular dermis.

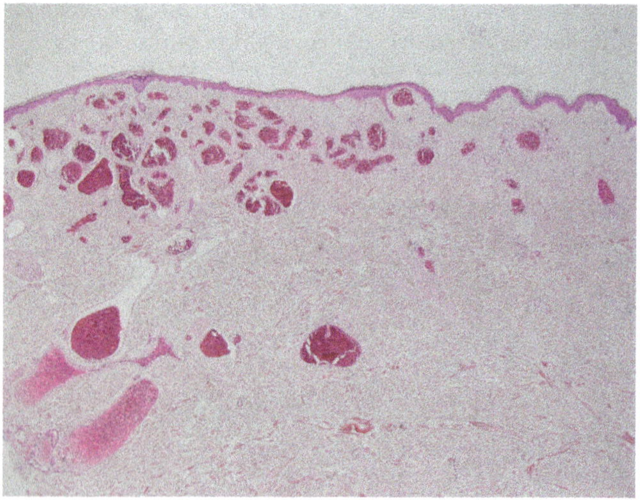

Capillary malformation (port-wine stain). There are thin-walled capillaries and postcapillary venules scattered throughout the superficial and deep dermis.

Acral arteriovenous malformations (aAVMs) have been considered "cirsoid" aneurysmal dilatations of cutaneous arterial structures or vascular channels comparable to the fibromuscular vessels of the **Sucquet-Hoyer canal** (Table 11-8B). Sucquet-Hoyer canals are most prominent in the fingers and toes and are involved in shunting of blood for temperature regulation. Although less prominent, they are also present in the face and oral mucosa. Clinically, aAVM is a relatively common acquired lesion primarily affecting middle-aged to elderly adults with a male predominance and a peak incidence in the fourth and fifth decades of life.

Table 11-8B. Acral Arteriovenous Malformation

Clinical Features
Most common in individuals 30 to 50 years of age
Affects men more after than women
Head and neck, acral sites
Red or purple papules
Usually solitary, 4-6 mm (≤ 3 cm)
Cutaneous or mucosal
Histopathologic Features
Well circumscribed, not encapsulated
Aggregates of thick-walled and thin-walled vessels
Variation in vessel caliber
Single layer of bland endothelium in vessels but occasional hobnail features present
Vessel walls contain fibrous tissue with occasional small smooth muscle component
A true arterial component usually present
Differential Diagnosis
Cherry angioma
Lobular capillary hemangioma
Venous lake
Angioleiomyoma

These lesions present as single red or violaceous papules ranging in size from 1 mm to 3 cm with an average of 4 to 6 mm in the head or neck region and less commonly involve the fingertips and mucosa. Most lesions are asymptomatic; however, enlargement, pain, or pruritus may occur. Occasionally, aAVMs are associated with angiolymphoid hyperplasia with eosinophilia, verruciform xanthoma, and basal cell carcinoma.

Microscopically, aAVM lesions are well circumscribed and unencapsulated. They are composed of an intimate admixture of thick-walled and thin-walled blood vessels distributed within the superficial and middle dermis. The proportion of thick-walled to thin-walled vessels is variable, although the former typically predominates. The vessels may be closely approximated to and dispersed between the cutaneous and mucosal adnexa. The lining endothelium is typically bland. Occasionally, the endothelial cells protrude into the vessel lumen in a "hobnail" fashion. Thrombi, often showing organization and recanalization, are an occasional finding. Girard and colleagues described direct communication between arteries and veins in a subset of their cases. Inflammation is an infrequent feature; when present, it is described as a mixed, chronic inflammatory cell infiltrate associated with accentuation of fibrous changes within vessel walls. Elastin stains typically show vessels with finely fibrillar elastinophilic fibers scattered throughout their walls, alternating with a true arterial component with an internal elastic lamina.

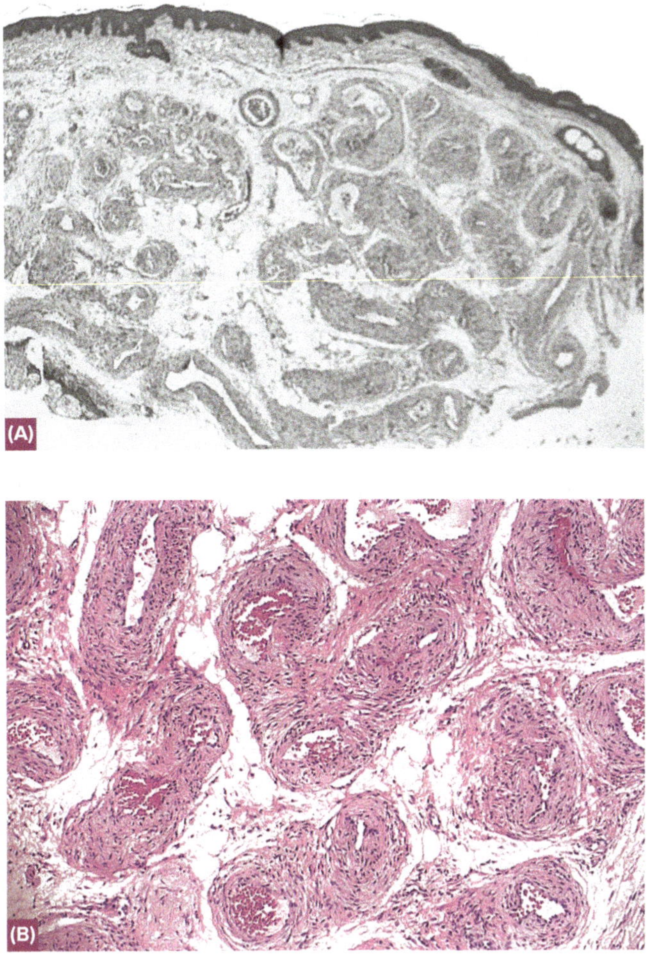

Acral arteriovenous malformation (acral arteriovenous hemangioma). (A) These lesions are well circumscribed and unencapsulated. They are composed of an intimate admixture of thick-walled and thin-walled blood vessels distributed within the superficial and middle dermis. **(B)** Some of the vessels resemble arteries.

Capillary malformation is distinguished from **aAVM** clinically by a typically larger size and an initial macular presentation. Although both lesions frequently involve the head and neck region, aAVM is typically a solitary papule. While capillary malformations are typically present at birth, aAVMs initially present much later in life (fourth to fifth decades of life). Microscopically, a component of the vessels of aAVM contains thick smooth muscle walls, unlike the thin capillary and postcapillary venules of capillary malformation.

ANSWER 11-9: A.

This is a **glomeruloid hemangioma** (GH), which is a rare vascular lesion that derives its name from its distinctive histologic resemblance to renal glomeruli and occurs in the setting of **POEMS syndrome**, a multisystem disorder consisting of polyneuropathy, organomegaly, endocrinopathy, M-protein development, and particular skin alterations (Table 11-9A). The cutaneous manifestations of POEMS syndrome include hyperpigmentation, hypertrichosis, hyperhidrosis, scleroderma-like skin thickening, and hemangiomas. Many patients with POEMS syndrome show overlapping features with **multicentric Castleman disease** and its characteristic **angiofollicular lymphoid hyperplasia** of lymph nodes. There is a strong predilection for Japanese patients. The glomeruloid "hemangioma" is considered to be a reactive endothelial proliferation with a similar pathogenesis as

Quick Fact

Vascular Proliferations with Eosinophilic Globules

- Congenital hemangioma
  - PAS+ hyaline globules
- Glomeruloid hemangioma
  - PAS+ Ig
- Papillary hemangioma
  - PAS+ α_1-antitrypsin
- Kaposi sarcoma
  - PAS+ hyaline globules
- Kaposiform hemangioendothelioma
  - PAS+ hyaline globules
- Dabska tumor
  - PAS+ hyaline globules

Table 11-9A. Glomeruloid Hemangioma

Clinical Features
Japanese > other populations
Fifth to sixth decades of life
Multiple, punctate to a few millimeters, erythematous or violaceous papules
Most common sites: trunk and proximal limbs
Histopathologic Features
Conglomerates of capillaries within ectatic spaces, giving a glomerulus-like appearance
Generally bland endothelial cells
Occasional plump endothelial and stromal cells with pale cytoplasm, clear vacuoles, or eosinophilic globules
Little to absent inflammation
Differential Diagnosis
Acquired tufted angioma
Intravascular pyogenic granuloma
Intravascular papillary endothelial hyperplasia
Reactive angioendotheliomatosis
Endovascular papillary angioendothelioma (Dabska tumor)

reactive angioendotheliomatosis and is the result of circulating angiogenic factors from activated lymphocytes. These patients have circulating cryoproteins that, when in contact with endothelium of peripheral microvessels, stimulate their proliferation with widespread inspissated cryoproteins within vascular lumina.

Microscopically, **glomeruloid hemangiomas** are characterized by ectatic vascular spaces that contain intraluminal conglomerates of blood-filled capillary loops that are lined by flat endothelial cells. GHs frequently contain stromal cells and eosinophilic droplets between the capillary loops. The eosinophilic globules, which are PAS positive and diastase resistant, show polytypic immunoglobulin staining and presumably represent circulatory-derived immunoglobulins and other proteinaceous material. Mitoses are inconspicuous, numbering less than 1 per 10 hpf. Little, if any, inflammation is present.

Choice B could describe either **kaposiform hemangioendotheliomas** or **tufted angiomas (TA)**, which are believed to be variants of one another. Additionally, both conditions are associated with **Kasabach-Merritt syndrome** (thrombocytopenia and depletion of coagulation factors). TA is frequently associated with peripheral vascular clefts; however, there is no actual intravascular angiomatous proliferation, and TAs are devoid of eosinophilic globules.

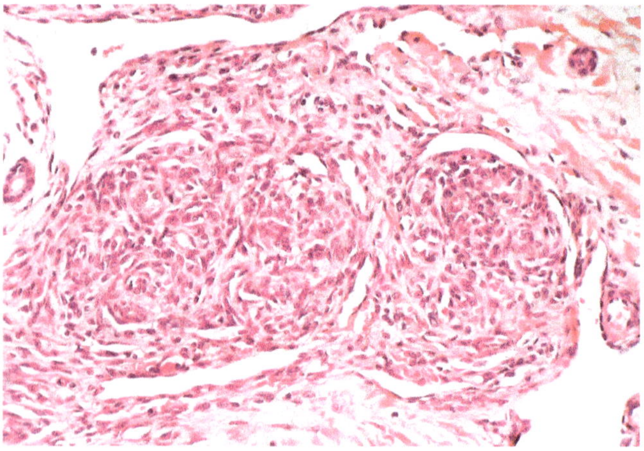

Tufted angioma. Crescentic cleft-like vessels are generally found at the periphery of some of the capillary tufts.

Option C describes **papillary intralymphatic angioendothelioma (PILA),** also known as **Dabska tumor** or **endovascular papillary angioendothelioma**, which in contrast to GH, shows intraluminal papillations lined by endothelium displaying some degree of pleomorphism and a hobnail or "head of a matchstick" appearance. The vascular channels of Dabska tumor are more primitive, and endothelial cells appear to float free as single cells or clumps within vascular lumina. Both lesions contain PAS-positive globules, but Dabska tumors frequently contain scattered and intrapapillary lymphocytic infiltrates. The hemorrhage and necrosis of more cellular lesions of Dabska tumor are not features of GH.

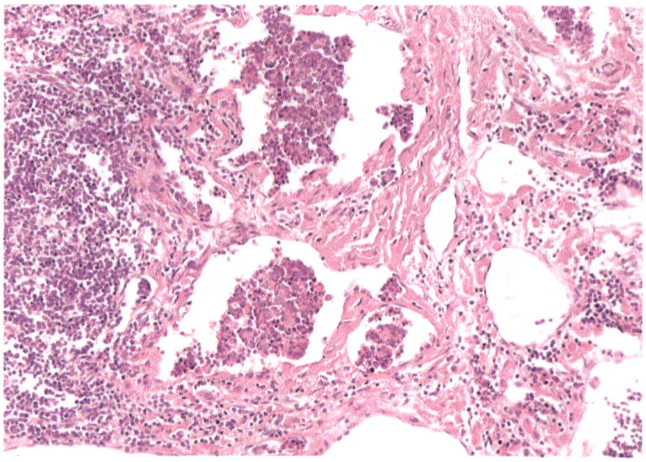

Papillary intralymphatic angioendothelioma (endovascular papillary angioendothelioma; Dabska tumor). Intraluminal papillary structures are lined by multilayered endothelial cells that show atypia. The clumps of cells appear to float free in the lumina.

Option D describes a **pyogenic granuloma (PG),** which may rarely occur intravascularly but does not show the glomeruloid appearance of GH.

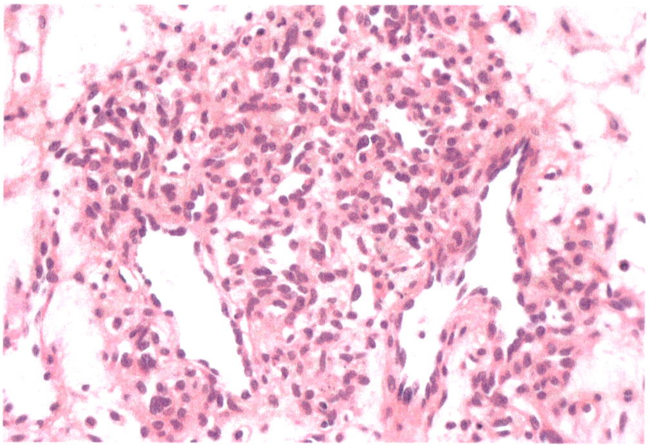

Pyogenic granuloma (lobular capillary hemangioma). In the final stage, some vessels progressively transform into veins. Initially, one or two such veins dominate each lobule, but later extensive "venulization" of the entire lesion takes place.

ANSWER 11-10: B.

This is a classic example of a **pyogenic granuloma (PG)**, which is a common vascular lesion often designated as **lobular capillary hemangioma** because of its lobular architecture at scanning power magnification. However, the latter designation is misleading because a lobular architecture may be seen in many other vascular tumors. Moreover, the neoplastic nature of PG is clearly questionable, hence many authors prefer to restrict the term "**hemangioma**" to vascular tumors proper and thus favor the use of the somewhat outdated but

Quick Fact

Vascular Tumors with Lobular Architecture

- Infantile hemangioma
- Congenital hemangioma
- Tufted angioma
- Pyogenic granuloma
- Papillary hemangioma
- Cherry hemangioma
- Acroangiodermatitis

universally understood term PG. The most common sites for PG are the fingers, face, and oral cavity. In the oral cavity, lesions may be seen on the gingiva, lips, and tongue. The term **granuloma gravidarum** or **pregnancy tumor** applies to a PG arising on the gingival surface during pregnancy. Whereas oral mucosal PGs favor female patients (2:1), cutaneous lesions affect both genders equally. In one study, PGs from pregnant women showed no immunoreactivity for estrogen and progesterone receptor proteins. Also, epidemiologic data are against a hormonal influence for cutaneous lesions. PG most commonly arises in association with trauma; however, it may also develop on capillary, venous, and arteriovenous malformations (ie, port wine stains [PWSs], cavernous malformations, and arteriovenous malformations [AVMs]). There is an association with medications such as antiretroviral therapy, retinoids, and minocycline. The phenomenon of satellite lesions arising after surgical removal, laser excision, or trauma to a PG is well known. The rapid growth of PG may result from decreased apoptosis associated with increased expression of the Bcl-2 family of apoptotic-regulatory proteins.

Microscopically, the typical PG contains variably cellular but cytologically bland lobular capillary proliferations with variable mitotic activity. The overlying epidermis is flattened, forms a peripheral collarette, and frequently shows erosion. Edema, hemorrhage, fibrin, necrosis, and neutrophilic infiltrates are frequent. Initially there is a compact vascular proliferation of solid, largely collapsed vascular structures. Later, there is a frank evolution into vascular structures with a multilobular arrangement and regular-appearing lumina with larger intralobular thin-walled stellate vessels.

In the final stage, there is a progressive transformation of some vessels into veins and intra- and interlobular fibrosis ensues. PGs have also occurred intravenously and in subcutaneous tissue. Intravenous PG extends into the vascular lumina as polypoid lesions that connect with the wall of the vein by a fibrovascular stalk.

The clinical differential diagnosis includes amelanotic melanoma, eccrine poroma, and glomus tumor. The histological differential diagnosis includes **tufted hemangioma (TA)**; however, TA lacks the nodular and exophytic character and intralobular open stellate vessels of PG.

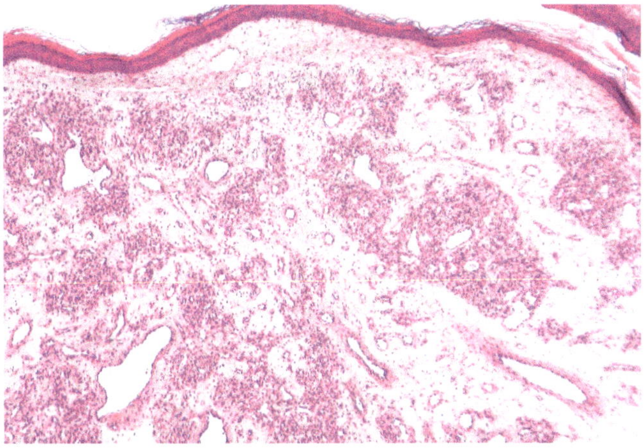

Pyogenic granuloma (lobular capillary hemangioma). With time, the vascular structures show less cellular multilobular arrangements and regular-appearing lumina with larger intralobular thin-walled stellate vessels.

ANSWER 11-11: A.

This is a classic depiction of an **epithelioid hemangioma**, also known as **angiolymphoid hyperplasia with eosinophilia**. The most common sites are the ear, forehead, and scalp. Uncommonly, the trunk, extremities, hands, oral mucosa, and penis may be involved. Disseminated lesions have also been reported. Most lesions are intradermal, but deeper extension into the subcutaneous tissue may occur presenting as a nodule. Peripheral blood eosinophilia is present in a minority of cases. Lesions are usually asymptomatic, but on occasion, there may be tenderness, pulsation, pruritus, or bleeding, either spontaneously or after minor trauma. EH is an entity that has evolved since the 1960s and carried various designations. Moreover, EH had been confused with **Kimura disease**, a condition that differs clinically and histopathologically from EH and is now viewed as a separate entity. With respect to the pathogenesis, whether EH is a reactive vascular proliferation versus a primary benign vascular tumor has not been resolved. HHV-8 has not implicated in the pathogenesis of EH. Microscopically these lesions are composed of mixed nodular lymphohistiocytic infiltrates with scattered eosinophils and numerous vessels of varying diameter lined by plump endothelial cells. These endothelial cells are characteristically enlarged, cuboidal to tombstone in shape, and contain large vesicular nuclei with abundant eosinophilic to amphophilic cytoplasm. Cytoplasmic vacuoles may be present and, when large, may distort the nucleus and protrude into the vascular lumina. These endothelial cells express common endothelial markers (CD31, CD34, von Willebrand factor) and may express simple epithelial keratins such as K19 and K7 focally. Thick-walled vessels with muscular media may be surrounded by or infiltrated by myxoid or mucoid material. Occasional thrombi may be seen, and mitotic activity is generally inconspicuous to absent. Kimura disease lacks the characteristic epithelioid endothelial cell of EH and is usually noted in young Asian males. Large subcutaneous masses typically develop in the parotid and submandibular regions. Commonly, the patient has associated manifestations, such as lymphadenopathy, blood eosinophilia, and increased serum levels of immunoglobulin (IgE). Distinctive histologic features of Kimura disease include a florid lymphocytic infiltrate with prominent lymphoid follicles, germinal center vascularization, germinal center necrosis, sclerosis, and marked eosinophilia with or without eosinophil abscess formation. Kimura disease is considered to be the result of an immunologic reaction of an allergic or autoimmune nature. **Juvenile temporal arteritis** recently has been speculated to be an accessory lesion of Kimura disease. **Epithelioid hemangioendothelioma (EHE)** is an angiocentric tumor often suggesting metastatic carcinoma that may also be mistaken for EH. Vascular differentiation in EHE is more primitive than that seen in EH and occurs primarily at the cellular level with the formation of vacuoles and most importantly intracellular lumina ("**blister cells**"). These lesions are often desmoplastic, relatively noninflammatory, and frequently associated with a chondromyxoid matrix. EHE is associated with a novel t(1;3) translocation (*WWTR1*-CAMTA1 fusion gene), which is not present in EH or angiosarcoma.

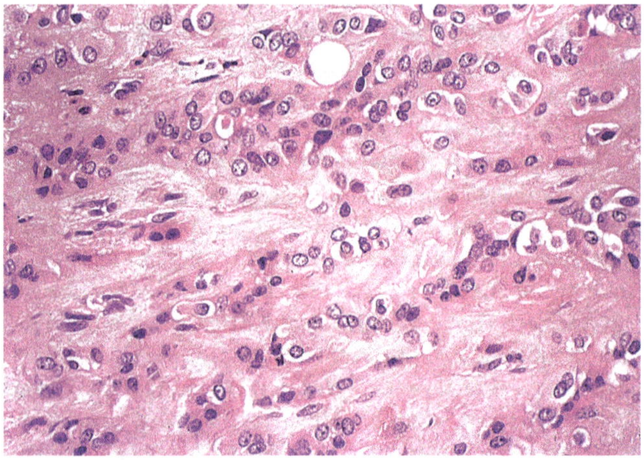

Epithelioid hemangioendothelioma. Cords of epithelioid cells in a fibrous stroma. Scattered lumen-like structures are present that eccentrically displace the nucleus ("blister cells"). Note the similarities to an infiltrative carcinoma.

Compared with EH, **epithelioid angiosarcoma** generally has conspicuous cytologic atypia, frequent mitotic figures, and piling up of cells and lacks the inflammatory infiltrate of EH, although rare angiosarcomas may display substantial infiltrates. Solid areas of EH may resemble epithelioid angiosarcoma and even more so EHE. However, epithelioid angiosarcoma is generally a highly malignant-appearing tumor that is more apt to be mistaken for poorly differentiated carcinoma than a lesion of EH. Both EHE and epithelioid angiosarcoma may also express cytokeratins in addition to vascular markers.

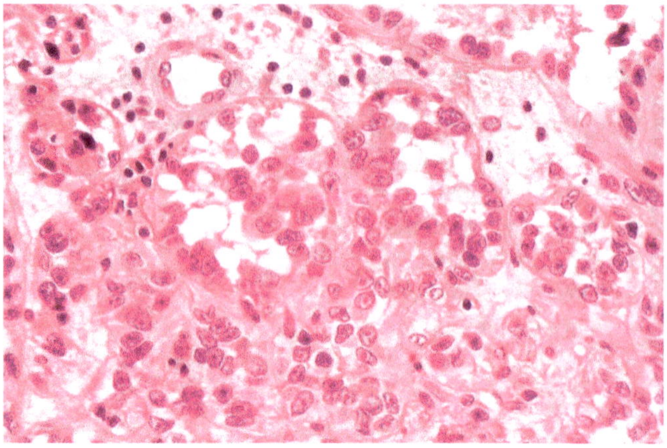

Epithelioid angiosarcoma. Large atypical epithelioid endothelial cells protrude into vascular spaces.

Hobnail hemangioma (aka **targetoid hemosiderotic hemangioma**) is a benign vascular lesion that typically presents on the extremities as a raised violaceous plaque. Microscopically anastomotic vessels lined by slightly crowded plump endothelial cells that protrude into the lumen characterize the lesion. Nucleoli and mitoses are sparse or absent.

ANSWER 11-12: B.

All of the answer choices are characterized by lobular vascular proliferations. **Eruptive cherry angiomas** have been reported in association with solid organ transplantation, chronic graft versus host disease, primary biliary cirrhosis, and exposure to various chemical compounds, including cyclosporine, 2-butoxyethanol (glycol ether solvent), bromides, sulfur mustard gas, and nitrogen mustard. **Cherry angioma** (aka **senile hemangioma**) is the most common adult vascular tumor and most commonly presents on the trunk or extremities and increase in number with age (Table 11-12A). Cherry angiomas are usually raised, dome-shaped lesions that exhibit an epidermal collarette. They manifest fairly well-defined lobules composed of thin-walled dilated vascular channels that are largely confined to the papillary dermis. The vascular channels in general are capillary to venular. The vascular lobules are separated by fibrous septa that vary in thickness depending on the age of the lesion. The entities to be considered in the differential diagnosis of cherry hemangioma include **pyogenic granuloma (PG)** (Choice A) and **bacillary angiomatosis (BA)** because of the lobular architecture and epidermal collarets. PG contains a fibromyxoid matrix and scattered neutrophils. Additionally, the vessels of PG may have more of an elongated slit-like appearance. Cherry angioma does not show the endothelial proliferation noted in PG or the inflammatory infiltrates of neutrophils, granular debris, and epithelioid endothelium observed in BA. A Warthin-Starry stain will highlight clumps of organisms in BA. Clinically, pyogenic granuloma is a rapidly growing polypoid tumor that is ulcerated in most cases. These tumors eventually regress completely over time.

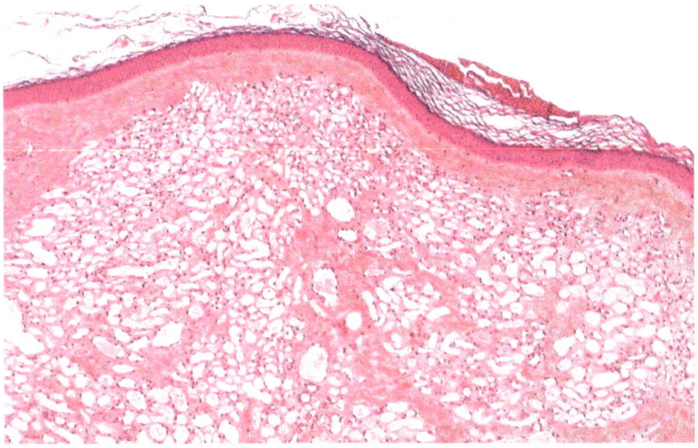

Cherry hemangioma. The histology consists of numerous lobules of moderately dilated capillaries lined by flattened endothelial cells. The stroma is edematous with homogenization of collagen.

Choice C represents **papillary hemangioma (PH),** which is a recently described vascular tumor of the head and neck area. The lesion presents as a bluish papule of 3 to 20 mm in diameter. The ages of patients have ranged from 2 to 77 years, but the majority of cases have been older than age 55 years. Only one patient among the 11 reported cases manifested lesional recurrence 10 years after diagnosis. Microscopically, all reported lesions have been remarkably similar to **noninvoluting congenital hemangioma (NICH)** as evidenced by papillary architecture and protrusion of capillary lobules into large, thin-walled vessels with prominent lumina. The papillae exhibit a fibrous core that contains bland capillaries. Endothelial cells containing intracytoplasmic eosinophilic PAS-positive hyaline globules line the outer surfaces of the aforementioned capillaries. These hyaline globules contain **α_1-antitrypsin** and **lambda immunoglobulin light chains**. Although the vascular proliferation is arranged in a lobular configuration, the vessels are not round but elongated with papillary architecture. One case reported as a glomeruloid hemangioma, unassociated with POEMS syndrome, has been reclassified as PH. Another closely related variant previously reported as **endovascular papillary angioendothelioma** (Dabska tumor) of the lip shows some resemblance to PH, but intracellular hyaline globules were not evident.

Table 11-12A. Cherry Hemangioma

Clinical Features
Prevalent lesion that increases in frequency with age
Often multiple involving trunk and extremities
Well-defined 2-mm papules
Bright red to dusky purple
Histopathologic Features
Dome shaped
Epidermal collarettes
Lobular vascular proliferation
Lobules containing thin-walled vascular channels, variable cellularity
Lobules often separated by fibrous septa
Differential Diagnosis
Pyogenic granuloma
Acral arteriovenous malformation
Venous malformation

Papillary hemangioma (PH) must be differentiated from **noninvoluting congenital hemangioma (NICH), glomeruloid hemangioma (GH), intravascular papillary endothelial hyperplasia (IPEH),** and **endovascular papillary angioendothelioma (papillary intralymphatic angioendothelioma or Dabska tumor)**. PH differs from NICH because it is an acquired lesion. Furthermore, the papillary architecture appears more diffuse and the intracytoplasmic hyaline globules more numerous and localized at the outer surface of the papillae in PH compared with NICH. Contrary to GH, PH reported thus far has never affected patients with POEMS syndrome. The capillary loops of GH are smaller and arranged in a more organoid glomeruloid fashion. IPEH is characterized by thin, elongated papillae demonstrating fibrin in the early stage of development and in later stages shows acellular hyaline collagen. Bland endothelial cells that do not contain hyaline globules line these papillae. In endovascular papillary angioendothelioma (Dabska tumor), the papillations are lined by columnar-appearing endothelial cells.

Choice D is an example of **acroangiodermatitis (AAD)**, which is an infrequent reactive vasoproliferative condition most commonly associated with venous stasis (Table 11-12B). First described by Mali in 1965, the importance of AAD relates to its striking resemblance to **Kaposi sarcoma (KS)**, hence the synonym pseudo-KS. The clinical lesions of acroangiodermatitis are scaly, violaceous plaques, papules, and nodules. In chronic venous insufficiency of the lower extremities, the lesions are most numerous over the extensor surfaces of the toes and foot. They tend to spare areas of the foot where direct pressure, either extrinsic or intrinsic, is applied. Areas of sparing include points where adjacent digits contact each other or a shoe. Lesions may also occur on the lateral aspect of the ankle and anterior lower leg. Surrounding tissues are edematous and show changes of stasis dermatitis. AAD arising in the setting of **arteriovenous malformations (AVM)** presents a similar clinical picture and is usually limited to the extremity involved by the AVM. Microscopically, reactive epidermal hyperplasia and compact hyperkeratosis are frequent features of AAD. The most striking histologic changes involve the papillary and superficial to mid-reticular dermis. A proliferation of small blood vessels with dilated, round lumina are distributed throughout the dermis in a loose, vaguely lobular

Table 11-12B. Acroangiodermatitis

Clinical Features
- Chronic venous insufficiency
- Venous stasis
- Extremity with arteriovenous malformation or hemodialysis shunt
- Middle age or older
- Younger distribution with congenital or acquired arteriovenous causes
- Scaly, violaceous papules, plaques, and nodules
- Distal lower extremities, particularly extensor foot and toes
- Accompanying stasis dermatitis

Histopathologic Features
- Epidermal acanthosis and compact hyperkeratosis
- Proliferation of small blood vessels with dilated, round lumina
- Upper half of the dermis
- Dermal edema and variable fibrosis
- Extravasated erythrocytes and hemosiderin, especially perivascular
- Inconspicuous mononuclear inflammatory infiltrate

Differential Diagnosis
- Kaposi sarcoma
- Pyogenic granuloma, dermal type

arrangement. The vessels tend to be relatively uniform in size and regular in contour. The endothelial cells are plump and one cell layer in thickness. The cytologic features are bland. The neovascular proliferation is superimposed on a background of dermal edema, fibrosis, erythrocyte extravasation, and hemosiderin deposition. Extravasated erythrocytes and sometimes exuberant hemosiderin deposits are most commonly distributed in superficial perivascular patterns.

The microscopic features of **AAD** are distinctly different from those of **Kaposi sarcoma**. The vessels of AAD are arranged in a lobular pattern; have round, regular contours; are centered in the papillary dermis; and show no tendency to localize about preexisting dermal structures. KS, in contrast, shows a haphazard arrangement of slit-like vascular spaces disposed about dermal structures. The inflammatory infiltrate in KS is more pronounced than that of AAD and contains greater numbers of plasma cells. Also, the lobular pattern of vascular proliferation may be quite pronounced and may vaguely mimic the vascular proliferation of dermal **pyogenic granuloma** or **cherry hemangioma**. The microvessels of PG are closely organized unlike to spaced microvessels of AAD. Cherry hemangioma lacks the extensive dermal fibrosis and hemosiderin of AAD. Additionally, the round vessels of cherry hemangioma are larger and more dilated.

ANSWER 11-13: D.

All of the answer choices consist of slit-like vascular proliferations characterized by varying degrees of infiltration through the dermal collagen. This is classic presentation for **targetoid hemosiderotic hemangioma** (**THH**), also known as **hobnail hemangioma** (Table 11-13A). These vascular proliferations are benign and possibly reactive in nature. Late lesions may show only a purple-brown, slightly elevated papule, likely secondary to trauma or thrombosis and may not be a constant feature. Hobnail hemangioma occurs in diverse sites, favoring the proximal upper and lower extremities (particularly the thigh) and the trunk. Overall, on low-power magnification, it gives a stratified or biphasic appearance with superficial ectatic vessels containing intraluminal papillary projections lined by epithelioid "hobnail" endothelial cells, and angulated, often collapsed, inconspicuous, anastomosing, thin-walled vessels criss-crossing the deep dermis. These plump endothelial cells may occasionally pile up and even obliterate vascular lumina.

Table 11-13A. Targetoid Hemosiderotic Hemangioma

Clinical Features
- Wide age distribution; childhood to elderly
- Diverse sites
- Annular target-like lesion: central violaceous papule surrounded by a pale rim and a more peripheral expanding ecchymotic ring

Histopathologic Features
- Early Lesions
  - Widely dilated, irregular, thin-walled vascular lumina in the superficial dermis
  - Endothelial cells flat to epithelioid
  - Intraluminal papillary projections usually lined by a single layer of epithelioid endothelial cells
  - Narrower, more angulated and inconspicuous vessels "dissecting" collagen bundles of the deeper reticular dermis
  - Dermal edema, red blood cell extravasation, hemosiderin, little lymphocytic inflammation
- Later lesions
  - Collapsed lumina
  - Extravascular spindle cells
  - Narrow, angulated, thin-walled vessels crisscross the dermis in "dissection" of collagen
- Variable hemosiderin deposition
- Expression of D2-40 in endothelial cells

Differential Diagnosis
- Early Kaposi sarcoma
- Lymphangioma-like Kaposi sarcoma
- Acquired progressive lymphangioma
- Retiform hemangioendothelioma

The deep vessels tend to be oriented around adnexal structures such as eccrine coils. Other features include dermal edema, often-intense red blood cell extravasation, hemosiderin deposition, and an inconspicuous to mild inflammatory infiltrate. Intraluminal fibrin thrombi may be present. Spindle cells often appear in close approximation to the vascular proliferation. Immunohistochemically, the endothelial cells express CD31 and D2-40 but react variably with CD34, von Willebrand factor, *Ulex europaeus* lectin 1, and VEGFR-3. They do not express HHV-8, excluding **Kaposi sarcoma** from the differential diagnosis. One study has shown continuity in vessels lined by endothelial cells of blood and lymphatic phenotypes, suggesting the existence of microshunts between blood and lymphatic vessels. THH is benign, may be removed by local excision or excisional biopsy, and typically does not recur.

In regard to the differential diagnosis, **THH** appears histopathologically as an atypical vascular proliferation with resemblance to **acquired progressive lymphangioma (APL), patch-stage Kaposi sarcoma, retiform hemangioendothelioma,** and **lymphangiosarcoma**. The clinical setting is helpful in differentiating these lesions because THH occurs as a solitary small lesion in healthy individuals.

Acquired progressive lymphangioma (APL) is clinically distinct from THH and occurs as well-demarcated dermal plaques that are larger in size than THH and often reach considerable proportions (Table 11-13B). APL is an entity that has undergone a nosologic evolution over three decades. We prefer the term **APL** because of the antinomy between benign and lymphangioendothelioma. As with hemangioendothelioma, **lymphangioendothelioma** should designate lesions with borderline or low-grade malignant status. APL is a rare entity that may offer diagnostic difficulty with **low-grade angiosarcoma** and the **lymphangioma-like form of KS**. Sites of involvement are diverse and include the head, neck, oral mucosa, trunk, breast, buttock, shoulder, forearm, thigh, and foot. Multiple sites of involvement, both synchronous and asynchronous, are documented. APL may occur after trauma to the affected area, including a report of APL arising in a traumatized birthmark, as well as at the site of a tick bite. Clinical lesions are well-demarcated dermal plaques that range in color from dull pink to dusky to violaceous. The lesion borders are usually clearly delineated from the surrounding uninvolved skin. Most lesions tend to pursue a relatively static clinical course, slowly increasing in size over a period of years. There are no reports of malignant transformation. Clinical recurrence after excision has not been reported. Microscopically, the lesions are dermal and may occasionally show full-thickness dermal involvement and may involve superficial subcutaneous tissue. The unifying histologic features identified in all cases are jagged, irregularly shaped vascular channels distributed between dermal collagen bundles, similar to THH. The thin-walled vessels tend to be arranged in horizontal array, and the endothelial lining is one cell layer in thickness. The cytologic features tend to be bland, although occasional plump or hyperchromatic endothelial cells are observed. Hobnail cytomorphology, when present in APL, is only focal and not as prominent a feature as that observed in the typically smaller THH. Pronounced cytologic atypia is not a feature of APL. Mitotic activity is absent. The most specific finding is that the vascular spaces are typically empty but may contain a faintly eosinophilic, proteinaceous material, consistent with lymphatic fluid. Immunohistochemical studies have been inconsistent, and not useful in distinguishing APL from other benign and malignant vascular proliferations. The HHV-8 genome has not been found in the single case of APL studied with PCR.

Table 11-13B. Acquired Progressive Lymphangioma

Clinical Features
Men and women equally affected
Childhood to elderly
Diverse sites
Well-demarcated dermal plaques, dull pink to violaceous
Variable size (3-30 cm)
Slow enlargement over time
Histopathologic Features
Variable degree of dermal involvement, favoring the upper half
Thin-walled, irregular vascular channels "dissecting" collagen
Bland endothelial cells
Scant or absent mononuclear inflammatory infiltrate
Lack of plasma cells, extravasated erythrocytes, and hemosiderin
Differential Diagnosis
Low-grade angiosarcoma
Lymphangioma-like Kaposi sarcoma
Lymphatic malformation

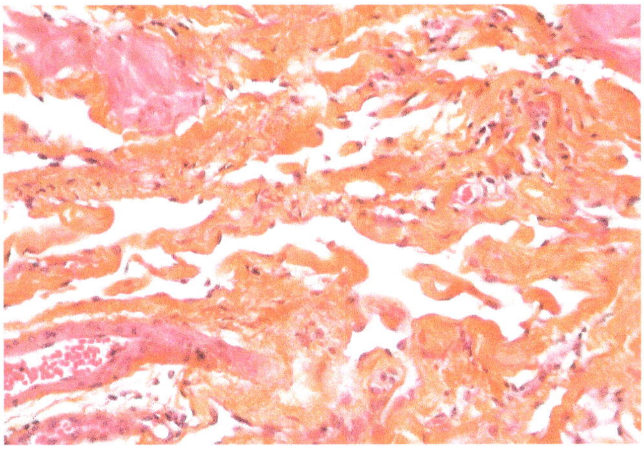

Acquired progressive lymphangioma (benign lymphangioendothelioma). Thin-walled, infiltrative, staghorn-shaped vessels devoid of red blood cells.

Four variants of **Kaposi sarcoma** have been characterized (Table 11-13C). The **classic form** is a rare indolent disease affecting predominantly elderly men of Mediterranean, Eastern European, and Jewish origins. The **endemic form** affects both children and adults from Central Africa and is often aggressive with disseminated disease. The **iatrogenic form** is described in transplant recipients treated with immunosuppressive drugs. The final **epidemic form** is associated with HIV-1 infection, affects predominantly homosexual men, and often progresses rapidly with disseminated or visceral involvement (or both). Outside of Africa, KS is seen classically in elderly individuals and secondary to AIDS. Lesions of KS are typically multiple and of variable size.

Table 11-13C. Kaposi Sarcoma

Clinical Features
Clinical forms of Kaposi sarcoma
Classic (European)
Predominantly men, older than age 50 years
Ashkenazi Jews; Mediterranean descent
Distal lower extremities
Relatively indolent clinical course
African (endemic)
Males, younger age distribution
Nodular, florid, infiltrative, lymphadenopathic subgroups
AIDS-associated (epidemic)
Homosexual men more than other risk groups
Upper half of the body
Early lesions, small, pink to light purple
Disseminated disease
Immunosuppression
Organ transplant recipients
Disseminated disease
Rare variants
Stewart-Treves–like syndrome developing years after ipsilateral radical mastectomy
Lymphangioma-like variant with bulla-like clinical appearance
Histopathologic Features
Patch stages
Inconspicuous, irregular, angulated blood vessels
Upper to entire reticular dermis
Promontory sign
Lymphocytic perivascular infiltrate, plasma cells
Plaque stage
Vessels fill the dermis and involve the superficial subcutis
Obvious spindle cells
Slit-like spaces containing erythrocytes
Extravasated erythrocytes, hemosiderin, apoptotic endothelial cells, hyaline globules
Nodular (or tumor) stage
Extensive spindle cell infiltrate in fascicles and sheets
Numerous slit-like spaces in sieve-like pattern, containing erythrocytes
Mitotic figures, variable numbers
All stages
Expression of lymphatic endothelial markers, HHV-8 (LANA-1)

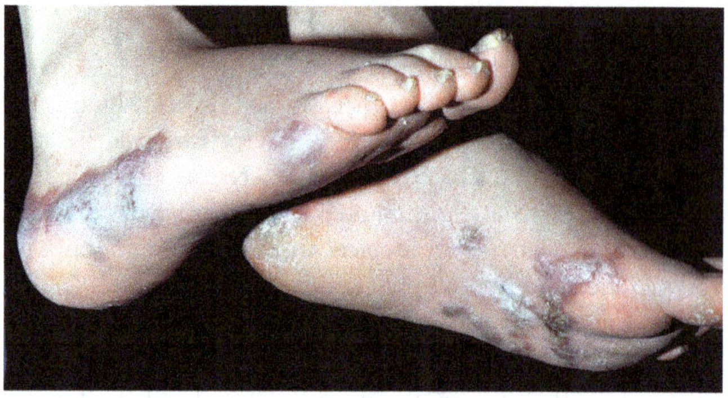

Classic Kaposi sarcoma of the feet. Brownish to blue nodules and plaques, partially hyperkeratotic on the soles and lateral aspects of the feet. This is a typical localization of early classic KS. (Reproduced, with permission, from Wolff K, Johnson RA, Saavedra AP. *Fitzpatrick's Color Atlas and Synopsis of Clinical Dermatology*. 7th ed. New York, NY: McGraw-Hill Education; 2013.)

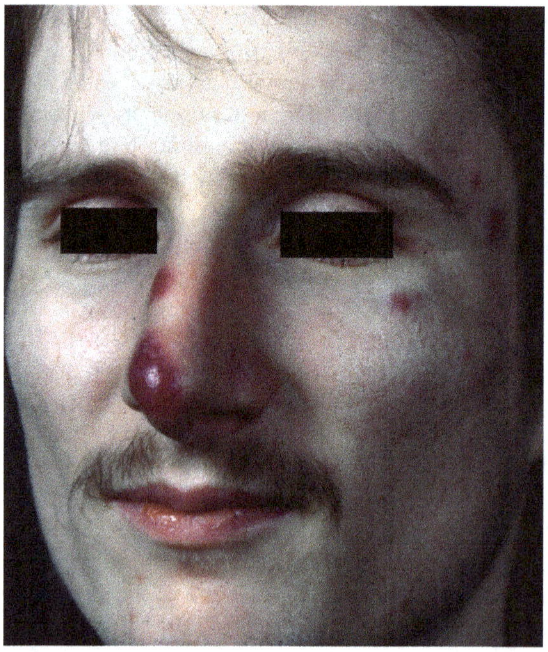

HIV/AIDS-associated Kaposi sarcoma. Bruise-like purplish macules and nodules are present in the face of this 25-year-old male homosexual with AIDS. Early involvement of the face is typical for HIV/AIDS-associated KS. (Reproduced, with permission, from Wolff K, Johnson RA, Saavedra AP. *Fitzpatrick's Color Atlas and Synopsis of Clinical Dermatology*. 7th ed. New York, NY: McGraw-Hill Education; 2013.)

It is now established, by in situ hybridization and immunohistochemistry, that **HHV-8** (or **KS-associated herpesvirus**) is present in the spindle cells and a subset of endothelial cells, at all stages and in all forms of the disease. This observation strongly indicates a role for this agent in the pathogenesis of KS. The histopathologies of cutaneous lesions associated with the various clinical forms of KS are essentially identical and are described together in accordance with their stage at presentation. The stages of KS include patch, plaque, and nodular. Although only patch stage KS shares histopathological features with THH (hobnail hemangioma), the histopathology of plaque and tumor stage KS are discussed below.

In **patch-stage KS**, the earliest features are inconspicuous, and on initial review, they may often be considered nondiagnostic or inflammatory. The earliest histologic manifestations essential for the recognition of KS include subtle microvascular alterations largely confined to the superficial half of or the entire reticular dermis. These critical findings are a proliferation of small, irregular, or jagged microvessels about normal or ectatic dermal vascular channels and adnexal structures. These newly formed vessels may protrude into a vascular lumen or surround and partially isolate normal dermal structures, a feature referred to as the **promontory sign**. In some lesions, these microvessels aggregate into clusters that resemble small hemangiomas. The endothelium may be inconspicuous or plump, a single layer in thickness, and shows little or no atypia or mitotic activity. Irregular, branching, thin-walled bland vascular channels may be seen dissecting between collagen bundles. These neovascular structures tend to be contiguous with preexisting dermal blood vessels. In well-developed patch-stage lesions, KS involves the entire dermis. Numerous extravasated red blood cells and hemosiderin pigment are typically present in the interstitial spaces.

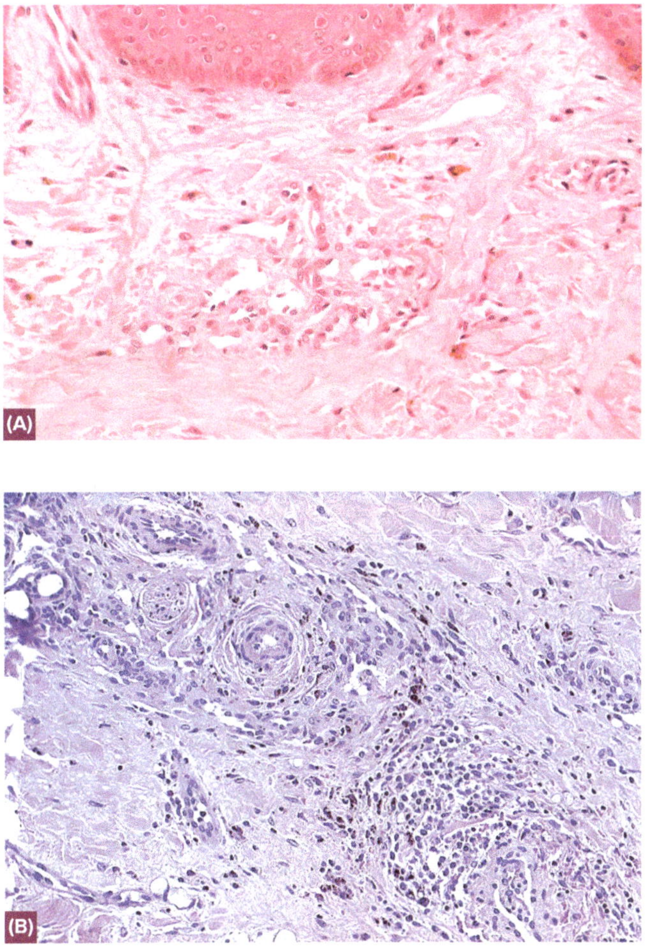

Kaposi sarcoma, patch stage. (A) This lesion exhibits irregular vascular channels and hemosiderin deposits. **(B)** Newly formed vessels may protrude into a vascular lumen or surround and partially isolate normal dermal structures, a feature referred to as the promontory sign. The angulated thin-walled lumina are the clue for the diagnosis.

Plaque-stage KS shows further progression of the neoplastic process with diffuse and more densely cellular involvement of the entire dermis and superficial subcutaneous tissue. The most characteristic feature of this stage is a significant spindle cell component. These relatively bland spindle cells are dispersed between dermal collagen bundles and around preexisting dermal vessels. Between these spindle cells, irregular clefts or slit-like spaces are formed, creating new, angulated vascular channels that contain small numbers of erythrocytes. The disposition of erythrocytes with a square box–like morphology in a linear single-file pattern between these spindle cells is highly characteristic of KS and has been termed "vascular slits." Hemosiderin deposits and **hyaline globules** are more prominent than in patch-stage KS. The vasoproliferative changes of the patch stage persist at the periphery of plaques. The predominantly lymphocytic, perivascular inflammatory infiltrate persists along with its component of plasma cells.

Nodular KS shows an even more pronounced proliferation of spindle cells into intersecting fascicles and sheets. Amid the spindle cell proliferation, slit-like vascular spaces containing erythrocytes are conspicuous. The spindle cells show a degree of cytologic atypia that generally ranges from mild to moderate. Frank anaplasia of the spindle cell component is distinctly uncommon and is more frequently described in the endemic African form of KS. Apoptotic cells, hyaline globules, and hemosiderin deposition are all readily visible. Mitotic figures vary in number but may be frequent. The dermal lymphoplasmacytic inflammatory infiltrate persists, and at the periphery of the nodules, ectatic blood vessels and lymphatics are generally noted.

Lymphangiomatous or **lymphangioma-like variants of KS** have been reported as both a focal and predominant clinicopathologic pattern in otherwise typical KS. These lesions may also closely mimic THH. The process usually involves the entire dermis and often extends into the superficial subcutaneous tissue. Angulated, irregular, narrow to ectatic, thin-walled vascular channels lined by a single layer of flattened, bland endothelium interconnect and dissect collagen bundles. The majority of the vascular spaces lack red blood

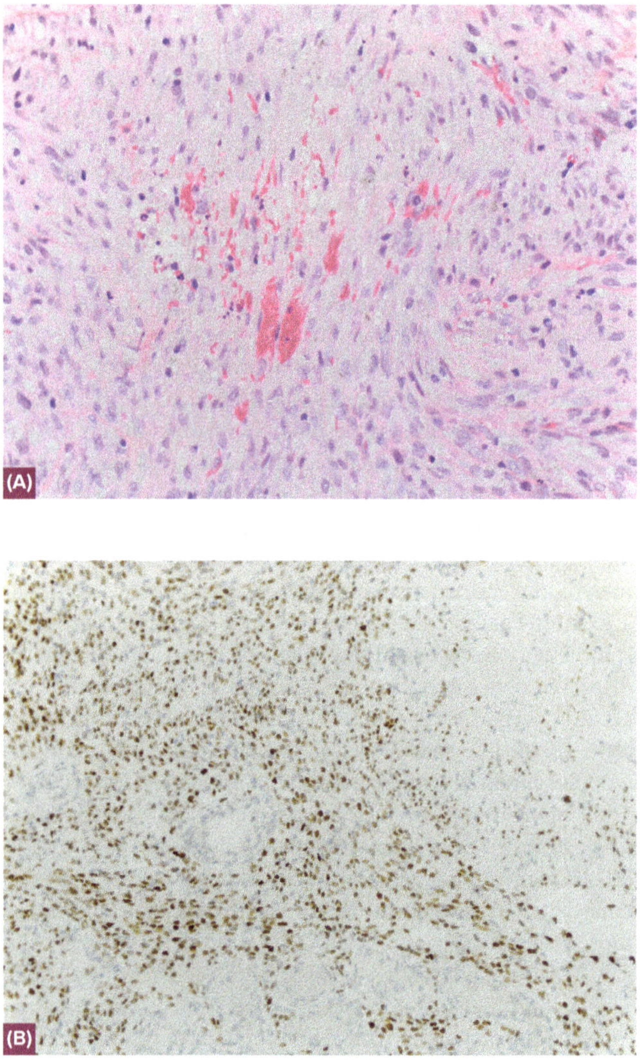

Kaposi sarcoma, tumor stage. (A) The compact spindle cell proliferation mimics other soft tissue sarcomas. Note the extensive red blood cell extravasation. **(B)** There is strong and diffuse nuclear immunostaining for HHV8 (LANA).

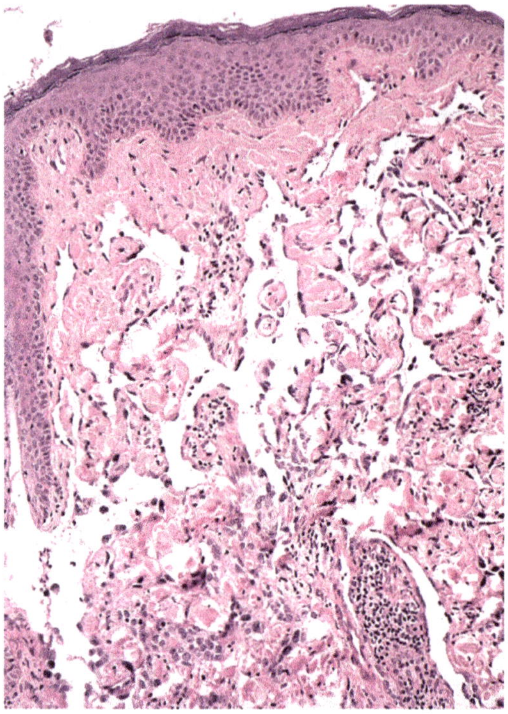

Kaposi sarcoma, lymphangiomatous variant. Highly irregular dilated vascular spaces dissect collagen and surround other blood vessels.

cells. Features typical of KS, such as a significant inflammatory infiltrate, extravasated erythrocytes, hemosiderin, and hyaline globules, have not been reported. Occasional cases show sparse numbers of spindle cells in close association with the vascular elements, but these cells are never a prominent feature.

THH shares histologic features with patches of **KS**. These similarities include angulated vascular lumina dissecting collagen bundles; erythrocyte extravasation; hemosiderin deposition; and, in late lesions, the presence of spindle cells. Differential features are present, however, and in particular, whereas the scanning magnification appearance of THH shows stratification, and KS tends to be "bottom heavy." The papillary intraluminal projections and epithelioid endothelial cells of early lesions of THH are not features of KS. THH typically lacks plasma cells and is more apt to show significant erythrocyte extravasation and hemosiderin. Apoptotic endothelial cells may be seen in early KS but do not seem to be a feature of THH. Despite all of these features, the overlap in morphologic features of THH and KS may be so great that clinicopathologic correlation is necessary to separate the lesions. Immunohistochemistry may be of help because, contrary to KS, HHV-8 is not demonstrated in THH.

Retiform Hemangioendothelioma (RH) is a recently described vascular tumor that is considered a well-differentiated and **low-grade angiosarcoma** usually presenting on the extremities of young adults. Although this tumor is prone to recurrences, metastatic spread appears to be very uncommon. Only one case with lymph node metastasis has been reported, and no deaths have occurred. Microscopically, there is a continuum between THH and RH. RH tumor has a predominantly subcutaneous location and is composed of ill-defined, arborizing, thin-walled vessels lined by a monotonous population of small protuberant hobnail endothelial cells. The vascular architecture is reminiscent of rete testis. Frequently, the tumor is surrounded by lymphocytic infiltrate, and in some instances, lymphocytes are present within the lumina of the neoplastic vessels. Solid areas exhibiting epithelioid or spindled endothelial cells may be present. THH may be confused with RH. In contrast to RH, THH is a more circumscribed superficial lesion. Also, it lacks the retiform architecture of RH.

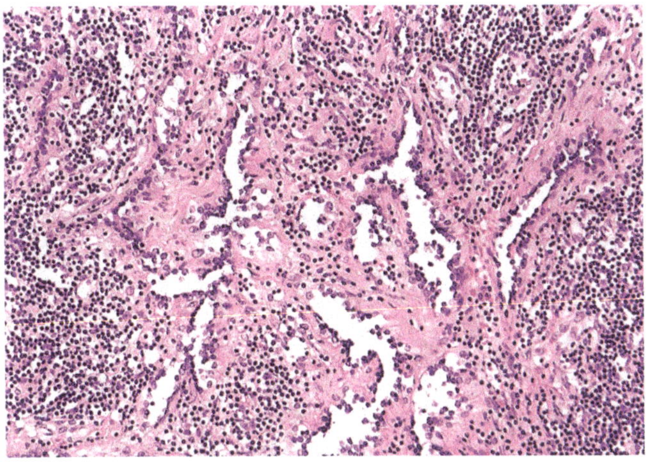

Retiform hemangioendothelioma. Branching and arborizing blood vessels are reminiscent of rete testis. Note the piling up of plump "hobnail" endothelial cells.

ANSWER 11-14: A.

Microvenular hemangiomas (MVH) have a characteristic histologic appearance of small, irregularly branching, dermal blood vessels, often with the appearance of collapsed venules (Table 11-14A). The vessels impart an infiltrative growth pattern throughout the dermis with a desmoplastic stromal response. Inflammation, dermal hemorrhage, and hemosiderin are scant or absent. The endothelial cells may be plump but lack cytologic atypia. A very similar, if not identical, appearing angioma arising in young women under the hormonal influence of pregnancy or hormonal contraceptives has been referred to as **microcapillary hemangioma** (MCH). MVHs present as solitary, small, red to purple plaques or nodules of the extremities of middle-aged patients. The natural history is usually brief, as most lesions involute during a

Table 11-14A. Microvenular Hemangioma

Clinical Features
Young to middle-aged adults
Extremities most common site
Small, purple to red plaques or nodules
Histopathologic Features
Irregular branching, small blood vessels
Inconspicuous lumina
Variable degree of desmoplasia
Scant or absent inflammatory infiltrate
Differential Diagnosis
Stasis change
Scar
Early Kaposi sarcoma
Sclerosing hemangioma or dermatofibroma

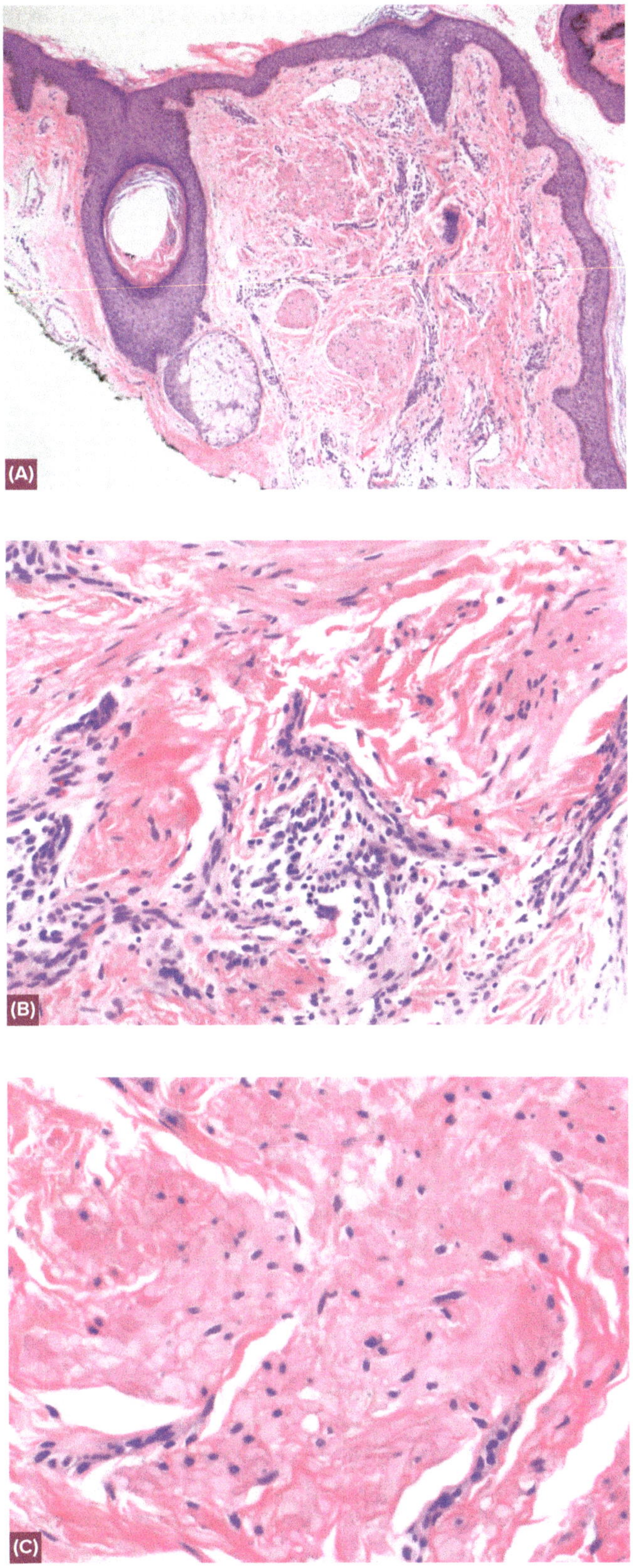

Microvenular hemangioma. (A) There are numerous irregularly branching, dermal blood vessels scattered throughout the dermis. The vessels have a collapsed appearance. **(B)** The vessels exhibit an infiltrative pattern of growth throughout the dermis. **(C)** Vessels are seen permeating arrector pili muscles.

Table 11-14B. Comparison of Histologic Features in MVH, KS, THH, and PG

	MAJOR CLINICAL FEATURES	IRREGULAR ANASTO-MOSING VASCULAR SPACES	CYTOLOGIC AND IMMUNO-HISTOCHEMICAL FEATURES OF ENDOTHELIAL CELLS	CELLULARITY	INFLAMMATION	HEMOSIDERIN
Microvenular hemangioma	Single, small, purple to red lesions favoring the extremities of young to middle-aged adults	1 +	Normal to plump HHV-8 – (+ in one case)	1-2 +	0 to sparse lymphocytic	0-1 +
Kaposi sarcoma (patch stage)	Usually multiple, pink to purple, broad, flat lesions favoring the lower extremities of elderly men in the classic form; more disseminated in the AIDS-associated form	4 +	Cells lining vessels normal; others spindle-shaped, hyperchromatic with variable atypia HHV-8 +	0-1 +	Sparse perivascular lymphocytes and plasma cells	0-3 +
Targetoid hemosiderotic hemangioma	Single, small, annular, often target-like lesions on the trunk and extremities of young to middle-aged adults	2-3 + with epithelioid fronds in early lesions	Normal to epithelioid HHV-8 –	1-2 +	0 to sparse lymphocytes (and variable but often intense red cell extravasation)	3-4 +
Pyogenic granuloma	Single or multiple, rapidly growing lesions of the skin or mucosal surfaces of individuals of all ages	0-1 +	Normal HHV-8 –	3-4 +	0-4 + Intense acute and chronic inflammation associated with ulcerated lesion	0-1 +

few weeks to months, but some lesions have persisted as long as 4 years. MVH is generally considered benign; however, rare HHV8 positivity introduces early Kaposi sarcoma into the differential diagnosis. Reported associations include **Wiskott-Aldrich syndrome, acute myelogenous leukemia,** and **POEMS syndrome.**

The histopathological differential diagnosis includes **stasis changes**, **reactive angiogenesis in scars**, **early KS**, **targetoid hemosiderotic hemangioma** (THH), and **pyogenic granuloma** (Table 11-14B). With the exception of pyogenic granuloma, these entities classically exhibit red blood cell extravasation, unlike MVH. **Stasis change** is clinically distinct from MVH, typically present on the distal lower extremities of an individual with chronic venous insufficiency. **Immature scars**, in contrast to MVH, show irregularly arranged fibroblastic and vascular proliferations often associated with erythrocyte extravasation, hemosiderin deposition, and an inflammatory infiltrate that may contain a few plasma cells. Early **Kaposi sarcoma** can be excluded by the clinical setting and the absence of angulated, irregular vascular spaces enveloping preexisting dermal blood vessels (promontory sign), plasma cells, hyaline (eosinophilic) globules, and a spindle cell component. **Targetoid hemosiderotic hemangioma** exhibits marked anastomosing of the vascular spaces. The vascular channels are typically dilated compared to the collapsed vessels of MVH. **Pyogenic granuloma** may exhibit anastomosing vessels lined by plump endothelial cells, but is arranged in lobules and surrounded by round small caliber capillaries. They frequently contain numerous neutrophils and a myxoid stroma.

ANSWER 11-15: C.

These tumors are **tufted angiomas (TA),** which are generally considered to be a distinct clinicopathologic entity. However, there are a number of clinical and morphologic observations that suggest that **kaposiform hemangioendothelioma (KHE)** may be a more aggressive form of TA or represents part of the spectrum of a single vascular condition. This is based on their common association with the **Kasabach-Merritt syndrome**, their morphologic overlap or association in the same patient, and the common expression of lymphatic markers (ie, D2-40). KHE is composed of larger, often interconnecting, lobules or sheets of vascular elements commonly with an infiltrative pattern. The spindling of tumor cells is more pronounced and diffuse in KHE, and there is much more extensive D2-40 staining. The relationship between TA and **PG (lobular capillary hemangioma)** has also merited discussion because of morphologic resemblance (ie, lesions reported as dermal PGs have been purported to be TA). TA generally presents as a macule, patch, or plaque of up to several centimeters and lacks ulceration, edema, inflammation, and a collarette, whereas PG presents as a small, easily bleeding papule or nodule with an epidermal collarette and contains numerous intralobular open stellate vessels. The scattered nature and crescentic peripheral vessels of TA tufts are fairly characteristic. Although the progressive nature of TA may invoke consideration of a **low-grade angiosarcoma** or **Kaposi sarcoma**, the clinicopathologic features and particularly the early onset of most cases allow distinction. **Glomeruloid hemangioma** may also be similar to TA, but the systemic manifestations of POEMS (polyneuropathy, organomegaly, endocrinopathy, monoclonal gammopathy, and skin changes) syndrome and the characteristic intracytoplasmic periodic acid-Schiff (PAS)–positive eosinophilic bodies allow distinction.

ANSWER 11-16: C.

This patient is presenting with **Kasabach-Merritt syndrome (KMS)**, characterized by life-threatening profound **thrombocytopenia** and **consumption coagulopathy**. This phenomenon is believed to be associated with the patient's vascular tumor, which in this case is a **kaposiform hemangioendothelioma (KHE)**. These lesions may exhibit locally aggressive behavior and lymph node involvement by contiguous spread. However, no patients have developed distant metastases. These multinodular tumors are composed of nodules or sheets of spindle cells that are connected and surrounded by dense hyalinized fibrous tissue. Such nodules exhibit elongated or crescent-shaped vascular spaces and spindle cells with minimal cytologic atypia. On occasion, rounded vascular lumina lined by attenuated endothelial cells may be observed. Platelet aggregates and fibrin thrombi may be present within vascular lumina, even in cases with normal platelet counts. Among the spindle cell areas, one may encounter fairly discrete aggregates of cytologically bland epithelioid endothelial cells (glomeruloid clusters). The latter cells often contain hemosiderin and **hyaline globules**. Some tumor lobules are thus partitioned into spindle cell areas and round glomeruloid clusters, realizing a "nodules in the nodule" pattern. Well-formed vascular channels are often nested at the periphery of tumor nodules and may also be surrounded by crescentic slit-like vessels. In general, the mitotic rate is low and often less than 3 mitoses per hpf. Inflammatory cell infiltrates containing lymphocytes and plasma cells are usually absent. The spindle cells comprising the tumor are positive for CD34, D2-40, and VEGFR-3 and are generally negative for von Willebrand factor and *Ulex europaeus* lectin. Actin-positive cells are mainly located in the center of the lobules and glomeruloid areas. HHV8 is consistently negative in these tumors. The coagulation disorder associated with these tumors is often of sudden onset and is accompanied by increase in the volume of the vascular tumor, which becomes tense, edematous, and ecchymotic or purpuric. With therapeutic intervention to restore the platelet levels, these vascular lesions often diminish rapidly in size but fail to show complete tumor regression. It has recently been shown that the tumors associated with KMS are almost always KHE or tufted angiomas (TA) rather than infantile hemangiomas (IH) as had previously been suggested.

> **Quick Fact**
>
> **Vascular Tumors Associated with Kasabach-Merritt Syndrome**
>
> - Tufted angioma
> - Kaposiform hemangioendothelioma

The histopathological differential diagnosis includes **Kaposi sarcoma (KS), infantile hemangioma (IH), tufted angioma,** and **spindle cell hemangioma.** In contrast to **KS**, KHE generally affects younger individuals; presents as a deep solitary mass; shows no association with HHV-8, HIV, or immunodeficiency; and is frequently associated with KMS. KHE does not show the diffusely infiltrative and multicentric pattern or the lymphoplasmacytic infiltrates noted in KS. In addition, KHE exhibits epithelioid cell aggregates, a feature not typically observed in KS. KHE differs from **infantile hemangioma** by demonstrating nodules of spindle cells with slit-like vascular channels (resembling KS), frequent hemosiderin deposition, and positive expression of VEGFR-3 and D2-40 but not GLUT-1. **Tufted angioma** is distinguished from KHE by discrete cellular nodules containing typical vascular channels and lacking prominent fascicles of spindle cells. In addition, there is intervening normal dermis between the tumor islands in tufted angioma. **Spindle cell hemangioma (SCH)** has a predilection for the extremities, particularly distally, often involving the hands and feet (Table 11-16A). Typically arising in the dermis or subcutaneous tissue, SCH presents as either solitary or multiple, asymptomatic nodules that gradually increase in size or number over a period of months or years and often eventuate in extensive disease. Clinically, the tumors may be several millimeters to centimeters in diameter and generally appear as small, circumscribed, red to red-brown nodules that on sectioning show variably sized cystic, hemorrhagic spaces. On occasion, a phlebolith may be present and "pop out" from these cavities. More than half of cases of SCH are entirely or partially intravascular, being associated with large vessels and often thick-walled veins. Microscopically, **spindle cell hemangioma** is characterized by a nodular appearance with two distinctive components: (1) thin-walled, "cavernous" blood vessels that are separated by thin fibrous septa and are sometimes filled with organizing thrombi and phleboliths and (2) solid, cellular areas composed predominantly of spindle cells. The proportion of cavernous spaces to areas of spindle cells is variable. The spindle cells may form a network of slit-like spaces or may form short fascicles between the dilated "cavernous" vessels. Small aggregates of plump, epithelioid cells are commonly interspersed among the spindle cells. Isolated or focally numerous intracytoplasmic clear vacuoles are often present, usually in association with the epithelioid areas. On occasion, these vacuolated cells may line vascular spaces. Cytologic atypia and mitotic activity are inconspicuous. These tumors also lack immunohistochemical expression of HHV8.

Table 11-16A. Spindle Cell Hemangioma

Clinical Features
- Men = women
- Any age, often in the third and fourth decades of life
- Favors the extremities, particularly distal
- Solitary or multiple, circumscribed, red to red-brown nodules
- Gradually increase in size or number
- Association with large vessels; many cases entirely or partially intravascular
- Cystic hemorrhagic cavities, occasionally with a phlebolith
- Associations with Maffucci disease, varicose veins, and congenital lymphedema

Histopathologic Features
- Cavernous, thin-walled blood vessels
- Organizing thrombi and phleboliths
- Solid, cellular areas of spindled cells
- Network of slitlike spaces
- Short fascicles
- Plumper, more epithelioid cells, occasionally vacuolated
- Relative lack of cytologic atypia and mitotic activity

Differential Diagnosis
- Kaposi sarcoma
- Nodular venous and malformation

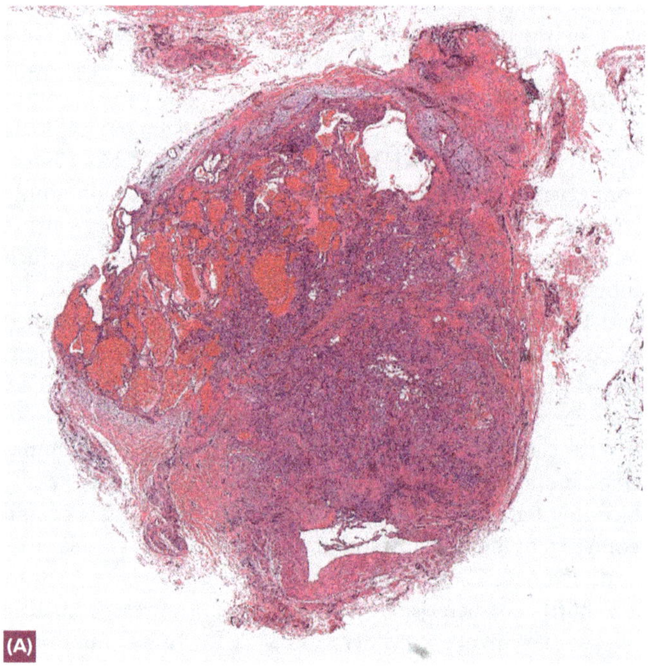
(A)

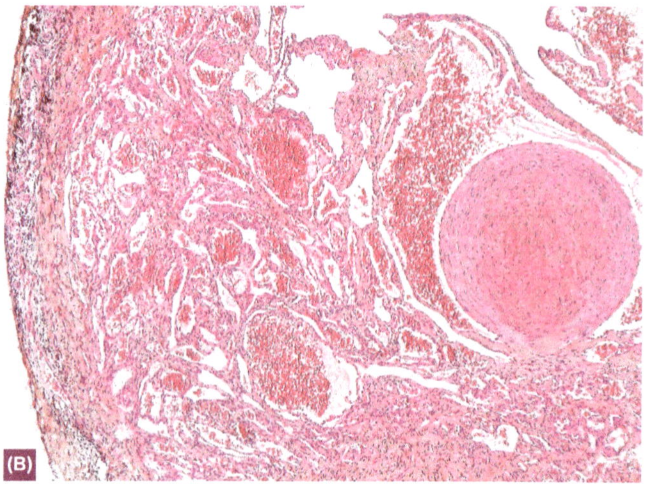
(B)

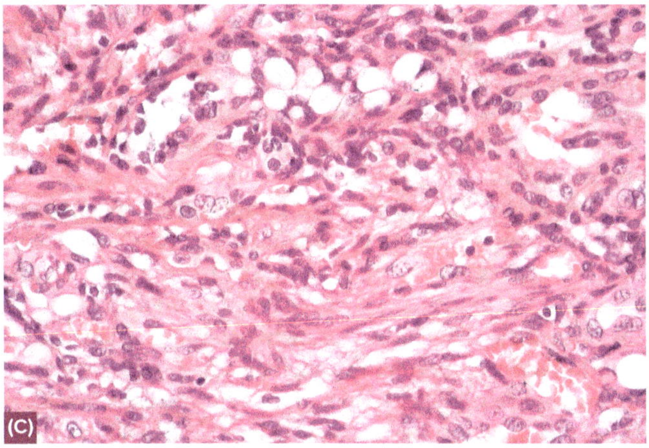

Spindle cell hemangioma. (A) The lesion is a well circumscribed vascular nodule composed of cavernous and highly cellular areas. **(B)** Cavernous vascular channels with an adjacent spindle cell proliferation. Note the large thrombus on the right. **(C)** A solid area composed of spindle cells.

ANSWER 11-17: A.

This is an example of a **spider angioma (arterial spider)** which is a common cutaneous lesion often seen as an incidental finding in healthy children. Some of these lesions persist into adulthood and may occur as acquired manifestations of pregnancy, hepatic cirrhosis, and thyrotoxicosis. The principal finding is an erythematous central punctum often slightly elevated, pulsatile on diascopy, and the source of an array of peripherally radiating fine vessels. The spider angioma typically blanches with pressure and upon release refills rapidly with blood flow originating from its center.

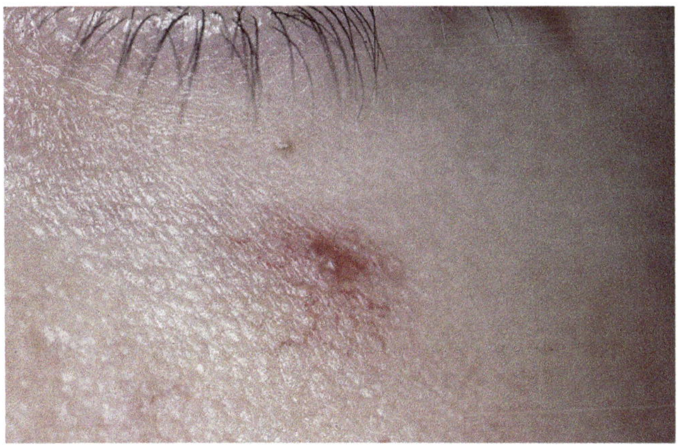

Spider nevus (spider angioma). Two small red papules from which telangiectasias radiate. Upon compression, the lesion blanches completely. (Reproduced, with permission, from Wolff K, Johnson RA, Saavedra AP. *Fitzpatrick's Color Atlas and Synopsis of Clinical Dermatology*. 7th ed. New York, NY: McGraw-Hill Education; 2013.)

Solitary or multiple arterial spiders occur, and they may be numerous, particularly in **chronic liver disease**. The most common sites are the face, particularly the upper infraorbital cheeks, neck, trunk, and hands. Microscopically, there is a central arteriole in the superficial dermis that demonstrates branching into smaller anastomosing venules and capillaries. Rarely, the wall of the central arterial vessel may contain glomus cells. Choices B, C, D, and E describe the clinical presentations of **infantile hemangioma, pyogenic granuloma, port-wine stain/Sturge-Weber syndrome,** and **angiokeratomas of Fordyce,** respectively.

ANSWER 11-18: A.

Papillary intralymphatic angioendothelioma (PILA), also known as **Dabska tumor** or **endovascular papillary angioendothelioma,** is an exceedingly rare vascular tumor of "borderline" or low-grade malignancy that most commonly occurs in children. These tumors classically present as enlarging cutaneous lesions, 4 to 9 cm in diameter, occurring as either a diffuse swelling or an intradermal tumor on the head, neck, and extremities. Local recurrence and lymph node metastasis may occur. **Dabska tumor (PILA)** affects mainly the skin and subcutis, but individual cases have been reported to involve the spleen, skeletal muscle, and bone. PILA may be associated with or develop in lymphatic or venous malformations or lymphedema.

Microscopically, the most characteristic feature of PILA is dilated lymphatic–like vessels containing intraluminal papillary structures. The latter structures are lined by endothelial cells showing minimal to moderate cytologic atypia and little or no mitotic activity. The endothelial cells are cuboidal to columnar with apically situated nuclei manifesting a hobnail or "matchstick-like" appearance. Clear intracytoplasmic vacuoles may be present in tumor cells reminiscent of **epithelioid hemangioma** and **epithelioid hemangioendothelioma**, but the cytoplasm is not eosinophilic or amphophilic. The associated matrix of the papillations may appear eosinophilic and hyalinized or suggest a hyaline globule on transverse sections. The basal part of the cytoplasm of the matchstick-like cells seems to merge imperceptibly with the hyalin core of the papillae. Papillary formations resembling renal glomeruli may also be seen. Tumor cells appear to float free in the lumina around **hyaline globules**, in clumps, or as single cells. The globules have the staining characteristics and ultrastructural appearance of basement membrane and contain collagen type IV. Hemorrhage, cholesterol clefts, and necrosis may be present. Lymphocytes may infiltrate the endothelial cells. The latter association suggests that the endothelial cells of PILA show differentiation toward "high" endothelial cells of post-capillary venules with attraction of lymphocytes mediated by intercellular adhesion molecule 1 (ICAM-1). However, immunohistochemical staining for lymphatic markers (D2-40 and VEGFR-3) and the presence of lymphatics or an LM adjacent to PILA suggest a lymphatic phenotype for PILA.

The histopathological differential diagnosis includes **lymphatic malformation**, **intravascular papillary endothelial hyperplasia (Masson lesion)**, **angiosarcoma**, **glomeruloid hemangioma,** and **retiform hemangioendothelioma.** In general, these lesions all share with PILA varying degrees of papillary endothelial cell proliferation within the vascular lumens. **Lymphatic malformations (LM)** are composed of variably dilated lymphatic vessels usually present either at birth or within the first few years of life. Various clinical types of LM have been reported over the years under a variety of terms, including **lymphangioma simplex**, **lymphangioma circumscriptum**, **cavernous lymphangioma,** and **cystic hygroma**, the last entity perhaps being a macrocystic (widely dilated lymphatic spaces) variant of LM occurring on typical clinical sites. LM typically have a deep component. Generalized LM (**lymphangiomatosis**) is exceedingly rare. Lymphatic malformations may suggest PILA because of cystic spaces on gross sectioning and scanning microscopic examination and lymphocytic infiltrates but fails to show the proliferative endothelial features of PILA. Occasionally, small clusters of free floating endothelial cells may be seen within the vascular spaces in LM.

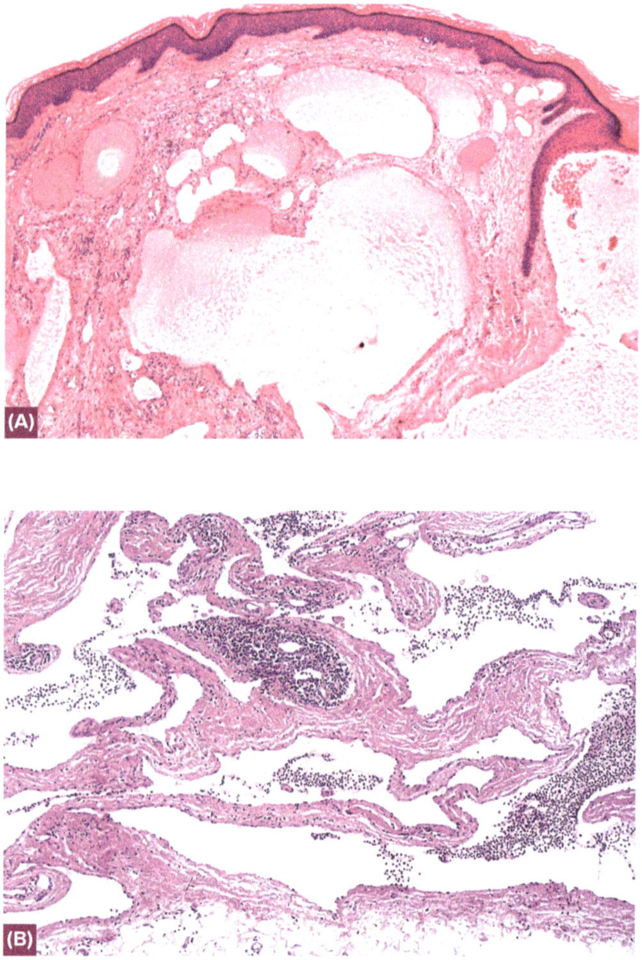

Lymphatic malformation. (A) Lymphangioma circumscriptum. Large lymphatic lumens impinging upon the epidermis. Note that the lumina contain proteinaceous material and lack red blood cells. **(B)** Cavernous lymphatic malformation. Widely dilated lymphatic channels are surrounded by fibrous tissue and lymphocytic infiltrates.

Intravascular papillary endothelial hyperplasia (Masson lesion) occurs in patients of all ages and occurs at diverse sites, but with a predilection for the head and neck and the extremities, particularly the fingers. The typical presentation is that of a slowly enlarging, often tender, blue to red, deep dermal to subcutaneous swelling or mass. Microscopically, these lesions show conspicuous intravascular papillary structures composed of cores of fibrin and lined by endothelial cells that are generally flattened in appearance. However, at times, endothelial cells may be plump with slightly enlarged nuclei, endothelial proliferation may be conspicuous on occasion, and may virtually fill the lumina of some blood vessels. Mitotic figures are generally absent or rare. A characteristic feature in most cases is the presence of an underlying thrombotic matrix that appears to be undergoing organization. The papillary projections result from the endothelialization of fragmented thrombotic material and the ingrowth of anastomosing capillaries. Immunohistochemically, Masson lesion shows a pattern of reactivity similar to that of organizing thrombi. In contrast to PILA, intravascular papillary endothelial hyperplasia (Masson lesion) has a generally flattened endothelial lining (not piled up clusters) and an underlying thrombotic matrix and lacks the lymphocytic infiltrate of PILA.

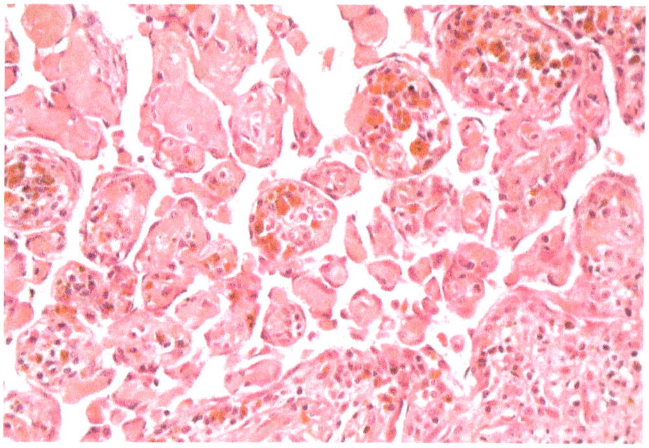

Intravascular papillary endothelial hyperplasia (Masson lesion). Papillary fronds with thin endothelial cells and fibrinous/collagenous cores.

Glomeruloid hemangioma (GH) is a rare vascular lesion that derives its name from its distinctive histologic resemblance to renal glomeruli and occurs in the setting of **POEMS syndrome**, a multisystem disorder consisting of polyneuropathy, organomegaly, endocrinopathy,

M-protein development, and particular skin alterations. Microscopically, these lesions are characterized by ectatic vascular spaces that surround intraluminal conglomerates of blood-filled capillaries. The microvessels within latter glomerulus-like structures are lined by flat endothelial cells. Some GHs may exhibit striking numbers of eosinophilic droplets. Similar cells, which may be immature endothelial cells, are interspersed as stromal cells between the capillary loops. The **eosinophilic globules**, which are PAS positive and diastase resistant, show **polytypic immunoglobulin staining** and presumably represent circulatory-derived immunoglobulins and other proteinaceous material. Mitoses are inconspicuous, numbering less than 1 per 10 hpf. Little, if any, inflammation is present. Compared with the flattened endothelium of GH, PILA demonstrates intraluminal papillations lined by endothelium with a hobnail or matchstick appearance. The vascularity in PILA is more primitive, and the endothelial cells within lumina may appear to float free as single cells or in clumps. The hemorrhage, cholesterol clefts, and necrosis of more cellular lesions of PILA are not usually observed in GH.

Angiosarcoma is extremely rare in childhood; it also differs from PILA by showing conspicuous cytologic atypia with piling up of the endothelial cells, frequent mitotic figures, and dissection of collagen bundles. The endothelial cells of angiosarcoma typically contain prominent nucleoli.

Finally, **retiform hemangioendothelioma (RH)** may share many features with PILA, including hobnail- and matchstick-like endothelial cells and papillations. However, whereas these papillations are only focal in RH, PILA presents with conspicuous papillary tufts and more dilated vascular lumina and typically lacks the arborizing rete testis–like appearance of RH. Nonetheless, the striking morphologic similarities between PILA and RH have suggested that these two lesions may be categorized under the term **hobnail hemangioendothelioma**. It seems, however, that besides differences in patient age and tumor location, some phenotypic differences also exist between these two lesions because PILA constantly express D2-40, which is found only in a minority of RH cases. Further studies are needed, however, to clarify this point because the number of cases studied is small.

ANSWER 11-19: A.

Angiosarcoma is a rare, malignant endothelial tumor that arises in skin, soft tissue, breast, bones, liver, and other viscera (Table 11-19A). **Cutaneous angiosarcoma** is the most common form of angiosarcoma. The prognosis for angiosarcoma is poor. In one series of 72 patients with angiosarcoma of the face and scalp, 36 died within 15 months of presentation. In the skin, angiosarcoma most commonly arises in the scalp and face of elderly individuals, with men affected more frequently than women. Angiosarcoma may also occur in the setting of chronic lymphedema, often developing in a lymphedematous upper extremity as a late sequela of radical mastectomy as described by Stewart and Treves. Other causes of lymphedema (idiopathic, filarial, traumatic), congenital

Table 11-19A. Angiosarcoma

Clinical Features
- Clinical settings for cutaneous angiosarcoma
  - Scalp and face of the elderly—men more affected than women
  - Postmastectomy (Stewart-Treves syndrome) and other causes of chronic lymphedema
  - Postradiation therapy
  - Foreign bodies
  - Arteriovenous fistulas and vascular grafts
  - Metastatic from an occult tumor of heart or aorta
- Ill-defined, red to violaceous patches, plaques, and nodules
- Extension well into adjacent, normal-appearing skin
- Satellite lesions
- Local recurrence and distant metastases

Histopathologic Features
- Angiomatous
  - Individual or widely anastomosing vessels in dissection of collagen bundles
  - Variably atypical endothelial cell lining, one or more layers
  - Mixed inflammation, often with plasma cells
  - Hemosiderin, variable extent
  - Lymphangiomatous-appearing areas, minimal cytologic atypia
- Spindled
  - Bundles of spindled cells
  - Cleft-like spaces containing erythrocytes
  - Syncytium of cells with insignificant blood vessel formation
- Undifferentiated or epithelioid
  - Circumscribed nodules
  - Sheets of epithelioid-appearing cells
  - Intracytoplasmic lumen formation
  - Cytologic atypia
  - Prominent mitotic activity
  - Starry-sky pattern in a subgroup of epithelioid angiosarcoma

Differential Diagnosis
- Kaposi sarcoma
- Lymphangioma-like Kaposi sarcoma
- Hemangiopericytoma
- Epithelioid angiosarcoma
- Poorly differentiated carcinoma
- Malignant melanoma
- Epithelioid hemangioendothelioma
- Composite hemangioendothelioma

hereditary lymphedema (**Milroy disease**), and morbid obesity have also been implicated. Ionizing radiation has been linked to the development of angiosarcoma, with cases developing in the breast after radiation for breast cancer, in the abdominal region after irradiation of pelvic tumors, and on the face after irradiation of a congenital hemangioma. These **radiation-associated angiosarcomas** exhibit **amplifications in the *MYC* gene.** This may be documented via either FISH or immunohistochemistry (nuclear staining). Rarely, angiosarcoma arises in association with foreign material (bullets, shrapnel, retained surgical sponges, gouty tophus) and with arteriovenous fistulae and vascular grafts. Angiosarcoma metastatic to the skin is exceedingly rare but can herald the presence of an occult tumor of an internal site such as the heart and the aorta.

Clinically, angiosarcoma generally appears as ill-defined, asymptomatic, red to violaceous patches, plaques, or nodules. Satellite lesions are frequent. Angiosarcoma frequently presents with multifocal disease, and there is a tendency toward both local recurrence and distant metastasis. The clinical appearance of angiosarcoma varies somewhat according to the degree of histologic differentiation. Histopathologically, more **undifferentiated angiosarcoma** lesions may grow rapidly, with fungating and ulcerative appearances. Undifferentiated angiosarcoma lesions may appear epithelioid and are high-grade neoplasms that generally affect deep, usually intramuscular, soft tissue and rapidly develop metastases. Cutaneous occurrence has been reported, although a few of the described cases had a distinctly better prognosis than other undifferentiated angiosarcoma. Such cutaneous tumors perhaps may fall into the spectrum of **epithelioid hemangioendothelioma.**

Microscopically, cutaneous angiosarcoma extensively infiltrates the dermis, with microscopic involvement extending well beyond the clinically apparent boundaries. The epidermis may be normal, atrophic, or ulcerated. Direct epidermal invasion or involvement of the papillary dermis does not usually occur. Three distinct patterns of proliferation have been described: angiomatous, spindled, and undifferentiated. Individual tumors are composed of varying proportions of each pattern.

In angiomatous areas, vascular spaces that are distinctly individual or widely anastomosing are dispersed between dermal collagen bundles in a dissecting fashion. The endothelium may be one to several cell layers in thickness and shows variable degrees of cytologic atypia. A mixed inflammatory response often containing plasma cells is usual. Hemosiderin deposition is variable. Some lymphedema-associated tumors have a lymphangiomatous appearance with irregular vascular channels devoid of erythrocytes dissecting dermal collagen bundles. The endothelium in these areas may be attenuated and show only subtle cytologic atypia. These foci are usually interspersed with more classic angiosarcomatous areas.

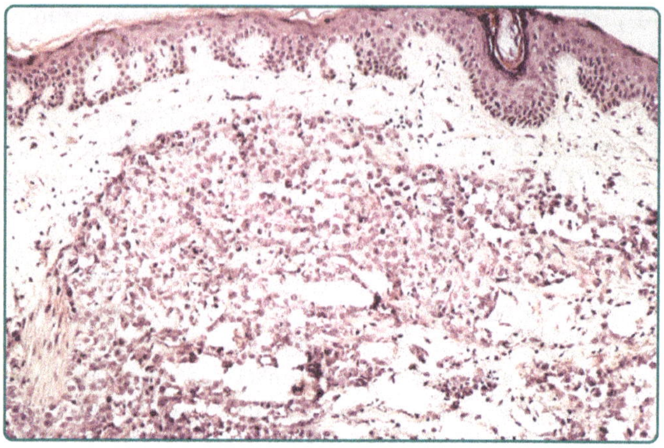

Angiosarcoma, well-differentiated angiomatous type. Irregular, thin-walled anastomosing vascular spaces dissect collagen throughout the dermis. (Reproduced, with permission, from Goldsmith LA, Katz SI, Gilchrest BA, Paller AS, Leffell DJ, Wolff K, eds. *Fitzpatrick's Dermatology in General Medicine*. 8th ed. New York, NY: McGraw-Hill Education; 2012.)

In spindle cell areas, spindled tumor cells are arranged in bundles that traverse the dermis in multiple directions, often enveloping adnexal structures. Cleft-like spaces and cracks containing erythrocytes are formed. The tumor may appear as a syncytium of cells without significant blood vessel formation. Undifferentiated areas are usually encountered as circumscribed nodules within more characteristic areas of angiosarcoma. Solid sheets of "epithelioid" tumor cells with abundant acidophilic cytoplasm and large, atypical nuclei expand the dermis. Lumen formation is usually only evident at the intracytoplasmic level. Intralesional hemorrhage may be prominent; this may not only obscure the diagnosis of angiosarcoma, but with the addition of **endothelial papillary hyperplasia (Masson lesion)**, may appear as an organizing hematoma. A starry-sky histologic pattern has been noted in a subgroup of **epithelioid angiosarcomas.** Recently, risk stratification of cutaneous angiosarcoma has been proposed based on the presence of necrosis, epithelioid features, and patient age older than 70 years. Tumor depth also has been correlated with the risk of local recurrence.

Studies of angiosarcoma have indicated variable blood vascular or lymphatic differentiation; consequently, the histogenesis of angiosarcoma has remained controversial. Ultrastructurally, angiosarcoma generally shows features of endothelial cells, and cases often suggest blood vessel differentiation. Angiosarcoma may react with *Ulex europaeus* lectin 1, vimentin, and laminin (a constituent of basal lamina). CD31 and CD34 may react weakly and favor areas with greater vascular differentiation. Markers of lymphatic endothelial cells (VEGFR-3, Podoplanin/D2-40, LYVE-1) are expressed in a subset of angiosarcoma, representing approximately half of the cases. Furthermore, the immunohistochemical pattern of angiosarcoma may vary within tumors, suggesting mixed differentiation of both blood vascular and lymphatic endothelium. Further clarification of the histogenesis must await the development of additional endothelial markers or progress in molecular biology. Tumors with extensive epithelioid cytomorphology (**epithelioid angiosarcoma**) may express cytokeratin.

In regard to the differential diagnosis, **atypical vascular lesions (AVL) associated with prior radiation exposure** may closely mimic well-differentiated angiomatous angiosarcomas. While these tumors are not considered malignant, overt angiosarcomas have been documented to arise within the vicinity of these lesions. Therefore, if feasible, it is recommended to completely excise these tumors. Unlike radiation-associated angiosarcomas, these tumors lack *MYC* amplification. The typical clinical presentation of AVL ranges from small erythematous/violaceous papules or nodules to large plaques with discoloration. Tumors may measure 0.1 to 20 cm; however, average 0.5 cm in diameter. Unlike radiation-associated angiosarcomas, which typically arise 6 years after exposure, AVLs arise within an average of 3.5 years status-post radiation. Microscopically, AVL is characterized by a fairly well-circumscribed vascular proliferation confined within superficial to mid dermis. The vessels are composed of complex anastomosing and focally dilated vascular spaces. Occasionally, the vessels may exhibit a dissecting growth pattern within dermal collagen. The endothelial cells are hyperchromatic and exhibit varying degrees of "hobnail" cytomorphology.

Quick Fact

- **Radiation-Associated Angiosarcoma**
  - *MYC*-positive amplification
- **Radiation-Associated Atypical Vascular Lesion**
  - *MYC* negative

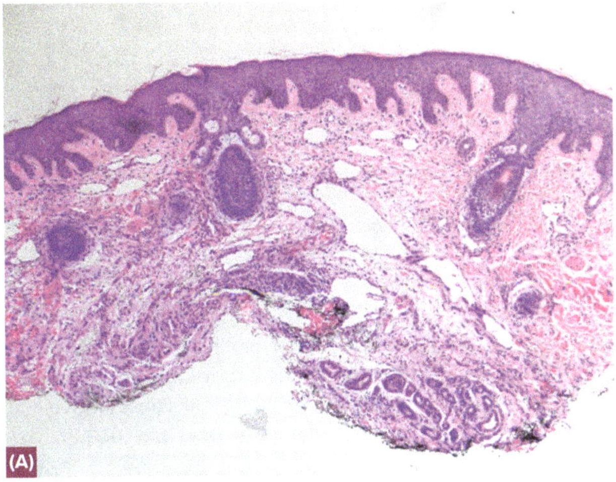

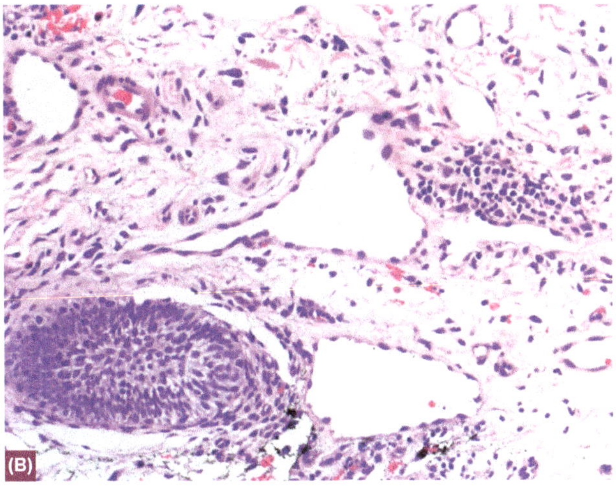

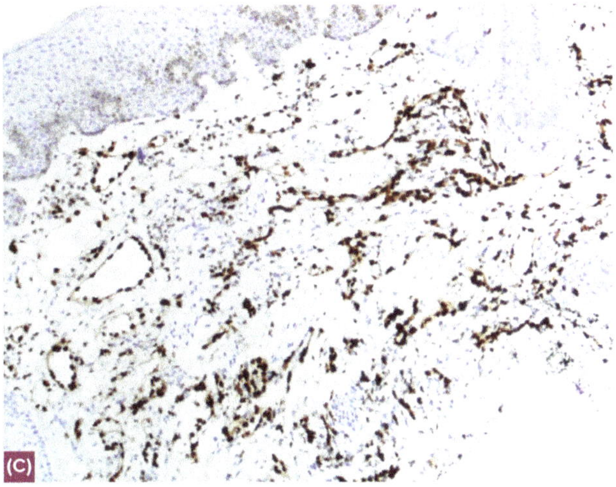

Atypical vascular lesion (AVL) associated with radiation exposure. (A) There are numerous anastomosing vascular channels infiltrating the dermis. **(B)** The dilated vessels are lined by plump hyperchromatic endothelial cells; however, these cells do not "pile up" or exhibit prominent nucleoli. **(C)** Immunohistochemical staining for ERG reveals the increased density of anastomosing vessels throughout the dermis.

ANSWER 11-20: E.

Congenital hemangioma (CH) designates a vascular malformation of intrauterine onset, which contrary to **infantile hemangioma (IH)** is fully developed at birth and does not exhibit postnatal growth. Despite the designation "hemangioma," CH is a **vascular malformation**. At least two subgroups of CH are recognized: **rapidly involuting congenital hemangioma (RICH)** and **noninvoluting congenital hemangioma (NICH)**. The patient in question most likely has a noninvoluting congenital hemangioma. There is an equal gender ratio of CH in contrast to the female preponderance of infantile hemangioma.

Clinically, **RICH** presents as raised violaceous tumors with central depression, ulceration, or scarring often with

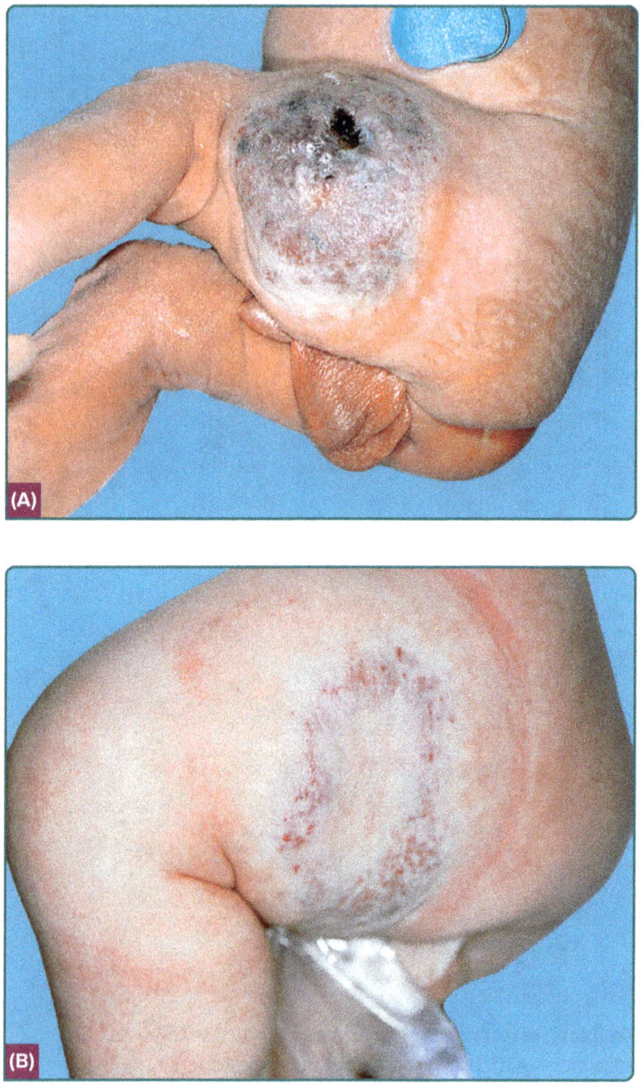

Rapidly involuting congenital hemangioma on left thigh. (A) Note central ulceration, violaceous color, and pale periphery. Fast-flow vessels were detected on Doppler examination. **(B)** Rapid regression at age 2 months. (Reproduced, with permission, from Goldsmith LA, Katz SI, Gilchrest BA, Paller AS, Leffell DJ, Wolff K, eds. *Fitzpatrick's Dermatology in General Medicine*. 8th ed. New York, NY: McGraw-Hill Education; 2012.)

coarse telangiectasias and a pale peripheral rim. These lesions are usually localized to the head and neck and extremities and range from 1 to 15 cm in diameter. They are warm on palpation. On magnetic resonance imaging (MRI), the lesions occupy the dermis and subcutis and sometimes extend into the underlying muscles. They contain large and irregular high-flow vessels with arterial aneurysms on ultrasonography and MRI. Such lesions commonly involute rapidly in 6 to 14 months.

NICH presents at birth as round to oval plaque-like or slightly raised lesions of pink to purple color often with telangiectasias. They are also warm on palpation and contain high-flow vessels. They lack the central depression or scar of RICH. NICH persists indefinitely with some alteration in color or size over time.

Some CHs exhibit characteristics of both RICH and NICH. For example, some CHs may suggest RICH at birth because of rapid involution that is ultimately incomplete and eventuates in a stable persistent process consistent with NICH.

Microscopically, **RICH** are characterized by a proliferation of capillaries grouped in lobules of variable sizes. Their lumina are small and round or irregular; however, a larger thin-walled vascular channel is often seen in the center of the lobules. The lobules are separated by fibrous tissue containing large tortuous vessels with irregular contours composed of thin-walled (veins or lymphatics) and thick-walled (arterial) channels. The centers of such lesions contain areas of fibrous tissue devoid of capillary lobules suggesting lesional involution. Thrombi, hemosiderin deposits, and calcifications may be present. **NICH** generally shows larger lobules of capillaries with irregular lumina. Endothelial cells have lymphocyte-like, dark, round nuclei protruding into the lumen with a hobnail pattern. Mild anisokaryosis is frequent. The cytoplasms focally contain **eosinophilic hyaline inclusions** similar to those observed in **papillary hemangiomas (PH)** and **glomeruloid hemangiomas (GHs)**; however, the material is hyaline and not a_1-antitrypsin or immunoglobulin, respectively. The complex branching and folding of lobular vessels sometimes results in a papillary appearance. Perilobular fibrosis and interlobular vascular networks are less developed than in RICH. Some of the vascular lobules of NICH protrude into large veins or lymphatic-like vessels.

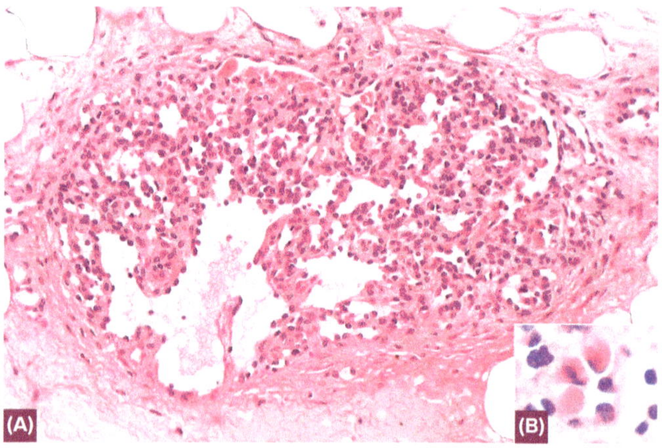

Congenital hemangioma. (A) Noninvoluting congenital hemangioma generally demonstrates larger lobules of capillaries with irregular lumina. **(B)** Endothelial cells (*inset*) have lymphocyte-like, dark, round nuclei protruding into the lumen with a hobnail pattern.

Quick Fact

- **Infantile Hemangioma**
  - Develops after delivery
  - GLUT-1 positive
- **Congenital Hemangioma**
  - Present at birth
  - GLUT-1 negative

Except for a single case of RICH, neither RICH nor NICH express GLUT-1, the specific marker of infancy hemangioma. Actin-positive smooth muscle cells may ensheathe individual capillaries as in IH but more characteristically form a poorly organized network about the capillaries

In regard to the differential diagnosis, the main entities to consider are **infantile hemangioma** and **pyogenic granuloma**. Intrauterine onset and lack of postnatal progression allow distinction of congenital hemangioma from the more common infantile hemangioma and from pyogenic granuloma. During its proliferative phase, infantile hemangioma lacks the interlobular fibrous tissue and large tortuous vessels of RICH. Involuting hemangiomas are generally less cellular than NICH and do not demonstrate hobnail nuclei and hyaline eosinophilic inclusions. The feeding and draining vessels of IH lobules have a high media-to-lumina ratio, contrasting with the intralobular thin-walled stellate vessels of congenital hemangioma. Contrary to RICH and NICH, infantile hemangiomas express GLUT-1 in almost all instances. Pyogenic granulomas commonly arise following traumatic injury and frequently ulcerate. Microscopically, they also exhibit a lobular pattern of vascular proliferation; however, numerous scattered neutrophils are typically present in a myxoid matrix.

ANSWER 11-21: C.

Distinguishing between benign and malignant mesenchymal neoplasms can be a difficult task with serious impact on patient management and prognosis. In general, there are several concepts to consider when evaluating soft tissue proliferations. While many tumors may exhibit one or more features associated with malignancy, it is the summation of all of these features that tends to predict the biological behavior of the proliferation. The features associated with malignant behavior include infiltrative pattern of growth, high cellularity, cellular pleomorphism, high mitotic rate with atypical mitotic figures (tripolar and quadripolar), tumor cell necrosis, and vascular invasion.

Well-circumscribed tumors tend to behave in a more indolent fashion than infiltrating tumors. In some cases, benign proliferations may exhibit a partially infiltrative pattern of growth; however, tumors with extensive permeation of the fat, fascia, or skeletal muscle are generally considered malignant. In general, malignant tumors tend to be more cellular than benign tumors. Overall, normal mesenchymal cells are less differentiated than those seen in epithelium. The most common cell type seen is the spindle cell, in which case establishing the line of differentiation (ie, fibroblast, smooth muscle, neural, fat, etc) may be very difficult by histomorphology alone and require adjunct immunohistochemical stains. There are two general categories of malignant mesenchymal neoplasms (**sarcomas**): monomorphous and pleomorphic. **Monomorphous sarcomas** are typically composed of cells that appear identical to one another. These malignant tumors tend to be locally aggressive, are clonal, and are associated with specific chromosomal translocations that create potent growth-promoting oncogenes. An example of this type of malignant mesenchymal tumor is **dermatofibrosarcoma protuberans** which is associated with a t(17;22) chromosomal translocation. When evaluating tumors with a monomorphous cytomorphology, it is imperative to evaluate for mitotic rate (including atypical mitoses), infiltrative pattern of growth, and foci of tumor necrosis. **Pleomorphic sarcomas** are composed of cell populations with marked variability in size and shape. These tumors tend to be polyclonal with numerous different mutations throughout the tumor cell population. These tumors are generally considered the least differentiated and behave aggressively with both local recurrence and distant metastasis. The best example of pleomorphic sarcoma is **malignant fibrous histiocytoma (MFH)**. Originally, the "MFH" category of soft tissue sarcomas contained five subcategories, including pleomorphic, angiomatoid, myxoid, inflammatory, and giant cell variants. Once the most commonly diagnosed malignant soft tissue tumor, the pleomorphic variant of "MFH" has been critically reevaluated. Using ultrastructural and immunohistochemical techniques, it has been shown that many tumors once designated as the pleomorphic variant of "MFH" are not histiocytic in nature and actually represent a diverse group of tumors that have in common marked cytologic pleomorphism, high mitotic rate, and frequent tumor cell necrosis. The criteria used to diagnose "MFH," including cytologic pleomorphism, multinucleated giant cells, and storiform cellular pattern, are not reproducible, and this diagnosis became a "wastebasket" for pleomorphic tumors. If pleomorphic tumors are thoroughly sampled and examined, most can be precisely diagnosed. In some cases a diagnosis of **high-grade pleomorphic sarcoma, not otherwise specified,** may be appropriate. Only if the pathologist strives for precise categorization of pleomorphic tumors will relevant clinical correlation be possible. Although many turn out to be sarcomas, such as pleomorphic variants of rhabdomyosarcoma, leiomyosarcoma, or liposarcoma, it is important to realize that cellular pleomorphism alone is not enough to establish a diagnosis of malignancy. Benign mesenchymal tumors frequently exhibit cellular pleomorphism, in which case the changes are referred to as **"senescent atypia."** It is believed that these tumor cells are locked into a nondividing state, and therefore it is critical to search for mitotic activity and tumor cell necrosis in these tumors. Examples of these benign pleomorphic tumors include **pleomorphic fibroma, pleomorphic lipoma, "ancient" schwannoma (degenerated neurilemoma), dermatofibroma with "monster" cells (atypical fibrous histiocytoma),** and **cutaneous symplastic leiomyoma**. Lastly, the anatomic compartment involved by the tumor also correlates with behavior and prognosis. Many tumors with a malignant histomorphology that are confined to the dermis exhibit little to no risk for distant metastasis. Examples include **atypical fibroxanthoma** (**AFX**) and **pilar leiomyosarcoma**. Many have recommended that the latter be referred to as **"atypical" leiomyomatous tumor** due to the seemingly benign clinical course.

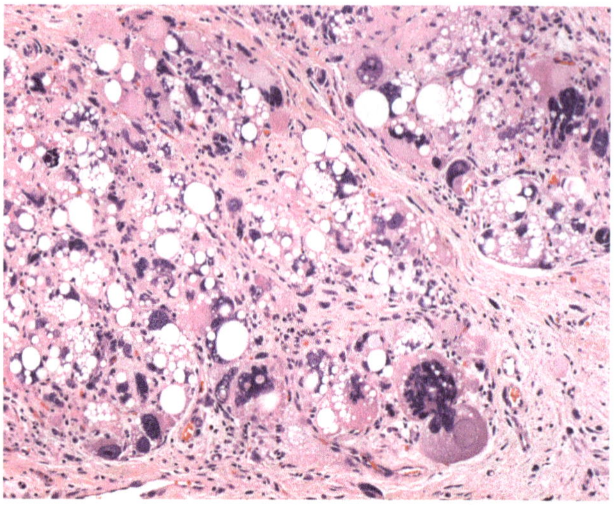

Pleomorphic liposarcoma. There are numerous pleomorphic multivacuolated lipoblasts. The cells are large and contain numerous mitotic figures, some of which are atypical.

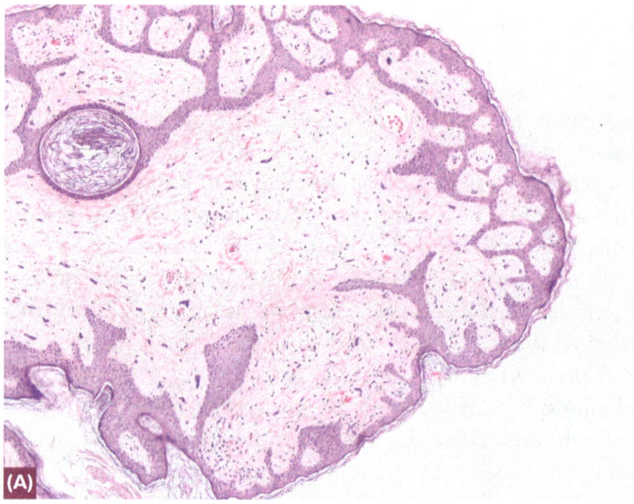

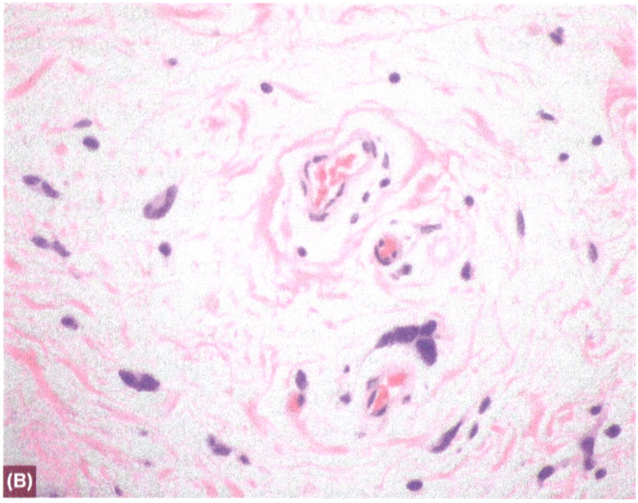

Pleomorphic fibroma. (A) This tumor is essentially a fibroepithelial polyp (skin tag) with bizarre pleomorphic fibroblasts characteristic of "senescent atypia." **(B)** Many of the cells are multinucleated, but are small and lack mitotic activity.

ANSWER 11-22: D.

This is a classic example of a **keloid**. Both **keloids** and **hypertrophic scars** begin as granulation tissue that gradually results in the accumulation of collagen with the maturation of myofibroblasts and an eventual decrease in dermal cellularity (Table 11-22A). Histopathologically, the defining feature of mature keloids is the characteristic thick rope-like bands of hyalinized collagen. The thick collagenous bands typically have a fibrillar appearance. Clinically, **keloids** are easily distinguished from **hypertrophic scars** by their tendency to gradually increase in size to extend beyond the site of initial injury. Additionally, there is a tendency for keloids to locally recur after excision. Hypertrophic scars tend to regress over time. It is not uncommon for scars to demonstrate small foci of keloidal collagen, in which case diagnostic distinction is best deferred to the clinical impression. **Dermatofibroma** is a firm 0.5- to 1-cm nodule most commonly arising on the lower extremities of female patients; however, these common tumors may arise at any site. The overlying skin may be flesh-colored to pigmented and tethers to the underlying dermis with lateral compression (dimple sign). Microscopically, dermatofibromas are typically more cellular than keloids. They are characterized by a storiform dermal proliferation of dendritic cells whose processes can be seen wrapping around the peripheral collagen bundles of normal size. Keloids also exhibit cellularity around collagen bundles, but their collagen bundles are much larger. The dendritic cells of dermatofibroma are positive for factor XIIIa by immunohistochemistry. Some paucicellular dermatofibromas may be indistinguishable from scars since these dendritic cells are also important in scar formation. **Fibroepithelial polyps**, also known as **skin tags** or **acrochordons**, are polypoid, soft, often slightly hyperpigmented, and attached by a thin fibrovascular stalk

Table 11-22A. Differences Between Keloids and Hypertrophic Scars

	KELOID	HYPERTROPHIC SCAR
Age	Especially third decade	Any
Onset after injury	Delayed[a]	Immediate
Growth beyond border of original wound	Yes	No
Spontaneous regression	Rare	Occasional
Recurrence	Common	Rare
Distorted shape	Common	Rare
Histopathology	Thick, hyalinized collagen	Fascicles of myofibroblasts arranged haphazardly
Treatment response	Poor	Good

[a]May occur spontaneously.

Source: Reproduced, with permission, from Goldsmith LA, Katz SI, Gilchrest BA, Paller AS, Leffell DJ, Wolff K, eds. *Fitzpatrick's Dermatology in General Medicine*. 8th ed. New York, NY: McGraw-Hill Education; 2012.

Table 11-22B. Fibroepithelial Polyp

Clinical Features
Commonly involve the skin of the neck and axillary area of middle-aged and elderly adults
Frequently multiple
1-15 mm in size
Polypoid, soft, and attached by a thin fibrovascular stalk
Often slightly hyperpigmented
Histopathologic Features
Polypoid with a collagenous core of loosely textured to dense sclerotic collagen
Soft fibromas are larger with adipose tissue
Epidermis may show features of lichen simplex chronicus or seborrheic keratosis
Differential Diagnosis
Seborrheic keratosis
Nevus lipomatosus superficialis
Angiofibroma
Pedunculated nevus

(Table 11-22B). They are most common on the face and intertriginous areas of middle-aged and elderly adults and are frequently multiple. They range in size from 1 mm to more than 1 cm. Not uncommonly, fibroepithelial polyps twist about their stalk and infarct, causing a change in color from tan to black. Microscopically, fibroepithelial polyps are composed of a polypoid portion of normal skin with dilated vessels and are devoid of adnexal structures. Lesions arising around the waist and proximal extremities frequently contain lobules of fat and are referred to as **soft fibromas** or **fibrolipomas**. **Juvenile hyaline fibromatosis** is an extremely rare disease that affects young children and is characterized by the deposition of an amorphous, hyaline material. Siblings are often affected, and the disease shows an autosomal recessive pattern of inheritance. This disorder may also be associated with impaired intellect, gingival hypertrophy, flexural contractures, and bone lesions. It represents an inherited abnormality of collagen metabolism rather than a neoplastic process. The gene for this disease is located on chromosome 4q21 and encodes capillary morphogenesis protein 2 (CMG2), which is involved in basement membrane assembly. The onset of this disease is usually before 5 years of age; however, new lesions may continue to develop during adulthood. Patients develop multiple exophytic lesions ranging from small papules measuring several millimeters to large masses many centimeters in diameter. The lesions have a predilection for the head, neck, and upper trunk. They are slow growing and usually asymptomatic. However, some patients develop multiple disfiguring nodules that require multiple surgical procedures over many years. Microscopically, these tumors are poorly circumscribed and show variable but usually low cellularity. Separating strands of bland appearing fibroblasts are ribbons of glassy hyaline eosinophilic material. Fibroblasts are sometimes surrounded by prominent clear halos caused by retraction artifact. The bands of homogeneous eosinophilic material,

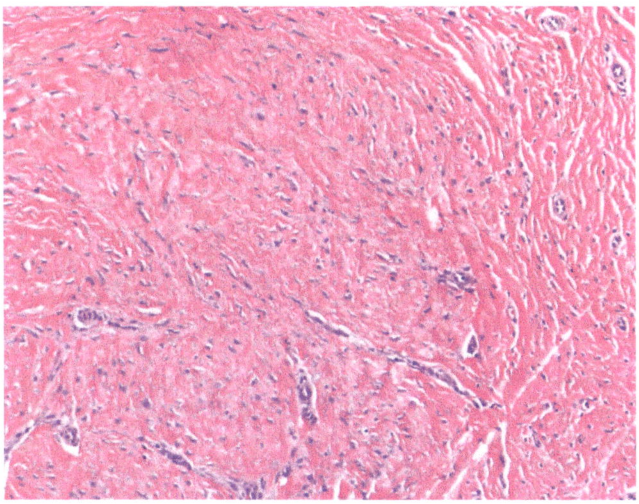

Hypertrophic scar. There is dense fibrillar collagen admixed with an increased number of vessels; however, thick ropey bundles of "keloidal" collagen are absent.

the defining feature of this disorder, stain with periodic acid-Schiff (PAS) and Alcian blue stains. The key distinguishing features from keloid include clinical presentation and family history. Additionally, the bands of amorphous hyaline material lack the fibrillar appearance of keloidal collagen.

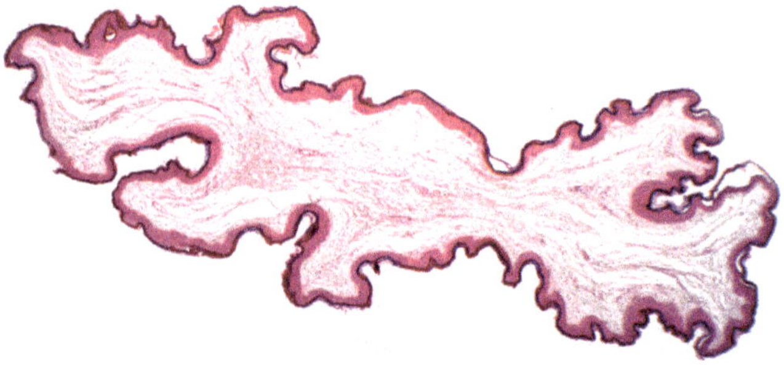

Fibroepithelial polyp with squamous epithelium surrounding loose collagenous stroma devoid of adnexal structures.

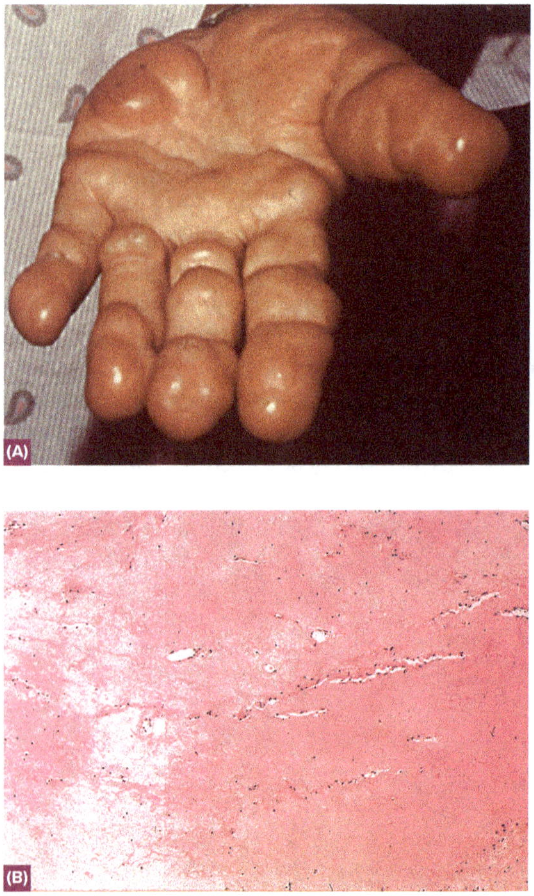

Juvenile hyaline fibromatosis. (A) Tumors involving the hand. Both hands were affected. **(B)** This unusual and rare lesion is characterized by paucicellular ribbons of glassy hyaline eosinophilic material and few vessels. (Part **(A)** reproduced, with permission, from Goldsmith LA, Katz SI, Gilchrest BA, Paller AS, Leffell DJ, Wolff K, eds. *Fitzpatrick's Dermatology in General Medicine*. 8th ed. New York, NY: McGraw-Hill Education; 2012.)

ANSWER 11-23: E.

Angiofibromas are fibrous proliferations composed of stellate cells and dilated thin-walled blood vessels. The composite stellate cells often are multinucleated resembling ganglion cells or radiation fibroblasts. Concentric fibrosis surrounding adnexal structures is a characteristic feature. The lesional cells are positive for CD34 and factor XIIIa via immunohistochemistry, but are consistently negative for S100. **Angiofibromas** are associated with three distinct clinical presentations (Table 11-23A). Solitary lesions of the central face are referred to as **fibrous papules**, most commonly arise on the nose, and may be clinically mistaken for basal cell carcinoma. Multiple lesions arising circumferentially around the glans penis are referred to as **pearly penile papules**. This condition is most common in African Americans and uncircumcised patients. Lesions may arise in the vulvar region, where they are simply referred to as angiofibromas. There is no association with HPV and should not be confused for condylomata. Smooth, shiny, flesh-colored nodules that arise from the nail folds are referred to as **periungual fibromas**. They range in size from a few millimeters to more than 1 cm. They usually present in the peripubertal period. The presence of multiple facial lesions, particularly the nasolabial folds, and periungual fibromas should prompt a careful family history and clinical examination for evidence of **tuberous sclerosis complex**. Periungual fibromas are seen in approximately half of patients with this disorder. Historically, the multiple facial lesions of tuberous sclerosis have been previously referred to as **adenoma sebaceum** in the literature. This is a misnomer since sebaceous glands are not a microscopic component. They develop at birth or in early childhood and may be the first sign of disease. Clinical recognition of these lesions as a manifestation of tuberous sclerosis is important because spontaneous mutations are believed to account for approximately two-thirds of patients. Tuberous sclerosis complex is an autosomal dominant neurocutaneous syndrome caused by mutations in the *TSC1* (hamartin) or *TSC2* (tuberin) gene. Central nervous system manifestations include mental retardation, epilepsy, glial hamartomas, and subependymal nodules and subependymal giant cell astrocytomas. Systemic manifestations include cardiac rhabdomyomas, angiomyolipomas of the kidney, renal cysts, and carcinomas, as well as pulmonary lymphangioleiomyomatosis and fibrous dysplasia of bone. Mucocutaneous lesions commonly seen in tuberous

Table 11-23A. Angiofibromas

Central face in child with stigmata of tuberous sclerosis = **facial angiofibroma (adenoma sebaceum)**
Shiny papule on face, especially nose with clinical appearance often mistaken for basal cell carcinoma = **fibrous papule**
Tiny papules on the glans penis = **pearly penile papules**

sclerosis include facial angiofibromas (adenoma sebaceum), ungual and periungual fibromas, café-au-lait spots, large hypomelanotic macules (ash-leaf spots or thumbprint-shaped lesions) and confetti-like macules, forehead fibrous plaques, gingival fibromas, molluscum pendulum, and connective tissue nevi (shagreen patch). Lastly, **acquired digital acral fibrokeratoma** is a related lesion that occurs mostly in adults and most frequently on the fingers; however, it is also seen on the toes, palms and soles, and feet. Fibrokeratomas are small (<1.5 cm) nodules that range from slightly elevated to protuberant lesions that often are exophytic with a narrow base. The overlying epidermis usually is verrucous and hyperkeratotic. A traumatic etiology has been discussed, although convincing evidence is lacking. Microscopically, fibrokeratoma is composed of dense hyalinized and irregularly arranged collagen bundles with variable numbers of fibroblasts. Sparse to numerous thin-walled vessels may be present. Vessels and collagen bundles are characteristically arranged perpendicular to the overlying epidermis. Elastic tissue stains usually fail to show elastic fibers.

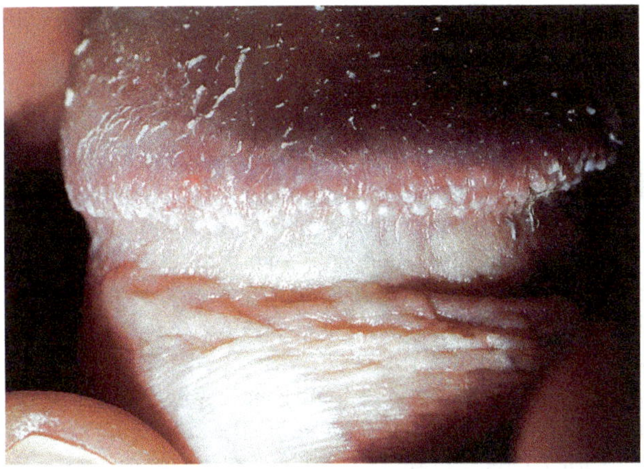

Pearly penile papules. Pink (skin-colored), 1- to 2-mm papules are seen regularly spaced along the corona of the glans penis. These structures, which are part of the normal anatomy of the glans, are commonly mistaken for condylomata or molluscum contagiosum. (Reproduced, with permission, from Wolff K, Johnson RA, Saavedra AP. *Fitzpatrick's Color Atlas and Synopsis of Clinical Dermatology*. 7th ed. New York, NY: McGraw-Hill Education; 2013.)

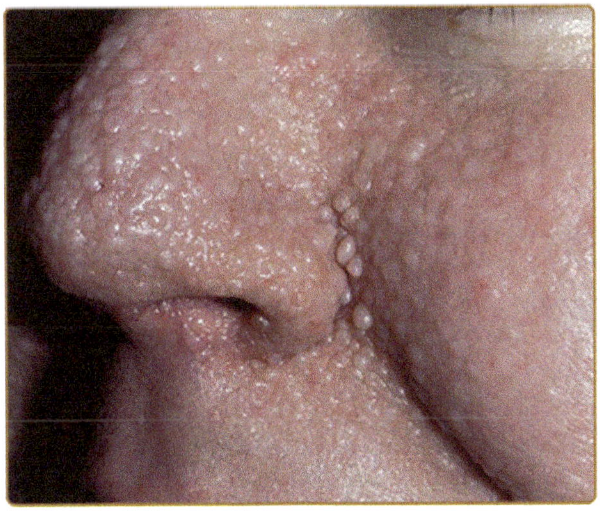

Multiple facial angiofibromas (adenoma sebaceum) in the alar grooves with tuberous sclerosis complex. (Reproduced, with permission, from Goldsmith LA, Katz SI, Gilchrest BA, Paller AS, Leffell DJ, Wolff K, eds. *Fitzpatrick's Dermatology in General Medicine*. 8th ed. New York, NY: McGraw-Hill Education; 2012.)

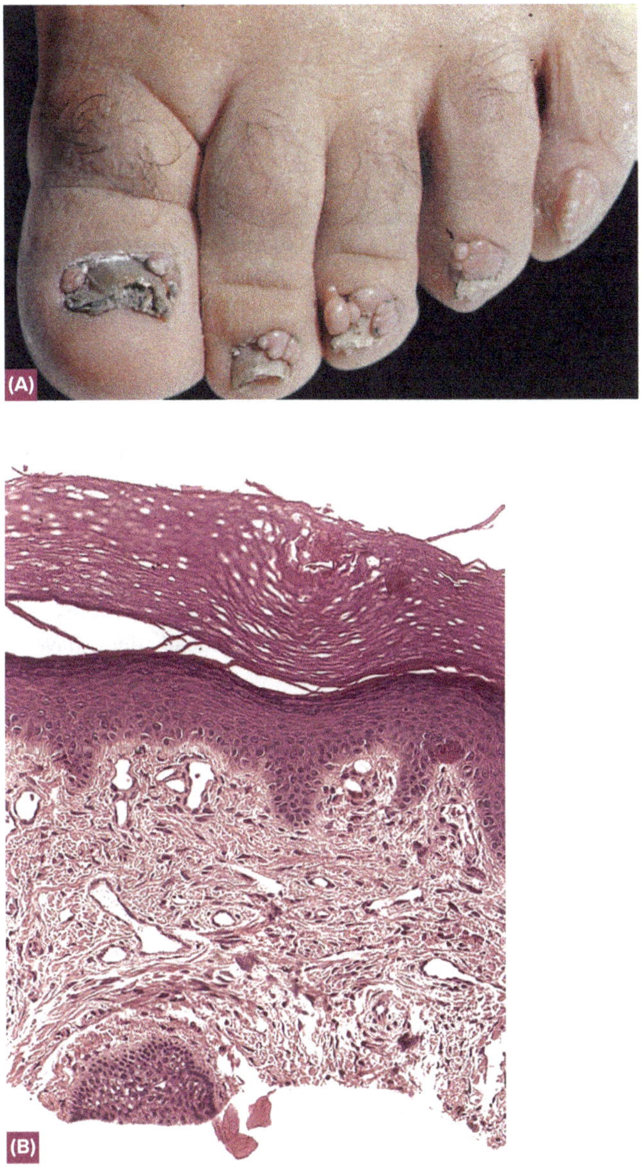

Periungual fibroma. (A) Multiple periungual and subungual fibromas on the toes in a patient with tuberous sclerosis complex. **(B)** The epidermis shows acanthosis and hyperkeratosis. The underlying dermis is expanded by dense collagen associated with stellate cells and a few ecstatic vessels. (Part **(A)** reproduced, with permission, from Goldsmith LA, Katz SI, Gilchrest BA, Paller AS, Leffell DJ, Wolff K, eds. *Fitzpatrick's Dermatology in General Medicine*. 8th ed. New York, NY: McGraw-Hill Education; 2012.)

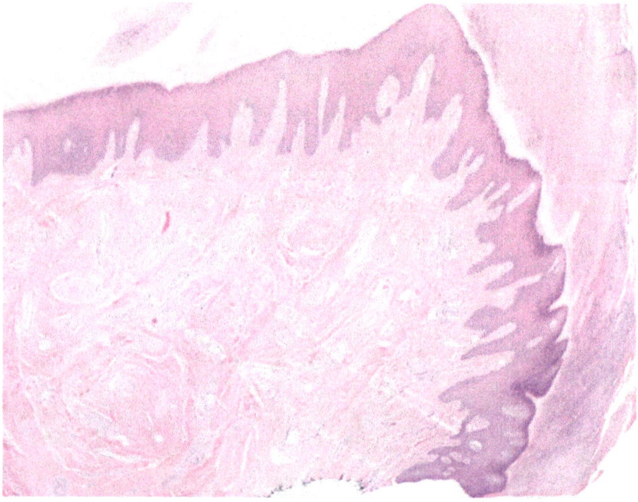

Acquired digital fibrokeratoma. There is verrucous epidermal proliferation overlying a markedly fibrotic dermis, in which dilated vessels and collagen bundles are oriented perpendicular to the epidermal surface.

ANSWER 11-24: B.

This is an example of **storiform collagenoma (sclerotic fibroma)**, which most often occurs in young and middle-aged adults as a solitary slow-growing nodule on the head and neck and upper extremities, usually measuring less than 1 cm in diameter (Table 11-24A). Recurrence is not a feature. Multiple lesions are associated with **Cowden disease**, an autosomal dominant familial cancer syndrome, in which patients have an inherited deletion of the PTEN tumor suppressor gene. There is a special susceptibility for breast, thyroid, endometrial, and gastrointestinal cancers, and the skin lesions are important markers. Skin lesions may appear first in childhood and develop over time. They consist of **trichilemmomas, translucent punctate keratoses of the palms and soles, hyperkeratotic flat-topped papules on the dorsa of the hands and forearms,** and **papules and papillomas of the mucous membranes**. Microscopically, these storiform collagenomas are symmetric and well circumscribed but unencapsulated. They are composed of paucicellular hyaline collagen containing numerous cleft-like spaces. Cellularity varies; however, most tumors contain only rare scattered fibroblasts interposed between collagen bands. The clefts are randomly oriented and impart a storiform pattern at low magnification. The tumor tends to expand and efface the overlying epidermis. **Giant cell collagenoma** is a variant with multinucleated giant cells with bizarre shapes. A summary of differential features for spindle cell tumors with a storiform pattern is provided in Table 11-24B. The histopathological differential diagnosis includes **tuberous xanthoma, dermatomyofibroma, keloid,** and **sclerosing perineurioma. Tuberous xanthomas** are firm, painless, red-yellow nodules that can coalesce to form multilobated tumors. They are strongly associated with hypercholesterolemia and usually develop in pressure areas, such as the extensor surfaces of the knees, the elbows, and the buttocks. Microscopically, they are composed of dermal storiform sclerosis similar to storiform collagenoma, but with foamy macrophages (xanthoma cells) in between the collagen bundles. The xanthoma cells are positive for CD68. **Keloids** can be distinguished by the association of typical hypertrophic scar and poor circumscription. Storiform collagenoma shows more uniform hyalinization compared with keloid. **Sclerosing perineuriomas (storiform perineurial fibroma),** typically seen in the hands, may closely mimic storiform collagenoma but typically arises within the subcutis and contain very delicate wavy spindled cells with long processes. The cells are EMA(+), CD34(+), and S100(−) (Table 11-24C). **Dermatomyofibroma** usually presents as a pale pink or hypopigmented plaque on the upper trunk or neck of adolescents and young adults, particularly females

Table 11-24A. Storiform Collagenoma

Clinical Features
Young and middle-aged adults
Usually <1cm
Slow-growing nodule in the head and neck region and upper extremities
Multiple collagenomas associated with Cowden disease
Histopathologic Features
Symmetric, well circumscribed but unencapsulated
Paucicellular hyaline collagen with numerous cleft-like spaces
Rare scattered fibroblasts between collagen bands
Clefts impart a storiform pattern to the tumor
Differential Diagnosis
Dermatofibroma
Myofibroma
Keloid

Table 11-24B. Tumors with Storiform Pattern

Confined to dermis with overlying epithelial hyperplasia = **dermatofibroma**
Less uniform storiform pattern mixed with fascicles parallel to epidermis = **dermatomyofibroma**
Extensive infiltration of fat and CD34+ = **dermatofibrosarcoma protuberans**
Marked atypia, sun-damaged skin, minimal infiltration of fat = **atypical fibroxanthoma**
Marked atypia, significant infiltration subcutaneous fat = **pleomorphic sarcoma, sarcomatoid carcinoma, melanoma**
Storiform pattern produced by cleft-like spaces in paucicellular hyaline nodule = **storiform collagenoma**

Table 11-24C. Soft Tissue Perineurioma

Clinical Features
Middle-aged adults
Predilection for extremities and trunk
Skin-colored soft tissue nodules and tumors
Histopathologic Features
Dermal or subcutaneous mass
Well circumscribed, but without thin capsules
Interweaving fascicles and whorls
Delicate, elongated spindle cells
Cracking or lamination of collagen fibers
Differential Diagnosis
Neurofibroma
Dermatofibrosarcoma protuberans
Myoepithelioma
Sclerotic fibroma

Table 11-24D. Dermatomyofibroma

Clinical Features
Pale pink or hypopigmented plaque
Upper trunk
Adolescents and young adults, usually girls and young women
Histopathologic Features
Fascicles oriented parallel to the skin surface
Grenz zone
Composite cells are myofibroblasts with eosinophilic cytoplasm
Significant extension into fat and subcutaneous tissue is not seen
Differential Diagnosis
Dermatofibroma
Dermatofibrosarcoma protuberans (plaque stage)

(Table 11-24D). Lesions may resemble keloid or plaque-like dermatofibrosarcoma protuberans (DFSP), grow slowly over many years, and attain a size of up to 5 cm. Surgical excision appears curative in the small number of cases reported. Dermatomyofibromas exhibits a band-like configuration in the reticular dermis with a grenz zone sparing the superficial dermis. The composite lesional cells are arranged in fascicles oriented parallel to the surface. Adnexal structures tend to be spared. Prominent extension into subcutaneous tissue is usually not seen, although focal involvement of subcutaneous fat is present in some cases. The composite cells are uniformly CD34(−), smooth muscle actin(+) myofibroblasts with eosinophilic cytoplasm. Although these lesions can be cellular and mitotically active, cytologic atypia is not present. The overlying epidermis is frequently hyperplastic rather than attenuated.

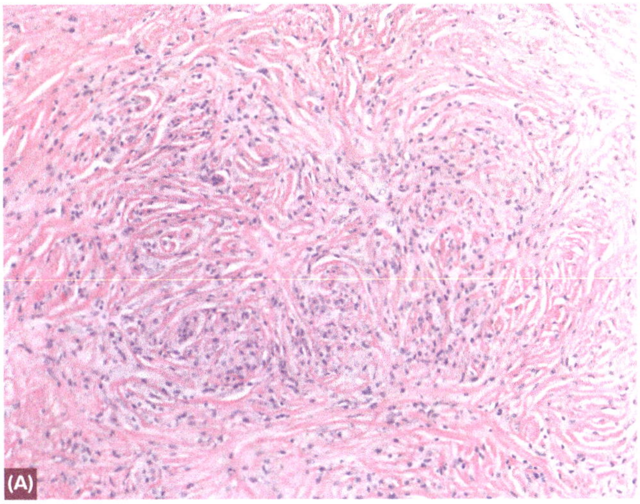

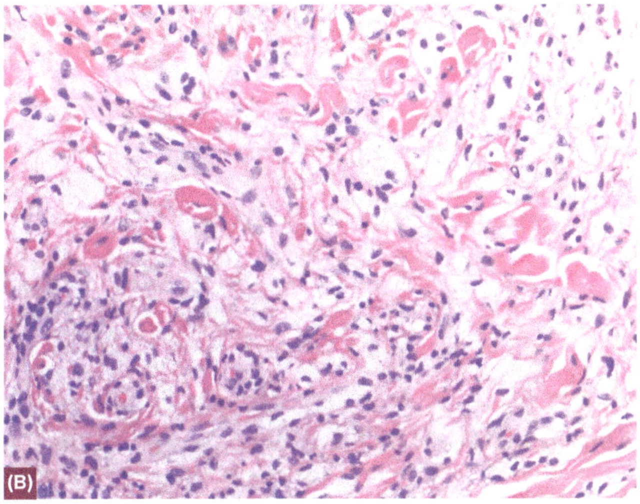

Tuberous xanthoma. (A) Note the storiform sclerotic nodule in the dermis. **(B)** The interstitial spaces are filled with foamy macrophages (xanthoma cells) containing large amounts of lipid.

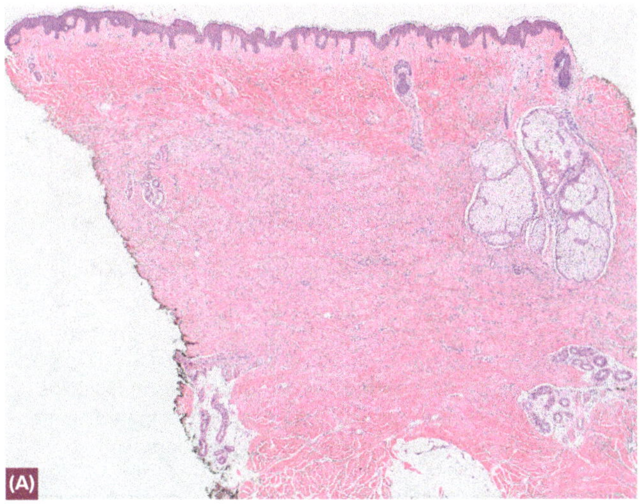

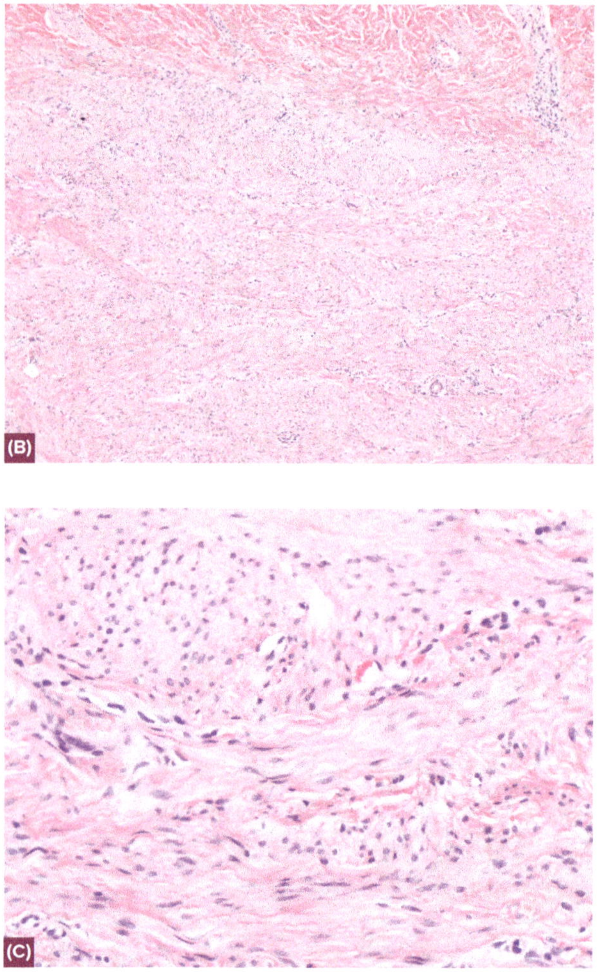

Dermatomyofibroma. (A) The tumor exhibits a plaque-like growth pattern in the reticular dermis with a grenz zone sparing the papillary dermis. Note the sparing of adnexal structures. **(B), (C)** The tumor is composed of horizontal fascicles of spindled cells with a myoid appearance.

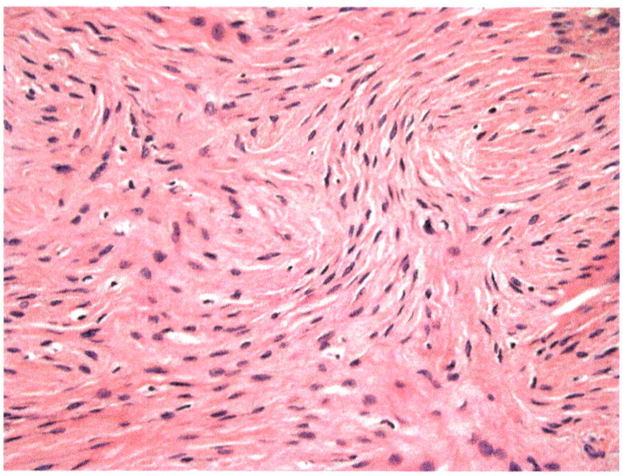

Soft tissue sclerosing perineurioma. Interweaving fascicles with a vague storiform pattern composed of elongated, slender, wavy, spindle cells with dissecting collagen fibers.

ANSWER 11-25: D.

Fibroma of tendon sheath is a tumor of unclear pathogenesis (Table 11-25A). It is seen most frequently on the hands and feet of young adults, particularly men. Most tumors are painless, slowly growing nodules or masses on a finger, measuring less than 3 cm in diameter. Attachment to the tendon or tendon sheath can usually be demonstrated at the time of surgery. Up to 25% of tumors may recur after surgical excision. Serious functional impairment is almost never seen. Microscopically, these tumors are well circumscribed and show variable cellularity. They are composed of uniform spindled fibroblasts and myofibroblasts with slender, tapered nuclei arranged in short fascicles. Paucicellular tumors may be markedly hyalinized and demonstrate concentric whorls of dense eosinophilic collagen. A characteristic feature is the presence of slit-like vascular channels that appear compressed by surrounding stroma. The presence of CD68+ multinucleated giant cells in occasional tumors suggests the existence of a morphologic spectrum with **giant cell tumor of tendon sheath (GCTTS)** (Table 11-25B). In fact, cellular tumors with giant cells may be difficult, if not impossible, to distinguish from **GCTTS.** The presence of slit-like vessels and tumor cells arranged in short fascicles favors fibroma of tendon sheath. These features, together with overall circumscription of the tumor, allow distinction from **fibromatosis**, which clinically presents as multiple small nodules coalescing into fibrous bands on the palmar and plantar surfaces. **Superficial fibromatosis** may also occur on the penis. Some cellular cases of fibroma of tendon sheath may show similarities to fibromatosis; however, the clinical presentation and site are different. The fibromatoses are a family of fibroblastic proliferations sharing similar histopathology, an infiltrative pattern of growth, and a tendency to recur after excision. Tumors located at some sites show the capacity for locally aggressive and destructive growth; however, these tumors never metastasize. The clinical behavior of fibromatoses is very site dependent; however, in general, superficial

Table 11-25A. Fibroma of Tendon Sheath

Clinical Features
- Young to middle-aged men
- Slow-growing, painless nodule of hands and feet
- 25% recur after excision

Histopathologic Features
- Well circumscribed
- Variably cellular, composed of fibroblasts and myofibroblasts in short fascicles
- Slit-like vascular spaces

Differential Diagnosis
- Giant cell tumor of tendon sheath
- Angioleiomyoma
- Fibromatosis

Table 11-25B. Giant Cell Tumor of Tendon Sheath

Clinical Features
- Predilection for young women
- Fingers, much less commonly in the toes
- Slowly growing painless mass, <3cm
- May recur after excision

Histopathologic Features
- Multilobulated
- Varying proportions of histiocytoid mononuclear cells, osteoclast-like multinucleated giant cells, xanthoma cells, chronic inflammatory cells, hemosiderin-laden macrophages, collagenized stroma
- Multinucleated cells may be difficult to find
- Mitotic figures may be present

Differential Diagnosis
- Fibroma of tendon sheath
- Dermatofibroma
- Epithelioid sarcoma
- Giant cell tumor of soft tissues

fibromatoses such as palmar and plantar fibromatosis are less aggressive than deep fibromatoses such as **desmoid fibromatosis**. Many patients with **palmar fibromatosis (Dupuytren contracture)** eventually develop flexion contracture with significant functional impairment (Table 11-25C). Flexion causes characteristic puckering of skin overlying the tumor. Fasciectomy with surgical division of the fibrous bands or complete removal of the lesion often are performed to give functional improvement. **Plantar fibromatosis (Ledderhose disease)** differs from its palmar counterpart by its tendency to occur in younger age groups and is less commonly associated with functional impairment. Plantar fibromatosis may cause minor discomfort when walking but rarely causes contractures. However, there is a significant tendency for local recurrence. **Penile fibromatosis (Peyronie disease)** is considered by some a form of fibromatosis (Table 11-25D). Middle-aged and older men develop a slowly enlarging fibrous thickening of the penis, usually on the dorsum. With time, pain and curvature of the penis develop, which are exacerbated by erection. The pathogenesis and relationship to other forms of fibromatosis are poorly understood; however, it seems probable that Peyronie disease has an inflammatory basis, possibly vasculitic in nature. In addition, association with diabetes mellitus and veno-occlusive dysfunction has been reported. Microscopically, **superficial fibromatosis** involves mainly fibrotendinous and subcutaneous tissue and appear to proceed through several histologic stages as the lesion ages. Early lesions tend to be more cellular, more mitotically active, and composed of extremely long fascicles of plump myofibroblasts with wavy nuclei. Later-stage lesions are much less cellular, less mitotically active, and tend to have more abundant hyalinized stromal collagen. Intermediate-stage lesions (when biopsy is most common) contain features of both phases in alternating areas. Histopathologically, the plantar form of the disease tends to be more uniformly hypercellular at all stages in the disease process. Both palmar and plantar fibromatoses are often more cellular than their deep soft tissue counterparts, a feature that often causes diagnostic concern.

Table 11-25C. Palmar and Plantar Fibromatosis

Clinical Features
- Palmar fibromatosis
- Both hands are commonly involved
- Small nodule that progressively enlarges to form a cordlike band that causes puckering of overlying skin
- Flexion contracture and functional impairment of the hand
- Plantar fibromatosis
- Occurs in younger age groups
- May cause minor discomfort when walking
- Rarely associated with functional impairment

Histopathologic Features
- Interlacing fascicles with wavy collagenous stroma
- Tumor cells are spindle shaped; tapering or vesicular nuclei
- Early lesions are fairly cellular, mitotically active, and composed of plumper myofibroblasts
- Later stage lesions are less cellular, less mitotically active, with more abundant hyalinized collagen
- Plantar form tends to be more cellular

Differential Diagnosis
- Fibrosarcoma
- Desmoid fibromatosis

Table 11-25D. Penile Fibromatosis

Clinical Features
- Middle-aged and older males
- Slowly enlarging fibrous thickening of the penis, usually on the dorsum
- Pain and curvature of the penis, exacerbated by erection

Histopathologic Features
- Chronic inflammation in early lesions
- Scar-like fibrous proliferation as lesion ages
- Calcification and metaplastic ossification in some cases

Differential Diagnosis
- Cicatrix

Multinucleated giant cells are also seen in some cases of superficial fibromatoses; however, the infiltrative pattern of growth (rather than nodular) and a tendency to recur after excision separate this entity from fibroma of tendon sheath and giant cell tumor of tendon sheath. Many cases of fibroma of tendon sheath show foci indistinguishable from **hyalinized forms of nodular fasciitis**, suggesting that at least some fibromas of tendon sheath represent old, "burned-out" fasciitis. **Nodular fasciitis** is typically characterized by loosely arranged fibroblasts with a "tissue-culture" appearance and an inflammatory background. The stroma typically has a pale myxoid appearance with abundant dermal mucin. Distinction of some cases from hyalinized forms of nodular fasciitis may be somewhat arbitrary. **Angioleiomyoma** may resemble fibroma of tendon sheath at low-power magnification; however, the vessels of angioleiomyoma have thick walls with smooth muscle cells radiating from them. The tumor cells of angioleiomyoma will be SMA+ and desmin+. A summary of differential feature for spindle cell tumors containing dense fibrous tissue is provided in Table 11-25E.

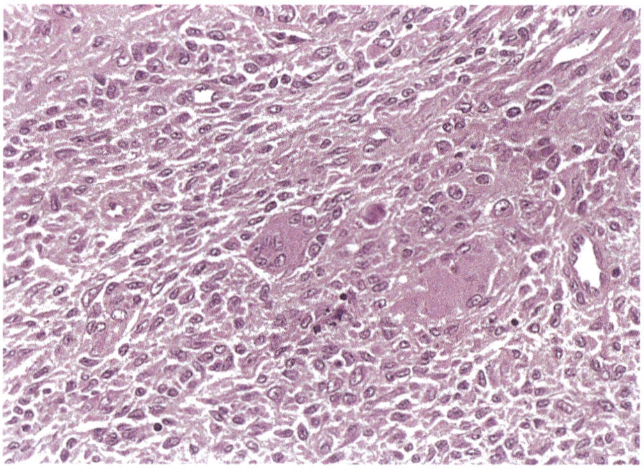

Giant cell tumor tendon sheath. The tumor is composed predominantly of sheets of histiocytic mononuclear cells and osteoclast-like multinucleated giant cells within variable amounts of amorphous collagenous stroma. In addition, xanthoma cells, chronic inflammatory cells, and hemosiderin-laden macrophages may be present.

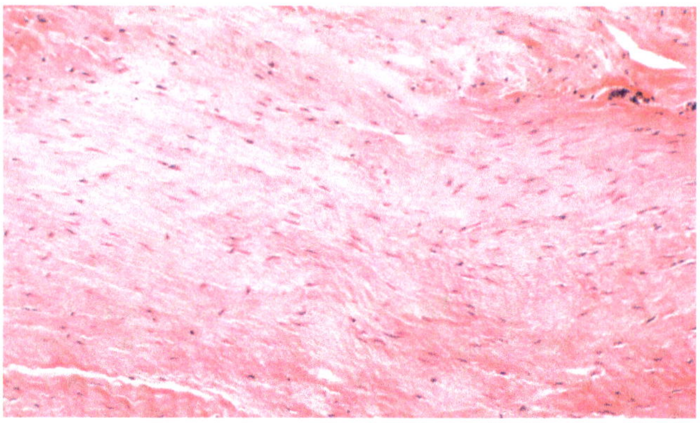

Plantar fibromatosis. The composite cells are spindled-shaped, often with wavy nuclei and are arranged in interlacing fascicles within very dense collagenous stroma.

Table 11-25E. Tumors Composed of Fibrous Tissue

Tumor composed of cellular "herringbone" fascicles with atypia, necrosis, high cellularity, necrosis and mitoses = **fibrosarcoma**
Paucicellular tumor with dense hyalinized collagen and spindled or wavy nuclei = **fibromatosis, knuckle pad, Peyronie disease**
Dense fibrous tissue with lobules of orderly bands of collagen parallel to the epidermis separated by blood vessels = **hypertrophic scar**
Features of hypertrophic scar with thick bands of glassy collagen = **keloid**
Tumor of hand or feet in young patient composed of spindled to epithelioid cells, with palisading around foci of calcification = **calcifying aponeurotic fibroma**
Exophytic lesion on hand with irregular thick bundles of collagen and variable numbers of blood vessels = **acral fibrokeratoma and periungual fibroma**

ANSWER 11-26: B.

Dermatofibroma (benign fibrous histiocytoma) is a very common dermal tumor that presents as a firm papule or nodule on the limbs and trunk, oftentimes following minor trauma (Table 11-26A). The face is rarely involved. The overlying skin may be flesh colored to pigmented and tethers to the underlying dermis with lateral compression (**dimple sign**). Most tumors are smaller than 1.5 cm. Dermatofibroma is a remarkably heterogeneous tumor with many variants described (Table 11-26B). Recognition of some variants of dermatofibroma is critical because they may mimic malignant neoplasms. The pathogenesis is unknown, and it is controversial if it is a reactive or neoplastic process. Clonal cytogenetic abnormalities have been identified in some cases of dermatofibroma. Microscopically, this tumor varies tremendously with regard to cellularity, vascularity, hemorrhage or hemosiderin deposition, degree of sclerosis (a feature of later-stage lesions), and types of accompanying cells (eg, giant cells, atypical cells, lipid-laden histiocytes). Attention to the characteristic growth pattern at scanning magnification is critical to recognizing variants of dermatofibroma. At low power, dermatofibromas are symmetric and fairly well demarcated, but not encapsulated, round to lens-shaped nodules centered in the reticular dermis and may occasionally extend deep into the subcutis

Table 11-26A. Dermatofibroma

Clinical Features
Young to middle-aged adults
Papule or nodule, most tumors <1.5 cm
Overlying skin may be erythematous or hyperpigmented, with borders gradually fading to normal skin color
"Dimple sign"
May persist for many years; some may regress spontaneously
Recurrence is infrequent after excision, except in the cellular, atypical, and aneurysmal variants
Histopathologic Features
Symmetric
Well circumscribed but not encapsulated
Most tumors confined to dermis or minimal extension into subcutaneous tissue
Tightly whorled fascicles in a storiform pattern
Fibrohistiocytic cells entrap preexisting collagen bundles
Lymphocytes, xanthoma cells, histiocytes, multinucleated giant cells
Touton-type giant cells may be seen in variable numbers
Overlying epidermis is acanthotic with basilar hyperpigmentation
Differential Diagnosis
Dermatofibrosarcoma protuberans
Leiomyosarcoma (for cellular variant)
Vascular tumors (for aneurysmal variant)

Table 11-26B. Variants of Dermatofibroma

Aneurysmal fibrous histiocytoma
Hemosiderotic histiocytoma
Atypical fibrous histiocytoma ("dermatofibroma with monster cells")
Epithelioid fibrous histiocytoma
Cellular variant
Palisading variant
Clear cell variant

along the fibrous septa; however, infiltration of fat lobules and entrapment of adipocytes is minimal or absent. The characteristic cell is the dermal dendritic cell, which frequently appears spindled in the plane of sectioning. The common denominator for this family of tumors is the presence of tightly whorled fascicles of these dendritic/spindle cells arranged in a storiform or pinwheel pattern. The most specific finding is ill-defined peripheral margins with trapping of bundles of dermal collagen at the lateral edges (**collagen wrapping**). In addition to these dendritic/spindle cells, scattered hemosiderin-laden macrophages, lipophages (xanthoma cells), and multinucleated cells (typically of Touton type) are seen. The lipid presumably reflects extravasated platelets and the hemosiderin a breakdown product of extravasated red blood cells. Frequently, the overlying epidermis is acanthotic with basilar hyperpigmentation, often suggesting a lentigo or seborrheic keratosis. In contrast, epidermal effacement may be seen over some lesions. In some cases, a striking induction of hair follicles may mimic basal cell carcinoma. A narrow grenz zone is often present. Occasional mitoses may be seen. While these features usually make for a straightforward diagnosis, small biopsies from the center of the lesion may be difficult to distinguish from **dermatofibrosarcoma protuberans (DFSP).**

In regard to the variants of dermatofibroma, recurrence is infrequent after excision of the classical type, but the aneurysmal and cellular variants recur in 20% to 25% of cases, especially if marginally or incompletely excised. The aneurysmal variant often shows rapid growth and can attain large size, causing clinical concern. Clinically, **aneurysmal fibrous histiocytoma** often is mistaken for a melanocytic or vascular neoplasm owing to its red-brown color secondary to hemorrhage and hemosiderin deposition. The **epithelioid fibrous histiocytoma** is noted for often being polypoid. Rare metastases of some variants, especially **cellular fibrous histiocytoma** and **atypical fibrous histiocytoma (dermatofibroma with monster cells)**, have been reported. Some dermatofibromas are highly vascular and have been designated **sclerosing hemangioma** in the past. Examples with extensive hemosiderin deposition have been designated **hemosiderotic dermatofibroma,** which may represent an early evolutionary stage of aneurysmal benign fibrous histiocytoma. **Aneurysmal fibrous histiocytoma** is an important variant to recognize because it is frequently misdiagnosed as a vascular proliferation (ie, Kaposi sarcoma, angiosarcoma) Histopathologically, aneurysmal fibrous histiocytoma tends to be very cellular with characteristic cleft-like or gaping pseudovascular spaces containing red blood cells, lacking an endothelial lining. The cleft-like spaces often have an artifactual appearance, giving the impression that the histotechnician cut the section using a dull blade. Examination of the periphery of the tumor shows features typical of dermatofibroma, with characteristic wrapping of collagen by lesional cells. **Atypical fibrous histiocytoma (dermatofibroma with monster cells)** denotes a variant with pleomorphic cells and bizarre giant cells. Although mainly dermal, approximately one-third of the lesions extend into the subcutis. Some cases also show worrisome features usually not seen in dermatofibroma such as unusually large size (>2 cm) and geographic necrosis. There is a variable proportion of pleomorphic cells with plump, spindle, or polyhedral cells with large hyperchromatic, irregular, or bizarre nuclei. Multinucleated giant cells are often present with bizarre nuclei and foamy, sometimes hemosiderin-rich cytoplasm. The background often shows classical features of dermatofibroma such as a storiform growth pattern and entrapped hyaline collagen bundles, especially at the periphery. Mitotic activity is variable, and atypical mitoses are sometimes seen. In the largest reported series, 2 of 59 patients developed metastases, although referral bias may have occurred in this study. **Epithelioid fibrous histiocytoma** is an underrecognized variant of dermatofibroma comprised largely of polygonal or rounded often binucleated cells with abundant eosinophilic cytoplasm. This variant is often exophytic with a collarette. The nuclei often are vesicular with small nucleoli. As with many variants of dermatofibroma, the periphery of the lesion often shows typical features of dermatofibroma. Perhaps the most problematic variant of dermatofibroma is **cellular fibrous histiocytoma**. This variant shows a more densely cellular fascicular growth pattern and may infiltrate fat in a limited fashion, causing confusion with DFSP or leiomyosarcoma. An admixture of inflammatory, foam cells, and giant cells often is present but sparse. Necrosis may be present, and normal mitoses are common. In difficult cases, immunohistochemistry may be helpful. The tumors are typically positive for factor XIIIa, stromelysin, and D2-40. While CD34 may be focally weakly positive in dermatofibroma, it is strongly diffusely positive in DFSP. Smooth muscle actin is positive in a majority of cases of dermatofibroma; however, other smooth muscle markers (desmin and caldesmon) are negative. The cellular variant must be distinguished from DFSP and leiomyosarcoma. Fascicular growth of eosinophilic spindled cells with ovoid to cigar-shaped nuclei, perinuclear vacuoles, and smooth muscle actin and desmin expression are characteristic of leiomyosarcoma. Extensive infiltration into fat in a sieve-like pattern and CD34 immunoreactivity are characteristic of DFSP. The presence of inflammatory cells, multinucleated giant cells, Touton-type giant cells, and xanthoma cells are supportive of dermatofibroma. Expression of factor XIIIa in dermatofibroma may aid in the differential diagnosis. **Aneurysmal fibrous histiocytoma** may be confused with vascular tumors such as **spindle cell hemangioma** and **Kaposi sarcoma**. The presence of slit-like vessels and immunoreactivity for endothelial markers such as CD31 favors a vascular tumor and not a dermatofibroma, which contains artifact-like pseudovascular spaces without an endothelial cell lining. The presence of thick-walled muscular vessels or organizing thrombi favors spindle cell hemangioma. Examining the periphery of aneurysmal fibrous histiocytoma shows characteristic entrapment of collagen fibers. This feature is particularly helpful in the distinction from Kaposi sarcoma (KS). The spindle cells of KS are positive for HHV8, whereas dermatofibromas are consistently negative. **Epithelioid fibrous histiocytoma** may be confused with melanocytic lesions, including epithelioid nevi, and **Spitz nevus** in particular. A junctional component and immunoreactivity for S-100 protein establish the diagnosis of a melanocytic tumor. A simple iron stain may be helpful in confirming iron pigment in dermatofibroma, in contrast to melanin pigment in melanocytic nevi.

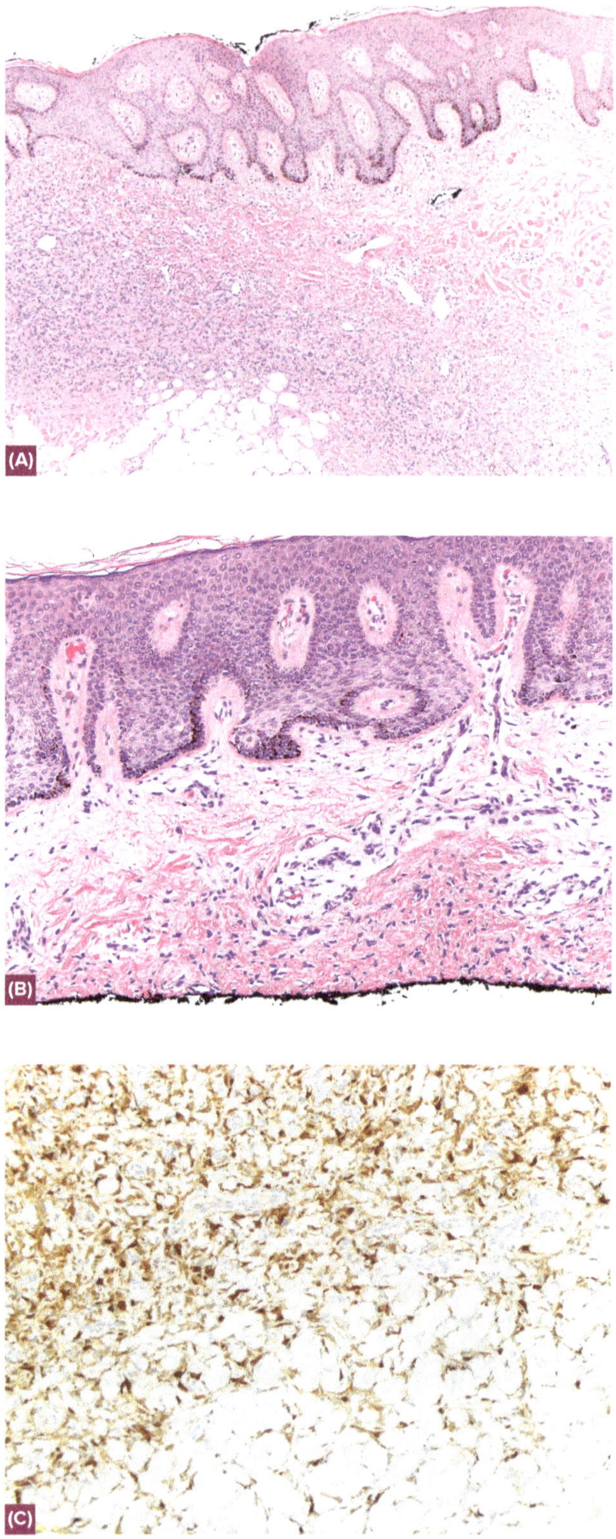

Dermatofibroma. (A) There is a dermal spindle cell proliferation with induction (acanthosis and hyperpigmentation) of the overlying epidermis. The cells approach but do not infiltrate the subcutaneous fat. **(B)** The basal keratinocytes within the epidermis may contain abundant melanin pigment and may be mistaken for lentigo on superficial biopsies. **(C)** The spindle cells express factor XIIIa via immunohistochemistry.

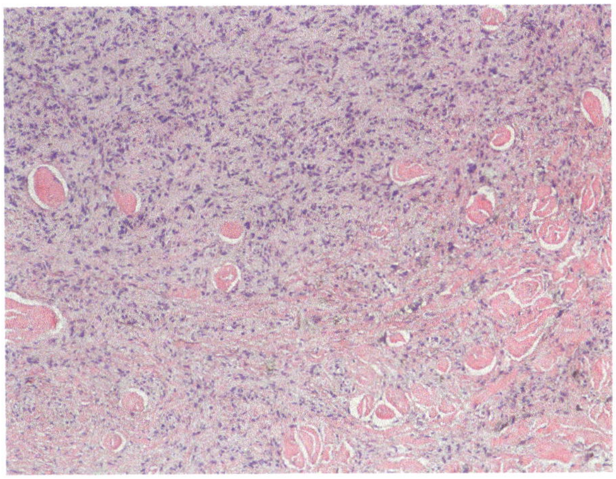

Dermatofibroma, high power. Note the tightly whorled fascicles of dendritic/spindle cells with extensive wrapping of collagen bundles at the periphery. Scattered hemosiderin-laden macrophages are also present.

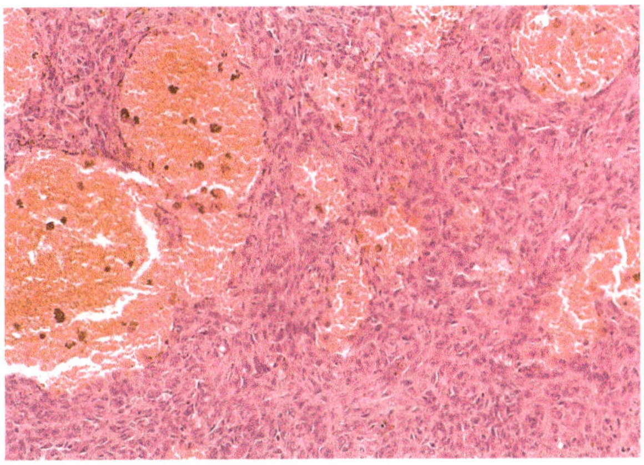

Aneurysmal fibrous histiocytoma is very cellular with characteristic cleft-like hemorrhagic pseudovascular spaces. Note the areas containing hemosiderin.

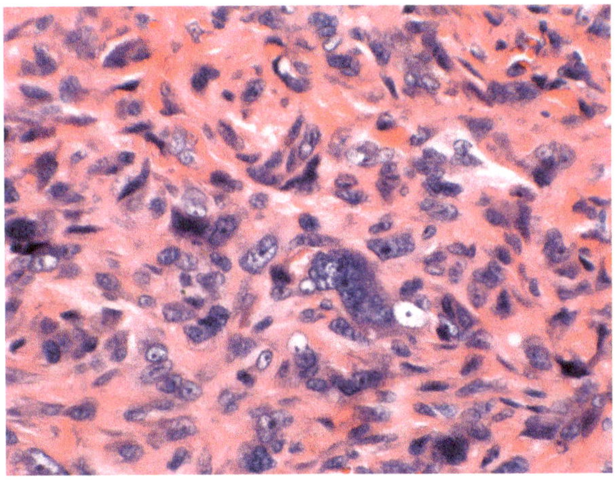

Atypical fibrous histiocytoma (dermatofibroma with monster cells). This variant shows scattered bizarre giant cells and cells with unusually plump nuclei superimposed on an otherwise typical dermatofibroma.

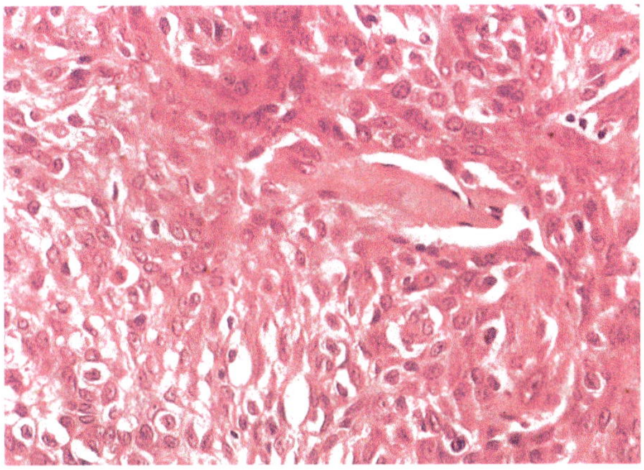

Epithelioid fibrous histiocytoma. This variant of dermatofibroma is composed of polygonal or rounded cells with abundant eosinophilic cytoplasm.

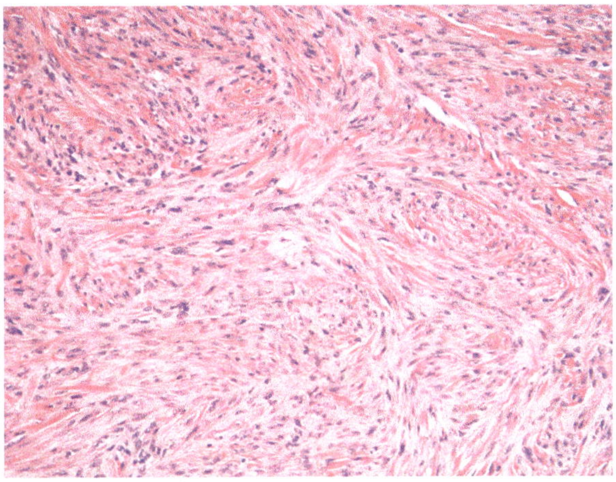

Cellular fibrous histiocytoma (cellular dermatofibroma). This hypercellular variant exhibits a fascicular pattern of growth and may rarely result in distant metastasis.

ANSWER 11-27: D.

Atypical fibroxanthoma is characterized by a highly pleomorphic histologic phenotype that is usually associated with benign biological behavior (Table 11-27A). Despite its seemingly malignant histologic features, atypical fibroxanthoma has little, if any, potential for metastasis and essentially is a benign tumor when strict diagnostic criteria are applied. Given the differences in behavior of atypical fibroxanthoma compared with other pleomorphic tumors, particularly **melanoma** and **spindle cell squamous cell carcinoma**, the pathologist must always approach atypical fibroxanthoma as a diagnosis of exclusion. These tumors almost exclusively arise in the sun-damaged skin of old adults, such as the face, bald scalp, superior ears, and forearms. Additionally, patients typically have a history of multiple squamous cell and basal cell carcinomas. Microscopically, the tumors are relatively symmetric, well-circumscribed, exophytic proliferations at

Table 11-27A. Atypical Fibroxanthoma

Clinical Features
- Sun-damaged skin of adults
- Head and neck
- Frequently rapidly enlarging, usually <1.5 cm
- Mistaken for squamous cell carcinoma, basal cell carcinoma clinically

Histopathologic Features
- Well circumscribed, symmetric at scanning magnification
- Located in the dermis with minimal extension in to subcutaneous tissue
- Marked nuclear pleomorphism, prominent nucleoli, hyperchromasia, and frequent multinucleated giant cells
- Mitoses are numerous and frequently atypical
- No necrosis or vascular invasion

Differential Diagnosis
- Squamous cell carcinoma
- Melanoma
- Pleomorphic sarcomas
- Metastasis

scanning magnification. The bulk of the tumor is located in the dermis; however, some tumors show very superficial extension into subcutaneous fat. Tumors involving the superficial dermis may exhibit a grenz zone between the epidermis and the neoplasm or extend to the dermal-epidermal interface, often with ulceration. Intraepidermal pagetoid spread is not seen, and the presence of intraepidermal malignant cells should raise the possibility of **melanoma** or **pleomorphic/spindle cell squamous cell carcinoma** with pagetoid spread. An epidermal collarette is quite common but is a nonspecific finding. The lesional cells range from highly pleomorphic bizarre forms with marked hyperchromasia and irregular nuclear outlines to more uniform spindled cells. Most cases show marked nuclear pleomorphism, prominent nucleoli, hyperchromasia, and frequent bizarre multinucleated tumor giant cells. Mitoses are often numerous and frequently atypical. Tumor cells often are arranged in a focally storiform pattern. Some tumors show a relatively monomorphic fascicular pattern that mimics **leiomyosarcoma**. Inflammatory cells, especially lymphocytes and histiocytes, including lipidized cells, are frequently seen within the tumor. Multinucleated giant histiocytes, including Touton-type giant cells, are also commonly noted. Importantly, however, necrosis and vascular or perineural invasion are not seen. The diagnosis of atypical fibroxanthoma must be carefully approached as a diagnosis of exclusion because all other tumors considered in the differential diagnosis are metastasizing malignant neoplasms. If strict criteria are followed, atypical fibroxanthoma may be regarded as benign neoplasms cured by simple excision. An unequivocal diagnosis of atypical fibroxanthoma should not be rendered in cases with atypical features. Atypical features that portend potential aggressive behavior include significant extension into adipose tissue, necrosis, and vascular invasion. Deeply invasive tumors raise the possibility of pleomorphic sarcomas including **leiomyosarcoma** (SMA+, desmin+), **pleomorphic liposarcoma** (S100+), **malignant peripheral nerve sheath tumor** (CD56+, PGP9.5+, S100+/−), and **pleomorphic rhabdomyosarcoma** (myoglobin+, MyoD1+, SMA+, desmin+). Immunohistochemical

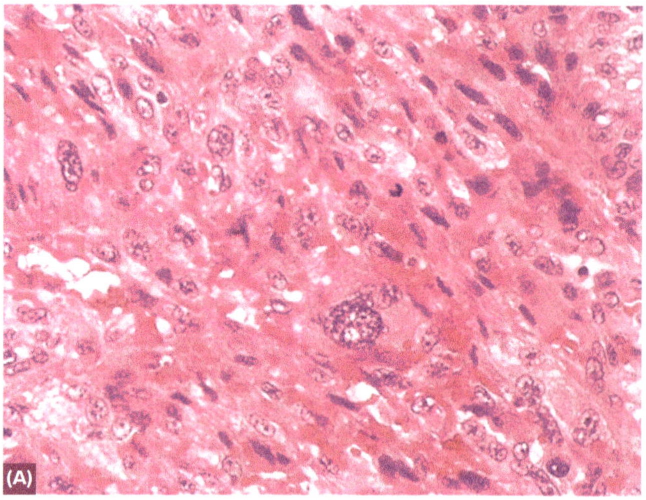

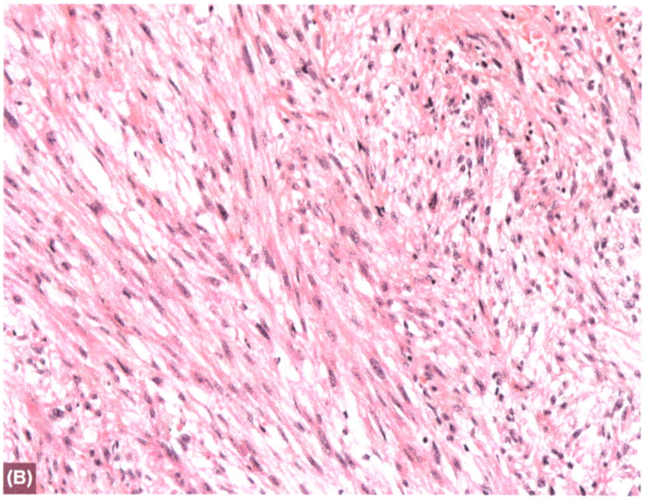

Atypical fibroxanthoma. (A) The composite cells range from highly pleomorphic bizarre forms with marked hyperchromasia and irregular nuclear outlines. **(B)** Occasional cases are composed of more uniform spindled cells. Mitoses are often numerous and frequently atypical. The tumor cells are often arranged in a storiform or fascicular pattern. (Reproduced, with permission, from Barnhill RL, Crowson NA, Magro CM, Piepkorn MW. *Dermatopathology*. 3rd ed. New York, NY: McGraw-Hill Education; 2010. Courtesy of Dr. A. Folpe, Mayo Clinic, Rochester, MN.)

studies may be helpful in the differential diagnosis. These studies should never be used to "rule-in" a diagnosis of atypical fibroxanthoma; rather, they are used to rule out other tumors. By definition, AFX is negative for S100 and cytokeratin. Nonspecific markers that are commonly expressed include vimentin, CD10, CD99, calponin, CD68, CD163, α_1-antitrypsin, and α_1-antichymotrypsin. Reactivity with cytokeratins, p63, and p40 suggests **spindle cell squamous cell carcinoma**, perhaps the most common simulant of atypical fibroxanthoma. Because atypical fibroxanthoma arises in severely sun-damaged skin, the presence of actinic keratosis or squamous cell carcinoma in situ in the same biopsy should not reflexively lead to a diagnosis of pleomorphic squamous cell carcinoma but nevertheless should be sought carefully. Keratin immunoreactivity is helpful in this situation. It is not surprising that atypical fibroxanthoma may coexist with other tumors related to sun exposure, especially basal cell carcinoma and squamous cell carcinoma. **Pleomorphic or spindle cell melanoma** must also be considered in the differential diagnosis of atypical fibroxanthoma. The epidermis should be examined for atypical intraepidermal malignant melanocytes and precursor lesions. Immunoreactivity for S-100 protein and HMB45 or Melan-A/MART-1 suggest melanoma; however, it should be kept in mind that HMB45 and Melan-A/MART-1 results are often negative in spindle cell or pleomorphic melanomas. It should be noted that scattered Langerhans cells and histiocytes immunoreactive for S-100 protein are commonly present within atypical fibroxanthoma and must be distinguished from immunoreactivity in tumor cells. Spindle cell variants of **angiosarcoma** may also rarely simulate atypical fibroxanthoma. In most cases, careful histologic evaluation reveals more typical areas of angiosarcoma, with dissecting vascular channels lined by hyperchromatic cells. Demonstration of CD31 expression is diagnostic of spindled forms of angiosarcoma, although as with S-100 protein, care must be taken not to mistake CD31-positive intralesional macrophages for reactive tumor cells. Tumors with morphologic and immunophenotypic features of AFX but exhibit the atypical features described above are best categorized and treated as a **superficial form of malignant fibrous histiocytoma.**

ANSWER 11-28: D.

Dermatofibrosarcoma protuberans (DFSP) is a locally aggressive fibroblastic neoplasm, which affects individuals over a wide age range, from children to the elderly, but occurs most commonly in young and middle-aged adults (Table 11-28A). The tumor presents as a slowly enlarging plaque and subsequent nodule that is frequently present for many years before diagnosis. After long periods of stable size or slow growth, tumors may enlarge rapidly. The most commonly affected sites are the trunk and proximal extremities. The extent of tumor infiltration of the underlying tissue is

Table 11-28A. Dermatofibrosarcoma Protuberans

Clinical Features
- Most common in young and middle-aged adults
- Slowly enlarging nodule or plaque
- Trunk and proximal extremities
- Tumors may enlarge rapidly
- Recurrence rate (20%) depends on wide local excision with generous free margins
- Occasional tumors metastasize

Histopathologic Features
- Diffuse infiltration of subcutaneous tissue with entrapment of fat creating a sieve-like pattern
- Uniform population of cells with spindled nuclei, scant cytoplasm
- Whorled or storiform pattern
- Inflammatory cells and xanthoma cells are absent or sparse
- Mitotic rate is usually <5 mitoses per 10 high-power fields
- Variants: myxoid change, fibrosarcoma-like areas, giant cell fibroblastoma-like foci, dendritic melanin-containing cells, myoid nodules

Differential Diagnosis
- Cellular dermatofibroma
- Neurofibroma
- Pleomorphic sarcoma
- Myxoid liposarcoma
- Myxofibrosarcoma

frequently underestimated, making surgical removal with tumor-free margins difficult. Tumors with uninvolved surgical margins of 3 cm or greater have a lower recurrence rate (20%) than tumors with narrower margins. Surgical clearance via Mohs micrographic surgery has been shown to offer the lowest recurrence rate. Although it has been difficult to estimate the incidence of metastatic disease, occasional tumors metastasize. Metastases seem to occur almost exclusively in recurrent lesions that have undergone **fibrosarcomatous transformation** after multiple excisions. The overall incidence of metastases appears to be less than 0.5%.

Microscopically, these tumors tend to be localized to the reticular dermis and subcutis, usually sparing the superficial papillary dermis. The epidermis frequently is unremarkable, but ulceration may occur. At scanning magnification, there is diffuse infiltration of subcutaneous tissue with entrapment of fat by tumor cells, resulting in a sieve-like or honeycomb pattern. The tumor is composed of a remarkably uniform population of cells with relatively small oval or spindled nuclei and scant pale cytoplasm, arranged in a whorled or storiform pattern. In general, this storiform pattern is maintained throughout the tumor. DFSPs usually have prominent cellularity, and this cellularity is usually greatest near the center of the lesion. The tumor cells strongly and diffusely express CD34, and are negative for factor XIIIa, D2-40, and stromelysin. This monomorphous cellular appearance is attributed to a t(17;22) chromosomal translocation which leads to the expression of a fusion gene consisting of the PDGF B-chain gene (*PDFGB*) and the collagen gene *COL1A1*. Autocrine stimulation of the PDGF receptor PDGFR by *PDGFB* appears to play a role in tumor cell proliferation. Interestingly the tyrosine kinase inhibitor imatinib mesylate appears to inhibit these signals and has been used successfully in various studies, leading to its approval for the treatment of unresectable or metastatic dermatofibrosarcoma. Multinucleate cells, xanthoma cells, and inflammatory cells are generally sparse or absent, unlike **dermatofibromas**. The mitotic rate is usually less than 5 mitoses per 10 high-power fields. Although most DFSPs are remarkably similar histopathologically with a monomorphous cellular appearance, some tumors display heterogeneity, including extensive myxoid change, hyalinization, fibrosarcoma-like areas, and giant cell fibroblastoma–like foci. Although it has been thought that tumors with a significant amount of fibrosarcoma-like areas have a worse prognosis, this does not appear to be true for lesions that have received appropriate surgical therapy. DFSP containing scattered dendritic melanin-containing cells have been termed **pigmented DFSP** or **Bednar tumor**. Although these cells are S100, Melan-A, and HMB45 positive, the lesional spindle cell population is negative for these markers, distinguishing the tumor from a spindle cell melanoma.

Although traditionally categorized separately, **DFSP** and **giant cell fibroblastoma** are now thought to represent histopathologic variants of the same entity since they both share a t(17;22) chromosomal translocation (Table 11-28B). Additionally, these tumors share a similar prognosis and immunohistochemical profile. Giant cell fibroblastoma typically occurs in much younger patients and features a myxoid matrix and pseudovascular spaces lined by floret-like giant cells. For small biopsy specimens, the main differential diagnosis is cellular dermatofibroma. Hyperplastic pigmented epidermal rete, inflammatory cell infiltrates, foam cells, and entrapment of collagen all favor dermatofibroma. **Paucicellular DFSPs** can be very difficult to distinguish from superficially biopsied **dermatofibromas** in which the characteristic infiltration of fat is not appreciated. Fortunately, the clinical appearance of dermatofibroma, that is, a small firm hyperpigmented nodule, is quite different from the gross appearance of DFSP. Thus, clinical information may be helpful in difficult cases. For equivocal tumors in which the base of the lesion is not visualized, it is prudent to request reexcision so that the entire lesion may be examined. Nearly all cases of DFSP are immunoreactive for CD34, an attribute helpful in distinguishing DFSP from dermatofibroma, which is positive for factor XIIIa, D2-40, and stromelysin. It should be recognized that cellular dermatofibromas may contain a reactive collar of CD34-positive cells, and care should be taken not to misdiagnose such cases as DFSP. DFSP may mimic **neurofibroma,** particularly in small biopsies. Careful search for more cellular areas with a storiform pattern usually leads to the correct diagnosis. Immunostaining for S-100 protein is very helpful because DFSP, unlike virtually all neurofibromas, is not immunoreactive with this marker. **Pleomorphic sarcomas** may also have a prominent storiform pattern. Although focal pleomorphism may occur in DFSP, marked pleomorphism favors a pleomorphic sarcoma. DFSP with extensive myxoid change may mimic **myxoid liposarcoma**; however, "chicken wire" vasculature and the lipoblasts are diagnostic of liposarcoma. Extensive sampling of DFSP with myxoid change almost always reveals areas with more typical histologic features. Scattered cells with marked pleomorphism, pseudolipoblasts, and characteristic arcuate vessels distinguish **myxofibrosarcoma** from **myxoid DFSP.**

Table 11-28B. Giant Cell Fibroblastoma

Clinical Features
Young children, particularly boys
Asymptomatic subcutaneous lesions of the trunk, groin, and lower extremities
30%-50% of cases recur after surgical excision
Histopathologic Features
Irregular pseudovascular spaces lined by multinucleated giant cells
Hypocellular hyalinized ribbons of collagenous tissue
Diffuse spindle cells
Storiform pattern resembling dermatofibrosarcoma protuberans in some cases
Differential Diagnosis
Vascular tumor or hemangioma
Dermatofibrosarcoma protuberans
Giant cell angiofibroma

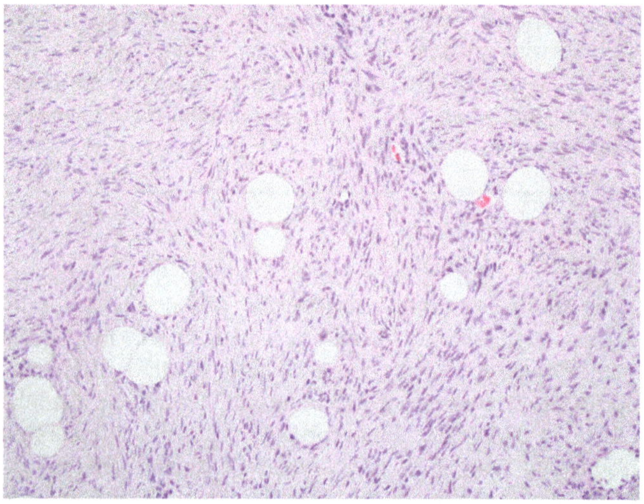

Dermatofibrosarcoma protuberans. There is a storiform (haphazardly arranged) spindle proliferation with scattered foci of entrapped fat.

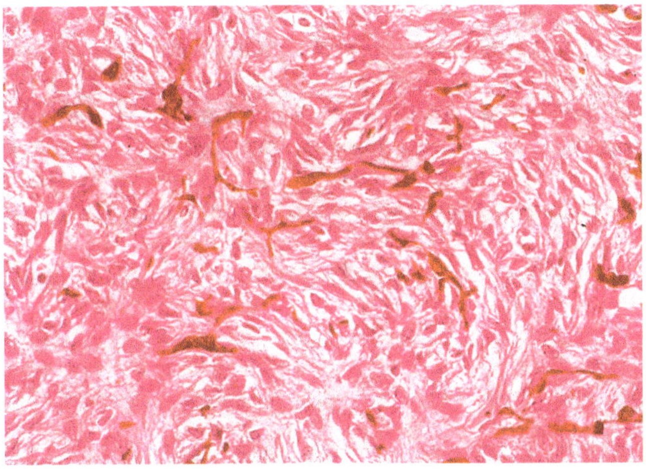

Pigmented DFSP (Bednar tumor). This tumor contains scattered pigmented dendritic melanocytes. Otherwise, the tumor is chiefly composed of typical monomorphous spindled fibroblasts.

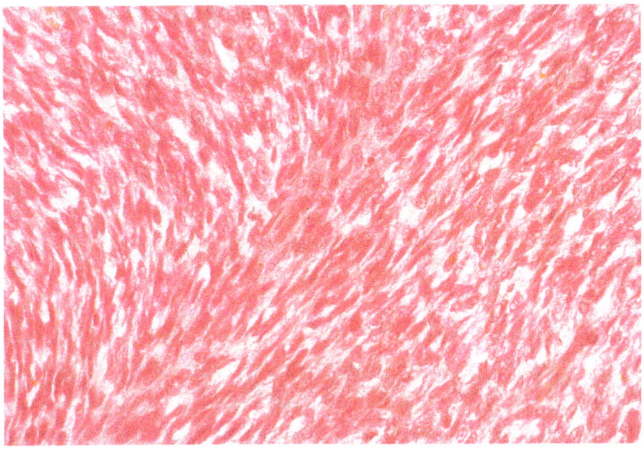

Dermatofibrosarcoma protuberans (DFSP) with fibrosarcomatous change. This DFSP shows areas identical to fibrosarcoma. Tumors with a significant degree of fibrosarcoma-like areas following multiple re-excisions may have a worse prognosis.

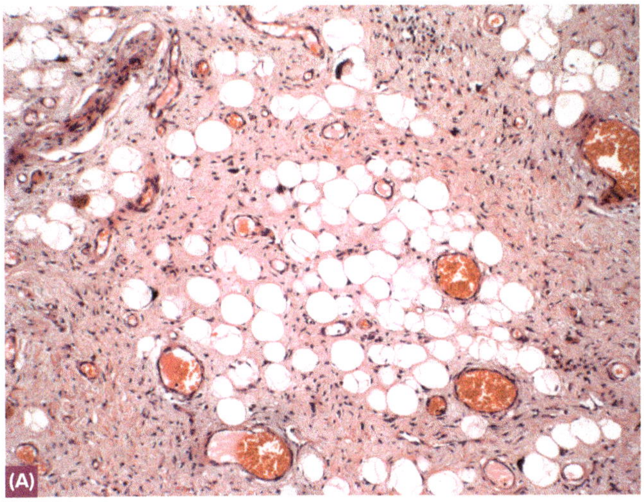

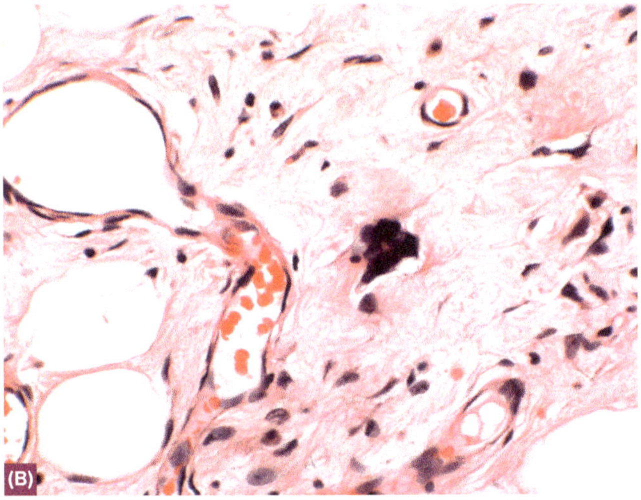

Giant cell fibroblastoma. (A) Scanning magnification shows pseudovascular spaces separated by ribbons of fibrous tissue consisting of fibroblastic spindle cells, which diffusely infiltrate the subcutaneous tissue. **(B)** High-power view of multinucleated floret-like giant cells.

ANSWER 11-29: A.

Infantile digital fibromatosis (inclusion body fibromatosis) occurs nearly exclusively in young children and infants (Table 11-29A). Most occur in children under 1 year of age, and one-third are present at birth. Approximately one-third of patients have multiple tumors that may affect both hands and feet, and these may be asynchronous. Most tumors are smaller than 2 cm, asymptomatic, and tend to be located

Table 11-29A. Infantile Digital Fibromatosis

Clinical Features
Asymptomatic dermal or subcutaneous nodule, <2 cm
Involvement of fingers and toes, especially lateral aspect
Sparing of the great toe and thumb
More than half recur after excision
Spontaneous regression in most cases
Rare cases in adults and at extradigital sites
Histopathologic Features
Poorly circumscribed
Sweeping fascicles of (myo)fibroblasts
Pathognomonic eosinophilic inclusions, stain with trichrome and PTAH (phosphotungstic acid-hematoxylin)
Differential Diagnosis
Dermal scar
Dermatofibroma

on the lateral aspect of the digit. Rare tumors with identical pathologic features have been observed in adults. In this population, the lesion tends to occur in nondigital locations. Because recurrence is common after excision and most of these lesions regress eventually without therapy, only clinical follow-up of these lesions is warranted unless functional compromise or symptoms dictate otherwise. Microscopically, the tumor is poorly circumscribed and composed of interlacing bundles of fibroblasts and myofibroblasts in variably collagenous stroma. Lesions may be located primarily in the dermis or extend deeply into the subcutaneous tissue, even to periosteum. Nuclei are uniform, spindled, and somewhat wavy. The pathognomonic intracytoplasmic eosinophilic (often orange-red) inclusions vary from a fraction of the size of a red blood cell to several times larger and are frequently located next to the nucleus. The inclusions may be rare or numerous. Staining with trichrome or smooth muscle actin is helpful to identify inclusions in cases in which they are difficult to locate on routine hematoxylin and eosin (H&E) staining.

The other answer choices are soft tissue tumors that also characteristically affect children. **Fibrous hamartoma of infancy** is a distinctive fibrous proliferation that occurs most often in children younger than 2 years of age and shows a predilection for boys (Table 11-29B). Approximately 15% of the tumors are present at birth. The patient presents with an ill-defined subcutaneous mass usually in the shoulder, upper arm, or axillary region. Less common sites include extremities, pubic area, and scrotum. Most tumors are smaller than 5 cm, may develop slowly or rapidly, and may be mobile or adherent to muscle or fascia. These tumors are not prone to spontaneous regression if followed clinically or recurrence after surgical excision. Microscopically, the tumors are situated in the deep dermis, are unencapsulated but relatively circumscribed, and are composed of four distinctive elements: (1) fascicles of pale eosinophilic spindle cells of varying width; (2) organoid nests of primitive appearing, round to spindled cells within a myxoid background. The myxoid matrix is Alcian blue positive, and staining is abolished with hyaluronidase pretreatment; (3) mature fat dispersed in varying amounts; (4) scar-like fibrous tissue. These four elements may be present in varying proportions. The spindle cells appear to be composed of actin-positive myofibroblasts and fibroblasts.

Table 11-29B. Fibrous Hamartoma of Infancy

Clinical Features
Children <2 years of age with a predilection for boys
15% of tumors are present at birth
Slowly or rapidly growing ill-defined subcutaneous mass
Shoulder, upper arm, or axillary region
Usually no spontaneous regression
No recurrence after surgical excision
Histopathologic Features
Fascicles of eosinophilic spindle cells
Organoid nests of primitive appearing round to spindle cells within a myxoid matrix, mature fat dispersed in varying amounts
Scar-like fibrous tissue
Differential Diagnosis
Infantile myofibromatosis
Connective tissue nevus

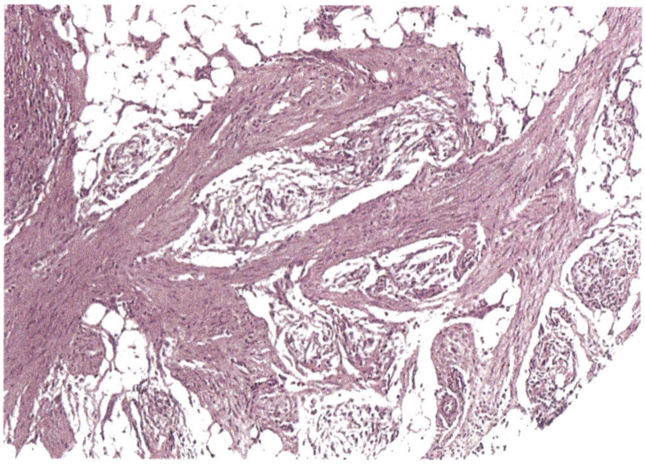

Fibrous hamartoma of infancy. Note the fascicles of palely eosinophilic spindle cells, organoid nests of primitive cells within a myxoid background, and fat.

Plexiform fibrohistiocytic tumor characteristically occurs in the upper extremities of boys and young men (Table 11-29C). This tumor is considered to be a low-grade neoplasm because of the potential for local recurrence as well as even metastasis. It is characterized by an alternating arrangement of nodules and fascicles of fibroblastic cells which interdigitate and entrap subcutaneous adipose tissue, similar to **dermatofibrosarcoma** and **giant cell fibroblastoma**. In addition to fascicles, there are characteristic nodules of histiocytes and multinucleated giant cells, mimicking

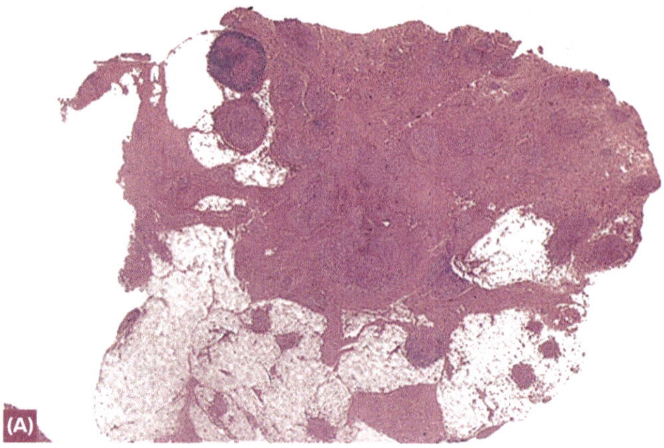

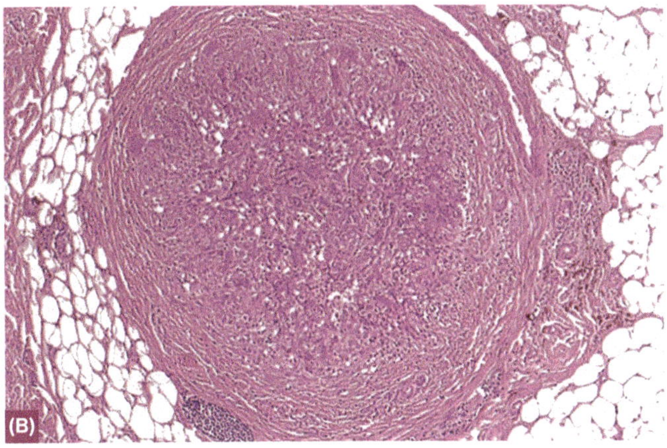

Plexiform fibrohistiocytic tumor. (A) Scanning magnification shows fascicles of fibroblastic cells arranged in a complex plexiform pattern. **(B)** High-power view shows nodular aggregates of histiocyte-like cells associated with osteoclast-like multinucleated forms surrounded by fibrous tissue.

granulomatous inflammation. Although mitoses are rare and cytologic atypia and necrosis are absent, lymphovascular invasion may be seen. Recognition of both fascicles of fibroblastic cells and histiocytic nodules is essential for a correct diagnosis.

Table 11-29C. Plexiform Fibrohistiocytic Tumor

Clinical Features
- Mainly children and young adults; more common in girls and young women
- Ill-defined, slow-growing nodule or mass, usually between 1 and 3 cm
- Upper extremity in nearly two-thirds of patients, particularly the shoulder and forearm
- 38% recur after excision; rare nodal or lung metastases

Histopathologic Features
- Fascicles of fibroblastic cells arranged in a complex plexiform pattern
- Aggregates of histiocyte-like cells, often with osteoclast-like multinucleated cells and associated lymphocytes
- Hemorrhage common in histiocytic nodules
- Pleomorphism is usually not present, and mitoses are rare

Differential Diagnosis
- Infectious process
- Primary granulomatous disease
- Fibromatosis
- Fibrous hamartoma of infancy
- Giant cell tumor of tendon sheath
- Giant cell tumor of soft tissues

Angiomatoid fibrous histiocytoma (AFH) was once considered a subtype of **malignant fibrous histiocytoma** due its high cellularity; however, two large studies have shown AFH to have a local recurrence rate of only 12% and a metastatic rate of 1% to 5% (Table 11-29D). For these reasons, the World Health Organization has reclassified AFH as a **fibrohistiocytic tumor of intermediate malignancy** rather than as a fully malignant sarcoma. Microscopically, these tumors are well circumscribed and composed of multiple nodules and sheets of uniform epithelioid to spindled cells with abundant eosinophilic cytoplasm and uniform ovoid vesicular nuclei. These nodules tend to be distributed in a densely collagenous stroma often containing hemosiderin pigment. The tumor is frequently surrounded by a pseudocapsule, and a cuff of chronic inflammatory cells that may be dense and associated with germinal center formation is present at the periphery of the tumor. The presence of hemorrhagic spaces lined by neoplastic cells may suggest a vascular neoplasm; however, the tumor cells are uniquely CD68+, desmin+, SMA−, and also negative for vascular markers (ie, CD31, CD34). A variety of growth patterns, including sheets, whorls, and short fascicles are typically seen in AFH, often within a given patient. Although AFH is typically cytologically bland, occasional cases may show striking pleomorphism, which has not been shown to have clinical significance. Aneurysmal and hemosiderotic variants of **dermatofibroma** may resemble AFH due to prominent pseudovascular change, hemorrhage, and hemosiderin deposition. Careful examination of **aneurysmal fibrous histiocytomas (aneurysmal dermatofibroma)** shows

Table 11-29D. Angiomatoid Fibrous Histiocytoma

Clinical Features
- Median age, 14 years
- Slowly enlarging deep dermal of subcutaneous growth
- Constitutional symptoms
- Local recurrence rate of 12% and metastasis rate of 1%-5%

Histopathologic Features
- Well-circumscribed multiple nodules and sheets of uniform epithelioid to spindled cells
- Cells show abundant eosinophilic cytoplasm and uniform vesicular nuclei
- Dense collagenous stroma, often with hemosiderin
- Usually shows pseudocapsule and cuff of chronic inflammatory cells, sometimes with germinal centers
- Hemorrhagic spaces lined by neoplastic cells

Differential Diagnosis
- Vascular tumors
- Aneurysmal and hemosiderotic variants of dermatofibroma
- Lymph node metastasis

the characteristic infiltration of spindled cells among preexisting collagen bundles, as well as a more polymorphous cell population, with siderophages and foamy macrophages. The characteristic cell of aneurysmal fibrous histiocytoma is also a spindled cell rather than the distinctly histiocytoid cell of AFH. All dermatofibromas lack a dense pseudocapsule.

Giant cell fibroblastoma is considered a variant of dermatofibrosarcoma that typically occurs younger patients and features a myxoid matrix and pseudovascular spaces lined by floret-like giant cells.

Infantile myofibromatosis is a disease of infants and young children with a predilection for boys. Some cases appear to be inherited, mostly in an autosomal dominant pattern. The disease may be limited to a single lesion, or multifocal lesions involving bones and viscera, particularly the lungs and gastrointestinal tract, may be present. Early literature emphasized cases with systemic involvement, giving the false impression that this was the most common form of the disease. Larger series have concluded that the **solitary myofibromas** predominate (Table 11-29E). Immunohistochemical and ultrastructural evidence suggest that these tumors are myofibroblastic in origin. Adults may be affected by tumors that are histopathologically similar to infantile myofibromatosis; however, multiple lesions are rare in this population. For this reason, the tumors are termed **adult solitary myofibromas**. Clinically, skin and soft tissue lesions tend to be smaller than 3 to 4 cm and often present in the perinatal period as small subcutaneous or soft tissue nodules or a poorly defined swelling. The head, neck, and trunk are the most common sites of skin and soft tissue involvement. Because lesions may recur after surgical excision and most lesions eventually show spontaneous regression if left untreated, close clinical follow-up after diagnosis is a reasonable clinical approach. Children with multiple lesions often show involvement of bones. Patients with visceral involvement, particularly lung and gastrointestinal tract, have a worse prognosis, with a potentially fatal outcome. The adult solitary myofibroma usually presents as a solitary subcutaneous nodule or mass in a wide variety of sites, but a head and neck location is most common. Visceral involvement is not seen in adults. Recurrence is rare.

Microscopically, the tumors are well circumscribed but unencapsulated and are composed of two distinct elements that are present in varying proportions. First, broad, sweeping fascicles or whorled nodules of myoid-appearing spindle cells with bland nuclei and abundant eosinophilic cytoplasm resembling myofibroblasts are present. The second component is characterized by more cellular areas of primitive small round to spindled cells with scant cytoplasm. This primitive cellular

Table 11-29E. Infantile Myofibromatosis and Solitary Myofibroma

Clinical Features
- Mainly infants and young children
- Predilection for boys
- Subcutaneous or soft tissue nodule, <3-4 cm
- Head and neck and trunk are the most common sites
- Lesions may recur after surgical excision
- Many lesions show spontaneous regression
- Minority of patients have bone or visceral involvement

Histopathologic Features
- Circumscribed but unencapsulated
- Sweeping fascicles or whorls of spindled cells with bland nuclei and abundant eosinophilic cytoplasm
- More cellular zones of smaller round to spindled cells with scant cytoplasm associated with hemangiopericytoma-like vascular pattern
- Necrosis, vascular invasion, and mitoses may be present

Differential Diagnosis
- "Infantile hemangiopericytoma"
- Fibromatosis
- Fibrous hamartoma of infancy

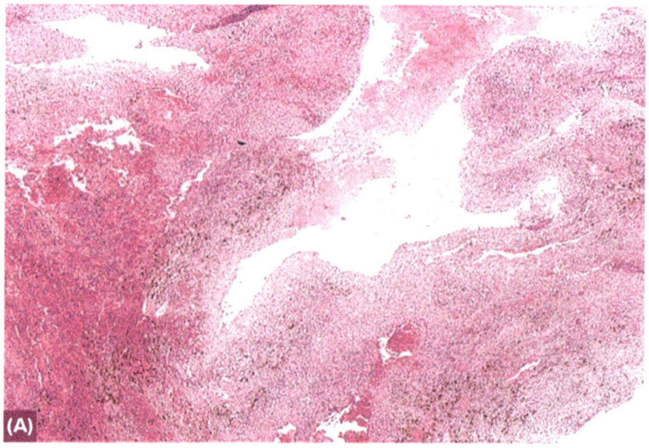

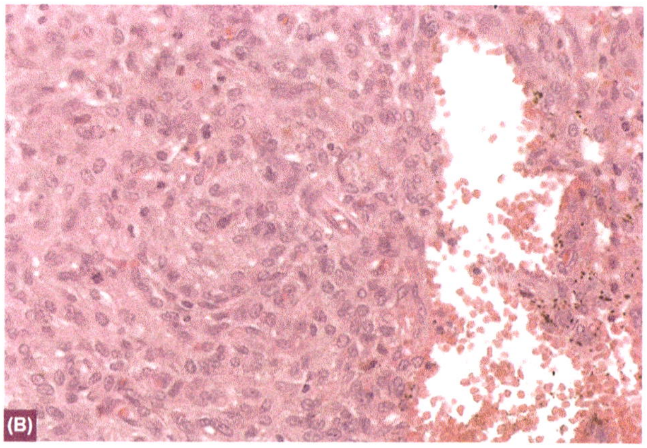

Angiomatoid fibrous histiocytoma. (A) At low magnification, this tumor shows large hemorrhagic spaces that may suggest a vascular neoplasm. **(B)** Higher magnification shows the tumor to be composed of highly cellular sheets of uniform epithelioid to spindled cells with abundant eosinophilic cytoplasm and uniform ovoid vesicular nuclei. These cells are not reactive for endothelial markers.

component is often associated with a hemangiopericytoma-like pattern of branching vessels (**"stag-horn vessels"**). A distinctly zonal appearance is seen in most myofibromas, with the myoid zones typically present at the periphery of the lesion and the primitive zones more centrally located. Several features may lead to a mistaken diagnosis of malignancy; necrosis, vascular invasion, and mitoses may be present. The spindled cells usually stain with actin. Solitary myofibroma of adults is histopathologically similar to the infantile form, except that there is often only a small component of primitive cells with a hemangiopericytoma-like vascular pattern. Stromal hyalinization, sometimes with a pseudochondroid appearance, is quite common. The distinctive zonal architecture of childhood myofibromas is seen less often in adult cases. The biphasic pattern of myofibroma also allows differentiation from **fibromatosis. Fibrous hamartoma of infancy** contains fascicles of myofibroblasts that are similar to those seen in **infantile myofibromatosis**. The former is distinguished by the presence of distinctive whorled organoid nests of primitive spindled cells in myxoid stroma as well as areas of disorderly fibrosis and mature adipose tissue. Most important is the recognition that mitoses, necrosis, and vascular invasion may be observed in infantile myofibromatosis and are not indicative of a malignant neoplasm. Vascular invasion is also a feature in up to one-third of adult lesions. A summary of fibrous and fibrohistiocytic tumors arising in children is provided in Table 11-29F.

Table 11-29F. Fibrous and Fibrohistiocytic Tumors in Children

Tumor of finger or toes composed of myofibroblasts in fascicles, characteristic eosinophilic inclusions = **infantile digital fibromatosis**
Biphasic tumor composed of sweeping or whorled fascicles of myofibroblasts alternating with hemangiopericytoma-like areas = **infantile myofibromatosis**
Paucicellular nodules composed of ribbons of PAS+ glassy hyaline eosinophilic material = **juvenile hyaline fibromatosis**
Biphasic tumor composed of anastomosing bands of fibrous tissue and nodular aggregates of histiocyte-like cells resembling granulomas, creating a plexiform pattern = **plexiform fibrohistiocytic tumor**
Myxoid tumor with giant cells lining pseudovascular spaces, CD34+ = **giant cell fibroblastoma**
Tumor of hand or feet composed of spindled to epithelioid cells, with palisading around foci of calcification cells = **calcifying aponeurotic fibroma**
Tumor composed of fascicles of eosinophilic spindle cells, distinctive organoid nests within a myxoid background, mature fat dispersed and fibrous tissue = **fibrous hamartoma of infancy**

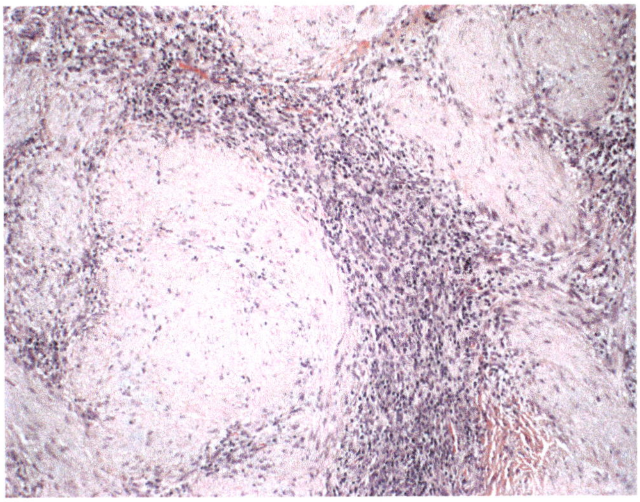

Myofibroma(tosis). These tumors, especially in children, show distinct zonation, usually with a peripheral rim of distinctly myoid-appearing spindled cells, and a central region of less mature, hemangiopericytoma-like cells.

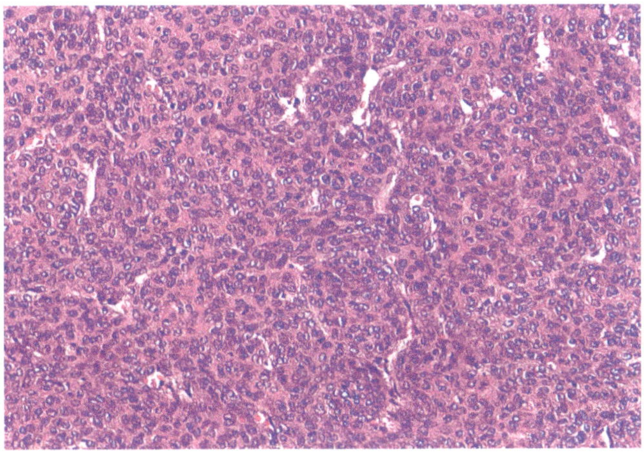

Myofibroma(tosis). The primitive cellular component often is associated with a hemangiopericytoma-like pattern of branching vessels.

ANSWER 11-30: B.

Nodular fasciitis is a reactive myofibroblastic proliferation notorious for being misinterpreted as a sarcoma (Table 11-30A). On the other hand, sarcomas may also be misinterpreted as nodular fasciitis, resulting in patients not receiving appropriate therapy promptly. To complicate matters, this reactive proliferation shows a variety of distinct histologic patterns. Most lesions are rapidly growing, often painful, subcutaneous or deep soft tissue masses, usually several centimeters in greatest dimension. Comparable lesions may arise primarily in the dermis. Alarmed patients often present with the history of a mass growing rapidly over the course of a week to several weeks, and some patients even testify to lesions growing "overnight." It must be emphasized, however, that some examples of nodular fasciitis

Table 11-30A. Nodular Fasciitis

Clinical Features
- Rapidly growing and often tender
- Subcutaneous or deep soft-tissue masses, usually several centimeters in greatest dimension
- Young adults
- Upper limb, particularly the forearm
- In children, most lesions in the head and neck region
- Recurrence is rare

Histopathologic Features
- May be well circumscribed or show infiltrative borders
- Cellularity varies within the tumor
- Areas of low cellularity have a distinctive myxoid, feathery background
- Short to broad, sweeping fascicles, focal storiform pattern
- "Tissue-culture" myofibroblasts with vesicular nucleus with occasional prominent nucleoli
- Essentially no cytologic atypia
- Mitoses may be abundant
- Inflammatory cells and multinucleated osteoclast-like giant cells may be seen
- Ganglion-like cells in proliferative fasciitis

Differential Diagnosis
- Fibromatosis
- Sarcoma, particularly low-grade myxofibrosarcoma and fibrosarcoma

are reported to have been present for an extended period, and such history does not exclude this diagnosis. Most patients are young adults; however, the overall age range is wide. The upper limb, particularly the forearm, is the most common site of involvement. In children, most lesions are seen in the head and neck region. **Cranial fasciitis**, a distinctive form of nodular fasciitis seen in infants, involves the soft tissue of the scalp and may erode into underlying bone. Recurrence is observed in 1% to 2% of cases and is most likely a result of inadequate surgical excision of growing lesions. Biopsy material from recurrent tumors must be reevaluated carefully to ensure that the original lesion was diagnosed correctly. Microscopically, this process most commonly involves the fascia and subcutaneous fat, but a rare dermal variant has also been described. Lesions may be either well circumscribed or show infiltrative borders. At low power, the cellularity varies from one area to another. Areas of low cellularity have a distinctive microcystic or myxoid background, creating a loosely textured "feathery" appearance. Cells in both the cellular and paucicellular zones tend to be arranged in broad, sweeping, and interlacing fascicles. A storiform pattern may be seen focally. There is a granulation tissue–like proliferation of vessels with small thin-walled capillaries and venules admixed with larger feeder vessels. The dominant cell types are fibroblasts and myofibroblasts with a spindled shape and vesicular nuclei and occasional prominent nucleoli. Many of these cells show abundant tapering eosinophilic cytoplasm with frequent stellate forms. Their morphology has been likened to fibroblasts grown in tissue culture. Mitoses may be abundant but are never atypical. Pleomorphism and nuclear hyperchromasia are absent. Variable numbers of acute and chronic inflammatory cells are usually seen. Multinucleated osteoclast-like giant cells are often present, particularly in children and in intravascular lesions. Long-standing examples of nodular fasciitis may show abundant hyalinized matrix, with only focal areas of more typical, cellular histology. The majority of cases of nodular fasciitis show immunoreactivity for smooth muscle actin and muscle specific actin with a characteristic "tram-track" pattern; however, reactivity for desmin is usually not seen, although sometimes this may be affected by the antibody used. The spindle cells are also negative for CD34. The immunohistochemical profile and ultrastructural characteristics support a myofibroblastic origin for nodular fasciitis. Recurrent nodular fasciitis is rare, and pathologic material from patients with recurrent lesions must be examined critically and the original diagnosis carefully reassessed.

The differential diagnosis includes **dermatofibroma, fibromatosis,** and **fibrosarcoma** for older hyalinized forms of nodular fasciitis, and cutaneous **myxoma, myxofibrosarcoma,** and **myxoid liposarcoma** for the early myxoid forms of nodular fasciitis. Because of rapid growth, high mitotic activity, and a frequently infiltrative pattern, nodular fasciitis is often mistaken for a malignant neoplasm. The low-power pattern of nodular fasciitis, with distinctive alternating cellular and paucicellular "feathery" myxoid zones, taken with the bland cytologic features, establishes the correct diagnosis. At higher power, "tissue culture" fibroblast-like cells with vesicular nuclei, absence of nuclear hyperchromasia, together with absence of atypical mitoses (tripolar or quadripolar), help exclude a diagnosis of sarcoma. Areas of dermal nodular fasciitis showing storiform patterns may be indistinguishable from **dermatofibroma**.

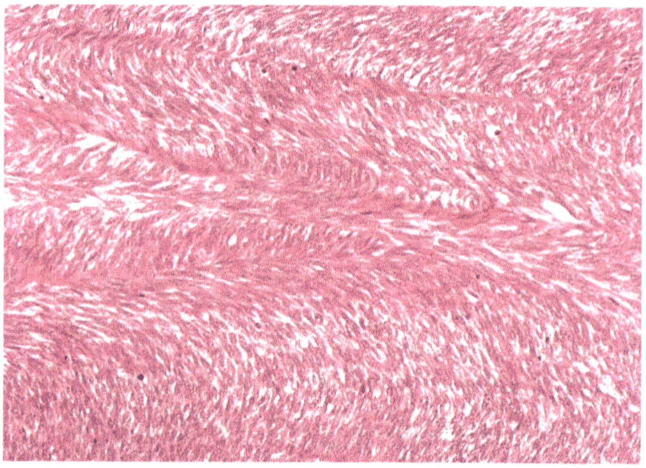

Fibrosarcoma. This tumor is composed of strikingly uniform spindled cells arranged in a herringbone configuration. Numerous mitotic figures are present throughout the tumor.

Nodular fasciitis is discriminated from dermatofibroma based on the other characteristic of "feathery" arrangements of uniform fibroblasts in broad, sweeping fascicles; myxoid alteration; and depth typical of nodular fasciitis. In addition, nodular fasciitis does not show collagen wrapping by tumor cells, a feature characteristic of dermatofibroma. **Fibromatosis** is more uniformly cellular and fascicular, is associated with more abundant dense collagen, and lacks the myxoid areas seen in nodular fasciitis. The fibroblasts in fibromatosis are more uniform and tend to have wavy nuclei. **Fibrosarcoma** was once considered the most common adult sarcoma, but since the introduction of immunohistochemistry and molecular techniques has essentially disappeared from the medical literature (Table 11-30B). Microscopically, fibrosarcoma is much more cellular, lacks the loose "feathery" pattern seen in nodular fasciitis, and is characterized by a herringbone fascicular pattern.

Cutaneous myxoma and **angiomyxoma** are benign tumors most commonly arising at acral sites, on the head, neck, and genital regions (Table 11-30C). Although myxomas are typically solitary lesions, numerous lesions may be the initial presentation of **Carney complex**, which is an autosomal dominant condition characterized by three major components: myxomatous masses (cardiac myxomas, cutaneous myxomas, myxoid fibroadenomas of the breast), spotty pigmentation of the skin (lentigines, blue nevi), and endocrine disorders (primary pigmented nodular adrenocortical disease, large cell calcifying Sertoli cell tumor of the testes, and pituitary adenomas). These tumors tend to be poorly circumscribed, paucicellular, and myxoid masses composed primarily of extracellular matrix, with a few scattered cells with a bland stellate to spindled cytomorphology. The absence of cytologic atypia is critical to exclude a **myxoid pleomorphic sarcoma**. Although small vessels may be abundant in

Table 11-30B. Fibrosarcoma

Clinical Features
- Adult form: deep-seated, slow-growing mass in the thigh or trunk
- Infantile form: children younger than 2 years of age, often congenital, superficially located
- Prognosis of infantile fibrosarcoma is much better than for the adult form

Histopathologic Features
- Uniform spindled cells arranged in herringbone fascicles
- Nuclei are slender with uniform chromatin and small, inconspicuous nucleoli
- Cytoplasmic borders not distinct
- High-grade tumors may have marked nuclear pleomorphism
- Hemangiopericytoma-like vascular spaces common in infantile tumors

Differential Diagnosis
- Fibromatosis
- Nodular fasciitis
- Malignant peripheral nerve sheath tumor
- Monophasic synovial sarcoma

Table 11-30C. Superficial Angiomyxoma and Cutaneous Myxoma

Clinical Features
- May be associated with the Carney complex
- Head and neck region of adults
- Slow-growing dermal or subcutaneous nodule, <3 to 4 cm
- May recur after surgical resection

Histopathologic Features
- Poorly circumscribed, paucicellular
- Myxoid matrix with widely scattered bland stellate and spindle fibroblasts
- Thin-walled blood vessels, lymphocytes, and neutrophils in varying numbers
- Mitoses may be seen
- Frequent association with epithelial proliferation, particularly cysts

Differential Diagnosis
- Low-grade myxofibrosarcoma
- Myxoid liposarcoma
- Aggressive angiomyxoma

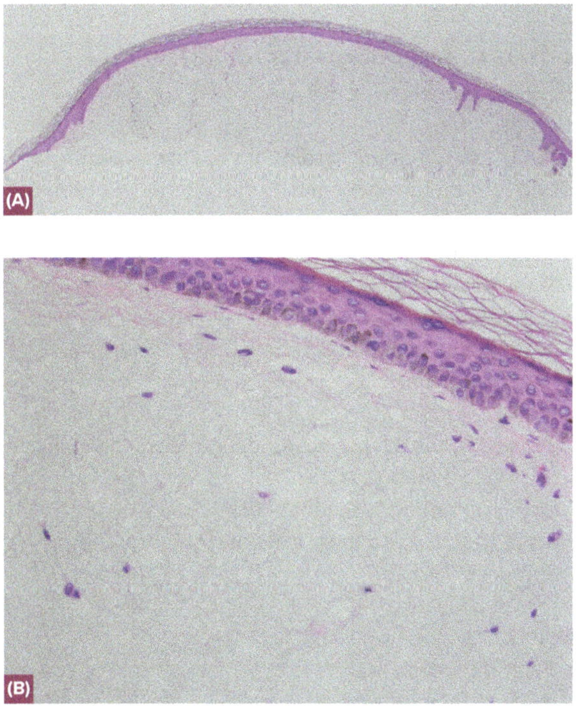

Cutaneous myxoma. (A) There is a poorly circumscribed, paucicellular, myxoid mass in the dermis. **(B)** Rare scattered stellate fibroblasts are present throughout the myxoid stroma.

angiomyxoma, the presence of thick-walled, curvilinear vessels should prompt concern for **myxofibrosarcoma**. A unique form of angiomyxoma with predilection for the pelvic region in women is referred to as **aggressive angiomyxoma**, due to a tendency for local recurrence following excision despite the fact the tumor does not invade the adjacent tissues.

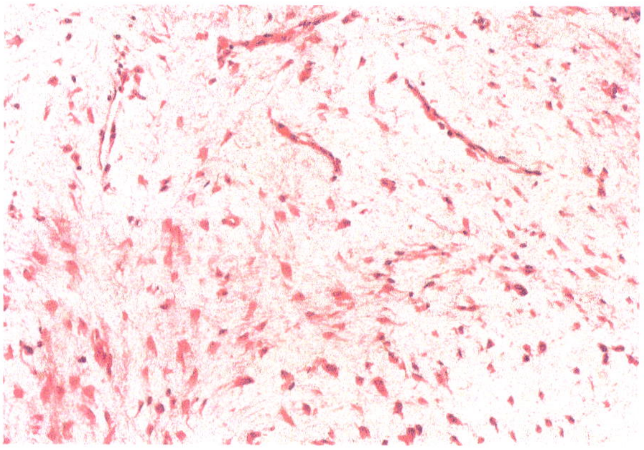

Superficial angiomyxoma. Typical myxoid paucicellular tumor with bland cytomorphology and thin-walled vessels.

Myxofibrosarcoma (formerly **myxoid malignant fibrous histiocytoma**) is occasionally misdiagnosed as nodular fasciitis (Table 11-30D). It is commonly seen on the arms and legs of older adults. It shows a spectrum of differentiation with good correlation between histologic grade and prognosis; low-grade tumors have little metastatic potential. Overall survival is 60% to 70% for all grades. Recurrence is common, with 57% within 5 years, as shown in a recent large study. At the well-differentiated end of this spectrum (low-grade), the tumor is typically hypocellular with scattered hyperchromatic spindle cells in a myxoid background. The most defining features of **low-grade myxofibrosarcoma** include a multilobular pattern of growth, true nuclear atypia, and thick-walled arcuate (or curvilinear) vessels with surrounding stromal condensation. **High-grade myxofibrosarcoma** may resemble other poorly differentiated **pleomorphic sarcomas**, such as malignant fibrous histiocytoma. Most importantly, high-grade myxofibrosarcoma appears to have the same prognosis as malignant fibrous histiocytoma. Occasionally, tumor cells in myxofibrosarcoma may have vacuolated cytoplasms and indented nuclei, mimicking lipoblasts. However, the cytoplasm contains mesenchymal mucin rather than lipid and will stain positively with Alcian blue. This tumor is distinguished from nodular fasciitis by characteristic curvilinear vessels and the presence of cells with atypical hyperchromatic nuclei and vacuolated cytoplasm that may resemble lipoblasts.

Table 11-30D. Myxofibrosarcoma

Clinical Features
- Usually located in the extremities of elderly adults
- Often located in subcutaneous tissue or deep dermis
- Correlation between histologic grade and prognosis; low-grade tumors have little metastatic potential
- Overall survival, 60%-70%

Histopathologic Features
- Myxoid hypocellular areas composed of acid mucopolysaccharide
- Arcuate vessels in myxoid areas
- Cells within the myxoid areas are spindled and stellate with atypical nuclei
- Mucin-containing "pseudolipoblasts"
- Abrupt transition to more cellular or high-grade pleomorphic areas

Differential Diagnosis
- Nodular fasciitis
- Benign myxomas
- Superficial angiomyxoma
- Myxoid liposarcoma
- Low-grade fibromyxoid sarcoma

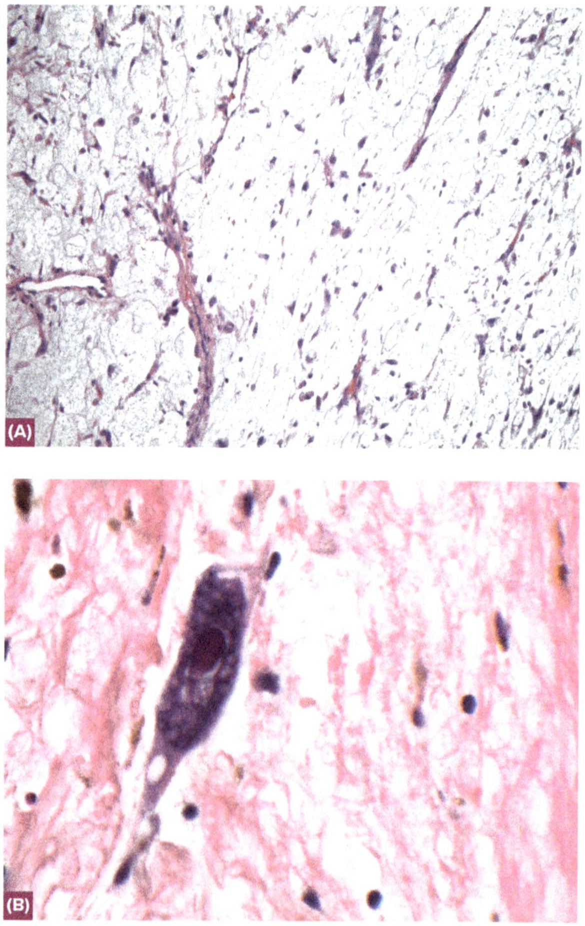

Myxofibrosarcoma. (A) Note the myxoid stroma and characteristic arcuate or curvilinear blood vessels with surrounding stromal condensation. **(B)** Scattered bizarre pleomorphic (lipoblast-like) cells are present in a myxoid background.

Myxoid liposarcoma arises in the deep soft tissues of the proximal lower extremity therefore this diagnosis should be made with caution when only a dermal-based lesion is present. These tumors exhibit a distinctive "chicken-wire" vasculature, distinct from the characteristic arcuate vessels of **myxofibrosarcoma**. A summary of differential findings for spindle cell tumors with a myxoid matrix is provided in Table 11-30E.

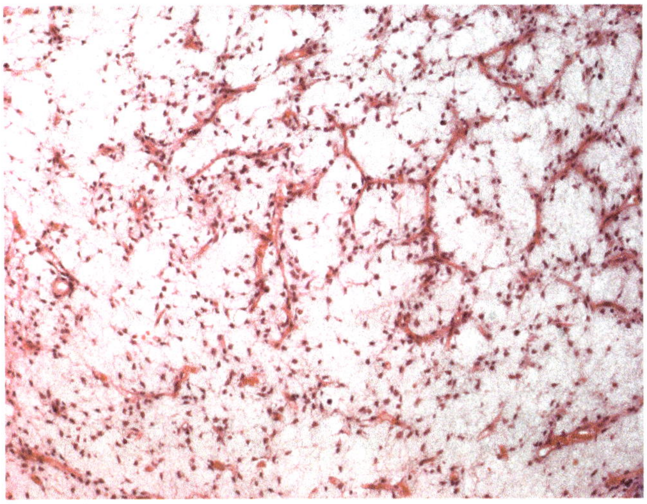

Myxoid liposarcoma. Arborizing "chicken wire" vasculature and bland mesenchymal cells and rare lipoblasts (not visualized).

Table 11-30E. Tumors with a Prominent Myxoid Component

Curvilinear vessels, atypical cells, pseudo-lipoblasts = **myxofibrosarcoma**
Tissue culture fibroblasts within tumor with myxoid feathery zones alternating with hypercellular zones = **nodular fasciitis**
Myxoid tumor in child with giant cells lining pseudo-vascular spaces, CD34+ = **giant cell fibroblastoma**
Paucicellular nodule with very bland stellate and spindled cells, inflammatory cells and thin-walled blood vessels = **myxoma, angiomyxoma**
Paucicellular tumor with myxoid areas admixed with whorled collagenous component, very bland cells = **low-grade fibromyxoid sarcoma (Evan tumor)**

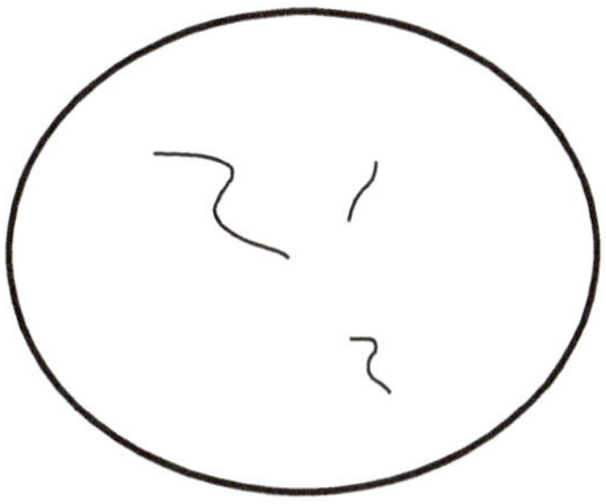

Myxoma. Small thin-walled vessels.

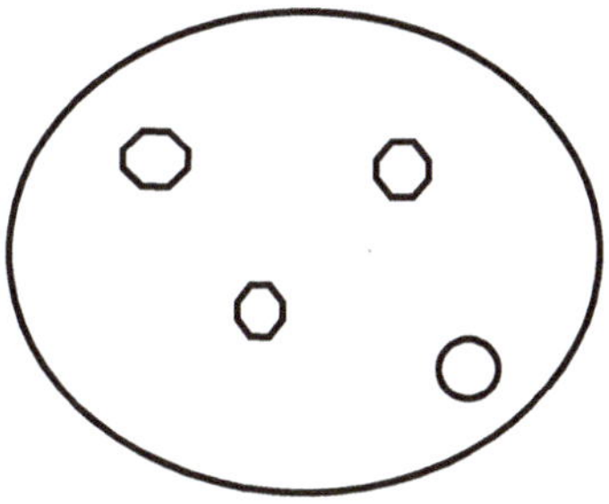

Aggressive angiomyxoma: Round thick-walled vessels.

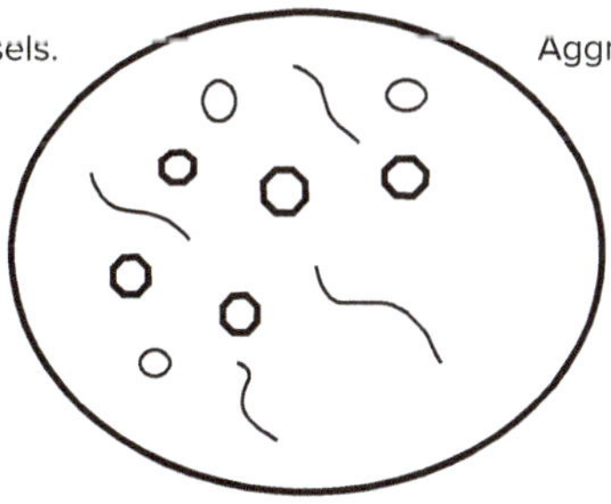

Nodular fasciitis: Granulation tissue–like vessels with small capillaries and larger "feeder" vessels. Exhibits foci of both hypo- and hypercellularity with scattered inflammatory cells.

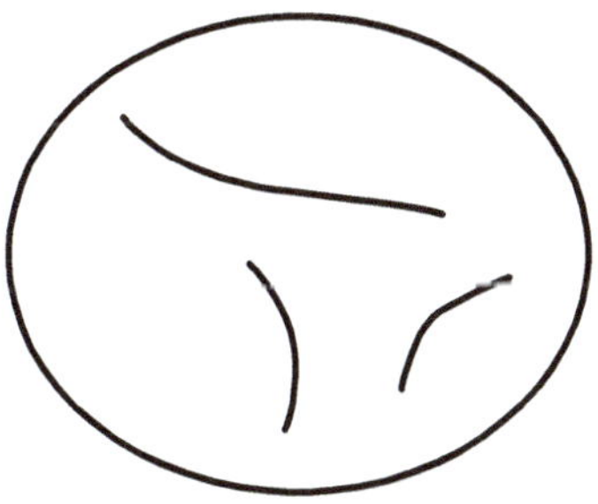

Myxofibrosarcoma: Curvilinear thick-walled vessels.

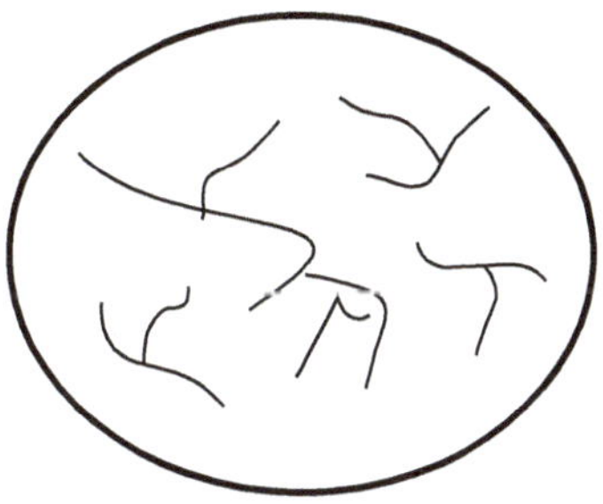

Myxoid liposarcoma: Arborizing "chicken wire" network of thin-walled vessels.

ANSWER 11-31: C.

Epithelioid sarcoma (ES) is an uncommon yet distinctive malignancy of uncertain pathogenesis (Table 11-31A). Recognition of this tumor is critical because it may be mistaken for a benign granulomatous process or infection. Tumors are most commonly located in the distal extremities, particularly the hand and fingers, of young adult men. Ulceration of the skin overlying superficial tumors is common. A "**proximal type" of epithelioid sarcoma** has also been described, in which case the tumor closely resembles a poorly differentiated carcinoma and frequently shows rhabdoid features. They are typically confined to the deep soft tissues of the pelvis, perineum, and genitals. Deep-seated tumors tend to be slow growing and show a multifocal growth pattern of local spread. Most tumors are a few centimeters in size at the time of presentation. Despite the initial clinical appearance of a single localized mass, pathologic examination often documents multifocal spread along tendons, nerves, and fascial structures in a serpiginous fashion. The characteristic early multifocal spread of this tumor and propensity for multiple recurrences demands early radical surgery. Metastases, usually to lymph nodes and lung, develop in at least 50% of patients. Even when this tumor appears localized clinically, early multifocal locoregional spread is often present, making surgical control a challenge. Patients often have multiple recurrences, and 5-year survival has been reported at approximately 50%. A recent study found 5- and 10-year disease-free survival rates of 34% and 17%, respectively. Prognosis correlates with tumor size, recurrence, and extent of tumor necrosis. Men tend to fare worse than women, and tumors in the distal extremities tend to do better than proximal and more centrally located tumors. Microscopically, **epithelioid sarcomas** frequently are multifocal with a plexiform and diffusely infiltrative pattern. They are composed of spindled to round cells with abundant eosinophilic cytoplasm and relatively uniform medium-sized nuclei. The spindled and epithelioid areas tend to gradually merge and have similar nuclear and cytoplasmic characteristics. A characteristic finding in approximately 40% to 50% of cases is tumor cells arranged in a palisade around areas of necrosis. This feature may lead to confusion with a granulomatous or necrobiotic process. Some tumors show a marked chronic inflammatory infiltrate, further contributing to this confusion. Cellular discohesion, producing a pseudovascular pattern, is also a common finding. Numerous mitoses are common. Epithelioid sarcoma has a propensity for neural and tendon sheath invasion. The tumor is immunoreactive for keratins, vimentin, and EMA. Approximately 50% of cases are CD34+. Loss of nuclear expression for INI-1 has been described in the majority of tumors studied. Immunoreactivity for keratins varies from focal to diffuse, but is present invariably. In regard to the differential diagnosis, distinguishing epithelioid sarcoma from necrobiotic granulomatous processes, such as **granuloma annulare, necrobiosis lipoidica,** and **rheumatoid nodule**, and **infection** may be difficult, particularly in small biopsies. Keratin immunoreactivity distinguishes epithelioid sarcoma from any of these granulomatous diseases. CD34 positivity is also not a feature of granulomatous diseases. Tumors that are discohesive form cleft-like pseudovascular spaces, and show intracytoplasmic vacuole formation may be mistaken for an epithelioid vascular neoplasm. Expression of specific vascular markers, such as CD31, ERG, or Fli-1 protein, establishes the diagnosis of a vascular neoplasm such as **epithelioid hemangioendothelioma** or **epithelioid angiosarcoma.** In fact, a rare low-grade vascular neoplasm with close histopathologic resemblance to epithelioid sarcoma, known as **epithelioid sarcoma-like hemangioendothelioma**, may be extremely difficult to distinguish from to ES. The importance of these vascular specific markers cannot be emphasized enough in establishing the correct diagnosis with potentially significant differences in prognosis. It should be noted that epithelioid angiosarcoma, epithelioid hemangioendothelioma, and epithelioid sarcoma–like hemangioendothelioma are also quite frequently immunoreactive for keratin and that both true vascular tumors and epithelioid sarcomas express CD34. The presence of overlying squamous cell carcinoma in situ, intercellular

Table 11-31A. Epithelioid Sarcoma

Clinical Features
- Most commonly located in the extremities, particularly in the hand and fingers
- Young adults males more often than females
- Tend to be slow growing and multifocal
- Propensity for multiple recurrences
- Metastases develop in 50%, usually to lymph nodes and lung
- Poor long-term prognosis

Histopathologic Features
- Spindled to round cells with abundant eosinophilic cytoplasm
- Palisade around areas of necrosis
- Some tumors show a marked chronic inflammatory infiltrate
- Immunoreactivity for keratins, vimentin, and epithelial membrane antigen

Differential Diagnosis
- Primary necrobiotic granulomatous processes (granuloma annulare, necrobiosis lipoidica, rheumatoid nodule)
- Granulomatous infection
- Giant cell tumor of tendon sheath
- Epithelioid angiosarcoma and epithelioid hemangioendothelioma
- Squamous cell carcinoma
- Melanoma
- Synovial sarcoma

bridges, and squamous pearls all help distinguish squamous cell carcinoma from epithelioid sarcoma. **Squamous cell carcinomas** are positive for p63, which is universally negative on ES. **Melanoma** is distinguished by the presence of melanin, associated melanoma in situ, or other precursor melanocytic lesions. In problematic cases, the immunohistochemical profile of melanoma allows distinction from epithelioid sarcoma; melanomas are, in general, nonreactive for keratins; immunoreactive for S-100 protein; and, at least when epithelioid, frequently express MART-1 or HMB45. Although both epithelioid sarcoma and **synovial sarcoma** show epithelial differentiation and express cytokeratin, they otherwise share almost no clinical or pathologic features and are therefore easily distinguished. **Plexiform fibrohistiocytic tumor (PFHT)** is considered a low-grade malignancy that occurs in children and young adults. Microscopically, PFHT is composed of plexiform fascicles of fibroblastic cells and well-defined histiocytic nodules with frequent multinucleated giant cells. Unlike PFHT, the spindled and epithelioid areas of ES tend to gradually merge and have similar nuclear and cytoplasmic characteristics. The spindled cells of PFHT are positive for vimentin and SMA. The histiocytic nodules are positive for CD68. There is no expression of S100, cytokeratin, CD45, Factor VIII, or desmin.

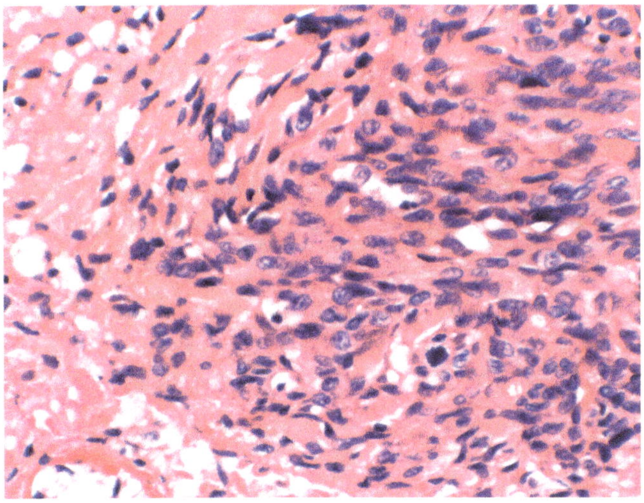

Epithelioid sarcoma. High magnification shows the neoplastic cells are round to spindled with abundant eosinophilic cytoplasm and relatively uniform nuclei.

ANSWER 11-32: B.

Lipomas are common and comprise up to 5% of all benign tumors and 25% to 50% of all soft tissue tumors (Table 11-32A). They are most common in the fifth and sixth decades of life. They occur anywhere but most are subcutaneous. The head and neck, arm, and upper thorax are often affected; lesions of the lower leg and hand are distinctly uncommon. Up to 7% are multiple; the latter are often more common in younger men. Solitary lesions affect men and women equally. Most are smaller than 5 cm in diameter. Fewer than 1% recur; recurrence suggests incomplete excision or possibly a more aggressive lipomatous lesion that has been misdiagnosed. Microscopically, lipomas are composed of lobules of mature adipose tissue enclosed in a thin fibrous capsule. The adipocytes are uniform in size and appearance. Fibrous tissue and scattered capillaries may also be present. Several histologic variants are recognized depending on the secondary features, such as myxoid change (**myxolipoma**) or fibrosis (**fibrolipoma**). Occasional cases have metaplastic bone or cartilage. Tumors embedded within a chondromyxoid stroma are referred to as **chondroid lipomas** (Table 11-32B). Degenerative changes, including foamy macrophages, lymphocytes, myxoid change, and calcification, may be seen. Multiple karyotypic abnormalities have been described, including rearrangement of chromosome bands 12q13-15, resulting in deregulation of the *HMGA2* gene, loss of material from or rearrangement of chromosome 13, and aberrations of chromosome band 6p21. In regard to the differential diagnosis, adipose tissue hypertrophy is similar but

Table 11-32A. Lipoma

Clinical Features
Adults
Upper body, but wide distribution
Histopathologic Features
Mature adipose tissue
Encapsulated
Differential Diagnosis
Angiolipoma
Lipomatosis
ALT/WDL

Table 11-32B. WHO Classification of Benign Adipocytic Tumors

Lipoma
Lipomatosis
Lipomatosis of nerve
Lipoblastoma or lipoblastomatosis
Angiolipoma
Myolipoma
Chondroid lipoma
Extrarenal angiomyolipoma
Spindle cell lipoma or pleomorphic lipoma
Hibernoma

lacks the circumscription of a lipoma or a capsule. However, some cases cannot be distinguished histopathologically based on sampling. **Nevus lipomatous superficialis** is a rare lesion of young adults most commonly presenting as unilateral lesions on the lower trunk or gluteal region. These are skin-colored papules that may coalesce into plaques with a cerebriform surface up to 10 cm in diameter. Single and multiple lesions occur; multiple lesions occur in younger patients and often are grouped in a zonal distribution on the buttock. Solitary lesions overlap clinically and histopathologically with **soft fibromas (fatty skin tags/fibrolipomas)**. Only rare recurrences are reported. Histopathologically, variable amounts of mature adipose tissue are present within the papillary dermis. This often is clustered around blood vessels of the superficial dermal vascular plexus, which may be increased in number. The overlying epidermis may be normal, acanthotic, or hyperkeratotic. A variable degree of myxoid change is often seen, and the histologic features of nevus lipomatous superficialis overlap significantly with dermal **spindle cell lipomas**. **Nodular-cystic fat necrosis** is a rare lesion of uncertain origin that may be confused with lipoma. It occurs in adolescent boys and middle-aged women, may be related to trauma, and consists of infarcted adipose tissue with well-preserved cell outlines and no nuclei contained within a thin fibrovascular capsule. It may occasionally show degenerative changes, including hyalinized pseudomembranes, which may resemble amyloid, and dystrophic calcifications. The absence of nuclei distinguishes it from lipoma. **Well-differentiated liposarcoma (WDL)** (aka **atypical lipomatous tumor** [ALT]) is the most important lesion to exclude. **Liposarcomas** are generally defined by the presence of enlarged hyperchromatic cells within irregular fibrous septa (**lipoblasts**), are often greater than 5 cm in size, and commonly are located in the thigh and retroperitoneum.

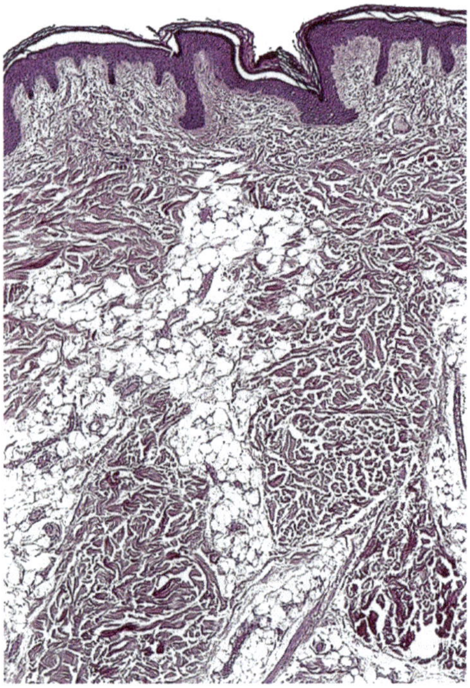

Nevus lipomatosus superficialis. A polypoid lesion containing mature adipose tissue that extends into the papillary dermis. When single, differentiation from a skin tag with herniation of adipose tissue may be impossible but is of little clinical significance.

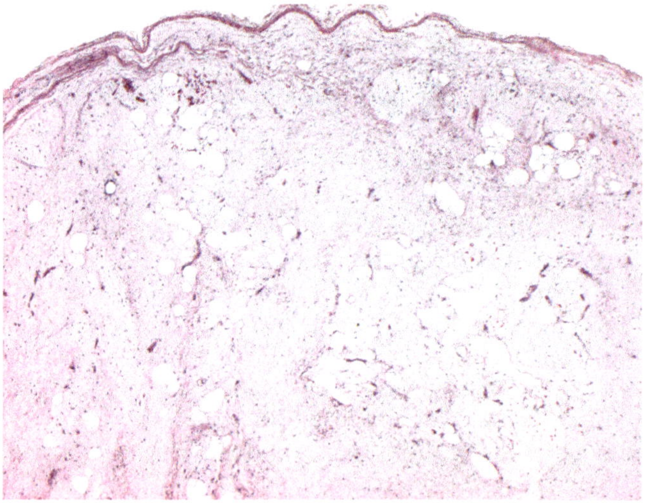

Myxolipoma. Abundant myxoid matrix may obscure the lipogenic nature of the tumor.

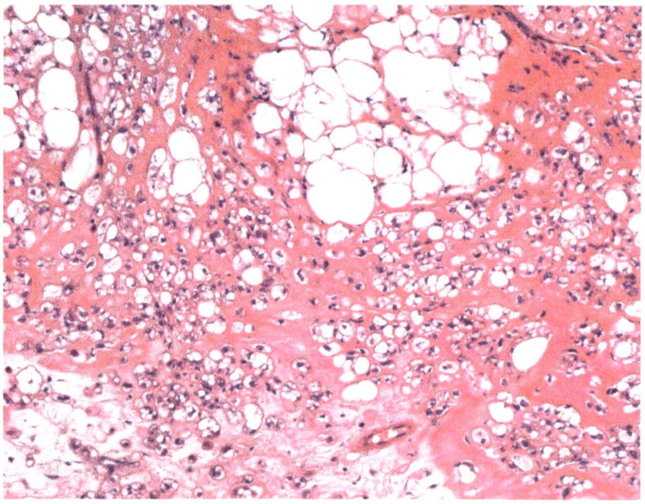

Chondroid lipoma. Vacuolated cells simulating lipoblasts arranged in nests admixed with adipocytes within a myxochondroid matrix.

ANSWER 11-33: A.

Compared with conventional lipomas, **angiolipomas** are one-fifth as common, occur at a younger age (17-24 years), are more commonly multiple, and often are painful (Table 11-33A). They occur most commonly in the forearm or on the trunk

Table 11-33A. Angiolipoma

Clinical Features
Young adults
Painful, often multiple
Upper body
Histopathologic Features
Mature adipose tissue
Capillaries (mainly peripheral)
Fibrin thrombi
Differential Diagnosis
Lipoma
Hemangioma
Angiomyolipoma

Table 11-33B. Hibernoma

Clinical Features
Young adults
Upper back
Histopathologic Features
Granular cells
Vacuolated cells
Mature adipose tissue
Differential Diagnosis
Lipoma

but also in similar locations as lipomas. Clinically, they may be firmer than lipomas, usually measure less than 2 cm, and are always subcutaneous. Angiolipomas are benign and cured by simple excision. Microscopically, the lesion is encapsulated and composed of mature adipose tissue and a variably prominent capillary network that is often denser at the periphery. The vessels may have a complex branching pattern and prominent pericytes. Fibrin microthrombi are present in almost all cases (seen in image B within the question). Examples in which the vascular component comprises the bulk of the lesion are known as **cellular angiolipomas**. The differential diagnosis includes **conventional lipoma, spindle cell lipoma, benign capillary hemangioma,** and **possibly early Kaposi sarcoma**. The normal karyotype of subcutaneous angiolipoma as well as its distinct clinical and morphologic features suggest a different pathogenesis from pure conventional lipomas. In cases with few capillaries, distinction from conventional lipoma may be difficult. The presence of fibrin thrombi may be helpful. Highly vascular lesions may be confused with hemangioma or even Kaposi sarcoma. In contrast to angiolipoma, **Kaposi sarcoma** has more poorly formed vascular spaces, solid aggregates of spindle cells, and hyaline globules and is poorly circumscribed. In **hemangiomas**, the capillaries radiate out from a central larger vessel, but in angiolipoma, the capillaries are located peripherally and radiate inward. **Spindle cell lipomas** with prominent vascularity may be similar but present in older individuals, are solitary, and have organized arrays of spindle cells often associated with hyaline collagen bundles. **Hibernomas** are tumors of brown fat (Table 11-33B). They arise usually in young to middle-aged adults (average age, 36 years) and are commonly located in the thigh, shoulder, and axilla. They are most often subcutaneous, well circumscribed, and measure up to 19 cm in diameter (mean, 10 cm). Occasional examples are intramuscular. **Hibernomas** are benign. Grossly, they usually have a yellow-brown, lobulated cut surface. Microscopically, three cell types are characteristically present. Intermediate-sized polygonal cells with abundant granular, eosinophilic cytoplasm, and centrally placed nuclei are often most common. Slightly larger cells with multiple cytoplasmic vacuoles that do not indent the centrally placed nucleus are also present. The third cell type resembles a mature adipocyte with a large, solitary vacuole displacing the nucleus off to the side. Four histologic variants are recognized. The **"typical" hibernoma** is composed of the aforementioned three cell types in varying proportions. The **"lipoma-like"** variant consists of only scattered hibernoma cells among white fat. The **"spindle cell"** variant combines the features of hibernoma and spindle cell lipoma. Last, the **"myxoid"** variant exhibits hibernoma cells in a myxoid matrix. The importance of these variants lies only in their recognition, not in their clinical behavior. The ultrastructural features differ from those of mature adipose tissue and include abundant mitochondria, basal lamina, and micropinocytotic vesicles. A summary of the differential features of the various forms of benign and malignant lipomatous neoplasms is provided in Table 11-33C.

Table 11-33C. Generalized Approach to Tumors of Adipose Tissue

Mature Adipose Tissue	
No other features	Lipoma
Thrombosed capillaries	Angiolipoma
Spindled cells, collagen, myxoid change	Spindle cell lipoma
Floret cells and spindle cells	Pleomorphic lipoma
Chondroblast-like cells and lipoblasts	Chondroid lipoma
Smooth muscle	Myolipoma
Brown fat	Hibernoma
Immature Adipose Tissue	
Young patient	Lipoblastoma
Older patient, presence of lipoblasts	Liposarcoma

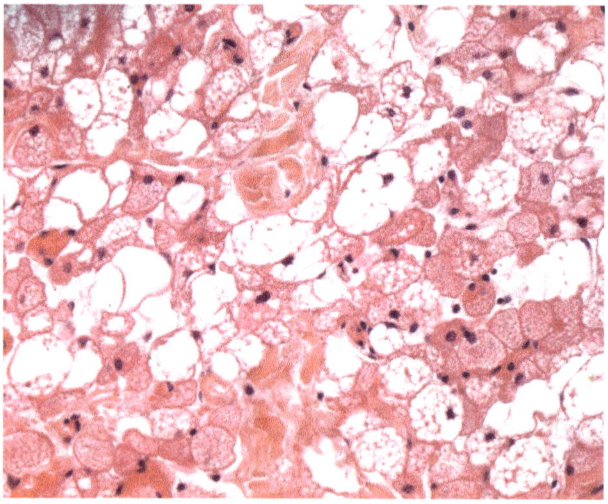

Hibernoma. Mixture of granular eosinophilic cells, multivacuolated cells, and mature adipocytes.

ANSWER 11-34: C.

Spindle cell lipoma occurs predominantly as a solitary subcutaneous mass in the shoulder and posterior neck of men between the ages of 45 and 70 years (Table 11-34A). A significant minority of cases arise on the face. Local recurrence is rare. Multiple spindle cell lipomas are rare and may mimic **Madelung disease (symmetrical lipomatosis)**. Familial and nonfamilial cases have been reported, with no risk of progression to liposarcoma. Both **spindle cell lipomas** and **pleomorphic lipomas** show karyotypic aberrations of 16q and 13q. Grossly, the lesions of spindle cell lipoma are circumscribed and average 4 cm in size (range, 1-14 cm). Microscopically, they are usually well demarcated and composed of variable amounts of mature adipose tissue, uniform spindle cells in a myxoid matrix, and thick (ropey) bundles of refractile collagen. Cases with little to no adipose tissue occur and are often mistaken for benign nerve sheath tumors (ie, **neurofibroma, schwannomas**). The spindle cells are small, with a single elongated nucleus and slender bipolar cytoplasmic processes. These cells stain positively for CD34 and are often oriented along bundles of collagen or form very short fascicles that are interspersed with the adipocytes. Mitoses are rare. It must be emphasized that otherwise typical spindle cell lipomas may contain lipoblasts. Cases with increased vascular areas and marked pseudoangiomatous degeneration have been described. Exceptional cases may contain bone or cartilage. When multiple spindle cell lipomas occur, the tumors become more cellular as the disease progresses, often with features of **pleomorphic lipoma**. Although pleomorphic cells are not present in classic spindle cell lipomas, it is well recognized that spindle cell and pleomorphic lipomas comprise a histologic spectrum of a single biologic entity. As such, hybrid lesions are not uncommonly encountered. The differential diagnosis includes **angiolipoma, classic pleomorphic lipoma, neurofibroma, myxoid liposarcoma, well-differentiated liposarcoma,** and **solitary fibrous tumor.** The characteristic age, gender, and site are very helpful in making the diagnosis of spindle cell lipoma. Heavily vascular cases may be mistaken for angiolipoma. **Pleomorphic lipomas** share a similar clinical presentation to spindle cell lipoma (Table 11-34B). Microscopically, they are circumscribed nodules composed of a mixture of variably sized adipocytes with a varying number pleomorphic enlarged cells. These cells contain moderate amounts of eosinophilic cytoplasm, are often multinucleated, and often have nuclei arranged in a circumferential pattern that has resulted in the term **floret cell.** The chromatin can be fine or smudgy and hyperchromatic. Rare **lipoblasts**, with cytoplasmic vacuoles indenting the nucleus, can also be found. Scarce mitoses may be present, but necrosis is not observed.

Table 11-34A. Spindle Cell Lipoma

Clinical Features
- Men
- Subcutaneous
- Shoulders, upper back, face

Histopathologic Features
- Mature adipose tissue
- Bland spindle cells
- Ropey collagen
- Mucinous background
- Mast cells

Differential Diagnosis
- Pleomorphic lipoma
- Neurofibroma
- ALT/WDL
- Solitary fibrous tumor

Table 11-34B. Pleomorphic Lipoma

Clinical Features
- Men
- Subcutaneous
- Shoulders, upper back, face

Histopathologic Features
- Mature adipose tissue
- Bland spindle cells
- Floret cells
- Rare lipoblasts

Differential Diagnosis
- Spindle cell lipoma
- ALT/WDL
- Solitary fibrous tumor

Quick Fact

Short List of CD34+ SPINDLE CELL Tumors

- Spindle cell lipoma
- Pleomorphic lipoma
- DFSP
- Solitary fibrous tumor
- Benign nerve sheath tumors

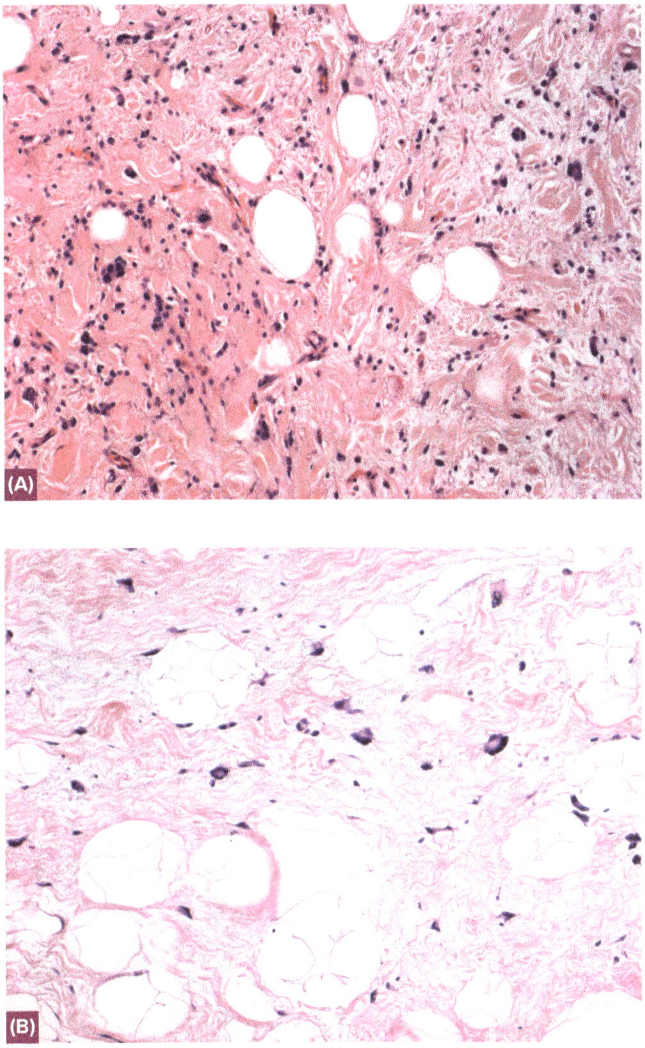

Pleomorphic lipoma. (A) Mature adipocytes and multinucleated floret-like cells. **(B)** The background may exhibit ropey collagen and rare mature adipocytes, or may be variably myxoid.

As mentioned previously, cases with a prominent spindle cell component may be confused with **neurofibroma**. However, in spindle cell lipoma, the nuclei are not as wavy, and the spindle cells are negative for S-100 (the adipocytes will be positive for S-100). Cases with a prominent myxoid background may be mistaken for **myxoid liposarcoma**. However,

Table 11-34C. Solitary Fibrous Tumor

Clinical Features
- Most common in pleura and soft tissues
- Rare in skin, with predilection of head and neck region
- Middle-aged and elderly patients
- Local recurrence described in skin tumors; 5%-10% of soft tissue and pleural tumors show aggressive behavior

Histopathologic Features
- Broad range of morphologic patterns
- Usually well-circumscribed with alternating hyper- and hypocellular areas
- Frequently prominent vascular network with branching hemangiopericytoma-like "Stag-horn" pattern
- Perivascular hyalinization and background of abundant, thick, hyalinized collagen
- Typically spindled or plump cells with minimal atypia, permeating between collagen bundles
- Occasionally adipocytic and myxoid areas
- CD34+/STAT6+ expression via immunohistochemistry

Differential Diagnosis
- Dermatofibroma
- Dermatofibrosarcoma protuberans

spindle cell lipoma has very monotonous spindle-shaped cells and abundant thick collagen, lacks the characteristic "chicken wire" vascular pattern, and usually lacks lipoblasts. Cellular cases may be mistaken for **well-differentiated liposarcoma (atypical lipomatous tumor)** or **sclerosing liposarcoma**. Well-differentiated liposarcoma may contain thick bundles of collagen but has a less uniform appearance, with large atypical cells clustered around fibrous septa. Well-differentiated liposarcomas are positive for MDM2 and CDK4 by immunohistochemistry, whereas pleomorphic and spindle cell lipomas are negative. Finally, very cellular lesions may resemble **solitary fibrous tumor** (Table 11-34C). Solitary fibrous tumors may contain mature adipose tissue and exhibit a similar immunohistochemical profile (so-called **lipomatous hemangiopericytoma**). However, spindle cell lipoma lacks the characteristic staghorn-like vessels of solitary fibrous tumor. In addition, the spindle cells of solitary fibrous tumor are more often curved rather than straight, do not form discrete fascicles, and are often less associated with either ropey collagen or a myxoid background. Lastly, solitary fibrous tumors uniquely exhibit nuclear expression of STAT6 via immunohistochemistry.

Dermatofibrosarcoma protuberans (DFSP) is also a CD34+ spindle cell proliferation that may exhibit histopathologic overlap with spindle cell lipoma. The presence of a

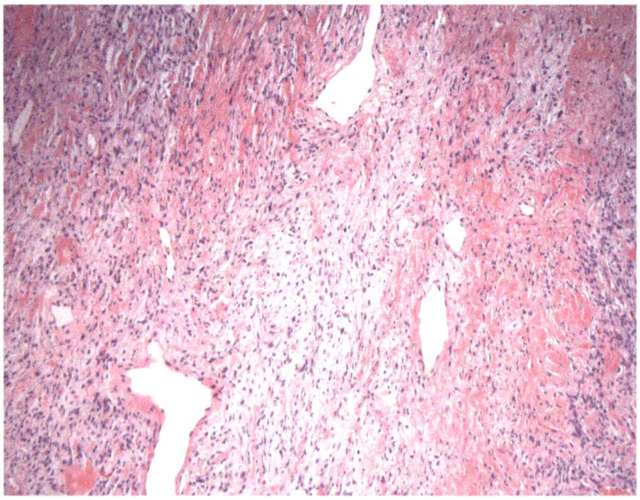

Solitary fibrous tumor. Alternating hyper- and hypocellular areas are present, with a prominent vascular network in a background of thick hyalinized stroma. The spindle cells will be positive for CD34.

diffuse infiltrative proliferation of spindle cells in a storiform pattern with adnexal entrapment by tumor cells is a feature that favors DFSP. Spindle cell lipoma is typically composed of an even distribution of spindle cells, ropey keloidal-like collagen, and fat. Spindle cell lipoma should lack adnexal structures. The diagnostic distinction on superficial biopsies may be extremely difficult and complete excision may be required for definitive diagnosis.

ANSWER 11-35: C.

Liposarcoma is the most common soft tissue sarcoma in adults and accounts for approximately 20% of all mesenchymal malignancies. Liposarcomas are most common in deep soft tissues, especially the thigh and retroperitoneum; however, they also occur, albeit relatively infrequently, in subcutaneous sites and rarely even in the dermis. The current WHO classification includes one neoplasm in the intermediate category and five categories of malignant fatty neoplasms with incorporation of relevant genetic findings (Table 11-35A).

The solitary entity within the intermediate (locally aggressive) category is **atypical lipomatous tumor/well-differentiated liposarcoma** (ALT/WDL) (Table 11-35B). Five distinct variants are recognized in the malignant category: **myxoid liposarcoma, round cell liposarcoma, pleomorphic liposarcoma, dedifferentiated liposarcoma,** and **mixed liposarcoma.** Despite this formal segregation, functionally, it is convenient to regard them as kindred entities, with dedifferentiated liposarcoma representing a unique biologic event occurring exclusively within ALT or WDL and myxoid or round cell liposarcoma representing a spectrum of the same entity. Taken together, most series show a male predominance and a mean age of 50 years (range, 30-80 years). However,

Table 11-35A. WHO Classification of Malignant Adipocytic Tumors

Malignant Behavior:
Well differentiated liposarcoma (i.e. retroperitoneal) = amplification ring from the long arm of chromosome 12 (*MDM2, CDK4*)
Dedifferentiated liposarcoma = amplification ring from the long arm of chromosome 12 (*MDM2, CDK4*)
Myxoid liposarcoma = t(12;16)(q13;p11) or t(12;22)(q13;q12)
Round cell liposarcoma = t(12;16)(q13;p11) or t(12;22)(q13;q12)
Pleomorphic liposarcoma = complex chromosomal abnormalities
Mixed type liposarcoma = t(12;16)(q13;p11) plus 6q deletions
Intermediate Malignant Behavior:
Atypical lipomatous tumor (i.e. extremity) = amplification ring from the long arm of chromosome 12 (*MDM2, CDK4*)
Lipoblastoma = 8q11–13 rearrangement

Table 11-35B. Atypical Lipomatous Tumor/ Well-Differentiated Liposarcoma

Clinical Features
Adults
Proximal extremities (for atypical lipomatous tumor)
Histopathologic Features
Mature adipose tissue with variably sized adipocytes
Hyperchromatic stromal cells
Lipoblasts
Differential Diagnosis
Lipoma
Pleomorphic lipoma
Lipoblastoma

myxoid or round cell tumors tend to occur 10 years earlier than well-differentiated and pleomorphic tumors.

Well-differentiated liposarcoma (WDL) of deep soft tissues is a well-recognized entity. When the same lesion occurs subcutaneously or in an intramuscular location, the preferred term is atypical lipomatous tumor (ALT) since this distinction indicates a markedly better prognosis. However, both terms (ALT and WDL) describe lesions identical both morphologically and karyotypically, thus the different terms are essentially synonyms. ALT/WDL occurs in adults of either gender, mainly in the fourth to eighth decades of life. Subcutaneous tumors are well circumscribed, 2 to 20 cm in diameter (mean 10 cm), and have a predilection for the upper and lower limb girdles. In subcutaneous lesions, recurrence is relatively infrequent. Metastases do not occur in an otherwise conventional well-differentiated liposarcoma and local recurrence rates are significantly lower in tumors confined to extremity (compared to retroperitoneum). However, dedifferentiation may take place in deep and rarely superficial lesions with subsequent metastatic potential.

Microscopically, these lesions superficially resemble lipomas. However, the adipocytes vary in size, and fibrous septae containing hyperchromatic pleomorphic stromal cells are often present. A varying number of monovacuolated or multivacuolated lipoblasts may be seen.

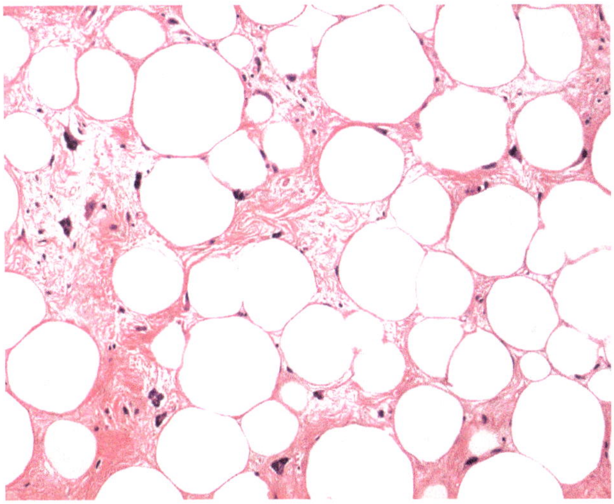

Well-differentiated liposarcoma/atypical lipomatous tumor. Variably sized adipocytes with scattered hyperchromatic stromal cells.

It is important to emphasize that the presence of **lipoblasts** does not make, and is not required, for a diagnosis of liposarcoma. Lipoblasts are strictly defined by the presence of single or multiple discrete, optically clear, round, and sharply demarcated cytoplasmic vacuoles that indent an enlarged hyperchromatic nucleus. A single lipoblast is present in the center of the illustration for this question.

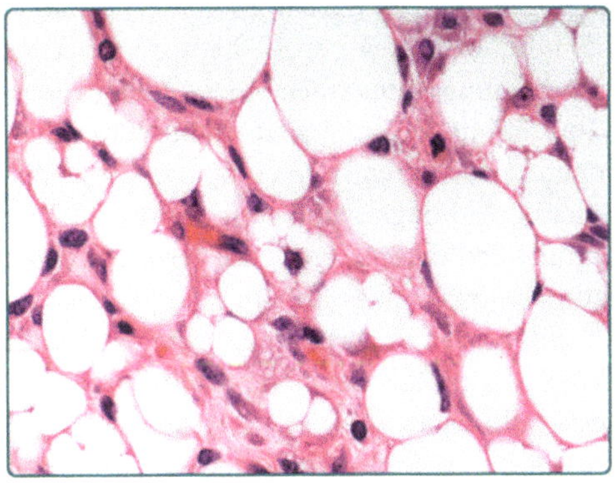

Lipoblast. Note the multiple clear cytoplasmic vacuoles indenting the enlarged hyperchromatic nucleus. *Fitzpatrick's Dermatology in General Medicine*, 8e. Chapter 129. Neoplasms of Subcutaneous Fat. EFIGURE 129-9.5

Cytogenetically, WDLs are associated with a ring or giant chromosome derived from the long arm of chromosome 12q13-15, leading to amplification of the proto-oncogenes MDM2 and CDK4.

In regard to the differential diagnosis, it must be emphasized that a number of entirely benign adipocytic tumors, such as **lipoblastoma** and **pleomorphic lipoma,** may contain lipoblasts. Thus, the presence of lipoblasts does not equate to a diagnosis of malignancy. With this in mind, the differential diagnosis includes benign, reactive, and malignant processes. The differential diagnosis includes **lipoma, pleomorphic lipoma, spindle cell lipoma, lipoblastoma, xanthomatous reactions, fat necrosis, diffuse neurofibroma,** and **dermatofibrosarcoma protuberans (DFSP).** The hyperchromatic stromal cells distinguish this tumor from a lipoma. Pleomorphic lipomas have a rather well-defined clinical context of well-circumscribed subcutaneous masses on the neck and upper back measuring less than 10 cm. Additionally, pleomorphic lipomas contain multinucleated floret-like cells rather than the smudgy atypical stromal cells observed in WDL/ALT. Spindle cell lipomas have distinctive ropey (thick bundles of) collagen and usually lack lipoblasts. Pleomorphic and spindle cell lipomas are negative for MDM2 and CDK4.

Lipoblastomas may be identical to WDL/ALT, but generally occur in young males less than 7 years of age, when the diagnosis of liposarcoma is indeed rare (Table 11-35C). Lipoblastoma typically occurs as a multilobulated mass on the extremities, is confined to the subcutis, and measures less than 5 cm in diameter. Although 15% to 20% of lesions recur (usually of the diffuse type), no metastases or deaths have been reported. Histopathologically, lipoblastoma may be almost identical to well-differentiated or myxoid liposarcomas. At low power, the tumor is distinctly lobulated or nested.

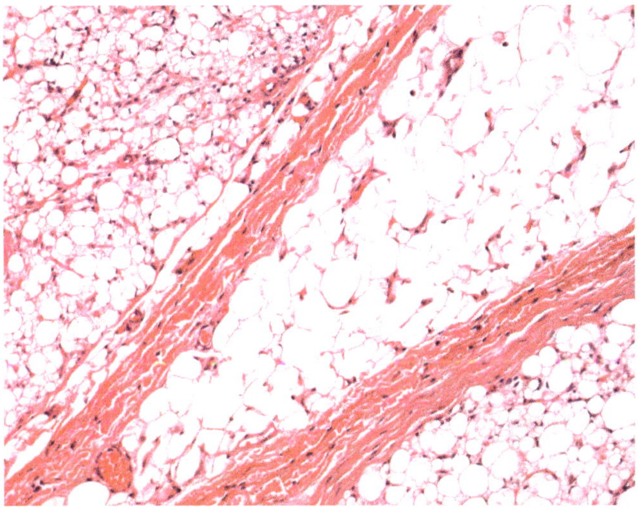

Lipoblastoma. Fibrous septa dividing fatty tumor into lobules with varying degrees of maturation.

Table 11-35C. Lipoblastoma

Clinical Features
Children
Boys > girls
Extremities
Localized or diffuse
Histopathologic Features
Lipoblasts
Lobular growth pattern
Mature adipose tissue
Differential Diagnosis
ALT/WDL

At high power, numerous lipoblasts, a rich plexiform capillary network, and a myxoid matrix resemble myxoid liposarcoma. Lesions with mature adipocytes interspersed with lipoblasts and spindled or stellate mesenchymal cells resemble WDL/ALT. In general, however, nuclear atypia is absent in contrast to that in liposarcoma. Maturing lipoblastomas display few lipoblasts but still have distinct lobularity and possibly increased vascularity. Fibrous septa may be pronounced. Signet ring and multivacuolated lipoblasts are both present. In contrast to liposarcomas, rearrangements of chromosome 8 are often found cytogenetically. Although lipoblastomas are asymptomatic and lack metastatic potential, they may cause dysfunction of other organ systems due to mass effect. Complete surgical excision with clinical follow-up is the preferred therapy. Like pleomorphic lipoma and spindle cell lipoma, lipoblastomas are negative for MDM2 and CDK4 expression.

Xanthomatous reactions have numerous foamy cells rather than cells with large, fat vacuoles (adipocytes); are associated with inflammation; and lack atypia. Likewise, fat necrosis shows aggregates of foamy histiocytes and lacks atypia.

Dedifferentiated liposarcoma usually presents as a longstanding, painless mass exhibiting a recent increase in size. Dedifferentiation may occur in either the primary WDL/ALT (90%) or in a recurrence (10%) generally in deep soft tissues, though rarely in superficial anatomic sites. Up to 50% of dedifferentiated liposarcomas recur and at least 15% metastasize. Microscopically, dedifferentiated liposarcoma is a malignant adipocytic neoplasm that morphologically exhibits an abrupt transition from WDL to nonlipogenic sarcoma.

The dedifferentiated component is often a high-grade sarcoma but may also be a low-grade spindle cell or myxoid sarcoma. Some are composed mainly of dedifferentiated areas with a largely obscured or absent well-differentiated component. The dedifferentiated component may display heterologous differentiation, generally toward **rhabdomyosarcoma, osteosarcoma,** or **chondrosarcoma.** Recently, the degree of cellularity and mitotic activity required for the diagnosis of dedifferentiation has come under question. Traditionally, dedifferentiated liposarcoma consists of a combination of WDL and a cellular nonlipogenic sarcoma having significant mitotic activity (at least 5 mitotic figures per 10 high-power fields [hpf]). A diagnostic dilemma arises when WDLs contain areas whose cellularity and mitotic rate are increased but lower than in the classically defined dedifferentiated component of dedifferentiated liposarcoma. Although some consider this finding to represent "low-grade dedifferentiation," this term has come under recent scrutiny because it has no effect on patient survival and may be best regarded as part of the spectrum of findings within ALT/WDL. If only the dedifferentiated component is sampled, the histopathological differential diagnosis would include other forms of **pleomorphic sarcoma (ie, malignant fibrous histiocytoma, pleomorphic rhabdomyosarcoma, leiomyosarcoma)**. Identification of a well-differentiated component or immunohistochemistry for MDM2 and CDK4 can be key to the diagnosis.

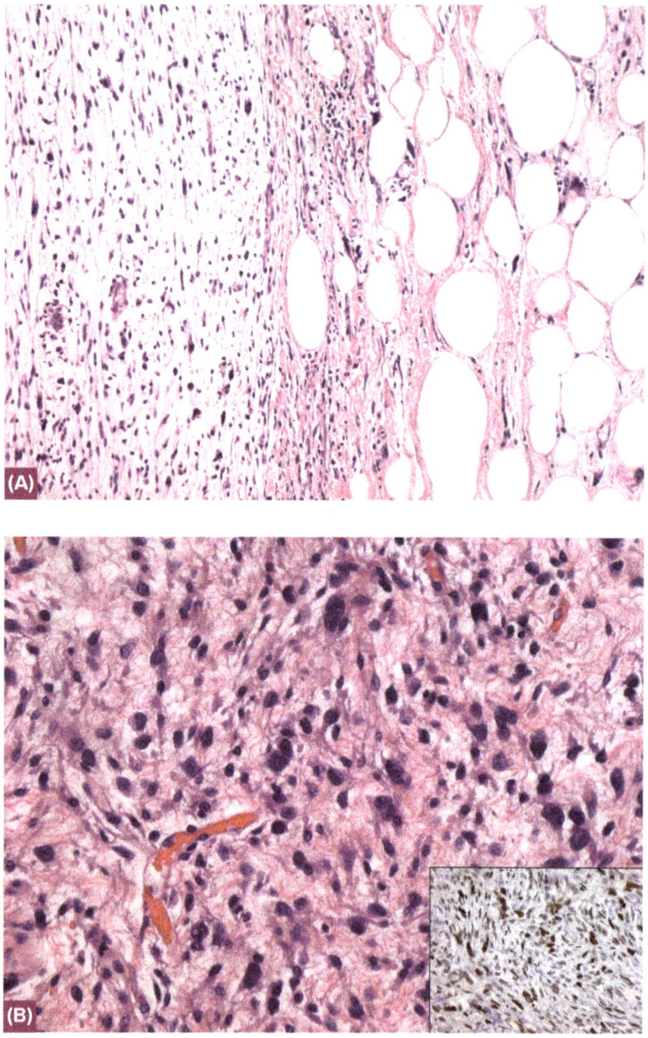

Dedifferentiated liposarcoma. (A) Abrupt transition from well-differentiated liposarcoma (right) to dedifferentiated liposarcoma (left). **(B)** The dedifferentiated component is nonlipogenic. Immunohistochemical expression of MDM2 is confirmatory (inset).

Table 11-35D. Myxoid Liposarcoma/Round Cell Liposarcoma

Clinical Features
Adults
Proximal extremities (for atypical lipomatous tumor)
Histopathologic Features
Mature adipose tissue
Myxoid matrix
Lipoblasts, often signet ring like
Chicken wire–like capillary network
Differential Diagnosis
Myxofibrosarcoma

Table 11-35E. Pleomorphic Liposarcoma

Clinical Features
Adults
Deep soft tissues
Histopathologic Features
Pleomorphic cells
Spindle cells
Lipoblasts
Differential Diagnosis
Myxofibrosarcoma
Pleomorphic lipoma
Pleomorphic rhabdomyosarcoma

Myxoid liposarcoma and **round cell liposarcoma** are related tumors that occur almost exclusively in the deep soft tissues of the proximal lower extremity (Table 11-35D). **Pure myxoid liposarcoma** consists of a uniform myxoid matrix, a characteristic "chicken wire–like" plexiform capillary network, numerous small relatively bland spindle cells, and a variable number of small lipoblasts. The most characteristic feature is the capillary network. The capillaries are evenly spaced, thin-walled, and slightly curved. Round cell change in myxoid liposarcoma **(round cell liposarcoma)** is characterized by a significant increase in cellularity, with nuclear overlapping and obscuring of the capillaries. The cells are smaller than adipocytes and have enlarged hyperchromatic nuclei and prominent nucleoli. The cytoplasm may be scant or vacuolated. The quantity of round cell differentiation has prognostic significance, with tumors exhibiting 5% to 25% round cell component displaying a lower rate of metastasis than those exceeding 25% (metastasis rate, 35% vs 58%). Cytogenetically, myxoid or round cell liposarcoma almost always has a t(12;16) (q13;p11) translocation that fuses the transcription factor gene *CHOP* on chromosome 12 to the *TLS/FUS* gene on chromosome 16. These liposarcomas are negative for MDM2 and CDK4 expression via immunohistochemistry. The dermatopathologist should be highly wary of making a diagnosis of myxoid/round cell liposarcoma when no deep-seated mass is present.

Pleomorphic liposarcomas are the least common type of liposarcoma; they occur most often in elderly individuals, and subcutaneous examples are especially rare (Table 11-35E). These tumors generally exhibit three morphologic pictures: a high-grade pleomorphic spindle cell sarcoma containing scattered multivacuolated lipoblasts, a cellular neoplasm containing sheets of bizarre pleomorphic monovacuolated as well as multivacuolated lipoblasts, and an epithelioid variant composed of sheets of pleomorphic epithelioid cells with distinct cell borders. The prognosis for patients with dermal pleomorphic liposarcomas appears to be substantially better than that of patients with more deeply seated lesions, based on a small number of reported cases. Cytogenetically, the majority of pleomorphic liposarcomas display complex karyotypes. The differential diagnosis for pleomorphic liposarcoma includes

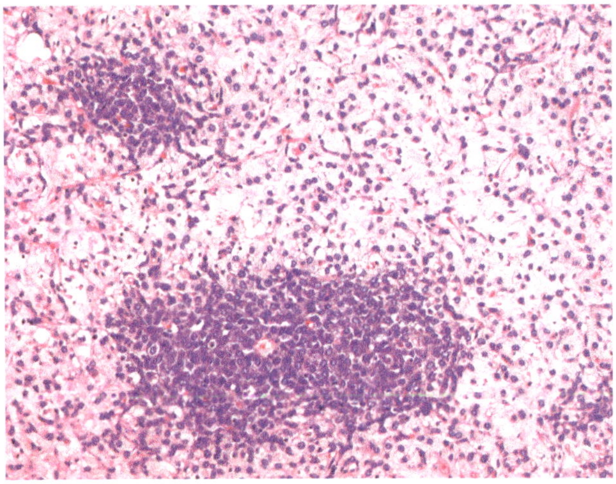

Round cell liposarcoma. Myxoid liposarcoma with its characteristic "chicken wire–like" vascular network. Note the nodular accumulations of small basophilic round cells, conferring a poor prognosis. A few scattered lipoblasts may be identified.

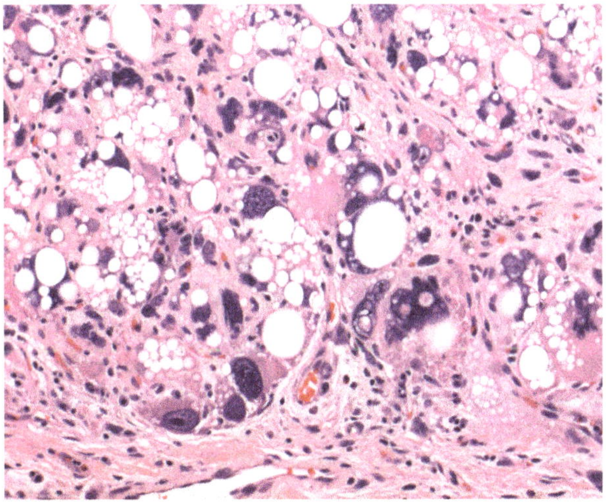

Pleomorphic liposarcoma. Numerous pleomorphic multivacuolated lipoblasts.

other pleomorphic high-grade sarcomas, such as pleomorphic rhabdomyosarcoma. The identification of lipoblasts is key. The epithelioid morphology in these pleomorphic tumors may closely simulate other malignant epithelial neoplasms, mainly adrenal cortical carcinoma. In this context, immunohistochemical stains must be interpreted prudently because overlap between these two entities may be seen, with focal expression of Melan-A and pan-keratin. Inhibin immunoreactivity, however, has not been reported in pleomorphic liposarcoma. The immunohistochemical profile of pleomorphic liposarcoma in nonlipogenic regions is heterogeneous; however, reactivity with S-100 protein in lipoblasts may also be helpful.

ANSWER 11-36: B.

This is a **Becker nevus**, containing a component of irregularly arranged smooth muscle bundles in the reticular dermis interspersed with collagen, adipocytes, and adnexa, consistent with a **congenital smooth muscle hamartoma**. Smooth muscle hamartomas of the skin are rare congenital lesions presenting in children up to 18 years old. In contrast, smooth muscle neoplasms occur mainly but not exclusively in adults. Clinically, smooth muscle hamartomas are most common on the torso; measure up to 10 cm in diameter; and may or may not occur in association with **Becker nevus**, a hamartoma most common in males and exhibits hyperpigmentation and hypertrichosis. Becker nevus is not clinically present at birth, but tends to arise during puberty and is associated with ipsilateral breast and limb hypoplasia and skeletal defects. Histopathologically, these hamartomas are composed of well-ordered noncohesive fascicles of smooth muscle arranged in various directions within the dermis and subcutaneous tissue. Adipocytes may also be present unusually high in the dermis. There may be an artifactual cleft between the lesion and the surrounding dermis. Smooth muscle is positive for smooth muscle actin (SMA) and desmin via immunohistochemistry. Becker nevus will additionally contain increased pigmentation within keratinocytes but normal numbers of melanocytes. **Pilar leiomyomas** are also composed of smooth muscle, but the muscle bundles tend to form a single mass, in contrast with hamartomas where the bundles are discrete and surrounded by ordered collagen (Table 11-36A). The smooth muscle bundles have no association with regional hair follicles. **Accessory nipple** is histopathologically identical to smooth muscle hamartoma and requires clinical correlation for diagnostic distinction. **Dermatomyofibroma** typically presents as a plaque on the trunk or upper limb girdle of female patients. Microscopically, there is an ill-defined proliferation of bland spindle-shaped myofibroblasts arranged in horizontal parallel fascicles with sparing of the adnexal structures. The tumor cells are positive for smooth muscle actin and vimentin, but are negative for desmin, CD34, and factor XIIIa. **Nevus lipomatosus superficialis** is a rare hamartoma characterized by ectopic adipocytes in the upper dermis.

Table 11-36A. Pilar Leiomyoma

Clinical Features
Adults
Skin, nipple
Painful, often multiple
Histopathologic Features
Fasciculated
Spindle shaped (sometimes epithelioid)
Boxcar-shaped nuclei
Eosinophilic cytoplasm
Differential Diagnosis
Leiomyosarcoma
Benign fibrous histiocytoma
Dermatofibrosarcoma protuberans

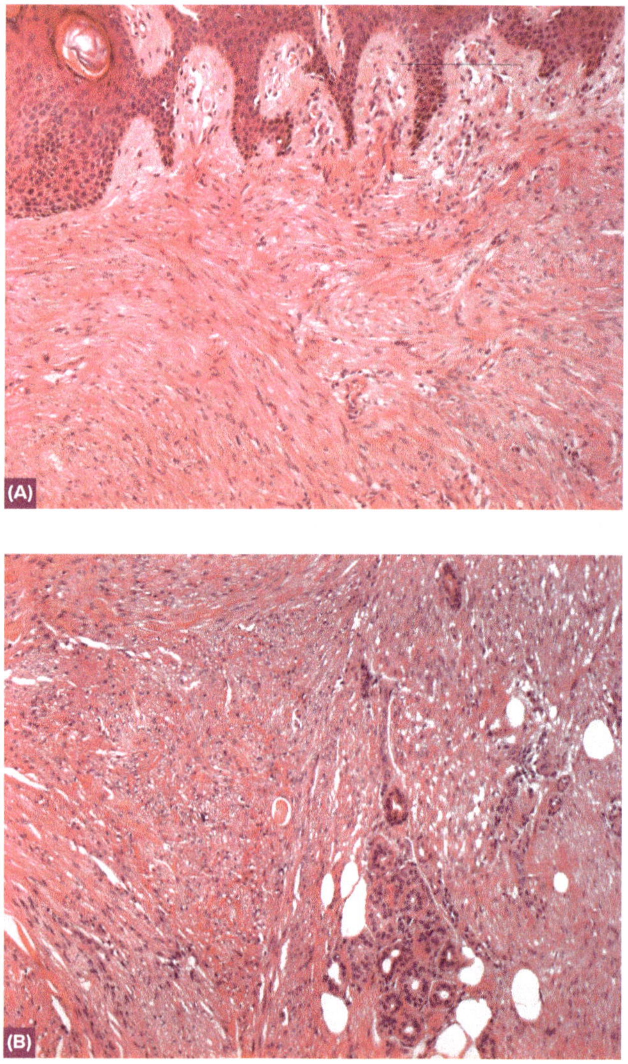

Pilar leiomyoma. (A) Solid areas with short, intersecting fascicles of bland spindled cells with eosinophilic cytoplasm and box-car (or pill shaped) blunt ended nuclei. **(B)** At the deep aspect, the tumor entraps adnexal structures.

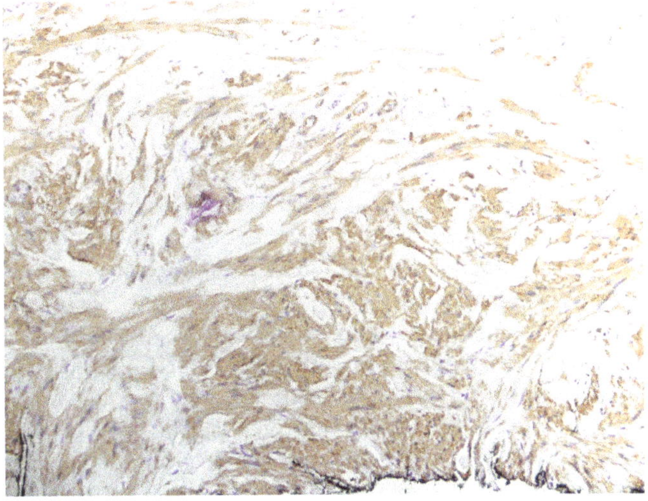

Pilar leiomyoma. Immunohistochemical expression of desmin.

ANSWER 11-37: A.

There is a spindle cell proliferation with a fascicular growth pattern. The tumor cells contain elongated nuclei with round or blunt ends ("box car nuclei") and abundant eosinophilic cytoplasm. Numerous mitotic figures are present. The immunohistochemical findings are consistent with smooth muscle differentiation. Based on the tumor location, the findings are consistent with an **atypical leiomyomatous tumor**. Smooth muscle tumors occur mainly but not exclusively in adults. The WHO classification of smooth muscle tumors is provided in Table 11-37A. Just like normal smooth muscle, the cells express smooth muscle actin, desmin, and caldesmin via immunohistochemistry. Determining the prognosis of these lesions may be a difficult task for the pathologist. While cytologic atypia is usually seen in malignant smooth muscle tumors, it may also be present in benign tumors (**symplastic leiomyoma**). Additionally, infiltrative growth and lack of circumscription may be seen in both benign and malignant tumors. The most important features of malignancy are mitotic rate (>1 mitoses per 10 high-power fields [40×]) and tumor necrosis. Ki-67, an immunohistochemical marker of cell division, typically reveals nuclear staining in greater than 10% of tumor cells in malignancy. Prognosis is very dependent on site. Extremely bland lesions in some sites may still carry a risk for recurrence, although this may occur late.

Smooth muscle tumors of the skin and subcutaneous tissues can be divided into **pure leiomyomas** and those arising in association with vascular structures, namely **angioleiomyomas**. Pure leiomyomas have no gender preference and generally arise in early adulthood. They can be separated into those that arise in the skin and those associated with the external genitalia (including the nipple, vulva, and scrotum). Leiomyomas of the skin arise from the erector pilae muscles and tend to occur on the extensor surface of the extremities and the trunk. These **pilar leiomyomas** are often multiple, painful, firm reddish-brown papules or nodules, commonly smaller than 2 cm in diameter. **Familial leiomyomatosis**, in which multiple cutaneous and uterine leiomyomas occur, is an autosomal dominant condition, with a predisposition to an aggressive form of renal cell carcinoma. Nipple lesions are similar and arise from areolar smooth muscle. **Genital leiomyomas** arise from dartos or vulvar smooth muscle. They are solitary, painless, well-circumscribed masses that may grow up to 15 cm in diameter and may be located in the subcutaneous tissue. Separation of dermal and genital leiomyomas is most important for prognosis. Small, solitary dermal leiomyomas tend to not recur. Patients with multiple dermal leiomyomas often experience recurrence (50%) and tend to develop subsequent lesions. Patients with genital leiomyomas tend usually to be disease free after 5 years of follow-up, but longer follow-up has shown the development of recurrences after periods as long as 15 years. **Angioleiomyomas** are solitary, often painful, subcutaneous, well-circumscribed nodules arising in adults (average age, 47 years) with a predilection for women (Table 11-37B). They occur mainly in the lower extremities, especially the lower leg and foot. The lesion is benign and only rarely recurs.

Table 11-37A. WHO Classification of Smooth Muscle Tumors

Angioleiomyoma
Deep leiomyoma
Genital leiomyoma
Leiomyosarcoma

Table 11-37B. Angioleiomyoma

Clinical Features
Adults; female predominance
Lower extremities
Painful, often solitary
Histopathologic Features
Well circumscribed
Blood vessels
Smooth muscle of vessel walls in irregular concentric bundles
Three variants: solid, cavernous, venous
Stromal hyalinization
Myxoid change
Differential Diagnosis
Leiomyoma
Leiomyosarcoma
Hemangioma

Microscopically, dermal **pilar leiomyomas** are composed of numerous fascicles of smooth muscle and variable amounts of collagen arranged randomly throughout the dermis or subcutaneous tissue. They are unencapsulated and infiltrative; involvement of hair follicles and adnexal glands is typical. The cells have abundant eosinophilic cytoplasm that may have a perinuclear vacuole; the nuclei are oval with blunt ends and evenly dispersed chromatin. **Genital leiomyomas** are larger, usually better circumscribed, and centered in the subcutaneous tissues. They may have a pseudocapsule, focal calcifications, and stromal myxoid change. Any mitotic activity in a smooth muscle tumor with any degree of nuclear atypia should raise the suspicion of malignancy. **Angioleiomyomas** are well-circumscribed solid masses composed of coalesced vessels with prominent walls consisting of smooth muscle and collagen. They are commonly located in the subcutis. The vascular lumina are usually compressed, but they are occasionally large and dilated. The muscle of the vessel walls forms irregular, often concentric bundles that merge with those of their neighbors. Stromal hyalinization or myxoid change is common. Rarely, mature adipose tissue is present, possibly resembling **angiomyolipoma**. Angiomyolipoma is a rare triphasic tumor composed of both smooth muscle, fat, and vessels that stains positive for HMB45. Unlike retroperitoneal tumors, there is no association with tuberous sclerosis in cutaneous angiomyolipomas. Atypia, mitoses, and necrosis are not seen.

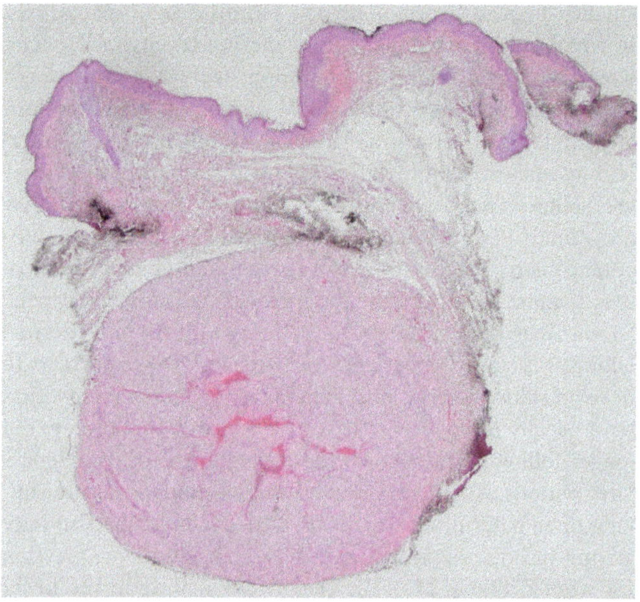

Angioleiomyoma. There is a deep dermal nodule composed of spindle cells with centrally located vessels.

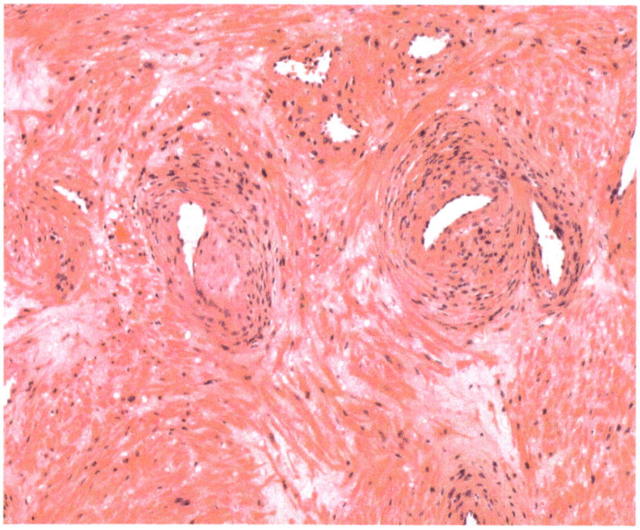

Angioleiomyoma. Bland smooth muscle fibers intimately merge with smooth muscle cells in the walls of blood vessels. Note the absence of mitotic activity, necrosis, and cytologic atypia.

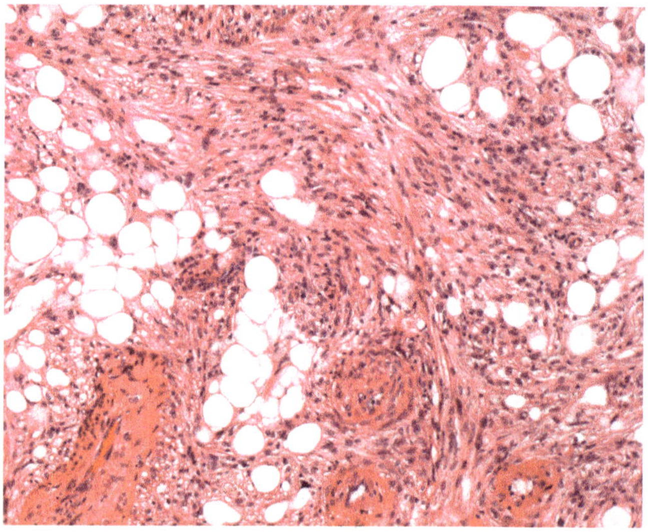

Angiomyolipoma. Typical triphasic histopathology exhibiting mature adipocytes, smooth muscle, and thick-walled vessels. These tumor cells express HMB45 by immunohistochemistry. Unlike retroperitoneal tumors, there is no association with tuberous sclerosis.

Myolipoma is an uncommon neoplasm occurring in adults but only infrequently arising in subcutaneous tissue. Although deep lesions have reached 25 cm in diameter, subcutaneous lesions were smaller (~5 cm) and well circumscribed. The tumor is an intimate mixture (in varying proportions) of mature adipose tissue interspersed with well-differentiated smooth muscle, resembling a sieve. A prominent vascular component is absent. The muscle cells form only short, irregular fascicles, in contrast to the long fascicles present in **leiomyomas**. The smooth muscle is reactive for both actin and desmin. No recurrences have been reported.

Some benign smooth muscle tumors may exhibit significant cytologic atypia and are analogous to the **"symplastic" leiomyoma** of the uterus. In these cases, careful inspection for mitotic activity and tumor necrosis is essentially to confirm benignity.

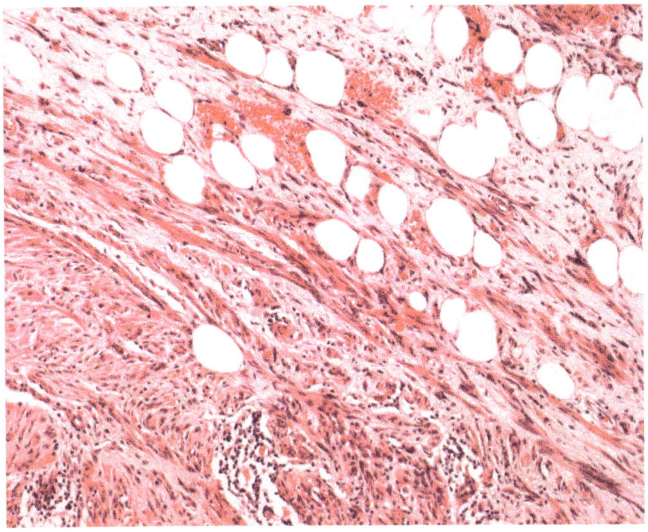

Myolipoma. Admixture of mature adipocytes and smooth muscle. No significant vascular component is present.

Superficial leiomyosarcoma (ie, dermal and subcutaneous) is most common between the ages of 40 and 80 years, although it has also been described in teenagers and children (Table 11-37C). These lesions are most common in the proximal extremities, especially the lower extremity, and generally are smaller than 5 cm in maximum diameter. Dermal tumors are believed to arise from erector pilae muscles and subcutaneous tumors from blood vessels. The prognosis is highly dependent on the size and anatomic compartment. In general, tumors smaller than 5 cm in diameter have a much better prognosis. Up to 40% of dermal-confined tumors recur, but metastasis is extremely rare. For this reason, some authorities prefer the term **"atypical leiomyomatous tumor"** for dermal-confined tumors. In contrast, when the tumor arises from the subcutis, it should be referred to and treated as a sarcoma, as such lesions metastasize in up to 50% of cases. For **subcutaneous leiomyosarcomas**, aneuploidy may be an additional unfavorable prognostic feature. Microscopically, leiomyosarcomas, particularly of the dermis, may closely resemble their benign counterparts with well-formed fascicles of spindle cells with abundant eosinophilic cytoplasm and elongated, blunt-ended nuclei. The nuclei may be more vesicular and have nucleoli. The fascicles typically run at right angles to each other. Unlike leiomyomas, most tumors display some pleomorphism, mitotic activity, or necrosis; however, well-differentiated tumors may be difficult to differentiate from leiomyomas. Dermal lesions are often highly infiltrative; by contrast, subcutaneous lesions appear more circumscribed.

The distinction of **leiomyosarcoma** from **leiomyoma** can be difficult (especially **symplastic leiomyomas**) (Table 11-37D). In general, leiomyosarcomas occur in an older age group and more commonly in the proximal extremity. Certainly, tumors that extend widely into the subcutis are larger than 2 cm, have more than 1 mitosis per 10 hpf, or necrosis should be considered malignant. In some cases, absolute distinction may not be possible, and in these cases, this uncertainty should be expressed in the report using such terms as **smooth muscle tumor of uncertain malignant potential. Dermatofibrosarcoma protuberans (DFSP)** has a storiform pattern rather than fascicles, more wavy nuclei, and reactivity for CD34. Primary cutaneous leiomyosarcoma should be distinguished from **metastatic leiomyosarcoma** originating in deeper visceral tissues, which is one of the more common deep tissue sarcomas to metastasize to skin. Cutaneous metastases typically present as painless firm nodules under an intact, normal-appearing epidermis. The scalp is the most common cutaneous site of involvement of metastatic leiomyosarcoma; metastases are generally of higher histologic grade.

Table 11-37C. Leiomyosarcoma

Clinical Features
Adults
Extremities
Dermal or subcutaneous
Histopathologic Features
Smooth muscle
Mitoses
Atypia
Necrosis
Differential Diagnosis
Leiomyoma
Benign fibrous histiocytoma
Dermatofibrosarcoma protuberans
Spindle cell rhabdomyosarcoma
Malignant melanoma
Granular cell tumor
Metastasis

Table 11-37D. Features Useful in Distinguishing Cutaneous Leiomyoma from Leiomyosarcoma

	LEIOMYOMA	LEIOMYOSARCOMA
Peak age (years)	20-50	30-80
Size	Trunk, extensor surfaces	Proximal lower extremities
Number	Often multiple	Solitary
Depth	More superficial	Usually extend deep
Size	Usually <2 cm	Often larger
Necrosis	Rare	Common
Mitoses	Rare (<1/10 hpf)	Often (>3/10 hpf)

ANSWER 11-38: A.

During their histogenesis, cutaneous neural tumors either recapitulate or retain to a variable extent the architectural arrangement and cytologic components of the **normal peripheral nerve**. Therefore, familiarity with the normal histology of the peripheral nerve is essential for the correct characterization of neural tumors. In short, the structural organization of the peripheral nerve follows a hierarchical arrangement of different compartments. The basic unit is the nerve fiber, which is composed of an **axon (neurite)** and the surrounding **Schwann cells**. Axons are cytoplasmic extensions of neurons that are located in the central nervous system (CNS) or in the sympathetic ganglionic chain. **Naked axons** are positive for PGP9.5 via immunohistochemistry. Axons become myelinated by multiple periaxonal rotation of the surrounding S100+ Schwann cells, thus creating a concentric layer of cytoplasmic membranes. **Unmyelinated nerve fibers** develop by invagination of the axons into the cytoplasm of the Schwann cells. In the next architectural compartment, several nerve fibers form nerve fascicles that are surrounded by a sheath, called a **perineurium**. The space within the perineurium is referred to as the **endoneurium**. The perineurium is composed of a specialized cell type, the **perineurial cell**, that is EMA+ and in continuity with the pia-arachnoidal lining of the CNS. Besides the nerve fibers, the endoneurium also contains fibroblasts, capillaries, and mast cells. In the final organizational compartment, numerous nerve fascicles are grouped into nerve bundles that are held together by a protective sheath referred to as the **epineurium**. The epineurium is made up of fibroblasts, collagen, and adipose tissue, but fine vascular structures also penetrate its wall. The sensory nerves are connected to various types of sensory corpuscles (eg, pacinian, meissnerian, Vater-Pacini, and Krause) that are differentiated to specific sensory perceptions.

ANSWER 11-39: B.

Neuromas represent hamartomatous proliferations of the nerve sheath components in which there is an approximate recapitulation of the normal structural arrangements of the peripheral nerve. The constituent fibers have an axon-to-Schwann cell ratio close to the normal (1:1), which makes this group of tumors distinct from other **nerve sheath neoplasms**. From an etiologic standpoint, neuromas can be classified as spontaneous and traumatic types. The spontaneous type has two main forms: a solitary, encapsulated type (**solitary palisaded encapsulated neuroma**) and a multiple, nonencapsulated type (Table 11-39A). Spontaneous neuromas are considered to be a form of primary hyperplasia of the nerve fibers without apparent antecedent tissue injury. **Traumatic neuromas** develop after sharp or blunt trauma of the peripheral nerve, resulting in a partial or complete transection of the continuity of the nerve fibers. After transection of the nerve fiber, the distal end undergoes **Wallerian degeneration**, and the fibers from the proximal end try to regenerate and reunite with the distal end. This attempt at regeneration often fails due to the severity of the damage and results in an unorganized, irregular overgrowth of regrowing nerve fibers from the proximal end of the nerve. Traumatic neuromas developing after a complete transection of the nerves are called **amputation neuromas** and are reactive proliferations rather than true hamartomas or neoplasms.

Table 11-39A. Palisaded and Encapsulated Neuroma

Clinical Features
Usually solitary
Predilection for the face of adults
Nondescript skin-colored papule or nodule suggesting a dermal nevus
Histopathologic Features
Well-circumscribed nodule with incomplete encapsulation
Spindled cells arranged in short fascicles
Well-developed palisading of nuclei is usually not present
Differential Diagnosis
Schwannoma
Leiomyoma
Neurotized nevus
Other spindle cell melanocytic tumors

Clinically, **palisaded encapsulated neuroma (PEN)** develops in adults (mean age, 45.5 years) with an approximately equal ratio of both genders. Most lesions (close to 90%) manifest on the face, but they can occur anywhere on the body. The lesions are solitary, small (2-6 mm), skin-colored, firm or rubbery, dome-shaped, asymptomatic papules. There is no known association with neurofibromatosis or multiple endocrine neoplasia (MEN syndromes). Multiple, nonencapsulated neuromas on the other hand usually manifest as part of **multiple endocrine neoplasia syndrome type 2B (MEN 2B)**. In this syndrome, there are numerous soft, skin-colored or pink papules and nodules around the mucosal orifices, mainly around the lips, but in the oral cavity as well. This manifestation is also referred to as **multiple mucosal neuromas**. Other components of this syndrome include pheochromocytoma and medullary thyroid carcinoma. **Traumatic neuromas** can occur at any age or in either gender but are obviously more prevalent in people working certain professions that make the individual prone to acute and chronic injuries (Table 11-39B). Thus, there is some predilection for the extremities. They are usually solitary, skin-colored, often broad-based, firm papules and nodules at the sites of previous injury or trauma. They may be asymptomatic, but older lesions often become sensitive and painful on pressure. Lancinating pain is considered

Table 11-39B. Traumatic Neuroma

Clinical Features
May occur at any site after trauma
Small skin-colored nodule or mass
Often painful
Histopathologic Features
Circumscribed but unencapsulated
Mass composed of axons and Schwann cells admixed with fibrous tissue
Differential Diagnosis
Neurofibroma
Perineurioma

characteristic for **amputation neuromas**. A special form of traumatic neuroma is the **supernumerary digit**, which occurs on the lateral-volar aspect of the hand in newborns and young infants. These lesions represent amputation neuromas at the site of an extranumerary digit separated in utero. Despite the term, they do not contain bone or cartilage of a true digit.

Microscopically, **palisaded encapsulated neuroma (PEN)** is a well-circumscribed, round or oblong nodule located in the dermis that occasionally has a polypoid configuration. The tumor is composed of tightly woven fascicles often separated by clear clefts. The cells in the fascicles are uniformly spindle shaped with eosinophilic cytoplasm and ovoid or wavy nuclei. Mitotic figures are rare or absent. There is often parallel arrangement of the nuclei in a given fascicle suggestive of a palisading pattern, although this is not a constant feature. Classic Verocay bodies are not present. There is no appreciable fibrosis, chronic inflammation, or granulomatous reaction within the tumor. A thin, capsule-like structure separates the tumor from the surrounding dermis. However, this capsule is often incomplete near the epidermal aspect of the lesion. A connection with adjacent nerves can usually be demonstrated on serially sectioned specimens. Variants of palisaded encapsulated neuroma with a plexiform or multinodular growth pattern and highly vascular stroma have been reported. The morphologic features of spontaneous neuromas, in either solitary or multiple settings, are similar, with the exception of histologic encapsulation.

Traumatic or **amputation neuromas** are usually well-defined nodular lesions located in the dermis or subcutis. The tumors are encased by a fibrous sheath, which is often incomplete at the distal end, where the regenerating fibers may infiltrate the adjacent stroma. The tumor nodules are composed of a chaotic tangle of regenerating nerve fascicles of various sizes and shapes separated by fibrous tissue; variable chronic inflammation; or less often, granulomatous reaction. Mucinous changes are common in early lesions, especially in the regenerating perineurial spaces. The regenerated individual fibers have a nearly normal structural organization of typical Schwann cells, perineurial cells, and centrally located axons.

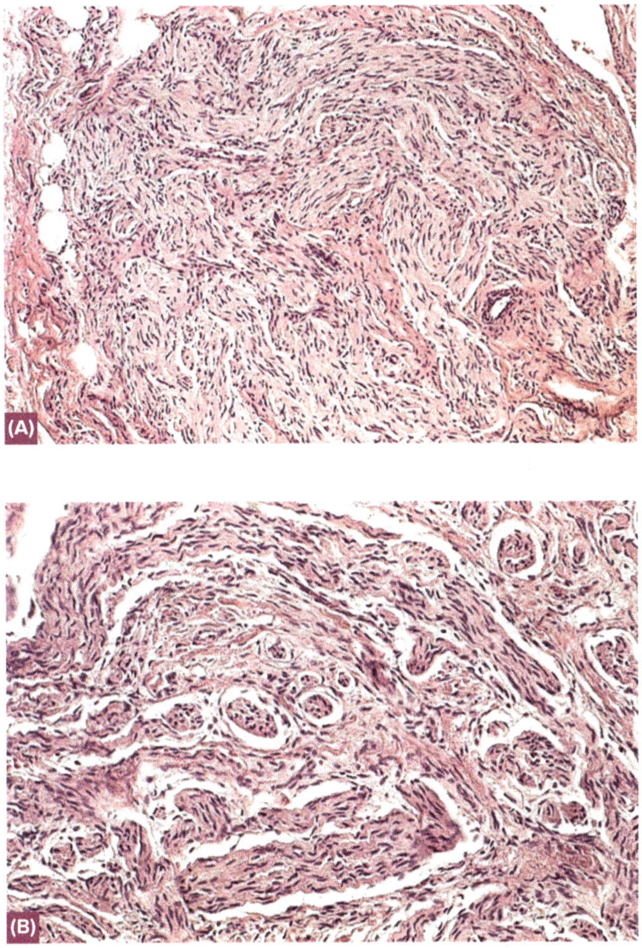

Traumatic neuroma. (A) The regenerating nerve fascicles have haphazard arrangement and are embedded in a markedly fibrotic stroma. **(B)** There is prominent variation in the size and shape of the fascicles, which are separated by scar tissue.

Immunohistochemically, **palisaded encapsulated neuroma** and **traumatic neuroma** share several features. The constituent cells of the fascicles stain for S-100 protein. In traumatic neuroma, the perineurial cells in the surrounding sheaths are positive for epithelial membrane antigen (EMA). In palisaded encapsulated neuroma, only the outer capsule reacts for this antigen, confirming a perineurial cell participation. Silver impregnation, neural filament, and PGP9.5 stains reveal that the fascicles are rich in axons in both lesions. In traumatic neuroma, the axons follow the normal longitudinal arrangement in the proximal part of the tumor, but they become haphazardly and irregularly arranged toward the distal end. Prominent myelinization is often present, as detected by antibodies to myelin basic protein and CD57.

In regard to the differential diagnosis, **palisaded encapsulated neuroma** must be differentiated from other peripheral nerve sheath tumors, particularly **schwannoma**, as well as non-nerve sheath proliferations such as **angioleiomyoma**. **Solitary schwannomas** contain **Antoni A** and **Antoni B type tissues** with **Verocay bodies** and are most often devoid of axons by special stains. **Neurofibroma** may also be considered on cytologic grounds; however, the haphazard architecture contrasts the orderly appearance of palisaded encapsulated neuroma. **Neurofibromas** do not displace surrounding adnexal structures, unlike PEN and schwannomas. **Angioleiomyomas** are well-circumscribed smooth muscle tumors that may occasionally mimic palisaded encapsulated neuroma, but the cytologic features of each are distinct. Smooth muscle cells of angioleiomyoma have a more eosinophilic, fine fibrillary cytoplasm and blunt-ended nuclei with a "bubbly" chromatin pattern. Thick-walled vessels are usually present. Axons are typically absent. Plexiform or multinodular variants of palisaded encapsulated neuromas should be differentiated from plexiform variants of neurofibroma, schwannoma, and fibrohistiocytic tumors.

Traumatic neuroma can be differentiated easily from the other variants of neuromas based on the presence of scar and chronic inflammation and a history of previous trauma. Painful plantar nodules, often referred to as **Morton neuromas**, are no longer considered true neuromas but rather localized forms of interdigital neuritis with a complex etiology.

ANSWER 11-40: E.

Neurofibromas are complex proliferations of the various components of the neuromesenchyme, including Schwann cells (S100+), endoneurial fibroblasts (vimentin+), perineurial cells (EMA+), mast cells (CD117+), and axons (PGP9.5) (Table 11-40A). In this complex proliferation, however, the proportion of each cell type varies, giving rise to broad histologic appearances. Because axons do not duplicate, their relative proportion to the other cell components is less than the usual 1:1 axon-to-Schwann cell ratio of the normal nerve. **Neuromas** (hamartomas) also tend to have a 1:1 axon-to-Schwann cell ratio. The main histopathologic types of neurofibromas include the sporadic cutaneous type, deep-seated encapsulated type, diffuse type, pigmented type, and plexiform type. Furthermore, other rare variants also exist, including atypical (cellular), sclerosing, and lipomatous types. Neurofibromas containing dendritic cells and hyperplastic Pacinian corpuscles have also been described.

Clinically, **sporadic neurofibromas** are relatively common lesions in adults and affect both genders equally. They are soft or rubbery, dome-shaped or polypoid, skin-colored or tan papules or nodules. They may display a **"button hole" sign** on pinching. They are usually asymptomatic, but the pedunculated forms may become irritated. A few lesions in a single patient, provided there are no other stigmata present, does not indicate **neurofibromatosis**; however, they still can be part of this syndrome. Contrary to this, the plexiform variant is considered pathognomonic for **neurofibromatosis type 1 (von Recklinghausen disease)**. The diffuse, deep-seated, and pigmented variants may also be more common in neurofibromatosis.

Table 11-40A. Neurofibroma

Clinical Features
Skin-colored or tan polypoid papule or nodule
Soft or rubbery
May involve any cutaneous site
Plexiform pattern—pathognomonic of neurofibromatosis
Histopathologic Features
Spindle cell proliferation, wavy nuclei with tapered ends
Often significant fibrosis
Occasional mucinous stroma
In general, not encapsulated
Mast cells are common
Plexiform variant is similar but with complex "wormlike" growth pattern
Differential Diagnosis
Neurotized nevus
Schwannoma
Trichodiscoma and related tumors
Dermatofibroma
Smooth muscle neoplasms
Hypertrophic scar

Whereas common solitary neurofibromas grow slowly and follow a benign course, the deep-seated, diffuse, and plexiform variants may cause local infiltration and organ displacement. The plexiform type also has an increased probability of malignant transformation into **malignant peripheral nerve sheath tumors**. The typical presentation of **plexiform neurofibroma** is a bag-like or twisted rope-like dermal or subcutaneous mass, often associated with redundant skin folds, hyperpigmentation, and hirsutism. Besides plexiform neurofibroma, the other important clinical stigmata of neurofibromatosis include conjunctival **Lisch nodules**, **café-au-lait spots, bilateral axillary freckling**, numerous superficial and deeply located **diffuse neurofibromas**, and various soft tissue, bone, endocrine, and other types of neoplasms.

Microscopically, common solitary cutaneous **neurofibromas** are round, oblong, or polypoid nodules in the dermis. Although they are well circumscribed, they are not encapsulated. The tumor is composed of proliferating delicate spindle cells with indistinct cytoplasmic membranes. The nuclei are wavy, with tapered ends and an evenly distributed chromatin pattern ("jumping dolphins"). Mitotic figures should not be present. The cells are embedded in a fibrillary pale-pink collagenous stroma. The cellularity varies from densely cellular to a loosely arranged pattern. The stroma can be markedly fibrotic, edematous, myxomatous, and even vascular. Compression of surrounding fibrous tissue may mimic the presence of a true capsule; however, the fibrous tissue is often less organized and prominent compared with the capsule of **schwannoma**. The cutaneous adnexa are surrounded but spared by the tumor. Mast cells are present in variable numbers throughout the lesion. Entrapped small nerve twigs, tactile body-like structures, or pigmented dendritic cells may be observed. Although nuclear palisading can occur, Verocay bodies are not characteristic findings. When neurofibromas develop in the deeper and larger nerves, they initially remain encapsulated due to confinement by the perineurium. These types are sometimes referred to as intraneural neurofibromas. In the deep-seated and diffuse types, the spindle cell proliferation is poorly defined and usually involves the subcutaneous fat. The tumor otherwise has similar features to the solitary type. The intraneural and diffuse (extraneural) growth patterns may be present in the same lesion. **Plexiform neurofibromas** are composed of interconnecting bundles and fascicles of markedly expanded nerves that are usually surrounded by a fibrous encapsulation of the epineurium and adjacent connective tissue. The superficial part, however, is usually not encapsulated, and the proliferating fascicles blend into the surrounding dermis. The individual fascicles display variable cellularity and often show edematous and mucinous changes. Cytologically, the cells are similar to those described in the solitary superficial form. In neurofibromatosis type 1, plexiform and diffuse growth patterns may coexist.

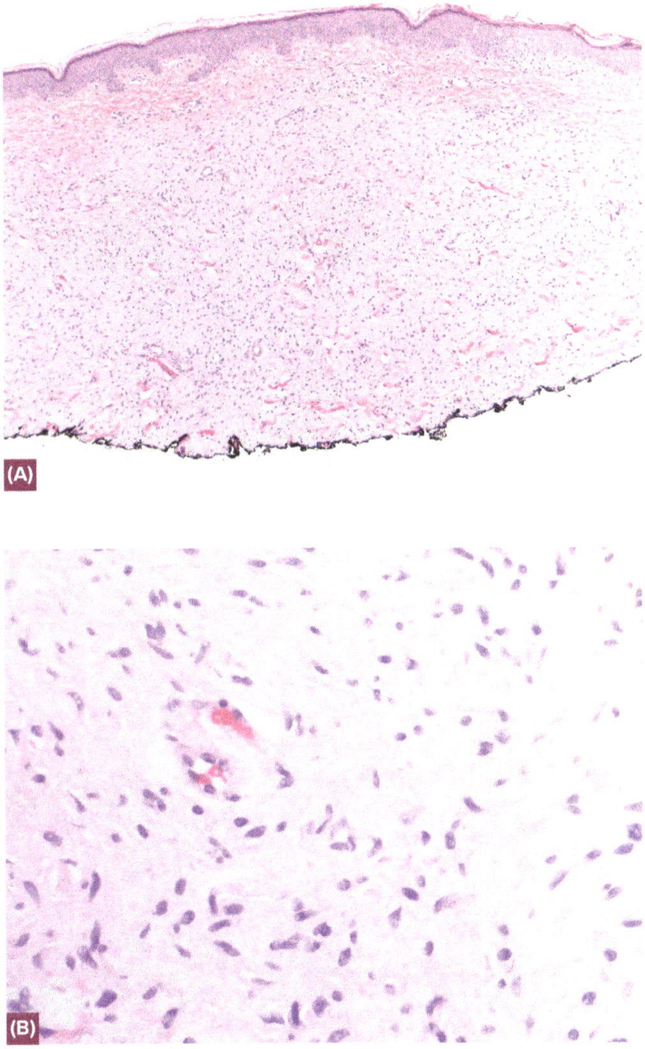

Neurofibroma. (A) A well-defined but non-encapsulated dermal nodule composed of spindle cells. Scattered blood vessels are present as well as rare entrapped dermal collagen bundles. **(B)** The slender spindle cells are haphazardly arranged in a fine fibrillary matrix. The cells have indistinct cell membranes and curved and tapered nuclei ("jumping dolphins").

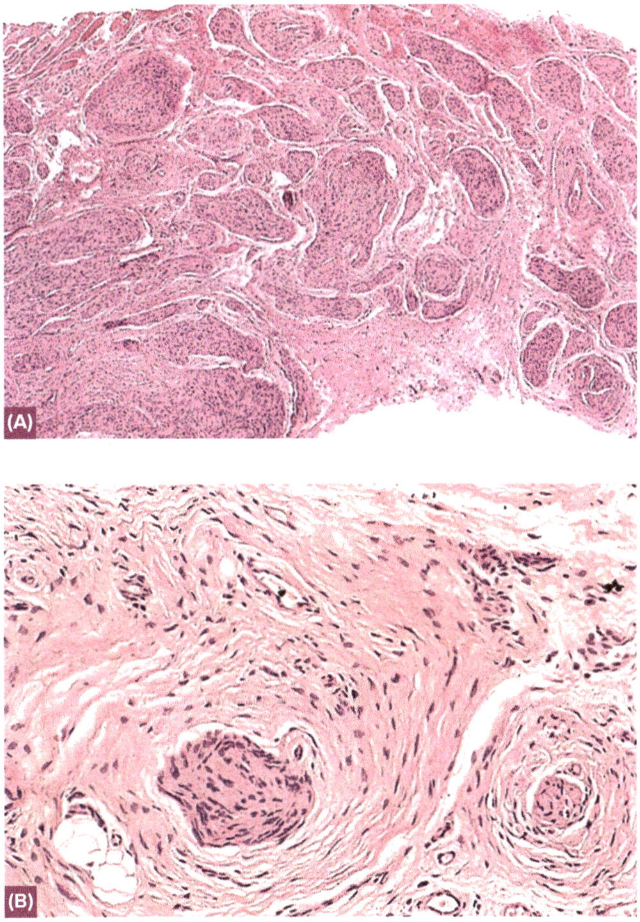

Plexiform neurofibroma, superficial type. (A) Interconnecting nerve fascicles of various size and shape infiltrating the dermis. **(B)** The spindle cells in a whirling pattern are embedded in a variably fibromatous stroma.

Cytologic atypia in neurofibroma is a rare but often a troubling finding. If not associated with increased cellularity or mitotic activity, isolated pleomorphism appears to have little clinical significance. An increased density of atypical cells, including areas of organized fascicular growth, necrosis, or mitotic activity, should raise concern for transformation to **malignant peripheral nerve sheath tumor (MPNST).**

Although the determination of malignant transformation is principally a morphologic exercise, strong expression of p53 or Ki-67 by the atypical cells may also favor development of MPNST (malignant peripheral nerve sheath tumor/malignant transformation of neurofibroma).

Immunohistochemically, the cells in **neurofibroma** variably express antigens, depending on the predominant cell types. These include S-100 protein and collagen type IV for Schwann cells, EMA for perineurial cells, vimentin for fibroblasts and Schwann cells, and neurofilament and myelin basic protein for axons and myelin sheaths, respectively. Axons may be scattered singly within the tumor, or clustered with similarity to small nerve twigs. **Pigmented neurofibroma** contains HMB45-positive cells, and the dendritic cells of the peculiar variant of dendritic cell neurofibroma with pseudorosettes express CD57.

In regard to the differential diagnosis, the **solitary superficial type of neurofibroma** must be differentiated from other spindle cell neoplasms that are not encapsulated, such as **dermatofibroma, hypertrophic scar, neurotized intradermal melanocytic nevus,** and **traumatic neuroma**. **Diffuse deep-seated neurofibromas** and **pigmented neurofibromas** may be confused with **dermatofibrosarcoma protuberans** and **common blue nevus. Plexiform neurofibroma**, which has the greatest clinical relevance because of its common association with **von Recklinghausen disease** and the increased possibility of malignant transformation, should be separated from **plexiform schwannoma** and **plexiform fibrohistiocytic tumor**. Each of these can be differentiated relatively easily with the help of immunohistochemical markers (Table 11-40B).

Table 11-40B. Histopathologic Diagnostic Features of Common Cutaneous Neural Neoplasms

FEATURE	TRAUMATIC NEUROMA	PALISADED, ENCAPSULATED NEUROMA	SOLITARY SUPERFICIAL NEUROFIBROMA	SOLITARY SCHWANNOMA	CLASSIC NERVE SHEATH MYXOMA	CELLULAR NEUROTHEKEOMA
Growth pattern	Well circumscribed at the proximal end, irregular at the distal end	Well circumscribed, nodular, rarely plexiform	Relatively well defined, but with infiltrative margins	Well circumscribed, nodular	Lobulated or plexiform	Fascicular or irregular sheaths and nests
Encapsulation	Partially by fibrous sheath	Yes, by perineurium	None	Yes, perineurium	Yes, partially by perineurium	None
Architecture	Unorganized tangles of regenerating fascicles	Compactly arranged fascicles, separated by clefts	Variable matrix from the fine fibrillary to dense fibrotic	Antoni A type: hypercellular Antoni B type: hypocellular	Hypocellular, myxoid matrix	Solid proliferation of epithelioid or spindled cells
Cytologic features	Spindled cells with tapered, wavy nuclei	Spindled cells with tapered, wavy nuclei	Spindled cells with tapered, wavy nuclei, plump fibroblasts, mast cells	Spindled cells with tapered, wavy nuclei, mast cells	Stellate, spindled, and giant cells	Large epithelioid or spindled cells
Nuclear palisading and Verocay bodies	None	Variable palisading	Rarely	Yes	None	None
Nerve fibers	Irregularly arranged axons	Relatively well-organized axons	Rare, scattered axons	None or only at the origin	None	None
Other important features	Extensive fibrosis, rarely inflammation, macrophages	No fibrosis or inflammation	Fibrosis, myxoid, and vascular changes	Hemorrhage, thrombosis, hyalinization, cytologic atypia (ancient changes)	Mild cytologic atypia	Variable atypia, rare mitotic figures

ANSWER 11-41: D.

The biopsy reveals an encapsulated nodule consisting of hypercellular and hypocellular types of tissues. Characteristic nuclear palisading and Verocay bodies with adjacent edematous stroma are present. The findings are consistent with **schwannoma** (Table 11-41A). **Schwannomas** (aka **neurilemomas**) are considered true nerve sheath neoplasms because they are composed almost entirely of proliferating **Schwann cells**. The Schwann cell proliferation takes place within the confines of the **perineurium** and displaces the remainder of the normal nerve fibers to the periphery of the tumor. This histogenesis explains the three main features of schwannomas: the exclusive Schwann cell component, encapsulation, and the virtual lack of axons within the tumor. There are four main types of schwannomas: (1) the common solitary type, which is almost invariably a benign neoplasm; (2) the ancient type, which represents a degenerated variant of the common type with senescent cytologic atypia; (3) the plexiform type, which displays cytologic features similar to the common type but that has a distinct growth pattern; (4) and the cellular type, a benign, hypercellular lesion that mimics a malignancy and is prone to recurrence. Malignant transformation of a benign schwannoma (**malignant schwannoma**) is extremely rare. This lesion is now usually designated as **malignant peripheral nerve sheath tumor (MPNST)**. Other less common variants, such as pigmented (psammomatous melanotic), glandular, epithelioid, and neuroblastoma-like, have also been reported.

Clinically, common **solitary schwannomas** are tumors of adulthood; however, although rare, unusual congenital variants have been documented. There is no significant predilection for either gender. The lesions are usually solitary tumors, but rarely they can occur as multiple lesions, designated as **neurilemmomatosis (schwannomatosis).** Whereas cutaneous

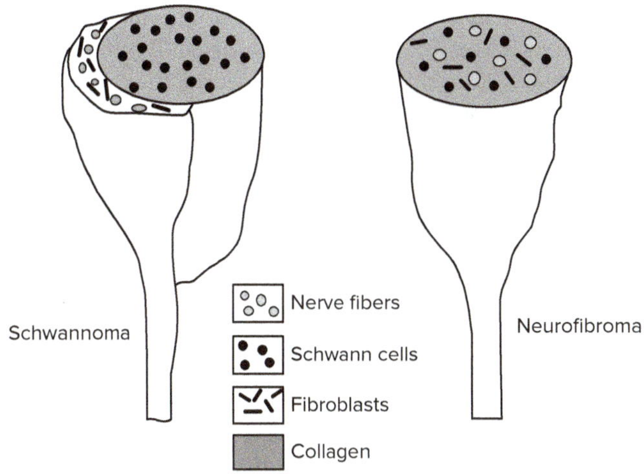

Modified from Poirier J, Gray F, Escourolle R: *Manual of Basic Neuropathology*, 3rd edition. Philadelphia, PA: Saunders/Elsevier; 1990

solitary schwannoma rarely can be part of neurofibromatosis type 1, bilateral schwannomas of the vestibular nerve are more common in **neurofibromatosis type 2**. The tumors have a predilection for the flexor aspects of the extremities, followed by the head and neck and mediastinum, but even the internal organs can be involved. The average size of the tumors ranges between 1.5 and 3 cm, but extreme growth may occur, especially in body cavities. The usual appearance is that of a skin-colored or pink-yellow, deep dermal or subcutaneous well-defined nodule that may be partially movable. Although the lesion in general is asymptomatic, it may be slightly painful or tender on palpation. Sensory or motor impairment may occur, but it is extremely rare. The cutaneous tumors grow slowly after an almost invariably benign course, but they may encompass adjacent tissues and organs, necessitating their removal. **Pigmented (melanotic) schwannomas** are a rare variant that may occur sporadically or in association with lentigines, cutaneous and visceral myxomas, blue nevi, and endocrine hyperactivity in patients with **Carney complex**. A subset of pigmented melanotic schwannomas carries a risk of metastatic potential.

Microscopically, common **solitary schwannomas** are ovoid or round tumors located in the deep dermis or subcutis. They are well delineated by a thin, fibrous capsule. Two main histologic patterns are considered characteristic of schwannomas: the Antoni type A and type B patterns. The **Antoni type A** pattern refers to a solid proliferation of Schwann cells forming compactly arranged fascicles and cords. The ovoid nuclei of the spindled Schwann cells are often arranged in a parallel fashion, referred to as **palisading**. When two rows of palisaded nuclei are separated by an acellular collagen-rich matrix, the resulting structures are designated as **Verocay bodies**. Although nuclear palisading is nonspecific and may occur in other soft tissue tumors (ie, **neurofibroma, dermatofibroma, leiomyoma**), it is quite common in schwannomas. Verocay bodies superficially resemble tactile bodies, but they do not have a sensory innervation. The cells constituting cellular

Table 11-41A. Schwannoma

Schwannoma
Clinical Features
Deep dermal or subcutaneous nodule
Up to 3 cm
May be painful
Predilection for flexor surface of extremities and head and neck
Histopathologic Features
Well-circumscribed, encapsulated, spindle cell proliferation
Alternating Antoni A and B areas
Palisaded nuclei
Cystic or myxoid degeneration is common
Thickened hyalinized vessel walls
Differential Diagnosis
Neuromas
Smooth muscle neoplasms
Melanocytic neoplasms with spindle cell phenotype

Antoni type A areas do not display significant cytologic atypia, and mitotic figures are absent or extremely rare. **Antoni type B** tissue shows various degrees of cystic, edematous, or myxoid degeneration associated with vascular changes, namely thickened and hyalinized vessel walls, and fibrosis. Thrombosis of the vessels, hemosiderin deposition, adjacent chronic inflammatory infiltrate, and increased numbers of mast cells are common. The degenerating cells often display variable nuclear atypia and pleomorphism, but mitotic figures are usually absent. If the tumor is thoroughly sampled, its nerve origin can be recognized, as a rule, around the periphery of the lesion.

Ancient schwannoma is composed almost entirely of Antoni type B tissue. The degenerating cells may display prominent cytologic atypia, but other features of malignancy are absent (ie, invasive growth pattern, mitoses, tumor cell necrosis).

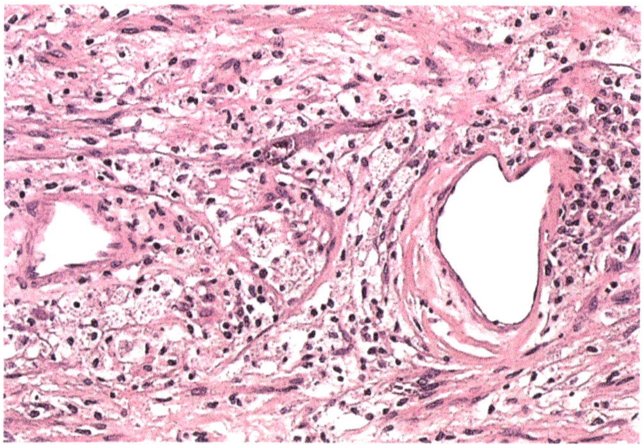

Ancient schwannoma. The lesion is composed of extensive Antoni B type areas with degenerative changes characterized by stromal edema, vascular abnormalities, chronic inflammation, and foamy macrophages. Cytologic atypia in the form of floret-like cells with smudgy nuclear chromatin are a common feature (not visualized).

Cellular schwannoma is usually a tumor of the mediastinum, retroperitoneum, or deep soft tissue. It is exceedingly rare in the skin. The tumor is a hypercellular mass of spindle-shaped cells that form intertwining fascicles and cords. Mild to moderate cytologic atypia and low mitotic rate (5 per 20 high-power fields [hpf]) are characteristic. Atypical mitotic figures, necrosis, and invasion are absent.

Plexiform schwannoma is predominantly composed of Antoni type A tissue. The proliferating cells form interconnecting fascicles and nodules extensively involving the dermis and subcutis. The proliferation, however, remains mainly within the confines of the capsule. Mild to moderate cytologic atypia is common, but mitotic figures are rare or absent. In contrast to the **plexiform neurofibroma**, this tumor is not considered pathognomonic of neurofibromatosis even though it has been reported in association with neurofibromatosis type 2. Its malignant transformation is uncommon.

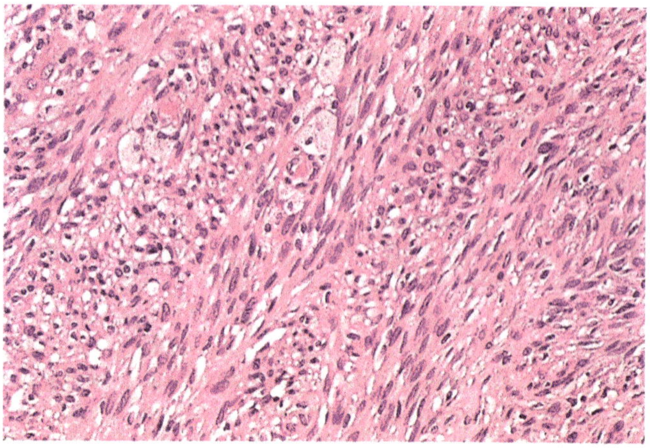

Cellular schwannoma. A compact fascicular proliferation of spindle cells with variable cytologic atypia and rare mitoses are seen.

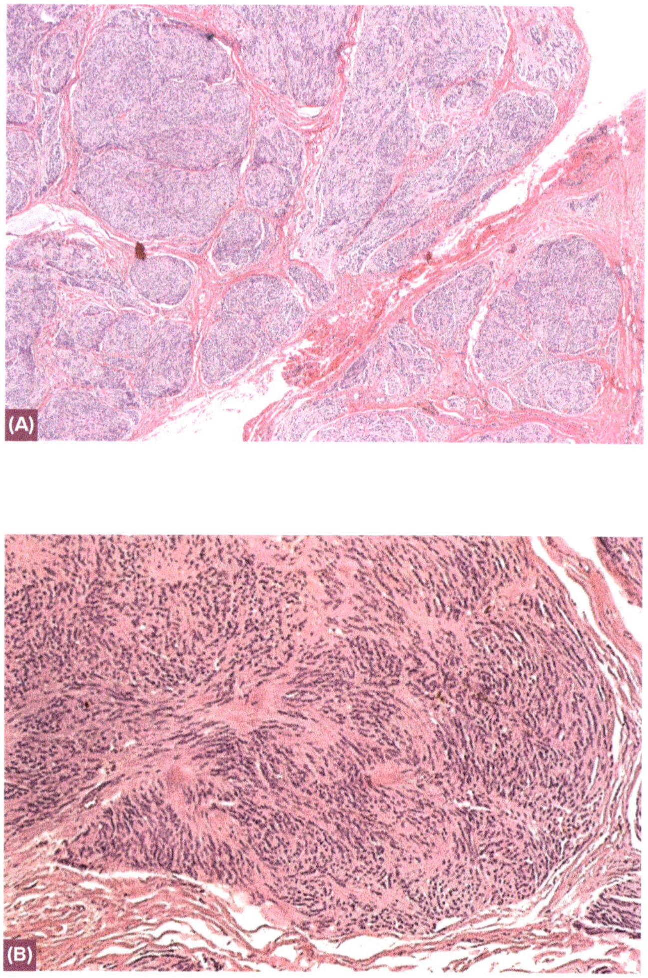

Plexiform schwannoma. (A) Interconnecting hypercellular nodules and fascicles infiltrating the dermis. **(B)** The individual fascicles are composed mainly of Antoni A type of tissue with common nuclear palisading and Verocay bodies.

Pigmented (melanotic) schwannomas contain melanin pigment, often in abundance. The lesional cells may be epithelioid, spindled, or enlarged with prominent nucleoli. The marked atypia characteristic of most melanomas is absent. Tumors of the Carney complex usually have psammoma bodies and admixed adipose tissue. **Epithelioid schwannoma** are uncommon but can mimic a malignancy due to the unusual morphologic features and low-level mitotic activity. The circumscribed growth pattern, relative uniform cytology, absence of atypical mitotic figures, and lack of necrosis favor a benign lesion. Collagen, especially type IV, is commonly produced by both spindled and epithelioid schwannoma cells and may provide a clue to the histogenesis. In rare cases, collagen production may manifest as rosette-like structures, or large, obscuring nodules. Malignant transformation of an ordinary solitary schwannoma is considered an exceedingly rare phenomenon. When present, however, the malignancy may manifest as epithelioid MPNST or angiosarcoma.

Immunohistochemically, schwannomas stain strongly for S-100 protein and type IV collagen in the Antoni type A areas. The capsule is positive for EMA, supporting perineurial cell participation. Stains for axons either by silver impregnation or by immunohistochemistry (PGP9.5) usually show residual parent nerve fibers in the capsule and a lack of axons in the tumor itself except at the periphery if the nerve of origin is present.

ANSWER 11-42: A.

The term **neurothekeoma** refers to a spectrum of neoplasms of uncertain histogenesis, which despite the name usually do not display definitive features of nerve sheath lineage (Table 11-42A). At one end of the spectrum are **hypocellular neurothekeomas** associated with abundant myxomatous stroma. In the past, these have been referred to as **classic nerve sheath myxomas** or **mature nerve sheath myxomas** because ultrastructurally and immunohistochemically some displayed characteristics of nerve sheath differentiation. At the other end of the spectrum are hypercellular tumors composed of immature cells in a collagenous stroma with only either minimal or absent myxoid quality. Such lesions displayed distinctly different features and were often designated **cellular neurothekeomas** or **immature nerve sheath myxomas.**

As more studies of these lesions have become available, the emerging concept is that a spectrum of myxoid (hypocellular), cellular, and mixed variants of neurothekeoma exist. To date, there remains inconsistency in the literature regarding whether **nerve sheath myxoma** should be included in the morphologic spectrum of **neurothekeoma.** Neurothekeomas (hypocellular, mixed, and cellular forms) may demonstrate multiple lines of mesenchymal differentiation, including histiocytic, myoid, and myofibroblastic, and peripheral nerve sheath lineage. Thus, their histogenesis remains controversial.

Clinically, neurothekeomas show a predilection for younger adults (second to third decades of life), with a female preponderance, and are found at any body site but mainly in the head and neck areas. These tumors are firm, pink or red-brown papules and nodules that usually are smaller than 3 cm in diameter. All variants are commonly asymptomatic, but on occasion, they may become sensitive or tender. They are benign lesions but may recur if they are incompletely excised.

Table 11-42A. Nerve Sheath Myxoma (Neurothekeoma)

Clinical Features
- Young to middle-aged adults
- Female predominance
- Predilection for head and neck and upper extremities
- Skin-colored papules or nodules

Histopathologic Features
- Lobules and fascicles of spindled cells within myxoid matrix
- Cells may be epithelioid or multinucleated
- Cellular variant is much more densely cellular with less myxoid matrix
- Atypia and mitoses may be present

Differential Diagnosis
- Neurofibroma
- Melanocytic neoplasms (especially Spitz tumor)
- Melanoma, especially neurotropic and myxoid variants
- Fibrohistiocytic neoplasms: juvenile and adult xanthogranuloma
- Smooth muscle neoplasms

Microscopically, **neurothekeoma** is most commonly a well-circumscribed tumor composed of nests or small clusters of spindled or epithelioid cells embedded in a variably myxoid or collagenous matrix. The myxoid ground substance may be abundant, similar to **nerve sheath myxoma**, relatively sparse, or intermediate. Some neurothekeomas are ill-defined, often infiltrative lesions occupying much of the dermis and even extending to the subcutis. The growth patterns are fascicular, plexiform, nodular, or nested, but a combination of these patterns may also occur. The tumor is mainly composed of epithelioid cells with large, ovoid nuclei; ample eosinophilic cytoplasm; and indistinct cytoplasmic membranes. The chromatin is often concentrated around the nuclear membrane, and there is a small, prominent nucleolus. Spindle-shaped cells with plump or ovoid nuclei are also common, especially when the cells form nests or whorls. When present, myxoid material is usually accumulated around the individual cell nests. In **cellular neurothekeomas**, individual cells or larger nests may be separated by thick bundles of hyalinized collagen. Alternatively, fascicles of cells may surround collagen bundles, mimicking dermatofibroma. Other stromal changes, including lymphocytic inflammation and angioplasia, may occur. Occasionally, the overlying epidermis shows mild to moderate melanocytic hyperplasia. A direct association with nerve twigs is difficult to demonstrate. Mitotic figures are usually rare and varying degrees of cytologic atypia may be seen. Although increased tumor size, nuclear pleomorphism, and mitotic activity may generate concern, these features do not appear predictive of recurrence. True malignant variants are rare, if they exist at all. Immunohistochemically, myxoid and cellular forms of neurothekeoma show a variable and inconsistent expression of antigens. If one lumps **nerve sheath myxoma** into the category of **myxoid neurothekeoma**, there appears to be a spectrum of immunohistochemical expression patterns between hypocellular, myxoid lesions and cellular lesions. The lesional cells of **nerve sheath myxoma/myxoid neurothekeoma** react strongly to S-100 protein and collagen type IV, variably to GFAP, and less intensely to neuron-specific enolase and CD57. When the capsule is preserved, a reaction to EMA is often present. Neurofilament stain for axons is usually negative. The myxomatous stroma is strongly positive for acidic mucopolysaccharides. **Mixed neurothekeomas** and **cellular neurothekeomas** show positive expression for NKI/C3, PGP9.5, microphthalmia transcription factor (MiTF), neuron-specific enolase (NSE), and type IV collagen. Expression of smooth muscle actin and CD57 (Leu-7) less frequently observed. GFAP is negative. The cells do not or only focally and weakly express S-100.

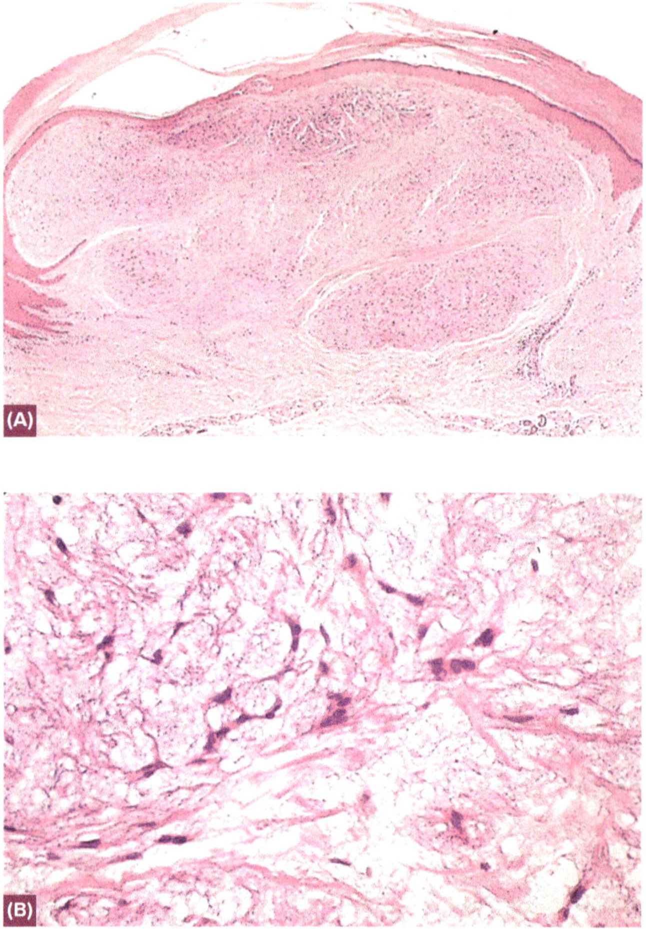

Nerve sheath myxoma. (A) Well-defined dermal nodules and fascicles with myxomatous stroma. **(B)** The mucinous stroma contains scattered spindle, polygonal, and stellate-like cells. These tumors are positive for S100.

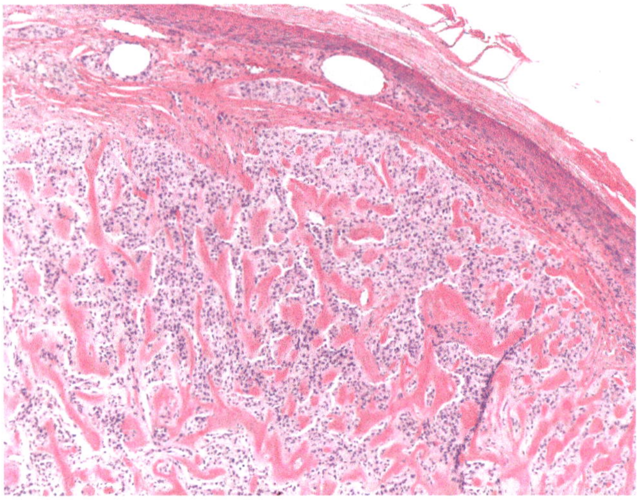

Cellular neurothekeoma. The tumor is composed of fascicles and nests infiltrating in between dermal collagen without prominent myxomatous change. The tumor cells have eosinophilic cytoplasm and large vacuolated nuclei. Rare mitoses are present.

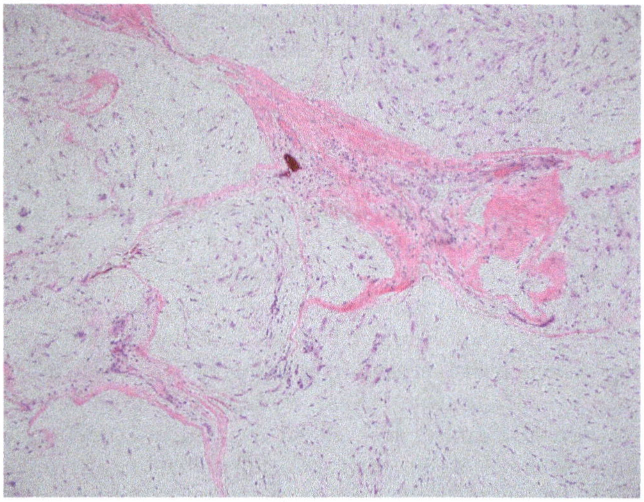

Myxoid neurothekeoma. There are asymmetric lobules of paucicellular myxoid material. There are scattered spindle cells arranged in a storiform pattern.

The histopathological differential diagnosis includes **granular cell tumor, Spitz nevus,** and **malignant peripheral nerve sheath tumor (MPNST). Granular cell tumors** are typically solitary tumors with a strong predilection for

Table 11-42B. Granular Cell Tumor

Clinical Features
Adults, predilection for women
May occur at almost any site, predilection for tongue
Extremely rare malignant counterpart is often large, deep seated, and unlikely to be encountered by dermatopathologist
Histopathologic Features
Ill-defined infiltrative tumors
Large cells with abundant finely granular eosinophilic cytoplasm
Often associated with pseudoepitheliomatous hyperplasia, particularly in mucosal locations
Criteria for malignancy are not well established but include large size and mitotic activity
Differential Diagnosis
Xanthoma
Reticulohistiocytoma
Adult-type rhabdomyoma
Alveolar soft part sarcoma
Metastatic Leydig cell tumor and granular cell variant of renal cell carcinoma

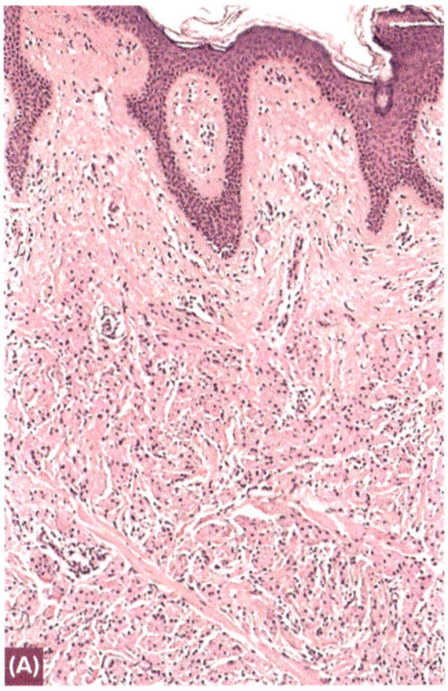

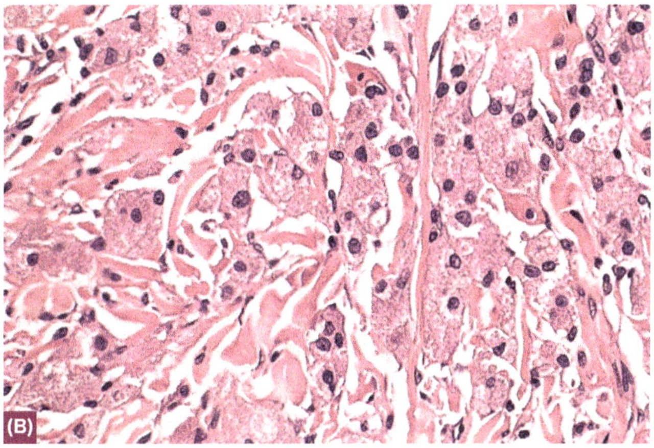

Granular cell tumor. (A) Indistinct, eosinophilic tumor cells forming nests and cords infiltrate the dermis and subcutis. The overlying epidermis is often acanthotic. **(B)** The tumor cells have a polygonal shape; indistinct cytoplasmic membranes; and uniformly small, round nuclei. The cytoplasm has a characteristic fine granular appearance. The tumor cell granules are positive for S100, CD68, and PASd.

women (Table 11-42B). Multifocality is most common in African American women. Although these tumors commonly arise in the skin, the tongue and oral mucosa are the most common sites. Microscopically, **granular cell tumors** are distinctive, consisting of fascicles or sheets of polygonal cells with abundant, granular, eosinophilic cytoplasm and small, often hyperchromatic, centrally placed nuclei. The granules can be highlighted with a PASd histochemical stain and S100 immunohistochemical stain. Ultrastructurally the granules correlate with lysosomes. The overlying epidermis characteristically shows marked pseudoepitheliomatous hyperplasia, often mimicking well-differentiated squamous cell carcinoma or a verruca. Although the tumor cells show immunohistochemical evidence of neural differentiation (S100+ and NSE+), they also express histiocytic markers CD68 and α_1-antitrypsin (but not lysozyme).

Dermal Spitz nevi may closely resemble cellular neurothekeoma histopathologically. Additionally, both Spitz nevi and cellular neurothekeomas express MITF. If scattered mitoses are present, a **spitzoid melanoma** may fall within the differential diagnosis. The distinction can be easily made with an S100 stain. While **Spitz nevi** strongly and diffusely express S100, **cellular neurothekeomas** are either negative or only focally and weakly positive for S100.

Malignant peripheral nerve sheath tumor (MPNST) is the malignant counterpart of neurofibroma and rarely schwannoma (Table 11-42C). Microscopically, an infiltrative densely cellular spindle cell population arranged in sweeping fascicles characterizes these tumors. Cytologic atypia and mitotic activity greater than 4 per 10 hpf are common. Intratumoral hemorrhage and geographic necrosis are particularly common in high-grade tumors. Interestingly, these tumors lose S100 expression in approximately 50% of cases. Although it is a well-established entity in soft tissues, this diagnosis should be approached with extreme caution in the skin, as it is indistinguishable from the much more common **spindle cell melanoma**. Features favoring MPNST over spindle cell melanoma include an absent intraepidermal component, a preexisting history of **neurofibromatosis**, and tumor association with a preexisting neurofibroma. Interestingly, S100 expression is lost in approximately 50% of MPNSTs. They are also negative for Melan-A, HMB45, and MITF.

Table 11-42C. Malignant Peripheral Nerve Sheath Tumor

Clinical Features
- Only rarely involves skin
- Often associated with neurofibromatosis

Histopathologic Features
- Spindle cells with wavy nuclei
- Cellular areas alternating with less cellular myxoid zones is characteristic
- Increased cellularity adjacent to blood vessels
- Only 50% of tumors are immunoreactive for S-100 protein
- Tumors may show heterogeneous differentiation (ie, rhabdomyoblastic, cartilaginous, osseous)

Differential Diagnosis
- Spindle cell melanoma, especially neurotropic melanoma
- Monophasic synovial sarcoma
- Fibrosarcoma

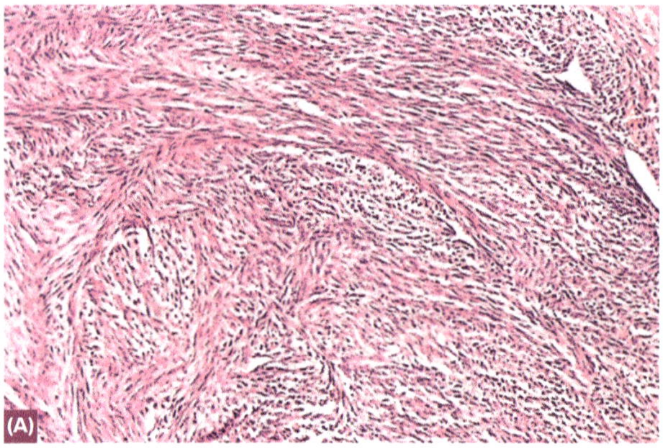

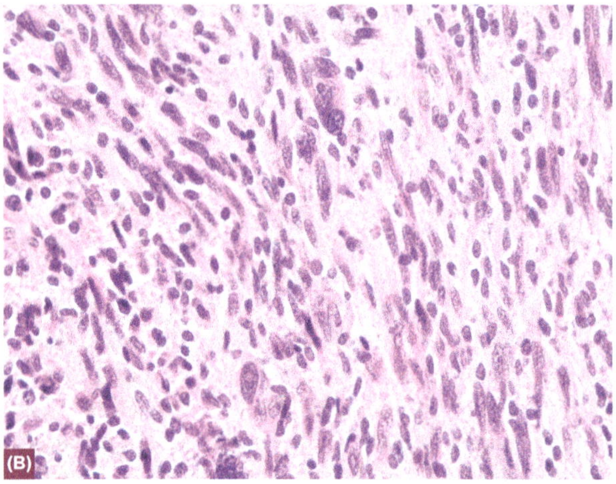

Malignant peripheral nerve sheath tumor. (A) The tumor is composed of intersecting and "sweeping" fascicles of spindle cells. **(B)** The tumor cells show marked cytologic pleomorphism, nuclear atypia, and increased mitotic rate.

ANSWER 11-43: D.

Although the cells of **primary neuroendocrine carcinoma of the skin (PNECS)** and the normal Merkel cell, which is a specialized receptor cell of touch located in the basal layer of the epidermis, share several morphologic, immunohistochemical, and ultrastructural features, there is little evidence for a direct histogenetic relationship between the two. Furthermore, other extracutaneous neuroendocrine tumors also display similar features; therefore, the conceptually more unifying term **PNECS** is preferred over **Merkel cell carcinoma** (Table 11-43A). PNECS is most common in late adulthood, and it is slightly more prevalent in Caucasians. The tumor involves mainly the head and neck areas, followed by the extremities and the buttocks. The usual appearance is a pink-red or violaceous, firm, dome-shaped solitary nodule that grows rapidly. Ulceration may occur. Although rare spontaneous regression has been reported, the usual biologic course is that of an aggressively growing, quickly metastasizing tumor with a usually fatal outcome. The local recurrence rate is approximately 40% and the overall 5-year survival rate for distant disease (stage IV) is 11%. Although a staging system has been proposed by the AJCC, the 5-year survival for stage I disease is only 81%. Wide local excision combined with adjuvant radiotherapy may improve locoregional control of the disease as well as relapse-free survival. Sentinel lymph node biopsy is recommended due to the high incidence of lymph node metastasis. The precise pathogenesis is unknown; however, there is a higher incidence in patients with chronic UV radiation exposure and immunosuppression. Recently the presence of **Merkel cell polyomavirus (MCV)** has been found in a significant subset of these tumors suggesting an infectious etiology.

Microscopically, **PNECS** appears as a poorly defined dermal mass, frequently infiltrating the subcutaneous fat, fascia, and muscle. Although it may show various growth patterns, a sheet-like growth is the most common, followed by the nested and trabecular types. Characteristically, the edge of

Table 11-43A. Neuroendocrine (Merkel Cell) Carcinoma of Skin

Clinical Features
- Predilection for head and neck of older adults
- Solitary rapidly growing nodule

Histopathologic Features
- Small, round, blue cell tumor
- Often nested or trabecular growth pattern
- High mitotic rate and frequent single-cell necrosis, often zonal necrosis
- Squamous differentiation not infrequently seen

Differential Diagnosis
- Metastatic small cell carcinoma of lung and other sites
- Lymphoma and leukemia
- Small cell melanoma

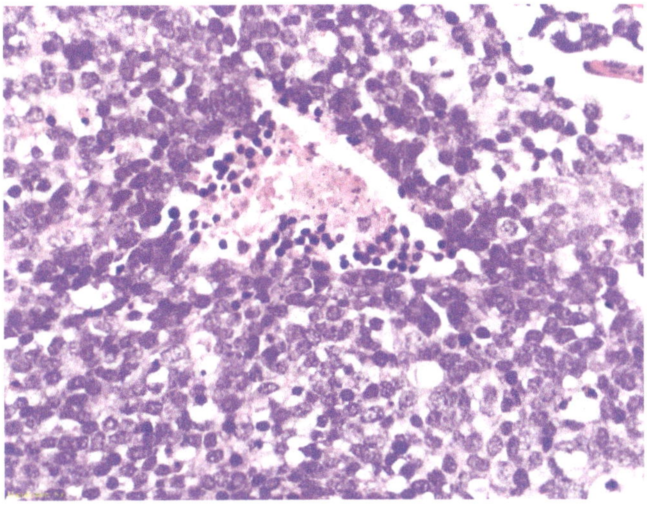

Merkel cell carcinoma (PNECS). The tumor is composed of small round cells with basophilic nuclei and scant cytoplasm. The nuclear chromatin is finely granular. Numerous mitoses and necrotic tumor cells are present. The nuclei assume conformity to adjacent cell nuclei referred to as nuclear molding. This finding is a clue to neuroendocrine differentiation, since these cells do not contain significant concentrations of structural keratin proteins.

the tumor shows a trabecular-infiltrating pattern. The tumor is composed of monotonously uniform, small, round to oval cells that are about two to three times larger than mature lymphocytes. The nuclei are ovoid with finely dispersed chromatin and distinct nuclear membranes. Nucleoli are usually not prominent. Mitotic figures are abundant. The cytoplasm is scant and faintly amphophilic. Extensive necrosis, including individual cell necrosis, and characteristic crush artifact are common in PNECS. Immunohistochemically, PNECS demonstrates a characteristic paranuclear, globular-appearing (so-called dot-like) reaction to low-molecular-weight keratins and cytokeratin 20. This staining pattern corresponds to the ultrastructurally seen distribution of paranuclear whorls of intermediate filaments. The cells also commonly express EMA. In addition, there is expression of various neuroendocrine markers, including chromogranin A, synaptophysin, somatostatin, calcitonin, vasoactive intestinal peptides, and others. These peptides are associated with the ultrastructurally demonstrable membrane-bound dense-core secretory granules. The tumor may also express neuron-specific enolase, neurofilament, and CD56. S-100 protein expression is characteristically negative. Immunohistochemical expression for p53 and p63 may also be present, the latter of which may portend a clinically aggressive course. Similar to **Ewing sarcoma (primitive**

Table 11-43B. Immunohistochemical Differential Diagnostic Features of Small Round Cell Cutaneous Tumors

	S-100	CK	CEA	EMA	LCA	VIM	CHG	SYN-7	Leu-7	DES	AC	NSE	NF	CD99 (013)	CK20
PNECS (Merkel cell tumor)	–	+	–	+	–	–	+	+	–	–	–	+	+/–	NK	+
PNET (neuroblastoma)	–	–	–	–	–	+	+/–	+/–	+/–	–	–	+	+/–	+	–
Malignant lymphoma	–	–	–	–	+	+	–	–	–	–	–	–	+	–	–
Poorly differentiated eccrine carcinoma	+/–	+	+	+	–	–	–	–	–	–	–	–	–	NK	NK
Small cell melanoma	+	–	–	–	–	+	–	–	–	–	+	–	–	NK	–
Embryonal rhabdomyosarcoma	+/–	–	–	–	–	+	–	–	+	+	–	–	–	Most–	–
Neuroblastoma	–	–	–	–	–	+	+/–	+/–	+/–	–	–	+	+	–	–
Small cell carcinoma	–	+	–	+	–	–	+	+	–	–	+	–	–	–	–

Key: +, present; –, absent; +/–, variably present; NK, not known.
AC = actin; CEA = carcinoembryonic antigen; CHG = chromogranin; CK = cytokeratin; DES = desmin; EMA = epithelial membrane antigen; LCA = leukocyte common antigen; NF = neural filaments; NSE = neuron-specific enolase; PNECS = primary neuroendocrine carcinoma of the skin; PNET = primitive neuroectodermal tumor; S-100 = S-100 protein; SYN = synaptophysin; VIM = vimentin.

neuroectodermal tumor (PNET)), CD99 and Fli-1 can be expressed in PNECS. Unlike Merkel cell carcinoma, Ewing sarcoma/PNET harbors t(11:22) in the majority of cases. A subset of PNECS stain for terminal deoxynucleotidyl transferase (TdT), which may result in confusion with lymphoma.

In regard to the differential diagnosis, a broad spectrum of small, round, blue cell tumors of various histogeneses may be confused with **PNECS.** These include **metastatic small cell carcinoma of the lung, poorly differentiated adnexal carcinoma, lymphoblastic lymphoma, primary or metastatic neuroblastoma, primary or metastatic Ewing sarcoma/ PNET, melanoma,** and **poorly differentiated squamous cell carcinoma.** These entities can usually be differentiated with the help of immunohistochemistry. In general, diffuse paranuclear reactivity for cytokeratin 20, absence of cytokeratin 7 and TTF-1, and expression of neurofilament favor **PNECS** over **metastatic pulmonary small cell carcinoma.** The main immunohistochemical differential diagnostic features are summarized in Table 11-43B.

BIBLIOGRAPHY

1. Acebo E, Val-Bernal JF, Arce, F. Giant intravenous glomus tumor. *J Cutan Pathol.* 1997;24:384–389.
2. Akhtar S, Oza KK, Wright J. Merkel cell carcinoma: report of 10 cases and review of the literature. *J Am Acad Dermatol.* 2000;43:755–767.
3. Alcalay J, Sandbank, M. The ultrastructure of cutaneous venous lakes. *Int J Dermatol.* 1987;26:645–646.
4. Allen PJ, Busam K, Hill ADK, et al. Immunohistochemical analysis of sentinel lymph nodes from patients with Merkel cell carcinoma. *Cancer.* 2001;92:1650–1655.
5. Allen PW. The fibromatoses: a clinicopathologic classification based on 140 cases. Part I. *Am J Surg Pathol.* 1977;1:255–270.
6. Aman P, Ron D, Mandahl N, et al. Rearrangement of the transcription factor gene CHOP in myxoid liposarcomas with t(12;16) (q13;p11). *Genes Chromosomes Cancer.* 1992;5(4):278–285.
7. Antonescu CR, Dal Cin P, Nafa K, et al. *EWSR1-CREB1* is the predominant gene fusion in angiomatoid fibrous histiocytoma. *Genes Chromosomes Cancer.* 2007;46:1051–1060.
8. Arai E, Kuramochi A, Tsuchida T, et al. Usefulness of D2-40 immunohistochemistry for differentiation between kaposiform hemangioendothelioma and tufted angioma. *J Cutan Pathol.* 2006;33:492–497.
9. Argenyi ZB, Cooper PH, Santa Cruz D. Plexiform and other unusual variants of palisaded encapsulated neuroma. *J Cutan Pathol.* 1993;20:34–39.
10. Argenyi ZB, LeBoit PE, Santa Cruz D, et al. Nerve sheath myxoma (neurothekeoma) of the skin: light microscopic and immunohistochemical reappraisal of the cellular variant. *J Cutan Pathol.* 1993;20:294–303.
11. Argenyi ZB, Santa Cruz D, Bromley C. Comparative light-microscopic and immunohistochemical study of traumatic and palisaded, encapsulated neuromas of the skin. *Am J Dermatopathol.* 1992;14:504–510.
12. Argenyi ZB. Immunohistochemical characterization of palisaded encapsulated neuroma. *J Cutan Pathol.* 1990;17:329–335.
13. Argenyi ZB. Recent developments in cutaneous neural neoplasms. *J Cutan Pathol.* 1993;20:97–108.
14. Asiolo S, Righi A, Volante M, et al. p63 expression as a new prognostic marker in Merkel cell carcinoma. *Cancer.* 2007;110:640–647.
15. Ballaux F, Debiec-Rychter M, De Wever I, et al. Chondroid lipoma is characterized by t(11;16)(q13;p12-13). *Virchows Arch.* 2004;444(2):208–210.
16. Barnhill RL, Dickersin GR, Nickeleit V, et al. Studies on cellular origin of neurothekeoma: clinical, light microscopic, immunohistochemical, and ultrastructural observations. *J Am Acad Dermatol.* 1991;25:80–88.
17. Barnhill RL, Mihm MC. Cellular neurothekeoma: a distinctive variant of neurothekeoma mimicking nevomelanocytic tumors. *Am J Surg Pathol.* 1990;14:113–120.
18. Bartuma H, Hallor KH, Panagopoulos I, et al. Assessment of the clinical and molecular impact of different cytogenetic subgroups in a series of 272 lipomas with abnormal karyotype. *Genes Chromosomes Cancer.* 2007;46(6):594–606.
19. Bauland CG, van Steensel MA, Steijlen PM, et al. The pathogenesis of hemangiomas: a review. *Plast Reconstr Surg.* 2006; 117:29e–35e.
20. Beham A, Badve S, Suster S, et al. Solitary myofibroma in adults: clinicopathological analysis of a series. *Histopathology.* 1993; 22:335–341.
21. Berenguer B, Mulliken JB, Enjolras O, et al. Rapidly involuting congenital hemangioma: clinical and histopathologic features. *Pediatr Dev Pathol.* 2003;6:495–510.
22. Bhattacharjee P, Hui P, McNiff J. Human herpesvirus-8 is not associated with angiolymphoid hyperplasia with eosinophilia. *J Cutan Pathol.* 2004;31:612–615.
23. Bienaime A, Rojat-Habib MC, Hesse S, et al. Giant vascular tumour in an adult: tufted angioma or kaposiform hemangioendothelioma. *Ann Dermatol Venereol.* 2006;133:553–556.
24. Billig R, Baker R, Immergut M, Maxrud W. Peyronie's disease. *Urology.* 1975;6:409–418.
25. Billings SD, Folpe AL Diagnostically challenging spindle cell lipomas: a report of 34 "low-fat" and "fat-free" variants. *Am J Dermatopathol.* 2007;29(5):437–442.
26. Billings SD, Folpe AL, Weiss SW. Do leiomyomas of deep soft tissue exist? An analysis of highly differentiated smooth muscle tumors of deep soft tissue supporting two distinct subtypes. *Am J Surg Pathol.* 2001;25(9):1134–1142.
27. Binh MB, Guillou L, Hostein I, et al. Dedifferentiated liposarcomas with divergent myosarcomatous differentiation developed in the internal trunk: a study of 27 cases and comparison to conventional dedifferentiated liposarcomas and leiomyosarcomas. *Am J Surg Pathol.* 2007;31(10):1557–1566.
28. Bisceglia M, Attino V, Bacchi CE. Metastasizing "benign" fibrous histiocytoma of the skin: a report of two additional cases and review of the literature. *Adv Anat Pathol.* 2006;13:89–96.
29. Bobos M, Hytiroglou P, Kostopoulos I, et al. Immunohistochemical distinction between Merkel cell carcinoma and small cell carcinoma of the lung. *Am J Dermatopathol.* 2006;28:99–104.
30. Bode-Lesniewska B, Frigerio S, Exner U, et al. Relevance of translocation type in myxoid liposarcoma and identification

of a novel EWSR1-DDIT3 fusion. *Genes Chromosomes Cancer.* 2007;46(11):961–971.
31. Boon LM, Mulliken JB, Enjolras O, et al. Glomuvenous malformation (glomangioma) and venous malformation: distinct clinicopathologic and genetic entities. *Arch Dermatol.* 2004; 140:971–976.
32. Boye E, Yu Y, Paranya G, et al. Clonality and altered behavior of endothelial cells from hemangiomas. *J Clin Invest.* 2001; 107:745–752.
33. Brasanac D, Janic D, Boricic I, et al. Retroperitoneal kaposiform hemangioendothelioma with tufted angioma-like features in an infant with Kasabach-Merritt syndrome. *Pathol Int.* 2003;53:627–631.
34. Brenn T, Fletcher CD. Cutaneous epithelioid angiomatous nodule: a distinct lesion in the morphologic spectrum of epithelioid vascular tumors. *Am J Dermatopathol.* 2004;26:14–21.
35. Brock JE, Perez-Atayde AR, Kozakewich HPW, et al. Cytogenetic aberrations in perineurioma: variation with subtype. *Am J Surg Pathol.* 2005;29:1164–1169.
36. Brouillard P, Boon LM, Mulliken JB, et al. Mutations in a novel factor, glomulin, are responsible for glomuvenous malformations ("glomangiomas"). *Am J Hum Genet.* 2002;70:866–874.
37. Browning J, Frieden I, Baselga E, et al. Congenital, self-regressing tufted angioma. *Arch Dermatol.* 2006;142:749–751.
38. Chang SE, Roh KH, Lee MW, et al. Microvenular hemangioma in a boy with acute myelogenous leukemia. *Pediatr Dermatol.* 2003;20:266–267.
39. Christenson LJ, Stone MS. Trauma-induced simulator of targetoid hemosiderotic hemangioma. *Am J Dermatopathol.* 2001;23:221–223.
40. Chu CY, Hsiao CH, Chiu HC. Transformation between kaposiform hemangioendothelioma and tufted angioma. *Dermatology.* 2003;206:334–337.
41. Coates SJ, Ogunrinade O, Lee HJ, Desman G. Epidermotropic metastatic epithelioid sarcoma: a potential diagnostic pitfall. *J Cutan Pathol.* 2014 Aug;41(8):672–676.
42. Coindre JM, Hostein I, Maire G, et al. Inflammatory malignant fibrous histiocytomas and dedifferentiated liposarcomas: histological review, genomic profile, and MDM2 and CDK4 status favour a single entity. *J Pathol.* 2004;203(3):822–830.
43. Coindre JM, Mariani O, Chibon F, et al. Most malignant fibrous histiocytomas developed in the retroperitoneum are dedifferentiated liposarcomas: a review of 25 cases initially diagnosed as malignant fibrous histiocytoma. *Mod Pathol.* 2003;16(3):256–262.
44. Cribier B, Noacco G, Peltre B, et al. Stromelysin 3 expression: a useful marker for the differential diagnosis dermatofibroma versus dermatofibrosarcoma protuberans. *J Am Acad Dermatol.* 2002;46:408–413.
45. Dal Cin P, Kools P, Sciot R, et al. Cytogenetic and fluorescence in situ hybridization investigation of ring chromosomes characterizing a specific pathologic subgroup of adipose tissue tumors. *Cancer Genet Cytogenet.* 1993;68(2):85–90.
46. Dal Cin P, Sciot R, de Wever I, et al. Cytogenetic and immunohistochemical evidence that giant cell fibroblastoma is related to dermatofibrosarcoma protuberans. *Genes Chromosomes Cancer.* 1996;15:73–75.
47. Davis DA, Scott DM. Lymphangioma-like Kaposi's sarcoma: etiology and literature review. *J Am Acad Dermatol.* 2000;43:123–127.
48. De Hertogh G, Bergmans G, Molderez C, et al. Cutaneous cellular fibrous histiocytoma metastasizing to the lungs. *Histopathology.* 2002;41:85–86.
49. de Visscher SA, van Ginkel RJ, Wobbes T, et al. Epithelioid sarcoma: still an only surgically curable disease. *Cancer.* 2006;107:606–612.
50. Debelenko LV, Perez-Atayde AR, Mulliken JB, et al. D2-40 immunohistochemical analysis of pediatric vascular tumors reveals positivity in kaposiform hemangioendothelioma. *Mod Pathol.* 2005;18:1454–1460.
51. Dei Tos AP. Liposarcoma: new entities and evolving concepts. *Ann Diagn Pathol.* 2000;4(4):252–266.
52. Deraedt K, Vander Poorten V, Van Geet C, et al. Multifocal kaposiform haemangioendothelioma. *Virchows Arch.* 2006; 448:843–846.
53. Deyrup AT, McKenney JK, Tighiouart M, et al. Sporadic cutaneous angiosarcomas: a proposal for risk stratification based on 69 cases. *Am J Surg Pathol.* 2008;32:72–77.
54. Domanski HA, Carlen B, Jonsson K, et al. Distinct cytologic features of spindle cell lipoma. A cytologic-histologic study with clinical, radiologic, electron microscopic, and cytogenetic correlations. *Cancer.* 2001;93(6):381–389.
55. Dotto JE, Glusac EJ. p63 is a useful marker for cutaneous spindle cell squamous cell carcinoma. *J Cutan Pathol.* 2006; 33(6):413–417.
56. Downs-Kelly E, Goldblum JR, Patel RM, et al. The utility of fluorescence in situ hybridization (FISH) in the diagnosis of myxoid soft tissue neoplasms. *Am J Surg Pathol.* 2008;32(1):8–13.
57. Enjolras O, Mulliken JB, Boon LM, et al. Noninvoluting congenital hemangioma: a rare cutaneous vascular anomaly. *Plast Reconstr Surg.* 2001;107:1647–1654.
58. Enjolras O, Picard A, Soupre, V. Congenital haemangiomas and other rare infantile vascular tumours. *Ann Chir Plast Esthet.* 2006;51:339–346.
59. Erdag G, Qureshi HS, Patterson JW, et al. Solitary fibrous tumors of the skin: a clinicopathologic study of 10 cases and review of the literature. *J Cutan Pathol.* 2007;34:844–850.
60. Evans HL, Baer SC. Epithelioid sarcoma: a clinicopathologic and prognostic study of 26 cases. *Semin Diagn Pathol.* 1993; 10:286–291.
61. Evans HL. Atypical lipomatous tumor, its variants, and its combined forms: a study of 61 cases, with a minimum follow-up of 10 years. *Am J Surg Pathol.* 2007;31(1):1–14.
62. Evans HL. Multinucleated giant cells in plantar fibromatosis. *Am J Surg Pathol.* 2002;26:244–248.
63. Fanburg-Smith JC, Michal M, Partanen TA, et al. Papillary intralymphatic angioendothelioma (PILA): a report of twelve cases of a distinctive vascular tumor with phenotypic features of lymphatic vessels. *Am J Surg Pathol.* 1999;23:1004–1010.
64. Felipo F, Vaquero M, del Agua C. Pseudotumoral encapsulated fat necrosis with diffuse pseudomembranous degeneration. *J Cutan Pathol.* 2004;31(8):565–567.
65. Feng H, Shuda M, Chang Y, et al. Clonal integration of a polyomavirus in human Merkel cell carcinoma. *Science.* 2008; 319:1096–1100.
66. Fergin PE, MacDonald DM. Naevus superficialis lipomatosus. *Clin Exp Dermatol* 1980;5:365–367.
67. Fetsch JF, Laskin WB, Hallman JR, et al. Neurothekeoma: an analysis of 178 tumors with detailed immunohistochemical data

and long-term patient follow-up information. *Am J Surg Pathol.* 2007;31:1103–1114.

68. Fetsch JF, Laskin WB, Miettinen M. Nerve sheath myxoma: a clinicopathologic and immunohistochemical analysis of 57 morphologically distinctive, S-100 protein- and GFAP-positive, myxoid peripheral nerve sheath tumors with a predilection for the extremities and a high local recurrence rate. *Am J Surg Pathol.* 2005;29:1615–1624.
69. Fetsch JF, Michal M, Miettinen M. Pigmented (melanotic) neurofibroma. A clinicopathologic and immunohistochemical analysis of 19 lesions from 17 patients. *Am J Surg Pathol.* 2000;24:331–343.
70. Fetsch JF, Miettinen M, Laskin WS, et al. A clinicopathologic study of 45 pediatric soft tissue tumors with an admixture of adipose tissue and fibroblastic elements, and a proposal for classification as lipofibromatosis. *Am J Surg Pathol.* 2000; 24:1491–1500.
71. Fetsch JF, Miettinen M. Sclerosing perineurioma: a clinicopathologic study of 19 cases of a distinctive soft tissue lesion with a predilection for the fingers and palms of young adults. *Am J Surg Pathol.* 1997;21:1433–1442.
72. Fetsch JF, Sesterhenn IA, Miettinen M, et al. Epithelioid hemangioma of the penis: a clinicopathologic and immunohistochemical analysis of 19 cases, with special reference to exuberant examples often confused with epithelioid hemangioendothelioma and epithelioid angiosarcoma. *Am J Surg Pathol.* 2004;28:523–533.
73. Fiore M, Grosso F, Lo Vullo S, et al. Myxoid/round cell and pleomorphic liposarcomas: prognostic factors and survival in a series of patients treated at a single institution. *Cancer.* 2007;109(12):2522–2531.
74. Fletcher CD, Akerman M, Dal Cin P, et al. Correlation between clinicopathological features and karyotype in lipomatous tumors. A report of 178 cases from the Chromosomes and Morphology (CHAMP) Collaborative Study Group. *Am J Pathol.* 1996;148(2):623–630.
75. Fletcher CDM, Theaker JM, Flanagan A, et al. Pigmented dermatofibrosarcoma protuberans (Bednar tumor): melanocytic colonization or neuroectodermal differentiation? A clinicopathologic and immunohistochemical study. *Histopathology.* 1988;13:631–643.
76. Fletcher JA, Kozakewich HP, Schoenberg ML, et al. Cytogenetic findings in pediatric adipose tumors: consistent rearrangement of chromosome 8 in lipoblastoma. *Genes Chromosomes Cancer.* 1993;6(1):24–29.
77. Florence E, Schrooten W, Verdonck K, et al. Rheumatological complications associated with the use of indinavir and other protease inhibitors. *Ann Rheum Dis.* 2002;61:82–84.
78. Folpe AL, Fanburg-Smith JC, Miettinen M, et al. Atypical and malignant glomus tumors: analysis of 52 cases, with a proposal for the reclassification of glomus tumors. *Am J Surg Pathol.* 2001;25:1–12.
79. Folpe AL, Lane KL, Paull G, et al. Low-grade fibromyxoid sarcoma and hyalinizing spindle cell tumor with giant rosettes: a clinicopathologic study of 73 cases supporting their identity and assessing the impact of high-grade areas. *Am J Surg Pathol.* 2000;24:1353–1360.
80. Folpe AL, Morris RJ, Weiss SW. Soft tissue giant cell tumor of low malignant potential: a proposal for the reclassification of malignant giant cell tumor of soft parts. *Mod Pathol.* 1999; 12:894–902.
81. Folpe AL, Veikkola T, Valtola R, et al. Vascular endothelial growth factor receptor-3 (VEGFR-3): a marker of vascular tumors with presumed lymphatic differentiation, including Kaposi's sarcoma, kaposiform and Dabska-type hemangioendotheliomas, and a subset of angiosarcomas. *Mod Pathol.* 2000;13:180–185.
82. Franke FE, Steger K, Marks A, et al. Hobnail hemangiomas (targetoid hemosiderotic hemangiomas) are true lymphangiomas. *J Cutan Pathol.* 2004;31:362–367.
83. Frieden IJ, Haggstrom AN, Drolet BA, et al. Infantile hemangiomas: current knowledge, future directions. Proceedings of a Research Workshop on Infantile Hemangiomas, April 7–9, 2005. *Pediatr Dermatol.* 2005;22:383–406.
84. Friedlander SF, Ritter MR, Friedlander M. Recent progress in our understanding of the pathogenesis of infantile hemangiomas. *Lymphat Res Biol.* 2005;3:219–225.
85. Fukunaga M. Expression of D2-40 in lymphatic endothelium of normal tissues and in vascular tumours. *Histopathology.* 2005;46:396–402.
86. Furlong MA, Fanburg-Smith JC, Miettinen M. The morphologic spectrum of hibernoma: a clinicopathologic study of 170 cases. *Am J Surg Pathol.* 2001;25(6):809–814.
87. Garzon MC, Enjolras O, Frieden IJ. Vascular tumors and vascular malformations: evidence for an association. *J Am Acad Dermatol.* 2000;42:275–279.
88. Garzon MC, Huang JT, Enjolras O, et al. Vascular malformations. Part II: associated syndromes. *J Am Acad Dermatol.* 2007; 56:541–564.
89. Garzon MC, Huang JT, Enjolras O, et al. Vascular malformations: part I. *J Am Acad Dermatol.* 2007;56:353–370; quiz 371–354.
90. Gebhard S, Coindre JM, Michels JJ, et al. Pleomorphic liposarcoma: clinicopathologic, immunohistochemical, and follow-up analysis of 63 cases: a study from the French Federation of Cancer Centers Sarcoma Group. *Am J Surg Pathol.* 2002;26(5):601–616.
91. Gengler C, Coindre JM, Leroux A, et al. Vascular proliferations of the skin after radiation therapy for breast cancer: clinicopathologic analysis of a series in favor of a benign process: a study from the French Sarcoma Group. *Cancer.* 2007;109:1584–1598.
92. Gessain A, Duprez R. Spindle cells and their role in Kaposi's sarcoma. *Int J Biochem Cell Biol.* 2005;37:2457–2465.
93. Goh SG, Calonje E. Cutaneous vascular tumours: an update. *Histopathology.* 2008;6:6.
94. Goldblum JR, Reith JD, Weiss SW. Sarcomas arising in dermatofibrosarcoma protuberans: a reappraisal of biologic behavior in eighteen cases treated by wide local excision with extended clinical follow up. *Am J Surg Pathol.* 2000;24:1125–1130.
95. Gollard R, Weber R, Kosty MP, et al. Merkel cell carcinoma: review of 22 cases with surgical, pathologic, and therapeutic considerations. *Cancer.* 2000;88:1842–1851.
96. Goodlad JL, Fletcher CDM. Intradermal variant of nodular fasciitis. *Histopathology.* 1991;17:569–571.
97. Goodlad JR, Mentzel T, Fletcher CDM. Low-grade fibromyxoid sarcoma: clinicopathologic analysis of eleven new cases in support of a distinct entity. *Histopathology.* 1995;26:229–237.
98. Gouillou L, Gebhard S, Salmeron S, et al. Metastasizing fibrous histiocytoma of the skin: a clinicopathologic and immunohistochemical analysis of three cases. *Mod Pathol.* 2000;13:654–660.
99. Grabellus F, von Winterfeld F, Sheu SY, et al. Unusual aggressive course of a giant cell tumor of soft tissue during immunosuppressive therapy. *Virchows Arch.* 2006;448:847–851.

100. Groger M, Niederleithner H, Kerjaschki D, et al. A previously unknown dermal blood vessel phenotype in skin inflammation. *J Invest Dermatol.* 2007;127:2893–2900.
101. Grubb RL 3rd, Franks ME, Toro J, et al. Hereditary leiomyomatosis and renal cell cancer: a syndrome associated with an aggressive form of inherited renal cancer. *J Urol.* 2007; 177(6):2074–2079; discussion 2079–2080.
102. Gruman A, Liang MG, Mulliken JB, et al. Kaposiform hemangioendothelioma without Kasabach-Merritt phenomenon. *J Am Acad Dermatol.* 2005;52:616–622.
103. Gu M, Sohn K, Kim D, et al. Metastasizing dermatofibroma in lung. *Ann Diagn Pathol.* 2007;11:64–67.
104. Guerin D, Calonje E, McCormick D. Superficial angiomyxoma: clinicopathological analysis of 26 cases of a distinctive cutaneous tumour with a tendency for recurrence (abstract). *J Pathol.* 1995;176(Suppl):51A.
105. Guo H, Garcia RA, Perle MA, et al. Giant cell tumor of soft tissue with pulmonary metastases: pathologic and cytogenetic study. *Pediatr Dev Biol.* 2005;8:718–724.
106. Gutzmer R, Kaspari M, Herbst RA, et al. Absence of HHV-8 DNA in hobnail hemangiomas. *J Cutan Pathol.* 2002;29:154–158.
107. Halling KC, Scheithauer BW, Halling AC, et al. p53 expression in neurofibroma and malignant peripheral nerve sheath tumor. An immunohistochemical study of sporadic and NF1-associated tumors. *Am J Clin Pathol.* 1996;106:282–288.
108. Hallor KH, Mertens F, Jin Y, et al. Fusion of the *EWSR1* and *ATF1* genes without expression of the MITF-M transcript in angiomatoid fibrous histiocytoma. *Genes Chromosomes Cancer.* 2005;44:97–102.
109. Hameed M. Pathology and genetics of adipocytic tumors. *Cytogenet Genome Res.* 2007;118(2–4):138–147.
110. Hanks S, Adams S, Douglas J, et al. Mutations in the gene encoding capillary morphogenesis protein 2 cause juvenile hyaline fibromatosis and infantile systemic hyalinosis. *Am J Hum Genet.* 2003;73:791–800.
111. Harris MN, Desai R, Chuang TY, et al. Lobular capillary hemangiomas: an epidemiologic report, with emphasis on cutaneous lesions. *J Am Acad Dermatol.* 2000;42:1012–1016.
112. Hashimoto H, Daimaru Y, Enjoji M. S-100 protein distribution in liposarcoma. An immunoperoxidase study with special reference to the distinction of liposarcoma from myxoid malignant fibrous histiocytoma. *Virchows Arch A Pathol Anat Histopathol.* 1984;405(1):1–10.
113. Henry F, Quatresooz P, Valverde-Lopez, JC, et al. Blood vessel changes during pregnancy: a review. *Am J Clin Dermatol.* 2006;7:65–69.
114. Hicks J, Dilley A, Patel D, et al. Lipoblastoma and lipoblastomatosis in infancy and childhood: histopathologic, ultrastructural, and cytogenetic features. *Ultrastruct Pathol.* 2001;25(4):321–333.
115. Hiruta N, Kameda N, Tokudome T, et al. Malignant glomus tumor: a case report and review of the literature. *Am J Surg Pathol.* 1997;21:1096–1103.
116. Hogewoning CJ, Bleeker MC, van den Brule AJ, et al. Pearly penile papules: still no reason for uneasiness. *J Am Acad Dermatol.* 2003;49:50–54.
117. Hollowood K, Fletcher CD. Soft tissue sarcomas that mimic benign lesions. *Semin Diagn Pathol.* 1995;12(1):87–97.
118. Hornick JL, Bosenberg MW, Mentzel T, et al. Pleomorphic liposarcoma: clinicopathologic analysis of 57 cases. *Am J Surg Pathol.* 2004;28(10):1257–1267.
119. Hornick JL, Fletcher CD. Criteria for malignancy in nonvisceral smooth muscle tumors. *Ann Diagn Pathol.* 2003;7(1):60–66.
120. Hornick JL, Fletcher CD. PEComa: what do we know so far? *Histopathology.* 2006;48(1):75–82.
121. Hornick JL, Fletcher CDM. Cellular neurothekeoma: detailed characterization in a series of 133 cases. *Am J Surg Pathol.* 2007;31:329–340.
122. Hornick JL, Fletcher CDM. Soft tissue perineurioma: clinicopathologic analysis of 81 cases including those with atypical histologic features. *Am J Surg Pathol.* 2005;29:845–858.
123. Huang HY, Antonescu CR. Epithelioid variant of pleomorphic liposarcoma: a comparative immunohistochemical and ultrastructural analysis of six cases with emphasis on overlapping features with epithelial malignancies. *Ultrastruct Pathol.* 2002;26(5):299–308.
124. Huang, HJ, Lal P, Qin J, et al. Low-grade myxofibrosarcoma: a clinicopathologic analysis of 49 cases treated at a single institution with simultaneous assessment of the efficacy of 3-tier and 4-tier grading systems. *Hum Pathol.* 2004;35:612–621.
125. Hudnall SD, Chen T, Brown K, et al. Human herpesvirus-8-positive micro-venular hemangioma in POEMS syndrome. *Arch Pathol Lab Med.* 2003;127:1034–1036.
126. Ide F, Kusama K. Endovascular papillary hemangioma of the lip. *J Oral Pathol Med.* 2002;31:565–566.
127. Ikediobi NI, Iyengar V, Hwang L. Infantile myofibromatosis: support for autosomal dominant inheritance. *J Am Acad Dermatol.* 2003;49(Suppl):S148–S150.
128. Jensen K, Wilkinson B, Wines N, et al. Procollagen 1 expression in atypical fibroxanthoma and other tumors. *J Cutan Pathol.* 2004;31:57–61.
129. Johnson MD, Jacobs AH. Congenital smooth muscle hamartoma. A report of six cases and a review of the literature. *Arch Dermatol.* 1989;125(6):820–822.
130. Kaddu S, McMenamin ME, et al. Atypical fibrous histiocytoma of the skin: clinicopathologic analysis of 59 cases with evidence of infrequent metastasis. *Am J Surg Pathol.* 2002; 26:35–46.
131. Kaddu S, McMenamin ME, Fletcher CD. Atypical fibrous histiocytoma of the skin: clinicopathologic analysis of 59 cases with evidence of infrequent metastasis. *Am J Surg Pathol.* 2002;26:35–46.
132. Kadono T, Kishi A, Onishi Y, et al. Acquired digital arteriovenous malformation: a report of six cases. *Br J Dermatol.* 2000;142:362–365.
133. Kahn HJ, Bailey D, Marks A. Monoclonal antibody D2-40, a new marker of lymphatic endothelium, reacts with Kaposi's sarcoma and a subset of angiosarcomas. *Mod Pathol.* 2002; 15:434–440.
134. Kamino H, Reddy VB, Gero M, et al. Dermatomyofibroma. A benign cutaneous plaque-like proliferation of fibroblasts and myofibroblasts in young adults. *J Cutan Pathol.* 1992;19:85–93.
135. Kanitakis J, Chouvet B. Expression of p63 in cutaneous metastases. *Am J Clin Pathol.* 2007;128(5):753–758.
136. Kao GF, Laskin WB, Olsen TG. Solitary cutaneous plexiform neurilemmoma (schwannoma): a clinicopathologic, immunohistochemical and ultrastructural study of 11 cases. *Mod Pathol.* 1986;2:20–26.
137. Katta R, Bickle K, Hwang L. Pyogenic granuloma arising in port-wine stain during pregnancy. *Br J Dermatol.* 2001;144: 644–645.

138. Kilpatrick SE, Doyon J, Choong PF, et al. The clinicopathologic spectrum of myxoid and round cell liposarcoma. A study of 95 cases. *Cancer.* 1996;77(8):1450–1458.
139. Kishimoto S, Takenaka H, Shibagaki R, et al. Glomeruloid hemangioma in POEMS syndrome shows two different immunophenotypic endothelial cells. *J Cutan Pathol.* 2000;27:87–92.
140. Kishimoto S, Takenaka H, Shibagaki R, et al. Verruciform xanthoma arising in an arteriovenous haemangioma. *Br J Dermatol.* 1998;139:546–548.
141. Kossard S, Kumar A, Wilkinson B. Neural spectrum: palisaded encapsulated neuroma and verocay body poor dermal schwannoma. *J Cutan Pathol.* 1999;26:31–36.
142. Larralde M, Gonzalez V, Marietti R, et al. Pseudo-Kaposi sarcoma with arteriovenous malformation. *Pediatr Dermatol.* 2001;18:325–327.
143. Laskin WB, Fetsch JF, Miettinen M. The "neurothekeoma": immunohistochemical analysis distinguishes the true nerve sheath myxoma from its mimics. *Hum Pathol.* 2000;31:1230–1241.
144. Leech SN, Kolar AJO, Barrett PD, et al. Merkel cell carcinoma can be distinguished from metastatic small cell carcinoma using antibodies to cytokeratin 20 and thyroid transcription factor 1. *J Clin Pathol.* 2001;54:727–729.
145. Leroy K, Dumas V, Martin-Garcia N, et al. Malignant peripheral nerve sheath tumours associated with neurofibromatosis type 1: a clinicopathologic and molecular study of 17 patients. *Arch Dermatol.* 2001;137:908–913.
146. Levy JA. A new human herpesvirus: KSHV or HHV8? *Lancet.* 1995;346:786.
147. Li CP, Lee FY, Hwang SJ, et al. Spider angiomas in patients with liver cirrhosis: role of vascular endothelial growth factor and basic fibroblast growth factor. *World J Gastroenterol.* 2003;9:2832–2835.
148. Liapis H, Dehner LP, Gutmann DH. Neurofibroma and cellular neurofibroma with atypia: a report of 14 tumors. *Am J Surg Pathol.* 1999;23:1156–1158.
149. Lin BT-Y, Weiss LM, Medeiros LJ. Neurofibroma and cellular neurofibroma with atypia: a report of 14 tumors. *Am J Surg Pathol.* 1997;21:1443–1449.
150. Lisovsky M, Hoang MP, Dresser KA, et al. Apolipoprotein D in CD34-positive and CD34-negative cutaneous neoplasms: a useful marker in differentiating superficial acral fibromyxoma from dermatofibrosarcoma protuberans. *Mod Pathol.* 2008;21:31–38.
151. Llombart B, Monteagudo C, Lopez-Guerrero JA, et al. Clinicopathological and immunohistochemical analysis of 20 cases of Merkel cell carcinoma in search of prognostic markers. *Histopathology.* 2005;46:622–634.
152. Lyons LL, North PE, Mac-Moune Lai F, et al. Kaposiform hemangioendothelioma: a study of 33 cases emphasizing its pathologic, immunophenotypic, and biologic uniqueness from juvenile hemangioma. *Am J Surg Pathol.* 2004;28:559–568.
153. Ma HJ, Zhao G, Shi F, et al. Eruptive cherry angiomas associated with vitiligo: provoked by topical nitrogen mustard? *J Dermatol.* 2006;33:877–879.
154. Macarenco RS, Zamolyi R, Franco MF, et al. Genomic gains of COL1A1-PDFGB occur in the histologic evolution of giant cell fibroblastoma into dermatofibrosarcoma protuberans. *Genes Chromosomes Cancer.* 2008;47(3):260–265.
155. Mager JJ, Westermann CJ. Value of capillary microscopy in the diagnosis of hereditary hemorrhagic telangiectasia. *Arch Dermatol.* 2000;136:732–734.
156. Makino E, Yamada J, Tada J, et al. Cutaneous angiolipoleiomyoma. *J Am Acad Dermatol.* 2006;54(1):167–171.
157. Martinez AE, Robinson MJ, Alexis JB. Kaposiform hemangioendothelioma associated with nonimmune fetal hydrops. *Arch Pathol Lab Med.* 2004;128:678–681.
158. Matsuyama A, Hisaoka M, Hashimoto H. Angioleiomyoma: a clinicopathologic and immunohistochemical reappraisal with special reference to the correlation with myopericytoma. *Hum Pathol.* 2007;38(4):645–651.
159. Mautner VF, Lindenau M, Baser ME, et al. Skin abnormalities in neurofibromatosis 2. *Arch Dermatol.* 1997;133:1539–1543.
160. McKenney JK, Weiss SW, et al. CD31 expression in intratumoral macrophages: a potential diagnostic pitfall. *Am J Surg Pathol.* 2001;25(9):1167–1173.
161. McMenamin ME, Fletcher CD. Reactive angioendotheliomatosis: a study of 15 cases demonstrating a wide clinicopathologic spectrum. *Am J Surg Pathol.* 2002;26:685–697.
162. McNiff JM, Cowper SE, Lazova R, et al. CD56 staining in Merkel cell carcinoma and natural killer-cell lymphoma: magic bullet, diagnostic pitfall, or both? *J Cutan Pathol.* 2005;32:541–545.
163. Megahed M. Histopathological variants of neurofibroma: a study of 114 lesions. *Am J Dermatopathol.* 1994;16:486–495.
164. Meis JM, Enzinger FM. Myolipoma of soft tissue. *Am J Surg Pathol.* 1991;15(2):121–125.
165. Meis-Kindblom JM, Sjogren H, Kindblom LG, et al. Cytogenetic and molecular genetic analyses of liposarcoma and its soft tissue simulators: recognition of new variants and differential diagnosis. *Virchows Arch.* 2001;439(2):141–151.
166. Mendlick MR, Nelson M, Pickering D, et al. Translocation t(1;3)(p36.3;q25) is a nonrandom aberration in epithelioid hemangioendothelioma. *Am J Surg Pathol.* 2001;25:684–687.
167. Mentzel T, Calonje E, Fletcher CDM. Dermatomyofibroma: additional observations of a distinctive cutaneous myofibroblastic tumour with emphasis on differential diagnosis. *Br J Dermatol.* 1993;129:60–73.
168. Mentzel T, Kutzner H. Reticular and plexiform perineurioma: clinicopathological and immunohistochemical analysis of two cases and review of perineurial neoplasms of skin and soft tissues. *Virchows Arch.* 2005;447:677–682.
169. Miettinen M, Fetsch JF. Evaluation of biological potential of smooth muscle tumours. *Histopathology.* 2006;48(1):97–105.
170. Miettinen M, Fetsch, JF. Distribution of keratins in normal endothelial cells and a spectrum of vascular tumors: implications in tumor diagnosis. *Hum Pathol.* 2000;31:1062–1067.
171. Murphey MD, Carroll JF, Flemming DJ, et al. From the archives of the AFIP: benign musculoskeletal lipomatous lesions. *Radiographics.* 2004;24(5):1433–1466.
172. Nakamura T. Apoptosis and expression of Bax/Bcl-2 proteins in pyogenic granuloma: a comparative study with granulation tissue and capillary hemangioma. *J Cutan Pathol.* 2000;27:400–405.
173. North PE, Kahn T, Cordisco MR, et al. Multifocal lymphangioendotheliomatosis with thrombocytopenia: a newly recognized clinicopathological entity. *Arch Dermatol.* 2004;140:599–606.
174. North PE, Mihm MC Jr. Histopathological diagnosis of infantile hemangiomas and vascular malformations. *Facial Plast Surg Clin North Am.* 2001;9:505–524.

175. North PE, Waner M, Buckmiller L, et al. Vascular tumors of infancy and childhood: beyond capillary hemangioma. *Cardiovasc Pathol.* 2006;15:303–317.
176. North PE, Waner M, James CA, et al. Congenital nonprogressive hemangioma: a distinct clinicopathologic entity unlike infantile hemangioma. *Arch Dermatol.* 2001;137:1607–1620.
177. North PE, Waner M, Mizeracki A, et al. GLUT1: a newly discovered immunohistochemical marker for juvenile hemangiomas. *Hum Pathol.* 2000;31:11–22.
178. O'Connell JX, Wehrli BM, Neilsen GP, et al. Giant cell tumors of soft tissue: a clinicopathologic study of 18 benign and malignant tumors. *Am J Surg Pathol.* 2000;24:386–395.
179. Oliveira AM, Dei Tos AP, Fletcher CD, et al. Primary giant cell tumor of soft tissues: a study of 22 cases. *Am J Surg Pathol.* 2000;24:248–256.
180. Onishi Y, Ohara, K. Angiolymphoid hyperplasia with eosinophilia associated with arteriovenous malformation: a clinicopathological correlation with angiography and serial estimation of serum levels of renin, eosinophil cationic protein and interleukin 5. *Br J Dermatol.* 1999;140:1153–1156.
181. Ordóñez NG. Granular cell tumor: a review and update. *Adv Anat Pathol.* 1999;6:186–203.
182. Ortiz-Rey JA, Gonzalez-Ruiz A, San Migue P, et al. Hobnail haemangioma associated with the menstrual cycle. *J Eur Acad Dermatol Venereol.* 2005;19:367–369.
183. Page RN, King R, Mihm MC Jr, et al. Microphthalmia transcription factor and NKI/C3 expression in cellular neurothekeoma. *Mod Pathol.* 2004;17:230–234.
184. Parsons A, Sheehan DJ, Sangueza OP. Retiform hemangioendotheliomas usually do not express D2-40 and VEGFR-3. *Am J Dermatopathol.* 2008;30:31–33.
185. Patel RM, Goldblum JR, Hsi ED. Immunohistochemical detection of human herpes virus-8 latent nuclear antigen-1 is useful in the diagnosis of Kaposi sarcoma. *Mod Pathol.* 2004;17:456–460.
186. Perez-Montiel MD, Plaza JA, Dominguez-Malagon H, et al. Differential expression of smooth muscle myosin, smooth muscle actin, h-caldesmon, and calponin in the diagnosis of myofibroblastic and smooth muscle lesions of skin and soft tissue. *Am J Dermatopathol.* 2006;28(2):105–111.
187. Phillips JA, Dixon JE, Richardson JB, et al. Glomeruloid hemangioma leading to a diagnosis of POEMS syndrome. *J Am Acad Dermatol.* 2006;55:149–152.
188. Prasad V, Fishman SJ, Mulliken JB, et al. Cutaneovisceral angiomatosis with thrombocytopenia. *Pediatr Dev Pathol.* 2005;8:407–419.
189. Raddaoui E, Donner LR, Panagopoulos I. Fusion of the *FUS* and *ATF-1* genes in a large, deep-seated angiomatoid fibrous histiocytoma. *Diagn Mol Pathol.* 2002;11:157–162.
190. Rahman N, Dunstan M, Teare MD, et al. The gene for juvenile hyaline fibromatosis maps to chromosome 4q21. *Am J Hum Genet.* 2002;71:975–980.
191. Rao VK, Weiss SW. Angiomatosis of soft tissue. An analysis of the histologic features and clinical outcome in 51 cases. *Am J Surg Pathol.* 1992;16:764–771.
192. Remstein ED, Arndt CAS, Nascimento AG. Plexiform fibrohistiocytic tumor: clinicopathologic analysis of 22 cases. *Am J Surg Pathol.* 1999;23:662–670.
193. Requena L, Kutzner H, Mentzel T, et al. Benign vascular proliferations in irradiated skin. *Am J Surg Pathol.* 2002;26:328–337.
194. Requena L, Sangueza OP. Cutaneous vascular anomalies. Part I. Hamartomas, malformations, and dilatation of preexisting vessels. *J Am Acad Dermatol.* 1997;37:523–549.
195. Robson AM, Calonje E. Cutaneous perineurioma: a poorly recognized tumour often misdiagnosed as epithelioid histiocytoma. *Histopathology.* 2000;37:332–339.
196. Roh HS, Kim YS, Suhr KB, et al. A case of childhood epithelioid hemangioendothelioma. *J Am Acad Dermatol.* 2000;42:897–899.
197. Rongioletti F, Rebora A. Cutaneous reactive angiomatoses: patterns and classification of reactive vascular proliferation. *J Am Acad Dermatol.* 2003;49:887–896.
198. Roses DF, Valensi Q, Latrenta G, et al. Surgical treatment of dermatofibrosarcoma protuberans. *Surg Gynecol Obstet.* 1986; 162:449–452.
199. Satti MB. Tendon sheath tumours: a pathological study of the relationship between giant cell tumour and fibroma of tendon sheath. *Histopathology.* 1992;20:213–220.
200. Schmid H, Zietz C. Human herpesvirus 8 and angiosarcoma: analysis of 40 cases and review of the literature. *Pathology.* 2005;37:284–287.
201. Schwartz RA, Fernandez G, Kotulska K, et al. Tuberous sclerosis complex: advances in diagnosis, genetics, and management. *J Am Acad Dermatol.* 2007;57:189–202.
202. Sciot R, Akerman M, Dal Cin P, et al. Cytogenetic analysis of subcutaneous angiolipoma: further evidence supporting its difference from ordinary pure lipomas: a report of the CHAMP Study Group. *Am J Surg Pathol.* 1997;21(4):441–444.
203. Sheehan M, Roumpf SO, Summerlin DJ, et al. Spindle cell hemangioma: report of a case presenting in the oral cavity. *J Cutan Pathol.* 2007;34:797–800.
204. Shyong EQ, Gorevic P, Lebwohl M, et al. Reactive angioendotheliomatosis and sarcoidosis. *Int J Dermatol.* 2002;41:894–897.
205. Sigel JE, Goldblum JR. Solitary fibrous tumor of the skin. *Am J Dermatopathol.* 2001;23:275–278.
206. Sirvent N, Coindre JM, Maire G, et al. Detection of MDM2-CDK4 amplification by fluorescence in situ hybridization in 200 paraffin-embedded tumor samples: utility in diagnosing adipocytic lesions and comparison with immunohistochemistry and real-time PCR. *Am J Surg Pathol.* 2007;31(10):1476–1489.
207. Skelton HG, Williams J, Smith KJ. The clinical and histologic spectrum of fibrous perineuriomas. *Am J Dermatopathol.* 2001;23:190–196.
208. Smith TA, Easley KA, Goldblum JR. Myxoid/round cell liposarcoma of the extremities. A clinicopathologic study of 29 cases with particular attention to extent of round cell liposarcoma. *Am J Surg Pathol.* 1996;20(2):171–180.
209. Suarez A, Johnson-Jahangir H, Desman G, Avarbock A. Post-radiation atypical vascular proliferation on the head of a young woman: a diagnostic challenge. *Dermatol Online J.* 2015 Jun 16;21(6).
210. Sur M, AlArdati H, Ross C, et al. TdT expression in Merkel cell carcinoma: potential diagnostic pitfall with blastic hematological malignancies and expanded immunohistochemical analysis. *Mod Pathol.* 2007;20:1113–1120.
211. Suurmeijer AJ, Fletcher CD. Papillary haemangioma. A distinctive cutaneous haemangioma of the head and neck area containing eosinophilic hyaline globules. *Histopathology.* 2007;51:638–648.
212. ten Heuvel SE, Hoekstra HJ, van Ginkel RJ, et al. Clinicopathologic prognostic factors in myxoid liposarcoma: a retrospective study

of 49 patients with long-term follow-up. *Ann Surg Oncol.* 2007;14(1):222–229.

213. Tennant LB, Mulliken JB, Perez-Atayde AR, et al. Verrucous hemangioma revisited. *Pediatr Dermatol.* 2006;23:208–215.
214. Tos AP. Classification of pleomorphic sarcomas: where are we now? *Histopathology.* 2006;48(1):51–62.
215. Tronnier M, Vogelbruch M, Kutzner, H. Spindle cell hemangioma and epithelioid hemangioendothelioma arising in an area of lymphedema. *Am J Dermatopathol.* 2006;28:223–227.
216. Ushiima M, Tsuneyoshi M, Enjoji M. Dupuytren's type fibromatosis. A clinicopathologic study of 62 cases. *Acta Pathol Jpn.* 1984;34:991–1001.
217. Vanni R, Fletcher CD, Sciot R, et al. Cytogenetic evidence of clonality in cutaneous benign fibrous histiocytomas: a report of the CHAMP study group. *Histopathology.* 2000;37:212–217.
218. Velez D, Delgado-Jimenez Y, Fraga J. Solitary glomeruloid haemangioma without POEMS syndrome. *J Cutan Pathol.* 2005;32:449–452.
219. Virgili A, Trincone S, Zampino MR, et al. Acroangiodermatitis of amputation stump. *Eur J Dermatol.* 2003;13:402–403.
220. Wang AR, May D, Bourne P, et al. PGP9.5: a marker for cellular neurothekeoma. *Am J Surg Pathol.* 1999;23:1401–1407.
221. Wang HW, Trotter MW, Lagos D, et al. Kaposi sarcoma herpesvirus-induced cellular reprogramming contributes to the lymphatic endothelial gene expression in Kaposi sarcoma. *Nat Genet.* 2004;36:687–693.
222. Wassef M, Vanwijck R, Clapuyt P, et al. Vascular tumors and malformations, classification, pathology and imaging. *Ann Chir Plast Esthet.* 2006;51:263–281.
223. Watabe H, Kashima M, Baba T, et al. A case of unilateral dermatomal cavernous haemangiomatosis. *Br J Dermatol.* 2000;143:143.
224. Watanabe C, Koga M, Honda Y, et al. Juvenile temporal arteritis is a manifestation of Kimura disease. *Am J Dermatopathol.* 2002;24:43–49.
225. Waters BL, Panagopoulos I, Allen EF. Genetic characterization of angiomatoid fibrous histiocytoma identifies fusion of the *FUS* and *ATF-1* genes induced by a chromosomal translocation involving bands 12q13 and 16p11. *Cancer Genet Cytogenet.* 2000;121:109–116.
226. Weinreb I, Howarth D, Latta E, et al. Perivascular epithelioid cell neoplasms (PEComas): four malignant cases expanding the histopathological spectrum and a description of a unique finding. *Virchows Arch.* 2007;450(4):463–470.
227. Woodruff JM. Pathology of tumors of the peripheral nerve sheath in type I neurofibromatosis. *Am J Med Genet (Semin Med Genet).* 1999;89:23–30.
228. Xu H, Edwards JR, Espinosa O, et al. Expression of a lymphatic endothelial cell marker in benign and malignant vascular tumors. *Hum Pathol.* 2004;35:857–861.

CHAPTER 12

Lymphoid, Leukemic, and Other Cellular Infiltrates

QUESTION 12-1.

Which general statement regarding T-cell pseudolymphoma is INCORRECT?

A) These lesions both clinically and histopathologically may resemble mycosis fungoides and may occasionally exhibit clonality via T-cell-receptor rearrangement analysis.
B) The natural history of T-cell pseudolymphoma is that of a chronic dermatosis that either transforms into lymphoma or eventually resolves spontaneously.
C) These lesions may be histopathologically characterized by nodular dermal infiltrates with scattered large CD30+ T cells.
D) T-cell pseudolymphoma is immunohistochemically defined by lost expression of pan-T-cell markers CD2, CD5, or CD7.
E) Reported associations include HIV disease, UV-light exposure, and various medications.

QUESTION 12-2.

A 66-year-old Caucasian male presents with irregular, well-circumscribed, confluent, yellowish-red patches with slight scaling on the trunk or buttocks. The lesions have been present for over 10 years. A biopsy is performed and the findings are illustrated below. Immunohistochemical staining reveals the infiltrate to be composed predominantly of CD3+, CD2+, and BF1+ T cells. The intraepidermal CD4 to CD8 ratio is 4:1 and the dermal CD4 to CD8 ratio is 10:1. There is preserved expression of CD5; however, there is a marked reduction in CD7 expression in the realm of 90%. Which of the following statements regarding this patient's condition is INCORRECT?

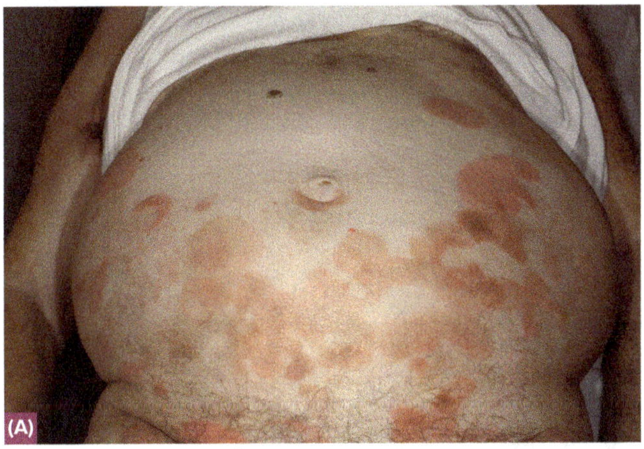

(A)

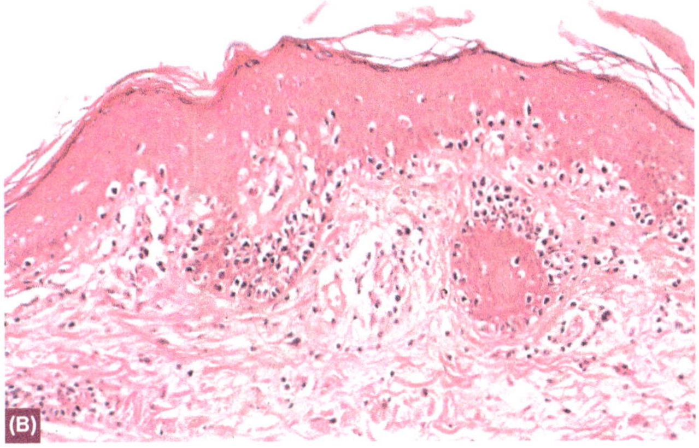

(B)

A) This patient has the *d'emblée form* of mycosis fungoides.
B) High-power examination will reveal the infiltrate to be composed predominantly of small lymphocytes with cerebriform nuclei.
C) This condition has a propensity to involve sun-protected sites such as the trunk or buttocks.
D) These patches will gradually progress to plaques and/or nodular tumors.
E) These lesions frequently contain intraepidermal clusters of lymphocytes without Langerhans cells.

QUESTION 12-3.

A 65-year-old male presents with plate-like thickening of the skin on the neck and chest and loose poikilodermatous folds in the axillary and scapular areas. A biopsy of the loose skin is performed and the findings are illustrated below. Immunohistochemistry reveals the small lymphoid cells to be of the CD3+, CD4+, CD8–, CD30– T-helper phenotype. The giant cells express CD163, lysozyme, and CD68. Elastic stain reveals a marked reduction of elastic fibers in the dermis. Fragmented elastic fibers are identified within the multinucleated giant cells. T-cell-receptor rearrangement analysis reveals clonality. Which of the following diagnoses is CORRECT?

A) Granulomatous mycosis fungoides
B) Pagetoid reticulosis
C) Granulomatous slack skin disease
D) Large plaque parapsoriasis
E) Small plaque parapsoriasis

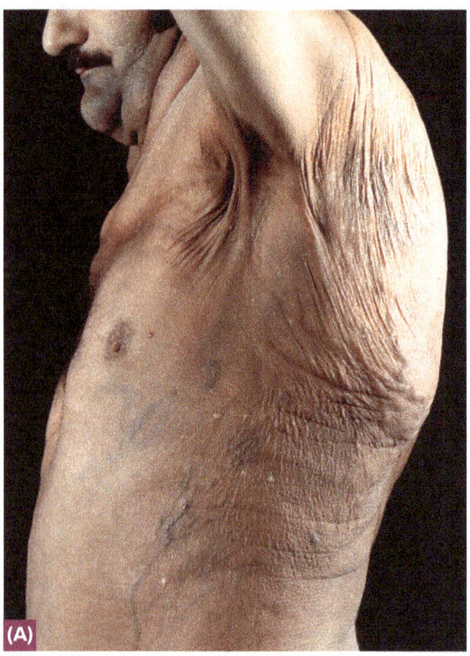
(A)

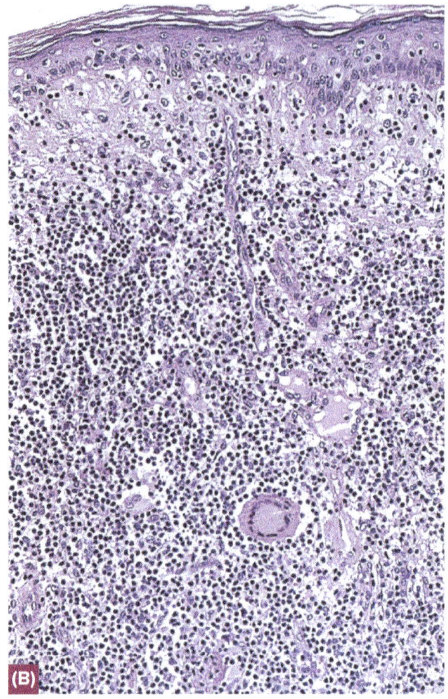
(B)

Part **(A)** reproduced, with permission, from Wolff K, Johnson RA, Saavedra AP. *Fitzpatrick's Color Atlas and Synopsis of Clinical Dermatology*. 7th ed. New York, NY: McGraw-Hill Education; 2013.

QUESTION 12-4.

A 38-year-old male presents with an erythematous plaque on the forehead that is studded with comedo-like pustules. Additionally, there is alopecia of the eyebrow. The lesion has been present for two years. A biopsy is performed and the findings are illustrated below. Langerhans cell clusters are noticeably absent within the follicular epithelium. The follicular infiltrates are composed of small lymphocytes with cerebriform nuclear contour irregularity and the perifollicular infiltrates consist of small- to medium-sized lymphocytes admixed with plasma cells and eosinophils. Immunohistochemical staining reveals the follicular infiltrate to be composed predominantly of CD3+, CD2+, BF-1+, CD4+, CD8– T cells with reduction in CD7 expression in the realm of 70%. Alcian blue stain reveals no dermal mucin within the hair follicle. Which of the following statements regarding this condition is INCORRECT?

A) This is a variant of mycosis fungoides with a significantly poorer progression free, disease free, and overall survival than classic mycosis fungoides and displays outcomes more similar to those seen in tumor stage mycosis fungoides.
B) These lesions are typically recalcitrant to UV-light therapy.

C) The absence of dermal mucin within the follicular epithelium is associated with a markedly improved clinical outcome.
D) Occasionally the infiltrates of this condition may contain scattered CD30+ immunoblast-like cells.
E) Gene expression profiling studies have shown that these lymphocytic infiltrates tend to express genes associated with typical mycosis fungoides of advanced stage with poor prognosis.

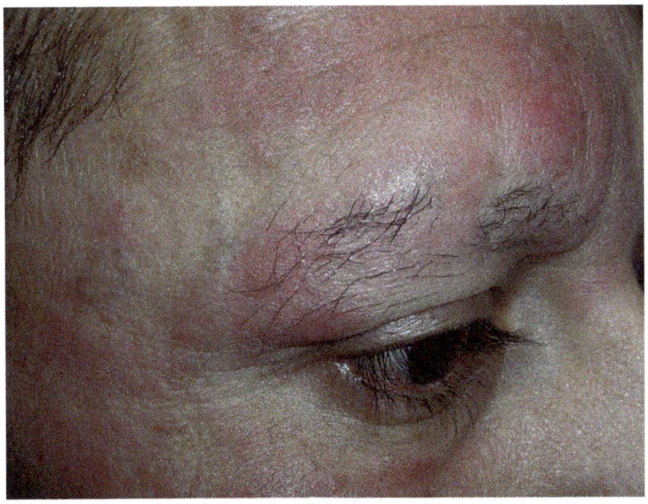

Reproduced, with permission, from Usatine RP, Smith MA, Mayeaux EJ Jr, Chumley HS, eds. *Color Atlas of Family Medicine*. 2nd ed. New York, NY: McGraw-Hill Education; 2012.

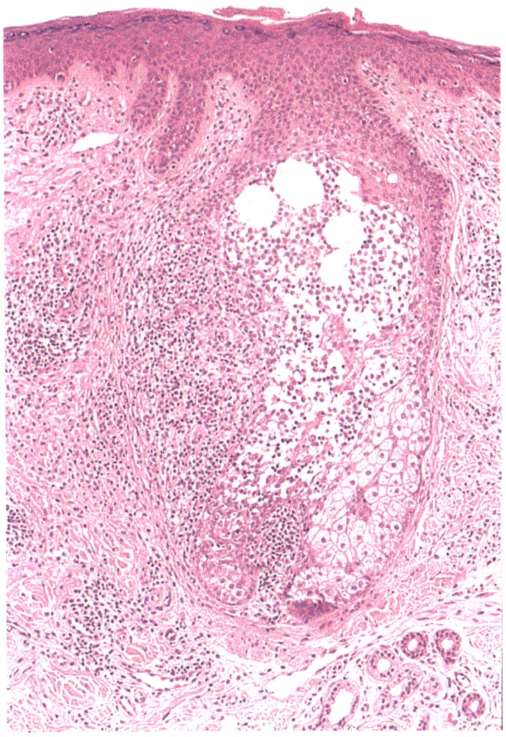

QUESTION 12-5.

A 67-year-old male patient presents with intense pruritus, erythroderma, scaling, edema, palmoplantar hyperkeratosis, hair loss, onychodystrophy, and diffuse enlargement of lymph nodes. A skin biopsy and peripheral blood smear are examined and the findings are illustrated below. Immunohistochemical staining of the skin biopsy reveals the lymphoid cells to be CD2+, CD3+, CD4+, CD5+, CD45RO+, CD8−, and CD30−. Peripheral blood analysis reveals greater than 1000 lymphoid cells per mm^3 with nuclear contour irregularity. Flow cytometry of the peripheral blood reveals a strikingly elevated CD4+ T-cell population resulting in a significantly increased CD4/CD8 ratio (>10). T-cell-receptor rearrangement analysis of the peripheral blood detects a clonal rearrangement. Which of the following diagnoses is CORRECT?

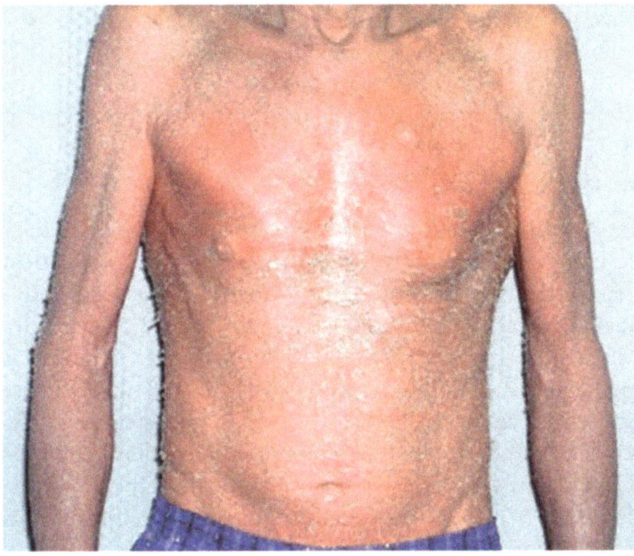

Reproduced, with permission, from Lichtman MA, Shafer JA, Felgar RE, Wang N. *Lichtman's Atlas of Hematology*. New York, NY: McGraw-Hill; 2007.

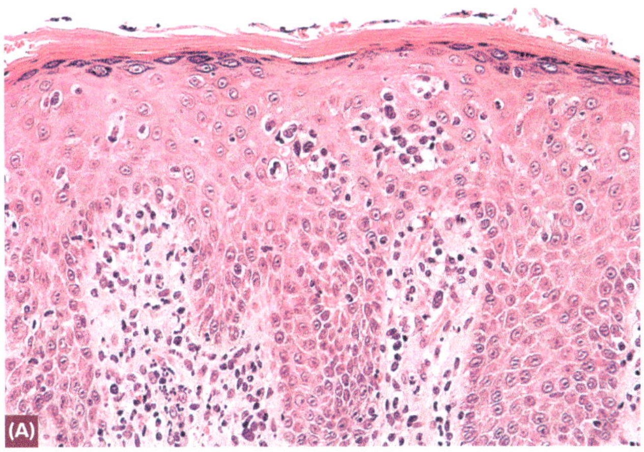

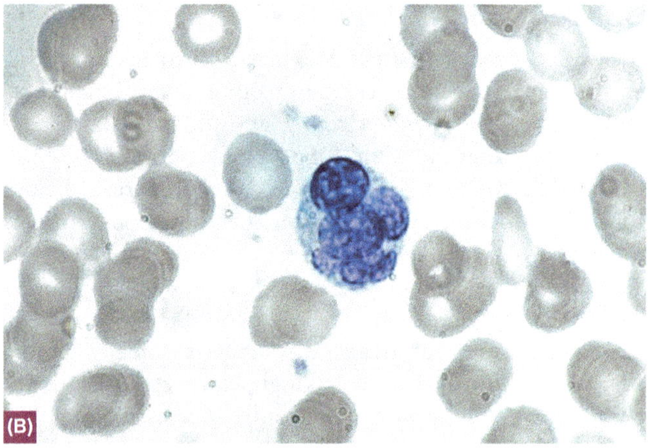

(B)

A) Erythrodermic mycosis fungoides
B) Sézary syndrome
C) Idiopathic erythroderma
D) Erythrodermic drug eruption
E) Generalized atopic dermatitis

QUESTION 12-6.

A 30-year-old patient presents with a few papulonodular lesions on the posterior thigh and popliteal fossa. The patient reports that similar lesions have formed in the past but spontaneously resolved. You notice that the healed lesions have left behind hyperpigmented varioliform scars. A biopsy is performed and the findings are illustrated below. There are superficial and deep nodular infiltrates with sparing of the epidermis (grenz zone). An immunohistochemical stain for CD30 reveals positive staining in approximately 40% of the infiltrate. Which of the following statements regarding this condition is INCORRECT?

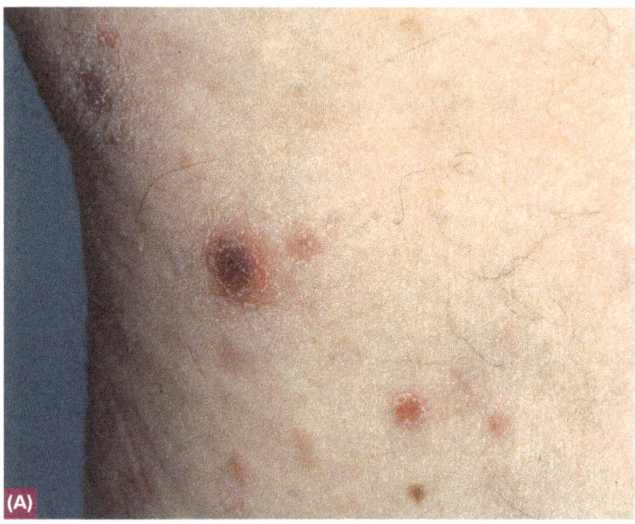

(A)

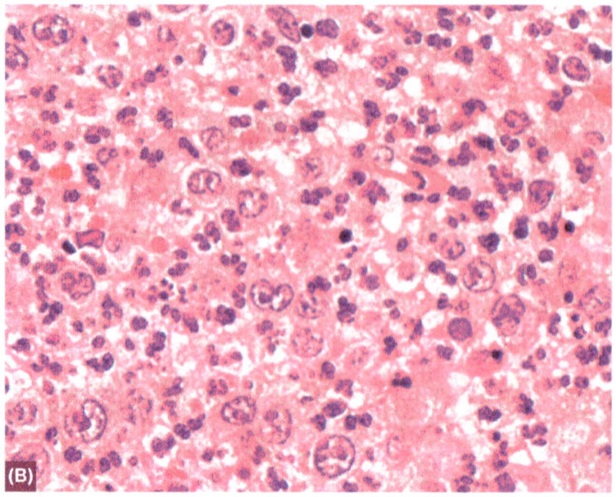

(B)

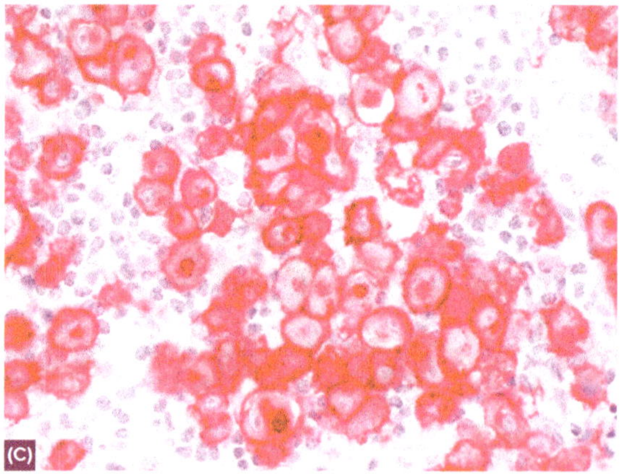

(C)

A) This is a benign condition that in approximately 10% to 20% of cases is associated with the development of a second malignant lymphoma such as mycosis fungoides, Hodgkin lymphoma, or anaplastic lymphoma.
B) High mitotic activity within the large cell population is indicative of anaplastic large cell lymphoma.
C) In addition to CD30+, the immunophenotype of the large cells is most likely CD3+, CD4+, CD8–, granzyme+, TIA-1+.
D) This condition may rarely contain only small lymphocytes with significant epidermotropism.
E) The 5-year survival from this condition is greater than 90%.

QUESTION 12-7.

A 57-year-old male presents with fever, night sweats, weight loss, and the sudden onset of multiple ulcerated nodules on both lower extremities. The lesions have been present for over 2 months and have been progressively enlarging. A CT scan reveals hilar lymphadenopathy and hepatosplenomegaly. A biopsy of one of the leg lesions is performed and the findings are illustrated below. The large cells account for greater than 75% of the total cellular infiltrate. Immunohistochemical staining reveals the tumor cells to be CD3+, CD30+, CD4+, granzyme+, TIA1+, MUM1+, EMA+, and ALK+. There is negative staining for CD8, CD56, CLA, and EBER (EBV). Tumor cytogenetics reveals a t(2;5) chromosomal translocation. The patient expires before any treatment can be initiated. Which of the following diagnoses is CORRECT?

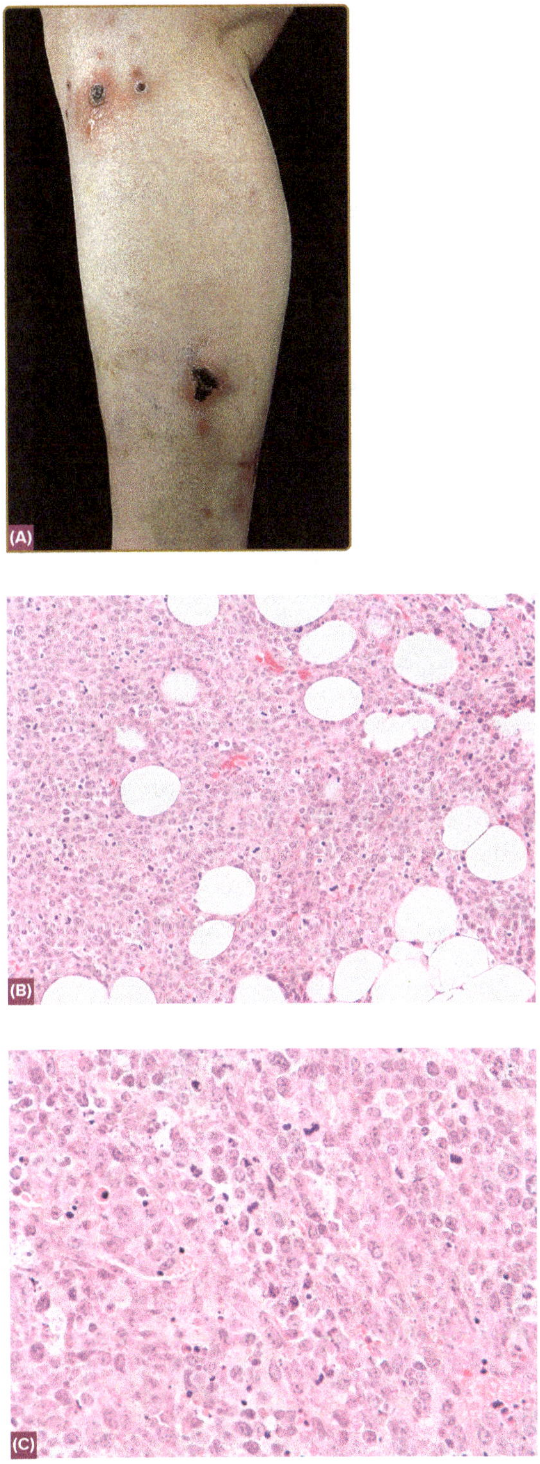

Reproduced, with permission, from Goldsmith LA, Katz SI, Gilchrest BA, Paller AS, Leffell DJ, Wolff K, eds. *Fitzpatrick's Dermatology in General Medicine*. 8th ed. New York, NY: McGraw-Hill Education; 2012.

A) Primary cutaneous anaplastic large cell lymphoma
B) Extranodal NK/T-cell lymphoma
C) Systemic anaplastic large cell lymphoma
D) Type C lymphomatoid papulosis
E) Large transformation of mycosis fungoides

QUESTION 12-8.

A patient with systemic lupus erythematosus presents with erythematous, firm, subcutaneous nodules on the right lower extremity. The lesions have been persistent over a period of 9 months. One of the nodules is ulcerated. A punch biopsy is performed and the findings are illustrated below. Immunohistochemistry reveals the lesional cells to be BF1+, CD2+, CD3+, CD4–, CD8+, CD5+, CD43+, CD56–, T1A-1+, granzyme+, perforin+, and EBER-. Clonal rearrangement of the α/β T-cell-receptor is found. Which of the following diagnoses is CORRECT?

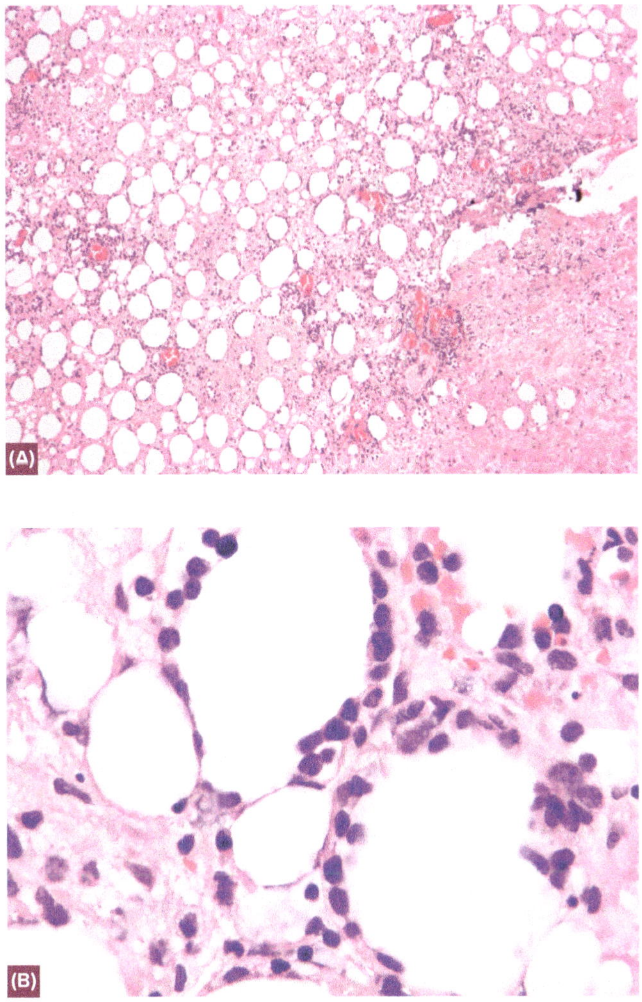

Parts **(A)** and **(B)** reproduced, with permission, from Kantarjian HM, Wolff RA, Koller CA. *The MD Anderson Manual of Medical Oncology*. 2nd ed. New York, NY: McGraw-Hill Education; 2011.

A) Subcutaneous panniculitis–like T-cell lymphoma
B) Lupus profundus
C) Subcutaneous gamma/delta lymphoma
D) Erythema nodosum
E) Tumor stage mycosis fungoides

QUESTION 12-9.

A patient presents with a skin-colored nodule without ulceration on the trunk. A biopsy is performed and the findings are illustrated below. Eosinophils, plasma cells, and histiocytes are admixed within the infiltrate. Immunohistochemistry reveals the tumor cells to have a CD3+, CD4+, CD8–, CD30–, T-helper phenotype. Rare scattered CD20+ B cells are present. CD21 stain is negative for dendritic cell networks within the lymphoid nodules. There is a slight loss of CD5 and CD7 expression. Clonal rearrangement of *TCR* genes is detected. Which of the following diagnoses is CORRECT?

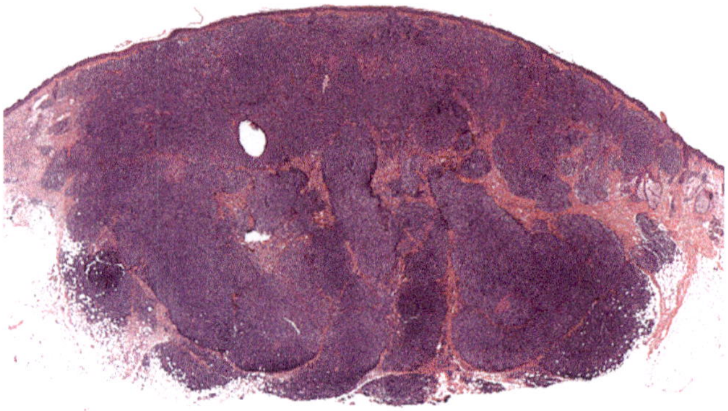

A) B-cell pseudolymphoma
B) Mycosis fungoides
C) Primary cutaneous anaplastic large cell lymphoma
D) Primary cutaneous CD4+ small- to medium-sized pleomorphic T-cell lymphoma
E) Low-grade B-cell lymphoma, marginal zone type

QUESTION 12-10.

An elderly patient with chronic idiopathic pancytopenia presents with contusiform, bruise-like, disseminated plaques on the head and trunk. A biopsy is performed and the findings are illustrated below. Immunohistochemistry reveals a CD20–, CD3–, CD4+, CD8–, CD56+, CD123+, TCL1+, EBV-, MPO-, CD14–, CD11c- immunophenotype. No clonal rearrangement of TCR genes is detected. Systemic workup reveals circulating malignant cells, as well as lymph node, bone marrow, and central nervous system involvement. The patient succumbs to the disease within 2 years. Which of the following diagnoses is CORRECT?

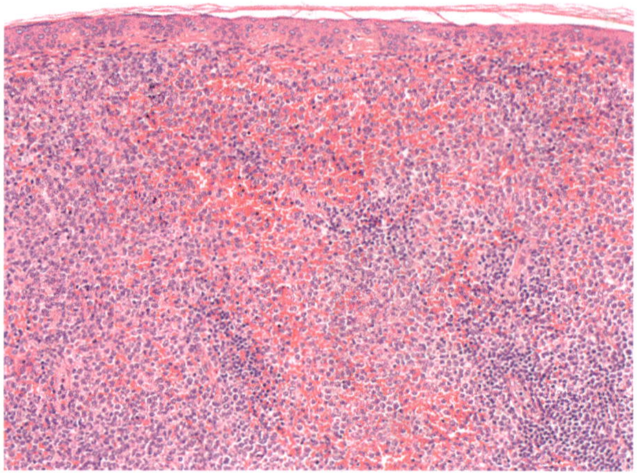

A) Diffuse large B-cell lymphoma, leg type
B) Anaplastic large cell lymphoma
C) Leukemia cutis (acute myelogenous leukemia)
D) Plasmacytoid dendritic cell tumor
E) Tumor stage mycoses fungoides

QUESTION 12-11.

A patient with a recent diagnosis of Lyme disease presents with a solitary red-purple nodule with a smooth surface on the earlobe. A biopsy is performed and the findings are illustrated below. Immunohistochemistry reveals a mixed CD3+ and CD20+ infiltrate (2:1 ratio). Additionally, the germinal center–like foci contain intact CD21+ dendritic cell networks colonized by CD10+, Bcl6+, Bcl2− lymphoid cells. Kappa and lambda staining reveals rare scattered cells in a ratio of 5:1. Ig-gene rearrangement analysis reveals a polyclonal infiltrate. Which of the following diagnoses is CORRECT?

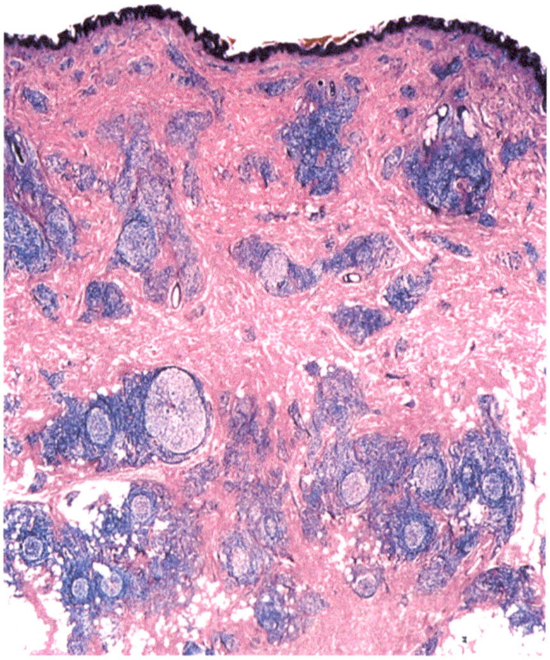

A) Primary cutaneous marginal zone type
B) Lymphocytoma cutis
C) Primary cutaneous CD4+ small- to medium-sized pleomorphic T-cell lymphoma
D) Erythema chronicum migrans
E) Primary cutaneous diffuse large B-cell lymphoma

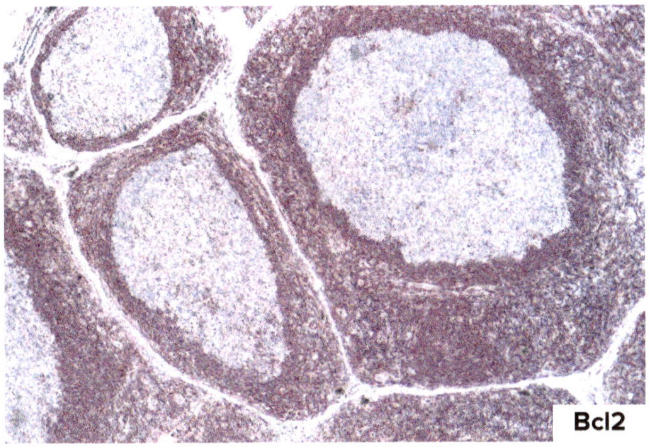
Bcl2

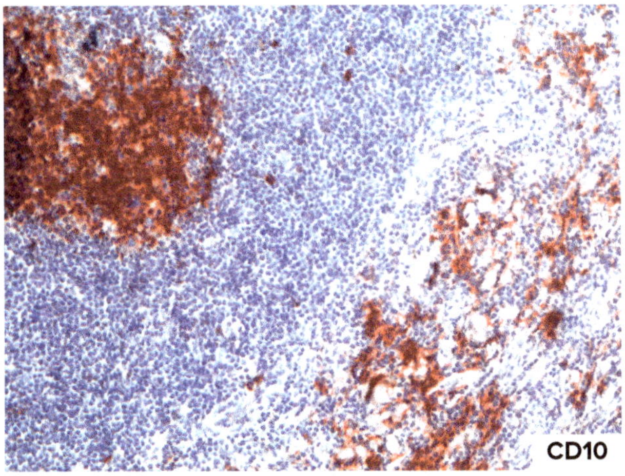
CD10

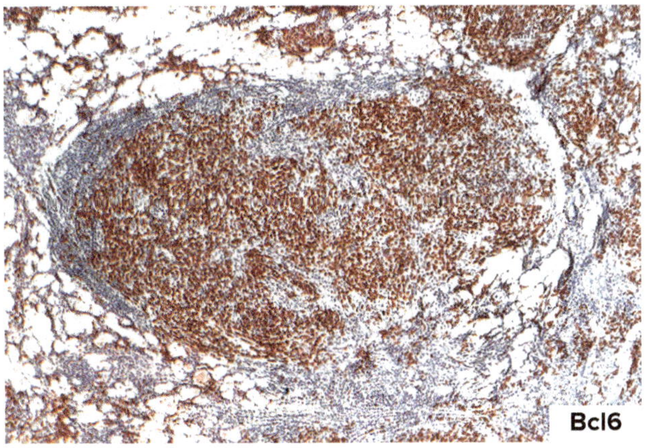
Bcl6

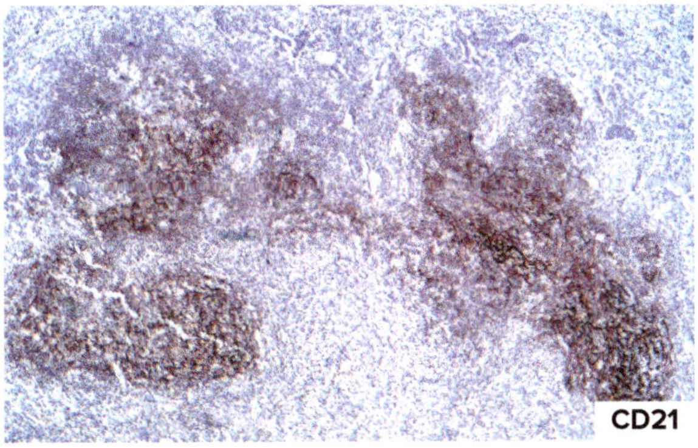
CD21

QUESTION 12-12.

Normal B lymphocytes undergo various stages of maturation to effectively mount humoral immunity. Recognizing the cytomorphology characteristic of these stages is important in understanding and distinguishing normal reactive lymphoid infiltrates from lymphomas. Which of the following statements regarding the main pathways of B-cell differentiation is INCORRECT?

A) In the bone marrow, stem cells give rise to B-precursor cells (lymphoblasts).
B) Rearrangement of immunoglobulin (Ig) genes does not occur until B cells have entered the germinal center.
C) Upon antigen stimulation, naive B lymphocytes transform into proliferating cells with a blastic appearance and eventually become plasma cells or centroblasts.
D) In activated germinal centers, centroblasts undergo a high rate of somatic mutations and cell divisions in effort to enhance antibody affinity to specific antigens, whereas centrocytes are nondividing cells.
E) Postgerminal center B cells enter the marginal zone and have the capacity to mature into plasma cells.

QUESTION 12-13.

A patient presents with agminated, reddish papules and plaques surrounded by erythematous patches on the forehead. A biopsy is performed and the findings are illustrated below. Immunohistochemistry reveals the lymphoid cells within and around the nodules to express CD20, whereas a minor peripheral population of lymphoid cells expresses CD3. Which of the following diagnoses is CORRECT?

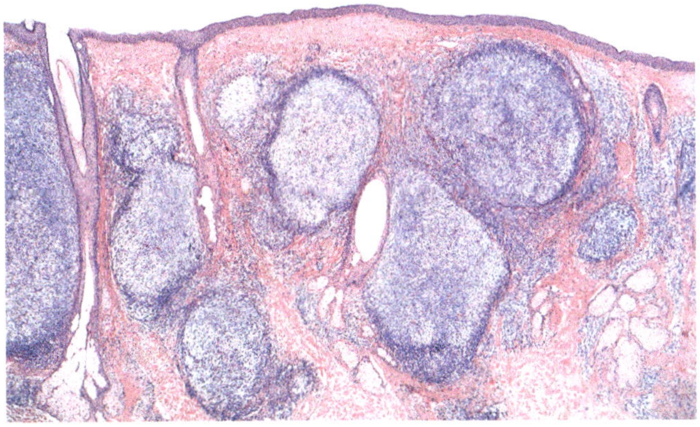

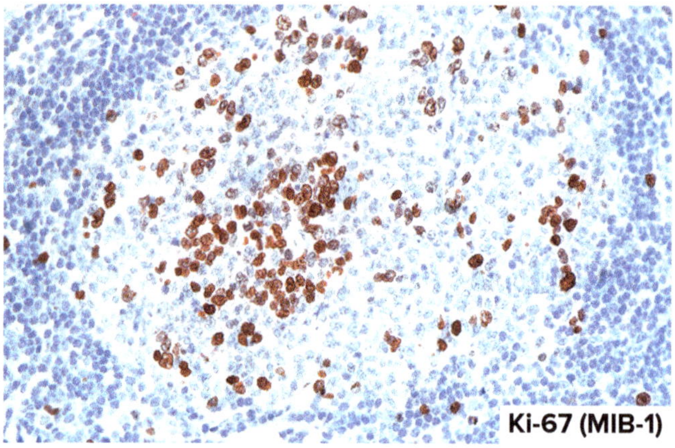

A) B-cell pseudolymphoma
B) Primary cutaneous marginal zone lymphoma
C) Diffuse large B-cell lymphoma, leg type
D) Primary cutaneous follicle center cell lymphoma
E) CD4+ small- to medium-sized pleomorphic T-cell lymphoma

QUESTION 12-14.

A patient presents with a reddish-brown plaque on the right upper extremity. A biopsy is performed and the findings are illustrated below. In image #1, reactive follicles can be vaguely recognized. Image #2 highlights the cells surrounding the germinal centers, and image #3 highlights a germinal center. Immunohistochemistry reveals a CD20+, CD79a+, CD5−, CD10−, Bcl-6−, and Bcl-2+ phenotype of the parafollicular cells as well as a few cells within the germinal center. CD21 reveals foci of dendritic cell lysis within the germinal centers. Kappa and lambda staining are illustrated below. Which of the following diagnoses is CORRECT?

A) Primary cutaneous follicle center cell lymphoma
B) Benign cutaneous lymphoid hyperplasia
C) Primary cutaneous marginal zone lymphoma
D) Diffuse large B-cell lymphoma
E) Mantle cell lymphoma

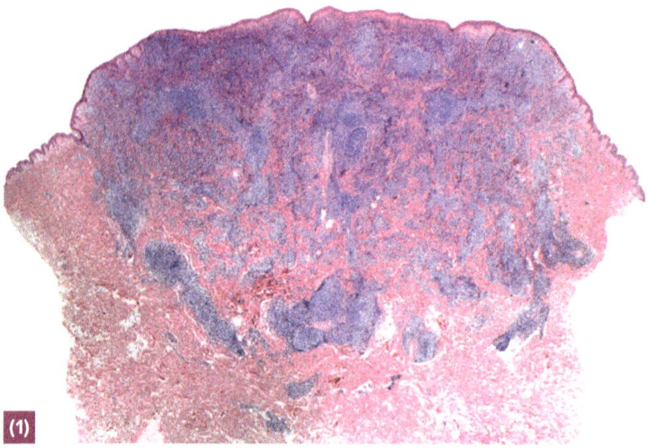
(1)

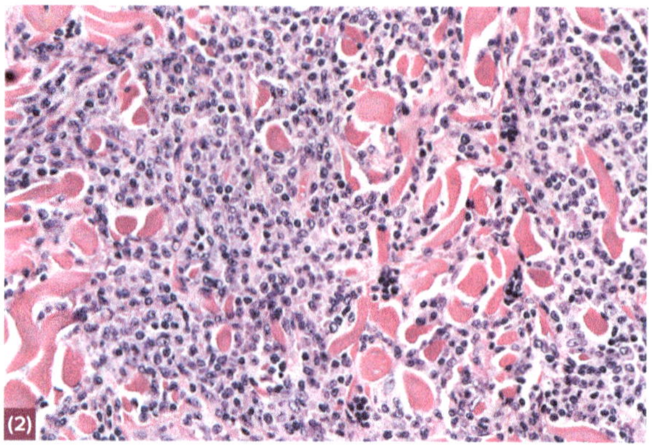
(2)

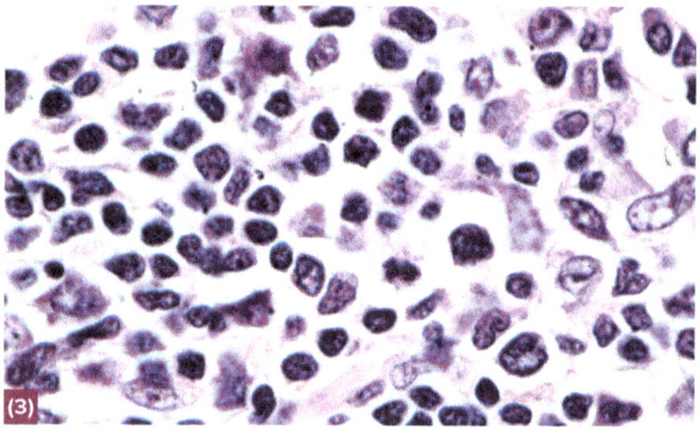
(3)

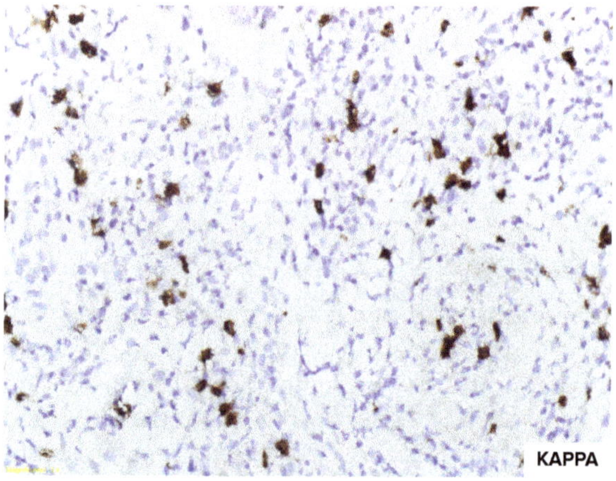

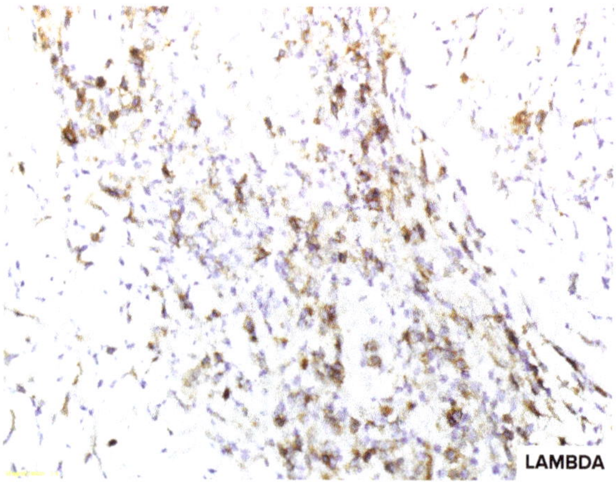

QUESTION 12-15.

A 75-year-old female patient presents several reddish nodules and tumors on the right leg. A biopsy is performed and the findings are illustrated below. Immunohistochemistry reveals a CD20+, CD79a+, Bcl2+, MUM1+, CD5−, CD10−, and CD30−. Rare scattered cells are positive for Bcl6 as well as CD3. CD21 reveals an absent network of dendritic cells. Kappa and lambda are negative. Fluorescent in situ hybridization studies reveal deletions of 9p21. Despite appropriate therapy, the patient quickly passes away. Which of the following diagnoses is CORRECT?

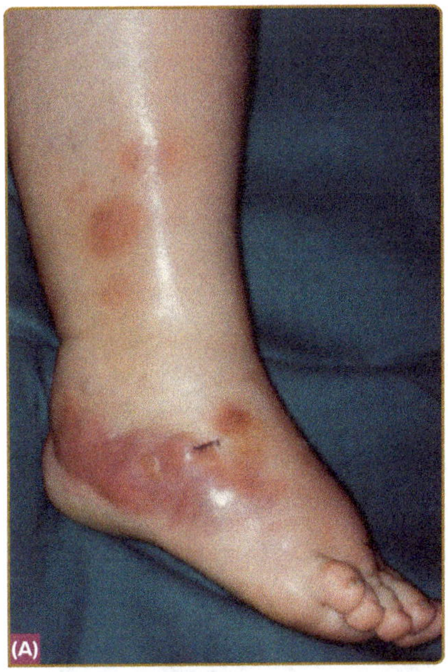

(A)

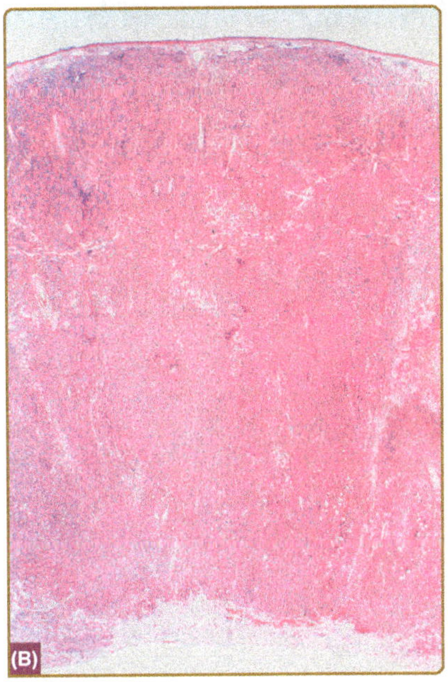

(B)

Reproduced, with permission, from Goldsmith LA, Katz SI, Gilchrest BA, Paller AS, Leffell DJ, Wolff K, eds. *Fitzpatrick's Dermatology in General Medicine*. 8th ed. New York, NY: McGraw-Hill Education; 2012.

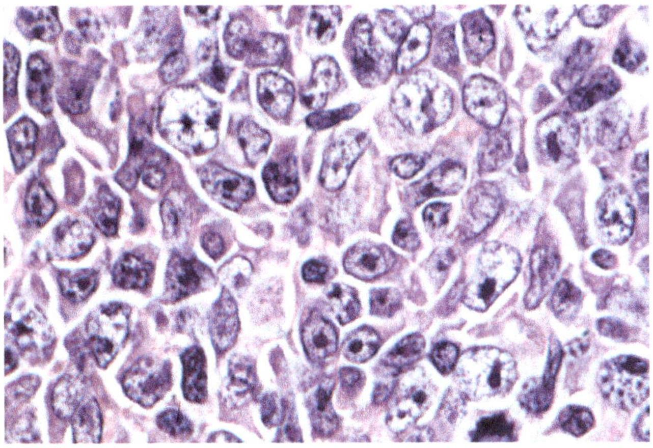

A) Chronic lymphocytic leukemia (small cell lymphoma)
B) Primary cutaneous diffuse large B-cell lymphoma, leg type
C) Primary cutaneous follicle center cell lymphoma
D) Anaplastic large cell lymphoma
E) Granulocytic sarcoma

QUESTION 12-16.

A 50-year-old male patient with chronic eczematous dermatitis presents with widespread areas of purpura involving the areas of dermatitis accompanied by generalized painless lymphadenopathy and peripheral lymphocytosis. A skin biopsy is performed and the findings are illustrated below. The infiltrate exhibits a CD20+, CD23+, CD3−, CD43+, and CD5+ immunophenotype. Which of the following statements regarding this patient's condition is INCORRECT?

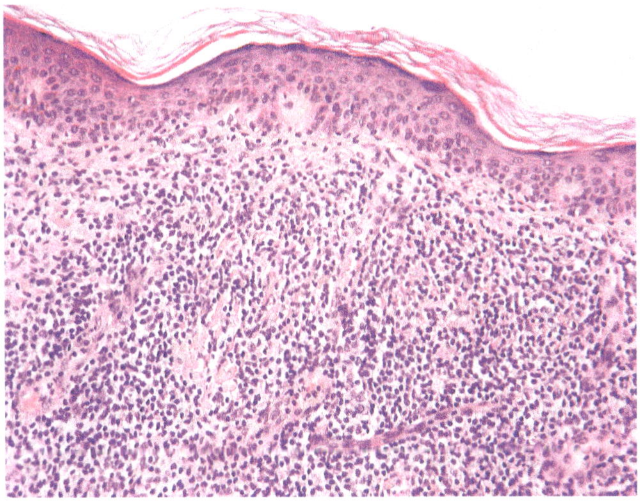

A) This patient has a form of circulating leukemia involving the skin.
B) This condition is associated with numerous aggressive squamous cell carcinomas.

C) This condition typically follows an indolent course followed an abrupt large cell transformation with a poor prognosis.
D) This condition is associated with hypogammaglobulinemia leading to recurrent infections
E) Expression of CD38 and Z-chain–associated protein kinase-70 (ZAP-70) is associated with a favorable prognosis.

QUESTION 12-17.

A patient is referred to you from the hematology/oncology service with generalized, painful, erythematous to violaceous, slightly elevated papules and nodules. There is a recent history of Sweet syndrome and a bone marrow biopsy revealing a dominance of blasts. A skin biopsy is performed and the findings are illustrated below. The infiltrate exhibits a CD20–, CD3–, CD4+, CD8–, CD56+, CD45+, CD68+, CD11c+, lysozyme+, myeloperoxidase+, and CD123– immunophenotype. Which of the following diagnoses is CORRECT?

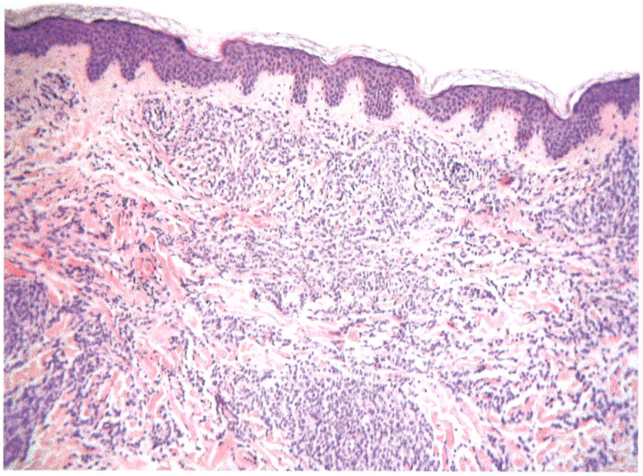

A) Acute myelogenous leukemia cutis
B) Hematodermic neoplasm
C) Granulocytic sarcoma
D) Chronic myelogenous leukemia cutis
E) NK/T-cell lymphoma

QUESTION 12-18.

Which of the following statements regarding cutaneous metastases is INCORRECT?

A) Tumors associated with vascular invasion (ie, melanoma, renal cell carcinoma, thyroid follicular carcinoma, and choriocarcinoma) are more frequently associated with distant metastases and frequent involvement of the scalp.
B) The most common cutaneous metastasis in women is breast adenocarcinoma.
C) The most common cutaneous metastases in men are lung adenocarcinoma and melanoma.
D) An important histopathologic feature supportive of primary cutaneous origin includes connection of the tumor with the epidermal surface or adnexal structures.
E) Cutaneous metastases of adenocarcinoma typically express p63 and D2-40, in contrast to primary cutaneous tumors, which are negative.

QUESTION 12-19.

A 69-year-old female patient presents with the rapid onset of a flaming-red rash associated with skin edema and dimpling. A biopsy is performed and the findings are illustrated below. Which of the following statements regarding this condition is INCORRECT?

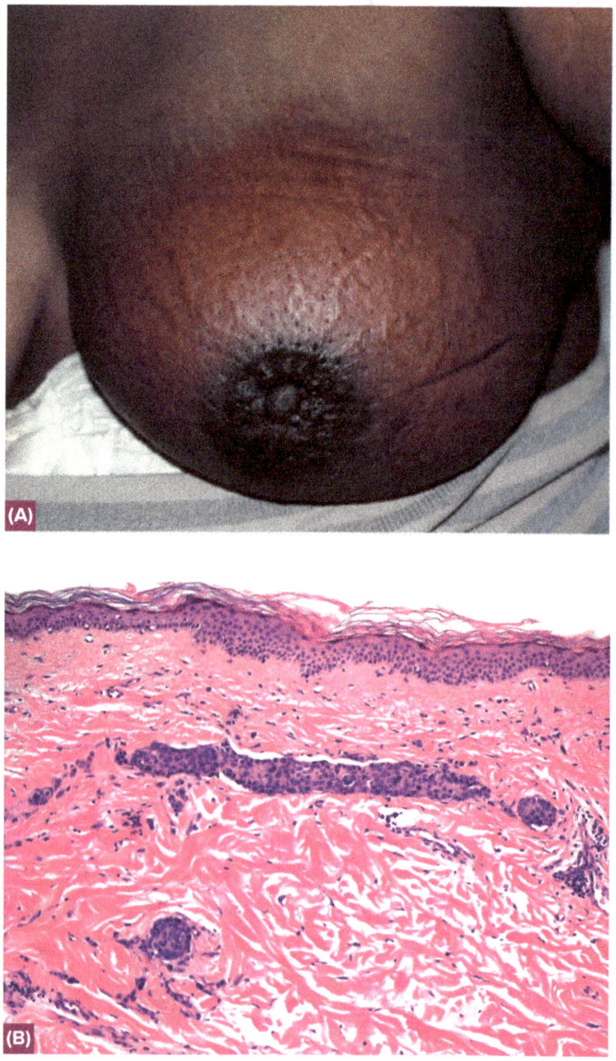

Part **(A)** Used with permission of Dr. Marilyn Leitch.

A) The elongated nest of epithelium in the dermis will be surrounded by a row of D2-40+ cells via immunohistochemistry.
B) This patient has stage IIIB breast adenocarcinoma.
C) The epithelial cells in the dermis will most likely be negative for p63 and positive for CK7, estrogen receptor, progesterone receptor, and GCDFP-15.
D) This patient has mammary Paget disease.
E) This patient should be worked up for metastatic adenocarcinoma.

QUESTION 12-20.

A 76-year-old male presents with a localized cluster of discrete, firm, nontender, flesh-colored nodules on the back. The lesions are of recent onset and rapidly grew to their current size; however, have remained stable for the past several weeks. A biopsy is performed and the findings are illustrated below. The tumor immunophenotype is CK7+, TTF1+, EMA+, CEA+, p63−, CK20−, CDX2−, CK19−, CK17−, CK5/6−, GCDFP15−, and mammaglobin−. Which of the following diagnoses is CORRECT?

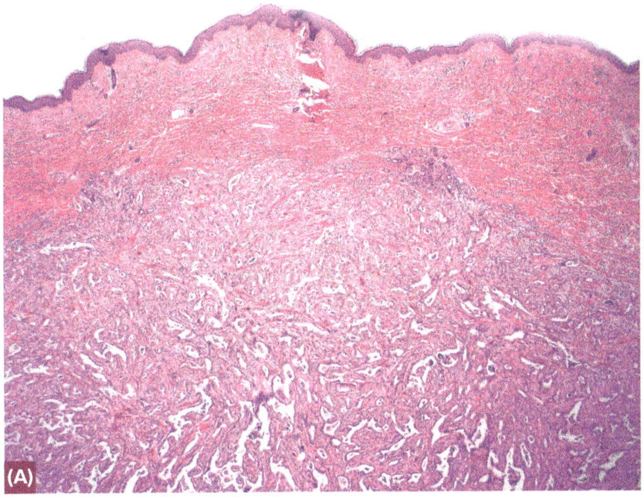
(A)

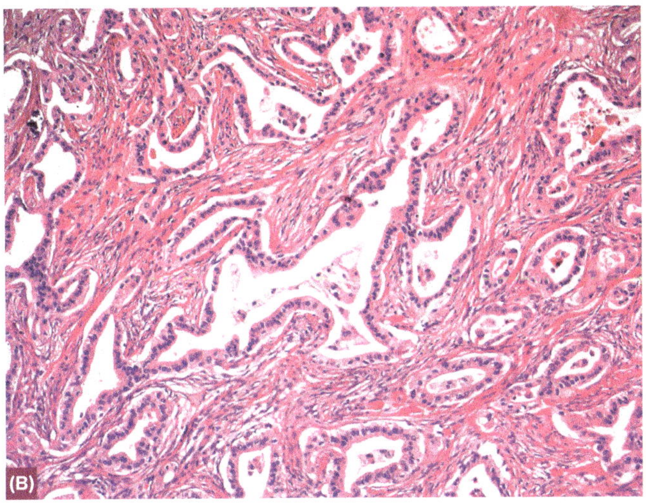
(B)

A) Metastatic lung adenocarcinoma
B) Metastatic mammary carcinoma
C) Metastatic lung squamous cell carcinoma
D) Metastatic pancreatobiliary adenocarcinoma
E) Eccrine ductal adenocarcinoma

QUESTION 12-21.

An elderly female patient presents with a flesh-colored pedunculated nodule around the umbilicus. A biopsy is performed and the findings are illustrated below. The tumor immunophenotype is pan-CK+ (AE1/AE3), CK20+, CK7+, CEA+, CDX2+, CK17−, TTF1−, p63−, ER−, CA125−, and GCDFP-15−. Which of the following diagnoses is CORRECT?

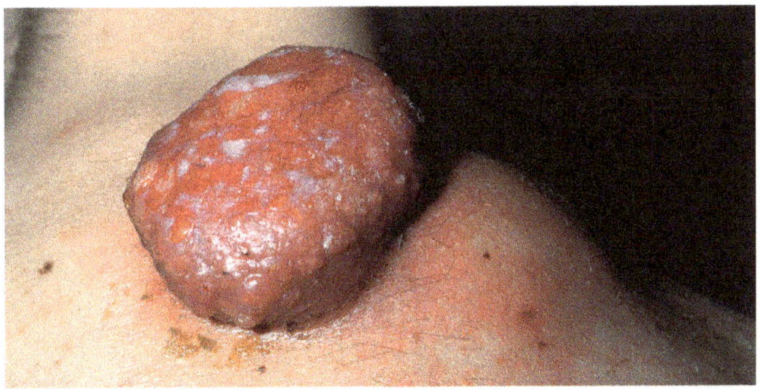

Reproduced, with permission, from Wolff K, Johnson RA, Saavedra AP. *Fitzpatrick's Color Atlas and Synopsis of Clinical Dermatology*. 7th ed. New York, NY: McGraw-Hill Education; 2013.

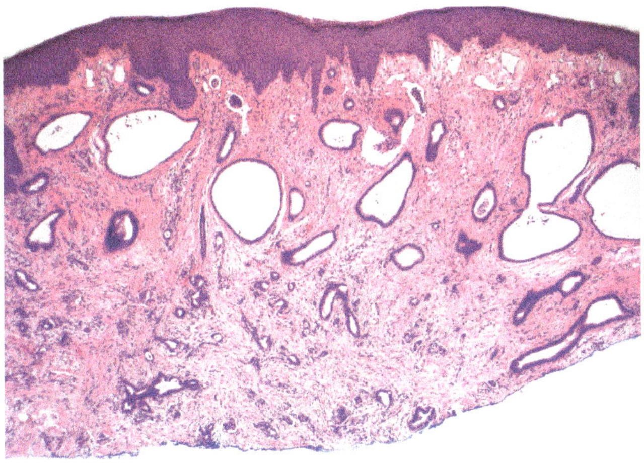

A) Metastatic urothelial carcinoma
B) Metastatic colorectal adenocarcinoma
C) Metastatic well-differentiated gastric adenocarcinoma
D) Metastatic lung adenocarcinoma
E) Metastatic endometrial adenocarcinoma

QUESTION 12-22.

An elderly female patient presents with a violaceous nodule on the scalp. A biopsy is performed and the findings are illustrated below. The immunophenotype of the tumor cells pan-CK+ (AE1/AE3), CAM 5.2+, EMA+, CD10+, vimentin+, carbonic anhydrase IX+, CK5/6–, CK7–, CK20–, CEA–, p63–, hCG–, PLAP–, S100–, and HMB45–. PAS and Sudan black stains are positive for glycogen and lipid, respectively. Which of the following diagnoses is CORRECT?

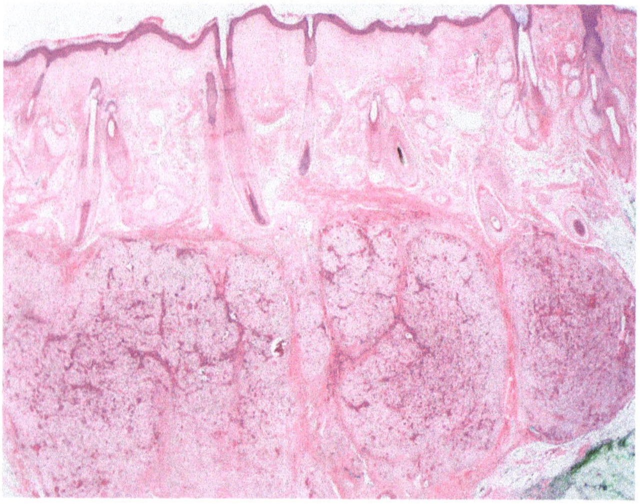

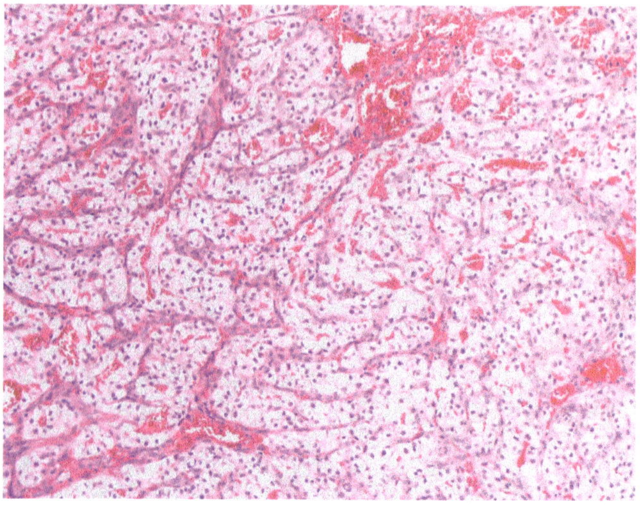

A) Metastatic choriocarcinoma
B) Cutaneous PEComa
C) Clear cell hidradenoma
D) Metastatic renal cell carcinoma
E) Sebaceous carcinoma

QUESTION 12-23.

A 19-year-old female patient presents with flesh-colored cutaneous nodules involving the scalp. A biopsy is performed and the findings are illustrated below. Immunohistochemical stains reveal the tumor cells to be TTF1+, CK7+, thyroglobulin+, ER–, PR–, CK20–, CK17–, CK19–, CDX2–, GCDFP15–, CA125–, hCG–, and uroplakin–. Which of the following diagnoses is CORRECT?

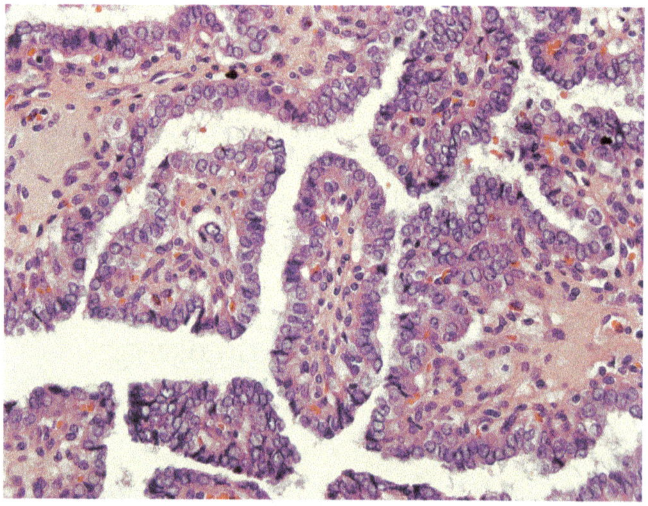

Reproduced, with permission, from Brunicardi FC et al, eds. *Schwartz's Principles of Surgery*. 9th ed. New York, NY: McGraw-Hill; 2010.

A) Metastatic papillary serous carcinoma of the ovary
B) Metastatic pancreatobiliary adenocarcinoma
C) Metastatic lung adenocarcinoma
D) Metastatic papillary thyroid carcinoma
E) Metastatic papillary urothelial carcinoma

QUESTION 12-24.

A 76-year-old female patient presents with several small flesh-colored nodules in an umbilical scar. A biopsy is performed and the findings are illustrated below. The tumor immunophenotype is CK20+, CK7+, CEA+, CDX2+, CA125+, ER–, PR–, mammaglobin–, GCDFP15–, p63–, and D2-40–. Which of the following diagnoses is CORRECT?

A) Metastatic mucinous adenocarcinoma of the ovary
B) Metastatic poorly differentiated gastric adenocarcinoma
C) Metastatic urothelial carcinoma
D) Metastatic poorly differentiated colonic adenocarcinoma
E) Metastatic mammary adenocarcinoma

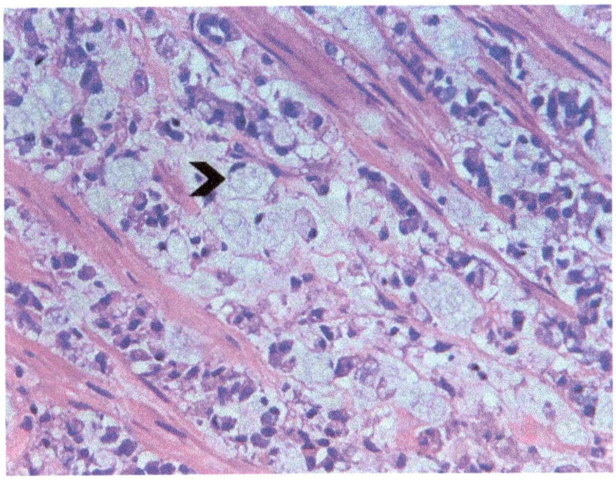

Reproduced, with permission, from Kemp WL, Burns DK, Travis Brown TG. *Pathology: The Big Picture*. 8th ed. New York, NY: McGraw-Hill Education; 2008.

QUESTION 12-25.

A 76-year-old male presents with widespread flesh-colored nodules on the chest. A biopsy is performed and the findings are illustrated below. The tumor immunophenotype is CK7+, TTF1+, chromogranin+, synaptophysin+, CD56+, CK20−, CAM 5.2−, CD45−, vimentin−, FLI1−, and myoD1−. Which of the following diagnoses is CORRECT?

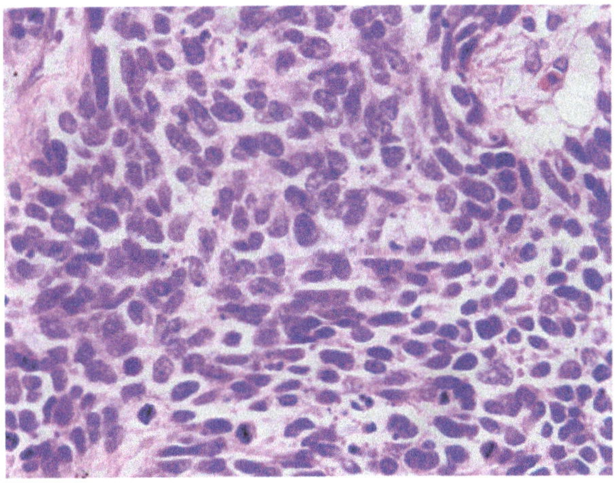

Reproduced, with permission, from Kantarjian HM, Wolff RA, Koller CA. *The MD Anderson Manual of Medical Oncology*. 2nd ed. New York, NY: McGraw-Hill Education; 2011.

A) Merkel cell carcinoma
B) Metastatic Ewing sarcoma
C) Metastatic small cell carcinoma of the lung
D) Metastatic neuroblastoma
E) Metastatic rhabdomyosarcoma

ANSWERS

ANSWER 12-1: D.

T-cell pseudolymphoma (aka **T-cell dyscrasia**) is a controversial diagnostic category of T-cell infiltrates that are characterized by chronic dermatoses of unknown significance (Table 12-1A). These infiltrates may be band like (resembling **mycosis fungoides**) or diffuse/nodular with scattered large CD30+ T cells (resembling **anaplastic large cell lymphoma**). In general, these eruptions share histopathologic features with both reactive inflammatory conditions and lymphoma; therefore, oftentimes represent an equivocal diagnosis of lymphoma (cannot be ruled out). There is a vast number of conditions that some have argued should be included in the band-like category (ie, **large plaque parapsoriasis, pityriasis lichenoides chronica, alopecia mucinosa, pigmented purpuric dermatosis, actinic reticuloid,** and **chronic dermatitis of HIV disease**). The incidence of transformation into **mycosis fungoides** is extremely variable among these conditions. In general, there is extremely low risk for **pityriasis lichenoides chronica** and **pigmented purpuric dermatosis**; however, there is a significant risk for **large plaque parapsoriasis** and **alopecia mucinosa**. There is currently much debate as to whether these high-risk conditions actually represent a form of indolent mycosis fungoides. A few authors have proposed the designation "**endogenous T-cell dyscrasia**" for these

Table 12-1A. T-Cell Pseudolymphoma

Clinical Features
- Broad spectrum: patchy or nodular lesions, erythroderma
- No progression, no extracutaneous spread

Histopathologic Features
- Two main patterns: band-like infiltrate with or without epidermotropism
- Nodular infiltrate
- Small lymphocytes, nuclear pleomorphism possible, but not prominent
- Admixture of eosinophils

Immunohistochemical Features
- CD3+, CD4+ T cells intermingled with CD3+, CD4−, CD8+ T cells
- No loss of T-cell antigens
- Few CD30+ T cells can be present in some cases

Differential Diagnosis
- Small cell pleomorphic T-cell lymphoma
- CTCL: mycosis fungoides, Sézary syndrome Chronic eczema

conditions, especially the high-risk entities. When these infiltrates are associated with medications, they are referred to as **lymphomatoid drug eruptions** or **drug-associated reversible T-cell dyscrasias** (Table 12-1B). Withdrawal of the offending medication leads to resolution of the eruption; however, the time course to resolution may be prolonged. Microscopically, where **mycosis fungoides** is associated with lymphocyte epidermotropism and minimal to no spongiosis and keratinocyte dyskeratosis, the band-like **T-cell pseudolymphomas** exhibit significant spongiosis with Langerhans cell–rich vesicles and/or true interface activity with variable keratinocyte dyskeratosis. Both conditions may contain atypical small lymphocytes with cerebriform nuclear contour irregularity (**Sézary cells**); however, these cells are found in much smaller numbers in pseudolymphoma (Table 12-1C).

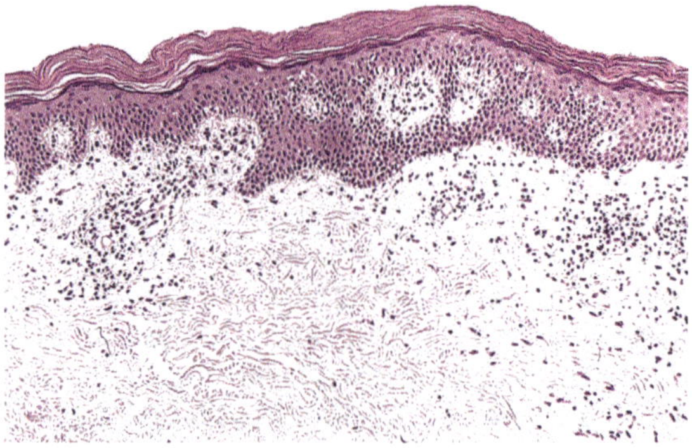

Lymphomatoid hypersensitivity reaction (mycosis fungoides–like drug eruption) in a patient on amitriptyline. A band-like dermal lymphocytic infiltrate is present and shows haphazard epidermotropism with minimal spongiosis; in other areas not shown, the epidermis was spared, unlike mycosis fungoides, where epidermal involvement is continuous in shave biopsy specimens.

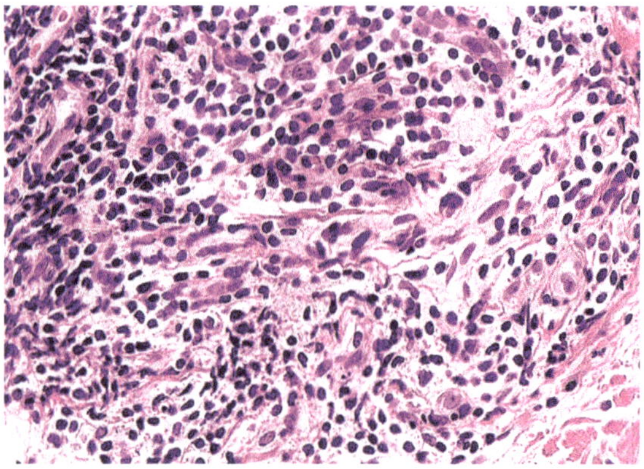

Lymphomatoid vascular reaction in a patient on diazepam. A perivascular and transmural infiltrate of mature and transformed lymphocytes is present and is unaccompanied by vascular fibrin deposition.

Table 12-1B. Drugs Implicated in Pseudolymphoma

ACE inhibitors
Alpha antagonists
Anticonvulsants
Antidepressants
Benzodiazepines
Beta-blockers
Calcium channel blockers
H_1 Antagonists
H_2 Antagonists
Lithium
Lipid-lowering agents
Nonsteroidal anti-inflammatory agents
Phenothiazines
Sex steroids

Table 12-1C. Histologic Features of the Lymphomatoid Hypersensitivity Reaction

MYCOSIS FUNGOIDES-LIKE PATTERN OF LYMPHOMATOID HYPERSENSITIVITY	FEATURES COMMON TO MYCOSIS FUNGOIDES AND LYMPHOMATOID HYPERSENSITIVITY
Infiltration of the epidermis by mildly atypical lymphocytes or by cells with a comparable cytomorphology to the small- and intermediate-sized atypical dermal lymphocytes	Dermal Sézary cells Atrophy
Sézary cells	Vascular ectasia
Directed pattern of epidermal infiltration with maximal involvement of suprapapillary plates/adnexae[a]	Dermal fibrosis, either vertical or laminated
Vesiculation[a]	
Papillary dermal edema[a]	
No Pautrier microabscesses	
Vascular fibrin deposition[a]	

[a]Histologic features characteristic of delayed-type hypersensitivity reactions.

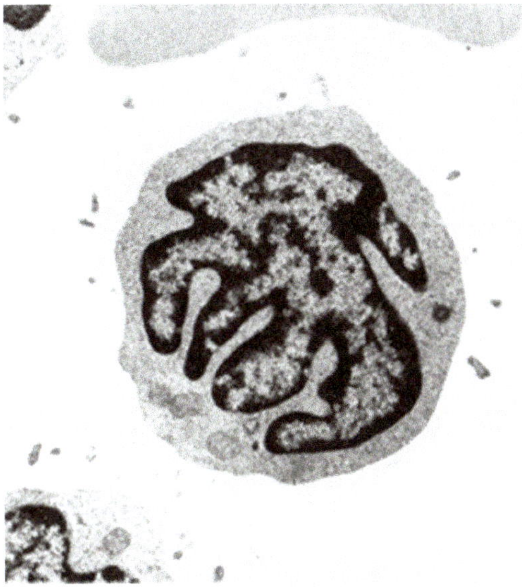

Sézary cell. Electron microscopy. Characteristics of the small lymphocyte with high nuclear to cytoplasmic ratio and cerebriform nuclear contour irregularity. (Reproduced, with permission, from Lichtman MA, Shafer JA, Felgar RE, Wang N. *Lichtman's Atlas of Hematology*. New York, NY: McGraw-Hill; 2007.)

In regard to the immunohistochemical phenotype, **mycosis fungoides** is associated with marked reduction in expression of pan-T-cell markers (CD2, CD5, and/or CD7). In **T-cell pseudolymphoma**, expression of these markers may be reduced but generally no more than 50%. T-cell-receptor rearrangement (TCR) analysis may reveal clonality in both mycosis fungoides and T-cell pseudolymphoma; however, much less often in the latter. In essence, TCR clonality is a sensitive marker for mycosis fungoides with limited specificity.

The **CD30+ pseudolymphomas** are diffuse or nodular dermal infiltrates containing large atypical CD30+ cells that may mimic **anaplastic large T-cell lymphoma** both clinically and histopathologically. The accompanying infiltrates may be mixed with scattered eosinophils, plasma cells, and neutrophils. The most common exogenous causes include medications or arthropod bites. Although generally regarded as a form of CD30+ lymphoproliferative disease, lymphomatoid papulosis could be considered an endogenous form due to the waxing and waning nature of its papular eruptions.

ANSWER 12-2: A.

Mycosis fungoides (MF) is a **peripheral T-cell lymphoma** initially and preferentially presenting in the skin with distinct clinical and histopathologic features (Table 12-2A). It is the most common type of cutaneous lymphoma. This lymphoma usually affects individuals in the fifth to seventh decades of life, but MF may also develop in children. There is a male preponderance. The disease starts with irregular, well-circumscribed, yellowish-red patches with pityriasiform scaling, mostly located on sun-protected sights such as the trunk or buttocks. UV light is toxic to lymphocytes and is frequently used to treat these lesions and may result in **poikiloderma**. These patches are persistent and usually take several years to develop into elevated plaques and tumors in the advanced stage. Progression to a large cell morphology and formation of nodular tumors that may undergo ulceration is referred to as **large cell transformation** of MF. It is associated with an aggressive clinical course. Moreover, extracutaneous spread to lymph nodes and visceral organs may occur in advanced stages (**Sézary syndrome**). The sudden multifocal eruption of tumors without preceding patches or plaques was formerly referred to as the *d'emblée*

Table 12-2A. Mycosis Fungoides

Clinical Features	
Irregular patches with pityriasiform scaling in early stage	
Evolution to plaques and nodular tumors in later stages	
Disease progression over years, in some patients with involvement of lymph nodes and internal organs	
Histopathologic Features	
Early stage: perivascular lymphocytic infiltrate with small lymphocytes with round or cerebriform nuclei	
Subepidermal edema and proliferation of postcapillary venules	
Admixture of eosinophils and plasma cells	
Plaque stage: dense subepidermal infiltrate with significant epidermotropism of single cells or cell clusters forming	
Pautrier microabscesses	
Tumor stage: nodular dense infiltrate, blast transformation, often loss of epidermotropism	
Immunohistochemical Features	
CD4+, CD2+, CD3+, CD5+, CD7+, CD8−, CD30−, CD45RO+	
Loss of T-cell antigens in plaque and tumor stages	
Differential Diagnosis	
MF patch stage:	Small and large plaque parapsoriasis
MF plaque stage:	Chronic eczema Sézary syndrome Pagetoid reticulosis Cutaneous CD8+ cytotoxic lymphoma
MF tumor stage:	CD30+ or CD30− pleomorphic large T-cell lymphoma

form of MF. According to the WHO-EORTC and WHO classifications, this form belongs to the group of peripheral T-cell lymphoma that is unspecified due to the lack of preceding patches and plaques.

Microscopically, in the early **patch stage of MF**, a perivascular or band-like subepidermal or periadnexal infiltrate is observed. The infiltrate may be relatively scant. In addition to lymphocytes, eosinophils and a few plasma cells may be present. Fibroplasia of the papillary dermis, resulting in what has been termed "wiry" collagen, is often present. This fibrosis is reflective of the chronicity of the eruption. **Epidermotropism,** mostly of single cells or small clusters of lymphoid cells, is present to a variable degree. **Epidermotropism** is defined by the infiltration of lymphocytes into the epidermis unaccompanied by inflammatory changes such as spongiosis or dyskeratotic keratinocytes. The presence of halo cells—that is, intraepidermal (epidermotropic) lymphocytes with a clear cytoplasmic rim—is a useful feature but is not always present. Single or small clusters of lymphocytes disposed along the junctional zone is a common finding and is referred to as **lining up**. Both **halo cells** and **lining up** of cerebriform lymphocytes are present in the image in question. Spongiosis is usually minimal or absent, but it may be present, and this finding should not exclude a diagnosis of MF. Additionally, interface changes may also be present. When these changes are present, the diagnostic distinction between **MF** and **T-cell pseudolymphoma** may be extremely difficult if not impossible. Patch-stage lesions in otherwise advanced MF show typical features with epidermotropism of clearly atypical cells. In **plaque stage MF,** there is usually a dense, band-like subepidermal infiltrate with significant epidermotropism of single cells or cell clusters forming **Pautrier microabscesses.** The term microabscesses is a misnomer and could be replaced by "collections" or "aggregations". These clusters do not contain Langerhans cells, indicative of epidermal infiltration independent of antigenic stimulation.

Common features of patch and plaque MF are subepidermal fibrosis and the admixture of eosinophils, plasma cells, macrophages, and dermal dendritic cells. The regression of lesions

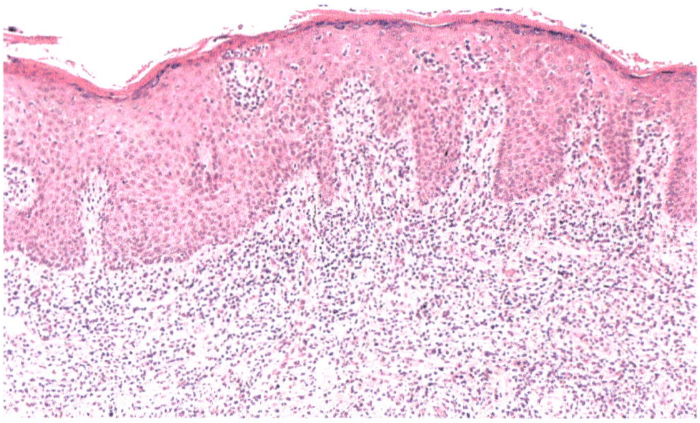

Mycosis fungoides, plaque stage. Band-like dense lymphocytic infiltrate in the upper and middle dermis. Significant epidermotropism with formation of Pautrier microabscesses.

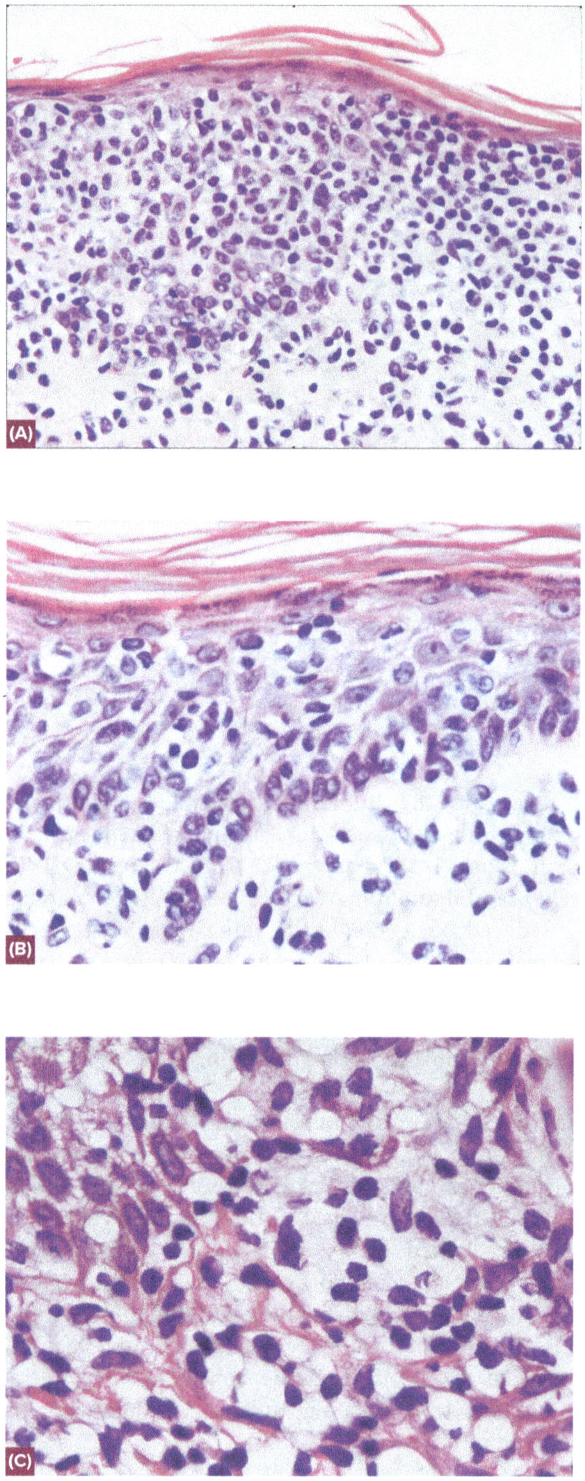

Mycosis fungoides, plaque stage. (A) There is a band-like lymphocytic infiltrate lining up along the dermal-epidermal junction. Scattered epidermotropic lymphocytes are present in the epidermis surrounded by a clear halo. There is little spongiosis or interface change. The lymphocytes exhibit severe nuclear contour irregularity (cerebriform nuclei). **(B)** Scattered Pautrier microabscesses are present throughout the epidermis. **(C)** The lymphocytes exhibit cerebriform nuclei (severe nuclear contour irregularity).

of MF may result in a nonspecific picture of **poikiloderma** or the presence of epidermal effacement and atrophy, telangiectasia, pigment incontinence, and papillary dermal thickening and fibroplasia. Such morphologic changes may be the defining histologic findings in treated lesions of MF. In addition, after light and psoralen therapy, focal keratinocyte necrosis and other changes associated with photoirritation may be observed.

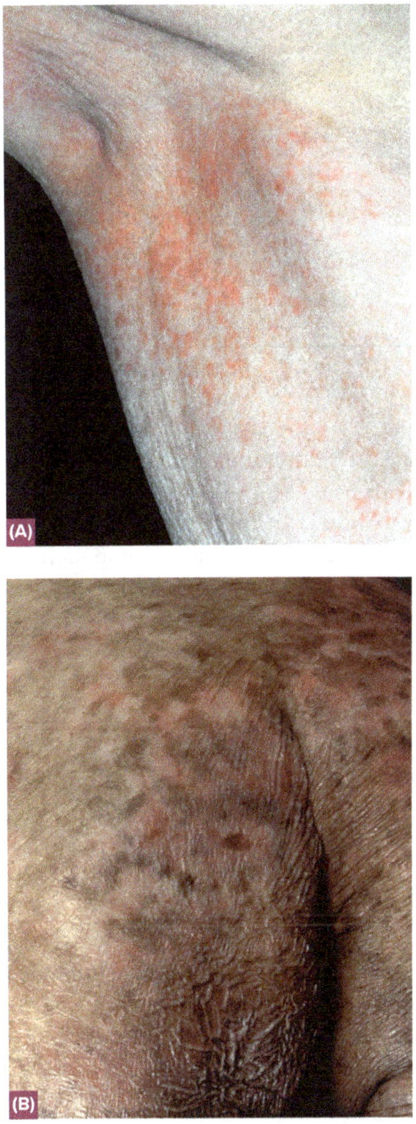

Mycosis fungoides: poikilodermatous lesions. (A) Small reticulated, confluent papules mixed with superficial atrophy give the impression of poikiloderma. **(B)** Poikiloderma in mycosis fungoides can also result from treatment. This patient had been treated with electron beam. (Reproduced, with permission, from Wolff K, Johnson RA, Saavedra AP. *Fitzpatrick's Color Atlas and Synopsis of Clinical Dermatology*. 7th ed. New York, NY: McGraw-Hill Education; 2013.)

In **tumor stage mycosis fungoides**, the infiltrate is nodular, and in addition to the predominantly horizontal spread seen in the earlier stages, vertical growth takes place, sometimes with progressive loss of epidermotropism.

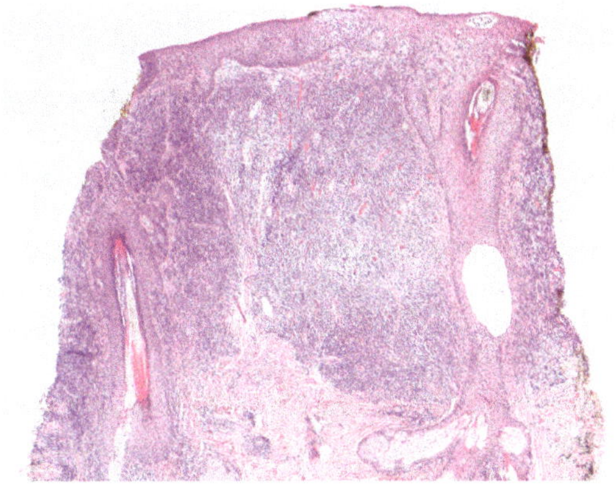

Tumor stage of mycosis fungoides showing a dense infiltrate involving all layers of the dermis. Only focal epidermotropism is seen.

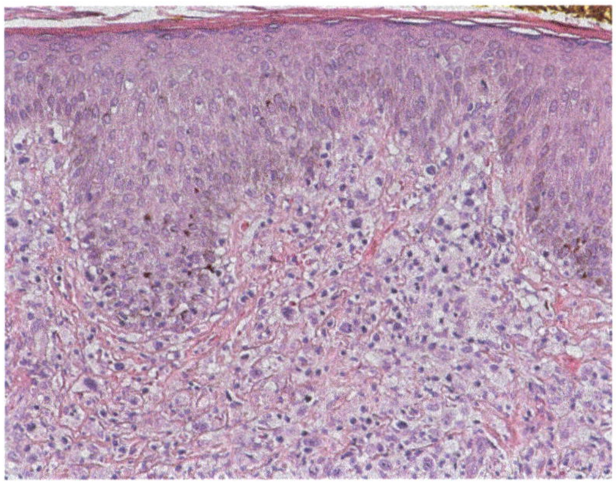

Large cell transformation of mycosis fungoides. Greater than 25% of the tumor cells exhibit a large pleomorphic cytomorphology.

Cytomorphologically, the infiltrates in MF are composed of predominantly small lymphocytes with round or cerebriform nuclei in the patch and plaque stages. With tumor progression, overtly neoplastic medium-sized to large lymphoid cells with pleomorphic nuclei account for an increasingly larger percentage of the infiltrate. **Immunoblasts** and **anaplastic cells** may be observed in transformed MF. **Large cell transformation** is generally defined by the presence of greater than 25% of the tumor cells exhibiting a large cytomorphology. While these large cells may be CD30+, large cell transformation is defined independent of CD30 expression.

Quick Fact

Large cell transformation of MF = >25% of the tumor cells exhibiting large pleomorphic cytomorphology.

The characteristic immunophenotype in classic MF is CD3+, CD4+, CD45RO+, CD8−, CD30−, and βF1+ (TCRβ+). In reactive inflammatory conditions, the intraepidermal CD4 to CD8 ratio is approximately 1:2 and the dermal CD4 to CD8 ratio is approximately 2:1. In classic CD4+ MF, the concentration of both intraepidermal and dermal CD4+ T cells is significantly increased. Rare cases display a CD3+, CD4+, CD8+ cytotoxic/suppressor T-cell phenotype or a CD4+, CD8−, or a CD56+ phenotype. CD8+ MF and CD56+ cases often manifest with hypo- or hyperpigmented patches and plaques but behave biologically similar to classic CD4+ MF. Poikiloderma is also a common feature of CD56+ variants of MF. Loss of T-cell antigens such as CD2, CD5, or CD7 is commonly found, with CD7 being expressed in only one-third of the lesions. In the tumor stage, an aberrant phenotype with loss of several T-cell antigens and occurrence of CD30+ expression are common findings (Table 12-2B).

The staging system for mycosis fungoides is based on the particular skin findings and findings of extracutaneous disease.

- Stage IA disease (as defined by the tumor, node, metastases blood [TNMB] system): Patchy or plaque-like skin disease involving less than 10% of skin surface area (T1 skin disease)
- Stage IB: Patchy/plaque-like skin disease involving 10% or more of the skin surface area (T2 skin disease)
- Stage IIB disease: Tumors are present (T3 skin lesions)
- Stage III disease: Generalized erythroderma is present
- Stage IVA1 disease: Erythroderma and significant blood involvement occur
- Stage IVA2 disease: Lymph node biopsy result shows total effacement by atypical cells (LN4 node)
- Stage IVB disease: Visceral involvement (ie, liver, lung, bone marrow) occurs

Table 12-2B. Antigens and Antibodies for the Immunophenotypic Evaluation of Cutaneous T-Cell Lymphoproliferative Disorders

CD	ANTIBODY	SPECIFICITY
CD2	Leu5, OKT11	T Lymphocytes
CD3	Leu4, OKT3	Mature thymocytes, peripheral T lymphocytes
CD4	Leu3, OKT4	Helper/inducer T cells, some macrophages
CD5	Leul, OKT1, Lyt2	T Lymphocytes; less than 5% of B lymphocytes
CD7	Leu9, WT1	T Lymphocytes
CD8	Leu2, OKT8	Suppressor/cytotoxic T cells
CD30	Kil, BerH2	Reed-Sternberg cells, Hodgkin cells, large cell anaplastic lymphoma, plasma cells
CD 43	MT-1	T Lymphocytes, monocytes, myeloid cells
CD45RO	UCHL-1	T Lymphocytes, monocytes, myeloid cells
CD56	NCAM	Natural killer (NK) cells
TIA-1	Granule-associated cytotoxic molecule	Cells with cytotoxic activity
βF1	T-cell-receptor α/β chain	T Lymphocytes
TCR δ	T-cell-receptor γ/δ chain	T Lymphocytes

ANSWER 12-3: C.

This is a classic example of **granulomatous slack skin disease.** Granulomatous reactions are present in about 2% of various cutaneous lymphomas, including both cutaneous T- and B-cell lymphomas. The granulomatous component in the dermal infiltrate can vary from a few giant cells to prominent epithelioid granulomas. The **granulomatous variant of mycosis fungoides (MF)** represents the most common cutaneous T-cell lymphoma (CTCL) with granulomatous features. **Granulomatous MF** and **granulomatous slack skin (GSS)** display overlapping histopathologic features but differ clinically by the development of bulky skin folds resembling **cutis laxa** in GSS. Due to the unique clinical features, GSS is listed as a separate subtype of MF in the WHO-EORTC classification. In addition to classic MF, the other variants of mycosis fungoides recognized by the WHO-EORTC include **follicular MF** and **pagetoid reticulosis.**

Characteristic clinical manifestations of **granulomatous slack skin disease (GSS)** include poikilodermatous patches in the flexural areas (the groins and axillae) that evolve to pendulous, bulky folds of skin resembling cutis laxa. The age of onset is between the second and fifth decades of life in most instances, but GSS may also begin in childhood. The course is typically indolent and slowly progressive, but some patients are at risk for the development of **secondary systemic CD30+ anaplastic large cell lymphomas** or **Hodgkin lymphoma**. Microscopically, most biopsies of GSS show a diffuse infiltrate composed of predominantly small lymphocytes and scattered large multinucleated giant cells are present in the dermis. These giant cells contain up to 30 peripherally located nuclei and display **emperipolesis** (ie, phagocytosis of lymphoid cells). Also, epidermotropism is usually limited or absent in GSS. There is an almost complete loss of elastic fibers, and fragments of the elastic fibers can be found as small inclusions in the cytoplasm of the giant cells (**elastophagocytosis**). There is overlap with the histopathologic features of granulomatous MF; therefore the clinical presentation is extremely important in making the diagnostic distinction. The small lymphoid cells express a CD3+, CD4+, CD8−, CD30− T-helper phenotype. The giant cells are of monocyte or macrophage derivation and thus express histiocytic markers such as CD163, lysozyme, and CD68. Clonal TCR gene rearrangement is commonly found.

In **granulomatous mycosis fungoides (GMF),** patients clinically present with erythematous or hyperpigmented patches and plaques commonly on the trunk. The clinical presentation of skin lesions in GMF is not indicative of the histopathologically detected granulomatous features. The loose skin folds of GSS are absent. Microscopically, there is a diffuse infiltrate of small and occasionally medium-sized lymphocytes and sarcoid-like granulomas throughout the entire dermis. Histiocytic giant cells are often present. Epidermotropism of lymphocytes is absent in almost half of the biopsies, limiting their value as a diagnostic marker in GMF. Remarkably, infiltration of the vessel walls of large veins by small lymphocytes and even by large multinucleated histiocytic giant cells is found in one-third of cases. Immunophenotyping reveals in most cases a CD4+ T-helper phenotype, but CD8+ cases have been observed. In the vast majority, a clonal T-cell population can be demonstrated by polymerase chain reaction (PCR), which may be a useful adjunctive diagnostic marker in the discrimination of GMF from inflammatory granulomatous disorders such as **sarcoidosis**. However, a very important diagnostic consideration is the **interstitial granulomatous drug reaction**, which may closely resemble granulomatous MF, including in the context of T-cell clonality and a reduction in the expression of CD7. GMF exhibits a therapy-resistant slowly progressive course. However, extracutaneous spread or development of a second lymphoproliferative disease occurs in a subset of patients. Prognosis in GMF is worse than in classic nongranulomatous MF, with a disease-specific 5-year survival rate of 66%. A subset of GMF with onset in childhood has been referred to as **juvenile granulomatous CTCL**. These patients appear to be at high risk for the development of a second lymphoid neoplasm.

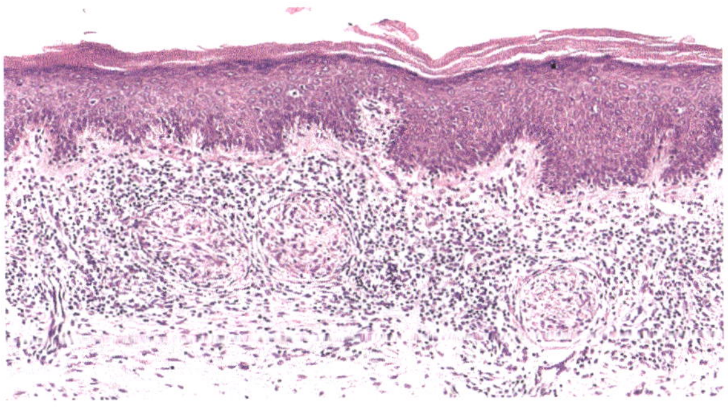

Granulomatous mycosis fungoides with epithelioid granulomas and numerous small lymphocytes embedded in fibrosis.

Pagetoid reticulosis (PR) is a distinct subtype of MF that can be regarded as a circumscribed, unilesional, low-grade malignant form. In 1939, Woringer and Kolopp reported a solitary plaque-like lesion on the arm of a 6-year-old boy. The term *PR* was introduced later by Braun-Falco and colleagues. Only the localized form should be referred to as *PR*, according to the WHO-EORTC classification. The disseminated form of PR described in 1931 by Ketron and Goodman is no longer referred to as PR and corresponds to **classic MF, primary cutaneous aggressive CD8+ cytotoxic T-cell lymphoma,** or **gamma delta-positive cutaneous T-cell lymphoma.** Clinically, PR presents as a solitary psoriasiform or bowenoid, erythematous, scaling, or crusty plaque with acral localization exhibiting slow centrifugal growth over years. In contrast to classic MF, PR does not disseminate or spread to extracutaneous sites. Microscopically, the epidermis shows marked psoriasiform hyperplasia with para- and ortho-hyperkeratosis. Characteristically pronounced epidermotropism of atypical **haloed** lymphoid cells with convoluted and hyperchromatic nuclei and clear cytoplasm manifest a sponge-like disaggregation of the epidermis. Mitotic figures are rare. A perivascular or diffuse band-like infiltrate of small cerebriform lymphocytes is present in the upper dermis. Immunohistochemically, PR displays a heterogeneous spectrum of phenotypes, including CD8+/CD4+, CD4+/CD8−, and CD30+. Clonal *TCR* gene rearrangement is found in most cases. The clinical differential diagnosis includes solitary lesions of psoriasis, Bowen disease, extramammary Paget disease, and lichen simplex chronicus. Histopathologically, PR must be differentiated from other epidermotropic neoplasms such as **classic MF, lymphomatoid papulosis (type B), primary cutaneous CD8+ aggressive epidermotropic T-cell lymphoma,** as well as from epithelial neoplasms with a pagetoid pattern **(Paget disease)** and **malignant melanoma.**

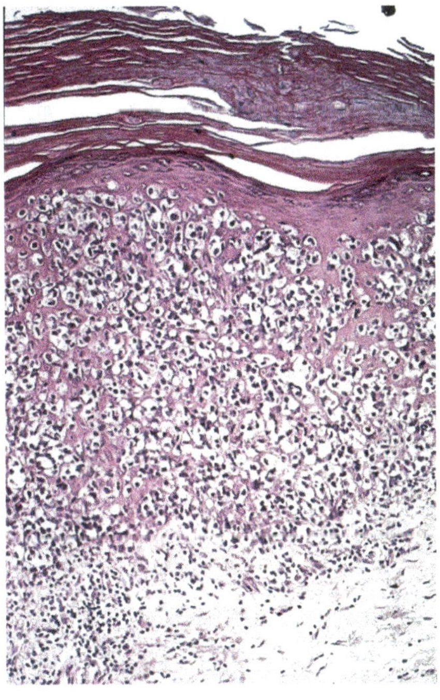

Pagetoid reticulosis. Sponge-like disaggregation of epidermis by epidermotropic haloed atypical lymphoid cells.

The **parapsoriasis** group of dermatoses, although described more than 100 years ago, is still controversial in regard to their relation with MF. Parapsoriasis is composed of both large plaque and small plaque types. It has been well documented that a subset of patients with **large plaque parapsoriasis (LPP)** shows progression to overt MF. Thus, some authors consider LPP as variant of MF with usually very slowly progressive course and low-grade potential for evolution to conventional MF. In **large plaque parapsoriasis** (aka **parapsoriasis en grandes plaques**), relatively few large (>10 cm in diameter), irregularly shaped, reddish, and fairly well-demarcated lesions with pityriasiform scaling are located on the trunk, extremities, or both. In contrast to LPP, **small plaque parapsoriasis (SPP)** behaves biologically similar to a chronic benign inflammatory disorder. In our opinion, SPP does not represent a precursor of MF. Clinically, **small plaque parapsoriasis** (aka **digitate dermatosis, chronic superficial dermatitis**) is characterized by oval or digitate patches 2 to 6 cm in diameter that are preferentially located on the lateral parts of the trunk and show a reddish or yellowish surface with pseudoatrophic wrinkling and slight pityriasiform scaling. The prognosis for patients with SPP is exceptionally good without any influence on survival. Fatal outcome of SPP has so far not been reported.

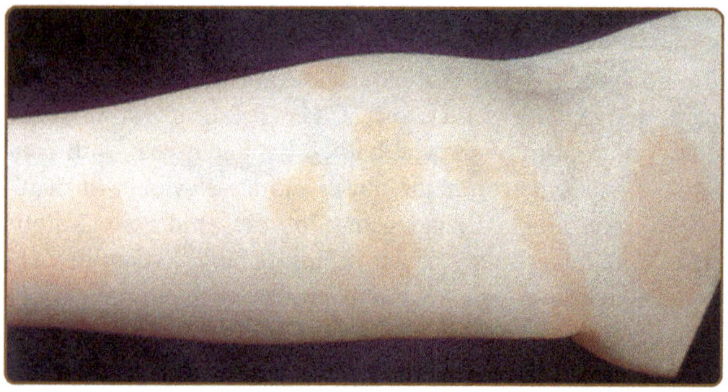

Large plaque parapsoriasis. Irregular-shaped patches of variable size on the arm of a 16-year-old girl. (Reproduced, with permission, from Goldsmith LA, Katz SI, Gilchrest BA, Paller AS, Leffell DJ, Wolff K, eds. *Fitzpatrick's Dermatology in General Medicine*. 8th ed. New York, NY: McGraw-Hill Education; 2012.)

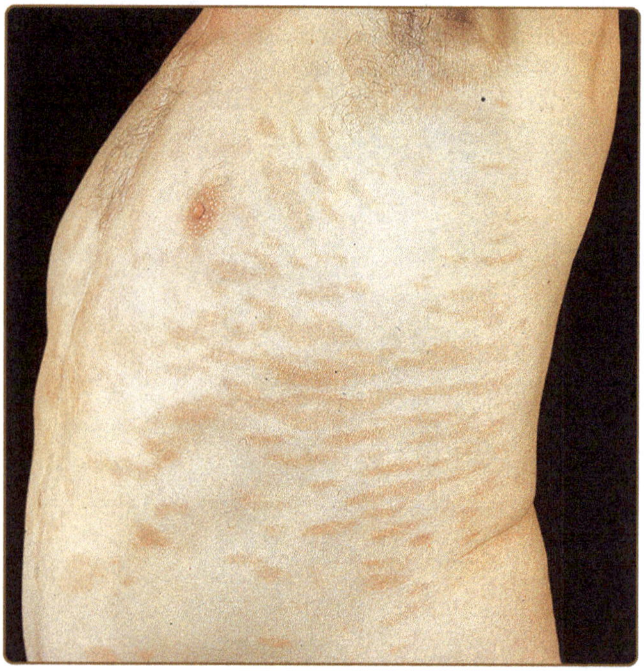

Small plaque parapsoriasis (digitate dermatosis). Typical "fingerprint" patches on the flank. Note that their length often exceeds their width. (Reproduced, with permission, from Goldsmith LA, Katz SI, Gilchrest BA, Paller AS, Leffell DJ, Wolff K, eds. *Fitzpatrick's Dermatology in General Medicine*. 8th ed. New York, NY: McGraw-Hill Education; 2012.)

Microscopically, the epidermis shows slight acanthosis with patchy parakeratosis. Scant perivascular infiltrates of small lymphocytes may be seen in the upper dermis, with or without subtle single-cell epidermotropism. In general, a few eosinophils are present, but plasma cells are not observed. Immunohistochemically, the infiltrate in SPP and LPP is mainly composed of CD4+, CD8–, and CD45RO+ T cells intermingled with a few CD8+ cells. While SPP typically preserves expression of pan-T-cell markers (CD2, CD3, CD5, and CD7) via immunohistochemistry, it is not uncommon to see a partial reduction, especially in CD7, in LPP. Clonal rearrangement of *TCR* genes is found occasionally in SPP and LPP.

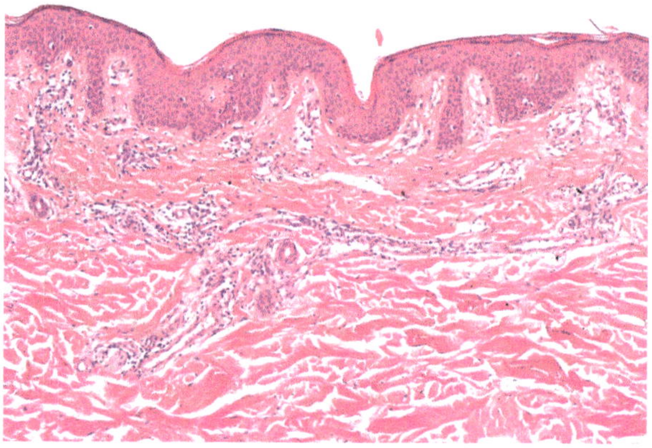

Parapsoriasis (small plaque form). Sparse perivascular lymphocytic infiltrate. No significant epidermotropism is seen. Subtle acanthosis and focal parakeratosis are present. Immunohistochemistry will reveal preserved expression of pan-T-cell markers (CD3, CD5, and CD7).

The major differential diagnosis of **SPP** and **LPP** includes **early-stage MF** and **chronic eczema**, which usually cannot be distinguished on histopathologic grounds alone. Additional information, including clinical presentation and course of the disease, are needed for the diagnosis. However, in some cases, only the stable course of the condition without progression allows one to differentiate parapsoriasis from MF retrospectively.

ANSWER 12-4: C.

Mycosis fungoides (MF) exhibits a broad spectrum of clinical, histopathologic, and immunophenotypic variants. Most variants behave in a clinically comparable fashion to classic MF. **Folliculotropic MF** and **granulomatous MF** as well as **pagetoid reticulosis (PR)** differ clinically in terms of presentation and prognosis. **Folliculotropic MF** is a subtype of MF that is defined by the perifollicular localization and folliculotropism of neoplastic lymphocytes that may or may not be accompanied by mucin deposits in the hair follicles (**follicular mucinosis**). Follicular MF is associated with a significantly poorer progression-free, disease-free, and overall survival than classic mycosis fungoides and displays outcomes more similar to those seen in tumor stage mycosis fungoides. Patients with follicular MF often are older than 40 years of age and present with erythematous papules, plaques, and comedo-like lesions involving the upper trunk and head and neck (most commonly the face). Unlike other forms of MF, follicular MF is typically nonresponsive to UV-light therapy, hence the predilection for involvement at sunexposed sites.

Microscopically, the neoplastic lymphocytes are small to medium sized and demonstrate prototypic cerebriform and hyperchromatic nuclei. The perifollicular infiltrates often consist of small- to medium-sized lymphocytes admixed with plasma cells and eosinophils. A granulomatous reaction may be observed, especially if follicle rupture has occurred. Dermal mucin may or may not be present within the hair follicle. The immunophenotype of the neoplastic lymphocytes is CD3+, CD4+, and CD8−. Absent or reduced expression of pan-T-cell markers (CD2, CD5, and CD7) is typical. Occasionally large CD30+ immunoblasts may be present scattered throughout the infiltrate.

The differential diagnosis includes **follicular mucinosis/alopecia mucinosa** and **follicular eczema**. Follicular eczema is most commonly seen in atopic patients and contains intrafollicular spongiotic vesicles containing mixtures of normal lymphocytes and Langerhans cells. Dermal mucin is typically absent in these lesions. The terms **alopecia mucinosa** and **follicular mucinosis** have often been used synonymously in the literature, creating much confusion. The term **follicular mucinosis** is simply a histological reaction pattern characterized by intrafollicular lymphocytic infiltrates and the accumulation of dermal mucin within the follicular epithelium. These findings may be seen in a variety of reactive conditions including **Ofuji disease, HIV-associated eosinophilic folliculitis, *Pityrosporum* folliculitis,** and **arthropod bite reactions.** The lymphocytes of these infiltrates lack the nuclear contour irregularity of MF and exhibit preserved expression of pan-T-cell antigens. **Alopecia mucinosa** refers to a **T-cell pseudolymphoma/dyscrasia** where the risk of transformation into **mucinous follicular MF** is unknown. **Secondary alopecia mucinosa** may arise in patients with **Sézary syndrome**, most likely representing **folliculotropic MF**. Microscopically, in addition to intrafollicular mucin, the follicular lymphocytic

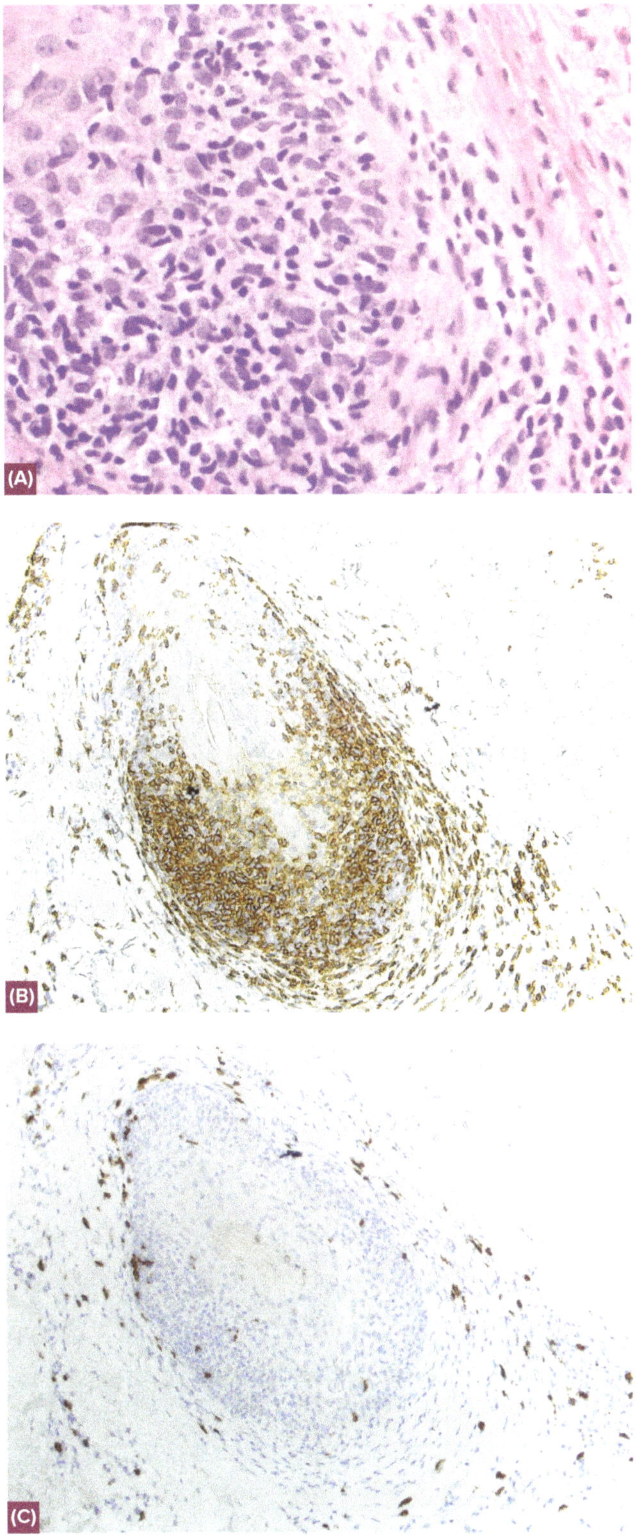

Follicular mycosis fungoides. (A) There is extensive lymphocytic folliculotropism without spongiosis of the outer root sheath epithelium. The lymphocytes exhibit significant nuclear contour irregularity. **(B)** Immunohistochemical stain for CD3 highlights the T-cell infiltrate. **(C)** Immunohistochemical stain for CD7 reveals a marked reduction in expression in the tumor cells in the realm of 99%.

infiltrates exhibit varying degrees of nuclear contour irregularity and reduced expression of pan-T-cell markers. **Idiopathic alopecia mucinosa** arising as solitary lesions in young adults typically has an indolent course; however, multiple lesions in older patients typically progresses to frank **follicular MF** with a poor prognosis. Approximately half of cases will exhibit clonality via T-cell-receptor rearrangement analysis. Several studies have shown that no consistent clinical, histological, or molecular findings allow distinction between idiopathic alopecia mucinosa and mucinous follicular mycosis fungoides; therefore these patients should be followed closely for evolution to follicular MF.

It is worth mentioning that a similar scenario exists for atypical lymphocytic infiltrates involving the sweat glands. **Syringotropic MF** is a very rare variant of MF that presents with a specific histomorphologic pattern that shows small lymphocytes with cerebriform nuclei and preferential involvement of the sweat glands and ducts with associated epithelial hyperplasia reminiscent of **Sjögren-associated lymphoepithelial lesions.** There may also be involvement of hair follicles, leading to circumscribed alopecia without follicular mucinosis. Patients presenting with more localized disease and mild lymphoid atypia may represent a form of syringotropic T-cell pseudolymphoma/dyscrasia referred to as **syringolymphoid hyperplasia with alopecia.** Similarly, the risk of progression to overt **syringotropic MF** cannot be determined via clinical, histopathological, or molecular findings.

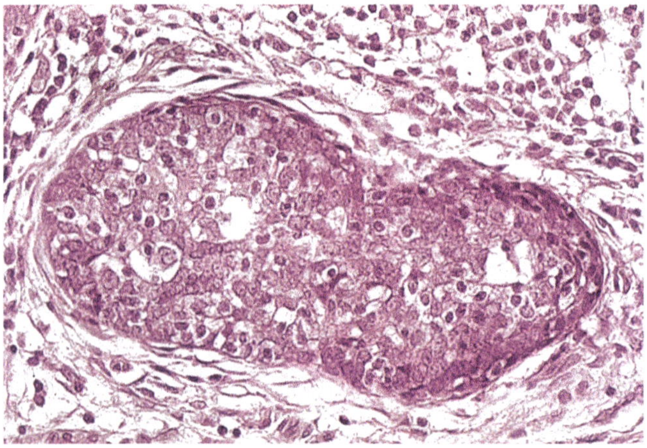

Syringotropic mycosis fungoides showing atypical lymphocytes within and around sweat gland structures.

ANSWER 12-5: B.

This is a classic case of **Sézary syndrome (SS)** (Table 12-5A). The skin biopsy reveals epidermotropism of lymphoid cells and formation of Pautrier microabscesses. The peripheral blood smear shows a classic cerebriform lymphocyte exhibiting nuclear hyperchromasia and gyrate nuclear contours. **Sézary syndrome** is a leukemic and erythrodermic peripheral T-cell non-Hodgkin lymphoma with distinct clinical features, circulating tumor cells, and lymphadenopathy. It is listed as a separate entity in the WHO-EORTC classification. Sézary syndrome is characterized by an erythroderma with intense pruritus, scaling, and edematous swelling of the skin; palmoplantar hyperkeratosis; hair loss; onychodystrophy; and enlargement of lymph nodes. Infiltration of bone marrow is a rare event; hence, the skin being the originating source of circulating lymphoma cells. SS affects patients in their fifth to seventh decades of life. The prognosis is worse than in MF, with a 5-year survival rate of 24%. **Large cell transformation** may occur in the skin with ulcerated tumors or in the lymph nodes. In the advanced stages, tumorous infiltration may result in **leonine facies.** In most cases, a nonspecific perivascular or band-like infiltrate with or without atypical lymphocytes is observed. Epidermotropism of atypical lymphocytes with formation of Pautrier microabscesses (ie, collections) is found in only up to 40% of biopsies therefore systemic workup is essential in establishing the diagnosis. Lymph nodes may show dermatopathic changes without histopathologic signs of involvement by tumor cells. Specific involvement is characterized by the effacement of lymph nodes by small cerebriform tumor cells. In transformation of SS to a **high-grade peripheral T-cell lymphoma,** dense sheets of large lymphoid cells with pleomorphic nuclei or **immunoblasts** are found in cutaneous tumors or lymph nodes. Immunophenotypically, the lymphoid cells express CD2+, CD3+, CD5+, CD45RO+, CD8−, and CD30−. There is clonal rearrangement of TCR genes in most of the cases in skin infiltrates, peripheral blood, and tumor-affected lymph nodes.

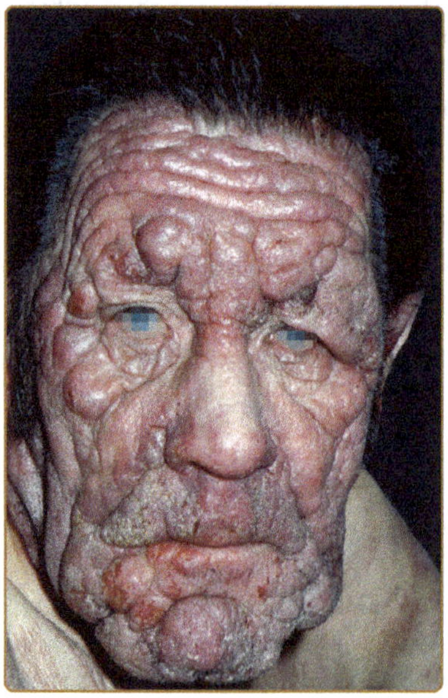

Leonine facies. The facial skin is coarse with thickened folds of the face, eyelids, and scalp. This clinical finding is not unique to mycosis fungoides and may be seen in a variety of conditions including lepromatous leprosy, systemic amyloidosis, and lichen myxedematosus. (Reproduced, with permission, from Goldsmith LA, Katz SI, Gilchrest BA, Paller AS, Leffell DJ, Wolff K, eds. *Fitzpatrick's Dermatology in General Medicine*. 8th ed. New York, NY: McGraw-Hill Education; 2012.)

In regard to the differential diagnosis, the main considerations are **erythrodermic mycosis fungoides, idiopathic erythroderma, erythrodermic psoriasis, generalized erythrodermic eczema,** and **erythrodermic drug eruption.** Based on the histopathologic features of a skin biopsy alone, **Sézary syndrome** cannot be distinguished from **erythrodermic MF,** as clinical evidence of systemic lymphoma is needed for a diagnosis of SS. Similar clinical and histopathologic changes are seen in the **idiopathic erythroderma ("pre-Sézary syndrome")**, generalized eczema, and drug reactions. **Generalized eczema** and **erythrodermic drug reactions** typically contain eosinophils and lack cerebriform lymphocytes, immunophenotypic abnormalities, and TCR clonality (Table 12-5B). One exception to this rule is with **lymphomatoid erythrodermic drug eruptions.** Cessation of the offending medication results in resolution of the erythroderma. **Idiopathic erythroderma** is a condition in which the patient's clinical, histopathologic, and peripheral blood findings are atypical but equivocal for SS; therefore some may argue that this condition belongs in the **endogenous T-cell dyscrasia/pseudolymphoma** category. Some of these patients progress to SS. CD8+ cases of erythroderma must be differentiated from **actinic reticuloid.** Detection of clonal rearrangement of *TCR* genes in the skin and peripheral blood, demonstration of at least 1000/mm^3 Sézary cells, and the presence of a strikingly elevated CD4+ T-cell population resulting in a significantly increased CD4/CD8 ratio (>10) are useful diagnostic criteria for the distinction of SS from other forms of erythroderma.

Table 12-5A. Sézary Syndrome

Clinical Features
Pruritic erythroderma with edematous swelling of the skin
Palmoplantar hyperkeratosis
Alopecia and onychodystrophy
Lymphadenopathy
Histopathologic Features
Band-like infiltrate and edema in the upper dermis
Epidermotropism with Pautrier abscesses in only 40% of the biopsies
Small lymphocytes with or without convoluted or cerebriform nuclei
Immunohistochemical Features
CD2+, CD3+, CD5+, CD8–, CD30–, CD45RO+
Peripheral blood: >1000 Sézary cells/mm^3; CD4/CD8 ratio >10
Differential Diagnosis
Red man syndrome/idiopathic erythroderma
Generalized (atopic) eczema
Drug reactions
Mycosis fungoides

Table 12-5B. Drugs Associated with Erythroderma

Acetylsalicylic acid
Sulfasalazine
Fenbufen
Oxytetracycline
Gentamicin
Nystatin
Ketoconazole
Sulfonamides
Cotrimoxazole
Clofazimine
Quinidine
Captopril
Timolol
Minoxidil
Phenobarbital
Methotrexate
Granulocyte-macrophage colony-stimulating factor
Etretinate

Quick Fact

- **Erythrodermic MF**
  - Diffuse MF confined to skin
- **Sézary syndrome**
  - Diffuse MF with peripheral blood involvement
- **Idiopathic erythroderma**
  - Equivocal for MF
- **Erythrodermic drug eruption**
  - +/– Lymphomatoid features

ANSWER 12-6: B.

This is a classic example of **Type A lymphomatoid papulosis (LYP). Primary cutaneous CD30+ lymphoproliferative disease (LPD)** represents a spectrum of low-grade cutaneous T-cell lymphoma (CTCL) (Table 12-6A). These entities are characterized by highly atypical (ie, pleomorphic and anaplastic) tumor cells that express CD30 (Ki-1) antigen. **CD30+ lymphoproliferative disease (LPD)** consists of **lymphomatoid papulosis (LYP), primary cutaneous (CD30+) anaplastic large cell lymphoma (CD30+ pcALCL)**, and so-called borderline cases. All forms of CD30+ LPD have a tendency for spontaneous regression of tumoral lesions but also recurrences and exhibit a favorable prognosis, with 5-year survival rates of over 90%.

LYP is a lymphoproliferative disease with a benign course but is nonetheless characterized by tumor cells with a histologic appearance suggesting malignancy. It is a chronic,

Table 12-6A. Lymphomatoid Papulosis

Clinical Features
- Recurrent, often grouped papulonodular self-regressing eruptions
- Preferential localization on the trunk and extremities
- Healing often with hyper- or hypopigmented scars
- Course over years or decades

Histopathologic Features
- Superficial and deep, wedge-shaped dermal infiltrate
- Medium-sized or large pleomorphic lymphoid cells with atypical mitoses, that are scattered (type A), epidermotropic (MF-like, type B), or in cohesive sheets (type C)
- Numerous small lymphocytes, neutrophils, and eosinophils admixed
- Ulceration

Immunohistochemical Features
- CD3+, CD4+, CD5+, CD8–, CD30+, TIA-1+, granzyme+, Ki-67+

Differential Diagnosis
- Primary cutaneous CD30 anaplastic large cell lymphoma
- Pityriasis lichenoides varioliformis et acuta
- Bite reaction, infestation
- Pseudolymphoma

recurrent disease with papulonodular lesions that undergo spontaneous regression after several weeks, sometimes leaving behind hypo- or hyperpigmented varioliform scars. The lesions are located mainly on the trunk and extremities. Their number can range from only a few grouped lesions to hundreds of disseminated lesions. LYP mainly affects individuals in the third and fourth decades of life, with a slight male preponderance. Despite its malignant histopathologic appearance, the disease may persist over many years or decades as an indolent process. A subset of patients (~10%-20%) develop a second malignant lymphoma such as **mycosis fungoides (MF), Hodgkin lymphoma, nodal anaplastic large cell lymphoma** (ALCL), or **cutaneous ALCL.** Molecular studies indicate a clonal relationship between the tumor cells in LYP and these secondarily developing lymphomas in some, but not all, patients.

Microscopically, the features vary considerably in **LYP** and depend on the stage of the disease. The most common histopathologic presentation (80% of cases) is that of **type A LYP.** The fully developed lesion is typified by a wedge-shaped dermal mixed cellular infiltrate. Cytomorphologically, the infiltrate is composed of scattered medium- or large-sized pleomorphic or anaplastic lymphoid cells admixed with numerous neutrophils and eosinophils; mitoses are commonly observed. Epidermotropism is typically absent. In **type C LYP**, cohesive sheets of tumor cells with only limited numbers of neutrophils and eosinophils are found. Large numbers of CD30+ cells are present, but do not exceed 75% of the total infiltrate. Rarely, an epidermotropic infiltrate of small- to medium-sized tumor cells indistinguishable from MF is present and defines the **type B LYP** variant. Despite the delineation of these three histologic types of LYP, one must recognize that there is a considerable overlap and that the composition of the lesions may vary from lesion to lesion in any individual patient.

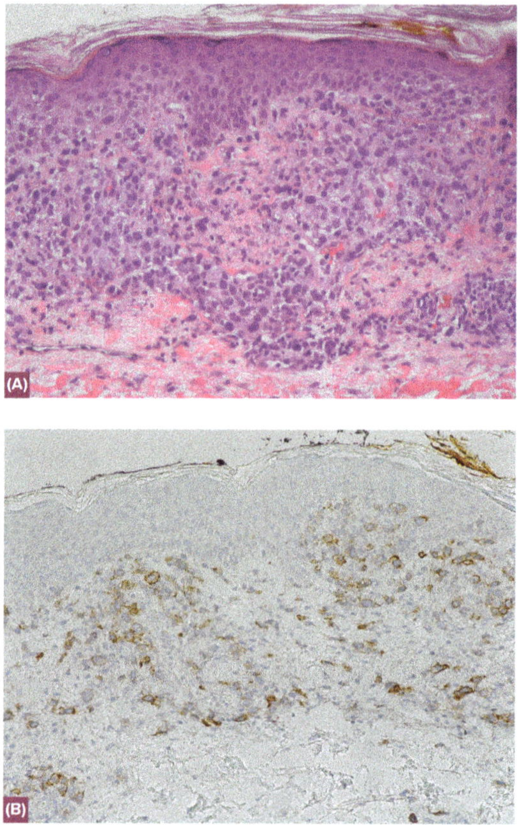

Lymphomatoid papulosis, Type A. (A) There is a superficial infiltrate composed of large pleomorphic mononuclear cells admixed with small lymphocytes and scattered macrophages. **(B)** The large cells express CD30.

In regard to the immunohistochemical phenotype, the large proliferating cells in LYP are activated helper T cells and express CD3+, CD4+, CD5+, CD8–, CD15–, EMA–, and CD30+ (Ki-1) as the immunophenotypic hallmark. Interestingly, although CD4+, the lesional cells are typically positive for cytotoxic markers TIA-1 and granzyme. Ki-67 may reveal an extremely high mitotic index; however, this finding has no correlation with clinical course. MUM1 and TRAF-1 are expressed in the vast majority of LYP cases and represent adjunctive differential diagnostic markers because they are expressed only in a minority of **primary cutaneous anaplastic large cell lymphoma (pcALCL).** Expression of fascin by tumor cells in LYP may be associated with an increased risk for the development of a second lymphoma. Clonal rearrangement of *TCR* genes can be demonstrated in fresh-frozen tissue but may not be detected in archival specimens, thus limiting its diagnostic value.

In regard to the differential diagnosis, **LYP** clinically resembles **pityriasis lichenoides et varioliformis acuta (PLEVA)** (aka **Mucha-Habermann disease**), but the latter lesions microscopically show pronounced epidermal changes with necrotic keratinocytes, exocytosis of CD8+ lymphocytes, and a lack of large anaplastic CD30+ cells. **Arthropod bite reactions** may occasionally contain small- to medium-sized CD30+ activated lymphocytes; however, these cells are typically small in number and scattered a solitary units compared to clusters. In addition, **viral infections** (ie, herpesvirus, molluscum contagiosum) and infestations (ie, **scabies**) may harbor CD30+ atypical-appearing lymphoid cells and thus may be misinterpreted as LYP.

> **Quick Fact**
>
> **Lymphomatoid papulosis (CD30+) is CD4+ but expresses cytotoxic markers granzyme and TIA-1"**

ANSWER 12-7: C.

Unlike **primary cutaneous large cell lymphoma (pcALCL)**, which typically has an excellent prognosis, cutaneous involvement by **systemic anaplastic large cell lymphoma (sALCL)** represents advanced disease and a poor prognosis. Although systemic workup is required for definitive diagnostic distinction, a few clinical, molecular, and immunophenotypic differences may be helpful in establishing the correct diagnosis. **Primary cutaneous anaplastic large cell lymphoma (pcALCL)** typically presents as a solitary tumor or multiple large nodular or tumoral lesions confined to one anatomic region. These tumorous lesions occur on normal-appearing skin without preceding patches or plaques and tend to ulcerate. Mostly patients in their fifth to sixth decades of life are affected, with a male-to-female ratio of 2:1. Nevertheless, pcALCL may also occur in children. Up to 20% to 25% of tumoral lesions have been reported to undergo spontaneous regression. Cutaneous involvement by **sALCL** typically presents as numerous scattered cutaneous nodules, accompanied by "B-symptoms" (night sweats, fever, weight loss), and distal lymph node or parenchymal involvement. Although regional lymphadenopathy may be seen in areas draining tumors of pcALCL, distant lymph node involvement is diagnostic of sALCL. In general, ALCLs are one of the most common forms of CTCL arising in transplant recipients.

Microscopically, **pcALCL** and **sALCL** are essentially identical with nodular dermal infiltrates often extending into the subcutis. The morphologic hallmarks are large, pleomorphic, anaplastic, and immunoblastic cells with large, irregularly shaped nuclei and dispersed chromatin; one or multiple nucleoli; and abundant pale or eosinophilic cytoplasms. Multinucleate giant cells with nuclei arranged in annular configurations are characteristic. Tumor cells are disposed in dense cohesive sheets reminiscent of melanoma or an undifferentiated carcinoma. Clusters of small reactive lymphocytes and eosinophils are found within and around the tumor. In neutrophil-rich variants of ALCL, the tumor cells are obscured by a profuse infiltrate of neutrophils. Cases with **pseudoepitheliomatous hyperplasia** of the overlying epidermis mimicking keratoacanthoma have been described.

In regard to the immunophenotype, the most striking feature of ALCL is expression of CD30 by the large anaplastic cells. T-cell–associated antigens (CD43, CD45RO) are expressed with variable loss of pan-T-cell antigens (CD2, CD3, CD5, CD7). In contrast to systemic ALCL, primary cutaneous forms may lack EMA expression and typically express the cutaneous lymphocyte antigen (CLA, HECA-452). CLA expression can, however, be seen in nodal ALCLs that disseminate to the skin. They may express CD4, perforin, TIA1, and granzyme, similar to **lymphomatoid papulosis.** In addition, expression of homeobox gene *HOXC5,* as well as lack of MUM1 and TRAF-1 expression, is found in pcALCL, in contrast to LYP and sALCL. ALK (p80) and the t(2;5) chromosomal translocation are usually absent in pcALCL. Clonal rearrangement of *TCR* genes is found in most patients with pcALCL and sALCL.

Other than **pcALCL**, the differential diagnosis includes **lymphomatoid papulosis, large cell transformation of mycosis fungoides, large cell transformation of Sézary syndrome, CD30-negative large cell peripheral T-cell lymphoma type unspecified,** and **extranodal NK/T-cell lymphoma. Lymphomatoid papulosis** clinically presents as scattered waxing and waning papules. The Type C variant of LYP most closely resembles ALCL histopathologically; however, the large anaplastic cell population typically accounts for less than 75% of the total cellular infiltrate. Both conditions share similar immunophenotypes (CD3+, CD30+, CD4+, granzyme+, and TIA1+). Occasionally, clinical correlation is required for definitive diagnosis. **Large cell transformation of MF** or **Sézary syndrome** typically presents with enlarging scattered tumor masses without and with systemic involvement, respectively. These tumor cells may express CD30; therefore preexisting history of mycosis fungoides or Sézary syndrome may be the only finding enabling the correct diagnosis. **Extranodal NK/T-cell lymphomas** typically present with either nasopharyngeal or subcutaneous involvement. Cutaneous lesions may be the primary or secondary manifestation of the disease. In regard to the nasal type, ulcerated papulonodular lesions extending onto the cutaneous surface from the nasopharynx are the most prevalent clinical manifestations. Typically there is gradual destruction of the midline face by this tumor. Systemic symptoms, including fever, malaise, and weight loss, are noted commonly. In addition, hemophagocytic syndrome may be observed. Most NK/T-cell lymphomas have an aggressive course. The median survival time is 12 to 15 months. Microscopically, the dermal and often subcutaneous infiltrates display an angiocentric and angiodestructive growth pattern with necrosis and ulceration. The lymphocytes are of variable size but are mostly medium sized. Like ALCL, these tumors may contain a mixed inflammatory infiltrate of eosinophils, plasma cells, and macrophages. The true NK lymphomas express CD2; cytoplasmic CD3 (CD3 epsilon); CD56; and cytotoxic proteins T1A-1, granzyme B, and perforin. EBER+ (EBV) is found in nearly all cases of secondary cutaneous NK lymphomas (ie, nasal type), but rarely in primary cutaneous forms (ie, subcutaneous). NK lymphomas exhibit a germ-line configuration; however, in the NK-like T-cell lymphomas, clonal TCR rearrangement can be detected, defining a critical discriminatory factor separating NK lymphoma from NK-like T-cell lymphoma. In addition, in the NK T-cell lymphomas, there is surface expression of CD3. The polyclonal CD3 used on paraffin-embedded tissue cannot reliably discriminate between CD3 epsilon and surface CD3; hence, both NK and NK-like T-cell lymphomas may show CD3 expression on routine immunohistochemical staining for CD3 on paraffin-embedded tissue.

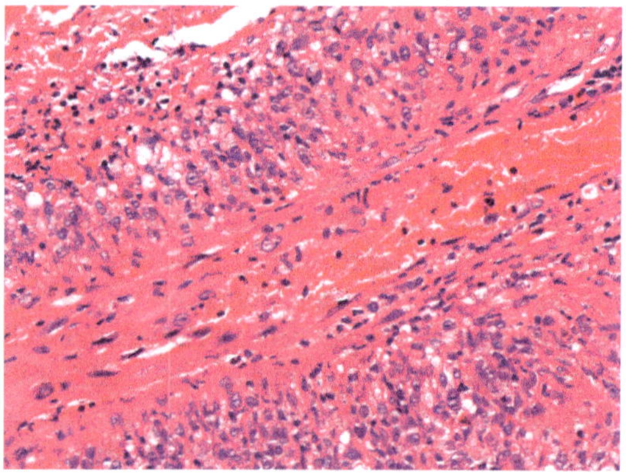

Extranodal natural killer/T-cell lymphoma, nasal type. Angiocentric and angiodestructive growth of atypical lymphoid cells is seen.

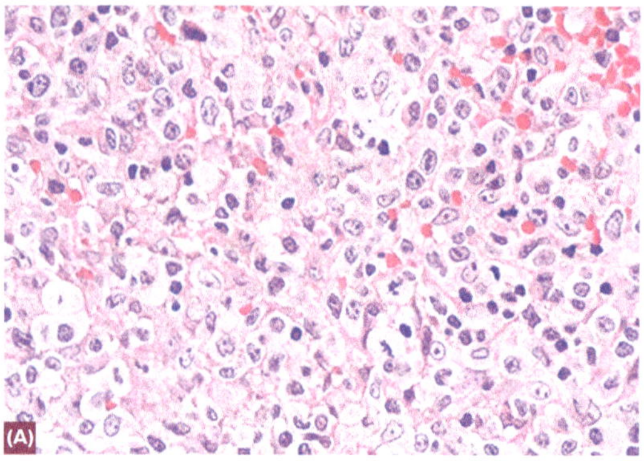

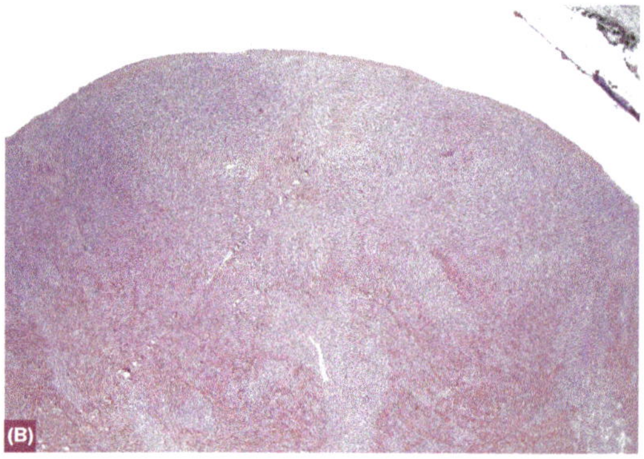

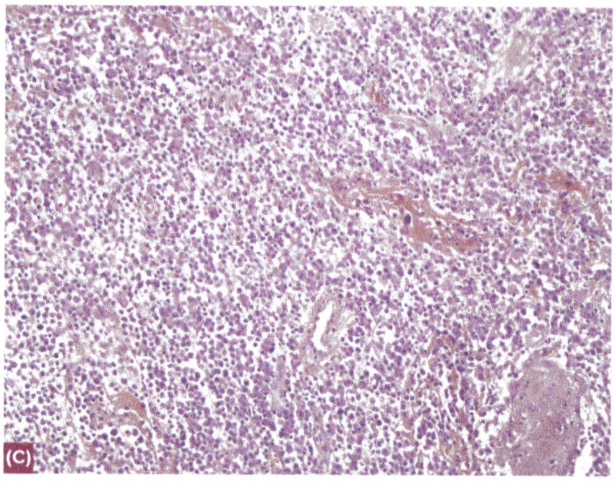

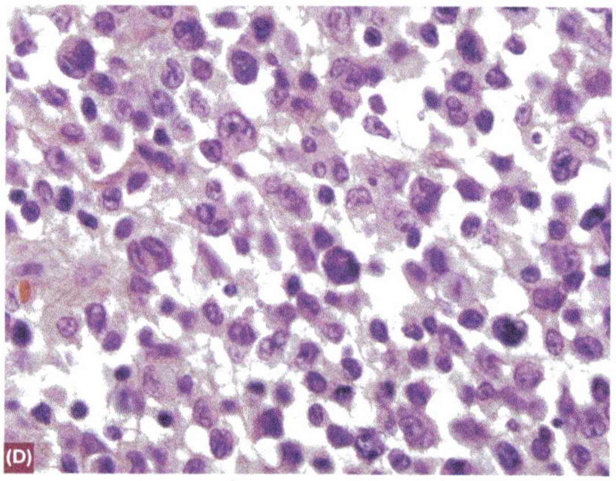

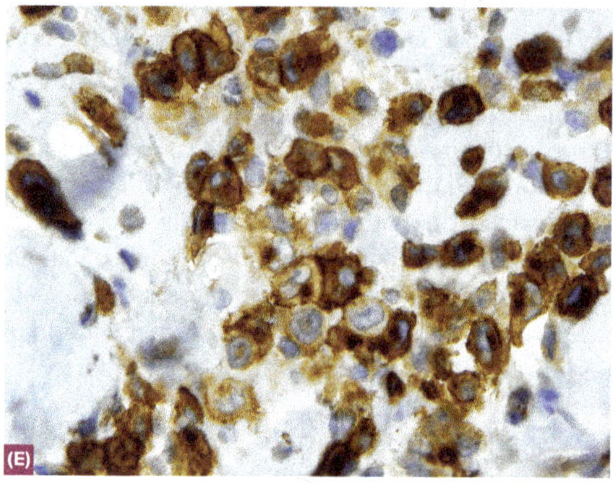

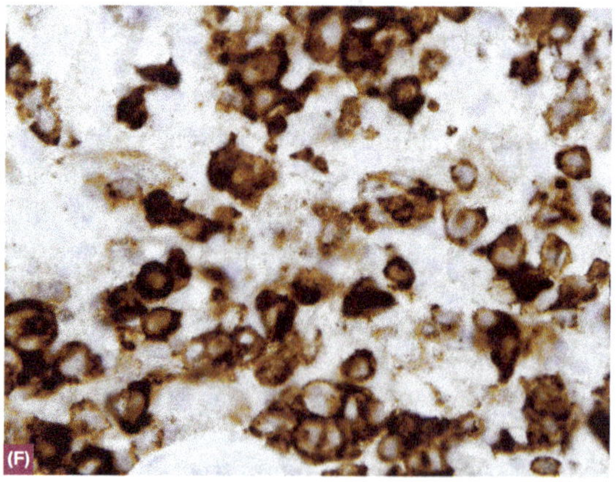

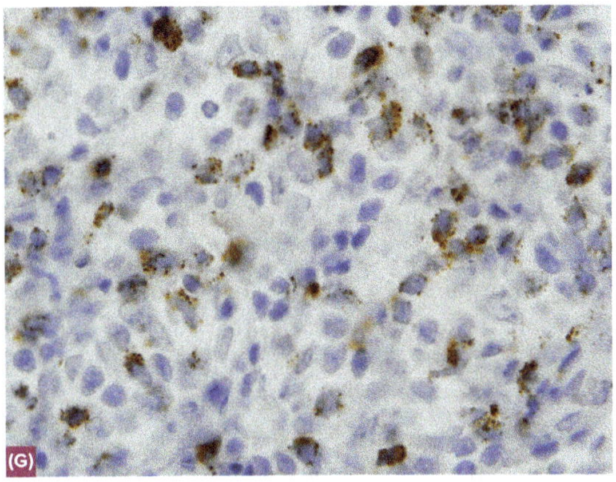

Primary cutaneous anaplastic large cell lymphoma. **(A)** Cohesive sheets of large anaplastic lymphoid cells. **(B)** This patient presented with an ulcerating tumor nodule of a few weeks' duration. An effacing superficial and deep nodular infiltrate with associated ulceration of the surface is seen. **(C)** and **(D)** The cells that make up the infiltrate are large and pleomorphic, including the presence of classic binucleated (Reed Sternberg like) and multinucleated cells with a horseshoe arrangement of nuclei. **(E)** The tumor cells express CD30 in cytoplasmic membrane and perinuclear Golgi patterns. **(F)** The tumor cells are extensively epithelial membrane antigen positive. **(G)** The tumor cells are granzyme positive. Note the granular staining within the tumor cells.

ANSWER 12-8: A.

According to the WHO-EORTC classification and the 2008 WHO classification, **subcutaneous panniculitis–like T-cell lymphoma (SPTCL)** is defined by its primary subcutaneous localization and the alpha/beta TCR+ as well as cytotoxic (CD8+, TIA1+, granzyme+, perforin+) phenotype (Table 12-8A). SPTCL presents clinically as panniculitis mimicking **erythema nodosum**, with erythematous, firm subcutaneous nodules favoring the legs. The lesions are persistent and may become ulcerated. Systemic signs may be present. In a subset of patients, a **hemophagocytic syndrome** may accompany SPTCL. The course is usually slowly progressive. Prognosis of SPTCL is favorable, with 5-year survival rate of 82%.

The diagnostic criteria include the primary subcutaneous location and a growth pattern of lymphoid infiltrates simulating a lobular panniculitis. Extensive hyaline necrosis may be present, mimicking **lupus profundus**. Cytomorphologically, the tumor cells may be small, medium, or large in size and pleomorphic. Margination (rimming) of lipocyte inner membranes by tumor cells is a common but nonspecific finding. The tumor cells have a cytotoxic T-cell profile (CD2+, CD3+, CD5+, CD4+, CD8+, CD43+, T1A-1+, granzyme B+, perforin+). By definition, they are TCR α/β+ (βF1+). There is no association with Epstein-Barr virus (EBV).

Table 12-8A. Subcutaneous Panniculitis–like Lymphoma

Clinical Features
- Subcutaneous nodules simulating panniculitis with or without ulceration
- Preferential localization: trunk, extremities (legs)

Histopathologic Features
- Subcutaneous infiltrate simulating lobular panniculitis
- Small or medium-sized to large pleomorphic lymphoid cells
- Rimming of fat cells by proliferating (Ki-67+) lymphoid cells

Immunohistochemical Features
- Various phenotypes:
  - T cell: CD3+, CD4−, CD5+, CD8+, CD30−, TIA-1+, Ki-67+
  - TCR α/β (βF1+): usually rather indolent course

Differential Diagnosis
- γ/δ (TCRδ-1+) subcutaneous T-cell lymphoma
- NK/T-cell lymphoma
- Panniculitis, especially lupus panniculitis
- Cytophagic histiocytic panniculitis

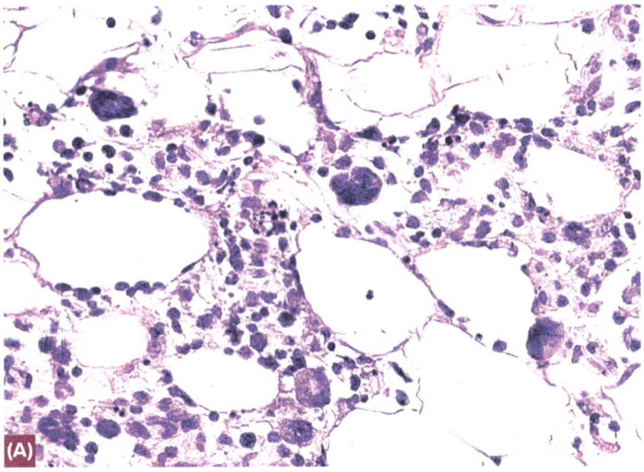

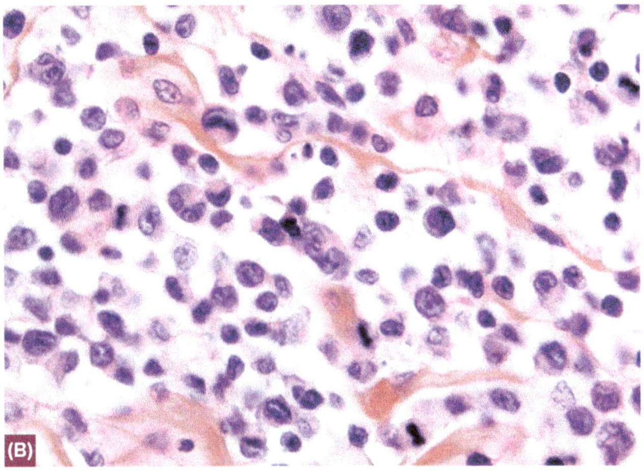

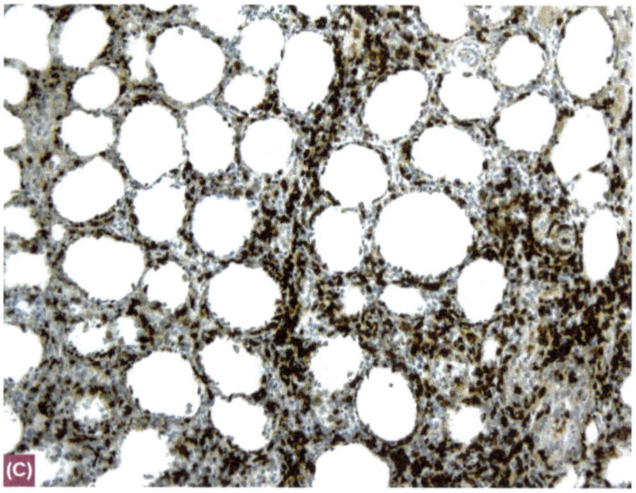

Subcutaneous panniculitis–like T-cell lymphoma. **(A)** Infiltration of subcutaneous fat tissue by small- to medium-sized pleomorphic cells surrounding adipocytes and internal rimming of the adipocyte membranes. **(B)** There is permeation of the interstitial spaces of the fat by small- to intermediate-sized lymphocytes. In many cases, the cells may appear only mildly atypical. **(C)** Subcutaneous panniculitis–like T-cell lymphoma is a tumor of cytotoxic CD8 lymphocytes in the majority of cases. Illustrated here is a CD8 preparation showing extensive staining.

In regard to the differential diagnosis, SPTCL must be differentiated from **subcutaneous gamma/delta (γ/δ+) T-cell lymphoma**, which exhibits a poor prognosis. The two entities are essentially identical both clinically and histopathologically. Tumor cells of subcutaneous γ/δ+ T-cell lymphoma exhibit a CD3+ CD56+ phenotype and are often CD4+, CD8– (double negative). They are also EBER– (EBV). By definition, they do not express betaF1 but are TCR-delta positive. *TCR* gamma genes are clonally rearranged. Isochromosome 7q is a common genetic abnormality. Among the nonneoplastic disorders, the differential diagnosis includes **atypical lymphocytic lobular panniculitis; lupus panniculitis (lupus profundus)**; and other forms of inflammatory panniculitis, especially **histiocytic cytophagic panniculitis**. The latter is a reactive process associated with a number of systemic diseases and presents with a hemorrhagic diathesis owing to **hemophagocytosis** in the absence of a lymphoproliferative disease. **Atypical lymphocytic lobular panniculitis** is a distinct form of subcutaneous T-cell dyscrasia (pseudolymphoma) characterized by clonal infiltrates of T cells whereby lymphoid atypia is mild, density of infiltration is low, and there is minimal to absent necrosis. This condition may potentially correspond to the waxing and waning phase that may presage subcutaneous panniculitis–like T-cell lymphoma. **Lupus profundus** contains abundant mucin and lacks clonality via TCR. Additionally, most cases will exhibit overlying features discoid lupus erythematosus.

ANSWER 12-9: D.

Primary cutaneous CD4+ small- to medium-sized pleomorphic T-cell lymphoma (SM-PTL) predominantly consists of small- to medium-sized pleomorphic tumor cells that do not express CD30 and differs from other entities within the group of primary cutaneous T-cell lymphoma because of its excellent prognosis. Clinically, SM-PTL manifests as skin-colored or red-brown nodules without ulceration. The prognosis is favorable for solitary lesions, with a 5-year survival of more than 90%. Unlike solitary tumors, presentations with multiple widespread tumors are associated with aggressive behavior and have been likened to d'emblée mycosis fungoides.

Microscopically, there is a nodular dense monomorphous lymphocytic infiltrate. Epidermotropism is usually absent or only focally present. The monomorphous infiltrate extends throughout the entire dermis and is composed of small- to medium-sized lymphocytes with pleomorphic moderately chromatin-dense nuclei and a small cytoplasmic rim. Eosinophils, plasma cells, and histiocytes may be admixed, and granulomatous features may be present. Clusters of B cells are commonly noted. In regard to the immunophenotypic and genotypic features, the tumor cells have a CD3+, CD4+, CD8−, CD30− T-helper phenotype. There may be loss of T-cell antigens. One recent study has reported PD1 expression within tumor cells. CD21+ dendritic cell networks with germinal center–like foci are absent. Clonal rearrangement of *TCR* genes has been detected in almost all cases reported and may be useful in the distinction of SM-PTL from **B-cell pseudolymphoma.**

In regard to the differential diagnoses, **SM-PTL** must be distinguished from **mycosis fungoides** by the absence of patches and plaques and the lack of epidermotropism. **B-cell pseudolymphoma** differs from SM-PTL by the lack of clonality and lack of T-cell antigen loss. B-cell pseudolymphoma is typically composed of a mixture of B and T cells with a ratio less than 1:1.5. Additionally, unlike SM-PTL, pseudolymphoma contains germinal center–like foci with CD21+ dendritic cell networks. **Low-grade B-cell lymphoma, marginal zone type,** is composed of an infiltrate dominated by B cells (>1.5:1, B- to T-cell ratio). **Anaplastic large cell lymphoma** presents with similar nodules and sheets of lymphoid cells, however, is composed of large cells that are CD30+.

ANSWER 12-10: D.

This lymphoma had originally been referred to as **blastic NK-cell lymphoma** and **CD4+, CD56+ hematodermic neoplasm**; however, recent studies have demonstrated that it is the neoplastic counterpart of plasmacytoid dendritic cells (PDCs); therefore it has been renamed **plasmacytoid dendritic cell neoplasm** in the 2008 WHO classification.

Clinically, the disease usually presents with contusiform, bruise-like disseminated plaques and nodules. The trunk and head are the most common sites, and mucosal involvement is common. Usually, there is already systemic involvement at the time of diagnosis with circulating malignant cells, lymph node and bone marrow involvement, and CNS infiltrates. The course is aggressive, with rapid dissemination and fatal outcome within 2 years of diagnosis. In some patients, the disease develops in the setting of preexisting **myelodysplastic syndrome.**

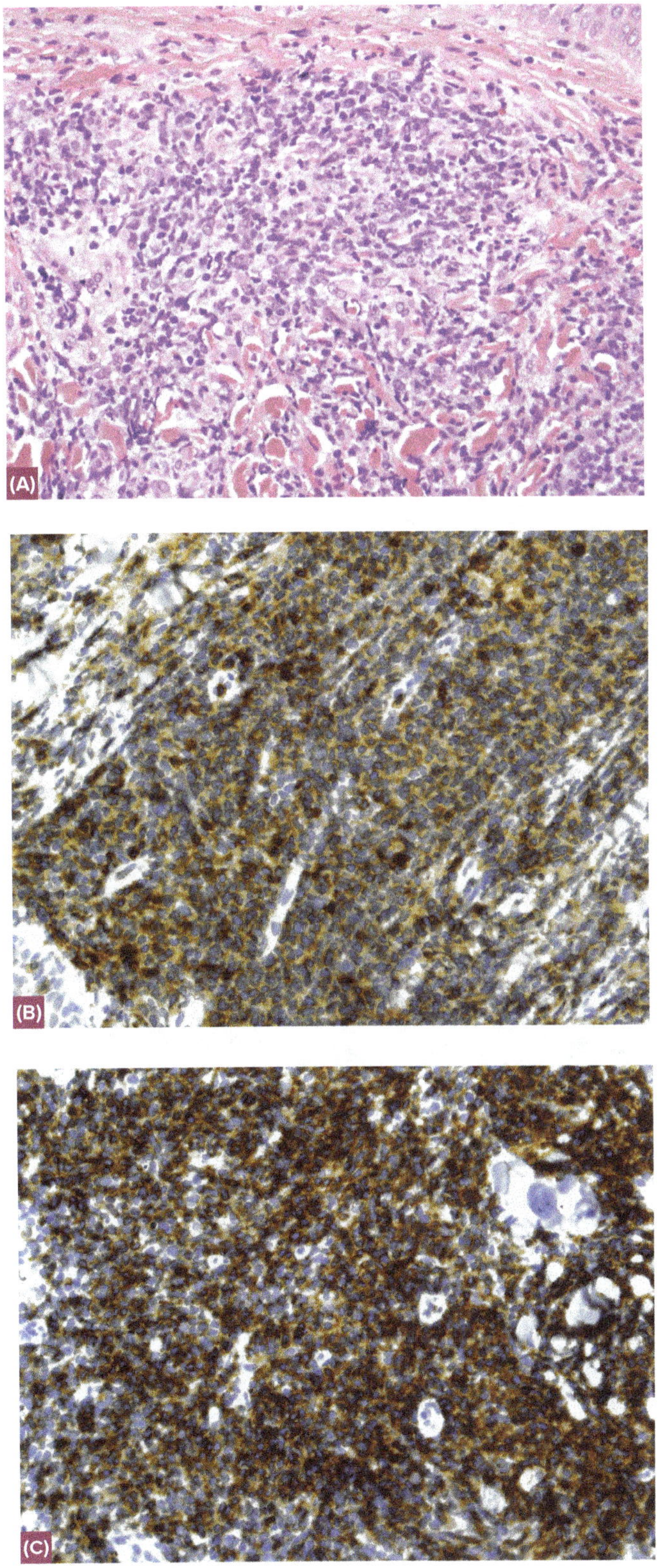

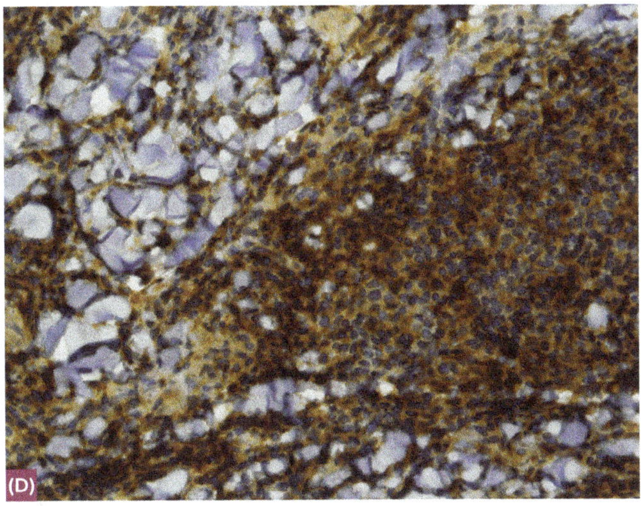

Plasmacytoid dendritic cell tumor (CD4+, CD56+ hematodermic neoplasm). (A) There is a striking interstitial and angiocentric infiltrate composed of a monomorphic infiltrate of small- to intermediate-sized mononuclear cells with a finely dispersed chromatin and inconspicuous nucleoli. The cytoplasms are minimal. There is a paucity of other inflammatory elements. **(B)** The tumor cells which define this neoplasm have a highly characteristic phenotypic profile which includes CD4 positivity. **(C)** Characteristically the tumor cells express CD56 and **(D)** CD123.

Microscopically, there is a monomorphous sheet–like infiltrate of blast cells that is band like in the upper and mid-dermis with column-like extensions into the deeper dermis and subcutis. Neither a grenz zone nor epidermotropism of tumor cells is observed. The tumor cells display nuclei with fine-dispersed chromatin and a sparse cytoplasm. Extravasated erythrocytes are found within the tumorous infiltrates. The tumor cells express CD4, CD56, CD123, and TCL-1 but are negative for T- and B-cell as well as myeloid-monocytic markers. There usually is no clonal rearrangement of TCR detectable. There is no association with EBV. The tumor cells express other plasmacytoid dendritic cell markers such as myxovirus protein (MXA), CD123, CD83, and BDCA-2. In addition, there may be expression of CD2 and CD7.

In regard to the differential diagnosis, the neoplasm has to be distinguished from specific infiltrates of **myeloid/monocytic leukemia,** which express myeloid-monocytic markers such as CD14, CD11c, and MPO, but are negative for TCL-1 in most cases. Immunophenotyping with CD20 and CD3 is useful to differentiate plasmacytoid dendritic cell neoplasms from **B-cell** and **T-cell lymphomas**, respectively.

ANSWER 12-11: B.

This is a classic example of **B-cell pseudolymphoma** (aka **lymphocytoma cutis, benign cutaneous lymphoid hyperplasia**) (Table 12-11A). In the recent past, many lymphoid proliferations that were classified previously as **cutaneous**

B-cell lymphoid hyperplasia (pseudolymphoma) have been reclassified as **low-grade malignant B-cell lymphomas** with a favorable clinical behavior. The term **cutaneous B-cell lymphoid hyperplasia** is still used, but it is not a specific diagnosis. It is descriptive and refers to a heterogeneous spectrum of diseases that simulate malignant B-cell lymphomas clinically, histopathologically, or both.

The classical clinical presentation of a **cutaneous B-cell lymphoid hyperplasia** is erythematous or red-brown to red-purple solitary nodules with a smooth surface. Agminated lesions in a region or disseminated papules may be observed rarely. Favored sites of involvement are the face (cheek, nose, earlobe), mammary area, and scrotum. Children and adults may be affected. The course of cutaneous B-cell lymphoid hyperplasia varies. The lesions may resolve with or without treatment. Various stimuli may induce lesions of cutaneous B-cell lymphoid hyperplasia, including **insect bites**, persistent nodules of **scabies**, **drugs** (antidepressant therapy), **vaccinations**, injections of antigens for hyposensitization, and **tattoos**. Cases of cutaneous B-cell lymphoid hyperplasia are often associated with infection by *Borrelia burgdorferi* (***Borrelia*-induced lymphocytoma**). In many cases, however, a precise cause is not found.

Microscopically, these lesions are characterized by relatively symmetrical, rather well-circumscribed nodular infiltrates within the dermis and sometimes within the subcutaneous fat. As a rule, the infiltrates are denser in the upper part of the dermis than in the lower part (however, in ***Borrelia*-associated lymphocytoma cutis** the infiltrate has usually a "bottom-heavy" arrangement). Germinal centers are usually present; however, rarely a nonfollicular pattern without formation of germinal centers can be observed. An important diagnostic criterion is the mixed character of the infiltrate. Although lymphocytes, especially small ones, are nearly always predominant, eosinophils, plasma cells, histiocytes, and giant cells are often found as well. The epidermis is not involved and is usually separated from the infiltrates of inflammatory cells by a thin zone composed of normal collagen bundles (grenz zone). Adnexal structures are also spared.

These histopathologic features frequently represent responses to infectious agents such as *B burgdorferi*, but other etiologies may be responsible. **Drug-associated cutaneous lymphoid hyperplasia** (most commonly associated with antidepressant therapy) usually reveal a mycosis fungoides–like pattern, but can occasionally also induce histopathologic features similar to lymphocytoma cutis. It should be emphasized that a "pseudolymphomatous" appearance does not necessarily mean that a tumor is benign; rarely, malignant nonlymphoid tumors may present with histopathologic features simulating a lymphoproliferative disorder (ie, **lymphoepithelial-like carcinoma, pseudolymphomatous angiosarcoma**).

Table 12-11A. Cutaneous B-Cell Lymphoid Hyperplasia

Clinical Features
- Preferential locations (Borrelia-induced lymphocytoma): nipple, earlobe, scrotum
- Solitary (or rarely multiple) nodules
- Both children and adults affected

Histopathologic Features
- Nodular, "top-heavy," mixed cell infiltrates
- Small lymphocytes predominate, plasma cells, eosinophils, and histiocytes
- Reactive lymphoid follicles frequently present

Immunohistologic Features
- CD20+
- CD79a+
- Polyclonal pattern (κ+, λ+)
- Bcl-2– (germinal center cells)
- CD10–, Bcl-6– (outside lymphoid follicles); CD10+, BCL6+ (within lymphoid follicles)
- Regular pattern of CD21+ follicular dendritic cells
- CD3+ reactive cells

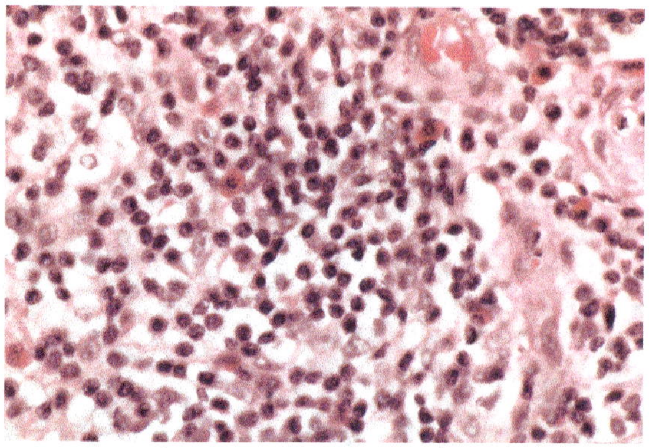

Benign cutaneous B-cell lymphoid hyperplasia. Mixed-cell infiltrate with small lymphocytes, lymphoplasmacytoid cells, eosinophils, and histiocytes.

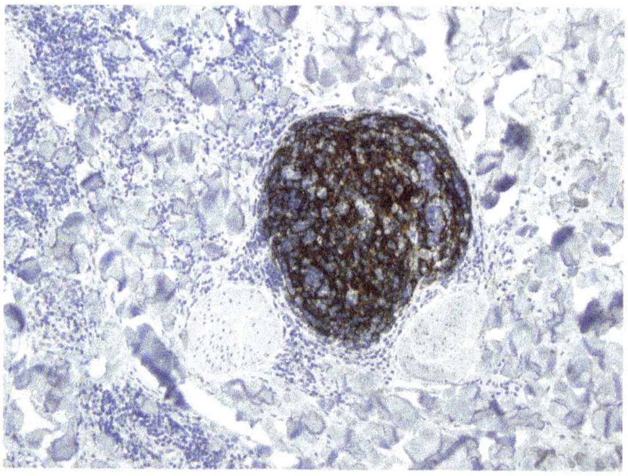

Preserved CD21 dendritic network. Network of dendritic reticulum cells as identified by expression of CD21 in this reactive germinal center. Note how the network is complete. B-cell lymphomas typically exhibit infiltration of the germinal centers with resultant lysis (disruption) of the network.

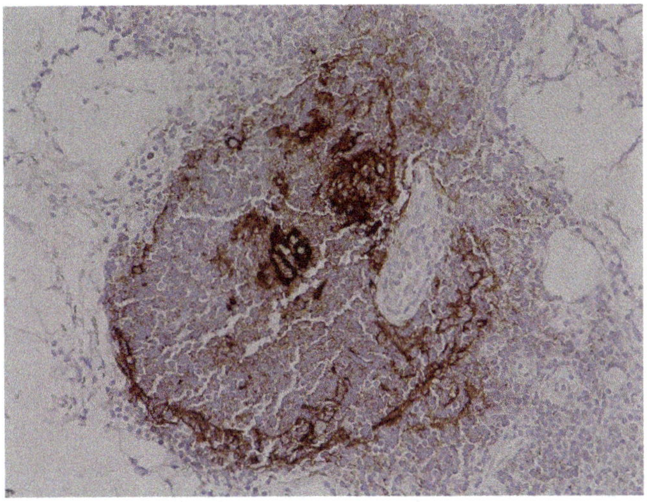

Lysis of CD21+ dendritic cell network. In this example of primary cutaneous marginal zone lymphoma, the lymphoma cells infiltrate the germinal center and disrupt the dendritic cell network.

Immunohistological investigations reveal the presence of B-cell compartments (CD20+) surrounded by T-cell aggregations. The T cells (CD3+, CD45RO+) should always predominate in a ratio no less than 1.5:1 (T- to B-cell ratio). When a predominance of B cells is present, **low-grade B-cell lymphoma** should be highly suspect. Cases with germinal center formation (CD10+, Bcl6+, Bcl2−) are associated with a regular network of dendritic reticulum cells (CD21+). Analysis of Ig-light chain expression usually discloses a polyclonal proliferation of B cells that express both κ and λ light chains. The normal kappa to lambda ratio ranges from 5:1 to 1:1. Any staining ratio greater or less should be considered clonally restricted (kappa and lambda, respectively). Very few systematic molecular studies have been performed. Polyclonal Ig-gene rearrangements are observed as a rule (Table 12-11B).

In regard to the differential diagnosis, certain clinical features may be helpful in the differentiating benign versus malignant B-cell infiltrates of the skin. Whereas benign B-cell lymphoid hyperplasias often present as a single papule or nodule with a smooth surface on a special location (ie, earlobe, nipple, genital area), lymphomas tend to be associated with clusters of papules, plaques, and tumors that may be ulcerated. B-cell lymphoid hyperplasia occurs frequently in children, in contrast to **cutaneous B-cell lymphomas (CBCLs)**. In B-cell lymphoid hyperplasia, there may be a history of a causative event (ie, drug intake, *B burgdorferi* infection), but in lymphomas, the cause is usually obscure. The histopathologic differentiation of cutaneous B-cell lymphoid hyperplasia from malignant CBCLs is one of the most difficult problems in diagnostic dermatopathology. As a rule, but not in all cases, cellular infiltrates in cutaneous B-cell lymphoid hyperplasia are relatively symmetrical, rather well circumscribed, and more dense in the upper part of the dermis than in the lower part ("top heavy"). In contrast, infiltrates in malignant B-cell

Table 12-11B. Histopathologic Criteria: B-Cell Cutaneous Lymphoid Hyperplasia Versus Malignant B-Cell Lymphoma

Cutaneous B-Cell Hyperplasia	Malignant B-Cell Lymphoma
Symmetry	Asymmetry
Wedge-shaped pattern	Lack of wedge-shaped pattern
Involvement of upper part of the dermis usually greater than that of the lower dermis	Involvement of the lower part of the dermis equal or greater than that of the upper dermis
Adnexal structures spared	Adnexal structures often obliterated
Lymphoid follicles with normal mantle zone	Lymphoid follicles devoid of mantle zone
Tingible body macrophages present in lymphoid follicles	Tingible body macrophages absent or reduced in lymphoid follicles

neoplasms are more massive, asymmetrical, poorly circumscribed, and are frequently more or less equally distributed in the superficial and deep dermis or more dense in the lower part of the dermis and subcutaneous fat ("bottom heavy"). There is a mixed character of the infiltrate in B-cell cutaneous lymphoid hyperplasia. In addition to lymphocytes, eosinophils, plasma cells, histiocytes, and giant cells are often present, but similar features can be observed in many low-grade malignant B-cell lymphomas, especially **marginal zone lymphoma**. Nuclear atypia is found more frequently in malignant lymphomas. However, in low-grade B-cell lymphomas nuclear atypia may be minimal or absent. The histopathologic features of distinct lymphoid follicles with germinal centers, which have been misinterpreted in the past as characteristic criteria of a benign inflammatory process, are not reliable for the differential diagnosis of B-cell lymphoma versus pseudolymphoma. Reactive follicles are also frequently present in lymphomas (**follicle center cell lymphoma** and **marginal zone lymphomas**). Unlike benign cutaneous lymphoid hyperplasia, infiltrating lymphoma cells in low-grade B-cell lymphoma disrupt the CD21+ dendritic cell networks of the germinal centers. Other findings helpful in the differential diagnosis are the tendency of the cellular infiltrates in cutaneous lymphoid hyperplasia to spare the epithelium of adnexa, in contrast to lymphomas, in which the adnexal epithelium structure is frequently infiltrated by neoplastic infiltrates, and the presence of tingible bodies (lymphocytic nuclear debris engulfed by macrophages) in germinal centers in cutaneous lymphoid hyperplasia but not in neoplastic follicles in lymphomas.

Immunohistochemical features are very important for the differential diagnosis. Whereas malignant populations of B lymphocytes usually show a monoclonal restriction to either κ or λ immunoglobulin light chain, benign infiltrates exhibit a polyclonal pattern with expression of both light chains. Unfortunately, however, there are several cases of B-cell lymphoproliferative disorders, both benign and malignant, in which the cells do not express immunoglobulins (or expression cannot be demonstrated in routinely fixed, paraffin-embedded specimens). Counter intuitively, a useful clue for the diagnosis of **follicle center cell lymphoma** is the diminished proliferative activity of malignant follicular cells as outlined by the Ki67/MIB-1 antibody (<50% of cells positive). Reactive germinal centers, in contrast, show a high proliferation (almost 100% of cells positive). About 80% of follicle center cell lymphomas and 15% to 30% of high-grade malignant B-cell lymphomas in the lymph nodes are characterized by the t(14;18) translocation, which is associated with overexpression of the *Bcl2* protein. By contrast, studies of cutaneous cases have shown that t(14;18) is very rare, and expression of Bcl2 can be observed only in a small minority of cases. Thus, in the skin, Bcl2 expression cannot be used as a criterion for the differentiation of follicle center cell lymphoma from B-cell pseudolymphoma with a follicular pattern. CD10 and Bcl6 expression outside of the follicles may be useful in differentiating follicle center cell lymphomas (CD10+ and/or Bcl-6+ interfollicular clusters can be found in these cases) from cutaneous B-cell lymphoid hyperplasias (no interfollicular clusters of CD10+ or Bcl6+ cells). Low-grade malignant lymphomas of B-cell lineage may show aberrant expression of some T-cell–associated markers most commonly CD43. CD5 is a pan-T-cell marker that reacts with the cells of most cases of B-cell **chronic lymphocytic leukemia (CLL)**. Normal B lymphocytes are CD43 negative, but several low-grade B-cell lymphomas are CD43 positive. The detection of an aberrant phenotype of the B lymphocytes (CD20+, CD5+, CD43+) is considered a sign of malignancy.

Concerning molecular analyses, the detection of a polyclonal pattern of immunoglobulin genes rearrangement using the PCR favors a diagnosis of cutaneous B-cell lymphoid hyperplasia, but a monoclonal rearrangement is usually (but not always) associated with malignancy. However, it must be stressed that cutaneous B-cell lymphomas do not always show a monoclonal pattern by PCR. It is important to emphasize that there are clear exceptions to each of the above-mentioned criteria. The diagnosis must therefore be based on a constellation of clinical, histopathologic, immunohistochemical, and molecular features, including follow-up information.

ANSWER 12-12: B.

To understand the different cytomorphologic appearances of the cells and their neoplastic counterparts, it is necessary to be familiar with the main pathways of B-cell differentiation. In the bone marrow, stem cells give rise to B-precursor cells (**Pre-pre-B cells**). They are the earliest detectable stage of B-cell differentiation: rearrangement of the immunoglobulin heavy chain gene has already begun, but immunoglobulins are not yet produced. **Pre-B cells**, in contrast, reveal intracytoplasmic μ heavy chain; they do not express surface Ig. Morphologically, the B-precursor cells appear as **lymphoblasts**. The end stage of antigen-independent B-cell differentiation is the mature, **naive B lymphocyte**. They have rearranged Ig genes. Upon antigen stimulation, naive B lymphocytes transform into proliferating cells with a blastic appearance (early primary response). These subsequently evolve into antibody-secreting **plasma cells**. In other instances, naive B lymphocytes transform into **centroblasts** that colonize the dendritic network of dendritic reticulum cells and form **germinal centers** (late primary response, secondary response). In **germinal centers**, a high rate of somatic mutations takes place to enhance the affinity of produced antibodies for the specific antigens. Germinal center cells whose somatic mutations have resulted in decreased affinity for the antigen die rapidly and are eliminated from the germinal center by macrophages (**"tingible-body" macrophages**). Additional B-cell subtypes with characteristic morphologic features are the **marginal zone cells** and the **mantle cells** of the inner follicle mantle. **Marginal zone cells** are closely related to monocytoid B cells. The position of marginal zone cells in the B-cell differentiation pathway is not completely clear, but they have the capacity to mature into plasma cells and appear to display specific homing patterns (**extranodal marginal zone lymphoma, MALT-type lymphoma**).

Principal Cell Types of the B-Cell Series

LYMPHOBLASTS. These are uniform-appearing, medium-sized cells with round, oval, or indented nuclei; fine chromatin; inconspicuous nucleoli; and scanty cytoplasm. These cells are found in **precursor B-lymphoblastic lymphomas.**

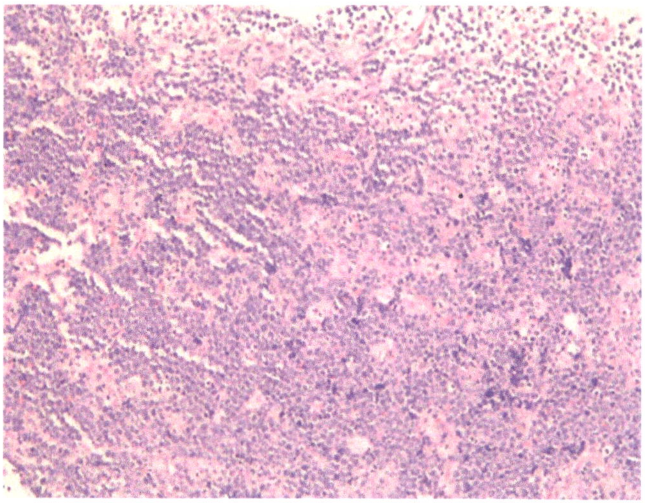

Burkitt lymphoma. This lymphoma is characterized by malignant B lymphoblasts. (Reproduced, with permission, from Lichtman MA, Shafer JA, Felgar RE, Wang N. *Lichtman's Atlas of Hematology*. New York, NY: McGraw-Hill; 2007.)

SMALL LYMPHOCYTES, B TYPE. These are small lymphocytes, usually with round nuclei, dense chromatin, and a small rim of cytoplasm. These cells correspond to those that are found in **B-cell chronic lymphocytic leukemia** (CLL).

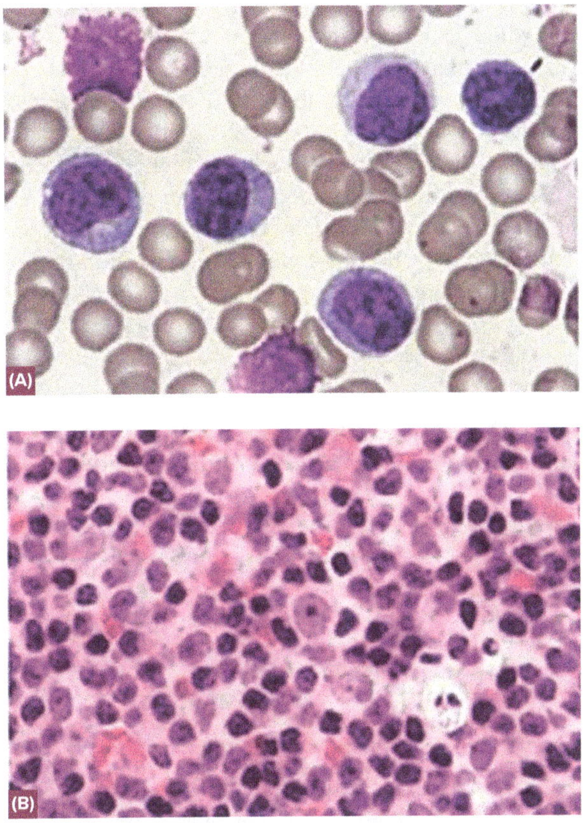

Chronic lymphocytic leukemia. Blood films. (A) Blood film. Marked increase in small lymphocytes. Smudge cells (lymphocyte nuclear remnant) characteristic of the tendency of lymphocytes to be disrupted by the shear forces during the preparation of the blood film. Occasional nuclear abnormalities evident. **(B)** Marrow film. Marrow replaced by diffuse infiltrate of small leukemic lymphocytes. Nuclear shapes sometimes irregular. Note occasional large prolymphocytes with prominent nucleoli. (Reproduced, with permission, from Lichtman MA, Shafer JA, Felgar RE, Wang N. *Lichtman's Atlas of Hematology*. New York, NY: McGraw-Hill; 2007.)

LYMPHOPLASMACYTOID CELLS AND PLASMA CELLS. Lymphoplasmacytoid cells are smaller than typical mature plasma cells. The nucleus resembles the nucleus of small lymphocytes, and the cytoplasm is abundant and basophilic, as in plasma cells.

The typical mature plasma cells are also known as the Marschalko-type plasma cells. They are characterized by a round, frequently eccentrically located, nucleus that exhibits the often-mentioned "cartwheel" or "clock face" pattern of chromatin distribution. The abundant cytoplasm is strongly basophilic and may show a paranuclear halo. Lymphoplasmacytoid cells and plasma cells are found in **marginal zone lymphomas** and **plasmacytomas.**

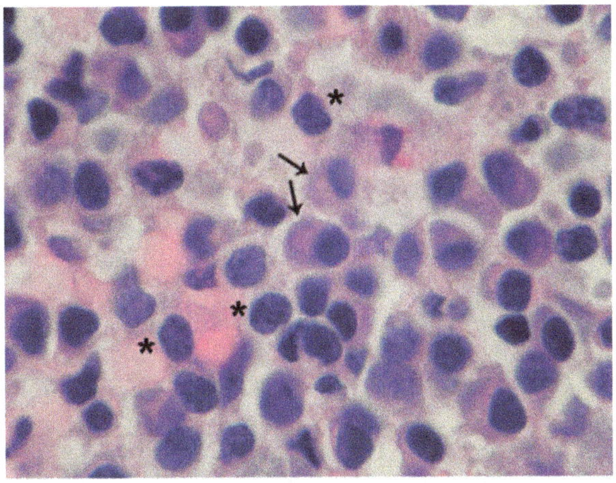

Waldenström macroglobulinemia (in lymph nodes this cellular infiltrate would be called lymphoplasmacytic lymphoma). Marrow biopsy shows a diffuse infiltrate of lymphocytes and plasmacytoid lymphocytes (asterisks), and plasma cells (arrows). The pink globules are composed of immunoglobulin, referred to as Russell bodies. (Reproduced, with permission, from Lichtman MA, Shafer JA, Felgar RE, Wang N. *Lichtman's Atlas of Hematology*. New York, NY: McGraw-Hill; 2007.)

GERMINAL CENTER CELLS. Two main types of lymphoid cells can be distinguished:

(1) **Centroblasts:** Large cells with a narrow rim of cytoplasm and oval, vesicular nuclei containing one or more distinctive nucleoli, typically situated near the nuclear membrane.
(2) **Centrocytes:** Smaller cells with irregular, sometimes cleaved nuclei, a fine chromatin pattern, and small nucleoli. The cytoplasm can be rarely identified.

The neoplastic counterparts of centroblasts and centrocytes are seen mainly in **follicle center lymphomas.**

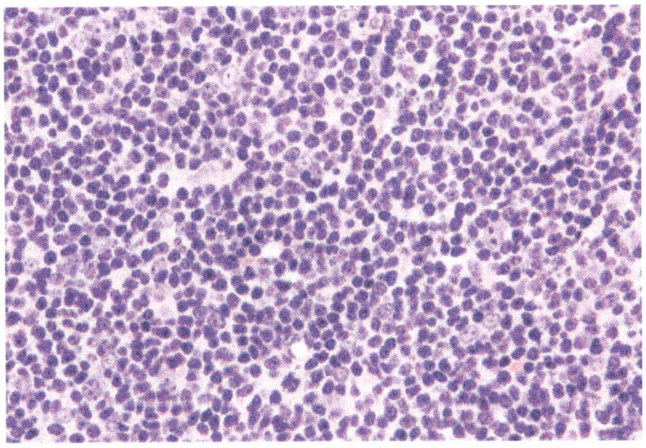

Follicular lymphoma. Lymph node biopsy. High-power view of the central portion of a neoplastic follicle showing small, cleaved cell cytology (centrocytes) as the predominant cell type. (Reproduced, with permission, from Lichtman MA, Shafer JA, Felgar RE, Wang N. *Lichtman's Atlas of Hematology*. New York, NY: McGraw-Hill; 2007.)

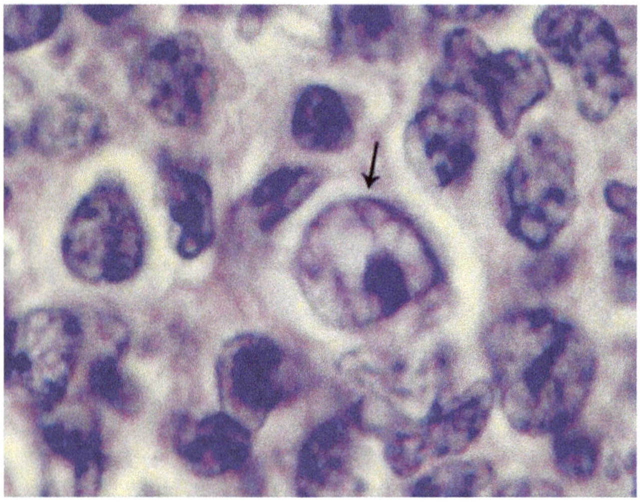

Follicular lymphoma. Lymph node biopsy. Admixed among the centrocytes are scattered large cells with prominent nucleoli called centroblasts (arrow). (Reproduced, with permission, from Lichtman MA, Shafer JA, Felgar RE, Wang N. *Lichtman's Atlas of Hematology*. New York, NY: McGraw-Hill; 2007.)

IMMUNOPHENOTYPIC FEATURES. The most useful B-cell markers are CD20 and CD79a, which detect nearly all lymphoid infiltrates of B-cell lineage. Large cell lymphomas of B-cell type (ie, **diffuse large B-cell lymphoma**) may reveal partial loss of one or more B-cell–associated antigens. Whereas malignant B-cell populations usually show a clonal restriction to either κ or λ light chain, benign infiltrates exhibit a polyclonal expression pattern of both light chains. Unfortunately, however, there are several cases of B-lymphoproliferative disorders, both benign and malignant, in which the cells do not express Ig or the Ig cannot be detected. In low-grade malignant lymphomas of B-cell lineage, aberrant expression of some T-cell–associated markers can be observed. CD5 reacts with the cells of **B-cell chronic lymphocytic leukemia** and of **mantle cell lymphoma.** Another abnormal pattern of reactivity that may be indicative of a low-grade malignant B-cell lymphoma is the coexpression of CD20 and CD43 (benign infiltrates of B lymphocytes are CD43 negative). Germinal center cells can be detected by the use of CD10 and Bcl-6 monoclonal antibodies. In **follicle center cell lymphomas**, CD10 and Bcl-6-positivity can be found also in interfollicular areas. Antibodies directed against the follicular dendritic reticulum cells (CD21, CD35) demonstrate the network of dendritic reticulum cells in reactive and malignant germinal centers. The assessment of proliferative activity with MIB-1 antibody may be useful in identifying areas with the greatest likelihood of containing tumor and in detecting the transformation from a low-grade lymphoma to high-grade "blastic" disease. In this context, it must be emphasized that neoplastic follicles in follicular lymphoma are characterized by a lesser degree of proliferation than reactive ones and that a reduced proliferation of cells within follicles is a diagnostic criterion of follicular lymphoma. Cutaneous B-cell lymphomas almost always show a distinct T-cell population, with a B- to T-cell ratio no less than 1:1.5. A summary of the various antibodies that are useful for the diagnosis of cutaneous B-cell lymphomas is provided in Table 12-12A.

MOLECULAR GENETIC ANALYSIS. B-lymphoid malignancies can be studied using specific probes detecting rearrangements of the Ig heavy- or light-chain genes. Microdissection of tumor areas may increase the sensitivity and specificity of the molecular analysis. However, a negative result does not exclude a diagnosis of malignant lymphoma. Specific translocations and numerical aberrations can be detected by fluorescence in situ hybridization (FISH) methods; however, in primary cutaneous B-cell lymphomas, only a minority of cases displays specific features by FISH.

Table 12-12A. Immunohistology: Antibodies Useful for the Diagnosis of Cutaneous B-Cell Lymphomas

CLUSTER/ ANTIBODY	SPECIFICITY
CD20	B lymphocytes
CD79a	B lymphocytes
Ig	B lymphocytes
CD5	T lymphocytes, B-CLL
CD10	Germinal center cells, common ALL antigen
CD43	T lymphocytes, monocytes
CD138	Plasma cells
MIB-1	Proliferating cells
CD21	Dendritic reticulum cell
Bcl-2	Bcl-2 protein
Bcl-6	Germinal center cells
MIB-1/Ki67	Proliferating cells
TdT	Precursor B lymphocytes
CD34	Precursor B lymphocytes
CD30	Activated B and T lymphocytes
CD68	Histiocytes
MUM-1	Multiple myeloma antigen 1
Cyclin D1	Activation or overexpression of cyclin D1 (mantle cell lymphoma)

CLASSIFICATION. Patients with involvement by cutaneous B-cell lymphomas (CBCLs) can be divided into the following groups:

(1) **Primary CBCLs**: Cutaneous disease alone with no evidence of extracutaneous manifestations after complete staging procedures have been performed.
(2) **Secondary CBCLs**: Extracutaneous disease and subsequent development of skin lesions
(3) **Concurrent CBCLs**: Extracutaneous disease at the same time as the skin lesions are diagnosed

Clinicopathologic correlation is extremely important in the accurate interpretation of CBCL. Adequate staging procedures should include examination of the entire integument, laboratory investigation, chest radiography, ultrasound examination of superficial lymph nodes and abdomen, computed tomography, and bone marrow biopsy.

Primary CBCLs comprise a broad spectrum of lymphomas with characteristic clinical, histopathologic, immunophenotypic, and molecular genetic findings. Thus, it is important that the various subtypes are appropriately classified as separate entities. It is also evident that lymphomas arising in lymph nodes and primary CBCLs, which may show similar or identical morphologic features, are different with respect to pathogenesis and clinical outcome. CBCLs only rarely exhibit the typical cytogenetic and molecular alterations characteristic of node-based B-cell lymphomas. The classification system proposed in 2005 by the WHO and EORTC can be applied satisfactorily for all CBCLs (Table 12-12B).

Secondary CBCLs can be observed in all types of B-cell lymphomas of lymphoid organs after dissemination and involvement of the skin. These lymphomas usually reveal the histopathologic features, immunology, and genetic features of the original lymphoma. The prognosis is usually poor. Of special interest for dermatopathologists are specific skin infiltrates in **B-cell chronic lymphocytic leukemia** and **B-lymphoblastic lymphoma.**

Table 12-12B. Joint World Health Organization–European Organization for Research and Treatment of Cancer Classification of Cutaneous B-Cell Lymphomas

Primary cutaneous marginal zone B-cell lymphoma
Primary cutaneous follicle center lymphoma
Primary cutaneous diffuse large B-cell lymphoma, leg type
Primary cutaneous diffuse large B-cell lymphoma, other
Intravascular large B-cell lymphoma

ANSWER 12-13: D.

Primary cutaneous follicle center lymphomas are defined as neoplasms of B cells composed of germinal center cells showing a follicular or less commonly a diffuse pattern with a mixture of **centrocytes** (cleaved follicle center cells) and **centroblasts** (large noncleaved follicle center cells) (Table 12-13A). Clinically, patients present with solitary or grouped reddish papules, plaques, or tumors that may be surrounded by erythematous patches. Preferential locations are the scalp and forehead or the back. Recurrences are observed in about 50% of patients. Dissemination to extracutaneous sites is rare, and follow-up data suggest that these patients have a favorable prognosis after adequate treatment (5-year survival, 95%).

Microscopically, these lymphomas are characterized by nodular or less frequently diffuse infiltrates commonly involving full-thickness dermis and often extending into the subcutaneous fat. Epidermotropism is usually not observed. A follicular pattern with germinal centers is found in a majority of cases. The rare diffuse growth pattern does not exhibit germinal center formation. Sometimes, however, follicular structures are present at the periphery of diffuse infiltrates.

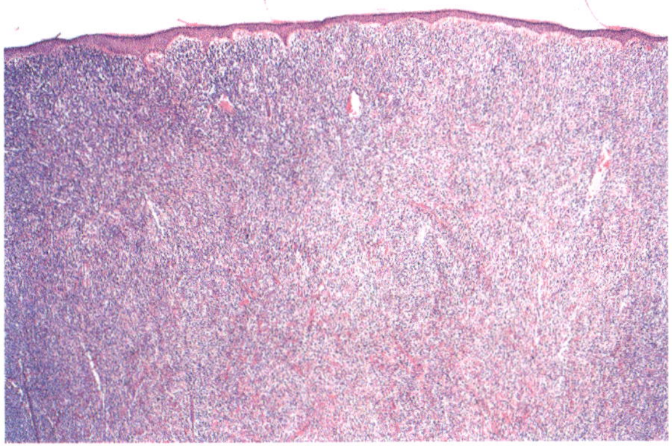

Primary cutaneous follicle center cell lymphoma with a diffuse growth pattern (less common presentation). Diffuse proliferation composed predominantly of centrocytes. Neoplastic follicles are not present.

The neoplastic cells consist mainly of centrocytes and centroblasts, but centrocytes usually clearly predominate. In cases with a prominent follicular pattern, the interfollicular areas contain small lymphocytes with a T-cell phenotype and histiocytes, as well as small clusters of follicular (neoplastic) cells.

Unlike **nodal follicular lymphomas** where an increased percentage of centroblasts correlates to a higher grade and worse prognosis, **primary cutaneous follicle center cell lymphomas** behave the same regardless of cellular composition. Therefore, it is not recommended to grade primary cutaneous follicle center cell lymphomas. In cases with a diffuse pattern of growth, the cytomorphologic appearance may be that of a **diffuse large B-cell lymphoma**. However, the clinical features and prognosis of these cases are similar to those of other cutaneous follicle center lymphomas, and they should not be

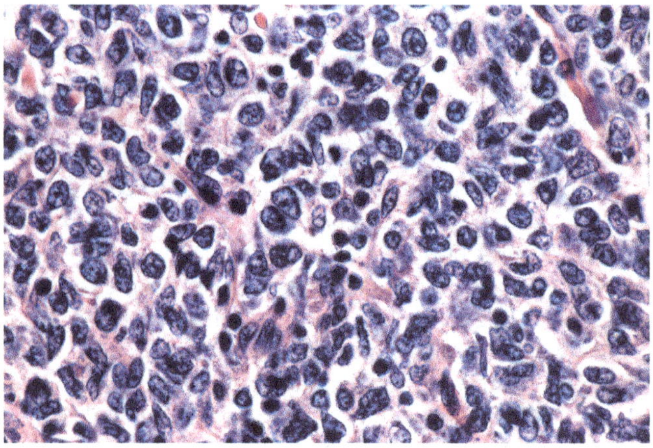

Primary cutaneous follicle center cell lymphoma. Large centroblasts predominate admixed with a few small centrocytes. The centrocytes are small to medium cells with irregular "cleaved" nuclei that often show nuclear indentations and grooves without any nucleoli. The cells contain scant cytoplasm and the nuclei appear twisted with a "stretched taffy"–like appearance. In contrast, centroblasts (large noncleaved cells) are larger cells with scant to moderate cytoplasm and round to oval nuclei with open chromatin and distinct nucleoli.

Table 12-13A. Follicle Center Cell Lymphoma

Clinical Features
- Preferential locations: head, back
- Solitary or regionally localized patches, papules, plaques, and tumors
- Favorable prognosis (5-year survival, 95%)

Histopathologic Features
- Nodular or rarely diffuse infiltrates
- Follicular, mixed, or diffuse pattern of growth
- Mixture of germinal center cells: centroblasts and centrocytes
- Predominance of large centrocytes in cases with diffuse pattern of growth

Immunohistochemical Features
- CD20+
- CD79a+
- CD21+ (dendritic cell lysis by tumor cells)
- CD5−
- Bcl-2−/+
- Bcl-6+
- CD10 +/−

Differential Diagnosis
- Cutaneous lymphoid hyperplasia
- Marginal zone B-cell lymphoma
- Large B-cell lymphoma, leg type

classified as large B-cell lymphomas. A variant of cutaneous follicle center lymphoma with predominant spindle cell morphology has been described. This variant may simulate other cutaneous spindle cell malignant neoplasms, such as sarcomas and spindle cell melanoma, among others.

In regard to the immunophenotype and genotype, the tumor cells express monotypic surface Ig and B-cell–associated antigens. They are CD5 and CD43 negative. In practically all cases with a follicular pattern and in the majority of cases with a diffuse pattern, neoplastic B lymphocytes are positive for Bcl-6 (both within and outside of germinal centers). Staining for CD10 is positive within the germinal centers in a smaller percentage of cases. The finding of CD10-positive or Bcl-6-positive cells in clusters outside follicular structures is considered a criterion of malignancy. Unlike **nodal follicular lymphomas**, Bcl-2 is usually negative, but they are frequently positive only in a minority of tumor cells. It is important to keep in mind that normal T-cells are Bcl-2+ and therefore one must compare Bcl2 expression with CD20+ and CD3+ cells. Staining with markers detecting proliferating cells (ie, Ki-67/MIB-1) shows that neoplastic follicles are characterized by a reduced proliferation compared with reactive germinal centers. Within the follicular areas, the organized network of CD21+ dendritic reticulum cells is present, but outward infiltration from the germinal center results in areas of lysis and irregularity (**dendritic cell lysis**). Clonal Ig gene rearrangement can be demonstrated in many cases. The interchromosomal (14;18) translocation, which has been shown to be very common in **nodal follicular lymphomas**, is extremely rare in **primary cutaneous follicle center lymphoma**. Despite the similar morphologic features, the differences in Bcl-2 protein expression and incidence of t(14;18) between nodal and cutaneous follicular lymphomas suggest that different mechanisms may be involved in the pathogenesis of these neoplasms.

The major differential diagnosis in cases of **primary cutaneous follicle center lymphomas** with follicular pattern is **benign cutaneous lymphoid hyperplasia** with follicular structures (B-cell pseudolymphoma). Benign cutaneous lymphoid hyperplasia contains a predominance of T cells, contains intact CD21+ dendritic cell networks within its germinal centers, and expresses Bcl-6 and CD10 within germinal center lymphocytes only. The diffuse variant of follicle center lymphoma should be differentiated from diffuse large B-cell lymphomas that are usually Bcl-2 and MUM-1 positive and often show a predominance of immunoblasts. **Marginal zone lymphoma** is also in the differential diagnosis. Both are characterized by reactive polyclonal follicle centers infiltrated by monoclonal lymphoma cells disrupting the CD21+ dendritic cell networks. However, it may be difficult or impossible to differentiate the neoplastic cells (centrocyte-like cells) in marginal zone lymphoma from the centrocytes in follicular lymphoma. Marginal zone lymphomas contain peripheral lymphoplasmacytic cells with either kappa or lambda light chain restriction. CD4+ small- to medium-sized pleomorphic T-cell lymphoma is composed predominantly of CD4+, PD1+ T cells without germinal center formation.

ANSWER 12-14: C.

Marginal zone B-cell lymphoma (aka **MALT lymphoma, cutaneous immunocytoma**) is a low-grade malignant lymphoma with morphologic evidence of differentiation into cells of the marginal zone that display tissue-specific homing patterns (Table 12-14A). Primary cutaneous MZL is closely related to MALT lymphomas. Clinically these tumors present as recurrent, localized, red to reddish-brown papules, plaques, and tumors located predominantly on the trunk and upper extremities are observed. The prognosis is excellent (5-year survival, 98%). In a few European cases, an association with *B burgdorferi* infection has been well demonstrated. However, other cases from different parts of the world have been negative, suggesting a regional variability of association of *B burgdorferi* with marginal zone lymphomas (MZL) and other cutaneous B-cell lymphomas.

Microscopically, MZLs show patchy, nodular, or occasionally diffuse infiltrates involving the dermis and superficial subcutaneous fat. The epidermis is not involved. A characteristic pattern can be observed at scanning magnification: nodular infiltrates, usually containing reactive germinal centers surrounded by a pale-staining population of small- to medium-sized cells with indented nuclei, inconspicuous nucleoli, and abundant pale cytoplasms (question images B and C; aka **marginal zone cells** or **monocytoid B cells**). In addition, **plasma cells** (at the margins of the infiltrate), **lymphoplasmacytoid cells**, small lymphocytes, and occasional large blasts are observed. Eosinophils are also a common finding. In some cases, there may be a granulomatous reaction with epithelioid and giant cells. Some cases of MZL present with predominance of lymphoplasmacytoid cells or plasma cells, showing features that were classified in the past as **cutaneous immunocytoma** or **cutaneous plasmacytoma**.

Table 12-14A. Marginal Zone B-Cell Lymphoma

Marginal Zone B-Cell Lymphoma
Clinical Features
Preferential location: upper extremities, trunk
Solitary or localized papules, plaques, and tumors
Excellent prognosis (5-year survival, 98%)
Histopathologic Features
Nodular or rarely diffuse infiltrates
Nodules of reactive B lymphocytes surrounded and partially infiltrated by neoplastic marginal zone cells
Plasma cells are frequent
Reactive lymphoid follicles are usually present
Some cases show predominance of lymphoplasmacytoid cells (formerly cutaneous immunocytoma) or plasma cells (formerly cutaneous plasmacytoma)
Immunohistologic Features
Cytoplasmic Ig+ (60-65%)
CD20+; CD79a+
CD21+ (dendritic cell lysis)
CD5−
CD10−
Bcl-6−
Bcl-2+
Differential Diagnosis
Cutaneous lymphoid hyperplasia
Follicle center cell lymphoma

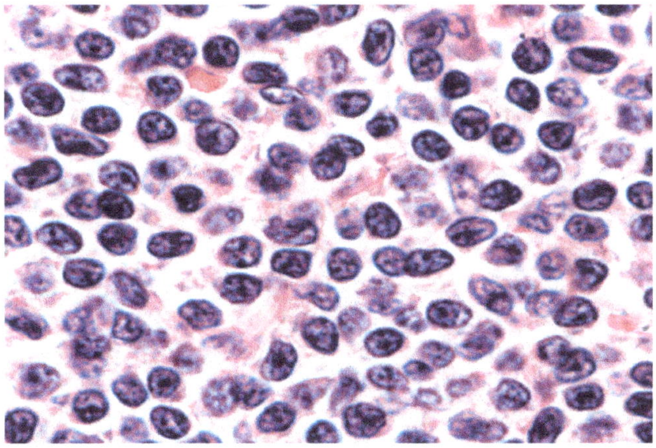

Primary cutaneous marginal zone B-cell lymphoma with predominance of lymphoplasmacytoid lymphocytes (formerly immunocytoma).

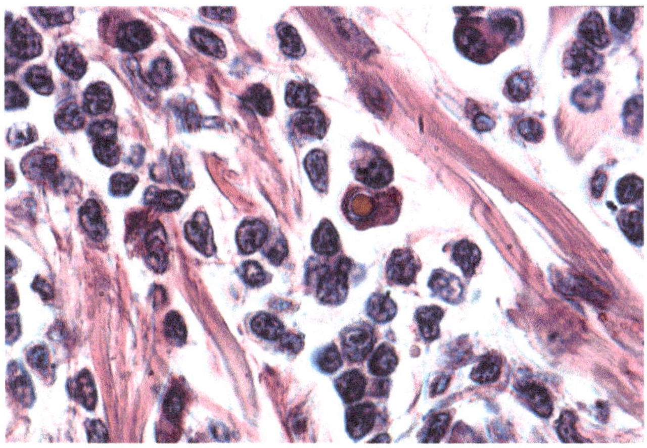

Primary cutaneous marginal zone B-cell lymphoma with predominance of lymphoplasmacytoid lymphocytes (formerly immunocytoma). Intranuclear globular periodic acid-Schiff–positive inclusion (Dutcher body).

In regard to immunophenotype, the marginal zone cells (monocytoid B cells) reveal a CD20+, CD79a+, CD5−, CD10−, Bcl−6−, and Bcl−2+ phenotype. Unlike **follicle center cell lymphoma** where the lymphoma cells arise within the germinal centers and disrupt the CD21+ dendritic cells

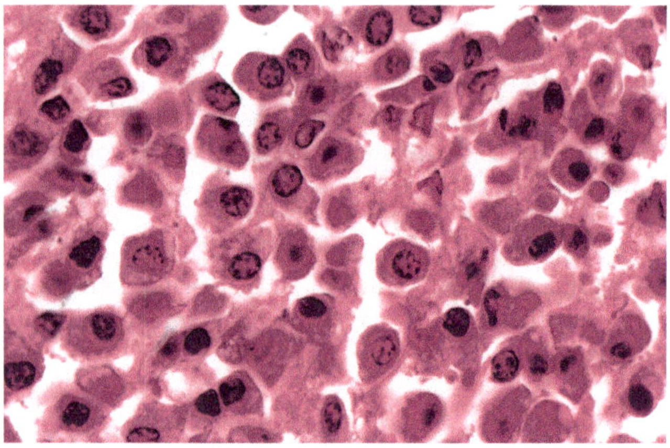

Primary cutaneous marginal zone B-cell lymphoma with prominent plasma cell differentiation (formerly cutaneous plasmacytoma). The predominant cell population consists of Marschalko type cells and atypical plasma cells.

networks, **marginal zone lymphoma** cells infiltrate into the germinal centers causing CD21+ dendritic cell lysis. In the vast majority of cases, a monoclonal distribution of Ig light chains can be observed (especially in the plasma cells). Immunohistochemical staining with kappa and lambda is a very useful tool in assessing for light chain restriction (clonality). Normal "reactive" kappa to lambda ratios range from 5:1 to 1:1. Ratios greater than 5:1 (kappa to lambda) are considered kappa restricted, and ratios less than 1:1 (kappa to lambda) are considered lambda restricted. This assessment is done by comparing the percentage of staining cells in a specific cellular focus within corresponding kappa- and lambda-stained sections. The case in question is clearly lambda light chain restricted. A clonal Ig heavy chain gene rearrangement can be observed in the majority of cases. Genetic studies have shown features similar to other extranodal MALT lymphomas.

In regard to the differential diagnoses, **MZL** can be confused with **lymphocytoma cutis**, which is characterized by a polyclonality of B cells. Additionally, **lymphocytoma cutis (benign cutaneous lymphoid hyperplasia)** lacks CD21+ dendritic cell lysis of germinal centers by tumor cells as well as light chain restriction. MZL must be distinguished from **follicle center lymphoma**. As already pointed out, whereas MZL may show follicles that are reactive, and is characterized by an interfollicular proliferation of centrocyte-like cells, in follicle center lymphoma, the neoplastic follicles reveal malignant morphologic and immunophenotypic features. **Mantle cell lymphoma**, which is not well defined in the skin and has been observed only in exceptional cases, is composed of relatively uniform, small- to medium-sized lymphocytes with irregular nuclear contours. Because of the cytologic similarities, it may be very difficult to differentiate this lymphoma from MZL. Neoplastic mantle cells express CD5 and cyclin D1 (both negative in cutaneous MZL), and the *Bcl-1* gene rearrangement can frequently be documented. Cases classified in the past as cutaneous **immunocytoma** represent variants of cutaneous MZL with a predominance of lymphoplasmacytoid cells and plasma cells. In these cases, the histology often reveals more monotonous infiltrates with large sheets of small lymphoid, lymphoplasmacytoid cells, and plasma cells, which contain cytoplasmic Ig. It has also been proposed that cases classified previously as **primary cutaneous plasmacytoma** (monoclonal proliferations of plasma cells that develop in the skin in the absence of bone marrow involvement) are variants of MZL. In fact, some patients with lesions classified as cutaneous plasmacytoma have presented with recurrent lesions showing histopathologic features of MZL. **Diffuse large B-cell lymphoma** lacks a nodular architecture, rarely contains germinal centers, and is composed of large pleomorphic cells.

ANSWER 12-15: B.

Diffuse large B-cell lymphomas are a group of aggressive malignant lymphomas that contain a predominant population of large B cells. About 80% of cases of **primary cutaneous large B-cell lymphoma, leg type**, develop on the legs (hence the term) of elderly patients (Table 12-15A). The clinical features are variable. Solitary or multiple reddish-brown or violaceous tumors are localized to one or sometimes both lower legs. Ulceration can be found. The disease predominantly affects older women (>70 years of age). Relapses and extracutaneous involvement are common. The prognosis is more unfavorable than that in the other primary cutaneous B-cell lymphomas, and the 5-year survival rate is approximately 55%.

Microscopically, the tumor is characterized by dense and diffuse (rather than nodular) infiltrates within the dermis and subcutis. Infiltration of the epidermis (epidermotropism) simulating a T-cell lymphoma can be observed rarely. Germinal centers are typically absent. Cytomorphologically, the neoplastic cells resemble either immunoblasts or centroblasts. There are many mitotic figures. A "starry sky" pattern with tingible body macrophages is sometimes present. Surface Ig or cytoplasmic Ig can be demonstrated in some cases. The neoplastic cells are CD20+, CD79a+ (loss of antigen expression can be observed), Bcl-2+, and most specifically MUM-1+. In many cases, a proportion of neoplastic cells are positive for Bcl-6. CD10 is typically negative. Molecular studies have revealed that cutaneous large B-cell lymphoma, leg type, is characterized by the monoclonal proliferation of postgerminal center B lymphocytes. Deletion of 9p21 is associated with aggressive biological behavior.

In regard to the differential diagnosis, **diffuse large B-cell lymphoma, leg type**, must be distinguished from **large cell anaplastic lymphoma,** which consists of CD3+, CD30+ large T cells with irregularly shaped nuclei admixed with giant cells resembling Reed-Sternberg (RS) cells. In this context, it must be emphasized that there is a variant of large B-cell

Table 12-15A. Large B-Cell Lymphoma, Leg Type

Clinical Features
Preferential location: lower leg
Solitary or multiple tumors
Older females predominate
5-year survival, ~55% (with multiple lesion; higher survival with solitary lesion)
Histopathologic Features
Diffuse growth pattern
Large cells with round nuclei (features of immunoblasts and centroblasts)
High mitotic rate; sometimes "starry-sky" pattern
Immunohistologic Features
CD20+
CD79a+
CD10 −/+ (mainly CD 10−)
Bcl-6 +/−
Bcl-2+
MUM-1+
Differential Diagnosis
Follicle center lymphoma, diffuse type
Granulocytic sarcoma
Large cell anaplastic lymphoma
Histiocytic tumors
Metastases

lymphoma that is characterized by anaplastic B lymphocytes positive for CD30. This variant should not be included in the group of CD30-positive anaplastic large cell lymphoma but should rather be classified among the large B-cell lymphomas. Diffuse variants of **follicle center cell lymphoma** are typically negative for MUM1 and Bcl-2 and are positive for Bcl-6 and occasionally CD10. **Granulocytic sarcoma**, histiocytic neoplasms, metastases, and other nonhematopoietic tumors can be excluded not only by morphology but also by applying a panel of monoclonal antibodies. **Chronic lymphocytic leukemia (small cell lymphoma)** also presents with diffuse infiltrates; however, the cells are small and monotonous and express CD5 in addition to pan-B-cell markers.

ANSWER 12-16: E.

Chronic lymphocytic leukemia (B-CLL) is a B-cell neoplasm and the most frequent form of leukemia in Western countries, accounting for nearly 25% of all leukemias with an estimated annual age-adjusted incidence of three to five per 100,000 persons (Table 12-16A). The median age at diagnosis is approximately 70 years, and the disease affects men twice as frequently as women. Patients typically present with peripheral lymphocytosis, painless lymphadenopathy, and hypogammaglobulinemia. Complications include recurrent infections,

Table 12-16A. Leukemic Skin Infiltrates of Chronic Lymphocytic Leukemia

Clinical Features
Most common form of leukemia in adults
Older than 60 years old
Men and women affected equally
Red or violaceous macules, papules, and nodules
Often ulcerated, large nodules
Located on face, scalp, trunk, and extremities
Sometimes at site of herpes zoster and herpes simplex scars
Histopathologic Features
Patchy perivascular and periadnexal lymphoid infiltrate
Nodular or diffuse infiltrate
Band-like infiltrate in the upper and middle dermis
May involve subcutaneous tissue
Immunophenotype
CD5+, CD19+, CD20+, CD23+; CD38+ equals a worse prognosis
Monoclonal expression of either κ or γ chain
Molecular Biology
Clonal rearrangement of Ig heavy (IgH)
Differential Diagnosis
Immunocytoma
Cutaneous B-cell lymphoma
Cutaneous B-cell pseudolymphoma
Lymphocytic infiltration Jessner-Kanof
Mycosis fungoides

aggressive squamous cell carcinomas, and **Richter transformation. Richter transformation** is serious complication seen in approximately 5% of cases and is characterized by transformation into **diffuse large B-cell lymphoma** with aggressive biological behavior and little response to chemotherapy. Specific skin lesions of CLL occur in approximately 8% of patients with CLL. The reported incidence of cutaneous lesions ranges from 4% to 45% if one takes into account nonspecific findings including purpura, ecchymoses, and maculopapular eruptions. The lesions are solitary, or more often multiple, red or violaceous macules, papules, or nodules. Large nodules may become necrotic and ulcerated. The lesions tend to occur on limited areas of the body mainly the trunk, extremities, face, and scalp, but often spread and become generalized. Specific cutaneous infiltrates arising at the site of **herpes zoster** and **herpes simplex** scars are common. These lesions may be a temporary phenomenon and frequently regress without treatment. Frequently the leukemic cells will colonize active lesions of dermatitis. In patients with CLL, infection with *B burgdorferi* may also trigger the development of specific cutaneous infiltrates at sites typical for **lymphocytoma cutis** such as the nipple, scrotum, and earlobe. In addition, a predilection for specific infiltrates to arise at the site of **squamous cell carcinoma, basal cell carcinoma,** and **actinic keratosis** has been observed. The clinical lesions may have striking variations in their morphologic features and distribution. Atypical manifestations may present as chronic paronychia, subungual nodules, plaques on the volar surface of the hands and fingers, finger clubbing with periosteal bone destruction, and papulovesicular eruptions. Involvement of the mucous membranes is rare. The prognosis of patients with specific skin lesions is probably not affected by skin involvement.

Microscopically, three main patterns of skin infiltrates can be distinguished in CLL: a superficial and deep perivascular and periadnexal infiltrate, a nodular-diffuse infiltrate, and a band-like infiltrate. Extensive involvement of the subcutaneous tissue is usually seen, particularly in large nodular lesions. A grenz zone of normal dermis is seen between the uninvolved epidermis and the dermal infiltrate, although the infiltrate occasionally extends close to the dermal-epidermal junction, with isolated epidermotropic lymphoid cells. Occasionally, a subepidermal bullous separation, accompanied by edema of the superficial dermis, may be present. Less commonly, leukemic infiltrates may invade the walls of blood vessels. Cyclic lymphocytic vasculitis associated with CLL has been reported. A granulomatous reaction composed of epithelioid and giant cells may occur, especially in skin infiltrates at sites of previous herpes infections. At higher magnification, the infiltrate is monomorphous and composed mainly of small- to medium-sized lymphocytes with a round nucleus and dense nuclear chromatin. Eosinophils, neutrophils, and plasma cells may also be present in the infiltrate.

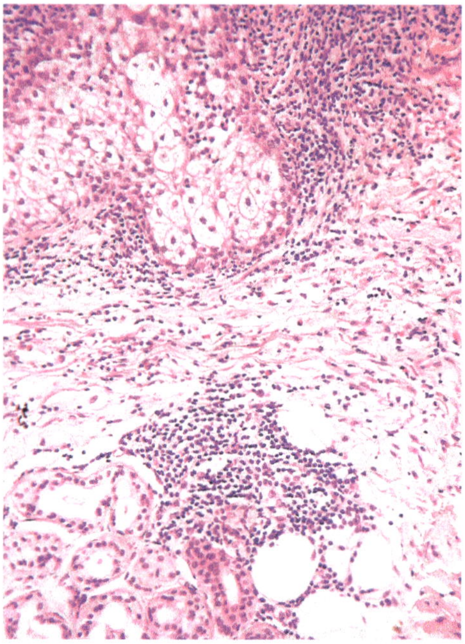

Chronic lymphocytic leukemia (B-CLL). There is a periadnexal infiltrate of small- to medium-sized lymphoid cells. Note the presence of eosinophils.

B-CLL cells are characterized by a CD19+, CD20+, CD43+, CD23+, and CD5+ immunophenotype. The detection of a monoclonal restriction to either κ or λ immunoglobulin light chain is an important feature of malignant cells in B-CLL. The neoplastic cells express monoclonal surface IgM or surface IgM and surface IgD. Demonstration of light-chain restriction may be difficult in formalin-fixed tissue and frozen sections are usually required for optimal analysis. Expression of CD38 and Z-chain–associated protein kinase-70 (ZAP-70) is associated with a worse prognosis. Clonal rearrangement of Ig heavy (IgH) is demonstrable in most cases.

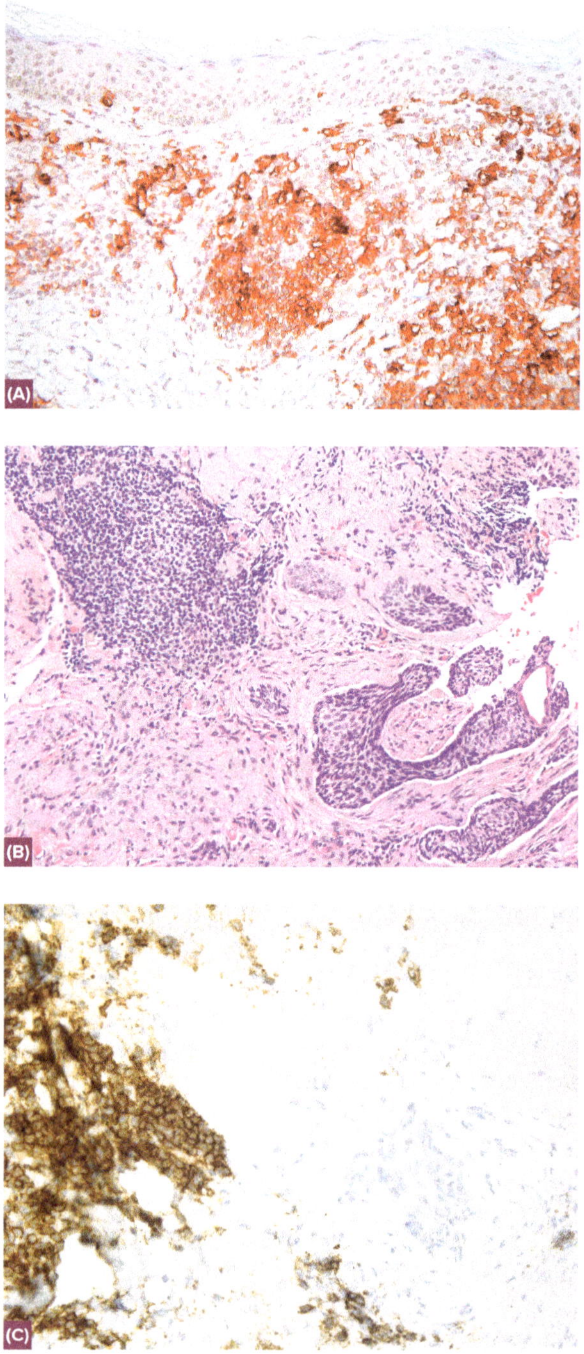

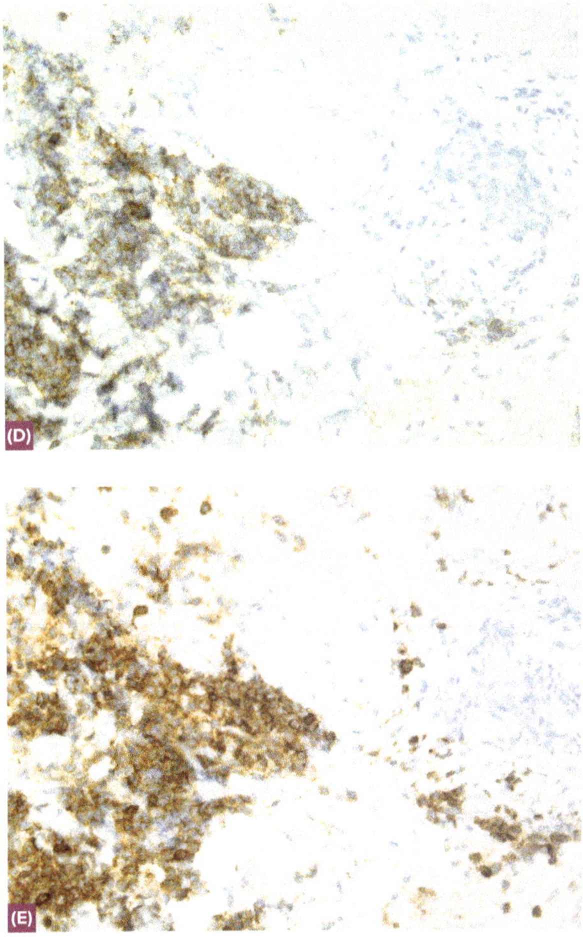

Chronic lymphocytic leukemia (B-CLL). (A) Perivascular pattern of infiltrate of CD20+ cells. **(B)** Chronic B-CLL. In this collage, one sees a well-differentiated small lymphocytic infiltrate that was found peripheral to an infiltrating basal cell carcinoma. The lymphocytes showed a typical chronic lymphocytic leukemia phenotypic profile composed of **(C)** CD20 positivity, **(D)** CD23 positivity, and **(E)** CD5 positivity.

ANSWER 12-17: A.

This is a classic example of **acute myeloid leukemia cutis (Table 12-17A)**. The French-American-British (FAB) classification of leukemias is based on the morphologic appearance of bone marrow and blood leukemic blasts, supplemented by cytochemical and immunohistochemical stains (Table 12-17B).

Acute granulocytic (myeloid) leukemia (AML) (M0-M3) accounts approximately for 40% to 50% of all acute leukemias, with the incidence of the different FAB types reported as 18% for M1, 28% for M2, and 8% for M3. Demonstration of the accumulation of blasts resulting from the block in differentiation characteristic of AML is the essential requirement for diagnosis. The AML types differ with respect to cell line and degree of differentiation. All cases should be negative for CD3 and CD20 (T- and B-cell markers). In AML with minimal evidence of myeloid differentiation (M0) or without maturation (M1), the predominant cell is undifferentiated by light microscopy, is peroxidase negative, and expresses CD34, CD33, and CD117 but lacks CD15. In AML with maturation (M2), myeloblasts with granules and promyelocytes account for more than 50% of nucleated cells (CD15+, CD33+, often CD34+, and CD117+). **Acute promyelocytic leukemia** (APL, M3) is recognized by a predominance of promyelocytes. Leukemia cutis lesions have been reported to occur in up to 10% of patients with AML subtypes M0 to M3. M4 through M7 represents myelomonocytic, monocytic, erythrocytic, and megakaryocytic differentiation, respectively. **Myelomonocytic leukemia (AMMoL, FAB M4)** represents about 25% of all cases of acute nonlymphocytic leukemia. In AMMoL, both granulocytic and monocytic precursors are present in varying proportions, and each cell line accounts for at least 20% of nucleated bone marrow cells. Leukemic mucocutaneous lesions are found in 13% to 27% of patients. **Acute monocytic leukemia (AMoL, FAB M5)** accounts

Table 12-17A. Leukemic Skin Infiltrates of Acute Myeloid Leukemias

Clinical Features
Erythematous papules and nodules
Usually widespread, mainly on the trunk
Sometimes solitary nodule
Ulceration may occur
Gingival involvement, especially in AMoL
Aleukemic leukemia cutis may occur
Histopathologic Features
Nodular or diffuse infiltrates of atypical myeloid cells
Subcutaneous tissue mostly involved
Grenz zone mostly present
Medium to large mononuclear cells with large nuclei (myeloblasts and myelocytes, AML)
Medium-sized or large mononuclear cells with indented or kidney-shaped nuclei (AMMoL, AMoL)
Thin rows of neoplastic cells between collagen bundles ("Indian file")
Concentric layering of neoplastic cells around blood vessels
Mitotic figures frequent
Immunohistochemistry
Predominant reactivity for lysozyme, myeloperoxidase, CD68, CD74, CD43, CD45
Differential Diagnosis
Metastatic carcinoma
Malignant melanoma
Merkel cell carcinoma
B-lymphoblastic lymphoma
Sweet syndrome
Cutaneous extramedullary hematopoiesis

Table 12-17B. French-American-British Classification of Leukemias

Acute Leukemias
M0 Acute myeloid leukemia with minimal evidence of myeloid differentiation
M1 Acute myeloid leukemia without maturation
M2 Acute myeloid leukemia with maturation
M3 Acute promyelocytic leukemia
M4 Acute myelomonocytic leukemia
M5 Acute monocytic leukemia
M6 Acute erythroleukemia
M7 Acute megakaryoblastic leukemia
Acute lymphoblastic leukemia
Chronic Leukemias
Chronic myeloid leukemia
Chronic lymphocytic leukemia
T-cell prolymphocytic leukemia
Adult T-cell leukemia/lymphoma
Hairy cell leukemia
Chronic myelomonocytic leukemia

for approximately 10% of all cases of acute nonlymphocytic leukemia. Extramedullary disease is more common in AMoL (M5) than in other subtypes of leukemia and is associated with a worse prognosis. Leukemic skin infiltrates are present in 10% to 30% of patients with AMoL (M5). Lastly, acute myelogenous leukemia is associated with various paraneoplastic conditions such as **Sweet syndrome** and **pyoderma gangrenosum.**

Clinically, the skin lesions acute myelogenous leukemia are erythematous or violaceous, slightly elevated papules or nodules. The gums are involved in about 18% and 60% of patients with M4 and M5, respectively. In M4, infiltrations of tumor cells into scars of previous sites of catheter placement, trauma, burns, and herpes simplex is characteristic.

Microscopically, biopsy specimens from specific skin lesions of AML show a dense leukemic infiltrate in the upper and deep dermis that usually extends to the subcutaneous tissue. It is generally separated from the epidermis by a narrow grenz zone, although the dermal-epidermal interface may be obliterated. The infiltrates typically surround the dermal blood vessels, hair follicles, and sweat glands. Transmural infiltration of dermal blood vessels and intravascular collections of atypical myeloid cells may be found. In some instances, the vessel is not only permeated by leukemic cells but may show evidence of vascular compromise as evidenced by red blood cell extravasation in concert with mural and/or luminal fibrin deposition. Typically, the leukemic myeloid cells spread between the collagen bundles and permeate the interstitial spaces of the fat lobule. The infiltrate of AML is composed predominantly of medium-sized or large atypical **myeloblasts** and **myelocytes** with round or oval basophilic nuclei and prominent nucleoli. Immature atypical myeloid cells with bizarre nuclei are frequently present. Also, there may be admixtures of polymorphonuclear leukocytes, although the numbers are small. Mitotic figures are a consistent finding in the infiltrate of AML.

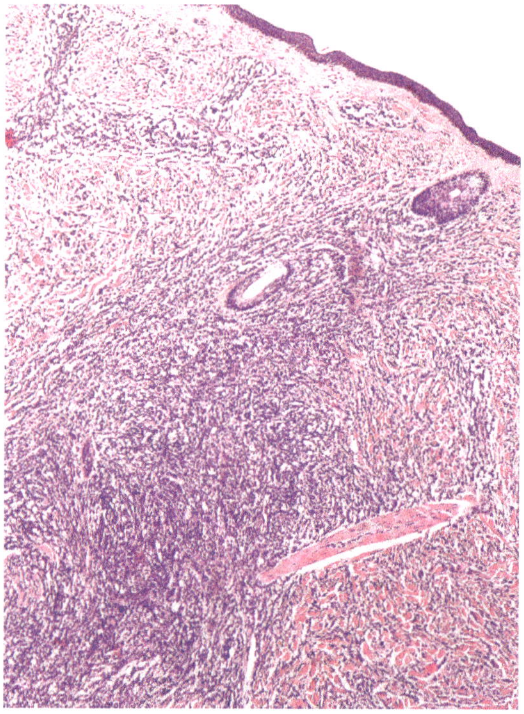

Acute myelomonocytic leukemia (AMMoL, M4). Diffuse infiltrate of atypical cells in the dermis.

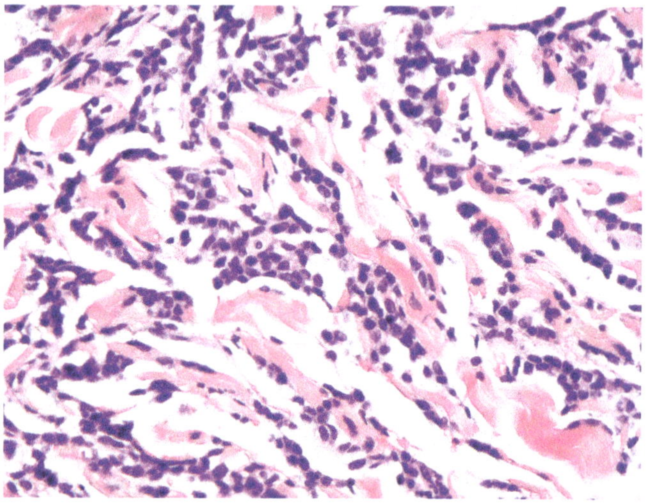

Acute myelomonocytic leukemia (AMMoL, M4). Rows of atypical cells migrating between collagen bundles.

In regard to the histochemical and immunohistochemical profiles, staining for lysozyme and myeloperoxidase usually shows positivity in specific infiltrates of AML subtypes.

However, staining for chloroacetate esterase is variable and may be negative in some M1 to M3 subtypes of AML. In addition, neoplastic cells are usually positive for CD68. Cells of M4 show variable staining with chloroacetate esterase, CD4 and CD117. The leukemic infiltrate in most cases of AMoL (M5) shows strong reactivity for CD4 positive. Expression of CD56 has been reported in specific skin infiltrates of some patients with AML. CD56 expression in AML has been associated with an increased incidence of leukemia cutis and a poor prognosis.

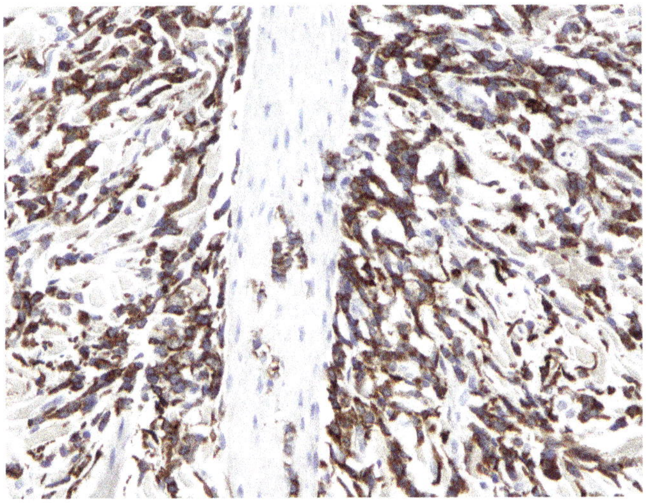

Acute myelomonocytic leukemia (AMMoL, M4). Atypical myeloid cells show strong reactivity for lysozyme.

In regard to the differential diagnosis, a tumor showing both CD4 and CD56 positivity may be confused with **CD4+, CD56+ hematodermic neoplasm (plasmacytoid dendritic cell neoplasm)**. These tumors have a highly characteristic immunophenotypic profile that includes CD4, CD56, and CD123 positivity. Nevertheless, some cases of AMoL may be CD123 positive. Perhaps the most useful differentiating stains are CD68 and lysozyme, which are negative in CD4+, CD56+ hematodermic neoplasms. **Chronic myeloid leukemia (CML)** is a disorder of hematopoietic stem cells accounting for 15% of adult leukemias (Table 12-17C). The median age at presentation is between 50 and 60 years. The majority of patients present in the chronic phase with relatively stable disease. Unpredictably, the disease eventually transforms into accelerated and blastic phases, becoming AML and more resistant to treatment. CML was one of the first diseases in which a specific chromosomal abnormality was identified, a Philadelphia (Ph') chromosome resulting from the t(9;22)(q34;q11) chromosomal translocation. Juvenile CML, a rare malignancy in childhood, is characterized by a rapidly progressive course. Specific (ie, neoplastic) skin lesions in CML are uncommon, with a reported incidence of 2% to 8%. The lesions are erythematous papules, plaques, or nodules. They occur anywhere on the skin and may be generalized in distribution. Occasionally, only a single lesion is present. Circinate erythematous annular plaques and nodules have been described in a few patients with juvenile CML. Microscopically, a dense nodular to diffuse infiltrate is present in the dermis composed of pleomorphic granulocytes in various stages of differentiation, including atypical myelocytes, metamyelocytes, eosinophilic metamyelocytes, and neutrophils. The neutrophils characteristically exhibit dysplastic features characterized by hyperlobation, nuclear lobe asymmetry, and hypogranularity. In CML, leukemic cells strongly stain for CD43, CD45, CD68, lysozyme, and myeloperoxidase. In addition, the presence of CD56 expression in specific skin infiltrates of CML has been reported. **Granulocytic sarcoma** is an extramedullary tumor mass composed of immature cells of the myeloid series that may occur specifically as a manifestation of AML, in the course of **myelodysplastic syndrome**, or as an isolated tumor in patients without evident hematologic disorders. The disease has been reported to occur in 2% to 8% of patients with acute nonlymphoblastic leukemia. Since the patient in question had bone marrow involvement before the onset of cutaneous findings, the condition is best classified as acute myelogenous leukemia cutis. Granulocytic sarcoma would be appropriate if the tumor originated as a solitary mass in the skin. When cut, the tumor nodules characteristically reveal a yellow-green coloration caused by the high concentration of myeloperoxidase, which changes color on exposure to air. The trunk, head, and extremities are the most commonly affected sites.

Table 12-17C. Leukemic Skin Infiltrates of Chronic Myeloid Leukemia

Clinical Features
Age 50-60 years
Rare juvenile form
Erythematous papules, plaques, or nodules
Almost any location
Histopathologic Features
Dense nodular to diffuse infiltrate
Subcutaneous tissue frequently involved
Pleomorphic infiltrate
Atypical myelocytes, metamyelocytes, and neutrophils
Immunohistochemistry
Predominant reactivity for lysozyme, myeloperoxidase, CD43, CD45, CD68

The diagnosis of leukemic myeloid skin infiltrates may be extremely difficult with routine histologic examination. The histopathologic differential diagnosis includes **cutaneous B-cell lymphoma, cutaneous lesions of Hodgkin disease, malignant histiocytosis, lymphomatoid papulosis, metastatic undifferentiated carcinomas, Merkel cell carcinoma**, and various benign dermatoses (ie, **granuloma faciale, erythema elevatum diutinum, mastocytosis, secondary**

syphilis, acute febrile neutrophilic dermatosis [**Sweet syndrome**], and **neutrophilic eccrine hidradenitis**). The histopathologic differentiation may be problematic, and a clinicopathologic correlation is important in establishing a diagnosis. Leukocyte common antigen (CD45) helps exclude poorly differentiated carcinomas. Positive staining for lysozyme, myeloperoxidase, chloroacetate esterase, and CD68 favors the diagnosis of a specific skin infiltrate of myeloid leukemia. Cutaneous lesions of **Hodgkin lymphoma** express CD30, CD15, CD25, and HLA-DR and are negative for CD45R. The tumor cells of **B-cell lymphoma** express B-cell–associated antigens. **Lymphomatoid papulosis** is of T-cell origin with a CD3+, CD4+, CD8–, and CD30+ phenotype. The presence of immature myeloid cells and dysplastic-appearing neutrophils are indicative of malignancy and should be differentiated from benign neutrophilic infiltrates. **Erythema elevatum diutinum** is ruled out by the presence of leukocytoclastic vasculitis. Neutrophils with rare leukocytoclastic debris are hallmarks of **acute febrile neutrophilic dermatosis (Sweet syndrome)**. Sweet syndrome is typically characterized by a benign neutrophilic infiltrate, but in a biopsy taken from a patient with AML, the dermal infiltrate may contain atypical leukemic cells especially in regard to those cells lying in close apposition to blood vessels. It should be kept in mind that vasculitis composed of leukemic cells, referred to as **leukemic vasculitis**, may accompany the leukemic skin infiltrates and is generally associated with an aggressive clinical course.

ANSWER 12-18: E.

Cutaneous metastases reflect the biologic behavior and population-based incidence of their associated primary tumors. The greatest incidence of cutaneous metastases is therefore in the fifth, sixth, and seventh decades of life, and the incidence and distribution of cutaneous metastases are correlated with gender. The results from two different studies evaluating the incidence of primary tumors in women and men with skin metastases are present in Table 12-18A.

Table 12-18A. Sites of Origin of Skin Metastases

PRIMARY SITE	WOMEN (%)	MEN (%)
Breast	69/70.7	2/2.4
Large intestine	9/1.3	19/11
Melanoma	5/12	13/32.3
Lung	4/2	24/11.8
Ovary	4/3.3	
Sarcoma	2/0	3/0
Uterine cervix	2/0.7	
Pancreas	2/0.3	2/0.8
Oral cavity	1/2.3	12/8.7
Bladder	1/1.3	2/2.4
Kidney	0/0	6/4.7
Stomach	0/0.7	6/0.8
Esophagus	0/0	3/2.4
Salivary gland	0/0	2/0
Prostate		1/0
Unknown primary site	0/3	0/8.7

SOURCES: Data from Brownstein and Helwig/Lookingbill et al.

Cutaneous metastases can take a variety of forms and occur in a variety of locations, but these forms and locations are not entirely specific either for the type of tumor or the site of the primary malignancy. Metastatic tumors frequently are flesh-colored nodules or plaques; multiple lesions are more common than solitary lesions, and sometimes multiple lesions are distributed in a zosteriform pattern.

In general, metastases are seen most often in the vicinity of the primary tumor. **Squamous cell carcinomas** of the head and neck tend to metastasize to regional actinically damaged skin, and it may be impossible to distinguish such metastases from primary cutaneous squamous cell carcinomas. **Breast** and **lung cancers** frequently metastasize to the chest wall. Abdominal tumors, such as those arising in the **gastrointestinal (GI) tract, ovary,** or **bladder**, most often metastasize to the abdominal wall. **Umbilical metastases** are called **Sister Mary Joseph nodules** after the nursing superintendent credited with first noting their significance, and they usually result from intraabdominal malignancies, including tumors from the stomach, colon, pancreas, and male and female genitourinary tract. Local metastases may also develop at the site of scars from previous surgical incisions, usually within 1 year of the procedure; in needle biopsy tracts; or in unrelated surgical or traumatic scars. Metastases to distant cutaneous sites have been most frequently associated with melanoma and primary carcinomas of the lung and breast. Tumors associated with **vascular invasion** are more frequently associated with distant metastases. Such tumors include **melanoma, renal cell carcinoma, thyroid follicular carcinoma,** and **choriocarcinoma. Scalp metastases** are disproportionately common in **renal cell** and **thyroid carcinomas**. Metastatic tumors were the third most common malignant cutaneous tumors of the scalp (12.8%) in a recent series from Taiwan. The time of onset of a cutaneous metastasis is variable and reflects the characteristics of the underlying malignancy. However, when a cutaneous metastasis does occur, it usually portends a poor prognosis. **Epithelioid sarcoma** is a sarcoma that occurs on the extremities of young adults and is characterized by a long clinical course of local recurrences and distant metastases.

As a general approach to cutaneous metastases, correlation with clinical history of prior malignancy is critical to proper classification. In some instances cutaneous metastasis may be the first manifestation of disease. If possible, comparison of the histopathological features of the tumor in question with the prior known malignancy is ideal for more precise classification. When a prior malignancy is unknown, the first approach should be establishing the type of neoplasm (**sarcoma** versus **carcinoma**) and the tumor architectural growth pattern and differentiation (spindle cell, squamous nests, glandular cords and nests, open glands, papillary structures, mucinous glands, clear cells or signet ring cells, or neuroendocrine). In regard to **squamous cell carcinomas**, when dermal tumors are present without connection to the overlying epidermal surface or hair follicles, or if squamous cell carcinoma in situ is not present, it should be communicated in the pathology report that a cutaneous metastasis of squamous cell carcinoma cannot be excluded. In regard to adenocarcinomas of the skin, a primary cutaneous origin can be established if the malignancy arises in association with a benign adnexal neoplasm. However, certain forms of **primary cutaneous sweat gland adenocarcinoma** are not associated with a benign precursor counterpart, making distinction from visceral metastasis difficult.

Immunohistochemistry is very helpful in establishing the origin of dermal-based malignancies. The pathologist's general approach to a metastatic tumor when the origin is not obvious is to first determine the immunophenotype that correlates with the cell line of differentiation (**pan-cytokeratin = carcinoma, CD45 = lymphoma, S100 + melan-A = melanoma, or vimentin = sarcoma**) and then to more narrowly classify the process by expression of various classes of antigens. Squamous epithelium is typically positive for p63 and glandular epithelium characteristically expresses CEA; therefore these markers are helpful in distinguishing their malignant counterparts. Primary cutaneous squamous and adnexal tumors (benign and malignant) express p63 and D2-40 in most cases. In contrast, visceral glandular metastases to skin are typically negative for these markers. As a reminder, p63 is expressed in all cutaneous epithelia (epidermis, hair follicles, and sweat glands) with the exception of apocrine sweat glands. However, exceptions exist and an expanded panel of immunostains should be performed to establish the precise lineage and origin of the tumor. It is worth noting that malignant tumors may not express detectable amounts of certain antigens characteristically expressed by their related cells of origin (ie, failure of some large cell lymphomas to express CD45RB [leukocyte common antigen, LCA]), and tumors may express antigens not usually seen in their cells of origin (ie, vimentin expression in many spindle cell squamous cell carcinomas) and cytokeratin (CK) expression in epithelioid angiosarcomas. Because of these considerations, in most cases when immunohistochemical data are desired, a panel of multiple markers should be applied to confirm or refute the diagnosis or narrow the differential diagnosis. This panel should be chosen in light of a probable diagnosis or reasonable differential diagnosis constructed on the basis of clinical and histopathologic features, and the panel should include markers chosen to both confirm and refute specific diagnoses.

Quick Fact

Squamous cell carcinomas (primary cutaneous and metastatic) = p63+
Primary cutaneous adnexal tumors = p63+*
Metastatic adenocarcinoma = p63−**

***Exception is apocrine tumors, which may be p63−**
****Exception is metastatic urothelial carcinomas, which are p63+"**

ANSWER 12-19: D.

Metastatic mammary adenocarcinoma accounts for 71% of cutaneous metastases in women and 2.4% of cutaneous metastases in men. This difference is attributed primarily to the difference in gender-specific prevalence of primary breast cancer. This patient has **inflammatory breast adenocarcinoma,** which is considered at least stage IIIB. Clinically, these patients present with the rapid onset of reddening of a large portion of the breast skin with edema and dimpling (**peau d'orange**). The breast feels warm to palpation and may be swollen. Microscopically, this condition is characterized by obstruction of lymphatic by metastatic carcinoma. Frequently foci of invasive adenocarcinoma may be seen infiltrating between dermal collagen bundles. Clusters of tumor cells can be identified within lymphatic spaces by an immunohistochemical stain for D2-40, which will highlight lymphatic endothelial cells surrounding the tumor clusters. Other presentations of **metastatic mammary adenocarcinoma** frequently occur on the trunk, but they are seen with lower frequency on other parts of the body such as the upper extremities and scalp These other presentations of metastatic mammary carcinoma include **en cuirasse metastases (encasement in armor)** characterized by diffuse morpheaform induration of the skin resulting from dermal sclerosis in association with tumor cells. **Telangiectatic metastases** are composed of clustered, violaceous papulovesicles that may demonstrate pigmentation so prominent as to resemble metastatic melanoma. Telangiectatic metastases demonstrate tumor cells in blood vessels as well as lymphatics. The obstructed lymphatics are more superficial than the obstructed lymphatics in inflammatory carcinoma. **Metastatic tumors of the inframammary crease** may present as exophytic nodules suggestive of a primary squamous or basal cell carcinoma or may simulate intertriginous dermatitis. **Alopecia neoplastica** is a form of scarring alopecia that results from a neoplastic process such as metastatic breast carcinoma. Alopecia neoplastica is characterized by alopecia, a smooth surface, and erythema in some instances. Alopecia neoplastica

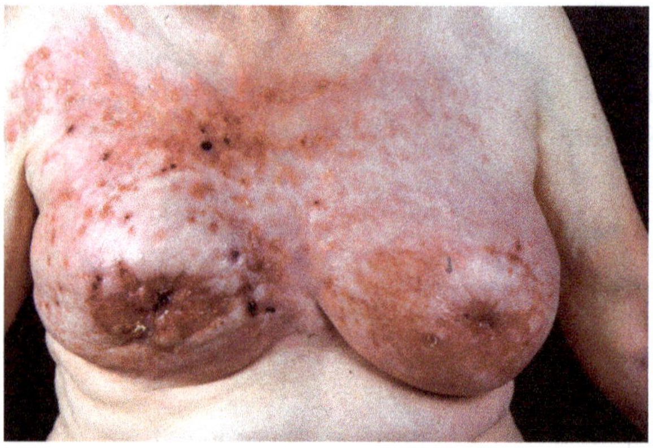

Metastatic breast cancer: cancer en cuirasse. Both breasts are hard upon palpation—like an armor plate. There are multiple small and large, ulcerated nodules and there is a background of erysipelas-like erythema (carcinoma erysipelatodes). (Reproduced, with permission, from Wolff K, Johnson RA, Saavedra AP. *Fitzpatrick's Color Atlas and Synopsis of Clinical Dermatology*. 7th ed. New York, NY: McGraw-Hill Education; 2013.)

may be the initial presentation of a tumor, primary or metastatic, and must be distinguished from other forms of scarring alopecia. Although infiltrating ductal carcinoma is the most common form of primary and metastatic breast cancer, breast cancer can have many other patterns, including lobular, tubular, cribriform, mucinous, and medullary variants.

The histopathology of breast carcinoma metastatic to the skin may closely resemble the corresponding histologic pattern of the primary tumor. Some clinical patterns of cutaneous metastasis reflect additional histopathologic features that may develop in the metastasis. In **inflammatory mammary adenocarcinoma**, tumor cells fill dermal lymphatics, and in some cases, lymphatics in the subcutaneous fat. **Telangiectatic mammary adenocarcinoma** has tumor cells in more superficially located lymphatics and blood vessels congested with erythrocytes. In **nodular mammary adenocarcinoma metastases**, some stromal fibrosis may be present, but tumor cells predominate. In contrast, **cancer en cuirasse** is characterized by a smaller proportion of tumor cells set in a prominent fibrous stroma and **alopecia neoplastica** by dermal fibrosis, an infiltrate of tumor cells, and loss of hair follicles.

Tumor cells of primary and metastatic **infiltrating ductal mammary adenocarcinoma** are variably pleomorphic. The tumor cells infiltrate their stroma in sheets or cords that sometimes demonstrate glandular structures, signet ring cells, or both.

Tumor cells of **infiltrating lobular mammary adenocarcinoma** are small round to ovoid cells with scant cytoplasms, eccentric nuclei with little pleomorphism, and few mitoses.

Intracytoplasmic lumina are more frequent in lobular carcinoma than in infiltrating ductal carcinoma and are best seen with histochemical special stains such as the PAS–Alcian blue stain or with immunohistochemical stains such as

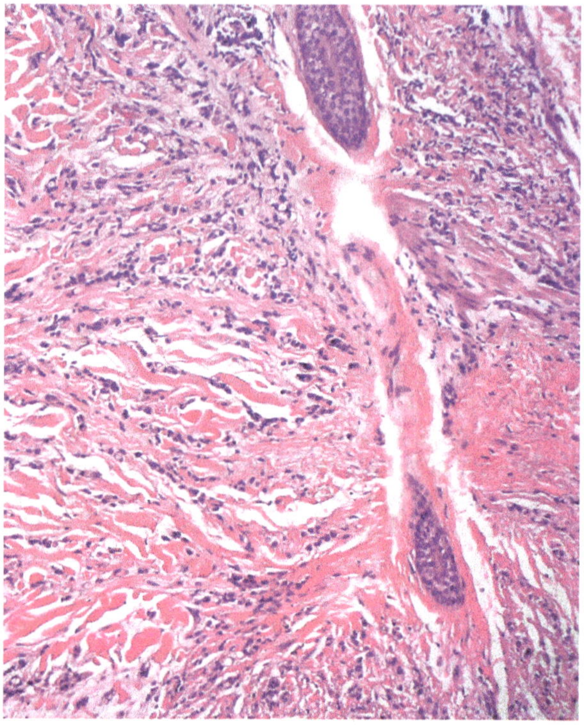

Metastatic infiltrating ductal breast carcinoma, low power. Infiltration of tumor cells in single file and small clusters between dermal collagen bundles results in a resemblance to granuloma annulare.

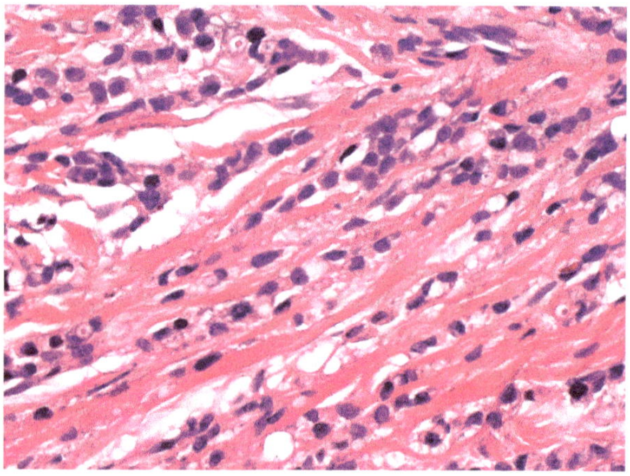

Metastatic infiltrating lobular breast carcinoma, high power. Single-file rows of tumor cells with cytological atypia and intracytoplasmic duct formation.

antibodies to EMA. Lobular carcinomas are characteristically negative for E-cadherin. The single-file pattern of infiltration associated most often with lobular carcinoma consists of cords of cells arranged in one-cell width files in a fibrotic stroma. Focal areas with this pattern of infiltration may also be seen in ductal adenocarcinoma. **Mucinous carcinoma** (also referred to as **colloid** or **mucoid carcinoma**) consists of islands of uniform, small epithelial cells with hyperchromatic nuclei and a cribriform or papillary pattern floating in lakes of mucin. It can be difficult or impossible to distinguish **primary cutaneous mucinous carcinoma** from **visceral mucinous carcinoma** metastatic from the breast or GI tract on the basis of histology, but immunohistochemistry can be very useful in this regard. Other patterns of primary breast cancer, such as alveolar, solid, tubular, tubulolobular, cribriform, and medullary, are seldom seen in cutaneous metastases.

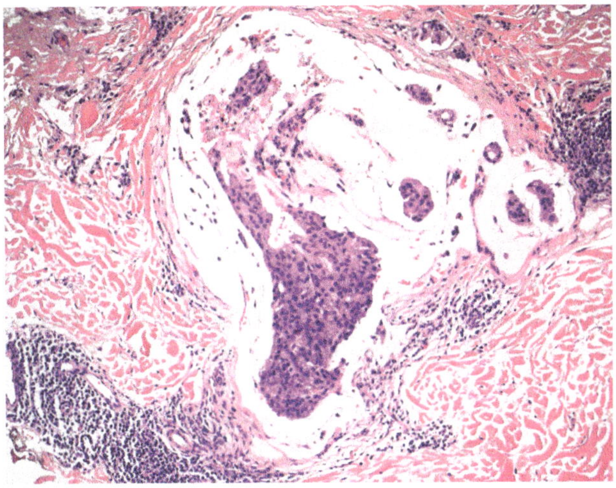

Metastatic mucinous breast carcinoma. Nests of relatively bland tumor cells float in pools of mucin.

In regard to the differential diagnosis, the various patterns of breast carcinoma each have their own list of conditions from which a cutaneous metastasis must be distinguished. A history of primary breast carcinoma is helpful, but patients may have more than one malignancy, so care must be taken not to overlook alternative cutaneous primary or metastatic tumors. In 1874, Paget first noted the association of breast carcinoma and "long persistent eczema" of the nipple and areola, now known as **Paget disease** of the breast.

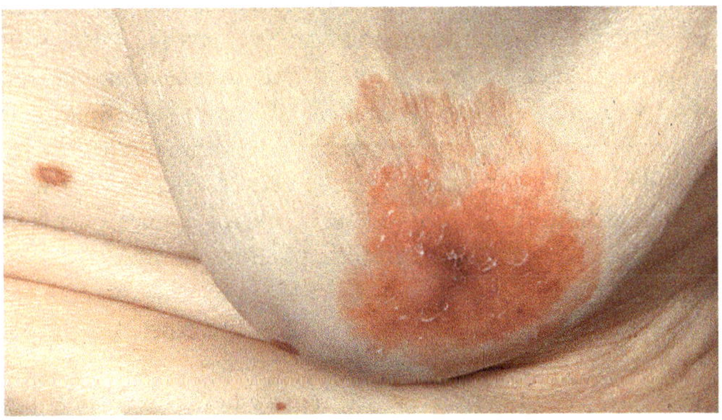

Mammary Paget disease. A sharply defined psoriasiform plaque that has obliterated the areola and nipple. There was a lump in the breast and a small axillary mass. (Reproduced, with permission, from Wolff K, Johnson RA, Saavedra AP. *Fitzpatrick's Color Atlas and Synopsis of Clinical Dermatology*. 7th ed. New York, NY: McGraw-Hill Education; 2013.)

Mammary Paget disease is almost exclusively associated with underlying **ductal mammary adenocarcinoma** (ER+, PR+, HER/neu+), either in situ or invasive. The tumor cells are believed to migrate along the lactiferous ducts into the epidermal surface. The cells exhibit the typical immunophenotype of mammary adenocarcinoma.

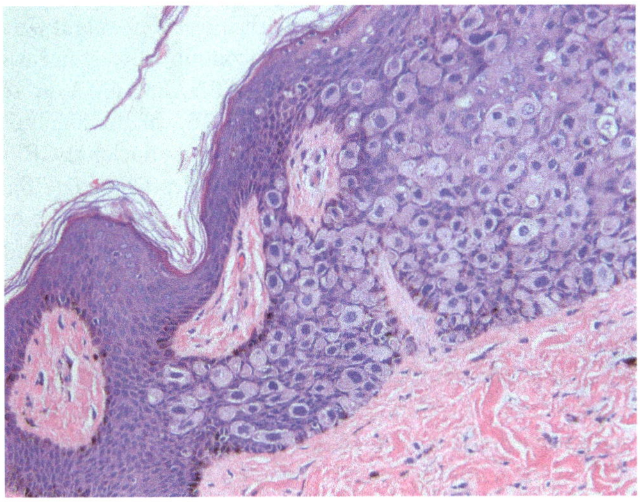

Paget disease of the nipple (mammary Paget disease). Note the neoplastic cells within the epidermis (right upper corner), with pleomorphic, hyperchromatic nuclei and abundant eosinophilic cytoplasm. Paget disease of the nipple indicates the presence of an underlying ductal carcinoma (in situ or invasive). (Reproduced, with permission, from Kemp WL, Burns DK, Travis Brown TG. *Pathology: The Big Picture*. 8th ed. New York, NY: McGraw-Hill Education; 2008.)

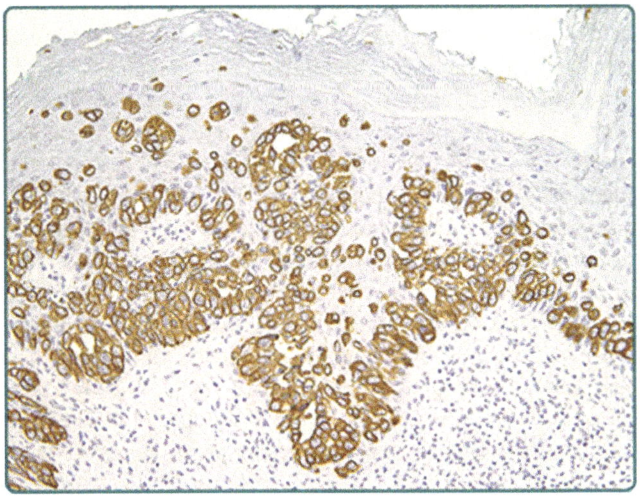

Mammary Paget disease, cytokeratin 7 stain. (Reproduced, with permission, from Goldsmith LA, Katz SI, Gilchrest BA, Paller AS, Leffell DJ, Wolff K, eds. *Fitzpatrick's Dermatology in General Medicine*. 8th ed. New York, NY: McGraw-Hill Education; 2012.)

A process clinically and histologically similar to **mammary Paget disease** may involve the skin of areas outside the breast. Although **extramammary Paget disease** may be a primary adnexal carcinoma, this process sometimes represents epidermal extension of primary visceral carcinomas. **Extramammary Paget disease** may involve the vulva, male genital area, perianal area, and rarely the axilla, external ear, and eyelid. Mammary carcinomas and Paget disease of the breast commonly express low-molecular-weight CKs, including CAM5.2 and CK7. Many primary and some rare metastatic breast tumors also express high-molecular-weight CKs such as CK5/6. CK20 expression is uncommon. Breast tumors often express pankeratin markers (eg, AE1/AE3), EMA, gross cystic disease fluid protein-15 (GCDFP-15), mammaglobin/MGB1, polyclonal-CEA but not usually monoclonal-CEA, and estrogen (ER) and progesterone receptors (PR). The presence of mammaglobin, GCDFP-15, and progesterone or estrogen receptors and the absence of CK20, m-CEA, and TTF-1 differentiate most metastatic breast cancers from adenocarcinomas metastatic from other common primary sites, especially if ovarian cancer can be excluded clinically (ie, ovarian cancer can exhibit tremendous phenotypic overlap with breast cancer). It is important to evaluate all metastatic mammary adenocarcinomas for ER, PR, and C-erb2 (HER2/neu) because these findings impact therapy. Fibrotic nodules with diffuse infiltration by sheets and cords of uniformly atypical cells may suggest dermatofibroma, sarcoma, and small cell or desmoplastic melanoma. Unlike mammary carcinoma, these tumors will express Factor XIIIa, vimentin, TTF-1, and S100, respectively. **Malignant adnexal neoplasms** with eccrine or apocrine differentiation may express also CAM5.2, CK7, CK5/6, and other high and low-molecular-weight CKs, EMA, CEA, mammaglobin, GCDFP-15, S-100 protein, and estrogen and progesterone receptors, contributing to the often considerable difficulty of distinguishing between primary or metastatic sweat gland carcinomas and metastatic breast cancer. Cutaneous adenocarcinomas can be taken as primary in cases in which an in situ component can be demonstrated. Many, but not all, primary sweat gland carcinomas contain an in situ component that may be highlighted by basal cell and myoepithelial markers such as p63, CK 5/6, and calponin. Unfortunately, **primary cutaneous apocrine adenocarcinomas** are characteristically negative for p63, which makes sense since the breast is essentially a modified apocrine sweat gland. **Metastatic mammary carcinomas** are almost always negative for p63. A number of recent articles have suggested that a p63-positive, CK 5/6-positive, and CK20-negative immunophenotype strongly favors a primary adnexal tumor over a metastasis from a noncutaneous primary tumor.

ANSWER 12-20: A.

This is an example of **metastatic lung adenocarcinoma** composed of open glandular structures. In older case series, cutaneous metastases from lung carcinoma represent 12% to 24% of cutaneous metastases in men and 2% to 4% in women. More recent series have shown an increase in cutaneous metastases from lung cancer in women, reflecting the increasing incidence of primary lung cancer in women. Although only 1.5% of patients with lung cancer develop cutaneous metastases, such metastases are noted before the lung primary tumor in 52% to 60% of patients. The chest, back, and abdomen are the most frequent sites of cutaneous metastasis of lung cancer, followed by the scalp and neck. The most common clinical presentation of cutaneous metastatic lung cancer is a localized cluster of discrete, firm, nontender, flesh-colored nodules of recent onset and rapid growth to a certain size followed by a stationary period. Some cutaneous metastases from the lung have a vascular appearance clinically, suggesting hemangioma, pyogenic granuloma, or Kaposi sarcoma.

Microscopically, the carcinomas of the lung most commonly observed as cutaneous metastases are **adenocarcinoma** (30%), **squamous cell carcinoma** (30%), **large cell undifferentiated carcinoma,** and **small cell neuroendocrine (oat cell) carcinoma**. Metastatic pulmonary adenocarcinomas are usually moderately differentiated tumors that may include small tubular and glandular structures and scattered, individual tumor cells containing intracytoplasmic mucin. The tumor cells tend to have pleomorphic, hyperchromatic nuclei with numerous mitotic figures. The immunophenotypic profile is typically CK7+, TTF1+, CEA+, CK20−, CDX2−, p63−, GCDFP15−, and mammaglobin−. TTF1 is a specific marker for either **lung adenocarcinoma, lung neuroendocrine carcinoma (small cell carcinoma),** and **thyroid carcinomas (papillary and follicular).** The differential diagnosis for metastatic lung adenocarcinoma is with other visceral adenocarcinomas such as those originating from the large intestine, pancreatobiliary tract, endometrium, or breast. These tumors are negative for TTF-1. **Primary cutaneous eccrine ductal adenocarcinoma** would be positive for p63 and negative for TTF-1.

Metastatic squamous cell carcinomas from the lung are usually moderately to poorly differentiated. The tumor cells are dispersed in solid sheets and islands of epithelial cells with varying degrees of keratinization and intercellular bridges, often with only a small number of whorls of squamous cells (pearls). More atypical features of the keratinizing cells may include large, bizarre cells, spindle cells, and clear cells with abundant mitotic figures. Central necrosis may occur in larger foci of tumor. The immunophenotypic profile of lung squamous cell carcinoma is CK5/6+, p63+, vimentin−/+, CK7−, TTF-1−, CK20−, and CDX2−. Therefore, diagnostic distinction from squamous cell carcinomas originating from other sites requires systemic workup and clinical correlation. It is worth mentioning that squamous carcinomas of the lung frequently show spindle cell features. Neoplastic spindle cells in squamous carcinomas primary to the lung and many other locations often coexpress keratin and vimentin, and these carcinomas may express predominantly vimentin. Expression of p63 may provide evidence that a vimentin-positive, keratin-negative primary or metastatic spindle cell malignancy is a carcinoma rather than a sarcoma.

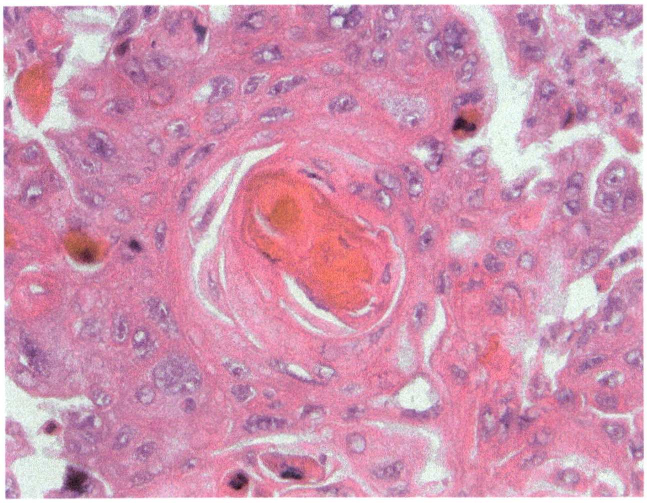

Squamous cell carcinoma of the lung. Squamous cell carcinoma is one of the major forms of carcinoma, occurring within many organs including the mouth, upper respiratory tract, and lungs. In the center of the photomicrograph is a keratin pearl, a characteristic feature of a well or moderately differentiated squamous cell carcinoma.

Large cell undifferentiated carcinomas consist of sheets of large pleomorphic tumor cells with abundant cytoplasms, prominent nucleoli, and numerous mitoses. The giant cell variant has monster cells with bizarre nuclei and cells that frequently contain leukocytes. The clear cell variant is composed of sheets and islands of clear cells without other forms of differentiation. Large cell undifferentiated carcinomas from the lung are usually positive for AE1/AE3, CK5/6, and p63 and negative for CK20, S-100 protein, and LCA (CD45). They are variable with regard to CK7, EMA, and CEA and may coexpress vimentin. Large cell undifferentiated carcinomas must be differentiated from **sarcomas** such as **rhabdomyosarcoma**, which is positive for myoid markers such as desmin, MyoD1, and myogenin; **lymphoma**, which is usually positive for LCA (CD45); and **melanoma**, which is positive for S-100 protein and often for MART-1 and HMB-45.

ANSWER 12-21: C.

This is an example of **metastatic well-differentiated gastric adenocarcinoma** with an open glandular pattern. Adenocarcinomas of the gastrointestinal tract are among the most frequent visceral tumors to metastasize to the skin in both men and women, accounting for 11% to 19% of cutaneous metastases in men and 1.3% to 9% in women. Carcinoma of the large intestine is usually discovered before the cutaneous metastasis. Cutaneous metastases from gallbladder and bile duct **(biliary carcinomas)** have been noted at the time that the initial tumor was recognized and as late as 40 years after resection of the primary tumor. These tumors may also frequently present with a well-differentiated open glandular pattern. Cutaneous metastases from the **gastric adenocarcinomas** and **pancreatic adenocarcinomas** usually occur before the discovery of the primary tumor. The usual sites of metastases from GI carcinomas are the abdominal wall, the perineum, and the umbilicus (**Sister Mary Joseph nodule**). In one series, 10% of metastases to the abdominal wall occurred in the umbilicus, and 28% of those tumors were of gastric origin. **Esophageal carcinomas** occasionally metastasize to the skin. These are usually squamous cell carcinomas that metastasize to the upper trunk and neck as single or multiple nodules, but distant metastases and metastases of esophageal adenocarcinomas have also been reported. Clinically, cutaneous metastases from the colon and rectum **(colorectal adenocarcinomas)** may present as flesh-colored sessile or pedunculated nodules, inflammatory carcinoma, grouped vascular nodules, or occasionally a nodular and inflamed perianal lesion suggestive of hidradenitis suppurativa. Tumor colonization of prior surgical scars is common. Colorectal carcinoma may also metastasize to a colostomy site. Gastric, pancreatic, and gallbladder carcinomas that metastasize to the skin usually present as nodules, sclerodermoid plaques, or **Sister Mary Joseph nodules.**

Microscopically, cutaneous metastases of **colorectal carcinomas** are predominantly well-differentiated, mucin-secreting adenocarcinomas that may have a pattern of **mucinous carcinoma** in some cases. The tumors characteristically contain central foci of gritty tumor necrosis. Poorly differentiated metastases are less common, but on rare occasions, metastatic colorectal carcinomas may be so anaplastic that it is difficult to discern that they are of epithelial origin.

Cutaneous metastases from the stomach are typically of two distinct varieties (**well-differentiated gastric adenocarcinoma** and **poorly differentiated "signet ring" gastric adenocarcinoma**). The patient in question has a **metastatic well-differentiated gastric adenocarcinoma** presenting as a Sister Mary Joseph nodule and is characterized by variable-sized glands lined by cytologically atypical cells infiltrating the dermis. Immunohistochemistry is extremely helpful in establishing the site of origin for adenocarcinomas in the vast majority of cases. Many primary and metastatic gastrointestinal carcinomas (including pancreas, hepatic, and bile duct) express homeobox transcription factor CDX2, which is not usually expressed by primary tumors of the breast, lung, skin, prostate, or urothelium, but they may rarely be expressed by adenocarcinomas of the ovary, endometrium, and kidney. Ovarian tumors are usually positive for CA125 and endometrial adenocarcinomas are usually positive for ER and PR. Gastric adenocarcinomas commonly express p-CEA, m-CEA,

Table 12-21A. Immunohistochemical Markers for Cutaneous Metastases

		IMMUNOHISTOCHEMICAL MARKERS	
ORIGIN	HISTOPATHOLOGY	POSITIVE	NEGATIVE
Breast	Ductal	CK7, estrogen-R, progesteron-R, GCDFP-15, CEA, *c-erb*B-2, mammaglobin, E-cadherin	CK20, CK5/6
	Lobular carcinoma	CK7, estrogen-R, progesteron-R, GCDFP-15, CEA, EMA, mammaglobin	S100, E-cadherin, podoplanin, P63
	Inflammatory carcinoma	CD31, podoplanin	
	Telangiectatic carcinoma	CD31	Podoplanin
	Mammary Paget disease	MUC1, CK7	MUC2, MUC5AC, CK20
Lung	Squamous cell carcinoma	CK5/6	CK7, CK20, TTF-1, CEA
	Adenocarcinoma	CK7, TTF-1, Ber-EP4, CEA Surfactant, apoprotein A	CK5/6, CK20
	Oat-cell carcinoma	TTF-1, CAM5.2, CK8/18, Ber-EP4, ENS	CK7, CK20, CD99
	Mesothelioma	CK5/6, calretinin, vimentin	CEA, TTF-1, S100, CD31
Colorectal	Adenocarcinoma	CK20, CEA, mucin, CDX2	CK7
Small intestine	Squamous cell carcinoma	CK20, EMA, AE1/AE3	CK7
	Adenocarcinoma	CEA, EMA	
Stomach	Adenocarcinoma	CK20, CEA, EMA, CDX2, HIK1083	CK7+/CK7−
Esophagus	Squamous cell/ adenocarcinoma	CK5/6, Ber-EP4	CK7, CK20
Mouth	SCC	Ber-EP4	
Liver	HCC	Alpha-fetoprotein, polyclonal CEA, Hep Par 1, arginase-1	All CKs, EMA, monoclonal CEA
Biliary system	Adenocarcinoma	CK7, CK20	CDX2
Pancreas	Adenocarcinoma	CA19.9, CK7, CK8, CK18, CK19	CK20
Kidney	RCC	AE1/AE3, MNF116, CD31, RCC-Ma (>2/3), vimentin, CD10, EMA, S100, adipophilin, PAX8	Inhibin, melan-A, TTF-1, CK7, CK20
Bladder–urethra	Transitional carcinoma	CK7, CK19, CK20, CK14 (50%), thrombomodulin, uroplakin III, CD10	
Prostate	Adenocarcinoma	PSA, prostatic acid phosphatase, AMACR (p504s), ERG transcription factor	CK7, CK20, thrombomodulin
Testis	Choriocarcinoma	Beta-HCG	
Ovary	Carcinoma	CA.125, CK7, PAX8	CK20 (except some mucinous variants)
Cervix and vagina	Carcinoma	CK7, EMA+/EMA−	CK20, CEA
Endometrium	Carcinoma	CK7, PAX8	CK20, P63, podoplanin

Table 12-21A. Immunohistochemical Markers for Cutaneous Metastases *(continued)*

		IMMUNOHISTOCHEMICAL MARKERS	
ORIGIN	**HISTOPATHOLOGY**	**POSITIVE**	**NEGATIVE**
Thyroid	Papillary Follicular	Thyroglobulin, TTF-1, PAX8 (50%)	
	Anaplastic	Thyroglobulin+/thyroglobulin−	
	Medullary	Calcitonin	Thyroglobulin, PAX8
Carcinoid tumors	Enterochromaffin carcinoma	NSE, chromogranin, synaptophysin Argentaffin and CDX2 (intestinal origin) TTF-1 (pulmonary origin)	CK5/6, CK7, CK20, p63
Neuroblastoma		NSE, chromogranin, synaptophysin	CD99, desmin, myogenin
Soft tissue sarcomas	Leiomyosarcoma	SMA, desmin	
	Rhabdomyosarcoma	MYOD1, vimentin, myogenin, leukocyte common antigen (CD45)	Desmin, SMA
	Angiosarcoma	CD31, CD34, ERG transcription factor, podoplanin, MYC amplification epithelioid variant: CKs, EMA	
	Chondrosarcoma	CD99, vimentin, S100 (focal), podoplanin, YKL-40, SMA, desmin, CAM5.2	AE1/AE3, SMA, CD117
	Ewing sarcoma	Vimentin, NSE, CD99, LEU7/CD57, FLI1 protein	Podoplanin
	Osteosarcoma	EZRIN, SMA, *c-erb*B-2 (50%)	
Salivary glands	Adenoid cystic carcinoma	CKs, CEA, S100, CD117/CKIT, SMA, vimentin (myoepithelial component)	
	Mucoepidermoid carcinoma	CK5/6, EMA, CEA	
Laryngeal and thracheal	Carcinoma	AE1/AE3, p53	
Nasopharynx	Carcinoma	RNA of EBV	
Glioblastoma		GFAP, EGFR+/EGFR−, vimentin YKL-40	Neurofilaments, HMB45, melan A, CKs, cocktail
Medulloblastoma		Synaptophysin NSE	Neurofilaments
Meningioma		Vimentin, EMA, S100, progesteron-R, CKs, CEA	
Adrenocortical	Carcinoma	NSE, inhibin, synaptophysin (focal), A103, chromogranin, calretinin	Melan A, CD10

AMACR, alpha-methylacyl-CoA racemase; beta-HCG, beta-human chorionic gonadotropin; Hep Par 1, hepatocyte paraffin 1; CEA, carcinoembryonic antigen; EMA, epithelial membrane antigen; GCDFP, gross cystic disease fluid protein; NSE, neuron-specific enolase; PSA, prostate-specific antigen; RCC-ma, renal cell carcinoma marker; SMA, smooth muscle actin.

Source: Reproduced with permission from Alcaraz I, Cerroni L, Rütten A, et al: Cutaneous metastases from internal malignancies: a clinicopathologic and immunohistochemical review, *Am J Dermatopathol.* 2012 Jun;34(4):347–393.

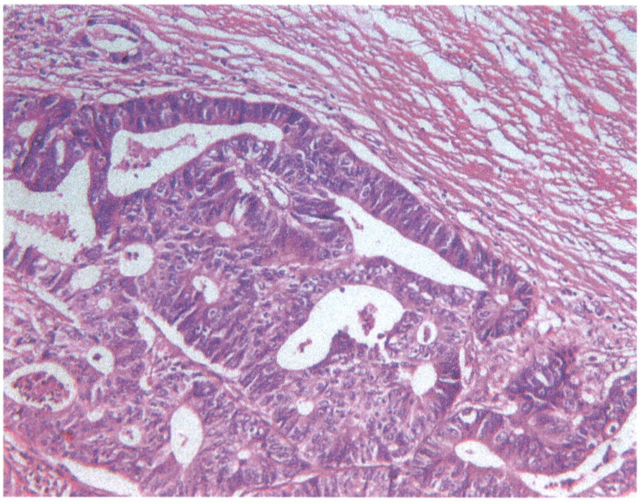

Metastatic colorectal adenocarcinoma. Note the tightly packed glands with focal areas containing gritty tumor necrosis (lower left corner). (Reproduced, with permission, from Kemp WL, Burns DK, Travis Brown TG. *Pathology: The Big Picture*. 8th ed. New York, NY: McGraw-Hill Education; 2008.)

AE1/AE3, and low-molecular-weight CKs such as CAM5.2, but gastric carcinomas are highly variable in their CK7- and CK20-staining patterns. Positive staining (when present) for CDX2, m-CEA, and CK20 and lack of reactivity with mammaglobin, GCDFP-15, or estrogen or progesterone receptors can help distinguish metastatic gastric adenocarcinomas, including signet ring carcinomas, from metastatic breast cancer. The differential expression of CK7 and CK20 has been well documented in various forms of visceral malignancy (see table below). As a general rule, tumors above the diaphragm are CK7+/CK20–, tumors of the gastrointestinal tract are CK7–/CK20+ (variable staining in the stomach, pancreas, and bile ducts), and tumors of the genitourinary tract are CK7+/CK20+.

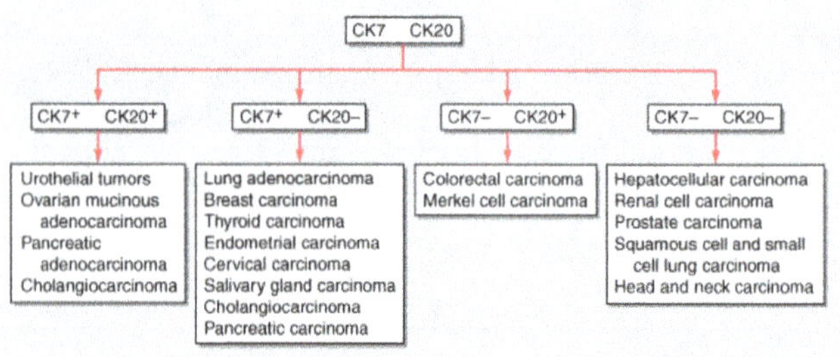

The differential expression of CK7 and CK20. Additional differential markers are listed in Table 12-21A. (Reproduced, with permission, from Longo DL, Fauci AS, Kasper DL, Hauser SL, Jameson JL, Loscalzo J, eds. *Harrison's Principles of Internal Medicine*. 18th ed. New York, NY: McGraw-Hill Education; 2011.)

ANSWER 12-22: D.

This is an example of metastatic carcinoma with a clear cell cytomorphology. In this case the tumor is a **metastasis of clear cell renal cell carcinoma.** A total of 4.6% of cutaneous metastases have been reported to originate from the kidney. Metastases from the kidney are seen more frequently in men than in women. Cutaneous metastases from renal cell carcinoma may be the first sign of the malignancy, but alternatively may occur 10 or more years after resection of the primary tumor. They may occur as local metastases, often in surgical scars, or as distant metastases. Metastases from renal cell carcinoma are seen most commonly on the head and neck, particularly the scalp. Renal cell carcinoma may metastasize as solitary or widespread dermal nodules. The nodules can be flesh colored, but they are more commonly violaceous with prominent vascularity resembling Kaposi sarcoma or pyogenic granuloma.

Microscopically, the most common renal cell carcinomas are clear cell adenocarcinomas. Metastatic nodules in the dermis are composed of large polyhedral cells with clear to finely granular cytoplasm and a central nucleus with little pleomorphism. The cells are arranged in sheets and cords with some gland formation and often a papillary component. The tumor cells are embedded in a delicate, highly vascular stroma containing extravasated erythrocytes and hemosiderin.

In regard to the differential diagnosis, renal cell carcinoma must be differentiated from other clear cell carcinomas that occasionally metastasize to the skin. These include primary tumors of the lung, liver, ovary, endometrium, cervix, and vagina. Primary tumors of the skin that may resemble renal cell carcinoma include **clear cell hidradenoma (eccrine acrospiroma), sebaceous tumors,** and **PEComas**. In contrast to renal cell carcinoma, clear cell hidradenoma is usually multilobular and has prominent ductal structures. It is not associated with prominent vascularity, hemorrhage, or hemosiderin deposition. Sebaceous tumors are not as vascular as renal tumors and have fine, vacuolated cytoplasms. PEComas (perivascular epithelioid cell tumor) are rare neoplasms related to angiomyolipoma and the "sugar" tumor of the lung. Unlike their noncutaneous counterparts, cutaneous PEComas are not associated with tuberous sclerosis. They are consistently positive for HMB45. Additionally, **amelanotic melanomas** are positive for HMB45 and S100. The clear cytoplasm in hidradenomas and PEComas is attributed to glycogen, therefore would be bright pink on PAS staining and negative for lipid with oil red O or Sudan black stains. The clear cytoplasm of sebaceous glands is attributed to lipid, therefore is negative on PAS stain. The cytoplasm of clear cell renal cell carcinomas contains high concentrations of both glycogen and lipid, therefore is positive for both PAS and lipid stains (oil red O and Sudan black). Renal cell carcinomas usually stain with broad-spectrum anti-CK antibodies such as AE1/AE3 and with antibodies to low-molecular-weight CKs (CAM 5.2), EMA, and vimentin but not for CK5/6, p63, CK7, CK20, CEA, or S-100 protein. Vimentin expression is

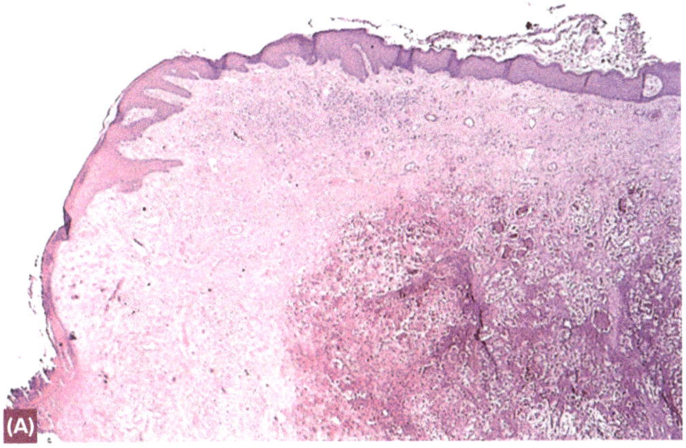

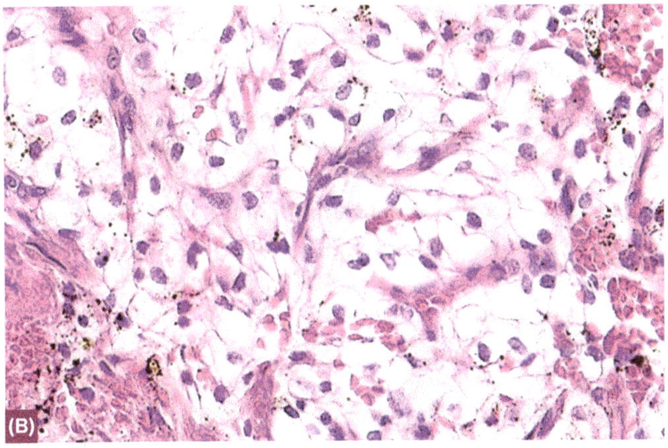

Metastatic clear cell adenocarcinoma from the kidney. **(A)** Well-demarcated nodule of tumor in the reticular dermis with clear cell and prominent extravasation of erythrocytes. **(B)** Sheets and cords of clear cells embedded in a delicate vascular stroma with some extravasated erythrocytes and hemosiderin deposition.

much less common in hidradenomas than in renal cell carcinomas. Hidradenomas may focally express CK7 and CEA, as may other clear cell carcinomas from other locations such as the lung. Sebaceous carcinomas stain with antibodies to broad-spectrum CKs, low-molecular-weight CKs including CAM 5.2 and CK7, and EMA but not usually with specific or monoclonal antibodies to CEA. Primary hidradenomas and sebaceous neoplasms stain with antibodies to p63, CK5/6, and D2-40 (podoplanin), and most metastatic renal carcinomas do not stain with these antibodies. Many metastatic renal carcinomas express CD10, but this antigen is also expressed by many primary cutaneous tumors, especially sebaceous tumors. Carbonic anhydrase IX (CA-IX) appears to be more specific but is also less sensitive than CD10 as a marker for metastatic renal carcinoma to the skin. **Choriocarcinomas** frequently present as a consequence of a metastasis, and involvement of the skin is not uncommon. Choriocarcinomas are usually gestational tumors composed of **cytotrophoblasts**, which are large, cuboidal cells with vesicular nuclei and pale cytoplasms, and **syncytiotrophoblasts**, which are large cells with irregular nuclei and basophilic cytoplasms. Clusters of cytotrophoblasts are surrounded by sheets and cords of syncytiotrophoblasts in a plexiform pattern resembling chorionic villi. Choriocarcinomas express human chorionic gonadotropin (hCG), PLAP, and with a recently described marker Mel-CAM/CD 146.

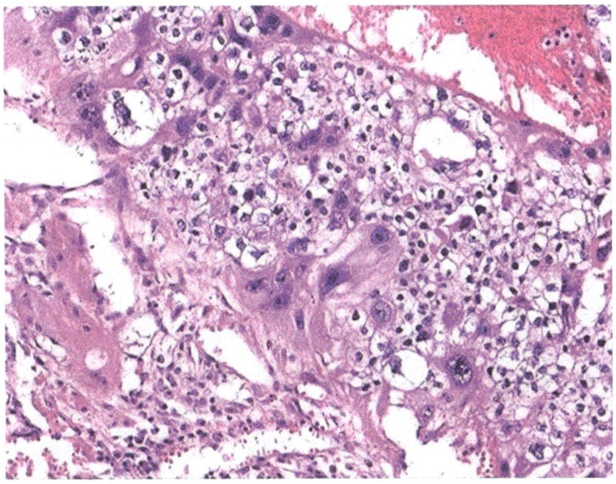

Metastatic choriocarcinoma. The tumor has a plexiform growth pattern and is composed of both cytotrophoblasts with pale/clear cytoplasm and syncytiotrophoblasts with anaplastic cytomorphology and eosinophilic cytoplasm. Extensive hemorrhage is typically present. The tumors typically lack the arborizing vasculature of clear cell renal cell carcinoma. They are strongly positive for hCG and PLAP and negative for CA-IX. (Reproduced, with permission, from Kantarjian HM, Wolff RA, Koller CA. *The MD Anderson Manual of Medical Oncology*. 2nd ed. New York, NY: McGraw-Hill Education; 2011.)

ANSWER 12-23: D.

This is a classic example of metastatic adenocarcinoma with papillary architecture, consistent with **papillary thyroid adenocarcinoma**. Various forms of thyroid carcinoma occasionally metastasize to the skin, especially the scalp. Of particular note, papillary thyroid carcinoma metastases have been described after intervals as long as 20 to 30 years. Thyroid carcinoma metastases may be flesh-colored or red-violet cutaneous nodules, often involving the scalp and abdomen. **Thyroid follicular carcinoma** metastases may be pulsatile or manifest bruits.

Microscopically, **papillary thyroid carcinoma** has an infiltrative pattern that consists of tubulopapillary structures with occasional psammoma bodies and dark, eosinophilic-staining colloid. The "orphan-Annie" nuclei of papillary carcinoma of the thyroid are large, ovoid, ground glass–appearing, and grooved nuclei with small nucleoli. **Follicular thyroid carcinoma** has trabeculae and follicles with intraluminal colloid. TTF-1 stains the nuclei of all types of thyroid carcinomas as well as many lung cancers. Positive staining for thyroglobulin and negative staining for CEA distinguish nonmedullary (nonneuroendocrine) thyroid cancer from most lung cancers. The combined expression of TTF1+ and thyroglobulin+ is very specific for metastatic papillary and follicular thyroid carcinomas.

The differential diagnosis of metastatic tumors to the skin with a papillary configuration includes papillary carcinomas of the thyroid and ovary, which may have psammoma bodies, as well as papillary carcinoma from the GI tract, kidney, lungs, ovary, endometrium, and papillary transitional cell carcinomas of the bladder. Differentiated follicular carcinoma of the thyroid has a unique appearance because of the colloid in the follicles and round glandular structures. Metastases from the urinary bladder usually occur after recognition of the primary tumor and most often on the trunk and extremities. Less common presentations of metastases include zosteriform lesions, warty papules, and inflammatory plaques. Transitional cell carcinoma of the bladder (**urothelial carcinoma**) may present as nests or sheets with squamous differentiation or more commonly as papillary fronds with varying thicknesses of atypical epithelial cells covering a fine fibrovascular core. The metastatic tumor cells may be located in the dermis in between collagen bundles or sometimes associated with a desmoplastic stroma, in the subcutaneous fat, or in the lumina of vessels. Most urothelial carcinomas express p63, D2-40, and high-molecular-weight CKs such as CK5/6 and 34BE12, making their distinction from squamous cell carcinomas or primary cutaneous adenocarcinomas difficult. However, most urothelial carcinomas stain positively for both CK7 and CK20. This CK7+/CK20+ pattern is also seen in many pancreatic and some mucinous ovarian carcinomas but is uncommon in other settings. Uroplakins are a family of transmembrane proteins present only in urothelia. Expression of uroplakins may be specific for urothelial carcinomas, but as with many other tissue-specific markers, uroplakin expression is reduced or absent in many high-grade and metastatic lesions. In women, papillary genital tract tumors that most commonly metastasize to the skin have ovarian (4%) and endometrial (4%) origin. A cutaneous metastasis from the ovary may be the initial manifestation of disease, but metastases from the endometrium usually occurs after recognition of the primary tumor. The trunk and pelvic areas are the primary sites of cutaneous metastases for each of these tumors, and ovarian metastases may involve the umbilicus and prior surgical scars. **Metastatic ovarian papillary serous adenocarcinoma** resembles papillary tumors from other sites such as the colon, thyroid gland, stomach, and lung. Psammoma bodies may be observed in both ovarian carcinoma and papillary carcinoma of the thyroid gland. Serous ovarian adenocarcinomas often stain with CK7 and estrogen and progesterone receptors but usually not with CK20, CDX2, CEA, or GCDFP-15, which facilitates distinction from colorectal adenocarcinomas (which are usually CK7 and ER negative and CK20, CDX2, and CEA positive) and breast carcinoma (which is GCDFP-15 positive). **Endometrial papillary serous adenocarcinomas** resemble serous ovarian adenocarcinomas with respect to immunophenotype except that CEA staining and coexpression of CKs and vimentin are common. Thyroid papillary carcinomas usually stain for a broad range of low- and high-molecular weight CKs, including CK7, but also for relatively specific markers such as thyroglobulin and TTF-1.

ANSWER 12-24: A.

This is an example of **metastatic poorly differentiated "signet ring" adenocarcinoma.** This type of adenocarcinoma commonly arises from the stomach; however, it may less commonly arise from metastases from the ovary or endometrium. Poorly differentiated mammary and urothelial metastases with mucinous differentiation should also be included in the differential diagnosis. **Mucinous ovarian carcinomas** vary considerably in their microscopic appearance and may be difficult to distinguish from endocervical, colorectal, gastrointestinal, and breast carcinomas. Microscopically, anaplastic cells that infiltrate a loose or fibrotic stroma characterize signet-ring adenocarcinoma. The tumor cells contain intracytoplasmic mucin, which pushes the nucleus to an eccentric location. Many mucinous ovarian tumors have an intestinal phenotype and express antigens such as CK20, CDX2, and villin. Significant expression of CK7 and CA125 with weaker and less diffuse staining for CK20 favors a **mucinous ovarian carcinoma** over a true **intestinal mucinous carcinoma**, but exceptions exist. CA125 is also negative in most breast cancers. Urothelial carcinomas are positive for CK7 and CK20, but also typically express p63 and D2-40.

ANSWER 12-25: C.

This is an example of a **"small blue cell" tumor**, consistent with **neuroendocrine carcinoma of the lung (small cell carcinoma). Small cell neuroendocrine carcinomas** are composed of islands, trabeculae, and sometimes rosettes of mildly pleomorphic cells that are somewhat larger than lymphocytes, with scant cytoplasms and hyperchromatic nuclei. There are frequent mitoses, and crush artifact is a common characteristic of these cells. Immunohistochemistry is essential in deciphering the origins of the poorly differentiated tumor. Small cell neuroendocrine carcinomas of the lung are usually positive for AE1/AE3 and with antibodies to low molecular CKs in a punctate pattern. These tumors often stain for the neuroendocrine markers synaptophysin and chromogranin. The most specific positive markers in regard to pulmonary origin are TTF1 and CK7. CK20 and neurofilament protein staining in a punctuate perinuclear pattern is much more common in **Merkel cell carcinomas** than in neuroendocrine carcinomas of the lung, and CK7 staining is less common in Merkel cell carcinomas than in lung carcinomas. Positive staining for CK7 and TTF-1 and negative staining for CK20 and neurofilament protein favors metastatic small cell carcinoma of lung origin over Merkel cell carcinoma. Small cell carcinomas from areas other than the lung and skin such as the gut, uterine cervix, and salivary glands may also express TTF-1 and less commonly CK20. Although positive staining with antibodies to CD56 is often used to help identify **natural killer (NK) cell lymphomas**, many neuroendocrine carcinomas, including primary neuroendocrine carcinomas of the lung and Merkel cell carcinomas, stain strongly with antibodies to CD56. Many Merkel cell carcinomas also stain with antibodies to terminal deoxynucleotidyl transferase (TdT), a DNA polymerase that is usually considered to be sensitive and specific antibody for blastic hematologic malignancies. It is not clear at this time whether neuroendocrine malignancies of other organ systems express TdT.

The differential diagnosis of **small cell neuroendocrine carcinoma of the lung** includes a variety of small round cell tumors, including **cutaneous adnexal carcinomas** (p63+), **primary** or **metastatic melanoma** (S100+, Melan-A+), primary or other metastatic neuroendocrine tumors such as **Merkel cell carcinoma** primary to the skin (TTF-1-, CK20+) and neuroendocrine carcinomas metastatic from another organs, **malignant lymphoma** (CD45+), **Ewing sarcoma** (Fli-1+), and **rhabdomyosarcoma** (myoD-1+).

BIBLIOGRAPHY

1. Aguilera NSI, Tomaszewski MM, Moad JC, et al. Cutaneous follicle center lymphoma: a clinicopathologic study of 19 cases. *Mod Pathol.* 2001;14:828.
2. Akhtar S, Oza KK, Wright J. Merkel cell carcinoma: report of 10 cases and review of the literature. *J Am Acad Dermatol.* 2000;43:755–767.
3. Al-Abbadi MA, Almasri NM, Al-Quran S, Wilkinson EJ. Cytokeratin and epithelial membrane antigen expression in angiosarcomas: an immunohistochemical study of 33 cases. *Arch Pathol Lab Med.* 2007;131:288–292.
4. Alkhayat H, Hong CH. Cutaneous metastases from non-small cell lung cancer. *J Cutan Med Surg* 2006;10:304–307.
5. Alwaheeb S, Ghazarian D, Boerner SL, Asa SL. Cutaneous manifestations of thyroid cancer: a report of four cases and review of the literature. *J Clin Pathol.* 2004;57:435–438.
6. Amador A, Monforte NG, Bejarano N, et al. Cutaneous metastasis from hepatocellular carcinoma as the first clinical sign. *J Hepatobiliary Pancreat Surg.* 2007;14:328–330.
7. Ansai S, Mitsuhashi Y, Kondo S, Manabe M. Immunohistochemical differentiation of extra-ocular sebaceous carcinoma from other skin cancers. *J Dermatol.* 2004;31:998–1008.
8. Assaf C, Gellrich S, Whittaker S, et al. CD56 lymphoproliferative disorders of the skin: a multicenter study of the Cutaneous Lymphoma Project Group of the European Organization for Research and Treatment of Cancer (EORTC). *J Clin Pathol.* 2006.
9. Assaf C, Gellrich S, Whittaker S, et al. CD56-positive haematological neoplasms of the skin: a multicentre study of the Cutaneous Lymphoma Project Group of the European Organisation for Research and Treatment of Cancer. *J Clin Pathol.* 2007;60:981.
10. Assaf C, Hirsch B, Wagner F, et al. Differential expression of TRAF1 aids in the distinction of cutaneous CD30-positive lymphoproliferations. *J Invest Dermatol.* 2007;127:1898
11. Attygalle A, Al-Jehani R, Diss TC, et al. Neoplastic T cells in angioimmunoblastic T-cell lymphoma express CD10. *Blood.* 2002;99:627.
12. Azoulay S, Adem C, Pelletier FL, et al. Skin metastases from unknown origin: role of immunohistochemistry in the evaluation of cutaneous metastases of carcinoma of unknown origin. *J Cutan Pathol.* 2005;32:561–566.
13. Bahrami S, Malone JC, Lear S, Martin AW. CD10 expression in cutaneous adnexal neoplasms and a potential role for differentiating cutaneous metastatic renal cell carcinoma. *Arch Pathol Lab Med.* 2006;130:1315–1319.
14. Baratta A, Gorin RJ, Costa R. Sister Mary Joseph nodule: a case report. *Cutis.* 2007;80:469–472.
15. Barrionuevo C, Anderson VM, Zevallos-Giampietri E, et al. Hydroa-like cutaneous T-cell lymphoma: a clinicopathologic and molecular genetic study of 16 pediatric cases from Peru. *Appl Immunohistochem Mol Morphol.* 2002;10:7.
16. Barry Delongchamps N, Peyromaure M, Debre B, Zerbib M. Renal cancer presenting as an isolated cutaneous metastasis. *Prog Urol.* 2004;14:538–539.
17. Bauza A, Redondo P, Idoate MA. Cutaneous zosteriform squamous cell carcinoma metastasis arising in an immunocompetent patient. *Clin Exp Dermatol.* 2002;27:199–201.
18. Bekkenk MW, Geelen FA, van Voorst Vader PC, et al. Primary and secondary cutaneous CD30(+) lymphoproliferative disorders: a report from the Dutch Cutaneous Lymphoma Group on the long-term follow-up data of 219 patients and guidelines for diagnosis and treatment. *Blood.* 2000;95:3653.
19. Bekkenk MW, Vermeer MH, Jansen PM, et al. Peripheral T-cell lymphomas unspecified presenting in

the skin: analysis of prognostic factors in a group of 82 patients. *Blood.* 2003;102:2213.

20. Benez A, Metzger S, Metzler G, et al. Aleukemic leukemia cutis presenting as benign-appearing exanthema. *Acta Derm Venereol.* 2001;81:45.
21. Bhargava R, Beriwal S, Dabbs DJ. Mammaglobin vs GCDFP-15: an immunohistologic validation survey for sensitivity and specificity. *Am J Clin Pathol.* 2007;127:103–113.
22. Bircan S, Candir O, Kapucoglu N, Baspinar S. The expression of p63 in basal cell carcinomas and association with histological differentiation. *J Cutan Pathol.* 2006;33:293–298.
23. Bobos M, Hytiroglou P, Kostopoulos I, et al. Immunohistochemical distinction between Merkel cell carcinoma and small cell carcinoma of the lung. *Am J Dermatopathol.* 2006;28:99–104.
24. Bornkessel A, Weyers W, Elsner P, Ziemer M. Epidermotropic metastases from squamous cell carcinoma of the lower female genital tract mimicking primary Bowen's carcinoma. *Am J Dermatopathol.* 2006;28:220–222.
25. Bostwick DG MA, Qian J, et al. Immunohistology of the prostate, bladder, testis and kidney. In: Dabbs D, ed. *Diagnostic Immunohistochemistry.* 2nd ed. New York, NY: Churchill Livingston; 2006:509–610.
26. Boutilier R, Desormeau L, Cragg F, et al. Merkel cell carcinoma: squamous and atypical fibroxanthoma-like differentiation in successive local tumor recurrences. *Am J Dermatopathol.* 2001;23:46–49.
27. Breccia M, Mandelli F, Petti MC, et al. Clinico-pathological characteristics of myeloid sarcoma at diagnosis and during follow-up: report of 12 cases from a single institution. *Leuk Res.* 2004;28:1165.
28. Brown HA, Macon WR, Kurtin PJ, et al. Cutaneous involvement by angioimmunoblastic T-cell lymphoma with remarkable heterogeneous Epstein-Barr virus expression. *J Cutan Pathol.* 2001;28:432.
29. Bruggemann M, White H, Gaulard P, et al. Powerful strategy for polymerase chain reaction-based clonality assessment in T-cell malignancies Report of the BIOMED-2 Concerted Action BHM4 CT98-3936. *Leukemia.* 2007;21:215.
30. Buechner S, Su WPD, Vardiman J. Cutaneous involvement by myeloid leukaemia. In: LeBoit PE, Burg G, Weedon D, Sarasin A, eds. *World Health Organization Classification of Tumours. Pathology & Genetics. Skin Tumours.* Lyon, France: IARC Press; 2006:211.
31. Buechner S, Su WPD. Acute (myelo-) Monocytic leukemia (AMoL, AMMoL). In: Burg G, Kempf W, eds. *Cutaneous Lymphomas.* Boca Raton, FL: Taylor & Francis; 2005:393.
32. Buechner S, Su WPD. Acute granulocytic (myeloid) leukemia (AML). In: Burg G, Kempf W, eds. *Cutaneous Lymphomas.* Boca Raton, FL: Taylor & Francis; 2005:389.
33. Buechner S, Su WPD. Chronic lymphocytic leukemia, B-cell type (B-CLL). In: Burg G, Kempf W, eds. *Cutaneous Lymphomas.* Boca Raton, FL: Taylor & Francis; 2005:375.
34. Buechner S, Su WPD. Chronic myeloid leukemia (CML). In: Burg G, Kempf W, eds. *Cutaneous Lymphomas.* Boca Raton, FL: Taylor & Francis; 2005:383.
35. Buechner S, Su WPD. Granulocytic sarcoma (Chloroma). In: Burg G, Kempf W, eds. *Cutaneous Lymphomas.* Boca Raton, FL: Taylor & Francis; 2005:403.
36. Buechner S, Su WPD. Hairy-cell leukemia (HCL). In: Burg G, Kempf W, eds. *Cutaneous Lymphomas.* Boca Raton, FL: Taylor & Francis; 2005:387.
37. Burg G, Jaffe ES, Kempf W, et al. WHO/EORTC classification of cutaneous lymphomas. In: LeBoit, P, Burg G, Weedon D, et al, eds. *World Health Organization Classification of Tumours. Pathology and Genetics of Skin Tumors.* Lyon: WHO IARC; 2006:166.
38. Burg G, Kempf W, Haeffner A, et al. From inflammation to neoplasia: new concepts in the pathogenesis of cutaneous lymphomas. *Recent Results Cancer Res.* 2002;160:271.
39. Burg G, Kempf W, Kazakov DV, et al. Pyogenic lymphoma of the skin: a peculiar variant of primary cutaneous neutrophil-rich CD30+ anaplastic large-cell lymphoma. Clinicopathological study of four cases and review of the literature. *Br J Dermatol.* 2003;148:580.
40. 1. Burg G, Kempf W. *Cutaneous Lymphomas.* 1st ed. New York, NY: Francis and Taylor; 2005.
41. Cabuk M, Inanir I, Turkdogan P, et al. Cyclic lymphocytic vasculitis associated with chronic lymphocytic leukemia. *Leuk Lymphoma.* 2004;45:811.
42. Calder KB, Coplowitz S, Schlauder S, Morgan MB. A case series and immunophenotypic analysis of CK20−/CK7+ primary neuroendocrine carcinoma of the skin. *J Cutan Pathol.* 2007;34:918–923.
43. Carlson JW, Nucci MR, Brodsky J, et al. Biomarker-assisted diagnosis of ovarian, cervical and pulmonary small cell carcinomas: the role of TTF-1, WT-1 and HPV analysis. *Histopathology.* 2007;51:305–312.
44. Cerilli L, Wick M. Immunohistology of soft tissue and osseous neoplasms. In: Dabbs D, ed. *Diagnostic Immunohistochemistry.* 2nd ed. New York, NY: Churchill Livingston; 2006:65–120.
45. Cerroni L, Arzberger E, Pütz B, et al. Primary cutaneous follicle center cell lymphoma with follicular growth pattern. *Blood.* 2000;95:3922.

46. Cerroni L, Borroni RG, Massone C, et al. Cutaneous B-cell pseudolymphoma at the site of vaccination. *Am J Dermatopathol.* 2007;29:538.

47. Cerroni L, El-Shabrawi-Caelen L, Fink-Puches R, et al. Cutaneous spindle-cell B-cell lymphoma. A morphologic variant of cutaneous large B-cell lymphoma. *Am J Dermatopathol.* 2000;22:299.

48. Cerroni L, Gatter K, Kerl H. *An illustrated guide of skin lymphomas.* 2nd ed. Oxford: Blackwell Publishing; 2004.

49. Cerroni L, Höfler G, Bäck B, et al. Specific cutaneous infiltrates of B-cell chronic lymphocytic leukemia (B-CLL) at sites typical for *Borrelia burgdorferi* infection. *J Cutan Pathol.* 2002;29:142.

50. Cerroni L, Kerl H. Primary cutaneous follicle center cell lymphoma. *Leuk Lymphoma.* 2001;42:891.

51. Cerroni L, Kerl H. The clinicopathologic spectrum of cutaneous B-cell lymphomas. *Prog Pathol.* 2001;5:1.

52. Cerroni L. Hemangiomas with a bad surprise. *Dermatology.* 2004;209:79.

53. Cessna MH, Zhou H, Perkins SL, et al. Are myogenin and myoD1 expression specific for rhabdomyosarcoma? A study of 150 cases, with emphasis on spindle cell mimics. *Am J Surg Pathol.* 2001;25(9):1150–1157.

54. Chan J. Tumors of the thyroid and parathyroid glands. In: Fletcher C, ed. *Diagnostic Histopathology of Tumors.* Vol 1, 3rd ed. New York, NY: Churchill Livingston; 2007:997–1098.

55. Chang S, Kim SH, Lim HK, et al. Needle tract implantation after sonographically guided percutaneous biopsy of hepatocellular carcinoma: evaluation of doubling time, frequency, and features on CT. *AJR Am J Roentgenol.* 2005;185:400–405.

56. Chang SS, Reuter VE, Heston WD, Gaudin PB. Comparison of anti-prostate-specific membrane antigen antibodies and other immunomarkers in metastatic prostate carcinoma. *Urology.* 2001;57:1179–1183.

57. Chang SS. Overview of prostate-specific membrane antigen. *Rev Urol* 2004;69(Suppl 10):S13–S18.

58. Chao C, Torosian M, Boraas M, et al. Local recurrence of breast cancer in the stereotactic core needle biopsy site: case reports and review of the literature. *Breast.* 2001;7:124–127.

59. Chen CH, Chao KC, Wang PH. Advanced cervical squamous cell carcinoma with skin metastasis. *Taiwan J Obstet Gynecol* 2007;46:264–266.

60. Chen QR, Vansant G, Oades K, et al. Diagnosis of the small round blue cell tumors using multiplex polymerase chain reaction. *J Mol Diagn.* 2007;9:80–88.

61. Cheuk W, Kwan MY, Suster S, Chan JK. Immunostaining for thyroid transcription factor 1 and cytokeratin 20 aids the distinction of small cell carcinoma from Merkel cell carcinoma, but not pulmonary from extrapulmonary small cell carcinomas. *Arch Pathol Lab Med.* 2001;125:228–231.

62. Chintamani M, Sharma R, Badran R, et al. Metastatic sweat gland adenocarcinoma: a clinicopathological dilemma. *World J Surg Oncol.* 2003;1:13.

63. Chiu CS, Lin CY, Kuo TT, et al. Malignant cutaneous tumors of the scalp: a study of demographic characteristics and histologic distributions of 398 Taiwanese patients. *J Am Acad Dermatol.* 2007;56:448–452.

64. Chu P, Arber DA. Paraffin-section detection of CD10 in 505 nonhematopoietic neoplasms. Frequent expression in renal cell carcinoma and endometrial stromal sarcoma. *Am J Clin Pathol.* 2000;113:374–382.

65. Chu P, Wu E, Weiss L. Cytokeratin 7 and cytokeratin 20 expression in epithelial neoplasms: a survey of 435 cases. *Mod Pathol.* 2000;13:962–972.

66. Chu PG, Weiss LM. Expression of cytokeratin 5/6 in epithelial neoplasms: an immunohistochemical study of 509 cases. *Mod Pathol.* 2002;15:6–10.

67. Chuang AY, DeMarzo AM, Veltri RW, et al. Immunohistochemical differentiation of high-grade prostate carcinoma from urothelial carcinoma. *Am J Surg Pathol.* 2007;31:1246–1255.

68. Chung JJ, Namiki T, Johnson DW. Cervical cancer metastasis to the scalp presenting as alopecia neoplastica. *Int J Dermatol.* 2007;46:188–189.

69. Cibull TL, Thomas AB, O'Malley DP, et al. Myeloid leukemia cutis: a histologic and immunohistochemical review. *J Cutan Pathol.* 2008;35:180.

70. Coffin CM, Belchis D. Immunohistology of pediatric neoplasms. In: Dabbs D, ed. *Diagnostic Immunohistochemistry.* 2nd ed. New York, NY: Churchill Livingston; 2006:611–636.

71. Cokonis CD, Green JJ, Manders SM. Primary carcinoid tumor of the skin. *J Am Acad Dermatol.* 2004;51:S146-8.

72. Colli C, Leinweber B, Müllegger R, et al. *Borrelia burgdorferi*-associated lymphocytoma cutis: clinicopathologic, immunophenotypic, and molecular study of 106 cases. *J Cutan Pathol.* 2004;31:232.

73. Comin CE, Saieva C, Messerini L. H-caldesmon, calretinin, estrogen receptor, and Ber-EP4: a useful combination of immunohistochemical markers for differentiating epithelioid peritoneal mesothelioma from serous papillary carcinoma of the ovary. *Am J Surg Pathol.* 2007;31:1139–1148.

74. Cooper L, Debono R, Alsanjari N, Al-Nafussi A. Merkel cell tumour with leiomyosarcomatous differentiation. *Histopathology.* 2000;36:540–543.

75. Cozzio A, Hafner J, Kempf W, et al. Febrile ulceronecrotic Mucha-Habermann disease with clonality: a cutaneous T-cell lymphoma entity? *J Am Acad Dermatol.* 2004;51:1014.

76. Crescentini F, Deutsch F, Sobrado CW, Araujo S. Umbilical mass as the sole presenting symptom of pancreatic cancer: a case report. *Rev Hosp Clin Fac Med Sao Paulo.* 2004;59:198–202.

77. Crum C, Lee Y, Genest D. Tumors of the female genital tract. Part C. Tumors of the placenta and gestational trophoblastic disease. In: Fletcher C, ed. *Diagnostic Histopathology of Tumors.* Vol 1, 3rd ed. New York, NY: Churchill Livingston; 2007:672–682.

78. Dabbs D, ed. *Diagnostic Immunohistochemistry.* New York, NY: Churchill Livingston; 2006.

79. Dabbs D. Immunohistology of metastatic carcinomas of unknown primary. In: Dabbs D, ed. *Diagnostic Immunohistochemistry.* 2nd ed. New York, NY: Churchill Livingston; 2006:180–226.

80. Dabbs D. Immunohistology of the breast. In: Dabbs D, ed. *Diagnostic Immunohistochemistry.* 2nd ed. New York, NY: Churchill Livingston; 2006:699–745.

81. Dahmoush L, Hijazi Y, Barnes E, et al. Adult T-cell leukemia/lymphoma. *Cancer.* 2002;96:110.

82. Damin DC, Lazzaron AR, Tarta C, et al. Massive zosteriform cutaneous metastasis from rectal carcinoma. *Tech Coloproctol.* 2003;7:105–107.

83. Danic D, Danic A. Head and neck squamous cell carcinoma skin metastases below of the diaphragm. *Acta Dermatovenerol Croat.* 2003;11:153–157.

84. Daniel L, Lechevallier E, Giorgi R, et al. Pax-2 expression in adult renal tumors. *Hum Pathol.* 2001;32:282–287.

85. de Leval L, Harris NL, Longtine J, et al. Cutaneous B-cell lymphomas of follicular and marginal zone types. Use of Bcl-6, CD10, Bcl-2, and CD21 in differential diagnosis and classification. *Am J Surg Pathol.* 2001;25:732.

86. Dearden C. T-cell prolymphocytic leukemia. *Med Oncol.* 2006;23:17.

87. DeCoteau JF, Butmarc JR, Kinney MC, et al. The t(2;5) chromosomal translocation is not a common feature of primary cutaneous CD30+ lymphoproliferative disorders: comparison with anaplastic large-cell lymphoma of nodal origin. *Blood.* 1996;87:3437.

88. DeLellis RA, Shin SJ. Immunohistology of endocrine tumors. In: Dabbs D, ed. *Diagnostic Immunohistochemistry.* 2nd ed. New York, NY: Churchill Livingston; 2006:261–300.

89. Dennis JL, Hvidsten TR, Wit EC, et al. Markers of adenocarcinoma characteristic of the site of origin: development of a diagnostic algorithm. *Clin Cancer Res.* 2005;11:3766–3772.

90. Di Como CJ, Urist MJ, Babayan I, et al. p63 expression profiles in human normal and tumor tissues. *Clin Cancer Res.* 2002;8:494–501.

91. Dobson CM, Tagor V, Myint AS, Memon A. Telangiectatic metastatic breast carcinoma in face and scalp mimicking cutaneous angiosarcoma. *J Am Acad Dermatol.* 2003;48:635–636.

92. Dodiuk-Gad R, Ziv M, Loven D, et al. Sister Mary Joseph's nodule as a presenting sign of internal malignancy. *Skinmed.* 2006;5:256–258.

93. Dotto JE, Glusac EJ. p63 is a useful marker for cutaneous spindle cell squamous cell carcinoma. *J Cutan Pathol.* 2006;33:413–417.

94. Drews R, Samel A, Kadin ME. Lymphomatoid papulosis and anaplastic large cell lymphomas of the skin. *Semin Cutan Med Surg.* 2000;19:109.

95. Dummer R, Kamarashev J, Kempf W, et al. Junctional CD8+ cutaneous lymphomas with nonaggressive clinical behavior: a CD8+ variant of mycosis fungoides? *Arch Dermatol.* 2002;138:199.

96. Eble J, Young R. Tumors of the urinary tract. In: Fletcher C, ed. *Diagnostic Histopathology of Tumors.* Vol 1, 3rd ed. New York, NY: Churchill Livingston; 2007:485–566.

97. Ehrig T, Billings SD, Fanburg-Smith JC. Superficial primitive neuroectodermal tumor/Ewing sarcoma (PN/ES): same tumor as deep PN/ES or new entity? *Ann Diagn Pathol.* 2007;11:153–159.

98. El Shabrawi-Caelen L, Kerl H, Cerroni L. Lymphomatoid papulosis: reappraisal of clinicopathologic presentation and classification into subtypes A, B, and C. *Arch Dermatol.* 2004;140:441.

99. Ellis I, Pinder S, Lee A. Tumors of the breast. In: Fletcher C, ed. *Diagnostic Histopathology of Tumors.* Vol 1, 3rd ed. New York, NY: Churchill Livingston; 2007:903–969.

100. El-Shabrawi-Caelen L, Cerroni L, Medeiros LJ, et al. Hypopigmented mycosis fungoides: frequent expression of a CD8+ T-cell phenotype. *Am J Surg Pathol.* 2002;26:450.

101. Erickson LA, Jin L, Nakamura N, et al. Clinicopathologic features and BRAF (V600E) mutation analysis in cutaneous metastases from well-differentiated thyroid carcinomas. *Cancer.* 2007;109:1965–1971.

102. Erickson LA, Papouchado B, Dimashkieh H, et al. Cdx2 as a marker for neuroendocrine tumors of unknown primary sites. *Endocr Pathol.* 2004;15:247–252.

103. Estrada-Chavez G, Vega-Memije ME, Lacy-Niebla RM, Toussaint-Caire S. Scalp metastases of a renal cell carcinoma. *Skinmed.* 2006;5:148–150.

104. Fereidooni F, Kovacs K, Azizi MR, Nikoo M. Skin metastasis from an occult esophageal adenocarcinoma. *Can J Gastroenterol.* 2005;19:673–676.

105. Fink-Puches R, Zenahlik P, Bäck B, et al. Primary cutaneous lymphomas: applicability of current classification schemes (European Organization for Research and Treatment of Cancer, World Health Organization) based on clinicopathologic features observed in a large group of patients. *Blood.* 2002;99:800.

106. Flaig MJ, Cerroni L, Schuhmann K, et al. Follicular mycosis fungoides. A histopathologic analysis of nine cases. *J Cutan Pathol.* 2001;28:525.

107. Fletcher C. Soft tissue tumors. In: Fletcher C, ed. *Diagnostic Histopathology of Tumors.* Vol 1, 3rd ed. New York, NY: Churchill Livingston; 2007:1527–1592.

108. Fletcher C. *Soft Tissue Tumors.* Vol 2, 3rd ed. New York, NY: Churchill Livingston; 2007:1592.

109. Folpe AL, Cooper K. Best practices in diagnostic immunohistochemistry: pleomorphic cutaneous spindle cell tumors. *Arch Pathol Lab Med.* 2007;131:1517–1524.

110. Folpe AL. MyoD1 and myogenin expression in human neoplasia: a review and update. *Adv Anat Pathol.* 2002;9:198–203.

111. Foschini MP, Eusebi V. Divergent differentiation in endocrine and nonendocrine tumors of the skin. *Semin Diagn Pathol.* 2000;17:162–168.

112. Fraggetta F, Pelosi G, Cafici A, et al. CDX2 immunoreactivity in primary and metastatic ovarian mucinous tumours. *Virchows Arch.* 2003;443:782–786.

113. Franco R, Fernandez-Vazquez A, Mollejo M, et al. Cutaneous presentation of follicular lymphomas. *Mod Pathol.* 2001;14:913.

114. Frazier SR, Kaplan PA, Loy TS. The pathology of extrapulmonary small cell carcinoma. *Semin Oncol.* 2007;34:30–38.

115. Fritzsche FR, Thomas A, Winzer KJ, et al. Co-expression and prognostic value of gross cystic disease fluid protein 15 and mammaglobin in primary breast cancer. *Histol Histopathol.* 2007;22:1221–1230.

116. Gabriele R, Borghese M, Conte M, Basso L. Sister Mary Joseph's nodule as a first sign of cancer of the cecum: report of a case. *Dis Colon Rectum.* 2004;47:115–117.

117. Gabriele R, Conte M, Egidi F, Borghese M. Umbilical metastases: current viewpoint. *World J Surg Oncol.* 2005;3:13.

118. Gallardo F, Costa C, Bellosillo B, et al. Lymphomatoid papulosis associated with mycosis fungoides: clinicopathological and molecular studies of 12 cases. *Acta Derm Venereol.* 2004;84:463.

119. Geho DH, Bandle RW, Clair T, Liotta LA. Physiological mechanisms of tumor-cell invasion and migration. *Physiology (Bethesda).* 2005;20:194–200.

120. Gellrich S, Rutz S, Golembowski S, et al. Primary cutaneous follicle center cell lymphomas and large B cell lymphomas of the leg descend from germinal center cells. A single cell polymerase chain reaction analysis. *J Invest Dermatol.* 2001;117:1512.

121. Gerami P, Guitart J. The spectrum of histopathologic and immunohistochemical findings in folliculotropic mycosis fungoides. *Am J Surg Pathol.* 2007;31:1430.

122. Gerami P, Shea C, Stone MS. Angiotropism in epidermotropic metastatic melanoma: another clue to the diagnosis. *Am J Dermatopathol.* 2006;28:429–433.

123. Gilliam AC, Wood GS. Cutaneous lymphoid hyperplasias. *Semin Cutan Med Surg.* 2000;19:133.

124. Giuffrida T, Kligora, GD G. Localized cutaneous metastases from an atypical fibroxanthoma. *Dermatol Surg.* 2004;30:1561–1564.

125. Gleizal A, Torossian JM, Wan DC, Beziat JL. Testicular carcinoma presenting as cutaneous nasal metastasis: case report and review of the literature. *Br J Oral Maxillofac Surg.* 2008;46(5):416–418.

126. Goldblum JR, Reith JD, Weiss SW. Sarcomas arising in dermatofibrosarcoma protuberans: a reappraisal of biologic behavior in eighteen cases treated by wide local excision with extended clinical follow up. *Am J Surg Pathol.* 2000; 24:1125–1130.

127. Goldstein N, Bosler D. Immunohistology of the gastrointestinal tract, pancreas, bile ducts, gallbladder and liver. In: Dabbs D, ed. *Diagnostic Immunohistochemistry.* 2nd ed. New York, NY: Churchill Livingston; 2006:442–508.

128. Gomaa AH, Yaar M, Bhawan J. Cutaneous immunoreactivity of D2-40 antibody beyond the lymphatics. *Am J Dermatopathol.* 2007;29:18–21.

129. Goodlad JR, Davidson MM, Hollowood K, et al. Primary cutaneous B-cell lymphoma and Borrelia burgdorferi infection in patients from the highlands of Scotland. *Am J Surg Pathol.* 2000;24:1279.

130. Goodlad JR, Krajewski AS, Batstone PJ, *et al.* Primary cutaneous follicular lymphoma. A clinicopathologic and molecular study of 16 cases in support of a distinct entity. *Am J Surg Pathol.* 2002;26:733.

131. Grange F, Beylot-Barry M, Courville P, et al. Primary cutaneous diffuse large b-cell lymphoma, leg type. Clinicopathologic features and prognostic analysis in 60 cases. *Arch Dermatol.* 2007;143, 1144.

132. Greisser J, Palmedo G, Sander C, et al. Detection of clonal rearrangement of T-cell receptor genes in the diagnosis of primary cutaneous CD30 lymphoproliferative disorders. *J Cutan Pathol.* 2006;33:711.

133. Groisman GM, Meir A, Sabo E. The value of Cdx2 immunostaining in differentiating primary ovarian

carcinomas from colonic carcinomas metastatic to the ovaries. *Int J Gynecol Pathol.* 2004;23:52–57.

134. Hafez H. Cutaneous pancreatic metastasis: a case report and review of literature. *Indian J Cancer.* 2007;44:111–114.

135. Haga R, Suzuki H. Rectal carcinoma associated with pagetoid phenomenon. *Eur J Dermatol.* 2003;13:93–94.

136. Haghighi B, Smoller BR, LeBoit PE, et al. Pagetoid reticulosis (Woringer-Kolopp disease): an immunophenotypic, molecular, and clinicopathologic study. *Mod Pathol.* 2000;13:502.

137. Hamada M, Toyoshima S, Duan H, Furue M. Pigmented cutaneous metastasis of mucinous carcinoma of the breast to the scalp mimicking malignant melanoma. *Eur J Dermatol.* 2006;16:592–593.

138. Hameed O, Humphrey PA. Immunohistochemistry in diagnostic surgical pathology of the prostate. *Semin Diagn Pathol.* 2005;22:88–104.

139. Hammar SP. Immunohistology of lung and pleural neoplasms. In: Dabbs D, ed. *Diagnostic Immunohistochemistry.* 2nd ed. New York, NY: Churchill Livingston; 2006:329–403.

140. Hasegawa T, Matsuno Y, Shimoda T, et al. Proximal-type epithelioid sarcoma: a clinicopathologic study of 20 cases. *Mod Pathol.* 2001;14:655–663.

141. Heath M, Jaimes N, Lemos B, et al. Clinical characteristics of Merkel cell carcinoma at diagnosis in 195 patients: the AEIOU features. *J Am Acad Dermatol.* 2008;58:375–381.

142. Hensley C, Caughman S. Neutrophilic dermatoses associated with hematologic disorders. *Clin Dermatol.* 2000;18:355.

143. Holm N, Flaig MJ, Yazdi AS, et al. The value of molecular analysis by PCR in the diagnosis of cutaneous lymphocytic infiltrates. *J Cutan Pathol.* 2002;29:447.

144. Holyoake T. Recent advances in the molecular and cellular biology of chronic myeloid leukaemia: lessons to be learned from the laboratory. *Br J Haematol.* 2001;113:11.

145. Hon C, Shek T, Liang R. Conjunctival chloroma (granulocytic sarcoma). *Lancet.* 2002;359:2247.

146. Huang HY, Shariat SF, Sun TT, et al. Persistent uroplakin expression in advanced urothelial carcinomas: implications in urothelial tumor progression and clinical outcome. *Hum Pathol.* 2007;38:1703–1713.

147. Hunt J, L B. Immunohistology of head and neck neoplasms. In: Dabbs D, ed. *Diagnostic Immunohistochemistry.* 2nd ed. New York, NY: Churchill Livingston; 2006:227–260.

148. Hwang JH, Alanen K, Dabbs KD, et al. Merkel cell carcinoma with squamous and sarcomatous differentiation. *J Cutan Pathol.* 2008;35(10):955–959.

149. Inamadar AC, Palit A, Athanikar SB, et al. Inflammatory cutaneous metastasis as a presenting feature of bronchogenic carcinoma. *Indian J Dermatol Venereol Leprol.* 2003;69:347–349.

150. Isaacs H, Jr. Fetal and neonatal neuroblastoma: retrospective review of 271 cases. *Fetal Pediatr Pathol.* 2007;26:177–184.

151. Ivan D, Hafeez Diwan A, Prieto VG. Expression of p63 in primary cutaneous adnexal neoplasms and adenocarcinoma metastatic to the skin. *Mod Pathol.* 2005;18:137–142.

152. Ivan D, Nash JW, Prieto VG, et al. Use of p63 expression in distinguishing primary and metastatic cutaneous adnexal neoplasms from metastatic adenocarcinoma to skin. *J Cutan Pathol.* 2007;34:474–480.

153. Izquierdo MJ, Pastor MA, Carrasco L, et al. Cutaneous metastases from Ewing's sarcoma: report of two cases. *Clin Exp Dermatol.* 2002;27:123–128.

154. Jass J. Tumors of the small and large intestines (including the anal region). In: Fletcher C, ed. *Diagnostic Histopathology of Tumors.* Vol 1, 3rd ed. New York, NY: Churchill Livingston; 2007:379–416.

155. Jensen K, Kohler S, Rouse RV. Cytokeratin staining in Merkel cell carcinoma: an immunohistochemical study of cytokeratins 5/6, 7, 17, and 20. *Appl Immunohistochem Mol Morphol.* 2000;8:310–315.

156. Jensen KC, Higgins JP, Montgomery K, et al. The utility of PAX5 immunohistochemistry in the diagnosis of undifferentiated malignant neoplasms. *Mod Pathol.* 2007;20:871–877.

157. Jun DW, Lee OY, Park CK, et al. Cutaneous metastases of pancreatic carcinoma as a first clinical manifestation. *Korean J Intern Med.* 2005;20:260–263.

158. Kadin ME, Carpenter C. Systemic and primary cutaneous anaplastic large cell lymphomas. *Semin Hematol.* 2003;40:244.

159. Kaimaktchiev V, Terracciano L, Tornillo L, et al. The homeobox intestinal differentiation factor CDX2 is selectively expressed in gastrointestinal adenocarcinomas. *Mod Pathol.* 2004;17:1392–1399.

160. Kakar S, Ferrell L. Tumors of the liver, gallbladder and biliary tree. In: Fletcher C, ed. *Diagnostic Histopathology of Tumors.* Vol 1, 3rd ed. New York, NY: Churchill Livingston; 2007:417–462.

161. Kanitakis J, Chouvet B. Expression of p63 in cutaneous metastases. *Am J Clin Pathol.* 2007;128:753–758.

162. Kargi A, Gurel D, Tuna B. The diagnostic value of TTF-1, CK 5/6, and p63 immunostaining in classification of lung carcinomas. *Appl Immunohistochem Mol Morphol.* 2007;15:415–420.

163. Karwowski JK, Nowels KW, McDougall IR, Weigel RJ. Needle track seeding of papillary thyroid carcinoma

from fine needle aspiration biopsy. A case report. *Acta Cytol.* 2002;46:591–595.

164. Kaufmann O, Fietze E, Mengs J, Dietel M. Value of p63 and cytokeratin 5/6 as immunohistochemical markers for the differential diagnosis of poorly differentiated and undifferentiated carcinomas. *Am J Clin Pathol.* 2001;116:823–830.
165. Kawabata H, Setoyama M, Fukushige T, et al. Spontaneous regression of cutaneous lesions in adult T-cell leukaemia/lymphoma. *Br J Dermatol.* 2001;144:434.
166. Kazakov DV, Burg G, Dummer R, et al. Cutaneous lymphomas and pseudolymphomas: newly described entities. *Recent Results Cancer Res.* 2002;160:283.
167. Kazakov DV, Burg G, Kempf W. Clinicopathological spectrum of mycosis fungoides. *J Eur Acad Dermatol Venereol.* 2004;18:397.
168. Kazakov DV, Kutzner H, Rutten A, et al. Carcinoid-like pattern in sebaceous neoplasms: another distinctive, previously unrecognized pattern in extraocular sebaceous carcinoma and sebaceoma. *Am J Dermatopathol.* 2005;27:195–203.
169. Kazakov DV, Mentzel T, Burg G, et al. Blastic natural killer-cell lymphoma of the skin associated with myelodysplastic syndrome or myelogenous leukaemia: a coincidence or more? *Br J Dermatol.* 2003;149:869.
170. Kazakov DV, Suster S, LeBoit PE, et al. Mucinous carcinoma of the skin, primary, and secondary: a clinicopathologic study of 63 cases with emphasis on the morphologic spectrum of primary cutaneous forms: homologies with mucinous lesions in the breast. *Am J Surg Pathol.* 2005;29:764–782.
171. Kempf W, KazakovDV, Burg G. Adult T-cell leukemia/lymphoma. In: Burg G, Kempf W, eds. *Cutaneous Lymphomas.* Boca Raton, FL: Taylor & Francis; 2005:215.
172. Kempf W, Kutzner H, Cozzio A, et al. MUM1 expression in cutaneous CD30 positive lymphoproliferative disorders: a valuable tool for the distinction between lymphomatoid papulosis and primary cutaneous anaplastic large-cell lymphoma. *Br J Dermatol.* 2008.
173. Kempf W, Levi E, Kamarashev J, et al. Fascin expression in CD30-positive cutaneous lymphoproliferative disorders. *J Cutan Pathol.* 2002;29:295.
174. Kempf W, Ostheeren-Michaelis S, Paulli M, et al. Granulomatous mycosis fungoides and granulomatous slack skin: a multicenter study of the Cutaneous Lymphoma Histopathology Task Force Group of the European Organization for Research and Treatment of Cancer (EORTC). *Arch Dermatol.* 2008.
175. Kempf W, Willemze R, Jaffe ES, et al. CD30+ T-cell lymphoproliferative disorders. In: LeBoit, P, Burg G, Weedon D, et al, eds. *World Health Organization Classification of Tumours. Pathology and Genetics of Skin Tumours.* Lyon: IARC Press; 2006:179.
176. Kempf W. CD30+ lymphoproliferative disorders: histopathology, differential diagnosis, new variants, and simulators. *J Cutan Pathol.* 2006;33(Suppl 1):58.
177. Kerl H, Fink-Puches R, Cerroni L. Clinical aspects of primary cutaneous B-cell lymphomas. *Rec Res Cancer Res.* 2002;160:294.
178. Kikuchi Y, Matsuyama A, Nomura K. Zosteriform metastatic skin cancer: report of three cases and review of the literature. *Dermatology.* 2001;202:336–338.
179. Kim YH, Willemze R, Pimpinelli N, et al. TNM classification system for primary cutaneous lymphomas other than mycosis fungoides and Sezary syndrome: a proposal of the International Society for Cutaneous Lymphomas (ISCL) and the Cutaneous Lymphoma Task Force of the European Organization of Research and Treatment of Cancer (EORTC). *Blood.* 2007;110:479.
180. Kimura N, Kimura I. Podoplanin as a marker for mesothelioma. *Pathol Int.* 2005;55:83–86.
181. Kloppel G, Klimstra D. Tumors of the exocrine pancreas. In: Fletcher C, ed. *Diagnostic Histopathology of Tumors.* Vol 1, 3rd ed. New York, NY: Churchill Livingston; 2007:463–484.
182. Kloppel G. Tumour biology and histopathology of neuroendocrine tumours. *Best Pract Res Clin Endocrinol Metab.* 2007;21:15–31.
183. Kodama K, Massone C, Chott A, et al. Primary cutaneous large B-cell lymphomas: clinicopathologic features, classification, and prognostic factors in a large series of patients. *Blood.* 2005;106:2491.
184. Lack E. Tumors of the autonomic nervous system (including paraganglia. In: Fletcher C, ed. *Diagnostic Histopathology of Tumors.* Vol 1, 3rd ed. New York, NY: Churchill Livingston; 2007:1763–1780.
185. Lee AH. The histological diagnosis of metastases to the breast from extramammary malignancies. *J Clin Pathol.* 2007;60:1333–1341.
186. Leinweber B, Colli C, Chott A, et al. Differential diagnosis of cutaneous infiltrates of B lymphocytes with follicular growth pattern. *Am J Dermatopathol.* 2004;26:4.
187. Lewis TB, Coffin CM, Bernard PS. Differentiating Ewing's sarcoma from other round blue cell tumors using a RT-PCR translocation panel on formalin-fixed paraffin-embedded tissues. *Mod Pathol.* 2007;20:397–404.
188. Liang H, Wu H, Giorgadze TA, et al. Podoplanin is a highly sensitive and specific marker to distinguish primary skin adnexal carcinomas from adenocarcinomas metastatic to skin. *Am J Surg Pathol.* 2007;31:304–310.

189. Liegl B, Leibl S, Gogg-Kamerer M, et al. Mammary and extramammary Paget's disease: an immunohistochemical study of 83 cases. *Histopathology.* 2007;50:439–447.

190. Lin CY, Lee CT, Huang JS, Chang LC. Transitional cell carcinoma metastasis to arm skin from the renal pelvis. *Chang Gung Med J.* 2003;26:525–529.

191. Lin JH, Lee JY, Chao SC, Tsao CJ. Telangiectatic metastatic breast carcinoma preceded by en cuirasse metastatic breast carcinoma. *Br J Dermatol.* 2004;151:523–524.

192. Lin JH, Lee JY. Primary cutaneous CD30 anaplastic large cell lymphoma with keratoacanthoma-like pseudocarcinomatous hyperplasia and marked eosinophilia and neutrophilia. *J Cutan Pathol.* 2004;31:458.

193. Lin X, Saad RS, Luckasevic TM, et al. Diagnostic value of CDX-2 and TTF-1 expressions in separating metastatic neuroendocrine neoplasms of unknown origin. *Appl Immunohistochem Mol Morphol.* 2007;15:407–414.

194. Liu HL, Hoppe RT, Kohler S, et al. CD30+ cutaneous lymphoproliferative disorders: the Stanford experience in lymphomatoid papulosis and primary cutaneous anaplastic large cell lymphoma. *J Am Acad Dermatol.* 2003;49:1049–1058.

195. Logani S, Oliva E, Arnell PM, et al. Use of novel immunohistochemical markers expressed in colonic adenocarcinoma to distinguish primary ovarian tumors from metastatic colorectal carcinoma. *Mod Pathol.* 2005;18:19–25.

196. Lopez-Tarruella Cobo S, Moreno Anton F, Sastre J, et al. Cuirasse skin metastases secondary to gastric adenocarcinoma. *Clin Transl Oncol.* 2005;7:213–215.

197. Lozzi GP, Massone C, Citarella L, et al. Rimming of adipocytes by neoplastic lymphocytes: a histopathologic feature not restricted to subcutaneous T-cell lymphoma. *Am J Dermatopathol.* 2006;28:9.

198. MacDonald D, Speight P. Tumors of the oral cavity. In: Fletcher C, ed. *Diagnostic Histopathology of Tumors.* Vol 1, 3rd ed. New York, NY: Churchill Livingston; 2007:215–238.

199. Magro C, Crowson AN, Kovatich A, et al. Pityriasis lichenoides: a clonal T-cell lymphoproliferative disorder. *Hum Pathol.* 2002;33:788.

200. Magro CM, Magro CM, Crowson AN, Kovatich AJ, Burns F. Drug-induced reversible lymphoid dyscrasia: a clonal lymphomatoid dermatitis of memory and activated T cells. *Hum Pathol.* 2003;34(2):119–129.

201. Magro CM, Morrison CD, Heerema N, et al. T-cell prolymphocytic leukemia: an aggressive T cell malignancy with frequent cutaneous tropism. *J Am Acad Dermatol.* 2006;55:467.

202. Magro CM, Nash JW, Werling RW, et al. Primary cutaneous CD30+ large cell B-cell lymphoma: a series of 10 cases. *Appl Immunohistochem Mol Morphol.* 2006;14:7.

203. Mao TL, Kurman RJ, Huang CC, et al. Immunohistochemistry of choriocarcinoma: an aid in differential diagnosis and in elucidating pathogenesis. *Am J Surg Pathol.* 2007;31:1726–1732.

204. Mao X, Lillington D, Scarisbrick JJ, et al. Molecular cytogenetic analysis of cutaneous T-cell lymphomas: identification of common genetic alterations in Sezary syndrome and mycosis fungoides. *Br J Dermatol.* 2002;147:464.

205. Marchevsky AM, Wick MR. Evidence-based guidelines for the utilization of immunostains in diagnostic pathology: pulmonary adenocarcinoma versus mesothelioma. *Appl Immunohistochem Mol Morphol.* 2007;15:140–144.

206. Marcoval J, Moreno A, Peyri J. Cutaneous infiltration by cancer. *J Am Acad Dermatol.* 2007;57:577–580.

207. Martel P, Laroche L, Courville P, et al. Cutaneous involvement in patients with angioimmunoblastic lymphadenopathy with dysproteinemia: a clinical, immunohistological, and molecular analysis. *Arch Dermatol.* 2000;136:881.

208. Massone C, El-Shabrawi-Caelen L, Kerl H, et al. The morphologic spectrum of primary cutaneous anaplastic large T-cell lymphoma: a histopathologic study on 66 biopsy specimens from 47 patients with report of rare variants. *J Cutan Pathol.* 2008;35:46.

209. Massone C, Kodama K, Kerl H, et al. Histopathologic features of early (patch) lesions of mycosis fungoides: a morphologic study on 745 biopsy specimens from 427 patients. *Am J Surg Pathol.* 2005;29:550.

210. Matutes E. Adult T-cell leukaemia/lymphoma. *J Clin Pathol.* 2007;60:1373.

211. Mazal PR, Stichenwirth M, Koller A, et al. Expression of aquaporins and PAX-2 compared to CD10 and cytokeratin 7 in renal neoplasms: a tissue microarray study. *Mod Pathol.* 2005;18:535–540.

212. McKenney JK, Heerema-McKenney A, Rouse RV. Extragonadal germ cell tumors: a review with emphasis on pathologic features, clinical prognostic variables, and differential diagnostic considerations. *Adv Anat Pathol.* 2007;14:69–92.

213. McLean SR, Shousha S, Francis N, et al. Metastatic ductal eccrine adenocarcinoma masquerading as an invasive ductal carcinoma of the male breast. *J Cutan Pathol.* 2007;34:934–938.

214. McNiff JM, Cowper SE, Lazova R, et al. CD56 staining in Merkel cell carcinoma and natural killer-cell lymphoma: magic bullet, diagnostic pitfall, or both? *J Cutan Pathol.* 2005;32:541–545.

215. Mentzel T, Scharer L, Kazakov DV, Michal M. Myxoid dermatofibrosarcoma protuberans: clinicopathologic, immunohistochemical, and molecular analysis of eight cases. *Am J Dermatopathol.* 2007;29:443–448.

216. Michaelis S, Kazakov DV, Burg G, et al. Extracutaneous transformation into a high-grade lymphoma: a potential pitfall in the management of patients with Sezary syndrome. *Int J Dermatol.* 2006;45:277.

217. Mimura T, Ito A, Sakuma T, et al. Novel marker D2-40, combined with calretinin, CEA, and TTF-1: an optimal set of immunodiagnostic markers for pleural mesothelioma. *Cancer.* 2007;109:933–938.

218. Molina Garrido MJ, Guillen Ponce C, Soto Martinez JL, et al. Cutaneous metastases of lung cancer. *Clin Transl Oncol.* 2006;8:330–333.

219. Moran C, Suster S. Tumors of the lung and pleura. In: Fletcher C, ed. *Diagnostic Histopathology of Tumors.* Vol 1, 3rd ed. New York, NY: Churchill Livingston; 2007:181–214.

220. Morand J, Lightburn E, Richard M, et al. Skin manifestations associated with myelodysplastic syndromes. *Rev Med Interne.* 2001;22:845.

221. Morgan K, Callen J. Sweet's syndrome in acute myelogenous leukemia presenting as periorbital cellulitis with an infiltrate of leukemic cells. *J Am Acad Dermatol.* 2001;45:590.

222. Mraz Gernhard S, Natkunam Y, Hoppe RT, et al. Natural killer/natural killer-like T-cell lymphoma, CD56+, presenting in the skin: an increasingly recognized entity with an aggressive course. *J Clin Oncol.* 2001;19:2179.

223. Mueller TJ, Wu H, Greenberg RE, et al. Cutaneous metastases from genitourinary malignancies. *Urology.* 2004;63:1021–1026.

224. Mullinax K, Cohen JB. Carcinoma en cuirasse presenting as keloids of the chest. *Dermatol Surg* 2004;30:226–228.

225. Mutter G, Ince TA. Tumors of the female genital tract. Part B. Endometrium. In: Fletcher C, ed. *Diagnostic Histopathology of Tumors.* Vol 1, 3rd ed. New York, NY: Churchill Livingston; 2007:652–671.

226. Nagao T, Gaffey TA, Olsen KD, et al. Small cell carcinoma of the major salivary glands: clinicopathologic study with emphasis on cytokeratin 20 immunoreactivity and clinical outcome. *Am J Surg Pathol.* 2004;28:762–770.

227. Nathanson SD. Insights into the mechanisms of lymph node metastasis. *Cancer.* 2003;98:413–423.

228. Navas IC, Ortiz-Romero PL, Villuendas R, et al. p16(INK4a) gene alterations are frequent in lesions of mycosis fungoides. *Am J Pathol.* 2000;156:1565.

229. Ng CS. Carcinoma erysipeloides from prostate cancer presenting as cellulitis. *Cutis.* 2000;65:215–216.

230. Nguyen TH. Mechanisms of metastasis. *Clin Dermatol.* 2004;22:209–216.

231. Nicholson SA, McDermott MB, Swanson PE, Wick MR. CD99 and cytokeratin-20 in small-cell and basaloid tumors of the skin. *Appl Immunohistochem Mol Morphol.* 2000;8:37–41.

232. Niiyama S, Satoh K, Kaneko S, et al. Zosteriform skin involvement of nodal T-cell lymphoma: a review of the published work of cutaneous malignancies mimicking herpes zoster. *J Dermatol* 2007;34:68–73.

233. O'Connell FP, Wang HH, Odze RD. Utility of immunohistochemistry in distinguishing primary adenocarcinomas from metastatic breast carcinomas in the gastrointestinal tract. *Arch Pathol Lab Med.* 2005;129:338–347.

234. Ohira S, Itoh K, Osada K, et al. Vulvar Paget's disease with underlying adenocarcinoma simulating breast carcinoma: case report and review of the literature. *Int J Gynecol Cancer.* 2004;14:1012–1017.

235. Olsen, E, Vonderheid E, Pimpinelli N, et al. Revisions to the staging and classification of mycosis fungoides and Sezary syndrome: a proposal of the International Society for Cutaneous Lymphomas (ISCL) and the cutaneous lymphoma task force of the European Organization of Research and Treatment of Cancer (EORTC). *Blood.* 2007;110:1713.

236. Ordonez NG. D2-40 and podoplanin are highly specific and sensitive immunohistochemical markers of epithelioid malignant mesothelioma. *Hum Pathol.* 2005;36:372–380.

237. Ordonez NG. Podoplanin: a novel diagnostic immunohistochemical marker. *Adv Anat Pathol.* 2006;13:83–88.

238. Ottinetti A, Colombo E, Dardano F, et al. Cutaneous metastasis of neuroendocrine carcinoma of the larynx: report of a case. *J Cutan Pathol.* 2003;30:512–515.

239. Pai KK, Pai SB, Sripathi H, et al. Epithelioid sarcoma: a diagnostic challenge. *Indian J Dermatol Venereol Leprol.* 2006;72:446–448.

240. Palmedo G, Hantschke M, Rütten A, *et al.* Primary cutaneous marginal zone B-cell lymphoma may exhibit both the t(14;18)(q32;q21) *IGH/BCL2* and the t(14;18)(q;32;q21) *IGH/MALT1* translocation: an indicator for clonal transformation towards higher-grade B-cell lymphoma? *Am J Dermatopathol.* 2007;29:231.

241. Park SG, Chang JY, Kim SH, Bang D. Cutaneous metastasis of choriocarcinoma: a case report. *J Korean Med Sci.* 2005;20:683–686.

242. Park SY, Kim BH, Kim JH, et al. Panels of immunohistochemical markers help determine primary sites

of metastatic adenocarcinoma. *Arch Pathol Lab Med.* 2007;131:1561–1567.

243. Parker DC, Folpe AL, Bell J, et al. Potential utility of uroplakin III, thrombomodulin, high molecular weight cytokeratin, and cytokeratin 20 in noninvasive, invasive, and metastatic urothelial (transitional cell) carcinomas. *Am J Surg Pathol.* 2003;27:1–10.
244. Passebosc-Faure K, Li G, Lambert C, et al. Evaluation of a panel of molecular markers for the diagnosis of malignant serous effusions. *Clin Cancer Res.* 2005;11:6862–6867.
245. Paydas, S, Zorludemir S. Leukaemia cutis and leukaemic vasculitis. *Br J Dermatol.* 2000;143:773.
246. Perna AG, Ostler DA, Ivan D, et al. Renal cell carcinoma marker (RCC-Ma) is specific for cutaneous metastasis of renal cell carcinoma. *J Cutan Pathol.* 2007;34:381–385.
247. Petrella T, Bagot M, Willemze R, et al. Blastic NK-cell lymphomas (agranular CD4+CD56+ hematodermic neoplasms): a review. *Am J Clin Pathol.* 2005;123:662.
248. Petrella T, Comeau MR, Maynadie M, et al. 'Agranular CD4+ CD56+ hematodermic neoplasm' (blastic NK-cell lymphoma) originates from a population of CD56+ precursor cells related to plasmacytoid monocytes. *Am J Surg Pathol.* 2002;26:852.
249. Petrella T, Maubec E, Cornillet-Lefebvre P, et al. Indolent CD8-positive lymphoid proliferation of the ear: a distinct primary cutaneous T-cell lymphoma? *Am J Surg Pathol.* 2007;31:1887.
250. Pimpinelli N, Olsen EA, Santucci M, et al. Defining early mycosis fungoides. *J Am Acad Dermatol.* 2005;53:1053.
251. Puri PK, Galan A, Glusac EJ, Cowper SE. Metastatic cutaneous carcinoid tumor mimicking an adnexal poroid neoplasm. *J Cutan Pathol.* 2008;35:54–57.
252. Quinn AM, Sienko A, Basrawala Z, Campbell SC. Extramammary Paget disease of the scrotum with features of Bowen disease. *Arch Pathol Lab Med.* 2004;128:84–86.
253. Quinn TR DL, Zembowicz A, Faquin WC. Cutaneous metastases of follicular thyroid carcinoma: a report of four cases and a review of the literature. *Am J Dermatopathol.* 2005;27:306–312.
254. Qureshi HS, Ormsby AH, Lee MW, et al. The diagnostic utility of p63, CK5/6, CK 7, and CK 20 in distinguishing primary cutaneous adnexal neoplasms from metastatic carcinomas. *J Cutan Pathol.* 2004;31:145–152.
255. Qureshi HS, Salama ME, Chitale D, et al. Primary cutaneous mucinous carcinoma: presence of myoepithelial cells as a clue to the cutaneous origin. *Am J Dermatopathol.* 2004;26:353–358.
256. Rasi A, Tajziehchi L, Shaianfar N. Metastatic carcinoma of the ovary presenting as zosteriform lesions. *Arch Iran Med* 2007;10:250–252.
257. Reddy S, Bang RH, Contreras ME. Telangiectatic cutaneous metastasis from carcinoma of the prostate. *Br J Dermatol.* 2007;156:598–600.
258. Regauer S. Extramammary Paget's disease—a proliferation of adnexal origin? *Histopathology.* 2006;48:723–729.
259. Reimann JD, Fletcher CD. Myxoid dermatofibrosarcoma protuberans: a rare variant analyzed in a series of 23 cases. *Am J Surg Pathol.* 2007;31:1371–1377.
260. Reis-Filho JS, Simpson PT, Martins A, et al. Distribution of p63, cytokeratins 5/6 and cytokeratin 14 in 51 normal and 400 neoplastic human tissue samples using TARP-4 multi-tumor tissue microarray. *Virchows Arch.* 2003;443:122–132.
261. Reis-Filho JS, Torio B, Albergaria A, Schmitt FC. p63 expression in normal skin and usual cutaneous carcinomas. *J Cutan Pathol.* 2002;29:517–523.
262. Renner R, Sticherling M. Sister Mary Joseph's nodule as a metastasis of gallbladder carcinoma. *Int J Dermatol.* 2007;46:505–507.
263. Requena L, Sangueza M, Sangueza OP, Kutzner H. Pigmented mammary Paget disease and pigmented epidermotropic metastases from breast carcinoma. *Am J Dermatopathol.* 2002;24:189–198.
264. Requena L, Santonja C, Stutz N, et al. Pseudolymphomatous cutaneous angiosarcoma: a rare variant of cutaneous angiosarcoma readily mistaken for cutaneous lymphoma. *Am J Dermatopathol.* 2007;29:342.
265. Resetkova E. Pathologic aspects of inflammatory breast carcinoma: part 1. Histomorphology and differential diagnosis. *Semin Oncol.* 2008;35:25–32.
266. Resnik KS, DiLeonardo M, Gibbons G. Clinically occult cutaneous metastases. *J Am Acad Dermatol.* 2006;55:1044–1047.
267. Rindi G, Kloppel G. Endocrine tumors of the gut and pancreas tumor biology and classification. *Neuroendocrinology.* 2004;80(Suppl 1):12–15.
268. Robak E, Robak T. Skin lesions in chronic lymphocytic leukemia. *Leuk Lymphoma.* 2007;48:855.
269. Rolz-Cruz G, Kim CC. Tumor invasion of the skin. *Dermatol Clin.* 2008;26:89–102, viii.
270. Russell-Jones R,Whittaker S. Sezary syndrome: diagnostic criteria and therapeutic options. *Semin Cutan Med Surg.* 2000;19:100.
271. Saad RS, Lindner JL, Lin X, et al. The diagnostic utility of D2-40 for malignant mesothelioma versus

pulmonary carcinoma with pleural involvement. *Diagn Cytopathol.* 2006;34:801–806.

272. Saeed S, Keehn CA, Morgan MB. Cutaneous metastasis: a clinical, pathological, and immunohistochemical appraisal. *J Cutan Pathol.* 2004;31:419–430.
273. Sandberg Y, Heule F, Lam K, et al. Molecular immunoglobulin/T-cell receptor clonality analysis in cutaneous lymphoproliferations. Experience with the BIOMED-2 standardized polymerase chain reaction protocol. *Haematologica.* 2003;88:659.
274. Santa Cruz D. Tumors of the skin. In: Fletcher C, ed. *Diagnostic Histopathology of Tumors.* Vol 2, 3rd ed. New York, NY: Churchill Livingston; 2007:1423–1526.
275. Santucci M, Pimpinelli N, Massi D, et al. Cytotoxic/natural killer cell cutaneous lymphomas. Report of EORTC Cutaneous Lymphoma Task Force Workshop. *Cancer.* 2003;97:610.
276. Sariya D, Ruth K, Adams-McDonnell R, et al. Clinicopathologic correlation of cutaneous metastases: experience from a cancer center. *Arch Dermatol.* 2007;143:613–620.
277. Sasaki E, Tsunoda N, Hatanaka Y, et al. Breast-specific expression of MGB1/mammaglobin: an examination of 480 tumors from various organs and clinicopathological analysis of MGB1-positive breast cancers. *Mod Pathol.* 2007;20:208–214.
278. Scarabello A, Leinweber B, Ardigo M, et al. Cutaneous lymphomas with prominent granulomatous reaction: a potential pitfall in the histopathologic diagnosis of cutaneous T- and B-cell lymphomas. *Am J Surg Pathol.* 2002;26:1259.
279. Scarabello A, Leinweber B, Ardigo M, et al. Cutaneous lymphomas with prominent granulomatous reaction. A potential pitfall in the histopathologic diagnosis of cutaneous T- and B-cell lymphomas. *Am J Surg Pathol.* 2002;26:1259.
280. Schoenlaub P, Sarraux A, Grosshans E, et al. Survival after cutaneous metastasis: a study of 200 cases. *Ann Dermatol Venereol.* 2001;128:1310–1315.
281. Schwartz RA, Wiederkehr M, Lambert WC. Secondary mucinous carcinoma of the skin: metastatic breast cancer. *Dermatol Surg.* 2004;30:234–235.
282. Shamsadin S, Esfandiarpoor I, Zeinali H, et al. Multifocal scalp hair loss. *Dermatol Online J.* 2006;12:24.
283. Sheridan T, Herawi M, Epstein JI, Illei PB. The role of P501S and PSA in the diagnosis of metastatic adenocarcinoma of the prostate. *Am J Surg Pathol.* 2007;31:1351–1355.
284. Shimizu S, Yasui C, Koizumi K, et al. Cutaneous-type adult T-cell leukemia/lymphoma presenting as a solitary large skin nodule: a review of the literature. *J Am Acad Dermatol.* 2007;57(Suppl):S115.
285. Shinohara S, Yamamoto E, Tanabe M, et al. Implantation metastasis of head and neck cancer after fine needle aspiration biopsy. *Auris Nasus Larynx.* 2001;28:377–380.
286. Siami K, McCluggage WG, Ordonez NG, et al. Thyroid transcription factor-1 expression in endometrial and endocervical adenocarcinomas. *Am J Surg Pathol.* 2007;31:1759–1763.
287. Siesling S, Elferink MA, van Dijck JA, et al. Epidemiology and treatment of extramammary Paget disease in the Netherlands. *Eur J Surg Oncol.* 2007;33:951–955.
288. Sigel JE, Skacel M, Bergfeld WF, et al. The utility of cytokeratin 5/6 in the recognition of cutaneous spindle cell squamous cell carcinoma. *J Cutan Pathol.* 2001;28:520–524.
289. Simon M, Flaig MJ, Kind P, et al. Large plaque parapsoriasis: clinical and genotypic correlations. *J Cutan Pathol.* 2000;27:57.
290. Sina B, Deng A. Umbilical metastasis from prostate carcinoma (Sister Mary Joseph's nodule): a case report and review of literature. *J Cutan Pathol.* 2007;34:581–583.
291. Sjodin A, Guo D, Hofer PA, et al. Mammaglobin in normal human sweat glands and human sweat gland tumors. *J Invest Dermatol* 2003;121:428–429.
292. Smith PD, Patterson JW. Merkel cell carcinoma (neuroendocrine carcinoma of the skin). *Am J Clin Pathol.* 2001;115(Suppl):S68–S78.
293. Snow S, Madjar D, Reizner G, et al. Renal cell carcinoma metastatic to the scalp: case report and review of the literature. *Dermatol Surg.* 2001;27:192–194.
294. Soslow R, Isacson C, Zaloudek C. Immunohistology of the female genital tract. In: Dabbs D, ed. *Diagnostic Immunohistochemistry.* 2nd ed. New York, NY: Churchill Livingston; 2006:699–745.
295. Sramek B, Lisle A, Loy T. Immunohistochemistry in ocular carcinomas. *J Cutan Pathol.* 2008.
296. Stanko C, Grandinetti L, Baldassano M, et al. Epidermotropic metastatic prostate carcinoma presenting as an umbilical nodule-Sister Mary Joseph nodule. *Am J Dermatopathol.* 2007;29:290–292.
297. Streubel B, Lamprecht A, Dierlamm J, et al. T(14;18)(q32;q21) involving *IGH* and *MALT1* is a frequent chromosomal aberration in MALT lymphoma. *Blood.* 2003;101:2335.
298. Streubel B, Scheucher B, Valencak J, et al. Molecular cytogenetic evidence of t(14;18)(*IGH;BCL2*) in a substantial proportion of primary cutaneous follicle center lymphomas. *Am J Surg Pathol.* 2006;30:529.

299. Streubel B, Simonitsch-Klupp I, Müllauer L, et al. Variable frequencies of MALT lymphoma-associated genetic aberrations in MALT lymphomas of different sites. *Leukemia.* 2004;18:1722.

300. Strickland-Marmol LB, Khoor A, Livingston SK, Rojiani A. Utility of tissue-specific transcription factors thyroid transcription factor 1 and Cdx2 in determining the primary site of metastatic adenocarcinomas to the brain. *Arch Pathol Lab Med.* 2007;131:1686–1690.

301. Striebel JM, Dacic S, Yousem SA. Gross cystic disease fluid protein-(GCDFP-15): expression in primary lung adenocarcinoma. *Am J Surg Pathol.* 2008;32:426–432.

302. Suh N, Yang XJ, Tretiakova MS, et al. Value of CDX2, villin, and alphamethylacyl coenzyme A racemase immunostains in the distinction between primary adenocarcinoma of the bladder and secondary colorectal adenocarcinoma. *Mod Pathol.* 2005;18:1217–1222.

303. Sur M, AlArdati H, Ross C, Alowami S. TdT expression in Merkel cell carcinoma: potential diagnostic pitfall with blastic hematological malignancies and expanded immunohistochemical analysis. *Mod Pathol.* 2007;20:1113–1120.

304. Swann MH, Yoon J. Merkel cell carcinoma. *Semin Oncol.* 2007;34:51–56.

305. Takeda Y, Tsuta K, Shibuki Y, et al. Analysis of expression patterns of breast cancer-specific markers (mammaglobin and gross cystic disease fluid protein 15) in lung and pleural tumors. *Arch Pathol Lab Med.* 2008;132:239–243.

306. Tamiolakis D, Antoniou C, Venizelos J, et al. Papillary thyroid carcinoma metastasis most probably due to fine needle aspiration biopsy. A case report. *Acta Dermatovenerol Alp Panonica Adriat.* 2006;15:169–172.

307. Tan KY, Ho KS, Lai JH, et al. Cutaneous and subcutaneous metastases of adenocarcinoma of the colon and rectum. *Ann Acad Med Singapore.* 2006;35:585–587.

308. Terada T, Sato Y, Furukawa K, Sugiura M. Primary cutaneous mucinous carcinoma initially diagnosed as metastatic adenocarcinoma. *Tohoku J Exp Med.* 2004;203:345–348.

309. Thurber SE, Zhang B, Kim YH, et al. T-cell clonality analysis in biopsy specimens from two different skin sites shows high specificity in the diagnosis of patients with suggested mycosis fungoides. *J Am Acad Dermatol.* 2007;57:782.

310. Tokura Y, Jaffe ES, Sander CA. Cutaneous adult T-cell leukaemia/lymphoma. In: LeBoit PE, Burg G, Weedon D, Sarasin A, eds. *World Health Organization Classification of Tumours. Pathology & Genetics. Skin Tumours.* Lyon, France: IARC Press; 2006:189.

311. Tomaszewski MM, Abbondanzo SL, Lupton GP. Extranodal marginal zone B-cell lymphoma of the skin: a morphologic and immunophenotypic study of 11 cases. *Am J Dermatopathol.* 2000;22:205.

312. Tornos C, Soslow R, Chen S, et al. Expression of WT1, CA 125, and GCDFP-15 as useful markers in the differential diagnosis of primary ovarian carcinomas versus metastatic breast cancer to the ovary. *Am J Surg Pathol.* 2005;29:1482–1489.

313. Toro JR, Liewehr DJ, Pabby N, et al. Gamma-delta T-cell phenotype is associated with significantly decreased survival in cutaneous T-cell lymphoma. *Blood.* 2003;101:3407.

314. Tot T. The value of cytokeratins 20 and 7 in discriminating metastatic adenocarcinomas from pleural mesotheliomas. *Cancer.* 2001;92:2727–2732.

315. Tsai HW, Yuan CC, Wang PH. Umbilicus as the only site of metastasis in recurrent ovarian cancer. *J Chin Med Assoc.* 2006;69:233–235.

316. Tsujita-Kyutoku M, Kiuchi K, Danbara N, et al. p63 expression in normal human epidermis and epidermal appendages and their tumors. *J Cutan Pathol.* 2003;30:11–17.

317. Ulbright TM. Germ cell tumors of the gonads: a selective review emphasizing problems in differential diagnosis, newly appreciated, and controversial issues. *Mod Pathol.* 2005;18(Suppl 2):S61–S79.

318. Ulmer A, Metzler G, Schanz S, et al. Dapsone in the management of "insect bite-like reaction" in a patient with chronic lymphocytic leukaemia. *Br J Dermatol.* 2007;156:172.

319. Unni K, Inwards C. Tumors of the osteoarticular system. In: Fletcher C, ed. *Diagnostic Histopathology of Tumors.* Vol 1, 3rd ed. New York, NY: Churchill Livingston; 2007:1593–1652.

320. Urso C, Bondi R, Paglierani M, et al. Carcinomas of sweat glands: report of 60 cases. *Arch Pathol Lab Med.* 2001;125:498–505.

321. Valbuena,JR, Herling M, Admirand JH, et al. T-cell prolymphocytic leukemia involving extramedullary sites. *Am J Clin Pathol.* 2005;123:456.

322. van Doorn R, Scheffer E, Willemze R. Follicular mycosis fungoides, a distinct disease entity with or without associated follicular mucinosis: a clinicopathologic and follow-up study of 51 patients. *Arch Dermatol.* 2002;138:191.

323. Vandergriff T, Krathen RA, Orengo I. Cutaneous metastasis of leiomyosarcoma. *Dermatol Surg.* 2007;33:634–637.

324. Vang R, Gown AM, Zhao C, et al. Ovarian mucinous tumors associated with mature cystic teratomas: morphologic and immunohistochemical analysis identifies a subset of potential teratomatous origin that shares

features of lower gastrointestinal tract mucinous tumors more commonly encountered as secondary tumors in the ovary. *Am J Surg Pathol.* 2007;31:854–869.

325. Varma M, Jasani B. Diagnostic utility of immunohistochemistry in morphologically difficult prostate cancer: review of current literature. *Histopathology.* 2005;47:1–16.
326. Vergier B, de Muret A, Beylot-Barry M, et al. Transformation of mycosis fungoides: clinicopathological and prognostic features of 45 cases. French Study Group of Cutaneious Lymphomas. *Blood.* 2000;95:2212.
327. Vidulich KA, Donley SE, Duvic M. Multinodular cutaneous spread in neuroendocrine tumor of the breast: an unusual presentation. *Am J Clin Dermatol.* 2007;8:379–383.
328. Volmar KE, Cummings TJ, Wang WH, et al. Clear cell hidradenoma: a mimic of metastatic clear cell tumors. *Arch Pathol Lab Med.* 2005;129:e113-6.
329. von den Driesch P, Coors EA. Localized cutaneous small to medium-sized pleomorphic T-cell lymphoma: a report of 3 cases stable for years. *J Am Acad Dermatol.* 2002;46:531.
330. Vonderheid EC, Bernengo MG, Burg G, et al. Update on erythrodermic cutaneous T-cell lymphoma: report of the International Society for Cutaneous Lymphomas. *J Am Acad Dermatol.* 2002;46:95.
331. Wang L, Vuolo M, Suhrland MJ, Schlesinger K. HepPar1, MOC-31, pCEA, mCEA and CD10 for distinguishing hepatocellular carcinoma vs. metastatic adenocarcinoma in liver fine needle aspirates. *Acta Cytol.* 2006;50:257–262.
332. Wang SQ, Mecca PS, Myskowski PL, Slovin SF. Scrotal and penile papules and plaques as the initial manifestation of a cutaneous metastasis of adenocarcinoma of the prostate: case report and review of the literature. *J Cutan Pathol.* 2008.
333. Watson KM, Mufti G, Salisbury JR, et al. Spectrum of clinical presentation, treatment and prognosis in a series of eight patients with leukaemia cutis. *Clin Exp Dermatol.* 2006;31:218.
334. Wenig B. Tumors of the upper respiratory tract. Part A. Nasal cavity, paranasal sinuses and nasopharynx. In: Fletcher C, ed. *Diagnostic Histopathology of Tumors.* Vol 1, 3rd ed. New York, NY: Churchill Livingston; 2007:83–149.
335. Werling RW, Yaziji H, Bacchi CE, Gown AM. CDX2, a highly sensitive and specific marker of adenocarcinomas of intestinal origin: an immunohistochemical survey of 476 primary and metastatic carcinomas. *Am J Surg Pathol.* 2003;27:303–310.
336. Wesche WA, Khare VK, Chesney TM, Jenkins JJ. Non-hematopoietic cutaneous metastases in children and adolescents: thirty years experience at St. Jude Children's Research Hospital. *J Cutan Pathol.* 2000;27:485–492.
337. Wick M. Immunohistology of melanocytic neoplasms. In: Dabbs D, ed. *Diagnostic Immunohistochemistry.* 2nd ed. New York, NY: Churchill Livingston; 2006:162–179.
338. Wick MR, Swanson PE, Patterson JW. Immunohistology of skin tumors. In: Dabbs D, ed. *Diagnostic Immunohistochemistry.* 2nd ed. New York, NY: Churchill Livingston; 2006:404–441.
339. Wick MR. Immunohistochemical approaches to the diagnosis of undifferentiated malignant tumors. *Ann Diagn Pathol.* 2008;12:72–84.
340. Wilkinson EJ, Brown HM. Vulvar Paget disease of urothelial origin: a report of three cases and a proposed classification of vulvar Paget disease. *Hum Pathol.* 2002;33:549–554.
341. Willemze R, Jaffe ES, Burg G, et al. WHO-EORTC classification for cutaneous lymphomas. *Blood.* 2005;105:3768.
342. Willemze R, Jaffe ES, Burg G, et al. WHO-EORTC classification for cutaneous lymphomas. *Blood.* 2005;105:3768.
343. Willemze R, Jansen PM, Cerroni L, et al. Subcutaneous panniculitis-like T-cell lymphoma: definition, classification, and prognostic factors: an EORTC Cutaneous Lymphoma Group Study of 83 cases. *Blood.* 2008;111:838.
344. Wong NS, Chang BM, Toh HC, Koo WH. Inflammatory metastatic carcinoma of the colon: a case report and review of the literature. *Tumori.* 2004;90:253–255.
345. Wood BL. Myeloid malignancies: myelodysplastic syndromes, myeloproliferative disorders, and acute myeloid leukemia. *Clin Lab Med.* 2007;27:551.
346. Wood GS, Kamath NV, Guitart J, et al. Absence of *Borrelia burgdorferi* DNA in cutaneous B-cell lymphomas from the United States. *J Cutan Pathol.* 2001;28:502.
347. Woodruff CA, Amrikachi M, Hsu S. Zosteriform metastatic transitional cell carcinoma. *Int J Dermatol* 2005;44:1028–1030.
348. Wu JJ, Huang DB, Pang KR, Tyring SK. Cutaneous metastasis to the chest wall from prostate cancer. *Int J Dermatol.* 2006;45:946–948.
349. Yada K, Kashima K, Daa T, et al. Expression of CD10 in basal cell carcinoma. *Am J Dermatopathol.* 2004;26:463–471.
350. Yamaguchi T, Ohshima K, Karube K, et al. Clinicopathological features of cutaneous lesions of adult T-cell leukaemia/lymphoma. *Br J Dermatol.* 2005;152:76.

351. Yamauchi K, Yasuda M. Comparison in treatments of nonleukemic granulocytic sarcoma. *Cancer.* 2002;94:1739.

352. Yang B, Tubbs RR, Finn W, et al. Clinicopathologic reassessment of primary cutaneous B-cell lymphomas with immunophenotypic and molecular genetic characterization. *Am J Surg Pathol.* 2000;24:694.

353. Yang DT, Holden JA, Florell SR. CD117, CK20, TTF-1, and DNA topoisomerase II-alpha antigen expression in small cell tumors. *J Cutan Pathol.* 2004;31:254–261.

354. Yang HI, Lee MC, Kuo TT, Hong HS. Cellulitis-like cutaneous metastasis of uterine cervical carcinoma. *J Am Acad Dermatol.* 2007;56(Suppl):S26–S28.

355. Yee KOBS. Chronic lymphocytic leukemia: diagnosis and treatment. *Mayo Clin Proc.* 2006;81:1105.

356. Yendluri V, Centeno B, Springett GM. Pancreatic cancer presenting as a Sister Mary Joseph's nodule: case report and update of the literature. *Pancreas.* 2007;34:161–164.

357. Yu H, Pinkus GS, Hornick JL. Diffuse membranous immunoreactivity for podoplanin (D2-40) distinguishes primary and metastatic seminomas from other germ cell tumors and metastatic neoplasms. *Am J Clin Pathol.* 2007;128:767–775.

358. Yu KJ, Lee HE, Ho HC, et al. Carcinoma erysipelatoides from squamous cell carcinoma of unknown origin. *Int J Clin Pract.* 2005;59:1104–1106.

359. Yurtsever H, Kempf W,Laeng RH. Posttransplant CD30+ anaplastic large cell lymphoma with skin and lymph node involvement. *Dermatology.* 2003;207:107.

360. Zalaudek I, Leinweber B, Richtig E, et al. Cutaneous zosteriform melanoma metastases arising after herpes zoster infection: a case report and review of the literature. *Melanoma Res.* 2003;13:635–639.

361. Zaloudek C. Tumors of the female genital tract. Part A. Ovary, fallopian tube and broad and round ligaments. In: Fletcher C, ed. *Diagnostic Histopathology of Tumors.* Vol 1, 3rd ed. New York, NY: Churchill Livingston; 2007:567–651.

362. Zehentner BK, Carter D. Mammaglobin: a candidate diagnostic marker for breast cancer. *Clin Biochem.* 2004;37:249–257.

363. Zelger B, Sepp N, Weyrer K, et al. Syringotropic cutaneous T-cell lymphoma: a variant of mycosis fungoides? *Br J Dermatol.* 1994;130:765.

364. Zembowicz A, Garcia CF, Tannous ZS, et al. Endocrine mucin-producing sweat gland carcinoma: twelve new cases suggest that it is a precursor of some invasive mucinous carcinomas. *Am J Surg Pathol.* 2005;29:1330–1339.

365. Zhang MQ, Lin F, Hui P, Chen ZM, et al. Expression of mucins, SIMA, villin, and CDX2 in small-intestinal adenocarcinoma. *Am J Clin Pathol.* 2007;128:808–816.

366. Ziemer M, Bornkessel A, Hahnfeld S, et al. 'Specific' cutaneous infiltrate of B-cell chronic lymphocytic leukemia at the site of a florid herpes simplex infection. *J Cutan Pathol.* 2005;32:581.

Index

Note: **Boldfaced** page numbers indicate the main topic of questions and answers.

www.ingramcontent.com/pod-product-compliance
Lightning Source LLC
LaVergne TN
LVHW080102011026
849160LV00013B/1013
* 9 7 8 0 0 7 1 4 8 9 2 2 5 *